Foundations
of Nursing
Second Edition

This book is dedicated to Elisabeth F. Williams, Senior Developmental Editor, at Thomson Delmar Learning. Her knowledge, professionalism, and caring have kept this author going. She is a great asset to the textbook publishing industry.

Foundations of Nursing

Second Edition

Lois White, RN, PhD

Former Chairperson and Professor
Department of Vocational Nurse Education
Del Mar College
Corpus Christi, Texas

THOMSON
™
DELMAR LEARNING   Australia Canada Mexico Singapore Spain United Kingdom United States

THOMSON

DELMAR LEARNING

Foundations of Nursing, Second Edition
by Lois White, RN, PhD

Vice President, Health Care Business Unit:
William Brottmiller
Editorial Director:
Cathy L. Esperti
Acquisitions Editors:
Matthew Filimonov and Melissa Martin
Senior Developmental Editor:
Elisabeth F. Williams
Editorial Assistant:
Patricia Osborn

Marketing Director:
Jennifer McAvey
Marketing Channel Manager:
Tamara Caruso
Marketing Coordinator:
Karen Summerlin
Production Director:
Karen Leet
Production Manager:
Barbara A. Bullock

Project Editor:
Natalie Wager
Art/Design Specialist:
Jay Purcell
Production Editor:
John Mickelbank
Technology Project Manager:
Victoria Moore
Technology Production Coordinator:
Sherry Conners

Library of Congress Cataloging-in-Publication Data

White, Lois.
    Foundations of nursing / Lois White.—2nd ed.
       p. cm.
    Includes bibliographical references and index.
    ISBN 1-4018-2692-X
    1.   Nursing—Handbooks, manuals, etc. 2. Holistic nursing—Handbooks, manuals, etc.
I.   Title.
    RT51.W44 2005
    610.73—dc22   2004012416

International Divisions List

Asia (including India):
Thomson Learning
60 Albert Street, #15-01
Albert Complex
Singapore 189969
Tel 65 336-6411
Fax 65 336-7411

Australia/New Zealand:
Nelson
102 Dodds Street
South Melbourne
Victoria 3205
Australia
Tel 61 (0)3 9685-4111
Fax 61 (0)3 9685-4199

Latin America:
Thomson Learning
Seneca 53
Colonia Polanco
11560 Mexico, D.F. Mexico
Tel (525) 281-2906
Fax (525) 281-2656

Canada:
Nelson
1120 Birchmount Road
Toronto, Ontario
Canada M1K 5G4
Tel (416) 752-9100
Fax (416) 752-8102

UK/Europe/Middle East/Africa:
Thomson Learning
Berkshire House
1680-173 High Holborn
London WC1V 7AA
United Kingdom
Tel 44 (0)20 497-1422
Fax 44 (0)20 497-1426

Spain (including Portugal):
Paraninfo
Calle Magallanes 25
28015 Madrid
España
Tel 34 (0)91 446-3350
Fax 34 (0)91 445-6218

Contents

SECTION II ADULT HEALTH NURSING

Unit 9 Essential Concepts

Unit 10 Nursing Care of the Client: Oxygenation and Perfusion

x   Contents

Chapter 42
Sexually Transmitted Diseases 1223

Unit 14 Nursing Care of the Client: Body Defenses

Chapter 43
Integumentary System 1237

Chapter 44
Immune System 1276

Unit 15 Nursing Care of the Client: Physical and Mental Integrity

Chapter 45
Mental Illness 1309

Chapter 52

Chapter 53

Chapter 54

Unit 18 Nursing Care of the Client: Childrearing

Chapter 55

Chapter 56

Contributors

Joy E. Ache-Reed, RN, MS
Assistant Professor of Nursing
Indiana Wesleyan University
Marion, Indiana
Chapter 11, Cultural Considerations

Carol A. Fetters Andersen, RN, MSN
Director of Mental Health Services
St. Anthony Regional Hospital and Nursing Home
Carroll, Iowa
Chapter 48, The Older Adult

Carma Andrus, RN, MN, CNS
Dauterive Primary Care Clinic
St. Martinville, Louisiana
Chapter 39, Sensory System

Diane R. Behrens, RNCS, MA, MSEd
Instructor
University of Saint Francis
Fort Wayne, Indiana
Chapter 44, Immune System

Susan L. Bredemeyer, RN, MS
Assistant Professor
Lutheran College of Health Professions
Fort Wayne, Indiana
Chapter 23, Assessment

Ali Brown, RN, MSN
Assistant Professor
College of Nursing
University of Tennessee
Knoxville, Tennessee
Chapter 8, Nursing Process/ Documentation

Gyl A. Burkhard, RN, BSN, MS
Instructor
OCM BOCES
Syracuse, New York
Chapter 36, Urinary System

Donna J. Burleson, RN, MS
Chair of Health Occupations
Cisco Junior College
Abilene, Texas
Chapter 1, Student Nurse Skills for Success

Ann H. Cary, RN, PhD, MPH, A-CCC
Professor and Coordinator, PhD in Nursing Program
College of Nursing and Health Sciences
George Mason University
Fairfax, Virginia
Chapter 3, Nursing History, Education, and Organizations

Diana L. Case, RN, MA, FNP
Neighborhood Health Clinic
Fort Wayne, Indiana
Chapter 30, Surgery

Judy Conlin
Chapter 18, Safety/Hygiene

Jan Corder, RN, DNS
School of Nursing
Northeast Louisiana University
Monroe, Louisana
Chapter 8, Nursing Process/ Documentation

Julie Coy, RNC, MS
Pain Consultation Service
The Children's Hospital
Denver, Colorado
Chapter 17, Rest and Sleep
Chapter 24, Pain Management

Gena Duncan, RN, MS, MSEd
Director of Associate Degree Program
University of Saint Francis
Fort Wayne, Indiana
Chapter 33, Cardiovascular System
Chapter 34, Hematologic and Lymphatic Systems

Mary Elias, RNC, BSN, CCE
Instructor
Practical Nursing Program
Ivy Tech State College
Fort Wayne, Indiana
Chapter 41, Reproductive System

Cheryl Erickson, RN, BSN, MA
Associate Professor
Lutheran College of Health Professions
Fort Wayne, Indiana
Chapter 23, Assessment

Mary Ellen Zator Estes, RN, MSN, FNP, APRN-BC, NP-C
Family Nurse Practitioner in Internal Medicine
Fairfax, Virginia *and*
Adjunct Faculty
School of Health Professions
Marymount University
Arlington, Virginia
Chapter 23, Assessment

Michael A. Fiedler, CRNA, MS
Assistant Professor
Applied Health Sciences
University of Alabama at Birmingham
Birmingham, Alabama
Chapter 29, Anesthesia

Mary Frost, RN, BSN
Covington, Louisiana
Chapter 15, Complementary/ Alternative Therapies

Norma Fujise, RN, C, MS
School of Nursing
University of Hawaii
Honolulu, Hawaii
Chapter 43, Integumentary System

Cathy Greer, RN, MS
Instructor
Lutheran College of Health Professions
Fort Wayne, Indiana
Chapter 30, Surgery

Margaret L. Griffin, RN, BSN, MS
Instructor
Lutheran College of Health Professions
Fort Wayne, Indiana
Chapter 43, Integumentary System

Susan Halley, RN, MS, FNP
Instructor of Nursing
Ball State University
Muncie, Indiana
Chapter 4, Legal and Ethical Responsibilities

Mary Jane Hamilton, RN, C, PhD
Professor of Nursing
Texas A&M University-Corpus Christi
Corpus Christi, Texas
Chapter 55, Basics of Pediatric Care

Beverly F. Hildebrand, RN, BSN, MS
Former Health Occupations Coordinator
Washington, Saratoga, Warren, Hamilton, & Essex Counties BOCES
Saratoga, New York
Chapter 36, Urinary System

Lucille Joel, RN, EdD, FAAN
Professor
College of Nursing
Rutgers, The State University of New Jersey
Newark, New Jersey
Chapter 5, The Health Care Delivery System

Janet Leah Joost, RN, BSN
Instructor
Front Range Community College
Boulder, Colorado
Chapter 32, Respiratory System

Denise M. Jordan, RN, BSN, MA
Instructor
Practical Nursing Program
Ivy Tech State College
Fort Wayne, Indiana
Chapter 4, Legal and Ethical Responsibilities

Janet E. Keith, RN, MSEd
Instructor
Practical Nursing Program
Ivy Tech State College
Fort Wayne, Indiana
Chapter 37, Musculoskeletal System

Vicki L. Khouli, RN, BSN, MA, IBCLC
Instructor
Practical Nursing Program
Ivy Tech State College
Fort Wayne, Indiana
Chapter 42, Sexually Transmitted Diseases

Mary E. A. Laskin, RN, CS, MN
Clinical Nurse Specialist
Surgical/Orthopedic Services
Kaiser Permanente
San Diego, California
Chapter 24, Pain Management

Celinda Kay Leach, RN, BS, MPH
Program Chair, Practical Nursing
Practical Nursing Program
Ivy Tech State College
Bloomington, Indiana
Chapter 31, Oncology

Sandra Liming, RN, MN
Nursing Instructor
North Seattle Community College
North Seattle, Washington
Chapter 41, Reproductive System

Judy Martin, RN, MS, JD
Nurse Attorney
Louisiana Department of Health and Hospitals
Health Standards Section
Baton Rouge, Louisiana
Chapter 4, Legal and Ethical Responsibilities

Linda McCuistion, RN, PhD
Assistant Professor
School of Nursing
Our Lady of Holy Cross College
New Orleans, Louisiana
Chapter 8, Nursing Process/ Documentation

Cheryl McGaffic, RN, PhD
Clinical Instructor
College of Nursing
The University of Arizona
Tucson, Arizona
Chapter 44, Immune System

Robin Theresa McKenzie, RN, MSN, CCRN
Assistant Chairman
Navy Medical Center
San Diego, California
Chapter 39, Sensory System

Betty Miller
Staff Development Coordinator
Meadowcrest Hospital
Gretna, Louisiana
Chapter 13, Loss, Grief, and Death

David K. Miller, RNC, BSN, MSEd
ICU/Medical–Surgical Manager
W.S. Major Hospital
Shelbyville, Indiana
Chapter 44, Immune System

Barbara S. Moffett, RN, PhD
Associate Professor of Nursing
School of Nursing
Southeastern Louisiana University
Hammond, Louisiana
Chapter 8, Nursing Process/Documentation

Mary Anne Mordcin-McCarthy, RN, PhD
Associate Professor and Director of the Undergraduate Program
College of Nursing
University of Tennessee–Knoxville
Knoxville, Tennessee
Chapter 8, Nursing Process/ Documentation

Barbara Morvant, RN, MN
Louisiana State Board of Nursing
Metairie, Louisiana
Chapter 4, Nursing History, Education, and Organizations

Joan Fritsch Needham, RNC, MS
Director of Education
DeKalb County Nursing Home
DeKalb, Illinois
Chapter 6, Arenas of Care
Chapter 13, Loss, Grief, and Death
Chapter 48, The Older Adult

Rebecca Osterhaut
Chapter 2, Holistic Care

Brenda Owens, RN, PhD
Associate Professor
School of Nursing
Louisiana State University Medical Center
New Orleans, Louisiana
Chapter 22, Medication Administration and IV Therapy

Raymond Phillips, RN, MS, CCRN
Clinical Nurse Specialist
Staff Development Coordinator
U.S. Naval Hospital
Rota, Spain
Chapter 39, Sensory System

Demetrius Porche, RN, CCRN, DNS
Associate Professor and Director
Bachelor of Science in Nursing
   Program
Nicholas State University *and*
Adjunct Assistant Professor
Tulane University
School of Public Health and Topical
   Medicine
New Orleans, Louisiana
Chapter 18, Safety/Hygiene
**Chapter 19, Infection Control/
   Asepsis**
**Chapter 20, Standard
   Precautions and Isolation**

Susan Reinhart, RN, MS
Assistant Professor
Department of Registered Nurse
   Education
Del Mar College
Corpus Christi, Texas
Chapter 45, Mental Illness

Suzanne Riche, RN
Charity School of Nursing
Delgado Community College
New Orleans, Louisiana
**Chapter 8, Nursing Process/
   Documentation**

**Kathy Rockwell, RN, BSN, MA,
   MSN, PNP**
Professor
Department of RN Education
Del Mar College
Corpus Christi, Texas *and*
Supervisor, Surgical Services
94th General Hospital
Seagoville, Texas
**Chapter 47, Responding to
   Emergencies**

Martha Ann Rust, RN, BSN, MSN
Instructor
Lutheran College of Health
   Professions
Fort Wayne, Indiana
**Chapter 38, Neurological
   System**

Mary Kay Schultz, RN, MSN, ANP
Instructor
Department of Nursing
Regis University
Denver, Colorado
Chapter 40, Endocrine System

Leslee R. Sinn, RN, BSN
Instructor
Front Range Community College
Boulder, Colorado
**Chapter 35, Gastrointestinal
   System**

Russlyn A. St. John, RN, MSN
Associate Professor & Coordinator,
   Practical Nursing
St. Charles Community College
St. Peters, Missouri
Chapter 40, Endocrine System

**Maureen Straight, RN, BSN,
   MSEd**
Regents College
Albany, New York
**Chapter 1, Student Nurse Skills
   for Success**

Susan Stranahan, RN, PhD
Chair, Nursing Department
Indiana Wesleyan University
Marion, Indiana
**Chapter 11, Cultural
   Considerations**

John M. White, PhD
Former Chairperson, Professor
Biology Department
Del Mar College
Corpus Christi, Texas
**Chapter 21, Fluid, Electrolyte,
   and Acid–Base Balance**

Donna Wofford RN, PhD
Professor
Department of RN Education
Del Mar College
Corpus Christi, Texas
**Chapter 56, Infants with Special
   Needs: Birth to 12 months**
**Chapter 57, Common Problems:
   1–18 years**

Lorrie Wong, RN, MS
School of Nursing
University of Hawaii
Honolulu, Hawaii
**Chapter 43, Integumentary
   System**

Rothlyn Zahourek, RN, CS, MS
Certified Clinical Nurse Specialist
Amherst, Massachusetts
**Chapter 15, Complementary/
   Alternative Therapies**

Procedure Contributors

Gaylene Bouska Altman, RN, PhD
Director, Learning Lab
Faculty, School of Nursing
University of Washington
Seattle, Washington

Sharon Aronovitch, RN, PhD, CETN
Regents College
Albany, New York

Dale D. Barb, MHS, PT
Academic Coordinator of Clinical Education
Department of Physical Therapy
Wichita State University
Wichita, Kansas

Theresa A. Barenz, RN, MN

Susan Weiss Behrend, RN, MSN
Fox Chase Cancer Center
Philadelphia, Pennsylvania

Patricia Buchsel, RN, MSN, FAAN
Clinical Instructor
School of Nursing
University of Washington
Seattle, Washington

Bethaney Campbell, RN,MN, OCN
University of Washington Medical Center
Seattle, Washington

Curt Campbell
Integrated Health Services of Seattle
Seattle, Washington

Jung-Chen (Kristina) Chang, RN, MN, Phd
University of Washington
School of Nursing
Seattle, Washington

Eileen M. Collins, MN, ARNP, CNOR
School of Nursing
University of Washington
Seattle, Washington

Cheryl L. Cooke, RN, MN
Student Services Coordinator
University of Washington
School of Nursing
Seattle, Washington

Valerie Coxon, RN, PhD
Affiliate Assistant Professor
School of Nursing
University of Washington
Seattle, Washington
Chief Executive Officer
NRSPACE Software, Inc.
Bellevue, Washington

Gayle C. Crawford, RN, BSN
Staff Nurse
University of Washington Medical Center
Seattle, Washington

Eleonor U. de la Pena, RN, BS
Northwest Asthma and Allergy Center
Seattle, Washington

Tom Ewing, RN, BSN
Hematology-Oncology
University of Washington Medical Center
Seattle, Washington

Amy Fryberger, RN, MN, ONC

Karrin Johnson, RN
Health Care Project Manager
NRSPACE Software, Inc.
Bellevue, Washington

Kimberly Sue Kahn, RN, MSN, FNP-C, CS, AOCN
University of Virginia
Portsmouth, Virginia

Catherine H. Kelley, RN, MSN, OCN
Chimeric Therapies, Inc.
Palatine, Illinois

Carla A. Bouska Lee, PhD, ARNP, FAAN
Clarkston College
Omaha, Nebraska

Kathryn Lilleby, RN
Clinical Research Nurse
Fred Hutchinson Cancer Research Center
Seattle, Washington

Joan M. Mack, RN, MSN, CS
Nebraska Medical Center
Omaha, Nebraska

Marianne Frances Moore, RN, MSN
Clarkson Hospital
Omaha, Nebraska

Susan Randolph, RN, MSN, CS
Manager, Transplant Services
Coram Healthcare
Parkerburg, West Virginia

Susan Rives, RN, BSN, OCN
CARE Center Coordinator
Martha Jefferson Hospital
Charlottesville, Virginia

Barbara Sigler, RN, MNEd, CORLN
Technical Publications Editor
Oncology Nursing Press, Inc.
Formerly: Clinical Nurse Specialist in Otolaryngology—Head and Neck Surgery
University of Pittsburgh Medical Center
Pittsburgh, Pennsylvania

Pam Talley, MN, PhD
University of Washington
School of Nursing
Seattle, Washington

Hsin-Yi (Jean) Tang, RN, MS, PhD
School of Nursing
University of Washington
Seattle, Washington

Robi Thomas, MS, RN, AOCN
Clinical Nurse Specialist for Oncology and the Pain Center
St. Mary's Mercy Medical Center
Grand Rapids, Michigan

Chandra VanPaepeghem, RN, BSN
University of Washington Medical Center
Seattle, Washington

Reviewers

Marilyn L. Adair, RN, MSN
Professor of Nursing
South Puget Sound Community
  College
Olympia, Washington

Donna Adams, RN, MSN
Instructor of Nursing
Grand Rapids Community College
Grand Rapids, Michigan

**Cynthia Francis Bechtel, MS, RN,
  CEN, EMT-I**
Associate Professor of Nursing
MassBay Community College
Southborough, Massachusetts

Emily Bond, RN, MSN, PhD
Professor of Nursing
Southeastern Louisiana University
Hammond, Louisiana

Angela M. Brewer, RN, BSN
Instructor of Nursing
Ivy Tech State College
Terre Haute, Indiana

Teresa L. Bryan, RN, MSN, C
Assistant Professor
Department of Associate Degree
  Nursing
Alcorn State University
Natchez, Mississippi

Sarah Covington, RN, MSN
Instructor of Nursing
Renton Technical College
Renton, Washington

Sheila Creason, BS, RN
VN Instructor of Nursing
Concorde Career Institute
North Hollywood, California

Marylou DeNatale, EdD, RN
University of San Francisco
School of Nursing
San Francisco, California

Jewel Diller, MS Ed, RN
Associate Professor
Practical Nursing Program
Ivy Tech State College
Fort Wayne, Indiana

Karen S. Edmondson, RN, MSN
University of South Carolina,
  Spartanburg
Spartanburg, South Carolina

Leota A. Ehm, BSN, RN
Former Practical Nursing Program
  Chair
Ivy Tech State College
Terre Haute, Indiana

Sally Flesch, PhD, RN
Professor and Former Department
  Chair
Black Hawk College
Moline, Illinois

Diane J. Gallagher, RN, BSN, MS
Hocking College
Nelsonville, Ohio

Ruth Gladen, RN, MS
Assistant Professor of Nursing
North Dakota State College of Science
Wahpeton, North Dakota

Nicole Harder, RN, MSN
Lecturer
Faculty of Nursing
University of Manitoba
St. Adolphe, Manitoba

Lisa C. Harris, RN, BSN
Adjunct Faculty
Spencerian College
Louisville, Kentucky

Susan Jewell, Med, BSN,
PN Chair
Ivy Tech State College
Sellersburg, Indiana

Trudy Ketterbach, RN
Coordinator
Practical Nursing Program
Tennessee Technology Center
Shelbyville, Tennessee

Suellen S. Klein, RN, MSN
Nursing Instructor
Lake Michigan College
Benton Harbor, Michigan

**Kathleen M. Larke, MEd, RNC,
  BC**
Nurse Educator
Middlesex Hospital
Portland, Connecticut

Patty Leary, MEd, RN
Allied Health Instructor
Mecosta Osceola Career Center
and
Instructor
Ferris State University, *and*
Staff
Kelsey Memorial Hospital ER
Lakeview, Michigan

Eloise T. Lewis, RN, BSN
Assistant Professor of Practical
  Nursing
Indiana Vocational and Technical
  State College
Columbus, Indiana

**Renee Martin-Thornton, MBA,
  RN**
Instructor of Nursing
Glendale Career College
Los Angeles, California

**Sally-Ann McDonald, RN, BSN,
  Midwife, Women's Health
  Nurse Pracitioner, IBLCE**
Professor of Nursing
Renton Technical College
Renton, Washington

**David K. Miller, RNc, CDE, BSN,
  MS Ed, CDE**
Professor of Nursing
Major Hospital
Hope, Indiana

Polly G. Moore, RN, DNS
Director of Nursing
Concorde Career Institute
San Diego, California

Carol Nelson, RN, MSN
Instructor of Nursing
Spokane Community College
Spokane, Washington

Preface

Foundations of Nursing, second edition, is a textbook developed to cover the entire curriculum of a practical/vocational nursing program (fundamentals, nutrition, growth and development, gerontology, mental health/mental illness, microbiology, personal/vocational adjustments, medical/surgical nursing, and maternal/pediatric nursing). Anatomy and physiology and medications are not included, but there is an anatomy and physiology review at the beginning of each medical/surgical system chapter. Pharmacology basics and medication administration are presented, though specific drugs are not discussed in detail. Critical thinking, presented in the first chapter, lays a foundation for the nursing process, which is presented in great detail.

The concept of holistic care is fundamental to this text. Throughout the book, boxes highlight special topics regarding life cycle considerations, client teaching, professional tips, community/home health care, infection control, cultural considerations, safety, and critical thinking.

Since the complete curriculum is covered, the student can see how the subject matter from the different areas is interrelated. Students will also find this text helpful by having all information in one book.

Organization

Foundations of Nursing, second edition, consists of 57 chapters grouped into 3 sections: Basic Nursing, Adult Health Nursing, and Maternal & Pediatric Nursing. These 3 sections are comprised of 18 units.

Basic Nursing

- **Unit 1: FOUNDATIONS**—discusses student nurse skills for success (including critical thinking, time management, study skills, and life organizing skills); holistic care; nursing history, education, and organizations; and legal and ethical responsibilities.
- **Unit 2: THE HEALTH CARE ENVIRONMENT**—describes the health care delivery system and arenas of care, focusing on the various settings in which practical/vocational nurses practice.
- **Unit 3: COMMUNICATION**—addresses the process of communication, how communication is used in the nurse/client relationship, and technical and legal aspects of documentation. Each component of the nursing process is explained in a clear, concise manner. The client teaching process is presented as a major nursing intervention for clients throughout the life cycle.
- **Unit 4: DEVELOPMENTAL AND PSYCHOSOCIAL CONCERNS**—describes the growth and developmental changes throughout the entire life cycle; cultural aspects and considerations; stress, adaptation, and anxiety; and loss, grief, and death, including postmortem care.

- **Unit 5: HEALTH PROMOTION**—addresses wellness concepts and complementary/alternative therapies. Basic nutrition, rest and sleep, and safety/hygiene are presented as methods of promoting health.
- **Unit 6: INFECTION CONTROL**—presents the chain of infection, describes various types of pathogenic microorganisms, and presents the concept of asepsis and aseptic technique along with Standard Precautions and isolation measures.
- **Unit 7: FUNDAMENTAL NURSING CARE**—thoroughly discusses fluid, electrolyte, and acid-base balance. Medication administration and IV therapy are presented in a nursing process format. Also included are legal considerations, dose equivalents, and dosage calculations. Assessment is covered in great detail, including head-to-toe physical assessment, nursing history, and functional assessment. Pain management covers causes of pain, transmission and perception, and nursing interventions for relieving pain. Caring for a client encountering diagnostic tests is thoroughly covered. The most commonly ordered diagnostic tests are explained in tables that provide the normal results and nursing considerations.
- **Unit 8: NURSING PROCEDURES**—basic, intermediate, and advanced procedures follow the nursing process format and are presented in a step-by-step fashion. Rationale is given for each step, and figures and multimedia links add to the clarity of the procedures.

Adult Health Nursing

- **Unit 9: ESSENTIAL CONCEPTS**—discusses the various types of anesthesia and the nursing care required for each. Surgery describes the perioperative care of clients. Oncology discusses the various types of cancer, the usual treatments, and the nursing care required.

The chapters in Units 10 through 14 each include an anatomy and physiology review and a presentation of each disorder, with medical/surgical management, nursing management, pharmacological, dietary, and activity aspects of treatment. The nursing process identifies subjective and objective data, possible nursing diagnoses, goals, interventions, and evaluation. A sample nursing care plan is found in each chapter in these units.

- **Unit 10: NURSING CARE OF THE CLIENT: OXYGENATION AND PERFUSION**—includes the respiratory system, cardiovascular system, and hematologic and lymphatic systems.
- **Unit 11: NURSING CARE OF THE CLIENT: DIGESTION AND ELIMINATION**—discusses the gastrointestinal system and urinary system.

- **Unit 12: NURSING CARE OF THE CLIENT: MOBILITY, COORDINATION, AND REGULATION**—covers the musculoskeletal system, neurological system, sensory system, and endocrine system.
- **Unit 13: NURSING CARE OF THE CLIENT: REPRODUCTIVE AND SEXUAL HEALTH**—includes the reproductive systems and sexually transmitted diseases.
- **Unit 14: NURSING CARE OF THE CLIENT: BODY DEFENSES**—discusses the integumentary system and immune system.
- **Unit 15: NURSING CARE OF THE CLIENT: PHYSICAL AND MENTAL INTEGRITY**—is concerned with substance abuse and the care of clients with common mental illnesses. Substance abuse describes substances which are commonly abused, the signs and symptoms of abuse, and treatments available.
- **Unit 16: APPLICATIONS**—describes how nursing knowledge is applied in emergencies and for the older adult. Specific information is provided for common emergencies. Bioterrorism is covered in some detail. Physiologic changes of aging are presented for each body system. A number of scenarios describing clients with multisystem problems assist students to see the integration of the body.

Maternal & Pediatric Nursing

- **Unit 17: NURSING CARE OF THE CLIENT: CHILDBEARING**—covers preconception education, prenatal care, fetal development, complications of pregnancy, the birth process, postpartum care, and care of the newborn.
- **Unit 18: NURSING CARE OF THE CLIENT: CHILDREARING**—presents the basics of pediatric care. Infants with special needs: birth to 12 months and common problems 1 to 18 years address the major situations of pediatric care.

Features

Each chapter opens with a **Making the Connection** box, which guides the reader to other key chapters related to the current chapter. This highlights the integration of the text material. Topics on *Delmar's Anatomy & Physiology CD-ROM* (order #0-7668-2415-2) and *Delmar's Heart & Lung Sounds CD-ROM* (order #0-7668-2416-0) are listed as appropriate. Procedures used for the care of clients with the disorders discussed in the chapter are identified as appropriate. **Learning Objectives** are provided to guide the readers' learning. A listing of **Key Terms** identifies important terminology for the student. These terms are bolded and defined at first use in the chapter.

The content of each chapter is presented in a nursing process format. Where appropriate, a **Sample Nursing Care Plan** is provided in the chapter. **Case Studies** are presented at the conclusion of the body systems and specialty chapters.

A bulleted list **Summary** and multiple-choice **Review Questions** at the end of each chapter assist the student in remembering and using the material presented. **References/Suggested Readings** allow the student to find the source of the material presented and also to find additional information concerning the topics covered. **Resources** are also listed and provide names, addresses, and telephone numbers of organizations specializing in a specific area of health care. Internet addresses are included as available.

Boxes used throughout the text emphasize certain points and provide specific types of information. The boxes are:

 LIFE CYCLE CONSIDERATIONS: provides information related to the care of specific age groups during the life span.

 CLIENT TEACHING: identifies specific items that the client should know related to the various disorders.

 PROFESSIONAL TIP: offers tips for the nurse to ensure quality care.

 COMMUNITY/HOME HEALTH CARE: describes factors to consider when providing care in the community or in a client's home, and adaptations in care that may be necessary.

 INFECTION CONTROL: indicates reminders of methods to prevent the spread of infections.

 CULTURAL CONSIDERATIONS: shares beliefs, manners, ways of providing care, communication, and relationships of various cultural and ethnic groups as a way to provide holistic care.

 COLLABORATIVE CARE: mentions members of the care team and their roles in providing comprehensive care to clients.

 DRUG ICON: highlights the pharmacological treatments and interventions that may be appropriate for certain conditions and disorders.

 SAFETY: emphasizes the importance of and ways to maintain safe care.

 CRITICAL THINKING QUESTIONS: encourages the student to use the knowledge gained to think critically about a situation.

Back matter includes a **Glossary of Terms.** The appendices include **NANDA Nursing Diagnoses; Recommended Childhood and Adolescent Immunization Schedule; Abbreviations, Acronyms, and Symbols;** and **English/Spanish Words and Phrases. Standard Precautions** are found on the inside back cover.

Teaching/Learning Package

The supplements package for *Foundations of Nursing*, second edition, will assist students in learning the information and procedures presented in the text. Also, the instructors will be assisted in planning and developing their classes for the most efficient use of time and resources.

- **Electronic Classroom Manager** (order #1-4018-2701-2) is a CD-ROM containing four components. PowerPoint® presentations aid instructors in lecture preparation and class presentation. An Image Library of over 800 illustrations and photographs used in the textbook may be easily printed or copied to create unique classroom handouts. An Instructor's Manual includes Instructional Approaches, Student Learning Activities, Resources, and Web Activities. A Computerized Testbank of over 1,200 questions on text material is also on the CD-ROM.
- **Study Guide** (order #1-4018-2693-8) provides additional review on all 57 chapters of *Foundations of Nursing*, with Key Term matching review questions, Abbreviation Review Exercises, Self-Assessment Questions, and Other Review Questions.
- **Procedures Checklist** (order #1-4018-2695-4) may be used to assist students in evaluating their comprehension and execution of the procedures contained within the core textbook.
- **Website**—accessible at no charge, this resource has information on workplace transition including job expectations and responsibilities; résumé, cover letter, and reference list preparation; job application; and interview preparation. Additional case studies and review exercises are also included. Visit www. delmarlearning.com/companions

Acknowledgments

Many people must work together to produce any textbook, but a comprehensive book such as this requires even more people with various areas of expertise. I would like to thank all of the contributors for their time and effort to share their knowledge gained through years of experience in both the clinical and academic settings.

The reviewers, I thank for their time spent critically reading the manuscript and providing the valuable suggestions that have added to this text. Thank you to the consultants Captain Alston Kirk, CHC, USN (retired), and John White, PhD, for providing their expertise in religions and anatomy and physiology respectively.

To my husband John, a huge thank you for his patience, understanding, and listening when problems arose and for some great suggestions to solve them.

I would like to acknowledge and sincerely thank the entire team at Thomson Delmar Learning who has worked to make this textbook a reality. Elisabeth F. Williams, senior developmental editor, is a jewel who works tirelessly and whose knowledge, guidance, humor, and attention to detail kept me motivated and on-track throughout this project. Her creative solutions to problems are a wonder to behold.

My thanks also go to the entire Thomson Delmar Learning team: Patricia Osborn, editorial assistant; Natalie Wager, project editor; Jay Purcell, art/design specialist; John Mickelbank, production editor; Sherry Conners, technology production coordinator; and Kate Kaufman, technology assistant. They have all worked diligently to bring this textbook to the faculty and students in practical/vocational nursing. My heartfelt thanks go to each person.

About the Author

Lois Elain Wacker White earned a diploma in nursing from Memorial Hospital School of Nursing, Springfield, Illinois; an Associate degree in Science from Del Mar College, Corpus Christi, Texas; a Bachelor of Science in Nursing from Texas A & I University–Corpus Christi, Corpus Christi, Texas; a Master of Science in Education from Corpus Christi State University, Corpus Christi, Texas; and a Doctor of Philosophy degree in education administration–community college from the University of Texas, Austin, Texas.

She has taught at Del Mar College, Corpus Christi, Texas, in both the Associate Degree Nursing program and the Vocational Nursing program. For 14 years she was also chairperson of the Department of Vocational Nurse Education. Dr. White has taught fundamentals of nursing, nutrition, mental health/mental illness, medical-surgical nursing, and maternal/newborn nursing. Her professional career has also included 15 years of clinical practice.

Dr. White has served on the Nursing Education Advisory Committee of the Board of Nurse Examiners for the State of Texas and the Board of Vocational Nurse Examiners, which developed competencies expected of graduates from each level of nursing. She maintains membership in the Texas Association of Vocational Nurse Educators, Sigma Theta Tau, American Nurses Association, and the National League for Nursing.

Dr. White has been listed in Who's Who in American Nursing. She currently serves on the Vocational Nursing Financial Aid Advisory Committee for the Texas Higher Education Coordinating Board. She has authored nine nursing textbooks.

How to Use this Text

This text is designed with you, the reader, in mind. Special elements and feature boxes appear throughout the text to guide you in reading and to assist you in learning the material. Following are suggestions for how you can use these features to increase your understanding and mastery of the content.

MAKING THE CONNECTION

Read these boxes before beginning a chapter to link material across the holistic care continuum and to tie new content to material you have already encountered.

LEARNING OBJECTIVES

Read the chapter objectives before reading the chapter content to set the stage for learning. Revisit the objectives when preparing for an exam to see which entries you can respond to with "yes, I can do that."

KEY TERMS

Review this list before reading the chapter to familiarize yourself with new terms and to revisit those terms you already know to link them to the content of the new chapter.

CRITICAL THINKING

Visit these boxes after reading the entire chapter to check your acquisition and understanding of the concepts presented.

PROFESSIONAL TIP

Use these boxes to increase your professional competence and confidence, and also to expand your knowledge base.

COMMUNITY/HOME HEALTH CARE

Read these boxes before making a home visit to a client with a given disorder. You can also use these boxes to prepare for client discharge to ensure that all necessary self-care topics have been covered with a client.

CULTURAL CONSIDERATIONS

Test your sensitivity to cultural and ethnic variations by scanning these boxes and incorporating their guidelines and suggestions into your practice. You may also want to ask yourself what biases or preconceptions you have about different cultural practices before reading a chapter and then read these boxes for information that may help you be more sensitive in your nursing care and approach to clients.

INFECTION CONTROL

When reading a chapter, stop and pay attention to these features and ask yourself, "Had I thought of that? Do I practice these precautions?"

CLIENT TEACHING

Read these boxes to gain insight into client learning needs related to the specific disorder or condition. You may want to make your own index cards listing these teaching guidelines to use when you are working with clients.

LIFE CYCLE CONSIDERATIONS

Use these boxes to increase your awareness of variations in care based on client age; this will help you deliver more effective and appropriate care.

SAFETY

Pause while reading to consider these elements and quiz yourself: "Do I take steps such as these to ensure my own and the client's safety? Do I follow these guidelines in every practice encounter?"

NURSING CARE PLAN

Use these features to test your understanding and application of the content presented. Ask yourself, "Would I have come up with the same nursing diagnoses? Are these the interventions that I would have proposed? What other interventions would be appropriate?"

REVIEW QUESTIONS

When you finish reading a chapter, use these questions to critically test your understanding of concepts covered. You might also read these questions before beginning a new chapter to gauge how much you already know or need to learn about the topic.

CASE STUDY

Read over these boxes within the text. Draw on the knowledge you have gained and synthesize information to develop your own educated responses to the case study challenges.

PROCEDURES

Reference the procedures as you read the chapters. Study the techniques, review the figures, and be prepared for your clinical days with questions of clarification for your instructor. View the multimedia resources indicated by the CD-ROM and video icons, to enhance your understanding of each procedure.

COLLABORATIVE CARE

These boxes explain which other health care professionals may be involved in the comprehensive care offered to clients. Review these boxes and ask yourself if you understand how your role as a nurse will complement the care provided by others on the health care team.

DRUG ICONS

These symbols draw your attention to information relating to the pharmacological management available for certain disorders. Review these sections to understand the pharmacological treatments appropriate for your clients' conditions.

SECTION I
BASIC NURSING

UNIT

1

Foundations

STUDENT NURSE SKILLS FOR SUCCESS

MAKING THE CONNECTION

Refer to the following chapters to increase your understanding of student nurse skills for success:

Basic Nursing
- **Communication**

- **Client Teaching**
- **Stress, Adaptation, and Anxiety**

LEARNING OBJECTIVES

Upon completion of this chapter, you should be able to:
- **Define key terms.**
- **Outline strategies for developing a positive attitude toward the learner role.**
- **Identify strategies for developing proficiency in basic skills.**
- **Identify learning-style methods that can be incorporated for effective study.**
- **Design a time-management plan.**
- **Design a personal study plan.**
- **Identify strategies for improving test-taking outcomes.**
- **Discuss the standards for critical thinking.**
- **Identify the six traits of a disciplined (critical) thinker.**
- **Complete a stress-reduction exercise using guided imagery.**

KEY TERMS

ability	learning disability
anxiety	learning style
attitude	mnemonics
attribute	opinion
critical thinking	perfectionism
disciplined	procrastination
encoding	reasoning
judgment	standards
learning	time management

LEARNING

Learning is defined as the act or process of acquiring knowledge and/or skill in a particular subject. An individual never stops learning. This is especially true in the field of nursing and health care. The amount of information within the health care domain has expanded exponentially in just the past several years. Consider, for example, the advances in drug therapies, complementary/alternative therapies, and genetics. By graduation, some of the information learned in the beginning of the program will have been displaced by new information and discoveries. We are living in the information age and have constant access to thousands of pieces of information through various media, including television and the Internet. Knowledge is never static. Learning also is not static, but, rather, is a lifelong process.

Individuals seek knowledge to effect some type of change. As a student, you are seeking knowledge to learn skills and to prepare yourself for a career in nursing. Referring to yourself as a learner implies that you are an active participant in the learning process, as opposed to a passive recipient of information. You bring to this new

INTRODUCTION

Welcome to practical/vocational nursing. You have chosen one of life's rewarding careers. The next few months of your life will be challenging, exhilarating, frustrating, and full of new experiences. When you consider the difficulty of the nursing program's admission process, being a member of this nursing class is no small achievement. The fact that you have survived the admissions process demonstrates that you are capable of overcoming the challenges that lie ahead. Balancing family, community, and school responsibilities may prove the most difficult task you have yet to face.

adventure yourself, your past experiences, your abilities, and your motivation to master the knowledge necessary to reach your goals. You have already learned much in your lifetime and are ready to continue the process. It is important that you take some time to think about the competencies needed for the role of learner. It is equally important to realize that *you* are in charge of developing the competencies that will enable you to learn.

The learning you are seeking will afford you the knowledge and skills necessary to become a nurse and, thus, to demonstrate your ability to competently provide care to clients who seek your professional talents. Nursing education is different from many other college majors in the turnaround time allowed for learning. Few other disciplines require the student to apply on Thursday that which was acquired on Monday. Nursing students must acquire a greater depth of understanding in a shorter amount of time; to achieve this, basic learning processes will need to be well developed.

This chapter addresses *how* you learn rather than *what* you learn. It focuses on competencies necessary to master the learning process: attitude, basic skills, learning style, time management, study strategies, critical thinking, and test-taking strategies. Assessing which habits you already practice and which ones you have yet to incorporate, internalize, and utilize will assist you in improving your process of learning. As you do so, your potential for attaining your goals will increase.

DEVELOP A POSITIVE ATTITUDE

Attitude is defined as a manner, feeling, or position toward a person or thing. In order to effect change in your behavior, you must first develop a positive attitude about this experience you are about to begin. You are in charge of setting yourself up for success. This is your opportunity to acquire the knowledge and skills that will make it possible for you to reach the goal of becoming a licensed practical/vocational nurse. You must develop a positive attitude toward yourself as a person and a learner, as well as a genuine desire to learn. To maintain this attitude late at night when you are struggling over the names of the latest drugs and writing client assessments, you must be convinced that you have the capability to complete your task, that some intrinsic factor will be able to support you in the pursuit of your goal. This positive self-attitude sustains the question "Why am I doing this?" Among the strategies you can practice to help you build a positive attitude are the following:

- Create positive self-images, and visualize yourself attaining your goals.
- Recognize your abilities.
- Identify realistic expectations.

Create Positive Self-Images

To begin to create a positive self-image, you must know those attributes that are unique to you. An **attribute** is a characteristic, either positive or negative, that belongs to you. For instance, some positive attributes that are typical to nurses include caring and compassion. Attributes are sometimes referred to as strengths and weaknesses. Whatever you call them, you must actively engage in listing and recalling these qualities about yourself. Divide a paper into two columns, with one headed positive and the other negative. List as many words describing your attributes as you can.

Which side has more entries? Did you start with the negative list? It is unfortunate that sometimes we can recall the negatives faster than the positives. We often speak about ourselves in negative terms, which creates negative self-images. For example, you may recall thinking some of the following: "I wish I were thinner . . . ," "I hope I can do this, I'm not very good at math." Neither of these statements draws a positive image of the speaker. You may need to lose 10 pounds, or improve your math skills, but these are not the total measure of your attributes. If they are the only qualities you recall, they might become the overall image you see of yourself. Regardless of where you started, you must concentrate on the positive side of the chart. You must actively recall your positive side at least as often as you recount the things that could be improved.

Begin to speak of yourself in positive terms and accept compliments from yourself! When an assignment is particularly difficult, you can refocus from "I hope I can do this. I have never been good at math" to "I can read and follow the chapter instructions on how to complete the problems." This simple restatement can sometimes make the difference between success or failure at attempts to acquire new knowledge.

The list does not have to stop at just the words you write today. Continue to practice and do periodic self-assessments. You will add more and more words to the positive side and begin to complement yourself more often. When things go awry, you will be able to draw on these positive attributes and know that you have these strengths.

Recognize Your Abilities

Recognizing your abilities is also an attitude builder. **Ability** can be defined as competence in an activity. An ability is something you can learn; competency is proficiency in a task. Your degree of competence as a nurse will depend on such factors as prior exposure, motivation, how often and with whom you practice, expectations of those things that you should be doing, and a willingness to laugh at attempts and learn from mistakes.

You have abilities and skills that you perform well. To acquire these things took courage, discipline, and hard work. Recalling these abilities and the ways you developed competency in them not only adds to your positive self-image, but also showcases your strengths. Begin by listing in two columns headed by "I am really good at" and "I avoid doing." Next, list all of the skills you need to be able to be "really good" at that task.

For example, maybe you wrote, "I am really good at cooking." Some skills you could have written are:

- *Arithmetic:* You must have an understanding of fractions and the relationships of parts to the whole.
- *Reading:* You must comprehend the words in the recipe in order to follow all the steps.
- *Prioritizing:* You must know with what to start in order to have all of the food ready at the same time.
- *Risk taking:* You may worry about whether your guests will like your dish, but you persist, confident in your ability to turn the raw ingredients into a delicious meal.

Now look at the other column. Maybe you wrote math. Mathematics is an ability you must develop in order to safely administer medications to your clients. If you view this skill only as something to avoid, you begin with a negative attitude toward an ability you will need. You are creating a negative image of yourself completing this task. Instead, look to your past experiences for your strengths; you may realize that you already possess much of the mathematical knowledge you need to correctly compute medication dosages. Realizing this puts a positive slant on this ability.

Now you must develop mathematical competency. Begin by listing the skills needed to perform mathematical operations. You must pay attention to details, understand the way parts relate to the whole, and have solid skills in arithmetic (addition, subtraction, division, and multiplication). Mathematics requires you to choose appropriate formulas to solve a variety of real-world problems. For example, to give the correct dose of medication to your client, you must know the correct formula to use for the calculation. This is a real-world problem for which you must both choose the correct formula and understand it. You must then accurately perform the arithmetic operations.

Identify Realistic Expectations

As mentioned earlier, developing a positive self-image is of primary importance to learning. Your expectations regarding how you will perform in the role as a learner will affect your attitude toward both yourself and learning. You have an expectation about the way you will progress through this program. Ideally, you will attend all classes, pass all exams, and graduate. Further, your current life responsibilities will cooperate with and support this plan. You will likely, however, encounter at least some obstacles. When you hit that first "speed bump" to your plan, your ability to look at the reality of your expectations will be important in regaining a positive focus. Consider the following example:

Marissa is a 25-year-old enrolled full time in a nursing program for the fall. She did well in high school and has already attended a college part time prior to this program. Marissa expects that she will get grades in the B and A range, as she did in prior course work. She works full time and has a 4-year-old daughter. When the class schedule is published, the times conflict with one of the days that she works. This will cause her to be 20 minutes late to work on that day. She has not shared with her employer that she is attending school. She has child care for her daughter, but the need to arrive at the clinical site at 7 A.M. means that she must rearrange her child care and that she will be 30 minutes late for clinical on Fridays. She does not tell her in-structors of her time constraints for child care. She has always needed quiet time for study and is a morning person. Marissa finds her reading assignments take twice as long as she had planned. With all her other responsibilities, her only time for study is after her daughter goes to bed. She has a family that lives close by, but she does not like to burden them with baby-sitting. She has always found a way to do things on her own in the past.

Marissa is a capable person, but her expectation of being able to control all the various facets of her life in perfect harmony is unrealistic. Maintaining a positive attitude while in the midst of the stress of completing all the tasks at hand is difficult, if not impossible, and the plan is often abandoned. In Marissa's case, abandoning the plan may mean abandoning her plans for school. Marissa's reality is that she cannot increase her time commitment by 30 hours of school work and keep everything else she does at the same level. She must set priorities with regard to the demands on her time, and she must identify realistic expectations for those things that she can accomplish.

When everything on your "to do" list cannot be completed, change the way you approach the list and realign your expectations. One way to do this is to ask for help. Asking for help is not a weakness, it is a success strategy. The most successful people are typically those who know when to ask for help and who have devised a plan to structure that help. In the previous example, Marissa needs to remove some of the stress related to work, childcare, and school commitments by informing her employer and instructors of her situation and asking for their help in guiding her to manage the many demands. Help may mean something as simple as talking to the employer about coming in 20 minutes late and working 20 minutes longer and asking a family member to take her daughter to the child-care place on Fridays.

If you do not set realistic expectations for yourself, you may fall victim to a positive attitude's biggest enemy, perfectionism. **Perfectionism** is an overwhelming expectation of being able to get everything done in a flawless manner. This is a setup for failure because it is a standard no one can live up to. Table 1-1 suggests some behaviors of perfectionists versus those of pursuers of excellence. Which list describes you most accurately? Remember to strive to be as realistic with your expectations as possible; be patient with yourself and ask for help when needed.

DEVELOP YOUR BASIC SKILLS

Reading, arithmetic and mathematics, writing, listening, and speaking are skills basic for success in academics and life. When you consider the importance of these basic skills, you must have a strong foundation in them to advance your knowledge beyond the level of memorization to comprehension and application. If you are struggling with these basic skills, you will have difficulty advancing. Developing these skills is basic to the habits of successful learners.

Reading

A large percentage of your program is in written format. To study effectively, you must be highly adept in the

TABLE 1-1 BEHAVIORS OF PERFECTIONISTS AND PURSUERS OF EXCELLENCE

PERFECTIONISTS	PURSUERS OF EXCELLENCE
• Reach for impossible goals	• Enjoy meeting high standards within reach
• Value themselves for what they do	• Value themselves for who they are
• Get depressed and give up	• Experience disappointment but keep going
• Are devastated by failure	• Learn from failure
• Remember mistakes and dwell on them	• Correct mistakes, then learn from them
• Can only live with being number one	• Are pleased with knowing they did their best
• Hate criticism	• Welcome criticism
• Have to win to maintain high self-esteem	• Do not have to win to maintain high self-esteem

basic skill of reading. To be competent in reading, you must be able to locate, understand, and interpret written information; determine the main idea or essential message; find the meanings for unknown or technical words; and judge the accuracy and plausibility of the writers.

Among the several strategies you can effectively implement in your reading and study plan to improve this skill are vocabulary building, comprehension, and reading level. Your basic skill of reading encompasses vocabulary building, which includes the skill of identification and understanding of both English and medical terminology. Investing in quality medical and English dictionaries is a good step to understanding both these languages. Another strategy is simply to take the time when reading to look up the words you do not know (Figure 1-1).

The primary reason for building a strong medical vocabulary is that words are the tools for thinking about and understanding your world, and you are entering the new world of nursing: You must therefore take the time to learn its language. Developing the habit of vocabulary building takes time initially, but as you persist in practicing this skill, your comprehension of the material will increase.

Comprehension goes beyond rote memorization. One sign of true comprehension is the ability to summarize the writer's message. When you summarize, you must state the material in your own words (Sotiriou & Phillips, 1999). Unless you understand the words you have read, you will not be able to advance your level of knowledge from rote memorization to comprehension. When you

are actively reading your nursing textbook and you realize that you are not understanding what you have read, you may find it helpful to use one, some, or all of the five strategies outlined in Table 1-2.

Reading level is another element of your reading skills. Reading level is not related to what you can understand, but, rather, refers to the length of the words and the sentences used in a text to explain, describe, and convey information. It does not have anything to do with your intelligence, but it has a great deal to do with the length of time it takes you to read.

Arithmetic and Mathematics

The next skill you must develop competency in is that of arithemtic and mathematics. To be competent in this skill, you must be able to perform basic computations using whole numbers, percentages, fractions, and decimals, and choose the appropriate formula to use. You will be responsible for correctly calculating dosages and safely administering medications to your clients. You must be able to recognize whether your calculations are correct and logical. In nursing, your mastery of mathematical basic skills cannot be overemphasized. Consider the following excerpt from a study of medication errors done in 1998 at a tertiary care teaching hospital; this excerpt underscores the importance of mathematical competency among nurses.

> Forty-two percent of dosage errors were considered to put the patient at risk for a serious or severe, preventable adverse outcome. Errors in decimal point placement, mathematical calculation, or expression of dosage regime accounted for 59.5% of the dosage errors. The dosage equation was wrong in 29.5% (Lesar, 1998).

Give yourself a reality check on your competency in mathematics and commit to improving those areas where you are weakest. You may want to investigate a resource such as the learning services center at your school, enlist the assistance of a tutor, or use a programmed-learning text to refresh your skills. There are also numerous texts written to assist nursing students in developing these essential skills. Consider also using computer-assisted instruction (CAI) programs or self-paced study modules to hone these skills. Whatever

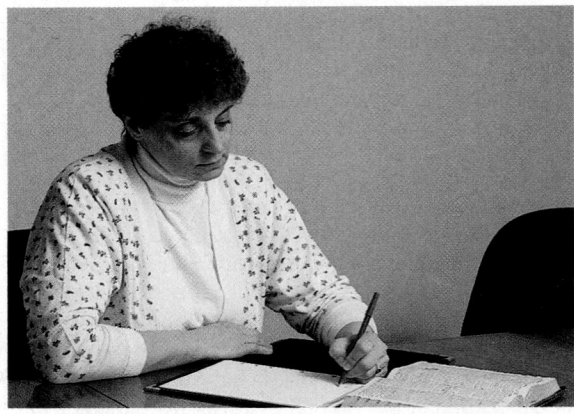

Figure 1-1 *Keep a notebook of new terms to expand your vocabulary. Review your notebook and try to use the words in practice daily.*

TABLE 1-2 STRATEGIES TO IMPROVE COMPREHENSION

STRATEGY	EXPLANATION
Reread	Do this after reading one section of the text, or even after one paragraph.
Define new words	Write the definitions of each new word in the margin of your text and then reread the paragraph. Use a small notebook to build your own glossary. Make your own flashcards for further study.
Visualize	Create mental pictures of the material you are reading. You may even want to draw a simple stick figure, and as you continue to read, adjust the picture.
Research	Many times the reason you are unable to comprehend the material presented is that you have insufficient background in the subject. A solution may be to consult another text that is specific to that knowledge base. Use a dictionary, anatomy and physiology text, general subject text (like a psychology text) or a nursing journal to increase your background knowledge in a subject area (Meltzer & Marcus-Palau, 1997).
Summarize	Use your own words to "tell" yourself what you just read and how this connects to what you are going to be doing. Ask yourself, "Why might I need to know this material?"

means you use, an honest assessment of your competency in mathematics and a commitment to improvement is essential to your practice in the profession.

Writing

In your role as a student and as a professional, you will need writing skills. To be competent in writing, you must be able to communicate thoughts and information clearly and completely using proper grammar, spelling, and punctuation. Contrary to popular opinion, the influx of the computer into health care has not removed the need for this skill. You will be writing client assessments, transfer summaries, discharge summaries, and client-teaching plans. The skill of writing can be practiced and improved.

Listening

The old saying "I know you can hear me, but are you listening?" can be applied to all of us. You must be listening, understanding, and processing information, as opposed to just hearing, when you are in class, as well as when you begin working with clients. To be competent in listening you must receive, interpret, and respond to verbal messages and other cues such as body language while attempting to both comprehend the information and evaluate the speaker. You may need to

polish up on ways that you can improve listening and evaluation skills to make the most of your class time. Class time is a time for listening. Listening effectively can make efficient use of this time to increase your comprehension of the content.

Among the many strategies that can be used to improve listening skills are the following:

- *Be interested in the subject.* Make a connection with the reason you are going to this lecture. What is the connection between the information and your need for the information? Have you read the material and come with questions about the subject?
- *Be open to the information.* When you hear a topic and immediately react with your instinct, you often miss the point and some aspect of the presentation you had not considered before. Listening does not automatically mean you will change your mind on topics, but it will allow you to evaluate and incorporate those aspects that are beneficial to you.
- *Do not be critical of the speaker.* Focus on the message, not the messenger. The speaker is not there as a member of a theatrical company to entertain you. The speaker's role is to impart information. It is up to you to concentrate on the information that you need to know and apply it properly.
- *Concentrate on the information.* Be present to the lecture. If you find yourself falling asleep, do muscle flexes or breathe deeply to try to stay alert and aware. Imagine test questions that might be asked on the information.
- *Evaluate the information.* Not every word is critical. Relate the information to what you know, where you may use it, and whether you agree with what is said. If you have difficulty with what is being said, use the next strategy to maintain your concentration.
- *Write down questions as you listen.* This allows you to follow the speaker to the end, and many of your questions may have been answered. If not, you have them written down and can refer later to the list. This promotes concentration on the information presented. You will not be distracted trying to remember questions you wanted to ask.

Speaking

Learning to speak or present in front of a group is one of the most-feared activities of many students. Yet as a nurse, you have entered one of the most "speaking"-oriented professions. You will communicate daily with clients, their families, instructors, peers, ancillary staff members, and the multiple members of the health care team. To be competent in speaking, you must be able to organize ideas and communicate them using verbal language in a tone, style, and level of complexity appropriate to the listener.

Most of the fear of speaking in public arises from our fear of appearing the fool. Many students will not ask questions during a lecture specifically because they believe themselves incapable of speaking clearly and identifying exactly the information they need. There is a saying, "There is no stupid question"; believe it. You must develop the confidence to speak up when you have a question; consider the potential consequences to your clients if you fail to clarify a medical order or question a procedure that is unclear.

Speaking

Thorough preparation is an important strategy for speaking about anything. Formulating multiple examples is one way of increasing your comfort level with the given information. For example, if you are asked to explain the way the pancreas produces insulin, you might draw the organ and indicate where the islets of Langerhans are. Or you may use a lock and key to explain the way insulin works to open the channels for glucose to enter the cells. You may trace a cracker as it travels through the body from teeth to cells and indicate just where and when insulin is utilized. Regardless of the specifics, creating multiple examples will assist you in thoroughly learning a topic and therefore creating a feeling of comfort about your knowledge of the subject.

The following strategies may help when you want to ask a question:

- *Understand why you are asking the question.* Instead of saying, "I don't understand," say, "I was with you on the physiology of the kidney until you reached the Bowman's capsule. Can you connect this particular part of the kidney with osmosis for me?" This puts you and the speaker in a positive light; you have not attacked the speaker's explanation, and you acknowledge your skill in listening. You are communicating what you need and asking the speaker to help by connecting the two concepts for you.
- *Know when to ask the question.* Writing down those topics on which you need further information may help you decide the correct time to ask a question. If the instructor begins by saying, "Today we will be speaking about pharmacokinetics," and you do not understand the word, stopping her before she has a chance to define the word may not be the most effective strategy. If instead you write down, "What does pharmacokinetics mean?" and listen for the meaning of that word in the context of the lecture, you will most likely hear clues as to the word's meaning. The instructor will use other words, such as *absorption*, *distribution*, *metabolism*, and *excretion* to describe what happens to a drug as it goes through the body. When an appropriate time in the presentation comes, review those things that have been said and clarify: "So, Prof. Z., am I correct when I say that pharmacokinetics has to do with the movement of drugs through all the systems of the body?" You will get your answer, and your instructor will know from your question that you have been listening.

You must speak clearly and articulate those things you need daily as you attend classes; listen to your instructors; listen to your clients; and transmit information to instructors, colleagues, support staff, doctors, and allied health care team members. Practice both the skills of listening and speaking equally and keep asking questions.

DEVELOP YOUR LEARNING STYLE

The term **learning style** refers to the ways you best receive, process, and assimilate information (knowledge) about a particular subject. In your life as a student, you have probably had both of the following experiences:

You attend class with Professor A for Course 100. The professor arranges the room casually in small groupings and breaks up class time to alternate short lectures with small group work. There is time for a hands-on demonstration of the principle along with actual work-related items used as examples. Professor A allows for student–teacher interchange of ideas and gives credence to experiences of the students during the class discussions. You leave the class exhilarated and with ideas, aware that this content connects with your

Learning Disabilities

According to the National Center for Learning Disabilities, Inc. (NCLD, 1999), 15% to 20% of the population have some form of learning disability. **Learning disability** is a generic term that refers to a heterogeneous group of disorders manifested as significant difficulties in the acquisition and use of listening, speaking, reading, writing, reasoning, or mathematical abilities.

Having a learning disability will not prohibit your success; you must, however, understand your different abilities. Find out the types of accommodations that will enhance your learning capabilities, and ask for those things that you need. Accommodations in postsecondary programs are mandated by the federal government; however, the onus to disclose, provide documentation, and request accommodations is on the student. Accommodations are determined on a case-by-case basis. Reasonable accommodations in the classroom may be as simple as having the instructor wear a microphone, being able to use a tape recorder or note taker, or requesting textbook tapes. In the clinical area, all reasonable accommodations are made within the confines of client safety and essential skills needed to participate in a program of study for nursing. A quiet work area and ear protectors may provide quiet for students who are hypersensitive to background noise. Using a computer for writing assignments, note taking in class, and studying may assist students who have difficulty writing. Getting a tutor who is skilled at working with students with learning disabilities may be another intervention to consider.

Whatever you suspect your needs to be, getting professional testing to ascertain whether you have a disability and to determine any specific accommodations you will need is crucial. Seek the assistance of your instructors, student service personnel, learning center personnel, or call the special education coordinator at the nearest high school. These resources will help you locate an accredited testing agency to provide you with further resources and documentation.

desired outcome. You plan a review of the notes with a fellow student you met in your class group. You continue to prepare throughout the course and prior to the final, on which you get a B.

The next day you attend Course 200 with Professor B. The room is arranged in rows. Professor B puts up the class outline on the overhead, lectures for 40 minutes, then allows 10 minutes at the end for questions. If you hand him a written question, he will answer it during the next class. You dread his boring presentation and wish that Professor B was more like Professor A. You really do not know anyone in the class with whom to study, you cannot understand the text, and your grades are in the low C to D range. You know you need this class for your major. You try to do your part, but you just can't "get into it."

Think about Professor A, who presents information in a variety of methods—short lecture, small group, hands-on demonstration. As a student, you can grasp the information from whichever method appeals to you. You come away feeling connected to the subject and your classmates and want to continue learning about the subject. You are rewarded for your efforts through the academic grade system.

Now consider Professor B, who knows just as much about the subject as does Professor A, but who presents it using only one method—lecture. Lecture is not your preferred learning style, and your ability to clarify your understanding through questions is limited by the class format. Your outcomes on tests are less rewarding, and you begin to avoid putting time into studying the subject all together. You end up thinking that you really do not do well in that subject and consider changing your major.

The difference in the outcomes of the two examples lies in the perceived role of the learner. In these examples, the student relied heavily on the *teacher's* ability to present material in the student's preferred learning style. Remember, *you* are in charge of your learning. Teacher presentations vary in ways that may not appeal to your primary learning style, but you can still learn the information. You must take charge of developing your abilities, increasing your awareness of your preferred learning styles, and implementing some simple strategies to enhance those styles. As you increase your skills in your preferred methods and strengthen those in your weaker ones, your outcomes will change.

Classification of Learning Styles

Learning styles are cognitive (mental) functions. They refer to the ways you perceive, remember, think, and solve problems: Their focus is *how* you learn as opposed to *what* you learn. Your preference for one style over another can be argued to be both genetic and developmental. Regardless, your awareness of the ways you best learn will affect your learning outcomes.

Learning styles are classified in many different ways. One classification method focuses on the route by which students best perceive and remember information: visual, auditory, or kinesthetic. These divisions are not mutually exclusive; we possess all three, and we use all of them to garner our information. Visual learners make up approximately 65% of the population, auditory

learners approximately 30%, and kinesthetic learners approximately 5% (Mind Tools, 1998).

Visual learners think in pictures. No matter how information is obtained (reading, hearing, or seeing), it is stored as visual images. This person says "I see" or "I get the picture." Auditory learners relate best to the spoken word and prefer class discussion and oral presentations. This person says "That sounds right" or "I hear you." Kinesthetic learners process and remember information well if they touch, imitate, and practice what they are studying. All of us have the capacity to learn in all three modes. You naturally gravitate to one over the others based on which style has lead to your greatest learning successes.

Another way to classify learning styles is according to brain-hemisphere dominance. The left hemisphere of the brain is associated with analytical activities, such as logic, structure, speech, reasoning, numbers, verbal expression, verification of data, and analysis of parts of the whole. The right side is associated with creativity and synthesizing parts to form a whole idea. The right side is also considered the more emotional side and links to insight, intuition, daydreams, visualization, music, rhythm, and color visualization.

We need both sides of the brain to function and learn. Numerous studies demonstrated that individuals with left-brain dominance are primarily auditory learners, and those with right-brain dominance are primarily visual. Additional studies show that right-brain–dominant learners process, recall, and retain more from information presented in computer-assisted instructional programs, whereas left-brain–dominant learners derive more success from a lecture format. To overlook or use one style to the exclusion of the other is using only part of your overall potential learning ability.

Strategies for Learning

By determining your preferred learning style, you will be able to adopt strategies to enhance that style when you study. You want to effectively move the required information into long-term memory and increase your knowledge level from memorization to comprehension and, finally, to application. To accomplish this you must know which strategies work with which learning styles. Refer to Table 1-3 and note all of the strategies listed that you consistently use in your study routine. Start with the style you previously ascertained to be your preferred learning style.

Are there strategies listed under your preferred style that you currently do not use? To enhance your acquisition of material, begin to incorporate these into your study plan. Are there strategies listed under any of the other styles that you could use when the material you are learning is especially difficult for you?

One way to incorporate more than one learning style into your study program is to employ a CAI program. Many texts now come with an accompanying disk designed to enhance learning style. Such disks may contain the total text along with testing materials, exercises that accompany the text, and/or resource material for the text. For example, several medical terminology packages come as program-instruction texts with disks and provide audio pronunciation in the computer programs. The student can read the text, manip-

TABLE 1-3 SAMPLE LEARNING STRATEGIES

VISUAL LEARNER	AUDITORY LEARNER	KINESTHETIC LEARNER
Takes notes in class	Reads aloud	Takes notes and rewrites them to condense
Writes notes in margin of book	Reads into a tape recorder and plays it back to self	Expresses self with hands, even while reading
Looks for reference books with pictures, graphs, and charts	Discusses ideas about class content with others	Handles visual aids during class
Draws own illustrations	Requests explanations of illustrations	Requests to do a demonstration

ulate the information on the computer, and hear the correct pronunciation.

When faced with a particularly difficult passage or concept, incorporate more than one style and one strategy to process the information. The more action you put into your learning methods, the more effective your time and outcomes will be. **Mnemonics,** words or phrases used to aid memory, may help. For example, ABC reminds you of airway, breathing, circulation.

DEVELOP A TIME-MANAGEMENT PLAN

Somewhere in your decision-making process to go to school, you decided you would have the time to do so. You now must make that a reality by actively engaging in a time-management plan. **Time management** is a system to help meet goals through problem solving. Practicing time-management strategies will not eliminate the need to perform tasks you do not like, but it will make doing so more manageable. Active application of time-management strategies will make a difference in what you can accomplish in the time you have.

Strategies for time management include the following:

• Analyzing your time commitments
• Knowing yourself
• Clarifying your goals
• Setting priorities and identifying one or two valued goals to achieve
• Disciplining yourself to adhere to the plan through changes and until the goal is reached

Analyze Time Commitments

To analyze your time commitments, start by listing them. Provide yourself with both a big-picture plan and a daily plan. Creating a year-at-a-glance calendar that lists all of your important time commitments can provide a quick illustration of the way the months ahead will be used. Start by putting in your graduation date in red capital letters. This will give you an instant visual reminder of your current goal. Next, using a pencil, insert all important dates, including holidays, birthdays, work, and organizational obligations. Remember to also include activities for those in your household that will require your partici-

pation, such as carpooling, special school programs, after-school activities, and child care. Use your academic program calendar as the source for the dates that classes, as well as vacations, begin and end, financial aid forms and tuition payments are due, and the like. Use your individual class schedules as the sources for dates of exams, special review or clinical days, field trips, or any other time commitments you must meet in order to complete the courses. This exercise will give you a big-picture view of your time commitments and will also point out any conflicts.

Conflicts are not impossible obstacles. Knowing about them in advance will allow you to take steps now to prioritize and reschedule. When prioritizing, think about delegating some tasks to other people. Do not always solve a conflict by removing those tasks you enjoy or that will renew you. Taking care of yourself during this time is very important. Never give up the time you need to refresh and renew, even if it is just a hot bath, a brisk 15-minute walk, or a dinner out with family and friends. Place yourself near the top of the priority list to complete your goal.

Each learner's big-picture map will differ. The struggle is to mesh your map with your other relationships and keep yourself toward the top of the list. One strategy is to prominently display your big-picture calendar in an area where all of the members of your household can see it—including and especially you. Everyone will then have the opportunity to see that they are on the list and that they contribute to helping you reach your goal.

The next step is daily planning. Using a week-at-a-glance planner helps illustrate more concrete expectations of those things you plan to do and the amount of time you actually have (Figure 1-2). You should include time to sleep, eat, drive, work, attend class, and study.

You may find that you must rearrange your schedule. This does not mean continuing to do all of the things you have listed but just on different days; rather, it means choosing two valued goals on which to work. *One goal must be to be a learner. The other will be unique to you.* This does not mean that you replace all other goals with these two valued goals. Rather, it means that these goals must take precedence when choosing ways to use your time. If you choose child care and learner as your most valued goals, you could refine them even further to complement each other. For example, you may opt to keep driving the carpool, but negotiate to drive every morning, because

PROFESSIONAL TIP

Time Wasters

Are you a time waster? We all sometimes behave in ways that sabotage the best of plans. Following are some examples of time wasters along with some strategies for helping you reclaim those wasted hours.

1. *Clutter:* Wisdom holds that you can save 1 hour each day by just clearing your work area of clutter and keeping it clean. This time can be put to good use in the form of study. Organize your study area so that when you arrive it is ready for work, and take a few minutes at the end of your session to prepare your area for the next session.

2. *Interruptions:* Intrusions into your study or work hours (from either people or things) can be real time wasters. Try the following:

• Learn to say "no." You do not have to agree to every request. Learn to pick your involvements carefully and according to those that are most important to you reaching your goals.

• Put your answering machine on, and turn the phone's ringer off. Delegate a time to listen and respond to messages after studying.

• Open your mail over the garbage can. Respond, delegate, or throw it out.

• Organize your papers. For instance, have a folder for each child's paper/notes. Keep your class notebooks, your calendar, and phone lists in one three-ring binder, so you have all your essentials together.

3. *Procrastination:* This refers to intentionally putting off or delaying something that should be done. **Procrastination** is a time waster because it does not afford effective use of time. Time management is not necessarily finishing everything at one sitting, but, rather, scheduling time to return to the task until you complete it; whereas procrastination is intentionally delaying the task without good cause or a plan to complete it in a time-efficient manner. Breaking the task down into manageable segments and rewards will encourage you to return to it again and again until it is complete.

4. *Perfectionism:* Very often we do not stick to a plan because it does not give us results immediately or does not give the results we expected. Perfectionism affects your time-management plan by prohibiting you from accepting anything less than perfection; it also damages your positive attitude of yourself by setting unrealistic expectations. Focus on your positive accomplishments, look for ways to improve, accept your failures, and build on your experiences.

	Monday	Tuesday	Wednesday	Thursday	Friday	Saturday	Sunday
7 AM	Work	Carpool	Carpool	Carpool	Clinical	House	
9 AM	Work	Class	Class	Class		House	Sunday school
11 AM	Work	Class	Class	Class		Chores	Church
1 PM	Work	Class	Class	Class			
3 PM	Work				Work	Work	
5 PM	Carpool Dinner				Work	Work	
7 PM					Work	Work	

Figure 1-2 *Week-at-a-Glance Calendar*

doing so will afford you 2 hours to study prior to class. You may then have to make child care arrangements for after school, which might mean asking your neighbor or contracting with an after-school program. You may also have to set aside 1 hour each evening to get everything laid out for the next day, a task you might ask someone else in the household to do each night so that you can gain an extra hour of study time. That extra hour, in turn, might mean that you dedicate Saturdays for nothing but family commitments. Regardless of the way you choose to solve such problems, the solutions must be designed to help you reach your goals.

Know Yourself

To develop your system, you must know yourself. You must be honest with yourself about your work habits and preferences. Consider the time of day when you are at your intellectual best. Is it early in the morning, or do you come alive at 10 P.M.? You must be able to focus and concentrate when you are studying. Deciding you are going to carpool in the morning to get to school early to study will not be effective if you cannot concentrate until after noon. If this is the case, it would be better to do the more mechanical and less intellectually demanding tasks, such as the shopping or laundry, in the 2 hours before class. Are you a person who is more left-brain oriented (logical, orderly, structured, and plays by the rules)? Then writing out lists of tasks and crossing them off may be your time-management strategy to stay on track. Perhaps you are a more right-brain personality (creative, resists rules, has own sense of time)? Scheduling your task within a specific time frame that has a time-sensitive goal/ reward at the end may assist you to use your available time more effectively.

Clarify Goals

Without setting goals, we cannot know whether we are making any progress. Goals are like grocery lists. Think about when you go to the store without a list. You may purchase many items, but when you get home you often discover that you did not get all the things you needed. If the next time you go to the store you make a list, you will likely get all the items you want.

Just like the grocery list, goals must be written down. They must be based on reality and broken down into manageable parts. Say your goal is to provide study time each week that will allow you to be successful in each unit exam of your program. This time will comprise the time you need to prepare and review material, prepare for clinical assignments, view information in the library, and practice new skills in the lab. As a rule, you will need 1 to 2 hours of study time for each hour you spend in class. If you are in class 12 hours per week, you will thus need to find 24 more hours to study; and if you are in clinical 6 hours 3 days per week for a total of 18 hours, you will need to fit in 36 hours of study. As a rough estimate, this would mean 12 class hours plus 24 study hours plus 18 clinical hours plus 36 preparation hours for a total of 90 hours per week (30 class hours plus 60 study hours) for the ideal study week and 30 hours (class attendance only) for a week without any study. So now you know what amount of time you are aiming for. You can now take this goal of 60 study hours per week and compare it to your written schedule and calendar to determine how to best arrange the demands on your time in order to meet your goals.

Set Priorities

Another part of setting goals is prioritizing tasks into general categories. Look at your daily calendar and list the general categories. Some examples might be as follows:

- Work
- Study
- Personal (eating, sleeping)
- Household chores (shopping, budget)
- Transportation (self, others)
- Supervising children
- Decision making (planning, outside organizational responsibility, time for self, time for spouse, friends, and children)

Next, rank these general categories in order of priority, keeping in mind that not everything is a primary priority. If you uncover conflicts, try to further clarify which items take top priority.

Another way to prioritize is to group tasks according to the time frame in which you wish them to be accomplished. To do this, divide a sheet of paper into three parts. Label the first part column A, the second, column

B, and the third, column C. Under column A, write "I must work on these tasks now." This list includes your priority tasks that need immediate attention. Under column B, write "I can do these after A is done." Under column C, write "I can delay, eliminate, or delegate these until after B is done" (Figure 1-3).

If you placed your entire list under column A, go back to your original two goals—one of which includes your new role as learner—and rethink your list. You must prioritize your activities in order to reach your goal. *You cannot be all things at all times to all people.* You also must know how to work smarter, not longer or harder, to remain focused on the priority task.

Discipline Yourself

The hardest strategy to commit to may be the last one. The idea that you must actively engage in using the plan sounds simple. In practice, the plan will not always work. When this happens, you may be tempted to abandon the plan instead of changing it. If the plan is not working, you must ascertain the reasons. Maybe you lack resources, have not scheduled enough time, or need to revisit and reevaluate your goals. Build time to plan into your weekly schedule. If you really want to use a time-management system, your ability to go back to the plan and revise it is very important.

DEVELOP A STUDY STRATEGY

Developing a study plan involves more than just buying a textbook and reading it. Several strategies that will assist you to study more efficiently and effectively follow.

Set Up the Environment

Where and when you study are as important as how. The fact that you assign a specific behavior to your study space will set you up for success. The space should fit your style. Do you like everything organized in neat spaces, or do you just need it near you? What type of lighting, seating, or noise level will assist or detract from your concentration? Consider your preferred learning style when setting up your study space. If you are a kinesthetic learner, you may want to put motion into your space by, for instance, using a treadmill in your study plan. You may want to spend a percentage of your study time sitting to read and take notes and then switch to walking or running on the treadmill to recite and reflect on the material. You will be increasing comprehension and making connections, all while walking 2 miles! Regardless of the way you arrange your space, take into consideration the type of learner you are and your biological and personality preferences.

Gather Your Resources

Your resources should all be easily accessible from your study space. In some homes, the kitchen table serves as the study space. If your study space serves more than one function, as would the kitchen table, consider keeping your study resources in a milk crate or box so they are portable yet readily at hand when needed.

Gathering your resources is your start to building a library of textbooks, which will serve you throughout

A	B	C
I must work on these tasks now	I can do these after A is done	I can delay, eliminate, or delegate until after B is done
school/study *child care* *self-care* *work*	*supervise children*	*organization* *shopping*

Figure 1-3 *Prioritizing Tasks*

your program. These resources become a reference library for you when you study. Some general resources to keep on hand include the following:

- A recent edition of an unabridged dictionary
- A medical dictionary
- An anatomy and physiology text

Additional resources you will need as you progress through your program may include texts on pharmacology, nutrition, and the nursing process. Depending on your personal knowledge base, you may need further resources in the foundation sciences—biology, psychology, and sociology. These areas serve as the knowledge base for your future profession.

Keeping your learning style in mind, consider purchasing accompanying workbooks or other study aids that come with the text and research CAI or videotapes available in your nursing program library. Using varied and multiple resources enhances your knowledge base and will increase your comprehension of the content. You must go beyond memorization, beyond amassing facts, to comprehension of this knowledge base in order to answer the questions on the exams. Keep in mind that you are studying for the program examination, the National Council Licensure Examination (NCLEX-PN)®, and, ultimately, to apply your knowledge base to provide safe, effective care to your clients.

Remember to use journals as resources. The articles and related client situations can assist you in understanding the application of content to the clinical area. Your ultimate goal is to apply your content information to client care. Consider getting a subscription to your nursing journal, *Journal of Practical Nursing* or *Practical Nursing Journal*. Nursing organizations such as the National Federation of Licensed Practical Nursing are also valuable resources, and many have websites, which you can visit.

Whatever resources you ultimately choose, gathering them and having your resources readily at hand are simple strategies that will make the time you have allotted for study more efficient and effective.

Minimize Interruptions

Interruptions to your study time decrease the actual time you can focus on the material and affect your concentration. Interruptions may also become your procras-

tination "triggers." If you allow your study time to be constantly interrupted, you will soon be doing something other than studying. At the very least, these interruptions minimize your efficient use of time. When you plan your time to study, do not set yourself up for interruptions. Look realistically at your time schedule and do not schedule your study time around the household's naturally busy times of the day—typically mornings, mealtimes, early evenings, and bedtimes.

This is where you put the strategies listed in the section on time management to work. If you have set aside a time and a space for study, make it known that you are not to be interrupted unless there is an emergency. Hang a sign on the door that reads, "Think before you knock." Planning on studying in 1- or 1½-hour blocks is also a way to cut down on interruptions. This is a reasonable time period for you to put the world on hold in order to accomplish your task.

Get to Know the Textbook

Your textbook is not intended to be read like the latest mystery novel, from beginning to end in one sitting. It has both directions on the way to use it (introduction, preface) and built-in references (glossary, appendix, summary questions). It is arranged in sections, each dealing with a major topic, and then subdivided into the parts (chapters) that make up the sum of that topic. Getting to know your textbook and its resources and the author's approach to writing may constitute the first part of your study plan. Having this information gives you some insight into the way the material has been grouped and connected.

Another author may have written the book in totally stand-alone chapters and may encourage students to review the table of contents and start anywhere they feel they need to. Self-instruction modules or texts in math often give students instructions to first take all of the posttests in the chapters, and as long as a certain score is reached, to go on. This is a means of giving students credit for knowledge already learned and facilitating recall of knowledge in preparation for new learning.

Take a look at various parts of this text. How is the information organized? What built-in references can assist you? Consider the cues given about the way to use this text to help you organize the big picture.

Set Up the Study Plan

Each time you enter your study space, your study plan should be with you. You should have a plan or a specific goal for that time. Each time you enter the space, bring a positive attitude toward reaching that goal. Your nursing course outline will drive your study plan. You will have a certain amount of material to cover in a specific time span. You first must know those things that are expected of you. Your course outline, curriculum, and instructors will give you this information.

As an example, consider a unit on vital signs, which is assigned to be completed in 1 week. The components of the unit include understanding the theory base about vital signs as well as learning the psychomotor skills involved in actually measuring these indicators. You are expected to acquire the knowledge by reading the chapter in the text, attending the lecture and demonstration, and practicing in the lab. You will be tested on your ability to apply your knowledge through a pencil-and-paper test and a redemonstration of your psychomotor skills. Now that you know the information you must cover, the sources of the information, and the way you will be tested, you can map out a study plan. Consider the following steps:

1. *Preview the material to be studied.* Your assigned reading from the text on the content of the unit may be contained in one chapter or may span several chapters. Always preview the assigned chapter(s). Often, the student reads only the pages assigned, thinking that this is the most efficient way to study. By not spending the 5 or 10 minutes to preview the entire chapter, the connections between the content may be lost. Previewing can be done very quickly by scanning the chapter headings, art, and tables.
2. *Consider the chapter heading.* The material about vital signs may be contained in a chapter labeled "Baseline Assessment" or "Measurement of Baseline Values" or "Physiologic Functions of the Body." All of these give you a cue as to what you are about to study.
3. *Read the objectives for the chapter.* The objectives list those things you should be able to do when you are finished learning the content of the chapter.
4. *Scan the vocabulary section and the end-of-chapter summary and questions.* Read the key terms and the summary and questions at the chapter's end. Doing so gives you an overview of the scope of the reading you will need to do and should take no more than 5 to 10 minutes.
5. *Set up your questions.* Beginning at the chapter objectives, write down those things you already know, questions about those things you must learn for each objective, and some additional resources that you think you should check. For example, in a chapter about vital signs, the initial page may look like the one in Figure 1-4. Jot down your current knowledge and your questions. The resources note relates to the reasons you are trying to learn this material. Connecting the material to your role in the profession is most important. You are now ready to read the chapter critically for the answers to your questions. You may uncover more and have more ques-

The Measurement of Vital Signs

At the completion of this chapter, you should be able to:

1. Describe the physiologic mechanisms controlling temperature, pulse, respiration, and blood pressure.

Temp = ?, Pulse = heart, Respiration = lungs, Blood pressure = arteries need to find out about temp.

2. Identify the normal range for vital sign measurements.

For adults? Children?

3. Select the appropriate equipment used to take vital signs.

Thermometer, stethoscope, blood pressure cuff

4. Demonstrate the correct psychomotor technique used in measuring vital signs.

I do this in the lab/get procedure from book or instructor? Ask in class.

5. Document the normal findings of the measurement of blood pressure.

Temp = 98.6, p = 60-80, bp = 120/80 I need to know this to be able to tell if the client is normal or having trouble.

Figure 1-4 *Start with the chapter objectives and devise questions and answers to determine those things you know and those things you will need to give more attention.*

tions at the end; but you have a plan and can move on to the next step.
6. *Read and take notes.* Answer your questions and check your vocabulary knowledge as you read.
7. *Reread when necessary.* Remember your basic skills and concentration.
8. *Reflect on the connections you can make between the material and client care.* Identify the reasons the information is important and the way you will use it.
9. *Recite or create your individual style cues.* This is where you will put your individual unique learning styles to work. Make up songs. Create mnemonics. Design flash cards for items that must be memorized. Try to create a logical connection when recalling information.
10. *Review or summarize the information.* Answer the objectives. Use your own words to answer your initial questions. Do you have more questions? Must you consult a second resource to answer them?
11. *End the session with a critical thinking question.* What would the client look like if his temperature were 103°F? What other body systems would be affected? What nursing measures might I use to support the client with this level temperature (e.g., monitor the client's fluid intake and output because the body

---

---

would be losing fluid as a result of the thermoregulation [sweating and evaporation that would reduce the temperature]), and why? Write these questions down in your notes. You will soon have a collection of "client scenarios" that you will be able to build on as you increase your knowledge base.

The preceding steps require skill in five areas: reading, rereading, reflecting, reciting, and review. With each step, you are engaging in the process of encoding the material. **Encoding** is thought of as actually laying down tracks in the areas of your brain. Each time you read, reread, reflect, recite, and review, you increase the depth of the tract, and your ability to recall and utilize the information increases. You move the information from short-term to long-term memory, and you increase your level of knowledge. The more senses and action you put into your study plan, the more you are able to utilize the information.

You move your level of knowledge from the memorization of a group of facts to the comprehension of the facts in a logical, organized fashion that allows you to relate the information to clients to whom you will provide care. Each time you sit down to study, this should be your goal. You can preview, question, and quickly outline the major points in the chapters before class. Listen to the lecture and take notes. Approach new material with the read, reread, reflect, recite, and review steps before moving on to the next topic.

Note Taking

Note taking is an action that connects you to the content of written material or a lecture presentation and will assist you in identifying the main ideas and their connection to the overall topic.

Keep materials for each of your classes or topics in a separate three-ring binder. Take notes on loose-leaf paper and write on one side only because this allows you to arrange your preview notes and lecture notes chronologically. You can also insert handouts from the class in the appropriate order as you receive them. Using this

method, you can also review notes against additional information you have from other resources to assist you when it is time to review for the examinations.

When you are taking notes from the text, read with a pencil in your hand to put yourself in the action mode. You will thus be ready to receive and process information. You may also take notes from text readings on your computer, which facilitates editing and rearranging material.

Before class, preview your chapter material and divide your paper, leaving a 3-inch border on the left side. From the assigned reading, identify the main topic to be covered, list the main section and the subheadings, and summarize the information in the left column. Then write your questions in this column. This prepares you for more active participation in the lecture; use the right column to take notes from the lecture.

Regardless of the way you choose to take notes, note taking while you study sets you up for connecting with the content. It positions you as an active participant in the learning process, and any time you increase your active participation in the learning process, you increase your learning.

When taking notes in class, listen attentively, lean forward, and concentrate on the information the speaker is imparting (Figure 1-5). Take notes on the following:

- The topic, as stated by the speaker; write it on the top of the page
- The main ideas and the details that support the topic
- The most important points, based on the speaker's organization and emphasis
- Other students' questions and the responses from the speaker, which are often the very questions you had

Look for visual and auditory cues from the speaker, for example, if the speaker says, "This is important" or writes steps on the board. Do not form an opinion of what is being said until you have heard the entire lecture. As stated earlier, a good strategy is to write your questions as you think of them. They may be answered by the time the lecture is over.

The purpose of note taking during a lecture is not to create a transcript of the information imparted, but, rather, to record what you understand. The combination of attending lecture, listening, and note taking can provide you with much knowledge that you will not have to learn elsewhere. Previewing the material to be covered further contributes to this dynamic. When taking notes, consider the following guidelines to make your note taking efficient and effective:

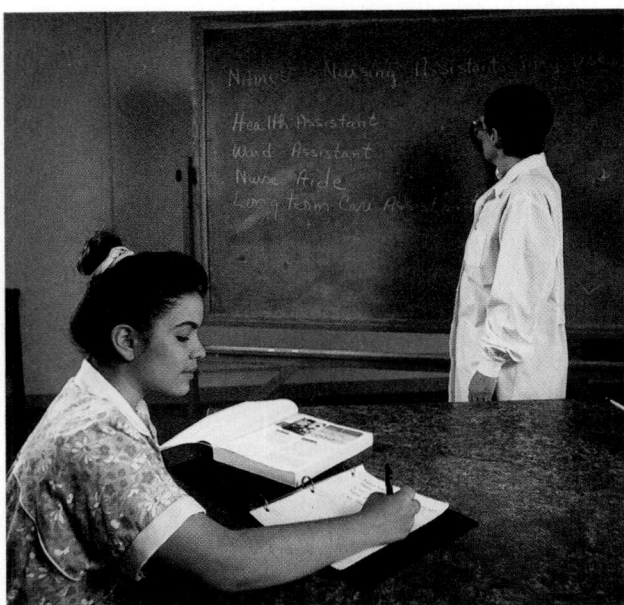

Figure 1-5 *Note taking is an important component of increasing your comprehension of the material.*

- Do not take notes with the intent of writing them over. This is a waste of time and, contrary to what you may expect, it does not improve recall.
- If your handwriting is sloppy, print or use a laptop computer.
- Condense the amount of actual writing you do by using symbols and abbreviations and leaving out everything but necessary words. For instance, instead of writing "If the client's blood pressure reading is greater than 140 systolic and 90 diastolic, . . ." write "If BP >140/90. . . ."
- Write definitions and mathematical formulas exactly as you heard them in lecture.
- In mathematics and science lab courses, write the process step by step exactly as explained. Indicate which formulas are used with which problems, for example

    "Use ratio/proportion for word problems."

- Pick an abbreviation system and stick to it.
- Review the notes as soon as possible after class. Many studies have demonstrated that even a brief review of notes after class increases retention of the material by 50%.

Prepare for Exams

The final plus of having a study plan is the ability to review for exams. Reviewing for exams is not studying all of the material over from the beginning. You will already have studied the subject matter you are going to cover on the exam; now, you are reviewing and recalling it through a series of exercises designed to increase your comprehension and facilitate application. Most nursing examinations are written at the comprehension or recall level. The NCLEX-PN® is written at the application level. On this exam you will not see many questions about naming where the pulse points are (comprehension, recall), for instance. You will instead find questions about which of the

pulse points of the body are most appropriate for assessing an infant (application). Making decisions about which fact or groups of principles you have learned will be the basis for most nursing examination questions.

Depending on the curriculum, you may have examinations every week or every month, a weekly quiz, a midterm, and a final. Regardless, you will know the schedule, and you must set aside review time for preparation. If you are to have weekly quizzes, you must build a time for review into your daily study plan. One way to do so is to set aside the last 30 minutes of each study session for review. Take each objective of your course outline and, without looking at your notes or text, turn them into questions and then answer them. If you are weak in one area, refer to your notes and devise a technique for recall, such as the use of flash cards, rhythms, mnemonics, pictures, or graphic drawings. Work through each of the objectives for the content that will be covered.

If your examinations are by unit, you must divide the material up over the time you will need to cover it, leaving at least 2 days for review and recall before the examination. Each of these review sessions will also serve as preparation for both your final examination and the NCLEX-PN®. As you are successful in each of your examinations and continue to see further connections in your clinical application, your depth as well as breadth of content mastery will increase.

PRACTICE CRITICAL THINKING

Most of this chapter thus far has been devoted to presenting strategies for the effective and efficient acquisition of knowledge. Your ultimate goal is to be able to use this knowledge to provide safe client care. To do so, you must go beyond the initial stage of simply acquiring information. In delivering nursing care, facts alone do not constitute a sufficient knowledge base for making sound decisions about client care. You must internalize these facts and be able to use them when presented with new situations.

In considering which actions you may need to take in a new situation, you must consider past experience and principles of care, postulate possible outcomes from a variety of interventions, and seek additional information from colleagues, clients, and resource materials. This process is called critical thinking, and it is what you will be expected to do with the knowledge you are acquiring.

The first step is to develop an understanding of **critical thinking**. A comprehensive definition is the **disciplined** (trained by instruction and exercise) intellectual process of applying skillful **reasoning** (use of the elements of thought to solve a problem or settle a question), imposing intellectual **standards** (a level or degree of quality), and self-reflective thinking as a guide to a belief or an action (Heaslip, 1994; Norris & Ennis, 1989; Paul, 1990).

Many students find the process of becoming responsible for their own thinking painful. You, along with many other students, may be uncomfortable when asked to defend your **opinions** (subjective beliefs) and **judgments** (conclusions based on sound reasoning and supported by evidence) or to decide what is important. Probably you would prefer to be told what you need to know.

Because practical/vocational nurses must make many decisions in the care of their clients, knowing how to make good decisions is essential.

Skills of Critical Thinking

Your abilities in the four basic skills of critical reading, critical listening, critical writing, and critical speaking can be measured by how well you achieve the universal intellectual standards (UIS). These standards are discussed in the next section.

Critical Reading

Reading for meaning is basic to the acquisition of knowledge from books. Study time is reduced, and information will be retained, leading to better results on tests. Use of a highlighter to mark the main ideas is often helpful. Those who do not read critically usually mark most of the page. Form a study group to compare the main ideas marked in the assigned material. When reviewing tests, note when misreading or misinterpretation was the cause of your incorrect answer. Make a conscious effort to identify your weaknesses.

As you prepare your assignments, have a dialogue with yourself:

- Before beginning to read, preview the material and ask yourself: What is it about; how is it related to what I already know; how it is organized; and are other resources required?
- As you are reading, ask yourself: Does it make sense; are all terms familiar or should I look them up; how is this related to what I already know; and can I summarize this section?
- After reading, ask yourself: Do I understand the main points; can I outline the main points; how will I use or apply this information; does something need to be clarified; and what questions are likely to be on the exam?

Critical Listening

Communication skills, especially listening skills, are greatly emphasized in the nursing curriculum. Many students do not have effective listening skills. Many persons have developed the habit of tuning in only occasionally to what is said, resulting in lost communication. Improve your listening skills by restating the points made in a discussion with another student and ask that student to give feedback about how accurately you have restated her position. As you listen, focus on what the speaker is saying, listen for key points, and make a note of anything that seems confusing to you (Figure 1-6).

Critical listening requires a conscious commitment to focus on the topic of discussion. Recognize things that

Figure 1-6 *Effective listening skills are essential to all client interactions.*

distract your attention. Attempting to take word-for-word notes, daydreaming, and focusing on the mannerisms or appearance of the speaker are common distractors. A good thinker is not afraid to identify weaknesses and strengths in order to improve.

Critical Writing

Basic to good thinking skills is the ability to state one's thoughts coherently, clearly, and concisely. Many students arrive at college unable to write well. The quality of thinking is improved by the discipline required to write well. Many students feel that writing is too revealing and are afraid to write down their thoughts. Writing is important for the improvement of thinking because it can be reviewed using the standards for critical thinking to evaluate the quality of the thinking reflected in the writing (Figure 1-7). These standards are discussed next.

Critical Speaking

Disciplined speaking is perhaps the most neglected skill. Examples of clear, logical, and accurate spoken communication are seldom heard. Oral communication is usually more spontaneous than written communica-

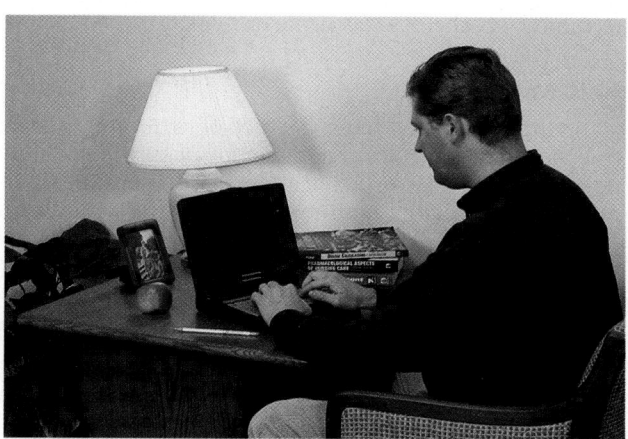

Figure 1-7 *Effective writing skills are integral to critical thinking.*

CRITICAL THINKING

Basic Skills

Of the four basic skills of critical thinking, which one are you able to do best? Why? How do you know?

tion and must be carefully presented. Ambiguous statements are misleading, and personal biases influence what the other person hears. Small group practice followed by feedback from the listeners can help a student assess and improve this skill.

Standards for Critical Thinking

Critical thinking relies on the use of intellectual standards for checking the quality of thinking (Elder & Paul, 2002). The first requirement is to become familiar with the Universal Intellectual Standards developed at The Center for Critical Thinking. These are used in this discussion because they provide a valid and reliable measure for the quality of thinking. Whether you are reading, listening, writing, answering test questions, or speaking, the standards of clarity, accuracy, precision, relevance, consistency, logic, depth, breadth, and fairness should be applied.

Clarity

Fundamental to quality thinking is the ability to think clearly. Clarity of thought means placing facts and ideas into a logical and coherent framework. The standard is the degree to which others can understand your position. Pay particular attention to the exact meaning of words. There will be many new terms and concepts in your nursing curriculum. Practice the proper use of these terms and apply concepts appropriately to improve clarity of thought and increased retention of content.

Think about the word *clarity*. There are several shades of meaning in the dictionary. Look up the word for yourself and decide which definition applies to the use of clarity in describing a standard for critical thinking.

Think about expressions you use frequently. Would someone from another part of the country understand them? The term *this evening* is common in some parts of the country. When would you expect someone who told you that she would visit "this evening?" In some places, the person might arrive in the early afternoon; in other places, at night. When speaking to clients, families, and other health team members, be sure that the words used clearly express the intended message. Do not assume that you understand a term; take time to verify the meaning. When a statement is unclear, it cannot be determined whether it is accurate or relevant.

Accuracy

Accuracy means being correct or true and within the proper parameters. The need for accurate calculation of a drug dose or accurate measurement of blood pressure can readily be understood. In the same way, the collection and interpretation of data must be accurate. Being accurate implies the use of some measuring instrument. Accuracy in thinking may be hard to conceptualize. When a person uses the term *hypertension* to mean someone who is anxious and very active instead of the actual meaning, an elevation of blood pressure above the accepted normal maximum, the standard of accuracy is not met. Students can improve their accuracy in thinking by writing new information in their own words and asking another student to interpret

what was written. Inaccurate information will become evident.

Accurate documentation of client care is essential to quality care. There are degrees of accuracy. For example, you might measure a client's temperature using a thermometer that can measure to the 0.01 degree, but this degree of accuracy is not necessary. On the other hand, when figuring a pediatric dosage, a difference of 0.01 is very important. A challenge to you is to learn the degree of accuracy required in given nursing situations.

Precision

Sometimes, students learn enough about a subject to be "in the ballpark," but not enough to hit a home run. The result is a general idea about a fact or idea, but not enough understanding to apply it. Precise thinking means that there is enough detail and specificity for a concept or word to be clearly understood in terms of its relationship to other concepts or words.

Relevance

Relevance refers to information connected to the issue as opposed to information that is not. Students may get sidetracked from the purpose of an exercise by failing to limit their discussion to the issue at hand. Their responses are not relevant. When studying, ask yourself how a particular concept is relevant to client care. It is also important to be able to recognize when sufficient relevant information is not available.

Consistency

Consistency is the appropriate use of principles and concepts. For instance, a particular nursing diagnosis based on specified indicators should be used when those indicators are present and never used when the indicators are not present.

Knowing the basic actions of epinephrine enables the nurse to predict client responses to the administration of the drug. It also helps the nurse understand that the client will have the same response when an increased secretion of epinephrine is released by the client's kidneys.

Logic

Thinking brings a variety of thoughts together in some order. Logic asks the question "Does this make sense?" Symptoms exhibited by clients can usually be understood based on knowledge of normal physiology and those changes produced by the client's disease or condition. For example, a client with a gall stone blocking the common bile duct is concerned because his stool is very light gray in color. Bile is the substance that colors the stool brown, so it follows that if there is no bile, the stool will not be brown. These two items make sense in combination.

When calculating a medication dosage, the standard of logic is extremely important. If the calculation answer is to give the client 200 pills of a certain medication, this is not logical; it does not make sense. Most likely, there is a missing decimal point, with the correct answer being two pills.

Depth

Students are often tempted to rely on the specific learning objectives as an indicator of which material they must master. This may result in a superficial understanding of the material. The ability to recognize the depth to explore concepts and ideas can be learned. Students should ask themselves, "What are the most significant factors; what are the complexities in this situation; what other problems may be involved?" These questions will guide the student to see other aspects that also need to be explored for a thorough understanding. Your instructor and the learning aids within your textbook are useful guides for identifying relevant information and the appropriate depth of knowledge required to make good clinical decisions.

Breadth

Breadth of thinking entails considering another point of view and asking if there is another way to look at the question or problem. Consider a pregnant woman, with a six-year-old son, who has been told she must stay in bed because of complications. The problem is broader than just the complication of the pregnancy. Who will care for the son, take him to school? Who will do the cooking, cleaning, laundry? Is this financially feasible? Can a mother or friend help out? Can the husband stay home? The narrow problem of a pregnancy complication has great breadth when the entire situation is considered.

Fairness

Everyone has a set of beliefs, opinions, and points of view. People tend to believe that what they think is true. Improving the quality of your thinking depends on your ability to identify the biases in your thinking and those biases present in the thinking of others. Following the standard of fairness will lead a person to question conclusions based on personal bias. When a nurse who responds to pain in a stoic manner assesses a person who responds to pain emotionally, the nurse may allow personal values to influence the assessment, with the result that the nurse provides inadequate pain relief for the client.

Reasoning and Problem-Solving

Although reasoning involves thinking, all thinking is not reasoning. Thinking is occurring when a person daydreams, jumps to conclusions, or decides to listen to music. However, these activities cannot be called reasoning. In order to effectively use reasoning, to figure things out, or to problem-solve, the student must become familiar with the components of reasoning. These components are purpose, the question at issue, assumptions, point of view, data and information, concepts, inferences and conclusions, and implications and consequences.

Purpose

All reasoning is directed toward some specific purpose. This is one aspect where reasoning is different from daydreaming. For the nursing student, the purpose of reasoning is to use the information learned in class to effectively solve client care problems.

The Question at Issue

The purpose of the reasoning process is to figure something out, answer a question, or solve some problem. This problem or question must be clearly stated. At the beginning of a study period, state clearly the problems presented by this particular material. Good clinical judgment begins with a clear statement of problems presented by each client.

Assumptions

Assumptions are ideas or things that are taken for granted. They are accepted as being true without examination. Assumptions may be helpful in problem-solving, but recognize them for what they are. An example of an assumption is that nursing makes a difference in the outcome of a client's illness. This is a necessary assumption for nurses to make in order to engage in problem-solving related to client care needs.

Assumptions that have proven reliable can help in decision making, while faulty assumptions may cause you to draw faulty conclusions and may lead to inadequate problem-solving. Learn to recognize your own assumptions and those of others. Never be afraid to challenge your own assumptions or to ask others to clarify the assumptions they are using.

Point of View

Each person reasons from his own point of view, which is influenced by previous experience, available information, the quality of thinking already acquired, and many other factors. All together these factors give each person a unique perspective and a unique way of thinking. Seek other points of view and evaluate their strengths and weaknesses. Each person sees things differently. An individual's point of view will determine what facts and information will be noticed, the importance given to the information, and even the acceptable solutions to the problem. Identify your own point of view and its limitations and acknowledge the right of others to have their own points of view (Figure 1-8).

Figure 1-8 *To be effective problem-solvers and critical thinkers, nurses must first take a good look at their own point of view.*

Data and Information

Data and information are the basic materials of reasoning. Be sure that all information and data are clear, accurate, and relevant to the question or problem at issue. Search for information that not only supports your position but also refutes it. Keep any claims or conclusions to those supported by the data you have collected.

Concepts

Identify concepts needed to explore the problem and the implications of each. The concepts (such as asepsis, pain, adaptation, and so on) important to nursing care must be part of the evidence supporting a nursing judgment.

Inferences and Conclusions

Reasoning requires interpretation of facts and information. The interpretation must be justified by the relevant facts. It must be supported by the data and information. Many times, students state opinions as judgments or inferences. This happens when inferences are based on assumptions and personal preferences rather than on the information.

Properly drawing judgments or inferences is basic to thinking well. For example, when the body's temperature goes above normal, the body's metabolic rate increases. Increased metabolism requires more oxygen for the tissues. More oxygen can be delivered to the tissues by increasing the heart rate. From these facts, it can infer that an elevated body temperature may result in an increased heart rate.

The product of reasoning is a conclusion regarding the problem. It is the answer to the question that began the process. The conclusion must be logical.

Implications and Consequences

The reasoning process usually produces more than one solution. Now it is necessary to examine the implications of each solution by thinking about the ease with which a solution can be applied, the ability of a person to carry out the required actions, or the risks involved. Look for both positive and negative consequences.

Consequences can result from action or inaction. It may not be possible to predict all consequences, but the possible outcomes should be examined as completely as possible.

Traits of a Disciplined Thinker

Reading the requirements of critical thinking in this chapter will not make anyone think critically. You can improve your own thinking by incorporating the idea that thinking about the quality of your own thinking in relation to UIS is a desirable goal. Improved thinking can not be acquired in a day or two. It takes time, effort, and disciplined practice. The result is well worth it, however. Consistent efforts to improve your thinking can result in the acquisition of the traits of a disciplined person (Center for Critical Thinking, 2002b). These traits, or habitual ways of thinking, can be recognized by others and enable a person to compete successfully in the high-tech world (Table 1-4).

Critical Thinking and the Nursing Process

A nursing education program is intended to help students develop the logic of nursing. In other words, you will learn to think like a nurse. The method nurses have adoped to implement the practice of nursing is called the nursing process. The nursing process applies the problem-solving process to the practice of nursing and requires critical thinking. When you find the relationship between the content of the textbooks and the logic of nursing, the study of nursing will be an exciting and challenging process. Using the nursing process will improve the quality of your thinking and using reasoning will enhance your use of the nursing process.

DEVELOP TEST-TAKING SKILLS

Testing is not studying; however, the skills you need for testing are similar to those needed for studying. The task involved in taking a test is not to pass it; to pass the test is the *outcome.* You cannot achieve the outcome if you do not perform the task. The task is to read the question, understand what the question is asking, and make a decision about a correct response.

To hone your test-taking behaviors, you must first perform a personal analysis with regard to your attitudes, preparation methods, and behaviors related to a testing situation. Only after you have identified these variables can you initiate strategies to improve your outcomes.

Attitude and Expectations

If you are like most students, you may feel quite anxious about taking a test. You may think of each test as the final chance to show your worth. Or you may consider receiving less than an A on an examination as being the same as failing. Neither of these is a reasonable

TABLE 1-4 TRAITS OF A DISCIPLINED THINKER	
TRAIT	**DESCRIPTION**
Faith in reason	Confident that interests of humankind are best served by giving free play to reason
	Values reasoning in self and others
	Has faith that people can learn to think for themselves, think coherently and logically, and come to reasonable conclusions
Intellectual humility	Aware of how much he does not know
	Sensitive to bias, prejudice, and limitations of own viewpoint
	Willing to examine beliefs and conclusions based on new evidence
	Respects thoughts and ideas of others
	Continually learning and improving own thinking
Intellectual courage	Addresses ideas, beliefs, or viewpoints causing strong negative emotions that have not received a serious hearing
	Recognizes that ideas considered dangerous are sometimes jusitified
	Willing to take unpopular positions based on reasoning
Intellectual integrity	Is true to own thinking
	Consistent in intellectual standards applied and does not change to suit circumstances or personal bias
	Admits discrepancies and inconsistencies in own thoughts and actions
	Practices what he advocates for others
Intellectual perseverance	Uses intellectual insights and truths despite difficulties and frustrations
	Pursues question or problem until conclusion is reached
	Adheres to rational principles
	Willing to struggle with confusion and unsettled questions over an extended time period to achieve deeper meaning
Intellectual empathy	Imaginatively puts self in place of others to genuinely understand them
	Able to reconstruct accurately the viewpoints and reasoning of others
	Remembers past occasions when he was wrong despite intense conviction of being right
Fair-mindedness	Considers all viewpoints
	Adheres to intellectual standards
	Is impartial

expectation for testing. Testing is a useful tool for both measuring your level of knowledge and showing what you still need to learn. Have you ever considered that receiving a grade of C on an examination usually indicates that you know 75% of all of the knowledge that was tested? And the knowledge on any given test does not represent all the knowledge you possess. Your attitude toward testing is very important if you are to improve your outcome. Maintain a reasonable expectation about both the purpose of the test and the meaning of your grade. This is often a key factor in improving your test performance.

Preparation

In analyzing your preparation for test taking, you must critically examine your study habits. Review the section in this chapter on study strategies and consider whether you are on task when it comes to your study habits. There may be some areas where you can improve. If you know of an area of weakness, make a conscious effort to develop this part of your preparation. Be reasonable in your expectations, and do not expect to see results overnight. Building your study habits takes time and persistence. Persevere and your outcome on tests will improve.

Next, consider the way you review for an examination. Do you cram the night before, or are you consistently planning for questions in your study plan and adding time for review of material before the examination? One strategy is to use the technique of note mapping to help you organize the material into manageable parts. Taking each part and developing a more detailed one-page outline that you can take with you to review for 15 to 20 minutes at a time is another method to try. Another suggestion is to change your

The 30-Second Vacation

For those of you who need an "anxiety buster," consider a "30-second vacation." The 30-second vacation is based on a guided imagery technique that is used often in the client care arena. This technique takes practice. Start by doing the following:

Sit in a comfortable spot where you will not be disturbed, close your eyes, and think of an event or a place that evokes a feeling of calmness (not necessarily happiness). This is an event or place that made you feel like everything was right with the world and with you. It can be from any time in your life.

It may take some time to settle on the right event or place. Relax and take a few minutes now and think.

Once you have it, don't tell anyone! This is your secret place, your place of peace, and when you go there, no one can find you.

Once you have selected this event or place, start to give it "life." To do this, you must begin to recall this event or place regularly. Practice doing so at the beginning of your study sessions, when you are stuck in traffic, when you are at the dentist, when you have something difficult to do, at the beginning of your test-taking exercises, or at the beginning of your real tests.

Each time you recall your event or place, give it more "life." Recall the time of day, the setting, the colors of that day. Was it raining, was it sunny, was it snowing? If it was raining, was it a summer rain or an autumn rain? Recall what you were wearing and what colors you had on. Were you alone or with others? Were you eating something? What did the food smell like?

study place and times. Instead of 1-hour sessions, break your review sessions into 30-minute recall sessions. You must draw an imaginary line between studying and reviewing. Studying is the learning of new knowledge; reviewing comprises recall, organization, and summary of information.

Do not study only just before the test. This is a poor technique. Approaching preparation in this manner serves only to put a few facts into short-term memory. Better to spend the time before the examination relaxing with a good book or good friends or at the spa or gym. You must be confident and rested and come to the testing area with that good feeling that results from doing something you like.

Consider the rest you get the night before the examination. Physical stamina is needed for concentration. If you cram for a test by "pulling an all-nighter," you are setting yourself up for possible errors on the examination. Be reasonable, revisit your study plan, and get adequate rest.

Next, consider whether you have enough energy to take the test. You can eat what you want, but eat. The

cells of the brain require glucose to function; this glucose is supplied in the calories you consume. Try not to increase caffeine intake immediately before a test because doing so may make you jittery.

Finally, ask yourself whether surrounding yourself with positive people helps keep you focused, or whether talking to students before a test only makes you more anxious. If the latter is the case, you should arrive with just enough time to walk into the testing room and you should not speak to anyone.

Minimize Anxiety

Anxiety is the physiologic response of the autonomic nervous system to a perceived stressful situation. As the situation becomes more stressful, the body's response increases. This affects the ability to process information and make rational choices. People are often not good at identifying what they are feeling and are often unaware of the degree to which stress affects the ability to take tests.

Develop a plan to deal with anxiety. Anxiety about performance is always present. Past experience with testing often contributes to the development of test anxiety. If the expectation regarding performance on a test is not mirrored in the grade we receive, our confidence in our ability is shaken, and we approach the whole experience with more and more anxiety.

To deal with anxiety, consciously develop an activity to counter the feeling that anxiety evokes. Some people listen to music, pace, or do deep breathing to combat feelings of stress and anxiety. All of these are good strategies, even if all of them cannot be done *while you are actually taking the test.*

Improve Test-Taking Skills

How do you improve your test-taking skills? You practice, practice, practice and analyze, analyze, analyze. Consider the following:

Treat every wrong answer as a treasure. Examine it and discover the secret of why you got it wrong.

This is the only way to know which errors you are making. Always request to review your examinations, and track your incorrect responses using the analysis worksheet presented in Figure 1-9. Initially when you review your tests, do not concern yourself with the content of the questions. Simply write the number of the question in the row that indicates the reason you got that question incorrect. You will also notice that there is a heavy black line before the last row of the worksheet. The first four rows represent what are known as *mechanical errors;* these can be eliminated by developing positive habits and revising current practices. You will notice after three or four quizzes that a pattern starts to emerge. Imagine that you just took a 100-question test and received a score of 60/100. You then use the worksheet to categorize your incorrect responses.

Of the 40 incorrect answers you provided, you see that 10 of them fell in "did not read carefully," 2 in "did not know the vocabulary," 7 in "inferred additional data," 4 in "identified priorities incorrectly," and 7 in "did not know the material." If you could eliminate the bad habits that resulted in the first 23 errors, this would

Test Question Analysis Worksheet

Reason for Incorrect Response	Test 1 Date	Test 2 Date
Did not read carefully (missed details, missed key words)		
Did not know the vocabulary (medical terminology, English vocabulary)		
Inferred additional data (made assumptions, "read into the question")		
Identified priorities incorrectly (placed events in wrong order)		
Did not know the material		

Figure 1-9 *Test Question Analysis Worksheet*

improve your test score immediately. Your grade would be 83/100. More important, tests would truly represent only what you did not know, not areas where bad habits resulted in poor test scores.

After you have identified your error patterns, you can work on developing the counterhabits that will eliminate them. Work first on the one that is the most glaring.

Read Carefully

Reading carefully is a test-taking behavior that must be practiced. The section on study strategies noted the value of scanning in looking for important words when you read. When you are reading a test question, however, you must *never* scan. Many students choose incorrect responses because they miss key words, scan the question for familiar terms, infer what the question is, or misinterpret words they read too quickly. Incorrect responses resulting from any of these actions represent poor reading habits rather than a substandard knowledge base. The following exercise will help improve your reading habits.

Exercise for Improving Your Literal Reading Skills

You will need:

- A timer (stove/egg)
- An NCLEX-PN® review text or any comparable question and answer book. It is important that you have the answers and the rationales for each answer in a review text.
- Two sheets of paper: one to take the test on and one to make your analysis worksheet
- Pencil or pen
- Dictionary

1. Pick a time and a place where there will be no interruptions for 20 minutes. You may neither speak to anyone nor get up to use any other resources. You are taking a test.
2. Randomly pick a page of the review book and choose five questions from that page. It does not matter whether you have studied the content in your program.
3. Set the timer for 5 minutes.
4. Start the test. Read each question out loud.
   a. If you read "over" a word, stop reading, make a mark next to that word, and begin again from the beginning.
   b. If you mispronounce a word, stop reading, make a mark next to that word, and begin again from the beginning.
   c. If you do not know the meaning of a word (English or medical), stop and look it up.
5. At the end of the question, restate what is being asked of you.
6. Read the choices, connect each to the question, and choose the most correct answer.
7. When the timer goes off, score your questions.
8. Analyze why you got questions correct or incorrect.
9. Repeat this exercise with five different questions three or four times a week.

The object of this exercise is not to finish all the questions, nor is it even to get all the answers right. Rather, the object is to consciously practice reading every word literally. Each time you do this exercise, you must treat it as a test—no food, no talking, no music, no interruptions. You must associate this type of reading with taking a test, so that each time you take a test, this literal reading habit is instinctual.

Know the Vocabulary

If vocabulary is your weak area, there is only one thing to do—learn the vocabulary. Look up the word (English and medical) in the appropriate dictionary, write the definition on the back of your analysis sheet, and review the definition during your next study session. Add additional time in your study plan for vocabulary building. Use additional modes of learning, such as audio or flash cards to master your vocabulary skills.

Do Not Infer Additional Data

The more experiences you have in life, the easier it is to infer additional data in any given situation. You must realize, however, that for the moment, the only relevant information is the information on the test paper—no more, no less. Based on that information alone and the given choices, you must decide on the correct responses. You base your decision on those things you have learned about the topic, on standards of care, on the nursing process, and on your base of knowledge. If you read into the question, you have in essence rewritten it and may not choose the correct answer. One strategy for overcoming this habit is to recognize whenever you begin to interject information upon getting to the last word in a question. In any such instance, you must stop, take some physical action to call your attention to the fact that you are adding information, and clear your mind—take a breath, clear your throat, wear a rubber band and snap it! Then start over again, concentrating on reading the question literally.

Identify Priorities Correctly

When questions concern priorities, ask yourself which of the given choices would result in serious consequences if not done first. When you are being questioned about procedural tasks, ask which of the given choices must be done before the others.

Know the Material

Not knowing the material represents a lack of knowledge base. Write down the content area of each of the questions you miss, then go back and review the concept or facts in question. If the same content areas are problematic over several tests, seek additional assistance from your instructor. You need clarification regarding your understanding of both the information and the questions.

Behaviors in the Testing Room

Setting yourself up in the testing room for a positive experience can make a difference in your outcome. Be sure to practice the following behaviors:

1. *Get a good seat.* Unless your seat is assigned, sit in an area that is quiet, has good light, and where you can "zone in" on the test and "zone out" the rest of the room. If you are a student who gets anxious when you are the last one left in the room, pick a seat in the front row and farthest from the door and turn your seat slightly toward the wall. You will be less apt to notice as people leave.
2. *Set the mood.* As you wait for the test to be passed out, take your 30-second vacation. Adopt the most positive attitude possible. Identify the task ahead of you. Take a breath and repeat the following:

   "I have prepared. I am able to read the questions, process the information, and, from the choices given, make the best choice and move on."

3. *Read—do not scan.* You must read literally every word in the question. Every word counts!
4. *Read the question to determine the following:*

   • *Who is the question about?* This will affect your chosen answer. If you automatically assume that all of the questions relate to the nurse, you may miss a question that asks you to decide those things the father might say to demonstrate his understanding of the discharge instructions, for example.

PROFESSIONAL TIP

LP/VN Services

Any time nursing services are provided by an LP/VN, the supervising RN must be on the premises or immediately available by telephone. Being available by an answering machine or service does not fall within the definition of "immediately available." The amount of supervision is a function of the setting. In home health care or long-term care settings, it is common practice for the supervising RN to be available by telephone rather than on the premises.

• *What is the question about?* You must determine to which part of the knowledge base the question refers. Is the question about the way to teach a 9-year-old diabetic to check his blood glucose? To answer this question, you must consider the learning style of the 9-year-old, his cognitive development and manual dexterity, and any significant others who should be involved in the session. The correct choice must support all of these principles.
• *When is the question about?* The time frame of the question is also significant in terms of the client's continuum of care. Is this the acute session? Is this a client who has had diabetes for 20 years and is now developing pulmonary vascular disease? Is this a new mother with her first child or a new mother with her fifth? Are you in the assessment phase of the nursing process, are you in the planning stage, or are you evaluating the effects of a treatment or a drug?
• *Where is the question about?* The focus of the nurse in the acute care institution is different from that of the nurse in the community clinic. This will affect your choice.

5. *Do not argue with the question.* Whether you agree with the question is irrelevant. The task is to read the question, put your mind to the question, and, given the choices offered, make your choice based on principles and the application of your knowledge base.
6. *Plan your time.* Do not spend an inordinate amount of time on one question. There are some things you will not know, and if you spend so much time on one question, you can sabotage your success on others. You can come back to any question, but you must be able to clear your mind of this question before moving on to tackle another. This is a good place for a 30-second vacation to put you back on task! If you cannot let a question go, you will be unable to concentrate on the next few questions and, very likely, will get several questions in a row incorrect. It is best to read, choose, and move on. Going back may work for paper-and-pencil tests during the nursing program, but the NCLEX-PN®, which you will take on computer for licensure upon completion of the nursing program, does not allow going back. Each question must be answered in the order presented.
7. *Do not panic.* When you come to a question that you cannot immediately answer, do not panic. Use your 30-second vacation to counter your anxiety and facilitate your ability to process. Recite again, "I have prepared, I am able to read, process, choose, and move on." Remember, the answer is on the paper.

YOUR PROGRAM IS ALMOST COMPLETED

Additional skills for success are required when you leave the protection of your nursing program. These include scope of practice/competence, tasks of the unlicensed assistive personnel (UAP), delegation, prioritizing care, and the nursing team.

Scope of Practice/Competence

Registered nurses (RNs) and licensed practical/vocational nurses (LP/VNs) are individually licensed. Although some overlap exists in the scopes of practice of the LP/VN and the RN, there are also some significant differences. LP/VNs are dependent practitioners, meaning that an RN, doctor, dentist, or some other health care provider must supervise them. Most often the supervisor is an RN.

In addition to a scope of practice, LP/VNs and RNs have scopes of competence. Within the scope of practice, there are tasks and responsibilities the individual may or may not be competent to implement. For example, it is within the scope of practice for the LP/VN to perform phlebotomy, but this task does not fall within the scope of competence of every LP/VN. The scope of competence expands as new skills are acquired, but all skills must fall within the scope of practice.

LP/VNs are qualified to care for clients with common illnesses and to provide basic and preventive nursing procedures. LP/VNs can participate in data collection, planning, implementation, and evaluation of nursing care in all settings. In most states, some specific activities are considered beyond the scope of practice of the LP/VN. These activities, with some variances by state, include the following:

• Client assessments (can collect data but not perform physical assessments)
• Independent development of the nursing care plan
• Triage, case management, or mental health counseling
• Intravenous chemotherapy
• Administration of blood and blood products
• Administration of initial doses of any intravenous medication
• Any procedures involving central lines

Tasks of the UAP

Unlicensed assistive personnel do not have a scope of practice. A task that falls within the protected scope of practice of any licensed profession (including registered nursing and licensed practical/vocational nursing) *cannot* be performed by a UAP. These personnel can perform only those health-related activities for which they have been determined competent to perform. These activities include the following:

• Activities of daily living (feeding, grooming, toileting, ambulating, dressing)
• Vital signs
• Venipuncture
• Glucometer use
• Mouth care and oral suctioning
• Care of hair, skin, and nails
• Electrocardiogram measurements
• Applying clean dressings without assessment
• Nonnursing functions (clerical work, transport, cleaning)

Duty Delegation

Delegation is the process of transferring to a competent individual the authority to perform a select task in a select situation. State provisions for the delegation of nursing tasks vary. Some states allow for the delegation of nursing tasks by an RN to both LP/VNs and UAP. In some states, LP/VNs may delegate certain nursing tasks to other LP/VNs or to UAP. Other states restrict delegation to licensed personnel only. It is *most* important to know what is allowed in your state. The National Council of State Boards of Nursing (NCSBN) website keeps a current listing of the address, telephone number, and website for each state board of nursing at www.ncsbn.org.

The licensed nurse retains accountability for the delegation. **Accountability** is defined as responsibility for actions and inactions performed by oneself or others. **Assignment**, another term frequently used to describe the transfer of activities from one person to another, involves the downward or lateral transfer of both responsibility and accountability for an activity.

At least one state differentiates between *delegating* nursing tasks to licensed nurses and *assigning* tasks to UAP. In New York, a nurse is not legally responsible for the process or outcome of care delegated to another licensed nurse. The nurse does remain responsible for tasks assigned to UAP, however. As an LP/VN, you are responsible for the decisions you make to delegate or assign tasks. Your knowledge of the client, activity, and worker will help you make sound decisions.

In most settings, RNs decide which nursing activities can be delegated or assigned to other licensed nurses

PROFESSIONAL TIP

Hierarchy

As defined in the Nursing Practice Acts, or in the state nursing board's rules and regulations, an LP/VN works under the direction of an RN, physician, or dentist. These are the professionals who will directly supervise your work. In some states, the language of the law indicates that "other health care providers" can supervise you. The question is, who are the other health care providers? In your state, must you follow orders written by a physician's assistant? A nurse practitioner? A physical therapist? The answers vary by state. It is critical that you know who can direct your nursing activities.

PROFESSIONAL TIP

Unlicensed Personnel

Much controversy surrounds the role of UAP. Concerns have been raised that unlicensed personnel are functioning as de facto licensed nurses in violation of Nursing Practice Acts. Further, serious questions exist about the cost savings and quality of care in light of increased reliance on UAP and a corresponding reduction in licensed nurses. Understanding the role and limitations of UAP is critical.

(RNs or LP/VNs) and to UAP. Registered nurses and LP/VNs must consider five factors when making the decision to delegate or assign duties:

1. *The potential for harm.* Certain nursing activities carry a risk for harming the client. Generally, the more invasive a procedure, the greater the potential for harm. Additionally, some activities carry a greater risk for certain kinds of clients (e.g., cutting the toenails of a diabetic). The greater the potential for harm, the greater the need for a licensed nurse to perform the activity.

2. *The complexity of the task.* The cognitive skills and psychomotor skills needed for different nursing tasks vary considerably. As the skills increase in complexity, the level of education and competence becomes more critical. Some activities require a level of nursing assessment and judgment that can be provided only by a licensed professional.

3. *The required problem solving and innovation.* As care is delivered, problems may develop. A successful outcome for the client may depend on a complex analysis of the problem and an individualized problem-solving approach. Alternatively, a simple activity may require special adaptation because of the client's condition. As problem solving increases in complexity and the need for innovation grows, so does the likelihood that a licensed nurse should provide the care.

4. *The unpredictability of the outcome.* A client's response to an activity may be very predictable. If the client is unstable or the activity is new for the client, however, client response may be unpredictable and unknown. As unpredictability increases, so does the need for a licensed nurse.

5. *The required coordination and consistency of the client's care.* Effective planning, coordination, and evaluation of client care requires the nurse to have direct client contact. The more stable the client and the more common the medical diagnosis, the more care can generally be delegated to support personnel. The need for a licensed nurse increases as the required coordination needed to delivery quality care increases.

The five rights of delegation provide further direction in making appropriate decisions about delegation. They are as follows:

1. *Right Task:* The nurse must determine whether the task should be delegated for a specific client.

2. *Right Circumstance:* Factors to consider include the client setting, availability of resources, client's condition, and other considerations.

3. *Right Person:* The nurse must ask the question, "Is the right person delegating the right task to the right person to be performed on the right client?"

4. *Right Direction/Communication:* A clear, concise description of the task should be conveyed, including all expectations for accomplishing the task.

5. *Right Supervision:* Appropriate monitoring, implementation, evaluation, and feedback must be provided.

Registered nurses are frequently responsible for delegating care and assigning clients to the other nursing staff. In some settings, however, LP/VNs make these decisions. LP/VNs should use the same guidelines to make decisions regarding delegating an activity to another LP/VN or assigning the task to UAP.

Prioritizing Care

Establishing priorities requires an understanding of the importance of different problems to the nurse, the client, the family, and other health care providers. For example, a client may be impatient to bathe because family is scheduled to visit. The nurse, however, does not want to remove the client's dressing for a bath until the physician has been able to examine the wound. Providing quality care while balancing such competing demands and ensuring completion of all tasks can be challenging.

Information obtained during the change-of-shift report is needed to appropriately establish priorities. This information can be useful in creating a worksheet identifying a list of tasks and target times for accomplishing these tasks. The time allotted for activities varies based on the condition of the client, the availability of support personnel, the availability of supplies, and a number of other factors. The effective use of time is important whether caring for one client, caring for a group of clients, or supervising the activities of others providing care.

Although it is useful to get an overview of the day's activities, the clinical setting can change quickly and frequently. This is especially true in acute care settings. The nurse must be flexible and continually evaluate and reorder the priorities of care.

Given the same assignment, nurses will not necessarily establish the priorities of care in exactly the same way. If working closely with an RN, you should determine the priorities as she views them. When supervising UAP, you must be clear about your priorities and expectations. Among the factors that can be examined when establishing priorities are the following:

- *Safety:* You should ascertain whether a safety situation must be addressed immediately. A client experiencing a cardiac arrest, a fall, an insulin reaction, and other situations presenting an imminent threat must be tended to first.
- *Timing:* Medications, tests, and vital signs are frequently ordered at specific times. Often, there is very little flexibility in shifting the times. In hospitals, medications, for example, must be given within a specified time frame, usually ½ hour before or after the established time.
- *Interdependence of events:* You must ascertain whether some activity must occur before another activity can take place. For example, a fasting blood sugar must be completed before the client receives either insulin or food; blood is drawn a specified time after the medication is given to ascertain the peak level of gentamyacin.
- *Client requests:* Quality care depends on meeting client needs. Some events—showers, bed changings, enema administration, and so on—can be scheduled after consulting with the client regarding personal preferences.
- *Availability of help:* If two people are needed to turn a client, ambulate a client, or provide other care, coordination of the health care team is essential for effective utilization of time. Ascertain which activities re-

quire assistance, then consult with coworkers about their availability.

• *Client's status:* Clients vary in the extent to which they can participate in their care. This factor influences the order of executing tasks and the length of time a task takes. A semi-independent client can be performing a task (e.g., bathing) with minimal assistance while the nurse attends to some other need.

• *Availability of resources:* If six clients are supposed to get out of bed and sit in chairs, and only two chairs are available, the clients clearly cannot get out of bed at the same time. Geri-chairs, wheelchairs, and other equipment are sometimes limited. Additionally, tasks may need to be delayed because supplies must be obtained from central supply.

Effectively organizing and establishing priorities with regard to care takes practice. Obtaining answers to certain questions when looking back at the day's events can help you hone this skill: Did you lack information that would have helped you prioritize more effectively? Did you fail to or inaccurately consider the client's status, the availability of help, or other factors? Did you establish priorities and set a schedule without getting client input? Did you fail to coordinate with coworkers? You will learn from experience. Both client and nurse feel the positive benefits of a day that flowed smoothly.

The Nursing Team

Within the nursing staff are different team members. Nursing staff includes nursing UAP, certified nurse assistants (CNAs), LP/VNs, RNs, and nurse practitioners (NPs). The roles, levels of education, skills, levels of independence, and lengths of education vary considerably (Figure 1-10). Familiarizing yourself with the roles of other nursing staff will help ensure that your practice conforms to the scope of practice as outlined by law.

Nursing UAP can have a number of different titles including UAP, patient care technician, clinical technician, and nursing assistant. These persons provide hands-on care to clients in addition to performing other duties. None of these personnel has a license to practice. Rather, training is provided by the employer and may last from 2 to 10 weeks. The tasks they are expected to perform are designated by the employer.

A CNA is also unlicensed. In contrast to other UAP, however, the curriculum and length of training to become a CNA are prescribed. As part of health care reforms in the long-term care setting, the primary employment setting of CNAs, a set curriculum of 100 hours duration must be completed to be certified.

LP/VNs work very closely with registered nurses. The LP/VN attends a 1-year program and must pass the National Council Licensure Examination for Practical Nurses (NCLEX-PN)®. The RN is educated in a 3-year hospital-diploma program, a 2-year college associate-degree program, or a 4-year college baccalaureate program and must pass the National Council Licensure Examination for Registered Nurses (NCLEX-RN®).

An NP is an RN who has obtained additional education (usually a master's degree) and is certified by the state. The role of the NP typically includes diagnosis and treatment of commonly occurring medical conditions.

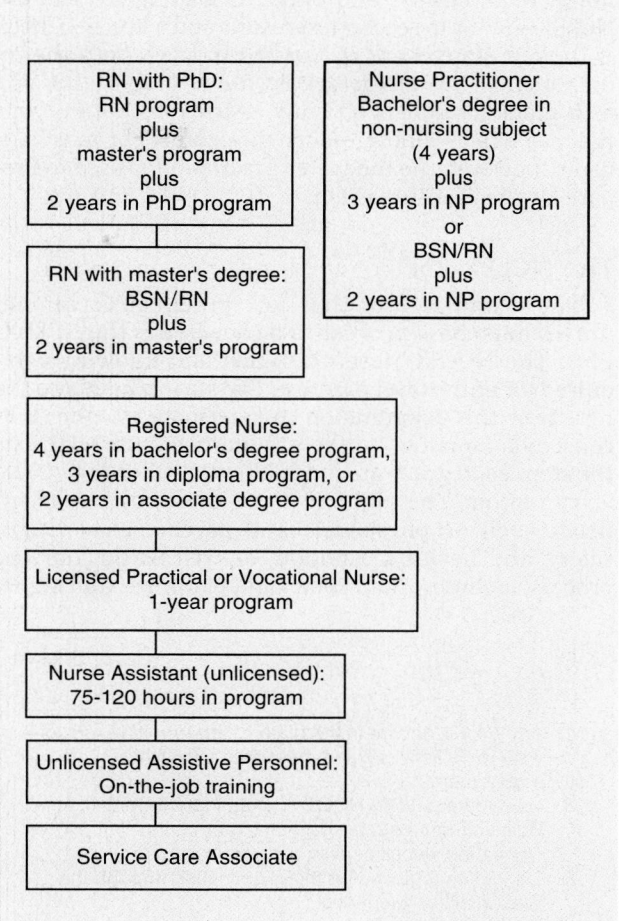

Figure 1-10 *Workplace Hierarchy*

Outpatient clinics frequently employ NPs. Increasingly, they are also found working in hospitals, long-term care facilities, and rehabilitation centers.

FROM STUDENT TO LP/VN

You have completed the licensed practical/vocational nursing educational program. Through formal education and clinical supervision, you have studied and learned the skills necessary to become competent in providing client care. Now you are ready to graduate and begin your career as a nurse.

Your first task as a graduate practical nurse is to take and pass the NCLEX-PN® examination and obtain your nursing license. After you have obtained your license, you can begin the search for a job. The effort required in the period of time between the job search and employment can be considered a job in and of itself. There are many tasks to complete and skills to master to land your first job as an LP/VN.

Examination and Licensure

In some states, you can begin work as a graduate LP/VN. A graduate LP/VN has completed the educational requirements and either is waiting to take the NCLEX-PN® or to receive test results and a license. Check with your state board of nursing to learn both the requirements for a temporary license to practice nursing as a graduate LP/VN and any restrictions put on your practice while working under this status. For most students, however, the time after graduation is used to prepare for the licensure exam.

The NCLEX-PN®

The examination that all practical/vocational nurses must pass in order to be licensed is the NCLEX-PN®. The NCLEX® tests the skills and knowledge required for entry-level practice. The state boards use the results of this examination to determine whether a license will be issued to the graduate. Figure 1-11 lists the steps each graduate must follow in order to take the examination. The NCLEX® tests knowledge of client needs such as physiologic and psychological needs, safety, and health promotion, as well as the nursing process, including data collection, planning, and imple-

1. Apply for licensure in the state or territory in which you wish to be licensed and meet their eligibility requirements.
2. Candidate gets an NCLEX® Examination Candidate Bulletin from the board of nursing or on the NCLEX® Candidate website (www.vue.com/nclex).
3. Candidate registers for the examination through the Web, mail, or telephone.
   Note: Candidates seeking licensure from Massachusetts must register through that jurisdiction. Follow registration instructions provided by that board of nursing.
4. The board of nursing will communicate the candidate's eligibility to test to Pearson Professional Testing. An Authorization to Test (ATT) will be sent by mail.
5. After receiving the ATT, an appointment to test can be made through the Web or by telephone.
6. On the appointed day, the candidate takes the test at a Pearson Professional Center.
7. Test results are transmitted to the designated board of nursing.
8. The board of nursing mails results to the candidate.

Figure 1-11 *Overview of Testing Process (Data from NCSBN, 2003b)*

PROFESSIONAL TIP

Temporary Permits

Although it is possible to work during the interim period between NCLEX-PN® testing and licensure, most employers will postpone hiring until after you have received your permanent nursing license. Therefore, do not be discouraged if you are unable to obtain employment as a graduate LP/VN during this period.

mentation. The test is administered via a computer using a method called computerized adaptive testing (CAT), wherein the computer selects the test questions as you take the examination. You must answer all of the questions as they are presented to you, and you may not skip questions. Most of the questions are four-option multiple choice in format.

In April 2003, alternate item formats were added to the NCLEX®. These alternate item formats include multiple choice requiring more than one response, fill-in-the-blank (must be spelled correctly), and identifying an area on a picture or graphic. The answers will be either correct or incorrect; no partial credit will be given (NCSBN, 2003a).

All LP/VN candidates answer a minimum of 85 questions and a maximum of 205 questions during the maximum 5-hour testing period (NCSBN, 2003b). The results are mailed to the candidate by the state board 1 month or less after the examination. Candidates may retake the examination; however, the National Council requires a wait of at least 91 days between testings. Your state board may have other policies related to retaking the exam.

Your License

After you have successfully passed the NCLEX®, you will be issued your nursing license from your state board. It is your responsibility to maintain your license according to your state's standards and inform your state board of any changes in name, address, and employment. Once licensed, you are ready to practice.

Summary

- Developing a positive attitude enhances your learning experience.
- Strategies for developing a positive attitude include creating a positive self-image, recognizing your abilities, and identifying realistic expectations for meeting those goals.
- Competency in the basic skills of reading, arithmetic and mathematics, writing, listening, and speaking is necessary.
- It is important to build your vocabulary and comprehension of medical terminology to better enable you to meet your clients' learning needs.
- Identifying your preference for a particular learning style will help you identify the strategies you need to be a successful student.
- Organizing your study space and decreasing interruptions will increase your efficiency and facilitate your sticking to your study plan.
- Several methods can be used to take notes. Note taking in lectures and from your text is a strategy to help you retain the information presented.
- Critical thinking is the ability to apply your knowledge base.
- Critical thinking is a disciplined way of thinking that the nursing student can begin to develop. The effective use of the nursing process depends on the ability to think well.
- Four basic intellectual skills are essential to quality thinking: critical reading, critical listening, critical writing, and critical speaking.

- Reasoning is the process of applying critical thinking to some problem to find an answer or to figure something out. Therefore, reasoning has a purpose.
- When students begin to be aware of their own thinking and begin to assume responsibility for it, they will begin to use their own logic to discover the logic of nursing. The result will be better learning and the ability to make high-quality decisions related to client care.
- Consistent attention to improving the quality of thinking will produce the traits of an educated person.
- Developing a strategy to minimize anxiety when taking tests will improve your performance.
- To successfully complete a test, read each question thoroughly, do not infer additional information, and identify priorities.

Review Questions

1. The sign of true comprehension of material is:
   a. the ability to repeat a paragraph word for word.
   b. memorization of the material.
   c. the ability to recite the material.
   d. the ability to summarize the material using your own words.

2. If you suspect you have a learning disability, it is important that you:
   a. ignore it; you will be able to work around it on your own.
   b. be tested to determine the assistance you will need to compensate for the disability.
   c. keep it to yourself; you will not be able to pass the program if you tell anyone about it.
   d. use it as an excuse to put less work into the program.

3. The best way to study is to:
   a. read only the assigned material.
   b. take notes in the lecture only.
   c. read, reread, reflect, recite, and review.
   d. read and attend lectures.

4. The best way to deal with any anxiety you may experience during a test is:
   a. jogging.
   b. listening to music.
   c. practicing deep breathing and imagery.
   d. asking for more time to take the test.

5. The person who has the ability to separate needed information from information not needed at the present time is practicing the standard for critical thinking called:
   a. logic.
   b. relevance.
   c. adequacy.
   d. significance.

References/Suggested Readings

Browne, M., & Keeley, S. (2000). *Asking the right questions: A guide to critical thinking* (6th ed.). Upper Saddle River, NJ: Prentice Hall College Division.

Center for Critical Thinking. (1997). *Critical thinking in living, working & learning (a real time video)* [Online]. Available: www.uncp.edu/home/vanderhoof/criticalthinking.ram

Center for Critical Thinking. (2002a). *A brief history of the idea of critical thinking* [Online]. Available: www.criticalthinking. org/University/univlibrary/cthistory.html

Center for Critical Thinking. (2002b). *Valuable intellectual traits* [Online]. Available: www.critcalthinking.org/University/univlibrary/intraits.html

The Center for New Discoveries in Learning Personal Learning Style Inventory/School Smart Kids. (1998). *Newsletter;* Vol. 1, No. 4 [Online]. Available: www.howtolearn.com/ndil3.html

Chaffee, J. (2000). *Thinking critically* (6th ed.). Boston: Houghton Mifflin College.

Chopra, D. (1997, May–June). How can I keep up? *Natural Health, 208.*

Dale, E. (1954). *Audiovisual methods in teaching,* New York: Dryden.

Elder, L., & Paul, R. (2002). *Universal intellectual standards* [Online]. Available: www.criticalthinking. org/University/univlibrary/unistan.html

Facionè, N. (2000). *Critical thinking assessment in nursing education programs: An aggregate data analysis.* Millbrae, CA: California Academic Press.

Guffey, M. E. (1998). *Five steps to better critical thinking, problem-solving and decision-making skills* [Online]. Available: www.westwords.com/GUFFEY/critical.html

Ham, K. (2001). *From LPN to RN—Bridges for role transitions.* Philadelphia: W. B. Saunders.

Heaslip, P. (1994, November). Defining critical thinking. *Dialogue: A Critical Thinking Newsletter for Nurses, 3.*

Higbee, K. (2001). *Your memory: How it works and how to improve it* (2nd ed.) Indianapolis, IN: Macmillan.

Holkeboer, R., and Walker, L. (1999). *Right from the start.* Belmont, CA: Wadsworth.

Knudsvig, G., & Smith, E. (1998). *Critical thinking: Building the basics.* Belmont, CA: Wadsworth.

Korchek, N., & Sides, M. B. (1998). *Successful test-taking: Learning strategies for nurses* (3rd ed.). Philadelphia: Lippincott Williams & Wilkins.

Kurfiss, J. (1988). *Critical thinking: Theory, research, practice and possibilities.* Washington, DC: Association for the Study of Higher Education. (ASHE-ERIC Higher Education Report No. 2.)

Lesar, T. S. (1998). Errors in the use of medication dosage equations. *Archives of Pediatric Adolescent Medicine, 152*(4), 340–344.

Martin, C. (2002). The theory of critical thinking of nursing. *Nursing Education Perspectives, 23*(5), 243–247.

Meltzer, M., & Marcus-Palau, S. (1997). *Learning strategies in nursing: Reading, studying and test taking* (2nd ed.). Philadelphia: W. B. Saunders Company.

Mind tools: How your learning style affects your use of mnemonics (1998) [Online]. Available: www.mindtools.com/mnem1sty.html

National Center for Learning Disabilities, Inc. (NCLD). (1999, January 24) [Online]. Information About Learning Disabilities. Available: www.ncid.org

National Council of State Boards of Nursing (NCSBN). (2003a). *Facts about alternative formats and the NCLEX examinations.* [Online]. Available: www.ncsbn.org/public/res/Innovative%20Items%20Secure.pdf

National Council of State Boards of Nursing (NCSBN). (2003b). *NCLEX examination candidate bulletin.* [Online]. Available:www.ncsbn.org/public/res/NCLEX%20Candidate%20Bulletin_NCS%20Pearson.pdf

Norris, S. P., & Ennis, R. H. (1989). *Evaluating critical thinking.* Pacific Grove, CA: Midwest.

Nosich, G. (2000). *Learning to think things through.* Upper Saddle River, NJ: Prentice Hall College Division.

Nugent, P. M., & Vitale, B. A. (2000). *Test taking techniques for beginning nursing students* (3rd ed.). Philadelphia: F. A. Davis.

Paul, R. (1990). *Critical thinking: What every person needs to survive in a rapidly changing world.* Rohnert Park, CA: Center for Critical Thinking and Moral Critique, Sonoma State University.

Paul, R., & Elder, L. (2000). *Critical thinking: Tools for taking charge of your learning and your life.* Upper Saddle River, NJ: Prentice Hall.

Paul, R., & Elder, L. (2002). *Helping students assess their thinking* [Online]. Available: www.criticalthinking.org/University/univlibrary/helps.html

Paul, R., & Willsen, J. (1993). *Critical thinking, from an ideal evolves an imperative.* Santa Rosa, CA: Foundation for Critical Thinking.

Rubenfeld, M. G., & Scheffer, B. (1998). *Critical thinking in nursing: An interactive approach* (2nd ed.). Philadelphia: Lippincott Williams & Wilkins.

Saucier, B., Stevens, K., & Williams, G. (2000). Critical thinking outcomes of computer-assisted instruction versus written nursing process. *Nursing and Health Care Perspectives, 21*(5), 240–246.

Schank, R. (2000). *Dynamic memory revisited* (2nd ed). Cambridge, UK: Cambridge University Press.

Sheehan, J. (2001). Delegating to UAPs—A practical guide. *RN, 64*(11), 65–66.

Smith, G. L., Davis, P. E., & Dennerll, J. T. (1999). *Medical terminology: A programmed systems approach* (8th ed.). Clifton Park, NY: Thomson Delmar Learning.

Sotiriou, P., & Phillips, A. (1999). *Steps to reading proficiency* (5th ed.). Belmont, CA: Wadsworth.

Resources

Center for Critical Thinking at Sonoma State University, P.O. Box 220, Dillon Beach, CA 94929, 707-878-9100, www.criticalthinking.org

The Center for New Discoveries in Learning, P.O. Box 1019, Windsor, CA 95492, 800-469-8653

The Center for New Discoveries in Learning Personal Learning Style Inventory/School Smart Kids Newsletter Vol. 1, No. 4, www.howtolearn.com

Choosing a College for Students with Learning Disabilities, www.ldresources.com

Closing the Gap, A Resource Directory, P.O. Box 68, 526 Main Street, Henderson, MN 56044, 507-248-3294, www.closingthegap.net

Directory of Adaptive Technology: Trace Research and Development Center, 5901 Research Park Boulevard, University of Wisconsin, Madison, WI 53719, 608-263-5408, http://trace.wisc.edu

Foundation for Critical Thinking, P.O. Box 220, Dillon Beach, CA 94929, 800-833-3645

Identifying Your Best Learning Styles, www.marin.cc.ca.us

Insight Assessment, 217 La Cruz Avenue, Millbrae, CA 94030, 650-697-5628, www.calpress.com

The Institute for Learning Sciences, Northwestern University, 1890 Maple Avenue, Evanston, IL 60201, 847-491-3500, www.ils.nwu.edu

International Center for the Assessment of Higher Order Thinking (ICA), 707-878-9100, www.criticalthinking.org/icat.html

Mind Tools: The Old School House, Yapton, West Sussex, United Kingdom BN18 ODU

Mind Tools: How Your Learning Style Affects Your Use of Mnemonics, www.mindtools.com/mnem1sty.html

National Center for Learning Disabilities, Inc., 381 Park Avenue South, Suite 1401, New York, NY 10016, 212-545-7510, 888-575-7373, www.ncld.org

National Council for Excellence in Critical Thinking, P.O. Box 220, Dillon Beach, CA 94929, 707-878-9100, www.critcalthinking.org/ncect.html

Socratic Arts, 732-888-8121, http://socraticarts.com

HOLISTIC CARE

MAKING THE CONNECTION

Refer to the following chapters to increase your understanding of holistic care:

Basic Nursing
- **Legal and Ethical Responsibilities**
- **Cultural Considerations**
- **Stress, Adaptation, and Anxiety**
- **Complementary/Alternative Therapies**
- **Basic Nutrition**

- **Safety/Hygiene**
- **Standard Precautions and Isolation**
- **Fluid, Electrolyte, and Acid-Base Balance**
Basic Procedures
- **Hand Hygiene**
- **Proper Body Mechanics**

LEARNING OBJECTIVES

Upon completion of this chapter, you should be able to:
- **Define key terms.**
- **Define health as it relates to the whole person.**
- **List and discuss the five aspects of total wellness.**
- **List and discuss Maslow's Hierarchy of Needs.**
- **Describe self-awareness and why it is important to nurses.**
- **Describe self-concept.**
- **Discuss the concept of personal responsibility for one's own illness.**
- **Discover personal attitudes about health and illness and take responsibility for personal well-being.**
- **Identify the components of a healthy lifestyle.**

KEY TERMS

attitude
body mechanics
culture
health
health continuum
holistic
homeostasis
intellectual wellness
Maslow's Hierarchy
  of Needs

physical wellness
psychological wellness
self-awareness
self-concept
sociocultural wellness
spiritual wellness
wellness

INTRODUCTION

As a nurse, you will be a professional caregiver. Your intimate contact with clients allows you the opportunity not only to provide physical and emotional support, but also to teach ways to take an active role in maintaining health.

You may have contact with hundreds of clients, each needing specialized treatment and care. The care you provide will vary from routine to critical to emergency. You will be part of a multidisciplinary team of caregivers that includes registered nurses, physicians, nursing assistants, physical therapists, respiratory therapists, laboratory technicians, dietitians, and social workers. All caregivers work together to promote and maintain client health.

Because the caregiver's goal is promoting and maintaining health, understanding the concept of health is paramount. Most simply, health means that an organism is performing its vital functions normally and properly (*Webster's*, 2000).

INTERRELATED CONCEPTS OF HEALTH

In 1948, the World Health Organization (WHO) was founded. The WHO, which functions as an arm of the United Nations, places particular emphasis on combating communicable diseases, educating health care workers, and improving the health of all people of the world. The WHO defines **health** as follows: "Health is a state of complete physical, mental, and social well-being and not merely the absence of disease or infirmity" (WHO, 1974).

Many people believe that health or wellness is only the absence of disease. In its truest form, however, health refers to the total well-being of the whole person.

Holistic Health

Holistic is a term derived from the Greek word *holos*, meaning "whole." Holistic health views the physical, intellectual, sociocultural, psychological, and spiritual aspects of a person's life as an integrated whole. These five aspects cannot be separated or isolated; anything that affects one aspect of a person's life also affects the other aspects. The environment within which a person lives and the manner whereby the person interacts with that environment are also considerations.

The American Holistic Nurses' Association (AHNA) (1994) describes health as the maintenance of harmony and balance among body, mind, and spirit. **Homeostasis** is the balance or stability that the body strives to achieve among these aspects of a person's life by continuous adaptation. Internal physiological homeostasis is a balance of the body's fluids.

Nurses must understand the integration of these aspects of a person's life in order to help clients through healing processes. Figure 2-1 illustrates the holistic perspective.

Holistic Care

Dossey (1998) reports that the use of holistic modalities is gradually becoming integrated into mainstream client care. The National Institutes of Health (NIH) established the National Center for Complementary and Alternative Medicine (NCCAM) to investigate holistic modalities. The NIH defines holistic care as care that "considers the whole person, including physical, mental, emotional, and spiritual aspects." The final goal of investigating holistic modalities is to allow the validated therapies to be further integrated into general client care.

Success in using holistic modalities in client care requires an awareness of a fundamental principle of holism: The nurse *facilitates* the client in attaining the best state for healing to occur. Among the holistic modalities most frequently used in nursing are the following:

- Biofeedback
- Exercise and movement
- Goal-setting
- Humor and laughter
- Imagery
- Journaling
- Massage
- Play therapy
- Prayer
- Therapeutic touch

Nurses must be open to new ideas and must not allow holistic modalities to become just another technology. They must work on developing personal healing qualities and become more aware of healing in their own lives. Among other qualities, a healer:

- Demonstrates awareness that self-healing is a continual process.
- Is familiar with self-development.
- Recognizes personal strengths and weaknesses.
- Models self-care.
- Demonstrates awareness that personal presence is as important as technical skills.
- Respects and loves clients.
- Presumes that clients know the best life choices.
- Guides clients in discovering creative options.
- Listens actively.
- Shares insights without imposing personal values and beliefs.
- Accepts client input without judgment.
- Views time spent with clients as an opportunity to serve and share (adapted from Dossey, 1998).

Nursing the Whole Person

Nursing the whole person, or holistic health care, is a comprehensive approach to health care. It considers physical, intellectual, sociocultural, psychological, and spiritual aspects, the response to illness, and the effect of illness on a person's ability to meet self-care needs. Also taken into account is the individual's responsibility for personal well-being. Teaching preventive care is always a focus.

Nurses work with people throughout life to promote wellness and prevent illness (Figure 2-2). The highest level of wellness should be the goal of each nurse and every client.

Wellness

Wellness is a responsibility, a choice, a lifestyle design that helps maintain the highest potential for personal health (Hill & Howlett, 1997). The **health continuum** is a way to visualize the range of an individual's health, from highest health potential to death (Figure 2-3).

Figure 2-1 *Holistic View of an Individual*

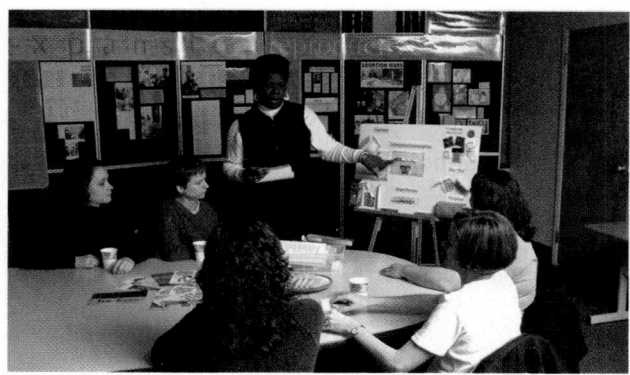

Figure 2-2 *Nurses work with clients of all age groups to encourage health and wellness.*

Figure 2-4 *Maslow's Hierarchy of Needs*

An individual's place on the continuum may change daily or even hourly depending on what is happening to that individual. Constant effort is required to balance all aspects of life and to maintain the highest level of health. A person at the highest level of wellness is one who demonstrates good physical self-care, emotional well-being, creative expression, and positive relationships with others.

Wellness incorporates physical, intellectual, sociocultural, psychological, and spiritual wellness. To provide holistic care, all aspects of the individual's wellness must be addressed.

Maslow's Hierarchy of Needs

Abraham Maslow developed a theory of behavioral motivation based on needs. This theory is often referred to as **Maslow's Hierarchy of Needs.** There are five levels in this hierarchy. The basic physiological needs must be met to maintain life. The rest of the needs are related to quality of life. They are safety and security, love and belonging, self-esteem, and self-actualization. The needs of the lower levels must be met before a person is motivated to meet the needs of the next higher level (Figure 2-4).

Many nursing programs use Maslow's Hierarchy of Needs as a basis for planning the care of clients. This ensures that basic physiological needs as well as the other needs are assessed and addressed in individualized care plans.

Physiological Needs

Although Maslow (1954) did not specifically identify the physiological needs, they are generally accepted to be the needs of oxygen, water, food, elimination, rest

(sleep)/activity (exercise), and sex. With the exception of sex, all of these needs must be met for the life of the individual to be maintained. Satisfying the sexual need, while not necessary for individual survival, is necessary for survival of the human race. The basic physiological needs must be met before higher-level needs become motivators of behavior. For example, a person who is truly hungry is motivated by that need, and behavior is focused on getting food.

Safety and Security Needs

The next level, safety, encompasses the needs for shelter, stability, security, physical safety, and freedom from undue anxiety. Safety needs include both physical and emotional aspects. Illness is often a threat to safety because the stability of life is disrupted.

Love and Belonging Needs

The third level of the hierarchy, love and belonging, incorporates not only giving but also receiving affection. Having friends and participating with others in groups and organizations are two ways to meet these needs. Meeting these needs is extremely important for mental health.

Self-Esteem Needs

The needs of the self-esteem level are met by achieving success in work and other activities. Recognition from others increases self-esteem and feelings of pride in one's accomplishments.

Self-Actualization Needs

Self-actualization is the highest level of the Maslow hierarchy. A person who has met these needs is confi-

Figure 2-3 *Health Continuum*

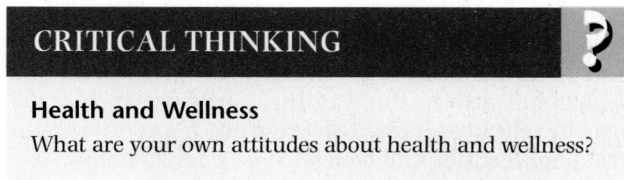

CRITICAL THINKING

Health and Wellness
What are your own attitudes about health and wellness?

dent, self-fulfilled, and creative; looks for challenges; and sees beauty and order in the world.

Maslow contends that because most people are so busy meeting the physiological and safety and security needs, little time or energy is left to meet the love and belonging, self-esteem, and self-actualization needs; thus, most people are less than satisfied at higher levels of the hierarchy. Even when the lower two levels are met without much trouble, many people have personalities and attitudes that make meeting the needs of the three higher levels difficult, if not impossible.

An individual does not move steadily up the hierarchy. As life situations change, a person's unmet needs change, and behavior is motivated by different levels of the hierarchy. For example, if a person who is working to meet the self-esteem need is suddenly laid off at work, the safety and security need of providing financially for self and family suddenly becomes the unmet need that motivates that person's behavior.

PROVIDING QUALITY CARE

The first step in providing quality client care is to be aware of yourself. What kind of personality do you have? Is your self-concept positive, or do you have self-doubts and lack self-confidence? What are your beliefs and attitudes? Knowing the answers to such questions will help you in your role as caregiver.

The next step is taking care of your own needs (see the preceding section on Maslow's Hierarchy of Needs). When you attend to the needs in your own life, you are then free to concentrate on caring for others. Your example of self-care inspires clients to have confidence that you will provide quality care. Thus, self-care is a factor in your effectiveness as a caregiver.

Self-Awareness

Self-awareness is consciously knowing how the self thinks, feels, believes, and behaves at any specific time. Being self-aware is a constant process that is focused on the present. A person's thoughts, feelings, and beliefs are interrelated and greatly influence behavior. Being self-aware influences a person in several ways.

Self-awareness may make a person uncomfortable. Awareness allows the person to either accept or alter feelings, beliefs, and behavior. One can learn to be self-aware. Begin now to concentrate on becoming aware of your thoughts and actions. Take note of your reactions to any given situation. What makes you anxious? What makes you happy? Listen to yourself when you respond to questions and when you visit with friends. Realize that everyone has strengths and weaknesses. Focus on your strengths. Spend your energies on today. Do not dwell on past mistakes; rather, try to learn from them, and then forget them. Stop periodically and pay attention to what you feel and believe. Listening not only to the words one speaks but also to the way the words are spoken assists in self-awareness. Use the word *I*, and take ownership of feelings and beliefs. Say, "I am so happy," instead of "That makes me happy."

Self-awareness is extremely important for nurses. Nurses must understand themselves so that their personal feelings, attitudes, and needs do not interfere with providing quality client care. The nurse who is self-aware is more likely to make decisions in response to the client's needs rather than the nurse's own needs. For example, student nurses—and even experienced nurses—are often anxious about caring for a specific client. By taking some time to practice self-awareness, the nurse might discover that the anxiety stems from never having performed the procedure in question. The nurse can then deal directly with the situation by reviewing the procedure and requesting assistance from an instructor or supervisor. All decisions about client care must be made in response to the client's needs, not the nurse's needs.

Development of Self-Concept

Self-concept is how a person thinks or feels about himself. These thoughts and feelings come from the experiences the person has with others and reflect how the person thinks others view him.

Self-concept begins forming in infancy. An infant whose needs are met feels satisfied and good. Experiences, both positive and negative, influence a person's self-concept (Figure 2-5). Interactions with significant others, such as parents, extended family, and friends, have a great impact on self-concept. This is true not only during the developing years, but also throughout life. Because of its influence on client care, it is important for the nurse to be aware of how her own self-concept has developed. Self-concept develops through feedback from others. The nurse is responsible for providing feedback that will not negatively affect the client's self-concept.

An individual who is constantly ignored or who receives messages such as "Don't bother me," "Can't you do anything right?", or "You don't have any sense" may very well begin to view himself in these terms, with the likely result being a negative self-concept. On the other hand, a person who is shown caring and who hears messages such as "Let me help you in a minute," "Let's try it this way," or "Have you thought about . . . ?" will move toward a positive self-concept.

Figure 2-5 *Self-concept and self-esteem can be enhanced by learning new skills.*

SELF-CARE AS A PREREQUISITE TO CLIENT CARE

The most effective means to teach wellness is by positive example. By first practicing good health habits as a nursing student, you will become, by example, an important factor in your clients' overall well-being and good health. Remind yourself and your clients that health is a personal choice and that each person has control over his or her own wellness.

You will be helping clients recognize how their own actions can prevent many of the conditions that cause illness. Choosing to exercise regularly, to eat a balanced diet, to eat breakfast each day, to control fat content, and to select from the basic food groups are good rules for wellness. Choosing to not smoke, to practice moderation in the use of alcohol, to avoid all nontherapeutic drugs, and to practice safe sex can help prevent many of the conditions that cause disease and death.

While emphasizing health promotion and client education, the nurse must also encourage and respect the client's responsibility for wellness. This respect allows the client to become an active partner in, rather than a passive recipient of, health care. It is not enough to tell a client *what* can be done to improve health; the nurse must also be prepared to explain *why*. If a client understands the reason behind an action, the likelihood of compliance increases.

Just as you are aware of yourself as a whole person with many components, help your clients see themselves and their health care as more than physical health. Help clients understand how physical, intellectual, sociocultural, psychological, and spiritual health are all related and can lead to an overall sense of well-being. This is the full meaning of holistic care.

Physical Wellness

Physical wellness refers to a healthy body that functions at an optimal level. To achieve physical wellness a person must practice good grooming; use proper body mechanics; have good posture; refrain from smoking and the use of drugs and alcohol; and have adequate nutrition, sleep, rest, relaxation, and exercise.

Grooming

The nurse communicates a message of health and well-being by being clean and neatly dressed (Figure 2-6). A daily bath or shower and the use of a deodorant form the basis of good grooming. Hair should be clean, combed, and neatly styled. Perfume should not be worn, because it may be offensive to clients. Frequent brushing, regular dental checkups, and avoiding refined sugars helps control dental caries.

While important for client safety, good hand hygiene is also crucial to the nurse's wellness. Antiseptic hand lotion can be used to prevent cracked, dry skin. Fingernails should be kept short, because long nails not only harbor dirt and microorganisms but can also scratch clients.

Standard Precautions have been established by the Centers for Disease Control and Prevention (CDC) in Atlanta, Georgia. These precautions are designed to pro-

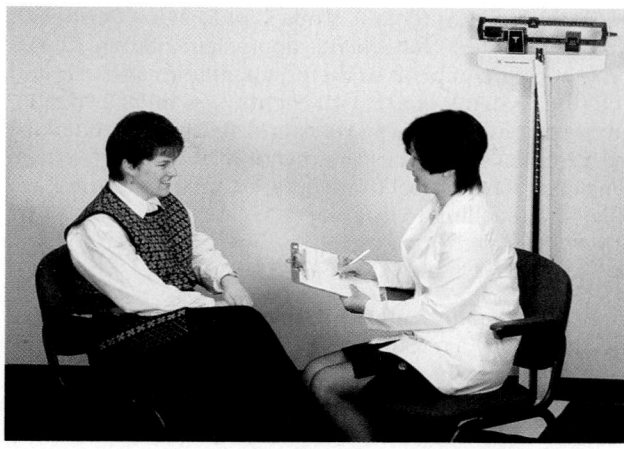

Figure 2-6 *The well-groomed nurse sends a message of health and well being.*

tect all health care workers and their clients from the transmission of communicable disease. Good hand hygiene is an integral part of Standard Precautions. As soon as you have been taught the skill of hand hygiene practice it. Make it a part of your daily life. Encourage your clients to establish good hand hygiene habits.

Jewelry, which can harbor bacteria, and excessive makeup are both inappropriate for the nurse in uniform. Clothing should be clean and free of stains and wrinkles. Clients will have confidence in the nurse who maintains a professional appearance and who practices good hygiene.

Body Mechanics

Wellness involves more than just good grooming practices. It also requires proper **body mechanics,** (i.e., using the body in the safest and most efficient way to move or lift objects). The use of proper body mechanics is very important because many of the skills and tasks you will perform as a nurse involve lifting or moving clients or objects. Bending, lifting, or stooping can cause injury if done incorrectly. One of the first skills you will study involves the practice of proper body mechanics to prevent physical disability, including safe methods for bending, lifting, and moving.

Posture

Good posture is the basis for proper body mechanics. Good posture means the ability to carry oneself well and in correct body alignment. Posture can also send messages about a person. A person who stands with feet spread apart and with hands on hips, for example, may be perceived as aggressive or authoritative, whereas one who holds the arms tightly folded over the chest may be viewed as closed minded.

Observe those around you as they communicate with others. Notice the differences in posture. Does the person who stands in good alignment, with shoulders back and head up, convey self-confidence and capability? Does the individual whose shoulders are drooped and head bowed convey depression, sadness, or lack of self-confidence?

As you continue your studies and begin client care, you will realize that clients appreciate having nurses who appear confident in their own abilities and decision making. When you are with clients, you must be particularly careful of the way you stand. Remember that your posture sends messages about your attitude and feelings. The client should feel that you are confident, caring, relaxed, and willing to listen.

Smoking

Smoking contributes to many health hazards and illnesses. It may also be personally offensive to clients. The odor of smoke on clothing or the breath (halitosis) may precipitate allergic reactions or lead to a feeling of nausea in some clients. Most health care facilities have strict rules about smoking. Many facilities are "smoke free." The nurse should never smoke in a client's room. Furthermore, great care should be taken to ensure that no offensive tobacco odors remain if the nurse uses or is in close proximity to tobacco products. In each situation, every effort should be made to enforce all safety rules for clients and visitors. "No smoking" signs should be posted and strictly enforced when oxygen is in use.

Drugs and Alcohol

A frightening trend in the United States is the increasing rate of alcohol and drug abuse. Drug abuse has become so widespread within the health professions that impaired caregiver programs have been implemented. Many states now provide access to treatment for the impaired nurse through the state board of nursing. Drug abuse can begin very insidiously when a nurse says to herself "I'll borrow a pill just this once for my headache." The second time is easier, and the downward spiral begins.

A nurse should never give or make a drug available to anyone without the written order of a physician or other person who can legally prescribe medications, such as a nurse practitioner. If you believe that a colleague is abusing drugs, you have an obligation to let your supervisor know so the colleague can receive help through the impaired nurse program in your state. If you become addicted, you have a duty to your clients, your peers, and yourself to accept help through a recovery program.

LIFE CYCLE CONSIDERATIONS

Nutrition

- Children's appetites vary with their growth spurts and growth plateaus.
- Healthy eating habits should be established during childhood.
- The amount of food eaten generally declines in the elderly person.
- Proper food choices are more important than quantity for the elderly person.

Nutrition

Nursing is emotionally, mentally, and physically demanding. Nurses must be able to think clearly and work efficiently. A balanced diet, including fruits and vegetables, whole grains and cereals, milk and milk products, and meats or other protein foods, is required for optimal body function.

Nursing students may be tempted to skip meals, omit breakfast, eat snacks, and follow fad diets. This is never a wise practice. While you are in school, your success depends on you functioning at your best. Skipping meals, especially breakfast, leaves a person tired, weak, and hungry. It is impossible to think efficiently when hungry. Remember Maslow's Hierarchy of Needs: The need for food must be satisfied before you will be motivated to meet the need to learn or to study.

Always eat a balanced breakfast. Pastries and coffee, although satisfying in the moment, elevate the blood sugar level only for a short while before the level plummets. This reaction leaves a person drained, irritable, and hungrier than before. Try to avoid snacking on junk foods, which contain empty calories, or those having very little nutritional value. Instead, plan to eat fruit or high-protein snacks.

Plan a routine for mealtimes, and stick to it. Doing so helps prevent the urge to binge on unhealthy snacks. Also, drink plenty of water. Water is the body's most important nutrient (Figure 2-7). A human being can survive for weeks without food but only for a few days without water. By weight, approximately 60% of the adult body is water. In order to maintain proper fluid balance and to facilitate the elimination of body wastes, it is necessary to drink plenty of fluids. Most authorities agree that the average adult needs six to eight (8-ounce) glasses

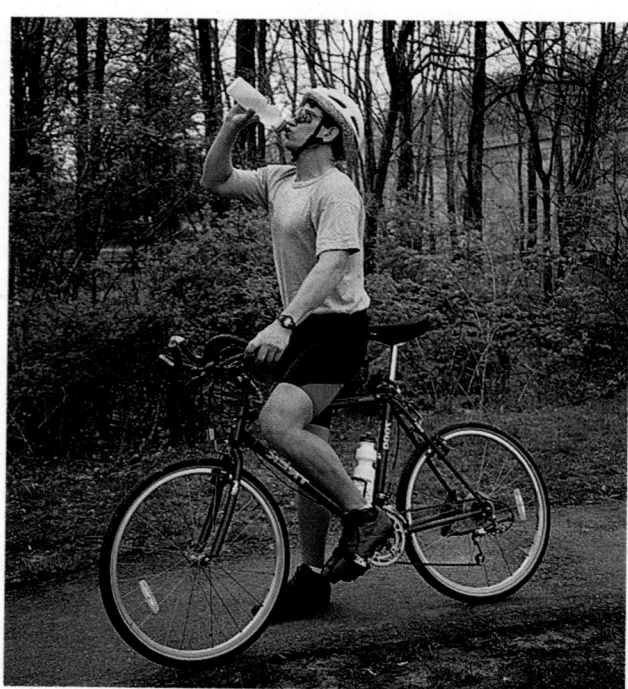

Figure 2-7 *Drinking plenty of water is an important element of proper nutrition.*

CLIENT TEACHING

Tips on Maintaining Proper Nutrition
- Read product labels.
- Avoid foods high in fat, sugar, and salt.
- Work to maintain or attain your ideal weight.
- If you drink alcohol, do so in moderation.
- Always eat breakfast.
- Make between-meal snacks healthy, such as raw fruits and vegetables.

of water each day. It is important to maintain a balance in the diet for optimal wellness.

Sleep, Rest, Relaxation, and Exercise

Wellness implies more than eating balanced meals, avoiding harmful substances, and practicing good grooming. Wellness also means taking time to enjoy yourself. It means making time for sleep, rest, relaxation, and exercise.

Sleep is time for the body to replenish its energy reserves and to heal itself. The amount of time needed may vary with the individual or even with the day. One person may need 8 hours of sleep after a heavy workday but need only 6 hours after a less strenuous day. An infant, of course, needs more sleep than does a young adult. Sleep is necessary to allow the body's organs to function at their most minimal levels. This period of rejuvenation for the body is necessary for total wellness.

Rest, meaning conscious freedom from activity and worry, is just as important as sleep. Rest is a time of inner quiet and physical inactivity. Only when a person is relaxed and at inner peace can that person rest.

Relaxation means doing something for the fun of it. That which is relaxing to one person may not be relaxing to another. Examples of relaxation activities include reading a novel, reading to children, playing cards or other games, fishing, painting, or sewing or other handwork.

Many experts agree that the best rest follows planned exercise. During exercise, heart rate and breathing increase, circulation improves, and muscles stretch. Exercise is also a time to free the mind of anxiety-producing thoughts. Sometimes after a day's work, a brisk walk frees the mind and allows the body to relax in preparation for rest.

Whichever form of exercise, rest, and relaxation is best for you, make time for it in each day. Rest and relaxation as well as regular sleep and exercise are essential ingredients for wellness and result in reduced fatigue and irritability and possibly increased resistance to colds, flu, and serious infections. Furthermore, the capacity to concentrate increases, which should make a significant difference in your studies.

Intellectual Wellness

Intellectual wellness is the ability to function as an independent person capable of making sound decisions. Such decisions are based on the individual's needs but at the same time take into account the needs of others. Clear thinking, problem-solving skills, good judgment, and the desire to continually learn are all qualities found in the person who is intellectually well.

Nursing requires making many decisions, some of which may mean life or death to the client. The nurse must have intellectual wellness to be able to make the best decisions possible with regard to client care.

Sociocultural Wellness

Sociocultural wellness is the ability to appreciate the needs of others and to care about one's environment and the inhabitants of it. As a nurse, you will care for clients of all ages and races who speak different languages and come from various cultural groups. Each client's **culture** (behavior, customs, and beliefs of the family, extended family, tribe, nation, and society) influences the way that person views wellness and responds to illness.

It is important that the nurse understand that while everyone's basic needs are the same, the ways that those needs are met may vary based on the client's culture. Today's population is working, playing, and contributing to society for more years than ever before. People are more health conscious, better educated, and more involved in making health choices than perhaps any previous generation. Nurses should encourage such involvement and work to dispel discrimination by accepting each person as an individual.

Psychological Wellness

Psychological wellness encompasses the enjoyment of creativity, the satisfaction of the basic need to love and be loved, the understanding of emotions, and the ability to maintain control over emotions. Emotions are an integral part of the balance sought in life and are important factors in the way a person relates to others. They are measures of inner thoughts and feelings and are apparent in actions or behaviors.

Wellness requires that individuals recognize emotions and control their reactions in various situations. By controlling their emotions, nurses help create a therapeutic environment within which to help clients.

Another aspect of emotional wellness is a positive attitude. An **attitude** is a feeling about people, places, or things that is evident in the way one behaves. It can be positive or negative. Many books have been written and hundreds of studies have described the role that a positive attitude plays in helping conquer illness. Many authorities believe having a positive attitude is at least as important as having the best treatment for an illness.

Nursing requires that you see the best in people during the worst of times. In order to survive and function well,

CULTURAL CONSIDERATIONS

Sociocultural Wellness

Nurses and nursing students come from various cultural backgrounds and are thus excellent resources for you to learn about cultural variations.

Self-Nurturing

- Develop activities that recharge the body, mind, and spirit.
- Make time for fun. Any activity that brings happiness or joy is beneficial.
- Schedule a few minutes each day to do at least one fun thing.

the nurse needs to see life as a challenge and as a gift to cherish and enjoy.

Because a positive attitude is so important when caring for your clients, it is vital that you share yours with them. An attitude can become a habit. If you repeatedly think positively, soon you will unconsciously find yourself seeing the positive aspects in any given situation. For example, you may find yourself at work when the usual number of staff does not show up. You can say to yourself at the beginning of your shift: "There is no way I will ever finish my work on time," or you can tell yourself, "This is the perfect opportunity to get organized early and work together as a team." Either way you will have the same number of staff members. But whereas having a negative attitude will increase your chances of being miserable and unsuccessful, having a positive attitude will help the day go smoother and increase the likelihood of your coworkers being cheerful and willing to help.

Having a positive attitude will also help you in your studies. It will help open your mind and will spill into your daily life, making that life more enjoyable.

Spiritual Wellness

Spiritual wellness manifests as inner strength and peace. Spirituality is a broader concept than religion and involves one's relationship with self, others, the natural order, and a higher power. It manifests as meaningful work, creative expression, familiar rituals, and religious practices

Tips for Wellness

Encourage clients to adopt the following tips for wellness:

- Eat healthy meals and healthy snacks.
- Eat breakfast.
- Do not use tobacco products.
- Exercise regularly.
- Do not use drugs.
- Do not drink alcoholic beverages or drink only in moderation.
- Focus on one problem at a time.
- Get enough sleep every night.
- Practice having a positive attitude.
- Think before speaking.
- Make a list of goals for each day.

(Wright, 1998). Spirituality involves finding meaning in everything, including life, illness, and death. Spiritual needs include love, meaning in life, forgiveness, and hope. The human spiritual dimension is a major healing force. It can mean the difference between life and death, wellness and illness (Dossey, Keegan, & Guzzetta, 2000).

Florence Nightingale spoke boldly about the importance of the spiritual aspect of client care. Dossey and Dossey (1998) state that the richness of a person's interactions with others correlates with positive health outcomes, and that practice of any religion correlates with greater health and increased longevity.

Nurses are not asked to take over the role of spiritual counselors. Rather, nurses are encouraged to integrate a holistic approach by extending love, compassion, and empathy; motivating clients to address spiritual issues; and suggesting how they might do so (Dossey & Dossey, 1998).

Cerrato (1998b) has two suggestions regarding nursing and spiritual wellness: (1) Nurses who have strong religious convictions should not impose those convictions on their clients, and (2) nurses should never assume that clients who have no religious interests have no interest in spiritual values. Clients not interested in religion can be encouraged to become involved in some humanitarian endeavor or to look at life's everyday wonders in a different way.

Because they play a key role in helping clients find hope and meaning in life, it is important that nurses understand spirituality. For many, religious practices are an expression of their spirituality. An important function for the nurse is to respect the religious beliefs of clients, provide clients with privacy to practice those beliefs, and make spiritual guidance available through the client's minister, priest, rabbi, or other representative, when requested.

NURTURE YOURSELF

The worthy and demanding profession of nursing requires unselfish caring for others. Those who select nursing as a career generally want to make a difference in people's lives. The demands of clients, employers, and coworkers can cause stress for the nurse. The nurse's personal life may also be a source of stress. Many caregivers do not know how to care for themselves. Those who do not nurture themselves will suffer stress symptoms and illnesses.

Persons who are well physically, intellectually, socioculturally, psychologically, and spiritually lead productive, creative lives. They are better able to meet life's challenges and to control their stressors. For nurses, wellness means practicing wellness habits daily. As role models for clients, nurses should be examples of the holistically healthy individual.

Personal Well-being

What are you doing or what can you do to take responsibility for your own well-being?

Summary

- Wellness includes physical, intellectual, sociocultural, psychological, and spiritual health.
- The keys to wellness are prevention and education.
- Each individual must learn to accept responsibility for his or her own wellness.
- The most effective means to reinforce teachings of wellness is by positive example.
- There are five levels in Maslow's Hierarchy of Needs: physiological, safety and security, love and belonging, self-esteem, and self-actualization.
- Self-awareness is important for nurses so their own needs do not interfere with providing quality client care.
- Nurses should get to know themselves by becoming aware of their thoughts, actions, and reactions to situations.
- Good posture is necessary for personal and client safety.
- Dental health is necessary for overall wellness and professionalism.
- Wellness tips include exercising regularly, getting enough sleep, and finding a quiet time each day for relaxing.
- A positive attitude is helpful in looking for the best in everyone.
- All nurses should learn to laugh at themselves and enjoy life's little pleasures.

Review Questions

1. Rest is defined as:
   a. sleeping.
   b. physical inactivity.
   c. playing games with family or friends.
   d. conscious freedom from activity and worry.

2. What responsibility does the nurse have who believes a colleague is abusing drugs?
   a. Report it to the supervisor.
   b. Ignore it; it is not the nurse's concern.
   c. Tell the colleague to stop or the nurse will call the police.
   d. Assist the nurse to receive help through the local drug treatment program.

3. What can be the result when breakfast is omitted?
   a. The person loses weight faster.
   b. The person is left tired, weak, and hungry.
   c. The person eats more at the noon and evening meals.
   d. The person's mind is sharper, and study time is more productive.

4. Positive or negative feelings about people, places, or things are called:
   a. culture.
   b. empathy.
   c. symptoms.
   d. attitudes.

5. The aspects of total wellness are:
   a. rest, exercise, and good grooming.
   b. physical, psychological, spiritual, intellectual, and sociocultural.
   c. self-awareness; rest; balanced, nutritious diet; good grooming; dental care.
   d. physiological; safety and security; love and belonging; self-esteem; self-actualization.

References/Suggested Readings

American Holistic Nurses' Association. (1994). AHNA Philosophy. *Journal of Holistic Nursing, 12*(3), 350–351.

Cerrato, P. (1998a). Understanding the mind/body link. *RN, 61*(1), 28–31.

Cerrato, P. (1998b). Spirituality and healing. *RN, 61*(2), 49–50.

Diluzio, J., & Spillane, E. (2002). Holistic nursing: Is it right for you? *RN, 65*(8), 32–35.

Dossey, B. (1997). *Core curriculum for holistic nursing.* Gaithersburg, MD: Aspen.

Dossey, B. (1998). Holistic modalities & healing moments. *AJN, 98*(6), 44–47.

Dossey, B. (2000). *Florence Nightingale: Mystic, visionary, healer:* Springhouse, PA: Springhouse.

Dossey, B., & Dossey, L. (1998). Attending to holistic care. *AJN, 98*(8), 35–38.

Dossey, B., Keegan, L., & Guzzetta, C. (2000). *Holistic nursing: A handbook for practice* (3rd ed.). Gaithersburg, MD: Aspen.

Dyer, E. (1998, April 6). Faith & healing. *Corpus Christi Caller-Times.*

Edlin, G., Golanty, E., & Brown, K. (2002). *Health and wellness* (7th ed.). Boston: Jones & Bartlett.

Frisch, N. C., Dossey, B., Guzzetta, C., Fristh, N., & Quinn, J. (2000). *AHNA standards of holistic nursing practice: Guidelines for caring and healing.* Gaithersburg, MD: Aspen.

Hill, S., & Howlett, H. (1997). *Success in practical nursing: Personal and vocational issues* (3rd ed.). Philadelphia: W. B. Saunders.

Hughs, C. (1997). Prayer and healing: A case study. *Journal of Holistic Nursing, 15*(3), 318.

Ivker, R. S. (2002). *Comparing holistic and conventional medicine.* [Online]. Available: http://ahha.org/articles/ivker.htm

Jerome, A., et al. (1992). Nurse self-awareness in therapeutic relationships. *Pediatric Nursing, 18*(2), 153–156.

Kahn, S., & Saulo, M. (1995). *Healing yourself.* Clifton Park, NY: Thomson Delmar Learning.

Kurzen, C. (2000). *Contemporary practical/vocational nursing* (4th ed.). Philadelphia: Lippincott, Williams & Wilkins.

Maslow, A. (1954). *Motivation and personality.* New York: Harper & Row.

National Institutes of Health (NIH). (2000). *Complementary & alternative medicine at the NIH* [Online]. Available: http://nccam.nih.gov/nccam/ne/newsletter/spring2000.

Rivera-Andino, J., & Lopez, L. (2000). When culture complicates care, *RN, 63*(7), 47–49.

Selye, H. (1956). *The stress of life.* New York: McGraw-Hill.

Taber's cyclopedic medical dictionary. (18th ed.) (1997). Philadelphia: F. A. Davis.

Walter, S. (1999). *Holistic health.* [Online]. Available: http://ahha.org/rosen.htm

Waughfield, C. (2002). *Mental health concepts* (5th ed.). Clifton Park, NY: Thomson Delmar Learning.

Webster's new world college dictionary (2000). Springfield, MA: Merriam-Webster.

World Health Organization. (1974). *Chronicle of WHO.* Geneva: Organization Interim Commission.

Wright, K. (1998). Professional, ethical, and legal implications for spiritual care in nursing. *Image: Journal of Nursing Scholarship, 30*(1)81–83.

Resources

American Holistic Health Association, Anaheim, CA 92817-7400, 714-779-6152, http://ahha.org

American Holistic Nurses' Association, P.O. Box 2130, Flagstaff, AZ 86003-2130, 800-278-AHNA (1461), www.ahna.org

National Center for Complementary and Alternative Medicine (NCCAM), P.O. Box 7923, Gaithersburg, MD 20898, 888-644-6226, http://nccam.nih.gov

Nurse Healers—Professional Associates International, Inc., 3760 South Highland Drive, Suite 429, Salt Lake City, UT 84106, 801-273-3399, www.therapeutic-touch.org

Videos

- *Holistic Nursing* (1996), American Holistic Nurses' Association, 800-278-2462
- *At the Heart of Healing: Expericing Holistic Nursing,* Kineholistic Foundation, 800-255-1914

NURSING HISTORY, EDUCATION, AND ORGANIZATIONS

MAKING THE CONNECTION

Refer to the following chapters to increase your understanding of nursing history, education, and organizations:

Basic Nursing
- **Legal and Ethical Responsibilities**

LEARNING OBJECTIVES

Upon completion of this chapter, you should be able to:
- **Define key terms.**
- **Define nursing as an art and a science.**
- **Identify major historical and social events that have shaped current nursing practice.**
- **Describe Florence Nightingale's impact on current nursing practice.**
- **Discuss the contributions of early nursing leaders in the United States.**
- **Discuss the impact of selected landmark reports on nursing education and practice.**
- **Define the role of the RN.**
- **Define the role of the LP/VN.**
- **Describe select nursing organizations and their purposes and functions.**
- **Differentiate between program approval and program accreditation.**

KEY TERMS

accreditation	morbidity
autonomy	mortality
clinical	nursing
didactic	primary care provider
empowerment	primary health care
health maintenance	staff development
organization	

INTRODUCTION

Nursing is the art and science of assisting individuals in learning to care for themselves whenever possible and of caring for them when they are unable to meet their own needs.

Nursing has developed into a scientific profession from an unorganized way of caring for the ill, resulting in change from mystical beliefs to sophisticated technology and caring. Nursing uses caring behaviors, critical thinking skills, and scientific knowledge.

Nursing focuses on the client's *response* to illness rather than on the illness. Nursing promotes health and assists clients move to a higher level of wellness, including assistance during a terminal illness with the maintenance of comfort and dignity during the final stage of life.

The development of nursing is traced through its rich history and the social forces that affected it. Nursing education and nursing organizations are also discussed in this chapter.

HISTORICAL OVERVIEW

A basic knowledge about the history of nursing is necessary to understand what nursing is today. The study of nursing history helps the nurse better understand the issues of **autonomy** (being self-directed), unity within the profession, education, supply and demand, salary, and current practice. Learning from the role models of history, nurses can increase their capacity to make positive changes in the present and set goals for the future.

The major reason for studying history is to learn from the past. By applying the lessons learned from history, nurses will continue to be a vital force in the health care system.

By studying nursing history, nurses learn how the profession has advanced from its beginnings. The process of enabling others to do for themselves is called **empowerment.** When nurses are empowered, they are autonomous. Historically, it has been difficult for nurses to achieve autonomy. Empowerment and autonomy are necessary for nursing to bring about positive changes in health care today. Personal power comes to individuals who are clear about what they want from life and who see their work as essential to the contributions they wish to make.

Evolution of Nursing

Nursing has evolved alongside human civilization. Although it is not possible to present a complete history of nursing and health care within the scope of this text, it is necessary for all nurses to have some understanding of their profession's heritage and of those pioneers who led the way on the path to modern nursing. Table 3-1 is a chronological listing of events in the evolution of nursing.

TABLE 3-1   HISTORICAL EVENTS INFLUENCING THE EVOLUTION OF NURSING

DATE	EVENT	DATE	EVENT
4000 B.C.	Primitive societies	1899	Founded: International Council of Nurses (ICN)
2000 B.C.	Babylonia and Assyria	1900	*American Journal of Nursing (AJN)* established
800–600 B.C.	Health religions of India		
700 B.C.	Greece: source of modern medical science	1903	New York: efforts fail to pass a nurse licensing law
460 B.C.	Hippocrates		
3 B.C.	Ireland: pre-Christian nursing		North Carolina: first state nurse registration law passes
A.D. 390	Fabiola: first hospital founded		
390–407	Early Christianity, deaconesses		Founded: Army Nurse Corps
711	Field hospital with nursing, Spain	1907	Thompson Practical Nursing School in Brattleboro, VT established
1096–1291	Military Nursing Orders (Knights Hospitalers of St. John in Jerusalem)	1910	Flexner report
1100	Ambulatory clinics, Spain (Moslems)	1911	Founded: American Nurses Association (ANA), formerly the Associated Alumnae
1440	First Chairs of Medicine, Oxford and Cambridge	1912	Founded: National League of Nursing Education, formerly the Superintendents' Society
1500–1752	Deterioration of hospitals and nursing, "dark ages of nursing"	1914	Mississippi is first state to license practical nurses
1633	Founded: Daughters of Charity		
1820	Florence Nightingale born	1917	Smith-Hughes Act passes (provided federal funds for practical nursing programs in vocational schools)
1836	Kaiserswerth, Lutheran Order of Deaconesses reestablished		
1841	Founded: Nursing Sisters of the Holy Cross	1918	Household Nursing Association School of Attendant Nursing in Boston, MA, established
1848	Women's Rights Convention, Seneca Falls, New York		
1854–1856	Crimean War	1920s	First prepaid medical plan established, Pacific Northwest
1859	Nightingale's *Notes on Nursing* published in England		Hospitals offer a prepaid plan
1860	Founded: first Nightingale School of Nursing, St. Thomas Hospital, London		Baylor Plan (prototype of Blue Cross) established
1861–1865	Civil War, United States	1921	Women get the right to vote
1861	Dorothea Dix appointed Superintendent of the Female Nurses of the Army	1923	Goldmark Report: Nursing and Nursing Education in the United States
1871	Founded: New York State Training School for Nurses, Brooklyn Maternity, Brooklyn, New York	1935	Social Security Act passes
		1941	Founded: Association of Practical Nursing Schools
1872	New England Hospital for Women's one-year program for nurses yields America's first trained nurse, Linda Richards	1942	Association of Practical Nursing Schools becomes National Association of Practical Nurse Education (NAPNE)
1873	Founded: first three Nightingale schools in United States: Bellevue (New York City), Connecticut, and Massachusetts General		Practical nursing curriculum planned and advocated across United States
1881	Founded: American Red Cross, by Clara Barton	1944	U.S. Department of Vocational Education commissions intensive study to differentiate tasks of the practical nurse
1892	Founded: Ballard School at YWCA Brooklyn, NY; first practical nursing school	1945	New York only state to have mandatory licensure law for practical nurses
1893	Founded: American Society of Superintendents of Training Schools for Nurses	1948	Brown Report: Future of Nursing

continues

TABLE 3–1 continued

DATE	EVENT	DATE	EVENT
1949	Founded: National Federation of Licensed Practical Nurses (NFLPN)	1973	Health Maintenance Organization Act
1952	National League of Nursing Education changes name to National League for Nursing (NLN)	1977	Rural Health Clinic Service Act
		1979	U.S. Surgeon General Report *Healthy People*
1955	Practical nursing established under (Title III) Health Amendment Act	1980	Omnibus Budget Reconciliation Act (OBRA)
	All states pass licensure laws affecting practical/vocational nursing	1982	Budget cut to Health Maintenance Organization Act
1959	National Association of Practical Nurse Education (NAPNE) changes name to National Association for Practical Nurse Education and Service (NAPNES)		Tax Equity Fiscal Responsibility Act (TEFRA)
		1983	Institute of Medicine Committee on Nursing and Nursing Education study
1960s	Established: Medicare and Medicaid	1987	Secretary's Commission on Nursing
1961	National League for Nursing establishes a Council for Practical Nursing Programs	1990s	Health care reform
		1991	U.S. Dept. Health and Human Services *Healthy People 2000*
	Surgeon General's Consultant Group	1996	Certification Examination for Practical and Vocational Nurses in Long-term Care
1965	First nurse practitioner program, pediatric	1997	Established: NLN Accrediting Commission (NLNAC)
	ANA position paper on entry into practice		
1966	Educational opportunity grants for nurses	2000	U.S. Dept. Health and Human Services *Healthy People 2010*
1970	Secretary's commission to study extended roles for nurses		

Primitive Times

Primitive humans may very well have derived early nursing care practices from observing the animal world. Many animals care for their sick and injured. For example, wild turkeys feed their young wild berries to ward off the chill of inclement weather, much as we use vitamin C (found in wild berries) today; the snipe (a small bird) has been observed splinting an injured leg with sticks and straw; many animals eat grass as an emetic when they have stomach problems. Early humans were closely associated with the animals.

Early Civilizations

Nursing dates back to 4000 B.C. to the primitive societies where mother–nurses worked with priests. The use of wet nurses in Babylonia and Assyria is recorded in 2000 B.C.

Ancient Greece

Temples to honor Hygiea, the goddess of health, were built by the ancient Greeks. These temples, religious institutions governed by priests, were more like health spas than hospitals. Priestesses (who were not nurses) attended to those visiting the temples. Nursing was done by women in the homes.

Hippocrates, a Greek physician born in 460 B.C., is considered the father of medicine. He used a system of physical assessment, observation, and record keeping in his care of the sick. Hippocrates wrote about many aspects of medicine, including anatomy, physiology, pathology, diagnosis, prognosis, mental illness, gynecology, obstetrics, surgery, client-centered care, bedside ob-

servation, hygiene, and professional ethics. Case histories that he wrote are still used as examples today. His emphasis on the importance of caring for the client laid a foundation for nursing. The Hippocratic Oath, taken by physicians today, is based on his principles.

Roman Empire

The first hospitals were established in the Eastern Roman Empire (Byzantine Empire). Fabiola, disciple of St. Jerome, was responsible for introducing hospitals in the West. These were primarily religious and charitable institutions sheltered in monasteries and convents. The caregivers who volunteered their time to nurse the sick had no formal training in therapeutic modalities.

Middle Ages

Hospitals in large Byzantine cities of the medieval era were staffed primarily by paid male assistants and male nurses. This was not true in the rural parts of the Eastern Roman Empire and in the West, where nursing was viewed as a natural nurturing job for women.

In Western Europe, medical practices remained basically unchanged until the 11th and 12th centuries. At that time formal medical education for physicians was required in a university setting, but other caregivers were not required to receive any formal education or training.

Renaissance

Interest in the arts and sciences emerged during the Renaissance (A.D. 1400–1550). This was also the time of many geographic explorations by Europeans, which resulted in the expansion of the world.

Universities were established because of a renewed interest in science, but there were no formal nursing schools. Social status and customs encouraged women to stay at home and attend to the traditional role of nurturer/caregiver.

Industrial Revolution

The Industrial Revolution led to a proliferation of factories, where conditions for the workers were deplorable. Grueling work, long hours, and unsafe conditions prevailed in the workplace, and the health of laborers received little attention.

The Royal College of Surgeons in London and other medical schools were founded in 1800. Male barbers in France also functioned as surgeons by performing leeching, giving enemas, and extracting teeth.

It was still considered unseemly in the mid-1800s for women to be nurses, even though some hospitals (almshouses) relied on women to bathe the poor, make beds, and scrub floors. Most nursing care was still performed in the home by female relatives of the ill.

Religious Influences

Religion had a strong influence on the development of nursing beginning in India in 800–600 B.C.. The religious influence prospered in Greece and Ireland in 3 B.C. with male nurse–priests.

Theodor Fleidner, a pastor in Kaiserswerth, Germany in 1836, revived the Lutheran Order of Deaconesses to care for the sick in a hospital he had founded. He established the first real school of nursing to educate the deaconesses in the care of the sick. These deaconesses of Kaiserswerth became famous because they were the only ones formally trained in nursing. Pastor Fleidner had a profound influence on nursing through Florence Nightingale, who received her nurse's training at the Kaiserswerth Institute.

Religious orders were established by the Catholic Church to care for the sick and poor. Only nurses who functioned within a religious order were approved by society. The need for nurses in the mid-19th century and changing social conditions set the stage for Florence Nightingale's reforms (discussed following).

The order of the Nursing Sisters of the Holy Cross was founded in LeMans, France, by Father Bassil Moreau in 1841. Also in 1841, four sisters were brought to Notre Dame in South Bend, Indiana by a Father Sorin. These sisters established St. Mary's Academy in Bertrand, Michigan, in 1844. In 1855, the school was moved to Notre Dame and became known as Saint Mary's College, which later had a strong influence on the emerging role of women (Wall, 1993).

Florence Nightingale

The founder of modern nursing is Florence Nightingale (1820–1910), who grew up in a wealthy, upper-class family in England. Unlike other young women of her era, Nightingale was educated in Greek, Latin, mathematics, history, and philosophy. She always had an interest in relieving suffering and caring for the sick, but social mores of her time made it impossible for

Figure 3-1 *Florence Nightingale in the Crimea (Courtesy of Pfizer, Inc.)*

her to consider caring for others because she was not a member of a religious order. After receiving encouragement from a family visitor, Dr. Samuel Gridley Howe, however, she became a nurse over the objections of society and her family.

Upon completion of a 3-month course of study at Kaiserswerth Institute, Nightingale worked to reform health care. Britain's war in the Crimea presented her with the opportunity to volunteer with 38 other nurses to serve in the battle-site hospital (Figure 3-1). The physicians in charge assigned the nurses to nonclient care duties. Florence Nightingale persisted in advocating cleanliness, good nutrition, and fresh air. When battle casualties mounted, the nurses had a chance to prove their worth. They worked around the clock, caring for the wounded, carrying oil lamps to light their way in the darkness. The symbol of the oil lamp is still used today in nursing and is the reason Florence Nightingale is called the "Lady with the Lamp." The implementation of her principles in the areas of nursing practice and environmental modifications resulted in reduced **morbidity** (illness) and **mortality** (death) rates during the war.

Nightingale worked to further develop the public's awareness of the need for educated nurses and forged the future of nursing education as a result of her experiences in training nurses to care for British soldiers. At St. Thomas' Hospital in London, she established the Nightingale Training School of Nurses. This was the first school for nurses providing both theory-based knowledge and clinical experience. She fundamentally changed both the public's perception of nursing and the method for educating nurses. Some of Nightingale's unique beliefs about nursing and nursing education were the need for the following:

- A holistic framework inclusive of illness and health
- A theoretical basis for nursing practice
- A liberal education as a foundation of nursing practice
- An environment that promotes healing
- A body of nursing knowledge distinct from medical knowledge (Macrae, 1995)

She introduced many other concepts that are still used today, although they were unique in her day. Specifically, Nightingale recommended (1) a systematic method of assessing clients; (2) individualized care based on the client's needs and preferences; and (3) confidentiality.

Recognizing the influence of environmental factors on health, she recommended that clean surroundings, fresh air, and light would improve the quality of care (Nightingale, 1969). She believed that nurses should be formally educated and function as client advocates (Selanders, 1994). She is credited with being the originator of modern nursing because many of these beliefs and concepts are still advocated in nursing schools today.

The Civil War and Nursing

During the Civil War (1861–1865), America's need for nurses increased dramatically. The Sisters of the Holy Cross were the first to respond to the need for nurses, with 12 sisters caring for wounded soldiers. By the end of the war, 80 sisters had cared for soldiers in Illinois, Missouri, Kentucky, and Tennessee (Wall, 1993).

Nursing care was also provided by the Sisters of Mercy, Daughters of Charity, Dominican Sisters, and the Franciscan Sisters of the Poor. These sisters, although influenced by the roles assigned to women during the 19th century, were willing to take risks when human rights were threatened (Wall, 1993). Other women also volunteered to care for the soldiers of both the Union and Confederate armies. These women implemented sanitary conditions in field hospitals and performed various other duties.

Dorothea Dix (1802–1887), was the first woman ever appointed to an administrative position by the federal government when she was made Superintendent of the Female Nurses of the Army in 1861. Her recruitment efforts procured more than 2,000 women to care for the sick in the Union Army. Following the Civil War, she concentrated on reforming the treatment of the mentally ill (Mohr, 2002).

Clara Barton (1821–1912), who volunteered her nursing services during the Civil War, organized the Red Cross in the United States in 1881.

The Women's Movement

The beginnings of social unrest started in 1848 with the Women's Rights Convention in Seneca Falls, New York. Women were not considered equal to men, women did not have the right to vote, and society did not value education for women. With suffrage, the rights of women and the nursing profession were advanced. More women

were being accepted into colleges and universities by the mid-1900s, but there were only a few university-based nursing programs available.

Nursing Pioneers and Leaders

The contributions of many outstanding nurses through the years made nursing what it is today. Nursing pioneers and leaders established public health nursing, rural health care services, and advanced nursing education. Some of these women are discussed following. Note that the term *trained nurse* was used historically to mean the same as *registered nurse*.

Linda Richards

In 1873, Linda Richards (1841–1930) was awarded the first diploma from an American training school for nurses. She established numerous hospital-based training schools for nurses and introduced the practice of keeping nurses' notes and physicians' orders as part of medical records. She also instituted the practice of nurses' wearing uniforms. While working as the first Superintendent of Nurses at Massachusetts General Hospital, she showed that trained nurses gave better care than nurses without formal nursing education.

Mary Mahoney

Mary Mahoney (1845–1926) was America's first African American professional nurse. She was a noted nursing leader who encouraged respect for cultural diversity. Today, the ANA bestows the Mary Mahoney Award to recognize individuals who have made significant contributions toward improving relationships among the various cultural groups.

Adelaide Nutting

As a nursing educator, historian, and scholar, Adelaide Nutting (1858–1947) actively campaigned for the university education of nurses. She was the first nurse appointed as a university professor.

Lavinia Dock

Another influential leader in nursing education, Lavinia Dock (1858–1956) graduated from Bellevue Training School for Nurses in 1886. She worked at the Henry Street Settlement House in New York City, caring for the indigent. Dock wrote one of the first nursing textbooks, *Materia Medica for Nurses*. Also, she was the first editor of the *American Journal of Nursing* (*AJN*) and wrote many other books.

Isabel Hampton Robb

Isabel Hampton Robb (1860–1910) was the founder of the Superintendents' Society in 1893 and the Nurses' Associated Alumnae of the United States and Canada in 1896 (Figure 3-2). She knew it was important for nurses to participate in professional organizations and to work for unity across the profession on important issues. She worked to establish both the American Nurses Association (ANA) and the National League of Nursing

Figure 3-2 *Isabel Hampton Robb (Photo courtesy of the American Nurses Association)*

Figure 3-3 *Nurses at the Henry Street Settlement in New York City (Photo courtesy of Visiting Nurses Service of New York)*

Education, the predecessor of the National League for Nursing (NLN). As an early supporter of the rights of nursing students, she urged that there be shorter working hours and stressed the role of the nursing student as a learner instead of an employee.

Lillian Wald

Lillian Wald (1867–1940) spent her life providing nursing care to poor people. She founded public health nursing with the establishment of the Henry Street Settlement Service in 1893 (Figure 3-3) in New York City (Silverstein, 1994). Wald was the first community health nurse, and also established a school of nursing. As a tireless reformer, she worked to:

• Improve housing conditions in tenement districts
• Establish education for the mentally challenged
• Pass more lenient immigration regulations
• Initiate change of child labor laws and founded the Children's Bureau of the U.S. Department of Labor

Mary Breckenridge

In 1925, Mary Breckenridge (1881-1965) introduced a decentralized system of delivering health care to rural America. This system for providing primary nursing care services in the Kentucky Appalachian Mountains, called the Frontier Nursing Service, lowered the childbirth mortality rate in Leslie County, Kentucky, from the highest in the nation to below the national average.

Mamie Hale

The Arkansas Health Department hired Mamie Hale in 1942 to upgrade the educational programs for midwives. A graduate of Tuskegee School of Nurse-Midwifery, she gained the support of public health nurses, granny midwives, and obstetricians. Through education, she decreased illiteracy and superstition among those functioning as midwives. Hale's efforts improved mortality rates for both infants and mothers (Bell, 1993).

PRACTICAL NURSING PIONEER SCHOOLS

Women who cared for others, but who had no formal education, often called themselves "practical nurses." Formal education for practical nursing began in the 1890s. The first schools were Ballard School, Thompson Practical Nursing School, and Household Nursing Association School of Attendant Nursing.

Ballard School

In 1892, the Ballard School, funded by Lucinda Ballard, was opened in New York City by the YWCA. It offered several courses for women, one of which was practical nursing. The 3-month course in simple nursing care focused on the care of infants, children, elders, and disabled persons in their own homes. The course included cooking, nutrition, basic science, and basic nursing procedures. When the YWCA was reorganized in 1949, the school closed.

Thompson Practical Nursing School

Thomas Thompson of Brattleboro, Vermont, left money in his will to help women who were making shirts for the army and were receiving only $1 per dozen. His executor, Richard Bradley, saw the need for nursing service and, in 1907, established a practical nursing school in Brattleboro. It is still operating today and is accredited by the NLN.

Household Nursing School

In 1918, a group of women in Boston were concerned about providing nursing care for people who were sick at home. After talking with Richard Bradley, they opened the Household Nursing Association School of Attendant Nursing. The name was later changed to Shepard-Gill School of Practical Nursing. It closed in 1984.

NURSING IN THE 20TH CENTURY

The beginning of the 20th century brought about changes that have greatly influenced contemporary nursing. Several landmark reports about medical and nursing education, early insurance plans, the establishment of visiting nurse associations and their use of protocols, and health care initiatives are discussed following.

Flexner Report

In 1910, Abraham Flexner, supported by a Carnegie grant, visited the 155 medical schools in the United States and Canada. The goal of the resulting Flexner report, which was based on his findings, was to impose accountability for medical education. Flexner's study resulted in the closure of inadequate medical schools, consolidation of schools with limited resources, creation of nonprofit status for remaining schools, and establishment of medical education in university settings that was based on standards and strong economic resources.

Seeing the value and impact of the Flexner report on medical education, Adelaide Nutting, together with colleagues from the Superintendents' Society, presented a proposal to the Carnegie Foundation in 1911 to study nursing education. That study was never done.

In 1906, Richard Olding Beard established a 3-year diploma school of nursing at the University of Minnesota under the College of Medicine.

Early Insurance Plans

At the turn of the 20th century, the concepts of third-party payments and prepaid health insurance were instituted. Third-party payment is the payment by someone other than the recipient of health care (usually an insurance company) for the health care services provided. Prepaid medical plans were started in lumber and mining camps of the Pacific Northwest, where employers contracted for medical services, for which they paid a monthly fee. As the first president of the

Figure 3-4 *A Baby Being Weighed by a Student Nurse and a Junior League Volunteer in 1929 (Photo courtesy of Touro Infirmary Archives, New Orleans, LA)*

National Organization for Public Health Nursing, Lillian Wald suggested that a national health insurance plan be established.

Visiting Nurses Associations

In 1901, Lillian Wald suggested that Metropolitan Life Insurance Company enter into an agreement with the Henry Street Settlement to provide visiting nursing services to its policyholders. One form of managed care began as Wald worked with Metropolitan to expand the services of the Henry Street Settlement to other cities.

Nurses providing care in the home had experienced greater autonomy of practice than did hospital-based nurses (Figure 3-4). This led to discord among physicians regarding the scope of medical practice versus the scope of nursing practice. Some physicians encouraged nurses to do whatever was necessary to care for the sick at home, whereas other physicians believed nurses were going to take over their practice.

In 1912, the Chicago Visiting Nurse Association developed a list of standing orders for nurses to follow when providing home care. When the nurse did not have specific orders from a physician these orders were to direct the nursing care of client. This established the groundwork for nursing protocols.

Blue Cross and Blue Shield

The main impetus for the growth of insurance plans was the Depression. The philosophy in the United States of health care for all further contributed to the growth of insurance plans. In 1920, American hospitals offered a prepaid hospital plan, which became the prototype for Blue Cross.

The American Hospital Association laid the groundwork for an insurance company to provide benefits to subscribers when hospitalized. This eventually became Blue Cross. The American Medical Association developed Blue Shield to provide subscribers reimbursement for medical services.

The federal government became involved in health care delivery in 1935 when the Social Security Act was passed. It provided for benefits for elderly persons, child welfare, and federal funding for training health care personnel, among other things. During World War II, the U.S. government extended the benefits of military personnel to include their dependents and health care for veterans.

Landmark Reports in Nursing Education

Several reports were issued concerning nursing education and practice during the first half of the 20th century. Three of these reports, the Goldmark, the Brown, and the Institute of Research and Service in Nursing Education, are discussed following.

Goldmark Report

In 1918, Adelaide Nutting approached the Rockefeller Foundation for support of nursing education reform. They provided funding, and, in 1919, the Committee for the Study of Nursing Education was established to investigate the training of public health nurses. A social worker, Josephine Goldmark, served as the secretary to the committee and developed the method of collecting data and the analysis for a small sampling of the 1,800 schools of nursing then in existence.

The Goldmark report, entitled *Nursing and Nursing Education in the United States*, was published in 1923. Goldmark identified that the major weakness of the hospital-based training programs was that the needs of the institution (service delivery) were put before the needs of the student (education). The apprenticeship form of education along with nursing tradition put the needs of the client before the learning needs of the student.

Limited resources, low admission standards, poorly trained instructors, lack of supervision, and failure to correlate clinical practice with theory were identified by the study as major inadequacies in nursing education. The report concluded that nursing education should take place in the university setting if nursing was to be on equal footing with other disciplines.

Brown Report

In 1948, the social anthropologist, Esther Lucille Brown, published *Nursing for the Future and Nursing Reconsidered: A Study for Change.* The Brown report, published 26 years after the Goldmark report, identified many of the same problems in hospital nursing education, including the fact that nursing students were still being used for service by the hospitals, resources were inadequate, and authoritarianism still prevailed.

Brown understood that the proper intellectual climate for educating professional nurses would be the university setting. Visionary nurse educators were securing libraries, laboratories, and clinical facilities as necessary learning resources. Nurse leaders were implementing professional endeavors such as research and publication.

Institute of Research and Service in Nursing Education Report

The 1950s addressed different aspects of nursing. Post World War II, a deficit in the supply of nurses coincided with an increased demand for nursing services. Hospitals were closed as a result of the nursing shortage. Other factors contributing to the scarce supply of nurses were the long hours combined with a heavy workload, low esteem of nursing as a profession, and low salaries.

The Institute of Research and Service in Nursing Education Report resulted in the establishment of practical nursing under Title III of the Health Amendment Act of 1955. There was a proliferation of practical nursing schools in the United States following this report.

Other Health Care Initiatives

In the 1960s, health care services were provided to the elderly and the indigent populations through the federal programs of Medicare and Medicaid.

The Nurse Training Act was passed in 1964, to provide federal funds to expand the enrollment in schools of nursing. Federal funds were made available to construct nursing schools and provide student loans and scholarships to nursing students.

The Health Maintenance Organization Act of 1973 provided an alternative to the private health insurance industry. **Health maintenance organizations** (HMOs) are prepaid health plans that provide primary health care services for a preset fee and focus on cost-effective treatment methods. **Primary health care** refers to the client's point of entry into the health care system and includes assessment, diagnosis, treatment, coordination of care, education, preventive services, and surveillance.

In 1977, the National Commission for Manpower Study resulted in amendments to Title XVIII of the Social Security Act, which provided payment for rural health clinic services. Anne Zimmerman, former President of the ANA, had the bill amended to substitute the term **primary care providers** (health care providers whom a client sees first for health care) for *physician extenders,* which allowed nurse practitioners to be paid directly for their services. This represented the first time that nurses could be directly reimbursed for care they rendered.

Costs and Quality Controls

During the 1970s, the rapid escalation of health care expenditures made the cost-control systems of various federal health programs inadequate. The 1982 Tax Equity Fiscal Responsibility Act (TEFRA) was passed in response to the $287 billion spent on health care in 1981. At the same time that the federal government was trying to control costs with TEFRA and prospective payment legislation, concern was also growing regarding the quality of health care.

Although business and industry embraced quality control systems in the 1940s and 1950s, the health care industry failed to see the need for such controls until the 1980s. The Joint Commission on Accreditation of Healthcare Organizations (JCAHO) in the late 1980s emphasized monitoring for quality of outcomes, rather than process. This changed the system from a static quality assurance system to a dynamic quality improvement program. The JCAHO (1996) views quality of care as an ongoing process that continuously looks for ways to improve the care provided.

Figure 3-5 *Nurses Making a Presentation Before a State Legislature (Photo courtesy of the New York State Nurses Association)*

CRITICAL THINKING

Learning from Experience

Think of some lessons you have learned from the past. Can you identify some life experiences that have taught you something? List two things you have learned from these experiences or situations.

Health Care Reform

With an ever-increasing number (over 60 million) of Americans being uninsured or underinsured, health care access and costs became a major focus of attention in the 1990s (Edelman & Mandle, 2002). Children are especially at risk for having their health care neglected, with one in five children in the United States being uninsured (Baker, 1994).

Nursing as a profession has made great strides in affecting federal and state health care legislation (Figure 3-5). Hospitals are moving away from the controlling, bureaucratic entities they once were and instead are more often being characterized by an environment of shared governance, where nurses have a voice in both clinical and administrative decision making. Nurses now serve as case managers and collaborate with physicians and other health care providers.

Advocates are working to obtain prescriptive privileges for all advanced practitioners.

NURSING EDUCATION

Educational programs that prepare graduates to take a licensing examination must be approved by a state board of nursing. These boards approve entry-level programs to ensure the safe practice of nursing by setting minimum educational requirements and guaranteeing that graduates of the program are eligible candidates to take a licensing examination. Candidates in the United States must pass the National Council Licensure

Examination (NCLEX®) before a state board of nursing will issue a license to practice nursing.

Types of Programs

There are two types of entry-level nursing programs available in the United States: licensed practical or vocational nurse (LPN or LVN) and registered nurse (RN). An entry-level educational program is one that prepares graduates to take a licensing examination. Graduates of licensed practical/vocational programs take the NCLEX® for practical nurses (NCLEX-PN®), and graduates of registered nurse programs take the NCLEX® for registered nurses (NCLEX-RN®).

Postgraduate programs prepare nurses to practice in various roles as advanced-practice registered nurses (APRNs). Statutory provisions for APRNs vary from state to state.

Licensed Practical/Vocational Nursing

Licensed practical nurses (LPNs) or licensed vocational nurses (LVNs, as they are called in Texas and California) work under the supervision of an RN or other licensed provider such as a physician or dentist. The LP/VN, like the RN, was first trained in hospitals. The Smith Hughes Act passed by Congress in 1917 gave impetus to the formation of vocational-school–based practical nursing programs. In 1998, there were 1,205 practical/vocational nursing programs in the United States producing 38,732 graduates (NLN, 2000b).

Programs are state approved and in some cases also have accreditation by the NLN. **Accreditation** is a process by which a voluntary, nongovernmental agency or organization appraises and grants accredited status to institutions and/or programs or services that meet predetermined structure, process, and outcome criteria. These educational programs are generally 1 year in length and provide both **didactic** (systematic presentation of information) and **clinical** (observing and caring for living clients) experience. The education is focused on basic nursing skills and direct client care. Although most clinical experience is in hospitals, long-term care facilities, physicians' offices, home health agencies, and ambulatory care facilities are also used.

Admission generally requires a high school diploma or General Education Development (GED) certificate. Schools may require a preentrance examination that assesses such skills as math, reading, and writing.

Once licensed, the LP/VN is prepared to work in structured settings such as hospitals, long-term care, home health, medical offices, and ambulatory care facilities. Just as the RN has been delegated duties previously considered the domain of the physician, the LP/VN has been assigned duties once considered the domain of the RN. Many hospitals offer programs that provide levels of advancement for the LP/VN.

The National Federation of Licensed Practical Nurses, Inc. has written standards of nursing practice for the LP/VN. They are listed in Table 3-2.

Registered Nursing

Registered nurses are graduates of state-approved and, in many cases, NLN-accredited programs. They are

TABLE 3-2 NURSING PRACTICE STANDARDS FOR THE LICENSED PRACTICAL/VOCATIONAL NURSE

Education
The licensed practical/vocational nurse:

1. Shall complete a formal education program in practical nursing approved by the appropriate nursing authority in a state.
2. Shall successfully pass the National Council Licensure Examination for Practical Nurses.
3. Shall participate in initial orientation within the employing institution.

Legal/Ethical Status
The licensed practical/vocational nurse:

1. Shall hold a current license to practice nursing as an LP/VN in accordance with the law of the state wherein employed.
2. Shall know the scope of nursing practice authorized by the Nursing Practice Act in the state wherein employed.
3. Shall have a personal commitment to fulfill the legal responsibilities inherent in good nursing practice.
4. Shall take responsible actions in situations wherein there is unprofessional conduct by a peer or other health care provider.
5. Shall recognize and commit to meet the ethical and moral obligations of the practice of nursing.
6. Shall not accept or perform professional responsibilities that the individual knows (s)he is not competent to perform.

Practice
The licensed practical/vocational nurse:

1. Shall accept assigned responsibilities as an accountable member of the health care team.
2. Shall function within the limits of educational preparation and experience, as related to the assigned duties.
3. Shall function with other members of the health care team in promoting and maintaining health, preventing disease and disability, caring for and rehabilitating individuals who are experiencing an altered health state, and contributing to the ultimate quality of life until death.
4. Shall know and utilize the nursing process in planning, implementing, and evaluating health services and nursing care for the individual patient or group.
   a. Planning: The planning of nursing includes:
      1) Assessment of health status of the individual patient, the family, and community groups
      2) Analysis of the information gained from assessment
      3) Identification of health goals
   b. Implementation: The plan for nursing care is put into practice to achieve the stated goals and includes:
      1) Observing, recording, and reporting significant changes that require intervention or different goals

   2) Applying nursing knowledge and skills to promote and maintain health, to prevent disease and disability, and to optimize functional capabilities of an individual patient
   3) Assisting the patient and family with activities of daily living and encouraging self-care as appropriate
   4) Carrying out therapeutic regimens and protocols prescribed by an RN, physician, or other persons authorized by state law
   c. Evaluation: The plan for nursing care and its implementations are evaluated to measure the progress toward the stated goals and will include appropriate persons and/or groups to determine:
      1) The relevancy of current goals in relation to the progress of the individual patient
      2) The involvement of the recipients of care in the evaluation process
      3) The quality of the nursing action in the implementation of the plan
      4) A reordering of priorities or new goal setting in the care plan
5. Shall participate in peer review and other evaluation processes.
6. Shall participate in the development of policies concerning the health and nursing needs of society and in the roles and functions of the LP/VN.

Continuing Education
The licensed practical/vocational nurse:

1. Shall be responsible for maintaining the highest possible level of professional competence at all times.
2. Shall periodically reassess career goals and select continuing education activities that will help to achieve these goals.
3. Shall take advantage of continuing education opportunities that will lead to personal growth and professional development.
4. Shall seek and participate in continuing education activities that are approved for credit by appropriate organizations, such as the NFLPN.

Specialized Nursing Practice
The licensed practical/vocational nurse:

1. Shall have had at least one year's experience in nursing at the staff level.
2. Shall present personal qualifications that are indicative of potential abilities for practice in the chosen specialized nursing area.
3. Shall present evidence of completion of a program or course that is approved by an appropriate agency to provide the knowledge and skills necessary for effective nuirsng services in the specialized field.
4. Shall meet all of the standards of practice as set forth in this document.

(Reprinted with permission of the National Federation of Licensed Practical Nurses, Inc.)

prepared for entry into practice in one of three ways: associate degree nursing programs, hospital diploma programs, or baccalaureate degree nursing programs.

Associate Degree Program Associate degree programs are offered through community colleges and are

typically 2 years in length. They may also be offered as an option at 4-year–degree-granting universities. The graduate receives an Associate Degree in Nursing (ADN). In 1998, there were 899 associate degree programs producing 50,394 graduates (NLN, 2000b). This represents 59% of nurse graduates that year. Traditionally, program content reflects basic skill preparation and emphasizes clinical practice in the hospital setting. Because of a decreasing use of hospital beds, however, students are now likely to spend a higher number of clinical hours in community-based institutions (e.g., ambulatory settings, clinics, or schools).

Diploma Program Diploma nursing programs are offered by hospitals and are typically 3 years in length. Most are now affiliated with colleges or universities that grant college credit for select courses. Graduates of these programs receive a diploma from the hospital rather than a college degree.

Program content historically prepared the graduate in basic nursing skills particularly suitable for hospitalized clients. Now, however, most diploma schools also use community-based settings such as physicians' offices, visiting nurse services, clinics, and health departments for clinical experiences.

Although prominent in the early history of nursing education, the 93 diploma nursing programs still operating in 1998 produced 3,443 graduates (NLN, 2000b). This represents 4% of nursing graduates that year; however, 24% of RNs working in 1996 were initially educated in diploma programs (U.S. Department of Health and Human Services [USDHHS], 1996).

Baccalaureate Degree Program Baccalaureate degree programs are offered through colleges and universities and are typically 4 years in length. The graduate receives a Bachelor of Science in Nursing (BSN). These programs emphasize a broader preparation for practice, not only in hospital settings but also for autonomous and collaborative practice. In 1998, 549 baccalaureate programs produced 31,010 nursing graduates (NLN, 2000b). This represents 37% of the nursing graduates that year.

Continuing Education and Staff Development

Once a nurse is in practice, both continuing education and staff development are used to maintain the needed knowledge and skills for continuing practice.

Nurses are responsible for their own continuing education. Continuing education offers both personal and professional growth to the nurse and constitutes an essential dimension of lifelong learning. In some states, license renewal depends on acquiring continuing education units (CEUs) according to the board of nursing's rules. Lifelong learning is essential to career development and competency achievement in nursing practice.

Staff development generally occurs in the setting of employment and is described as the delivery of instruction to assist nurses to achieve the goals of the employer. It is guided by the accreditation standards of the JCAHO and ANA's *Standards for Nursing Staff Development* (ANA, 1990).

Orientation is an important organizational tool for both recruitment and retention. The sessions typically occur at the beginning of employment and whenever positions or roles change. The sessions include information unique to the institution of employment, such as philosophy, goals, policies and procedures, role expectations, facilities, resources and special services, and assessment and development of competency with equipment and supplies used in the work setting.

In-service education occurs after orientation and throughout employment. It supports the nurse in acquiring, maintaining, and increasing skills to fulfill assigned responsibilities.

Trends in Nursing Education

Trends in nursing education reflect issues in nursing, nursing education, delivery of care, and the public's health. At the heart of many of these trends are two fundamental issues: competency development and delivery of care.

Competency Development

The debate about multiple education levels for entry into nursing practice will continue. Demonstration of basic competency by all entry-level graduates regardless of education is likely to gain great support from nursing. It allows for not only consensus about the outcome (competency) but also diversity (innovation) about the process. Many changes in nursing education are being stimulated by competency development.

Delivery of Care

The demand for nursing care will continue to be driven by a larger aging population that uses long-term care and home health services. Other changes will include expansion of primary and preventive care to focus on health promotion and wellness; an increased use of ambulatory care services because they are less expensive; increased complexity of health care delivery, which requires well-educated nurses; and increased demand to provide health services such as prenatal care, well child clinics, adolescent clinics, and neighbor care clinics to underserved populations (such as inner-city residents).

Managed care arrangements are the delivery systems of the future. They emphasize wellness, health promotion, and disease prevention. More and more factors contributing to disease point to health behaviors as preventive interventions. The Healthy People 2010 goals, focus areas, and leading health indicators can be found on the Web at www.health.gov.

NURSING ORGANIZATIONS

Nursing organizations exist for LP/VNs and RNs. Some organizations also welcome as members those who are interested in nursing but who are not nurses. There are also many specialty nursing organizations.

All nurses should maintain membership in a nursing organization. The organizations represent the nurses to the public; to legislative bodies, both state and national; to federal agencies; and to all health care facilities. Through these organizations, nurses' concerns about workplace issues are addressed, high standards of practice are fostered, ethics codes are established, continuing education programs are certified and provided, and nurses' general welfare is protected. It is a professional obligation to be a participating member of a nursing organization. There is strength in unity. Table 3-3 provides pertinent information about selected nursing organizations.

National League for Nursing

The original organization, established in 1893, was named The American Society of Superintendents of Training Schools for Nurses. The last name change,

National League for Nursing, was made in 1952. Because of the growth of practical/vocational nursing programs, the NLN established a Department of Practical Nursing Programs (now called Council of Practical Nursing Programs, [CPNP]) in 1961. The NLN offers accreditation services to all nursing programs through an independent subsidiary called the National League for Nursing Accrediting Commission (NLNAC) (National League for Nursing, 2002a).

TABLE 3–3   SELECTED NURSING ORGANIZATIONS

ORGANIZATION	DESCRIPTION
National League for Nursing (NLN)	Established: 1893 as The American Society of Superintendents of Training Schools for Nurses. 1952 name changed to National League for Nursing. Purpose: To advance quality nursing education that prepares the nursing workforce to meet the needs of diverse populations in an ever-changing health care environment Activities: • Accredit (through voluntary participation from schools) nursing education programs • Conduct surveys to collect data on education programs • Provide continuing-education programs • Offer testing services, including: Achievement tests for use in nursing schools Preadmission testing for potential nursing students Membership: • Open to any individual (nurse or nonnurse) or agency interested in improving nursing services or nursing education Publication: • *Nursing Education Perspectives*
National Association for Practical Nurse Education and Service, Inc. (NAPNES)	Established: 1941 Purpose: To improve the quality, education, and recognition of nursing schools and LP/VNs in the United States Activities: • Provide workshops, seminars, and continuing-education programs • Evaluate and certify continuing-education programs of others • Provide individual student professional liability insurance program • Inform legislatures and public on LP/VN issues • Authorize those who pass the Certification Examination for Practical and Vocational Nurses in Long-term Care (CEPN-LTC)™ to use the initials *CLTC* Membership: • LP/VNs • RNs, physicians, and caregivers in all fields • Practical/vocational nursing students Publications: • *Journal of Practical Nursing* • *NAPNES Forum*
National Federation of Licensed Practical Nurses, Inc. (NFLPN)	Established: 1949 Purpose: • Provide leadership for LP/VNs • Foster high standards of practical/vocational nursing education and practice • Encourage continuing education • Achieve recognition for LP/VNs • Advocate effective utilization of LP/VNs • Interpret role and function of LP/VNs

continues

TABLE 3–3 continued

ORGANIZATION	DESCRIPTION
National Federation of Licensed Practical Nurses, Inc. (NFLPN) *(continued)*	• Represent practical/vocational nursing • Serve as central source of information on practical/vocational nursing education and practice Activities: • Promote continuing education of LP/VNs; evaluate programs for CEU credit • Offer IV and gerontology certification • Establish principles of ethics • Offer members an opportunity to participate in activities of the organization • Keep members informed on matters of interest and concern • Offer members best type of low-cost insurance • Represent and speak for LP/VNs in Congress • Encourage fellowship among LP/VNs • Develop mutual understanding and good will among members, other allied health groups, and the general public Membership: • Three-tier concept of local, state, and national enrollment • LP/VNs • Practical/vocational nursing students • Affiliate (person who has an interest in the work of NFLPN but is neither an LP/VN nor an LP/VN student) Publication: • *Practical Nursing Journal*
American Nurses Association (ANA)	Established: 1911 Purpose: To work for the improvement of health standards and availability of health care service for all people, foster high standards for nursing, stimulate and promote the professional development of nurses, and advance their economic and general welfare. Activities: • Establish standards for nursing practice • Establish a professional code of ethics • Develop educational standards • Promote nursing research • Oversee a credentialing system • Influence legislation affecting health care • Protect the economic and general welfare of registered nurses • Assist with the professional development of nurses (i.e., by providing continuing education programs) Membership: • Registered nurses only • Federation of state nurses' associations • Individual, by joining respective state nurses' association Publications: • *American Journal of Nursing (AJN)* • *American Nurse*
National Council of State Boards of Nursing, Inc. (NCSBN)	Established: 1978 Purpose: Provide an organization through which boards of nursing act and counsel together on matters of common interest and concern affecting the public health, safety, and welfare, including the development of licensing examinations in nursing Activities: • Develop and administer licensure examinations for registered nurse and licensed practical/vocational nurse candidates • Conduct job analyses that provide data required to support the NCLEX® examinations and the test development process *continues*

TABLE 3–3 continued

ORGANIZATION	DESCRIPTION
National Council of State Boards of Nursing, Inc. (NCSBN) *(continued)*	• Maintain a national disciplinary data bank • Monitor and analyze issues and trends in public policy, nursing practice, and nursing education that impact nursing regulation • Serve as the national clearinghouse of information on nursing regulation • Offer educational conferences and regional meetings Membership: • Boards of nursing in the 50 states, the District of Columbia, and five United States territories • No individual membership Publications: • *Issues* • *NCLEX-PN® Program Reports* • *NCLEX-RN® Program Reports*

Data from *About ANA* (Online), by American Nurses Association, 2002b, Available: www.ana.org/about/summary/99hodact.htm; *History of NAPNES,* by National Association for Practical Nurse Education and Service, Inc., 1998, Silver Spring, MD: Author; *All About NFLPN* (Online), by National Federation of Licensed Practical Nurses, 2000, Available: www.nflpn.org/allaboutnflpn.htm; *Bylaws,* by National League for Nursing, 1995, New York: Author; *About NLN* (Online), by National League for Nursing, 2000a, Available: www.nln.org/info-default.htm; *About the National Council* (Online), by National Council of State Boards of Nursing, Inc., 1999, Available: www.ncsbn.org/files/aboutnc

National Association of Practical Nurse Education and Service, Inc.

Originally called the Association of Practical Nurse Schools, this organization was dedicated exclusively to practical nursing. The multidisciplinary membership planned the first standard curriculum for practical nursing. The name was changed to the National Association of Practical Nurse Education (NAPNE) in 1942. In 1945, they established an accrediting service for practical/vocational nursing schools. This service has been discontinued for some years. In 1959, the name was changed to the National Association of Practical Nurse Education and Service (NAPNES, 1998).

PROFESSIONAL TIP

Professional Memberships
Every nurse should become involved in a nursing organization. Membership means more political clout for passing legislation to improve health care for all citizens and to improve the profession of nursing.

Nursing students must stay abreast of current issues and meet with local nursing leaders to discuss health care reform, alternative health care delivery models, and other issues. Then as graduates, they will be able to share this information with both the public and legislators.

National Federation of Licensed Practical Nurses, Inc.

The National Federation of Licensed Practical Nurses (NFLPN) was founded in 1949 by a group of LPNs who recognized that to gain status and recognition in the health field and to have a channel through which they could officially speak and act for themselves, they needed an organization of their own. Since 1991, affiliate membership (lacking the rights to vote and hold office) has been available to anyone who is interested in the work of NFLPN but who is neither a practicing LP/VN nor an LP/VN student. The NFLPN is the official organization for LP/VNs (NFLPN, 2002).

American Nurses Association

The ANA represents registered nurses through its constituent state organizations. The ANA fosters high standards of nursing practice, promotes the economic and general welfare of nurses in the workplace, projects a positive and realistic view of nursing, and lobbies Congress and regulatory agencies on health care issues affecting nurses and the public (ANA, 2002b).

National Council of State Boards of Nursing

The National Council of State Boards of Nursing (NCSBN) was established in 1978 to assist member boards, collectively and individually, to promote safe and effective nursing practice in the interest of protecting public health and welfare. They have developed the NCLEX-PN® and NCLEX-RN® to test the entry-level nursing competence of candidates for licensure as

LP/VNs and RNs (National Council of State Boards of Nursing, 1999).

In 1996, they began administration of the first large-scale, national certification examination available to LP/VNs. It is named the Certification Examination for Practical and Vocational Nurses in Long-Term Care (CEPN-LTC™). Those who pass the examination are certified in long-term care and are authorized by NAPNES to use the initials *CLTC* to signify their new status (National Council of State Boards of Nursing, 1996).

Summary

- Nursing is the art and science of assisting people in learning to care for themselves whenever possible and of caring for them when they are unable to meet their own needs.
- By studying nursing history, the nurse is better able to understand such issues as autonomy, unity within the profession, supply and demand, salary, education, and current practice, and can thus promote the empowerment of nurses.
- Nursing's early history was heavily influenced by religious organizations and the need for nurses to care for soldiers during wartime.
- Florence Nightingale forged the future of nursing practice and education as a result of her experiences in training nurses to care for soldiers.
- Early American leaders, the professional organizations, and the landmark reports of nursing determined the infrastructure of current nursing practice.
- Influential nursing leaders such as Lillian Wald, Isabel Hampton Robb, Adelaide Nutting, and Lavinia Dock were instrumental in the advancement of nursing education and practice.
- Other nursing leaders such as Mary Breckenridge, Mary Mahoney, and Linda Richards made important contributions to both nursing education and practice.
- In 1923, the Goldmark Report concluded that for nursing to be on equal footing with other disciplines, nursing education should occur in the university setting.
- The Brown Report (1948) addressed the need for nurses to demonstrate greater professional competence by moving nursing education to the university setting.
- The Health Maintenance Organization Act of 1973 provided an alternative to the private health insurance industry.
- Title III of the Health Amendment Act of 1955 resulted in the establishment of practical nursing.
- Types of programs that currently prepare nurses for entry level practice are practical/vocational, diploma, associate degree, and baccalaureate degree.

Review Questions

1. The founder of modern nursing is considered to be:
   a. Lillian Wald.
   b. Dorothea Dix.
   c. Florence Nightingale.
   d. The Nursing Sisters of the Holy Cross.

2. The first practical nursing school was:
   a. Ballard School.
   b. Thompson Practical Nursing School.
   c. Bellevue Training School for Nurses.
   d. Household Nursing Association School of Attendant Nursing.

3. Practical nursing was established under:
   a. Bureau of Medical Services, 1908.
   b. Health Maintenance Organization Act of 1973.
   c. Title III of the Health Amendment Act of 1955.
   d. Nursing and Nursing Education in the United States, 1923.

4. The nursing organization that accredits schools of nursing is:
   a. ANA.
   b. NLN.
   c. NFLPN.
   d. NAPNES.

5. The National Council of State Boards of Nursing began administering a national certification examination available to the LP/VN. It is for:
   a. licensure.
   b. acute care.
   c. accreditation.
   d. long-term care.

References/Suggested Readings

American Nurses Association. (1990). *Standards for nursing staff development.* Kansas City, MO: Author.

American Nurses Association. (1991). *American Nurses Association bylaws.* Washington, DC: Author.

American Nurses Association. (2002a). *Mission statement* [Online]. Available: www.nursingworld.org/about/mission.htm

American Nurses Association. (2002b). *About ANA* [Online]. Available: www.ana.org/about/summary/99hodact.htm

Anglin, L. T. (2000). Historical perspectives: Influences of the past. In J. Zerwekh (Ed.), *Nursing today: Transitions and trends* (3rd ed.). Philadelphia: W. B. Saunders.

Baker, C. M. (1994). School health: Policy issues. *Nursing & Health Care, 15*(4), 178–184.

Bell, P. (1993). "Making do" with the midwife: Arkansas' Mamie O. Hale in the 1940s. *Nursing History Review*, 155–169.

Calhoun, J. (1993, March). The Nightingale pledge: A commitment that survives the passage of time. *Nursing & Health Care*, 14(3), 130–136.

Cushing, A. (1995, Summer). A historical note on the relationship between nursing and nursing history. *International History Nursing Journal*, 1(1), 57–60.

Dossey, B. (1995). Endnote: Florence Nightingale today. *Critical Care Nursing*, 15(4), 98.

Edelman, C. L., & Mandle, C. L. (2002). *Health promotion throughout the lifespan* (5th ed.). St. Louis, MO: Mosby.

Estabrooks, C. A. (1995). Lavinia Lloyd Dock: The Henry Street years. *Nursing History Review*, 3, 143–172.

Guide to Nursing Organizations. (2000). *Nursing2000*, 30(5), 54–56.

Humphreys, K. (2002). Guide to 2002 nursing organizations. *Nursing 2002*, 32(5), 46–48.

Joint Commission on the Accreditation of Healthcare Organizations. (1996). *Accreditation standards and scoring guidelines for hospital-based mental health*. Oak Brook Terrace, IL: Author.

Macrae, J. (1995). Nightingale's spiritual philosophy and its significance for modern nursing. *Image: Journal of Nursing Scholarship*, 27(1), 8–10.

Mason, D. J., & Leavitt, J. K. (1995). The revolution in health care: What's your readiness quotient? *AJN*, 95(6), 50–54.

Mohr W. (2003). *Johnson's psychiatric–mental health nursing: Adaptation and growth* (5th ed.). Philadelphia: Lippincott Williams & Wilkins.

National Association for Practical Nurse Education and Service, Inc. (1998). *History of NAPNES*. Silver Spring, MD: Author.

National Council of State Boards of Nursing, Inc. (1996). *Creating new national certification examination for LPN/VNs* [Online]. Available: www.ncsbn.org/files/publications/annual reports/ar1996/creatnc.asp

National Council of State Boards of Nursing Inc. (2001). *About the National Council* [Online]. Available: www.ncsbn.org/

National Federation of Licensed Practical Nurses. (2002). *All about NFLPN* [Online]. Available: www.nflpn.org/allabout-nflpn.htm

National League for Nursing. (1995). *Bylaws*. New York: Author.

National League for Nursing. (1998). Research Department Communication. New York: Author.

National League for Nursing. (2002a). *About NLN* [Online]. Available: www.nln.org/aboutnln/info-history/htm

National League for Nursing. (2000b). *Unofficial, unpublished data from 1998*. Research Department Communication. August 15, 2000.

Nightingale, F. (1969). *Notes on nursing: What it is and what it is not*. New York: Dover.

Ogren, K. (1994). The risk of not understanding nursing history. *Holistic Nursing Practice*, 8(2), 10.

Secretary's Commission on Nursing. (1988). *Final report*. Washington, DC: Department of Health & Human Services.

Selanders, L. C. (1994). *Florence Nightingale: An environmental adaptation theory*. Newberry Park, CA: Sage.

Silverstein, N. G. (1994). Lillian Wald at Henry Street, 1893–1895. In P. L. Chinn (Ed.), *Developing the discipline: Critical studies in nursing history and professional issues*. Gaithersburg, MD: Aspen.

U.S. Department of Health and Human Services. (1996). *The registered nurse population*. Washington, DC: Author.

U.S. Department of Health & Human Services. (2001). *Healthy People 2010*. [Online]. Available: www.health.gov/healthypeople/About/hpfact.htm

Wall, B. (1993). Grace under pressure: The nursing sisters of the Holy Cross, 1861–1865. *Nursing History Review*, 71–88.

Wolf, P. (2003). Guide to nursing organizations. *Nursing 2003*, 33(5), 50-52.

Resources

American Nurses Association (ANA), 600 Maryland Avenue SW, Suite 100 West, Washington, DC 20024-2571, 202-651-7000, 800-274-4ANA (262), www.ana.org

National Association of Practical Nurse Education and Service, Inc. (NAPNES), 8607 2nd Avenue #404A, Silver Spring, MD 20910, 301-588-2491 www.napnes.org

National Council of State Boards of Nursing, Inc. (NCSBN), 676 North St. Clair Street, Suite 550, Chicago, IL 60611-2921, 312-787-6555, www.ncsbn.org

National Federation of Licensed Practical Nurses, Inc. (NFLPN), 893 U.S. Highway 70 West, Suite 202, Garner, NC 27529, 800-948-2511, www.nflpn.org

National League for Nursing (NLN), 61 Broadway, 33rd Floor, New York, NY 10006, 212-363-5555, 800-669-1656, www.nln.org

LEGAL AND ETHICAL RESPONSIBILITIES

MAKING THE CONNECTION

Refer to the following chapters to increase your understanding of legal and ethical responsibilities:

Basic Nursing
- **Student Nurse Skills for Success**
- **Nursing Process/Documentation**

- **Cultural Considerations**
- **Loss, Grief, and Death**

LEARNING OBJECTIVES

Upon completion of this chapter, you should be able to:
- **Define key terms.**
- **Describe the difference between public law and civil law.**
- **State the purpose and identify various sources of standards of practice.**
- **Discuss the difference between intentional and unintentional torts.**
- **Discuss ways that informed consent impacts nursing practice.**
- **Discuss the concept of advance directives.**
- **Describe the purpose and correct utilization of an incident report.**
- **Discuss ways the nurse can reduce personal liability.**
- **Identify the benefits of having one's own malpractice insurance policy.**
- **List steps to be taken when suspecting a colleague of being impaired by drugs or alcohol.**
- **Describe the major ethical principles that have an impact on health care.**
- **Explain the link between ethics and values and the process involved in reconciling the potential conflicts between them.**
- **Relate the ethical code developed by the National Federation of Licensed Practical Nurses daily nursing practice.**
- **Identify the rights of the client as established by the American Hospital Association.**
- **Discuss the roles of the nurse as client advocate and whistleblower in the delivery of ethical nursing care.**

KEY TERMS

active euthanasia
administrative law
advance directive
assault
assisted suicide
autonomy
battery
beneficence
bioethics
civil law
client advocate
confidential
constitutional law
contract law
criminal law
defamation
deontology
durable power of attorney for health care
ethical dilemma
ethical principle
ethical reasoning
ethics
euthanasia
expressed contract
false imprisonment
felony
fidelity
formal contract
fraud
Good Samaritan law
impaired nurse

implied contract
incident report
informed consent
justice
law
liability
libel
living will
malpractice
material principle of justice
misdemeanor
negligence
nonmaleficence
nursing practice act
passive euthanasia
peer assistance programs
privacy
public law
restraint
slander
standards of practice
statutory law
teleology
tort
tort law
utility
value system
values
values clarification
veracity
whistleblowing

INTRODUCTION

Nursing, which embodies a concern for the client in every aspect of life, encompasses a great responsibility—one that requires knowledge, skill, care, and commitment. As society and technology change, the issues affecting nursing practice also change. We continue to recognize the importance of the right to decide what is best for one's self, informed consent, and belief in the client's bill of rights; however, difficult issues, such as advance directives, do-not-resuscitate (DNR) orders, and impaired nurses, now must be faced by the nursing profession. The delivery of ethical health care is becoming an increasingly difficult and confusing issue in contemporary society. Nurses are committed to respecting their clients' rights in terms of providing health care and treatment. This desire to maintain clients' rights, however, often conflicts with professional duties and institutional policies. Nurses must thus learn to balance these potentially conflicting perspectives to achieve the primary objective—the care of the client. This chapter provides a general overview of many legal and ethical concepts that affect nursing.

BASIC LEGAL CONCEPTS

Because it is useful to have working definitions of some basic legal concepts before applying them to a health care setting, a discussion of pertinent legal concepts follows.

Definition of Law

Laws are decisions about conduct that guide the interactions of people. Laws are necessary, binding, and enforceable so people can live and work together. When laws are broken, a penalty is incurred.

The word **law** is derived from an Anglo-Saxon term meaning "that which is laid down or fixed." The two types of law are **public law,** which deals with the individual's relationship to the state, and **civil law,** which deals with relationships among individuals.

Sources of Law

The four sources of public law at the federal and state levels are constitutional, statutory, administrative, and criminal. At the federal and state levels, the three sources of civil law are contracts, torts, and protective/reporting laws.

Public Law

Constitutional law, set forth in the U.S. and state constitutions, defines and limits the powers of government. **Statutory law** is enacted by legislative bodies. State boards and professional practice acts, such as nursing practice acts, are created and governed under statutory laws.

Administrative law (regulatory law) is developed by those persons appointed to governmental administrative agencies. These persons are entrusted with enforcing the statutory laws passed by the legislature. Administrative law gives state boards of nursing the power to make rules and regulations governing nursing as set forth in the nursing practice acts. In these administrative rules, nursing boards delineate the specific processes for educational programs; licensure; grounds for disciplinary proceedings; and the establishment of fees for services and for penalties rendered by the board.

Criminal law, the most common example of public law, addresses acts or offenses against the safety or welfare of the public. Under criminal law, there are two types of crime: **felony** (a crime of a serious nature that is usually punishable by imprisonment at a state penitentiary or by death, or a crime violating a federal statute that involves punishment of more than 1 year incarceration) and **misdemeanor** (offense less serious than a felony that may be punishable by a fine or a sentence to a local prison for less than 1 year). Table 4-1 outlines the types of public law.

Civil Law

Civil law addresses crimes against a person(s) in matters such as contracts, torts, and protective/reporting law (Table 4-2). Most cases of malpractice fall under the civil law of torts (Flight, 2004).

TABLE 4-1 TYPES OF PUBLIC LAW

TYPE	FEDERAL EXAMPLES	STATE EXAMPLES
Constitutional law	U.S. Constitution Civil Rights Act	State Constitutions
Statutory law	None	Various state boards and professional practice acts
Administrative law	Social Security Act National Labor Relations Act	Rules and regulations of various state boards
Criminal law	Controlled Substance Act Homicides	Criminal codes (defining manslaughter, murder criminal negligence, rape, illegal possession of drugs, fraud, theft, assault, and battery)

TABLE 4-2 TYPES OF CIVIL LAW

TYPE	FEDERAL EXAMPLES	STATE EXAMPLES
Contract law	None	Business contracts with clients Employment contracts
Torts	Federal Torts Claims Act	State Torts Claims Act (allows claims against the state) Assault Battery Defamation (libel and slander) Fraud False imprisonment Invasion of privacy Negligence (common law claim) Malpractice statutes (professional liability)
Protective/reporting laws	Child Abuse Prevention and Treatment Act Privacy Act of 1974	Good Samaritan Law Abuse statutes (domestic violence, child, elderly) Age of consent statutes (medical treatment, drugs, sexually transmitted disease) Americans with Disabilities Act Living will legislation Involuntary Hospitalization Act Abortion statute

Contract law is the enforcement of agreements among private individuals. The three essential elements in a legal contract are:

- Promise(s) between two or more legally competent individuals that state what each individual must do or not do
- Mutual understanding of the terms and obligations the contract imposes on each individual
- Compensation for lawful actions performed

Contract terms may be agreed on in writing or orally; however, a **formal** (written) **contract** cannot be changed legally by an oral agreement. An **expressed contract** gives, in writing, the conditions and terms of the contract. An **implied contract** acknowledges a relationship between parties for services.

In accord with U.S. Contract Law, the nurse is legally required to:

- Follow the employer's policies and standards unless they conflict with state or federal law.
- Complete the terms of contracted service with the employer.
- Respect the rights and responsibilities of other health care providers, especially to promote continuity of client care.

Along with these legal responsibilities, the nurse has a right to expect:

- Adequate and qualified assistance in providing care
- Reasonable and prudent conduct from the client
- Compensation from the employer for services rendered
- A safe work environment with the necessary resources to render services

- Prudent, reasonable conduct from other health care providers

A **tort** is a civil wrong committed by a person against another person or property (Zerwekh & Claborn, 2003). **Tort law** is the enforcement of duties and rights among individuals independent of contractual agreements.

The protective/reporting law may be considered criminal law, depending on classification by the state. Two examples of protective law are The Americans with Disabilities Act (ADA) and the Good Samaritan Laws.

The ADA was passed by the U.S. Congress in 1990. It prohibits discrimination in employment, public services, and public accommodations on the basis of disability. The ADA defines a disability as a physical or mental impairment that substantially limits one or more of the major life activities.

All 50 states and the District of Columbia have enacted **Good Samaritan** laws, which protect health care providers by ensuring immunity from civil **liability** (obligation one has incurred or might incur through any

PROFESSIONAL TIP

Good Samaritan Laws

Good Samaritan laws vary in coverage from state to state and may be amended periodically by legislation. It is the responsibility of caregivers to know the law for their respective jurisdictions (Brown, 1999).

act or failure to act) when care is provided at the scene of an emergency and the caregiver does not intentionally or recklessly cause the client injury (Brown, 1999).

The Good Samaritan law applies only in emergency situations, usually those outside the hospital setting. It stipulates that the health care worker must not be acting for an employer or receive compensation for care given. There is also a federal Good Samaritan law that protects health care providers who voluntarily give care to a person in distress during an airplane flight (Brown, 1999).

In most states, health care professionals are not required to stop at the scene of accidents. If they do stop, however, they are held to higher standards than is a layperson. Health care professionals are expected to use their specialized body of knowledge when providing care. They are expected to act as would most other professionals with the same background and education.

THE LAW AND NURSING PRACTICE

Nursing practice falls under both public law and civil law. In all states, nurses are bound by rules and regulations stipulated by the **nursing practice act** as determined by the legislature.

Public laws are designed to protect the public. When these laws are broken, a nurse can be punished by paying a fine, losing her license, or being incarcerated. For example, a nurse guilty of diverting drugs, which is a crime against the state, could lose her license to practice and could be sent to jail.

Civil laws deal with problems occurring between a nurse and a client. For example, if a nurse catheterizing a client perforates the bladder the client has sustained injury. No law affecting the population as a whole has been broken, but the client may bring a civil suit against the nurse. The client may receive compensation for injuries, but the nurse receives no jail time.

Multistate nursing practice has become a pressing issue with telehealth, transporting of clients across state lines, and employment by staffing companies operating in several states (Ventura, 1999b). The NCSBN, in 1997, endorsed a model of nursing regulations for RNs and LP/VNs now called the Nurse Licensure Compact that allows nurses licensed in one of the compact states to practice in any of the compact states. Nurses are licensed in their state of residence. When necessary, disciplinary action may be taken by any of the compact states against a nurse, even when licensed by another compact state. The 15 states that have passed the legislation and have implemented this compact are Arizona, Arkansas, Delaware, Idaho, Iowa, Maine, Maryland, Mississippi, Nebraska, North Carolina, North Dakota, South Dakota, Texas, Utah, and Wisconsin. Three states—Indiana,

New Jersey, and Tennessee—are writing their rules for implementation (NCSBN, 2002).

Standards of Practice

State boards of nursing have the responsibility of regulating nursing practice and setting educational guidelines for the programs. They stipulate who may practice nursing in their respective states through licensure. The related criteria usually involve graduating from a state-approved program, passing the National Council Licensure Exam (NCLEX)®, and meeting certain legal and moral standards. The boards have authority to bring disciplinary action against a nurse for violation of its rules and regulations. Disciplinary action may include revocation or suspension of the nurse's license and/or a fine.

From the nursing practice acts, guidelines have been developed to direct nursing care. These guidelines are called **standards of practice** or standards of care.

Standards of practice are also derived from other sources. Professional organizations such as the American Nurses Association (ANA) for the registered nurse (RN) and the National Federation of Licensed Practical Nurses (NFLPN) for the LP/VN have also developed standards of practice. Nursing care planning books especially for specialized areas, are other resources for practice standards.

Policy and procedure manuals also represent standards of practice. Each facility has identified specific ways of performing procedures such as collecting specimens, passing medications, and inserting catheters. Nurses employed by the facility are expected to follow the guidelines in the policy and procedure manuals. For situations not covered in the policy and procedure manuals, the nurse is expected to exercise good judgment. In other words, the nurse is expected to act in a reasonable and prudent manner.

What is meant by reasonable and prudent? In nursing, it means that the nurse is expected to act as would other nurses at the same professional level and with the same amount of education or experience. If most nurses respond to a particular situation in a certain way, and the nurse in question does too, the nurse is acting in a reasonable and prudent manner; however, if most nurses respond differently than the nurse in question, the nurse is not be behaving in a reasonable and prudent manner and can be held responsible or liable for damages. Liability is determined by whether the standards of practice were adhered to.

Legal Issues in Practice

Many aspects relating to nursing practice and areas of nursing are subject to liability, including physician's orders, floating, inadequate staffing, critical care, and pediatric care.

Physician's Orders

The physician is in charge of directing the client's care, and nurses are to carry out the physician's orders for care, unless the nurse believes that the orders are in error or would be harmful to the client. In this case, the physician must be contacted to confirm and/or clarify the orders. If the nurse still believes the orders to be inappropriate, the nursing supervisor should be immedi-

---

PROFESSIONAL TIP

Nursing Practice Act

Nursing practice acts state those things that the nurse can and cannot do.

ately contacted and why the orders are not being carried out put in writing. A nurse who carries out an erroneous or inappropriate order may be held liable for harm experienced by the client. *Nurses are responsible for their actions regardless of who told them to perform those actions.*

Floating

Nurses sometimes are asked to "float" to an unfamiliar nursing unit. The supervisor should be informed about a float nurse's lack of experience in caring for the type of clients on the new nursing unit. The nurse should be given an orientation to the new unit and will be held to the same standards of care as are the nurses who regularly work on that unit.

Inadequate Staffing

The Joint Commission on Accreditation of Healthcare Organizations (JCAHO) has established guidelines for determining the number of staff needed for any given situation (staffing ratios) (JCAHO, 2002). When there are not enough nurses to meet the staffing ratio and provide competent care, substandard care may result, placing clients at physical risk and the nurse and institution at legal risk. The nurse in this situation should provide nursing administration with a written account of the situation. *A nurse who leaves an inadequately staffed unit could be charged with client abandonment.*

Critical Care

Because the monitors used in critical care units are not infallible, constant observation and assessment of clients are required. This makes a 1:1 or a 1:2 nurse–client ratio imperative. Furthermore, equipment must be checked regularly and on a schedule by the biomedical department.

Pediatric Care

Legislation in each state requires that suspected child abuse or neglect be reported. Legal immunity is provided to the person who makes a report in good faith. When suspected child abuse or neglect is not reported by health care providers, legal action, civil or criminal, may be filed against them.

NURSE–CLIENT RELATIONSHIP

Situations can develop between a nurse and a client that may require legal intervention. The types of torts that may arise are discussed following.

Torts

When a case is brought against a nurse, it is usually a civil action that falls under tort law. Torts can be intentional or unintentional (Table 4-3). The person who commits an intentional tort violates the civil rights of another

TABLE 4-3 SELECTED TORTS: DEFINITIONS AND EXAMPLES

TYPE OF TORT	DEFINITION	EXAMPLE
Intentional		
Assault	Threaten or attempt to touch another person.	Tells client he will be tied in bed if he tries to get out.
Battery	Unconsented touching.	A treatment is performed against the client's will.
False imprisonment	Unwarranted restriction of the freedom of an individual.	A client who is of sound mind and is not in danger of inflicting injury on self or another is restrained.
Quasi-intentional		
Invasion of privacy	All individuals have the right to privacy and may bring charges against any person who violates this right.	Information is disclosed about a client that is considered private or photographs taken without client consent
Defamation (libel and slender)	Verbal (slander) or written (libel) remarks that may cause the loss of an individual's reputation.	A statement is made that could either ruin the client's reputation or cause the client to lose his or her job.
Unintentional		
Negligence	Failure to use such care as a reasonably prudent person would use under similar circumstances, which leads to harm.	Client's property is lost. A medication error occurs. A client is burned from the improper use of equipment. A change in the client's condition is not observed and/or reported. Inaccurate count of sponges in the operating room is taken.
Malpractice	Failure of a professional to use such care as a reasonably prudent member of the profession would use under similar circumstances, which leads to harm.	An inaccurate nursing diagnosis is made and the wrong treatment is imlemented. Physician's orders are not followed. Physician's clearly erroneous order is not questioned.

individual knowingly and willfully. Examples of intentional torts are assault and battery, defamation (libel and slander), fraud, false imprisonment, and invasion of privacy. Unintentional torts are those actions that cause harm to the client resulting from carelessness or negligence by the nurse. If found liable, the nurse generally must pay monetary damages. Prison terms are rare.

Intentional Torts

Assault and battery, defamation, fraud, false imprisonment, and invasion of privacy are types of intentional torts.

Assault and Battery Assault and battery are in fact two separate terms. **Assault** is the threat to do something that may cause harm or be unpleasant to another person. **Battery** is the unauthorized or unwanted touching of one person by another.

The key elements in assault are fear and intimidation. The person assaulted must believe that the threat can and will be carried out; for example, a client confined to a wheelchair is told, "If you do not finish your meal, you are going to sit there all night." The client complies because he believes the health care worker will leave him to sit there. The client knows the worker is in a position to carry out this threat.

Consent is the key factor in battery. People have the right to be free of unwanted handling of their person. Striking a client, performing a procedure without the client's consent, and forcing a person to take medication he does not want are all battery. Any unwanted touching can be construed as battery.

Defamation Defamation is using words to harm or injure the personal or professional reputation of another person. If the words are written down, they constitute **libel.** If the information is communicated verbally to a third party, it constitutes **slander.**

Negative or derogatory comments that are untrue leave the nurse no defense against charges of defamation. If comments are true, the relevance of the information is important. The most common examples of this tort are giving out inaccurate or inappropriate information from the medical record; discussing clients, families, or visitors in public areas; or speaking negatively about coworkers (Zerwekh & Claborn, 2003).

Fraud Fraud is a wrong that results from a deliberate deception intended to produce unlawful gain. Common forms of fraud in health care include deceit in obtaining or attempting to obtain a nursing license (Flight, 1998) and illegal billing.

False Imprisonment False imprisonment refers to making the client wrongfully believe that she cannot leave a place. Any means used to confine a client or to restrict movement can be considered a restraint and a form of false imprisonment. This includes threats, physical restraints such as wrist or vest restraints, locked doors, side rails, geriatric chairs, and psychotropic drugs. A common example of this tort is telling a client not to leave the hospital until the bill is paid (Zerwekh & Claborn, 2003).

A dilemma arises when a client decides to leave the health care facility and no discharge order has been written. If the health care problem has not been resolved, the nurse may feel that it is not in the best interest of the client to leave. A client of sound mind has the right to make this decision, regardless of what others think is best. Detaining the individual could bring charges of false imprisonment.

Documentation is very important in these situations, including the client's reasons for leaving the facility and any teaching or interventions related to the situation. Facility policy usually requires that the client sign a form indicating that he is leaving against medical advice (AMA), which releases the facility of any liability. If the client refuses to sign the AMA form, the client's refusal should be documented, and the nursing supervisor and the client's physician should be notified.

Any device used to restrict movement is called a **restraint.** To prevent possible charges of false imprisonment, carefully assess the situation and include the client or significant other in the care planning process. If it is decided that a restraint is needed, the purpose and use of the restraint should be explained, including how the restraint fits into the plan of care, the length of time the restraint may be necessary, and the expected outcome. Document the planning session in the client's medical record.

Documentation must show that the client:

- Is assessed every 15 minutes (JCAHO, 2000)
- Is toileted
- Receives food and water
- Has position changes

In acute care settings, restraints can generally be applied temporarily as a nursing measure for client safety; however, in most states, a physician's order must be immediately obtained. In long-term care settings, a physician's order is required before utilizing any restraints.

Invasion of Privacy Privacy includes the right to be left alone, to choose care based on personal beliefs, to govern body integrity, and to choose when and how sensitive information is shared (Badzek & Gross, 1999). People are entitled to **confidential** (nondisclosure of information) health care. All information gathered from working with

---

CULTURAL CONSIDERATIONS

Assault and Battery Charges

To prevent assault and battery charges, note the following:

- Respect the client's cultural values, beliefs, and practices with regard to "touching."
- African Americans sometimes view touching another person's hair as offensive.
- Asian Americans usually do not touch others during conversations. Touching someone on the head is considered disrespectful because the head is considered sacred.
- European Americans employ handshakes for formal greetings.
- Hispanic Americans are very tactile and may embrace and shake hands when greeting one another.
- Native Americans prohibit touching a dead body. This may leave the offender open to charges of assault.

a client or from his medical records must be kept confidential. Therefore, a client's health status may not be discussed with a third party, unless either the client is present and has given verbal permission or permission has been obtained in writing. This does not apply to nurses discussing a client's health status with other health care workers involved in the care of the client.

Invasion of privacy occurs when a person's private affairs become public knowledge without the person's permission. Photographing a client without his consent is an invasion of privacy, as is failure to pull curtains to shield the client when performing personal or intimate care.

Discussing clients in public areas is a common mistake made by health care personnel. When talking in the cafeteria or in the elevator it is difficult to know who may overhear what is said. The client's job or family situation may be compromised, depending on the nature of the information. For example, news of an abortion, positive HIV status, or venereal disease may be socially damaging. *Clients or their health care status should never be discussed in public areas or with anyone not directly involved in the care of the client.*

To protect the client's privacy, permission should be obtained before going through a client's belongings, doors should be kept closed and curtains pulled when providing personal care, and people not involved in the performance of a procedure should not be invited to watch unless the client has given permission. Clients cannot be photographed or videotaped without their permission, and a release form must be signed. Nursing students should never use a client's full name on care plans, case studies, or other assignments. Only initials should be used to protect the client's privacy in case the papers are lost. The client's chart and other materials should not be left lying around, allowing a client's private information to become public knowledge.

Since the time of Florence Nightingale, nurses have been practicing and advocating clients' basic right to privacy and confidentiality. Now there is a federal regulation covering these aspects. On April 14, 2003, the Health Insurance Portability and Accountability Act (HIPAA) privacy regulations went into effect. Protected health information (PHI) includes all health care information that can be traced to or identified with a specific individual (Ziel & Gentry, 2003).

The rules now protect how client health care information is stored and transferred and prescribe to whom it can be revealed. Also, clients are given the right to access their health care records, amend health care information, and obtain a list of who has seen their health care records (Trossman, 2003; Frank-Stromborg & Ganschow, 2002). Clients must be given a written notice by hospitals, physicians, pharmacies, and other covered entities of their privacy practices (Ziel & Gentry, 2003; Frank-Stromborg & Ganschow, 2002). When a state's law is more stringent than HIPAA regulations, the state's law will prevail.

Unintentional Torts

Negligence and malpractice are considered unintentional torts.

Negligence **Negligence** is a general term referring to negligent or careless acts on the part of an individual who is not exercising reasonable or prudent judgment. All nurses, including student nurses, are expected to use good judgment when providing client care. For example, side rails should not be left down on confused clients' beds, and puddles and spills should be cleaned up immediately to prevent falls, rather than waiting for housekeeping. Any person, even without the specialized knowledge required for nursing, could make these judgments. When a nurse fails to protect a client in such a situation or in one requiring similar judgment, the nurse could be found negligent.

Malpractice Negligent acts on the part of a professional can be termed **malpractice**, or professional negligence. Malpractice relates to the conduct of a person while acting in a professional capacity.

Not meeting the standards of care, not doing what a reasonable and prudent nurse would do in similar circumstances, results in negligent or careless acts on the part of a nurse. A nurse can be charged with malpractice for acts committed or acts omitted. Failing to properly assess a client or act on the assessment information are examples of omission. Giving a client the wrong medication and improperly performing a procedure resulting in client injury are acts of commission.

Malpractice differs from negligence in that anyone can be accused of negligence; only professionals can be accused of malpractice. Several factors must hold true for a nurse to be found guilty of malpractice (professional negligence):

- The nurse owed a special duty to the client; that is, a nurse–client relationship existed.
- The nurse failed to meet the standards of care.
- The injury occurred as a direct result of the nurse's action or inaction.
- Damage such as physical or emotional pain, suffering, monetary losses, or medical expenses must be proved. If there is not damage, the plaintiff is not entitled to an award (Lee, 2000).

The prudent nurse is protected by adhering to facility policy and procedure and attempting to meet the standards of care at all times.

Legal Risk

Nurses today are more likely to have problems for violating statutes (i.e., laws and regulations) than to be sued for malpractice (Infante, 2000). Two common sources of statutory liability are federal antifraud laws and state reporting requirements. Statutory liability may lead to criminal charges rather than just civil penalties (Infante, 2000). The best protection against statutory liability is to learn about the federal and state laws and regulations that apply to the nurse's particular practice setting. A good resource is the facility's risk manager.

Federal Antifraud Laws

The federal government has:

- Expanded the list of activities that constitute fraud.
- Imposed new criminal sanctions on violators.

- Increased the budget for investigating and prosecuting these activities.

Infante (2000) lists as examples of fraudulent activities the following:

- Billing for services either unnecessary or not provided
- Falsifying care plans
- Forging physician's signature
- Filing false cost reports
- Falsifying or omitting information about a client's condition to obtain reimbursement

State Reporting Requirements

Nurses are required to report cases of suspected child abuse or neglect in every state (Infante, 2000). Most states also require nurses to report cases of suspected elder abuse and neglect (Morris, 1998). Infante (2000) identifies some criminal acts that must be reported. Many states require that:

- Police are notified of known or suspected cases of rape.
- Reports of gunshot or stab wounds are made.

Some states require that clients who have taken narcotics or who have a blood alcohol level higher than the legal limit for driving be reported (Ventura, 1999c).

These laws are not only for the general public but also for health care providers. If a suspected abuser is a health care provider, many states require that the event be reported to the agency that licenses that professional (Morris, 1998). Also, many states require nurses to report *any* provider who acts unprofessionally or is incompetent (Infante, 2000).

Professional Discipline

More than 5,000 nurses (RNs and LP/VNs) are annually disciplined for professional misconduct in the United States (LaDuke, 2000). That is, the nurses are found to have violated existing laws or regulations that govern a nurse's practice. LaDuke (2000) suggests that a nurse:

- Should *immediately* seek representation by an attorney specializing in professional misconduct and discipline if under investigation
- Is not obligated to talk to *any* investigator without an attorney present
- Know and understand the applicable state nursing practice act and established standards of care
- Look closely at the disciplinary process and ask questions to promote understanding

Sanctions

Boards of nursing determine and issue sanctions for nurses found to have demonstrated professional misconduct. Monetary damages are not generally awarded to consumers. A sample of sanctions from which boards of nursing may choose, includes:

- Warn, censure, or reprimand the licensees
- Impose a fine
- Place on probation or set a condition of licensure
- Limit the license
- Suspend the license

- Revoke the license
- Dismiss the complaint

Disciplinary Data Banks

The National Council of State Boards of Nursing (NCSBN) maintains a Disciplinary Data Bank (DDB), as do many other professional organizations. The purpose of these data banks is to facilitate the communication of information about unsafe practitioners. In 1990, Congress created the National Practitioner Data Bank (NPDB) to improve the quality of health care by encouraging the identification and discipline of health care professionals (mostly physicians and dentists) who engage in incompetent and unsafe behavior.

As part of the Health Insurance Portability and Accountability Act (HIPAA) of 1996, the Healthcare Integrity and Protection Data Bank (HIPDB) was implemented in 1999. This data bank collects and discloses certain final adverse actions taken against nurses at all levels of practice, other licensed practitioners, and unlicensed persons who provide health care services or are involved in the health insurance business (Health Resources and Services Administration, 2000).

Documentation

The source of information regarding the client's clinical history is the medical record, or the chart. The chart should accurately reflect diagnosis, treatment, testing, clinical course, nursing assessment, and intervention. According to the law, "If it was not charted, it was not done." When a chart ends up in court, this is the standard the jury applies in determining what happened and who is at fault.

Medications should not be charted before they are given. This constitutes a direct violation of the standards of practice for documentation and medication administration. The standard of practice is that medications are documented *after* they are administered. All client care, including treatments, is documented after being provided.

Documentation must be objective and accurate. The nurse should describe what is seen and done. Nurses' notes should reflect facts, not inferences or opinions, about the client. It is not enough to chart nursing assessment or identified problems; any actions taken, including nursing interventions and physician's orders implemented, must also be documented.

Entries must be neat, legible, spelled correctly, written clearly, and signed or initialed. It is illegal to change a chart.

INFORMED CONSENT

Informed consent refers to a competent client's ability to make health care decisions based on full disclosure of the benefits, risks, potential consequences of a recommended treatment plan, and alternate treatments, including no treatment, and the client's agreement to the treatment as indicated by the client's signing a consent form. This detailed explanation, provided by the physician, lets the client make intelligent decisions about treatment options. Consent to treatment also protects health care workers from unwarranted charges of battery.

Nurses must obtain consent for nursing procedures. Each client, on admission, signs a general care consent form. The nurse is obligated to explain what is to be done to the client and to receive at least implied consent, as indicated by lack of objection on the part of the client. Individuals who are declared incompetent are assigned a guardian or someone who has power of attorney to make heath care decisions and give consent for treatment. The physician is responsible for obtaining consent for medical or surgical treatment. The discussion about the risks and benefits of treatment generally takes place when the nurse is not present, often in the physician's office. The client usually decides on the basis of the discussion whether to accept the treatment recommendation. Confusion arises, however, because nurses are often delegated the duty of collecting the signature on the informed consent form. *Student nurses should neither ask the client to sign a consent form nor witness a consent form.*

When a nurse has a client sign the informed consent form, the nurse is verifying the following three things:

1. The client's signature is authentic.
2. The client has the mental capacity to understand what was discussed with the physician.
3. The client was not coerced into signing the form.

The client should not sign the form if the client still has questions or if the nurse is unsure about the client's understanding. The nurse should document the client's

lack of understanding and contact the physician. Further clarification must come from the physician.

Clients older than age 18 may give consent for their own health care. Parents or guardians give consent for minor children. In most states, minors who live on their own, are married, become pregnant, or require treatment for sexually transmitted diseases, substance abuse, or mental illness, may give consent for themselves.

Complex situations occur when minors refuse treatments to which parents have consented, or parents refuse consent or treatment that has been deemed medically necessary for their minor children. The court has had to intervene in such cases. In situations such as these, the child may be made a ward of the court and decision making temporarily taken away from the parents. An example would be the child of Jehovah's Witnesses who needs a blood transfusion but whose parents refuse treatment on the basis of religious beliefs.

A typical consent form (Figure 4-1) is used to obtain client permission for the performance of invasive medical, surgical, or diagnostic procedures, such as surgery, cardiac catheterization, or HIV testing. Consent for procedures that are not invasive can be either given verbally or implied. Consent is implied when the client cooperates with the procedure offered. For example, if the orderly says, "Mr. Garza, I am here to take you for your hand x-ray," and Mr. Garza gets into the wheelchair, consent is implied by Mr. Garza's cooperation.

ADVANCE DIRECTIVES

An **advance directive** is a written instruction for health care, recognized under state law, related to the provision of care when the individual is incapacitated. Advance directives emphasize the client's right to self-determination. These instructions about health care preferences regarding life-sustaining measures may indicate who is to make health care decisions for the client if he becomes unable to do so for himself.

A client of sound mind has the right to make all health care decisions and even reverse previous decisions. When a situation arises and the person becomes incapable of making decisions, advance directives guide

TO THE PATIENT: You have the right as a patient to be informed about your condition and the recommended surgical, medical, or diagnostic procedure to be used so that you may make the decision whether or not to undergo the procedure after knowing the risks and hazards involved. This disclosure is not meant to scare or alarm you, but is simply an effort to make you better informed so you may give or withhold your consent to the procedure. Any questions or concerns you may have with respect to the proposed procedure, its risks, complications, or benefits should be directed to your treating physician.

I (we) voluntarily request Dr. _____ as my physician, and such associates, technical assistants and other health care providers as they may deem necessary to treat my condition, which has been explained to me as: _____

I (we) understand that the following surgical, medical, and/or diagnostic procedures are planned for me, and I (we) voluntarily consent and authorize these procedures: _____

I (we) understand that my physician may discover other or different conditions which require additional or different procedures than those planned. I (we) authorize my physician, and such associates, technical assistants, and other health care providers, to perform such procedures which are advisable in their professional judgment.

I (we) [DO] [DO NOT] consent to the use of blood and blood products as deemed necessary.

I (we) understand that no warrant or guarantee has been made to me as a result or cure.

Just as there may be risks and hazards in continuing my present condition without treatment, there are also risks and hazards related to the performance of the surgical, medical, and/or diagnostic procedures planned for me. I (we) realize that common to surgical, medical, and/or diagnostic procedures is the potential for infection, blood clots in veins and lungs, hemorrhage, allergic reactions, and even death. I (we) realize that the following risks and hazards may occur in connection with this particular procedure:

(Additional Consent Information On Back.)

INITIAL: _____

CHRISTUS SPOHN HEALTH SYSTEM

DISCLOSURE AND CONSENT
MEDICAL AND SURGICAL PROCEDURES
PATIENT CARE SERVICES

2704980   NEW: 05/82   REVISED: 10/99

3025

I (we) understand that anesthesia involves additional risks and hazards, but I (we) request the use of anesthetics for the relief and protection from pain during the planned and additional procedures. I (we) realize the anesthesia may have to be changed, possibly without explanation to me (us).

I (we) understand that certain complications may result from the use of any anesthetic, including respiratory problems, drug reaction, paralysis, brain damage, or even death. Other risks and hazards which may result from the use of general anesthetics range from minor discomfort to injury to vocal cords, teeth, or eyes. I (we) understand that other risks and hazards resulting from spinal or epidural anesthetics include headache, chronic pain, remote possibility of nerve injury, hematoma, infection, septic and aseptic meningitis, nausea, vomiting, itching, and urinary retention.

I (we) consent to the photographing of the operations or procedures to be performed, including appropriate portions of the body, for medical, scientific, or educational purposes, provided my identity is not revealed by descriptive texts accompanying the picture.

I (we) consent to the disposition by hospital authorities of any tissues or parts which may be removed.

I (we) have been given the opportunity to ask questions about my conditions, alternative forms of anesthesia and treatment, risks of non-treatment, the procedures to be used, and the risks and hazards involved, and I (we) believe that I (we) have sufficient information to give this informed consent.

My physician has discussed the alternatives, risks and benefits, of the proposed procedures. I (we) certify that this form has been fully explained to me; that I (we) have read it or have had it read to me; that the blank spaces have been filled in, and that I (we) understand its contents.

_____
PHYSICIAN'S SIGNATURE

DATE: _____ TIME: _____ A.M./P.M.

_____
Witness (Signature of witness/print name of witness)

_____
Patient/Other Legally Responsible Person
(Minor patient and parent/guardian signature)

Figure 4-1 *Disclosure and Consent—Medical and Surgical Procedures (Courtesy CHRISTUS Spohn Health System, Corpus Christi, TX)*

CLIENT TEACHING

Advance Directives

- Advance directives should be discussed with the family and physician so that everyone understands the client's wishes and conflicts are less likely to occur at a later time.
- An advance directive may be changed by the client as long as the client is competent.

family members concerning those kinds of treatment that should or should not be allowed. Advance directives permit those involved in the decision-making process to know what the client prefers. Although these instructions are best put in writing, this is not always done. Sometimes, health care preferences are shared verbally with family members or friends. Verbal instructions can be interpreted differently by different people, creating difficulty for all involved—the physician, the health care facility, and the family. Thus, it is best to get this information in writing. When an advance directive indicates that the client does not wish to have cardiopulmonary resuscitation (CPR) performed in the event of cardiac arrest, the physician must write a DNR order, also referred to as a "No Code."

Health care facilities that receive Medicaid or Medicare monies are required to offer the opportunity to complete advance directives to all competent clients on admission. The client should be told about the availability and purpose of a living will and durable power of attorney for health care (discussed following). If desired, assistance in completing these documents is to be offered to the client. The medical record must show that the client was offered the opportunity to complete these documents, and documentation must indicate decisions made or not made at that time. Clients cannot be discriminated against for not signing an advance directive, nor can they be coerced into signing an advance directive.

Durable Power of Attorney for Health Care

A **durable power of attorney for health care** (DPAHC) is a legal document designating who may make health care decisions for a client when that client is no longer capable of decision making. This health care representative, appointed by the client, is expected to act in the best interests of the client. This appointment can be revoked any time the competent client chooses.

For example, if a client becomes comatose and the prognosis is poor, the health care representative having DPAHC can either give consent for certain types of treatment or withhold consent for treatment, even if the lack of treatment results in the client's death. Only when the client is no longer competent to make health care decisions is the DPAHC activated.

The person who has a regular power of attorney does not have the same authority about health care issues.

CRITICAL THINKING

Advance Directives

How would you explain advance directives to your family? To a friend?

The right to make health care decisions must be specified in the power of attorney agreement, or a DPAHC must be signed (Figure 4-2). A person who stands to benefit from the client's estate cannot be appointed health care representative.

Living Will

A **living will** is a legal document that allows a person to state preferences about the use of life-sustaining measures in case she is unable to make her wishes known. These preferences can be expressed either with a living will or a Life-Prolonging Procedure Declaration. These documents allow the client to specify, in advance, those life-sustaining measures that are to be done or not done. Food, fluids, and comfort measures are generally continued, and the person is not abandoned; however, artificial means of sustaining life, such as ventilators or feeding tubes, are not to be used.

Although not all states currently recognize living wills, the client's requests should be given due weight when making health care decisions. The nurse must be knowledgeable about living will legislation in her state. A sample living will is shown in Figure 4-3.

A Life-Prolonging Procedure Declaration stating that the person wants all possible procedures done to delay the dying process, including the use of ventilators, is available in some places.

INCIDENT REPORTS

An **incident report** is a risk management tool used to describe and report any unusual event that occurs to a client, visitor, or staff member. It is used by the facility to identify or track problem areas and to alert the legal department to possible lawsuits. An incident report is not a punitive device, although it is often perceived that it is.

Incident reports are completed to document such events as falls, medication errors, forgotten treatment, injuries—anything that happens out of the ordinary. An incident report may also be called a variance report or an occurrence report. The following three examples illustrate the types of occurrences that should be documented in an incident report.

- Mrs. Duncan had blood drawn for various laboratory tests. It was later discovered that the laboratory work had been ordered on Mrs. Falson, not Mrs. Duncan. The requisition had been stamped with the wrong name.
- Mrs. Barnes was given Lasix 20 mg po at 9 A.M. When reviewing the physician's orders, the evening nurse discovered that Losec 20 mg had been ordered. Mrs. Barnes received the wrong medication.

Part I. Durable Power of Attorney for Health Care

- If you do NOT wish to name an agent to make health care decisions for you, write your initials in the box

[Initials]

This form has been prepared to comply with the "Durable Power of Attorney for Health Care Act" of Missouri.

1. Selection of agent. I appoint:
Name:_____
Address:_____
_____
Telephone:_____
as my Agent.

It is suggested that only one Agent be named. However, if more than one Agent is named, anyone may act individually unless you specify otherwise.

2. Alternate Agents. Only an Agent named by me may act under this Durable Power of Attorney. If my Agent resigns or is not able or available to make health care decisions for me, or if an Agent named by me is divorced from me or is my spouse and legally separated from me, I appoint the person(s) named below (in the order named if more than one):

First Alternate Agent	Second Alternate Agent
Name:_____	Name:_____
Address:_____	Address:_____
_____	_____
Telephone:_____	Telephone:_____

This is a Durable Power of Attorney, and the authority of my Agent shall not terminate if I become disabled or incapacitated.

Part I. Durable Power of Attorney for Health Care (Continued)

3. Effective date and durability. This Durable Power of Attorney is effective when two physicians decide and certify that I am incapacitated and unable to make and communicate a health care decision.

- If you want ONE physician, instead of TWO, to decide whether you are incapacitated, write your initials in the box to the right.

[Initials]

4. Agent's powers. I grant to my Agent full authority to:

A. Give consent to, prohibit, or withdraw any type of health care, medical care, treatment, or procedure, even if my death may result;

- If you wish to AUTHORIZE your Agent to direct a health care provider to withhold or withdraw artificially supplied nutrition and hydration (including tube feeding of food and water), write your initials in the box to the right.

[Initials]

- If you DO NOT WISH TO AUTHORIZE your Agent to direct a health care provider to withhold or withdraw artificially supplied nutrition and hydration (including tube feeding of food and water), write your initials in the box to the right.

[Initials]

B. Make all necessary arrangements for health care services on my behalf, and to hire and fire medical personnel responsible for my care;

C. Move me into or out of any health care facility (even if against medical advice) to obtain compliance with the decisions of my Agent; and

D. Take any other action necessary to do what I authorize here, including (but not limited to) granting any waiver or release from liability required by any health care provider, and taking any legal action at the expense of my estate to enforce this Durable Power of Attorney.

5. Agent's Financial Liability and Compensation. My Agent acting under this Durable Power of Attorney will incur no personal financial liability. My Agent shall not be entitled to compensation for services performed under this Durable Power of Attorney, but my Agent shall be entitled to reimbursement for all reasonable expenses incurred as a result of carrying out any provision hereof.

Part II. Health Care Directive

- If you DO NOT WISH to make a health care directive, write your initials in the box to the right, and go to Part III.

[Initials]

I make this HEALTH CARE DIRECTIVE ("Directive") to exercise my right to determine the course of my health care and to provide clear and convincing proof of my wishes and instructions about my treatment.

If I am persistently unconscious or there is no reasonable expectation of my recovery from a seriously incapacitating or terminal illness or condition, I direct that all of the life-prolonging procedures which I have initialed below be withheld or withdrawn.

I want the following life-prolonging procedures to be withheld or withdrawn:

| • artificially supplied nutrition and hydration (including tube feeding of food and water) . . . . | Initials |

- surgery or other invasive procedures. . . . . [Initials]
- heart-lung resuscitation (CPR) . . . . [Initials]
- antibiotic. . . . . [Initials]
- dialysis. . . . . [Initials]
- mechanical ventilator (respirator). . . . . [Initials]
- chemotherapy. . . . . [Initials]
- radiation therapy. . . . . [Initials]
- all other "life-prolonging" medical or surgical procedures that are merely intended to keep me alive without reasonable hope of improving my condition or curing my illness or injury. . . . . [Initials]

However, if my physician believes that any life-prolonging procedure may lead to significant recovery, I direct my physician to try the treatment for a reasonable period of time. If it does not improve my condition, I direct the treatment be withdrawn even if it shortens my life. I also direct that I be given medical treatment to relieve pain or to provide comfort, even if such treatment might shorten my life, suppress my appetite or my breathing, or be habit forming.

IF I HAVE NOT DESIGNATED AN AGENT IN THE DURABLE POWER OF ATTORNEY, THIS DOCUMENT IS MEANT TO BE IN FULL FORCE AND EFFECT AS MY HEALTH CARE DIRECTIVE.

Part III. General Provisions Included in the Directive and Durable Power of Attorney

YOU MUST SIGN THIS DOCUMENT IN THE PRESENCE OF TWO WITNESSES. IN WITNESS WHEREOF, I have executed this document this_____day of _____, year____.

_____
Signature

Print name _____
Address _____

The person who signed this document is of sound mind and voluntarily signed this document in our presence. Each of the undersigned witnesses is at least eighteen years of age.

Signature_____	Signature_____
Print name _____	Print name _____
Address _____	Address _____

ONLY REQUIRED FOR PART I — DURABLE POWER OF ATTORNEY

STATE OF MISSOURI   )
) as
_____OF _____   )

On this _____day of _____, year_____, before me personally appeared to me known to be the person described in and who executed the foregoing instrument and acknowledged that he/she executed the same as his/her free act and deed.

IN WITNESS WHEREOF, I have hereunto set my hand and affixed my official seal in the County of _____, State of Missouri, the day and year first above written.

_____
Notary Public

My Commision Expires:

Figure 4-2 *Durable Power of Attorney for Health Care and Health Care Directive (Reprinted with permission of the Missouri Bar)*

Sample Living Will

Declaration made this _____ day of _____, year_____.
I, _____, willfully and voluntarily make known my desire that my dying not be artificially prolonged under the circumstances set forth below, and I do hereby declare:

If at any time I have a terminal condition and if my attending or treating physician and another consulting physician have determined that there is no medical probability of my recovery from such condition, I direct that life-prolonging procedures be withheld or withdrawn when the application of such procedures would serve only to prolong artificially the process of dying, and that I be permitted to die naturally with only the administration of medication or the performance of any medical procedure deemed necessary to provide me with comfort care or to alleviate pain.

It is my intention that this declaration be honored by my family and physician as the final expression of my legal right to refuse medical or surgical treatment and to accept the consequences for such refusal.

In the event that I have been determined to be unable to provide express and informed consent regarding the withholding, withdrawal, or continuation of life-prolonging procedures, I wish to designate, as my surrogate to carry out the provisions of this declaration:

Name: _____
Address: _____
_____ Zip Code: _____
Phone: _____

I wish to designate the following person as my alternate surrogate, to carry out the provisions of this declaration should my surrogate be unwilling or unable to act on my behalf:

Name: _____
Address: _____
_____ Zip Code: _____
Phone: _____

Additional instructions (optional):

I understand the full importance of this declaration, and I am emotionally and mentally competant to make this declaration.
Signed: _____

Witness 1:
    Signed: _____
    Address: _____

Witness 2:
    Signed: _____
    Address: _____

Figure 4-3 *Sample Living Will (Reprinted by permission of Partnership for Caring, 1620 Eye Street NW, Suite 202, Washington, DC 20006)*

- Mrs. Gomez was visiting her daughter, who had just given birth to the family's first grandchild. While walking down the hall, Mrs. Gomez slipped and fell, injuring her right hip.

The previous examples are incidents or variances that occur in health care settings. For each situation, an incident report must be completed and channeled to the risk management department. Risk management convenes representatives from various departments, such as nursing administration, dietary services, environmental safety, and others, to review the incident reports. This group tries to identify those factors, if any, that contributed to the incident. Examples of questions asked include "Can the causal factors be eliminated or reduced?" "Does the possibility of a lawsuit exist as a result of the incident?" and "What can be done to prevent this incident from occurring again?"

Incident reports are filed by the person who was responsible for, who discovered, or who witnessed the incident. The report should state what was observed, as opposed to what is supposed. It should be concise and factual. In the third example given previously, if the nurse did not witness the actual fall, the correctly worded report would read: "Mrs. Gomez found lying on floor outside room 222. Several puddles of liquid found under and around her; paper cup lying nearby." An incorrect, presumptuous, and potentially damaging report might read: "Mrs. Gomez tripped and fell outside room 222. She slipped in a puddle of water." Mrs. Gomez may have spilled the cup of water she was carrying during the fall; however, this second note implies that Mrs. Gomez slipped in water that was already on the floor, thus implicating the facility.

Incident reports should include a description of the care given to the client or individual and the name of the physician who was notified. The incident should be charted in the client's medical record, but the incident report should not be referred to in any way. Although the incident report is not a part of the medical record, the details described in the medical record and in the incident report should be the same.

When completing an incident report, the nurse should be sure to include the date and time of the incident as well as assessments and interventions. The time that family members and physicians were notified should also be included. The nurse should refer to nursing administration policy and procedure regarding follow-up documentation.

LIABILITY INSURANCE

Many nurses assume the insurance provided by their employer is adequate and they do not need their own malpractice or liability insurance. This attitude may leave a nurse vulnerable both professionally and personally (Laduke & Biondo, 2003).

Nurses assert they are knowledgeable and competent health care providers. Health care consumers hold nurses accountable for their actions, resulting in nurses being named as defendants in malpractice suits. Under the doctrine of *Respondeat Superior,* employers are responsible for the actions of their employees; however, if policy was violated and the employer has to pay damages, the employer has the right to sue the nurse to recover the loss. Also, this responsibility stops when the employee leaves work.

A professional liability policy provides the nurse with an attorney who will represent that nurse in court. The needs of an individual nurse will be secondary to an attorney representing the facility or a group of employees. The individual nurse is better represented in court by private counsel.

Friends and family members ask nurses for assistance and advice in health care matters. They seek this advice because of their experience and knowledge. Family members or friends might bring a law suit against the nurse later depending on the results of the advice. The nurse is accountable for the advice given even though no money was exchanged for information or services.

The nurse needs legal representation if the situation ends up in court, which is costly as are judgments against the nurse. The nurse is protected with a professional liability insurance policy that provides legal representation and pays the judgments.

Liability protection comes in two forms: the claims made policy and the occurrence policy. The claims made policy covers claims made while the policy is in effect. The nurse is not covered if a claim is made after the policy is terminated. An occurrence policy protects the nurse for events taking place during the active period of the policy even if a claim is filed after the policy is terminated. The occurrence policy seems to provide better protection for the nurse. Check if there is coverage for disciplinary claims (Sloan, 2002a).

Whether nurses should carry individual liability insurance is often debated. Some health care professionals and attorneys believe this practice encourages lawsuits. The benefits and cost of buying professional liability insurance must be compared against the loss of personal assets and cost of potential legal fees. When buying liability insurance the company's reputation should be investigated. Many nursing organizations offer group professional liability insurance. Sloan (2002a) suggests that nurses must assess their liability risk by considering their employment status (employee, independent contractor, or borrowed servant [agency nurse]), employer (well financed, having financial hardship, government), and area of specialty (ED, critical care, and obstetrics are considered high-risk settings).

IMPAIRED NURSE

A sensitive issue in nursing today is the impaired nurse. By definition, an **impaired nurse** is a nurse who is habitually intemperate or is addicted to the use of alcohol or habit-forming drugs. Although job performance may not be immediately compromised, substance abuse does eventually interfere with clinical judgment and performance. The chemical dependency rate among nurses is no higher than in the general population (Trinkoff et al., 2000).

In cases of impaired health care workers, the primary concern is client care. As a client advocate, the nurse cannot let loyalties to coworkers interfere with duty to the client. It is difficult reporting a coworker. No one wants to be a squealer. In many states, however, the board of nursing requires nurses to report impaired coworkers. Nurses suspected of being under the influence of drugs or alcohol must be reported to the proper authority at the place of employment. The second consideration is getting help for the impaired nurse and taking action to correct the problem.

When a coworker is suspected of diverting drugs or abusing alcohol, the nurse should:

1. Document the dates, times, and observed behavior. It is critical to be specific and descriptive of what was observed. For example:

   March 10, 2003. C.D. working 3–11 shift. Client A and Client B verbalized unrelieved postoperative pain. Documentation by C.D. stated both clients were comfortable after administration of Demerol 75 mg IM to each client. Narcotic count at shift change satisfactory.

   March 11, 2003. Client C and Client D verbalized unrelieved pain. Documentation by C.D. indicated both clients stated pain was relieved after administration of Demerol 100 mg IM. Narcotic count at shift change okay.

   March 12, 2003. Narcotic count listed 1 Demerol 100-mg syringe as broken and 1 Demerol 75-mg syringe as wasted, "client changed her mind." C.D. signed the narcotic sheet.

   or

   April 13, 2003. S.L. working the night shift. Strong odor of alcohol on his breath.

   April 14, 2003. S.L. observed walking with unsteady gait, speech is slurred, strong odor of alcohol on breath.

2. Report concerns to the supervisor and provide a copy of the documentation about the incidents. The supervisor is responsible for confronting the suspected employee. Intoxication requires immediate removal from the clinical area. In other situations, the supervisor will devise a plan before confronting the nurse.
3. Do not approach or confront the coworker yourself. The impaired coworker may become defensive and deny the problem or make threats. Also, once aware that someone is suspicious, the nurse may become more secretive, making detection less likely. Frequently, the nurse will leave one facility and go to another, repeating the same pattern.

Some employers offer an employee assistance program to rehabilitate the impaired nurse. In addition, most states have **peer assistance programs** (rehabilitation programs designed to provide an impaired nurse with referrals, professional and peer counseling support groups, and assistance and monitoring for reentry into nursing). These peer assistance programs operate under the guidance of the state nurses association in conjunction with the board of nursing. The goals of assistance programs are to protect the public from impaired nurses, provide the needed assistance to the impaired nurse, and assist the nurse to reenter nursing by monitoring the nurse's compliance. The peer counselor helps the impaired nurse develop a contract for treatment. Compliance is monitored, and confidentiality is ensured. Successful completion of the program allows the nurse to return to the practice setting.

Participation in these programs is optional. A nurse choosing not to cooperate, however, may be terminated, and the board of nursing may impose sanctions, including revoking the license to practice.

CONCEPT OF ETHICS

Ethics is the branch of philosophy concerned with determining right from wrong on the basis of knowledge rather than on opinions. Ethics deals with one's responsibilities (duties and obligations) as defined by logical argument. It is *not* a religious dogma. Ethics looks at human behavior—what people do in what circumstances. But ethics is not merely philosophical in nature; ethical persons put their beliefs into action.

Health Care and Ethics

Bioethics is the application of general ethical principles to health care. Every area of health care, including direct care of clients, utilization of staff, and allocation of finances is affected by ethics.

Ethics raises questions but does not provide easy answers. Ethical practice has more importance in health care today for several reasons. Some of these reasons are:

- An increase in technology. Advanced technology creates situations involving complicated issues, such as:

  - Newborns are surviving at earlier gestational ages, and many have serious health problems.

  - People are living much longer than ever before.

  - Organ transplants and use of bionic body parts are becoming more common.
- Changing of our society. Family structure is moving to more single-parent families and nonrelated groups living together as families.
- Clients are more knowledgeable about their health and health care, resulting in a consumer-driven system.

ETHICAL PRINCIPLES

Ethical principles are widely accepted codes generally based on the humane aspects of society that direct or govern actions. Ethical decisions reflect what is best for the client and society. Table 4-4 summarizes the major ethical principles. Each principle is discussed in detail in the following paragraphs.

The nurse can become more systematic in solving ethical conflicts by using ethical principles. They can be used as guidelines in analyzing dilemmas and can serve as justification (rationale) for resolving ethical problems.

Autonomy

The principle of **autonomy** refers to the individual's right to choose and the individual's ability to act on that choice. Each person's individuality is respected. This respect is a dominant value in U.S. society.

TABLE 4-4 OVERVIEW OF ETHICAL PRINCIPLES	
PRINCIPLE	**EXPLANATION**
Autonomy	Respect individual's right to self-determination; respect individual liberty
Nonmaleficence	Cause or do no harm to another
Beneficence	Do good to others and maintain a balance between benefits and harms
Justice	Distribute equitable potential benefits and risks
Veracity	Tell the truth
Fidelity	Do what one has promised

Nurses must respect the client's right to decide and must protect those clients who are unable to decide for themselves. The ethical principle of autonomy respects the individual's right to self-determination for a competent person. The right to autonomy rests on the client's competency to decide; however, the legal definition of competency varies among states.

Informed consent is based on the client's right to make choices. Respecting autonomy means the nurse accepts client choices, even choices not in the client's best interests or choices that conflict with the nurse's values. Examples of autonomous client behavior that can hinder recovery or treatment include:

- Smoking after a diagnosis of emphysema or lung cancer
- Refusing to take medication

PROFESSIONAL TIP

Autonomy

- Competent clients have a right to self-determination, even if their decisions may result in self-harm.
- Probably one of the most difficult things for nurses to accept is that clients are ultimately responsible for themselves; they will do what they want to do.

COMMUNITY/HOME HEALTH CARE

Client Autonomy

With the increased acuity level of clients cared for in the home setting, home health nurses face ever-increasing ethical challenges because they have less control over what the client does on a day-to-day basis at home.

- Continuing to drink alcohol after being diagnosed with cirrhosis of the liver
- Refusing to receive a blood transfusion because of religious beliefs

Nonmaleficence

Nonmaleficence is the obligation to cause no harm to others. Harm can be physiological, psychological, financial, social, and/or spiritual. Included are both the risk of harm and intentional harm. The principle of nonmaleficence when guiding treatment decisions asks the question "Will this treatment modality cause more harm or more good to the client?" There may not be a clear-cut answer. Consider these factors when choosing a treatment:

- A reasonable expectation of benefit
- Lack of excessive pain, expense, or other inconvenience

The nurse practices according to professional and legal standards of care when following the principle of nonmaleficence. Nonmaleficence is considered a fundamental duty of health care providers. The Vocational Nurses's Pledge (Table 4-5), The Practical Nurse's Pledge (Table 4-6), and the Nightingale Pledge (Table 4-7) all profess the same basic philosophy of nursing care. Some clinical examples of nonmaleficence are:

- Preventing medication errors (including drug interactions)
- Being aware of potential risks of treatment modalities
- Removing hazards (e.g., obstructions or water on the floor that might cause a fall)

Beneficence

Beneficence is the duty to promote good and to prevent harm. Beneficence is often viewed as the core of nursing practice. The nurse nurtures the client and incorporates the desires of the client into the plan of care. Sometimes, it is difficult to determine what is "good," es-

TABLE 4-5   VOCATIONAL NURSE'S PLEDGE

God being my Witness and Judge and the Light whereby my life is patterned, do solemnly pledge myself to keep the following vows:

I shall endeavor in all ways so to live and to conduct myself, at home and abroad, that my vocation shall be uplifted in the eyes of all people.

I shall help to elevate the standards of my vocation by doing my work, where ever I may be, at least a little better on each tomorrow than I was able to do it on each today.

I shall put the welfare of my patients above all else.

I shall not engage in idle talk about other vocational nurses, professional nurses, or doctors, for we are united in our care of the patient and gossip destroys unity.

So let me live that I may be of service to Him Who "so loved the world that He gave His only begotten Son that whosoever believeth in Him should not perish but have everlasting life."

Author unknown: Used for more than 35 years by the Department of Vocational Nurse Education, Del Mar College, Corpus Christi, TX.

TABLE 4-6   PRACTICAL NURSE'S PLEDGE

Before God and those assembled here, I solemnly pledge:

To adhere to the code of ethics of the nursing profession.

To cooperate faithfully with the other members of the nursing team and to carry out faithfully and to the best of my ability the instructions of the physician or the nurse who may be assigned to supervise my work.

I will not do anything evil or malicious and I will not knowingly give any harmful drug or assist in malpractice.

I will not reveal any confidential information that may come to my knowledge in the course of my work.

And I pledge myself to do all in my power to raise the standards and the prestige of practical nursing.

May my life be devoted to service, and to the high ideals of the nursing profession.

Reprinted with permission of the National Association for Practical Nurse Education and Services Inc., Silver Springs, MD.

pecially when doing good causes the client discomfort. For example, a client who has had a serious stroke may resist performing range-of-motion exercises and become angry at the nurse for insisting. The nurse knows the long-term value of these exercises, yet perceives the client's physical and psychological pain.

Justice

The principle of **justice** is based on the concept of fairness extended to each individual. The major health-related issues of justice involve the way people are treated and the way resources are distributed.

This principle directs that unless there is a justification for unequal treatment, all people must be treated equally. The **material principle of justice** is the rationale for determining those times when there can be unequal allocation of scarce resources. This concept specifies that resources may be allocated according to:

- Need
- Individual effort
- The individual's merit (ability)
- The individual's contribution to society

TABLE 4-7   NIGHTINGALE PLEDGE

I solemnly pledge myself before God and in the presence of this assembly: To pass my life in purity and to practice my profession faithfully.

I will abstain from whatever is deleterious and mischievous, and will not take or knowingly administer any harmful drug.

I will do all in my power to maintain and elevate the standards of my profession, and will hold in confidence all personal matters committed to my keeping, and all family affairs coming to my knowledge in the practice of my profession.

With loyalty will I endeavor to aid the physician in his work, and devote myself to the welfare of those committed to my care.

The Veterans Affairs (VA) Medical Centers are an example of the application of the material principle of justice (according to the individual's contribution to society). Only those who served their country by joining the military are eligible to receive health care through the VA in acute care, ambulatory, and psychiatric facilities.

Veracity

Veracity means truthfulness (neither lying nor deceiving others). There are many forms of deception: intentional lying, partial disclosure of information, or nondisclosure of information. Veracity often is difficult to achieve. Telling the truth may not be hard, but deciding how much truth to tell may be very hard. Exceptions to truth-telling are sometimes upheld by the principle of nonmaleficence, when the truth does greater harm than good. The act of giving placebo medications is an example of when telling the truth does greater harm than good.

Fidelity

Fidelity, which is the ethical foundation of nurse–client relationships, means faithfulness and keeping promises.

Clients have a right to expect nurses to act in their best interests. The nurse's function as a **client advocate** (a person who speaks up for or acts on behalf of the client) upholds the principle of fidelity. Fidelity is demonstrated when nurses:

- Share the client's wishes with other members of the health care team.
- Keep their own personal values from influencing their advocacy for clients.
- Support the client's decision, even if it conflicts with their own preferences.

Within the nurse–client relationship, nurses are to be loyal to their responsibilities, maintain privacy, keep promises, and meet clients' reasonable expectations. Nurses also have a duty to be faithful to themselves. The nurse may question who is owed fidelity when conflict between commitments occurs. Remaining client centered may help clarify the question, but it may not resolve the conflict. For example, if the mother of a frightened teenage girl tried to pressure the nurse into revealing the results of the daughter's pregnancy test after the daughter had already requested that her mother not be told, although the nurse may believe that the mother has the girl's best interests at heart, the nurse must protect the client's right to privacy.

ETHICAL THEORIES

Ethical theories have been debated since the time of Plato and Aristotle. Ethical theories can be used to analyze ethical problems, but no theory by itself can provide the "correct" answer to any ethical conflict. Common ethical theories include teleology, deontology, situational theory, and caring-based theory.

Teleology

Teleology is an ethical theory that states that the value of a situation is determined by its consequences.

The criterion for determining the value of an action is the outcome of an action, not the action itself. An example would be immunizations—receiving an injection is not "good," but preventing the illness is.

A basic concept of teleology is the principle of **utility,** which states that an act must result in the greatest positive benefit for the greatest number of people involved. Thus, any act can be ethical if it delivers positive results. All alternatives are assessed for potential outcomes, both negative and positive. The action selected results in the most benefits and the least harm for all involved. Minority and individual rights may be ignored for the benefit of the masses.

 Safety: Immunizations
- The outcome of immunizations is the prevention of given illnesses in the individual and, thus, the prevention of the spread of those illnesses to the community.
- The greatest good for the greatest number of persons is achieved with immunizations.

Deontology

Deontology is an ethical theory that considers the intrinsic significance of an act itself as the criterion for determination of good. A person must consider the motives of the individual performing the act, not the consequences of the act. For example, health care researchers might risk the well-being of a person participating in an experimental procedure for the sake of finding a drug that will save many people from suffering.

Situational Theory

The situational theory holds that there are no set norms, rules, or majority-focused results. Each situation must be considered individually, with an emphasis on the uniqueness of the situation and a respect for the person involved. Decisions made in one situation cannot be generalized to another situation (Pappas, 2000).

Caring-Based Theory

Caring-based theory is founded on the idea that ethical decisions are not made based on principles but are made with respect to relationships, communication, caring, responsiveness, and a desire not to hurt others. Caring-based theory focuses on emotions, feelings, and attitudes. This theory is sometimes referred to as the "voice of care" and is contrasted with the "voice of justice." Justice and caring are not considered mutually exclusive and can, in fact, be complementary (Beare & Myers, 1998).

ETHICS AND VALUES

Ethics and values which are closely related, which both enlightens and complicates the nurse's balancing the ethical principles of the client with those of the health care profession. Nurses must understand their own values in order to practice ethically. **Values** influence the development of beliefs and attitudes rather than behaviors, although they often indirectly influence behaviors. A **value system** is an individual's collection of inner beliefs that guides the way the person acts and helps determine the choices the person makes in life. Although nearly nothing in life is value free, the impact of values on decisions and resultant behaviors is often not considered. Values are similar to the act of breathing; one does not think about them until a problem arises.

Nurses often care for clients whose value systems conflict with their own. For example, a client with a value system of "grin and bear it" may be insulted by a nurse's attempts to offer pain medications. In order to ascertain those things that are meaningful to the client, the nurse must have an understanding of the client's value system (Figure 4-4). Furthermore, nurses must be aware of their own values, especially when they conflict with the values of clients.

Values Clarification

Values clarification is the process of analyzing one's own values to better understand those things that are truly important. Values clarification can increase nurses' self-awareness and help them better care for clients whose values differ from their own. Raths, Harmin, and Simon's (1978) classic work *Values and Teaching*, explained their theory of values clarification and three-step process of valuing, as follows:

- *Choosing:* Beliefs are chosen freely (without coercion)
- *Prizing:* The beliefs selected are cherished.
- *Acting:* The selected beliefs are demonstrated consistently through behavior.

Figure 4-4 *Clients' values determine those things that are meaningful to them.*

Because values are individual and not universal, the nurse should not impose personal values on clients. Providing ethical nursing care is directly related to the nurse's values. For example, the nurse who strongly values the sanctity of life may experience an ethical conflict when caring for a terminally ill client who refuses treatment that might extend life for a short time.

CODES OF ETHICS

Professions determine ethical behavior for their members. Several nursing organizations have developed codes as guidelines for ethical conduct. The Code for Licensed Practical/Vocational Nurses, developed by the National Federation of Licensed Practical Nurses, Inc. (NFLPN), is presented in Table 4-8. This code, providing motivation for establishing, maintaining, and elevating

TABLE 4-8 THE CODE FOR LICENSED PRACTICAL/VOCATIONAL NURSES

1. Know the scope of maximum utilization of the LP/VN as specified by the nursing practice act and function within this scope.
2. Safeguard the confidential information acquired from any source about the patient.
3. Provide health care to all patients regardless of race, creed, cultural background, disease, or lifestyle.
4. Refuse to give endorsement to the sale and promotion of commercial products or services.
5. Uphold the highest standards in personal appearance, language, dress, and demeanor.
6. Stay informed about issues affecting the practice of nursing and delivery of health care and, where appropriate, participate in government and policy decisions.
7. Accept the responsibility for safe nursing by keeping oneself mentally and physically fit and educationally prepared to practice.
8. Accept responsibility for membership in NFLPN and participate in its efforts to maintain the established standards of nursing practice and employment policies which lead to quality patient care.

From Nursing Practice Standards for the Licensed Practical/Vocational Nurse, by National Federation of Licensed Practical Nurses, Inc. (NFLPN), 1996, Garner, NC: Author. Copyright 1996 by Author. Reprinted with permission.

professional standards, was adopted by NFLPN in 1961 and revised in 1979 and in 1998. Each LP/VN entering the profession inherits the responsibility to adhere to the standards of ethical practice and conduct as set forth in this code.

A Code for Nurses was developed by both the International Council of Nurses (ICN) and the American Nurses Association (ANA) for the ethical conduct of registered nurses (See the ANA website for their code at www.nursingworld.org/ethics/chcode.htm). A code of ethics identifies broad principles for determining and evaluating nursing care but is not legally binding. Most state boards of nursing have authority to reprimand nurses for unprofessional conduct resulting from violation of the ethical code.

CLIENT RIGHTS

Culture defines rights and obligations. The dominant culture in the United States, however, holds the ethnocentric perspective that our rights and values are shared globally.

Clients have certain rights that apply regardless of the setting for delivery of care. These rights include, but are not limited to, the right to:

- Make decisions regarding their care (Figure 4-5)
- Be actively involved in the treatment process
- Be treated with dignity and respect (Figure 4-6)

Figure 4-6 *Clients have the right to dignity and respect and may keep personal articles in their rooms.*

Clients in short-term acute care agencies or extended care facilities are entitled to certain rights. The American Hospital Association (AHA) adopted *A Patient's Bill of Rights* in 1973. It identifies the rights and responsibilities of clients receiving care in hospitals (Table 4-9). This document was revised in 1992 providing health care workers with guidelines for treating clients ethically and encouraging all health care providers to protect the rights of clients.

COMMUNITY/HOME HEALTH CARE

The Client's Rights

The client's rights as outlined in Table 4-9 should be respected regardless of the setting for delivery of care. For care delivered in the home environment, for instance, the home health care nurse should discuss the client's rights with the client during the initial assessment (Figure 4-7).

ETHICAL DILEMMAS

When two or more ideals or values are in conflict, there is an **ethical dilemma.** In an ethical dilemma, a choice is to be made between the conflicting ideals or values. Questions remain in some cases, even after the dilemma seems to have been settled. Areas where ethical dilemmas frequently occur are euthanasia, refusal of treatment, and scarcity of resources.

Figure 4-5 *Clients have the right to information that will enable them to make decisions regarding their care.*

Figure 4-7 *A home health nurse explains a client's rights.*

TABLE 4-9 A PATIENT'S BILL OF RIGHTS

Introduction

Effective health care requires collaboration between patients and physicians and other health care professionals. Open and honest communication, respect for personal and professional values, and sensitivity to differences are integral to optimal patient care. As the setting for the provision of health services, hospitals must provide a foundation for understanding and respecting the rights and responsibilities of patients, their families, physicians, and other caregivers. Hospitals must ensure a health care ethic that respects the role of patients in decision making about treatment choices and other aspects of their care. Hospitals must be sensitive to cultural, racial, linguistic, religious, age, gender, and other differences as well as the needs of persons with disabilities.

The American Hospital Association presents *A Patient's Bill of Rights* with the expectation that it will contribute to more effective patient care and be supported by the hospital on behalf of the institution, its medical staff, employees, and patients. The American Hospital Association encourages health care institutions to tailor this bill of rights to their patient community by translating and/or simplifying the language of this bill of rights as may be necessary to ensure that patients and their families understand their rights and responsibilities.

Bill of Rights*

1. The patient has the right to considerate and respectful care.

2. The patient has the right to and is encouraged to obtain from physicians and other direct caregivers relevant, current, and understandable information concerning diagnosis, treatment, and prognosis. Except in emergencies when the patient lacks decision-making capacity and the need for treatment is urgent, the patient is entitled to the opportunity to discuss and request information related to the specific procedures and/or treatments, the risks involved, the possible length of recuperation, and the medically reasonable alternatives and their accompanying risks and benefits. Patients have the right to know the identity of physicians, nurses, and others involved in their care, as well as when those involved are students, residents, or other trainees. The patient also has the right to know the immediate and long-term financial implications of treatment choices, insofar as they are known.

3. The patient has the right to make decisions about the plan of care prior to and during the course of treatment and to refuse a recommended treatment or plan of care to the extent permitted by law and hospital policy and to be informed of the medical consequences of this action. In case of such refusal, the patient is entitled to other appropriate care and services that the hospital provides or transfer to another hospital. The hospital should notify patients of any policy that might affect patient choice within the institution.

4. The patient has the right to have an advance directive (such as a living will, health care proxy, or durable power of attorney for health care) concerning treatment or designating a surrogate decision maker with the expectation that the hospital will honor the intent of that directive to the extent permitted by law and hospital policy. Health care institutions must advise patients of their rights under state law and hospital policy to make informed medical choices, ask if the patient has an advance directive, and include that information in patient records. The patient has the right to timely information about hospital policy that may limit its ability to implement fully a legally valid advance directive.

5. The patient has the right to every consideration of privacy. Case discussion, consultation, examination, and treatment should be conducted so as to protect each patient's privacy.

6. The patient has the right to expect that all communications and records pertaining to his/her care will be treated as confidential by the hospital, except in cases such as suspected abuse and public health hazards when reporting is permitted or required by law. The patient has the right to expect that the hospital will emphasize the confidentiality of this information when it releases it to any other parties entitled to review information in these records.

7. The patient has the right to review the records pertaining to his/her medical care and to have the information explained or interpreted as necessary, except when restricted by law.

8. The patient has the right to expect that, within its capacity and policies, a hospital will make reasonable response to the request of a patient for appropriate and medically indicated care and services. The hospital must provide evaluation, service, and/or referral as indicated by the urgency of the case. When medically appropriate and legally permissible,or when a patient has so requested, a patient may be transferred to another facility. The institution to which the patient is to be transferred must first have accepted the patient for transfer. The patient must also have the benefit of complete information and explanation concerning the need for, risks, benefits, and alternatives to such a transfer.

9. The patient has the right to ask and be informed of the existence of business relationships among the hospital, educational institutions, other health care providers, or payers that may influence the patient's treatment and care. The patient has the right to obtain information as to the existence of any professional relationships among individuals, by name, who are treating him.

10. The patient has the right to consent to or decline to participate in proposed research studies or human experimentation affecting care and treatment or requiring direct patient involvement, and to have those studies fully explained prior to consent. A patient who declines to participate in research or experimentation is entitled to the most effective care that the hospital can otherwise provide.

11. The patient has the right to expect reasonable continuity of care when appropriate and to be informed by physicians and other caregivers of available and realistic patient care options when hospital care is no longer appropriate

12. The patient has the right to be informed of hospital policies and practices that relate to patient care, treatment, and responsibilities. The patient has the right to be informed of available resources for resolving disputes, grievances, and conflicts, such as ethics committees, patient representatives, or other mechanisms available in the institution. The patient has the right to be informed of the hospital's charges for services and available payment methods.

The collaborative nature of health care requires that patients, or their families/surrogates, participate in their care. The effectiveness of care and patient satisfaction with the course of treatment depend, in part, on the patient's fulfilling certain responsibilities. Patients are responsible for providing information about past illnesses, hospitalizations, medications, and other matters related to health status. To participate effectively in decision making, patients must be encouraged to take responsibility for requesting additional information or clarification about their health status or treatment when they do not fully understand

continues

TABLE 4-9   continued

information and instructions. Patients are also responsible for ensuring that the health care institution has a copy of their written advance directive if they have one. Patients are responsible for informing their physicians and other caregivers if they anticipate problems in following prescribed treatment.

Patients should also be aware of the hospital's obligation to be reasonably efficient and equitable in providing care to other patients and the community. The hospital's rules and regulations are designed to help the hospital meet this obligation. Patients and their families are responsible for making reasonable accommodations to the needs of the hospital, other patients, medical staff, and hospital employees. Patients are responsible for providing necessary information for insurance claims and for working with the hospital to make payment arrangements, when necessary.

A person's health depends on much more than health care services. Patients are responsible for recognizing the impact of their lifestyle on their personal health.

Conclusion

Hospitals have many functions to perform, including the enhancement of health status, health promotion, and the prevention and treatment of injury and disease; the immediate and ongoing care and rehabilitation of patients; the education of health professionals, patients, and the community; and research. All these activities must be conducted with an overriding concern for the values and dignity of patients.

*These rights can be exercised on the patient's behalf by a designated surrogate or proxy decision maker if the patient lacks decision-making capacity, is legally incompetent, or is a minor.

A Patient's Bill of Rights was first adopted by the American Hospital Association (AHA) in 1973. This revision was approved by the AHA Board of Trustees on October 21, 1992. Copyright 1992 by the American Hospital Association, 840 North Lake Shore Drive, Chicago, IL 60611. Printed in the U.S.A. All rights reserved. Reprinted with permission of the American Hospital Association.

Euthanasia

The word *euthanasia* comes from the Greek word *euthanatos*, which literally means "good, or gentle, death." In current times, **euthanasia** refers to intentional action or lack of action that causes the merciful death of someone suffering from a terminal illness or incurable condition.

Active euthanasia refers to taking specific action to hasten a client's death, such as removing a client who is in a vegetative state from a respirator. **Passive euthanasia** is working with the client's dying process. An example is not putting in a feeding tube to provide nourishment when the client cannot or will no longer eat.

Assisted suicide is a form of active euthanasia where another person provides a client with the means to end his own life. Some nurses look on assisted suicide as violating ethical principles on which the practice of nursing is based, whereas other nurses see assisted suicide as an ethical dilemma. For example, in answer to the question "Does assisted suicide violate the principle of autonomy?" it might be argued that *refusing* to assist a suicide violates a client's autonomy. Regardless of personal viewpoint, assisted suicide is still illegal.

Refusal of Treatment

The principle of autonomy is the basis of a client's right to refuse treatment. Only after treatment methods and their consequences have been explained can the client refuse treatment. The values of most health care providers are challenged when a client refuses treatment.

Honoring the refusal of treatments that a patient does not desire, that are disproportionately burdensome to the patient, or that will not benefit the patient is ethically and legally permissible (Curtin, 1995).

One possible ethical dilemma in this area relates to the use of ventilators for clients who would otherwise die. These clients continue to breathe as long as they are connected to the machine. What are the physical, emotional, psychological, and fiscal costs? What quality of life is prolonged by technology?

Scarcity of Resources

The use of expensive services is being closely examined because of the emphasis on containing health care costs. For example, the length of a hospital stay and the number of office visits allowed for individual clients are already set by many third-party payers. The availability of goods (such as organs) contributes to a scarcity of resources.

Clients often wait extended periods to receive donated organs. Allocating scarce resources is a major ethical dilemma: Who should receive the benefit of such a scarce and precious resource as a living organ? How should the determination be made? Currently, organ recipient selection is based on objective criteria such as organ availability, the degree of the recipient's need, donor/recipient match, and the recipient's readiness to comply with a lifetime of drug therapy and follow-up care. Should only objective criteria be used in determining who receives a donated organ, or should moral judgments also be made?

ETHICAL DECISION MAKING

Ethical questions (dilemmas) are not easy to answer. **Ethical reasoning** is the process of examining the issue in a methodical manner. Ethical decisions should not be made based on emotions. Ethical decision making is used in situations where conflicts of rights and duties exist.

Kinsella (2001) identifies eight steps to guide ethical decision making:

1. Recognize the ethical dimension of the issue.
2. Identify the parties involved, their relationships to each other, and their rights and responsibilities.
3. Examine the values involved, what ideals or principles are at issue.

Providing Ethical Care

- Find out about the client's wishes. Listen more than talk. (For example, it might be helpful to ask "If your heart stopped, would you want us to try to start it again?")
- Assess the client's understanding of the illness and treatment options available.
- Allow time for the client to explore values and to communicate.
- Facilitate communication of the client's desires to family and other health care providers.

Figure 4-8 *Ethics Committee Meeting (Photo courtesy of Photodisc)*

4. Compare benefits and burdens (positives and negatives) for each option.
5. Evaluate similar cases or ask colleagues about situations of ethical decision making.
6. Discuss, if possible, the issue with the relevant others.
7. Check legal and organizational policies so the decision meets legal, professional, and organizational standards.
8. Assess your comfort level with the decision, if uncomfortable reconsider.

NURSING AND ETHICS

Because nurses are accountable for protecting the interests and rights of the client, quality nursing practice involves making ethical decisions. Each practice setting has its own set of ethical concerns. Nurses must balance their ethical responsibilities to each client with their professional obligations.

Ethics Committees

Providing ethical health care requires both dialogue among health care providers and self-examination by each care provider. Many health care agencies now recognize the need for a systematic manner for discussing ethical concerns (Figure 4-8). Multidisciplinary committees (also referred to as institutional ethics committees) constitute one arena for dialogue regarding ethical dilemmas. Ethics committees can serve as a forum for discussion of ethical issues and lead to policies and procedures for preventing and resolving dilemmas.

Ethical Decision

An 80-year-old woman is in a persistent vegetative state as a result of a cardiovascular accident. She has always talked about "someday" signing a living will requesting that heroic measures not be taken, but her family wants "everything to be done that can be done." Whose wishes should prevail? What ethical principles would come into play in this decision process?

Nurse as Client Advocate

The nurse's first step in acting as a client advocate is to develop a meaningful relationship with the client. The nurse is then able to make decisions with the client based on the strength of the relationship. The nurse's primary ethical responsibility is to protect clients' rights to make their own decisions.

Nurse as Whistleblower

Whistleblowing refers to calling public attention to the unethical, illegal, or incompetent actions of others. The ethical principles of veracity and nonmaleficence are the basis for whistleblowing. Professionals are expected to monitor coworkers' abilities to perform their duties safely. Although nurses are expected to "blow the whistle" on incompetent health care providers, many are reluctant to do so because there are inherent risks in whistleblowing. Haddad (1999b) identifies some of the questions a person should consider before reporting unethical or incompetent behavior:

- Has the behavior in question created or is it likely to create serious harm?
- Have I gathered all appropriate information, and am I competent to judge this behavior?
- Do others confirm my information and judgment?
- Have all internal resources been exhausted to resolve the problem?
- Is it likely that past wrongdoing will be corrected or future damage prevented after the problem is reported?
- Is the harm created by whistleblowing likely to be less than the harm done by the behavior in question?

The False Claims Act (FCA) encourages whistleblowers to report evidence of fraud against the federal government (Polston, 1999; Sloan, 2002b).

Protection of privacy to whistleblowers is provided by federal law and state laws (to varying degrees). The fear of reprisal and the inclination to protect one's coworkers may keep a nurse from fulfilling the ethical obligation to report substandard behaviors.

Summary

- Laws are rules that guide personal interaction. They are derived from several sources and can be classified as public or civil.

- Within most states, the nursing practice act indicates the scope of practice for nurses. Standards have been developed to guide nursing practice.
- The nurse must be familiar with client rights. Care must be taken not to falsely imprison a client or violate the client's right to privacy.
- The client's chart is a legal document and should accurately reflect client status and care. Entries should be neat and timely.
- Informed consent is more than just signing a form. It requires a competent client understanding the risks, benefits, and alternatives to treatment.
- Whether to purchase malpractice insurance is a personal decision, but having one's own policy provides both coverage off the job and individual legal counsel.
- Incident reports are a risk management tool. They are not meant to be used for punitive purposes.
- Advance directives are instructions about health care preferences. They both protect the rights of the client and guide the family through difficult decisions.
- Ethics examines human behavior—those things that people do under a given set of circumstances.
- There is a connection between acts that are legal and acts that are ethical. Nursing actions are to be both legal and ethical.
- Ethical decisions are based on principles such as autonomy, nonmaleficence, beneficence, justice, veracity, and fidelity.
- Because ethics and values are so closely associated, nurses must explore their own values in order to acknowledge the value systems of their clients.
- Ethical codes that have been developed by nursing organizations such as the NFLPN, the ICN, and the ANA establish guidelines for the ethical conduct of nurses with clients, coworkers, society, and the nursing profession.
- The Patient's Bill of Rights is designed to guarantee ethical care of clients.
- The roles of client advocate and whistleblower enable nurses to protect their clients' rights and ensure the ethical and competent actions of their peers within the nursing profession.

Review Questions

1. Standards of practice are:
   a. different for each school of nursing.
   b. guidelines to direct nursing care.
   c. not legally binding.
   d. specific criteria on how to perform procedures.

2. The situation that violates client privacy is:
   a. copying information from the chart for a case study.
   b. discussing client status with clinical instructor.
   c. shutting the door and closing the curtain during a procedure.
   d. talking in the cafeteria about an interesting client.

3. Informed consent occurs when the:
   a. nurse discusses the surgical procedure with the client.
   b. client gives consent verbally.
   c. client understands the risks, benefits, and alternatives to treatment.
   d. client signs the consent form.

4. Nurses would use the Code for Licensed Practical/Vocational Nurses to:
   a. solve an ethical dilemma.
   b. develop a nursing care plan.
   c. seek an answer to a client care problem.
   d. understand the professional expectations required of them.

5. An ethical dilemma is a:
   a. choice to be made between right and wrong.
   b. problem with two equally unsatisfactory solutions.
   c. series of problems that the nurse encounters in each client care situation.
   d. problem the nurse cannot solve without the intervention of a physician.

References/Suggested Readings

American Hospital Association. (1992). *A patient's bill of rights.* Chicago: Author.

Awong, L., & Miles, A. (1998a). When an adolescent wants to forgo therapy. *AJN, 98*(7), 67–68.

Awong, L., & Miles, A. (1998b). When the physician disregards the patient's expressed wishes. *AJN, 98*(2), 71.

Badzek, L., & Gross, L. (1999). Confidentiality and privacy: At the forefront for nurses. *AJN, 99*(6), 52–54.

Bandman, E. L., & Bandman, B. (2001). *Nursing ethics through the life span* (4th ed.). Norwalk, CT: Appleton-Lange.

Beare, G., & Myers, J. (1998). *Adult health nursing* (3rd ed.). St. Louis, MO: Mosby.

Beyea, S., & Nicoll, L. (1999). Using ethical analysis when there is no research. *AORN Journal, 69*(6), 1261–1263.

Brooke, P. (2003). How good a SAMARITAN should you be? *Nursing 2003, 33*(6), 46–47.

Brown, S. (1999). Good Samaritan laws: Protection and limits. *RN, 62*(11), 65.

Curtin, L. (1995). Nurses take a stand on assisted suicide. *Nursing Management, 26*(5), 71–76.

Daly, B. (1999). Ethics: Why a new code? *AJN, 99*(6), 64–66.

Dempski, K. (2000). Serving as an expert witness. *RN, 63*(2), 65–68.

Douglas, R., & Brown, H. (2002). Attitudes toward advance directives. *Journal of Nursing Scholarship, 34*(1), 61–65.

Dunn, D. (1999). Exploring the gray areas of informed consent. *Nursing99, 29*(7), 41–44.

Edge, R., & Groves, J.R. (1999). *The ethics of health care: A guide for clinical practice* (2nd ed.). Clifton Park, NY: Thomson Delmar Learning.

Flick, C. (2002). Organ donation: A delicate balance. *RN, 65*(12), 43–46.

Flight, M. (2004). *Law, liability, and ethics* (4th ed.). Clifton Park, NY: Thomson Delmar Learning.

Flores, J. (2002). What if you're named in a lawsuit? *RN, 65*(12), 65–68.

Fowler, M. (1999). Ethics: Relic or resource? The code for nurses. *AJN, 99*(3), 56–58.

Frank-Stromborg, M., & Ganschow, J. (2003). How HIPAA will change your practice. *Nursing 2002, 32*(9), 54–57.

Gebbie, K. (2001). Privacy: The patient's right. *AJN, 101*(6), 69–73.

Haddad, A. (1998). Ethics in action. *RN, 61*(3), 21–24.

Haddad, A. (1999a). Ethics in action, *RN, 62*(7), 23–26.

Haddad, A. (1999b). Ethics in action, *RN, 62*(1), 23–26.

Health Resources and Services Administration, U.S. Department of Health and Human Services. (2000). *Fact sheet on the Healthcare Integrity and Protection Data Bank.* [Online]. Available: www.npdb-hipdb.org/pubs/fs/nh017fs.pdf

Helm, A., & Kihm, N. (2001). Is professional liability insurance for you? *Nursing 2001, 31*(1), 48–49.

Higginbotham, E. (2003). Does error + injury = negligence? *RN, 66*(5), 67–68.

Hill, S., & Howlett, H. (2001). *Success in practical nursing: Personal and vocational issues* (4th ed.). Philadelphia: W. B. Saunders.

Infante, M. C. (2000). Malpractice may not be your biggest legal risk. *RN, 63*(7), 67–73.

Joint Commission on Accreditation of Healthcare Organizations (JCAHO). (2002). *Accreditation Manual for Hospitals.* Oakbrook Terrace, IL: Author.

Joint Commission on Accreditation of Healthcare Organizations (JCAHO). (2000). *Restraint standards* [Online]. Available: www.jcaho.org/standard/restraint/restraint_stds.html

Keepnews, D. (2000). A systems approach to health care errors. *AJN, 100*(6), 77–78.

Kennedy-Schwarz, J. (2000). The "ethics" of instinct. *AJN, 100*(4), 71–73.

Kinsella, L. (2001). Truth telling in patient care: Resolving ethical issues. *Nursing 2001, 31*(12), 52–55.

LaDuke, S. (2000). The effects of professional discipline on nurses. *AJN, 100*(6), 26–33.

LaDuke, S., & Biondo, T. (2003). Protect your future with personal liability insurance. *Nursing 2003, 33*(2), 52–53.

Lee, N. G. (2000). Proving nursing negligence. *AJN, 100*(11), 55–56.

Maltz, A. (2001). Keeping pace with new patient privacy rules. *RN, 64*(9), 71–74.

Mock, K. D. (2001). Keep lawsuits at bay with compassionage care. *RN, 64*(5), 83–86.

Morris, M. R. (1998). Elder abuse: What the law requires. *RN, 61*(8), 52.

National Council of State Boards of Nursing, Inc. (2000). *NCSBN welcomes two more states to the nurse licensure compact.* [Online]. Available: www.ncsbn.org.public/nurselicensurecompact/nurselicensurecompact_index.htm

National Council of State Boards of Nursing, Inc. (2000). Why disciplinary databanks? Why the National Practitioner Data Bank (NPDB)? [Online]. Available: www.ncsbn.org/files/ publications/issues/vol171/ddb.171

National Council of State Boards of Nursing, Inc. (2002). What boards of nursing do . . . and what you can do [Online]. Available: www.ncsbn.org/public/regulation/boards_of_

National Federation of Practical Nurses, Inc. (NFLPN). (1996). *Nursing practice standards for the licensed practical/vocational nurse.* Garner, NC: Author.

News (2000). Health care fraud in Hawaii. *AJN, 100*(1), 21.

Nguyen, B. (1999). Protecting nurse whistleblowers. *AJN, 99*(12), 71.

Pappas, A. (2000). Ethical issues. In J. Zerwekh & J. Claborn (Eds.), *Nursing today: Transitions and trends.* (3rd ed.). Philadelphia: W. B. Saunders.

Polston, M. (1999). Whistleblowing: Does the law protect you? *AJN, 99*(1), 26–31.

Professional Update. (2000). JCAHO to amend its new restraint standards. *RN, 63*(7), 14.

Raths, L., Harmin, M., & Simon, S. (1978). *Values and teaching* (2nd ed.). Columbus, OH: Merrill.

Salladay, S. (1998). Ethical problems. *Nursing98, 28*(7), 30.

Sheehan, J. P., & Sullivan, G. H. (2001). Test your knowledge of the disciplinary process. *RN, 64*(8), 71–74.

Showers, J. (2000). What you need to know about negligence lawsuits. *Nursing2000, 30*(2). 45–48.

Sloan, A. (1999). Whistleblowing: There are risks! *RN, 62*(7), 65–68.

Sloan, A. (2001). The national data bank nurses need to know about. *RN, 64*(7), 65–69.

Sloan, A. (2002a). Liability insurance: Is your coverage adequate? *RN, 65*(10), 69–72.

Sloan, A. (2002b). Whistleblowing: Proceed with caution, *RN, 65*(1), 67–70.

Sloan, A., & Vernarac, E. (2001). Impaired nurses: Reclaiming careers. *RN, 64*(2), 58–63.

Sullivan, G. H. (2000). Keep your charting on course. *RN, 63*(5), 75–79.

Trinkoff, A. M., Zhou, Q., et al. (2000). Workplace access, negative proscriptions, job strain, and substance use in registered nurses. *Nursing Research, 49*(2), 83.

Trossman, S. (2003). Protecting patient information. *AJN, 103*(2), 65–68.

U.S. Department of Health and Human Services (2001). *National standards to protect the privacy of personal health information,* [Online]. Available: www.hhs.gov/acr/hipaa

Ventura, M. (1999a). Staffing issues. *RN, 62*(2), 26–30.

Ventura, M. (1999b). The great multistate licensure debate. *RN, 62*(5), 58–62.

Ventura, M. (1999c). When information must be revealed. *RN, 62*(6), 61.

White, L., & Duncan, G. (2001). *Medical surgical nursing: An integrated approach.* (2nd ed.). Clifton Park, NY: Thomson Delmar Learning.

Wolfe, S. (1999). Ethics on the job: A survey, quality vs. cost. *RN, 62*(1), 28–33.

Zerwekh, J., & Claborn, J. C. (2003). *Nursing today: Transitions and trends* (4th ed) Philadelphia: W. B. Saunders.

Ziel, S., & Gentry, K. (2003). Ready? HIPAA's here. *RN, 66*(2), 67–70.

Zollo, M. B., & Derse, A. (1997). The abusive patient: Where do you draw the line? *AJN, 97*(2), 31–35.

Resources

Partnership for Caring, 1620 Eye Street NW, Suite 202, Washington, DC 20006, 202-296-8071, 800-989-9455, www.partnershipforcaring.org

Living Wills, Films for the Humanities and Sciences, P.O. Box 2053, Princeton, NJ 08543-2053, 800-257-5126, www.films.com

The Living Bank International, P.O. Box 6725, Houston, TX 77265, 800-528-2971, www.livingbank.org

National Association for Practical Nurse Education and Service, Inc. (NAPNES), 8607 2nd Avenue #404A, Silver Spring, MD 20910, 301-588-2491, www.napnes.org

National Federation of Licensed Practical Nurses, Inc. (NFLPN), 893 U.S. Highway 70 West, Suite 202, Garner, NC 27529, 800-948-2511, www.nflpn.org

United Network of Organ Sharing (UNOS), 1100 Boulders Parkway, Suite 500, P.O. Box 13770, Richmond, VA 23225-8770, 888-894-6361, 804-330-8541, www.unos.org

The Health Care Environment

THE HEALTH CARE DELIVERY SYSTEM

MAKING THE CONNECTION

Refer to the following chapters to increase your understanding of the health care delivery system:

Basic Nursing
- **Legal and Ethical Responsibilities**

- **Arenas of Care**
- **Wellness Concepts**

LEARNING OBJECTIVES

Upon completion of this chapter, you should be able to:
- **Define key terms.**
- **Describe the three levels of service in the U.S. health care delivery system.**
- **Identify the members of the health care team and their respective roles.**
- **Describe the differences among financial programs for health care services and reimbursement.**
- **Explain the factors that influence health care delivery.**
- **Identify the challenges to providing care.**
- **Describe nursing's role in meeting the challenges within the health care system.**
- **Discuss the emerging trends and issues for the health care delivery system.**

KEY TERMS

capitated rate	Medigap insurance
comorbidity	preferred provider
exclusive provider	organization
organization	prescriptive authority
fee-for-service	primary care
health care delivery	primary care provider
system	primary health care
health maintenance	prospective payment
organization	secondary care
managed care	single-payer system
medical model	single point of entry
Medicaid	tertiary care
Medicare	

INTRODUCTION

A **health care delivery system** is a method for providing services to meet the health needs of individuals. The U.S. health care delivery system is experiencing dramatic change. The once economically thriving health care institutions now search for ways to survive. Health care providers seek cost-effective ways to deliver a larger range of services to consumers, who are demanding greater accessibility to quality affordable health care services. The increase in consumerism is fueled by the Internet, regulatory changes, the rising popularity of nontraditional therapies, and frustration of clients and their families feeling they have been mistreated by the system (Haugh, 1999).

Because nursing is a major component of the U.S. health care delivery system, nurses must understand the changes occurring within the system, and nursing's role in shaping those changes. This chapter explores the levels of health care services available, the settings offering those services, and the members of the health care team. The economics of health care, the challenges within the health care delivery system, and nursing's role in meeting those challenges are also addressed.

LEVELS OF HEALTH CARE SERVICES

Health care services are classified into three levels: primary, secondary, and tertiary. Table 5-1 provides an overview of the levels of care. The trend is toward holistic care (i.e., care of the entire person, including physiological, psychological, social, intellectual, and spiritual aspects).

Primary Care

The major purposes of **primary care** are to promote wellness and prevent illness or disability. Care is coordi-

TABLE 5-1   LEVELS OF HEALTH CARE SERVICES

TYPE OF CARE	DESCRIPTION	EXAMPLES
Primary	*Goal:* To decrease the risk to a client (individual or community) for disease or dysfunction *Explanation:* General health promotion Protection against specific illnesses	Teaching Lifestyle modification for health (e.g., smoking cessation, nutrition counseling) Referrals Immunization Promotion of a safe environment (e.g., sanitation, protection from toxic agents)
Secondary	*Goal:* To alleviate disease and prevent further disability *Explanation:* Early detection and intervention	Screenings Acute care Various therapies Surgery
Tertiary	*Goal:* To minimize effects and permanent disability associated with chronic or irreversible conditions *Explanation:* Restorative and rehabilitative activities to attain optimal level of functioning	Education and retraining Provision of direct care Environmental intervention (e.g., advising on necessity of wheelchair accessibility for a person who has experienced a cerebrovascular accident [stroke])

nated by the office of the primary care provider, usually a family practice physician, pediatrician, internal medicine physician, or family nurse practitioner. The U.S. health care system traditionally focused on treating illness rather than promoting wellness. Now, however, the focus is on health-promoting behaviors such as regular exercise, reducing fat in the diet, monitoring cholesterol level, and reducing air pollution. Wellness promotion activities may be directed toward the individual, the family, or the community.

Under the traditional **medical model**, our health care delivery system was not a *health* care system at all, but, rather, an *illness* care system. Services were directed toward care after disease or disability developed rather than preventive aspects of care. Today, however, there is more of an emphasis on the holistic promotion of wellness and on the preventive aspects of care.

Secondary Care

Services within the realm of **secondary care**—diagnosis and treatment—occur after the client exhibits symptoms of illness. Acute treatment centers (hospitals) still constitute the predominant site for the delivery of these health care services, but there is a growing movement to provide diagnostic and therapeutic services in locations that are more easily accessed by the population. These are often satellite care centers of a major hospital, where holistic care is promoted.

Tertiary Care

Restoring an individual to the state of health that existed before the development of an illness is the purpose of **tertiary** (rehabilitative) **care**. When a person is unable to regain previous functional abilities, the rehabilitation goal is to reach the optimal level of health possible. For example, a client regains partial use of an arm after experiencing a stroke. Restorative care is holistic in that the physiological, psychological, social, and spiritual aspects of the person are all addressed in the provision of care.

HEALTH CARE DELIVERY SYSTEM

The intricate U.S. health care delivery system involves many providers, consumers, settings, personnel, and services.

Providers/Consumers

Health care services in the United States are delivered by public (including official and voluntary), public/private, and private sectors. Consumers are the individuals who receive the health care services.

Public Sector

Tax monies fund public agencies, and these agencies are accountable to the public. Official (or governmental) agencies and voluntary agencies make up the public sector.

The U.S. Public Health Service (USPHS), the major agency that oversees the actual delivery of care services, is administered by the U.S. Department of Health and Human Services (USDHHS). Table 5-2 lists the USPHS agencies and their purposes. The Veterans Administration (VA), also financed by tax monies, has hospitals and clinics providing services to veterans of the armed services.

The states vary in the public health services provided. Generally, activities of local health departments are coordinated by a state department of health.

Local services provide immunizations, maternal–child care, and control of infectious and chronic diseases.

TABLE 5-2 AGENCIES OF THE U.S. PUBLIC HEALTH SERVICE

AGENCY	PURPOSE
Health Resources and Services Administration (HRSA)	Furnish health-related information; control programs of health care for the homeless; people with human immunodeficiency virus (HIV) and acquired immunodeficiency syndrome (AIDS); rural health care; organ transplants; and employee occupational health
Food and Drug Administration (FDA)	Protect the public from unsafe drugs, food, and cosmetics
Centers for Disease Control and Prevention (CDC)	Study and control the transmission of communicable diseases
National Institutes of Health (NIH)	Conduct research and education about specific illnesses
Alcohol, Drug Abuse, and Mental Health Administration (ADAMHA)	Serve as clearinghouse for information on substance abuse and mental health issues
Agency for Toxic Substances and Disease Registry (ATSDR)	Keep registry of certain diseases Provide information on toxic agents Study mortality and morbidity on defined population groups
Indian Health Service (IHS)	Furnish health care services to Native Americans, including health promotion, nutrition, maternal–child health, disease prevention, alcoholism, suicide prevention, and substance abuse
Agency for Health Care Research and Quality (AHRQ)	Serve as main source of federal support for research related to quality of health care delivery

Voluntary agencies also constitute an important part of the public sector of the health care delivery system. These not-for-profit agencies (e.g., the National Federation of Licensed Practical Nurses [NFLPN], the American Nurses Association [ANA], the National League for Nursing [NLN], and the American Medical Association [AMA]) can exert significant legislative influence. Other voluntary agencies, such as the American Diabetes Association and the American Heart Association, provide educational resources to health care providers and the general public. Voluntary agencies receive funds from individual contributions, membership dues, and corporate philanthropy.

Public/Private Sector

A blending of the public and private sectors in many areas of health care has gradually occurred following the inception of Medicare and the diagnosis-related groups (DRGs), discussed in an upcoming section. Federal regulations guide both the care provided to clients in private nonprofit and for-profit agencies by private physicians and the reimbursement to both the agencies and the physicians.

Private Sector

The private sector of the health care delivery system is composed mainly of independent health care agencies and providers, who are reimbursed on a **fee-for-service** basis (the recipient directly pays the provider for services as they are provided). Fee-for-service clients may have private insurance or use their own financial resources to pay for the services.

Settings

The various settings where health care is delivered include acute care hospitals, extended care facilities, outpatient settings, home health care agencies, schools, and hospice, which are discussed in Chapter 6, Arenas of Care.

Personnel and Services

Many personnel and services exist within the various health care settings. Large hospitals provide the greatest number of services. Other health care settings may provide some but not all of these same services. The service departments most commonly found in the various settings include nursing units, specialized client care units, diagnostic departments, therapy departments, and support services.

HEALTH CARE TEAM

Health care services are delivered by a multidisciplinary team (Figure 5-1). Table 5-3 lists the various health care team members, their educational requirements, and their roles. Nurses work daily with other team members, so they must understand the role of each team member.

Nurses have various roles when assisting clients to meet their needs. Table 5-4 identifies the most common nursing roles. Nurses function in independent, interdependent, and dependent roles. In the independent role, the nurse requires no direction or order from another health care professional (e.g., in deciding that a client's

Figure 5-1 *Members of the health care team work together for the benefit of the client.*

TABLE 5-3 HEALTH CARE TEAM MEMBERS

TEAM MEMBER	EDUCATION	FUNCTION/ROLE
Nurse (LP/VN, RN, and APRN)	LP/VN: 1 year RN: 2 to 4 year APRN (Advanced Practice Registered Nurse): 1 to 3 years post-RN	Emphasize health (wellness) promotion Use a holistic approach to assist clients in coping with illness or disability by providing nursing care, health and health care education, and discharge planning Formulate nursing diagnoses to guide plan of care Address the needs of the client (individual, family, or community) Assist physician Functions may vary by state and specialization
Physician (medical doctor [MD])	8+ years	Formulate medical diagnoses and prescribe therapeutic modalities Perform medical and surgical procedures
Dentist (both doctor of dental surgery [DDS] and doctor of dental medicine [DMD])	8+ years	Diagnose and treat conditions affecting the mouth, teeth, and gums Perform preventive measures to promote dental health
Registered pharmacist (Rph)	5 to 6 years	Prepare and dispense drugs for therapeutic use May be involved in client education
Physician's assistant (PA)	2 years (plus a master's degree for PA licensure, required in many states)	Provide medical services under the supervision of a physician
Registered dietitian (RD)	4+ years	Plan diets to meet special needs of clients Promote health through nutrition education and counseling May supervise preparation of meals
Social worker (SW)	4 years	Assist clients with psychosocial problems (e.g., financial, housing, marital) Make referrals to other facilities and support groups May assist with discharge planning
Respiratory therapist (RT)	2 years	Provide various therapeutic treatments for respiratory illnesses Administer pulmonary function tests
Physical therapist (PT)	4 years	Work with clients experiencing musculoskeletal problems Assess client's strength and mobility Perform therapeutic measures (e.g., range of motion, massage, application of heat and cold) and teach new skills (e.g., crutch walking)
Occupational therapist (OT)	4 years	Work with clients who have functional impairment to teach skills for activities of daily living
Speech therapist	4 years	Assist clients who have speech impairments to speak understandably or to learn another method of communication
Chaplain	8 years	Assist clients in meeting spiritual needs Provide individual counseling and support to families Conduct religious services

TABLE 5-4 NURSING ROLES

ROLE	DESCRIPTION
Caregiver: LP/VN and RN	Traditional and most essential role Function as nurturer Provide direct care Be supportive Demonstrate clinical proficiency Promote comfort of client
Teacher: LP/VN and RN	Provide information Serve as counselor Seek to empower clients in self-care Encourage compliance with pre-scribed therapy Promote healthy lifestyles Interpret information
Advocate: LP/VN and RN	Protect the client Provide explanations in client's language Act as change agent Support client's decisions
Manager: LP/VN and RN	Make decisions Coordinate activities of others Allocate resources Evaluate care and personnel Serve as a leader Take initiative
Expert: RN	Advanced practice clinician Conduct research Teach in schools of nursing Develop theory Contribute to professional literature Provide testimony at governmental hearings and in court
Case manager: RN	Track client's progress through the health care system Coordinate care to ensure continuity
Team member: LP/VN and RN	Collaborate with others Use excellent communication skills

edematous arm should be elevated). In the interdependent role, the nurse works in collaboration with other health care professionals, (e.g., in a client care conference where several members of the health care team together plan ways to meet the client's needs). In the dependent role, the nurse requires direction from a physician or dentist, (e.g., medications must be ordered by a physician or dentist before a nurse may administer them to the client). The degree of autonomy nurses ex-

perience is related to client needs, nurse expertise, and practice setting.

HEALTH CARE ECONOMICS

Cost has been the primary motivation of the reform movement in health care. Control of costs has shifted from the health care providers to the insurers, with the result being increasing constraints on reimbursement. The predominant method of paying health care costs was for years, fee for service, with little incentive for cost-effective delivery of care. All that is changing.

The U.S. health care system's financial base is composed of both public and private funding, resulting in administrative costs for health care reimbursement that are higher in this country than in countries with a **single-payer system** (a model wherein the government is the only entity to reimburse health care costs, such as in Canada). Health care expenditures in the U.S. are higher than any other nation, and most cost-containment measures have been ineffective in slowing the expenditure growth (Schieber, Poullier, & Greenwald, 1997). Despite the enormous expenditure of public funds, the United States has not found a way to provide health care coverage for all its citizens. Figure 5-2 shows the sources of the nation's health dollars in 2000.

Private Insurance

The private insurance model is the basis for the system of financing health care services in the United States. Private insurance companies constitute one of the largest sectors of the health care system. Currently, more than

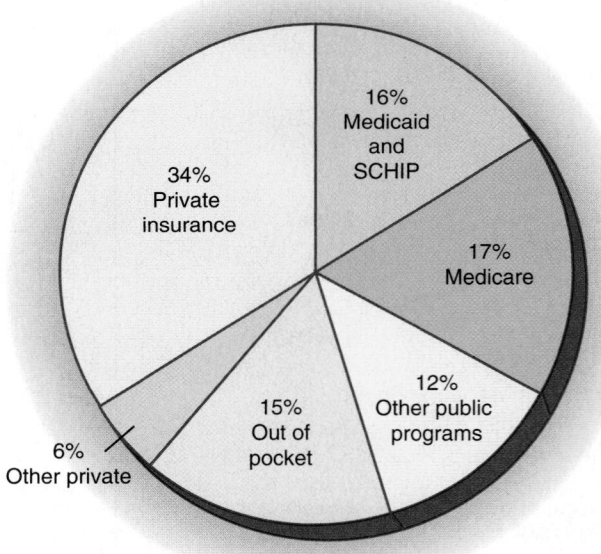

Figure 5-2 *Source of the Nation's Health Dollar in 2000. *Note: "Other Public" includes workers' compensation, public health activity, Department of Defense, Department of Veterans Affairs, Indian Health Service, state and local government hospital subsidy, and school health. (Figures from Health Care Financing Administration, 2002c.)*

1,000 private insurance companies exist (Feldstein, 1999). Payment rates to health care providers vary among insurance companies.

In the United States, insured individuals pay substantial monthly premiums for insurance coverage having high deductibles for health care services. For many, these costs may prove barriers to procuring necessary insurance coverage and health services. In addition, insurers will no longer pay for services that *they* deem unnecessary, effectively taking client care decisions out of the hands of physicians. The quality of care provided is now being monitored not only by providers (physicians), but also by third-party payers (insurance companies) and, ever increasingly, by consumers.

Medigap insurance to pay for costs not covered by Medicare is purchased from private insurance companies. Congress has restricted it to a basic plan with nine possible expansions (Abrams et al., 2000). Nursing home care costs are covered 39% by private insurance, about 10% by Medicare, and 48% by Medicaid (CMS, 2002a). Long-term care insurance benefits vary greatly depending on the insurance company.

Managed Care

Managed care is a system of providing and monitoring care wherein access, cost, and quality are controlled before or during delivery of services. Delivering services in the most cost-efficient manner possible is the goal of managed care. Managed care organizations combine financing and delivery of health care and try to control costs by monitoring delivery of services and restricting access to expensive procedures and providers.

Managed care was designed to provide coordinated services emphasizing prevention and primary care. The rationale behind managed care is to give consumers preventive services delivered by a **primary care provider** (a health care provider whom a client sees first for health care; typically, a family practitioner, internist, or pediatrician). The primary care provider is responsible for managing or coordinating all care of a client when illness makes referrals necessary. This approach is supposed to result in less expensive interventions.

Although managed care has existed for years, only within the past 20 years has it enjoyed national prominence. In 1973 the Health Maintenance Organization Act implemented two mandates. First, federal grants and loans were made available to **health maintenance organizations** (HMOs) (prepaid health plans that provide primary health care services for a preset fee and that focus on cost-effective treatment measures) that complied with strict federal regulations instead of the less-restrictive state requirements. Second, large employers were required to provide employees with an HMO option for health care coverage. From the beginning, HMOs have been a viable alternative to the traditional fee-for-service system.

Managed care is not a place but, rather, an organizational structure with several variations. One such variation is the HMO, which is both provider and insurer. Other variations are **preferred provider organizations** (PPOs), wherein members must use providers within the system in order to obtain full reimbursement but may use other providers for lesser reimbursement, and **exclusive provider organizations** (EPOs), wherein care must be delivered by the providers in the plan in order for clients to receive any reimbursement. In the past decade, there has been a great shift on the part of the population from private insurance to HMOs and PPOs (Feldstein, 1999).

Health Maintenance Organizations

Health maintenance organizations often maintain primary health care sites (although not necessarily) and commonly employ provider professionals. They use **capitated rates** (preset flat fees based on membership in, not services provided by, the HMO), assume the risk of clients who are heavy users, and exert control over the use of services. HMOs have used advanced practice registered nurses (APRNs) as primary care providers and precertification programs to limit unnecessary hospitalization. They also emphasize client education for health promotion and self-care.

Another common feature of HMOs is the practice of **single point of entry** (entry into the health care system through a point designated by the plan), through which primary care is delivered. **Primary health care** is the client's point of entry into the health care system and includes assessment, diagnosis, treatment, coordination of care, education, preventive services, and surveillance. It covers all of the services provided by a family practitioner (nurse or physician) in an ambulatory setting. Primary care providers (PCPs) are "gatekeepers" to the health care system by deciding which, if any, referrals to specialists are needed by the client. HMOs purposely limit direct access to specialists to reduce costs. Managed care plans assume much of the risk of providing health care and, therefore, encourage wise use by both providers and consumers. In 1976, there were 175 HMOs in the United States; by 2002 there were 650 (Centers for Education and Research on Therapeutics [CERTS], 2003).

Preferred Provider Organizations

The most common managed care systems are PPOs. A PPO is a contractual relationship between providers, hospitals, insurers, employers, and third-party payers forming a network wherein providers negotiate with group purchasers to provide health services for a specific population at a preset cost (Feldstein, 1999). Care received within the network is associated with the highest reimbursement; care received outside the network is associated with lower reimbursement, with the client paying the difference. Preferred provider organizations have been very popular in the United States. In fact, the number of PPOs has increased from fewer than 10 in 1981 to 1,070 in 2003 (First Mark, 2003).

Exclusive Provider Organizations

Exclusive provider organizations create a network of providers (such as physicians and hospitals) and offer the incentive of consumer services for little or no copayment if the network providers are used exclusively. If a member receives treatment outside of the network, no benefit is paid. For instance, a member who becomes ill and receives treatment while visiting relatives in another state would receive no benefits for the treatment.

Federal Government Plans

With the advent of Medicare and Medicaid in 1965, the federal government became a third-party payer for health care services. The Health Care Financing Administration (HCFA) is a federal agency that regulates Medicare, Medicaid, and Children's Health Insurance Program (CHIP) expenditures.

With the ultimate goal of curtailing spending for hospitalized Medicare recipients, the federal government created diagnosis-related groups (DRGs) to categorize the average cost of care for each diagnosis. A prospective payment system was then created based on the DRGs. **Prospective payment** is a predetermined rate paid for each episode of hospitalization based on the client's age and principal diagnosis and on the presence or absence of surgery and **comorbidity** (simultaneous existence of more than one disease process in an individual). Hospitals are reimbursed the predetermined amount regardless of the actual cost of providing services to the client. The prospective payment system, originally designed for Medicare, has been adopted by other agencies and insurance companies.

Medicare

In 1965, **Medicare** (Title XVIII) was signed into law as an amendment to the Social Security Act. It was originally intended to protect those older than 65 years from excessive health care costs. In 1972, Medicare was modified to also cover permanently disabled individuals and those with end-stage renal disease. The federal government through the Centers for Medicare and Medicaid Services (CMS) administers Medicare. Medicare Part A covers inpatient hospital care, home health care, and hospice care. It may pay for care in a skilled nursing facility but, there are many restrictions, and coverage criteria changes frequently. Medicare Part B partially covers costs for physician services, outpatient rehabilitation, and certain services and supplies not covered by Part A.

Limited skilled care and rehabilitation services in certified long-term care facilities may be paid if the client and the services provided meet specific criteria. Intermittent visits for skilled health care by a registered nurse may be reimbursed to certified home health care agencies. In 2003, it is estimated that Medicare will spend $254.8 billion for the care of its 40.7 million enrollees (CMS, 2002b).

Medicaid

Medicaid (Title XIX) pays for health services for low-income families with dependent children, the aged poor, and the disabled (Abrams, Beers, & Berkow, 2000). It is financed by both federal and state funds but is administered by the states. Each state determines who is "medically indigent" and qualifies for public monies, so services provided vary from state to state. Medicaid is the primary health financing program for disabled individuals and low-income families. This means-tested program provides funds only when all other financial resources have been exhausted. Services covered include physician services, inpatient and outpatient hospital care, diagnostic services, skilled nursing care, rural health clinic services, and home health services. States may choose to cover other services, such as dental, vision, and prescription drugs. Medicaid will spend an estimated $158.7 billion in 2003 (CMS, 2002b). It is the principal source of financial assistance for long-term care and pays for skilled home health care in all states. The optional benefit of personal care in the home is also covered in 29 states. There are 40.4 million beneficiaries enrolled in Medicaid (CMS, 2002b).

Children's Health Insurance Program

The Children's Health Insurance Program was created in 1997 as part of the Balanced Budget Act. The program is designed to provide health care to uninsured children, many of whom are members of working families that earn too little to afford private insurance on their own but earn too much to be eligible for Medicaid. It is a partnership between the federal and state governments to cover previously uninsured children. The states administer the program.

FACTORS INFLUENCING HEALTH CARE

Despite cost-containment efforts (such as DRGs, established by the federal government, and managed care, established by the insurers), the U.S. health care system still has problems with issues of access, cost, and quality. These issues are important for nurses to understand and are integral to any effort toward health reform.

Cost

Cost is a driving force for change in the health care system, as shown by the number of managed care plans, greater use of outpatient services, and shorter hospital stays. Maximum profits with minimum costs are the market forces dominating the current changes in the health care system.

PROFESSIONAL TIP

Impact of Prospective Payment System and DRGs

- Decreased length of client stay in hospitals
- More emphasis on preventive care
- Increased concern about consumer's (client's) response to care
- Increased number of critically ill clients in hospitals
- Clients sicker upon discharge from hospital
- Increase in outpatient care
- Client and family more responsible for care
- Greater need for home health care
- Mergers or closures of hospitals because of inordinate competition

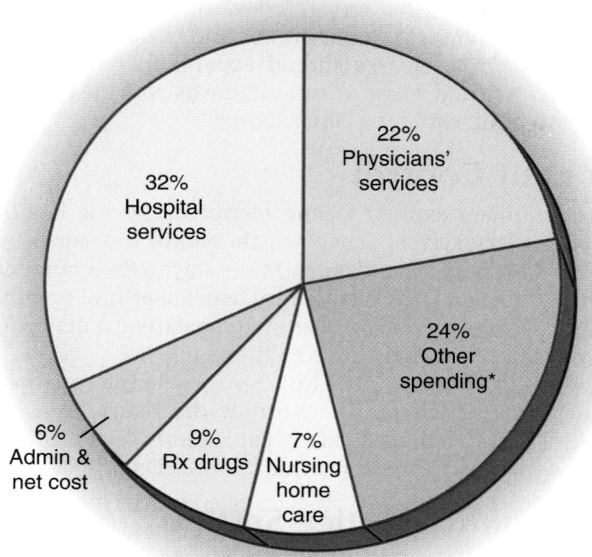

Figure 5-3 *Health Care Expenditures in 2000. (Note: "Other spending" included dental services, other professional services, home health, durable medical products, over the counter medicines and sundries, public health, research, and construction. (Figures from Health Care Financing Administration, 2002c.)*

The cost of providing health care has risen dramatically during the past 15 years. The U.S. government spends more on health care per person than does any other country. The use of federal funds for health care means that resources are not available for other areas of need, such as education, housing, and social services (Grace, 2001). Figure 5-3 illustrates health care expenditures.

The most cost-efficient programs in terms of administration are Medicare and Medicaid (HCFA, 1998). Private agencies and organizations are subcontracted to administer these programs. In contrast, some private small business plans use more than 40 cents of each dollar for administration. The cost of employee health care benefits is thus an expensive commitment for small businesses.

Three major factors increase the cost of health care: (1) an oversupply of specialized providers (fees are raised to maintain provider income in light of fewer clients); (2) a surplus of hospital beds (empty beds are a cost liability); and (3) the passive role assumed by most consumers (when someone else pays the bill, consumers typically are less concerned about cost) (Feldstein, 1999). Other factors contributing to the high cost of health care are the aging population, the increased number of people with chronic illnesses, and the proliferation of health-related lawsuits and the associated use of unnecessary services (e.g., additional diagnostic testing). Advanced technology has allowed more people to survive formerly fatal illnesses.

Access

Related to the issue of cost is that of access to health care services, which carries serious implications for the functioning of the health care system. Health care for many people is crisis oriented and fragmented because of

the high costs. Numerous people in the United States are unable to gain access to health care services because of inadequate or no insurance; thus, illness among these people may progress to an acute stage before intervention is sought. Their access is typically through emergency departments during acute illnesses. Emergency room and acute care services are very expensive compared to prevention and early intervention.

Medicare covers only a small portion of the medically indigent. The many underinsured individuals are neither poor nor old but are those who have jobs lacking adequate health care benefits or middle-class unemployed Americans. In addition to poverty and unemployment, other factors can hinder a person's ability to obtain insurance and/or health care services, including the following:

- Lack of insurance provision by employer because of prohibitive costs
- High costs of obtaining individual insurance
- Certain preexisting conditions
- Cultural barriers
- Shortages of health care providers in some geographic areas (especially rural or inner-city areas)
- Limited access to ancillary services (e.g., child care and transportation)
- Status as single-parent or two-income family, making it difficult for parents to take time from work to transport children to health care providers

Quality

Lee, Soffel, & Luft (1997) report that 30% to 40% of diagnostic and medical procedures performed in this country are unnecessary. This inappropriate use of resources can be traced to several factors, including:

- The litigious environment and resultant tendency toward defensive practice (e.g., ordering all possible tests instead of only those that the provider deems truly necessary)
- The widely held American belief that more is better
- Lack of access to and continuity of services and the subsequent misuse of acute care services

Quality may be sacrificed in an attempt to provide universal access to services in a cost-effective manner. For example, hospitals that reduce the number of nurses

---

CULTURAL CONSIDERATIONS

Barriers to Health Care Services

Certain cultural beliefs and values may prevent individuals from seeking health care. These may include the following:

- Belief in divine healing
- Refusal of care on holy days
- Belief that the individual taking the ill person to a health care facility is responsible for the ill person for the rest of that person's life after recovery
- Belief that illness is a result of sins committed in previous life
- View of prayer as a tool for deliverance from illness
- Belief that illness is God's punishment

(downsizing) risk endangering quality. Safety and quality are often compromised by inappropriately substituting unqualified personnel for LP/VNs and RNs in direct client care. The quality of care in hospitals decreases with cross-training of staff, greater use of unlicensed personnel, and reduction of full-time positions for nurses.

CHALLENGES WITHIN THE HEALTH CARE SYSTEM

The major challenges facing the U.S. health care delivery system, which also impact the control of costs, include the public's disillusionment with providers; consumers' and providers' loss of control over health care decisions; changing practice settings; decreased use of hospitals; vulnerable populations; and ethical issues.

Disillusionment with Providers

Greed and waste have been identified as major problems of the U.S. health care system (Maraldo, 2001). The cause of these problems is irrelevant to the public. Reform success means starting with public expectations of eliminating the greed of providers and the waste in the health care system. Furthermore, people in the United States have become suspicious of health care providers. The high level of esteem in which medicine has traditionally been held has eroded over the past few years. Consumers, increasingly tired of paying the high cost of care, are questioning medical practices and fees (Zerwekh & Claborn, 2000); however, the public is not as disillusioned with nurses. As reported in the *American Journal of Nursing* (AJN), a November 1999 Gallup poll reported that almost three-quarters of those surveyed rated the honesty and ethics of nurses as "high" or "very high" (Health Care News, 2000). Nursing received higher ratings than any other profession, including other health care professionals. *Nurse Week* and Sigma Theta Tau International commissioned another survey. It revealed that 92% of the public trusts health information provided by registered nurses.

Positive Perception of Nurses

Nurses are viewed as part of the solution, not the problem. If nurses were allowed to use their skills, the public believes they would significantly enhance quality and reduce costs. One survey (ANA, 1993a) asked consumers about receptivity to nurses' having expanded responsibilities. Respondents supported **prescriptive authority** (legal recognition of the ability to prescribe

---

CRITICAL THINKING

Perception of Nurses

What factors do you think have contributed to a positive perception of nurses? A negative perception? What can you do specifically to promote positive images of nursing to the public?

---

medications) for RNs and endorsed the role of nurses in performing physical examinations and managing minor acute illnesses. Nurses should expand their focus on holistic care and spend as much time as possible on prevention of illness and wellness issues.

Loss of Control

Consumers express feeling terrorized by the health care delivery system. They feel they have lost personal control over their health care. Many stay in their current jobs because of their health care benefits or give up employment mobility out of fear of being denied a new policy because of preexisting conditions.

Providers feel they have lost control over the care they provide to their clients. Increasingly, the insurance companies or the managed care organizations decide which care can and cannot be provided to the client.

Changing Practice Settings

Most nurses practice in hospitals and will continue to do so in the future. The increasing presence of severely ill clients requires that nurses who work in hospitals possess technical expertise, critical thinking skills, and interpersonal competence. Outside the hospital setting, there is an ever-increasing need for nurses in different areas of practice. Home health services, in particular, will need to continue expanding in order to meet the growing needs of the steadily increasing elderly population (Hull, 1997). Social and political changes are affecting nurses by creating the need for expanded services and settings. More nurses will be needed in the future because:

- The increasing elderly population requires more health care services.
- Admissions to nursing homes is increasing.
- The number of homeless individuals is increasing rapidly.

Reforms may displace some nurses from their current jobs. The demand for greater access to health care services will create many more jobs. More nurses will be needed for primary care, extended care, home care, and public health.

Decreased Hospital Use

In the early 20th century, hospital focus was providing care to those who had no caregivers in the family or community. These early institutions provided care, not cure (Grace, 2001). In the mid-1940s the focus of hospitals changed because of technology and the 1946 Hill–Burton Act, which funded the renovation and construction of hospitals. This resulted in sizable oversupply of hospital beds. To keep the hospital beds occupied, everyone was put in the hospital, for everything from a complete physical examination to specific diagnostic testing to acute care or surgery, and health care costs escalated.

The demand for hospital beds steadily increased from 1945 to 1982. After 1982, there was a steady decline in hospital admissions and the average length of stay (Grace, 2001). In 1995, there were 23.7% fewer inpatient days than in 1985 (Feldstein, 1999). Many small hospitals have closed because they could no longer compete with the large hospitals.

Hospitals are still the center of the U.S. health care system. They employ a majority of health care workers. Fewer clients are in hospitals today because of earlier discharge and the large number of procedures performed in outpatient settings. Clients hospitalized today need more nursing care because of their complex needs and severity of illness. Additional factors that have contributed to the decreased hospital population include:

- Greater availability of outpatient facilities and services
- Advances in technology
- Expectations/demands of third-party payers

The changes in reimbursement practices resulted in hospital restructuring (also referred to as redesigning and reengineering). Examples include mergers with larger institutions; development of integrated systems that provide a full range of services focusing on continuity of care, such as preadmission, outpatient, acute inpatient, long-term inpatient, and home care; and the substitution of multiskilled workers for nurses.

Vulnerable Populations

Meeting the health care needs of underserved populations is especially challenging. Groups that may be unable to gain access to health care services include children, the elderly, people with AIDS, rural residents, and the homeless and others living in poverty. Increasing poverty strains hospitals because Medicaid can no longer meet the needs of the medically indigent.

Our current health care system neglects the overall needs of children who are more likely than adults to be uninsured or underinsured. Children who are covered by health insurance have a greater degree of well-being.

Many parents have their children immunized only when the children are ready to start school, because immunization is a requirement for entry into the public school system. Preventive health care emphasizing early immunization should be encouraged and made available to children of all ages.

Rural areas have fewer health care providers and facilities than urban areas. Approximately 45% of those older than age 65 live in rural areas (Vrabec, 1995). Many people in rural areas have no health insurance because they tend to be self-employed or work for small businesses.

As of December 2000, the CDC estimated that 339,000 persons in the United States were living with AIDS (CDC, 2002a). It is estimated that at least 40,000

COMMUNITY/HOME HEALTH CARE

Cost of Home Health Care

- Since the advent of Medicare and Medicaid, home health care has grown rapidly. Because it is much less costly to provide home care, clients are sent home to recuperate.
- Expenditures for health care in the home are greatly increasing.

LIFE CYCLE CONSIDERATIONS

Health Care for Children

- Approximately one-third of the 71,731,000 children younger than age 18 who live in poverty are younger than 6 years of age (U.S. Census Bureau, 2002).
- Seven million of the 11 million children who are uninsured could have health care coverage today (RWJF, 2001).
- Six out of 10 parents whose children may qualify for Medicaid or State Children's Health Insurance Program (SCHIP) do not believe these programs apply to them (RWJF, 2001).
- Belief that their children do not qualify is highest in households where both parents work or when annual income is $25,000 or more (RWJF, 2001).
- By 1996, 90% or more of toddlers had received the most critical doses of vaccines for children by age 2 (CDC, 2002b).
- Nine percent fewer poor children complete the full series of immunizatons (National Academies, 2002).
- Each day 11,000 babies are born who will need immunizations (National Academies, 2002).
- Federal funds supporting the immunization network are shrinking (CDC, 2002b).

new infections occur each year (CDC, 1998). It is spreading most rapidly among women, children, and intravenous drug users and their sexual partners. Additional funding is necessary, and outpatient care settings (such as home care, hospices, and clinics) must be expanded to care for those affected.

The homeless and others living in poverty are often mobile, having no permanent address. They may not know which services are available to them or how to access the system except through inner-city hospitals. This creates a significant financial burden on these health care agencies. Illegal aliens, because of fears of being arrested and deported, may enter emergency departments under false identities and in acute distress, receive treatment, and then disappear.

Ethical Issues

The United States is struggling with the ethical issue of cost containment versus compassionate care. According to Hicks and Boles (1997), no country can provide all citizens with every health care service they need or desire. The U.S. health care delivery system has a dilemma of needs being greater than available resources. Difficult choices must be made to determine which needs are met and which remain unmet.

The national mentality, reflected in the expectation that everything must be done to save a dying person, has created an enormous drain on health care resources. There will be much debate about the ethics of decisions made about how scarce resources are to be allocated. Nurses must strongly advocate for just and ethical distribution of resources.

NURSING'S RESPONSE TO HEALTH CARE CHALLENGES

The United States will continue to seek ways to reform health care. There will be increasing implications for nursing. Some nurses feel threatened, but others are excited about changing the health care system into something better. The nursing profession responded to these challenges by proposing a plan for reform.

Nursing's Agenda for Health Care Reform

In 1991, in response to high cost, limited access, and eroding quality affecting the U.S. health care system, the nursing community wrote a public policy agenda that was endorsed by more than 70 organizations. *Nursing's Agenda for Health Care Reform* (ANA, 1991) provides a framework for health care policy changes and establishes a legislative program, through which to implement these changes. A major aspect of the proposal is that health care services be delivered in familiar, easily accessible, and consumer-friendly environments. Another essential aspect is that consumers are empowered in the area of self-care. A study in Maryland shows that universal coverage is feasible and will also save a substantial amount of money (Health Care News, 2000). A one-payment system with lower administrative costs accounts for the monetary savings.

Standardization of Care

A move toward standardization of care is another approach to the challenges of the health care delivery system. The Agency for Health Care Policy and Research (AHCPR) was established in December 1990, with the specific charge of reaching consensus within the medical/health care community about the diagnosis and treatment of certain illnesses and diseases. The AHCPR aspires to identify standards of diagnosis and treatment for high-volume, expensive disease conditions to which the health care community can be held. Currently, 18 AHCPR-published guidelines are available to the public and should be integral to nursing practice.

Advanced Practice

Advanced-practice nursing developed as nursing became more complex and specialized. Nurse practition-

ers (NPs), clinical nurse specialists (CNSs), certified nurse midwives (CNMs), and other advanced practice registered nurses (APRNs) have provided primary health care services to individuals since the late 1960s. Many of these individuals would have had inadequate or no access to services (Boyd, Lowes, Guglielmo, & Slomski, 2000). The APRN has advanced skills and in-depth knowledge in specific areas of practice (Stafford & Appleyard, 2001). Although there are differences among various advanced-practice roles, all APRNs are experts who work with clients to promote health and prevent disease.

There are more than 80,000 APRNs in the United States (Boyd et al., 2000). Advanced-practice nurses are moving toward independent practice. Advanced-practice nurses prescribe less-expensive diagnostic tests, have client visits comparible in length to that of physicians, and charge less for services because of the lower cost of professional liability insurance (Boyd et al., 2000). The single biggest obstacle to APRN practice is that most people are unaware of what APRNs can offer.

Currently, all states award APRNs some type of prescriptive authority (Pearson, 2000). In 10 states, this authority is complete and unrestricted and includes all classes of drugs (Pearson, 2000).

Public vs. Private Programs

The competition between the public and private sectors has encouraged quality and progress. Each setting has benefits as well as obstacles for health care recipients.

Public dollars are needed to help the poor and those who have no health care benefits through the workplace. To prevent the health care system from becoming a two-tiered process based on personal resources, both the poor and nonpoor and the privileged and nonprivileged should be enrolled in the same programs. Minimal national standards should be set, but local planning and implementation should be promoted.

The U.S. philosophy of states' rights is an obstacle to having national standards. Some consistency in the cost of services from coast-to-coast is needed with some local adjustments allowed.

Public Health

In the past decade, public health has visibly deteriorated. Immunizations, environmental concerns (conditions that may affect health), prenatal care, and analysis of the prevailing disease patterns in a community are included in public health services. Current public health problems include:

LIFE CYCLE CONSIDERATIONS

Rural Elders

Health care barriers experienced by elderly persons living in rural areas include the following:

- Lower Medicare reimbursement rates for rural hospitals than for urban hospitals contributed to the closure of some rural hospitals
- Fewer health care providers availabile
- Greater travel distances to obtain services

CRITICAL THINKING

Health Care System

Even with the advantages of technology, biomedical research, and state-of-the-art clinical equipment and facilities, many consider the U.S. health care system to be in crisis. From your perspective, is the health care system in a state of strength or weakness? Explain your response.

- Prevalence of overweight population
- Emergence of drug-resistant strains of tuberculosis and other infections
- Presence of toxic environmental conditions

Community Health

Prevention and primary care are the focus of community-based care. Nursing has a rich legacy of contributing community aid, as demonstrated by the work of pioneers such as Mary Breckenridge and Lillian Wald.

ISSUES AND TRENDS

As various trends appear, the delivery of health care services will continue to change. The challenge is to improve the nation's delivery of health care services by preserving nursing integrity. Nursing must be involved from the beginning of any change. Factors that will continue to shape reform of the health care delivery system include:

- Aging of the U.S. population
- Increasing population diversity
- More single-parent families and children living in poverty
- Growth of outpatient care and a greater demand for primary care providers
- Technological advances resulting in more services in outpatient settings (including the home)
- More states using managed care to provide the medically indigent with services
- Incentives for those participating in preventive activities
- Federal funds for health care provider education requiring service to underserved populations and areas
- Managed care dominating service delivery
- Focus on quality improvement

Summary

- The three levels of health care services are classified as primary, secondary, and tertiary.
- Health care services are financed and delivered by the public (official, voluntary, and nonprofit agencies), public/private, and private sectors.

- The health care team is composed of nurses, nurse practitioners, physicians, physician's assistants, pharmacists, dentists, dietitians, social workers, various therapists, and chaplains.
- Managed care organizations seek to control health care costs by monitoring the delivery of services and restricting access to costly procedures and providers.
- The primary federal government insurance plans are Medicare, which provides health care coverage for elderly persons and disabled persons; Medicaid, which is administered with the states to provide health care services for the poor; and CHIP, which provides health care to uninsured children.
- To achieve equity for all Americans, health care reform must address the three critical issues of cost, access, and quality of health care services.
- The challenges that the health care delivery system must overcome are the public's disillusionment with providers; provider and consumer loss of control over health care decisions; the decreased use of hospitals; the change in practice settings; ethical issues; and the health care needs of vulnerable populations.
- The Agency of Health Care Policy and Research aims to identify therapeutic standards to which the health care community can be held.
- A primary goal of the nursing profession is to provide health care services emphasizing prevention and primary health care, which will help reduce costs and increase the quality of health care.

Review Questions

1. When the goal of a health care service is to decrease the risk to clients for a disease or dysfunction, the type of care is called:

    a. primary.
    b. tertiary.
    c. exclusive.
    d. secondary.

2. Identified members of the health care team include:

    a. nurses, pharmacists, chaplains.
    b. nurses, physicians, ward clerks.
    c. therapists, housekeeping personnel, dietitians.
    d. dentists, social workers, maintenance personnel.

3. The primary federal government insurance plan(s) is (are):

    a. Medicaid and welfare.
    b. Medicaid and Social Security.
    c. Medicaid and diagnosis-related groups.
    d. Medicare and Children's Health Insurance Program.

4. The nursing role that protects the client and supports the client's decisions is:

    a. teacher.
    b. advocate.

c. caregiver.

d. team member.

5. The major health care problem for children is:

a. living in poverty.

b. having no transportation.

c. receiving substandard health care.

d. not receiving immunizations as infants.

References/Suggested Readings

Abrams, W. B., Beers, M. H., & Berkow, R. (Eds.). (2000). *The Merck manual of geriatrics* (3rd ed.). Whitehouse Station, NJ: Merck Research Laboratories.

American Nurses Association. (1991). *Nursing's agenda for health care reform*. Kansas City, MO: Author.

American Nurses Association. (1993a, September). *Consumers willing to see a nurse for routine "doctoring" according to Gallup poll* [news release]. Washington, DC: Author.

American Nurses Association. (1995). Managed care: Challenges and opportunities for nursing. *Nursing facts* (Item PR-27). Washington, DC: Author.

Boyd, L., Lowes, R., Guglielmo, W., & Slomski, A. (2000). Advanced practice nursing today. *RN, 63*(9), 57–62.

Centers for Disease Control and Prevention (CDC). (1998). *Combating Complacency—HIV Prevention, Geneva '98. Trends.* [Online] Available: www.cdcnpin.org

Centers for Disease Control and Prevention (CDC). (2002a). *HIV/AIDS Surveillance Report* [Online]. Available: ftp://ftp/cdcnpin.org/Surveillance/SurvRep/2002/nasrl3ol.pdf

Centers for Disease Control and Prevention (CDC). (2002b). *IOM Report—Calling the shots: Immunization finance policies and practice* [Online]. Available: www.cdc.gov/nip/registry/ss/irc-2001p24.pps

Centers for Education and Researach on Therapeutics (CERTS). (2003). *Annual Report.* [Online]. Available: http://certs/hhs/gov/aboutcerts/annualreports/year2/y2certs.pdf

Centers for Medicare & Medicaid services (2000). *The state of the Children's Health Insurance Program.* [Online] Available: www.cms.hhs.gov/schip/wh0700.pdf

Centers for Medicare & Medicaid Services (CMS). (2002a). *Program information,* June 2002, ed. [Online]. Available www.cms.hhs.gov/chart/series/sec1.pdf

Centers for Medicare & Medicaid Services (CMS). (2002b). *Program information,* June 2002, ed. [Online]. Available: www.cms.hhs.gov/chart/series/sec2.pdf

Dochterman, J., & Grace, H. K. (Eds.). (2001). *Current issues in nursing* (6th ed.). St. Louis, MO: Mosby.

Feldstein, P. J. (1999). *Health care economics* (5th ed.). Clifton Park, NY: Thomson Delmar Learning.

First Mark. (2002). *Preferred provider organizations list.* [Online]. Available: www.firstmark.com/fmkcat/ppo.htm

Grace, H. K. (2001). Can medical costs be contained? In J. Dochterman, & H. K. Grace (Eds.), *Current issues in nursing* (6th ed.). St. Louis, MO: Mosby.

Grace, H. K., & Brock, R. M. (2001). Solving the health care dilemma: What will work? In J. Dochterman & H. K. Grace (Eds.), *Current issues in nursing* (5th ed.). St. Louis, MO: Mosby.

Haugh, R. (1999). The new consumer. *Hospital Health Network, 73*(12), 30–34, 36.

Health Care Financing Administration (HCFA). (1998). *Medicare and Medicaid expenses, 1997* [Online]. Available: www.hcfa.gov/pubforms/finance/97/ch2n1216.htm

Health Care Financing Administration (HCFA). (2002c). The nation's healthcare dollar: 2000 [Online]. Available: www.hcfa.gov/stats/nhe-oact/tables/chart.htm

Health Care News. (2000). Maryland group shows universal coverage can work. *AJN, 100*(8), 20.

Hicks, L. L., & Boles, K. E. (1997). Why health economics? In C. Harrington & C. L. Estes (Eds.), *Health policy and nursing: Crisis and reform in the U.S. health care delivery system* (2nd ed.). Boston: Jones & Bartlett.

Hull, K. (1997). Hospital trends. In C. Harrington & C. L. Estes (Eds.), *Health policy and nursing: Crisis and reform in the U.S. health care delivery system* (2nd ed.). Boston: Jones & Bartlett.

Lee, P. R., Soffel, D., & Luft, H. (1997). Costs and coverage: Pressures towards health care reform. In P. Lee, C. Estes, & N. Ramsay (Eds.), *The nation's health* (5th ed.). Boston: Jones & Bartlett.

Maraldo, P. J. (2001). Nursing's agenda for health care reform. In J. Dochterman & H. K. Grace (Eds.), *Current issues in nursing* (6th ed.). St. Louis, MO: Mosby.

National Academies. (2002). *Strengthening America's vaccine safety net* [Online]. Available: www.national-academies.org/includes/shots.htm

News. (2000). High public esteem for nurses. *AJN, 100*(1), 26.

Pearson, L. J. (2000). Annual legislative update: How each state stands on legislative issues affecting advanced nursing practice. *Nurse Practitioner, 25*(1), 16.

Peck, S. P. (2001). Community nursing centers: Implications for health care reform. In J. Dochterman & H. K. Grace (Eds.), *Current issues in nursing* (6th ed.). St. Louis, MO: Mosby.

Schieber, G. J., Poullier, J. P., & Greenwald, L. M. (1997). U.S. health expenditure performance: An international comparison and data update. In C. Harrington & C. L. Estes (Eds.), *Health policy and nursing: Crisis and reform in the U.S. health care delivery system* (2nd ed.). Boston: Jones & Bartlett.

Stafford, M., & Appleyard, J. (2001). Clinical nurse and nurse practitioners. In J. Dochterman & H. K. Grace (Eds.), *Current issues in nursing* (6th ed.). St. Louis, MO: Mosby.

The Robert Wood Johnson Foundation (RWJF). (2001). *About covering kids* [Online]. Available: www.coveringkids.org/about

U.S. Census Bureau. (2002). *Poverty 2000* [Online]. Available: www.census.gov/hhes/poverty/poverty00/tables00.html

Vrabec, N. J. (1995). Implications of U.S. health care reform for the rural elderly. *Nursing Outlook, 43*(6), 260–265.

Zerwekh, J., & Claborn, J. C. (2000). *Nursing today: Transitions and trends.* (3rd ed.). Philadelphia: W. B. Saunders.

Resources

American Academy of Ambulatory Care Nursing, East Holly Avenue, Box 56, Pitman, NJ 08071-0056 806-256-2350 www.aaacn.org

American Nurses Association (ANA), 600 Maryland Avenue SW, Suite 100 West, Washington, DC 20024-2571, 800-274-4ANA (262), www.ana.com

National Federation of Licensed Practical Nurses, Inc. (NFLPN), 1418 Aversboro Road, Garner, NC 27529, 800-948-2511, www.nflpn.org

ARENAS OF CARE

MAKING THE CONNECTION

Refer to the following chapters to increase your understanding of areas of care:

Basic Nursing
- **Legal and Ethical Responsibilities**
- **Cultural Considerations**
- **Loss, Grief, and Death**

- **Assessment**
- **Pain Management**
Adult Health Nursing
- **The Older Adult**

LEARNING OBJECTIVES

Upon completion of this chapter, you should be able to:
- **Define key terms.**
- **List three reasons why there has been a significant change in the growth of nonacute care services.**
- **Distinguish among licensure, certification, and accreditation.**
- **Describe the role of the LP/VN as a member of the interdisciplinary health care team in various health care settings.**
- **Discuss the types of clients that would benefit from participation in a rehabilitation program.**
- **Identify the responsibilities of the LP/VN in acute care, rehabilitation, long-term care, home care, and hospice.**
- **List the various types of long-term care services.**

INTRODUCTION

The traditional arenas for providing care have been physicians' offices and acute care hospitals. Many nonacute arenas of health care are now available, including long-term care, outpatient settings, home health care, and hospice, with rehabilitation provided in any of these. Table 6-1 describes arenas of care, services provided, and the nurse's role. Most of these facilities must be licensed and certified and some have accreditation.

KEY TERMS

accreditation	licensure
adult day care	long-term care facility
assisted living	rehabilitation
certification	respite care
hospice	subacute care

LICENSURE, CERTIFICATION, AND ACCREDITATION

Several methods have been designed to ensure that the agency, facility, or service meets minimal standards of care. **Licensure** is a mandatory system of granting licenses according to specified standards and is regulated by each state. **Certification** is a voluntary process that establishes and evaluates compliance with rules and regulations but is required for any provider who seeks reimbursement from government funds. Because government funding is regulated by the federal government, certification rules are generated by the federal government. **Accreditation** is an additional confirmation of quality and generally indicates that the delivery of care and service is above minimum standards.

Licensure

All health care facilities must be licensed. A designated agency (often the Department of Public Health) is

TABLE 6-1　HEALTH CARE ARENAS

ARENA	SERVICES PROVIDED	NURSE'S ROLE
Acute care hospital	Diagnosis and treatment of illnesses (chronic and acute) Acute inpatient services Diagnostic procedures Surgical interventions Ambulatory care services Critical (intensive) care Rehabilitative care	Provide ongoing assessment Caregiver and educator Maintain client safety Coordinate care and collaborate with other health care providers Initiate discharge planning
Extended-care (long-term care) facilities (e.g., nursing homes, skilled nursing facilities)	Intermediate and long-term care for people who have chronic illnesses and are unable to care for themselves Restorative and rehabilitative care until client is ready for discharge home	Plan and coordinate care Provide care directed toward meeting basic needs (e.g., nutrition, hydration, comfort, elimination) Administer medications, treatments, and other therapeutic modalities Provide teaching and counseling
Outpatient (clinics, physician's offices, ambulatory treatment centers)	Treatment of illness (acute and chronic) Diagnostic testing Select surgical procedures	*Traditional role:* Prepare client for examination Check vital signs Assist with diagnostic tests *Expanded role:* Perform physical (or mental status) examination Provide teaching and counseling In some settings, advanced practice registered nurses (APRNs) act as primary care providers
Home health care agencies	Wide range of services, including curative and rehabilitative	Provide skilled nursing care Coordinate health-promotion activities (e.g., education)
Hospice	Care of individuals who have terminal illnesses Improve the quality of life until death	Promote comfort measures Provide pain control Support grieving families Educate family/client
Schools (school-based clinics [SBCs])	Federally funded to provide physical and mental health services in middle and high schools	Coordinate health-promotion and disease prevention activities Provide health education Treat minor illnesses
Community nursing centers	Direct access to professional services	Promote health and wellness Treat client's responses to health problems
Adult daycare centers/programs	Maintain safety for clients Provide social experiences Monitor health	Provide safe environment Encourage socialization Health assessment and promotion
Rural primary care hospitals (RPCHs)	Stabilize clients until they are physiologically able to be transferred to more skilled facilities	Perform assessments and provide emergency care
Industrial clinics	Maintain safety and health of workers	Conduct ongoing screenings Provide preventive services (e.g., tuberculosis testing) Coordinate health-promotion activities Provide education for safety Provide urgent care as needed Maintain health records

responsible for licensing health care facilities in each state. Annually each facility is visited by a team of surveyors to determine if the facility complies with the rules and regulations of the state. Any area of noncompliance results in severe sanctions and financial penalties for the institution. A limited amount of time is given to the facility to correct any deficiencies. The facility may lose its license to operate if residents' lives or well-being are threatened.

Certification

Any facility that chooses to be reimbursed by government funds, Medicare, and Medicaid must be certified. Regulations must be met for certification to be granted. State agencies perform this function under contract with CMS. In some states the long-term care survey for licensure and certification is done concurrently. The states have generally adopted the federal regulations but in some cases exceed federal regulations. Certification may not be granted to the facility not complying with regulations, resulting in no reimbursement from Medicare or Medicaid.

Accreditation

Accreditation is a voluntary (not required by law) process. Standards are issued by accrediting organizations, whereas rules and regulations are issued by state/federal licensure and certification agencies. The Joint Commission on Accreditation of Healthcare Organizations (JCAHO) has long been accrediting hospitals and skilled nursing facilities. The Commission on Accreditation of Rehabilitation Facilities (CARF) has been accrediting comprehensive inpatient rehabilitation programs since 1966. Rehabilitation facilities may seek accreditation from both groups.

ACUTE CARE HOSPITAL

Large acute care hospitals provide the greatest number of services. Other health care settings may provide some but not all of these services. The service departments most commonly found in acute care hospitals include nursing units, specialized client care units, diagnostic departments, therapy departments, and support services.

Nursing Units

Nursing units are composed of client rooms, where most nursing care is provided. Units often serve one particular type of client, such as cardiac, orthopedic, diabetic, surgical, pediatric, or obstetric. The nurse responsible for the unit may be called by several different titles, such as unit coordinator, nurse manager, or head nurse. Registered nurses (RNs), licensed practical/vocational nurses (LP/VNs), and nursing assistants provide the nursing care.

Specialized Client Care Units

Specialized units provide nursing care for specific needs of the clients. The LP/VN may work in these areas depending on experience, education, the size and loca-

tion of the hospital, and the number of RNs available. Examples of specialized units include the following:

- Emergency department (ED): Provides care to clients involved in all types of accidents and those confronted with medical emergencies such as heart attack or stroke
- Intensive care unit (ICU): Provides care to critically ill clients until they are stabilized and can be managed with routine nursing interventions on a regular nursing unit
- Coronary care unit (CCU): Provides care to clients who have had a heart attack or who have had heart surgery such as coronary artery bypass or valve replacement
- Mental health unit: Provides care to clients who are having difficulty with relationships, coping with everyday demands, or dealing with a crisis
- Psychiatric unit: Provides care to clients diagnosed as having mental illness
- Rehabilitation unit: Provides care to clients who must learn to regain the highest level of self-care possible following injury, accident, or illness
- Dialysis unit: Provides care to clients who need dialysis because of renal failure
- Hospice unit: Provides both care to clients who are dying and support to their families; may be a unit in a hospital or a freestanding unit
- Outpatient unit: Provides care to clients when admission to the hospital is unnecessary
- Home care: Provides care to clients in their homes when professional supervision and/or minimal care is required; has been added to many hospitals to provide continuity of care
- Client education unit: Provides teaching to clients, either individually or in groups, about specific client conditions or other health-related issues

Surgical Units

Care of the client just before, during, and after surgery is performed by the operating room (OR) and recovery room (RR) personnel. In addition to the main surgical unit, many hospitals also have a day surgery/ambulatory surgery unit. Clients come in a couple of hours before their scheduled surgeries and leave when recovered from the anesthesia. Total length of stay is shorter than 24 hours.

Diagnostic Departments

Diagnostic departments provide specialized tests that assist the physician in making a diagnosis.

Clinical Laboratory

Clinical laboratory personnel examine specimens of tissues, feces, and body fluids, such as blood, sputum, urine, amniotic fluid, and spinal fluid. Testing assesses values of normal components and of any abnormal components of these specimens.

Radiology (Nuclear Medicine)

X-ray studies are performed in the radiology department, along with computed tomography (CT) scans, mammography, ultrasound, arteriograms, venograms, echo-cardiograms, and magnetic resonance imaging (MRI).

Other Diagnostic Services

Other diagnostic services may include the following:

- Sleep center: Provides observation, testing, and monitoring of clients as they sleep, to identify sleep-related problems
- Electroencephalography (EEG): Records brain waves and ascertains electrical activity in the brain
- Electrocardiogram (EKG): Records electrical activity in the heart
- Electromyogram (EMG): Records electrical activity in body muscles

Therapy Departments

The function of the various therapy departments is to provide specialized treatments and/or rehabilitation services to clients to improve functional level in a specific area. Most hospitals have respiratory therapy and physical therapy departments. Some large teaching hospitals also have occupational therapy and speech therapy departments.

Support Services

Support services meet various other needs in providing care to clients.

Pharmacists mix and dispense medications to the various client care units. Nurses then administer the medications to the clients.

Dietitians supervise food preparation for all clients. They specifically choose the foods and calculate the amounts for special diets and provide client teaching for those clients on special diets.

Social workers help clients deal with psychosocial problems, providing assistance in areas such as housing, finances, and referrals to support groups.

Chaplains provide individual counseling to clients and support to families and assist clients in meeting spiritual needs.

The admission department handles the admission process by preparing necessary paperwork and ensuring that the ordered preadmission laboratory testing and x-rays are performed.

The business office oversees insurance and financial affairs upon client discharge from the health care agency.

Medical records, also called health information systems, maintains and stores all medical records for every client cared for by the health care agency.

Housekeeping and maintenance keep the physical facilities and equipment clean, in good repair, and in proper working order.

Role of the LP/VN

There are many opportunities for LP/VNs in acute care hospitals. They provide direct client care on the general nursing units. This may include assisting with personal hygiene and ambulation, checking vital signs, and administering medications and IV therapy. LP/VNs perform client assessments and work with RNs to formulate nursing diagnoses and write plans of care. After some years of experience and additional education in specific areas,

LP/VNs may work in specialized client care units, such as ICU, CCU, dialysis, and home care, as previously described.

LONG-TERM CARE

Long-term care refers to the various services provided to individuals having an ongoing need for health care. Traditionally, long-term care has meant a community-based nursing home licensed for skilled or intermediate care. The rights of residents of long-term care facilities are regulated by the Omnibus Budget Reconciliation Act (OBRA) of 1987 (Table 6-2). There is a great demand for this level of care, and there is also a market for other levels of long-term care. It is estimated that by the year 2030, more than 8 million seniors will be residing in nursing homes (American Health Care Association [AHCA], 1998). Currently 1.5 million persons live in 17,000 nursing homes. Of the residents, 90% are older than age 65, with 24% older than age 85 (AHCA, 1998).

The growing population of elderly persons has caused tremendous changes in health care delivery. Various housing options are now part of the package of services available. The least restrictive level of care, appropriate for the client's needs, is generally the most cost effective. The Joint Commission on Accreditation of Healthcare Organizations (JCAHO) has established standards for pain assessment and treatment in long-term care facilities (JCAHO, 2000).

Long-Term Care Facilities

A **long-term care facility** may be licensed for either intermediate care or skilled nursing care. Long-term care facilities provide services to individuals who have continuing health care needs but are not acutely ill, yet cannot function independently at home. Intermediate care facilities (ICFs) may be certified for Medicaid funding, but are not certified for reimbursement from Medicare. Skilled nursing facilities (SNFs) are eligible to be certified by both Medicare and Medicaid, but not all facilities choose to do so. These facilities were formerly called rest homes, nursing homes, or convalescent centers. An *extended care facility* (ECF) is any facility that provides care for a long period of time and could refer to either an intermediate or skilled facility. Every facility that receives government funds from any source is required by law to comply with OBRA regulations. It is estimated that 2 of 5 persons in the United States will need long-term care some time in their lives (AHCA, 1998).

Today's restorative philosophy of care directs the interdisciplinary team, which emphasizes assisting the client (usually called resident) to attain and maintain the highest level of physical, mental, and psychosocial function. The approach is holistic with family members part of the care team.

Many facilities have special units for the care of residents with specific problems, such as Alzheimer's, diabetes, and respiratory disorders.

Subacute Care

Subacute care is a concept designed to provide services for clients who are out of the acute stage of their illnesses but who still require ongoing treatments, skilled

TABLE 6-2   RESIDENT'S RIGHTS—LONG-TERM CARE

This is an abbreviated version of the Resident's Rights as set forth in the Omnibus Budget Reconciliation Act. This document must be given to all residents and/or their families prior to admission to any long-term care facility.

1. **The resident has the right to free choice, including the right to:**
   - choose an attending physician
   - full advance information about changes in care or treatment
   - participate in the assessment and care planning process
   - self-administration of medications
   - consent to participate in experimental research
2. **The resident has the right to freedom from abuse and restraints, including freedom from:**
   - physical, sexual, mental abuse
   - corporal punishment and involuntary seclusion
   - physical and chemical restraints
3. **The resident has the right to privacy including privacy for:**
   - treatment and nursing care
   - receiving/sending mail
   - telephone calls
   - visitors
4. **The resident has the right to confidentiality of personal and clinical records.**
5. **The resident has the right to accommodation of needs including:**
   - choices about life
   - receiving assistance in maintaining independence
6. **The resident has the right to voice grievances.**
7. **The resident has the right to organize and participate in family and resident groups.**
8. **The resident has the right to participate in social, religious, and community activities including the right to:**
   - vote
   - keep religious items in the room
   - attend religious services
9. **The resident has the right to examine survey results and correction plans.**
10. **The resident has the right to manage personal funds.**
11. **The resident has the right to information about eligibility for Medicare/Medicaid funds.**
12. **The resident has the right to file complaints about abuse, neglect, or misappropriation of property.**
13. **The resident has the right to information about advocacy groups.**
14. **The resident has the right to immediate and unlimited access to family or relatives.**
15. **The resident has the right to share a room with the spouse if they are both residents in the same facility.**
16. **The resident has the right to perform or not perform work for the facility if it is medically appropriate for the resident to work.**
17. **The resident has the right to remain in the facility except in certain circumstances.**
18. **The resident has the right to personal possessions.**
19. **The resident has the right to notification of change in condition.**

(As determined by Omnibus Budget Reconciliation Act [OBRA] of 1987)

nursing, and monitoring. The clients have complex medical needs. It is intended to fill the gap between the acute care hospital and the traditional long-term care facility (AHCA, 2000).

Subacute care facilities are usually part of a freestanding long-term care facility. Services may include intensive rehabilitation therapies, postsurgical services, wound and pain management, care for clients with acquired immunodeficiency syndrome (AIDS), oncology care, peritoneal dialysis, ventilator care, intravenous therapy, nutritional support, and cardiac monitoring. Many subacute care units specialize in one or two of these areas. Clients stay from 20 to 30 days. Thorough discharge planning with client teaching are essential components to the plan of care.

Continuing Care Retirement Communities

Continuing Care Retirement Communities (CCRCs) are designed to provide continuous care as the individual's health care needs change. Such levels are:

- Independent living apartments on the premises with housekeeping services and meals provided

- **Assisted living**—a combination of housing and services for those who need help with ADLs
- Full Care—short-term for persons recovering from a temporary disorder or permanent for long-term illnesses such as Alzheimer's disease. The CCRC health care facility may be licensed as either intermediate or skilled

Usually, a fee is charged upon entry and then a monthly fee. The client must show proof of adequate financial resources for acceptance into the system. The residents are secure knowing they will receive care for the rest of their lives. Most CCRCs want individuals to enter the system when they can live independently in the apartments. The CCRC health care facility may be certified for Medicaid for clients who exhaust their financial resources; it may also be certified for Medicare for clients qualified to receive such services. Neither Medicaid nor Medicare will pay for the independent living or assisted living areas of a CCRC.

Assisted Living

Assisted living provides housing and services for those who require assistance with ADLs. No nursing care is provided. These persons cannot live alone but do not need 24-hour care. The individual's independence and freedom of choice are maintained. This care may be available in a freestanding facility or as part of a long-term care facility or CCRC as previously described. The monthly fee covers meals, rent, utilities, housekeeping services, assistance with ADLs, health promotion, exercise programs, and transportation (Assisted Living Federation of America [ALFA], 2002).

There are an estimated 25,000 assisted living residences in the United States with 800,000 residents (ALFA, 2003; NCAL, 2001). The typical resident is a female (single or widowed) 82 years old or older (ALFA, 2003). Assisted living residences are licensed by the state. Costs range from $1,000 to $3,000 per month and are mainly paid from personal funds (NCAL, 2001).

Adult Day Care

Adult day care centers may be freestanding, located in a private home, or as a separate part of a long-term care facility. It is a protective setting for adults who are unable to stay alone but who do not need 24-hour care. A variety of services are provided. The centers are usually open 5 days a week and serve two or three meals. The daily or hourly fee does not include meals. Services may be comprehensive offering nursing care and some rehabilitation or limited to socialization. Working persons whose spouse or parent living with them cannot be left alone often use these services. Fifty percent of day care clients have some degree of cognitive impairment (NADSA, 2001).

Respite Care

Respite care may be offered by long-term care facilities, adult day care centers, or in private homes. It provides a break to caregivers for a few hours a week, for an occasional weekend, or for longer vacations. Supervision, meals, and planned activities are included.

Foster Care

Foster homes for individuals unable to live independently yet who do not require care in a health care facility are being investigated in some states. These homes are similar to the foster home concept for children.

Role of the LP/VN

Long-term care facilities probably offer more career opportunities for the LP/VN than any other type of health care described in this chapter. Small facilities may use the LP/VN as supervisor during the evening or night shift. The LP/VN might have charge of one unit with an RN as house supervisor in larger facilities. The nurse needs good assessment skills and the ability to make nursing judgments based on assessment findings. The LP/VN may also be expected to coordinate and supervise the work of nursing assistants. LP/VNs may take the Certification Examination for Practical and Vocational Nurses in Long-Term Care (CEPN-LTC™) given by the National Council of State Boards of Nursing (NCSBN). Those who pass the examination are certified in long-term care and may use the initials "CLTC" to signify their certification.

OUTPATIENT CARE

Outpatient care includes services provided without actually admitting the client to a health care facility. Same-day surgery (in and out within 24 hours) may be found as a unit in an acute care hospital or as a freestanding facility. Various clinics and treatment centers offer diagnostic testing, chemotherapy, physical therapy, and other services.

Role of the LP/VN

The major role of LP/VNs is preparing the client for the treatment or procedure, checking vital signs, answering questions, and doing discharge teaching. They may also assist with the test or procedure.

HOME HEALTH CARE

Home care is the fastest growing segment of health care and encompasses many services delivered to persons in their homes. Clients may receive IV therapy, chemotherapy, ventilator care, and parenteral nutrition at home. Nurse specialists often care for complicated cases involving wounds, diabetes, and respiratory or cardiac problems.

Medicare-certified agencies (7,747 in 1999) provide intermittent care to persons meeting the criteria for care (NAHC, 2001a). A registered nurse calls on the client a certain specified number of times each week to assess the client's condition, deliver skilled nursing care, and supervise the work of LP/VNs and unlicensed workers. Nursing assistants give personal care; check vital signs; and do positioning, transfers, and passive range-of-motion exercises. In addition, the agency may provide therapists and social workers to serve their clients, also on an intermittent basis. These services are time-limited by Medicare and are not reimbursable if the client does not require skilled care.

The home health agency may provide homemaker services for light housekeeping tasks, companion services, transportation for outpatient care, and pain management. The home health nurse must be aware of the availability of respite care for family members needing a break from the rigors of caregiving and may need to encourage them to do so. Client rights and responsibilities are listed in Table 6-3.

Role of the LP/VN

The role of the LP/VN in home care is expanding, with 40,849 LP/VNs working in home health care. Also, there are 129,304 RNs, 326,633 home care aides, and 14,098 physical therapists working in home care (NAHC, 2001). The LP/VN responsibilities vary among agencies. All nurses working in home care must have excellent assessment skills and a keen ability to identify actual and potential problems. Working with the family may be a greater challenge than meeting client needs. A major responsibility for the home health nurse is teaching the client and family. Clients with chronic health problems have ongoing needs after home health care is discontinued. They and their family caregivers must be taught the following:

TABLE 6-3 CLIENT RIGHTS AND RESPONSIBILITIES—HOME CARE

Clients receiving home health care services or their families possess basic rights and responsibilities. These include:

The right to:
1. be treated with dignity, consideration, and respect.
2. have their property treated with respect.
3. receive a timely response from the agency to requests for service.
4. be fully informed on admission of the care and treatment that will be provided, how much it will cost, and how payment will be handled.
5. know in advance if they will be responsible for any payment.
6. be informed in advance of any changes in care.
7. receive care from professionally trained personnel, to know their names and responsibilities.
8. participate in planning care.
9. refuse treatment and to be told the consequences of this action.
10. expect confidentiality of all information.
11. be informed of anticipated termination of service.
12. be referred elsewhere if denied services solely based on ability to pay.
13. know how to make a complaint or recommend a change in agency policies and services.

The responsibility to:
1. remain under a doctor's care while receiving services.
2. provide the agency with a complete health history.
3. provide the agency all requested insurance and financial information.
4. sign the required consents and releases for insurance billing.
5. participate in care by asking questions, expressing concerns, stating whether information is not understood.
6. provide a safe home environment in which care is given.
7. cooperate with the doctor, the staff, and other caregivers.
8. accept responsibility for any refusal of treatment.
9. abide by agency policies that restrict duties the staff may perform.
10. advise agency administration of any dissatisfaction or problems with care.

PROFESSIONAL TIP

Sharps Injuries in the Home

- Significantly more home health workers receive needle injuries than do hospital workers (Jagger & Perry, 2000).
- OSHA cannot regulate private homes.
- Home health employers are responsible for meeting OSHA requirements that are not site specific, including sharps with built-in injury protection.

The disease process
- Complications that may occur
- How to prevent complications
- Signs and symptoms of complications
- How to reduce risk factors, such as dietary adaptations and exercise programs

Medications
- Actions of medications
- Special administration guidelines, such as timing related to meals
- Side effects

Special skills
- Drawing up and administering insulin or other injectables
- Using a blood glucose monitor
- Changing dressings
- Monitoring vital signs
- Using special client care equipment, adaptive devices, and assistive devices

Documentation and communication
- How to keep records for nurse or physician visit; for example, blood glucose, blood pressure, and weight

- How and when to contact the home health nurse
- How and when to contact the physician
- How and when to contact emergency services

HOSPICE

Hospice is humane, compassionate care provided to clients who can no longer benefit from curative treatment and have 6 months or less to live. The special care is designed to provide sensitive support, allowing clients to be alert, pain-free, and have other symptoms managed so the last days are spent with dignity and quality of life at home or in a homelike setting. This is sometimes referred to as palliative care.

The first hospice in the United States began in 1974. Today, there are more than 3,000 programs that are estimated to serve 450,000 terminally ill clients and their families each year (Hospice Foundation of America [HFA], 2001).

The primary physician must refer the client to hospice. Care and support are provided to both client and family by a team consisting of the physician, nurses, counselors, therapists, social worker, aides, and volunteers. The team regards dying as a normal process and

PROFESSIONAL TIP

Hospice Settings

Hospice care may be implemented in a variety of settings: the client's home, a special area of hospitals or nursing homes, or freestanding inpatient facilities. Most clients receive care at home. In 1995, 77% of hospice clients died in their home, 19% died in an institutional facility, and 4% died in other settings (NHO, 1999).

Working in Various Facilities
What are the pros and cons related to working for an acute care hospital, home health agency, hospice, or long-term care facility?

does nothing to hasten or postpone death. Relief of pain and other distressing symptoms is provided. The client is supported to live as actively as possible until death. The family is supported to help them cope during the client's illness and in their bereavement after the client's death. Health care workers may also need support because the task of caring for the dying is often quite stressful.

Benefits for hospice are included in most private health care insurance, HMOs, and managed care; Medicare; and in 43 states plus the District of Columbia by Medicaid. Forty-four states have licensure laws for hospice programs. Some programs are certified voluntarily by Medicare and accredited by the JCAHO or Community Health Accreditation Program (CHAP) (HFA, 2001).

REHABILITATION

Rehabilitation is the process of helping individuals reach their optimal level of physical, mental, and psychosocial functioning. This is accomplished by modifying the effects of the disability, preventing complications, and increasing independence. The individual's self-esteem is increased, thus improving the quality of life. Rehabilitation works to increase the client's ability to complete the basic activities of daily living (ADLs) and the instrumental activities of daily living (IADLs). ADLs include grooming and hygiene, dressing, eating, mobility, and toileting. The IADLs include higher-level tasks such as using the telephone, household and money management, and driving a car. The goal is to teach clients to manage their own care when there is limited potential for regaining total independence.

The Interdisciplinary Health Care Team

An interdisciplinary health care team (IHCT) is the essential component to the rehabilitation process. Client and family are the focus and are encouraged to participate in the planning of care. The client determines the amount of family participation. The professional members of the team are selected based on the needs of the client. The physician, rehabilitation nurses, social workers, dietitians, physical and occupational therapists, a speech/language pathologist, recreational therapists, and mental health professionals are usually required to provide services.

Each discipline completes an assessment and shares this information at the care planning conference so that a consensus among members (including the client and family) can be reached. This avoids both duplication of services and fragmented care. A holistic approach is used so that the client's physical, mental, and psychosocial needs are identified.

Functional Assessment and Evaluation for Rehabilitation

Clients who need rehabilitation are screened before admission to a program. Assessments are completed by health care professionals whose services may be required by the client. The purpose of screening is to select the best setting for services. Criteria for admission to a program usually require that the client be:

• Medically stable
• Able to learn
• Able to sit supported for at least 1 hour per day and to actively participate in the program

Interdisciplinary programs may stipulate that the client has disabilities in two or more areas of function:

• Mobility
• Performance of ADLs
• Bowel and bladder control
• Cognition
• Emotional function
• Pain management
• Swallowing
• Communication

Several standardized assessment instruments are designed to evaluate cognition, speech and language, motor function, mobility, and the performance of ADLs. There are additional tools that identify the client's risk for pressure ulcer formation and potential for bowel and bladder management for incontinence. Refer to the AHCPR publication *Post-Stroke Rehabilitation, Clinical Guideline Number 16* for a complete description of assessment instruments.

Role of the LP/VN

Rehabilitation nursing is a specialty practice that requires specialized knowledge, skills, and attitudes. A sound knowledge base in the anatomy and physiology of the neurological, musculoskeletal, gastrointestinal, and urological systems is a prerequisite. The nurse must have excellent clinical skills in the areas of therapeutic positioning, range-of-motion exercises, transfers, ambulation, and ADLs. The nurse is responsible for planning measures to prevent complications, such as impaired skin integrity and contractures, and to implement interventions for dysphagia, incontinence, and other identified problems.

The nurse, as a member of the interdisciplinary team, may function as caregiver, client advocate, counselor, and coordinator of care. The nurse needs to understand the roles and responsibilities of each discipline and how to relate to each discipline.

Rehabilitation Settings

Rehabilitation takes place in a variety of settings. It begins during the acute stage of illness when the client's medical condition stabilizes. Rehabilitative services are often needed after discharge from acute care, necessitating transfer to a hospital inpatient program, an outpatient re-

SAMPLE NURSING CARE PLAN

THE CLIENT REQUIRING REHABILITATION

Mr. Jason, 65 years old, was admitted to a skilled nursing facility following hospitalization for a right cerebral hemisphere stroke. He is unable to purposefully change position without assistance. His gag reflex is weakened, swallowing is delayed, and there is coughing after swallowing. Mr. Jason has smoked for 50 years and is still doing so. Rehabilitation was initiated in the hospital. A feeding tube was put in place with the goal to assist Mr. Jason to regain his swallowing ability so the tube can be removed. Mr. Jason frequently expresses his discouragement with his dependency on the staff. He is married and lives in the community with his wife. Mr. Jason had been retired for 1 year before the stroke. Mrs. Jason works full time. Two adult children live in other states. Mrs. Jason hopes that her husband will regain adequate mobility skills so she can eventually take him home.

Nursing Diagnosis 1   *Impaired Physical Mobility* related to musculoskeletal, neuromuscular, and sensoriperceptual impairments as evidenced by inability to purposefully change position of body without assistance

Nursing Outcomes Classification (NOC)	**Nursing Interventions Classification (NIC)**
Ambulation: Walking	*Exercise: Ambulation*
Body Positioning: Self-Initiated	*Positioning*

PLANNING/GOALS	NURSING INTERVENTIONS	RATIONALE
Mr. Jason will maintain current level of range of motion in all joints.	Change position at least every 2 hours. Do passive range-of-motion exercises twice a day on affected extremities.	Prevents contracture formation and pressure ulcers. Hemiplegic limbs are flaccid immediately after stroke and then become spastic.
Mr. Jason will remain free of contractures.	Assist with active range-of-motion exercises on unaffected extremities. Teach to do self-range-of-motion exercises when condition permits.	Maintains joint mobility and prevents contracture formation, also increases strength and endurance.
Mr. Jason will begin program of progressive mobilization.	Teach Mr. Jason to move in bed: —Begin in supine position with the knees bent and feet flat in bed. —Raise the hips by pressing his heels down. —Stabilize the affected limb by nurse exerting pressure downward through the thigh just above the knee while assisting the client to lift the pelvis clear of the bed.	Increases the client's bed mobility. The recovery of a client with a stroke is dependent on the cooperative efforts of several interdisciplinary team members.
	Consult with physical therapist about program for progressive mobilization.	The physical therapist is an expert in mobility.

EVALUATION   Range of joint motion is preserved. No contractions noted. Progress in mobilization is achieved; movement in bed, transfers with 1 to 2 assists.

Nursing Diagnosis 2   *Impaired Swallowing* related to neuromuscular impairment as evidenced by weakened gag reflex, delayed swallowing, and coughing after swallowing

Nursing Outcomes Classification (NOC)	**Nursing Interventions Classification (NIC)**
Swallowing Status	*Swallowing Therapy*

continues

SAMPLE NURSING CARE PLAN

PLANNING/GOALS	NURSING INTERVENTIONS	RATIONALE
Mr. Jason will swallow without aspirating.	Consult with speech/language pathologist regarding video-recorded fluoroscopy for swallowing evaluation.	Makes a definitive diagnosis of impaired swallowing and is the basis for intervention.
	Serve semisolid foods of medium consistency. Use a commercial thickener for liquids. Avoid milk, citrus juices, and water.	Requires less manipulation in the mouth and allows concentration on swallowing rather than chewing. Liquids are more manageable when thickened. Milk and citrus juices stimulate production of saliva.
	Allow rest period before eating. Position client at 60- to 90-degree angle before, during, and for 1 hour after eating.	Decreases risk of aspiration.
	Maintain head in midline with neck slightly flexed.	Facilitates the passage of food through the pharynx.
	Face Mr. Jason, avoid haste.	Allows feeder to evaluate the eating process.
	Minimize distractions, keep conversation minimal.	Focuses the client's attention on eating.
	Allow Mr. Jason to see and smell food. Give verbal descriptions. Use regular metal teaspoon, give one-half teaspoon at a time.	Sensory cues promote awareness of eating.
	Place food on unaffected side of mouth. Teach to hold food in mouth, think about swallowing, and then swallow twice.	Buccal pocketing of food in the cheek on the affected side is common after a stroke.

EVALUATION   There are no signs of aspiration.

Nursing Diagnosis 3   *Situational Low **S**elf-Esteem* related to the functional impairments of inability to move and delayed swallowing as evidenced by verbal expression of discouragement

Nursing Outcomes Classification (NOC)	**Nursing Interventions Classification (NIC)**
Body Image	*Body Image Enhancement*
Hope	*Coping Enhancement*

PLANNING/GOALS	NURSING INTERVENTIONS	RATIONALE
Mr. Jason will verbalize acceptance of self, situation, and lifestyle changes.	Assess for signs of severe or prolonged grieving.	May indicate need for counseling.
	Assess client's interactions with significant others.	Others may reinforce the concepts of helplessness and invalidism.
	Listen in nonjudgmental fashion to comments about situation.	Builds trust and encourages verbalization of thoughts.

EVALUATION   Mr. Jason is progressing through all rehabilitation therapies and presents no signs of prolonged grieving.

habilitation program, a home rehabilitation program, or a skilled nursing facility. Entry into a rehabilitation program should reflect a consensus among the client, family or significant others, physician, and the rehabilitation program.

Hospital Inpatient Program

Hospitals may have a separate rehabilitation unit, or services may be available in a freestanding hospital specializing in rehabilitation services. The hospitals are staffed by a full range of rehabilitation professionals with RNs and a physician skilled in rehabilitation (physiatrist) available 24 hours a day. Hospital programs are generally more intense and comprehensive than programs in other settings, requiring greater physical and mental effort from the client.

Skilled Nursing Facility

The skilled nursing facility offering rehabilitation services may be hospital based or community based. Programs are similar to those offered in hospital settings, with a full range of services and health care professionals. Physician coverage varies, but professional nursing care is provided 24 hours a day. The program is usually less intense than a hospital program. Families should research the services available because they differ greatly from one facility to the next.

Outpatient Rehabilitation

Outpatient services offered by hospital-based rehabilitation programs range from occasional visits to three or four visits per week. Day hospital programs are another form of outpatient services but require the client to spend several hours per day for 3 to 5 days per week at the hospital. Availability of transportation is a prerequisite for all outpatient programs.

Home Rehabilitation

Some home health agencies provide a full scope of services, including nursing, all therapies, rehabilitation, and social services. The accessibility of services varies greatly depending on the availability of therapists in the area.

Summary

- There has been a significant increase in the growth of nonacute care settings.
- Medicare (federal funds) and Medicaid (state and federal funds) are major sources of health care payment, especially for the elderly and permanently disabled.
- Rehabilitation can be provided in a variety of settings.
- There is a need for the services and skills of the LP/VN in all health care services. Experience and additional education may be required for employment in special care settings.

Review Questions

1. Subacute care is most often provided:
   a. in a step-down unit of the hospital.
   b. in a special care unit of a skilled care facility.
   c. for clients who are terminally ill.
   d. for clients who require life support.

2. Which of the following clients would be most likely to benefit from rehabilitation services?
   a. Mr. J, 64 years old, had a stroke, is responsive and stable.
   b. Mrs. B, 89 years old, has Alzheimer's disease in the fourth stage.
   c. Miss Z, 26 years old, is recovering from pneumonia.
   d. Mr. K, 56 years old, has terminal cancer of the lung.

3. As a member of the interdisciplinary health care team, the LP/VN must be able to:
   a. participate in the planning of client care.
   b. plan the appropriate diet for clients.
   c. teach the new amputee how to walk with a prosthesis.
   d. provide alternative methods of communication for the client with recent stroke.

4. In the home health care setting, it is essential that the LP/VN possess skills in:
   a. advanced intravenous therapy.
   b. respiratory therapy treatments.
   c. physical assessment.
   d. planning and providing speech therapy.

5. In a long-term care facility, the LP/VN may serve as the:
   a. charge nurse of a unit.
   b. physical therapist.
   c. clinical nurse specialist.
   d. social worker.

References/Suggested Readings

American Association of Retired Persons (AARP). (1998). *A profile of older Americans.* Washington, DC: U.S. Department of Health and Human Services.

American Health Care Association (AHCA). (1998). *The looming crisis* [Online]. Available: www.ahca.org

American Health Care Association (AHCA). (2000). *Nursing facility subacute care: The quality and cost-effective alternative to hospital care* [Online]. Available: www.ahca.org/who/pubsubac.htm

Assisted Living Federation of America (ALFA). (2003). *What is assisted living?* [Online]. Available: www.alfa.org

Barker, E. (1999). Life care planning. *RN, 62*(3), 58–61.

Boon, T. (1998). Don't forget the hospice option. *RN, 61*(2), 30–33.

Bral, E. (1998). Caring for adults with chronic cancer pain. *AJN, 98*(4), 26–32.

Dochterman, J., & Bulechek, G. (2004). *Nursing Interventions Classification (NIC)* (4th ed.). St. Louis, MO: Mosby.

Feldkamp, J. (2002). The legal landscape of long-term care. *RN, 65*(4), 61–62.

Ferrell, B., & Coyle, N. (Eds.). (2001). *Textbook of palliative nursing*. Oxford: Oxford University Press.

Ferrell, B., & Coyle, N. (2002). An overview of palliative nursing care. *AJN, 102*(5), 26–31.

Grove, N. (1997). Helping families select a nursing home. *RN, 60*(3), 37–40.

Haddad, A. (2003). When should you suggest hospice? *RN, 66*(5), 27–30.

Hospice Education Institute (1999). *Definition of palliative care* [Online]. Available: www.hospiceworld.org

Hospice Foundation of America (HFA) (2001). *What is hospice?* [Online]. Available: www.hospicefoundation.org

Jagger, J., & Perry, J. (2000). Preventing sharps injuries in the home. *Nursing2000, 30*(12), 73.

Joint Commission on Accreditation of Healthcare Organizations (JCAHO). (2000). *Pain Assessment and Management Standards* [Online]. Available: www.jcaho.org/standard/pm_coll.html

Kennison, M. (1999). A case study in care. *RN, 62*(1), 46–48.

Kovner, C., & Harrington, C. (2003). Nursing care in assisted living facilities. *AJN, 102*(1), 97–98.

Lattanzi-Licht, M. E. (1998). *The hospice choice: In pursuit of a peaceful death*. New York: Simon and Schuster/Fireside.

Loeb, J., & Pasero, C. (2000). JCAHO standards in long-term care. *AJN, 100*(5), 22–23.

Mitty, E. (2003). Assisted living & the role of nursing, *AJN, 103*(8), 32–43.

Moorhead, S., Johnson, J., & Mass, M. (2004). *Nursing Outcomes Classification (NOC)* (3rd ed.). St. Louis, MO: Mosby.

National Adult Day Services Association (NADSA). (2001). *Adult day services fact sheet.* [Online]. Available: www.ncoa.org/nadsa/ADS_factsheet.htm

National Association for Home Care (NAHC). (2001a). *Basic statistics about home care.* [Online]. Available: www.nahc.org/consumer/hcstats.html

National Association for Home Care (NAHC). (2001b). *Hospice* [Online]. Available: www.nahc.org/HAA

Puopolo, A. (1999). Gaining confidence to talk about end-of-life care. *Nursing99, 29*(7), 49–51.

Resnick, B., & Fleishell, A. (2002). Developing a restorative care program: A five-step approach that involves the resident. *AJN, 102*(7), 91–95.

Skokal, W. (2000). IV push at home? *RN, 63*(10), 26–29.

The National Center for Assisted Living (NCAL). (2001). *Assisted living resident profile.* [Online]. Available: www.ncal.org/about/resident.htm

Ufema, J. (1999). Reflections on death and dying. *Nursing99, 29*(6), 56–59.

Waid, M. O. (1998). *Brief summaries of Medicare and Medicaid* [Online]. Available: www.hcfa.gov/medicare/ormedmed.htm

Resources

American Association of Homes and Services for the Aging (AAHSA), Suite 500, 901 E Street NW, Washington, DC 20004-2011, 202-783-2242, www.aahsa.org

American Association of Retired Persons (AARP), 601 E Street NW, Washington, DC 20049, 800-424-3410, www.aarp.org

American Health Care Association (AHCA), 1201 L Street NW, Washington, DC 20005, 202-842-4444, www.ahca.org

American Hospital Association (AHA), Chicago Headquarters (CH), One North Franklin, Chicago, IL 60606, 312-422-3000, www.aha.org

Assisted Living Federation of America, 11200 Waples Mill Road, Suite 150, Fairfax, VA 22030, 703-691-8100, www.alfa.org

Association of Rehabilitation Nurses (ARN), 4700 W. Lake Avenue, Glenview, IL 60025-1485, 800-229-7530, 847-375-4710, www.rehabnurse.org

Department of Health and Human Services (DHHS), 200 Independence Avenue, SW, Washington, DC 20201, 202-619-0257, 877-696-6775, www.hhs.gov/

Health Care Financing Administration (HCFA), 7500 Security Boulevard, Baltimore, MD 21244, 800-638-6833, www.hcfa.gov

Home Healthcare Nurses Association, 228 7th Street, SE, Washington, DC 20003, 202-546-4754, www.hhna.org

Hospice Association of America (HAA), 228 Seventh Street SE, Washington, DC 20003, 202-546-4759, www.nahc.org/HAA

Hospice Education Institute, 3 Unity Square, P.O. Box 98, Machiasport, ME 04656-8098, 800-381-1620, www.hospiceworld.org

Hospice Foundation of America (HFA), 2001 S Street NW #300, Washington, DC 20009, 800-854-3402, www.hospicefoundation.org

National Adult Day Services Association Inc. (NADSA), 8201 Greensboro Drive, Suite 300, McLean, VA 22102, 866-890-7357 www.nadsa.org/ncoa

National Association for Home Care (NAHC), 228 Seventh Street SE, Washington, DC 20003, 202-547-7424, www.nahc.org

National Citizens' Coalition for Nursing Home Reform, Suite 202, 1424 16th Street NW, Washington, DC 20036-2211, 202-332-2275, www.nccnhr.org

National Hospice and Palliative Care Organization (NHPCO), 1700 Diagonal Road, Suite 625, Alexandria, VA 22314, 703-837-1500, www.nhpco.org

National Rehabilitation Association, 633 S. Washington Street, Alexandria, VA 22314, 703-836-0850, www.nationalrehab.org

National Rehabilitation Information Center (NARIC), 4200 Forbes Boulevard, Suite 202, Lanham, MD 20706, 800-346-2742, www.naric.com

Communication

COMMUNICATION

MAKING THE CONNECTION
Refer to the following chapters to increase your understanding of communication:

Basic Nursing
- **Student Nurses Skills for Success**
- **Legal and Ethical Responsibilities**

- **Cultural Considerations**
- **Loss, Grief, and Death**
- **Assessment**

LEARNING OBJECTIVES

Upon completion of this chapter, you should be able to:
- **Define key terms.**
- **Discuss the process of communication and factors that influence it.**
- **Compare and contrast between verbal and nonverbal communication.**
- **Utilize therapeutic communication.**
- **Describe the psychosocial aspects of communication.**
- **Demonstrate proper telephone communication.**
- **Communicate effectively with clients and families.**
- **Communicate with special clients who are visually impaired, hearing impaired, speech impaired, unconscious, and non-English speaking.**
- **Communicate effectively with terminally ill clients and their families.**
- **Communicate effectively with other members of the health care team.**

KEY TERMS

active listening
aphasia
communication
congruent
dysarthria
dysphasia
empathy
feedback
hearing
listening
nonverbal
  communication

professional
  boundaries
proxemics
rapport
shift report
telehealth
telemedicine
telenursing
therapeutic
  communication
verbal communication

INTRODUCTION

Why study communication? Students in a nursing program have generally had a minimum of 17 years of communicating. Have you ever told another person a story and then heard the story repeated by someone else? Or have you ever played the game "telephone," where a message is whispered from one person to another and the last one states the message out loud? In both situations, when you hear the story or message again, it typically has changed from the original. When communicat-ing with a client, family, or another member of the health care team, it is important that the message be sent and received accurately.

This chapter addresses the process of communication; methods of communicating, including verbal and nonverbal communication; and factors that influence communication, such as age, culture, education, language, attention, emotions, and surroundings. Techniques that promote effective (therapeutic) communication are also described, as are barriers to communication, and examples of both are presented. Also explored are psychosocial aspects of communication, such as style, gestures, meaning of time, meaning of space, cultural values, and political correctness, and their importance to the health care system. Finally, communication with the client, family, and health care team as well as self-communication is discussed.

PROCESS OF COMMUNICATION

Communication is the process by which information is exchanged between the sender and receiver. The six aspects of communication are sender, message, method, receiver, feedback, and influences.

Sender

The person who has a thought, idea, or emotion to convey to another person is called the sender. Messages stem from a person's need to relate to others, to create meanings, and to understand various situations.

Message

The thought, idea, or emotion one person sends to another person is called the message. It is a stimulus produced by the sender and responded to by the receiver.

Method

The person sending the message must decide how to send the message. The method by which a message may be transmitted is verbal or nonverbal (Table 7-1).

Receiver

The physiological component involves auditory, visual, and kinesthetic processes. The person's psychological processes may enhance or hinder the receiving of messages. For example, anxiety may cause an individual to experience alterations in **hearing** (act or power of perceiving sounds), vision, or feeling.

The cognitive element is the "thinking" part of receiving. It involves interpreting stimuli and converting them into meaning, as in **listening** (interpreting sounds heard and attaching meaning to them).

Feedback

Feedback is a response from the receiver that enables the sender to verify that the message received was the message sent. When these are not the same, more messages are sent and received until the receiver understands the message sent by the sender.

Influences

Culture, age, emotions, language, and attention influence both the sender and receiver as well as the situation within which they find themselves. All of these elements together are called a person's frame of reference. These influences sometimes help communication, and sometimes they hinder communication. Figure 7-1 shows the process of communication with the influences affecting both the sender and receiver.

METHODS OF COMMUNICATION

There are two methods of communicating: verbally and nonverbally. Which is better? The answer is neither, or more accurately, it depends on what the sender is trying to communicate. Nonverbal aspects accompany virtually every spoken message. Since nonverbal communication is usually conveyed unconsciously by the sender, it is believed to be more honest than is verbal communication.

Verbal Communication

Verbal communication is the use of words, either spoken or written, to send a message. Methods of verbal communication include speaking, listening, writing, and reading.

TABLE 7-1 METHODS OF COMMUNICATION

SENDING	RECEIVING	DESCRIPTION	EXAMPLE
Verbal Speaking	Auditory		
	• Hearing	Receives auditory stimulus	Hears the client say, "My head hurts"
	• Listening	Interprets sounds heard and attaches meaning to them	Hears loud moaning in a client's room, and nurse checks if the client is in pain
Nonverbal or Verbal Writing Gestures Facial Expressions Body Posture Eye Contact Physical Appearance	Visual		
	• Sight	Receives a visual stimulus	Sees reddened area on heels
	• Reading		Documents on client's record
	• Observation	Interprets a visual stimulus by noting accompanying sounds	Makes note of moaning sounds when client turns to side and concludes that client has pain
	• Perception	Assigns meaning to a visual event	Decides client has pain when grimaces
Nonverbal Touch	Kinesthetic		
	• Procedure sensation	Performs nursing care	Gives the client a back rub
	• Caring sensation	Conveys emotional support	Places hand on client's shoulder

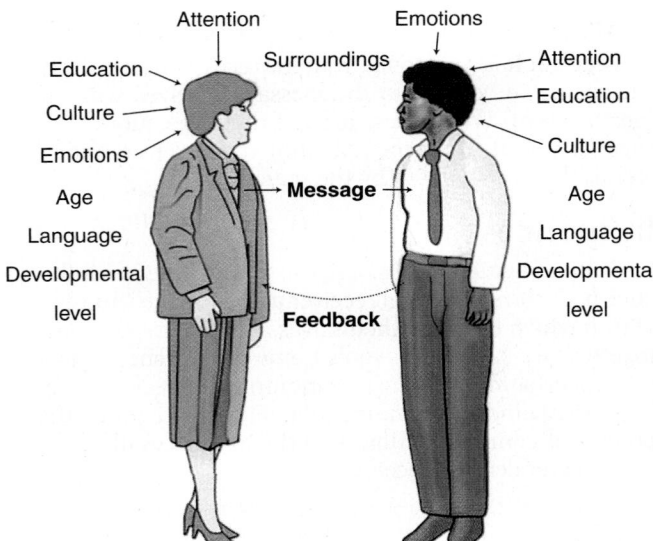

Figure 7-1 *Process of Communication with Influences Identified*

Speaking/Listening

Speaking is usually thought of as verbal communication, but the receiver of a spoken message must listen. For communication to take place both speaking and listening must occur. Have you ever spoken to someone in the same room with you and received a nonmeaningful, senseless response from that person, or no response at all? The other person probably was only hearing words but not listening to the message.

Communication experts say that people speak at a rate of 125 to 150 words per minute (WPM) but hear at a rate of 400 to 800 WPM. This extra time allows for distractions. Listeners are generally distracted because they are not concentrating on what is being said. Listening is one of the most difficult skills to learn and execute well.

Writing/Reading

The other method of verbal communication is writing. The receiver of the written message reads the words. The reader must understand the words and then attach meaning to them. With a written message there is generally no opportunity for immediate feedback. Therefore, great care should be taken to ensure clarity when composing a written message. A good example is charting. The physician may read the caregivers' notes after they have gone home, allowing no opportunity for immediate feedback. In such an instance, if the notes read that a client was "uncooperative," the physician would have little idea exactly what the caregiver meant. An entry of "refused to eat lunch, refused to get out of bed and sit in chair," however, is far more exact, illustrating the clarity in writing that is essential to good communication.

Nonverbal Communication

Nonverbal communication, or body language, is a method of sending a message without using speech or writing. Communication without words, is done in many ways including gestures, facial expressions, posture and gait, tone of voice, touch, eye contact, body position, and physical appearance.

Nonverbal communication, which is part learned behavior and part instinct is generally unconscious. Feelings are believed to be most honestly expressed nonverbally because there is little conscious control over nonverbal communication.

Clients are particularly sensitive to nonverbal messages and seem to believe them. Nurses must therefore make every effort to be aware of the nonverbal messages they may be sending to clients. Consider, for example, the nursing skills that are not pleasant yet must be done. How would the client feel if the nurse had a facial expression of disgust or revulsion when emptying a bed pan?

Nurses must also be aware of and sensitive to the client's nonverbal messages. Many clients do not want to bother "busy" nurses, so they say they are fine or do not need anything when in fact they do. The perceptive nurse will observe nonverbal signs such as clenched fists, stiff posture, or a frowning expression and know that something is not right. The nurse would then proceed with further assessment to determine the reason the client is sending those nonverbal clues.

Gestures

Gestures are often referred to as "talking with hands." Gestures may be used to help clarify a verbal message, to emphasize an idea, to hold another's attention, or to relieve stress. Fingertapping, fidgeting, or ring twisting generally indicates tension, nervousness, or impatience. Shaking a fist indicates anger, whereas pointing may be used to clarify directions.

Facial Expressions

Although some people have very expressive faces, others do not. A big smile is easily interpreted as indicating happiness. Eyebrows can be very expressive, showing surprise, worry, thoughtfulness, or displeasure. The manner in which the forehead is wrinkled also sends a message.

Nurses must be very aware of their own facial expressions, especially when caring for a client under "unpleasant" conditions, such as when a client is vomiting or suffering from bowel incontinence. An expression of displeasure manifested as a "curled-up" nose or disgust is easily identified by the client. The client, often already embarrassed at requiring such care, will be reassured and comforted by a nurse's facial expression indicating caring, concern, and empathy.

Posture and Gait

Good posture, with the head held up, and a purposeful gait are usually interpreted as meaning self-confidence, competence, and a positive self-image. Stooped shoulders, a downward-held head, and a shuffling gait generally convey low self-esteem, depression, lack of confidence, or apathy.

CULTURAL CONSIDERATIONS

Eye Contact

In some Asian cultures it is considered rude or disrespectful to make direct eye contact.

Tone of Voice

Tone of voice has been estimated to convey 23% of the context of a message. When the same words are said in different tones of voice, they can have very different meanings. Tone of voice might be pleasant, sincere, sorrowful, sarcastic, joyful, or angry.

Touch

Touch is a simple yet powerful form of nonverbal communication that even a newborn infant can understand. Touch can communicate caring, understanding, encouragement, warmth, reassurance, or affection. Of course, touch can also communicate anger, displeasure, or a lack or caring and understanding.

Many nursing tasks involve touching the client (i.e., bathing, dressing changes, ambulating). Touch, along with other nonverbal communication such as facial expression, posture, eye contact, and tone of voice, will convey the nurse's caring and acceptance. Most clients accept touch as an integral part of nursing care when it is done appropriately and professionally.

Eye Contact

Eyes, it is said, mirror the soul. Have you ever seen joy, sadness, pain, or laughter in someone's eyes? It is very difficult to control these messages of the eyes.

Eye contact is generally interpreted as indicating interest and attention, whereas lack of eye contact is thought to indicate avoidance, disinterest, or discomfort.

Body Position

Body position is often a good indicator of a person's attitude. For example, crossed arms generally indicate withdrawal, although the person could just be cold. Open body positions, with the arms held freely at the sides, are usually taken to mean a receptive attitude.

Physical Appearance

A person's physical appearance says a great deal about that person. A clean, neat, appropriately dressed individual conveys a positive self-image, knowledge, and competence. A dirty, sloppy, or inappropriately dressed person conveys the message of "I don't care how I look," with the potential implication of "maybe I am not too knowledgeable or competent," or "I am sloppy in what I do."

It is very important for every nurse to be clean, neat, and professionally dressed. Clients and families understand the nonverbal message that appearance conveys. Appearance does influence communication.

INFLUENCES ON COMMUNICATION

Communication involves more than just sending and receiving verbal and nonverbal messages. How a person sends or receives a message is influenced by such factors as age, education, emotions, culture, and language. Attention to the message and the surroundings are other influences. These factors must be taken into account for accurate communication to take place.

Age

Factors related to age affect communication. For instance, communicating with a child is different from communicating with an adult and depends on the child's age. Nonverbal communication, particularly touch, and facial expression can be understood by infants. Before learning to understand words, a child can interpret tone of voice and gestures. Preschool children respond well to communication involving toys or play situations. They should be allowed some choices, but no more than two alternatives should be offered. As the child's vocabulary increases, more verbal communication can take place.

Elderly persons may have some degree of hearing loss or a slowed response time. The nurse should face the elderly client when speaking and allow time for a response. The client should be addressed as "Mr." or "Ms." unless he or she asks to be called by his or her first name. These measures reflect respect to the individual from the caregiver (Figure 7-2).

Figure 7-2 *Face elderly clients when addressing them and allow adequate response time. A warm touch on the hand or arm will communicate caring and respect.*

Developmental Level

Age and developmental level do not necessarily go hand-in-hand. Individuals with mental retardation or developmental delays will communicate at their level of development, not at what is usually expected for their chronological age.

Education

Education is another strong influence on communication. Vocabulary generally increases as well as the ability to discuss and understand concepts and abstract ideas.

Emotions

A person's emotional state greatly influences how messages are sent or received. Someone who is very anxious or upset, for example, may not hear what is said or may interpret the message differently than the sender intended. This same person typically speaks in an abrupt manner, loudly, and in harsh tones. The depressed person, on the other hand, typically says very little, speaking only one or two words or in very short sentences.

Culture

Each culture has its own standards of communication, especially with regard to nonverbal behavior. In the United States, for example, eye contact is considered a sign of openness and honesty. Those of Spanish heritage, however, believe eye contact to be disrespectful. Similarly, in many parts of Europe, a kiss on the cheek between two men is accepted. People from other parts of the world, however, may look suspiciously on this behavior.

Language

Language certainly influences communication. Speaking the same language assists people in understanding each other, although regional accents or dialects of a language can inhibit communication and understanding. When verbal communication comes to a standstill, nonverbal communication is often employed to assist. Any nurse who works in an area where there is a predominant second language should learn a few words or phrases in that language to help put clients at ease and to facilitate their understanding.

Attention

The amount of attention each individual focuses on a given communication greatly affects the outcome. In selective listening, the receiver hears only what he wants or expects to hear. Pain or discomfort, physical or mental, may result in preoccupation, limiting the attention given to the communication.

Surroundings

Most people do not want to talk about the intimate details of their health care concerns in public (Figure 7-3). Thus, privacy should be provided. If the client occupies a room alone, the nurse should close the door; if the client shares a room, the nurse should take the client to a conference room or to another private place, if possible, to discuss personal information.

Figure 7-3 *Provide privacy when discussing personal or intimate health concerns with clients.*

The nurse should respect the client's current "home" (e.g., the hospital room) as she would any person's home, knocking on the door before entering the room, not sitting on the bed without permission, and asking before moving any personal articles. These simple courtesies show respect for the client as a person. When the client feels respected, communication is enhanced.

CONGRUENCY OF MESSAGES

It is important that verbal and nonverbal communications are in agreement, or **congruent.** Saying, "I really appreciate what you just did," in a pleasant tone of voice while smiling is congruent and clear; saying the same words in a disgusted tone of voice while frowning is incongruent and, thus, potentially unclear. The receiver may not know whether the sender is genuinely pleased with what was done or is displeased and being sarcastic. Messages such as these can confuse the receiver, who then may require feedback in order to correctly interpret the message.

It is important for the nurse to watch for congruency between verbal and nonverbal messages and to ask for clarification when incongruity exists.

LISTENING/OBSERVING

Listening and observing are two of the most valuable skills a nurse can have. These two skills are used to gather the subjective and objective data for the nursing assessment. Because the nursing diagnoses and nursing interventions are based on the assessment, it is imperative that the assessment be accurate.

The term **active listening** has been used to describe the behavior of listening and observing; it reflects the process of hearing spoken words and noting nonverbal behavior. It is listening for the meaning behind the words. This takes energy and concentration. To show undivided attention to the client, the nurse should be at eye level with the client, lean slightly forward toward the client, and make eye contact. In this position the nurse will be able to listen and observe more accurately.

Responses from the nurse such as "go on," "yes," "tell me more," "mmhm," or "what else?" communicate that the nurse is really listening and encourage the client to continue.

PSYCHOSOCIAL ASPECTS OF COMMUNICATION

The psychosocial aspects of communication are important for nurses to understand and then apply when caring for individual clients. Consideration of these aspects makes communication more effective.

The psychosocial aspects of communication include gestures, style, meaning of space, meaning of time, cultural values, and political correctness. These aspects are based on individuality and culture and influence the nurse–client relationship.

Gestures

Gestures are movements of the body to reflect a thought, feeling, or attitude. Some gestures are known globally, such as applause to indicate approval. Some gestures, however, have entirely different meanings in various countries. The nurse must be sensitive to cultural variances and exercise good judgment when caring for clients of different backgrounds and heritages.

Style

Each person has a style of communication reflecting the personality and self-concept of that person. According to Jack (2000), there are three common types of style: passive, aggressive, and assertive. Remember that a person's style of communication is learned and has been reinforced over the years. Because communication style is learned, it can be changed.

The stress, fear, and anxiety associated with being a client in the health care system may change a client's style to passive or aggressive.

Passive

The person using the passive style of communication is not able to share feelings or needs with others, has dif-

---

CULTURAL CONSIDERATIONS

Gestures

The meaning of gestures is not universal. For instance, in many places, a small circle made with the thumb and forefinger means "okay." This is not true in Japan and France, however, where this gesture means "money" and "zero," respectively. And in Brazil and Turkey, this gesture is a symbol for female genitalia and is considered an insult.

---

ficulty asking for help, does not stand up for himself, and is hurt and angry when others take advantage of him. This person has a weak, soft voice; uses apologetic words; makes little eye contact; and is often fidgety. The person with a passive style of communication will often go along with others without expressing a personal desire for an alternate plan of action. The client who is generally very compliant, asks for nothing, and gets little attention has a passive style of communication.

Aggressive

The person using the aggressive style of communication puts his own needs and feelings first. Communication is done in a haughty or angry manner. The voice is often demanding. This person works to control or manipulate others, shows no concern for anyone else's feelings, and has an attitude of superiority.

Assertive

The assertive person stands up for himself without violating the basic rights of others. True feelings are expressed in an honest, direct manner and others are not allowed to take advantage of him. The voice is firm and confident, and appropriate eye contact is made. Such a person also respects the rights, needs, and feelings of others; takes responsibility for the consequences of his actions; and behaves in a manner that enhances self-respect.

A person using the assertive style of communication effectively lets others know his thoughts, feelings, and needs. He also listens to and acknowledges the other person's thoughts, feelings, and needs. If the thoughts, feelings, or needs of the persons communicating are in conflict, a compromise acceptable to both can usually be worked out.

PROFESSIONAL TIP

When Clients Block Communication

In instances when clients block communication, keep the following things in mind:

- The client may not wish to discuss the topic introduced by the nurse or may not wish to talk at all. Everyone needs time alone to think.
- Accept and respect the client's desires to not communicate at a particular time.
- Let the client know that you are ready to listen whenever the client is ready to talk.

PROFESSIONAL TIP

Being Assertive

"I" messages—I think . . . , I expect . . . , I feel . . . , I need . . .—are excellent ways to begin practicing assertive communication. Such messages indicate ownership of the thought, feeling, or need—a fact with which no one can argue.

Meaning of Space

For many years Edward T. Hall (1959) studied **proxemics,** the study of space between people and its effect on interpersonal behavior. Hall says that like other animals, humans are territorial. Consider the following examples of human territoriality: People on a beach, mark territory with a towel or blanket; space is marked in waiting rooms, with a hat, jacket, luggage, or newspaper; students in a classroom generally sit in the same place and expect others to respect that space.

How much space do you prefer between yourself and another person? This distance usually varies with the person and the situation. The distance at which one person is comfortable with another person is influenced by age, gender of those interacting, and cultural values. Hall (1959) categorizes these comfort zones as intimate, personal, social, and public space, defined as follows:

- Intimate—touch to 18 inches; usually limited to family and close friends; necessary when performing most nursing procedures.
- Personal—18 inches to 4 feet; used with friends and coworkers; effective for many nurse–client interactions involving interviewing or data gathering.
- Social—4 to 12 feet; preferred distance with casual acquaintances.
- Public—12 feet or more; generally used with strangers in public places.

Comfort zone distances vary from person to person. While some people are comfortable being very close to the person with whom they are interacting, others prefer a greater distance. Nurses should always be aware of the client's spatial comfort level (Figure 7-4).

Much of nursing care involves touching the client, yet on admission, the nurse and client generally do not know each other. The nurse must move from the client's public space to the client's intimate space in a very short span of time to provide care. When care is given competently and professionally it helps the client feel more comfortable as the nurse occupies the client's intimate space.

Figure 7-4 *A distance of up to 4 feet is appropriate for interviewing and data gathering.*

Meaning of Time

In the United States, great emphasis is placed on schedules and being on time. Time is money. The clock is watched so individuals know where they are to be every hour of the day and night. When scheduled appointments are kept, the person is considered to be dependable.

Some cultures do not have an instrument for telling time. They have other ways of perceiving and dividing time. Some cultures know a day has passed because the sun has risen, set, and is rising again. Scheduling in these cultures often means "when we get around to it."

Cultural Values

It is important that the nurse be familiar with the cultural values of the people in the nurse's region of employment, especially when those values differ from the values of the dominant culture. For example, optimal health for all is the focus of the dominant U.S. culture. In some cultures, however, health is not a major concern, and little financial or political effort is dedicated to health. Likewise, individualism is stressed in our culture. In many other cultures, however, the social group, not the individual, is the primary focus.

As another example, consider that a number of cultural groups have learned to enjoy what they have and do not feel the need to keep working for some goal or material object. This contrasts with the dominant U.S. culture, where persons must work hard, achieve, and keep busy in order to be considered successful. Finally, in the dominant U.S. culture, cleanliness is closely related to optimal health and is a dominant value. Few cultural groups emphasize cleanliness in the way the U.S. culture does.

Political Correctness

Politically correct communication uses language that shows sensitivity to those who are different from oneself. It is intended to avoid the use of language that offends and to help eliminate prejudice. Terms that suggest inferior status for members of minority groups and terms that exclude older people, women, and those with handicaps are replaced by politically correct language. Prejudice and false ideas, which often lead to violence, are perpetuated by racist and bigoted language.

THERAPEUTIC COMMUNICATION

Therapeutic communication, sometimes called effective communication, is purposeful and goal directed, creating a beneficial outcome for the client. The focus of the conversation is the client, the client's problems, or the client's needs, not the problems or needs of the nurse.

Goals of Therapeutic Communication

Therapeutic communication has several goals or purposes. One or more of these goals guides each therapeutic communication between the nurse and client. The goals are to develop trust, obtain or provide information, show caring, and explore feelings.

Develop Trust

Clients and nurses are generally strangers when they first meet. The nurse then works to establish trust with each client. Examples of ways to build trust include answering questions honestly, responding to call lights promptly, and following through. When caring is shown, trust develops faster. Mutual trust established between client and nurse is termed **rapport.**

Obtain or Provide Information

The nurse obtains information from the client about general health and specific health problems. With this information the nurse can make an accurate assessment and plan of care.

The nurse provides information to the client from admission to discharge, beginning with the orientation of a new client to the hospital policies and routines. Sharing of information continues throughout the hospital stay as the nurse explains procedures, treatments, and tests; teaches the client self-care; clarifies instruction from other health care workers; and answers client questions. The discharge instructions constitute the final stage of information provision.

Show Caring

Two ways to show caring are offering a drink of water without being asked or fluffing a pillow. Knocking on the room door before entering and taking time to always greet the client by name are additional ways to show caring.

Explore Feelings

After rapport is established, the nurse can encourage the client to explore feelings. Many clients are anxious about their illness. Some have anxiety about being in the hospital and some fear the results of diagnostic tests. Some individuals will not admit they are anxious or fearful. The nurse is often able to help the client talk about feelings and reduce anxiety by using therapeutic communication techniques. Sometimes, only a clarifying statement is needed to alleviate fear or anxiety. Other times, fear and anxiety are reduced by allowing the client to talk.

Behaviors/Attitudes to Enhance Communication

Behaviors and attitudes that enhance therapeutic communication include warmth, active listening, car-

TABLE 7-2   WAYS TO SHOW CARING

ACTIVITY	STATEMENTS TO USE WITH ACTIVITY
Cover the client with a blanket.	"It feels chilly in here. Perhaps this blanket will help."
Assist the client to dress.	"I noticed you're having a little trouble getting your robe on. Perhaps I can help."
Serve a tray to the client.	"It's time to eat. I hope you're hungry because it really looks good."
Offer assistance.	"Here, let me help you. Perhaps together we can arrange these flowers."
Ask when leaving the room.	"Is there anything more I can do for you before I go?" or "I'm leaving now, but I'll be back in 20 minutes."
Move the client up in bed.	"You look so uncomfortable. Let me move you up in bed."
Make the client's bed.	"Now you have a nice fresh bed."
Regulate environmental temperature.	"It seems very warm in here. Perhaps if I turn the air conditioner up, it will help."
Turn the client in bed.	"Changing position really makes a difference, doesn't it?"
Straighten a pillow.	"Let me straighten your pillow for you."

ing, genuineness, empathy, acceptance and respect, and self-disclosure.

Caring

Caring is an attitude that enhances communication as well as a goal of therapeutic communication. Caring is the basis of a nurse–client relationship and makes the client feel important. The client can easily identify a caring attitude. Table 7-2 gives some examples of ways to show caring.

Keller and Baker (2000) identify four steps to help communicate a caring attitude to clients:

1. *Connect with the client.* Make eye contact; be at eye level when speaking to client; address client formally by the last name.
2. *Appreciate the client's situation.* Listen carefully; focus on what client is saying; acknowledge client's point of view; express concern.
3. *Respond to client needs.* Clarify what is being asked; respond in ordinary language; let client know what to expect.
4. *Empower the client.* Find out what client knows about condition and acknowledge opinions; work as partner to develop plan of care; allow choices as appropriate; encourage questions.

Warmth

Warmth, expressed predominantly by nonverbal communication, makes the client feel relaxed, welcomed, and unjudged.

Figure 7-5 *Active listening, concentrating on the interaction with the client, enhances communication.*

While touch is an important method to show warmth, it must be used appropriately. Society dictates the touching that is appropriate in various situations. Communication may be greatly enhanced by holding a client's hand or putting a hand on the shoulder. This touching provides a connection between the nurse and the client. Remember touch may not always be welcomed by the client.

Active Listening

As implied, listening is an active process requiring energy and concentration. It involves listening to the spoken words as well as being attentive to the nonverbal messages.

Responses from the nurses indicate that the nurse is really listening to the client. It is important that the nurse concentrate on the interaction at hand and not become distracted by other thoughts (Figure 7-5).

Genuineness

Effective communication is genuine. The nurse must be honest about personal feelings. Sometimes it is appropriate to cry with a client.

Genuineness means being truthful and not attempting to answer a question when the answer is not known. After admitting not knowing the nurse should offer to find the answer and then do so. Knowing that being genuine builds trust, the nurse must use good judgment about confronting a family member, client, another health care worker, or expressing negative thoughts.

Empathy

Empathy, the capacity to understand another person's feelings or perception of a situation, is an objective awareness of, or a sensitivity to, another person's feelings and thoughts. Although the nurse is not involved in the thoughts and feelings of the client, through empathy the nurse is able to understand and accept the feelings and thoughts of the client. Sympathy is different from empathy. In sympathy, the nurse shares in the feelings

and thoughts of the client. These feelings and thoughts are generally related to a loss.

Acceptance and Respect

Acceptance of clients as individuals with values and beliefs of their own is an attitude that enhances communication. Nurses must accept the fact that clients may have different values and beliefs. It is called being nonjudgmental when a client is accepted at face value.

Acceptance is shown by not expressing differing beliefs or values and by simply accepting the statements or complaints of clients. Clients then feel free to communicate and cooperate in their care.

After acceptance comes respect. In order to understand clients as unique individuals, they must be accepted in a nonjudgmental way. Acceptance and respect by the the nurse lets clients know they can be themselves and they will still receive quality nursing care, even though they have different values and beliefs than the nurse. Respect is shown when the nurse introduces herself and also addresses the client by name (preceded by "Mr.," "Mrs.," or "Ms.").

Self-Disclosure

Sharing something about yourself such as thoughts, expectations, feelings, or ideas is termed self-disclosure. It does not mean sharing personal problems. A nurse who shares something, such as personal future goals in nursing, is trusting the client with that knowledge. The client who feels trusted will trust the nurse, and therapeutic communication is augmented.

Techniques of Therapeutic Communication

Certain techniques promote therapeutic communication. These techniques should be learned and incorporated into the nurse's manner of communicating.

Clarifying/Validating

Clarifying or validating are used when the nurse is not sure of the meaning of a message. Clarifying is the technique used to understand verbal messages. For example:

"Do you mean . . . ?"

Validating is used to establish truth or accuracy. It is used for nonverbal as well as verbal messages. Examples are as follows:

"Are you saying that you did not get your medication today?"

"You are holding your side. Are you having pain there?"

Open Questions

Open questions encourage clients to express their own thoughts and feelings. *How, when, where,* and *what* are words with which to begin an open question. Open questions cannot typically be answered with "yes" or "no" or with just one or two words. For example:

"How has this medication affected your vision?"

"What did the doctor tell you about going home?"

Indirect Statements

An indirect statement calls for a response from the client. Because it is a statement and not a question, the client does not feel quizzed. Indirect statements allow the client to determine the direction of the conversation, thus helping the client maintain a feeling of independence. Examples of indirect statements are as follows:

"Tell me about your physical therapy today."

"You were telling me about. . . ."

Reflecting

Reflecting is repeating all or part of a message back to the sender. Often, reflecting focuses on feelings and helps the sender "hear" the message from the receiver. This allows the sender a chance to clarify the message and shows that the listener is trying to understand the message. Reflecting can be a very useful technique if not overused. Examples include the following:

Client: "I'm really nervous about my surgery tomorrow. My friend got an infection after her surgery. I'm very frightened."

Nurse: "You are anxious about your surgery and afraid of getting an infection?"

Paraphrasing

Paraphrasing is restating the message in the receiver's own words. This lets the sender know how the receiver interpreted the message. Clarification can then be done if necessary. The sender is aware that the receiver is listening and trying to understand the message. For example:

Nurse: "You are afraid that you might have complications from your surgery?"

Summarizing

Summarizing is stating in a sentence or two the major points of a conversation to let the sender know what was heard. The sender can then add more information or clarify what was originally heard. An example might be as follows:

"Let me see, we have discussed. . . ."

Focusing

Keeping communication focused on the topic being discussed can sometimes be difficult. Clients may wander off to other topics, or the topic may shift to the nurse. It is important to keep the focus on the client and not the nurse. For example the nurse could say:

"We can discuss that in a minute, right now I'd like to discuss. . . ."

"A minute ago you mentioned that you'd had an upset stomach after taking your medication. Tell me more about that."

Silence

Silence is one of the most difficult but effective techniques to use. In the dominant U.S. culture, most people are uncomfortable with silence and feel the need to fill

---

PROFESSIONAL TIP

Improve Communication Skills
Communication skills can be improved by:

- Minimizing distractions
- Making eye contact
- Listening
- Being patient
- Not interrupting
- Checking congruency of words spoken with nonverbal cues
- Using clear, easy-to-understand terminology and explaining medical terms when used
- Asking client to paraphrase important information

---

the gap by saying something. Silence can be a valuable therapeutic technique, allowing the client time to gather thoughts or check emotions. Silence also gives the nurse a chance to decide how best to continue the interaction. If the nurse employs behaviors to enhance communication during the silence, the client will often verbalize thoughts or feelings.

Barriers to Communication

Employing behaviors and attitudes to enhance communication will be of little use if the nurse also employs barriers to communication. Although the communication process is intense, it should not be threatening. The purpose in learning about things that block communication is to enable the nurse to identify them and avoid using them. Many mistakes can be corrected when identified. A simple "I'm sorry, I shouldn't have said that" will often take care of the situation. Practice helps sharpen communication skills. The most common barriers are discussed following.

Closed Questions

Questions that can be answered with "yes" or "no" or with only one or two words are considered closed. After the one- or two-word answer, communication is usually ended; there is no other avenue for the communication to follow. This type of question is appropriate in certain circumstances, however, such as when taking a health

---

PROFESSIONAL TIP

Therapeutic Communication
Practice the techniques of therapeutic communication with family, classmates, friends, and instructors. This may seem artificial and uncomfortable at first, but it will become easier with practice. If you begin using the techniques of therapeutic communication now, you will have incorporated them into your manner of communication by the time you begin clinical experience.

history or in an emergency. Examples of closed questions are as follows:

"Is the pain gone?"

"Did you sleep well?"

Clichés

Clichés are overused, trite phrases that are almost meaningless. They are impersonal and often used when individuals are at a loss for anything better to say. They are used without thinking of the impact on the other person and often seem disrespectful of the client's individual circumstances. Examples include the following:

"Hang in there, tomorrow is another day."

"It could be worse."

False Reassurance

False reassurance about the outcome of a situation is often used in an effort to cheer up the client regardless of the facts. False reassurance can be especially traumatic to a terminally ill client who may be desperate to believe assurances even if they are not founded in reality. An example of false reassurance is as follows:

"Don't worry, I'm sure everything will be fine."

Judgmental Responses

Judgmental responses are based on the nurse's personal value system and imply right or wrong. Such responses allow no room for further discussion. For example:

"You shouldn't feel that way."

"You ought to do. . . ."

Agreeing/Disagreeing or Approving/Disapproving

Whether the nurse is agreeing/approving or disagreeing/disapproving, offering an opinion implies that one belief is right and the other wrong. Clients are thus prevented from sharing their feelings and may feel pressured to express the same values and opinions as the nurse. One example is as follows:

"I wouldn't do it that way."

Giving Advice

Giving advice involves offering personal rather than professional opinion. When the nurse does this, the client's responsibility for making decisions is diminished. Furthermore, some clients may end up feeling unable to make their own choices and may therefore become more dependent on the nurse. One example might be:

"I think you should. . . ."

Stereotyping

Stereotyping occurs when individual differences are ignored and a person is automatically put into a specific category because they have certain characteristics. For example:

"Someone your age shouldn't worry about that."

"Boys aren't supposed to cry."

Belittling

Belittling conveys to a person that his thoughts or feelings really have no value, that it is silly to think or feel a certain way, or that he is no different from other individuals in similar circumstances. Examples include the following:

"Many people have it much worse."

"Yes, everyone feels like that."

Defending

Defending is a response to a feeling of being directly or indirectly threatened. The nurse may make statements in defense of self, another nurse, a doctor, or the health care facility. Defending implies that the client is not permitted to criticize or express feelings. This may be one of the most difficult communication barriers to overcome. No one likes to be criticized or to hear coworkers criticized. A natural first response is to defend why something was said, done, or not done. An example of defending is as follows:

"No one on this unit would say that."

Requesting an Explanation

It can be very intimidating for a client when a nurse asks for an explanation of behaviors, feelings, or thoughts. Often, the client does not know the "why." The usual results are increased anxiety, becoming defensive, and an end to communication. Examples are as follows:

"Why did you do that?"

"Why do you feel that way?"

Changing the Subject

An abrupt change of subject by the nurse generally indicates to the client that the nurse is uncomfortable or anxious about the topic under discussion. It often is used to avoid listening to a client's fear, distress, or problems and is interpreted by the client as a lack of interest.

Client: "I don't think I'll ever get well."

Nurse: "Isn't it a beautiful day?"

CRITICAL THINKING

Communication Barriers

Which barriers to communication do you use?

Join a classmate in pointing out the barriers that each of you use.

Discuss how each of you feel when confronted with these communication barriers.

What can you do to eliminate these communication barriers?

PROFESSIONAL BOUNDARIES

All communication with clients must take place within **professional boundaries** (the limits of the professional relationship that allow for a safe, therapeutic connection between the professional and the client). The nurse must abstain from obtaining personal gain at the expense of the client and refrain from inappropriate involvement in the client's personal relationships.

NURSE–CLIENT COMMUNICATION

One of the most important aspects of nursing care is communication. Good communication skills are essential whether the nurse is gathering admission information, taking a health history, teaching, or implementing care.

Nurses have both an ethical and moral responsibility to use any information gathered from the client in the client's best interest. Information that affects the health status or care of the client should be shared with other members of the health care team. All information concerning a client is confidential and should never be discussed in elevators, the cafeteria, the hallways, or other public places outside the health care facility.

Nurses' competence is often judged by their communication skills. Client satisfaction is increased by good communication, and increased client satisfaction leads to better compliance with the therapeutic regimen.

A key factor in the client's perception and evaluation of the health care services provided is communication.

Formal/Informal Communication

Formal communication is purposeful and is employed in a structured situation such as information gathering on admission or scheduled teaching sessions (Figure 7-6). Specific items covered in a planned sequence provide more information in the shortest amount of time.

Informal communication does not follow a structured approach, although it often reveals information that is pertinent to the client's care. For instance, a client may comment that the tape holding her bandage in place is irritating to her skin. This would lead the nurse to assess the wound area and take action to correct the problem. This interaction, although not planned or structured, was nonetheless helpful in ensuring quality nursing care.

Figure 7-6 *Formal Interaction, Admission Interview*

Social Communication

Everyday conversations with friends, family, and acquaintances are called social communication. Topics usually are those of interest to both parties and reflect the social relationship of the persons involved. Both people share information, feelings, and thoughts. Social communication provides a way to get acquainted with clients to learn about each other, and to begin a nurse–client relationship.

Although social communication is not considered therapeutic communication, it is used in the nurse–client relationship. It is nonthreatening and puts the client at ease, allowing the nurse to get to know the client and what is important to the client. Social communication is often interpreted by clients as expressions of caring on the part of the nurse—that is, the nurse cares enough about the client to spend time communicating as a person rather than as a nurse.

Interactions

Nurse–client interactions and relationships progress through three phases. The purpose of the interaction dictates the amount of time spent on each phase.

Introduction Phase

The introduction phase of any interaction is usually fairly short. After greeting the client by name, the nurse should introduce himself and define his role. Then expectations of the interaction are clarified, and mutual goals are set. A good format might be:

> "Good morning, Mrs. Ishdu. My name is Lorenzo Lopez. I am a student practical (vocational) nurse. I will be caring for you today and tomorrow. During this time, I will be teaching you some leg exercises that you will have to do after your surgery tomorrw."

Working Phase

The working phase generally constitutes the major portion of any interaction and is used to accomplish the goal or objective defined in the introduction. Feedback should always be asked for to ensure understanding on the part of the client. In the previously presented scenario, the client's demonstrating the leg exercises and verbalizing why the exercises are necessary would indicate understanding.

Termination Phase

The termination phase is the final phase of any interaction. Seldom do nurses have unlimited time to spend with one client, and there are several ways for the nurse to indicate the end of an interaction. The nurse may ask whether the client has any questions about the topic discussed. Summarizing the topic is another good way for the nurse to indicate closure.

Factors Affecting Nurse–Client Communication

As mentioned previously, factors such as age, education, emotions, culture, language, attention, and surroundings affect both parties in a communication. In nurse–client communications, additional factors relating to both the nurse and client also come into play. The nurse must be sensitive to these factors and avoid personal biases in order to provide appropriate nursing care.

Nurse

Many factors pertaining to the nurse influence nurse–client communication. The nurse's state of health, home situation, workload, staff relations, and past experiences as a nurse, can all impact the attitude, thinking, concentration, and emotions of the nurse. These all influence the way a nurse sends and receives messages. Self-awareness (an awareness of all these factors) is very important for the nurse when communicating.

Client

Factors related to the client that must be considered include social factors, religion, family situation, visual ability, hearing ability, speech ability, level of consciousness, language proficiency, and state of illness.

Hearing Ability If a hearing-impaired person is able to read, writing may be the easiest method of communication; however, many hearing-impaired persons have learned to speechread at least to some degree. This was formerly known as lipread. Communicating with a client who is hearing impaired requires time and patience.

The client may experience frustration when communicating. Such frustration generally stems more from trying to understand others rather than from trying to be understood. Face the client and speak slowly and deliberately using slightly exaggerated word formation. Gesturing can also be very effective. Check to see whether the client has a hearing aid and, if so, encourage its use during the communication.

Speech Ability **Dysphasia,** the impairment of speech, and **aphasia,** the absence of speech, are most commonly seen as the result of a stroke, although both can result from a brain lesion. Other neurological diseases such as Parkinson's disease may also cause dysphasia. A dysfunction of the muscles used for speech is termed **dysarthria,** which makes a person's speech dif-

CRITICAL THINKING

Communication and the Unconscious Client

Why should you communicate with an unconscious client?

How can you communicate with an unconscious client?

ficult, slow, and hard to understand. Dysphasia, aphasia, and dysarthria create communication problems.

The person with dysphasia has difficulty putting thoughts and feelings into words and sending messages. It should be noted, however, that seldom does the person with dysphasia have difficulty receiving and interpreting messages; thus, explanations should be given before doing anything. If the client can write, paper and pencil can be used for communication. A picture board, word board, letter board, or computer may also be employed. A person with speech impairments may feel frustrated and helpless. Establishing some method of communication for the client provides hope and maintains self-esteem while minimizing or preventing feelings of depression, anger, and hostility.

Level of Consciousness True communication cannot be accomplished with unconscious or comatose clients. It should be remembered, however, that unconscious or comatose clients may be able to hear even though they cannot respond. Caregivers should speak to these clients just as they would to alert clients. Always greet the client by name, identify yourself, and explain why you are in the room (i.e., what you are going to do). Then let the client know when you are leaving and, if possible, when you will return. Although one-sided, this interaction is critical to the client's care.

Language Proficiency The client's ability to communicate effectively through spoken language also influences the nurse–client interaction. Clients who do not speak English generally come from another culture. Learning about the other culture, especially about the values and beliefs, will help prevent the nurse from violating those values and beliefs.

A family member who speaks English could be used as an interpreter, as shown in Figure 7-7. When another health care worker on the nursing unit speaks the same language as does the client, that person could also be used as an interpreter as long as it does not interfere with his or her work. Speak directly to the client whether an interpreter is present or not. Make eye contact with the client and speak slowly and clearly. Use simple words and avoid slang and medical jargon.

Pictures or a two-language dictionary are often helpful. When another language is prevalent in the community, nurse's should learn some phrases in that language to use in client assessment and care. *Remember, gestures, facial expressions, and other nonverbal communication send messages without the use of language.*

Social Factors Socially acceptable health concerns, such as having the gallbladder or appendix removed or having the flu, are easy to discuss. It may be more difficult to communicate with a woman who is having a breast removed. The symbolic meaning of the breast

Figure 7-7 *A family member interprets communication with a non-English-speaking client.*

may make it difficult for the client to accept its removal and may influence how she relates to others. A person who is HIV positive or has another sexually transmitted disease may be very reluctant to discuss the illness.

Stage of Illness The stage of a client's illness may influence the client's desire to communicate with the nurse. Clients in the early stages of illness may be eager to learn all they can about the illness or may express anger and resentment at their current state of health.

Terminally ill clients may pose special challenges for the nurse. Most terminally ill clients know they are dying and are concerned about those whom they love. It is thus important for the nurse to have the client identify those persons the client considers to be "family." Family and nurses often struggle with effective communication techniques when speaking with one who is dying. Death is not a prime subject for discussion as it is often considered a defeat by health care workers. *Remember that silence and listening are both part of communication and can relay caring, compassion, and acceptance.*

Whenever a client begins talking about death the nurse must be willing to listen and take part in the con-

versation. Many times nurses hesitate to communicate with the terminally ill for fear they will say the wrong thing. The client who wishes to talk needs a good listener. Allow the client to guide the conversation. Listen and accept what the client says. Trying not to give advice may be very difficult to do.

The nurse and the family must work together to understand the ways that the terminally ill client communicates. It can take persistence and insight to identify and decipher some messages. "Listening" to the client's gestures and facial expressions helps facilitate understanding of messages.

Religion Communication can be difficult when religious beliefs conflict with those of the health care team. Members of some religions seek healing only through faith and not through conventional medical services, including not receiving blood transfusions.

When a client has a minister, priest, or rabbi visit, privacy should be provided if at all possible.

Family Situation Illness often unites family members around the client, but communication between the family and client may be strained if the family has not been close to or supportive of the client before the illness. The nurse must be careful not to discuss aspects of the client's condition or treatment in front of family members. It is usually best to ask family members to step out of the room when any nursing care is being given. This maintains the client's right to privacy and confidentiality.

If the client asks for a specific person to remain in the room, it is usually allowed unless specifically contraindicated.

Visual Ability Communicating with clients who are visually impaired may not seem to be a challenge at first; however, because the nonverbal part of any message, such as facial expressions, gestures, and other body language, is not able to be observed, an important part of every message is lost to the client.

Generally, persons who are visually impaired speak only when spoken to. Their speech is often loud when they are not sure where the other person is. Silence makes them uncomfortable.

When orienting a new client who cannot see, the nurse must include an explanation of "hospital sounds." Describe the room in detail and guide the client around the room if possible. Always speak and identify yourself when entering the room. Each step of a procedure as

---

PROFESSIONAL TIP

Caring for the Client Who Is Hearing Impaired

- Check to see whether the client wears a hearing aid. Be sure it is in working order and turned on.
- Make every effort to move the client to a setting with minimal background noise.
- Always face the client.
- Speak in a normal tone and at a normal pace.
- Determine whether the client uses sign language. If signing is used, enlist the assistance of an interpreter.
- Pay particular attention to nonverbal cues of the client and to your own nonverbal behavior.
- Provide a pen and paper to facilitate communication, if necessary.

PROFESSIONAL TIP

Caring for the Client Who Is Visually Impaired

- Look directly at the client when speaking.
- Use a normal tone and volume of voice.
- Advise the client when you are entering or leaving the room.
- Orient the person to the immediate environment; use clock hours to indicate positions of items in relation to the client.
- Ask for permission before touching the client.

well as any touching should be described before it is initiated. To prevent startling a client, always inform the visually impaired client before touching.

COMMUNICATING WITH THE HEALTH CARE TEAM

Because providing care to clients is a team effort, effective communication is necessary. This communication between team members may be oral or written, individual, group, or on computer.

Oral Communication

Oral communication takes place among all health care team members. To provide continuity of care to the client, all persons who provide that care communicate orally concerning that care.

Nurse–Student Nurse

Student nurses communicate not only with their clinical instructor but with the staff nurses too. How well staff nurses interact with student nurses depends on the experiences the staff nurses have had with other student nurses and also on how the staff nurses were treated as students. Student nurses are present in the clinical facility for very specific learning experiences, which are selected by the instructor and relate to classroom discussion. They will review client records, communicate with and care for their clients, and when possible observe others performing procedures. Depending on how far they have progressed through the nursing curriculum, students may be limited in their nursing activities. Communication between student nurses and staff nurses is essential because staff nurses are responsibile for the care of clients even though clients are assigned to

students. Usually a helping relationship develops between staff nurses and nursing students.

Nurse–Nursing Assistant

The nurse is responsible for assigning duties to the nursing assistants. A relationship of trust and mutual respect is established by answering questions and providing reasons for specific activities requested.

Nursing assistants are often much more comfortable and confident in providing bedside care. Therefore, they can be of considerable assistance to the new graduate (whether an LP/VN or RN). They often have creative solutions to problems and should be included in planning care.

Nurse–Nurse

Nurse–nurse communications can be either peer–peer or superior–subordinate communication. Peer–peer communication takes place many times every day. When each nurse uses effective communication with peers as well as clients, the unit runs more efficiently, and client care will be more effective. Superior–subordinate communication often occurs when the superior discusses client care to be performed by the subordinate. The way this communication is handled affects both the attitude of the subordinate and the client care given.

Nurse–Physician

Nursing education and expertise have evolved over the years to a professional level. Nurses are responsible for their own actions even when under the direction of a physician. Nurses have a duty to secure physician clarification of any order that is illegible or unclear, that violates hospital policy or procedure, or that is below the acceptable standard of care (Calloway, 2001).

Nurses must communicate openly and honestly with physicians, demonstrating competence in assessments, nursing skills, provision of quality care, reporting change in client status, and accurate documentation.

Nurse–Other Health Professionals

Communicate with professionals in other departments on a peer-to-peer basis. The focus of communication should be clarification of goals for each client and ways to meet those goals. Top-quality care is provided to clients by listening to those in other departments and establishing mutual respect for each other's area of expertise.

Group Communication

Client care conferences may be scheduled whenever the need arises or on a regular basis. Some conferences may be only for the staff of a specific nursing unit; others may include some members of other departments. Only persons directly involved with client care should be invited (Figure 7-8).

The objectives of the conference are established by the conference leader, who makes all necessary arrangements. The meeting site should be a conference room or other private place. One person should record the discus-

Figure 7-8 *Nurses work together to plan client care.*

sion. When the conference is about a particular client, only facts are to be documented on the client's chart. When the topic is general and not related to any one client, only a record of the discussion is needed.

Telephone

When a student nurse takes a telephone call, the call should be answered with the name of the department or floor and the student's full name and position (i.e., student nurse). If a message is taken, the student nurse should write it down and read it back to the caller, asking for the caller's name and for the caller to spell out his or her name. The student nurse must never give out any information about clients.

Shift Report

Vital to continuity of client care is the **shift report** (report about each client between shifts). An oral report is the most common. The charge nurse of the outgoing shift may report to all members of the incoming shift or only to the incoming charge nurse who, in turn, shares the information with the appropriate caregivers on the incoming shift.

Sometimes, the report is put on a tape recorder for the next shift. This allows no chance for feedback, which can be a disadvantage.

Another method is a "walking report." The outgoing nurse reports to the oncoming nurse on each client as they walk from bed to bed. This way the client is included and aware of the information provided to the next shift.

The shift report about each client should be complete and concise no matter which method is used. The report should be focused on the clients and given in an orderly manner. This is not the time for social conversation.

Written Communication

Most written communication relates to the client's chart. All aspects of a client's care are recorded on that client's chart.

Requisitions to x-ray or to physical or respiratory therapy and requests for laboratory services for a client are all forms of written communication. The reports resulting from these requests become part of the client's chart.

One type of written communication not pertaining to a specific client is the interdepartmental memo requesting equipment, supplies, maintenance, or housekeeping. Such documents are necessary to keep the nursing unit functioning efficiently and effectively.

Electronic Communication

Computers are being used extensively in the business offices of health care agencies and have been so for years. The introduction of computers into the departments of direct client care has been slower, however. Nonetheless, in many places, computers are used by client care departments to send requisitions to other departments and to receive test results. Some hospital pharmacies use computer programs that show safe dosages and drug interactions. There are also programs to aid physicians in diagnosing and treating some conditions. With the expanding use of computers in health care and the corresponding potential for increased use, it is important for all health care workers to have some knowledge about computers.

The Institute of Medicine (IOM) defines the computerized patient record (CPR) as an "electronic record that resides in a system specifically designed to support users through availability of complete and accurate data, practitioner reminders and alerts, clinical decision support systems, links to bodies of medical knowledge and other aids." This moves the client record from simply tracking client care to serving as a resource for health care delivery (Zolot, 1999).

As widespread use of the CPR is implemented many questions are being considered, including: How can changes to the data entered be prevented? How will charting errors be corrected? What happens when the computers are down? How will security be maintained? What are the legal implications of electronic or digital signatures? According to Zolot (1999), all client records must be confidential, accurate, secure, and protected from unauthorized access and disclosure, regardless of the form.

Telehealth

According to Hutcherson (2001), **telehealth** is using telecommunication equipment and communication networks to transfer health care information between participants at different locations. It can be used in almost every area of health care.

Telenursing, an element of telehealth, permits nurses to provide care through a telecommunication system. The simplest form has been used for years—the telephone. **Telemedicine,** another element of telehealth, permits physicians to provide care through a telecommunication system. Recognized subspecialties include teledermatology, teleoncology, telepathology, and teleradiology.

Two issues related to telehealth that are especially important to nursing include licensure and standards of practice. The National Council of State Boards of Nursing (NCSBN) developed a plan for multistate licensure through legal agreement (interstate compacts) between a group of states. In these agreements a nurse is licensed in one state but can practice nursing in any of the states in the compact. Before multistate licensure, nurses could participate in telenursing only within the state of their licensure. Practice standards for telenursing are in the process of being established. To assist nurses when providing telenursing care, the American Nurses Association (ANA) has developed some core principles for telehealth (ANA, 1999) and telehealth protocols (ANA, 2001).

The use of two-way video allows the client and health care provider to see, hear, and talk to each other. A stethoscope or otoscope (called peripherals) can be included in the hookup so that the sounds and visual images can be transmitted (Granade, 1997). This allows physician specialists in large medical centers to examine a client many miles away.

COMMUNITY/HOME HEALTH CARE

Use of Telenursing

- From the office, a home health nurse can watch a client at home change a dressing or self-administer insulin.
- During a video consult, a home health nurse might assist by manipulating the peripherals or actually performing a physical assessment.

PROFESSIONAL TIP

Telehealth Confidentiality

- Avoid sending or receiving client data by e-mail unless the computer has encryption capabilities.
- During a two-way video consultation, inform the client of any other people who are present in the room, but off camera. Try to ensure that only those persons who must know about the client's condition are present (Granade, 1997).

California and Arizona have both passed legislation requiring providers to obtain written and verbal informed consent before providing any nonemergency care via telemedicine. Oklahoma is also considering such legislation (Granade, 1997).

Nurses should document all activities, assessment findings, information provided by the client, and any instructions given to the client. All data transmissions (e.g., telemetry printouts or videotapes) should be stored in the client's record. Most telemedicine laws require that existing confidentiality rules be maintained.

COMMUNICATING WITH YOURSELF

People talk to themselves every day whether they admit it or not. Often, such communication takes the form of thoughts rather than spoken words. What people say to themselves influences their personalities and, therefore, how they interact with others. This self-talk may be positive or negative.

Positive Self-Talk

The practice of positive self-talk is key to positive self-esteem. You can send positive thoughts to yourself about yourself, but better yet, say the thoughts out loud. Thinking, saying, and hearing positive statements about oneself reinforces positive self-esteem. When you have had a difficult day, whether in the classroom or clinical area, remind yourself of your good attributes and accomplishments. Every day tell yourself out loud what you learned or what good care you gave to your client(s).

The desire to succeed is reinforced by positive self-talk. When things are not going well and frustration sets in, memories of success can serve as positive influences.

Positive affirmation is a positive thought or idea on which a person consciously focuses to produce a desired result. Positive affirmation can be used to change negative inner messages to positive messages. For instance, say, "I know I can pass this test" instead of saying, "I don't know if I can pass this test." Of course, positive affirmation cannot be a substitute for studying and preparing for the test. Positive affirmation merely serves to modify your attitude about the test—or about any other situation.

Negative Self-Talk

Whenever you say to yourself, "I can't do . . . ," you are decreasing your self-esteem with the negative self-talk. Negative self-talk may originate within you or may be a replay of things that others have said about you. Negative self-talk is self-destructive. Your self-image is lowered by your own criticism, and you begin to see yourself as a failure.

Summary

- Communication is influenced by factors such as age, education, emotions, culture, language, attention, surroundings, and past experience.

- Nonverbal messages are generally more accurate in communicating a person's feelings.
- Verbal and nonverbal messages must be congruent for clear communication to take place.
- Techniques of therapeutic communication should be practiced and incorporated into the nurse's communication.
- Barriers to communication should be identified and avoided when communicating.
- People have four comfort zones of closeness: intimate, personal, social, and public.
- Therapeutic communication is purposeful and goal directed.
- Psychosocial aspects of communication may hinder or aid communication.
- Most nurse–client interactions should involve therapeutic communication.
- Nurse–client communication is influenced by both the client and the nurse.
- The nurse is many times a role model for the family in terms of communicating with the terminally ill client.
- Accurate communication among the health care team is necessary for continuity of client care.

Review Questions

1. Mr. Reynolds is in the bathroom with the door partially closed. A nurse enters his room and says, "You will not be able to eat or drink after supper because of tests tomorrow," and then leaves. Did communication take place?

   a. No, there was no feedback.
   b. No, there was no eye contact.
   c. Yes, Mr. George had to hear the message.
   d. Yes, there was a sender, receiver, and message.

2. Which of the following are all examples of verbal communication?

   a. singing, dancing, smiling
   b. reading, writing, listening
   c. shaking hands, reading, grimacing
   d. whispering, making eye contact, answering

3. When a client says, "I'm not sure how I'll handle all this," which response of the nurse represents clarification?

   a. "Handle all this?"
   b. "Well, you can ask your sister to help."
   c. "Oh, you'll be able to handle things. You're an intelligent person."
   d. "I'm not sure I understand what it is you're concerned about being able to handle."

4. A critically ill client denies there is anything wrong and talks constantly about going home. The nurse should:

   a. listen but say nothing.
   b. acknowledge the client's wishes and hopes.
   c. advise the client that it will be impossible to go home.
   d. assist the client in planning when to return home.

5. A client tells the nurse that she would rather die than have chemotherapy. The nurse should report this communication to:

   a. the physician only.
   b. all nurses on the unit.
   c. the physician and charge nurse.
   d. no one; it is a confidential communication.

References/Suggested Readings

American Nurses Association. (1999). *Core principles on telehealth.* Washington, DC: Author.

American Nurses Association. (2001). *Developing telehealth protocols: A blueprint for success,* Washington, DC: Author.

Bailey, D., & Bailey, D. (1997). *Therapeutic approaches in mental health/psychiatric nursing* (4th ed.). Philadelphia: F. A. Davis.

Barry, P., Farmer, S. (2000). *Mental health and mental illness* (7th ed.). Philadelphia: Lippincott Williams & Wilkins.

Burtt, K. (1997, November/December). Nurses use telehealth to address rural health care needs, prevent hospitalizations. *The American Nurse, 21.*

Bush, K. (2001). Do you really listen to patients? *RN, 64*(3), 35–37.

Calloway, S. D. (2001). Preventing communication breakdowns. *RN, 64*(1), 71–74.

Chaffee, M. (1999). A telehealth odyssey. *AJN, 99*(7), 26–32.

Deering, C., & Jennings, D. (2002). Communicating with children and adolescents. *AJN, 102*(3), 34–41.

Estes, M. E. Z. (2002). *Health assessment & physical examination* (2nd ed.). Clifton Park, NY: Thomson Delmar Learning.

Fiesta, J. (1998). Failure to communicate. *Nursing Management, 29*(2), 22.

Frisch, N., & Frisch, L. (2002). *Psychiatric mental health nursing.* (2nd ed.). Clifton Park, NY: Thomson Delmar Learning.

Granade, P. (1997). The brave new world of telemedicine. *RN, 60*(7), 59–62.

Gravely, S. (2001). When your patient speaks Spanish—and you don't. *RN, 64*(5), 65–67.

Hall, E. (1959). *The silent language.* New York: Doubleday.

Hutcherson, C. (Sept. 30, 2001). Legal considerations for nurses practicing in a telehealth setting. *Online Journal of Issues in Nursing, 6*(3), manuscript 3. [Online]. Available: www.nursingworld.org/onjin/topic16/tpc16_3.htm

Jack, L. (2000). Effective communication. In J. Zerwekh & J. Claborn (Eds.), *Nursing today: Transition and trends* (3rd ed.). Philadelphia: W. B. Saunders.

Keller, V., & Baker, L. (2000). Communicate with care. *RN, 63*(1), 32–33.

Kübler-Ross, E. (1969). *On death and dying.* New York: MacMillan.

Kübler-Ross, E. (1975). *Death: The final stage of growth.* Englewood Cliffs, NJ: Prentice Hall.

Kübler-Ross, E. (1978). *To live until we say good-bye.* Englewood Cliffs, NJ: Prentice Hall.

Lyon, B. (2000). Conquering dysfunctional anxiety: What you say to yourself matters. *Reflections on Nursing Leadership, 26*(4), 33–35.

Milliken, M. (2004). *Understanding human behavior* (7th ed.). Clifton Park, NY: Thomson Delmar Learning.

Puopolo, A. L. (1999). Gaining confidence to talk about end-of-life care. *Nursing99, 29*(7), 49–51.

Rochman, R. (2000). Are computerized patient records for you? *Nursing2000, 30*(10), 61–62.

Tamparo, C., & Lindh, W. (2000). *Therapeutic communications for health professionals* (2nd ed.). Clifton Park, NY: Thomson Delmar Learning.

Thomas, N., & Thompson, J. (2003). Tomorrow's nurses need your help today. *RN, 66*(6), 51–53.

Waughfield, C. (2002). *Mental health concepts.* (6th ed.). Clifton Park, NY: Thomson Delmar Learning.

Zolot, J. S. (1999). Computer-based patient records. *AJN, 99*(12), 64–69.

Resources

American Health Information Management Association, 919 North Michigan Avenue, Suite 1400, Chicago, IL 60611- 1683, 312-787-2672, www.ahima.org

American Nurses Association, 600 Maryland Avenue SW, Suite 100 West, Washington, DC 20024-2571, 800-274-4ANA (161), www.nursingworld.org

Language Line Services, 1 Lower Ragsdale Frive Building 2, Monterey, CA 93940, 800-752-0093 Ext. 196, www.languageline.com

National Council of State Boards of Nursing, 676 North St. Clair Street, Suite 550, Chicago, IL 60611-2921, 312-787-6555, www.ncsbn.org

Office for the Advancement of Telehealth, 5600 Fishers Lane, Room 11A-55, Rockville, MD 20857, 301-443-0447, http://telehealth.hrsa.gov

NURSING PROCESS/ DOCUMENTATION

CHAPTER

8

MAKING THE CONNECTION

Refer to the following chapters to increase your understanding of the nursing process:

Basic Nursing
- **Holistic Care**
- **Legal and Ethical Responsibilities**

- **The Health Care Delivery System**
- **Communication**
- **Assessment**

LEARNING OBJECTIVES

Upon completion of this chapter, you should be able to:
- **Define key terms.**
- **Explain the nursing process.**
- **Describe the components of assessment.**
- **Describe the three types of nursing diagnoses.**
- **Discuss planning and outcome identification.**
- **Discuss the types of skills that nurses must possess in order to perform the nursing interventions during the implementation step of the nursing process.**
- **Identify factors that may influence evaluation.**
- **Explain how critical thinking and problem solving are related to the nursing process.**
- **Use the nursing process to provide safe, effective client care.**
- **Discuss the purposes of documentation in health care.**
- **Explain the principles of effective documentation.**
- **Describe various methods of documentation.**
- **Identify various types of documentation records.**
- **Document client care accurately and completely.**

KEY TERMS

actual nursing diagnosis
analysis
assessment
assessment model
assigning
charting by
  exception (CBE)
collaborative problems
comprehensive
  assessment
confidential
critical pathway
data clustering
defining characteristic
delegation
dependent nursing
  intervention
discharge planning
documentation
etiology
evaluation
expected outcome
focus charting
focused assessment
goal
health history
implementation
incident report
independent nursing
  intervention

initial planning
interdependent nursing
  intervention
Kardex
long-term goal
medical diagnosis
narrative charting
nursing audit
nursing care plan
nursing diagnosis
nursing intervention
Nursing Intervention
  Classification (NIC)
Nursing Minimum Data
  Set (NMDS)
Nursing Outcome
  Classification (NOC)
nursing process
objective data
ongoing assessment
ongoing planning
PIE charting
planning
point-of-care charting
primary source
problem-oriented
  medical record
process
protocol
risk nursing diagnosis

Continues

INTRODUCTION

The nursing process and documentation depend on each other for providing safe and effective client care. The nursing process lays out a plan of care that guides not only the care provided but also the accurate recording of that care. Documentation provides a legal record that all aspects of the nursing process were properly carried out and that professional standards of care, regulatory standards, and agency policies were met.

This chapter first explains the nursing process in general and then each step individually. The legal aspects, methods, and forms for documenting are explained. Many examples are provided throughout the chapter.

NURSING PROCESS HISTORY

The first reference to nursing as a "process" was in a 1955 journal article by Lydia Hall, yet the term *nursing process* was not widely used until the late 1960s (Edelman & Mandle, 2002). Johnson (1959), Orlando (1961), and Wiedenbach (1963) referred to the nursing process as a series of three steps: assessment, planning, and evaluation. Yura and Walsh (1967) identified four steps in the nursing process:

1. Assessing
2. Planning
3. Implementing
4. Evaluating

The term *nursing diagnosis,* was first used by Fry (1953). After the first meeting of the group now called the North American Nursing Diagnosis Association (NANDA) in 1974, nursing diagnosis was added as a separate step in the nursing process. Now, the steps of the nursing process are:

1. Assessment
2. Diagnosis
3. Planning and outcome identification
4. Implementation
5. Evaluation

THE NURSING PROCESS

A **process** is a series of steps or acts that lead to accomplishing some goal or purpose. According to Bevis,

"processes have three characteristics: (1) inherent purpose, (2) internal organization, and (3) infinite creativity" (1989). These characteristics are found in the nursing process. The **nursing process** is a systematic method for providing care to clients. The purpose is to provide individualized, holistic, effective client care efficiently. Although the steps of the nursing process build on each other, they are not linear. Each step overlaps with the previous and subsequent steps (Figure 8-1).

The nursing process is dynamic and requires creativity in its application. The steps are the same for each client situation, but the correlation and results will be different. The nursing process can be used with clients of all ages and in any care setting. It is also the organizing system for the National Council Licensure Examination for both practical/vocational nurses (NCLEX-PN®) and registered nurses (NCLEX-RN®).

Assessment

Assessment, the first step in the nursing process, includes systematic collection, verification, organization, interpretation, and documentation of data. The completeness and correctness of this data relate directly to the accuracy of the steps that follow. Assessment involves the following steps:

- Data collection from a variety of sources
- Data validation
- Data organization
- Data interpretation
- Data documentation

Purpose of Assessment

The purpose of assessment is to organize a database regarding a client's physical, psychosocial, and emotional health so that health-promoting behaviors and actual and/or potential health problems can be identified. The nurse ascertains the client's functional abilities, the absence or presence of dysfunction, normal activities of daily living and lifestyle patterns through assessment.

NURSING PROCESS

Figure 8-1 *Five Components of the Nursing Process: Assessment, Diagnosis, Planning and Outcome Identification, Implementation, and Evaluation. The arrows going down represent revisions.*

Identifying the client's strengths gives the nurse information about the abilities, behaviors, and skills the client can use during the treatment and recovery process. Assessment also provides an opportunity to form a therapeutic interpersonal relationship with the client. During assessment, the client can discuss health care concerns and goals with the nurse.

Types of Assessment

The information needed for assessment is usually determined by the health care setting and needs of the client. Three types of assessment are comprehensive, focused, and ongoing. A comprehensive assessment is most desirable when first determining a client's need for nursing care. Time limits or special circumstances may require an abbreviated data collection, as shown in a focused assessment. The assessment database can then be broadened through ongoing assessment.

Comprehensive Assessment A **comprehensive assessment** provides baseline client data including a complete health history and current needs assessment. It is usually completed upon admission to a health care agency. Changes in the client's health status can be measured against this database. It should include assessment of the client's physical and psychosocial health, perception of health, presence of health risk factors, and coping patterns.

Focused Assessment A **focused assessment** is limited to potential health care risks, a particular need, or health care concern. They are not as detailed as comprehensive assessments and are often used when short stays are anticipated (e.g., outpatient surgery centers and emergency departments), in specialty areas such as mental health settings, labor and delivery, or for screening for specific problems or risk factors (e.g., well-child clinics).

Ongoing Assessment When problems are identified during a comprehensive or focused assessment, follow-up is required. An **ongoing assessment** includes systematic monitoring of specific problems. This type of assessment broadens the database and allows the nurse to confirm the validity of data obtained during the initial assessment. Systematic monitoring allows the nurse to determine the client's response to nursing interventions and to identify any other problems.

Sources of Data

Although data are collected from a variety of sources, the client is considered the **primary source** of data (the major provider of information about a client). As much information as possible should be gathered from the client, using both interview techniques and physical examination skills. Sources of data other than the client are considered **secondary sources** and include family members, other health care providers, and medical records.

Types of Data

Two types of information are collected through assessment: subjective and objective. **Subjective data** are data from the client's (sometimes family's) point of view and include perceptions, feelings, and concerns. The primary method of collecting subjective data (also called symptoms) is the interview. The **health history,** a review of the client's functional health patterns prior to the current contact with the health care agency, provides much of the subjective data.

Objective data (also called signs) are observable and measurable data that are obtained through both standard assessment techniques performed during the physical examination (Figure 8-2) and the results of laboratory and diagnostic testing. Table 8-1 provides examples of both subjective and objective data.

Validating the Data

Objective data may add to or validate subjective data. Validation is a critical step that prevents misunderstandings, omissions, and incorrect inferences and conclusions (Figure 8-3). This process is particularly important if data sources are considered unreliable, such as when a client is confused or unable to communicate. If two sources provide conflicting data, further information or

Figure 8-2 *The nurse is gathering objective data by examining retinal structures.*

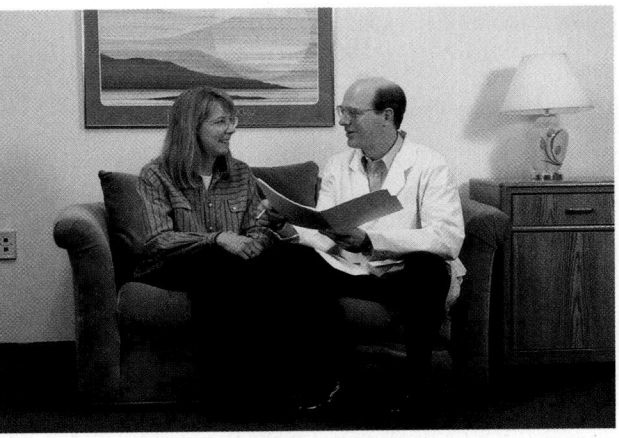

Figure 8-3 *This nurse is validating information collected from the client during assessment.*

TABLE 8-1	TYPES OF DATA	

DATA

An African-American male, age 79, comes to the emergency room because he cannot move his left arm. The client states "It happened about an hour ago when my headache got worse. Now I am nauseated and dizzy."

The nurse takes his vital signs: T 99, P 100, R 28, BP 168/96, and observes that he cannot move his left arm and his face is flushed.

TYPE OF DATA

Subjective	Objective
headache	T 99, P 100
nausea	R 28, BP 168/96
dizziness	cannot move left arm
	flushed face

clarification must be sought. Findings should also be compared with norms, and grossly abnormal findings should be rechecked and confirmed.

Organizing the Data

Collected data must be organized so as to be useful to the health care professional collecting the data and to others involved in the client's care. After being organized into categories, the data are clustered into groups of related pieces. **Data clustering** is the process of putting data together in order to identify areas of the client's problems and strengths. Many health care agencies use an admission assessment format, which assists the nurse in collecting and organizing data.

An **assessment model** is a framework providing a systematic way to organize data. A few of the many assessment models available to nurses are described following.

Hierarchy of Needs Maslow's hierarchy of needs proposes that an individual's basic needs (physiological) must be met before higher-level needs can be met. An initial assessment of all physiological needs followed by assessment of the higher-level needs is necessary when using this model.

Body Systems Model The body systems model organizes data collection according to tissue and organ function in the various body systems (e.g., respiratory, cardiovascular, gastrointestinal). Physicians frequently use this model, so it is sometimes called the "medical model."

Functional Health Patterns Gordon's Functional Health Patterns (Gordon, 1998) provides a framework for data collection focusing on 11 functional health patterns. These functional health pattern areas cluster information about a client's habitual patterns and any recent changes to determine if the client's current response is functional or dysfunctional. For example, the elimination pattern is assessed for a client who now has diarrhea several times a week. Data collection would be focused on elimination habits, diet, and fluid intake before the diarrhea began, and the effect of any changes on the client's functional ability and lifestyle. The 11 patterns are:

- Health perception/health management pattern
- Nutritional/metabolic pattern
- Elimination pattern
- Activity/exercise pattern
- Cognitive/perceptual pattern
- Sleep/rest pattern
- Self-perception/self-concept pattern
- Role/relationship pattern
- Sexuality/reproductive pattern
- Coping/stress-tolerance pattern
- Value/belief pattern (Gordon, 1998)

Theory of Self-Care Orem (2001) developed the theory of self-care based on a client's ability to perform self-care activities. Self-care, learned behavior with deliberate actions responding to need, includes activities an individual performs to maintain health. This theory focuses on the assessment of the client's ability to meet self-care needs and identifying existing self-care deficits. This theory is primarily concerned with illness states. The self-care essentials are:

- Maintenance of a sufficient intake of air
- Maintenance of a sufficient intake of water
- Maintenance of a sufficient intake of food
- Provision of care associated with elimination processes and excrements

- Maintenance of a balance between activity and rest
- Maintenance of a balance between solitude and social interaction
- Prevention of hazards to human life, human functioning, and human well-being
- Promotion of human functioning and development within social groups in accord with human potential, known human limitations, and the human desire to be normal (Orem, 2001)

Interpreting the Data

After data have been collected, the nurse can begin developing impressions or inferences about the meaning of the data. Organizing data in clusters helps the nurse recognize patterns of response or behavior. When data are placed in clusters, the nurse can:

- Distinguish between relevant and irrelevant data.
- Determine whether and where there are gaps in the data.
- Identify patterns of cause and effect.

Documenting the Data

Assessment data must be recorded and some reported. The nurse must decide which data should be immediately reported to the head nurse and/or physician and which data can just be recorded. Data reflecting a significant change from the normal (e.g., BP 180/100, severe difficulty in breathing, or a high level of anxiety) would need to be reported as well as recorded. Data that need only be recorded include the fact that prescribed medication relieved a headache and that an abdominal dressing is dry and intact.

It is essential for accurate and complete recording of assessment data to communicate information to other health care team members. The basis for determining quality of care is documentation, which includes data to support identified problems.

Diagnosis

The second step in the nursing process involves further **analysis** (breaking down the whole into parts that can be examined) and **synthesis** (putting data together in a new way) of the collected data. A list of nursing diagnoses is the result of this process. According to NANDA, a **nursing diagnosis**

is a clinical judgment about individual, family, or community responses to actual or potential health problems/life processes. A nursing diagnosis provides the basis for selection of nursing interventions to achieve outcomes for which the nurse is accountable. (NANDA, 2003)

The nursing diagnoses provide the basis for client care through the remaining steps.

Clients have both medical and nursing diagnoses. Table 8-2 compares the two categories of diagnoses. It is important to have a clear understanding of the nature of a nursing diagnosis as compared to a **medical diagnosis** (clinical judgment by the physician that identifies or determines a specific disease, condition, or pathological state). Table 8-3 compares selected nursing and medical diagnoses.

TABLE 8-2 COMPARISON OF NURSING AND MEDICAL DIAGNOSES

NURSING DIAGNOSIS	MEDICAL DIAGNOSIS
Recognizes situations that the nurse is licensed and qualified to treat.	Recognizes conditions the physician is licensed and qualified to treat.
Concentrates on the client's responses to health problems or life processes.	Concentrates on injury, illness, or disease processes.
Varies as the client's responses and/or health problems change.	Stays the same until a cure is realized or client dies.
Example: Nausea, Acute Pain, Acute Pain, Impaired Physical Mobility	**Example:** Cholelithiasis, Surgery, Cholecystectomy

TABLE 8-3 COMPARISON OF SELECT NURSING AND MEDICAL DIAGNOSES

NURSING DIAGNOSIS	MEDICAL DIAGNOSIS
Decreased Cardiac Output, Ineffective Breathing Pattern, Risk for Imbalanced Fluid Volume	Congestive heart failure
Impaired Physical Mobility	Meniere's disease
Death Anxiety	Lung cancer
Ineffective Airway Clearance	Chronic obstructive pulmonary disease
Ineffective Breathing Pattern Anxiety	

The nurse uses critical-thinking and decision-making skills in developing nursing diagnoses. These skills are discussed later in the chapter.

Components of a Nursing Diagnosis

The nursing diagnosis may be stated as a two-part statement or a three-part statement. The two-part statement is NANDA approved and used by most nurses because it is brief and precise. The three-part statement is often required of nursing students and is preferred by nurses who desire the diagnostic statement to include specific manifestations. Refer to the appendices for the list of NANDA-approved nursing diagnoses.

Two-Part Statement The first part, the actual nursing diagnosis, is a problem statement or diagnostic label describing the client's response to an actual or risk health problem or a wellness condition.

The second part is the **etiology,** the related cause or contributor to the problem, which is identified in the complete NANDA diagnosis description. The diagnostic label and etiology are linked by the term *related to* (R/T). Because the NANDA list of nursing diagnoses is constantly evolving, there may be times when no etiology is provided. In such cases, the nurse should attempt to describe likely contributing factors to the client's condition. Examples of a two-part nursing diagnosis statement are *Disturbed Body Image* R/T loss of left lower extremity and *Activity Intolerance* R/T decreased oxygen-carrying capacity of cells.

Three-Part Statement In a three-part statement, the first two parts are the diagnostic label and the etiology. The third part consists of **defining characteristics** (collected data, also known as signs and symptoms, subjective and objective data, or clinical manifestations). The third part is joined to the first two parts with the connecting phrase *as evidenced by* (AEB). An example of a three-part nursing diagnosis statement is *Ineffective Breathing Pattern* R/T pain AEB respiratory rate less than 11 and use of accessory muscles. Table 8-4 provides other examples.

Types of Nursing Diagnoses

Analysis of the collected data leads the nurse to make a diagnosis in one of three categories:

- An **actual nursing diagnosis** indicates that a problem exists; it is composed of the diagnostic label, related factors, and signs and symptoms. An example of an actual diagnosis is *Situational Low Self-esteem* R/T loss (first chair trumpet in band) AEB self-negating verbalization "I'm no good anymore."

TABLE 8-4 EXAMPLES OF NURSING DIAGNOSES WRITTEN AS TWO- AND THREE-PART STATEMENTS

TWO-PART STATEMENT	THREE-PART STATEMENT
Toileting *Self-care Deficit* R/T neuromuscular impairment	Toileting *Self-care Deficit* R/T neuromuscular impairment, right sided AEB inability to ambulate to the bathroom
Impaired Swallowing R/T mechanical obstruction	*Impaired Swallowing* R/T/mechanical obstruction AEB presence of tracheostomy tube
Impaired Urinary Elimination R/T urinary tract infection	*Impaired Urinary Elimination* R/T urinary tract infection AEB frequency and dysuria
Impaired Memory R/T fluid and electrolyte imbalance	*Impaired Memory* R/T fluid and electrolyte imbalance AEB inability to recall recent or past events
Impaired Home Maintenance R/T individual/family member disease or injury	*Impaired Home Maintenance* R/T individual/family member disease or injury AEB repeated lice infestations

- A **risk nursing diagnosis** (potential problem) indicates that a problem does not yet exist, but that specific risk factors are present. A risk diagnosis begins with the phrase *Risk for* followed by the diagnostic label and a list of the risk factors. An example of a risk diagnosis is *Risk for Situational Low Self-esteem;* risk factors include unrealistic self-expectations AEB receiving "B" in two college courses while working full-time (expected "A").
- A **wellness nursing diagnosis** denotes the client's statement of a desire to attain a higher level of wellness in some area of function. It begins with the phrase *Readiness for Enhanced* followed by the diagnostic label. For example, a wife who has been caring for her husband who had a stroke two months ago asks the nurse about meeting with other wives who are/have been in a similar situation. The nurse would make a wellness diagnosis of *Readiness for Enhanced Family Coping.*

Examples of the three types of diagnoses are shown in Table 8-5.

After formulation, the nursing diagnoses should be discussed with the client, but if this is not possible, the diagnoses may be discussed with family members. The list of nursing diagnoses is recorded on the client's record, and the remainder of the client's care plan is completed. The list of nursing diagnoses is dynamic, changing as more data are collected and as client goals and responses to interventions are evaluated.

Carpenito (2002) discusses situations in which nurses intervene in collaboration with other disciplines.

TABLE 8-5 TYPES OF NURSING DIAGNOSES

TYPE	EXAMPLE
Actual Diagnosis	*Perceived Constipation R/T faulty appraisal AEB expectation of passage of stool at same time every day*
Risk Diagnosis	*Risk for Aspiration R/T decreased cough and gag reflexes*
Wellness Diagnosis	*Readiness for Enhanced Spiritual Wellbeing*

She defines **collaborative problems** as "certain physiologic complications that nurses monitor to detect onset or changes in states. Nurses manage collaborative problems using physician-prescribed and nursing-prescribed interventions to minimize the complications of the events." She has identified 52 specific collaborative problems grouped under 9 generic problem categories. For example, under the generic collaborative problem category of *Potential Complication (PC): Respiratory* are the specific collaborative problems of "PC: Hypoxemia, PC: Atelectasis/pneumonia, PC: Tracheobronchial Constriction, and PC: Pneumothorax."

The collaborative problem statement *always* begins with *Potential Complication* or PC. This differentiates it from a nursing diagnosis. A benefit of using collaborative problem statements is that they identify, and thus keep the nurses aware of, the potential complications a client may encounter. As in the previous example, the specific potential complication for a client with a respiratory problem would be listed on the care plan.

Planning and Outcome Identification

Planning and outcome identification are the third step of the nursing process and include both establishing guidelines for the proposed course of nursing action to resolve the nursing diagnoses and developing the client's plan of care. After the nursing diagnoses and the client's strengths have been identified, planning begins.

The planning occurs in three phases: initial, ongoing, and discharge. **Initial planning** involves development of a preliminary plan of care by the nurse who performs the admission assessment and gathers the comprehensive admission assessment data. Progressively shorter stays in the hospital make initial planning very important to ensure resolution of the problems. **Ongoing planning** updates the client's plan of care. New information about the client is collected and evaluated and revisions made to the plan of care. **Discharge planning** involves anticipation of and planning for the client's needs after discharge.

The planning phase involves several tasks:

- Prioritizing the nursing diagnoses
- Identifying and writing client-centered long- and short-term goals and outcomes (outcome identification)
- Identifying specific nursing interventions
- Recording the entire nursing care plan in the client's record

Prioritizing the Nursing Diagnoses

Prioritizing the nursing diagnoses involves deciding which diagnoses are the most important and require attention first. Maslow's hierarchy of need is one of the most common methods of selecting priorities. After basic physiological needs (e.g., respiration, nutrition, temperature, hydration, and elimination) are met to some degree, the nurse can then consider needs on the next level of the hierarchy (e.g., safe environment, stable living condition, affection, and self-worth) and so on up the hierarchy until all of the nursing diagnoses have been prioritized.

Alfaro-LeFevre (1999) suggests a three-level approach to prioritizing client problems (nursing diagnoses):

- **First-level priority problems (immediate):**
  Airway problems
  Breathing problems
  Signs (vital sign problems)
- **Second-level priority problems (immediate, after treatment for first-level problems is initiated):**
  Mental status change
  Acute pain
  Acute urinary elimination problems
  Untreated medical problems requiring immediate attention (e.g., a diabetic who has not had insulin)
  Abnormal lab values
  Risks of infection, safety, or security (for client or others)
- **Third-level priority problems:**
  Health problems that do not fit in the above categories
  She also proposes that *sometimes* the priority order may change. For example, if acute pain causes breathing problems, managing the pain may have the higher priority; if abnormal lab values are life threatening, then they have a higher priority. Table 8-6 illustrates the prioritizing process.

TABLE 8-6 PRIORITIZING NURSING DIAGNOSES

NURSING DIAGNOSIS	PRIORITIZING METHOD	PRIORITY
Decreased Cardiac Output R/T altered heart rate rhythm	Maslow, physiologic	High
	Alfaro-LeFevre, cardiac/circulatory	High
Diarrhea R/T travel	Maslow, physiologic	High
	Alfaro-LeFevre, untreated medical problem	Moderate
Relocation Stress Syndrome R/T isolation from family/friends	Maslow, safety and security	Moderate
	Alfaro-LeFevre, risk to security	Moderate
Disturbed Sleep Pattern R/T daytime activity pattern	Maslow, safety and security	Moderate
	Alfaro-LeFevre, other health problems	Low
Ineffective Coping R/T inadequate resources available	Maslow, self-esteem	Low
	Alfaro-LeFevre, other health problems	Low

Identifying Outcomes

Outcome identification includes establishing goals and expected outcomes, which together provide guidelines for individualized nursing interventions and establish evaluation criteria to measure the effectiveness of the nursing care plan.

Goals A **goal** is an aim, intent, or end. Goals are broad statements that describe the desired or intended change in the client's condition or behavior. Client-centered goals are established in collaboration with the client when possible. Goal statements refer to the diagnostic label (or problem statement) of the nursing diagnosis. Client-centered goals ensure that nursing care is individualized and focused on the client.

A **short-term goal** is a statement that profiles the desired resolution of the nursing diagnosis over a short period of time, usually a few hours or days (less than a week). It focuses on the etiology part of the nursing diagnosis. A **long-term goal** is a statement that profiles the desired resolution of the nursing diagnosis over a longer period of time, usually weeks or months. It focuses on the problem part of the nursing diagnosis. Table 8-7 provides examples of short-term and long-term goals.

Expected Outcomes After the goals have been established, the expected outcomes can be identified based on those goals. An **expected outcome** is a detailed, specific statement describing the methods to be used to achieve the goal. It includes direct nursing care, client teaching, and continuity of care. Outcomes must be measurable, realistic, and time limited. Several expected outcomes may be required for each goal (Table 8-8). Then nursing interventions are formulated to enable the client to reach the goals.

Identifying Specific Nursing Interventions

A **nursing intervention** is an action performed by the nurse that helps the client achieve the results specified by the goals and expected outcomes. Nursing interventions refer directly to the related factors or the risk factors in nursing diagnoses. Nursing interventions that reduce or remove the related factors and risk factors resolve or prevent the problem.

There may be a number of nursing interventions for each nursing diagnosis. Nursing interventions are stated

TABLE 8-8 GOAL AND EXPECTED OUTCOMES

Nursing Diagnosis: *Impaired Urinary Elimination* R/T Urinary Tract Infection AEB Frequent Urination in Small Amounts

GOAL	EXPECTED OUTCOMES
Client will have improved urinary elimination.	Client will take antibiotic as ordered. By next visit, client will identify three factors to prevent a urinary tract infection. In 2 days, client will have a plan to increase water intake. By next visit, client will be urinating at least 150 mL at 2 hour or longer intervals.

Nursing Diagnosis: *Powerlessness* R/T Illness-Related Regimen AEB Nonparticipation in Care or Decision Making When Opportunities Are Provided

GOAL	EXPECTED OUTCOMES
Client will participate in care and decision making.	In 2 days, client will participate in one aspect of own care each day. Client will state preference in decision-making situation within 1 week.

in specific terms. Examples of nursing interventions are as follows:

- Assist client to turn, cough, and deep breathe q 2 h beginning at 0800, 4/15
- Teach cord care at 1000, 6/20
- Weigh client at 0700 each day

Interventions formulated for each diagnosis are recorded on the client's care plan. The list of interventions is also dynamic and may change as the nurse interacts with the client, assesses responses to interventions, and evaluates those responses.

Categories of Nursing Interventions

Nursing interventions are classified into one of three categories: independent, interdependent, or dependent. **Independent nursing interventions** are initiated by the nurse and do not require direction or an order from another health care professional. Most states' nursing

TABLE 8-7 SHORT- AND LONG-TERM GOALS

NURSING DIAGNOSIS: *DISTURBED BODY IMAGE R/T SURGERY FOR BREAST CANCER*

Short-term Goals (focus on etiology)	Long-term Goals (focus on problem)
Will verbalize loss of breast	Will verbalize acceptance of change in physical self
Will identify negative feelings about body	
Will touch chest where breast was	

Nursing Interventions

Differentiate among the three categories of nursing interventions: independent, interdependent, and dependent.

practice acts allow independent nursing interventions for activities such as daily living, health education, health promotion, and counseling. An example of an independent nursing intervention is elevating a client's edematous extremity.

Interdependent nursing interventions are implemented collaboratively by the nurse in conjunction with other health care professionals. For example, the nurse may assist a client to perform an exercise taught by the physical therapist.

Dependent nursing interventions require an order from a physician or another health care professional. Administration of a medication is an example of a dependent intervention. This intervention requires specific nursing knowledge and responsibilities, but it is not within the realm of legal practice for LP/VNs to prescribe medications. The nurse is responsible for knowing the classification, normal dosage, pharmacological action, contraindications, adverse effects, and nursing implications of the drug. Dependent nursing interventions must be governed by appropriate knowledge and judgment.

Recording the Nursing Care Plan

The **nursing care plan** is a written guide of strategies to be implemented to help the client achieve optimal health. Nursing care plans usually include components such as assessment, nursing diagnoses, goals and expected outcomes, and nursing interventions. The care plan is begun on the day of admission and is continually updated until discharge.

Care plans may be standardized, institutional, or computerized.

The standardized care plan is a printed guide for the care of clients with common needs. This care plan usually follows the nursing process format. It may be individualized by including handwritten notes for unusual problems.

Institutional nursing care plans are concise documents that become a part of the client's medical record after discharge. This care plan may simply include the nursing diagnoses, nursing interventions, and evaluation. Figure 8-4 provides an example of an institutional care plan.

Computers can generate both standardized and individualized nursing care plans. Appropriate diagnoses are selected from a menu, which lists possible goals and nursing interventions. Figure 8-5 is an example of a computerized nursing care plan.

Implementation

The fourth step in the nursing process is **implementation,** the performance of the nursing interventions identified during the planning phase. It also involves the **delegation** (process of transferring a select nursing task to a licensed individual who is competent to perform that specific task) of some nursing interventions to staff members or **assigning** a specific nursing task to assistive (unlicensed) personnel capable of competently performing the task. The nurse is accountable for appropriate delegation and supervision of care provided by unlicensed personnel.

Requirements for Effective Implementation

Implementation involves many skills, including assessing the client's condition before, during, and after each nursing intervention. Positive responses add information to the database to use when evaluating the intervention. Negative responses must be dealt with immediately.

Psychomotor, interpersonal, and cognitive skills are also needed to perform the planned nursing interventions. Psychomotor skills are used when handling medical

Nursing Diagnosis	Nursing Interventions	Evaluation
Ineffective Breastfeeding R/T deficient knowledge AEB inability to latch on to the maternal breast correctly	1. Teach various breastfeeding positions and techniques to encourage the infant.	1. Client tried the various positions and techniques.
	2. Stay with mother during feeding and assist as needed.	2. Client able to assist infant to latch on to breast correctly.
Risk for Constipation R/T abdominal muscle weakness and hemorrhoids	1. Assess daily for bowel movement frequency and consistency.	1. Bowel movement daily, very firm consistency.
	2. Encourage more fluid and fiber intake.	2. Asking for fruit between meals; drinking 8 oz water
	3) exercise	every 2 hours when
	4) Meds / order	awake.

Figure 8-4 *Handwritten Institutional Care Plan*

Client Name: Jane White   **Sex:** Female

Age: 77   **Temp:** 101.5   **BP:** 168/74   **Pulse:** 124   **O₂ Sat:** 89%

Client Health History

Ms. White has smoked two to three packs of cigarettes a day for the past 60 years. She was diagnosed with COPD 4 years ago and has required supplemental oxygen at 2 L/min for the past 18 months. Her chief complaints are increasing dyspnea on exertion and a cough, which is sometimes productive, yielding thick, green-yellow sputum. She states, "I don't know why I'm coughing up this awful stuff."

Assessment Findings

Respiratory Rate 38

Sonorous and sibilant wheezes on expiration in the posterior lung fields with superimposed coarse crackles heard in the right posterior lower lung field.

Unable to ambulate to the bathroom or complete other ADLs because of dyspnea

Nursing Diagnosis: *Ineffective **B**reathing Pattern* R/T diseased lungs, infection, and increased secretions AEB severe dyspnea, elevated blood pressure, and increased pulse

Goals: Ms. White will:

1. Have a normal respiratory rate.
2. Have clear lung sounds.
3. Be able to complete ADLs.
4. Increase oral fluid intake.

Planning and Intervention

Intervention	Rationale
1. Assist client in assuming a high Fowler's position	Maximizes thoracic cavity space, decreases pressure from diaphragm and abdominal organs, facilitates use of accessory muscles
2. Provide humidified, low flow (2 L/min) oxygen, as ordered	Provides some supplemental oxygen to improve oxygenation and makes secretions less viscous
3. Administer bronchodilators, as ordered	Reduces bronchospasm and improves air flow
4. Administer IV fluids and increase oral fluids (2000–3000 mL/day as tolerated), as ordered	Improves hydration, decreases secretions

5. Administer expectorants, as ordered	Decreases secretions of previously ineffective cough
6. Administer antibiotics, as ordered	Eradicates respiratory infection or pneumonia and reduces secretions and end inflammation
7. Administer xanthines (aminophylline, theophylline), as ordered	Decreases smooth muscle spasm and edema of the mucosa
8. Administer non-narcotic cough suppressants, as ordered	Coughing can lead to fatigue. It is important for COPD clients to get adequate rest and not become fatigued

Evaluation/Outcome

Client's breathing returns to a more normal pattern

Client is able to cough up secretions

Client is able to ambulate to bathroom and complete ADLs

Client is drinking at least 2000 mL/day of water

Nursing Diagnosis: *Impaired **G**as Exchange* R/T lower airway (alveolar) wall destruction preventing adequate exchange of gases of respiration and airway obstruction (secretions) preventing adequate oxygenation AEB severe dyspnea, tachypnea, elevated blood pressure, increased pulse, and decreased oxygen saturation

Goals: Ms. White will:

1. Have O2 saturation of 95%.
2. Have normal vital signs.

Planning and Interventions

Intervention	Rationale
1. Assist client in assuming a high Fowler's position	Decreases the work of breathing (at least through crisis period)
2. Administer medications to loosen secretions, as ordered	Decreases secretions of previously ineffective cough
3. Provide humidified, low flow (2 L/min) oxygen, as ordered	Improves oxygenation, moistens thick secretions

Evaluation/Outcome

Client's O₂ saturation is 94%

Client's vital signs in normal range

Figure 8-5   *Computer-Generated Nursing Care Plan*

equipment and performing skills such as changing dressings, giving injections, and helping a client perform range-of-motion (ROM) exercises.

Interpersonal skills are used when collecting data, providing information in teaching sessions, and offering support in times of grief.

Cognitive skills enable the nurse to make appropriate observations, understand the rationale for the activities performed, ask appropriate questions, and make decisions about those things that need to be done. Critical thinking is an important element within the cognitive domain. It helps the nurse analyze data, organize observations, and apply prior knowledge and experiences to current client situations.

Orders for Nursing Interventions

Nursing interventions are written as orders in the care plan and may be initiated by nurses, physicians, or from collaboration with other health care professionals. Interventions can be implemented on the basis of specific orders, standing orders, or protocols.

A **specific order** is an order written in a client's medical record by a physician or nursing care plan by the nurse especially for that individual client; it is not used for any other client.

A **standing order** is a standardized intervention written, approved, and signed by a physician that is kept on file within health care agencies to be used in predictable situations or in circumstances requiring immediate attention. Nurses implement standing orders after assessing the client and identifying the problem. A physician-initiated standing order on an inpatient unit might be a specific medication to be given for constipation.

A **protocol** is a series of standing orders or procedures that should be followed under certain specific conditions. It defines interventions that are permitted and circumstances under which the nurse can implement the measures. Health care agencies or individual physicians often use standing orders or protocols for preparing clients for diagnostic tests or for immediate interventions in life-threatening circumstances. Protocols prevent needlessly writing the same orders for different clients, saving valuable time.

Documenting and Reporting Interventions

The implementation step also involves documentation and reporting. Data to be recorded include the client's condition before the intervention, the specific intervention performed, the client's response to the intervention, and client outcomes. Documentation provides valuable communication among health care team members to ensure continuity of care and evaluate progress toward expected outcomes. Written documentation also provides data necessary for reimbursement.

Verbal communication between nurses generally occurs at the change of shift, when care responsibility changes. Nursing students must report relevant information to the nurse responsible for their clients when they leave the unit. Information that should be shared in the verbal report includes:

- Completed activities and those not completed
- Status of current relevant problems
- Assessment changes or abnormalities
- Results of treatments
- Diagnostic tests scheduled or completed (and results)

Both written and verbal communication must be objective, descriptive, and complete. It must include observations, not opinions and be stated or written to show an accurate picture of the client's condition. Communication of implementation activities is basic to client care and evaluation of progress toward goals.

Figure 8-6 *Relationship of Evaluation to the Other Components of the Nursing Process: Evaluation Impacts Every Component*

Evaluation

Evaluation, the fifth step in the nursing process, determines whether client goals have been met, partially met, or not met. When a goal is met, the nurse decides whether nursing interventions should stop or continue for the status to be maintained. When a goal is partially met or not met, the nurse reassesses the situation. The reasons the goal is not met and modifications to the plan of care are determined by more data collection. Reasons that goals are not met or are only partially met include:

- Initial assessment data were incomplete.
- Goals and expected outcomes were unrealistic.
- Time frame was not adequate.
- Nursing interventions were not appropriate for the client or situation.

Evaluation is a fluid process that depends on all the other components of the nursing process. As shown in Figure 8-6, evaluation affects, and is affected by, the other four parts. Table 8-9 shows how evaluation is woven into every component of the nursing process. Ongoing evaluation is essential for the nursing process to be implemented appropriately. As Alfaro-LeFevre (2004) states:

> When we evaluate early, checking whether our information is accurate, complete, and up-to-date, we're able to make corrections *early*. We avoid making decisions based on outdated, inaccurate, or incomplete information. Early evaluation enhances our ability to act safely and effectively. It improves our *efficiency* by helping us stay focused on priorities and avoid wasting time continuing useless actions.

THE NURSING PROCESS AND CRITICAL THINKING

Many skills are necessary when nurses use the nursing process as a framework for providing client care. Critical thinking is one. Critical thinkers ask questions, identify assumptions, evaluate evidence, examine alternatives, and seek to understand various points of view.

Critical thinking can be learned, just as other skills are learned. The skill of critical thinking is an especially vital tool for the nurse but is useful in all aspects of a

COMMUNITY/HOME HEALTH CARE

Standing Orders

Nurses in home health care agencies may have standing orders for administering certain medications or ordering laboratory tests when indicated.

TABLE 8-9 INTERACTION OF OTHER COMPONENTS OF THE NURSING PROCESS WITH EVALUATION	
NURSING PROCESS COMPONENTS	**EVALUATION QUESTIONS**
Assessment	Are data relevant to client needs?
	Are data obtained appropriately?
	Are data collected from many, varied sources?
	Is a systematic, organized method used to collect data?
	Is data collection complete?
Diagnosis	Are diagnoses based on the data collected?
	Is each nursing diagnosis complete?
	Are nursing diagnoses client centered and relevant?
	Do nursing diagnoses guide planning and implementation of care?
Planning and Outcome Identification	Are nursing diagnoses prioritized?
	Are expected outcomes relevant to nursing diagnoses?
	Are outcomes realistic?
	Are resources (also team members) used effectively and efficiently?
	Are care plans documented?
	Is care plan revised according to the client's needs?
Implementation	Is plan of care followed by all team members?
	Are necessary resources available?
	Do nursing actions assist client in meeting expected outcomes?
	Are expected outcomes achieved?
	Does documentation reflect client status and responses to nursing interventions?

COMMUNITY/HOME HEALTH CARE

Effectiveness of Care

In the home, the nurse can use the following questions to evaluate client achievement of expected outcomes:

- Were the goals realistic for client abilities and the time frame?
- Did external variables (e.g., finances, housing problems, impaired family dynamics) prevent goal achievement?
- Did the family have resources (e.g., money, transportation) necessary to meet the goals?
- Was care appropriately coordinated with other providers?

person's life. Examples of questions the nurse, as critical thinker, might ask at each step in the nursing process are listed in Table 8-10.

THE NURSING PROCESS AND DECISION MAKING

Every day, nurses make decisions. These decisions should be the best decisions possible based on reliable information, and made using critical thinking. Each step of the nursing process requires decisions.

Each decision, resulting from critical thought and reliable information, leads to appropriate nursing interventions for the client.

THE NURSING PROCESS AND HOLISTIC CARE

The broad base of nursing knowledge is derived from many fields, including natural science, social science, behavioral science, arts and humanities, and nursing science. With this broad knowledge base the nurse interacts with the client in a holistic manner. Referral and collaboration among nurses and other health care professionals contribute to holistic achievement of client goals.

In some settings, the traditional nursing care plan formulated solely by nurses has been replaced by plans that are developed by a multidisciplinary team and referred to as critical pathways. **Critical pathways** are comprehensive, standard plans of care for specific conditions.

DOCUMENTATION

The methods of recording and reporting information relevant to client care have developed as a response to standards of practice, legal and regulatory standards, institutional standards and policies, and society's norms.

Recording and reporting are the major ways health care providers communicate. The client's medical record is a legal document of all activities regarding client care. **Documentation** is any printed or written record of activities. In health care it should include:

- Changes in the client's condition
- The administration of tests, treatments, procedures, and client education; with the results of, or client's response to them.
- The client's response to an intervention
- The evaluation of expected outcomes
- Complaints from client or family

Purposes of Documentation

The two primary reasons for documentation are professional responsibility and accountability. The professional responsibility of all health care practitioners, documentation provides evidence of the practitioner's accountability to the client, the institution, the profession, and society. Other reasons are communication; legal and practice standards; education; reimbursement; research; and auditing.

TABLE 8-10	USE OF CRITICAL THINKING WITH THE NURSING PROCESS
STEP OF NURSING PROCESS	**SAMPLE CRITICAL THINKING QUESTIONS**
Assessment	What data are necessary to prevent, anticipate, or detect health problems? What data are necessary to manage or eliminate a client's health problems? From what other sources can data be obtained? How does the client view his health situation? How efficient is care delivery? What assumptions or biases does the nurse have?
Diagnosis	How can the data be put together and analyzed? Are there any gaps in the data? What health problems can be identified? What are the underlying causes of risk factors for the health problems? What are the client's strengths and resources? Which satisfactory aspects of the client's health could be improved?
Planning and Outcome Identification	What are the specific desired outcomes for this client? What interventions will detect or prevent health problems? Which interventions will manage the client's health problems? What interventions will promote optimum wellness and independence for the client? How can the desired outcomes be achieved in a cost-effective, timely manner? Who is best qualified to carry out the interventions? How much does the client wish to be involved?
Implementation	How ready is the health care giver to perform the interventions? What are the critical steps of this intervention? How can the intervention be altered to meet this client's needs yet maintain principles of safety? How does the client respond during and after the intervention? What is to be documented to monitor the client's progress toward the goals and outcomes?
Evaluation	Were the specific desired goals and outcomes met? If all were met, can these goals and outcomes be eliminated? If not met, how should the plan be modified (revised)? If revision of the plan, goals, or outcomes is necessary, what ongoing, continuous assessments (data) are required? Were assumptions or biases missed that affected the interventions? What other nursing diagnosis(es) may be appropriate? What additional outcomes and interventions should be considered?

Communication

Documentation is a communication method that confirms the care provided to the client and clearly outlines all important information regarding the client. Thorough documentation provides:

- Accurate data to plan care and ensure continuity of care
- Communication to health care team members involved in the client's care
- Evidence of things done to or for the client, the client's response, and revisions made in the plan of care
- Evidence of compliance with professional practice standards
- Evidence of compliance with accreditation criteria (e.g., those of the Joint Commission on Accreditation of Healthcare Organizations [JCAHO])
- A resource for reimbursement, education, and research and audit
- A written legal record to protect the client, institution, and practitioner

The client's medical record contains documents for recordkeeping. The type of documents that constitute the medical record in a given health care institution is determined by that institution. Table 8-11 outlines the content of the documents generally found in a client's record.

Practice and Legal Standards

The focal issue in many malpractice cases is failure to document appropriately (Springhouse, 1999). *The medical record is a legal document, and in a lawsuit, it is the record that serves as the description of exactly what happened to a client.* In 80% to 85% of client care lawsuits, the determining factor in providing proof of significant events is the medical record (Iyer & Camp, 1999). The legal aspects of documentation require:

- Writing, legible and neat
- Spelling and grammar, properly used
- Authorized abbreviations
- Time-sequenced, and factual descriptive entries

State Nursing Practice Acts State nursing practice acts establish guidelines to ensure safe practice and to demonstrate accountability to society. The standards of care set forth in the practice acts are based on the nursing process components and require documentation as evidenced of compliance. Nurses must be familiar with the practice act of the states in which they work.

Joint Commission on Accreditation of Healthcare Organizations (JCAHO) The JCAHO surveys health care facilities who voluntarily apply for accreditation to measure compliance with its standards for providing safe health care. Eligibility for Medicare, Medicaid, and private funding reimbursement depends on JCAHO accreditation.

The JCAHO requires documented evidence of an individualized plan of care (JCAHO, 1998). The JCAHO's standards require:

- The involvement of the client or family in the development of the plan, which must be documented in the medical record

TABLE 8-11 DOCUMENTS OF THE CLIENT MEDICAL RECORD

DOCUMENT	CONTENT
Face Sheet	*Demographic data:* name, client's identifying number, address, telephone number, date of birth, place of birth, sex, race, marital status, religion, name and address of closest relative, social security number, admission date and hour, type of admission
	Financial Data: expected payer(s), insured's name and sex, client relationship to insured, employer's name and location, group name, insurance group number, insured's policy number
	Clinical Data: admitting diagnosis, admitting diagnosis-related group (DRG), client's advance directive (if has one)
	Discharge Data (to be entered by the physician on discharge of client): name of attending physician, discharge date and hour, principal diagnosis and other diagnoses, external cause of injury code, procedures and dates, operating physician(s), disposition of client
Medical History and Physical Examination	Client's description of chief complaint, present and past illnesses, personal and family histories, and review of systems as elicited by the physician, findings of physician's assessment of all body systems
Nursing Admission Assessment	Data from interview and physical assessment performed by the nurse
Physician's Orders	Physician's written or verbal orders to admit, to direct client's diagnostic and therapeutic course, and to discharge
Consultation Report	Findings of a physician whose opinion or advice is requested by another physician for evaluation and/or treatment of a client
Physician's Progress Notes	Provides a pertinent, chronologic report of the client's course in the hospital and reflects any changes in condition and response to treatment. May also contain notes by other members of the health care team (e.g., dietary or social service)
Laboratory Reports	Results from laboratory tests ordered by the physician
Radiology Reports	Radiologists interpretation of radiologic and fluoroscopic diagnostic services
Nuclear Medicine	Describes diagnostic studies and therapeutic procedures performed using radiopharmaceutical agents
Graphic Sheet	Various client parameters, most commonly: T, P, R, and BP. May also include weight, diet, I&O
Client Care Plan (Nursing Plan of Care)	Treatment plan including nursing diagnoses or problem list, client goals, nursing actions, and evaluation
Nurse's Progress Notes	Details care and treatments provided, client's response to care and treatments, achievement of expected outcomes that do not duplicate information on Flow Sheet (if used)
Flow Sheet	All routine interventions that can be indicated by a check mark or other simple descriptor
Medication Administration	Contains all medications administered orally, topically, by injection, inhalation, and infusion in one place; includes date, time, dosage, route of administration, and name of professional administering the drug. Routine, PRN, and single dose orders generally have separate sections.
Consent Forms	*Admission:* gives the insitution and physician permission to treat
	Surgical: explains the reason for and nature of the treatment, the risks, complications, alternate forms of treatment, no treatment, consequences of treatment or procedure. Sometimes surgical and anesthesia consents are separate so that responsibility is placed appropriately.
	Blood Transfusion: gives specific permission to administer blood or blood products
	Other: procedure specific consent forms, participate in research project, photography
Client Education Record	Describes the nurse's teaching to the client, family, or other caregiver and the learner's response
Health Care Team Record	Used by respiratory, physical therapy, dietary when physician's progress are used only by physicians
Nursing Discharge Summary	Contains brief summary of care provided, medications, teaching, and other instructions (e.g., return appointment, referrals), discharge status, and mode of discharge
Discharge Summary	Review of events describing the client's illness, investigation (diagnostic studies), treatment, response, and condition at discharge. Instructions to the client and plans for follow-up care as included.
Advance Directive	Both a living will and a durable power of attorney for health care are considered advance directives. Federal law requires that all clients be given written information about their rights so they can make decisions concerning medical care. An advance directive is not required to be n a client's medical record.
Other Documents	These may or may not be in a client's medical record: Operative report, Anesthesia report, Pathology report, Transfusion record, Rehabilitation report, Critical pathway, Restraint record, and Autopsy report.

- Interdisciplinary planning and implementation of all aspects of care

The reviewers during an accreditation survey look for evidence of an organized and systematic method of monitoring and evaluating client care by checking documentation in medical records. Documenting the steps of the nursing process ensures compliance with JCAHO's plan of care requirements.

Confidentiality The client record is **confidential** and is to be read only by those health care providers directly involved in the care of that client. The record should not be left where just anyone has access to it. Keep it in its proper storage place when not being used.

Informed Consent Informed consent is a competent client's ability to make health care decisions based on full disclosure of the benefits, risks, and potential consequences of a recommended treatment plan and of alternative treatments, including no treatment, and the client's agreement to the treatment. Informed consent can be given either orally or in writing. The law does not require written consent; however, written consent documents the process of informed consent, which could be crucial in the event of a lawsuit (Olson-Chavarriaga, 2000). The physician who will perform the procedure is responsible for obtaining the client's informed consent, but the nurse is often the one who actually has the client sign the form.

The nurse's signature as a witness on an informed consent form is vouching that the client or appropriate surrogate is the person signing and that the person signing understands that a consent form is being signed (Olson-Chavarriaga, 2000).

Advance Directives An advance directive (i.e., living will and durable power of attorney for health care) is written instructions about an individual's health care preferences regarding life-sustaining measures to guide family members and health care professionals as to those treatment options that should or should not be considered when the individual is no longer able to decide. This allows competent clients, to make end-of-life decisions and to choose the types of life-sustaining procedures they wish to be performed.

Reimbursement

The federal government requires peer review organizations (PROs) to monitor and evaluate the quality and appropriateness of care provided. Medical records are reviewed for documentation of intensity of services and severity of illness.

The diagnosis-related group (DRG) classification system changed the reimbursement process from a cost-per-case to a prospective payment system (PPS). With PPS, the medical record must have documentation supporting the DRG and the appropriateness of care. It also must show evidence of client and family education and discharge planning.

From the agency's perspective, when information in the medical record shows compliance with Medicare and Medicaid standards, reimbursement is maximized. Failure to document equipment or procedures used daily (e.g., feeding pump; daily weight, intake and output; intravenous therapy; drug additives) can result in reimbursement being denied.

Education

Health care students use the medical record as a tool to learn about disease processes, medical and nursing diagnoses, complications, and interventions. The results of laboratory and diagnostic testing and physical examinations provide valuable information about specific diagnoses and interventions.

Nursing students can enhance their critical-thinking skills by examining the records following in chronological order, health care team's plan of care, including the way it was developed, implemented, and evaluated, analyzing the results. All health care professionals including students must maintain confidentiality when reading any client's chart.

Research

The client's medical record is used by researchers to determine whether a client meets the research criteria

---

PROFESSIONAL TIP

The Importance of Communication

Important assessment information needing immediate intervention should be documented and communicated orally to the other practitioners involved in the client's care. Time must direct decision making when critical information is obtained.

PROFESSIONAL TIP

Consent from Sedated Clients

Sedated clients should never be asked or allowed to sign an informed consent. If the client is not capable of understanding the nature of and risks associated with the procedure, the consent is invalid, and the nurse and institution are legally at risk. Either wait for the client to be competent and free of sedation (usually 4 hours after administration of medication that alters the level of consciousness) or have a legally acceptable family member sign.

COMMUNITY/HOME HEALTH CARE

Documentation

Home health agencies also keep client medical records. They must also comply with state and federal regulations affecting health care, documentation, and reimbursement.

for a study. Documentation can also indicate a need for research. For example, if documentation shows an increased rate of falls on certain nursing units, researchers can look for and study the variables associated with the increased fall rate.

Nursing Audit

A **nursing audit** is a method of evaluating the quality of care provided to clients. A nursing audit can focus on implementation of the nursing process, on client outcomes, or on both in order to evaluate the quality of care provided. The nursing audit is follow-up evaluation that not only evaluates the quality of care of an individual client but also provides an evaluation of overall care given in that health care facility. During a nursing audit the evaluators look for documentation of all five components of the nursing process in the client records.

Each health care facility has an ongoing nursing audit committee to evaluate the quality of care given. The nursing audit committee reviews client records after discharge of the clients. They examine the records for data related to:

- Safety measures
- Treatment interventions and client responses to them
- Expected outcomes as basis for interventions
- Client teaching
- Discharge planning
- Adequate staffing

EFFECTIVE DOCUMENTATION PRINCIPLES

The health care facility (hospital, nursing home, home health agency), the setting within the facility (e.g., emergency room, perioperative unit, medical-surgical unit), and the specific client population (e.g., obstetric, pediatric, geriatric) determines different documentation requirements. Even so, the documentation of the client care provided must reflect the nursing process. General documentation guidelines are listed in Table 8-12.

Follow the Nursing Process

Nursing notes must be logical, focused, and relevant to care, and the outcomes must represent each phase in the nursing process (Glondys, 1999; Habel, 2000b). Nursing documentation based on the nursing process facilitates effective care because client needs can be traced from assessment, through identification of the problems

PROFESSIONAL TIP

Follow the Nursing Process

Document according to the nursing process to ensure compliance with nursing practice acts and with reimbursement and accreditation criteria.

TABLE 8-12 GENERAL DOCUMENTATION GUIDELINES

- Ensure that you have the correct client record or chart and that the client's name and identifying information are on every page of the record.
- Document as soon as the client encounter is concluded to ensure accurate recall of data (follow agency guidelines on frequency of charting).
- Date and time each entry.
- Sign each entry with your full legal name and with your professional credentials, per your institutional policy.
- Do not leave space between entries.
- If an error is made while documenting, use a single line to cross out the error, then date, time, and sign the correction (follow institutional policy); avoid erasing, crossing out, or using correction fluid.
- Never change another person's entry, even if it is incorrect.
- The first entry of the shift should be made early (e.g., at 7:30 A.M. for the 7–3 shift, as opposed to 11:30 A.M. or 12 P.M.). Chart at least every 2 hours, or per institutional policy.
- Use quotation marks to indicate direct client responses (e.g., "I feel lousy").
- Document in chronological order; if chronological order is not used, state why.
- Write legibly.
- Use a permanent-ink pen (black is usually preferable because it photocopies well).
- Document in a complete but concise manner by using phrases and abbreviations as appropriate.
- Document all telephone calls that you make or receive that are related to a client's case.

Adapted from *Health Assessment & Physical Examination* (2nd ed), by M.E.Z. Estes, 2002, Clifton Park, NY: Thomson Delmar Learning. Copyright 2002 by Thomson Delmar Learning. Adapted with permission.

to the care plan, implementation, and evaluation. A brief outline of the elements of the nursing process as they relate to documentation follows:

- *Assessment:* Assessment data related to an actual or potential health care need are summarized without duplication. With reassessment, any new findings or any changes in the client's condition (e.g., increased pain) are highlighted.
- *Nursing diagnosis:* NANDA terminology is used to identify the client's problem or need.
- *Planning and outcome identification:* The expected outcomes and goals of client care, as discussed with the client and communicated to members of the multidisciplinary team, should be documented on the care plan or critical pathway rather than in the progress notes.
- *Implementation:* After an intervention has been performed, observations, treatments, teaching, and related clinical judgments should be documented on the flow sheet and progress notes. Client teaching should include learning needs, teaching plan content, methods of teaching, who was taught, and the client's response.

- *Evaluation:* The effectiveness of the interventions in terms of the expected outcomes is evaluated and documented: progress toward goals; client response to tests, treatments, and nursing interventions; client and family response to teaching and significant events; questions, statements, or complaints voiced by the client or family.
- *Revisions of planned care:* The reasons for the revisions along with the supporting evidence and client agreement are documented.

Effective Documentation Elements

The elements for effective documentation are:

- Document accurately, completely, and objectively including any errors that occurred
- Note date and time
- Use appropriate forms
- Identify the client
- Write in ink
- Use standard abbreviations
- Spell correctly
- Write legibly
- Correct errors properly
- Write on every line
- Chart omissions
- Sign each entry

Accurate, Complete, and Objective

Record just the facts—exactly what you see, hear, and do. For example, "Two 4 × 4s completely soaked with yellow-green drainage in 20 minutes" is more accurate than "large amount of drainage." Never record opinions or assumptions. Chart relevant information relating to client care and reflecting the nursing process (Figure 8-7). *Remember, if it is not charted, it was not done.* It is difficult to prove in court that an aspect of client care was provided if it was not documented.

Document information promptly; the information is more likely to be accurate and complete. Important details may be forgotten if charting is left until the end of the shift, and those details may later become a legal issue. Chart medications immediately *after* administration. This prevents errors such as another nurse administering pain medication when the first dose was not charted.

Avoid subjective statements such as "client is uncooperative." Record the client's exact words using quotation marks, for example, *Client stated, "I don't want to take a bath, and I don't want any breakfast."*

Date and Time

Be sure each entry is dated and has a specific time. Especially note the exact time of sudden changes in a client's condition, nursing actions, and other significant events. Do not chart in blocks of time, such as 7 A.M. to 11 A.M. This is vague and sounds like the client has had no attention during that time frame.

When military time is used, there is no confusion between A.M. and P.M. entries. For this reason, many facilities use military time (Figure 8-8).

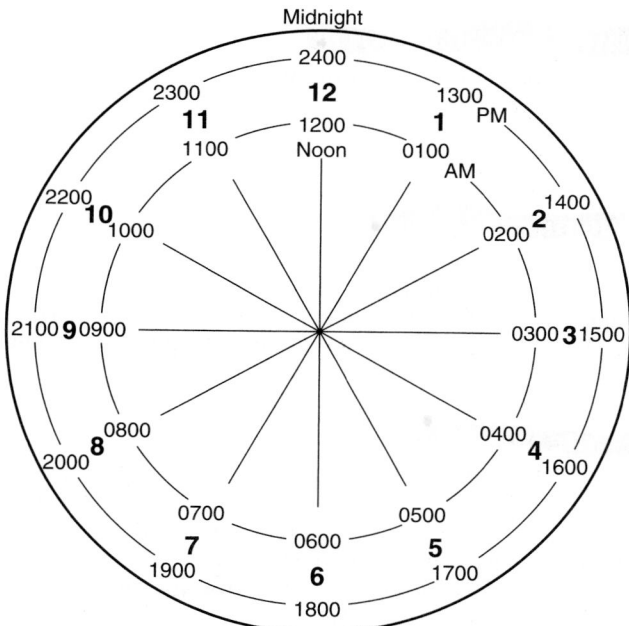

Figure 8-8 *Military time uses a 24-hour clock.*

NURSE'S PROGRESS RECORD

DATE	HOUR	PROGRESS NOTES
2/3/04	0815	Client verbalizes severe abdominal pain (8 on a 0–10 pain scale). Lying on Right side. States "I don't want to take a bath, and I don't want any breakfast". Abdomen distended. No bowel sounds ascultated. Acute Pain R/T no flatus passed since surgery. ————— L. White, RN
2/3/04	0820	Administered Prostigmin Injection 0.5 mg (1 mL of 1:2000 solution) given IM in left gluteus maximus. Assisted to Left side (Sim's position). ————— L. White, RN
2/3/04	0900	Client states "I passed some gas, the pain is much less now, about a 4 (on 0–10 pain scale). ————— L. White, RN

Figure 8-7 *Accurate, Complete, Objective Documentation*

NURSE'S PROGRESS RECORD

DATE	HOUR	PROGRESS NOTES
2/3/04	1100	*Late Entry (2/3/04—0900) Client crying after talking to mother on the telephone.————————L. White, RN*

Figure 8-9 *Recording a Late Entry*

If documentation cannot be done in a timely manner, explain the delay. For example, "chart in x-ray with client." When an entry must be added after notes are completed, follow the facility's policy for recording a late entry. Generally, the practice is to enter the date and time and note "Late Entry." This indicates that the entry is out of sequence. Then the date and time the entry should have been made is followed by the information to be recorded (Figure 8-9).

Use Appropriate Forms

Use the appropriate forms as required by the facility's policy manual. The forms used are not the same in every facility. Some facilities use flow sheets instead of progress notes.

Identify the Client

Each page of the client's record should have the client's name on it. This aids in preventing confusion and helps ensure that information is charted on the correct record. Many facilities use the addressograph to stamp the client's name on each page.

Write in Ink

The client's record is a permanent document, and information should be charted in ink or printed out from a computer. Only black ink should be used because it will photocopy well. Felt-tipped pens are not to be used, especially on forms with carbons, because they do not hold up under pressure to make a clear copy. Also, they often bleed through the paper.

Use Standard Abbreviations

Each health care facility has a list of approved abbreviations and symbols to be used in documenting information on its client records. This is to meet the JCAHO standards and the regulations in many states. Such a list prevents confusion. The use of some abbreviations causes ambiguity that could be misleading and endanger a client's health (Figure 8-10). Appendix C lists commonly used abbreviations.

Spell Correctly

Misspelled words on client records may be confusing and certainly convey a sense of unprofessionalism. They may generate questions about the quality of the care provided, increase the chance of liability, and produce a loss of the writer's credibility. When you are unsure of how to spell a word, *look it up*. Most units in a health care facility have a dictionary and other books to use as references.

PROFESSIONAL TIP

Abbreviations

Avoid abbreviations that can be misunderstood (Figure 8-10). For example, what does the abbreviation *Pt* mean? Does it refer to the patient, prothrombin time, physical therapy, or part-time? Refer to your institution's approved abbreviations listing.

MEDICATION ADMINISTRATION RECORD

MEDICATION   DATE: 3/02/04

MEDICATION	0701–1500	1501–2300	2301–0700
cyanocobalamin 20 mg	1400 *LW*		

Shift	Signature	Initials
0701-1500	*L White RN*	*LW*
1501-2300		
2301-0700		

Is this milligram or microgram?

It is less confusing to use mcg for microgram.

Figure 8-10 *Misleading Abbreviation*

Write Legibly

Legible handwriting is imperative for effective documentation. Sloppy writing hinders communication, and errors in client care can occur. Trying to decipher illegible writing wastes time. Illegible handwriting also creates a poor impression of the person who did the writing and damages that person's credibility. Print rather than use cursive writing; it is usually easier to read.

Correct Errors Properly

Promptly correct any error you make in documenting on a client's record. Know and follow your facility's policy for correcting errors. Generally, it is acceptable to draw a single line through the mistaken entry so that what was written can still be read. Above it carefully write "Mistaken Entry" followed by your initials and the date (Brooke, 2002; Pethtel, 2000; and Dumpel, James, & Phillips, 1999). The original entry must still be readable. *NEVER scratch out, erase, or use correction fluid (white-out)* on a mistaken entry. Using these methods makes it look as if something is trying to be hidden. Be sure the mistaken entry is still readable (Figure 8-11).

Write on Every Line

Fill each line completely. Leave no blank lines or partially blank lines. Draw a line through the empty part of the line (see Figure 8-12). This prevents others from inserting information later that may change the meaning of the original documentation. On forms, when information requested does not apply to a particular client, write "NA" (not applicable) or draw a line through the space. This indicates that every item on the form has been addressed.

Chart Omissions

Charting is supposed to show implementation of the medical and nursing plans of care. Whenever a part of the plan is omitted, document the reason why. For example, a treatment is not provided or medication is not administered because the client was in x-ray (Figure 8-12).

Sign Each Entry

Each entry on the nurse's notes (progress notes) is to be signed with your first name or initial, full last name, and professional licensure (i.e., LVN, LPN, RN). The signature should be at the end of the entry on the far right side. When there is not enough room on the last line of the documentation, draw a line from the last word to the end of the line and on the next line, leaving enough room to sign the entry at the far right.

For a long entry that will conclude on another page, record "(Continued on Next Page)" and sign your name. Begin the next page with "(Continued from Previous Page)", finish the entry, and sign your name (Figure 8-13).

Documenting a Medication Error

An incident report is required for all medication errors (discussed later). The medication given in error should be recorded on the Medication Administration Record (MAR) and in the nurse's progress notes. Remember, the purpose of the medical record is to report any care or treatment the client receives; this includes any errors made. Document in the nurse's notes the name and dosage of the medication; time it was given; client's response to the medication; time and name of the practitioner notified of the error; nursing interventions or medical treatment to counteract the error; and client's response to treatment. Do not mention that an incident report was completed.

Some health care facilities are now using a specific medication incident (variance) report for situations related to medications (Figure 8-14). This provides the facility with specific information to possibly change policies or procedures that will work to prevent medication incidents.

NURSE'S PROGRESS RECORD

DATE	HOUR	PROGRESS NOTES
2/3/04	0600	*Client verbalizes severe abdominal pain (8 on a 0–10 pain scale) when lying on ~~Left side~~ Right side.——L. White, RN*

Figure 8-11 *Mistaken Entry*

NURSE'S PROGRESS RECORD

DATE	HOUR	PROGRESS NOTES
2/3/04	0900	*Abdominal dressing not changed. Client in x-ray for a flat plate of the abdomen.——L. White, RN*

Figure 8-12 *Charting an Omitted Part of the Care Plan*

NURSE'S PROGRESS RECORD

DATE	HOUR	PROGRESS NOTES
2/3/04	1300	to assess client's knowledge of diabetes (Continued on next page) ———————————————— L. White, RN

NURSE'S PROGRESS RECORD

DATE	HOUR	PROGRESS NOTES
2/3/04	1300	(Continued from previous page) on the 3rd or 4th day post op ———————————————— L. White, RN

Figure 8-13 *Entry Continues on Another Page*

SYSTEMS OF DOCUMENTATION

Systems of recording and reporting data pertinent to client care have evolved primarily in response to demands that health care practitioners be held to societal norms, professional standards of practice, legal and regulatory standards, and institutional policies and standards. The documentation systems used today reflect specific needs and preferences of the many health care agencies.

Among the many systems used for documentation are the following:

- Narrative charting
- Source-oriented charting
- Problem-oriented charting
- PIE charting
- Focus charting
- Charting by exception
- Computerized documentation
- Critical pathways

Narrative Charting

Narrative charting, the traditional method of nursing documentation, is a chronologic account written in paragraphs that describe client status, interventions and treatments, and the client's response to treatments. This was the only method for documenting care before the advent of flow sheets.

Narrative documentation is the most flexible of all systems and is usable in any clinical setting. The relationship between nursing interventions and client's responses is clearly shown (Figure 8-15).

However, subjectivity is a common problem. Client problems may be difficult to track because the same information may not be consistently documented. The client's progress may be difficult to identify. Narrative charting often fails to reflect the nursing process.

Source-Oriented Charting

Source-oriented charting is a narrative recording by each member (source) of the health care team on separate documents. Each discipline uses a separate record, often resulting in fragmented care and time-consuming communication between disciplines.

Problem-Oriented Charting

Problem-oriented medical record (POMR) employs a structured, logical format and focuses on the client's problem. There are four critical components of POMR:

- Database (assessment data)
- Problem list (client's problems numbered according to when identified)
- Initial plan (outline of goals, expected outcomes, and learning needs and further data, if needed)
- Progress notes (charting based on the SOAP, SOAPIE, or SOAPIER format)

The format in which progress notes are to be written includes SOAP, SOAPIE, or SOAPIER.

- S: subjective data (what the client or family states)
- O: objective data (what is observed/inspected)
- A: assessment (conclusion reached on the basis of data formulated as client problem or nursing diagnosis)
- P: plan (expected outcomes and actions to be taken)

SOAPIE and SOAPIER refer to formats that add the following:

- I: implementation
- E: evaluation
- R: revision

An entry need not be made for each component of SOAP(IER) at every documentation (Figure 8-16); however, each problem must have a complete note every 24 hours if unresolved or whenever the client's condition changes.

Continuity of care is shown when the plan of care and interventions performed are documented together. Figure 8-16 shows an example of SOAPIE charting. Some physicians use this format when writing progress notes.

PIE Charting

After the SOAP format gained popularity, the Problem, Intervention, Evaluation **(PIE) charting** system was

Addressograph

Addressograph

CHRISTUS Health
QUALITY COMMITTEE
Medication Safety And Quality Report
Adverse Drug Event(Errors/Reactions)
Medical Record #
□ Male □ Female
Name:

Address:

Medication Error: any preventable event that may cause or lead to inappropriate medication use or patient harm, including prescribing, order communication, product labeling, packaging, compounding, dispensing, distribution, administration and use. (adapted from USP); any variance from the established process.

Instructions: Person discovering event completes Sections 1 through 13 according to facility policy and procedure. Forward to manager for additional review and investigation. Manager or analyst completes sections 14 through 19.

Event Number: _____ (# assigned by Risk Management)

1. FACILITY NAME _____

1. Diagnosis:

3. Date of Occurrence: ___/___/___ Time: ___:___ AM PM

Check if event occurred on: □ Holiday □ Weekends

4. Event Type: Variance Occurred to: □ Patient(01) □ Other(OT)

5. Type/Event Indicator:
□ Adverse Drug Reaction
□ Clinical (lab, vital signs)
□ Deteriorated Drug Errors (dispensing expired drug)
□ Documented Allergy
□ Drug-Disease Interaction
□ Dose Omission
□ Drug-Drug Interaction
□ Improper Dose
□ Drug-Food Interaction
□ Extra Dose
□ Narcotic Discrepancy
□ Frequency
□ Wrong Dosage Form
□ Resulting in Overdosage
□ Wrong Drug
□ Resulting in Under Dosage
□ Wrong Duration
□ IV Infiltration/Extravasation
□ Wrong Patient

□ Monitoring Error
(70.10)
(70.20)
(70.30)
(70.40)
(70.41)
(70.42)
(70.43)
(70.44)
(70.50)

□ Wrong Rate (77.10)
□ Too Fast (71.11)
□ Too Slow (71.12)
□ Wrong Route of Administration (71.20)
□ Wrong Strength/Concentration (71.30)
□ Wrong Technique (71.40)
□ Wrong Time (71.50)
□ Other (79.99)
(70.60)
(70.61)
(70.62)
(70.63)
(70.64)
(70.65)
(71.60)
(70.70)
(70.80)
(70.90)
(70.00)

6. Setting of initial event:(Dept. or unit)

7. Setting where event discovered: (Dept or unit)

8. Medication as Ordered: (Name, Dose, Route, Frequency)

9. Medication as Dispensed or Administered:

10. DESCRIPTION OF EVENT:

11. Patient Outcome: (Errors or reactions with ** to left of description require physician notification and notification of Risk Management according to facility policy and procedure)
□ No Error, but circumstances, policies or procedures that could lead to error (31.0)
□ Error occurred but medication did not reach patient.(i.e. dispensing error, caught in pharmacy or on delivery to unit) (32.1)
□ Error or reaction that reaches patient (32.2)
□ Medication reaches the patient but not administered (32.4)
□ ** Medication reaches the patient and is administered, no additional treatment, monitoring or intervention (32.3)
□ ** Increased patient monitoring only:(more frequent vital signs, laboratory tests ordered) (32.5)
□ **Treatment or intervention required:(meds ordered, procedures required) (33.1)
□ **Initial or prolonged hospitalization (33.2)
□ **Permanent patient harm (33.3)
□ **Near-death event (e.g., anaphylaxis, cardiac arrest) (33.4)
□ **Death (34.0)

12. Reported By: _____ Date: ___/___/___ Time: ___:___ AM PM Risk Mgmt notified? □Yes □No

13. Physician Notified □ Yes □ No By: _____ Date: ___/___/___ Time: ___:___ AM PM

THIS IS A COMMITTEE DOCUMENT & IS PRIVILEGED AND CONFIDENTIAL.

Sections 14 through 19 to be completed by Manager

14. Persons Involved (include name and phone, if appropriate, for purpose of followup or participation in possible root cause analysis)

Ordered Med: _____
□ Intern (A1) □ Resident(A2) □ Other Physician(A3)
□ Nurse Practitioner/Advanced Practice (C1)

Prepared/Administered Med: _____
□ Registered Nurse(C2) □ Licensed Practical Nurse(C3)
□ Pharmacy Technician (E) □ Pharmacist (B)
□ Other(H)

Dispensed Med: _____
□ Pharmacist(B) □ Other(H)

15. System Breakdown Points: Were any of the following items identified during error investigation? Check all that apply
□ Administration not documented (C1) □ Location(adjacent medications) (C27)
□ Allergy information not in chart (C2) □ Look alike/Sound alike product name/packaging (C28)
□ Allergy information not on MAR/Kardex (C3) □ Look alike/Sound alike patient name (C29)
□ Armband/name not checked (C4) □ MAR/Kardex incorrect, misleading or unclear (C30)
□ Abbreviations (C5) □ Medication not available at scheduled admin time (C31)
□ Automated dispensing device (C6) □ Medication stored in wrong drawer/location (C32)
□ Calculation error in pharmacy (C7) □ Multiple orders for same medication (C33)
□ Calculation error on nursing unit (C8) □ Order entry error (user error) (C18)
□ Change of shift (C9) □ Order not sent to/received by pharmacy (C34)
□ Computer system down (C10) □ Order overlooked/missed by pharmacy (C35)
□ Computer system functionality (C50) □ Order overlooked/missed by nursing (C36)
□ Decimal error(NOT Leading/Trailing Zeros) (C11) □ Order misinterpreted by pharmacy (C37)
□ Delayed dose (C12) □ Order misinterpreted by nursing (C49)
□ Documentation (C17) □ Order stamped/labeled for wrong patient (C19)
□ Error in stocking/restocking/cart fill/floor stock etc (C13) □ Order unclear or ambiguous (C38)
□ Handwriting (C14) □ Patient off unit (C39)
□ Illegible fax or NCR order copy (C15) □ Patient with stated allergy to medication given (C40)
□ Incomplete order (C16) □ Policy/procedure not followed (C41)
□ Insufficient staff (C20) □ Prepared in patient care area (C42)
□ Inexperienced staff (C21) □ Pump programmed incorrectly (C43)
□ Fatigue or extended shift (C22) □ Pump/Equipment failure (C44)
□ Lack of training (C23) □ Transfer patient /orders (C45)
□ Leading /Trailing zeros (C24) □ Transcription error (C46)
□ Labeling of drug incorrect or misleading (C25) □ Verbal order (C47)
□ Lack of knowledge (C26) □ Other (Explain in section 16) (C48)

16. Notes regarding investigation, action, recommendations for system improvement:

17. Nature of Injury:
(Check all that apply)
□ Abscess (44)
□ Amputation (06)
□ Anoxia (44)
□ Blister (50)

□ Blood Disorder (62)
□ Circulatory Impairment (11)
□ Dermatitis/Skin Disorder(29)
□ Deterioration in Condition(4)
□ Fever (24)
□ Headache (52)

□ Hearing Disorder (39)
□ Heart Attack (41)
□ Hematoma (51)
□ Infection (31)
□ Inflammation (27)
□ Phlebitis (19)

□ Respiratory Disorder/ Asphyxia/Choking (43)
□ Rupture (99)
□ Seizure (22)
□ Shock (Non-Electrical) (37)
□ Stroke (45)

□ Tissue Damage (61)
□ Visual Impairment (40)
□ Other (99)

□ No Injury Noted (48)

18. Does this injury involve one of these outcomes... (Check only one)
□ Burn (04)
□ Amputation (01)
□ Burn Injury (02)
□ Brain Damage (03)

□ Events Resulting in Disability (06)
□ Kidney Failure (11)

□ Loss of Hearing (13)
□ Loss of Eyesight (12)
□ Loss of Sensation (14)

□ Residual Paralysis (18)
□ Sepsis/ma After Admission (19)
□ Unexpected Death (20)

19. Manager Review: _____ Date: _____

20. Director/Administrator Review: _____ Date: _____

THIS IS A COMMITTEE DOCUMENT & IS PRIVILEGED AND CONFIDENTIAL.

Figure 8-14 *Medication Incident Report (Courtesy of CHRISTUS Spohn Hospital Shoreline, Corpus Christi, TX)*

NURSE'S PROGRESS RECORD

DATE	HOUR	PROGRESS NOTES
2/3/04	1630	Client 6 hours post op; awakens easily, oriented x 3. Abdominal dressing dry and intact. Denies pain but stated he felt nauseated and immediately vomited 50 mL of clear fluid. Attempted to ambulate to bathroom with assistance, but felt dizzy. Assisted to lie down in bed. Voided 250 mL clear, yellow urine in urinal. Client encouraged to turn in bed, cough, and deep breathe.————————————————L. White, RN
2/3/04	1650	Continues to feel nauseated. Tigan 250 mg given by mouth.——————————————————L. White, RN
2/3/04	1730	States he is no longer nauseated. Remains pain free. Properly demonstrated coughing and deep breathing.——— —————————————————————L. White, RN

Figure 8-15   *Narrative Charting*

NURSE'S PROGRESS RECORD

DATE	HOUR	PROGRESS NOTES
2/3/04	0730	#1 Pain S: Client states "The pain in my hip is so bad." O: Client states pain is 9 (0–10 scale); skin warm, moist, pale. Lying stiffly in bed with fists clenched. A: Acute Pain, needs medication for relief P: Check orders for analgesia; check vital signs; if within normal limits give analgesia as ordered; then recheck in 30 minutes for response.————————————L. White, RN
2/3/04	0740	#1 Pain O: BP 142/86, P 104, R 28 I: meperidine 75 mg IM in right gluteus maximus.——— —————————————————————L. White, RN
2/3/04	0810	#1 Pain S: Client states "The pain is better." O: Client states pain now 4 (0–10 scale); skin warm, dry, normal color. Lying relaxed in bed. A: Pain relieved P: Continue to monitor for pain E: Analgesic effective————————L. White, RN
2/3/04	0810	#2 Anxiety S: Client states "I'm still worried about the surgery on my hip." O: Client clutching sheet A: Anxiety R/T surgery the next day P: Encourage verbalization of concerns and feelings. Involve family in discussion of concerns, if client agreeable.——— —————————————————————L. White, RN

Figure 8-16   *SOAPIE Charting*

NURSE'S PROGRESS RECORD

DATE	HOUR	PROGRESS NOTES
2/3/04	0830	P #1: Disturbed Body Image R/T bilateral mastectomy—
		I #1: Encourage verbalization of feelings and concerns and
		remain alert for client's comments about body changes;
		encourage looking at surgical site when ready—
		E #1: Glanced at chest during dressing change. Continue
		encouraging client's involvement in dressing changes.—
		————————————————L. White, RN
2/3/04	0830	P #2: Ineffective Breathing Pattern R/T musculoskeletal
		impairment following mastectomy—
		I #2: Encourage use of incentive spirometer every 2 hours
		increasing level each day; assess breath sounds, rate, and
		quality of respirations every 4 hours; monitor O_2 saturation
		with pulse oximeter—
		E #2: Using incentive spirometer every 2 hours when
		awake, Breath sounds normal, respirations 20 shallow, O_2
		saturation 93%.————————————L. White, RN

Figure 8-17 *PIE Charting*

NURSE'S PROGRESS RECORD

DATE	HOUR	FOCUS	PROGRESS NOTES
2/3/04	1300	Deficient	D: Client states that she does not
		Knowledge R/T	understand why she has to take three
		medications	medications. "I don't like to take pills."
			A: Reason for each medication explained,
			dosages, and side effects.————
			R: Client verbalizes better understanding
			of her medications.————L. White, RN
2/3/04	1600	Abnormal	D: Client states that her period just
		vaginal bleeding	started and she is passing clots.
			A: One maxi pad saturated in 30 minutes.
			BP 110/68, P 100, R 20. No clots seen.
			Status reported to Dr. Medoffer and
			orders received. IV started with 20 G
			catheter, 1000 mL normal saline hung at
			100 mL/h. Continue monitoring bleeding
			and vital signs. Dr. Medoffer will see
			client in 1 hour.
			R: Client understands reason for IV.—
			————————————L. White, RN

Figure 8-18 *Focus Charting*

developed to streamline documentation. The main parts of this system are an integrated plan of care, assessment flow sheets, and nurse's progress notes. Figure 8-17 shows an example of PIE charting.

Focus Charting

Focus charting is a documentation system using a column format to chart Data, Action, and Response (DAR) (Smith, 2000b). Usually the focus is a nursing diagnosis, but it may also be:

- A sign or symptom (e.g., abnormal vaginal bleeding)
- An acute change in the client's condition (e.g., sudden increase in blood pressure)
- A special need (e.g., a discharge referral)

Data are the subjective and objective information describing the focus. Action is the nursing interventions. Response is the client's response to the interventions (Figure 8-18). The column format of this system is used within the progress notes but is easily distinguished from other entries.

Charting by Exception — Not good

Charting by exception (CBE) is a documentation system using standardized protocols stating what the expected course of the illness is, and only significant findings (exceptions) are documented in a narrative form. It assumes that client care needs are routine and predictable and that the client's responses and outcomes are also routine and predictable.

The rule of thumb related to charting "if it is not charted, it was not done" is replaced in CBE by the presumption that unless documented otherwise, all standardized protocols have been met and no further documentation is needed. Time spent by nurses documenting client care may be reduced, but according to Dumpel, James, & Phillips (1999), CBE is not in the best interest of the client, and according to DeWitt (2000), CBE is a ticket to the courtroom.

Computerized Documentation

Health care facilities have been using computers for many years to order diagnostic tests and medications and to receive results of diagnostic tests. Using a totally computerized client record is slowly being adopted. In terms of both time and finances, it is a huge commitment for a facility to plan for and make the change to computerized client records.

Issues to be addressed when considering computerized client records include data standards, vocabularies, security, legal issues, and costs.

- Data standards—include length of fields, how dates and times are shown, and ASCII or binary data.
- Vocabularies—the most commonly used are the combination of North American Nursing Diagnosis Association (NANDA) nursing diagnoses, Nursing Interventions Classification (NIC) nursing interventions, and Nursing Outcomes Classification (NOC) nursing outcomes.
- Security—includes privacy, confidentiality, who has access to which data, how errors are to be corrected, and protection against data loss
- Legal issues—electronic signatures
- Costs—include planning, hardware, software, and training for all users.

Nursing information systems (NIS) are various software programs that allow nursing documentation in an electronic record. These systems generally follow the components of the nursing process. The NIS works in conjunction with the hospital information system (HIS). Each NIS can be customized to fit a facility's documentation forms.

Decision-support systems are available to alert nurses, physicians, and pharmacists of client drug incompatibility, appropriate antibiotics based on culture and antibiotic susceptibility results, and adverse drug reactions. Another decision-support system uses assessment data to suggest possible nursing diagnoses, goals and outcome criteria, and interventions from which the nurse selects those appropriate for a specific client. A medical spell check is also available.

Bedside computer terminals allow the nurse to immediately document client assessments, medications given, and interventions performed; the nurse can also check care plans and revise if necessary, check test results, and many other functions. Timeliness, completeness, and the quality of nursing documentation are improved.

Voice-activated systems are available in some facilities. The nurse speaks into a special telephone handset, and the words appear on the computer screen. These are generally located at a central place rather than at the bedside.

Besides reducing documentation time and increasing accuracy, computerized charting increases legibility; stores and retrieves information quickly and easily; helps link diverse sources of client information; and uses standardized terminology, thus improving communication among health care departments. Planners for health care, researchers, lawyers, and third-party payers can quickly and easily retrieve information for their respective jobs.

Problems with computerized charting may occur if used incorrectly, and client information may be mixed up. When security measures are neglected, client confidentiality may be compromised. Users (e.g., nurses, physicians) should never share computer ID numbers or passwords with anyone. Many systems keep a record of what each user has done in the system.

To prevent these problems, users must also remember to log off to prevent unauthorized access by others. Users should also follow facility protocol for correcting errors, and keep monitors and print versions of client information where others cannot see the information (Habel, 2000b).

Information is temporarily unavailable when the computer system is "down" either for routine servicing or an unexpected failure. Processing time may be slow during peak usage times when too few terminals are available.

Point-of-Care Charting

Point-of-care charting is a computerized documentation system allowing health care providers to have immediate access to client information. The system permits input and retrieval of client data at the bedside with a handheld portable computer. This is especially useful for nurses working in home health care.

The advantages of point-of-care charting are related to the computer system efficiency, through which the following can be achieved:

- Operating costs are controlled.
- Existing information systems are complemented.
- Redundant data entry is eliminated.
- The practitioner has more one-on-one time for client care.
- Crucial client information is available to all health care providers in a timely fashion.

CRITICAL THINKING

Systems for Charting

Why are there so many systems for charting? Of what value is each?

Point-of-care charting enhances continuity of care by providing each health care practioner with client data. It also fosters compliance with accreditation and regulatory standards.

Critical Pathway

A **critical pathway** (care map) is a comprehensive preprinted interdisciplinary standard plan of care reflecting the ideal course of treatment for the average client with a given diagnosis or procedure, especially those with relatively predictable outcomes. They are generally not written for extremely complex client situations with less predictable outcomes.

The overall goal for critical pathways is to improve the quality and efficiency of client care. The sequence and timing of interdisciplinary activities is established, including assessments, consultations, diagnostic tests, nutrition, medications, activities, treatments, therapeutics, education, and discharge planning. Although nursing diagnoses as such are not generally included in a critical pathway, a nurse may identify nursing diagnoses and interventions for a specific client.

Health care facilities develop their own critical pathways. An interdisciplinary team, including nurses, physicians, dietary, rehabilitative services, social services, and others when needed, develops the critical pathway through consensus about the management of the identified case situation. This is a time-consuming task, but once written, a critical pathway can be revised based on a review of the variances.

Goals not met or interventions not performed within the established time frame are called **variances.** The nurse documents on a variance form why a goal is not met or an intervention is not performed (Klenner, 2000). Documentation becomes complicated when clients have more than two diagnoses or variations. Additional documentation forms are needed to complement the pathway.

FORMS FOR DOCUMENTATION

Forms for recording data include Kardex, flow sheets, nurse's progress notes, and discharge summaries. They are designed to facilitate record keeping and allow quick, easy access to information.

Kardex

A **Kardex** is a brief worksheet with basic client care information that traditionally is not part of the medical record. The Kardex is used as a reference throughout the shift and during change-of-shift reports. It comes in

COMMUNITY/HOME HEALTH CARE

Home Health Kardex

The home health Kardex also contains information related to family contacts, practitioners (physician), other services, and emergency referrals.

various sizes, shapes, and types, including computer-generated. The Kardex usually contains the following information:

- Client name, age, marital status, religious preference, physician, family contact with phone number
- Medical diagnoses: listed by priority
- Nursing diagnoses: listed by priority
- Allergies
- Medical orders: diet, medications, intravenous (IV) therapy, treatments, diagnostic tests and procedures (including dates and results), consultations, DNR (do-not-resusitate) order (when appropriate)
- Activities permitted: functional limitations, assistance needed in activities of daily living, and safety precautions

Flow Sheets

Flow sheets, with vertical or horizontal columns for recording date, time, and assessment data and intervention information, make it easy to track the client's changes in condition. Special equipment used in client teaching and IV therapy are other parts of the flow sheet. These forms usually contain legends identifying the approved abbreviations for charting data because they have small spaces for recording (Figure 8-19). Flow sheets must be completely filled out because blank spaces imply that something was not recognized, attempted, or completed.

Because they decrease the redundancy of charting in the nurse's progress notes, flow sheets are used as supplements in many documentation systems. They do not, however, replace the progress notes. Nurses still must document observations, client responses and teaching, detailed interventions, and other significant data in the progress notes.

Nurse's Progress Notes

Nurse's progress notes are used to document the client's condition, problems, and complaints; interventions; the client's response to interventions; and achievement of outcomes. Documents falling under the general heading of nurse's progress notes includes nurse's notes, personal care flow sheets, MAR, teaching records, vital sign records, intake and output forms, and specialty forms (e.g., diabetic flow sheet or neurologic assessment form). Progress notes can be either narrative or incorporated into a standardized flow sheet (Figure 8-19) to complement SOAP(IE), PIE, focus charting, and other documentation systems.

Discharge Summary

The client's illness and course of care are highlighted in the discharge summary. A narrative discharge summary in the progress notes includes:

- Client status on admission and discharge
- A brief summary of the client's care
- Intervention and education outcomes
- Resolved problems and continuing care needs for unresolved problems, including referrals
- Client instructions about medications, diet, food-drug interactions, activity, treatments, follow-up, and other special needs

The assessment portion (top right of figure):

	Date:	7-3 Time:	3-11 Time:	11-7 Time:
Neuro	Normal: alert, oriented to time, place, person, follows command, speech clear	WNL: ☐ *	WNL: ☐ *	WNL: ☐ *
Respiratory	Normal: Regular, unlabored symmetrical respirations, no abnormal lung sounds	WNL: ☐ *	WNL: ☐ *	WNL: ☐ *
Cardiovascular	Normal: Heart rhythm regular, peripheral pulses easily palpable and strong bilaterally, no edema, capillary refill brisk	WNL: ☐ *	WNL: ☐ *	WNL: ☐ *
Musculo-Skeletal	Normal: Full ROM of All joints, no weakness, steady balance and gait, handgrips equal	WNL: ☐ *	WNL: ☐ *	WNL: ☐ *
Nutrition	Normal: Consumes greater than 1/2 of solid food meals	WNL: ☐ *	WNL: ☐ *	WNL: ☐ *
G.I.	Normal: Abdomen soft, bowel sounds present all 4 quadrants, no nausea/vomiting, diarrhea/constipation Last BM:	WNL: ☐ *	WNL: ☐ *	WNL: ☐ *
G.U.	Normal: Voiding without difficulty, clear urine, no bladder distention	WNL: ☐ *	WNL: ☐ *	WNL: ☐ *
Skin	Normal: Skin warm, dry, intact, tugor elastic, oral cavity moist and intact Date of Last EZ Graph ___ Site: ___	WNL: ☐ *	WNL: ☐ *	WNL: ☐ *
Psychosocial	Normal: Thought processes logical, memory intact, behavior appropriate for situation	WNL: ☐ *	WNL: ☐ *	WNL: ☐ *
Incision	Normal: Incision clean, no redness, drainage Site: ___	WNL: ☐ *	WNL: ☐ *	WNL: ☐ *
Wound	Normal: Dry, no drainage, no odor Site: ___	WNL: ☐ *	WNL: ☐ *	WNL: ☐ *

Safety Assessment

STATUS: MENTAL/PHYSICAL
D E N
☐☐☐ (5) Confused/judgement impaired
☐☐☐ (5) Sensory impairment
☐☐☐ (5) Combative/aggressive
☐☐☐ (5) "Sundowners" syndrome
☐☐☐ (5) Noncompliance/uncooperative
☐☐☐ (5) Paralysis/amputee
☐☐☐ (5) Urgent/frequent elimination needs
☐☐☐ (10) Restraints in use
☐☐☐ (5) Weakness/debilitation/mobility impaired

MEDICATIONS
D E N
☐☐☐ (5) Diuretics
☐☐☐ (5) Laxatives/G.I. preps
☐☐☐ (3) Antihypertensives
☐☐☐ (3) Antiseizures
☐☐☐ (3) Sedative/hypnotics
☐☐☐ (3) Analgesics
☐☐☐ (3) Antipsychotics/antidepressants

HISTORY
D E N
☐☐☐ (5) Age greater than 60
☐☐☐ (5) History of previous falls
☐☐☐ (3) From nursing home
☐☐☐ (3) Has had sitter/companion at home

SAFETY LEVEL
D E N
☐☐☐ Level 1 (0-17)
☐☐☐ Level 2 (18-24)
☐☐☐ Level 3 (25 or greater)

TOTAL D ___ E ___ N ___

The intervention/flow sheet portion (bottom left of figure):

Date: ___

Nutrition:
Diet ☐   NPO ☐   Bath ☐   Sitz ☐
Hyperal ☐   Tube Fed ☐   Shower ☐

Hygiene:

	7-3	3-11	11-7
Oral Care	self ☐ assist ☐ Total	self ☐ assist ☐ Total	self ☐ assist ☐ Total
Shave	self ☐ assist ☐ Total	self ☐ assist ☐ Total	self ☐ assist ☐ Total
Peri Care	self ☐ assist ☐ Total	self ☐ assist ☐ Total	self ☐ assist ☐ Total

Other: ___   Comments: ___

Breakfast: All >1/2 ☐   <1/2 ☐   0 ☐
Lunch: All >1/2 ☐   <1/2 ☐   0 ☐
Dinner: All >1/2 ☐   <1/2 ☐   0 ☐
Snacks: All >1/2 ☐   <1/2 ☐   0 ☐

Tube Feeding Residuals

Time	Amount

	Intake						Output			
	PO	IV	NG & Flush	Enteral	Other	Urine	Ng/Emesis	Stool	Drains
7-3									
3-11									
11-7									
7-3 Total									
3-11									
11-7									
24hr/ Total									

Weight
Today:
Previous:

Vital/Signs

Time	T	P	R	B/P	P/S

CHRISTUS SPOHN HEALTH SYSTEM

FLOW SHEET - 24 HOUR RECORD
PATIENT CARE SERVICES

2705066

REV. 06/00

4010

Figure 8-19 Assessment and Intervention Flow Sheet (Courtesy of CHRISTUS Spohn Health System, Corpus Christi, TX)   continues

EDUCATION REASSESSMENT

Have the Education needs of the patient changed in past 24 hours? ☐ Yes ☐ No
Is the patient scheduled for any new test or procedure today? ☐ Yes ☐ No
Explanation given? ☐ Yes ☐ No
Patient/significant other verbalizes understanding: ☐ Yes ☐ No
Patient desires/requires education on: _____

Have Discharge Planning needs changed in past 24 hours? ☐ Yes ☐ No
If yes, send consult to Social Services and document changes below.

ALL EDUCATION MUST BE DOCUMENTED ON THE MULTIDISCIPLINARY EDUCATION FORM

TIME	PROBLEM #	PROGRESS NOTES

TIME	PROBLEM #	PROGRESS NOTES

PLAN OF CARE VERIFICATION

RN _____ Time _____

IV SITE ASSESSMENT		7-3 Time:	3-11 Time:	11-7 Time:
Normal: IV Patent; No redness, drainage or edema	Site #1: Start Date:	WNL: ☐ *	WNL: ☐ *	WNL: ☐ *
# of IVAC's in use _____	Site #2: Start Date:	WNL: ☐ *	WNL: ☐ *	WNL: ☐ *
IV Site Care per hospital standard ☐	Time:			
IV Tubing Change per hospital standard ☐	Time:			

IV Start:	Time	Attempts	Site	Needle Size	S	U
Site prep per Standard ☐					☐ ☐ ☐	☐ ☐ ☐

INITIALS	SIGNATURE	INITIALS	SIGNATURE

Figure 8-19, continued

Many facilities have a form itemizing discharge and client instructions. The form has a duplicate copy for the client, with the original being placed in the medical record. Figure 8-20 is an example of this form.

DOCUMENTATION TRENDS

Computerized charting is one of the most widespread trends in nursing documentation; however, computerized nursing documentation can demonstrate the quality, effectiveness, and value of the services nurses provide only if standardized databases are developed that ensure accuracy and precision of the information. The need to define and develop standard terminology for nursing data, nursing diagnoses, nursing interventions, and nursing outcomes is continually evolving.

Nursing Minimum Data Set

In 1985, Werley and Lang convened an invitational working conference to identify the elements that should be included in a **Nursing Minimum Data Set** (NMDS)

(elements that should be in clinical records and abstracted for studies on the effectiveness and costs of nursing care) (Werley & Lang, 1988). The three categories into which the 16 identified elements were grouped are:

1. *Demographics:* personal identification, date of birth, gender, race and ethnicity, and residence
2. *Service:* unique facility or service agency number, episode admission or encounter date, discharge or termination date, disposition of client, expected payer, unique health record number of client, and unique number of principal registered nurse provider
3. *Nursing care:* nursing diagnosis, nursing intervention, nursing outcome, and intensity of nursing care (Werley & Lang, 1988)

The development of standard terminology for the four nursing care categories: diagnoses, interventions, outcomes, and intensity is challenging. For example, automated information systems must be able to support cost-effective nursing practice with efficient, comprehensive documentation. The consistent use of a taxonomy pro-

Figure 8-20 *Discharge Summary (Courtesy of CHRISTUS Spohn Health System, Corpus Christi, TX)* moting validity and reliability is basic to standardizing databases. The NMDS, however, does not specify for any of the four elements a taxonomy such as NANDA (2003) nursing diagnoses, Nursing Interventions Classification (NIC), Nursing Outcomes Classification (NOC), or acuity ratings. Nursing must find consensus in terminology so clinical data can be included in the nursing care elements of an NMDS.

Nursing Diagnoses

The North American Nursing Diagnosis Association (NANDA) is recognized as the pioneer in diagnostic classification in nursing. The NANDA definition of a nursing diagnosis is: "A nursing diagnosis is a clinical judgment about individual, family, or community responses to actual or potential health problems or life processes" (NANDA, 2003). Currently, there are 167 approved nursing diagnoses classified into 46 classes and 13 domains.

Many diagnostic labels (nursing diagnoses) now have new descriptors. The word *altered* has been removed and a more specific term used. This allows for more specific documentation and for the nursing diagnoses to be linked to NIC and NOC. The nursing diagnoses are now listed in alphabetical order by the diagnostic concept, not by the first word of the nursing diagnosis (NANDA, 2003). For example: *Excess Fluid Volume* is found under "fluid." The entire listing can be found in Appendix A.

Each diagnosis has a label, definition, major and minor defining characteristics, and related factors. The diagnoses identify client states which can then be used to select interventions that are intended to achieve the desired outcomes.

In 1992, the NANDA terms were accepted into the Unified Medical Language System (UMLS). The UMLS was begun in 1986 by the National Library of Medicine as a way to help health professionals and researchers retrieve and integrate electronic biomedical information from a variety of sources (National Library of Medicine, 2000).

Nursing Interventions Classification

The **Nursing Interventions Classification (NIC)** is a comprehensive standardized language for nursing interventions organized in a three-level taxonomy. This taxonomy sorts, labels, and describes interventions used by nurses for various diagnostic categories. Initiated by a research team (Iowa Intervention Project, 1993) at the University of Iowa in 1987, the three-level taxonomy now comprises 7 domains, 30 classes, and 514 interventions. The seven domains are:

1. Physiological: basic
2. Physiological: complex
3. Behavioral
4. Safety
5. Family
6. Health system
7. Community

A nursing intervention is any direct care treatment that a nurse performs on behalf of a client (Gordon, 1998). These treatments include nurse-initiated treatments resulting from nursing diagnoses, physician-initiated treatments resulting from medical diagnoses, and performance

of the daily essential functions for the client who cannot do these.

Each nursing intervention has a label, a definition, a set of activities to carry out the interventions and a list of references. *Activities are not interventions and should not be identified as such in nursing information systems* (Dochterman & Bulechek, 2004).

Although continuing to evolve, this classification system already provides assistance in choosing interventions based on nursing diagnoses or problems. The NIC interventions have been incorporated into health care data sets and the computerized client medical record. The NIC is included in the *National Library of Medicine's Metathesaurus,* one of four knowledge sources for the UMLS (McCloskey & Bulechek, 1995).

Nursing Outcomes Classification

An outcome is a measurable individual, family, or community state, behavior, or perception that is measured along a continuum and is responsive to nursing interventions (The University of Iowa College of Nursing, 2001b).

The Iowa Outcomes Project being conducted at the University of Iowa has developed a taxonomy of client outcomes for nursing care, called **Nursing Outcomes Classification (NOC).** This classification system now comprises 330 outcomes grouped into 29 classes and 7 domains (Moorhead, Johnson, & Maas, 2004). The seven domains are:

1. Functional health
2. Physiologic health
3. Psychosocial health
4. Health knowledge and behavior
5. Perceived health
6. Family health
7. Community health

Each NOC outcome has the outcome label, the outcome definition, a list of indicators for measurement, a five-point measurement scale, and a list of references (Aquilino & Keenan, 2000). The NOC is included in the *National Library of Medicine's Metathesaurus for a Unified Medical Language* (NCVHS, 1999).

REPORTING

Reporting summarizes the current critical information pertinent to clinical decision making and continuity of care. Reporting, like recording, is based on the nursing process, standards of care, and legal and ethical principles. To verbally report in a well-organized efficient manner the nurse should consider the following questions:

- What to say
- Why to say it
- How to say it

Another critical element of reporting is listening. Reports require everyone present to participate. When receiving a report, enhance listening skills by eliminating distractions, putting thoughts and concerns aside, concentrating on those things being said, and not anticipating the presenter's next statements. The reporting process

Figure 8-21 *Nursing Rounds*

is integral to promoting continuity of client care. Some facilities tape record the end-of-shift report. Summary reports, walking rounds, telephone reports and orders, and incident reports are all types of reporting.

Summary Reports

Information pertinent to the client's needs and identified by the nursing process is outlined in summary reports. Summary reports commonly occur either at the change of shift when new caregivers arrive or when the client is transferred to another area. A summary report should include the following information in the order indicated:

1. Background data obtained from client interactions and assessment of the client's functional health patterns
2. Prioritized medical and nursing diagnoses
3. Identified client risks
4. Recent changes in condition or in treatments (e.g., new medications, elevated temperature)
5. Effective interventions or treatments of priority problems, inclusive of laboratory and diagnostic results (e.g., client's response to pain medication)
6. Progress toward expected outcomes
7. Adjustments in the plan of care
8. Client or family complaints

This logical and time-sequenced format follows the nursing process and thus provides structure and organization to the data. In order to provide continuity of care, the new caregiver must receive an accurate, concise report about those things that happened during the previous shift. Because client and family complaints usually generate questions and discussion, they should be addressed last.

Walking Rounds

Walking rounds can take the form of nursing rounds, instructor–student rounds, physician–nurse rounds, or multidisciplinary rounds. **Walking rounds** is when the members of the care team walk to each client's room and discuss progress and care with each other and with the client, as shown in Figure 8-21.

Nursing rounds are used most frequently by charge nurses as their method of report. The oncoming nurse is introduced to the client and the offgoing nurse discusses with the client and the on-coming nurse any changes in the plan of care. This is more time-consuming than a summary report, but gives the nurses and the client time to evaluate the effectiveness of care together.

Nursing rounds are also used for teaching when the instructor introduces the client to the student and they discuss the client's care together. The student's observation, communication, and decision-making skills can also be assessed by the instructor.

Nurse-physician rounds involve the physician and either staff nurse or the charge nurse. These rounds usually occur daily and allow the nurse, the physician, and the client to evaluate the effectiveness of care.

Multidisciplinary rounds involving all disciplines occur less frequently than other types of rounds, primarily because it is difficult to schedule everyone. Multidisciplinary rounds are done most commonly to discuss discharge planning or to supplement case conferences.

Telephone Reports and Orders

Nurses are expected to exhibit courtesy and professionalism when using the telephone.

When initiating a phone call, the nurse should organize the information to be reported or received. For example, the nurse should:

- Ensure that all lab results are back; if they are not, identify those that are missing and telephone the lab or check the computer to ascertain whether the results are available. Spell the client's name and provide the client's medical record number when calling the lab to minimize the chances of receiving results for the wrong client. Write down the tests and the results.
- Have the client's assessment data available, especially any significant data related to abnormal results.
- Minimize the chance of being interrupted during the call by informing the charge nurse or someone else at the nurses' station of the call.

State the reason for the call, for example, "I am calling Dr. Wojtal regarding the blood culture results for Mrs.

PHYSICIAN'S ORDER SHEET

DATE	HOUR	ORDERS
2/3/04	1420	Give Demerol 50 mg IM stat. ————————
		————————— T.O. Dr. Weng/L. White RN

Figure 8-22 *Documenting a Telephone Order*

Beacon." Be brief, listen carefully, and repeat the test results and any orders received from the physician.

The date and time the phone call was placed, the client data reported by the nurse, the name of the person with whom the nurse spoke, and whether an order was obtained should be recorded accurately in the client's record. Telephone orders should be charted and the nurse's progress notes updated immediately after the call to prevent another caregiver from writing an entry before the telephone orders have been written.

Figure 8-22 shows how to write a telephone order on the physician's order sheet: the entry is dated and timed; the order as given by the physician is recorded; the order is signed beginning with t.o. (telephone order); the physician's name is written; and the nurse's name is signed. If another nurse witnesses the phone order, that nurse's signature should follow the first nurse's signature.

The physician must countersign the order within a time frame specified by the facility's policy. The use of fax machines has decreased the need for lengthy or complicated telephone orders, saving time and minimizing errors. The physician should be phoned to confirm the physician's identity as the initiator of the fax orders. The physician must countersign the fax orders according to agency policy.

Incident Reports

Incident reports, also called occurrence reports or variance reports, document any unusual occurrence or accident in the facility. Incident reports are not a means of punishment, but ethical practice requires that an incident report be filed to protect the individual involved.

Incident reports are not only an internal device for the facility; they are required by federal, national, and state accrediting agencies. For legal reasons, nurses are often advised not to document the filing of an incident report in the nurse's notes.

An incident report serves two functions:

1. It informs the facility's administration of the incident and allows risk management personnel to consider ways to prevent similar occurrences in the future.

PROFESSIONAL TIP

Documenting an Incident

The incident should be factually documented in the nurse's notes, but the notes should not say "incident report filed."

2. It alerts the facility's insurance company to a potential claim and the possible need for investigation.

Incident report forms vary from one facility to another, but the following information must be recorded on the report:

*   The date, exact time, and place the nurse discovered the occurrence.
*   The person(s) involved in the occurrence, including witnesses.
*   The exact occurrences witnessed by the nurse (e.g., "Found the client sitting on the floor, client stated that . . . ," rather than "Client fell.").
*   The exact details and time sequence of what happened and the consequences for the persons involved.
*   The nurse's actions to provide care and the results of the nurse's assessment for injuries and client complaints.
*   The supervisor on duty who was notified and the time and name of the physician notified; if telephone orders were received from the physician, these should be documented as previously discussed and the orders implemented.
*   Never record personal opinions, assumptions, judgments, or conclusions about what happened; point blame; or suggest ways to prevent similar occurrences. Forward the incident report to the designated person defined in the facility's policy.

Iyer and Camp (1999) suggest writing a brief, accurate description of the incident and keeping it at home. The description should include details of the incident and the names of the people who were involved. Because lawsuits may take several years until the case goes to court, personal notes will help accurate recall of the incident. The notes may be read by the plaintiff's attorney and should reflect the same elements as the incident report.

Summary

*   The nursing process composed of five steps: assessment, diagnosis, planning and outcome identification, implementation, and evaluation, is an organized way to plan and deliver nursing care.
*   The nurse uses the assessment process to establish a database about the client, to form an interpersonal relationship with the client, and to provide the client with an opportunity to discuss health care concerns.
*   The second step in the nursing process involves further analysis and synthesis of the data and results in a list of nursing diagnoses.

- Nursing diagnoses identify knowledge unique to nursing, improve communication among nurses and other health care professionals, and promote individualized client care.
- Planning and outcome identification, the third step in the nursing process, involves prioritizing nursing diagnoses, identifying and writing goals and client outcomes, developing nursing interventions, and recording the plan of care in the client's record.
- The implementation step of the nursing process is directed toward meeting client needs, resulting in health promotion, prevention of illness, illness management, or health restoration.
- Evaluation, the fifth step in the nursing process, measures the effectiveness of nursing interventions by the examination of the goals and expected outcomes, which provide direction for the plan of care and serve as standards against which the client's progress is measured.
- Critical-thinking, decision-making, and holistic skills are important in the nursing process.
- Documentation provides a system of written records that reflect client care provided on the basis of assessment data and the client's response to interventions.
- Nurses are responsible for assessing and documenting that the client has an understanding of the treatment prior to the intervention.
- Accreditation and reimbursement agencies require accurate and thorough documentation of the nursing care rendered and the client's response to interventions.
- Effective documentation requires clear, concise, accurate recording of all client care and other significant events in an organized and chronological fashion representing each phase of the nursing process.
- Incident reports are used to document any unusual occurrence in a health care facility.

Review Questions

1. Mrs. Rose was admitted to your unit 2 hours ago. The following data are recorded on her chart. Which data are objective?

    a. temperature 102°F
    b. nausea
    c. headache
    d. pain in abdomen

2. The nursing care plan includes:

    a. collected documentation of all team members providing care for the client.
    b. physician orders, demographic data, and medication administration and rationales.
    c. client's nursing diagnoses, goals, expected outcomes, nursing interventions, and evaluation.
    d. client assessment data, medical treatment regimen and rationales, and diagnostic test results and significance.

3. Systematic documentation is critical because it:

    a. is done every hour.
    b. shows the care given by all health care providers.
    c. identifies the planning and implementation phases.
    d. presents in a logical fashion the care provided by nurses.

4. The person responsible for ensuring that the client understands the procedure or intervention and has signed the informed consent is the:

    a. nurse.
    b. physician.
    c. social worker.
    d. admission officer.

5. Documentation of the nursing care the client receives must:

    a. never have an error.
    b. be neatly spaced out.
    c. reflect the nursing process.
    d. be signed at the end of each shift.

References/Suggested Readings

Alfaro-LeFevre, R. (2002). *Applying nursing process* (5th ed.). Philadelphia: Lippincott Williams and Wilkins.

Alfaro-LeFevre, R. (2004). *Critical thinking and clinical judgment.* (3rd ed.). Philadelphia: W. B. Saunders.

American Nurses Association. (1991). *Standards of nursing practice.* Kansas City, MO: Author.

Aquilino, M., & Keenan, G. (2000). Having our say: Nursing's standardized nomenclature. *AJN, 100*(7), 33–38.

Bevis, E. O. (1989). *Curriculum building in nursing: A process* (3rd ed., Publication No. 15-2277). New York: National League for Nursing.

Beyea, L. (1996). *Critical pathways for collaborative nursing care.* Menlo Park, CA: Addison-Wesley Nursing.

Brooke, P. (2002). Legal questions: Documentation errors. *Nursing2002, 32*(1), 67.

Calloway, S. (2001). Preventing communication breakdowns. *RN, 64*(1), 71–74.

Carpenito, L. J. (2002). *Nursing diagnosis: Application to clinical practice* (9th ed.). Philadelphia: Lippincott Williams & Wilkins.

Celia, L. (2002). Keep electronic records safe! *RN, 65*(6), 69–71.

Chaffee, M. (1999). A telehealth odyssey. *AJN, 99*(7), 26–32.

Charting Tips. (1999). Documenting discharges and transfers in long-term care. *Nursing99, 29*(6), 17.

Charting Tips. (1999). Easy as PIE. *Nursing99, 29*(4), 24.

Clark, M. (1998). Implementation of nursing standardized languages NANDA, NIC, and NOC. *Online Journal of Issues in Nursing 2*(2) [Online]. Available: www.nursingworld. org

DeWitt, A. (2000). *Documentation: Legal principles of good charting,* Penumbra Seminars LLC. [Online]. Available: www.respiratorycase-online.com/doc_handoutPDF

Dochterman, J., & Bulechek, G. M. (2004). *Nursing interventions classification (NIC)* (4th ed.). St. Louis, MO: Mosby.

Dumpel, H., James, M., & Phillips, T. (1999). Charting by exception. *California Nurse,* June/July 1999, p. 9. [Online]. Available: www.califnurse.org/cna/junju99/9cnjj99.html

Dykes, P., & Wheeler, K. (Eds.) (1997). *Planning, implementing, and evaluating critical pathways,* New York: Springer.

Edelman, C. L., & Mandle, C. L. (2002). *Health promotion throughout the lifespan* (5th ed.). St. Louis, MO: Mosby.

Estes, M. E. Z. (2002). *Health assessment & physical examination* (2nd ed.). Clifton Park, NY: Thomson Delmar Learning.

Fry, V. S. (1953). The creative approach to nursing. *AJN, 53*(3), 301–302.

Gardner, P. (2002). *Nursing process.* Clifton Park, NY: Thomson Delmar Learning.

Glondys, B. (1999). *Documentation requirements for the acute care patient record.* Chicago, IL: American Health Information Management Association.

Gordon, M. (1998). Nursing nomenclature and classification system development. *Online Journal of Issues in Nursing.* [Online]. Available: www.nursingworld.org/ojin/tpc7/tpc7_1.htm

Gordon, M. (2002). *Manual of nursing diagnoses* (10th ed.). St. Louis, MO: Mosby.

Grane, N. B. (1995). Documenting a "harmless" medication error. *Nursing95, 25*(4), 80.

Gregory, K. (2000). Nurse the patient! *RN, 63*(9), 52–54.

Grulke, C. C. (1995). Seven ways to help a student nurse. *AJN, 96*(60), 24L.

Habel, M. (2000a). *Documenting patient care, Part 1.* [Online]. Available: www.nurseweek.com/cc/ce10a.html

Habel, M. (2000b). *Documenting patient care, Part 2.* [Online]. Available: www.nurseweek.com/cc/ce20a.html

Heery, K. (2000). Straight talk about the patient interview. *Nursing2000, 30*(6), 66–67.

Humphrey, C. J. (1998). *Home care nursing handbook* (3rd ed.). Gaithersburg, MD: Aspen.

Iowa Interventions Project. (1993). The NIC taxonomy structure. *Image: Journal of Nursing Scholarship, 25*(3), 187–192.

Iyer, P. W., & Camp, N. H. (1999). *Nursing documentation: A nursing process approach.* (3rd ed.). St. Louis, MO: Mosby.

Johnson, D. (1959). A philosophy for nursing diagnosis. *Nursing Outlook, 7,* 198–200.

Johnson, M. (1998). Overview of the Nursing Outcomes Classification (NOC). *Online Journal of Nursing Informatics, 2*(2) [Online]. Available: http://cac/psu.edu/~dxm12/OJNI.htm

Johnson, M., & Maas, M. (1998). Implementing the nursing outcomes classification in a practice setting. *Outcomes Management for Nursing Practice, 2*(3), 99–104.

Johnson, M., Bulechek, G., Dochterman, J., Maas, M., & Moorhead, S. (2001). *Nursing diagnoses outcomes & interventions, NANDA, NOC and NIC linkages.* St. Louis, MO: Harcourt Health Sciences.

Joint Commission on Accreditation of Healthcare Organizations. (1998). *1998 Hospital accreditation standards.* Oakbrook Terrace, IL: Author.

Klenner, S. (2000). Mapping out a clinical pathway. *RN, 63*(6), 33–36.

LaDuke, S. (2000). Spotlight: What you *really* do with this powerful documentation tool. *Nursing2000, 30*(6), 68.

Malestic, S. (2003). A quick guide to verbal reports. *RN, 66*(2), 47–49.

McCloskey, J. C., & Bulechek, G. M. (1995). Validation and coding of the NIC taxonomy structure. *Image: Journal of Nursing Scholarship, 27*(1), 43–49.

McCloskey, J. C., & Bulechek, G. M. (1998). Nursing interventions classification (NIC): Current status and new directions. *Online Journal of Nursing Informatics, 2*(2) [Online]. Available: http://milkman.cac.psu.edu/ndxm12/OJNI. html

McCloskey, J. C., & Maas, M. (1998). Interdisciplinary team: The nursing perspective is essential. *Nursing Outlook, 46*(4), 157–163.

McConnell, E. (1999). Charting with care. *Nursing99, 29*(10), 68.

Moorhead, S., Johnson, M., & Maas, M. (Eds.). (2004). *Nursing outcomes classification (NOC)* (3rd ed.). St. Louis, MO: Mosby.

National Committee on Vital and Health Statistics (HCVHS) Hearings on Medical Terminology and Code Development. (1999). *Health care terminology: Nursing outcomes classification, The University of Iowa* [Online]. Available: http://aspe.os.dhhs.gov/NCVHS/990518t4.htm

National Federation of Licensed Practical Nurses (NFLPN). (1996). *Nursing practice standards for the licensed practical/vocational nurse.* Garner, NC: Author.

National Library of Medicine. (2000). *Fact sheet, UMLS* [Online]. Available: www.nlm.nih.gov/pubs/ factsheets/umls. html

North American Nursing Diagnosis Association (NANDA) (2003). *Nursing diagnoses: Definitions & classifications 2003–2004.* Philadelphia: Author.

Oermann, M., & Huber, D. (1999). Patient outcomes: A measure of nursing's value. *AJN, 99*(9), 40–47.

Olson-Chavarriaga, D. (2000). Informed consent: Do you know your role? *Nursing 2000, 30*(5), 60–61.

Orem, D. E., Taylor, S. G., & Renpenning, K. (2001). *Nursing: Concepts of practice* (6th ed.). St. Louis, MO: Mosby.

Orlando, I. (1961). *The dynamic nurse–patient relationship.* New York: Putnam.

Ozbolt, J. (1998). *From minimum data to maximum impact: Using clinical data to strengthen patient care* [Online]. Available: http://cti.itc.virginia.edu/~spt2j/707materials/ozbolt98. htm

Pethtel, P. (2000). *Nursing documentation.* [Online]. Available: http://garnet.indstate.edu/ppethtel/chartingforweb

Raymond, L. (2001). How to chart for peer review. *RN, 64*(6), 67–70.

Raymond, L. (2002). Documenting for the "PROs." *Nursing 2002, 32*(3), 50–53.

Roberts, D. (2002). How to keep electronic health records private. *Nursing 2002, 32*(10), 95.

Rochman, R. (2000). Are computerized patient records for you? *Nursing 2000, 30*(10), 61-62.

Seaback, W. (2001). *Nursing process: Concepts & application.* Clifton Park, NY: Thomson Delmar Learning.

Sheehan, J. (2001). Delegating to UAPs—A practical guide. *RN, 64*(11), 65–66.

Smith, L. (2000a). How to use focus charting. *Nursing2000, 30*(5), 76.

Smith, L. (2000b). Safe computer charting. *Nursing2000, 30*(9), 85.

Smith, L. (2002). How to chart by exception. *Nursing20002, 32*(9), 30.

Springhouse. (1998). *Charting made incredibly easy.* Springhouse, PA: Author.

Springhouse. (1999). *Mastering documentation* (2nd ed.). Springhouse, PA: Author.

Stewart, K. (2001). Charting Tips: Documenting adverse incidents. *Nursing2001, 31*(3), 84.

Sullivan, G. (2000). Keep your charting on course. *RN, 63*(5), 75-79.

The University of Iowa College of Nursing (2001a). *Strengths of the nursing interventions classification.* [Online]. Available: http://coinfo.nursing.uiowa.edu/nic/strength.htm

The University of Iowa College of Nursing (2001b). *Nursing outcomes classification overview.* [Online]. Available: http://coinfo.nursing.uiowa.edu/noc/overview.htm

Thede, L. (2003). *Informatics and Nursing.* Philadelphia, PA: Lippincott Williams & Wilkins.

Thompson, C. (1995, May). Writing better narrative notes. *Nursing95, 25*(5), 87.

Tucker, S., Canobbio, M., Paquette, E., & Willis, M. (2000). *Patient care standards: Collaborative planning & nursing interventions* (7th ed.). St. Louis, MO: Mosby.

Werley, H. H., & Lang, N. M. (1988). The consensually derived nursing minimum data set: Elements and definitions. In H. H. Werley & N. M. Lang (Eds.), *Identification of the nursing minimum data set* (pp. 402–411). New York: Springer.

Wiedenbach, E. (1963). The helping art of nursing. *AJN, 63*(11), 54–57.

Wilkinson, J. M. (2001). *Nursing process and critical thinking.* (3rd ed.). Redwood City, CA: Addison-Wesley Nursing.

Wilkinson, J. M. (2000). *Nursing diagnosis handbook with NIC interventions and NOC outcomes.* (7th ed.). Englewood Cliffs, NJ: Prentice Hall.

Yocum, R. F. (2002). Documenting for quality patient care. *Nursing 2002, 32*(8), 58–63.

Yura, H., & Walsh, M. B. (1967). *The nursing process.* Washington, DC: Catholic University of America Press.

Resources

American Health Information Management Association, 233 North Michigan Avenue, Suite 2150, Chicago, IL 60601-5800, 313-233-1100, www.ahima.org

American Nursing Informatics Association (ANIA), PMB105, 10808 Foothill Boulevard, Suite 160, Rancho Cucamonga, CA 91730, www.ania.org

Center for Nursing Classification, NB 407, The University of Iowa, College of Nursing, Iowa City, IA 52252-1121, www.nursing.uiowa.edu

Medical Records Institute, P.O. Box 600770, 567 Walnut Street, Newton, MA 02460, 617-964-3923, www.medrecinst.com

North American Nursing Diagnosis Association (NANDA), 1211 Locust Street, Philadelphia, PA 19107, 800-647-9002, www.nanda.org

Nursing Diagnosis (journal), 1211 Locust Street, Philadelphia, PA 19107, 800-242-6757

CLIENT TEACHING

MAKING THE CONNECTION

Refer to the following chapters to increase your understanding of client teaching:

Basic Nursing
- **Legal and Ethical Responsibilities**
- **Communication**
- **Nursing Process/Documentation**

- **Life Cycle**
- **Cultural Considerations**
- **Stress, Adaptation, and Anxiety**

LEARNING OBJECTIVES

Upon completion of this chapter, you should be able to:
- **Define key terms.**
- **Explain the importance of client education in today's health care climate.**
- **Relate principles of adult education to client teaching.**
- **Identify common barriers to learning.**
- **Explain the ways that learning varies throughout the life cycle.**
- **Discuss the nurse's professional responsibilities related to teaching.**
- **Relate the teaching–learning process to the nursing process.**
- **Describe teaching strategies that make learning meaningful to clients.**

KEY TERMS

affective domain
auditory learner
cognitive domain
formal teaching
informal teaching
kinesthetic learner
learning
learning plateau
learning style

psychomotor domain
readiness for learning
self-efficacy
teaching
teaching–learning
  process
teaching strategies
visual learner

INTRODUCTION

Client education is an integral part of nursing care. The nurse is responsible to help the client identify learning needs and resources that will restore and maintain that client's optimal level of functioning. This chapter discusses the teaching–learning process, including barriers and responsibilities, and relates it to the nursing process.

THE TEACHING–LEARNING PROCESS

The **teaching–learning process** is a planned interaction that promotes behavioral change that is not a re-

sult of maturation or coincidence. **Teaching** is an active process wherein one individual shares information with another to facilitate learning and thereby promote behavioral changes. A teacher is someone who uses a variety of goal-directed activities to promote change by assisting the learner to absorb new information.

Learning is the process of assimilating information, resulting in behavior change. Knowledge is power. By sharing knowledge with clients, the nurse helps them achieve their maximum level of wellness. The teaching–learning process has the same basic steps as the nursing process: assessment, identification of learning needs (nursing diagnosis), planning, implementation of teaching strategies, and evaluation of learner progress and teaching efficacy. These steps are discussed in greater detail later in this chapter.

Edelman and Mandle (2002) describe the goal of health education as helping individuals achieve optimal states of health through their own actions. Often, deficient knowledge about the course of illness and/or self-care practices hinders the client's recovery or in practicing health-promoting behaviors. The nurse's role is to help bridge the gap between those things a client knows and those things a client needs to know to achieve optimal health.

Client teaching is done for a variety of reasons, including to:

- Promote wellness
- Prevent illness
- Restore health
- Facilitate coping abilities

Client education focuses on the client's ability to practice healthy behaviors. The client's ability to care for self is enhanced by effective education. Client education may:

- Improve quality of care
- Decrease length of hospital stays
- Decrease chance of hospital readmission
- Improve compliance with treatment regimens

These benefits are enhanced through nurses' continued active participation as client educators.

Formal teaching is planned and goal directed, but informal teaching can occur in any setting at any time.

Formal Teaching

Formal teaching takes place at a specific time, in a specific place, and on a specific topic. It is planned and goal directed (Figure 9-1). The teacher prepares the information and/or activities related to the topic. Formal teaching may take place in a class setting with several learners, or it may be performed one-on-one. For example, many health care facilities provide formal classes related to diabetes. The same basic information is necessary for all clients with diabetes.

Informal Teaching

Informal teaching takes place any time, any place, whenever a learning need is identified. While providing nursing care, nurses have many opportunities for informal teaching, such as answering the clients' questions and explaining care being given to the client. Informal teaching may also occur in the midst of formal teaching. A comment or question from a learner in a formal setting may trigger some informal teaching in response. For example, during a class on diet for the diabetic client, a question about dietary cholesterol may be asked. The response would be considered informal teaching because it was not the planned topic.

An understanding of learning domains, learning principles, learning styles, learning barriers, and teaching methods is helpful. These topics are discussed as follows.

Learning Domains

In his classic work, Bloom (1977) identifies three areas or domains wherein learning occurs: the **cognitive domain,** which involves intellectual understanding; the **affective domain,** which involves attitudes, beliefs, and emotions; and the **psychomotor domain,** which involves the performance of motor skills. Information is processed in each domain. Table 9–1 briefly outlines the three learning domains and provides clinical examples.

Figure 9-1   *Nurses engage in formal teaching with both individual and group clients. (Second photo coutresy of Bellevue Woman's Hospital, Niskayuna, NY)*

Nurses must be sensitive to all three learning domains when developing effective teaching plans and must use **teaching strategies,** or techniques to promote learning, that will tap into each of the domains. For instance, teaching a diabetic client how insulin works in the body falls within the cognitive domain; helping the same client learn how to use a glucose monitor falls within the psychomotor domain; and encouraging the client to view diabetes as only one aspect of the individual falls within the affective domain.

Learning Principles

Fundamental principles of learning can be used when teaching clients. Knowles, Holton, and Swanson (2000) cite four basic assumptions about adult learners, which are applicable to client education:

- *Assumption 1:* Personality develops in an orderly fashion from dependence to independence. *Nursing application:* Plan teaching–learning activities promoting client participation. This encourages independence and increases client control and self-care.
- *Assumption 2:* Learning readiness is affected by developmental stage and sociocultural factors. *Nursing application:* Conduct a psychosocial assessment before planning teaching–learning activities.
- *Assumption 3:* Previous learning experiences are a foundation for further learning. *Nursing application:* Perform

TABLE 9-1 LEARNING DOMAINS

DOMAIN	DEFINITION	EXAMPLE
Cognitive	Learning involving the acquisition of facts and data; used in decision making and problem solving	Client states the symptoms of possible complications
Affective	Learning involving attitude, emotion, and belief changing; used in making judgments	Client begins to accept the lifestyle changes required
Psychomotor	Learning involving gaining motor skills; used in physical application of knowledge	Client uses glucose monitor

a complete assessment to ascertain what the client already knows and build on that knowledge base.

- *Assumption 4:* Immediacy reinforces learning. *Nursing application:* Provide opportunities for immediate application of knowledge and skills and incorporate feedback as part of each nurse–client interaction.

Learning principles include relevance, motivation, readiness, maturation, reinforcement, participation, organization, and repetition.

Relevance

The material to be learned must be meaningful to the client, easily understood by the client, and related to previously learned information. Individuals must believe that they need to learn the information before learning can occur. If an individual sees the information as being personally valuable, the information is more likely to be learned. Because relevance is individually determined, the nurse must assess the personal meaning of learning for each client.

Motivation

The psychologist Bandura (1977) purports that **self-efficacy** (one's belief that one will succeed in attempts to change behavior) has a profound influence on motivation. If clients believe they will not achieve the goals, they will lack motivation to try. To maximize motivation, the nurse must keep the teaching–learning goals realistic by breaking the content down into small, achievable steps. For example, the cardiac client must see value in information about exercise, such as that the heart will be strengthened and the client will have more energy.

Readiness

The client should be able and willing to learn. Readiness is closely related to growth and development. For example, the client must have the requisite cogni-

tive and psychomotor skills for learning a particular task, and the client must comprehend the information. One indicator of learning readiness is if clients ask questions; another is if clients become involved in learning activities, such as participating in return demonstration of a dressing change. Some indicators of lack of client readiness are anxiety, avoidance, denial, and lack of participation in discussion, demonstration, or self-care activities.

Maturation

The client should be developmentally able to learn and have requisite cognitive and psychomotor abilities. Assess the client for characteristics that will hinder or facilitate learning, such as developmental stage. Assess the client's developmental stage. Do not automatically assume that a 34-year-old client has mastered the developmental tasks of earlier stages.

Maturity level greatly influences the client's ability to learn information. Each developmental stage is characterized by unique skills and abilities affecting the response to various teaching tools. Developmental stage greatly determines the type of data to be taught, the method(s) to be used, the vocabulary to be used, and the location of teaching. In addition to developmental stage, the nurse should also evaluate the client's cognitive skills, problem-solving abilities, and attention span.

Reinforcement

Feedback provided to the learner should be immediate and positive to reinforce the client's motivation and readiness to learn. For example, the client who is learning to apply a sterile dressing to an open wound should be told during the application of the dressing that it is being done correctly (if it is) and should be praised upon completion for learning so quickly (or whatever is appropriate). If some aspect of the dressing application is lack-

LIFE CYCLE CONSIDERATIONS

Ability to Learn

Remember that age is not always synonymous with developmental level; observation of behavior provides the clearest picture of developmental level.

ing, the nurse must maintain a positive approach in guiding the client to correctly perform the application.

Participation

The client's active involvement in the learning process promotes and enhances learning. Client involvement is relatively easy to monitor when a psychomotor skill is to be learned, as the client is actively involved in practicing a physical skill. Learning that takes place in the cognitive or affective domain is also most effective when active involvement of the client is encouraged. For example, the client who is to be on a low-fat diet can be involved in learning to self-regulate with regard to diet by reading labels of foods and planning menus of low-fat meals.

Organization

The material to be learned should incorporate previously learned information and be presented in sequence from simple to complex and from familiar to unfamiliar. Again using the example of the client learning about a low-fat diet, the nurse should begin the teaching session by finding out what the client knows about the nutrient content of foods and then proceed by helping the client learn to read food labels, then plan a meal, and plan a menu for a day and a week, and so forth.

Repetition

Retention of material is reinforced with practice, repetition, and presentation of the same material in a variety of ways. The more often the learner hears or sees the material, the greater the chance that the material will be retained.

It is good to keep in mind that a **learning plateau,** or peak in the effectiveness of teaching and depth of learning, will occur in relation to the client's motivation, interest, and perception of relevance of the material. Frequent reinforcement of learning through immediate feedback and continual reassessment of effectiveness will enhance the value of the learning process for both the teacher and the learner. Making the information-acquisition process as user friendly as possible also increases satisfaction and success. This can be done, by making learning as creative and interesting as possible and adopting a flexible approach to allow the learning process to be dynamic.

Learning Style

Each individual has a unique way of processing information. The manner whereby an individual incorporates new data is called **learning style.** Some people learn by processing information visually **(visual**

learner), others by listening to the words **(auditory learner),** and others by experiencing the information or by touching, feeling, or doing **(kinesthetic learner).** A variety of techniques, should be used, such as lecture, discussion, role play, modeling, games, return demonstration, imitation, problem solving, and question-and-answer sessions, to match various learning styles of clients. A good way to discover learning style is by asking the client, "What helps you learn?" or "What kinds of things do you enjoy doing?" Then teaching strategies can be matched to the client's learning style.

Barriers to the Teaching–Learning Process

The giving and receiving of information does not, in and of itself, guarantee that learning will occur. Several barriers can impede the teaching–learning process. In a nursing situation, the nurse, the client, or both may encounter one or more of these barriers. Learning barriers can be classified as either internal (psychological or physiological) or external (environmental or sociocultural). Examples of these barriers are listed in Table 9–2. To facilitate the learning process, the nurse must assess for the presence of learning barriers. Specific assessment information is presented later in this chapter.

Environmental Barriers

Both the nurse and client are subject to environmental barriers. As part of planning for a teaching session, the nurse should ensure necessary privacy and minimize interruptions and extraneous stimuli.

Sociocultural Barriers

When language is a barrier to the teaching–learning process, several steps can be taken to ensure that learning does take place, such as using pictures, providing printed material in the appropriate language, or using an interpreter. Even when the nurse and client both speak the same language, a language barrier may exist when clichés, health care jargon, or value-laden terms are used. Furthermore, the meanings that the nurse

TABLE 9-2 BARRIERS TO LEARNING

EXTERNAL BARRIERS	INTERNAL BARRIERS
Environmental • Lack of privacy • Extraneous stimuli • Interruptions	**Psychological** • Anxiety • Anger • Fear • Depression
Sociocultural • Language • Level of education • Values	**Physiological** • Pain • Oxygen deprivation • Fatigue • Hunger

and client attach to specific types of body language may differ depending on cultural influences. Nurses must be aware of their own value systems but focus client teaching within the client's value system. The client's level of education must be kept in mind, and words tailored to the client's educational level, without "talking down" to the client.

Psychological Barriers

Nurses may be anxious about client teaching. Knowing the client's learning needs and adequate preparation related to content, environmental and sociocultural aspects, and developmental ability of the client should alleviate some of this anxiety. What little anxiety is left will likely make the nurse more alert and sensitive.

Clients and families are often upset about the health situation. They may be anxious, angry, fearful, or depressed. In addition to the client's words, the nurse should pay attention to body language and behavior. If clients or family members are obviously angry, the nurse should acknowledge the anger by saying something like "You appear to be very angry about something. Tell me what you are feeling." Allowing clients and family members to express their emotions clears the air and allows learning to take place.

CULTURAL CONSIDERATIONS

Overcoming Sociocultural Barriers

• Use pictures whenever possible.
• Provide written material in the appropriate language.
• Use a culturally sensitive interpreter or a family member who understands health care terminology.
• Avoid the use of clichés, jargon, or value-laden terms.
• Learn about the client's cultural norms.
• Be aware of your own values.
• Tailor teaching (information and questions) to the client's ability to read and write.
• Have the client verbalize what has been understood from the teaching–learning session.

PROFESSIONAL TIP

Overcoming Psychological Barriers

• Recognize your own emotions related to client teaching.
• Assess for psychological barriers to learning.
• Acknowledge the client's emotions but do not respond in kind.

PROFESSIONAL TIP

Physiological Comfort and Learning

• Administer pain medication, as appropriate, before a teaching session to enable the client to concentrate on the information being presented.
• Plan teaching sessions when the client is not fatigued, as might be the case after a physical therapy session, for example.
• Ensure that the client is in a comfortable position and does not have to go to the bathroom.

Physiological Barriers

The physiological situation affects the client's ability to learn. The client who is struggling to breathe, for example, is unable to pay attention to any teaching. A teaching session should be planned for a time when the client is rested and free from pain.

Teaching Methods

Many different teaching methods can be used depending on the client's learning need and the applicable learning domain.

Teaching Methods Applicable in the Cognitive Domain

Effective methods for promoting cognitive learning include discussion, formal lecture, question-and-answer sessions, role play, and games/computer activities.

Discussion Discussions may involve the nurse and one or several clients who need to learn the same information. Active participation in the discussion is promoted. Group discussions allow peer support.

Formal Lecture In formal lectures, the teacher presents the information to be learned, and learner participation is usually minimal.

Question-and-Answer Sessions Question-and-answer sessions can take two forms. In one, the client's concerns are addressed by the client asking the questions and the nurse providing answers. In the other the nurse assists the client in applying the knowledge learned by asking the client questions that the client then answers (Figure 9-2).

Role Play Role play provides the client an opportunity to apply knowledge in a safe, controlled environment.

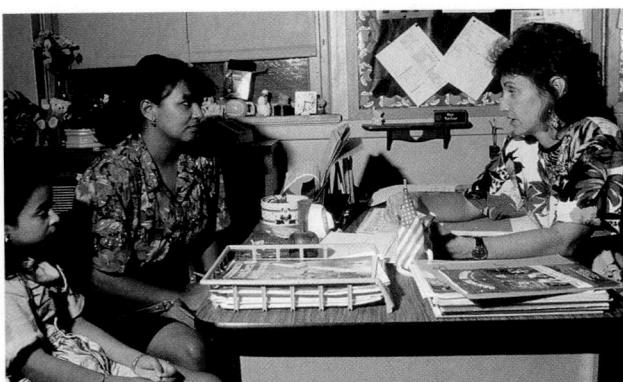

Figure 9-2 *A Question-and-Answer Session with School Nurse, Mother, and Child*

Figure 9-3 *Demonstrating Application of a Splint*

In role play, the nurse and client each assume a certain role in order to play out different possible scenarios. For instance, the nurse teaching a client sex education information intended for an adolescent may have the client assume the role of parent, while the nurse assumes the role of the teenager. The two can then engage in practice discussion sessions to prepare the client for the actual parent–teen discussion.

Games/Computer Activities Games and computer activities can be used to teach clients at a level that is appropriate for them. These methods allow the client to use the new information in various situations and to have fun while learning.

Teaching Methods Applicable in the Affective Domain

Role play and discussion are both effective methods for stimulating affective learning.

Role Play Role play allows expression of feelings, attitudes, and values in a safe, controlled environment. The client can try out different attitudes and values.

Discussion One-on-one discussion between nurse and client is effective for personal or sensitive topics related to values, feelings, attitudes, and emotions.

Teaching Methods Applicable in the Psychomotor Domain

Demonstration, supervised practice, and return demonstration assist the client to learn psychomotor skills.

Demonstration In demonstration, the nurse presents in a step-by-step manner the skill or procedure to be learned, explaining what is being done and why. In this way, the client sees not only the equipment and the way it is used, but also the nurse's attitude and behaviors (Figure 9-3).

Supervised Practice In supervised practice, the client uses the equipment and performs the skill or procedure while the nurse watches. The nurse gives suggestions or corrects the client as the practice proceeds. Repetition can continue until the client feels confident in performing the skill or procedure.

Return Demonstration In return demonstration, the client performs the skill or procedure without any coach-

ing from the nurse. Upon completion of the task, the nurse provides feedback and reinforcement to the client.

LIFELONG LEARNING

One basic assumption underlies teaching: *All people are capable of learning.* However, the ability to learn varies from person to person and from situation to situation. Learning needs and learning abilities change throughout life. The client's developmental stage and chronological age greatly influence the ability to learn. The principles of learning discussed earlier in this chapter are relevant to learners of all ages. Teaching approaches must be altered depending on the client's developmental stage and level of understanding. Specific information for children, adolescents, and older adults is described in the following sections.

LIFE CYCLE CONSIDERATIONS

Teaching Children

- Ensure that the child is comfortable.
- Encourage participation of caregiver.
- Assess the child's developmental level, learning readiness, and motivation. Do not equate age with developmental level.
- Assess the child's psychological status.
- Determine self-care abilities of the child.
- Use play, imitation, and role play.
- Use various visual stimuli, such as books, chalkboards, and videos, to share information and assess understanding.
- Use terms easily understood by the client and caregiver.
- Provide frequent repetition and reinforcement.
- Develop realistic goals consistent with developmental level.
- Remember that the goals of educating children are to improve cooperation, prevent excessive anxiety, and hasten the recovery process.

Children

Readiness for learning (evidence of willingness to learn) varies during childhood depending on maturation level. The nurse must work closely with the child's caretaker, especially when caring for young children.

Young children learn primarily through play. Incorporating play into teaching activities for children can therefore enhance learning (Figure 9-4). Puppets, coloring books, and toys can be effective teaching tools for the young child. Encourage the young child to be an active participant in the learning process.

Older children can also benefit from the use of art materials to express their emotions and their understanding of those things that are or will be happening to them. Using medical supplies (such as medicine cups or bandages), the child may play at giving medicine to a doll or putting a bandage on the doll like the bandage that will be put on the child. While the child is involved in play, the nurse is both teaching the child what to expect regarding treatment procedures and alleviating anxiety.

Adolescents

Individuals approaching adolescence are better able to understand relationships between things. Usually,

CLIENT TEACHING

Do As I Do

- Individuals learn from examples set by role models.
- Adolescents are very sensitive to any discrepancy between words and actions.
- Encourage parents to model the behaviors they wish their children to develop.

reading and comprehension ability have advanced, and the adolescent can understand more complex information. Because one of the strongest influences on the adolescent is peer support, group meetings are often useful in teaching. The nurse can often be a potent teacher as a role model.

Older Adults

Many physiological changes accompany aging. These changes cause some older adults to experience perceptual impairments in vision and hearing. The nurse must assess for these changes and adjust teaching materials accordingly. For example, providing large-print written material and verifying that the client hears all instructions and directions are strategies helpful in teaching older clients.

PROFESSIONAL RESPONSIBILITIES OF TEACHING

The nurse empowers clients in their self-care abilities through teaching. Teaching provides information to clients about health-promoting behaviors, specific disease processes, and treatment methods. Although each state has its own definition of nursing practice, teaching is a required function of nurses in most states. Redman (2001) cites National League for Nursing documents dating back to 1918 as stating that "the nurse is essentially a teacher and an agent of health."

Figure 9-4 *A, The nurse is at the child's level while the child learns about the instrument to be used in the examination; B, The nurse encourages a child to select a toy to help in teaching.*

LIFE CYCLE CONSIDERATIONS

Teaching Adolescents

- Respect the adolescent.
- Boost their confidence by seeking their input and opinions on health care matters.
- Encourage exploration of their own feelings.
- Be sensitive to peer pressure.
- Help adolescents identify and build on their positive qualities.
- Use language that is clear yet appropriate to the health care setting.
- Encourage independent and informed decision making by engaging them in problem-solving activities.

LIFE CYCLE CONSIDERATIONS

Teaching Older Adults

- Ensure that the client is comfortable. Fatigue, pain, a full bladder, or hunger can hinder learning.
- Assess the client's developmental level, motivation, and learning readiness.
- Assess the client for depression, anxiety, or denial, which can interfere with learning.
- Determine client's ability for self-care.
- Use words easily understood by the client.
- Avoid talking down to the client; a condescending, paternalistic manner hinders learning.
- Find the time of day when the client is most alert.
- Present material slowly using examples.
- Encourage client participation.
- Ask for feedback and listen actively.
- Provide feedback frequently.
- Assess for perceptual impairments and individualize teaching strategies accordingly:

For memory-impaired clients:
- Repeat material.
- Use different cues (spoken words, pictures, written materials, and symbols).

For visually impaired clients:
- Use large-print materials.
- Furnish a magnifying glass.
- Be sure prescription eyeglasses are worn.
- Arrange adequate lighting and reduce glare.

For hearing-impaired clients:
- Face the client when speaking.
- Use short sentences with words that are easily understood.
- Use gestures and demonstrate to reinforce verbal information.
- Eliminate distractions (activities or noises in the environment) as much as possible.

Providing client education is expected of all nurses. Freda (1997) is disturbed by reports that some nurses in the United States, however, are voluntarily giving up their client teaching responsibilities, mainly because of a perceived lack of time. If nurses give up their role as client educators to spend time performing additional tasks, nursing's worth to the health care system could greatly diminish. Client teaching requires the depth of information that only nurses possess; as such, it is one of the truly independent functions of nursing practice.

Client teaching is also required by several accrediting bodies, including the Joint Commission for Accreditation of Healthcare Organizations (JCAHO, 2002). The American Hospital Association's *Patient's Bill of Rights* (1992) calls for the client's understanding of health status and treatment approaches. Only clients who are well informed can give informed consent. Nurses assess clients' level of understanding about treatment methods and correct any knowledge deficits. The nurse often serves as an interpreter for the client by explaining, clarifying, and referring.

Teaching supports behavioral changes that lead to positive adaptation by the client. Teaching decreases the fear of change by reducing anxiety and anticipation stresses.

Client teaching is an essential nursing function in every practice setting. All clients require information about disease prevention, growth and development, safety, first aid, nutrition, and hygiene. The hospitalized client needs information about his condition, the expected treatment, and the environment of the health care facility. By the time of discharge, clients must also have information about postdischarge care related to medications, dietary modifications, activity, complication prevention, and rehabilitation plans.

Clients recovering at home and their families also have significant learning needs. A primary role of the home health nurse is to teach the client about caring for himself at home. This often involves teaching family members ways to provide care (Figure 9-5) and information about their illness, accident, or injury. They should also be taught ways to achieve and maintain a maximum state of wellness. Accurate teaching plans for the home-based client and family are established by assessing many factors, such as:

Support system
- Individuals available to help give care
- Caregivers' knowledge about necessary care

Environmental
- Home accessibility
- Space to meet special needs of the client
- Need for and availability of equipment and supplies
- Need for assistance with self-care activities

Figure 9-5 *The nurse teaches a family member how to provide care.*

- Need for information about environmental cleanliness related to health

Economic
- Ability to purchase medications, equipment, and supplies
- Available financial assistance

Community resources
- Area resources
- Awareness of and access to support services
- Respite for the family available

Self-Awareness

Several characteristics of nurses influence the outcome of the teaching–learning process. Nurse self-awareness with regard to the concepts discussed in the following sections is an all-important first step in teaching.

Knowledge Base

It is impossible for nurses to teach if they lack the knowledge or skills that are to be taught. Staying both current in knowledge and proficient in skills is the first step to maintaining efficacy and credibility as a teacher. Although it is impossible for one individual to be an expert in every area of nursing, knowing when to refer the client to others for teaching is an important critical-thinking skill.

Interpersonal Skills

Effective teaching is based on the nurse's ability to establish rapport with the client. The empathic nurse shows sensitivity to the client's needs and preferences. An atmosphere in which the client feels free to ask questions promotes learning. Activities that help establish an environment conducive to learning include:

- Showing genuine interest in the client
- Including the client in *every* step of the teaching–learning process

- Employing a nonjudgmental approach
- Communicating at the client's level of understanding

Documentation

The standard is for nurses to document client education. From a legal perspective, if the nurse teaches a client but does not document it, the teaching never occurred. Documentation of teaching facilitates accurate communication to other health care colleagues and promotes continuity of care.

Many different approaches can be used to document client teaching. Figure 9-6 is an example of a documentation form related to client teaching in an inpatient setting.

Because client education is a standard and essential component of nursing practice, each nurse must document the teaching interventions used and the client's response. Elements to be documented in all practice settings include:

- Content
- Teaching methods
- Learner(s) (e.g., client, family member, other caretaker)
- Client/family response to teaching activities

TEACHING–LEARNING AND THE NURSING PROCESS

The teaching–learning process and the nursing process are interdependent. Both are dynamic and comprise the same phases: assessment, diagnosis, planning, implementation, and evaluation.

Assessment

Primary (client) and secondary (family or significant other) sources are used by nurses to assess learning needs. Communication is the foundation of assessment related to learning. Factors to be considered include:

- Actual learning needs
- Potential learning needs
- Ability and readiness to learn
- Client strengths and limitations
- Previous experiences

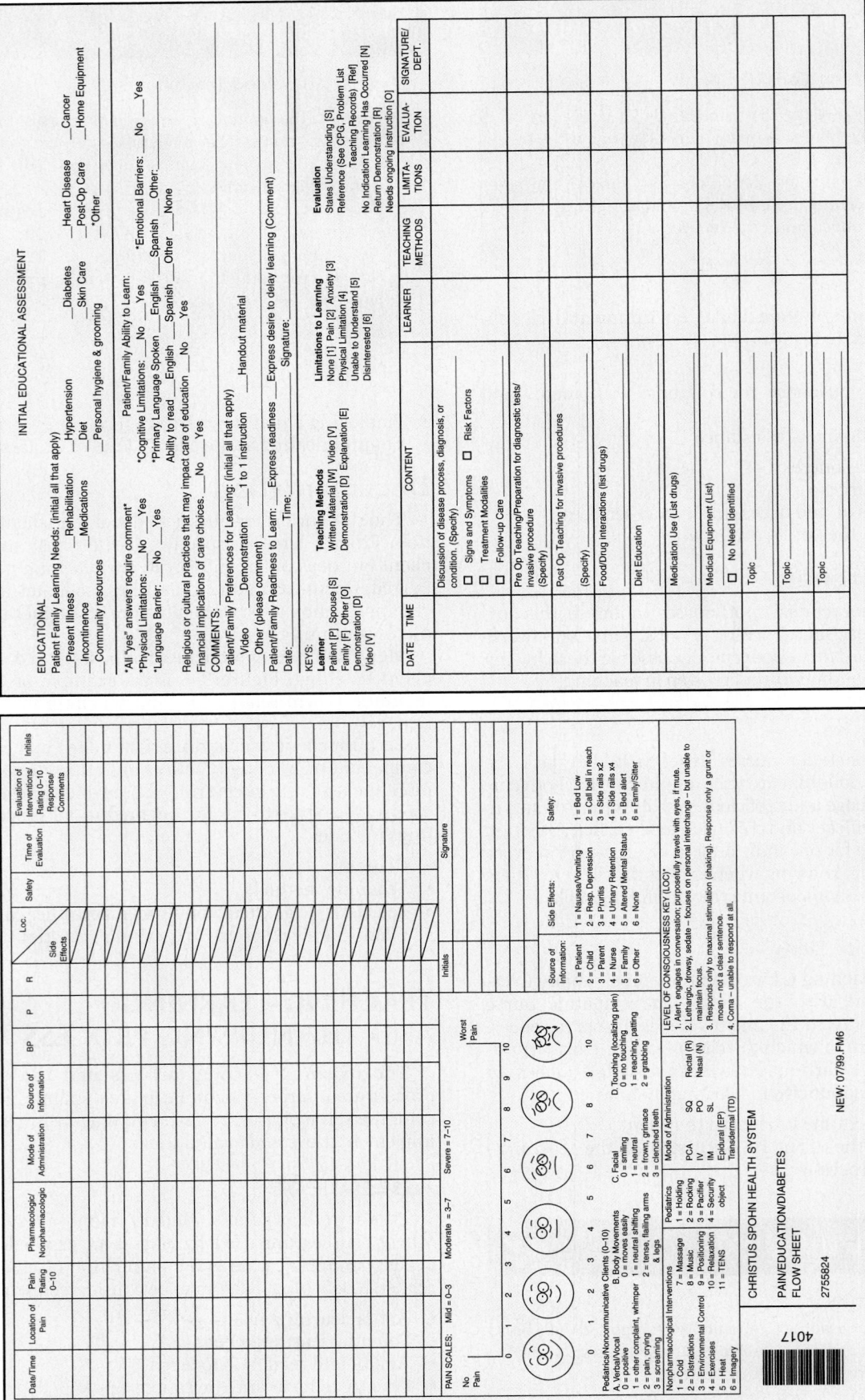

Figure 9-6 *Documentation Form for Client Teaching: Inpatient Setting Courtesy of CHRISTUS Spohn Health System, Corpus Christi, TX)* *continues*

INJECTION SITE:
RA – Right Arm
LA – Left Arm
RT – Right Thigh
LT – Left Thigh
RG – Right Gluteal
LG – Left Gluteal
RQ – Right Abdominal Quadrant
LQ – Left Abdominal Quadrant

Initial/Signatures

DIET:

For Documentation of Routine Blood Sugar Results i.e. BID, TID or AC and HS

DATE	AC Break-fast	AC Lunch	AC Dinner	AC HS Snack	2 A M	COMMENTS
Bld Glu						
Meter #						
Insulin Admin.						
Bld Glu						
Meter #						
Insulin Admin.						
Bld Glu						
Meter #						
Insulin Admin.						

Int.	#	Problem	Goal	Exp. Date of Resol.	Date Comp. Int.
		Alteration in Comfort	Comfort maintained		
		Injury Potential	Safety Maintained		
		Fever	Temp. within Normal Limits		
		Anxiety/Fear	Reduced Anxiety/Fear		
		Knowledge Deficit	Increased Understanding		
		Infection	Minimized/Absent Signs		
		Body Image Disturbance	Acknowledge Change		
		Fluid/Lyte Imbalance	Main. Fluid/Lyte Bal.		
		Impaired Gas Exchange	Main./Increase Gas Ex.		
		Ineffective Airway Clearance	Maintain Patient Airway		
		Ineffective Breathing Pattern	Maintain Patient Airway		
		Altered Tissue Perfusion	Optimal Tissue Perfusion		

DATE	AC Break-fast	AC Lunch	AC Dinner	AC HS Snack	2 A M	COMMENTS
Bld Glu						
Meter #						
Insulin Admin.						
Bld Glu						
Meter #						
Insulin Admin.						
Bld Glu						
Meter #						
Insulin Admin.						
Bld Glu						
Meter #						
Insulin Admin.						

Int.	#	Problem	Goal	Exp. Date of Resol.	Date Comp. Int.
		Impaired Skin Integrity	Regain Skin Integrity		
		Pot. For Skin Impairment	Skin Integrity Maintained		
		Activity Intolerance	Maintain/Increase Activity		
		Impaired Mobility	Imp. Function/ Mobility		
		Self Care Deficit	Improve ADL's		
		Altered Thought Process	Reduced Disorientation		
		Impaired Communication	Improve Communication		
		Constipation	Bowel Elim. With WNL		
		Diarrhea	Bowel Elim. With WNL		
		Incontinence	Maintain Bowel Integrity		
		Impaired Swallowing/ Chewing	Optimal Nutrition Status		
		Alteration in Nutrition	Optimal Nutrition Status		

Pain-Ed-Diabetes.FM6   09/16/99

DATE	TIME	CONTENT	LEARNER	TEACHING METHODS	LIMITA-TIONS	EVALUA-TION	SIGNATURE/ DEPT.
		Rehabilitation (Describe)					
		PT ___ TR ___ OT ___ Speech ___					
		Special Treatments (Describe)					
		Community Resources (Specify)					
		Diabetes Teaching □ DM Medication □ Insulin Adm. Techniques □ Diet Guidelines □ Hypoglycemia–Sx., Tx., Prev. □ Foot Care □ Sick Day Guidelines □ Refered to OP Diabetes Class					
		Explanation of safety program, level precautions, and wristband					
		Topic: Pain Management Information Sheet					
		Topic ___					
		Topic ___					
		Topic ___					
		Topic ___					
		Topic ___					
		Topic ___					
		Topic ___					
		Topic ___					
		Topic ___					

Figure 9-6, continued

Actual Learning Needs

Everyone who receives health care services has some need for learning. Client teaching may be indicated when a client:

- Asks for information to make decisions
- Requires new skills
- Desires to make lifestyle changes
- Is in an unfamiliar environment

The client's knowledge about the content to be taught must be evaluated. Previous knowledge can be used as a foundation for new concepts. The client's learning needs can be determined in a variety of ways, including:

- Asking the client directly
- Observing client behaviors
- Asking the client's family or significant others

The nurse must first address the client's immediate need for knowledge. For example, preoperative clients must be taught deep breathing exercises and leg exercises before surgery so they will be able to perform those exercises after surgery and thereby prevent potential complications. Incision care to be performed at home can be taught after surgery.

Potential Learning Needs

Potential learning needs are also assessed so that anticipatory planning can be done to prevent a relapse in the recovery process or to maintain wellness. Following are two scenarios with related potential learning needs noted:

- Mrs. Lougy is pregnant for the first time. *Potential learning need:* Infant care
- Mr. Harmon has diabetes and has just been told that he must take insulin daily. *Potential learning need:* Self-administration of insulin

Ability and Readiness to Learn

Assess the client for factors that will hinder or facilitate learning. Age does not determine developmental level. Behavior provides the best indication of developmental level. The client's cognitive skills and attention span, along with developmental level, all indicate a client's ability to learn.

PROFESSIONAL TIP

Learning Needs Assessment

Assess the client's learning needs by answering the following:

- Is the client uncertain about an upcoming procedure?
- Does the client know about medications, purposes, and side effects?
- Can the client describe necessary lifestyle modifications?
- Is the client able to correctly perform treatment procedures (e.g., colostomy irrigations, injections, blood glucose monitoring)?

CULTURAL CONSIDERATIONS

Learning and Culture

- Culture plays an important role in knowledge acquisition.
- Attitudes, which are derived from a cultural context, toward what is appropriate to learn and who should teach may require alterations in the nurse's approach.
- Sensitivity to cultural values affects every aspect of the teaching–learning process.

Readiness to learn is influenced by the client's ability to learn, the client's comfort, and the client's motivation (or lack of) to learn.

Client Strengths and Limitations

Identification of the client's strengths and limitations is the foundation for realistic expectations. Understanding the client's strengths and limitations allows the nurse to plan successful teaching–learning experiences. Determining a client's strengths assists the nurse to select appropriate teaching methods. For example, a client who has limited vision should not be given pamphlets or other reading material in small print from which to learn the intended information.

Previous Experiences

The client's knowledge base acquired from life experiences affects the client's attitude about learning and perception of the importance of the information to be learned. A client who has had several experiences of hospitalization will have both a basis of knowledge and feelings (positive and negative) about those experiences. Current attitudes about this hospitalization will be influenced by prior hospital experiences.

Nursing Diagnosis

Several nursing diagnoses are pertinent to the learning process. When lack of knowledge is the primary learning need, the diagnosis of *Deficient Knowledge (specify)* is applicable. For example:

- A client who is to use crutches for assisted ambulation may have the diagnosis of *Deficient Knowledge: Crutchwalking,* R/T lack of exposure AEB many questions and hesitancy to walk.
- A client who must give self-insulin and will be discharged soon may have a diagnosis of *Deficient Knowledge: Insulin Injection,* R/T lack of exposure AEB many questions.

Deficient Knowledge may also be a component of many other nursing diagnoses that encompass risk or impaired ability. For instance, *Risk for Constipation* may relate to a client's compromised health status; this risk may be modified or reduced through certain dietary changes and client education. A client having a diagnosis of *Feeding Self-Care Deficit* may need both assistance in cutting the food and opening containers related to present physical ability.

Planning

Learning does not just happen by chance—it is planned. An important part of planning is goal setting. The client and family or significant others should be involved in setting goals. Specific learning goals should include the following elements:

- Measurable behavioral change
- Time frame
- Methods and intervals for evaluation

Teaching–learning goals must be realistic (i.e., based on the abilities of the learner and the teacher).

Establishing teaching–learning goals involves setting priorities. One way to set priorities with regard to goals is to teach "need-to-know" content (that which is necessary for survival) before moving on to "nice-to-know" content. For example, Mrs. Stone, who is in her first trimester of pregnancy, must be taught guidelines for diet and exercise ("need-to-know" content); information about infant care ("nice-to-know" content at this time) can be given later in the pregnancy.

Planning involves considering the following:

- Why teach?
- What should be taught?
- How should teaching be done?
- Who should teach and who should be taught?
- When should teaching occur?
- Where should teaching occur?

Why Teach?

Client need is *why* teaching is done. The client may realize the need for knowledge about a given subject and ask for information or ask questions about the subject. The nurse should recognize the client's need for knowledge even when the client does not recognize that need. For example, the nurse should recognize that a preoperative client needs to know how to do deep breathing exercises and leg exercises after surgery. The nurse should then plan teaching for that purpose.

What Should Be Taught?

Determination of *what* to teach is accomplished through comprehensive assessment. The content to be taught depends greatly on the client's knowledge base, current health status, and readiness to learn.

How Should Teaching Be Done?

Deciding *how* to teach involves deciding which teaching strategies are best for the content and the client's learning style and abilities. The effective teacher uses methods that capture the client's interest. Teaching methods are often influenced by the teaching location. For example, videos can often be used effectively in inpatient settings; however, the same information may need to be presented with flipcharts or brochures in the home setting.

Who Should Teach and Who Should Be Taught?

Planning includes deciding *who* will teach the client. The nurse is the coordinator of the health care team's teaching activities. Responsibility for a comprehensive teaching approach rests with the nurse. The teaching plan greatly affects continuity of care. The "who" part of planning also relates to who should be taught. The nurse must determine who in addition to the client (e.g., family members, significant others) must be taught.

When Should Teaching Occur?

When to teach should be carefully considered. The nurse should recognize that every interaction with the client is an opportunity for teaching. When a client asks a question, it is an opportunity for teaching. These opportunities for teaching must be used. A client's motivation to learn is quickly destroyed when comments such as "Ask your doctor that" or "We'll talk about that later. Right now, take your medicine" are made. The best time for teaching is when the client is comfortable—physically and psychologically.

Where Should Teaching Occur?

Where teaching occurs must also be well planned. The location of teaching affects the quality of learning. Some factors to be considered in determining the location of teaching include privacy and equipment availability.

Implementation

Katz (1997) suggests several strategies to achieve successful client teaching, as outlined in the following sections.

Get and Keep the Client's Attention

Begin a teaching session by telling the client what will be taught and why it is important to the client. The client's interest can be held by varying the tone of voice and using assorted teaching methods to present the material. Making the abstract concrete by using realistic examples from the client's experience also helps keep the client's attention.

PROFESSIONAL TIP

Guidelines for Effective Client Teaching

- Assess the client's needs and knowledge.
- Organize content from the simple to the complex, building on what the client already knows.
- Be creative.
- Ensure a comfortable environment.
- Maintain a flexible approach.
- Use a variety of teaching methods.
- Relate material to client's prior knowledge.
- Encourage the client's active participation.
- Reinforce learning frequently.
- Provide immediate feedback.
- Provide for immediate application of knowledge or skill.
- Emphasize oral instructions with the written word and pictures.
- Expect learning plateaus.

Stick to the Basics

Because the average adult can remember only five to seven points at a time, the nurse must be specific about what the client is to learn. Simple, everyday language should be used, and the most critical information should be presented first.

Use Time Wisely

The nurse can incorporate teaching into client care by providing information during each nurse–client interaction. Involving the client's family and friends, allowing them to discuss the material with the client, is also helpful. The nurse should consider supplementing teaching with written material for the client and/or family to read; this provides time for the learners to review the material and then ask questions to clarify understanding.

Reinforce Information

Repetition creates habits; the nurse can take advantage of this by reviewing the material with the client and serving as a role model. For example, when teaching a client a procedure, the nurse must be sure to do it correctly each time and to avoid taking shortcuts. The nurse can reward the client by giving positive reinforcement such as a smile, a nod, or a few words of praise.

PROFESSIONAL TIP

Evaluation of Learning

- Did the client meet the goals and objectives?
- Can the client demonstrate skills?
- Did the client's attitude change?
- Can the client cope better?
- Does the family understand how to help?

PROFESSIONAL TIP

Evaluation of Teacher Effectiveness

- Were learning objectives stated in behavioral terms (i.e., easy to evaluate)?
- Was content presented clearly and at the client's level of comprehension?
- Did the nurse show interest in the client and in the material?
- Were a variety of teaching aids used?
- Were the teaching aids appropriate for the client and the content?
- Was the client encouraged to participate?
- Did the nurse give frequent feedback and allow for immediate return demonstration?
- Was the nurse supportive?

Evaluation

Evaluation of teaching–learning is a twofold process:

1. Determining what the client has learned
2. Assessing the nurse's teaching effectiveness

Evaluation of Client's Learning

In performing the continual process of evaluating what the client has learned, the nurse must determine whether a behavior change has occurred, whether the behavior change is related to learning activities, whether further change is necessary, and whether continued behavior change will promote health. The following strategies can be used to evaluate client learning:

- Asking questions
- Observation
- Return demonstration
- Written follow-up (e.g., questionnaires)

Evaluation of Teaching Effectiveness

A major purpose of evaluation is to assess the effectiveness of the teaching activities and to decide which modifications, if any, are necessary. If learning objectives are not met, teaching–learning activities must be reassessed and modified. Goals that are measurable and specific facilitate evaluation. Evaluating teaching effectiveness can be accomplished through:

- Feedback from the learner
- Feedback from colleagues
- Self-evaluation

Summary

- The teaching–learning process is a planned interaction that promotes behavioral change that is not a result of maturation or coincidence.
- Learning is the process of assimilating information that results in behavioral change.
- Three domains of learning are the cognitive (intellectual), the affective (emotional), and the psychomotor (motor skills).
- Learning readiness is affected by developmental and sociocultural factors.
- Elements of documenting client education include the content taught, the teaching methods used, the person(s) taught, and the response of the learners.
- Evaluation of the teaching–learning process involves: determining what the client has learned and assessing teacher efficacy.

Review Questions

1. Bloom identified three areas wherein learning occurs: the psychomotor domain, the affective domain, and the:

    a. attitude domain.

    b. cognitive domain.

c. emotional domain.

d. knowledge domain.

2. A clinical example of psychomotor learning is when a client:

a. changes the dressing on a leg ulcer.

b. states an acceptance of a chronic illness.

c. states the name and purpose of a medication.

d. chooses to change the type of exercise performed.

3. It is important for the nurse to be aware that learning needs:

a. change daily.

b. are the same for everyone.

c. change throughout the life cycle.

d. change as teaching approaches are modified.

4. Nurses are required to provide teaching by:

a. all state nursing practice acts.

b. the National League for Nursing.

c. the American Hospital Association.

d. the Joint Commission for Accreditation of Healthcare Organizations.

5. Because age is not synonymous with developmental level, the nurse, when preparing to teach a client, must:

a. teach everyone the same way.

b. set the goals for the client.

c. observe the client's behavior.

d. ask the client about self-efficacy.

References/Suggested Readings

American Hospital Association. (1992). *A patient's bill of rights.* Chicago: Author.

Bandura, A. (1977). *Social learning theory.* Englewood Cliffs, NJ: Prentice Hall.

Beare, P. G., & Myers, J. L. (1998). *Principles and practice of adult health nursing* (3rd ed.). St. Louis, MO: Mosby.

Bloom, B. S. (1977). *Taxonomy of educational objectives: The classification of educational goals, handbook I: Cognitive domain.* New York: Longman.

Bruccoliere, T. (2000). How to make patient teaching stick. *RN, 63*(2), 34–38.

Doak, C. C., Doak, L. G., & Root, J. H. (1996). *Teaching patients with low literacy skills* (2nd ed.). Philadelphia: Lippincott Williams & Wilkins.

Duffy, B. (1997). Using creative teaching process with adult patients. *Home Healthcare Nurse, 15*(2), 102–108.

Edelman, C. L., & Mandle, C. L. (2002). *Health promotion throughout the lifespan* (5th ed.). St. Louis, MO: Mosby.

Freda, M. (1997). Don't give it away. *MCN—The American Journal of Maternal/Child Nursing, 22*(6), 330.

Joint Commission for Accreditation of Healthcare Organizations. (2002). *Accreditation manual.* Chicago: Author.

Jubeck, M. E. (1994). Teaching the elderly: A commonsense approach. *Nursing94, 24*(5), 70–71.

Katz, J. R. (1997). Back to basics: Providing effective patient teaching. *AJN, 97*(5), 33–36.

Knowles, M. S., Holton, E. F., & Swanson, R. A. (2000). *The adult learner* (5th ed.). Houston: Gulf.

Mayer, G. G., & Rushton, N. (2002). Writing easy-to-read teaching aids. *Nursing2002, 32*(3), 48–49.

Messner, R. L. (1997). Patient teaching tips from the horse's mouth. *RN, 60*(8), 29–31.

Meyers, D. (1998). *Client teaching guides for home health care* (2nd ed.). New York: Aspen.

Muma, R. D., Lyon, B. A., & Newman, T. A. (Eds.). (1996). *Patient education: A practical approach.* New York: McGraw-Hill.

Redman, B. K. (2001). *The practice of patient education* (9th ed.). St. Louis, MO: Mosby.

Ruholl, L. (2003). Tips for teaching the elderly. *RN, 66*(5), 48–52.

Seley, J. J. (1994). 10 strategies for successful patient teaching. *AJN, 94*(11), 63–65.

Sodeman, W. A. (1999). *Instructions for geriatric patients* (2nd ed.). Philadelphia: W. B. Saunders.

Weissman, M., & Jasovsky, D. (1998). Discharge teaching for today's times. *RN, 61*(6), 38–40.

Winslow, E. (2001). Patient education materials: Can patients read them, or are they ending up in the trash? *AJN, 101*(10), 33–38.

UNIT
4

Developmental and Psychosocial Concerns

LIFE CYCLE

MAKING THE CONNECTION

Refer to the following chapters to increase your understanding of the life cycle:

Basic Nursing
- **Communication**
- **Basic Nutrition**
- **Safety/Hygiene**

Adult Health Nursing
- **Sexually Transmitted Diseases**
- **Mental Illness**
- **The Older Adult**

Maternal & Pediatric Health Nursing
- **Prenatal Care**

LEARNING OBJECTIVES

Upon completion of this chapter, you should be able to:
- **Define key terms.**
- **Discuss the basic concepts and principles of growth and development.**
- **Identify the factors influencing growth and development.**
- **Compare the major developmental theories.**
- **Discuss the importance of growth and development as a holistic framework for assessing and promoting health.**
- **Describe the important milestones for each developmental period.**
- **Discuss the specific nursing interventions relevant to each developmental stage.**

KEY TERMS

accommodation	menarche
adaptation	middle adulthood
adolescence	moral maturity
assimilation	neonatal stage
bonding	older adulthood
critical period	preadolescence
development	prenatal stage
developmental task	preschool stage
embryonic phase	puberty
fetal phase	school-age stage
germinal phase	self-concept
growth	spirituality
infancy	teratogenic substance
learning	toddler stage
maturation	young adulthood

INTRODUCTION

Individuals constantly change from conception to death. Physical growth, emotional maturation, psychological, cognitive, and moral development, and spiritual growth occur throughout life. Progress through each developmental stage influences health status. Quality nursing practice depends on a thorough understanding of developmental concepts. This chapter presents the eleven life cycle stages.

BASIC CONCEPTS OF GROWTH AND DEVELOPMENT

Development occurs continuously through the life span. Adults continue to have transition periods during which growth and development occur.

Growth is the measurable changes in the physical size of the body and its parts. Examples of growth are the changes in height, weight, bone density, and dental structure. Growth patterns can be predicted even though growth is not a steady process. The rate varies from periods of rapid growth to periods of slower growth. Rapid growth is most common in the prenatal, infant, and adolescent stages.

Development is the behavioral changes in skills and functional abilities. Thus, developmental changes are not as easily measured. **Maturation,** the process of becoming fully grown and developed, applies to the individual's physiological and behavioral aspects. It depends on biological growth, behavioral changes, and **learning** (assimilation of information resulting in a behavior change). During each life cycle stage, certain goals **(developmental tasks)** must be accomplished. These developmental tasks are the foundation for future learning.

The time of most rapid growth or development in a stage of the life cycle is called the **critical period.** An individual is most vulnerable to stressors during a critical period.

Growth, development, maturation, and learning are interdependent processes. The individual must be mature enough to grasp the concepts and make required behavioral changes for learning to occur. Physical growth is essential for many types of learning; for example, a child must have the physical ability to reach the door knob before learning to open the door. Likewise, cognitive maturation precedes learning.

Principles of Growth and Development

Individual abilities and talents contribute to each person's development as a unique entity. *The exact rate of development for any given individual cannot be predicted.* There are a few general principles relating to growth and development of all humans (Table 10-1).

The sequence of development is predictable, but performance of specific skills varies with each person. For example, not all infants roll over at the same age, but most roll over before they crawl.

Factors That Influence Growth and Development

Many factors such as heredity, health status, life experiences, and culture influence growth and development. A person's choices about health behaviors are also determined by these factors.

Heredity

Genetic information is passed from parents to children. An individual's genetic makeup determines not only physical characteristics such as skin color, facial features, hair texture, and body structure, but also a predisposition to certain diseases (i.e., sickle cell anemia, Huntington's disease). Heredity is the genetic blueprint for an individual's growth and development. The role of heredity is complex and not yet fully understood.

Health Status

Individuals experiencing wellness progress through the life cycle as expected. Achievement of developmental milestones can be delayed by illness or disability. Individuals with a chronic condition may meet developmental milestones, but later.

Life Experiences

The rate of growth and development can be influenced by life experiences. For example, a child whose family has few resources for food, shelter, and health care has a higher risk of lagging in physical and mental

TABLE 10-1 PRINCIPLES OF GROWTH AND DEVELOPMENT	
PRINCIPLE	**EXAMPLE**
Growth and development are orderly and predictable, occurring from:	Everyone goes through the same processes.
• *cephalocaudal* (head to toe)	Head larger at birth in relation to body.
	Head controlled before crawling and sitting occurs before walking.
• *proximodistal* (functions near midline develop before those distant)	Arm movements controlled before finger movements.
• *general to specific*	Sounds and noises made before words are spoken. Walking occurs before hopping or skipping.
Rate of growth and development:	Rapid growth in infancy and adolescence.
• is not consistent	Slower growth in school age and young adulthood.
• is individual	Slower-growing child will be smaller than others of the same age.
Each stage has specific characteristics.	Infants depend on others for survival.
	Adolescents search for their own identity.
Certain tasks must be accomplished in each stage.	Infants must develop trust so as adolescents they can establish individual identity.
Some stages are more critical than others.	First few weeks of pregnancy are critical for embryonic development.

CRITICAL THINKING

Heredity or Life Experiences

What is most important in determining a person's behavior: the person's genetic predisposition or the response of other people and socialization?

CULTURAL CONSIDERATIONS

Growth and Development

The time for mastery of such developmental tasks as speaking and toilet training is as dependent on cultural norms as it is on physiological development.

growth and development than a child whose family has plenty of resources.

Culture

Individuals are expected to master certain skills at each developmental period, but the age for mastery is determined partly by culture. For instance, some cultures expect mate selection at age 12 or 13, with the birth of a child soon after.

DIMENSIONS AND THEORIES OF HUMAN DEVELOPMENT

Nurses need to thoroughly understand growth and development so they can provide individualized care. Remember, *chronological age and developmental age are not the same.* An overview of the dimensions and major theories of human development follows.

Physiological Dimension

The physiological dimension of growth and development consists of physical size and functioning of the individual. It is influenced by the interaction of genetic predisposition, nutrition, the central nervous system (CNS), and the endocrine system.

Psychosocial Dimension

Growth and development's psychosocial dimension consists of feelings and interpersonal relationships. A positive **self-concept** (perception of one's self, including body image, self-esteem, and ideal self) is an important part of a person's happiness and success. Characteristics of an individual with a positive self-concept include:

- Self-confidence
- Willing to take risks
- Able to accept criticism and not become defensive
- Able to adapt to stressors
- Has innovative problem-solving skills

People with a positive self-concept believe in themselves and set goals they can achieve. Achieving the goals reinforces their positive self-concept.

An individual with a negative or poor self-concept, on the other hand, is likely to have low self-esteem, a lack of confidence, and difficulty setting and achieving goals. A person with a positive self-concept is more likely to change unhealthy habits (such as smoking and sedentary lifestyle) to promote health than someone with a negative self-concept.

Various psychosocial theories have been put forth to explain the development of self-concept. A discussion of various theories of personality development follows.

Theorists

Two major theorists of personality development are Sigmund Freud and Erik Erikson. Freud's theory is called the psychosexual theory (Table 10-2). He identified sexuality (anything that gives bodily pleasure) as the underlying motivation for behavior. He believed that all behaviors have meaning and that repressed sexual problems in childhood cause problems later in life. Excessive gratification or excessive frustration at any stage, he thought, may cause a fixation (preoccupation with the pleasures of that stage).

Erikson (1968) theorized that psychosocial development proceeds throughout life. His theory is known as the psychosocial theory. Erikson believed that each stage has a task to be mastered. His eight developmental stages of life are described in Table 10-3.

The interpersonal theory focuses on a person's relationships with those around him. Harry Stack Sullivan (1953) theorized that relationships with others influence personality development. Approval and disapproval from significant others shapes an individual's personality. An individual must complete six stages of development in order to form satisfying relationships with others, as shown in Table 10-4.

TABLE 10-2	**FREUD: STAGES OF PSYCHOSEXUAL DEVELOPMENT**	
STAGE	**AGE**	**DESCRIPTION**
Oral	Birth–1 year	Explores and receives pleasure with mouth and tongue
Anal	1 year–3 years	Control of elimination muscles
Phallic (Oedipal)	3 years–6 years	Attracted to opposite-sex parent
Latency	6 years–12 years	Identifies with same sex parent
Genital	12 years–adulthood	Develops sexual relationships

Data from *Civilization and Its Discontents,* by S. Freud, 1961, New York: Norton. Copyright 1961 by Norton.

TABLE 10-3   ERIKSON: STAGES OF PSYCHOSOCIAL DEVELOPMENT

STAGE	AGE	TASK TO MASTER	HOW TO ASSIST
Trust vs. mistrust	Birth–1 year	Establish a sense of trust.	Give consistent, affectionate care. Deficient, inconsistent care prevents trust development.
Autonomy vs. shame and doubt	1 year–3 years	Do things for self.	Provide praise, support, and encouragement to increase independence.
Initiative vs. guilt	3 years–6 years	Initiate activities and moral responsibility.	Answer questions and encourage creative activities. Threatening punishment or labeling behavior as "bad" leads to guilt and fear of doing wrong.
Industry vs. inferiority	6 years–12 years	Develop scholastic and social skills and self-esteem.	Recognize the child's accomplishments. Unrealistic expectations or excessively harsh criticism results in feelings of inferiority.
Identity vs. role confusion	12 years–18 years	Seek sense of identity and values.	Help decision making. Encourage active participation in home events. Assist with planning for the future.
Intimacy vs. isolation	18 years–30 years	Develop intimate relationship and choose career.	Teach how to establish realistic goals. Avoid ridiculing romances or job choices.
Generativity vs. stagnation	30 years–65 years	Establish a family and become productive.	Provide emotional support. Recognize accomplishments and provide appropriate praise.
Integrity vs. despair	65+ years	Accept one's life.	Encourage person to reminisce. Review contributions made by the individual.

Data from *Childhood and Society,* by E. Erikson, 1968, New York: Norton. Copyright 1968 by Norton; *American Nursing Review of Psychiatric and Mental Health Nursing Certification,* by N. Randolph, 1998, Springhouse, PA: Springhouse. Copyright 1998 by Springhouse.

TABLE 10-4   SULLIVAN: INTERPERSONAL MODEL OF PERSONALITY DEVELOPMENT

STAGE	AGE	DESCRIPTION
Infancy	Birth–1 year	Learn to rely on caregivers to meet needs and desires.
Childhood	1 year–6 years	Begin learning to delay immediate need for gratification of needs and desires.
Juvenile	6 years–9 years	Form fulfilling peer relationships.
Preadolescence	9 years–12 years	Relate successfully to peers of the same gender.
Early adolescence	12 years–14 years	Learn to be independent and form relationships with members of the opposite sex.
Late adolescence	14 years–21 years	Establish an intimate, long-lasting relationship with someone of the opposite sex.

Data from *Interpersonal Theory of Psychiatry,* by H. S. Sullivan, 1953, New York: Norton. Copyright 1953 by Norton.

Cognitive Dimension

The way a person thinks and understands the world shapes that person's perception, memory, attitude, action, and judgment and is the basis of cognitive theory. It develops as an individual progresses through life. Cognition is an adaptive process. Intelligent beings are able to change behavior in response to the demands of an ever-changing environment.

Jean Piaget (1963) studied the differences in children's thinking patterns at various ages and how they used intelligence to answer questions and solve problems. He theorized that children learn to think by playing.

Piaget (1963) lists four stages of intellectual development: sensorimotor, preoperational, concrete operations, and formal operations. Table 10-5 describes these stages. Each stage is characterized by the ways that the child interprets and uses the environment. There is great variation in age for each phase; ages are approximate.

Individuals learn by interacting with the environment using three processes: assimilation, accommodation, and adaptation. **Assimilation** is the process of taking in new experiences or information. **Accommodation** allows for adjustment of thinking to take in new information and increase understanding. **Adaptation** is the change resulting from assimilation and accommodation.

Moral Dimension

The moral dimension is a person's value system, which helps one differentiate right and wrong. Closely

TABLE 10-5 PIAGET: STAGES OF COGNITIVE DEVELOPMENT

STAGE	AGE	DESCRIPTION
Sensorimotor	Birth–2 years	Sense of cause and effect develops Learning develops from touching, tasting, and feeling Learns body movement and acquires language
Preoperational	2 years–7 years	Interprets objects and events in relation to self Begins using representational thought (symbolism) Imagination flourishes and use of language increases
Concrete Operational	7 years–12 years	Engages in inductive reasoning and concrete problem-solving
Formal Operational	12+ years	Engages in abstract reasoning and analytical problem-solving

Data from *The Origins of Intelligence in Children,* by J. Piaget, 1963, New York: Norton. Copyright 1963 by Norton.

TABLE 10-6 KOHLBERG: STAGES OF MORAL DEVELOPMENT

LEVEL AND STAGE	DESCRIPTION
Level I: Preconventional (Birth–9 years) Stage 1: *punishment and obedience orientation* Stage 2: *instrumental-relativist orientation*	Authority figures are obeyed to avoid punishment Views misbehavior in terms of damage done A deed is perceived as "wrong" if one is punished; the activity is "right" if one is not punished "Right" is relative, follows rules when in own interest
Level II: Conventional (9 years–13 years) Stage 3: *interpersonal concordance* Stage 4: *law and order orientation*	Maintains cordial interpersonal relationships Seeks approval of others through actions Respects authority. Believes in rules Feels "duty bound" to uphold laws
Level III: Postconventional (13+ years) Stage 5: *social contract orientation* Stage 6: *universal ethics orientation*	Understands laws of greatest good for greatest number Upholds laws protecting universal rights Understands the principles of human rights and personal conscience

Data from *Recent Research in Moral Development,* by L. Kohlberg, 1977, New York: Holt, Rinehart, & Winston. Copyright 1977 by Holt, Rinehart, & Winston.

related to emotional and cognitive development is **moral maturity** (the ability to independently decide for oneself what is "right"). Lawrence Kohlberg (1977) described a framework for understanding how individuals decide on a moral code.

According to Kohlberg, there are six stages of moral development. Each stage is built on the previous stage and becomes the foundation for the next stage. Moral development evolves relative to cognitive development. Individuals who think at higher levels have the reasoning skills on which to base moral decisions. Table 10-6 provides an overview of Kohlberg's stages of moral development. Kohlberg indicates that individuals move through the six stages sequentially, but not everyone reaches stages five and six (Kohlberg, 1977).

Spiritual Dimension

The spiritual dimension is described as a sense of personal meaning. The term *spirit* is derived from the Latin word meaning breath, air, and wind. Thus, spirit refers to whatever gives life to a person. **Spirituality** refers to relationships with one's self, others, and divine source or a higher power. It does not refer to a specific religion. Spirituality is developed throughout life.

TABLE 10-7	FOWLER: STAGES OF FAITH	
STAGE	AGE	CHARACTERISTICS
Prestage: *undifferentiated faith*	Infant	Trust, hope, and love compete with environmental inconsistencies or threats of abandonment.
Stage 1: *intuitive-projective faith*	Toddler and preschooler	Has no understanding of spiritual concepts but imitates parents' behaviors and attitudes about religion and spirituality.
Stage 2: *mythical-literal faith*	School-age child	Accepts existence of a deity. Religious and moral beliefs are symbolized by stories. Accepts concept of reciprocal fairness.
Stage 3: *synthetic-conventional faith*	Adolescent	Questions values and religious beliefs while attempting to form own identity.
Stage 4: *individuative-reflective faith*	Late adolescent and young adult	Assumes responsibility for own attitudes and beliefs.
Stage 5: *conjunctive faith*	Adult	Integrates other perspectives about faith into own definition of truth.
Stage 6: *universalizing faith*	Adult	Makes concepts of love and justice tangible.

Data from *Stages of Faith: The Psychology of Human Development and the Quest for Meaning*, by J. W. Fowler, 1995, New York: Harper & Row. Copyright 1995 by Harper & Row; *Johnson's Psychiatric–Mental Health Nursing: Adaptation and Growth* (5th ed.), by W. Mohr & B. S. Johnson, 2002, Philadelphia: Lippincott Williams & Wilkins. Copyright 2002 by Lippincott Williams & Wilkins.

Figure 10-1 *Holistic Nature of Individuals*

tions must be appropriate to each client's stage of development. Nursing's holistic perspective recognizes that an individual's development progresses throughout life. Progress, or lack thereof, in one dimension affects the other dimensions of development. Figure 10-1 shows the holistic nature of individuals.

Knowledge of growth and development is useful as guidelines for assessment. When developmental milestones are not met, prompt identification and comprehensive intervention is essential. For example:

- The infant who does not roll over, sit, or walk at expected times
- The adolescent girl who has not experienced menarche by the expected time
- The adult who fails to adjust to physiological changes

LIFE CYCLE STAGES

Eleven developmental stages will be discussed: prenatal, neonatal, infancy, toddler, preschooler, school-age, preadolescent, adolescent, young adult, middle adult, and older adult. The indications of growth and development in the physiological, psychosocial, cognitive, moral, and spiritual dimensions are discussed for each stage, along with pertinent nursing implications.

Prenatal Stage

The **prenatal stage** (development beginning with conception and ending with birth) is a critical time in growth and development and consists of three phases: germinal, embryonic, and fetal. The **germinal phase** begins with conception and lasts approximately 10 to 14 days. Rapid cell division and implantation of the fertilized egg in the uterine wall delineates this stage. In this very early stage, the CNS is already forming.

The **embryonic phase** (weeks 2 to 8 after conception) is marked by rapid differentiation of cells, development of the body systems, and growth. In this period the

The work of Erikson, Piaget, and Kohlberg all influenced Fowler's theory of spiritual development. Fowler's theory has a prestage and six distinct stages of faith development (Fowler, 1995). The sequence of stages remains the same, although the age at which individuals experience each stage varies. Table 10-7 outlines Fowler's theory.

Some clients seem to be unaware of their spiritual natures. The understanding of a client's spirituality is basic to nursing. Caring for the whole person is the distinguishing characteristic of a holistic nurse.

HOLISTIC FRAMEWORK FOR NURSING

A basic concept of nursing is to provide care to the whole person. So it is essential for nurses to know growth and development concepts. Nursing intervenembryo is most vulnerable for a spontaneous abortion (i.e., miscarriage).

The **fetal phase** (the intrauterine developmental period from 8 weeks to birth) is characterized by rapid growth and differentiation of body systems and parts.

Significance for Nursing

Early prenatal care is essential for a positive pregnancy outcome, with physical examinations and screenings throughout pregnancy.

Enhancing Wellness The primary environment affecting prenatal growth and development is the uterus.

The mother must provide a sufficient supply of nutrients. Women who consume an insufficient amount of protein during pregnancy have a high rate of preterm and low birth weight infants. Teaching must emphasize that vitamin supplements are *not* substitutes for adequate food intake. Other ways to promote prenatal health include:

- Screening (blood pressure, urine glucose, and albumin)
- Teaching (e.g., nutrition, self-care)
- Assisting economically disadvantaged clients to obtain prenatal care

Safety Concerns Any substances consumed by the mother affect the fetus, whether they are wholesome nutrients or deadly toxins. Cigarette toxic substances, including nicotine, cross the placenta and interfere with oxygen transport to the fetus. These toxins may result in fetal death, premature birth, retarded growth, and learning difficulties.

Alcohol use during pregnancy can result in **fetal alcohol syndrome** (FAS), a condition wherein fetal development is impaired, resulting in physical and intellectual problems. Alcohol consumption is most dangerous during the first 3 months of pregnancy, when the embryo's brain and other vital organs are developing. The effects of alcohol on the fetus are permanent. Fetal alcohol syndrome is considered to be the leading cause of mental retardation among infants, and the incidence continues to increase (Hockenberry-Eaton, 2003).

 Safety: Use of Tobacco and Alcohol During Pregnancy
No cigarette smoking is advised during pregnancy. All pregnant women should abstain from drinking alcohol, because a "safe" amount of alcohol consumption has not been determined.

There are many other teratogenic substances in addition to nicotine and alcohol. A **teratogenic substance** is anything that crosses the placenta and impairs normal growth and development. The Food and Drug Administration (FDA) requires that all manufactured drugs list the potential for causing birth defects. Illegal drug use by pregnant women is a very serious threat to the unborn.

Neonatal Stage

The **neonatal stage** (the first 28 days of life following birth) is a time of major adjustment to extrauterine life. The neonate (newborn) focuses energy on achieving equilibrium by stabilizing major body systems. Table 10-8 outlines neonatal development.

The neonate's activities are reflexive, consisting mainly of sucking, crying, eliminating, and sleeping. Reflexes play a major role in the neonate's ability to survive. The neonate progresses developmentally from a mass of reflexes to behavior that is more purposeful.

Adjusting to the parental figure(s) is the major psychological task of neonates. **Bonding,** the attachment between parent and child, begins when the parent and neonate make initial eye contact. Parent–neonate bonding is the foundation for trust necessary when developing future interpersonal relationships.

Significance for Nursing

A thorough assessment of the neonate is performed immediately after delivery. The neonate's reflexes should be evaluated at the same time or when the neonate is physiologically stable.

Soon after birth encourage the parents to cuddle the newborn, explain the neonate's interactive abilities, and encourage mutual eye contact between neonate and parents by showing parents how to hold the child in a position facing them.

Enhancing Wellness The most important nursing activity in promoting neonatal wellness is teaching. Other nursing interventions enhancing neonatal wellness are:

- Continually assess physiological status.
- Provide a warm environment.
- Monitor nutritional status.
- Provide a clean environment; teach parents that neonates need a clean environment, not a sterile one.
- Conduct screening tests; for example, the blood test for phenylketonuria (PKU).
- Promote *early* parent–neonate interaction.

Safety Concerns Because neonates depend totally on others to meet their needs, safety is a primary concern. Accidents are the primary cause of neonatal mortality (Fuller & Schaller-Ayers, 2000). One important method to prevent neonatal accident is to teach parents about using infant car seats. Under current federal law, neonates and infants must be secured in an approved infant car seat each time the child travels in a motor vehicle.

 Safety: Car Seats
A neonate should never be sent home from the hospital in a car unless an infant seat is available for the trip.

Infections are also a serious health risk to the neonate. Newborns should not be near anyone who has

CLIENT TEACHING

Pregnancy and Medications

Pregnant women should check labels of *all* medicines, especially over-the-counter, about potential effects on the fetus. Expectant mothers should question their practitioner about the safety of any drug taken during pregnancy.

TABLE 10-8   NEONATAL STAGE: GROWTH AND DEVELOPMENT

DIMENSION	CHARACTERISTICS	NURSING CONSIDERATIONS
Physiological	Heart takes over circulatory function from umbilical cord.	Accurately assess neonate's cardiovascular status.
	Gas exchange shifts from placenta to lungs.	Immediately after birth, hold the neonate's head lower than body to allow fluids that may block respiratory passages to drain.
	Respiratory reflexes are activated within seconds of birth.	Resuscitate immediately if spontaneous respirations do not occur.
	Neck and shoulder muscles are weak.	Support the neonate's head.
	Temperature-regulating mechanism is immature.	To conserve heat: • Dry neonate immediately after birth and place in a warmed bassinet and • Place a stockinette cap on neonate's head.
	Ossification (process of cartilage changing to bone) is incomplete.	Protect the anterior fontanel on neonate's skull.
	Visual acuity is poor, and visual focus is generally rigid.	Teach parents to be directly in front of the neonate (about 9–12 inches from child's face) when communicating.
Motor	Reflexes direct the majority of movement.	Teach parents to recognize neonate's protective reflexes.
	The full-term neonate has some limited ability to hold the head erect and is able to lift the head slightly when lying prone.	Support neonate's neck and head when lifting.
Psychosocial	Crying is the neonate's way of communicating. There is a reason for crying.	Teach parents about the dynamics of crying so that they neither label the neonate as "fussy" nor develop the misconception that they are inadequate caregivers.
	The bonding process begins shortly after birth.	Encourage parents to distinguish the various cries. Encourage parents to interact with the neonate during every contact (feeding, bathing, changing, cuddling).
Cognitive	Neonates learn through sensory experiences. Learning is enhanced in an environment providing stimuli without bombarding the neonate. Learning occurs by repeated exposure to stimuli.	Encourage parents to provide frequent sensory stimuli (touching, talking, looking the neonate in the eyes).

Data from *Health Assessment: A Nursing Approach* (3rd ed.), by J. Fuller and J. Schaller-Ayers, 2000, Philadelphia: Lippincott Williams & Wilkins. Copyright 2000 by Lippincott Williams & Wilkins; *Health Promotion Strategies through the Life Span* (7th ed.), by R. B. Murray and J. P. Zentner, 2001, Upper Saddle River, NJ: Prentice Hall. Copyright 2001 by Prentice Hall; *Whaley & Wong's Nursing Care of Infants and Children* (7th ed.), by M. Hockenberry-Eaton, 2003, St. Louis, MO: Mosby–Yearbook. Copyright 2003 by Mosby–Yearbook.

CLIENT TEACHING

Parents and Newborn

Parents need information about:

- Basic newborn needs
- Nutrition
- Infection control (especially hand hygiene and hygienic diaper changing practices)
- Care of the umbilicus
- Incorporating the newborn into the family unit
- Growth and development milestones in order to provide appropriate stimulation and have realistic expectations for their newborn

an infectious disease. It is essential that the neonate's skin integrity be maintained. Teach parents the importance of skin cleanliness. Diaper rash, a common skin problem for newborns and infants, is caused by the ammonia found in urine, which can burn and irritate the skin. In addition to changing wet diapers promptly, bathing and protective creams may be useful in preventing skin breakdown.

Infancy Stage

Infancy (development from the end of the first month to the end of the first year of life) is a period of continued adaptation, with rapid physiological growth and psychosocial development (Figure 10-2). Table 10-9 provides an overview of infant development.

Choice of Infant Feeding Method
There are some cultural sanctions against breastfeeding, and some cultures view bottle-feeding as a status symbol. Be sensitive to the client's cultural background and norms when discussing infant feeding.

Significance for Nursing

The nurse providing care to an infant must focus on safety, prevention of infection, and teaching parents about incorporating the child into the family. It is essential for parents and other caregivers to know the developmental milestones. Nursing care involves providing information, support, and reassurance to the parents.

Enhancing Wellness Nurses enhance infant wellness by teaching growth and development concepts to parents. Knowing the behavior to expect at certain ages both guides and reassures parents. Parents often need guidance about nutrition, protection from infection, and promotion of sleep.

An important factor enhancing infant wellness is providing adequate nutrients in a loving, consistent manner. Special formulas are available for infants who have PKU, are hypersensitive to protein, or experience fat malabsorption. Soy-based formulas are available for the infant who is lactose intolerant or allergic to regular formula. Infants who are formula fed usually have more subcutaneous fat. Whole cow's milk is not recommended for infants younger than 1 year of age. Human milk and commercially prepared formula are more easily digested.

Solid foods are usually introduced at 3 to 4 months of age. Rice cereal is the first solid food of choice because it causes the fewest allergic responses.

Infants are especially vulnerable to infections because the immune system is not fully matured.

 Infection Control: Hand Hygiene and Infant Care
Hand hygiene is most important to prevent the transmission of microorganisms. This is especially true when caring for infants, whose immune systems are still immature.

Immunizations are most important for infants. Nurses should advocate the administration of all recommended immunizations, which now include PCV to prevent invasive pneumococcal infections (Simmerman & Mauzy, 2001), and should confirm those received by the infant. Refer to the appendices for a recommended schedule for immunizations.

Information about normal sleep patterns of infants and how those patterns change with maturation is often needed by parents. To promote sleep, parents should:

• Provide a quiet room for the infant.

Figure 10-2 *This infant is exploring his world and is developing in both the physiological and cognitive dimensions.*

CLIENT TEACHING

Bottle-Feeding

• Assume a comfortable position and place the baby in a semireclining position, cradled close to your body.
• Never prop a bottle; choking may result.
• Use care if heating bottles. Do not warm bottles in the microwave; the hot liquid may burn the mouth and throat.
• Avoid using the bottle as a pacifier; this may result in tooth decay and may set the stage for overeating in the future.

CLIENT TEACHING

Preventing Infant Accidents

• To prevent vehicular accidents: Use infant seats and keep infants out of the paths of automobiles and other vehicles.
• To prevent burns: Keep infants away from open heaters, fireplaces, hot stoves, and matches.
• To protect from falls: Keep crib rails up at all times, never leave the infant lying unattended on furniture, and use protective gates and barriers to block stairways.
• To prevent drowning: Never leave the infant unattended near water (buckets, bathtubs, swimming pools).
• To prevent electrocution: Keep electrical cords out of the infant's reach and use plastic safety plugs to cover all electrical outlets.
• To prevent choking: Closely monitor the infant exploring the environment. During this oral phase, the infant tests out the environment and seeks pleasure through the mouth. Aspiration accidents are common, with infants choking on objects such as buttons and coins.

TABLE 10-9   INFANCY STAGE: GROWTH AND DEVELOPMENT

DIMENSION	CHARACTERISTICS	NURSING CONSIDERATIONS
Physiological	Physical growth is rapid. Birth weight usually triples by age 1 and length increases approximately 9 inches.	Advise parents of the developmental norms.
	All body systems move toward maturation.	Encourage parents to have recommended "well-baby" checkups.
	Teeth eruption begins at 4–6 months.	
	Brain grows rapidly (reaching approximately half the adult size).	
	Eyes begin to focus.	Provide visual stimulation.
Motor	Physical maturation allows for development of motor skills.	Teach parents anticipated ages for various motor skills to develop.
	Primitive reflexes are replaced by movement that is more voluntary and goal directed.	
	Motor skills develop rapidly:	
	• 6 months: rolls over voluntarily	
	• 8–10 months: crawls	
	• 8 months: sits alone	
	Grasping of objects, reflexive for the first 2–3 months, gradually becomes voluntary.	
Psychosocial	*Freud:* oral stage	Encourage parents to provide toys and objects for sucking and teething.
	Seeks immediate gratification of needs.	
	Receives pleasure and comfort through mouth, lips, and tongue.	
	Erikson: trust vs. mistrust stage	Encourage parents to feed promptly and consistently (feed on demand rather than a fixed schedule).
	A sense of self begins to develop.	
	Responds to caregiver's voice.	Promote trust by providing warmth, diapering, and comforting.
	Separation anxiety develops at approximately 6 months.	
Cognitive	*Piaget:* sensorimotor stage	Encourage parents to provide a variety of sensory stimuli: visual, sensory, auditory, and tactile (e.g., colorful mobiles; musical toys; soft, plush animals; rubbing, patting, and stroking of the infant's skin).
	Infant learns by interacting with the environment.	
	Language development includes babbling, repetition, and imitation.	Encourage caregivers to talk to the infant and to name objects that are the focus of the infant's attention.
	8–10 months says "mama" and "dada"	
Moral	*Kohlberg:* preconventional stage	Parents should start teaching (by role modeling) the difference between "right" and "wrong."
Spiritual	*Fowler:* stage of undifferentiated faith	Encourage caregivers to model the values they want the infant to learn.

Data from *Health Promotion Strategies through the Life Span* (7th ed.), by R. B. Murray and J. P. Zentner, 2001, Upper Saddle River, NJ: Prentice Hall. Copyright 2001 by Prentice Hall; *Whaley & Wong's Nursing Care of Infants and Children* (7th ed.), by M. Hockenberry-Eaton, 2003, St. Louis, MO: Mosby–Yearbook. Copyright 2003 by Mosby–Yearbook.

- Schedule feedings and other care activities during periods of wakefulness rather than drowsiness.
- Develop awareness to the unique sleep and rest periods of the infant.
- Provide comfort and security measures (e.g., rocking, singing).
- Establish routine times for sleep.

Safety Concerns Most infant injuries and deaths are related to motor vehicle accidents. The consistent and proper use of infant car seats is one of the most effective measures to ensure the infant's safety.

 Safety: Aiding a Choking Infant
Never use the Heimlich maneuver on a choking infant. Instead, use alternating back blows and chest compressions to dislodge the object.

Toddler Stage

The **toddler stage** begins at 12 to 18 months of age, when a child begins to walk alone, and ends at approximately 3 years of age. The family promotes language development and teaches toileting skills. The child becomes more independent, and temper tantrums often result when attempts at autonomy are prevented. This stage is often called "the terrible twos." The toddler's frequent use of the word *no* is an expression of developing autonomy.

Nurses greatly influence the quality of parent–child interaction when teaching parents developmental concepts. This information helps parents have realistic expectations of the toddler's behavior. Using firm limits consistently applied helps the toddler learn and provides parameters for safe, socially acceptable behavior. Table 10-10 outlines the toddler's growth and development.

Significance for Nursing

Nurses working with toddlers must be sensitive that children this age are often anxious and fearful in the presence of strangers. Establishing rapport by playing with the child helps alleviate stranger anxiety.

Fear and anxiety can make a hospital experience a negative one. The major stressor is separation from the parents. The unfamiliar environment is also a stressor for the toddler. Nurses can help reduce stress by teaching

Figure 10-3   *This toddler is learning the importance of washing his hands.*

both the child and parents about procedures. Anxiety is lessened through play.

Regular health examinations and immunizations are an essential part of health care for toddlers. Involve parents during examinations and immunizations. They can alleviate the toddler's stress by holding the child and talking calmly when the health care provider is present.

Enhancing Wellness Teaching involves both toddlers and their parents. Use play to establish an effective relationship with the child. Play is a valuable process for toddlers because it is the primary way they learn and socialize. When teaching, the nurse should be at the toddler's eye level and use words she can understand.

Respiratory infections are common health problems for toddlers. Parasitic diseases are also fairly common. Teach parents about preventive measures such as frequent handwashing with antibacterial soaps as in Figure 10-3. The nurse should also verify which immunizations are needed.

As the rate of growth slows, nutritional needs change. Toddlers need fewer calories than do infants. The required amounts of protein and fluids (Hockenberry-Eaton, 2003) also decrease. Most toddlers become picky about the foods they will eat, so it

---

PROFESSIONAL TIP

Health Care for Toddlers

- Explain what is being done in a calm voice.
- Alleviate anxiety with play (e.g., demonstrate a procedure on a doll or teddy bear; allow the child to handle equipment, such as a stethoscope, before using it on the child).
- Provide simple, short directions.
- Comfort the child after a painful procedure.
- Encourage active participation of parents.

TABLE 10-10 TODDLER STAGE: GROWTH AND DEVELOPMENT

DIMENSION	CHARACTERISTICS	NURSING CONSIDERATIONS
Physiological	Overall rate of growth slows. By 24 months of age, weight is usually four times that at birth. Brain grows rapidly. Bones in extremities grow in length. Physiological readiness for bowel and bladder control develops.	Instruct parents on need for vitamin D, calcium, and phosphorus. Explain timing for toilet training and need for consistency and patience.
Motor	Learns to walk, run, climb stairs, jump, ride a tricycle and throw a ball.	Have parents assess home environment for safety.
Psychosocial	*Freud:* anal stage Receives pleasure from contraction and relaxation of sphincter muscles. *Erikson:* autonomy vs. shame and doubt stage	Have parents avoid overemphasis on toilet training. Teach parents to encourage toddler's attempts at independence (e.g., trying to feed and dress self).
Cognitive	*Piaget:* preoperational stage Can follow simple directions. Thought processes are concrete. Able to anticipate future events. Child has short attention span. Child comprehends self as a separate entity. *Language:* At approximately 1 year of age, the child can make two-syllable sounds (e.g., ma-ma, da-da) By age 3, the child can form short sentences and has a vocabulary of approximately 900 words.	Instruct parents to give only one direction at a time. Use a calendar to show today's date and the number of days until a significant event. Teach caregivers importance of calling child by name. Have caregivers talk to child frequently but avoid "baby talk."
Moral	*Kohlberg:* preconventional stage Child learns to distinguish right from wrong.	Parents should be consistent in setting limits. Emphasize the significance of modeling desired behavior to the child.
Spiritual	*Fowler:* intuitive-projective stage of faith	Instruct parents to provide simple answers to questions related to religion, God, and church. Instruct on the importance of incorporating religious rituals and ceremonies into daily life.

Data from *Health Promotion Strategies through the Life Span* (7th ed.), by R. B. Murray and J. P. Zentner, 2001, Upper Saddle River, NJ: Prentice Hall. Copyright 2001 by Prentice Hall; *Whaley & Wong's Nursing Care of Infants and Children* (7th ed.), by M. Hockenberry-Eaton, 2003, St. Louis, MO: Mosby–Yearbook. Copyright 2003 by Mosby–Yearbook.

may be difficult to provide enough calcium and iron. Toddlers should consume an average of 2 to 3 cups of milk per day to ensure adequate calcium intake. Drinking more than a quart of milk per day increases the risk of developing anemia, because the child will be "full" and may not eat other foods (Hockenberry-Eaton, 2003). Nurses can play a key role in nutritional counseling for toddlers.

Safety Concerns Accidents (especially those involving automobiles) are the most frequent cause of disability and death among toddlers (Edelman & Mandle, 2002). The information regarding use of car seats for neonates and infants also applies to toddlers.

Another common type of accident among toddlers involves toys. As children gain new skills (Figure 10-4),

parents must reassess the safety of toys and the environments where the toddler might play.

 Safety: Toys for Toddlers
Parents should check toys for:
- Age appropriateness
- Sharp pieces or corners
- Small parts that can be swallowed
- Poisonous paint (e.g., lead-based paint)
- Flammable or toxic materials
- Manner in which toys are used

With their increased mobility and curiosity, toddlers are especially prone to accidental poisoning (Figure 10-5). Parents should thus child-proof the home and carefully observe the toddler.

CLIENT TEACHING

Toddler Nutrition

- Avoid using food as a reward because doing so encourages overeating.
- Do not serve large helpings; it may overwhelm the child, possibly resulting in a refusal to eat.
- Expect sporadic eating patterns (eating a lot one day and very little the next, or enjoying one food for several days and then suddenly refusing to eat that food).
- Avoid power struggles related to meals. It is counterproductive to establishing healthy eating habits to force a child to eat.
- Establish a mealtime routine and follow it; toddlers like rituals.
- Provide nutritional snacks to meet dietary requirements.

CRITICAL THINKING

Male/Female Stereotypes

Our society labels certain characteristics as "masculine" or "feminine." How do you think these stereotypes influence the development of young boys and girls in our society?

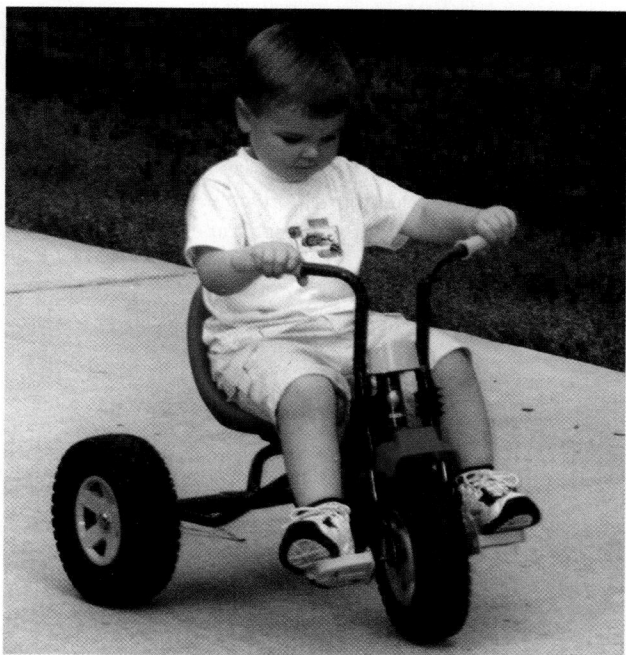

Figure 10-4 *This toddler's gross motor development had progressed so he can learn the new skill of riding his tricycle. Parents must be aware of safety hazards and provide a helmet for this child.*

Preschool Stage

Development from ages 3 to 6 years is called the **preschool stage.** During this stage, physical growth slows, and psychosocial and cognitive development accelerate. Table 10-11 outlines preschool development in detail.

During this period, curiosity increases, and the child is better able to communicate. Parents should be taught that the child's frequent use of the word *why* is necessary for normal psychosocial and cognitive development.

The child's world continues to expand outside the immediate home environment. The preschooler uses play to both learn about and develop relationships.

Significance for Nursing

Play is a tool that can be used by nurses to help reduce fear and anxiety in the preschooler. Play helps preschoolers reduce tension, learn about the environment, and incorporate socially defined expectations for behavior (Figure 10-6).

Enhancing Wellness It is important to communicate at the child's level of comprehension yet not talk down to the child. Include the child in decisions and activities as much as possible. During the preschool years, the child begins showing an interest in health. To promote the development of lifelong health-promoting lifestyles, the astute nurse capitalizes on this by making health education fun. Immunizations are major wellness intervention for preschoolers. At

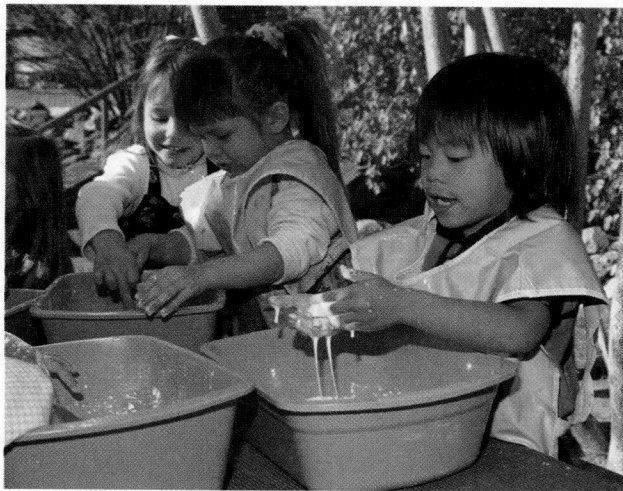

Figure 10-5 *Parents must ensure that all materials a child plays with are safe, nontoxic, and nonflammable.*

each checkup the nurse should verify that immunizations are up to date.

Safety Concerns Accidents are the leading cause of death among young children. Cognitive immaturity coupled with an eagerness to explore the environment lead to the preschooler's risk for accidents. Parents must understand the importance of teaching young children the meaning of the word *no.*

Common accidents among preschoolers include automobile accidents, falls, burns, animal bites, drowning, and ingestion of poisonous substances.

TABLE 10-11   PRESCHOOLER STAGE: GROWTH AND DEVELOPMENT

DIMENSION	CHARACTERISTICS	NURSING CONSIDERATIONS
Physiological	Physical growth slows; average weight at age 5 years is 45 pounds. Head size approximates that of an adult. Deciduous teeth come in fully; these "baby teeth" start to fall out about age 6 and will be replaced by permanent teeth.	Eats a variety of foods and larger meals.
Motor	Fine motor skills develop (e.g., can skip, throw a ball overhand, use scissors, tie shoelaces).	Emphasize providing a safe environment for play and exploration. Praise attempted independent activities.
Psychosocial	*Freud:* phallic stage Oedipal conflict leads to development of superego (conscience). *Erikson:* initiative vs. guilt stage	Self-control is learned by interacting with others.
Cognitive	*Piaget:* preoperational stage Vocabulary over 2,000 words. Play more reality based. Increased ability to communicate, increases socialization with peers.	Tell parents that children of this age learn through frequent use of the word *why.*
Moral	*Kohlberg:* preconventional stage A conscience begins to develop. Fears wrongdoing, and seeks parental approval.	Encourage parents to teach the child basic values, ideally by modeling. Encourage parents to provide consistent praise and acceptance of child.
Spiritual	*Fowler:* intuitive-projective stage of faith Not yet able to understand spiritual concepts but imitates parent's behaviors.	Teaching by example is the best approach for a child of this age.

Data from *Health Promotion Strategies through the Life Span* (7th ed.), by R. B. Murray and J. P. Zentner, 2001, Upper Saddle River, NJ: Prentice Hall. Copyright 2001 by Prentice Hall; *Whaley & Wong's Nursing Care of Infants and Children* (7th ed.), by M. Hockenberry-Eaton, 2003, St. Louis, MO: Mosby–Yearbook. Copyright 2003 by Mosby–Yearbook.

Figure 10-6 *Play is an important vehicle for socialization among preschoolers.*

CLIENT TEACHING

Promoting Wellness

- Encourage healthy lifestyles (nonsedentary activities, nutritious meals).
- Teach children appropriate hygienic measures.
- Schedule regular checkups.
- Keep immunizations up to date.
- Schedule dental checkups and encourage daily brushing and flossing.
- Teach safety precautions.
- Establish sleep patterns.
- Report any symptoms of illness to the health care provider.

TABLE 10-12 SCHOOL-AGE STAGE: GROWTH AND DEVELOPMENT

DIMENSION	CHARACTERISTICS	NURSING CONSIDERATIONS
Physiological	Steady physical growth (approximately 3–6 pounds and 2–3 inches per year). Body has an overall slimmer shape. CNS maturation is nearly complete. By age 12, all permanent teeth (except second and third molars) are present.	Emphasize to parents the need for a balanced diet to sustain growth requirements. Need daily dental hygiene (brushing and flossing) and regularly scheduled visits to the dentist. Change toothbrush every 3 months.
Motor	Motor control continues to develop. Less dependent on parents for activities of daily living.	Encourage participation in physical activities. Praise independent activities.
Psychosocial	*Freud:* latency stage Same-gender companions are preferred. *Erikson:* industry vs. inferiority stage Develops initiative and high self-esteem as manifested in school and sports. Less dependent on family.	To develop a sense of confidence, encourage child to: • Participate in group and individual activities Encourage parents to praise child's efforts.
Cognitive	*Piaget:* concrete operations stage Ability to cooperate with others and to see other points of view leads to more meaningful communication. Reasoning now logical and rational. Abstract thinking is not fully developed. The concept of time develops • Knows difference between past and present • Begins to learn to tell time Able to categorize, classify and order objects. Relationships between objects seen.	Encourage group activities. Remember child's level of comprehension.
Moral	*Kohlberg:* conventional stage Understands what is unacceptable behavior but may need assistance to choose between right and wrong.	Encourage parents to provide consistent limits. Emphasize modeling appropriate behavior. Praise appropriate behavior.
Spiritual	*Fowler:* mythical-literal stage Accepts deity existence. Beliefs are symbolized through stories.	Encourage parents to discuss their beliefs. Stories reinforce understanding of spiritual concepts.

Data from *Health Promotion Strategies through the Life Span* (7th ed.), by R. B. Murray and J. P. Zentner, 2001, Upper Saddle River, NJ: Prentice Hall. Copyright 2001 by Prentice Hall; *Health Promotion throughout the Lifespan* (5th ed.), by C. L. Edelman and C. L. Mandle, 2002, St. Louis, MO: Mosby–Yearbook. Copyright 2002 by Mosby–Yearbook.

The nurse should emphasize parental education about protecting preschoolers from potential hazards. The safety practices learned as a preschooler will be lifelong. Accident prevention can be best taught through modeling. Parents who always buckle their seatbelts in a car protect themselves and teach their children an important accident prevention measure.

School-Age Stage

During the **school-age stage** (development from the ages of 6 to 10 years), physical changes are slow, even, and continuous. Table 10-12 gives an overview of growth and development of the school-age child.

The world of a school-age child expands greatly. Participating in school activities, team sports, and play enlarges their social network. As they mature, play becomes more structured and less spontaneous. Communication increases, and an expanded vocabulary allows the expression of thoughts, needs, and feelings.

The school-age child's cognitive abilities expand, and academic, sporting, and social activities stimulate creativity.

Figure 10-7 *This school-age child has learned that safety equipment such as helmets, elbow pads, and knee pads helps protect her from injury.*

Significance for Nursing

Common health problems among school-age children are minor illnesses such as upper respiratory infections and accidents. Teaching health promotion is a major role when caring for school-age children.

Enhancing Wellness Nurses can promote healthy lifestyles among children in schools. This is a cost-effective way to teach wellness behaviors.

Safety Concerns School-age children often experience accidents during play. Common injuries relate to the use of skates, skateboards, and bicycles.

Safety: Accidents and Abductions
- Children must learn safety rules for riding toys (e.g., use of protective equipment, see Figure 10-7).
- Parents must frequently remind children of the danger of playing near traffic.
- Teach children to use caution with strangers because of the possibility of abduction.

Preadolescent Stage

Preadolescence (development from the ages of 10 to 12 years) is marked by rapid physiological changes having psychological and social implications. The child begins to experience hormonal changes that will result in the onset of **puberty** (the emergence of secondary sex characteristics). Girls generally experience puberty at a younger age than do boys—approximately 9 to 10 years of age, as compared to 10 to 11 years of age for boys (Edelman & Mandle, 2002). Table 10-13 provides an overview of preadolescent development.

In girls, breast development begins between the ages of 10 and 11. The release of estrogen during puberty stimulates further breast development. **Menarche** (onset of the first menstrual period) occurs about 2 years after breast buds appear. The first menstrual periods are usually scant, irregular, and ovulation may or may not

occur. The average age of menarche has declined over the past century in the United States and is now 12.8 years. This decline is probably caused by improved general health status (Hockenberry-Eaton, 2003).

The menstrual cycle has physiological and psychological changes occurring monthly. A girl's cycle usually is established in a regular pattern after the first 6 to 12 months. Nurses must remember that some girls may receive incorrect or inadequate information regarding menstruation. Client teaching should emphasize the physiological changes, emotional changes, and personal hygiene.

In preadolescent boys, the first signs of puberty are:

- Testicles enlarge
- Penis enlarges
- Scrotum becomes redder and thins
- Pubic hair grows

Significance for Nursing

Sensitivity is essential in working with the preadolescent. To increase sensitivity, the nurse should use a nonjudgmental approach and attend to the preadolescent's body language.

Enhancing Wellness Information about nutrition, activity and rest, and physiological changes is needed by the preadolescent. This client should be taught about the dramatic growth spurt, the sexual changes, and the psychosocial changes that characterize this life stage (Figure 10-8). Preparing the preadolescent for upcoming changes promotes physical and emotional health. Confirm that immunizations are current.

Safety Concerns The preadolescent is at risk for injury during play and sports activities.

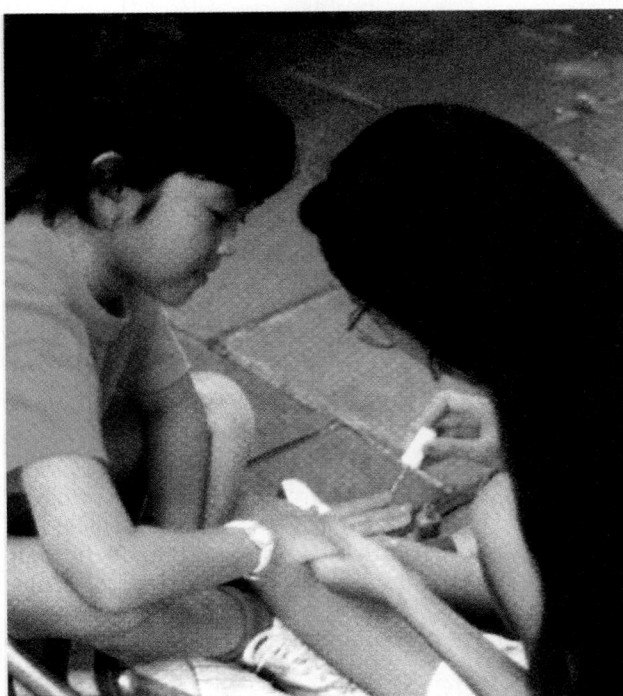

Figure 10-8 *Preadolescence is a time of gender role discovery and increasing independence.*

TABLE 10-13 PREADOLESCENT AND ADOLESCENT STAGE: GROWTH AND DEVELOPMENT

DIMENSION	CHARACTERISTICS	NURSING CONSIDERATIONS
Physiological	*Physiological changes:* Physical growth accelerates and is accompanied by changes in body proportion. Extremities grow first, then trunk and hips. *Endocrine changes:* Hypothalamus stimulates pituitary to secrete gonadotropins, causing reproductive maturity. Primary and secondary sex characteristics develop. Beginning of puberty is evidenced in girls by: • Breasts develop, • Pubic and axillary hair grows, • Menarche (onset of menses), and • Height increases. Beginning of puberty is evidenced in boys by: • Genitals develop, • Facial, pubic, and axillary hair grows, • Ejaculations occur at night, • Height increases, and • Voice deepens *Musculoskeletal changes:* Bones ossify. Muscle mass and strength increase. *Dental changes:* Last four molars erupt. *Integumentary changes:* Skin becomes thicker and tougher. Activation of sebaceous glands may lead to acne. Pubic hair appears.	Teach child and parents to expect growth spurts. Provide information and support about sexual changes. Encourage physical activities and adequate intake of calcium. Continue daily dental hygiene. Encourage sunscreen use and to avoid prolonged sunlight exposure. Support preadolescent experiencing acne.
Motor	Completely independent in performing self-care activities.	Encourage parents to allow some freedom of expression and choice.
Psychosocial	*Freud:* genital stage *Erikson:* identity vs. role diffusion stage The major task is to develop a sense of identity. A new body image develops. Intimacy with members of opposite gender is established. Primary support is the peer group. Often rebels against adult authority.	Provide sex education. Advise parents that rebellion is a normal developmental experience.
Cognitive	*Piaget:* formal operations stage Approach to thinking is logical, organized, and consistent. Most adolescents think in terms of cause and effect. Sees self as exceptional, special, and unique, and views self as being immune to problems. Tends to be extremely idealistic. Egocentric (self-centered) thinking is common, as is a view of self as omnipotent.	False sense of immunity ("It can't happen to me" attitude) has an impact on health behaviors. Advise about safe: • Sex practices • Driving practices (no driving with alcohol use) *continues*

TABLE 10-13 continued

DIMENSION	CHARACTERISTICS	NURSING CONSIDERATIONS
Moral	*Kohlberg:* postconventional stage The adolescent tends to support the morality of law and order in determining right from wrong. Adolescents begin to question and discard the status quo and to choose different values. Moral maturity depends on the context of the situation and the relationship. Own moral reasoning may be overcome by peer pressure.	Teach parents that questioning of values is normal. Teach assertiveness skills preadolescent can use when communicating with peers.
Spiritual	*Fowler:* synthetic-conventional stage The adolescent questions values and beliefs.	Curiosity about other religious beliefs is normal.

Data from *Health Promotion throughout the Lifespan* (5th ed.), by C. L. Edelman and C. L. Mandle, 2002, St. Louis, MO: Mosby–Yearbook. Copyright 2002 by Mosby–Yearbook; *American Nursing Review of Psychiatric and Mental Health Nursing Certification,* by N. Randolph, 1998, Springhouse, PA: Springhouse. Copyright 1998 by Springhouse.

Other areas in which to promote safety are development of healthy lifestyle, substance abuse prevention, and sex education.

Adolescent Stage

Adolescence (development from the ages of 13 to 20 years) begins with the onset of puberty. The individual undergoes the transition from child to adult as many physiological changes and rapid growth occur. The rapid changes occurring are not only physical; many psychosocial adjustments must also be made. Friendships become very important (Figure 10-9). Establishing a sense of personal identity takes up a great amount of the adolescent's psychic energy. Questions such as "Who am I?" and "What is *really* important?" are common ones among adolescents.

Most adolescents are very concerned with their appearance. The importance of physical attractiveness may cause eating disorders, such as anorexia nervosa (self-imposed starvation that results in a 15% loss of

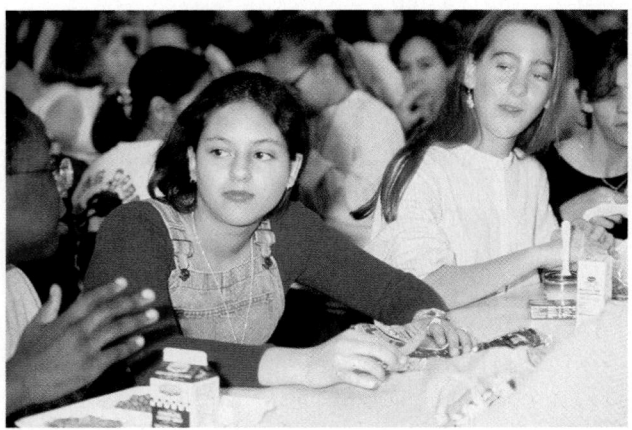

Figure 10-9   *Peer group is very important during adolescence.*

body weight), bulimia nervosa (episodic binge-eating followed by purging), or obesity (weight that is 20% or more above ideal body weight).

Significance for Nursing

Support the adolescent by providing information about the many bodily changes experienced during this developmental stage. Encourage adolescents to share health concerns with parents, but honor the adolescent's choice to keep sensitive information from parents. The confidentiality of the client as well as of those in a relationship with the client (sexual partners) must be protected.

Enhancing Wellness The adolescent's wellness is enhanced primarily through teaching. Areas to emphasize in health education for adolescents include nutrition, hygiene, developmental changes, sex education, and substance abuse prevention. Information is available from the American Academy of Pediatrics (AAP, 2002b).

Teaching adolescents about the physical changes they are undergoing is often done by school nurses (Figure 10-10).

Safety Concerns Unhealthy behaviors contribute to the three major causes of adolescent death: accidents, homicide, and suicide. The adolescent's risk for accidents increases because of:

• Impulsive behavior
• Feeling invulnerable to accidents

Figure 10-10 *Wellness promotion for the adolescent may include in-school seminars by school nurses, such as this one on AIDS prevention.*

PROFESSIONAL TIP

Working with Adolescents

- Use a nonjudgmental attitude to establish rapport when working with adolescents.
- Treat every adolescent in a respectful, dignified manner.
- Avoid using a condescending attitude when communicating with the adolescent.
- To form a collaborative partnership, treat the adolescent as an active participant in health care.
- Answer all questions honestly.
- Be sensitive to nonverbal clues. Adolescents are often too embarrassed to initiate discussion.
- Remember that the peer group is of major importance to the adolescent; use group settings.
- Demonstrate acceptance of the adolescent even when limits must be established.
- Questioning adult authority is a normal part of adolescence. Do *not* personalize such behavior. Nurses who do so become defensive and lose their interpersonal effectiveness and credibility with adolescents.

- Testing limits
- Rebelling

As a result, many adolescents engage in unhealthy behaviors such as smoking, consuming alcohol and other drugs, reckless driving, unprotected sexual activity, and violence.

Many adolescent health problems relate to sexual behaviors. For example, consider the following facts:

- Acquired immunodeficiency syndrome (AIDS) is the fifth leading cause of death (CDC, 2002a) of individuals between the ages of 24 and 44 years; many of these people were infected during their adolescent years.
- Approximately 3.75 million new cases of sexually transmitted diseases (STDs) are found in teenagers (CDC, 2001).
- Every year, about 1 million teenagers become pregnant (CDC, 2002b).

Teen pregnancy has a great effect on families and communities. Social programs providing resources to meet the needs of pregnant adolescents are decreasing. Many pregnant teens become trapped in a cycle of school failure (or dropout), limited employment opportunities, and poverty.

The pregnant adolescent needs information, expert prenatal care, and a supportive environment. Teaching must emphasize preventing STDs because the pregnancy is evidence of high-risk (i.e., unprotected) sexual activity. Almost 70% of 12th graders report having sexual intercourse, but less than half say they used condoms (AAP, 2002). It is estimated that 25% of students will develop an STD before high school graduation (AAP, 2002).

Nurses teaching safe-sex practices must be sensitive to cultural influences on sexual activity. A high risk of suicide is a major health problem during adolescence. The rate is higher among adolescent males than females. Suicide is often thought to be the only alternative to an overwhelming situation. Suicidal behavior can be traced to low self-esteem, lack of maturity, and resultant impulsive behaviors.

Assessment for suicide potential should always be direct questions about plans for harming or killing themselves. The following are signs of suicide risk in adolescents:

- Change in eating and sleeping habits
- Writing suicide notes
- Discussion of suicide
- Aggressive behavior
- Substance abuse
- Loss of interest in pleasurable activities
- Preoccupation with death
- Neglect of personal hygiene
- The giving away of treasured objects
- Marked personality change
- Verbal cues (e.g., "You won't have to worry about me much longer.")
- Fatigue, headache, stomachache
- Social withdrawal

When someone exhibits signs of suicide risk, contact a health care professional *immediately*. Most communities have a special suicide-prevention telephone line available.

 Safety: Suicide Prevention
- Never leave the suicidal adolescent alone.
- The best deterrent to suicide is close observation.

Another significant health problem for many adolescents is substance abuse. A common maladaptive way to cope with the stressors of adolescence is using alcohol or other drugs.

Sexually Active Adolescents

How would you provide care to sexually active adolescents if you think their behavior is immoral or "wrong"? Is it ethical for you to try to change their values so they become congruent with yours? Should you change your values to be congruent with those of the client?

Nurses can help adolescents make responsible, informed decisions before experimenting with drugs.

Young Adulthood Stage

Physical growth stabilizes during **young adulthood** (development from the ages of 21 years through approximately 40 years). The young adult still experiences physical and emotional changes, but at a slower rate than the adolescent. Table 10-14 outlines the development of young adults. This is a time of transition from adolescence to adulthood.

Pregnancy is experienced by many young adults. It is a time of transition and lifestyle adjustments. Women experience changes in self-concept during pregnancy and may need reassurance that this is normal.

TABLE 10-14   YOUNG ADULTHOOD: GROWTH AND DEVELOPMENT

DIMENSION	CHARACTERISTICS	NURSING CONSIDERATIONS
Physiological	*Physiological changes:* Physical growth stabilizes. Physical functioning is at an optimum and therefore less likely to be concerned with own health. Maturation of body systems is complete. *Cardiovascular changes:* Men are more likely to have an increased cholesterol level than are women. *Gastrointestinal changes:* After age 30, digestive juices decrease. *Musculoskeletal changes:* At approximately age 25, skeletal growth is complete. *Reproductive changes:* *Women:* Ages 20–30 are optimal years physically for reproduction. *Men:* Beginning at approximately age 24, male hormones slowly decrease (does not affect reproductive ability).	Teach importance of health-promoting behaviors. Encourage a healthy lifestyle.
Psychosocial	*Erikson:* intimacy vs. isolation stage Engage in productive work. Develops intimate relationships.	Emphasize need for social support as the person assumes new roles. Provide sex education information, including information on prevention of STDs.
Cognitive	*Piaget:* formal operations stage Problem-solving abilities are realistic. Manifest less egocentricism. Many engage in formal education.	
Moral	*Kohlberg:* postconventional stage Right and wrong are defined in terms of personal beliefs and principles.	Respect the person's value system and beliefs.
Spiritual	*Fowler:* individuative-reflective faith stage Assumes responsibility for own beliefs.	Encourage use of spiritual support system.

Data from *Adult Health Nursing* (3rd ed.), by P. G. Beare and J. L. Myers, 1998, St. Louis, MO: Mosby–Yearbook. Copyright 1998 by Mosby–Yearbook; *Health Promotion throughout the Lifespan* (5th ed.), by C. L. Edelman and C. L. Mandle, 2002, St. Louis, MO: Mosby–Yearbook. Copyright 2002 by Mosby–Yearbook.

Figure 10-11 *The assessment of this young adult's blood pressure is one part of enhancing this client's wellness.*

Significance for Nursing

Young adulthood is usually the healthiest time in a person's life. Consequently, concern for health is low, and wellness is taken for granted. Preventive measures fall into two categories:

* Developing health-promoting behaviors (e.g., lifestyle modification)
* Avoiding accident, injury, and violence

By teaching and counseling, the nurse plays an important role in each of these areas of health promotion (Figure 10-11). Other developmentally appropriate topics for the nurse to address are vocational counseling and relationship establishment.

Enhancing Wellness Decision making by young adults affects their health status. Young adults often take excessive risks, making them at greater risk for accidents, suicide, or homicide (Edelman & Mandle, 2002). Reckless driving, driving while intoxicated, and unprotected sex are examples that demonstrate a lack of fear by many young adults. Sexually transmitted diseases cause infection often resulting in reproductive dysfunction. Nurses should teach women how to perform a breast self-examination (BSE) monthly, and men must learn how to perform a testicular self-examination (TSE). The nurse should confirm currency of tetanus/diphtheria (Td) immunization.

Safety Concerns A health risk to many young adults is sunbathing. Exposure to the radiation resulting from direct sunlight or the lighting used in tanning salons is directly linked to skin cancer. According to the American Cancer Society (2003), 1.3 million new cases of nonmelanoma skin cancer are diagnosed every year. Nurses can teach and model safe behaviors related to sunbathing.

Middle Adulthood Stage

Middle adulthood (development from the ages of 40 to 65 years) is characterized by productivity and responsibility. Many physiological changes occur during middle adulthood. Table 10-15 lists the major changes experienced by the middle-aged person. Most activity revolves around family and work with success measured by family life and career accomplishments.

The major developmental task of middle adulthood concerns the conflict of generativity (a sense that one is making a contribution to society) versus stagnation (a sense of nonmeaning in one's life). An individual who

TABLE 10-15	MIDDLE ADULTHOOD: GROWTH AND DEVELOPMENT	
DIMENSION	**CHARACTERISTICS**	**NURSING CONSIDERATIONS**
Physiological	*Cardiovascular changes:* Decreased capacity for physical activity. Blood vessels lose elasticity. Hypertension (high blood pressure), coronary artery disease, and cerebral vascular accidents ("strokes") may appear.	Encourage to remain physically active. Teach lifestyle modifications related to cardiovascular health: • Quit smoking • Avoid secondary tobacco smoke • Practice good nutrition (low fat, low cholesterol) • Engage in physical activity.
	Neurological changes: Impaired sensation of heat and cold.	Explain age-related changes. Teach safety precautions regarding: • Exposure to sunlight, • Sensitivity to heat stroke, and frostbite
	Gastrointestinal changes: Slower gatrointestinal motility results in constipation.	Teach to: • Increase high-fiber food intake; drink more fluid, and • Maintain physical activity. Teach signs indicating dehydration.
	Genitourinary changes: Nephron units diminish in number and size; blood supply to kidneys diminishes.	Advise to maintain adequate fluid intake.

continues

TABLE 10-15 continued

DIMENSION	CHARACTERISTICS	NURSING CONSIDERATIONS
Physiological —continued	*Integumentary changes:* Wrinkles develop. Hair may thin and turn gray. *Musculoskeletal changes:* Bone mass and density decreases. Slight loss of height (1–4 inches) may occur. Generalized decrease in muscle tone; appearance becomes "flabby," and agility lessens, leading to an increased risk of injury. *Endocrine changes:* Reduced production of enzymes and increased hydrochloric acid, leading to acid indigestion and belching. *Reproductive changes:* *Women:* Estrogen and progesterone production cease at menopause. Secondary sex characteristics regress (decreased breast size, loss of pubic hair). Vaginal secretions decrease. *Men:* Testosterone level decreases as does the amount of viable sperm. Sexual energy declines, and it takes longer to achieve an erection, but it is sustained longer. Adapting to chronic diseases and sexual problems may diminish self-esteem.	Assess for body image alterations. Employ nonjudgmental listening. Advise about: • Need for increased calcium intake, • Decreasing caffeine and alcohol consumption, and • Effects of sedentary lifestyle on osteoporosis. Instruct about need for proper posture (especially when sitting), exercise, and adequate fluid intake. Advise about need for physical activity. Instruct client to: • Eat foods that are not spicy or fried • Avoid eating within 2 hours of bedtime. Teach age-related sexual/reproductive changes. Encourage responsible sexual behavior. Teach prevention of sexually transmitted diseases.
Psychosocial	*Erikson:* generativity vs. stagnation stage Those who have achieved generativity feel good about themselves and comfortable with their lives. Become involved in altruistic acts (volunteer work). Family roles may change (become caregiver to aging parents, become grandparent).	Provide support as aging occurs. Encourage involvement in community activities. Advise on the need to care for self while caring for others.
Cognitive	*Piaget:* Uses all stages, depending on the task. Able to reflect on the past and anticipate the future. Reaction time diminishes. Learning ability remains for motivated person.	Encourage clients who return to school or participate in other intellectually stimulating activities.
Moral	*Kohlberg:* postconventional stage	Be nonjudgmental when discussing values.
Spiritual	*Fowler:* conjunctive faith stage The middle-aged adults is able to appreciate others' belief systems. Middle-aged adults are less dogmatic about own beliefs. Religion is often a source of comfort.	Encourage use of spiritual support. Refer to clergy if desired by client.

Data from *Adult Health Nursing* (3rd ed.), by P. G. Beare and J. L. Myers, 1998, St. Louis, MO: Mosby–Yearbook. Copyright 1998 by Mosby–Yearbook; *Health Promotion throughout the Lifespan* (5th ed.), by C. L. Edelman and C. L. Mandle, 2002, St. Louis, MO: Mosby–Yearbook. Copyright 2002 by Mosby–Yearbook; *Health Assessment: A Nursing Approach* (3rd ed.), by J. Fuller and J. Schaller-Ayers, 2000, Philadelphia: Lippincott Williams & Wilkins.

Self-Care for Middle Adulthood

Self-care topics for the middle-aged adult include:

- Nutrition, exercise, and weight control
- Managing stress
- Recommendations for health screening (cholesterol, prostate exam, mammogram, Pap test)
- Changes related to aging

successfully resolves this developmental conflict is usually accepting of age-related changes.

Evaluation of one's life may lead to a midlife crisis, especially if the individual feels that little has been accomplished or self-expectations have not been met.

Significance for Nursing

Middle-aged adults constitute almost half the U.S. population (Edelman & Mandle, 2002). The baby-boom generation has entered this stage, and more nurses will be required to care for them.

Assist middle-aged clients in improving their health by identifying risk factors and providing early intervention. The major risk factors are primarily behavioral and environmental for adults in the middle years, so they can be changed. In assisting the middle-aged client to change unhealthy behaviors, the nurse can work on either a one-on-one or group basis.

Enhancing Wellness Encourage middle-aged adults to assume more responsibility for their own health by receiving influenza and pneumococcal immunizations as recommended by their physicians. Confirm currency of Td (tetanus/diphtheria) immunization.

Safety Concerns Middle adulthood is the time when lifelong unhealthy practices, such as smoking, being sedentary, and overuse of alcohol, begin to exhibit their adverse effects. Reversing these practices can greatly improve one's health status. Occupational health hazards are another significant problem.

Most middle-aged individuals have more leisure time for jogging, tennis, golf, or boating, resulting in an increased risk of injuries.

Older Adulthood Stage

Older adulthood is development occurring from age 65 until death. Table 10-16 provides an overview of growth and development in the older adult.

TABLE 10-16   OLDER ADULTHOOD: GROWTH AND DEVELOPMENT

DIMENSION	CHARACTERISTICS	NURSING CONSIDERATIONS
Physiological	Refer to the older adult chapter for a detailed discussion of physiological changes related to aging.	
Psychosocial	*Erikson:* integrity vs. despair stage Accepts own life as it is. A sense of worth is gained from helping others.	Seek the older person's advice. Identify and use the older adult's strengths. Advocate reminiscence. Encourage socialization with peers.
Cognitive	*Piaget:* formal operations stage No decline in IQ is associated with aging. Reaction time slows. *Memory:* Short-term: Capacity for recall decreases. Long-term: Capacity remains unchanged.	Allow time for responses. Watch for medication-induced confusion.
Moral	*Kohlberg:* postconventional stage Makes moral decisions to fit own principals and beliefs.	Support decision making. Respect values even when different from own.
Spiritual	*Fowler:* universalizing stage Generally satisfied with own spiritual beliefs and tends to act on beliefs.	Listen carefully to determine spiritual needs. Acknowledge losses and encourage appropriate grieving.

Data from *Women's Health: Instant Nursing Assessment,* by P. A. Firth and S. J. Watanabe, 1996, Clifton Park, NY: Thomson Delmar Learning. Copyright 1996 by Thomson Delmar Learning; *Health Promotion throughout the Lifespan* (5th ed.), by C. L. Edelman and C. L. Mandle, 2002, St. Louis, MO: Mosby–Yearbook. Copyright 2002 by Mosby–Yearbook; *Health Promotion Strategies through the Life Span* (7th ed.), by R. B. Murray and J. P. Zentner, 2001, Upper Saddle River, NJ: Prentice Hall. Copyright 2001 Prentice Hall.

COMMUNITY/HOME HEALTH CARE

Home Safety for Older Adults

Encourage the elderly client to make the home environment safe by:

- Ensuring adequate lighting
- Removing all throw or loose rugs
- Clearing all walking paths
- Having a handrail on all stairs
- Installing hand-holds in tubs and showers

Older adults have several psychosocial tasks to accomplish, including:

- Accepting own life as it is
- Finding meaningful activities
- Adjusting to any infirmities
- Coping with changes and losses
- Making preparations for death.

Significance for Nursing

Nursing care is important in assisting the aging person to develop a sense of well-being (Eliopoulos, 2001). Nurses working with elderly clients must be aware of their own attitudes, feelings, and beliefs about aging and understand how these may affect care provided to these clients.

Assessment of the older adult should include the client's background, family history, work history, achievements, and hobbies (Figure 10-12). Encourage clients to talk about their life experiences. Care is more likely to be individualized when the client's unique experiences and assets are recognized.

When clients express dissatisfaction and regrets about the past, listen in a nonjudgmental manner. Help older clients put disappointments into perspective by reviewing with them their achievements and accomplishments. Encourage family members to reminisce with the older client. Many nursing interventions for the older adult include introspection and reflection on their lives.

Figure 10-12 *These older adults maintain their self-esteem through volunteering to make quilts for those less fortunate.*

Life review (or reminiscence therapy) promotes a positive self-concept in older people (Heriot, 1999).

Enhancing Wellness Health-promotion activities should focus on maintaining functional independence and maximizing abilities and strengths. Independent, older adults are generally healthier. Specific topics for discussion with older clients are regular physical activity, use of leisure time, increased socialization, maintaining a positive mental attitude, and adequate nutrition. Many older people engage in more health-promoting behaviors than do younger people (Sapp & Bliesmer, 1999). Encourage the client to obtain influenza and pneumococcal immunizations as recommended and confirm currency of Td immunization.

Safety Concerns Falls pose a major health threat to elderly persons. Teach ways to minimize risk of falling. Confusion with complicated medication regimens causes problems for many elderly. Emerging technology is producing many assistive devices related to medication administration (Logue, 2002).

Summary

- Growth is the measurable changes in physical size, and development refers to behavioral changes in functional abilities and skills.
- Growth and development of an individual are influenced by heredity, life experiences, health status, and cultural expectations.
- Maturation is the process of becoming fully grown and developed both physically and behaviorally.
- Certain developmental tasks must be achieved during each developmental stage for normal development to occur.
- According to Freud, repressed sexual problems in childhood cause problems later in life.
- Erikson explains that psychosocial development is a series of conflicts occurring during eight stages of life.
- Piaget's theory cites four stages of cognitive development: sensorimotor, preoperational, concrete operations, and formal operations. Each stage is characterized by how the child interprets the environment.
- Kohlberg's theory describes six stages of moral development through which individuals develop a moral code to guide their behavior.
- Fowler's theory outlines six distinct stages of faith development. The sequence remains the same, but the age at which each stage is experienced varies.
- Promoting the health and safety of individuals at each stage of life is an important role for nurses.

Review Questions

1. The fact that development occurs in a proximodistal manner means that the infant is able to:

   a. crawl before he walks.
   b. raise his head before he is able to sit up.

    c.   move his arms before picking up an object with his fingers.

    d.   master psychological tasks before establishing a separate identity.

2.   The nurse knows that at birth the neonate's activities are:

    a.   reflexive.

    b.   adjusting.

    c.   purposeful.

    d.   continuing.

3.   Immunizations are important during:

    a.   infancy.

    b.   childhood.

    c.   adolescence.

    d.   entire life span.

4.   The nurse working with preadolescent children should:

    a.   offer opinions on the child's lifestyle choices.

    b.   provide an opportunity for the child to ask questions about health-related concerns.

    c.   finish the child's thoughts and sentences to avoid awkward silences.

    d.   give a lecture on all the changes to be expected in the next few years; nutrition; and personal hygiene.

5.   A great many health problems among adolescents are related to:

    a.   nutrition.

    b.   sexual behaviors.

    c.   activity/exercise.

    d.   sleep/rest behaviors.

References/Suggested Readings

American Academy of Child & Adolescent Psychiatry (AACAP). (1998a). *Teenagers with eating disorders* [Online]. Available: www.aacap.org/publications/factsfam/eating.htm

American Academy of Child & Adolescent Psychiatry (AACAP). (1998b). *Teen suicide* [Online]. Available: www.aacap.org/publications/factsfam/suicide.htm

American Academy of Pediatrics. (1998). Guidance for effective discipline. *Pediatrics, 101*(4), 723.

American Academy of Pediatrics. (2001). *2001 red book: Report of the Committee on Infectious Diseases* (24th ed.). Elk Grove, IL: Author.

American Academy of Pediatrics (AAP). (2002a). *Adolescent health.* [Online]. Available: www.aap.org/advocacy/washing/chiah/htm

American Academy of Pediatrics (AAP). (2002b). Puberty information for boys and girls [Online]. Available: www.aap.org/family/puberty.htm

American Cancer Society (ACS). (2003). *Cancer facts & figures 2003.* Atlanta, GA: Author.

Beare, P. G., & Myers, J. L. (1998). *Adult health nursing* (3rd ed.). St. Louis, MO: Mosby.

Bradley-Springer, L. (2001). HIV prevention: What works? *AJN, 101*(6), 45–48.

Centers for Disease Control and Prevention (CDC). (2001). *Tracking the hidden epidemics: Trends in STDs in the United States 2000.* [Online]. Available: www.cdc.govnchstp/dstd/Stats_Trends/Trends2000.pdf

Centers for Disease Control and Prevention. (2002a). *AIDS falls from top ten causes of death; teen births, infant mortality, homicides all decline; Updated 7-26-02* [Online]. Available: www.cdc.gov/od/oc/media/pressrel/r981007.htm

Centers for Disease Control and Prevention. (2002b). *Teen pregnancy* Updated 4-20-02 [Online]. Available: www.cdc.gov/nccdphp/teen.htm

Deering C, & Jennings, D. (2002) Communicating with children and adolescents. *AJN, 102*(3), 34–41.

Edelman, C. L., & Mandle, C. L. (2002). *Health promotion throughout the lifespan* (5th ed.). St. Louis, MO: Mosby.

Eliopoulos, C. (2001). *Gerontological nursing* (5th ed.). Philadelphia: Lippincott Williams & Wilkins.

Erikson, E. (1968). *Childhood and society.* New York: Norton.

Estes, M. E. Z. (2002). *Health assessment & physical examination* (2nd ed.). Clifton Park, NY: Thomson Delmar Learning.

Firth, P. A., & Watanabe, S. J. (1996). *Women's health: Instant nursing assessment.* Clifton Park, NY: Thomson Delmar Learning.

Forshner, L., & Garza, A. (1999). Childhood vaccines: An update. *RN, 62*(4), 32–36.

Fowler, J. W. (1995). *Stages of faith: The psychology of human development and the quest for meaning.* New York: Harper & Row.

Freud, S. (1961). *Civilization and its discontents.* New York: Norton.

Fuller, J., & Schaller-Ayers, J. (2000). *Health assessment: A nursing approach* (3rd ed.). Philadelphia: Lippincott Williams & Wilkins.

Guyton, A. C., & Hall, J. (2002). *Textbook of medical physiology* (10th ed.). Philadelphia: W. B. Saunders.

Hale, P. J. (2000). HIV, hepatitis, and sexually transmitted diseases. In M. Stanhope & J. Lancaster (Eds.), *Community & public health nursing* (5th ed.). St. Louis, MO: Mosby.

Heriot, C. S. (1999). Developmental tasks and development in the later years of life. In M. Stanley & P. Beare (Eds.), *Gerontological nursing: A health promotion/protection approach* (2nd ed.). Philadelphia: F. A. Davis.

Hockenberry-Eaton, M. (2003). *Whaley & Wong's nursing care of infants and children* (7th ed.). St. Louis, MO: Mosby.

Hogstel, M. (2001). *Gerontology: Nursing care of the older adult.* Clifton Park, NY: Thomson Delmar Learning.

Kimbell, S. (2001). Before the fall: Keeping your patient on his feet. *Nursing2001, 31*(8), 44–45.

Kohlberg, L. (1977). *Recent research in moral development.* New York: Holt, Rinehart, & Winston.

Levinson, D. (1978). *The seasons of a man's life.* New York: Knopf.

Logue, R. M. (2002). Self-medication and the elderly: How technology can help. *AJN, 102*(7), 51–55.

Mayo Clinic. (1998a). *Children's snacks: Don't ban them, plan them* [Online]. Available: www.mayohealth.org/mayo/9806/htm/snacks.htm

Mayo Clinic. (1998b). *Vegetarianism: Is it OK for children?* [Online]. Available: www.mayohealth.org/mayo/9807/htm/vegie.htm

Mohr, W. & Johnson, B. S. (2002). *Johnson's Psychiatric-mental health nursing: Adaptation and growth* (5th ed.). Philadelphia: Lippincott Williams & Wilkins.

Murray, R. B., & Zentner, J. P. (2001). *Health promotion strategies through the life span* (7th ed.). Upper Saddle River, NJ: Prentice Hall.

Piaget, J. (1963). *The origins of intelligence in children.* New York: Norton.

Randolph, N. (1998). *American nursing review of psychiatric and mental health nursing certification.* Springhouse, PA: Springhouse.

Sapp, M., & Bliesmer, M. (1999). A health promotion/protection approach to meeting elders' healthcare needs through public policy and standards of care. In M. Stanley & P. Beare (Eds.), *Gerontological nursing: A health promotion/prevention approach.* Philadelphia: F. A. Davis.

Simmerman, J. M., & Mauzy, C. L. (2001). Finally! Babies can get this vaccine. *RN, 64*(7), 28–32.

Sullivan, H. S. (1953). *Interpersonal theory of psychiatry.* New York: Norton.

Resources

American Academy of Pediatrics, 141 Northwest Point Boulevard, Elk Grove Village, IL 60007-1098, 847-434-4000, www.aap.org

American Association of Retired Persons, 601 E Street NW, Washington, DC 20049, 800-424-3410, www.aarp.org

American Foundation for Suicide Prevention, 120 Wall Street, 22nd floor, New York, NY 10005, 888-333-2377, www.afsp.org

American Society on Aging, 833 Market Street, Suite 511, San Francisco, CA 94103-1824, 415-974-9600, www.asaging.org

Centers for Disease Control and Prevention (CDC), 1600 Clifton Road NE, Atlanta, GA 30333, 404-639-3311, 888-246-2673, www.cdc.gov

Gerontological Society of America, 1030 15th Street NW, Suite 250, Washington, DC 20005, 202-842-1275, www.geron.org

National Institute of Child Health & Human Development NICHD Clearinghouse, P. O. Box 3006, Rockville, MD 20847, 800-370-2943, www.nichd.nih.gov/

Zero to Three: National Center for Infants, Toddlers and Families, 2000 M Street NW Suite 200, Washington, DC 20036, 202-638-1144, www.zerotothree.org

CULTURAL CONSIDERATIONS

MAKING THE CONNECTION

Refer to the following chapters to increase your understanding of cultural considerations and nursing:

Basic Nursing
- **Legal and Ethical Responsibilities**
- **Communication**
- **Wellness Concepts**

- **Complementary/Alternative Therapies**
- **Pain Management**

LEARNING OBJECTIVES

Upon completion of this chapter, you should be able to:
- **Define key terms.**
- **Describe the characteristics and components of culture.**
- **Discuss the impact of cultural beliefs on illness and health.**
- **Compare and contrast diverse health beliefs of major cultural groups in the United States.**
- **Describe cultural differences in relation to time and space.**
- **Identify nutritional preferences held by various cultural groups.**
- **Identify the general beliefs that account for the differences among religions.**
- **Describe the way that the nurse's religious beliefs or lack thereof can influence nursing care.**
- **Discuss the nurse's role in meeting the spiritual needs of the client and family.**
- **Analyze personal values and cultural beliefs.**
- **Perform a cultural assessment.**

INTRODUCTION

Every aspect of a person's life—including attitudes, values, and beliefs—is influenced by that person's culture. Behavior, including behavior affecting health, is culturally determined. Recognition of cultural differences and their impact on health care becomes even more critical as the population of the United States con-

KEY TERMS

acculturation	minority group
agnostic	oppression
atheist	race
cultural assimilation	religious support system
cultural diversity	spiritual care
culture	spiritual need
dominant culture	stereotyping
ethnicity	yin and yang
ethnocentrism	

tinues to diversify. Because nurses provide health care to culturally diverse client populations in various settings, knowledge of culturally relevant information is essential for delivery of competent nursing care. This chapter discusses the various concepts related to culture, the influence of culture on health, the relationships between culture and health beliefs, cultural aspects and the nursing process, and illnesses associated with ethnic groups.

CULTURE

Each individual is culturally unique. A person's culture, as influenced by life experiences, education, and creative thought, is the lens through which a person sees everything. The nurse needs a thorough understanding of concepts to provide holistic care.

In society, **culture** refers to an integrated dynamic structure of knowledge, attitudes, behaviors, beliefs, ideas, habits, customs, languages, values, symbols, rituals, and ceremonies that are unique to a particular group of people. This structure provides the group of people with a general design for living.

Individuals often acquire cultural beliefs unconsciously throughout the process of growth and maturation (Giger & Davidhizar, 2004). People are exposed to culture at an early age through the observance of traditions (established customary patterns of thought and behavior). Cultural beliefs, values, customs, and behaviors are transmitted from one generation to another through interaction, daily activities, and celebrations. For instance, the birth of a child is celebrated according to the family's cultural norms and customs, which may include prayers, blessings, special naming ceremonies, religious rites, and so forth. Parents, grandparents, and other elders all teach children cultural norms and expectations through demonstration, discussion, and role modeling (Figure 11-1).

Culture is not static, nor is it uniform among all members within a given cultural group. Culture represents adaptive dynamic processes learned through life experi-

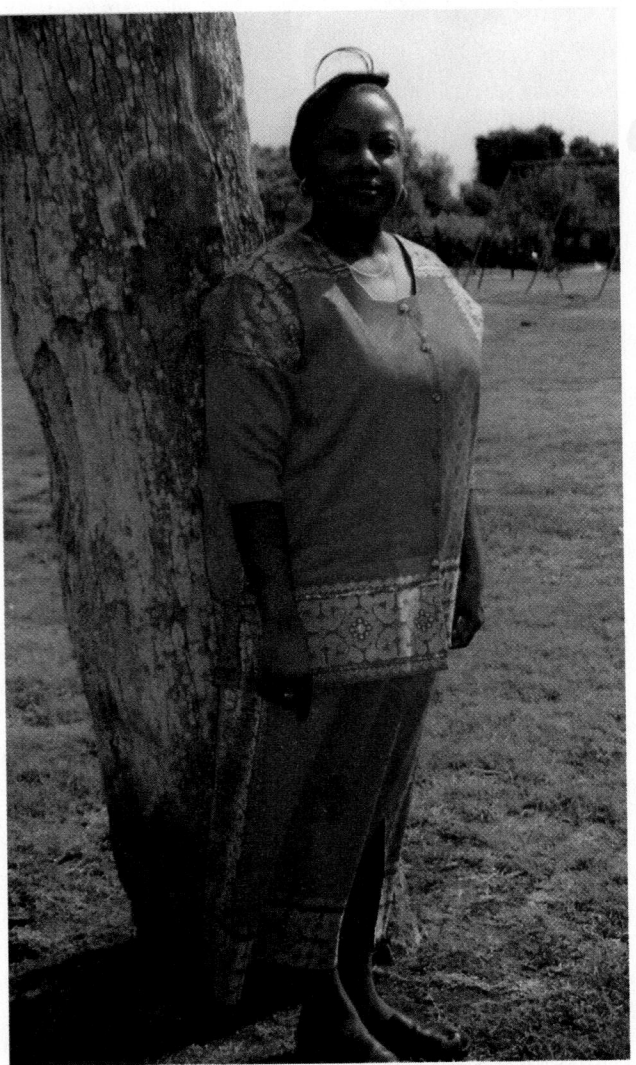

Figure 11-1 *This woman celebrates her African American heritage when wearing this ethnic dress. Photo courtesy of Tira Butler.*

CULTURAL CONSIDERATIONS

Sharing Culture

Cultural messages are transmitted in a variety of settings such as homes, schools, religious organizations, and communities. The various media, such as radio and television, are also powerful transmitters and shapers of culture.

ences. Diversity among and within cultural groups results from individual perspectives and practices. Consider, for example, the way that a family deals with a crisis. A crisis may cause a family that is part of a culture with a strong sense of responsibility to family and blood relatives to become closer; conversely, the same situation may cause a family that is from a culture that values independence and individuality to withdraw and create distance among its members. These reactions are rooted in the family's cultural background and heritage.

Ethnicity and Race

Ethnicity is a cultural group's perception of itself, or a group identity. Ethnicity is a common social heritage providing a sense of belonging that is passed from one generation to the next. Members of an ethnic group display their sense of identity through common traits and customs. Ethnic identity can be expressed in many ways, including dress; for instance, many African Americans display ethnic pride by choosing clothing that highlights their ethnic origin and shared heritage.

Race is a group of people with biological similarities. Members of a racial group have similar physical characteristics, such as facial features and color of hair, eyes, and skin. Racial and ethnic groups often overlap because the cultural and biological commonalities support one another (Giger & Davidhizar, 2004). The similarities of racial and ethnic group members reinforce a sense of identity and cohesiveness.

Cultural Diversity

Cultural diversity refers to the differences among people resulting from ethnic, racial, and cultural variations. A variety of rich cultural heritages exists within the United States. The sociopolitical climate is enriched by this vast potential of human resources with divergent viewpoints and behaviors. A diverse population provides varied ideas, viewpoints, and problem-solving approaches and an expectation of increased tolerance.

Living and working in such a culturally diverse society has some disadvantages. Problems arise when differences between and within cultural groups are not understood. Apprehension and turmoil often accompany people's expectations of others.

Some cultural groups have historically experienced prejudice or bias in the form of racism (discrimination based on race and biological differences). Individuals may experience sexism (discrimination based on gender) and classism (prejudice based on perceived social class). Society perpetuates these biases consciously or unconsciously. The underlying premise is that one way is superior and every other way is inferior. **Ethnocentrism,** the assumption of cultural superiority and inability to accept another culture's ways, results in oppression. When the rules, values, and ideals of one group are imposed on another group, it is termed **oppression.** Oppression is based on cultural biases, which stem from beliefs, expectations, and traditions.

Stereotyping is the belief that all people within the same ethnic, racial, or cultural group will act the same way, sharing the same beliefs and attitudes. Stereotyping results in labeling people according to cultural preconceptions, thereby ignoring individual identity.

The group whose values prevail within a given society is the **dominant culture.** The dominant culture of the United States is composed of white, middle-class Protestants of European ancestry. The European values have greatly influenced U.S. culture.

These dominant values may conflict with the values of minority groups. A **minority group** is a group of people constituting less than a numerical majority of the population. Such groups are often labeled and treated differently from others in the society. Minority groups are generally considered to have less power than the dominant group (Giger & Davidhizar, 2004).

When people assume the characteristics of the dominant culture, it is called **acculturation** (the process of learning beliefs, norms, and behavioral expectations of a group). **Cultural assimilation** happens when members of a minority group are absorbed by the dominant culture, taking on the characteristics of the dominant culture.

Culture's Components

Stewart identified five components of culture that establish the way people think about life (as cited in Lock, 1992):

- *Perception of self and the individual:* Refers to personal identity, respect for individuals, and value
- *Motivation:* Explains the methods and value of achievement
- *Activity:* Identifies the ways people organize and value work
- *Social relations:* Explains the structure and importance of gender roles, friendships, and class
- *Perception of the world:* Indicates the explanation of religious beliefs and life events

These concepts are particularly helpful to the nurse when planning care for a client from another cultural group. Self-identity, social relationships, work, success, and religion influence the cultural group's definition of health and illness and the response to health events. For example, if a culture values relationships more than work, the culture may sanction an extended period of illness and a lengthy time away from the employment site; however, if a culture measures achievement by output at work, illness may be interpreted negatively. Members of the latter culture may deny illness and delay seeking appropriate health care.

Culture's Characteristics

Spradley and Allender (2001) have identified five characteristics shared by all cultures:

- *Culture is not inherited or innate.* It is integrated throughout all the interrelated components. Motivations, activities, world views, relationships, and individuality are affected by consistent patterns of behavior and form a cohesive whole.
- *Culture is learned.* Behavior patterns are picked up as children imitate adults and develop actions and attitudes acceptable in society.
- *Culture is shared.* Behavioral patterns are not individually defined, but are defined, accepted, and practiced by everyone who belongs to the cultural group.
- *Culture is dynamic (constantly changing).* New ideas experienced by each generation may lead to different standards for behavior.
- *Culture is tacit (unspoken).* Everyone in the cultural group understands acceptable behavior. Cultural beliefs are widely known and adopted.

CULTURAL INFLUENCES ON HEALTH CARE BELIEFS AND PRACTICES

Culture influences health care decisions and practices, and determines the way we react to illness and pain. In cultures where raw foods are not consumed, for instance, the incidence of shigellosis may be lower than cultures where consumption of raw meat and fish is common. On the other hand, cultural taboos against eating protein during pregnancy have a harmful or destructive effect on fetal development. Cultural values define human responses to illness and determine whether an individual will seek professional care when ill and comply with prescribed treatment.

CULTURAL CONSIDERATIONS

Individuality

Remember that each person is first and foremost an individual, and second a member of a cultural group. Although similarities may exist within an ethnic or culture group, individual differences must be respected.

PROFESSIONAL TIP

Cultural Sensitivity

Nurses must be able to provide culturally appropriate care to a diverse population of clients. Cultural diversity presents special challenges for nurses who must provide care that is incongruent with personal beliefs and values. Nurses caring for clients who differ from themselves must remember to find out how the client views the event (illness), including the significance (meaning) that the client assigns the event. The nurse must honor individual differences.

Beliefs and patterns of behavior affect attitudes about various aspects of health. Beliefs about the definition of health; etiology (cause and origin of disease); health promotion and protection practices; and health practitioners and remedies are all influenced by cultural background. Clients tend to define wellness and illness in the context of their own culture (Estin, 1999).

Definition of Health

The most widely accepted definition of health, developed by the World Health Organization (WHO), states that health is not only the absence of disease, but also complete physical, mental, and social wellness. While this definition of health is broad enough to be global, the physical, mental, and social dimensions are culturally defined. Any deviation from that which is culturally understood to be normal health is considered illness. For example, a biological disease of immediate etiology might not be interpreted as an illness by some cultures; intestinal parasites are so common in some areas in Africa that the presence of ascaris in stools is considered normal. If a cultural group does not perceive certain symptoms or behaviors as illness, members are not likely to seek medical care when these symptoms appear. In this situation, disease conditions may persist untreated, resulting in permanent damage or even death.

Etiology

The noted medical anthropologist, Peter Morley, presents four views of the origin of disease: supernatural, nonsupernatural, immediate, and ultimate (Morley & Wallis, 1978). The supernatural view of disease traces diseases to metaphysical forces such as witchcraft, sorcery, and voodoo. An individual with this view might attribute illness to evil spirits or to a curse by a powerful spiritual person. The nonsupernatural view holds that diseases have an accepted cause-and-effect relationship, even though that relationship may lack scientific rationale. For example, people of many cultures believe that colic in an infant is caused by breast milk rendered impure when a nursing mother has sexual relations. In such cultures, sexual relations are prohibited for nursing mothers. The immediate view of disease traces diseases to known pathogenic agents, such as chickenpox is caused by *Herpes varicella*; and the ultimate view describes determinates for diseases, such as smoking resulting in lung cancer. Most cultural groups support a multietiologic origin, believing there may be three or four explanations as to why and how diseases occur.

Health Promotion and Protection

Strategies for achieving and maintaining good health vary by cultural group. For example, the dominant U.S. culture has come to endorse a low-fat, high-fiber diet; regular exercise; and appropriate immunizations as means to promote and protect health. Other cultures may place greater value on prayer, meditation, and restored relationships, particularly in those cultures where disease prevention and health maintenance are closely linked to beliefs about disease etiology. For example, disease prevention may require paying homage to ancestral spirits to avoid offending them and seeking their revenge through illness.

Practitioners and Remedies

Variety in health/illness care providers is a natural extension of culturally diverse concepts of etiology and definitions of health and illness. Standard medicine may not be accepted as treatment when a scientific rationale for the etiology of disease is not accepted by a cultural group. Alternative remedies and practitioners are often found in culturally diverse groups. In order to enhance client compliance with treatment regimens, health care providers must make efforts to base therapy and prescribe treatments that respect culturally traditional remedies. Clients who trace disease etiology to a supernatural cause are more likely to seek interventions from spiritual leaders or traditional healers.

The folk medicine system categorizes illnesses as either natural or unnatural (Giger & Davidhizar, 2004). The classification of an illness determines the type of treatment and healer used. Because the folk medicine system (also referred to as alternative medicine) can present challenges to nurses caring for clients from diverse cultures, knowledge of basic beliefs about illness, factors contributing to illness, and home remedies is necessary.

Folk healers are knowledgeable about cultural norms and customs (Edelman & Mandle, 2002). Table 11-1 lists both the various healers within the five dominant cultural groups in the United States (European American, African American, Hispanic American, Asian American, and Native American) and the common folk healing practices within these cultures. Nurses must be able to relate care and treatment to the client's cultural context and incorporate informal caregivers, healers, and other members of the client's support system as allies in treatment.

Beliefs of Select Cultural Groups

While the population of the United States encompasses innumerable ethnic groups, European Americans, African Americans, Hispanic Americans, Asian Americans, and Native Americans together represent a majority. These groups form the basis for the following brief discussion of specific health beliefs influenced by culture.

European American

In 2000, Americans of European descent represented 71% of the U.S. population (U.S. Census Bureau, 2001). The prevailing value system for many European Americans is based on what is referred to as the white, Anglo-Saxon, Protestant (WASP) ethic (Sue & Sue, 2003). This ethnic group traces its origins to the Caucasian Protestants who came to this country from Northern Europe more than 200 years ago. Values that still dominate the Caucasian American middle-class ethic include independence, individuality, wealth, comfort, cleanliness, achievement, punctuality, hard work, aggression, assertiveness, rationality, orientation toward the future, and mastery of one's own fate (Andrews & Boyle, 2003; Edmission, 1997).

TABLE 11-1   FOLK MEDICINE: HEALERS AND PRACTICES

CULTURAL GROUP	TRADITIONAL HEALERS	HEALING PRACTICES
European American	• Nurse • Physician	• Exercise • Medications • Modified diets • Amulets (charms to ward off evil or disease or to protect) • Religious healing rituals
African American	• Elderly women healers • "Community Mother" or "Granny" • "Root doctor" • Voodoo healer ("Mambo" or "oungan") • Spiritualist	• Herbs, roots, oils • Poultices • Religious healing through rituals (e.g., laying on of hands) • Talismans worn around the wrist or neck or carried in a pouch to ward off disease
Hispanic American	• Curandero • Espiritualista • Yerbero (herbalist) • Brujo (healer who uses witchcraft) • Sobadora • Santiguadora	• Hot and cold foods to treat some conditions • Herbal teas, such as manzanilla, to treat gastrointestinal problems, insomnia, and menstrual cramps • Prayers and religious medals • Massage • Azabache, a black stone, worn as a necklace or bracelet to ward off the "evil eye" • Among some Haitian mothers, the "three baths" ritual (bathing for the first 3 postpartum days in water boiled with special leaves)
Asian American	• Herbalist • Physician	• Hot and cold foods • Herbs, soups • Cupping, pinching, and rubbing • Meditation • Acupuncture • Acupressure • Application of tiger balm (a salve) to relieve muscular pains • Energy to restore balance between yin and yang
Native American	• Shaman • Medicine man/woman	• Plants and herbs • Medicine bundle or bag filled with herbs that have been blessed by a medicine man/woman during a healing ceremony • Sweet grass (herbs) burned to purify the ill person • Estafiate (dried leaves) boiled to produce a tea for treating stomach disorders • The Blessingway ceremony (a healing ritual conducted by the medicine man/woman) • In some Navajo tribes, sand paintings made by the medicine man/woman for diagnostic purposes

Data compiled from *Cultural Diversity and Community Health Nursing*, by C. Degazon, in *Community Health Nursing* (5th ed.), by M. Stanhope and J. Lancaster (Eds.), 2000, St. Louis, MO: Mosby–Yearbook; *Transcultural Nursing: Assessment and Interventions* (4th ed.), by J. Giger and R. Davidhizar, 2004, St. Louis, MO: Mosby–Yearbook; and Cultural Dimensions in Home Health Nursing, by D. Grossman, 1996, *AJN 96*(7).

CULTURAL CONSIDERATIONS

Subculture

Many Caucasian Americans do not belong to the mainstream culture, but, instead, belong to ethnic subcultures that hold strong values of their own (e.g., Irish, Jewish, German, Italian, Norwegian, Appalachian, and Amish subcultures).

Traditionally, most Caucasian Americans have wanted to be recognized as individuals rather than as members of groups. Thus, Caucasian Americans, unlike members of many other cultures, tend to be competitive rather than cooperative with each other. Mainstream American culture also values the nuclear family and its traditions (Luckmann, 1999).

African American

The African American population in 2000 represented 12% of the U.S. population (U.S. Census Bureau, 2001). African American ancestors came to North America from various African countries and the Caribbean as either free immigrants or slaves. The heterogeneous (different) cultural practices among African Americans today may be explained by the diverse countries of origin, disparate educational levels, income, occupations, and religious beliefs.

Traditional African societies may believe that disease is caused by disharmony in relationships. Discord may occur between a client and evil spirits, living relatives, or ancestral spirits. Restoration of harmony may be achieved through prayer, meditation, or other activities, such as wearing a charm, offering a gift, or confessing a wrong, leading to healing.

Disease may be viewed as sent by God or another higher power as a punishment for a serious infraction. Evil forces may be thought to account for illness in other cases. Healing may be found in home remedies and herbs, consultation with a local healer, or prayer.

Hispanic American

Hispanic Americans also represented 12% of the U.S. population in 2000 (U.S. Census Bureau, 2001). The majority of this group has origins in Mexico, Puerto Rico, and Cuba. Although the Spanish language is common to most Hispanics, cultural patterns vary according to the different countries of origin. The Hispanic American usually belongs to a large extended-family system within which females are seen as subservient to males but as having a major role in family cohesiveness (Giger & Davidhizar, 2004).

In Hispanic populations the influence of religion on culture is particularly evident. Most Hispanic Americans have roots in Catholicism blended with traditional Indian beliefs. Illness may be viewed as "an act of God" as punishment for sin, as the result of witchcraft or a curse by an enemy, or as having a natural cause. Diseases may be traced to an imbalance between "hot" and "cold" or "wet" and "dry" forces. Treatment depends on the cause. Western medicine is believed to be appropriate for some diseases, whereas the native healer (curandera) may be called on to intervene for illnesses having supernatural causes. Treatment may consist of religious ceremonies, herbal potions, or diets based on hot and cold foods.

Asian American

Asian Americans, representing 4% of the U.S. population in 2000 (U.S. Census Bureau, 2001), have origins in the Pacific Rim countries: China, Japan, Korea, Vietnam, Laos, the Philippines, and Cambodia. Generalization of a specific Asian culture is not possible; however, certain similarities do exist. Family relations are traced through males. Males as the head of household are the decision makers. Elders are revered and respected. Only physical complaints are acceptable, and maintaining eye contact is considered disrespectful (Estin, 1999).

Asians believe in yin (cold) and yang (hot) as etiology of disease. **Yin and yang** are opposing forces that yield health when in balance. An imbalance in these forces causes illness. Foods are identified as either hot or cold and are used in treatment. For example, if yang is overpowering yin, hot foods are avoided until balance is restored. Illness may be thought to be caused by supernatural powers such as God, ancestral spirits, or evil spirits. In this situation, healing is sought through prayer or treatment by a traditional healer. Many Asian Americans rely on acupuncture, herbal remedies, and cupping and burning. In cupping, the inside and rim of a cup are heated with a candle flame. Then the rim of the cup is applied directly to the client's skin. Blood is drawn to the surface of the skin as the cup cools, causing a bruised appearance. Cupping is used to draw out evil or illness in order to restore yin and yang. The nurse must be aware of these cultural practices so they are not viewed as abuse but, rather, as important cultural customs.

Native American

Native Americans represented 1% of the U.S. population in 2000 (U.S. Census Bureau, 2001). These peoples form a very diverse group, descending from more than 200 different tribes across the United States. Although many Native Americans have assumed Euro-American practices with regard to health, some still use traditional practices. Health is believed to result from a harmonious relationship with nature and the universe. Illness is frequently traced to a supernatural origin and discord with the forces of nature. Using witchcraft is believed to cause illness, and treatment may require the exorcism of evil spirits. Disease prevention may be achieved through prayer, charms, and fetishes (objects having power to protect or aid the owner). "Medicine men" are persons believed to have supernatural powers of healing. Health may be restored through herbal drinks, prayers, rituals, and ceremonies.

CULTURAL AND RACIAL INFLUENCES ON CLIENT CARE

Clients' cultural backgrounds and preferences influence the manner whereby they interact with other people and with the world around them. In an unfamiliar situation, such as admission to a health care setting, cultural differences may seem even greater. In these instances of stress, most people hold tightly to that which is familiar in order to protect themselves from the unknown. The nurse can show caring in such a situation by acknowledging the expression of these differences and encouraging the client to retain what is familiar. Providing opportunities for decisions in their care decreases the stress of unfamiliar situations.

The influences of culture and race can be viewed through the phenomena of communication, space and time orientation, social organization, and biological variations.

Communication

Although language is common to all human beings, not everyone shares the same language. This cultural difference can lead to misunderstanding and frustration. The nurse must realize that a client who speaks a different language or with an accent simply has a different means of expressing needs. When communication is restricted because of language differences, alternative methods of communication, such as gestures and flash cards, can be used.

PROFESSIONAL TIP

Non-native Speakers

When interacting with someone who does not understand English well, many people will try to compensate for the lack of understanding by speaking loudly. Speaking slowly, distinctly, and in a normal volume, making eye contact, and avoiding slang and medical jargon are effective measures to ensure communication.

Figure 11-2 *Family members may serve as interpreters to help clients who do not speak English understand procedures and instructions and to communicate the client's thoughts and questions to the nurse.*

The client's family may be able to assist when there is a block in communication. Family members can interpret procedures and instructions for the client and communicate the client's thoughts and questions to the nurse (Figure 11-2). If no family members are available, the hospital social worker may be able to find an interpreter.

Orientation to Space and Time

Orientation with regard to space and time represents two other culturally influenced variables that may affect a client's attitude toward care. Territoriality, or interpretation of personal space, is a pattern of behavior resulting from an individual's belief that certain spaces and objects belong to that person. The distance that a person prefers to maintain from another is determined by one's culture. In general, people of Arabic, Southern European, and African origin frequently sit or stand relatively close to each other (0 to 18 inches), whereas people of Asian, Northern European, and North American origin are more comfortable with a larger personal space (more than 18 inches).

Affection and caring behaviors are not communicated by touch in some cultures. For instance, among Asians, adults seldom touch one another, and the head is believed to be sacred. The nurse should thus not touch an Asian client's head without permission to do so. When working with clients from cultures where personal touch is viewed negatively, the nurse should use the universal sign of caring and acceptance: the smile.

People in U.S. society tend to be future oriented: They plan for the future, establish long-term goals, and, increasingly, are concerned with prevention of future illnesses. In daily life, they are oriented to time of day, constantly referring to clock time for everything from meal time to time of appointments with health care professionals as well as other obligations. The nurse must also be very attentive to time. Medications are given at scheduled times, and work begins and ends at specified times. Other groups that tend to be future oriented are Japanese, Jews, and Arabs. These groups tend to view time as a commodity for achieving future goals.

Not all cultural groups are future oriented, however. People of some cultures (e.g., Asians) may be oriented to the past. For Asians, this orientation is reflected in the roles that ancestor worship and Confucianism play in the present. Members of other cultural groups, such as Native Americans, tend to be present oriented. Many Native Americans do not own clocks, and they live one day at a time, showing little concern for the future (Giger & Davidhizer, 2004). Mexican Americans and African Americans often value relationships with people in the present more than in the future. African Americans tend to be present oriented in health care behaviors as well. They often express the fatalistic belief that "it's going to happen anyway, so why bother" and fail to seek medical attention until a disabling condition occurs. The African American culture often teaches flexible attention to schedules; whatever is happening currently is most important. Explanations about the necessity of time scheduling (e.g., the need for strict schedules for medication requiring therapeutic blood level maintenance) must be given to the client.

An individual's orientation to time may affect promptness or attendance at health care appointments, compliance with self-medication schedules, and reporting the onset of illness or other health concerns. Clients might not see the necessity for preventive health care measures if they experience no difference in their health today when they follow a special diet or exercise program. The nurse must both teach clients when timing is critical in health care situations and practice patience when working with people whose background differs from that of the dominant culture.

Social Organization

Social organization refers to the ways that cultural groups determine rules of acceptable behavior and roles of individual members. Examples of social organization include family structure, gender roles, and religion.

Family Structure

The definition of family has changed dramatically through the years. Until 1920 the norm was the "institutional family," which was organized around economic production and the kinship network. Marriage was not a romantic relationship but a functional one. Family loyalty and tradition were more important than individual romantic interests or goals. Responsibility was the chief value.

From 1920 to 1960, the norm was the "psychological family." Affairs were more private and less tied to the extended family. Family was based on fulfillment of the individual members and personal satisfaction in a nuclear, two-parent arrangement. Satisfaction was the chief value.

The social changes of the 1960s caused modifications in the family, including gender equality and personal freedom. The increased divorce rate may have resulted from the sexual revolution and the attitude that the individual deserves more and owes less to the family.

Today, no single family arrangement has a monopoly. Many types of families have emerged and are accepted. Flexibility is the chief value. Family no longer necessarily implies biological relation, but rather has come to mean members of a shared household who have similar values and participate in shared goals. Fawcett (1993) cites the following characteristics of family:

- Love and affection
- Caring and compassion
- Sense of belonging and connectedness

- History and linkage to posterity
- Rituals of rejoicing
- Sense of place
- Acceptance of members, including shortcomings
- Honor of elders
- System of earning and spending money
- Competent manner of parenting or caretaking
- Division of chores and labor

Systems theory states that families are considered to be interacting, interdependent individuals related by marriage, birth, or mutual consent. Examples of families with varying lifestyles today are two-parent nuclear, single-parent, blended (through remarriage), extended (including grandparents), cohabiting (couple having never married), gay or lesbian, divorced, adoptive, multi-adult, and mixed or interracial families.

Gender Roles

Gender roles vary according to cultural context (Figure 11-3). For example, in families organized around a patriarchal structure (with the man being the head of the household and chief authority figure), the husband/father is the dominant member. Such expectations are typically the cultural norm in Latino, Hispanic, and traditional Muslim families. The husband/father is the one who makes decisions regarding health care for all family members. Also, in such cultures, the wife is responsible for child care and household maintenance, whereas the father's role is to protect and support the family members.

Religion

Anthropologists have identified the strength of the influence of religion on culture. In many cases, culture and tradition have been maintained and preserved through religious beliefs. Religion often is the formal organizational structure for social behavior.

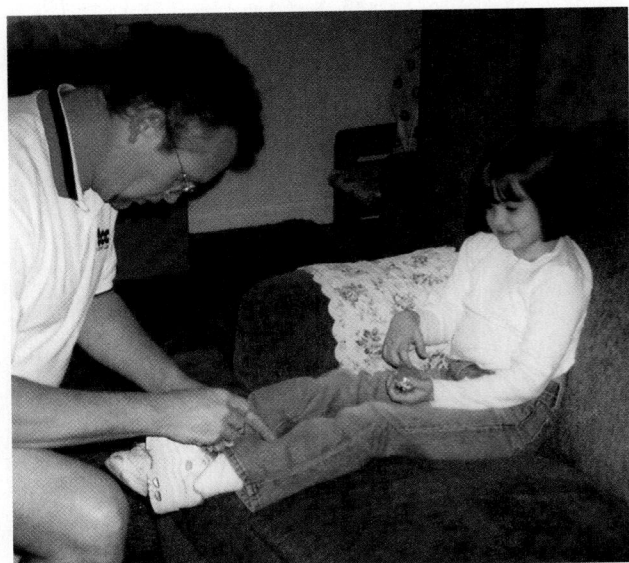

Figure 11-3 *Fathers assuming more responsibility in caring for children is one example of shifting gender roles.*

COMMUNITY/HOME HEALTH CARE

Culturally Sensitive Care

To provide culturally sensitive care in the home:

- Remember that the setting for care is not controlled by the health care provider but by the client and family.
- Be aware that the nurse is often viewed as a guest by the client and family. Social communication may be necessary to facilitate rapport.
- Be nonjudgmental about the home (e.g., presence of clutter and disarray).
- Display consideration and respect for the client. For example:
  —Before entering the home, wipe your feet.
  —Before washing your hands, ask permission to use the sink or bathroom.
  —Before moving the client's belongings, ask permission, then replace items when finished.
- Benefit from the home environment by assessing cultural values and norms. Clues to cultural values may include:
  —Possessions and decor on display in the home
  —Family roles and task assignment
  —Interactions among family members
  —Value placed on privacy and possessions

Figure 11-4 *Spiritual needs often increase when individuals are sick.*

Religious and spiritual beliefs are important in many individuals' lives. These beliefs can influence attitudes, lifestyle, and feelings about life, pain, and death. Some religions specify practices about diet, birth control, and appropriate medical care. Often, spiritual beliefs assume a greater significance at the time of illness than at other times in a person's life. These beliefs assist some people in accepting their illnesses and help explain illness for others. Religion can both help people live fuller lives and console or strengthen people during suffering and in preparation for death. Religion, by providing meaning to life and death, can supply the client, the family, and the nurse with a sense of security and strength during a time of need.

Spiritual needs are identified as an individual's desire to find purpose and meaning in life, pain, and death. To provide holistic care, the nurse must be attentive to the spiritual dimension of each client and assist the client in meeting spiritual needs (Figure 11-4).

While spiritual needs are recognized by many nurses, **spiritual care** (recognition of and assistance toward meeting spiritual needs) is often neglected. Spirituality is defined as an individual's search to find purpose and meaning in life. The goal of spiritual nursing care is to empower clients to identify and utilize their spiritual beliefs to cope with a health crisis. Among reasons that nurses give for failing to provide spiritual care are:

- Spirituality is a private matter.
- Uninformed about the religious beliefs of others.
- Have not identified their own spiritual beliefs.
- Meeting the spiritual needs of the client is a family or clergy responsibility, not a nursing responsibility.

Spiritual nursing care is appropriate when the nurse cares about the client's emotional, physical, and psychosocial health. The nursing diagnosis, *Spiritual Distress*, can be apparent in a client who is unable to practice religious or spiritual rituals because of illness or confinement in a health care institution.

The **religious support system** is a group of ministers, priests, nuns, rabbis, shamans, mullahs, or laypersons who are able to meet clients' spiritual needs. The nurse is responsible for working with these individuals and including them in the client care team.

Be aware of the general philosophies of clients' spiritual beliefs, and also be aware that some individuals do not believe in a higher being or practice a specific religion. **Agnostics** believe that the existence of God cannot be proved or disproved, whereas **atheists** do not believe in God or any other deity.

It is important to identify particular beliefs from various religions that can influence client care activities. Some of these beliefs concern holy day practices, dietary restrictions, birth, death, and organ donation.

Protestant Many separate denominations (more than 1,200) constitute the group known as Protestant. Protestant groups include such denominations as Baptist, Episcopal, Lutheran, Methodist, Presbyterian, and Seventh Day Adventist. The majority worship on Sunday, and their primary written reference is the Holy Bible.

Baptist Baptists believe that baptism is performed only after the believer reaches an age of understanding and confesses a personal acceptance of Jesus' saving work. Communion is a spiritual act symbolizing the suffering, death, and resurrection of the Lord.

Episcopal Episcopalians have a number of sacraments, including baptism, confession, communion, and anointing of the sick (Holy Unction). Holy Unction is most often given as a healing sacrament. They believe that a dying infant should be baptized, and a nurse may perform the rite. Usually an Episcopal priest administers these sacraments.

Lutheran Traditionally, Lutherans baptize infants and adults by sprinkling. Any baptized Christian may perform an emergency baptism. The Lutheran churches recognize two sacraments, baptism and Holy Communion. Holy Communion is understood to be the body and the blood of Jesus. It is often administered to the ill or those awaiting surgery. Central to Lutheran doctrine is the belief in "justification by faith." People are redeemed by God solely on the basis of God's grace, which they receive through faith in what God has done for them.

Methodist Methodists practice both infant and adult baptism. For them, religion is a matter of personal belief, and the conscience is used as a guide for living.

Presbyterian Presbyterians also practice baptism and communion, which is a remembering of the death of Jesus Christ for them. Salvation is believed to be a gift from God.

Seventh Day Adventist Seventh Day Adventists baptize individuals only after they reach an age of accountability. Some dietary restrictions are followed. Sunset on Friday to sunset on Saturday is observed as their Sabbath. Jobs or worldly pleasures are not pursued during this time.

Roman Catholic Priests perform various rites known as Sacraments (sacred) at various times in the life of the Catholic. Sacraments that might be encountered in the health care setting are baptism, the Eucharist (Communion), confession, and sacrament of the sick. Baptism, administered only once in the life of a Catholic, is believed to be absolutely necessary for salvation. A client preparing for communion is generally asked to abstain from food or drink an hour before the rite. Water and medications are allowed at any time. Confession is a sacrament for forgiveness of sins. It should be respected as a very private matter. The Sacrament of the Sick, in which the client is anointed with holy oil, was formerly given to someone near death and was called the "last rites."

Orthodox Orthodox churches show their love of God through worship liturgies. It is important that followers remain faithful to the teachings of the ancient church. Holy Unction, anointing the body with oil, is used for healing of both bodily and spiritual infirmities. Baptism is important, so in life-threatening situations an unbaptized child should have an emergency baptism.

Jehovah's Witness Receiving any blood or blood products, including plasma, is prohibited. Also, they will not eat anything containing blood. Blood volume expanders that are not derivatives of blood are permissible. To receive blood when a medical condition requiring blood transfusion is life-threatening, children have been made wards of the court. They hold a special observance of the Lord's Supper.

Mormon (Church of Jesus Christ of the Latter Day Saints) Mormons baptize at the age of eight years. When necessary, baptism of the dead is performed for adults. Mormons wear a special undergarment that symbolizes dedication to God. This may be worn under the hospital gown.

Christian Science Christian Scientists believe that illness will be eliminated through prayer and spiritual understanding. A critically ill Christian Scientist client may wish to have a Christian Science practitioner contacted to provide treatment through prayer. They usually do not use medicine, do not agree to surgical procedures, and do not accept blood transfusions.

American Indian Religions All life is sacred and all things are interconnected is the central belief of the various religions. Community importance is emphasized. The individual who is able to communicate with the spirits or the Great Spirit is the spiritual leader. There are no written religious books. Religious traditions are passed on orally and through participation in ceremonies and festivals. Illness may be the result of a sin or a spirit or god who is unhappy.

Judaism Judaism is both an ethnic identity and a religious faith. The religion is based on the five books of Moses called the Torah. Religion and culture are deeply interwoven in the Jewish faith, resulting in ritual, tradition, religious ceremony, and social laws.

There are three groups of Judaism: Orthodox, Conservative, and Reformed. They vary in how strictly they follow the traditions, but all share the fundamental teachings of Judaism. Orthodox Jews strictly observe all traditional practices. The Conservative group observes many of the traditional practices, and the Reformed group loosely interprets the traditions.

The spiritual leader of the Jewish congregation is the rabbi and the person to be informed when a client requests it.

The Jewish Sabbath, or day of worship, begins at sunset on Friday and ends at sunset on Saturday.

Circumcision is performed on the male infant eight days after birth. It may be done by the pediatrician or by the Mohel who may also be a rabbi.

Islam Islam is the religion of Muslims. Allah is the supreme deity, and Mohammed, the founder of Islam, is the chief prophet. The Muslim's day of worship lasts from sunset on Thursday to sunset on Friday. Some Muslims pray five times a day (after dawn, at noon, at mid-afternoon, after sunset, and at night). A bed or chair may be positioned facing southeast (in the continental United States) when a client requests that he face Mecca, the holy city of Islam. Muslim clients may wear an article of writing from the Koran on a piece of string around the neck, waist, or arm. This should not be removed or allowed to get wet. Rules of cleanliness involve eating with the right hand and cleansing self with the left hand after defecating or urinating. Hand medications or other materials to the Muslim client with the right hand so as not to offend them.

Some Islamic females wish to be clothed from head to ankle. They may prefer to undress one body part at a time during a physical examination and may refuse to be cared for by male nurses or physicians.

Buddhism Buddhism is a general term indicating a belief in Buddha, "the enlightened one." Nirvana, a state of greater spontaneity and inner freedom, is the goal of existence. When one achieves Nirvana, the mind has supreme purity, strength, and peace. Buddhism does not dictate any specific sacraments or practices. There are no special holy days or religious restrictions for therapy. Buddhists believe in reincarnation but not in healing through faith. The religious support system for the sick is the priest. Figure 11-5 shows the inside of a Buddhist temple.

Figure 11-5 *Inside of a Buddhist Temple (Photo courtesy of John White, Corpus Christi, TX)*

Hindu Hinduism has no common doctrines or creeds that keep Hindus together. They are free to worship one or more of their 320,000 gods. The Vedas are the Scripture of Hinduism. Reincarnation is central in Hindu thought. Freedom from the cycle of rebirth and death and entrance into what the Hindus, like the Buddhists, call Nirvana is the goal of existence. Hindu temples are dwelling places of deities and where offerings are brought. Some Hindus believe that illness is God's way of punishing a person for sins; others believe in faith healing.

Biological Variation

Biological variations distinguish one racial or cultural group from another. Easily identified biological variations include skin color, hair texture, eye shape, thickness of lips, and body structure (Degazon, 2000). Less obvious biological variations include enzyme differences and susceptibility to disease (Andrews & Boyle, 2003; Giger & Davidhizar, 2004). Enzyme differences account for varied responses of some groups to dietary and drug therapy (Table 11-2).

According to Kudzma (1999), drug metabolism is genetically determined, and race seems to affect the response. A drug is more efficient in clients who metabolize the drug rapidly. Sometimes, it may be metabolized too quickly for the full clinical effect to be achieved. When a drug is metabolized slowly, it is less effective, and the client experiences greater drug toxicity.

TABLE 11-2 BIOLOGICAL VARIATIONS

CULTURAL GROUP	BIOLOGICAL VARIATION
European American	• Liver enzyme differences cause caffeine to be metabolized and excreted faster. • Increased susceptibility for breast cancer, heart disease.
African American	• Isoniazid (drug used to treat tuberculosis) is metabolized rapidly, so quickly becomes inactive; occurs in approximately 60% of population. • Increased susceptibility for keloid formation, hypertension, lactose intolerance, sickle cell disease. • Higher doses of antihypertensive drugs (e.g., propranolol) must be administered to produce same effects as in European Americans.
Hispanic American	• Increased susceptibility for diabetes, lactose intolerance.
Asian American	• Isoniazid is metabolized rapidly, so quickly becomes inactive; occurs in approximately 85% to 90% of population. • Alcohol is rapidly metabolished resulting in excessive facial flushing and other vasomotor symptoms. • Increased susceptibility for hypertension, lactose intolerance. • Chinese men require half as much propranolol (antihypertensive drug) to produce same effects as in European American men.
Native American	• Isoniazid is metabolized rapidly, so quickly becomes inactive; occurs in approximately 60% to 90% of population. • Increased susceptibility for tuberculosis, diabetes, heart disease. • Rapid metabolism of alcohol results in excessive facial flushing and other vasomotor symptoms.

Data compiled from *Transcultural Nursing: Assessment and Intervention* (4th ed.), by J. Giger and R. Davidhizar, 2004, St. Louis, MO: Mosby–Yearbook; Cultural Diversity and Community Health Nursing, by C. Degazon, in *Community Health Nursing* (5th ed.), by M. Stanhope and J. Lancaster (Eds.), 2000, St. Louis, MO: Mosby–Yearbook; and *Transcultural Concepts in Nursing Care* (3rd ed.), by M. M. Andrews and J. S. Boyle, 1999, Philadelphia, PA: Lippincott Williams & Wilkins.

CULTURAL ASPECTS AND THE NURSING PROCESS

Each individual comes from a cultural background that, in some way, influences behavior and attitudes about health and illness. Personal attitudes and behaviors determine not only the ways that clients interpret

PROFESSIONAL TIP

Culturally Diverse Coworkers

Many nursing units have a mix of nationalities and cultures. While such a mix has the potential of improving nursing care, in practice it often leads to conflict and poor teamwork. The same cultural differences discussed in relation to clients may also be found among coworkers. Ways to successfully manage diversity in the workplace include:

- Be aware of your own biases, and strive to avoid stereotyping others.
- Be aware of the way the things you do and say affect others.
- Help others to be more sensitive and help correct misconceptions.
- Learn to welcome different opinions and viewpoints.
- Be open to feedback.

Nurses must cultivate a cultural consciousness. There must be a heightened sensitivity and awareness of the uniqueness and diversity of perspective each individual has to offer. Cultural awareness is essential in the process of providing appropriate, effective care (Mullins, 1999). As health care professionals, even if we cannot understand or accept particular cultural practices, it is important to show respect for them. This directly reflects how we value our own beliefs and practices.

CRITICAL THINKING

Culture and Health Practices

How has your culture influenced your beliefs about health practices?

If a client put an amulet (religious icon and necklace) around her newborn's neck, how would you approach this client to discuss your concern about the risk of strangulation?

health events and utilize health care, but also the ways that nurses interpret health events and provide health care. Health care providers should evaluate their personal views about health and illness before assessing and caring for clients from other cultural groups.

Assessment

Culturally sensitive nursing care begins with an examination of one's own culture and beliefs. It is followed by an assessment of the client's cultural beliefs and background.

Personal Cultural Assessment

Spradley and Allender (2001) suggest five areas to be examined when assessing one's own culture and the influence it has on personal beliefs about health care.

- Influences from own racial/ethnic background
- Usual verbal and nonverbal communication patterns
- Cultural norms and values
- Religious practices and beliefs
- Health practices and beliefs

They suggest that the nurse should identify information on each issue and then validate this information with another person(s) from the same cultural group.

Client Cultural Assessment

After examining one's own culture and the influences it may have had in developing personal beliefs about health and sickness, then assess the client's cultural background (Figure 11-6). Data about various cultures may be collected from members of the culture to be studied, from others familiar with the culture, or from the local library.

Six categories of information necessary for a comprehensive cultural assessment of the client are suggested by Spradley and Allender (2001).

- *Ethnic or racial background.* Where did the client group originate, and how does that influence the status and identity of group members?
- *Language and communication patterns.* What is the preferred language spoken, and what are the culturally based communication patterns?
- *Cultural values and norms.* What are the beliefs, values, and standards regarding education, roles, leisure, family functions, child-rearing, work, aging, death and dying, and rites of passage?
- *Biocultural factors.* Are there genetic or physical traits unique to the ethnic or racial group that predispose group members to certain conditions or illnesses?
- *Religious beliefs and practices.* What are the religious beliefs, and how do they influence roles, life events, health, and illness?
- *Health beliefs and practices.* What are the beliefs and practices regarding treatment, causes, and prevention of illnesses?

Nursing Diagnosis

Any nursing diagnosis may be appropriate for a client of any cultural group. When cultural variables are identified during assessment, the nurse should be as specific as possible when asking questions and determining appropriate nursing diagnoses, so that interventions can be individualized with respect to the client's cultural beliefs. For instance, *Decreased Cardiac Output* may be viewed by the nurse or physician as having a medical or physical cause, whereas the client may attribute the origin to an imbalance of yin and yang. Table 11-3 lists select nursing diagnoses that are most likely to have cultural implications.

Planning/Outcome Identification

Cultural variables must be taken into consideration when establishing goals and planning interventions. Care will be most effective when the client and family are active participants in planning care, and when cultural preferences are respected. Suggested goals to consider when cultural factors are involved include:

- Client will express health care needs to family and caregiver.

Cultural Asssessment Guide

Name _____

Other names or nicknames _____

Date of birth _____ Place of birth _____

Primary language _____ Other languages _____

Religious affiliation _____

How much do you identify with your cultural group? _____

To what ethnic group do you belong? _____

Describe your beliefs or customs about:

       Life _____

       Health _____

       Illness _____

       Death _____

How do you learn best? _____

       Reading _____ Listening _____ Watching _____

Does your religion or culture forbid any foods? _____

_____

Describe personal food preferences _____

Describe your family's dietary habits _____

How do your religious practices and beliefs affect your life when in good health? _____

_____

When in poor health? _____

Who provides your health care services or healing? _____

_____

What cultural health practices are you aware of, and which do you utilize? _____

_____

What cultural restrictions should your caregiver know? _____

_____

Describe how family members relate to and communicate with each other _____

_____

What or who is your primary source of health information? _____

_____

What other cultural beliefs would you like to share? _____

_____

Figure 11-6 *Cultural Assessment Guide*

TABLE 11-3 NURSING DIAGNOSES WITH CULTURAL IMPLICATIONS

Anxiety
Disturbed **B**ody Image
Ineffective **B**reastfeeding
Impaired Verbal **C**ommunication
Decisional **C**onflict (specify)
Ineffective **C**oping
Compromised Family **C**oping
Fear
Anticipatory **G**rieving
Ineffective **H**ealth Maintenance
Health-Seeking Behaviors (specify)
Noncompliance
Imbalanced **N**utrition: More Than Body Requirements
Pain
Ineffective **R**ole Performance
Disturbed **S**leep Pattern
Impaired **S**ocial Interaction
Spiritual Distress

CLIENT TEACHING

Culturally Sensitive Teaching Guidelines

Consider the following guidelines for teaching clients from diverse cultures:

- Identify the client's cultural background.
- Evaluate the client's current knowledge by asking the client to state what he knows about the topic.
- Identify the perception of need by asking the client and family what they need and want to learn.
- Observe interactions between the client and family to determine family roles and authority figures. Ask the client which family member they would like included in teaching and care sessions.
- Use language easily understood by the client, avoiding jargon and complex medical terms.
- Clarify your verbal and nonverbal messages with the client.
- Ask the client to repeat the information. Ask the client to do a return demonstration of the material taught.

- Client will maintain cultural health practices as appropriate.
- Client and family will understand the effect that health care beliefs have on health status.

Implementation

Cultural aspects are always a factor in a nursing care plan, and effective communication and client education are important nursing responsibilities that can enhance cultural understanding and appreciation. Interventions should be carried out in a manner that will respect, to the degree possible, the preferences and desires of the client. When a client does not speak or understand the native language well, the nurse should arrange to have an interpreter present to explain procedures and tests.

PROFESSIONAL TIP

Culturally Appropriate Care

- Respect clients for their beliefs.
- Be sensitive to behaviors and practices different from your own.
- Accommodate differences if they are not detrimental to the client's health. For example, a client might believe that eating onions will resolve his respiratory infection. While eating onions may not be therapeutic, it is also not likely to cause any health problems.
- Listen for cues in the client's conversation that relay a unique ethnic belief about prevention, etiology, transmission, or some other aspect of disease. For example, a client might say, "I knew I would be sick today. I heard an owl last night."
- Use the occasion to teach positive health habits if the client's practices are deleterious to good health. For example, when asked about her diet, a pregnant woman might reply that she never eats meat or eggs while pregnant because she believes that gaining too much weight will increase her risk of a difficult delivery. This situation offers the nurse an opportunity to provide nutritional instruction.

Evaluation

Evaluation should include feedback from the client and family to determine their reaction to the interventions. Revisions to the plan of care need to be made with client and family input, and alternative sources and resources brought in when needed to enhance communication and exchange of information. Nurses should also perform self-evaluations to identify their attitudes toward caring for clients from diverse cultures.

Summary

- Culture is composed of beliefs about relationships, motivation, activities, perception of the world and about self.
- Culture is learned, shared, integrated, unspoken, and dynamic.
- Beliefs about concepts of health, disease etiology, health promotion and protection, and practitioners and remedies are influenced by culture.
- Unlike opinions, preferences, and attitudes, which can change, cultural characteristics are deeply rooted and are thus difficult to change. Clients reflect their cultural and ethnic heritage every time they interact with the world around them.
- Culture is influenced by religion, which also affects practices and beliefs about health and illness.
- Spiritual and religious beliefs are important in many people's lives. They can influence lifestyle, attitudes, and feelings about illness and death.
- Individuality exists among all peoples; nurses should not make assumptions based on the client's religious and cultural affiliations.

SAMPLE NURSING CARE PLAN

THE FAMILY WITH INEFFECTIVE COPING

Mrs. Wong, an 82-year-old Asian American housewife, is in the hospital with severe nausea and vomiting related to recurrent breast cancer with bone metastasis treatment. Her appetite is decreasing, although she is able to drink some fluids.

At Mrs. Wong's insistence her husband of 61 years and their two grown daughters remain at her bedside. She does not bother the nurses for her basic care and insists that the oldest daughter bathe her and walk her to the bathroom. Mr. Wong leaves only to go home and shower. Both daughters remain when he goes home.

Mr. Wong looks exhausted and appears to have lost weight. The daughters try to relieve their father at night, but he insists on remaining at the bedside.

Mrs. Wong has her husband and daughters constantly massaging her back and legs but never voices discomfort. She changes position slowly and grimaces with each movement. Mrs. Wong lets her family talk for her. When questioned by the nurse she denies pain, but she complains of pain to her family. She does not sleep well.

Mrs. Wong's treatment plan is supportive. The hospital staff suggested the idea of hospice care when Mrs. Wong stated that she wants to go home.

Nursing Diagnosis 1   *Compromised Family Coping* related to prolonged disease or disability progression that exhausts the supportive capacity of significant people as evidenced by Mr. Wong's looking exhausted.

Nursing Outcomes Classification (NOC)
Family Coping
Family Normalization

Nursing Interventions Classification (NIC)
Family Involvement Promotion
Family Support
Family Mobilization

PLANNING/GOALS	NURSING INTERVENTIONS	RATIONALE
Family will plan a rotation schedule to meet each one's needs for rest and support while caring for Mrs. Wong.	Provide empathy and support for the husband and daughters. Provide family with unlimited visitation, adequate space for members who stay overnight, and privacy.	Family is very important in the life of the Asian American. A sense of obligation to intervene and assist is highly valued. Casual help from strangers is avoided.
	Assess family members for signs of fatigue or overexertion.	Self-control and self-sufficiency are highly valued. Asking for help would mean loss of face and dignity.
	Explore with husband and daughters other support persons who would be willing and accepted by Mrs. Wong to keep her company.	Prolonged periods of unrelieved vigil will exhaust family members.
	Develop trusting and respectful relationships with Mrs. Wong and family members.	Asian Americans tend to be reserved with those whom they view as being in authority.
Client and family will maintain open communication.	Encourage Mr. Wong to discuss realistic plans and expectations of daughters, including health care providers as needed.	Asians traditionally value authoritarian styles of leadership, where the father makes unilateral family decisions.
Family will provide care without compromising their own physical and emotional health.	Assess if basic physical and emotional needs of Mrs. Wong and family are being met focusing on nonverbal clues.	Silent communication and stoic reactions to pain and other uncertain situations is common. Direct expression of negative feelings is unusual.
	Monitor ability of family members to carry out treatment plan and provide safe care.	Care is provided by family members who are exhausted, which is a safety issue.

EVALUATION   Husband and eldest daughter remain at bedside during daytime hours. Youngest exchanges places with the father and eldest sister at night. Mrs. Wong is agreeable. The entire family meets with the primary care nurse to discuss the plan of care. Mr. Wong and his daughters continue to provide the physical care for Mrs. Wong. The daughters express gratefulness that their father is stronger and has taken on the leadership role.

- The focus of nursing care is to help clients maintain their own beliefs when in a health care crisis. Those personal beliefs can be used to strengthen coping patterns.
- It is an important aspect of nursing to understand client differences.
- Response to health and illness varies depending on cultural origin.
- Providing culturally appropriate care begins with an understanding of the nurse's own cultural beliefs.
- Prerequisite to providing appropriate nursing care is performing a cultural assessment.

Review Questions

1. A mother is observed breastfeeding her 4-year-old son, a client in the hospital. The nurses talk in the nursing station about why a mother would continue to breastfeed a 4-year-old. They state that the American way is better. The nurses are expressing:

   a. stereotyping.
   b. ethnocentrism.
   c. acculturation.
   d. cultural diversity.

2. The nurse knows that the religious group teaching that physical healing comes exclusively through prayers and readings is:

   a. Hindu.
   b. Roman Catholic.
   c. Christian Science.
   d. Seventh Day Adventist.

3. A blood transfusion would most likely be refused by:

   a. Buddhist.
   b. Orthodox.
   c. American Indian.
   d. Jehovah's Witness.

4. The nursing diagnosis that might be used for a client who is hospitalized and has religious practices that conflict with hospital procedure is:

   a. *Religious Guilt.*
   b. *Guilt and Misery.*
   c. *Spiritual Distress.*
   d. *Spiritual Depression.*

5. If a client says to the nurse, "I need to pray with my group leader to get well," the most appropriate response for the nurse is:

   a. "May I call your group leader for you and ask her to visit you?"
   b. "The medications and treatment will make you well."
   c. "Why do you think your group leader is needed to make you well?"
   d. "When you are released from the hospital, you can go to your group leader and pray."

References/Suggested Readings

Andrews, M. M., & Boyle, J. S. (2003). *Transcultural concepts in nursing care* (4th ed.). Philadelphia: Lippincott Williams & Wilkins.

Andrews, M. M., & Hanson, P. (1999). Religion, culture, and nursing. In M. M. Andrews & J. S. Boyle (Eds.), *Transcultural concepts in nursing care* (3rd ed.). Philadelphia: Lippincott Williams & Wilkins.

Boyle, J. S. (1999). Culture and community. In M. M. Andrews & J. S. Boyle (Eds.), *Transcultural concepts in nursing care* (3rd ed.). Philadelphia: Lippincott Williams & Wilkins.

Clark, M. (1999). *Community Health Nursing Handbook.* New York: Prentice Hall.

Davidhizar, R., Dowd, S., & Giger, J. (1998). Educating the culturally diverse health care student. *Nurse Educator, 23*(2), 38–42.

Degazon, C. (2000). Cultural diversity and community health nursing practice. In M. Stanhope & J. Lancaster (Eds.), *Community & public health nursing* (5th ed.). St. Louis, MO: Mosby.

Dochterman, J., & Bulechek, G. (2004). *Nursing Interventions Classification (NIC)* (4th ed.). St. Louis, MO: Mosby.

Doherty, W. (1992). Private lives, public values. *Psychology Today, 25*(3), 27–32.

Doswell, W., & Erlen, J. (1998). Multicultural issues and ethical concerns in the delivery of nursing care interventions. *Nursing Clinics of North America, 33*(2), 353–361.

Edelman, C., & Mandle, C. (2002). *Health promotion throughout the lifespan* (5th ed.). St. Louis, MO: Mosby.

Edmission, K. W. (1997). Psychosocial dimensions of medical–surgical nursing. In J. M. Black & E. Matassarin-Jacobs (Eds.), *Medical surgical nursing: Clinical management for continuity of care.* (5th ed.). Philadelphia: W. B. Saunders.

Estin, P. (1999). Spotting depression in Asian patients. *RN, 62*(4), 39–40.

Fawcett, C. (1993). *Family psychiatric nursing.* St. Louis, MO: Mosby.

Giger, J., & Davidhizar, R. (2004). *Transcultural nursing: Assessment and intervention* (4th ed.). St. Louis, MO: Mosby–Yearbook.

Gonzalez, R. (1999). ANA advocates more diversity in nursing. *AJN, 99*(11), 24.

Gravely, S. (2001). When your patient speaks Spanish—and you don't. *RN, 64*(5), 65–67.

Grossman, D. (1996). Cultural dimensions in home health nursing. *AJN, 96*(7), 33–36.

Kelz, R. (1997). *Delmar's English–Spanish pocket dictionary for health professionals.* Clifton Park, NY: Thomson Delmar Learning.

Kelz, R. (1999). *Conversational Spanish for health professionals* (3rd ed.). Clifton Park, NY: Thomson Delmar Learning.

Kirkpatrick, M., Brown, S., & Atkins, T. (1998). Using the internet to integrate cultural diversity and global awareness. *Nurse Educator, 23*(2), 15–17.

Kudzma, E. C. (1999). Culturally competent drug administration. *AJN, 99*(8), 46–51.

Lee, E. (Ed.). (1997). *Working with Asian Americans: A guide for clinicians.* San Francisco: Richman Area Multi-Services.

Leininger, M. (2001). *Transcultural nursing: Concepts, theories, research, and practice.* (3rd ed.). New York: Glencoe McGraw Hill.

Lock, D. (1992). *Increasing multicultural understanding: A comprehensive model.* Newbury Park, CA: Sage.

Louie, K. B. (1999). Health promotion interventions for Asian American Pacific Islanders. In L. Zhan (Ed.), *Asian voices* (pp. 3–13). Boston: Jones & Bartlett.

Luckmann, J. (1999). *Transcultural communication in nursing.* Clifton Park, NY: Thomson Delmar Learning.

Malone, B. (1998). Diversity, divisiveness and divinity. *American Nurse, 30*(1), 5.

Mazanec, P., & Tyler, M. K. (2003). Cultural considerations in end-of-life care. *AJN, 103*(3), 50–57.

McCaffery, M., & Pasero, C. (1999). Pain control. *AJN, 99*(8), 18.

Moorhead, S., Johnson, M., & Maas, M. (2004). *Nursing Outcomes Classification (NOC)* (3rd ed.). St. Louis, MO: Mosby.

Morley, P., & Wallis, R. (Eds.). (1978). *Culture and curing: Anthropological perspectives on traditional medical beliefs and practices.* Pittsburgh, PA: University of Pittsburgh Press.

Mullins, M. (1999). Cultural awareness. *OB/GYN Nurse Forum, 7*, 3.

NewsWatch (2000). Delay in seeking MI treatment is tied to social factors. *RN, 63*(10), 20.

North American Nursing Diagnosis Association (NANDA). (2003). *Nursing diagnoses: Definitions & classifications 2003–2004,* Philadelphia: Author.

Providing culturally competent care. (2001). *Travel Nursing Today (A supplement to RN)* Sept. 2001, pp. 26–32.

Purnell, L., & Paulanka, B. (2003). *Transcultural health care: A culturally competent approach* (2nd ed.). Philadelphia: F. A. Davis.

Rivera-Andino, J., & Lopez, L. (2000). When culture complicates care. *RN, 63*(7), 47–49.

Shelley, J. (2000). *Spiritual care: A guide for caregivers.* Downers Grove, IL: Inter Varsity.

Smith, L. (1998). Concept analysis: Cultural competence. *Journal of Cultural Diversity, 5*(1), 4–10.

Spector, R. (2000). *Cultural care: Guides to heritage assessment and health traditions* (2nd ed.). Upper Saddle River, NJ: Prentice Hall.

Spector, R. E. (2000). *Cultural diversity in health and illness* (5th ed.). Upper Saddle River, NJ: Prentice Hall.

Spradley, B. W., & Allender, J. A. (2001). *Community health nursing: Concepts and practice* (5th ed.). Philadelphia: Lippincott Williams & Wilkins.

Stanhope, M., & Knollmueller, R. (2000). *Handbook of community-based and home health nursing practice* (3rd ed.). St. Louis, MO: Mosby.

Stanhope, M., & Lancaster, J. (2000). *Community & public health nursing* (5th ed.). St. Louis, MO: Mosby.

Sue, D. W., & Sue, D. (2003). *Counseling the culturally diverse: Theory and practice* (4th ed.). New York: Wiley.

U.S. Census Bureau. (2001). *Population estimates.* [Online]. Available: www.census.gov/population/estimates/nation/intfile3-1.txt

U.S. Department of Commerce, Bureau of the Census. (1999). *Statistical abstract of the United States: 1999* (112th ed.). Washington, DC: U.S. Government Printing Office.

Resources

Cultural Diversity in Health Care (video), *American Journal of Nursing,* 345 Hudson Street, New York, NY 10014

Language Line Services, 1 Lower Ragsdale Drive, Building 2, Monterey, CA 93940, 800-752-0093 Ext. 196, www.languageline.com

12

STRESS, ADAPTATION, AND ANXIETY

MAKING THE CONNECTION

Refer to the following chapters to increase your understanding of stress, adaptation, and anxiety:

Basic Nursing
- **Holistic Care**
- **Communication**
- **Complementary/Alternative Therapies**

- **Infection Control/Asepsis**
- **Pain Management**

LEARNING OBJECTIVES

Upon completion of this chapter, you should be able to:
- **Define key terms.**
- **Describe how stress, adaptation, and anxiety affect health.**
- **Identify factors that contribute to the stress response.**
- **Describe the general adaptation syndrome.**
- **Detail the effects of stress on the whole individual.**
- **Explain intrinsic stressors in the change process.**
- **Describe the role of the nurse as a change agent.**
- **Discuss nursing interventions that promote positive adaptation to stress.**
- **Develop an individualized plan for managing stress.**

KEY TERMS

adaptation	depersonalization
adaptive energy	distress
adaptive measures	endorphin
anxiety	eustress
burnout	fight-or-flight response
catharsis	general adaptation
change	syndrome (GAS)
change agent	homeostasis
cognitive reframing	local adaptation
conditioning	syndrome (LAS)
crisis	maladaptive measures
crisis intervention	stress
defense mechanisms	stressor

INTRODUCTION

Stress and anxiety are universal experiences that can be either a catalyst for positive change or a source of discomfort and pain. Nurses help clients cope with the stress of illness, disability, injury, or treatment approaches. Caring for clients experiencing a high level of anxiety can also be stressful for the nurse. Successful stress management is necessary for everyone's well-being. This chapter discusses the major concepts related to stress and anxiety, including strategies for coping with stress.

STRESS

According to Hans Selye (1974), **stress** is a nonspecific response to any demand made on the body. Selye termed such demands **stressors.** Any situation, event, or agent that produces stress is a stressor. A stressor is a stimulus that evokes the need to adapt. Stressors can be internal or external. For example, pain is an internal stressor, whereas loss of a job is an external stressor.

Even pleasant events can be stressful when they evoke the need to adapt. Stressors themselves are neutral, neither good nor bad. It is the individual's *perception* of the stressor that determines whether the effect is positive or negative. Any event can be stressful, depending on how the person views the event.

Responses to Stress

Adaptive energy is the term Selye coined to describe the inner force an individual uses to respond or adapt to stress. All persons have adaptive energy, but the amount of adaptive energy varies. When an individual has used all of his adaptive energy, illness, disease, or even death may result, as he is no longer able to adapt. Reactions to stress are typically categorized as either general (affecting the entire body) or local (affecting only the involved body part).

General Adaptation Syndrome

Stressors cause structural and chemical changes in the body as the body attempts to maintain **homeosta-** **sis,** which is the balance or equilibrium among the physiologic, psychological, sociocultural, intellectual, and spiritual needs of the body. Selye called these responses to stressors the **general adaptation syndrome** (GAS).

Selye divided the GAS into three stages, as illustrated in Figure 12-1. In the first stage, crisis or alarm, the body readies itself to handle the stressors. The physiologic changes may result in symptoms such as cool, pale skin; shivering; and sweating of the palms and soles of the

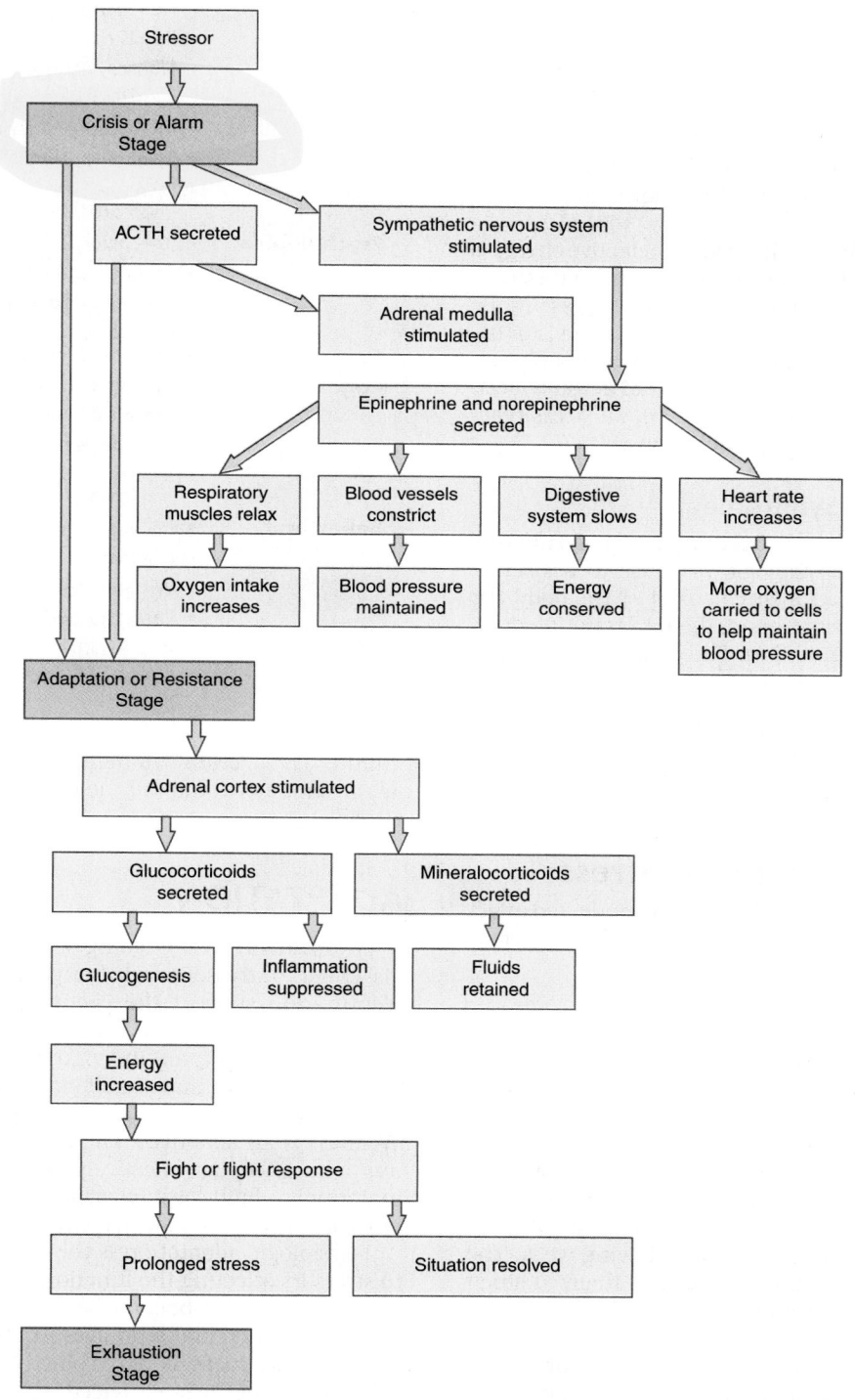

Figure 12-1 *Physiological Effects of the General Adaptation Syndrome (GAS) (Adapted from* Mental Health Concepts *[5th ed.], by C. Waughfield, 2002, Clifton Park, NY: Thomson Delmar Learning. Copyright 2002 by Thomson Delmar Learning.)*

TABLE 12-1 SIGNS AND SYMPTOMS OF STRESS

PROFESSIONAL TIP

Anticipatory Stress

Thoughts can be stressors that trigger the GAS, such as a person worrying about a situation. The body responds as if the person were *actually* experiencing the event, and the individual may feel ill, sweaty, nauseous, or very jittery.

TABLE 12-1 SIGNS AND SYMPTOMS OF STRESS

Physiologic	• Pulse rate increases
	• Blood pressure increases
	• Breathing is rapid, shallow
	• Blood thickens
	• Dizziness, sweaty palms
	• Headache
	• Pupils dilate
	• Nausea, change in appetite
	• Constipation or diarrhea
	• Increased urination
	• Twitching, trembling
	• Increased level of blood glucose and cortisol
Psychological	• Irritability
	• Feelings easily hurt
	• Sadness, depression
	• Feelings of pleasure and accomplishment reduced
Cognitive	• Impaired memory and judgment
	• Confusion, unable to concentrate
	• Poor decision making
	• Altered perceptions, delayed response
Behavioral	• Pacing, rapid speech
	• Insomnia
	• Withdrawal
	• Easily startled
Spiritual	• Alienation, social isolation
	• Feeling of emptiness

feet. Severe stress may cause dilated pupils, dry mouth, pounding heart, nausea, and diarrhea.

During the second stage, adaptation or resistance, the body attempts to defend against the stressor through the **fight-or-flight response.** The body becomes physiologically ready to defend itself by either fighting or fleeing from the stressor.

The third stage, exhaustion, occurs if adaptive energy is inadequate to deal with prolonged or overwhelming stress.

The physiologic reactions of the body are essentially the same no matter what the source of the stress. For example, an imagined stressor will have the same physiologic response (GAS) as if the stressor had actually been experienced. According to Selye (1976), all stress reactions exhibit similar physiologic reactions.

Local Adaptation Syndrome

Selye also described the **local adaptation syndrome** (LAS), which is the physiologic response to a stressor (e.g., trauma, illness) on a specific part of the body. For example, if a person cuts a hand, the LAS is initiated, inducing localized inflammation. The classic symptoms of inflammation (redness, swelling, and warmth) occur at the injured site. The LAS is usually a temporary process that resolves when the traumatized area is restored to its preinjury state; however, if the inflammation does not resolve with the LAS, the individual then experiences the GAS as the entire body becomes affected.

Signs and Symptoms of Stress

The signs and symptoms of stress are many and affect every dimension of a person. Common signs and symptoms of stress are outlined in Table 12-1.

Outcomes of Stress

Experiencing stress provides the individual with two possibilities: (1) an opportunity for personal growth or (2) the risk of disorganization and distress. When stressors are handled appropriately, adaptation is attained, and the body returns to normal.

The term **eustress** describes a type of stress resulting in positive outcomes. Consider for example, students who have an examination scheduled the following week. The stress over the impending test motivates them to study early, and they pass the examination. This stress was positive because it motivated them to study (an example of growth) and resulted in positive or desired outcomes.

Stressors evoking an ineffective response cause **distress.** For example, students who have a scheduled examination the next day put studying off until the last

minute. They "cram" all night, do not know the material, are not alert, and fail the examination; they experience distress.

ADAPTATION

Adaptation is an ongoing process whereby individuals adjust to stressors and change. The nurse's goal is to identify and support the client's positive adaptive responses. Adaptation is a holistic response that involves all dimensions of an individual. Individuals seek to maintain a steady state in all dimensions of life: physiologic, psychological, cognitive, social, and spiritual. Wellness is an adaptive state; that is, the well person is one who is coping effectively with stressors and thus maintains a high level of wellness. Adaptation may be physiologic, psychological, cognitive, social, or spiritual.

Physiologic adaptation is the way the body responds to stressors affecting the functioning of the body. It may involve the entire body (GAS) or only a specific area (LAS). An individual who lives in the mountains (high elevation) produces more red blood cells to carry enough oxygen to meet the body's needs. The chest also enlarges to allow the lungs to expand to accommodate the needed exchange of oxygen and carbon dioxide.

Psychological adaptation involves the use of defense mechanisms and learning to mentally accept new situations. A person's hardiness includes a sense of commitment, challenge, and control (Kobasa, 1979). A 55-year-old worker who suddenly finds himself unemployed will need to learn to adapt psychologically to the new situation and decide which steps to take next.

Cognitive adaptation involves education, communication, problem-solving ability, and perception of people and the world. A person gains these methods throughout life. For example, the high-school student will have a different perspective of the world and different problem-solving abilities than will this same individual as a college graduate.

Social adaptation involves social relationships with family, friends, and coworkers who may provide support in times of stress. A person unable to cope may withdraw socially. An example of social adaptation would be a family moving to a new town and making new friends and modifying relationships with existing friends.

Spiritual adaptation involves beliefs about a supreme being and a positive sense of life's purpose and meaning. These beliefs are a personal resource for coping with stressors. Following the loss of a loved one, for instance, a family's spirituality and sense of faith may undergo changes.

Coping Measures

Coping measures include all the ways an individual may react to stress. Stress is an automatic response, but individuals can learn to conserve their adaptive energy through conditioning. **Conditioning** occurs when a person is taught a behavior until it becomes an automatic response. Some individuals who are conditioned to do so can handle a great deal of stress, whereas others cannot handle even a small amount of stress. Other factors that affect an individual's ability to cope with stress are the following:

- Degree of danger perceived by the individual
- Immediate needs of the individual
- Amount of support from others
- Individual's belief in his own ability to handle the stressful situation
- Individual's previous successes and failures in coping
- Number of concurrent or cumulative stresses being handled by the individual (Waughfield, 2002)

Adaptive Measures

Measures for coping with stress that require a minimal amount of energy are called **adaptive measures.** They deal directly with the stressful situation or the

LIFE CYCLE CONSIDERATIONS

Coping Ability

An individual's ability to cope with stressors depends in part on age and developmental level.

CULTURAL CONSIDERATIONS

Adaptive Measures

Nurses must be sensitive to the fact that culture and ethnicity may influence an individual's choice of coping mechanisms. For instance, moaning and chanting may be an expected response to stress in some cultures; the nurse must be careful to view this behavior not as maladaptive, but as a culturally healthy response to a stressor.

symptoms thereof. Adaptive measures useful in dealing with stressful situations include:

- Using support people
- Relaxing to relieve tension
- Changing behavior
- Developing more realistic goals
- Solving problems

Defense Mechanisms

Just as the body has physiologic mechanisms (e.g., the immune system, the inflammatory response) to defend against infection and disease, the mind has psychological protective mechanisms. Most **defense mechanisms** are unconscious functions protecting the mind from anxiety. They are used to gain and maintain psychological homeostasis. The individual does not consciously decide to use a defense mechanism; it happens automatically.

Everyone uses defense mechanisms. Their use does not imply mental illness or psychosocial imbalance. Defense mechanisms are only considered maladaptive when they are the only way an individual responds to a threat or when they limit the individual's ability to function. Table 12-2 describes and gives examples of various defense mechanisms.

Maladaptive Measures

Measures used to avoid conflict and stress are considered **maladaptive measures,** because they prevent the individual from making progress toward resolving and accepting stress. They may include somatic disorders (transferring stress to an organ as pain), rituals, excessive use of alcohol or drugs, excessive eating, or withdrawal from reality.

PROFESSIONAL TIP

Defense Mechanisms

The nurse who is unfamiliar with defense mechanisms may be judgmental about clients who do not respond as the nurse expects. If the nurse tries to break through a client's denial (defense mechanism) too quickly by presenting reality, the client may be overwhelmed by anxiety and will panic.

TABLE 12-2   DEFENSE MECHANISMS

DEFENSE MECHANISM	DESCRIPTION	EXAMPLE
Denial	Refusal to acknowledge the reality of threatening situations despite factual evidence	A person with heart disease continues to eat fatty foods and fried foods, despite medical advice to the contrary.
Displacement	Transfer of feelings or reactions from one object to another object, usually one that is "safer"	A husband who is angry with his wife yells at the dog instead of dealing with his anger at his wife.
Projection	Attribution of one's own thoughts, feelings, or impulses to others	An adolescent who does not want to go with the crowd states, "My parents won't let me go."
Rationalization	Intellectual explanation or justification of ideas, feelings, or behavior	A student responds after failing a test that "The test had many trick questions on it; I really know the material."
Reaction formation	Expression of a feeling that is the opposite of one's real feeling	A client brings a gift to a nurse with whom he is really angry.
Regression	A return to a previous developmental level	A child who has not sucked her thumb in 2 years starts to do so again when admitted to the hospital.
Repression	The unconscious blocking from awareness of material that is painful or threatening	Adult's claim, despite evidence, that "I never got angry with my parents; we lived in love and harmony."
Suppression	A conscious or unconscious attempt to keep threatening or unpleasant material out of consciousness	Failure to remember a house fire during childhood.
Sublimation	Channeling of socially unacceptable impulses into socially acceptable activities	A young man who deals with aggression by playing football.

Adapted from *Psychiatric Mental Health Nursing* (2nd ed.), by N. Frisch and L. Frisch, 2002, Clifton Park, NY: Thomson Delmar Learning. Copyright 2002 by Thomson Delmar Learning.

Crisis

A crisis occurs when stressors surpass the ability to cope. A **crisis** (an acute state of disorganization) occurs when the usual coping mechanisms are no longer adequate. Crisis is characterized by extreme anxiety, disorganized behavior, and inability to function. A crisis is time limited because no one can stay in acute disequilibrium for a long time and experience the great discomfort. Given the time-limited nature of crisis, a client in crisis needs immediate intervention for a successful resolution. Crisis intervention is discussed later in this chapter.

Crisis can be a negative experience, but it can also present an opportunity for growth and learning. The outcome depends on each individual's perception and coping abilities. Nurses can guide clients to discover opportunities in the crisis and adapt in positive, healthy ways.

Stressful events do not always result in a crisis. A crisis is *not* a mental illness, even though persons experiencing the acute anxiety and discomfort fear for their sanity. Each crisis is unique to the individual; however, crises have common characteristics (Table 12-3).

TABLE 12-3   CRISIS CHARACTERISTICS

- A loss, actual or perceived, is a part of every crisis.
- A crisis occurs suddenly.
- A crisis has a known precipitating event.
- The situation is seen as overwhelming or life threatening.
- Communication becomes impaired.
- Usual coping skills cannot resolve the situation.
- Intervention is required to reestablish equilibrium.

Data from *Contemporary Psychiatric-Mental Health Nursing*, by H. S. Wilson, C. R. Kneisl, and E. Trigoboff, 2003, Upper Saddle River, NJ: Prentice Hall. Copyright 2003 by Prentice Hall.

ANXIETY

Anxiety is a subjective response that occurs when a person experiences a real or perceived threat to well-being; it is a diverse feeling of dread or apprehension. There is a close relationship between anxiety and stress. Anxiety is the psychological response to a threat, such as the worry that results when oversleeping on a work day. This worry can translate into stress (the person's physiologic response to a stimulus) by rushing, perspiring, and becoming careless. Anxiety can be an activator of stress *and* a response to stress: It is usually activated by stress and may lead to more stress. Anxiety is a major component of mental health disturbances.

The most common emotional (affective) response to stress is anxiety. Individuals feel anxious when they are threatened, even if the threat is only perceived. Anxiety occurs on a continuum; some degree of anxiety is beneficial as a motivator. A high level of anxiety, however, can overpower a person and diminish the ability to function and think. The person is less able to function as the level of anxiety increases (Figure 12-2). Table 12-4 describes the levels of anxiety.

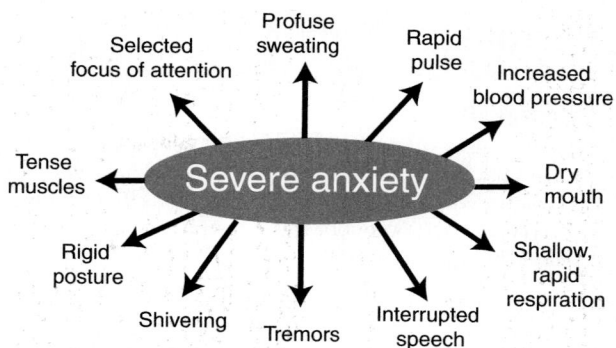

Figure 12-2 *Physical and Mental Responses to Severe Anxiety (From* Mental Health Concepts *[5th ed.], by C. Waughfield, 2002, Clifton Park, NY: Thomson Delmar Learning. Copyright 2002 by Thomson Delmar Learning.)*

EFFECTS OF AND ON ILLNESS

Anxiety often increases during illness and recovery. It is often difficult to determine whether illness or stress came first. Illness occurs when adaptive attempts are unsuccessful. Also, an ill person has fewer usable adaptive resources to cope with stressors. Some stressors may not directly cause disease, but stress is a substantial aspect in the onset and progress of many illnesses. Some disorders commonly associated with stress include:

- Arrhythmias
- Asthma
- Back pain
- Decreased libido
- Diabetes
- Eating disorders
- Eczema
- Emphysema
- Fertility problems
- Headache
- Hives
- Hypertension

TABLE 12-4 LEVELS OF ANXIETY		
ANXIETY LEVEL	**CHARACTERISTICS OF THE ANXIOUS PERSON**	**NURSING CONSIDERATIONS**
Mild	• Increased degree of alertness • Increased vigilance • Increased motivation • Readiness for action • Slight increase in vital signs	• Best time for client teaching.
Moderate	• Subjective distress (tension) • Decreased perception and attention • Alert only to specific information • Possible tendency to complain or argue • Possible headache, diarrhea, nausea, or vomiting	• Assist client in determining cause and effect between stressor and anxiety.
Severe	• Increased subjective distress • Feeling of impending danger • Selective attention • Distorted communication • Distorted perception • Feelings of fatigue	• Encourage verbalization. • Encourage motor activity (walking, exercise). • Give specific directions.
Panic	• Major perceptual distortion • Immobilization; inability to function • Feelings of terror • Possible harm to self and others	• Provide guidelines and limits. • Maintain client safety (both physical and psychological).

Data from *Interpersonal Relations in Nursing*, by H. E. Peplau, 1952, New York: Putnam. Copyright 1952 by Putnam; and *The Interpersonal Theory of Psychiatry*, by L. S. Sullivan, 1953, New York: Norton. Copyright 1953 by Norton.

- Impotence
- Irritable bowel syndrome
- Menstrual disorders
- Periodontal disease
- Psoriasis
- Ulcers
- Viral activation, herpes or HIV
- Weight gain or loss

The immune system is impaired during prolonged periods of stress. Steroid production increases as the body fights the perceived or actual threat. Steroids reduce the immune system's ability to function, and the body is less able to protect itself from disease.

All clients in a health care facility have a change in their routine, which may cause anxiety and stress. The unfamiliar environment, loss of control over their schedule, and dependence on others for care are issues with which these clients must cope. Each issue is a stressor requiring adaptation by the client to maintain homeostasis. Some clients do not have the adaptive energy to cope with the many changes and cope with their illness. Cues that a person may not be coping well to hospitalization include:

- Increased stress response
- High level of anxiety
- Increased use of coping mechanisms
- Inability to function
- Disorganized behavior

The person having "minor" surgery at an outpatient center, the adolescent being treated by the school nurse, or the employee being treated at an industrial clinic for a work-related injury may also experience client role stressors. Even clients who are treated in their homes may experience stressors from having a health care provider in their personal environment.

The greater the threat (or perceived threat), the higher the level of anxiety. Nurses must be sensitive to stress and many changes caused by illness. This reduces the risk of depersonalizing the client.

Depersonalization is the process of treating an individual as an object instead of a person. It takes away a client's individuality by treating him as a thing. Nursing

interventions focus on assisting the client to lessen feelings of loss of control.

CHANGE

Change, a dynamic process whereby an individual's response to a stressor leads to an alteration in behavior, is an inevitable part of life. Whether change is planned or unplanned, it is inevitable and constant. Change can be stressful to individuals and activate the GAS. Characteristics of change are that it:

- May be eustressful or distressful.
- Can be externally imposed or self-initiated.
- Can occur abruptly or have a gradual onset.
- Requires energy to effect, as well as to resist.

All health care providers should know how to initiate and cope with change. Critical-thinking and problem-solving skills are needed to effectively initiate and cope with change.

Types of Change

Change may be unplanned or planned. Unplanned change is unpredictable and may be imposed by others or by uncontrollable events (e.g., losing one's home in a fire). Planned change is a specific effort to modify a situation. A marriage is an example of a planned change. In addition to planned change and unplanned change, there are other types of change.

Developmental changes are physical and emotional alterations occurring at different stages of life. These are usually predictable and occur in a certain order. For instance, a baby will first learn to roll over, then crawl, then walk. The exact age will vary, but the sequence usually does not.

Accidental or reactive changes are adaptive responses to change imposed by others. This may include a change in one's working hours or a child's baseball game being rescheduled.

Covert changes are often subtle and occur without a person's conscious awareness. These might include a gradual shifting of responsibilities as new skills are acquired or developed at work.

Figure 12-3 *Through talking, listening, and touch, the nurse can help relieve the client's feelings of anxiety.*

Overt changes are obvious and identifiable, and an individual is aware they are occurring. They are usually not under an individual's direct control, such as the restructuring of one's place of employment, but must be adapted to and accepted in order to continue functioning effectively.

Resistance to Change

People tend to resist change because of the energy required to adapt, although energy is also required to resist change, or to maintain the status quo. The ability to tolerate (or even thrive on) change differs in individuals. There are no guarantees that change will lead to a positive outcome. Uncertainty regarding outcome is a major barrier to change.

It is risky to challenge one's own ideas or those of others by initiating change. Questioning is one of the first signs of the need for change. The nurse who wonders "Why?" "What if?" or "Why not?" will likely risk initiating change. Successful risk takers consider the costs and benefits of their ideas and the outcomes relative to available resources.

Because change is inevitable, nurses must learn ways to deal with change. Resistance looks like the individual is rejecting proposed new ideas without critically thinking about the proposal. Nurses must take time to research ideas and make informed decisions as to whether change is worthwhile. Coping with change calls for adaptability, flexibility, and resilience.

Nurse as Change Agent

The nurse often serves as a **change agent** (a person who intentionally creates and implements change). Change agents seek ways to make improvements using critical thinking to develop innovative, creative solutions.

Change should be planned by individuals who are proactive. The proactive individual initiates action rather than waiting for others to solve problems, make decisions, or become rescuers. Reactive persons, on the other hand, respond only to externally imposed change. Proactive nurses are change agents who often affect the entire health care system as well as individual clients.

Change agents work toward a positive outcome. Client education is a powerful tool for initiating change. The client is provided with an opportunity to change when taught a disease process, a treatment modality, or a lifestyle alteration. Learning results in behavioral changes. The change process is similar to the nursing process, in that change involves assessment, planning, decision making, implementation, and evaluation.

NURSING PROCESS

Nurses can be instrumental in helping clients both understand their anxiety and learn measures to cope with and control their feelings of stress.

Assessment

The nurse must first ascertain the anxious client's perception of the situation. This is accomplished by directly asking the client and then listening carefully to the client's response. Nurses must be aware of their own body language because the nurse's nonverbal behavior can affect the client's anxiety level. Anxiety is a subjective experience and cannot be directly observed. The nurse must therefore look for signs of anxiety (refer back to Table 12-4).

A thorough assessment of stress and anxiety levels includes asking the client about:

- Types or patterns of stressors
- Usual response to stressful situations
- Cause-and-effect relationships among stressors and thoughts, feelings, and behaviors
- History of successful coping

The client's coping abilities can be assessed in various ways. Open-ended questions can be used to ascertain previously used coping mechanisms. Some sample questions are:

- What is the problem?
- What have you tried before?
- How well did it work?

Appropriate nursing diagnoses and an effective plan of care can be established by identifying the client's coping abilities. Assessment provides the data necessary for identifying nursing diagnoses.

Nursing Diagnosis

Several nursing diagnoses may apply to clients experiencing anxiety; the most common of these are *Anxiety; Ineffective Coping; Ineffective Denial;* and *Powerlessness.* Additional North American Nursing Diagnosis Association (NANDA, 2003) diagnoses that may also apply include:

- *Impaired Adjustment*
- *Ineffective Role Performance*
- *Disturbed Thought Processes*
- *Defensive Coping*
- *Fear*
- *Post-Trauma Syndrome*
- *Impaired Social Interaction*
- *Spiritual Distress*
- *Hopelessness*

- *Fatigue*
- *Disturbed Sleep Pattern*

Planning/Outcome Identification

Involving clients in planning care is essential because helping clients learn to cope successfully is part of the empowerment process. Planning means exploring with the client self-responsibility issues. A major goal for working with an anxious client is to reduce anxiety so problem solving and learning can occur.

There may be many expected outcomes (goals) appropriate for clients experiencing stress or anxiety. A few basic goals are for the client to:

- Identify situations when stress and anxiety increase.
- Describe ways to decrease the effects of usual stressors.
- Identify positive and negative stressors in the client's life.
- Group stressors into categories: ones that can be eliminated, ones that can be controlled, and ones that cannot be controlled directly by self.
- Demonstrate correct use of select stress-management exercises (e.g., progressive muscle relaxation, guided imagery, thought stopping).
- Describe plan for managing stress, including lifestyle modifications.

 Safety: The Client Experiencing Panic
Never leave a panic-stricken client alone. The client with panic-level anxiety may harm self. Stay with this client or have someone else do so.

Implementation

Teaching is part of holistic nursing practice. Stress management methods can be taught to clients of every age and developmental stage in all health care settings.

A major step in improving self-care is to teach clients how to reduce their own stress level. Education gives clients options. Clients who understand their options can make informed decisions (Figure 12-4). Some of the many interventions that may assist the anxious clients follow.

Meet Basic Needs

Stress and basic physiologic needs are closely related. Anything interfering with the basic needs being met elicits the stress response, causing anxiety. Clients who are in pain, cold, or hungry have a higher anxiety level than when comfortable. The perception of pain increases with a higher level of anxiety. The nurse actually improves the potential for recovery by reducing client anxiety.

Minimize Environmental Stimuli

An individual's immediate environment can influence stress levels. The nurse should decrease environmental stimuli that may cause anxiety. Environmental stimuli can be reduced by:

- Closing the client's room door
- Turning the television off
- Reducing loudness of the telephone ringer or disconnecting the phone, if feasible
- Dimming the lights or closing the blinds

Figure 12-4 *The nurse discusses the options for care and provides the client with the information needed to plan effective lifestyle changes.*

- Limiting the number of visitors (unless isolation increases the client's anxiety)

Verbalize Feelings

Encouraging clients to express their feelings is especially helpful to reduce stress. Freud (1959) described the process of talking out one's feelings as a **catharsis.** People seem to instinctively know the value of "getting things off their chest." Verbalizing promotes relaxation because (1) a verbalized feeling becomes real, and an identified problem can be dealt with and (2) the activity of talking uses energy and reduces anxiety.

Involve Family/Significant Others

The type of intervention for managing stress is influenced by the client's developmental stage. All ages of children need and rely on their parents or caretakers for security and support (Fennell, 1999). Because families provide essential support for clients, it is important to include the entire family in the care of the client whenever possible (Figure 12-5) to decrease the stress level of everyone involved.

Family members who are anxious may have a negative impact on the client's health status. One way nurses must often help family members relax is to provide information and explanations. Researchers have concluded that both the client and family benefit from family presence during invasive procedures and resuscitation (Meyers, et al., 2000).

Use Stress-Management Techniques

A variety of stress-management techniques can easily be taught to clients, families, and significant others. Some of the most common approaches for managing stress are discussed following.

Exercise A powerful way to reduce anxiety is physical exercise. The need for incorporating exercise into one's lifestyle should be emphasized in client teaching. To establish an exercise program:

- Explore the different exercise programs available.
- Ask a health care provider about the safety of a specific exercise program.

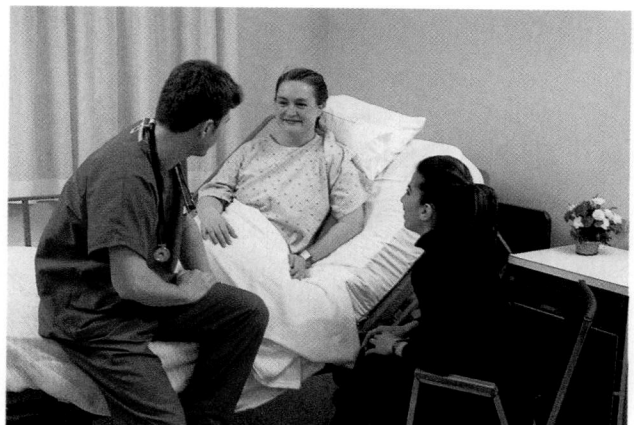

Figure 12-5 *The nurse encourages interaction between client and family members and significant others. This involvement helps ease the client's anxiety and keeps the family informed about the client's cares.*

- Set realistic goals.
- Select a routine allowing warm-up and cool-down periods.
- Take up activities that increase heart rate for a period of time.

If exercise is to reduce anxiety, it must be done on a regular, ongoing basis. Physiologic benefits of regular exercise are listed in Table 12-5 and include:

- Feelings of well-being are enhanced.
- Concentration and memory improve.
- Depression is lessened.
- Insomnia is lessened.

CLIENT TEACHING

Cognitive Reframing or Thought Stopping

- Listen to self-talk (thoughts).
- Identify negative self-talk.
- Do something physical when a negative thought is detected to stop the train of thought, such as clapping your hands or snapping a rubber band on your wrist.
- Replace the negative thought with one that is both realistic and positive.

   Like all other relaxation exercises, thought stopping becomes more effective with repetition.

- Dependence on external stimulants or relaxants is reduced.
- Self-esteem increases.
- Sense of self-control over anxiety is renewed.

Relaxation Techniques Several techniques can help individuals relax (Figure 12-6). Complementary and alternative interventions such as progressive muscle relaxation and guided imagery are useful in helping clients learn to relax. Meditation and hypnosis can also be very effective in inducing relaxation and relieving stress.

Cognitive Reframing or Thought Stopping Cognitive reframing is a technique based on Aaron Beck's (1976) theory that a person's emotional response to an event is determined by the meaning attached to it. For example, the client is likely to feel anxious if an event is perceived as threatening. The client will be less anxious if the interpretation of the event can be modified.

TABLE 12-5   PHYSIOLOGICAL BENEFITS OF EXERCISE

EFFECT OF EXERCISE	PHYSIOLOGICAL BENEFIT
Promotes metabolism of adrenalin and thyroxine	• Minimizes autonomic arousal and hypervigilance
Reduces musculoskeletal tension	• Decreases feelings of being tense and "uptight"
Improves circulation, resulting in better oxygenation of the brain	• Increases alertness and concentration, and leads to enhanced problem-solving ability
Stimulates **endorphin** (a group of opiate-like substances produced naturally by the brain) production	• Raises the body's pain threshold, and promotes a sense of well-being
Reduces cholesterol level	• Decreases the risk of atherosclerosis
Reduces blood pressure	• Decreases the risk of myocardial infarction (heart attack) and cerebral vascular accident (CVA) (stroke)
Stimulates elimination (through lungs, skin, bowels)	• Reduces toxin buildup in the body.

From *Nutrition, Exercise, and Movement,* by L. Keegan, 2000, in B. Dossey, L. Keegan, & C. Guzzetta (Eds.), *Holistic Nursing: A Handbook for Practice* (3rd ed.), Gaithersburg, MD: Aspen. Copyright 2000 by Aspen; and *Health Promotion and the Individual,* by C. Mandle and R. Gruber-Wood, 2002, in C. Edelman and C. Mandle (Eds.), *Health Promotion Throughout the Lifespan* (5th ed.), St. Louis, MO: Mosby. Copyright 2002 by Mosby.

Figure 12-6 *The nurse demonstrates the technique of progressive muscle relaxation in a client-education program.*

Reframing is used to alter one's perceptions and interpretations by changing one's thoughts.

Crisis Intervention

Some clients will be in an acute crisis state and require **crisis intervention,** a specific technique to help a person regain equilibrium. Crisis intervention views individuals as capable of personal growth and able to influence and control their own lives (Kneisl & Riley, 1996). The five steps of crisis intervention are:

1. Identify the specific problem, including the underlying issues.
2. Identify all possible options.
3. Examine possible outcomes for each option and select an option.
4. Implement the selected option.
5. Evaluate the overall effectiveness of the plan.

Clients sometimes need more assistance than the nurse is able to provide. Prompt consultation with or referral to other health care providers is necessary, such as:

- Psychiatric clinical nurse specialists
- Nurse psychotherapists
- Psychologists
- Psychiatrists
- Social workers
- Clergy or other counselors

Evaluation

Evaluation of the client's coping abilities must include client input. The nurse must evaluate client outcomes as well as nursing care. The family can also be a valuable source of information about the effectiveness of the stress-reduction approaches.

STRESS MANAGEMENT FOR THE NURSE

There are many stressors in nursing. It is essential that nurses learn to cope successfully with the stressors

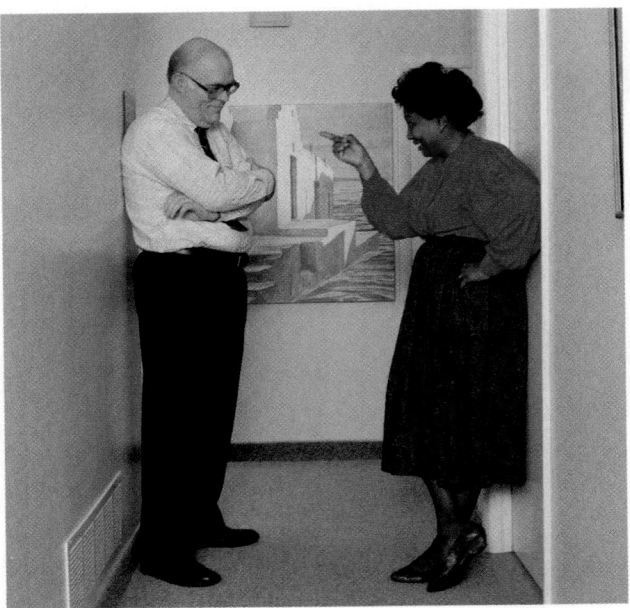

Figure 12-7 *Sharing a light and humorous moment with a friend is a wonderful way to relieve stress and regain perspective.*

(Figure 12-7). Nurses must cope successfully with stress to maintain their own wellness and to model healthy behaviors. Nurses must first be able to manage their own stress before helping clients learn to manage theirs. High stress levels among nurses often lead to **burnout,** a state of physical and emotional exhaustion occurring when caregivers use up their adaptive energy. Nurses experiencing such an overwhelming degree of stress often treat clients in a depersonalizing manner. These nurses also lack feelings of personal accomplishment. Burnout imposes a high price on individual nurses and on the profession as highly qualified professionals leave nursing. The quality of care declines as a result.

Several work-related factors can contribute to burnout:

- Heavy workload (critically ill clients)
- Interpersonal conflict in the work environment
- Mandatory overtime and "floating" to other units
- Little work-related social support

Stress management is the key to burnout prevention and recovery. A stress-management plan begins with

CRITICAL THINKING ?

Burnout

A client is exhibiting panic-level anxiety and should not be left alone. You are experiencing severe burnout because of very long work hours and recent stressful situations. Your stress level is so high that you feel you cannot stay in the room with this client. If you leave the room to find another nurse to stay with him, he may injure himself; if you stay, you risk your own emotional well-being. How do you deal with this situation?

TABLE 12-6	STRATEGIES FOR MANAGING PROFESSIONAL STRESS

STRATEGY	RATIONALE
Develop active support systems at work and away from work.	Non–health care provider friends help maintain a balance in life.
Use time management and decision-making methods.	Viewing personal needs as a priority encourages one to schedule time to meet those needs. Breaking down large tasks into small, realistic ones prevents being overwhelmed.
Focus on accomplishments.	Increases self-esteem.
Know personal limits.	Helps separate the important from the less important.
Avoid harmful substances.	Smoking, overeating, and intake of caffeine, alcohol, or other substances often increase stress and anxiety in the long run.
Nourish the body with healthy diet, exercise, and sleep.	A healthy mind and body is better able to handle stress.
Practice slow, focused breathing.	Muscle tension is alleviated with more oxygen in the blood.
Vary tasks between mental and physical activities.	Conserves energy, reduces fatigue, and maintains a sense of balance.
Maintain a sense of humor.	Helps keep a positive outlook; can be used to reframe a situation.

CRITICAL THINKING

Self-Care

Society often labels people who take care of themselves as selfish. Do you agree? Why or why not? Consider how taking care of yourself can help you be a better care provider. What are some specific things you can do now to take better care of yourself?

- *Commitment:* Become involved in what one is doing.
- *Challenge:* Perceive change as an opportunity for growth instead of an obstacle or threat.
- *Control:* Believe that one is directing what happens to oneself rather than feeling victimized and helpless.

According to studies (Kobasa, 1979; Kobasa, Maddi, & Kahn, 1982), persons having higher degrees of hardiness are healthier than those with low degrees of hardiness. When experiencing multiple stressors, such people develop fewer illnesses.

Many nurses must learn when to stop working and relearn the value of play. Nursing students, spending many hours working and studying, may need to schedule play time. The student nurse doing so is making a start on managing stress.

Summary

- Stress is an individual's physiologic response to a demand made on the body.
- Individuals experiencing prolonged periods of stress risk developing stress-related diseases.
- Anxiety, the psychological response to a real or perceived threat to the health and well-being of an individual, activates the stress response.
- An individual seeks equilibrium through adaptation. When adaptation is effective, homeostasis is maintained.
- The general adaptation syndrome (GAS), the physiologic response to stress, consists of three stages: alarm, resistance, and exhaustion. The GAS is the same whether the stressor is actual or imagined, present or potential.
- Major stressors for clients and their families are illness and hospitalization. To alleviate the stress of hospitalization, nursing interventions should reduce the client's feelings of unfamiliarity and loss of control.
- Change can be perceived as stressful because of a fear of failure, a threat to security, or a potential for loss of self-esteem.
- Burnout occurs when the nurse is overwhelmed by stress, resulting in physical, emotional, and behavioral dysfunction, including decreased productivity.
- A stress-management plan for nurses involves maintaining support systems; using time-management and decision-making skills; maintaining a sense of humor and knowing personal limits.

self-awareness. It is a continuous process, not the occasional use of a technique or exercise. Nurses often fail to take care of themselves, but it is essential that nurses learn to care for themselves.

There are many strategies to help nurses manage professional and personal stress, as outlined in Table 12-6.

Nurses who cultivate the hardiness factor will likely be resilient to stress. Kobasa (1979) put forth the concept of hardiness in the late 1970s. Hardiness consists of a set of attitudes, beliefs, and behaviors that make individuals more resilient (or hardy) to the negative effects of stress. The three components to stress hardiness are:

SAMPLE NURSING CARE PLAN

THE CLIENT EXPERIENCING SEVERE ANXIETY

Shari is a 38-year-old female in the emergency department of the local hospital. She paces, wrings her hands, and is tearful. She says she has chest pressure, palpitations, and shortness of breath. She is diaphoretic and her hands are trembling. Her blood pressure is 140/90, pulse 110, and respirations 30 and shallow. She says that her husband left her a month ago. She states, "I feel like I'm going crazy! My heart is racing and I can't sit still."

Assessment reveals autonomic hyperactivity (rapid pulse and respirations, elevated blood pressure), verbalized feelings of apprehension, restlessness, and going crazy.

Nursing Diagnosis: *Anxiety* related to situational crisis, threat to self-concept, and change in role status as evidenced by statement "I feel like I'm going crazy" and the fact that husband left her a month ago

Nursing Outcomes Classification (NOC)
Anxiety Control
Coping
Psychosocial Adjustment: Life Change

Nursing Interventions Classification (NIC)
Anxiety Reduction
Coping Enhancement
Simple Relaxation Therapy

PLANNING/GOALS	NURSING INTERVENTION	RATIONALE
Shari will identify effective coping mechanisms.	Establish a trusting relationship.	Reduces anxiety.
	Have Shari identify and describe physical and emotional feelings.	Is the first step in coping with anxiety.
	Help Shari relate cause-and-effect relationship between stressors and anxiety.	Enhances Shari's sense of power and control over the situation.
	Encourage Shari to use previously successful coping mechanisms.	Builds confidence in own coping abilities.
Shari will report that anxiety has lessened and is manageable.	Using therapeutic communication techniques, encourage Shari to talk about what has been happening in her life.	Clarifies situation by talking about it.
Shari will demonstrate relaxation skills.	Teach Shari relaxation techniques (such as cognitive reframing and imagery).	Counters the physiologic effects of the stress response (lower blood pressure, decreased heart rate, and respirations).

EVALUATION   Shari looks relaxed. Vital signs are within normal limits. Shari verbalizes that she feels calmer and no longer afraid that she is "going crazy."

Review Questions

1. The body's reaction to any demand made on it (stimulus) is called:
   a. stress.
   b. anxiety.
   c. stressor.
   d. stress response.

2. The general adaptation syndrome (GAS) is the:
   a. behavioral response to stress.
   b. sociocultural response to stress.
   c. psychological response to stress.
   d. physiologic response to stress.

3. The level of anxiety best for client learning is:
   a. no anxiety.
   b. mild anxiety.
   c. severe anxiety.
   d. moderate anxiety.

4. The purpose of the first stage of the GAS is to:
   a. alert the individual to danger.
   b. determine the cause of the danger.
   c. mobilize energy needed for adaptation.
   d. prevent the individual from having an unpleasant experience.

5. Coping mechanisms to avoid dealing directly with stress are called:

    a. adaptive measures.

    b. maladaptive measures.

    c. nonadaptive measures.

    d. progressive measures.

References/Suggested Readings

Aguilera, D. C. (1998). *Crisis intervention: Theory and methodology* (8th ed.). St. Louis, MO: Mosby.

Alfaro-LeFevre, R. (2004). *Critical thinking and clinical judgment* (3rd ed.). Philadelphia: W. B. Saunders.

American Institute of Stress (AIS). (2002a). *America's #1 health problem.* [Online]. Available: www.stress.org/problem.htm

American Institute of Stress (AIS). (2002b). *Job stress.* [Online]. Available: www.stress.org/job.htm

American Institute of Stress (AIS). (2002c). *Stress.* [Online]. Available: www.stress.org

Badger, J. M. (1995). Tips for managing stress on the job. *AJN, 95*(9), 31–33.

Beck, A. (1976). *Cognitive therapy and emotional disorders.* New York: International Universities Press.

Cullen, A. (1995). Burnout: Why do we blame the nurse? *AJN, 95*(11), 23–27.

Dochterman, J., & Bulechek, G. (2004). *Nursing Interventions Classification (NIC)* (4th ed.). St. Louis, MO: Mosby.

Fennell, M. E. (1999). Parents in the OR? You Bet! *RN, 62*(12), 38–40.

Freud, S. (1959). Inhibitions, symptoms and anxiety. In J. Strachey (Trans.), *The standard edition of the complete psychological works of Sigmund Freud* (Vol. 20). London: Hogarth.

Frisch, N., & Frisch, L. (2002). *Psychiatric mental health nursing.* (2nd ed.). Clifton Park, NY: Thomson Delmar Learning.

Keegan, L. (2000). Nutrition, exercise, and movement. In B. M. Dossey, L. Keegan, & C. E. Guzzetta (Eds.), *Holistic nursing: A handbook for practice* (3rd ed.). Gaithersburg, MD: Aspen.

Kneisl, C. R., & Riley, E. (1996). Crisis intervention. In H. S. Wilson & C. R. Kneisl (Eds.), *Psychiatric nursing* (5th ed., pp. 711–731). Menlo Park, CA: Addison-Wesley.

Kobasa, S. C. (1979). Stressful life events, personality and health. An inquiry into hardiness. *Journal of Personality and Social Psychology, 37*(1), 1–11.

Kobasa, S. C., Maddi, S. R., & Kahn, S. (1982). Hardiness and health: A prospective study. *Journal of Personality and Social Psychology, 45*(4), 839–850.

Lyon, B. L. (2000). Situational anger and self-empowerment. *Reflections on Nursing LEADERSHIP, 26*(3), 36–37.

Mandle, C. L., & Gruber-Wood, R. (2002). Health promotion and the individual. In C. L. Edelman & C. L. Mandle (Eds.), *Health promotion throughout the life-span* (5th ed.). St. Louis, MO: Mosby.

Mayo Clinic. (1999). Stress patrol: Stop tension in its tracks [Online]. Available: www.mayohealth.org/mayo/9912/htm/stress_patrol.htm

Mayo Clinic. (2000a). Dealing with co-worker conflict [Online]. Available: www.mayohealth.org/mayo/9704/htm/stre_1sb.htm

Mayo Clinic. (2000b). Workplace stress: Can you control it? [Online]. Available: www.mayohealth.org/mayo/9704/htm/stress.htm

Meyers, T. A., Eichhorn, D. J., Guzzetta, C. E., Clark, A. P., Klein, J. D., Taliaferro, E., & Calvin, A. (2000). Family presence during invasive procedures and resuscitation. *AJN, 100*(2), 32–40.

Moorhead, S, Johnson, M., & Maas, M. (2004). *Nursing Outcomes Classification (NOC)* (3rd ed.). St. Louis, MO: Mosby.

North American Nursing Diagnosis Association. (2003). *Nursing diagnoses: Definitions & classification, 2003–2004.* Philadelphia: Author.

Page, K. (2002). Panic attack. *Nursing2002, 32*(1), 88.

Peplau, H. (1952). *Interpersonal relations in nursing.* New York: Putnam.

Selye, H. (1974). *Stress without distress.* New York: New American Library.

Selye, H. (1976). *Stress in health and disease* (Rev. ed.). Boston: Butterworths.

Sullivan, H. S. (1953). *The interpersonal theory of psychiatry by H. S. Sullivan.* New York: Norton.

Talbott, S. W. (1997). Political analysis: Structure and process. In D. J. Mason, S. W. Talbott, & J. K. Leavitt (Eds.), *Policy and politics for nurses* (2nd ed., pp. 129–148). Philadelphia: W. B. Saunders.

U.S. Preventive Services Task Force (USPSTF). (2002). Screening for depression: Recommendations and rationale. *Annals of Internal Medicine, 136*(10), 760.

Waughfield, C. (2002). *Mental health concepts* (5th ed.). Clifton Park, NY: Thomson Delmar Learning.

Wilson, H. S., & Kneisel, C. R. (1996). *Psychiatric Nursing* (5th ed.). Menlo Park, CA: Addison-Wesley.

Wilson, H. S., Kneisel, C. R., & Trigoboff, E. (2003). *Contemporary Psychiatric-Mental Health Nursing.* Upper Saddle River, NJ: Prentice Hall.

Resources

American Holistic Nurses' Association, P.O. Box 2130, Flagstaff, AZ 86003-2130, 800-278-2462, www.ahna.org

American Institute of Stress, 124 Park Avenue, Yonkers, NY 10703, 914-963-1200, www.stress.org

International Stress Management Association, USA Branch, 638 St. Lawrence Avenue, Reno, NV 89509, www.stress-management-isma.org/ISMA-USA.html

MAKING THE CONNECTION

Refer to the following chapters to increase your understanding of loss, grief, and death:

Basic Nursing
- **Legal and Ethical Responsibilities**
- **Arenas of Care**

- **Cultural Considerations**
- **Complementary/Alternative Therapies**

LEARNING OBJECTIVES

Upon completion of this chapter, you should be able to:
- **Define key terms.**
- **Discuss the various losses that affect individuals at different stages of the life cycle.**
- **Identify characteristics of an individual experiencing grief.**
- **Compare and contrast adaptive grief and pathological grief.**
- **Discuss the stages of the normal grieving process.**
- **Describe the holistic needs of the dying person and family.**
- **Plan care for a dying client.**
- **Describe nursing responsibilities when a client dies.**
- **Discuss ways that nurses can cope with their own grief.**

KEY TERMS

algor mortis	life review
anticipatory grief	liver mortis
autopsy	loss
bereavement	maturational loss
breakthrough pain	mortuary
Cheyne-Stokes	mourning
respirations	palliative care
complicated grief	postmortem care
death rattle	resuscitation
disenfranchised grief	rigor mortis
dysfunctional grief	shroud
grief	situational loss
Health Care	traumatic imagery
Surrogate Law	uncomplicated grief
hospice	

INTRODUCTION

Individuals are constantly experiencing loss. Episodes of personal crisis, natural disaster, and terrorism result in the experience of loss. The nurse must be aware of the many ways individuals react and adapt to losses.

Individuals are faced with losses throughout the life cycle. Growth and development would not continue to progress without some losses.

Nurses encounter clients every day who are responding to grief associated with losses. An understanding of the major concepts related to loss and grieving is necessary for each nurse. Many people consider loss only in terms of death and dying. Because nurses also care for dying clients, this chapter includes information on meeting the special needs of terminally ill clients and their families.

LOSS

Loss is any situation, either potential, actual, or perceived, wherein a valued object or person is changed or is not accessible to the individual. Everyone experiences losses because change is a major constant in life. Loss can be actual (e.g., a child is lost in the woods) or anticipated (a diabetic client is faced with having a foot amputated). The loss can be tangible or intangible. For example, when a person is not selected for a job, the tangible loss is income, and the intangible loss is self-esteem.

Losses also occur as a person moves from one developmental stage to another. An example of such a **maturational loss** is the toddler who loses the bottle after learning to drink from a glass. A **situational loss** takes place in response to external events generally beyond the individual's control, such as losing a job when the company is bankrupt.

The four major categories of loss are loss of significant other, loss of aspects of self, loss of external objects, and loss of a familiar environment.

Loss of Significant Other

Losing a loved one is a very significant loss. Such a loss can result from moving to a different area, separation, divorce, or death.

Loss of Aspect of Self

Loss of an aspect of self can be physiological or psychological. Physiological loss includes loss of physical function or loss resulting from disfigurement or disappearance of a body part, as is the case with amputation or mastectomy. Loss of a physical aspect of self can result from trauma, illness, or a treatment methodology such as surgery. Psychological aspects of self that may be lost include a sense of humor, ambition, or enjoyment of life. These feelings of loss may result from life events such as losing a job or failing at a task that the individual deems important.

Loss of an External Object

Whenever an object that a person highly values is changed or damaged, or disappears, loss occurs. The type and amount of grieving depends on the significance of the lost object to the individual. For instance, an individual who loses a family heirloom in a fire may react not only to the lost financial value of the piece, but also to the lost sense of history and heritage that the piece represented.

Loss of Familiar Environment

The loss of a familiar environment occurs when a person moves away from familiar surroundings, for instance to another home or a different community, to a new school, or to a new job. A client who is hospitalized or institutionalized may also experience loss when faced with new surroundings. This type of loss evokes anxiety related to fear of the unknown.

GRIEF

Grief is a series of intense psychological and physical responses occurring after a loss. These responses are necessary, normal, natural, and adaptive responses to the loss. Loss moves the individual to the adaptive process of **mourning,** the period during which grief is expressed and integration and resolution of the loss occur. **Bereavement** is the period of grief that follows the death of a loved one (Figure 13-1).

Stages of Grief

Three stages of grief generally recognized are shock, reality, and recovery.

Shock Stage

The period of shock may last from only days to a month or more. The person may describe feeling

Figure 13-1 *Older adults may grieve intensely over the loss of a person or situation that has been a part of their lives for many years.*

"numb." It is an emotional numbness rather than a physical one.

Reality Stage

A painful experience begins when the individual consciously realizes the full meaning of the loss. Anger, guilt, fear, frustration, and/or helplessness may be the expressed reactions.

Recovery Stage

During the last stage, recovery, the loss is integrated into the reality of the individual's life. The person exhibits adaptive behaviors and begins to live again, doing things that were formerly enjoyed.

Types of Grief

Grief is a normal, universal, response to loss. Grief drains people, both physically and emotionally, and relationships often suffer. Different types of grief include uncomplicated ("normal"), anticipatory, dysfunctional, and disenfranchised grief.

PROFESSIONAL TIP

Successful Grieving

The person experiencing successful grieving will:

- Consciously recognize that a significant loss has occurred.
- Progress through the stages of grief.
- Use adaptive coping behaviors, such as interacting with others, participating in and completing tasks, and having a positive attitude.

Nurses assist many individuals to understand the normal grieving process. Nurses who understand all types of grief are better prepared to assist others.

Uncomplicated Grief

Uncomplicated grief is what many individuals would refer to as *normal grief*. Engle (1961) proposed the term **uncomplicated grief** to describe the grief reaction normally following a significant loss. Uncomplicated grief has a fairly predictable course that ends with relinquishing the lost object and resuming the duties of life.

The grieving person may feel angry, hopeless, or sad and may express feelings of depression. A person who is grieving may experience loss of appetite, weight loss, insomnia, restlessness, indecisiveness, impulsivity, and inability to concentrate or carry out daily activities.

Anticipatory Grief

Anticipatory grief is the occurrence of grief before an expected loss actually occurs. Anticipatory grief may be experienced by both the person's family and the terminally ill person. This process promotes early grieving, freeing emotional energy for adapting once the loss has occurred. Although anticipatory grieving may be helpful in adjusting to the loss, it also has some potential disadvantages. For example, in the case of the dying client, the family members may distance themselves and not be available for support. Also, if the family members have separated themselves emotionally from the dying client, they may seem cold and distant and, thus, not meet society's expectations of mourning behavior. This response can, in turn, prevent the mourners from receiving their own much-needed support from others (Pritchett & Lucas, 1997b).

Dysfunctional Grief

Dysfunctional grief is a demonstration of a persistent pattern of intense grief that does not result in reconciliation of feelings. The person experiencing dysfunc-

PROFESSIONAL TIP

Identifying Dysfunctional Grief

Normal and dysfunctional grief are differentiated in that the person experiencing dysfunctional grief is unable to adapt to life without the deceased person.

Dysfunctional grief can take several forms, specifically chronic grief, delayed grief, exaggerated grief, or masked grief.

Chronic grief is the inability to conclude grieving.

Delayed grief occurs when grief work does not take place at the time of loss.

Exaggerated grief describes the situation when grief is experienced as overwhelming.

Masked grief occurs when grief is covered up by maladaptive behaviors such as apathy, irritability, and unstable moods or a physical symptom such as loss of libido, with the person being unaware of the connection to the loss and grief.

tional (or pathological) grief does not progress through the stages of grief. The dysfunctionally grieving person cannot reestablish a routine. The professional caregiver must be aware of these behaviors and refer the pathologically grieving person to professional counseling.

Disenfranchised Grief

Disenfranchised grief is described as grief not openly acknowledged, socially sanctioned, or publicly shared. When an individual either is reluctant to recognize the sense of loss and develops guilt feelings or feels pressured by society to "get on with life," grief can become disenfranchised. An example of disenfranchised grief is extreme sadness over the loss of a pet when this mourning might be viewed by others as excessive or inappropriate. A mother's sadness over a miscarriage might also be considered disenfranchised grief because a lengthy period of mourning may not be publicly expected despite the mother's intense feelings of loss and despair.

Factors Affecting Loss and Grief

Variables affecting the intensity and duration of grieving are:

- Developmental stage
- Religious and cultural beliefs
- Relationship with the lost object
- Cause of death

Developmental Stage

Depending on the client's place on the age/development continuum, the grief response to a loss will be experienced differently. For example, a pregnant woman will, to some degree, experience loss after delivery of a first child (loss of freedom, independence, and self-focused life), even when the child is normal and healthy. Certain kinds of loss at key developmental points may have a profound effect on a person's ability to both work through the resulting grief and achieve the tasks of the given developmental stage. For example, an adolescent who has lost a parent may have difficulty forming an intimate relationship with members of the opposite sex.

Childhood Children vary in their reactions to loss and in the ability to comprehend the meaning of death. It is important to understand the way a child's concept of death evolves, because the concept varies with developmental level and may affect mastery of developmental tasks (Table 13-1).

Children who are grieving need honest explanations about death using terms they can understand.

Adolescence Physical attractiveness and athletic abilities are valued by most adolescents. Because adolescents seek approval of their peer group, when the adolescent suffers the loss of a body part or function, grief includes fear of being rejected. After a disfiguring accident, grief is usually very intense. Even though they have an intellectual understanding of death, adolescents believe themselves to be invulnerable and, thus, immune to death; they reject the possibility of their own mortality.

Early Adulthood In the young adult, grief is often precipitated by loss of role or status. For example, significant

LIFE CYCLE CONSIDERATIONS

Talking with Children about Death

- *Avoid the use of euphemisms.* For example, if a child is told that the deceased person has "gone away" the child may believe that the dead person will return. Also, a child may develop sleep phobia if told that the deceased is "asleep."
- *Do not overexplain.* Keep explanations concise and factual; do not offer lengthy explanations of medical conditions.
- *Use simple, concrete terms.* Young children are not able to conceptualize abstract ideas such as "grandma is in a better place now."
- *Show them.* Many young children understand something only when they see it. Take them to the funeral service and cemetery.

(Data from *The 1996 National Directory of Bereavement Support Groups and Services,* by M. M. Wong, 1996, Forest Hills, NY: ADM Publishing.)

CRITICAL THINKING

Perceptions of Death

Find a classmate from a different cultural background than yours. How does your classmate's perception of death differ from yours?

---

grief may be caused by unemployment or the breakup of a relationship. The concept of death in this age group primarily reflects spiritual beliefs and cultural values.

Middle Adulthood The potential for experiencing loss increases during middle adulthood. The death of parents often occurs during this developmental phase. As an individual ages, it can be especially threatening when peers die, because these deaths force acknowledgment of one's own mortality.

Late Adulthood Most individuals recognize the inevitability of death during late adulthood. It is challenging for elders to experience the death of age-old friends or to find themselves the last one of their peer group left living. Older adults often turn to their children and grandchildren as sources of comfort and companionship. Cultivating friendships in all age groups helps prevent loneliness and depression.

Religious and Cultural Beliefs

An individual's grief experience is significantly affected by religious and cultural beliefs. Every culture has rituals for care of the dying and beliefs about the significance of death. Other beliefs regarding an afterlife, redemption of the soul, a supreme being, and reincarnation can assist the individual in grief work.

TABLE 13-1   PERCEPTION OF DEATH BY CHILDREN AND ADOLESCENTS

DEVELOPMENTAL STAGE	PERCEPTION	POTENTIAL DEVELOPMENTAL DISRUPTIONS
Infancy, toddlerhood	• Unaware of death • Aware of changes in normal routine • Reacts to family's expressions of grief	• Death of primary caregiver during the first 2 years of life may have significant long-lasting psychosocial implications.
Preschool	• Believes death is a temporary separation • Reacts to the gravity of death as they see parents or others react	• Loss of either parent may have significant psychosocial implications, especially between ages 4 and 6 years (owing to *magical thinking,* wherein children may believe death is their fault). • Problems with development of sexual identity, depending on the gender of the parent lost, the child's identification with that parent, and the child's present state of sexual identity.
School-age	• Comprehends that death is inevitable and final • Conjectures about and is inclined to personify death ("the boogie-man")	• Potential nightmares. • Potential death-avoidance behaviors (e.g., hiding under the covers, leaving the lights on, closing closet doors). • Possible intense guilt and a sense of responsibility for the death.
Preadolescence and adolescence	• Acknowledges that death is final • Comprehends that death is inevitable • *Preadolescents:* may worry about dying; *adolescents:* seem to deny that they could die	• Loss of a parent may cause difficulty in forming an intimate relationship with members of the opposite sex.

Relationship with the Lost Person or Object

Generally, the grief experienced is more intense the more intimate the relationship was with the deceased. The risk for dysfunctional grieving is particularly great after the death of a child.

The death of a child is generally thought to be exceptionally painful because it upsets the natural order of things; parents do not expect their children to die before them.

Parents experiencing grief usually have intense responses and reactions (Figure 13-2). Parental grief is unique in that it encompasses both the loss of the perceived potential of that child and the loss of parental hopes for the child. Table 13-2 suggests some characteristics of parents of infants who have died.

The death of a sibling or parent can be a major challenge for children. Adults failing to understand the child's need to mourn may not recognize the child's feelings. Normal reactions of a child when a sibling dies as an infant, and nursing responses to these reactions, are given in Table 13-3.

Cause of Death

The intensity of the grief response also varies depending whether the cause of death was unexpected, traumatic, or a suicide.

Unexpected Death The bereaved have particular difficulty in achieving closure when the loss occurs as a result of an unexpected death. As Roach and Nieto (1997) state, any death is a traumatic experience to the surviving loved ones, even an anticipated death. Survivors are shocked and bereaved after an unanticipated death, such as an aneurysm, heart attack, or stroke. Usually, the bereaved can work through the grieving process without complications.

Traumatic Death **Complicated grief** is associated with traumatic death such as death by accident, violence, or homicide. Survivors are not necessarily predisposed to complications in mourning, but often have more intense emotions than those associated with normal grief.

Following a violent death, the bereaved may undergo **traumatic imagery** (imagining the feelings of horror felt by the victim or reliving the terror of the incident). Traumatic imagery is a common occurrence in cases of traumatic death. Such thoughts, coupled with intense

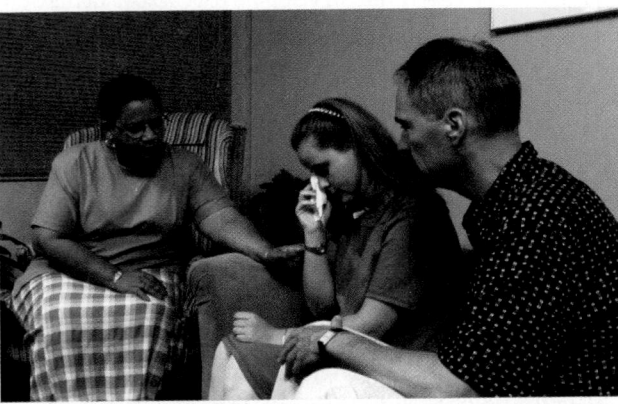

Figure 13-2 *This couple discusses grief over the loss of a child.*

TABLE 13-2	CHARACTERISTICS OF PARENTS WHEN A CHILD DIES
TYPE OF DEATH	**PARENTAL CHARACTERISTICS**
Spontaneous abortion (miscarriage) and stillbirth	• The mother, especially, may have feelings of intense sadness, guilt, or anger. If the loss occurs in early weeks of pregnancy, the death may be inadequately recognized by others. • The death may be regarded as a personal failure. • Parents may blame themselves or others. • Previous miscarriages may be relived and grieved. • If the condition of the infant was known, anticipatory grief may occur. • Grief may increase if ambivalent about being pregnant. • Despair may be greatest when the parents leave the hospital or birthplace without the baby.
Neonatal death	• Similar reactions as with stillbirth. • The bond between parents and infant intensifies the grief. • Both parents may have intense grief.
Sudden infant death syndrome (SIDS)	• Parents are in a state of shock. • Lack of knowledge and misinformation increases pain. • Because SIDS usually occurs during the first 6 months of life, parental bonding is complete. • May feel guilt. • Grief is acute; parents are not prepared for the loss. • May be engrossed with the details of the death.
Induced abortion	• Secrecy, guilt, and shame may accompany grief. • May have ambivalent feelings. • May find little support or comfort from others. • Feelings of despair and depression may be present when relief was expected. • If child was not wanted, no guilt may be felt.

From *Healing and the Grief Process*, by S. S. Roach and B. C. Nieto, 1997, Clifton Park, NY: Thomson Delmar Learning. Copyright 1997 by Thomson Delmar Learning.

TABLE 13-3   REACTIONS OF SIBLINGS AFTER INFANT DEATH

NORMAL REACTION	NURSING RESPONSE
• Fear loss of and separation from parents	• Reassure that parents will not leave them
• Guilt, because of feelings of jealousy and anger related to wishing that the infant would go away	• Reassure siblings that they did not influence the cause of death by providing information (at the appropriate level of understanding)
• Fear that parents' intense reactions will hinder parents' ability to take care of them	• Provide assurance that life will go on by continuing routine activities
• Fear of dying soon and concern over own health	• Persuade parents to avoid being overprotective, which will reinforce children's fears

Data adapted from "Supporting Families after Sudden Infant Death," by M. McClain and J. Shaefer, 1996, *Journal of Psychosocial Nursing and Mental Health Services*, 24(4), 30–34.

Figure 13-3 *The nurse provides support to this client to help him through the grief process.*

grief, can lead to post-traumatic stress disorder (PTSD) in the survivors. Nurses' awareness of the possibility of PTSD and alertness for the presence of symptoms is important. Symptoms may include:

• Chronic anxiety
• Psychological distress
• Sleep disturbances, such as recurrent, terror-filled nightmares

Only when this problem is identified and the survivors are encouraged to express their intense feelings will they be able to move through the normal, adaptive grieving process.

Suicide The loss of a loved one to suicide is frequently compounded by feelings of guilt by the survivors for failing to recognize clues that may have permitted the victim to receive help. The feelings of guilt and self-blame can change into anger at the victim for inflicting such pain. Having a suicide in the family may evoke feelings of shame. Survivors may be prohibited from successfully resolving their grief by the negative stigma of suicide.

Nursing Care of the Grieving Client

Although it is a painful process, clients must resolve the loss in their own way. As the client moves through the process of mourning, nurses can assist by providing support. Rodebaugh, Schwindt, and Valentine (1999) suggest that grief be thought of as a journey through four broad categories titled reeling, feeling, dealing, and healing. Clients are reeling when experiencing shock or disbelief. Feelings may be expressed in various emotions and behaviors. Dealing occurs when they begin to adapt to the loss. Things do not necessarily get better; they just

get different. Healing is when the loss becomes part of them, and the acute anguish lessens; it does not mean forgetting. People are changed by grief. Self-esteem is affected, new ways of coping are developed, and a new lifestyle without the deceased is begun.

Nurses can assist people to grieve by encouraging them to experience their feelings to the fullest in order to work through them. Providing support and explaining to the bereaved that it will take time to grieve the loss and to gain some closure to the relationship are both important nursing responsibilities (Figure 13-3).

Assessment

Determining the personal meaning of the loss is the beginning of a thorough assessment of the grieving client and family. The person's progress through the grieving process is another key assessment area. The stages of grieving are not necessarily mastered sequentially, but instead individuals may move back and forth through the stages of grief.

Nursing Diagnosis

The North American Nursing Diagnosis Association (NANDA) defines *Dysfunctional Grieving* as "extended, unsuccessful use of intellectual and emotional responses by which individuals, families, communities attempt to work through the process of modifying self-concept based upon the perception of loss" (NANDA, 2003). The other grieving diagnosis is *Anticipatory Grieving*, defined as "intellectual and emotional responses and behaviors by which individuals, families, communities work through the process of modifying self-concept based on the perception of potential loss" (NANDA, 2003).

Planning/Outcome Identification

When planning care for the grieving client, it is important to clarify the expected outcomes. Some expected goals for the person experiencing grief are:

- Accept the loss.
- Verbalize feelings of grief.
- Share grief with significant others.
- Renew activities and relationships.

Some of these expected outcomes will take a long time to achieve, and some must be achieved before others are mastered. For example, to accept the loss, the person must begin to share grief with others by verbalizing those feelings. Two of the expected outcomes are discussed below.

Acceptance of the Loss Individuals are able to reach some acceptance and resolution of feelings about the loss only by going through grief work. Often, people try to find some meaning in their situations. This search involves introspection, for which spiritual support may be therapeutic.

Renewal of Activities and Relationships The basis of grief work revolves around accepting the fact that the needs met by key people in life can be met by other people in other ways. Knowing that the deceased cannot be replaced, healing must occur so that new relationships may begin.

Implementation

Basic to therapeutic nursing care is an understanding of the significance of the loss to the client. The nurse must spend time listening to understand the client's perspective. Even if the client does not respond according to the nurse's belief system or expectations, the nurse must demonstrate acceptance. The nurse's nonjudgmental, accepting attitude is essential during the bereaved's expression of all feelings, including anger and despair. The nurse avoids personalizing and using defensive behaviors by communicating an understanding of the client's anger. The expression of grief is not only appropriate but also essential for therapeutic resolution of the loss.

Grieving people need reassurance, support, and counseling. One mechanism of support on a long-term basis is support groups. The nurse must be informed about the availability of such groups within the community in order to make appropriate referrals. Members of support groups have experienced similar losses. Discussions in support groups decrease the feelings of loneliness and social isolation that are so common in the grief experience.

Evaluation

People follow their own time schedule for grief work. Because it takes months or years for grief resolution, nurses usually do not have the opportunity to know when the bereaved family completes its grief work. The nurse does have a unique opportunity to lay the foundation for adaptive grieving by encouraging the family to verbalize their experience and share their feelings with significant others. The foundation for evaluation is the goals mutually established with client and family. It is important for nurses to teach grieving individuals that resolution of the loss is generally a process of lifelong adjustment.

DEATH

Historically, death has been considered as natural as birth, as simply the last stage of life. Significant changes in the perception of death have occurred in the last three decades. In some cases, dying and death are no longer simple matters but are issues involving ethical concerns and, in some cases, legal intervention by the court system.

Each person dies a unique death, just as each person lives a unique life. Death may be sudden and unexpected, caused by accident or heart attack, for example, or death may be prolonged, coming after a distressing long-term illness. For the older person who dies during sleep, death comes quietly. Those who choose to die on their own terms by suicide plan their deaths.

Health care workers must understand the ethical and legal issues surrounding dying and death. Understanding the stages of death and dying and the signs of impending death will help prepare the nurse to render sensitive, effective care, both to the client and family and to the client's body after death. Nurses must also come to terms with their own mortality and feelings about death if they are to provide comfort to dying clients and their families. Health care workers can learn a great deal about life from the dying client.

Legal Considerations

The *Patient Self-Determination Act* (PSDA) is part of the Omnibus Budget Reconciliation Act (OBRA) of 1990. This act provides a legal means for individuals to specify the circumstances under which life-sustaining measures should or should not be rendered to them. The individual's choices are identified in advance directives. An advance directive is any written instruction recognized under state law, including a durable power of attorney for health care or living will. The act applies to hospitals, home health agencies, long-term care facilities, hospice programs, and certain health maintenance organizations (HMOs). According to the PSDA, all clients entering the health care system through any of these organizations must be given information and the opportunity to complete advance directives if they have not already done so. In many states, just signing these documents may not be adequate for carrying out client wishes. They may also need to indicate their desires regarding intubation, artificial feeding, blood transfusions, chemotherapy, surgery, and transfer to the hospital (for residents in skilled care facilities).

Although a durable power of attorney for health care and living will are legal documents, they do not prevent **resuscitation** (support measures to restore consciousness and life). The medical record must have a written do-not-resuscitate (DNR) order from a physician if this is in agreement with the client's wishes and with the advance directives. In the absence of such an order, resuscitation will be initiated.

In many states a **Health Care Surrogate Law** is implemented when there is no advance directive. This law varies from state to state but basically provides a legal means for certain individuals to make decisions for the client when the client cannot do so. The spouse is the first person who would act in the interests of the client. Then children in the event there is no spouse.

Ethical Considerations

Death is often fraught with ethical dilemmas that occur almost daily in health care settings. Ethics committees in many health care agencies develop and implement policies to deal with end-of-life issues. These committees are interdisciplinary and may have clergy and attorneys as well as health care providers as members. Ethical decision making is a complex issue. Determining the difference between killing and allowing someone to die by withholding life-sustaining treatment methods is one of the most difficult dilemmas.

The American Nurses Association (ANA) distinguishes mercy killing (euthanasia or assisted suicide) and relieving pain. Euthanasia is viewed as unethical, whereas pain relief is a central value in nursing. The ANA's position is that increasing doses of medication to control pain in terminally ill clients is ethically justified, even at the expense of maintaining life (ANA, 1992).

Stages of Dying and Death

Elizabeth Kübler-Ross (1969, 1974) identified in her classic works five stages of dying that are experienced by clients and their families (Table 13-4). Every client does

TABLE 13-4	KÜBLER-ROSS' STAGES OF DYING AND DEATH
STAGE	**EXAMPLE**
Denial	*Verbal:* "No, I don't believe that." *Behavioral:* Client diagnosed with leukemia and refuses to consider treatment options.
Anger	*Verbal:* "Why me, why?" *Behavioral:* Client is demanding and demonstrates aggressive behavior.
Bargaining	*Verbal:* Client prays, "Please, just let me live to see my new grandbaby." *Behavioral:* Client makes deals with caregivers or god.
Depression	*Verbal:* "I just want to be alone." *Behavioral:* Client turns away and closes eyes.
Acceptance	*Verbal:* "I am ready. I feel at peace now." *Behavioral:* Client gets legal and financial affairs in order and says goodbye to family and friends.

Data from *On Death and Dying*, by E. Kübler-Ross, 1969, New York: Macmillan. Copyright 1969 by Macmillan.

PROFESSIONAL TIP

Care of the Dying Client

Dying was once considered to be a normal part of the life cycle. Today, it is often considered to be a medical problem that should be handled by health care providers. Technological advances in medicine have led to depersonalized and mechanical care of those who are dying.

Our highly technological world calls for application of high-touch interventions with the dying. In other words, appropriate care of the dying is administered by compassionate nurses who are both technically competent and able to demonstrate caring. Huizdos (2000) learned that death is not the enemy—lack of caring is.

not move through each stage sequentially. These stages are experienced for varying lengths of time and in varying degrees. The client may express denial, and then, a few minutes later, express acceptance of the inevitable, and then express anger. An important value of Kübler-Ross' work is that it has increased sensitivity to the dying client's needs.

Denial

During the first stage of dying, the initial shock can be very overwhelming, making denial a useful tool of coping. It is an essential, protective mechanism that may last for only a few minutes or may manifest for months.

In some clients, denial manifests as "doctor shopping" (not to imply that second opinions are not sometimes necessary) or insisting that there must have been a mix-up or mistake in the diagnostic tests. In other clients, denial manifests as simply avoiding the issue. Their daily routines are the same as though nothing in their lives has changed. Given time, most people will eventually move past the stage of denial.

Clients may choose to be selective in the use of denial. For example, clients try to protect certain family members or friends from the truth by using denial. Clients may also use denial from time to time to set aside thoughts of illness and death in order to focus on living.

Anger

Anger often follows the initial stage of denial. The client's security is threatened by the unknown, with the normal daily routines becoming disrupted. This stage is typically very difficult for family and caregivers because they often feel useless in terms of helping their loved one through the situation. Since the client has no control over the situation, anger is the response. The anger may be directed at self, God, others, the environment, and the health care system. In the client's eyes, whatever is done is not the right thing. Family members may be greeted with silence or with outbursts of anger. Their response, in turn, may be anger, guilt, or despair.

LIFE CYCLE CONSIDERATIONS

Reactions to Impending Death

- Persons of all ages generally experience the same feelings and emotions as they progress through a terminal illness.
- Persons of any age who have endured a long illness may view death as a release from their suffering.
- Persons of any age may find it difficult to reach acceptance if they have unfinished business.
- Many people receive satisfaction from **life review** (a form of reminiscence wherein a client attempts to come to terms with conflict or to gain meaning from life and die peacefully).
- Elderly clients may welcome death, especially if they have outlived everyone who was near and dear to them.

Bargaining

The client attempts to postpone or reverse the inevitable by bargaining. The client's bargaining represents an attempt to postpone death and usually has self-imposed limitations. For example, a client may ask to live long enough to see the first grandchild in exchange for giving money to a charity. Most clients bargain in silence or in confidence with their spiritual leader. It is not uncommon for a client to live long enough for some special event (a wedding or birth), then die shortly afterward.

Depression

Depression resulting from the realization that death can no longer be delayed is different from dysfunctional depression because it helps the client detach from life and makes it easier to accept death. Depression in this sense is a therapeutic experience for the dying person. Clients sometimes feel abandoned, as persons who were once friends begin to visit less and less, sometimes severing ties with the client even before death; this may compound the client's feelings of depression and hopelessness.

Acceptance

Every dying client may not reach the final stage, acceptance. Peace and contentment comes with acceptance. The client often expresses feeling that all that could be done has been done. It is important to reinforce the client's feelings and sense of personal worth. Many clients will make an effort to get all of their personal and financial affairs in order.

Sleep is required to fill a physical and emotional need, not to avoid reality. The client may limit visitors to those people with whom he feels comfortable and safe. The most significant forms of communication at this time are touch and moments of silence.

Nursing Care of the Dying Client

Nursing care of clients who are terminally ill or who are facing and preparing for their own death can be both challenging and rewarding. The death process is typically a very emotional time for clients and their families; compassionate and sensitive nursing care that respects clients' wishes as well as meets their physical needs can help bring peace and dignity to this natural process.

Assessment

A thorough assessment of the client's holistic needs is the basis for nursing interventions. Assessment of the dying client includes an ongoing collection of data regarding the strengths and limitations of the dying person and the family.

Nursing Diagnoses

The nurse's assessment of the dying client may lead to several diagnoses. One NANDA-approved nursing diagnosis that is applicable for many dying clients is *Powerlessness*, that is, "the perception that one's own action will not significantly affect an outcome; a perceived

CULTURAL CONSIDERATIONS

Rituals following Death

- Judaism practices burial of the dead within 24 hours. A 7-day period of mourning, called *Shiva*, begins the day of the funeral.
- In the Islamic faith, men wash the body of a man and women wash the body of a woman after death.
- Buddhists believe that after death, the body should not be disturbed by movement, talking, or crying.
- Hindus pour holy water into the mouth of the dying person. The eldest son arranges for the funeral and cremation within 24 hours of death. Embalming is forbidden.
- Jehovah's Witnesses believe that the soul dies with the body, but 144,000 will be resurrected at the end-time and will be born again as spiritual sons of God.
- Native Americans believe that the spirit lives on after death. Ancestor worship is practiced.

PROFESSIONAL TIP

Planning Care for the Dying Client

- Schedule time to spend with the client.
- Identify areas of special concern to the client and make referrals when appropriate (e.g., social worker consult for information on equipment rental).
- Promote and protect individual self-esteem and self-worth.
- Balance the client's needs for assistance and independence.
- Meet the physiological needs of the client and family.
- Respect the client's confidentiality.
- Provide factual information to the client and family and answer all questions.
- Offer to contact clergy or other spiritual leader.

(Adapted from Death and Dying, by K. Pritchett and P. Lucas. In *Psychiatric–Mental Health Nursing: Adaptation and Growth* (4th ed., p. 208), by B. S. Johnson (Ed.) (1997) Philadelphia: Lippincott Williams & Wilkins.)

lack of control over a current situation or immediate happening" (NANDA, 2003). Another response that is often experienced by the dying is described by the diagnosis **Hopelessness,** "a subjective state in which an individual sees limited or no alternatives or personal choices available and is unable to mobilize energy on own behalf" (NANDA, 2003). The client may also exhibit *Death Anxiety,* "apprehension, worry, or fear related to death or dying" (NANDA, 2003).

Planning/Outcome Identification

The major goals of nursing care are the physical, emotional, and mental comfort of the client. The goals of nursing care for the dying client are the same as those goals developed for all clients who are unable to meet their own needs. The dying client should be treated as a unique individual worthy of respect, instead of a diag-

PROFESSIONAL TIP

Information Gathered in Assessment of the Dying Client

- Client and family goals and expectations
- Client's awareness that illness is terminal
- Client's stage of dying
- Identification of support systems
- History of positive coping skills
- Client perception of unfinished business to be completed

(Adapted from Death and Dying, by K. Pritchett and P. Lucas, 1997. In *Psychiatric–Mental Health Nursing: Adaptation and Growth* (4th ed., pp. 206-207), by B. S. Johnson (Ed.), 1997, Philadelphia: Lippincott Williams & Wilkins.)

nosis to be cured. Many dying clients do not fear death but are anxious about a painful death or dying alone.

Promoting optimal quality of life includes treating the client and family with respect and providing a safe environment for expressing their feelings. Planning should focus on meeting the client's and family's holistic needs, as specified in the Dying Person's Bill of Rights (Figure 13-4). It is as relevant today as when it was written in 1975. When planning care, the nurse should make every effort to be sensitive to the rights of the dying client.

Implementation

The first priority is to communicate caring to the client and family. Powell (1999) found that the presence of a comforting nurse made a tremendous difference to the client. LaDuke (2001) suggests holding a client's or family member's hand and saying "I will not leave you." This assurance of the nurse's presence is a powerful way to show caring.

The nurse should approach the client in denial with understanding and the knowledge that moving between the stages of dying is enhanced by a trusting nurse–client relationship. Establishing rapport facilitates the client's verbalization of feelings (Figure 13-5). A safe environment established by the nurse allows the client to express those feelings being experienced. Nurses must understand that clients are not angry with them, but, rather, with the situation they are experiencing.

Terminally ill clients are often given **palliative care,** or care that relieves symptoms, such as pain, but does not alter the course of disease. A primary aim of palliative care is to help the client feel comfortable, safe, and secure. The nurse can do much to increase the client's feelings of safety by being available when needed. Holding the client's hand and listening are therapeutic

The Dying Person's Bill of Rights

- I have the right to be treated as a living human being until I die.
- I have the right to maintain a sense of hopefulness, however changing its focus may be.
- I have the right to be cared for by those who can maintain a sense of hopefulness, however challenging this might be.
- I have the right to express my feelings and emotions about my approaching death in my own way.
- I have the right to participate in decisions concerning my care.
- I have the right to expect continuing medical and nursing attention even though "cure" goals must be changed to "comfort" goals.
- I have the right not to die alone.
- I have the right to be free from pain.
- I have the right to have my questions answered honestly.
- I have the right not to be deceived.
- I have the right to have help from and for my family in accepting death.
- I have the right to die in peace and dignity.
- I have the right to retain my individuality and not be judged for my decisions, which may be contrary to beliefs of others.
- I have the right to expect that the sanctity of the human body will be respected after death.
- I have the right to be cared for by caring, sensitive, knowledgeable people who will attempt to understand my needs and will be able to gain some satisfaction in helping me face my death.

Figure 13-4 *The Dying Person's Bill of Rights (From* The Dying Person's Bill of Rights, *by A. J. Barbus, 1975, AJN, 75[1].)*

Figure 13-5 *Establishing a caring and trusting relationship helps the client come to terms with a terminal illness.*

measures. Ufema (1995a) suggests asking the client three questions: What do you want? From whom do you want it? and When do you want it? The client needs to know that he has the nurse's support as an advocate for his care and well-being.

Physiological Needs Physiological needs are essential for existence, according to Maslow's hierarchy of needs. Therefore, they must be met before all other needs. Areas that are often problematic for the terminally ill client are respirations; fluids and nutrition; mouth, eyes, and nose; mobility; skin care; and elimination.

Respirations Oxygen is frequently ordered for the client experiencing labored breathing. Suctioning may be needed to remove secretions that the client is unable to swallow.

Fluids and Nutrition Dying clients almost universally refuse food and fluids. It is believed that the dying client does not feel thirst and hunger. Although the issue of permitting dehydration in terminally ill clients is often met with great resistance, the literature supports the concept that forced nutrition has questionable value and may even exacerbate the client's condition (Taylor, 1995). Artificial nutrition often increases the client's agitation, increases the risk of aspiration pneumonia, and leads to increased use of limb restraints. Withholding of artificial nutrition is not painful, according to hospice nurses. The client's own wishes must always take precedence in every situation. Family members must be given truthful and accurate information when a comatose client has not previously made his wishes known. Withholding artificial nutrition for the person in an irreversible coma does not cause death; instead, it allows life to take its natural course (Taylor, 1995). The American Dietetic Association, the American Medical Association, and the ANA agree that it is ethically, legally, and professionally acceptable to discontinue nutritional support if that is the terminally ill client's request.

Mouth, Eyes, and Nose The only documented side effect of dehydration in the terminally ill client is oral discomfort (Taylor, 1995). The administration of oxygen and mouth breathing both increase the need for meticulous oral care. Saliva substitutes and moisturizers can be used to alleviate discomfort. Regular use of toothpaste and a toothbrush may be adequate. The tongue should be gently brushed. Offer ice chips and sips of favorite beverages frequently. Apply petroleum jelly to the lips. To maintain the client's comfort, oral care must be given every 2 to 3 hours.

If the eyes become irritated due to dryness, artificial tears will alleviate this discomfort. A cotton ball should be used to gently wipe the eye from inner to outer canthus (one wipe per cotton ball) to remove any discharge.

The nares may become dry and crusted. Oxygen given by cannula can further irritate the nares. A thin layer of water-soluble jelly applied to the nares will help alleviate discomfort. The elastic strap of the oxygen cannula should not be applied too tightly, lest it cause discomfort. If oxygen tubing is placed behind the ears, the area should be assessed for irritation.

Mobility Mobility decreases as the client's condition deteriorates. The client requires more assistance as he becomes less able to move about in bed or get out of bed. Physical dependence increases the risk of complications related to immobility, such as atrophy and pressure ulcers. These complications, which increase both cost of care and client discomfort, can be prevented by attentive nursing care.

Reposition the client at least every 2 hours. Remember that the client may have other disorders that contribute to discomfort related to mobility, such as arthritis or lung disease. Maintain body alignment with the use of pillows and other supportive equipment and use positioning techniques to facilitate ease of breathing. Perform passive range-of-motion exercises at least twice a day to prevent stiffness and aching of the joints. The client may wish to be in a reclining type of chair several times a day. Use a wheelchair to increase the client's environmental space and give the client more mobility, control, and independence.

Skin Care Prevention of pressure ulcers is a priority. They are painful, can cause secondary complications, and are costly to treat. Two preventive measures are passive range-of-motion exercises and regular repositioning. In addition, keeping the skin clean and moisturized will promote healthy tissue. Inspect the skin once or twice daily, with special attention paid to pressure points and areas where skin surfaces rub together. Gentle massages with soothing lotion are comforting. Bed baths are adequate if the client cannot get into the tub or sit in a shower chair.

Elimination Side effects of pain medications and a lack of physical activity may cause constipation. For clients with adequate oral intake, foods with high-fiber content and fluids can be effective preventive measures. Constipation can also be alleviated by administering suppositories, if necessary, and maintaining a scheduled time for bowel elimination. A commode with padded arms can be more comfortable than a toilet.

The client may become incontinent of bowel and bladder. After each incontinent episode, clean the skin with peri-washes, and apply a moisture barrier. Urine and fecal material on the skin will quickly lead to excoriation and skin breakdown.

Indwelling catheters are not a first choice for bladder management; however, for some clients, the discomfort of using a bedpan, getting out of bed to use the toilet or commode, or the need for frequent cleaning may cause agonizing pain. The benefits of a urinary catheter greatly outweigh the risks in such circumstances.

Comfort The primary activities for promoting physical comfort include pain relief, keeping the client dry and

clean, and providing a safe, nonthreatening environment. The nurse who has a caring, respectful attitude increases the client's psychological comfort. Fear of a painful death is almost universal. Pain is a subjective, personal experience, and the client is the best judge of the severity of the pain. Many, but not all, dying clients experience pain. The ANA states in its position statement on pain relief for the terminally ill that promotion of comfort is the major goal of nursing care (ANA, 1992). Comfort is to be maximized by managing pain and other causes of discomfort.

The client must know that caregivers accept and believe complaints of pain and that they will intervene to alleviate or prevent the pain. Ask the client to rate the pain on a scale from 0 to 10, with 0 being no pain, and 10 being severe pain. To maintain therapeutic blood level, medication must be given around the clock and not "as needed." A nonnarcotic analgesic may be effective in early stages for mild, intermittent pain. As the pain increases, the client may need to be started on morphine, titrated at increments until adequate pain relief is achieved without severe side effects. Finding the lowest dose and the longest interval that will relieve pain is called titrating the dose. The dosage that should be used is the one that controls the pain to the satisfaction of the client and that causes minimal side effects. For some clients, this may be 10 mg of oral morphine sulfate (MS) every 4 hours, while other clients may require 480 mg MS intravenously per hour. The dose is individual and continually assessed to remain therapeutic in controlling pain.

Monitor the client's responses with regard to pain rating and respiratory rate. For example, 10 mg MS given IM may afford pain relief, but if the respiratory rate drops from 12 to 6 per minute, the medication may need to be adjusted or changed. If the same dose given to another client provides minimal relief, and the client is alert and displays no change in respirations, the next dose should be increased (McCaffery & Pasero, 1999).

Monitor the client for **breakthrough pain,** or sudden, acute, temporary pain that is usually precipitated

---

COMMUNITY/HOME HEALTH CARE

Equipment To Increase Client Comfort

The following equipment can be rented and may qualify for payment by Medicare or private insurance:

- An electric hospital bed with overhead trapeze allows the client some control of the environment.
- A commode promotes the client's independence in elimination.
- A lifting device eases getting the dependent client out of bed.
- Handheld shower and chair for the bathtub or shower are helpful.
- Devices such as cushions for chairs and special mattresses for the bed provide comfort
- An overbed table for eating and other activities is useful.
- Comfortable chairs close to the bed facilitate visits of friends and family.

PROFESSIONAL TIP

Adjuvant Therapy

Adjuvant therapy may be effective. Nonsteroidal anti-inflammatory agents are beneficial for bone metastases; tricyclic antidepressants and anti-seizure medications for neurogenic pain, antidepressants for terminally ill clients, and steroids for headaches related to cerebral edema. Nonpharmacological techniques can be used along with medication. Relaxation techniques, guided imagery, massages, and repositioning may enhance the action of the medications.

by a treatment, a procedure, or by unusual activity of the client. A supplemental dose of medication is then required. If the precipitating factor is known (e.g., dressing changes), give medication 30 to 60 minutes before the procedure.

Physical Environment The client's comfort can be significantly increased by a soothing physical environment. Soft lighting may enhance vision. Complying with the client's request for a nightlight is also helpful in creating a pleasant and nonthreatening environment. If possible, the client should be offered the opportunity to have the bed or a chair near a window to increase the range of the environment. Since body temperature falls as circulation becomes more sluggish, a lightweight comforter will increase warmth without adding much weight. Help eliminate environmental odors by ensuring adequate ventilation, daily cleaning of the room, removal of leftover food, and frequent linen changes. Noise can be distracting and anxiety provoking, so the nurse and visitors should comply with the client's wishes with regard to the use of radio and television. The telephone can be removed from the room, if the client finds the ringing disturbing.

Psychosocial Needs Death presents a threat to one's psychological integrity, as well as to one's physical existence. The dying person is often tethered to tubes and electronic gadgetry in an intensive care unit. The client is held captive in a tangle of technology and is kept at a distance from the supportive presence and touch of family and friends.

Technology cannot replace concern, touch, compassion, or human companionship. By their presence, nurses and family can humanize the dying person's environment. Invite and encourage families to participate in the client's care, if they desire to do so and the client is willing.

For many clients, maintaining a well-groomed appearance is important. When the client can no longer make requests or give directions for care, caregivers should presume that the client would prefer to maintain the same grooming habits as were previously preferred. Shaving the male client's beard or cleaning and trimming the client's fingernails and toenails, for instance, will help the client maintain a well-groomed appearance and will also promote client dignity. Combing and brushing the hair not only improves appearance but is also a comforting and relaxing activity for many clients.

Dressing and undressing may become a cumbersome, frustrating, and fatiguing activity. The client who spends time up and about may choose attractive pajamas, housecoats, dusters, or exercise suits. Advise individuals who may be purchasing clothing for the client to select items that are loose fitting, have few fasteners, and are washable.

Spiritual Needs Nurses have the opportunity to play a major role in promoting the dying client's spiritual comfort.

Yet a survey on end-of-life care by Ferrell et al. (2000) showed that fewer than 35% of nurses described grief/bereavement support and the attention to spiritual needs as effective; however, 66% of nurses said that care of the dying was better than 5 years prior.

Dying clients are most vulnerable. The moral health and integrity of the broader community can be measured in part by the way we respond to their needs.

Dying persons may experience confusion, anger at their god, crises of faith, or other types of spiritual distress.

Dying is a personal and often a lonely process. Table 13-5 provides information on the views of various religions with regard to withdrawal of life support, death, and organ donation. Listen as a client expresses values and beliefs related to death. Therapeutic nursing interventions that address the spiritual needs of the dying client include:

- Use touch
- Play music
- Pray with the client
- Communicate empathy
- Contact clergy, if requested by the client
- Read religious literature aloud, at the client's request

Support for the Family The presence of the nurse is extremely important. It shows support and caring not only for the client but for the family as well. Family members may have increased guilt because of feelings of helplessness. LaDuke (2001) suggests encouraging family members to speak to, touch, read to, sing to, pray with, or just sit with the client. This can give family members a sense of purpose, ease feelings of helplessness, and provide more pleasant memories in the future.

Each family group has its unwritten rules, its leaders and followers, and its methods for coping with crises. The family's equilibrium is threatened by the impending death. If family members have limited coping skills and inadequate support systems, they need assistance and guidance from the caregivers. Nurses must remember that the rules and coping mechanisms used by the family may not always coincide with the values and beliefs of the staff and that the client's and family's wishes must be respected to the extent possible.

The relationship with the family does not always end with the client's death. Staff members may attend visitations, funerals, or memorial services. If a hospice was involved, the family may participate in a bereavement support program. If the client was a resident in a long-term care facility, family members may return to visit other residents with whom they became acquainted.

CLIENT TEACHING

Guidelines for Teaching a Family Caregiver

- Use adult-education principles.
- Frequently reinforce material.
- Provide information about the nature and extent of the disease process.
- Explain the purpose of palliative care yet maintain a sense of realistic hope.
- Reassure client and family by informing them of available community resources; tell them that they are not alone.
- Discuss steps for caregiver to follow if an emergency arises at home by providing written instructions, including persons to be contacted and important telephone numbers.

TABLE 13-5 RELIGIONS AND DYING AND DEATH ISSUES

RELIGION	LIFE SUPPORT WITHDRAWAL	DEATH	ORGAN DONATION
Judaism	Allowed under the right circumstances (when life support is serving only to impede a natural death).	• Suicide is forbidden. • Burial should occur within 24 hours. • Cremation is forbidden. • Autopsy is permitted if it will save future lives.	• Permitted because the procedure saves life. • Rejected by Orthodox Jews.
Islam	Permitted if only serving to prolong death or if client's condition is medically hopeless.	• Suicide is forbidden. • Relatives and friends are present. • Autopsy is permitted to solve a crime or provide further medical knowledge.	• Permitted.
Catholicism/Orthodoxy	Controversial; permitted if client's condition is hopeless.	• Prayers are offered at time of death. • Burial and cremation are permitted. • Autopsy is permitted.	• Permitted.
Protestantism	Permitted if client's condition is hopeless.	• Prayers are offered at time of death. • Burial and cremation are permitted. • Autopsy is permitted.	• Permitted, although may be rejected by some Baptists or Pentecostals.
Jehovah's Witness	Permitted if serving only to prolong death or if quality of life is nonexistent.	• Suicide is not approved. • Autopsy is permitted if legally necessary.	• Individual choice.
Buddhism	Acceptable for those on threshold of death.	• Suicide is criticized. • Cremation is common.	• Controversial.
Hinduism	Supported to allow a natural death.	• Prefer to die at home. • Embalming is forbidden. • Autopsy is discouraged. • Suicide is forbidden.	• Forbidden.
Mormons	A client or family decision.	• Cremation is discouraged. • Autopsy is a family decision.	• A family decision.
Native Americans	Life support is viewed as unnatural and, therefore, unnecessary.	• Complex beliefs about death and treatment of the body.	• Discouraged.

Data from *Health Assessment & Physical Examination* (2nd ed.), by M. E. Z. Estes, 2002, Clifton Park, NY: Thomson Delmar Learning. Copyright 2002 by Thomson Delmar Learning.

Learning Needs The nurse's role is to provide the client and family members with support and information. For example, they may not realize that the dying person should conserve energy. Family activities are best scheduled early in the morning or following a period of rest by the client. The nurse may need to point out to the family this type of commonsense approach, as simple interventions such as these can be overlooked during this highly charged emotional time.

Client and family learning needs may relate to:

• Information about physical condition and treatment regimen
• Anticipating a medical crisis
• Inexperience with the personal threat of death

• Unfamiliarity with what to do in case of an emergency outside of the hospital

Hospice Care **Hospice** is care for the terminally ill founded on the concept of allowing individuals to die with dignity surrounded by those who love them. Clients

CRITICAL THINKING

Caring for a Dying Client
Think about caring for a dying client. How can you prepare to care for a dying client?

enter hospice care either at home or in a hospice center, when aggressive medical treatment is no longer an option or when the client refuses further medical care.

Impending Death

There is no way to predict how long a client may be in the terminal stages of illness. A client may have signs of impending death and then rally to live several more days. Clients often live until a family member arrives for a last good-bye. The client who has had a long illness and is ready to die may need "permission" to die from a loved one, who says, "It's okay, you can go now." Some clients may not wish to die when anyone is present and will wait to take the last breath until alone in the room.

It is never easy for the family, even when death is expected. The family should be simply and thoroughly informed about what will happen before and after the client's death, including:

- Physical changes that occur just before and following death
- Death pronouncement
- Postmortem care
- Body removal

Impending death is signaled by a series of irrevocable events (Durham & Weiss, 1997):

- The lungs become unable to provide adequate gas diffusion.
- The heart and blood vessels become unable to maintain adequate tissue perfusion.
- The brain ceases to regulate vital centers.

Cheyne-Stokes respirations (breathing characterized by periods of apnea alternating with periods of dyspnea) most often herald pulmonary system failure. Secretions accumulate in the larynx and trachea, causing noisy respirations, often called the **death rattle.**

The heart fails in its pumping function, resulting in poor perfusion, ischemia, and cell death. The skin becomes cool and, possibly, very pale, cyanotic, jaundiced, or mottled. The pulse becomes rapid, irregular, weak, and thready. Death is several hours away if a peripheral pulse is strong and easily palpated. Cold, cyanotic extremities and irregular respirations indicate that death may be expected within an hour or two (Durham & Weiss, 1997).

Inadequate cerebral perfusion hinders the brain's ability to integrate vital functions. The client may be confused and lethargic and may respond only to direct visual, auditory, or tactile stimulation. Pupils no longer react to light and become fixed. The client may "talk" to dead loved ones. A frown or tight facial muscles may indicate pain or discomfort. A client in a coma will move only in response to deep pain. Analgesics should not be withdrawn from a conscious client in a coma.

The care of the client does not cease during this final stage of life. The nursing actions previously described should be continued. Tell the client in brief, simple terms what is happening as care is rendered. The family should be allowed and encouraged to continue their participation, if that is their wish. Caution family members that the dying client can hear even in the absence of verbal response, so all comments and conversation should continue to be respectful.

There may be other indications that death is near. The client may report seeing angels (Ufema, 1995b) or hearing beautiful music. These experiences should be accepted as a natural step in the process of dying. When the final breath is taken, the heart stops beating. Within a few minutes, cerebral death (the point at which brain cells die) occurs, and brain activity ceases.

Care after Death

Meeting the needs of the grieving family and caring for the deceased body are nursing responsibilities. Treat the body of the deceased with respect by maintaining privacy and preventing damage to the body. **Postmortem care** is given immediately after death but before the body is moved to the mortuary.

After death, several physiological changes occur. Body temperature decreases, resulting in a lack of skin elasticity **(algor mortis).** In order to avoid skin breakdown, the nurse must therefore use caution when removing tape from the body. **Liver mortis,** a bluish-purple discoloration of the skin is a by-product of red-blood-cell destruction. It usually begins within 20 minutes of death (Harvey, 2001). This discoloration occurs

---

COMMUNITY/HOME HEALTH CARE

When the Client Dies at Home (Preparing for an Expected Death)

Have the family prepare:

- A list of names and telephone numbers they wish to notify of the death including the name and telephone number of the funeral director.

Instruct the family:

- Whom to call (physician or hospice nurse or funeral director).
- Whom *not* to call (ambulance and emergency services).
- To record the time of death, last medications given, the condition of the client during the last few hours, and the last time the client was seen by the nurse.

PROFESSIONAL TIP

Postmortem Care

- Treat the body with dignity and respect.
- Bathe and put a clean gown on the body—and place an incontinent pad under the client's hips.
- Remove dressings and tubes, unless these must remain in place for an autopsy.
- Place the body in alignment with the head elevated.
- Place dentures in a denture cup and send with the body.
- Comb the client's hair.

in dependent areas of the body; the nurse should therefore elevate the head of the bed 30 degrees to prevent discoloration of the head and neck. If the body is moved on a stretcher, keep the head elevated on two pillows. **Rigor mortis,** the natural stiffening of muscles after death, begins about 4 hours after death. The funeral director will have the best results if embalming is completed before rigor mortis sets in (Harvey, 2001). Position the body in a natural position.

When preparing the body for family viewing, endeavor to make the body look natural and comfortable. This means preparing and positioning the body as previously described. According to Harvey (2001), if the client wore dentures, they should *not* be put in the deceased person's mouth. Jaw muscles relax after death, so dentures often fall out and are lost or broken. Put them in a hospital denture cup without water and send them with the body to the funeral director. After the family has viewed the body, place identification tags on the body's toe and wrist. Then place the body in a plastic or fabric **shroud** (a covering for the body after death), and tag the shroud. Next, transport the body to the morgue according to the agency's policy, where it is kept until it can be transported to a **mortuary** (funeral home). In some institutions, the body is kept in the room until the funeral director arrives. The nurse is also responsible for returning the deceased's possessions, such as jewelry, eyeglasses, clothing, and all other personal items, to the family.

Information for Funeral Director

Harvey (2001) explains information that is important to the funeral director when preparing the body. The cause of death influences which procedures are used. For example, a client with liver or renal failure has a high level of ammonia in the body. A special solution will have to be used because the ammonia neutralizes the formaldehyde generally used. If the client had tuberculosis (TB) or any other communicable disease, special procedures will be followed to prevent spreading the disease. If the client weighed more than 300 pounds (136 kg), the funeral director will need extra staff for transferring the body.

Legal Aspects

The physician is legally responsible for determining the cause of death and signing the death certificate in most states. In certain situations, the RN may be responsible for certifying the death. Nurses must know their legal responsibilities, as defined by their respective state boards of nursing.

Autopsy

An **autopsy** is the examination of the body after death, by a pathologist to determine the cause of death. It is mandated in situations where an unusual death has occurred. For example, a violent death or an unexpected death are circumstances necessitating an autopsy. For an autopsy to be performed in other situations, families must give consent. The funeral director must know whether an autopsy is to be performed.

Organ Donation

Organ donation for transplantation requires sensitivity and compassion from the health care team. Health care facilities must have a policy regarding the referral of a potential organ donor to appropriate organ procurement agencies. A staff member of the organ procurement agency is generally the person who speaks to the family about organ donation. When an organ(s) is to be donated, that person also coordinates the entire process, including finding organ recipients (Nursing Grand Rounds, 2000).

The organs and tissues that can be transplanted are:

- Liver
- Lungs
- Heart
- Kidneys
- Pancreas
- Skin
- Bones (middle ear bones and long bones)
- Corneas

Transplantation must occur within 4 to 5 hours for heart and lungs, 18 hours for liver and pancreas, and 72 hours for kidneys (Nursing Grand Rounds, 2000).

Care of the Family

The nurse provides invaluable support to the family of the deceased at the time of death. It is extremely important to inform the family of the circumstances surrounding the death. The nurse offers information about viewing the body and contacts support people (e.g., other relatives, clergy). The nurse may even help the family with decisions regarding transportation, a funeral home, and removal of the deceased's belongings. Sensitive and compassionate interpersonal skills are essential when providing information and support to families. Providing coffee, tissues, and light snacks are small gestures that convey sensitivity to the family and friends and are appreciated.

Nurse's Self-Care

Working with dying clients can evoke both a personal and a professional threat in the nurse. Grief is a common experience for nurses because many nurses are confronted with death and loss daily. Smith-Stoner and Frost (1998) describe a part of the psyche called the shadow self, where stresses are stored. Unresolved sadness is called shadow grief. Everyone has a shadow self and may have some shadow grief. Nurses often have a great deal of shadow grief, which, if not released, may cause illness and burnout. Frequent exposure to death can interfere with the nurse's effectiveness because of subsequent anxiety and denial.

Nurses are at particular risk for experiencing negative effects from caring for the dying, whether working in a hospital, a hospice, a long-term care facility, or the home. They may not wish to confront their grief and will often use some of the common defense mechanisms against grieving such as being strong, keeping busy, and suffering in silence. Nurses must talk about the intense emotions associated with caregiving instead of pretending that they do not experience grief. According to Smith-Stoner and Frost (1998), shadow grief may be

PROFESSIONAL TIP

Care for Yourself during Grief

- Do what nurses do well: care. Help the family and your feelings of helplessness will diminish.
- Plan time for your own grieving.
- Allow for crying to help ease the pain.
- Learn when to ask your coworkers for help.
- Express your feelings of grief to someone you can trust.
- Find support within your facility from counselors, support groups, and clergy.
- Use rituals to say good-bye to the deceased client and bring closure.

(Adapted from "Please Cry with Me: Six Ways to Grieve," by C. D. Reese, 1996, *Nursing96, 26*[8], 56.)

starting to overwhelm a person if that person experiences the following:

- A loss of energy, spark, joy, and meaning in life
- Detachment from surroundings
- A feeling of being powerless to make a difference
- Increased smoking or drinking

- Unusual forgetfulness
- Constant criticism directed toward others
- Consistent inability to get work done
- Uncontrolled outbursts of anger
- Perception of clients and their families as objects
- Surrender of hobbies or interests

To effectively cope with their own grief, nurses need education, support, and assistance when coping with the death of clients. The focus of staff education should be on ways to seek support, decreasing staff anxiety when working with grieving clients and families, and ways to provide support to coworkers. Smith-Stoner and Frost (1998) suggest the following ways to cope:

- Take time to cry with and for clients.
- Get physical: run, walk, bike, play tennis.
- Ask colleagues to help with tasks; do not try to be "Supernurse."
- Connect to a place of worship; pray.
- Look for joy in work. Laughter is a great healer.
- Create a caring circle of friends.
- Listen to music.

The nurse's own fears and doubts about death may surface and cause anxiety about feelings of mortality. Caring for the dying client and the client's family is emotionally draining, so nurses must remember to care for themselves.

SAMPLE NURSING CARE PLAN

THE CLIENT WITH A TERMINAL ILLNESS/CANCER OF THE LUNG

Mrs. Paoli, an 84-year-old widow, was diagnosed with cancer of the right lung 6 months ago. After a right lower lobectomy, she was discharged to a local skilled-care facility and planned to go home after completing her radiation therapy. After completing the treatments, Mrs. Paoli's condition began deteriorating. She did not want to go home so discharge plans were discontinued. Now she is frequently short of breath, has dyspnea, requires pain medication, and needs some assistance with activities of daily living because of fatigue. She frequently grimaces and says, "I hurt." Her nutritional intake is very little because of swallowing difficulties. Mrs. Paoli gets up only to use the commode. Her two adult children and four grandchildren live nearby and visit often. They want to assist their mother to get her affairs in order, but she resists their efforts. The family is trying to make Mrs. Paoli's remaining time as serene and comfortable as possible, but Mrs. Paoli often defies their attempts.

Nursing Diagnosis 1   *Chronic **Pain*** related to disease progression as evidenced by verbal statements, body language, and the need for pain medication

Nursing Outcomes Classification (NOC)
Pain: Disruptive Effects
Pain: Psychological Response
Pain Control

Nursing Interventions Classification (NIC)
Pain Management
Analgesic Administration
Active Listening

continues

SAMPLE NURSING CARE PLAN

PLANNING/GOALS	NURSING INTERVENTIONS	RATIONALE
Mrs. Paoli will verbalize relief from pain.	Give analgesics as ordered.	Administering regular doses of analgesics is more effective than waiting until the pain begins.
	Have client rate pain on a scale of 0 to 10, with 0 being no pain and 10 being severe pain, to assess the need for morphine. Give morphine as ordered, titrated at increments until adequate pain relief is achieved.	The client should be given analgesics when pain is experienced. Morphine is the drug of choice for severe pain associated with cancer.
	Monitor for signs of breakthrough pain. If the precipitating factor is known, give medication 30 to 60 minutes before the event. Medicate as soon as possible for unpredictable breakthrough pain.	Breakthrough pain is often precipitated by activity or stress and supplemental medication is required.
	Assure Mrs. Paoli that the nurses will help her manage the pain and keep it under control. Reposition frequently and give back massages for comfort. Assist with relaxation techniques if client agreeable.	Needs reassurance that everything possible will be done to manage the pain. Promotes psychological comfort.
	Monitor bowel elimination.	Pain medication often causes constipation.

EVALUATION   Mrs. Paoli's body language and verbal statements indicate freedom from pain.

Nursing Diagnosis 2   *Ineffective Breathing Pattern* related to diminished lung function as evidenced by dyspnea and shortness of breath

Nursing Outcomes Classification (NOC)
Respiratory Status: Airway Patency
Respiratory Status: Gas Exchange
Energy Conservation

Nursing Interventions Classification (NIC)
Airway Management
Respiratory Monitoring
Oxygen Therapy

PLANNING/GOALS	NURSING INTERVENTIONS	RATIONALE
Mrs. Paoli will be free from moderate or severe dyspnea.	Teach breathing exercises and effective coughing techniques.	Enhances gas exchange in the alveoli.
	Allow adequate time for physical activities. Postpone activity if dyspnea is present. Provide as much assistance as needed.	Physical exertion increases dyspnea.
	Administer low-flow oxygen if blood gases indicate need.	Effective only if indicated by blood gases.
	Encourage client to drink 8 to 10 glasses of fluid each day.	Liquifies respiratory secretions and promotes hydration.
	Humidify the air with a cold-water vaporizer.	Enhances breathing.
	Assess respiratory system frequently.	Identifies complications at early stages.

EVALUATION   Mrs. Paoli has mild dyspnea, which sometimes interferes with activities.

continues

SAMPLE NURSING CARE PLAN

Nursing Diagnosis 3 *Ineffective Coping* related to terminal illness as evidenced by inability to communicate effectively with family members and to accept their help

Nursing Outcomes Classification (NOC)
Decision Making
Information Processing
Psychosocial Adjustment: Life Change

Nursing Interventions Classification (NIC)
Coping Enhancement
Counseling
Support System Enhancement

PLANNING/GOALS	NURSING INTERVENTIONS	RATIONALE
Mrs. Paoli will express her feelings openly.	Consult Mrs. Paoli on all aspects of care. Give complete information. Provide opportunities to express feelings. Acknowledge Mrs. Paoli's feelings and let her know that crying and grieving are beneficial.	Allows Mrs. Paoli to express her feelings and validates those feelings as being normal and expected.
	Listen for clues indicating unfinished business that needs to be completed. Encourage the process of life review.	Life review is a process of reflection and pondering of one's past and accepting one's life as being meaningful and valuable.
Mrs. Paoli will maintain a satisfying relationship with her family.	Encourage family visits. Provide privacy.	Families need privacy in order to feel free to express their emotions.

EVALUATION   Mrs. Paoli still resists family's assistance.

Summary

- Loss is when someone (or something) of value is no longer available. It is a universal response.
- Grief is a psychological response to loss evidenced by deep sorrow and mental anguish.
- The difference between pathological and normal grief is the inability of the individual to adapt to life without the loved one.
- Kübler-Ross identified five psychological stages of the dying process: denial, anger, bargaining, depression, and acceptance.
- Complicated grief is associated with traumatic death such as suicide, accident, or homicide.
- Each person dies a unique death.
- Hospice care is an alternative to hospitalization when aggressive medical treatment is no longer an option.
- After death, the nurse's focus is on supporting the family and caring for the deceased body.
- Nurses must care for themselves in order to provide compassionate, quality care to the dying person and family.

Review Questions

1. Susan, age 11 years, was left with a distant relative 2 weeks ago. Her parents have not returned or called. Susan is experiencing a:

   a. physical loss.

   b. situational loss.

   c. maturational loss.

   d. anticipational loss.

2. A defining characteristic of the NANDA nursing diagnosis *Anticipatory Grieving* is:

   a. prolonged denial or depression.

   b. unsuccessful adaptation to loss.

   c. social isolation or withdrawal from others.

   d. an expression of distress at potential loss.

3. The purpose of the Patient Self-Determination Act is to:

   a. serve as an order for "do not resuscitate."

   b. designate a guardian for an incompetent client.

c. provide a means, instead of a will, to designate what is to be done with a person's property, money, and personal possessions.

d. provide a legal means for individuals to state those circumstances under which life-sustaining treatment should or should not be provided to them.

4. One of the major goals of hospice care is:

a. freedom from pain and other symptoms.

b. free care for all dying clients and their families.

c. to cure the client using very aggressive medical treatment.

d. to transfer all dying clients to the hospital when death is imminent.

5. Signs of impending death include:

a. flushed warm skin.

b. very slow regular pulse rate.

c. inability to hear.

d. Cheyne-Stokes respirations.

References/Suggested Readings

American Nurses Association (ANA). (1996). Promotion of comfort and relief of pain in dying patients. In *Compendium of ANA position statements.* Washington, DC: Author.

Andreas, L. (1998). Controlling pain: Keeping a dying patient comfortable. *Nursing98, 28*(1), 70.

Backer, B. A., Hannon, N. R., & Russell, N. A. (1994). *Death and dying: Understanding and care* (2nd ed.). Clifton Park, NY: Thomson Delmar Learning.

Barbus, A. J. (1975). The dying person's bill of rights. *AJN, 75*(1), 99.

Boon, T. (1998). Don't forget the hospice option. *RN, 61*(2), 30–33.

Boss, P. (2000). *Ambiguous loss: Learning to live with unresolved grief.* Cambridge, MA: Harvard University Press.

Bowlby, J. (1982). *Attachment and loss: Vol. 2. Separation anxiety and anger.* New York: Basic.

Bral, E. (1998). Caring for adults with chronic cancer pain. *AJN, 98*(4), 27–32.

Cerrudo, J. (1998). Letting go of Abuelo. *AJN, 98*(8), 53.

Corless, I., Germino, B., & Pittman, M. (Eds.). (1995). *A challenge for living: Death, dying, and bereavement.* Boston: Jones & Bartlett.

Corr, C., Nabe, C., & Corr, D. (2000). *Death and dying, life and living* (3rd ed.). Belmont, CA: Wadsworth.

Dineen, K. (2002). Gift of presence. *Nursing2002, 32*(7), 76.

Dochterman, J., & Bulechek, G. (2004). *Nursing Interventions Classification (NIC)* (4th ed.). St. Louis, MO: Mosby.

Durham, E., & Weiss, L. (1997). How patients die. *AJN, 97*(12), 41–46.

Edelman, C. L., & Mandle, C. L. (2002). *Health promotion throughout the lifespan* (5th ed.). St. Louis, MO: Mosby.

Egan, K., and Arnold, R. (2003). Grief and bereavement care. *AJN, 103*(9), 42–52.

Engle, G. L. (1961). Is grief a disease? *Psychosomatic Medicine, 23,* 18–22.

Estes, M. E. Z. (2002). *Health assessment & physical examination* (2nd ed.). Clifton Park, NY: Thomson Delmar Learning.

Ferrell, B. (1998a). End-of-life care. *Nursing98, 28*(9), 58.

Ferrell, B. (1998b). How can we improve care at the end of life? *Nursing Management, 29*(9), 41–43.

Ferrell, B., Virani, R., Grant, M., Coyne, P., & Uman, G. (2000). End-of-life care: Nurses speak out. *Nursing2000, 30*(7), 54–57.

Forbes, V. (1998). The dying game. *AJN, 98*(9), 50.

Frisch, N., and Frisch, L. (2002). *Psychiatric mental health nursing.* Clifton Park, NY: Thomson Delmar Learning.

Furman, J. (2000). Taking a holistic approach to the dying time. *Nursing2000, 30*(6), 46–49.

Furman, J. (2001). Living with dying: How to help family caregivers. *Nursing2001, 31*(4), 36–41.

Furman, J. (2002). What you should know about chronic grief. *Nursing2002, 32*(2), 56–57.

Harvey, J. (2001). Debunking myths about postmortem care. *Nursing2001, 31*(7), 44–45.

Haynor, P. (1998). Meeting the challenge of advance directives, *AJN, 98*(3), 27–32.

Hellwig, K. (2000). A family lesson in dying. *RN, 63*(12), 32–33.

Hooks, F. J., & Daly, B. J. (2000). Hastening death: Is a natural death always best? *AJN, 100*(5), 56–63.

Huizdos, D. (2000). The tie that binds: Hanging on by a shoelace. *AJN, 100*(7), 25.

Kübler-Ross, E. (1969). *On death and dying.* New York: Macmillan.

Kübler-Ross, E. (1974). *Questions and answers on death and dying.* New York: Macmillan.

Kübler-Ross, E. (1995). *Death is of vital importance: On life, death, and life after death.* Barrytown, NY: Station Hill.

Kübler-Ross, E. (1997). *Meaning of our suffering.* Barrytown, NY: Barrytown, Ltd.

Kübler-Ross, E. (1997a). *Death, the final stage of growth.* Old Tappan, NJ: Simon & Schuster.

Kübler-Ross, E. (1997b). *To live until we say good-bye.* Upper Saddle River, NJ: Prentice Hall Trade.

Kübler-Ross, E., and Kessler, D. (2001). *Life lessons: Two experts on death and dying teach us about the mysteries of life and living.* Carmichael, CA: Touchstone Books.

LaDuke, S. (2001). Terminal dyspnea & palliative care. *AJN, 101*(11), 26–31.

Lindemann, E. (1944). Symptomatology and management of acute grief. *American Journal of Psychiatry, 101,* 141–148.

Lynn, J., Schuster, J. L., & Kabcenell, A. (2000). *Improving care for the end of life: A sourcebook for health care managers and clinicians.* New York: Oxford University Press.

Mazanec, P., & Tyler M. K. (2003). Cultural considerations in end-of-life care. *AJN, 103*(3), 50–58.

McCaffery, M., & Pasero, C. (1999). *Pain: Clinical manual for nursing practice* (2nd ed.). St. Louis, MO: Mosby.

McClain, M. E., & Shafer, S. M. (1996). Supporting families after sudden infant death. *Journal of Psychosocial Nursing and Mental Health Services, 34*(4), 30–34.

McGowan, D. (1998). The right to say goodbye. *RN, 61*(5), 84.

Moorhead, S., Johnson, M., & Maas, M. (2004). *Nursing Outcomes Classification (NOC)* (3rd ed.). St. Louis, MO: Mosby.

North American Nursing Diagnosis Association. (2003). *Nursing diagnoses: Definitions and classification 2003–2004.* Philadelphia: Author.

Nursing Grand Rounds. (2000). Helping a family through the organ donation process. *Nursing2000, 30*(4), 52–55.

Paice, J. (2002). Managing psychological conditions in palliative care. *AJN, 102*(11), 36–42.

Panke, J. (2002). Difficulties in managing pain at the end of life. *AJN, 102*(7), 26–33.

Pitorak, E. (2003). Care at the time of death. *AJN, 103*(7), 42–51.

Popernack, M. (2000). Are we overlooking a hidden source of organs? *Nursing2000, 30*(1), 44–47.

Powell, C. (1999). Near death: A nurse reflects. *RN, 62*(4), 43–44.

Pritchett, K., & Lucas, P. (1997a). Death and dying. In B. S. Johnson (Ed.), *Psychiatric–mental health nursing: Adaptation and growth* (4th ed., pp. 206–207). Philadelphia: Lippincott Williams & Wilkins.

Pritchett, K., & Lucas, P. (1997b). Grief and loss. In B. S. Johnson (Ed.), *Psychiatric–mental health nursing: Adaptation and growth* (4th ed., pp. 199–218). Philadelphia: Lippincott Williams & Wilkins.

Puopolo, A. (1999). Gaining confidence to talk about end-of-life care. *Nursing99, 29*(7), 49–51.

Reese, C. D. (1996). Please cry with me: Six ways to grieve. *Nursing96, 26*(8), 56.

Roach, S. S., & Nieto, B. C. (1997). *Healing and the grief process.* Clifton Park, NY: Thomson Delmar Learning.

Rodebaugh, L., Schwindt, R., & Valentine, F. (1999). How to handle grief with wisdom, *Nursing99, 29*(10), 52–53.

Scanlon, C. (2003). Ethical concerns in end-of-life care. *AJN, 103*(1), 48–55.

Slade, J., & Lovasik, D. (2002). Understanding brain death criteria. *Nursing2002, 32*(12), 68–69.

Smalkin, P. (2001). Facing a mother's death. *Nursing2001, 31*(7), 51.

Smith-Stoner, M., & Frost, A. (1998). Coping with grief and loss: Bringing your shadow self into the light. *Nursing98, 28*(2), 49–50.

Smith-Stoner, M., & Frost, A. (1999). How to build your "hope skills." *Nursing99, 29*(9), 49–51

Spicer, T. (2003). Coping with grief when a patient dies. *Nursing2003, 33*(3), 32hn6.

Taylor, M. (1995). Benefits of dehydration in terminally ill clients. *Geriatric Nursing, 16*(6), 271–272.

Thompson, G. (2002). Taking the measure of a fathr's grief. *Nursing2002, 32*(3), 46–47.

Tutka, M. A. (2001). Near-death experiences: Seeing the light. *Nursing2001, 31*(5), 62–64.

Ufema, J. (1995a). How to help dying clients feel "safe." *Nursing95, 25*(9), 59.

Ufema, J. (1995b). Insights on death and dying. *Nursing95, 25*(11,12), 19, 22–23.

Ufema, J. (1999). Reflections on death and dying. *Nursing99, 29*(6), 56–59.

Ufema, J. (2000a). Death & dying: Bedside vigils. *Nursing2000, 30*(7), 26.

Ufema, J. (2000b). Death & dying: Seeking closure. *Nursing2000, 30*(8), 28.

Ufema, J. (2000c). Death & dying: Setting goals, withholding nutrition, will to die. *Nursing2000, 30*(9), 66–67.

Ufema, J. (2002). Insights on death and dying. *Nursing2002, 32*(10), 28–30.

Vanderbeek, J. (2000). Till death do us part: A firsthand account of family presence. *AJN, 100*(2), 44.

Virani, R., & Sofer, D. (2003). Improving the quality of end-of-life care. *AJN, 103*(5), 52–60.

Wong, M. M. (1996). *The 1996 national directory of bereavement support groups and services.* Forest Hills, NY: ADM.

Wong, M. M. (2001). *Understanding your grieving heart after a loved one's death.* Forest Hills, NY: ADM.

Zerwekh, J. (2003). End-of-life hydration—benefit or burden? *Nursing2003, 33*(2), 32hn1–32hn3.

Resources

American Nurses Association Center for Ethics and Human Rights, 600 Maryland Avenue, Suite 100 West, Washington, DC 20024, 800-274-4262, www.nursing world.org

Americans for Better Care of the Dying, 4125 Albemarle Street NW, Suite 210, Washington, DC 20016, 202-895-9485, www.abcd-caring.org

Association for Death Education & Counseling, 342 North Main Street, Hartford, CT 06117-2507, 860-586-7503, www.adec.org

Compassion in Dying Federation, 6312 SW Capitol Highway, Suite 415, Portland, OR 97201, 503-221-9556, www.compassionindying.org

Hospice Foundation of America, 2001 S. Street NW #300, Washington, DC 20009, 800-854-3402, www.hospice foundation.org

Last Acts, 325 West Huron, Suite 300, Chicago, IL 60610, 312-751-1297, www.lastacts.org

Partnership for Caring: America's Voices for the Dying, 475 Riverside Drive, Suite 1852, New York, NY 10115, 800-989-9455, www.partnershipforcaring.org

The National Hospice and Palliative Care Organization, 1700 Diagonal Road, Suite 625, Alexandria, VA 22314, 703-837-1500, www.nhpco.org

TransWeb, The Northern Brewery, 1327 Jones Drive, Suite 105, Ann Arbor, MI 48105, 734-998-7314, www.transweb.org

United Network for Organ Sharing, 1100 Boulders Parkway, P.O. Box 13770, Richmond, VA 23225-8770, 888-894-6361, www.unos.org

UNIT 5

Health Promotion

CHAPTER

14

WELLNESS CONCEPTS

MAKING THE CONNECTION

Refer to the following chapters to increase your understanding of wellness concepts:

Basic Nursing
- Cultural Considerations
- Loss, Grief, and Death

Adult Health Nursing
- Reproductive System
- The Older Adult

LEARNING OBJECTIVES

Upon completion of this chapter, you should be able to:
- Define key terms.
- Explain the importance of Healthy People 2010.
- Discuss the scope of prevention.
- Describe the benefits of using a genogram.
- Teach and follow the guidelines for healthy living.
- Make a teaching plan to promote and maintain wellness.

KEY TERMS

genogram
health
prevention
primary prevention

secondary prevention
tertiary prevention
wellness

INTRODUCTION

Individual adults have the responsibility for maintaining their own health, and parents are also responsible for maintaining their children's health and teaching them a healthy lifestyle. Health maintenance includes prevention of disease and early detection and treatment of disease, requiring constant effort focusing on all aspects of a person's life.

Simon (1992) quotes Dr. Wood Hutchinson, who in 1896 wrote in the *Journal of the American Medical Association* that "our system's philosophy might be condensed in the motto 'millions for health care and not a penny for prevention'." More than 100 years have passed and still less than 3 cents of each health dollar is spent on prevention and education.

The United States is 16th among nations in life expectancy yet is the world leader in medical science and education. We rank 24th in infant mortality and spend more for health care than any other country. Preventive medicine has not been incorporated by many doctors into their practices (Simon, 1992).

There is no profit in prevention. Insurance pays for diagnosis and treatment of illnesses, not health mainte-

nance, but often will not pay for preventive testing and treatment. Paying for clinical care makes illness the priority, not wellness.

HEALTH

The generally accepted definition of **health** from the World Health Organization (WHO) defines health as a state of complete physical, mental, and social well-being, not merely the absence of disease or infirmity.

Another concept of health focuses on motivation. The individual is motivated by joy and self-fulfillment and believes that health is the realization of potential, and illness is an obstacle in that realization.

Those who have an adaptive view of health are motivated by altering the risks in self or the environment through diet and exercise or by reducing exposure to environmental hazards. When the individual is unable to cope with the stresses and risks of daily life, illness results.

Some individuals are motivated by being able to meet responsibilities at home, at work, at play, and in the community: Their health focus is role performance. Health is considered achieved when the individual fulfills the responsibilities and obligations to family, job, and community.

Other individuals are motivated by the absence of disease: Theirs is a clinical health focus. As long as no disease is present, the individual considers himself healthy.

A person's definition of health influences personal health decisions and life choices.

WELLNESS

Wellness is defined as a state of optimal health wherein an individual maximizes human potential, moves toward integration of human functioning, has greater self-awareness and self-satisfaction, and takes responsibility for health. Floyd, Mimms, and Yelding-Howard (1995), Turner, Hoeger, and Hafen (2001), and Seiger, Vanderpool, and Barnes (2000) describe the behaviors exhibited by individuals in a state of wellness. These researchers outline seven areas of wellness: emotional, mental, intellectual, vocational, social, spiritual, and physical wellness. Various areas of wellness overlap and none is mutually exclusive.

Emotional Wellness

Emotions bridge the gap between body and mind. The individual who is emotionally well understands his own feelings and knows when to express them appropriately. This person accepts limitations, copes with stress in healthy ways, has the ability to adjust to change, is optimistic and happy, enjoys life, and shows respect and affection to others.

Mental Wellness

The person who is mentally well is alert, curious, clear thinking, open-minded, creative, logical, and accepting of others. This person also has a good memory, common sense, and a desire for continual learning.

Intellectual Wellness

Intellectual wellness is revealed by an ability to think, process information, and solve problems. The intellectually well person questions and evaluates information and situations, is creative, flexible, and open to new ideas, and learns from life experiences.

Vocational Wellness

The individual who is satisfied in school and/or job and who works in harmony with others enjoys vocational wellness (Figure 14-1).

Figure 14-1 *Vocational wellness means being content and satisfied with your occupation.*

Social Wellness

The person who shows affection, fairness, concern, and respect for others; communicates effectively; has satisfying relationships; and interacts well with others enjoys social wellness. This person has a network of friends and family, is a member of various organizations, and enjoys working together. Other behaviors exhibited are confidence, loyalty, honesty, and tolerance.

Spiritual Wellness

Spiritual wellness gives direction, meaning, and purpose to life through values, morals, and ethics. The spiritually healthy person has optimism, faith, and high self-esteem.

Physical Wellness

Physical wellness is seen in individuals who exercise regularly, eat a well-balanced diet, and have regular physical examinations. They avoid risky sexual behavior; try to limit exposure to environmental contaminants; and restrict the intake of alcohol, tobacco, caffeine, and drugs (Figure 14-2).

HEALTH PROMOTION

Health promotion is more than preventing illness: It means assisting individuals to better health, functioning, and well-being, and to maximize their potential. Health promotion focuses on choosing healthy behaviors rather than on eluding illness. The goal is for individuals to control and improve their health. Health pro-

CLIENT TEACHING

Suppressed Anger in Women

Research has shown that middle-aged women who suppress anger and have hostile attitudes may be at greater risk for developing cardiovascular disease (Matthews, 1998). Nurses can help such women minimize this risk by encouraging them to learn to express negative feelings constructively, to talk calmly about their feelings, to find other women who may share some of the same concerns and stressors, and to engage in regular exercise routines to relieve stress and tension.

CULTURAL CONSIDERATIONS

Spiritual Well-Being

Oman and Reed (1998) studied nearly 2,000 persons age 55 years and older for 5 years. They found that those persons who attended religious services were 24% less likely to have died in those 5 years than were those who did not attend services. This underscores the importance of religion and spiritual wellness to an individual's overall state of health.

Figure 14-3 *Families can engage in activities together to achieve wellness.*

Healthy People 2000

In 1980 and again in 1990, the U.S. Department of Health and Human Services (DHHS) released a list of objectives for disease prevention and health promotion in 22 priority areas (DHHS, 1990). More than 10,000 individuals representing 300 national organizations met in 1990 to develop the health objectives for the year 2000. More than 300 health objectives were drafted for the nation to achieve by the year 2000. These objectives were published in a document titled *Healthy People 2000: National Health Promotion and Disease Prevention Objectives,* which addresses three important issues:

- *Personal responsibility:* Each individual must be health-conscious and must practice informed, responsible, health behaviors.
- *Health benefits for all people:* Everyone must have health benefits for the nation to be healthy.
- *Health promotion and disease prevention:* Health care must change from a treatment focus to a prevention focus to increase the quality of life and to cut costs.

The overall goals included:

- Increasing the span of healthy life for Americans
- Reducing health disparities among Americans
- Achieving access to preventive services for all Americans

Figure 14-2 *Individuals must learn to achieve physical wellness in a manner that accommodates their lifestyle and physical abilities.*

motion is appropriate for the individual and the entire population.

The concept of self-responsibility is important to health promotion. No one else can make a person live a healthy life; self-responsibility is the only way to make changes. An individual can be given information relating to health and wellness, but only that person can change unhealthy or destructive habits. With the exception of small children, each individual must take responsibility for behaviors leading to health and wellness (Figure 14-3). Objectives for healthy living are outlined in the *Healthy People 2000* and *Healthy People 2010* documents issued by the federal government.

PROFESSIONAL TIP

Predictors of Healthy Aging

The most consistent predictors of healthy aging are low serum glucose, normal blood pressure, avoidance of smoking, and maintenance of target weight for height (Reed, 1998). To prevent disease in later years, young adults and even adolescents must keep these four factors in check. It is never too late to modify these four factors to improve health.

A sample of the objectives is found in Table 14–1. The entire document may be ordered from the U.S. Department of Health and Human Services, Washington, DC, DHHS Publication No. (PHS) 91–50212.

The DHHS (2000b) reported on the progress made in meeting the 319 objectives of *Healthy People 2000*. In 1997, 15% of the goals had been reached or surpassed, and progress had been made in another 44%. Eighteen percent had fallen short of target, 6% showed mixed re-

sults, and 2% showed no change. Eleven percent now have baseline data but no data to evaluate progress, and baselines have not yet been established for 3% of these goals (DHHS, Healthy People 2000b).

Healthy People 2010

The Healthy People 2000 Consortium met in November 1996 to discuss necessary improvements and

TABLE 14–1 SELECTED OBJECTIVES FROM *HEALTHY PEOPLE 2000* AND *HEALTHY PEOPLE 2010*				
OBJECTIVE	BASELINE	YEAR 2000 TARGET	REPORT	YEAR 2010 TARGET
Physical Activity and Fitness				
• Increase the proportion of people who engage regularly in light to moderate physical activity for at least 30 minutes per day	22% (1985)	30%	23% (1995) (+)	30%
• Increase the proportion of young people in grades 9 to 12 who participate in daily school physical activity	42% (1991)	50%	27% (1997) (−)	50%
Nutrition				
• Increase the proportion of people aged 2 years and older who meet the Dietary Guidelines average daily goal of no more than 30% of calories from fat	34% (1989–91)	30%	33% (1994–96) (−)	75%
• Reduce the prevalence of BMI at or above 30.0 among people ages 20 years and older	24% males 27% females (1976–80)	20% both groups	34% males 37% females (1988–94) (−)	15%
Tobacco				
• Increase the proportion of cigarette smokers ages 18 years and older who stopped smoking cigarettes for a day	34% (1986)	50%	45.8% (1995) (+)	75%
• Increase the proportion of worksites with a formal smoking policy that prohibits smoking or limits it to separately ventilated areas at the workplace	NA	NA	59% of worksites with 50 or more employees (1992)	100%
Substance Abuse				
• Decrease alcohol-related motor vehicle crash deaths	9.8/100,000 (1987)	5.5/100,000	6.5/100,000 (1997)	3.5/100,000
• Reduce drug-related deaths	3.8/100,000 (1987)	3/100,000	4.7/100,000 (−) (1998)	1.3/100,000
Family Planning				
• Reduce the proportion of individuals ages 15 to 17 who have ever had sexual intercourse	33% of males 27% of females (1988)	15%	27% of males 22% of females (1999)	15%
• Increase the proportion of all females ages 15 to 44 at risk of unintended pregnancy who use contraception	88.2% (1982)	95%	92.5% (1999)	95% (modified to "use effective contraception")
Mental Health and Mental Disorders				
• Reduce suicide rates	11.7/100,000 (1987)	10.5/100,000	11.3/100,000 (1996)	9.6/100,000 *continues*

TABLE 14-1   continued

OBJECTIVE	BASELINE	YEAR 2000 TARGET	REPORT	YEAR 2010 TARGET
Injury/Violence Prevention				
• Reduce firearm-related deaths	14.6/100,000 (1990)	11.6/100,000	13.5/100,000 (1996)	Fewer than 11.6/100,000
• Increase use of bicycle helmets of 9th- to 12th-grade students who ride bicycles		50%	8% (1995)	50%
Maternal, Infant, Child Health				
• Increase the proportion of all pregnant women who begin prenatal care in the first trimester of pregnancy	78.9% (1993)	90%	82.5% (1999)	90%
• Reduce the cesarean delivery rate	24.4/100 (1987)	15/100	21.8/100 (1999)	15/100
Cancer				
• Reduce cancer deaths		130/100,000	130/100,000 (1998) (=)	103/100,000
AIDS/HIV Infection				
• Confine annual incidence of diagnosed AIDS cases among adolescents and adults	29.8/100,000 (1994)		28/100,000 (1998) (+)	12/100,000
• Increase the proportion of those with positive HIV tests who return for counseling	72.5% (1989)	80%	83% (1995) (+)	none
Sexually Transmitted Diseases				
• Reduce prevalence of *Chlamydia trachomatis* infections among 14–24 year olds	12.5% (1996)	5%	10.9% (1998)	3%
• Eliminate sustained domestic transmission of primary and secondary syphilis	84% higher than 1997 (1990)	4/100,000	3.2/100,000 (1998) (+)	0.25/100,000
Immunizatons and Infectious Diseases				
• Reduce indigenous cases of vaccine preventable diseases				
–Diphtheria		0	4 (1997)	0
–Polio		0	0 (1997)	0
–Measles	3,058 (1988)	0	135 (1997)	0
–Rubella	225 (1988)	0	161 (1997)	0
–Mumps	4,866 (1988)	500	612 (1997)	0
–Pertussis	3,450 (1988)	1,000	6,568 (1997) (−)	2,000
• Increase proportion of contacts completing course of preventive therapy for tuberculosis	66.3% (1987)	85%	65.4% (1995) (−)	85%
Environmental Health				
• Reduce exposure of children age 6 and younger who are regularly exposed to tobacco smoke	39% (1986)	20%	27% (1997)	15%

(+) Exceeding target
(−) Receding from target
(=) Met target
Data from U.S. Department of Health & Human Services (DHHS), Public Health Service. (2000b). 1998–1999 Progress Review [On-line] Available: http://odphp.osophs.dhhs.gov/pubs/hp2000.

modifications to be made for Healthy People 2010 objectives. The consortium worked with a wide range of representatives of national membership organizations, state governments, managed care organizations, and private businesses through focus groups, public meetings, and the Healthy People 2010 website. Several themes emerged from the meetings and focus groups and were earmarked to be addressed in the revised objectives. These include the following:

- Need to address morbidity and mortality in setting objectives
- Value of packaging the 2010 document into different formats for multiple audiences
- Necessity of linking objectives to community-based health improvement initiatives
- Importance of using language that is understandable to the general public

Two goals for the 2010 objectives emerged as a result of these sessions: (1) "Increase Years of Healthy Life," which was retained from the Healthy People 2000 goal, and (2) "Eliminate Health Disparities," a stronger version of the Healthy People 2000 goal "Reduce Health Disparities." These two goals will be supported by four enabling goals concerned with promoting healthy behaviors, protecting health, achieving access to quality health care, and strengthening community prevention. A comparison of select 2000 objectives is presented in Table 14–1, along with baselines, targets, and 2010 objectives.

The 467 objectives for 2010 are grouped into 28 focus areas. New focus areas include disability; people with low income; race and ethnicity; chronic diseases; and public health infrastructure (DHHS, 2000a).

To expand the ability to track the objectives, new strategies are being developed to improve data collection, especially at the community level, and to improve the ability to measure access and quality of health services. *Healthy People 2010* was released in January 2000.

ILLNESS PREVENTION

Prevention (obstructing, thwarting, or hindering a disease or illness) incorporates both new and old ideas. The dietary laws, taboos, and traditions of various ethnic, cultural, and religious groups were begun for a reason. There is no reason not to practice the old ways if scientific research has not proven them incorrect or harmful. New methods of illness prevention emerge as technology expands and health awareness increases.

Preventive health should be practiced in all stages of life, beginning before conception with healthy parents and continuing through prenatal care and the life span. Interventions for disease prevention range from lifestyle changes that cost little or nothing to high-tech procedures that are very expensive.

Major changes are needed in health care delivery, funding, and insurance coverage before the full impact of illness prevention can be discovered. The health care system must insist on more research relating to prevention and must then apply the results of the research to insurance practices. Prevention practices must be supported and funded by the health care system in order for a change from illness treatment to illness prevention to occur. Enhanced health, longer life expectancy, and a pop-

ulation that functions better, feels better, and looks better will be the rewards of such a shift.

Types of Prevention

There are three types of prevention: primary, secondary, and tertiary. Primary prevention has not historically been supported by our health care system, whereas secondary and tertiary prevention have been, and still are, the main focus. They are also the most expensive.

Primary Prevention

Primary prevention includes all practices designed to keep health problems from developing. Primary prevention includes following recommended childhood immunization schedules, eating calcium-rich foods to prevent osteoporosis, and not smoking to prevent lung cancer. Every individual and health care provider should focus on primary prevention. It is usually the least expensive intervention and provides the greatest benefits.

Secondary Prevention

Secondary prevention refers to early detection, screening, diagnosis, and intervention to reduce the consequences of a health problem. An illness or disease is identified before the individual has any symptoms or functional impairment. Screening for tuberculosis and performing monthly breast self-examinations are both examples of secondary prevention. When no known methods of primary prevention exist for a specific disease or illness (such as breast cancer), the focus should be on performing self-examinations, having a regular physical exam, and testing.

Tertiary Prevention

Tertiary prevention refers to caring for a person who already has a health problem, which is treated after symptoms appeared to prevent further progression. For example, taking antibiotics for an ear infection should eliminate the infection. Furthermore, potential complications and the disability of hearing impairment are prevented. Rehabilitation is an important aspect of tertiary prevention; this refers to preventing deterioration of a person's condition and minimizing the loss of function. One example is providing range-of-motion exercises to a client who has had a stroke, to encourage circulation and maintain function in the extremities.

Prevention Health Care Team

The individual assisted by nurses and the primary physician make up the prevention health care team.

Individual

The center of the prevention health care team is the individual. The individual must combine the knowledge of preventive health care with behavioral changes necessary to live a healthier life.

Individuals should decide those things that they want and expect from health care. Clients must be honest with self, the nurses, and physician; be assertive and ask questions of the physicians and nurses; and be active, informed health care consumers. Ultimately, responsibility for health care rests with the individual.

Nurses

Nurses, especially nurse practitioners, often do the initial health screening in clinics and physicians' offices. This provides a great opportunity to inquire about the preventive health habits and lifestyle of the client. Nurses can use their excellent listening skills to give clients time to discuss health care habits and ask questions. Nurses are also great teachers of preventive health habits and health promotion activities.

Primary Physicians

Primary physicians usually are family practitioners, internists, or pediatricians. These are the family doctors seen on a regular basis. They have the opportunity and obligation to discuss and inquire about preventive health habits. They refer clients to specialists for specific problems when necessary. When the problem is resolved, the client returns to the primary physician for further care.

FACTORS AFFECTING HEALTH

The many factors affecting health can be categorized into four broad topics:

- Genetics and human biology
- Environmental influences
- Personal behavior
- Health care

Genetics and Human Biology

Inherited traits and the way the human body functions have an impact on an individual's state of health and wellness. An individual's genetic makeup may include inherited disorders, such as sickle-cell anemia, or chromosomal anomalies, such as Down syndrome. Both of these may ultimately affect the individual's quality of life and level of health.

Human biology affects health because normal body functioning prevents some illnesses and makes us more susceptible to others. Many of these effects are produced by the female and male hormones, estrogen and testosterone, respectively (Hoffman, 1996) (Table 14–2).

TABLE 14-2   EFFECTS OF ESTROGEN AND TESTOSTERONE ON SPECIFIC TISSUES

	HORMONE	
TISSUE	ESTROGEN (FEMALE)	TESTOSTERONE (MALE)
Cardiovascular	• Increases arterial dilation • Causes vascular spasms • Improves cardiac function	• Increases size of heart
Liver	• Inhibits production of triglycerides, low-density lipoprotein (LDL) (bad) cholesterol, and free glucose • Decreases drug metabolism, prolonging action	• Produces triglycerides, LDL (bad) cholesterol, and free glucose • Increases drug metabolism, shortening action
Fat	• Encourages fat deposits in breasts, hips, and thighs and suppresses the movement of fat from these areas	• Encourages fat deposits in the abdomen
Gastrointestinal	• Slows motility and favors formation of gallstones	
Respiratory	• Increases respiratory rate and basal body temperature	
Musculoskeletal	• Enhances bone density	• Ensures bone density and strength
Immune	• Enhances antibody production and suppresses T cell-mediated processes (prevents rejection of sperm and fetus)	
Blood	• Suppresses red blood cell (RBC) development • Lowers hemoglobin (Hgb) level • Increases coagulation	• Increases RBC development • Increases Hgb level
Integumentary	• Enhances skin vitality • Increases collagen and water content	• Promotes body hair

Data from Our Health, Our Lives, *by E. Hoffman, 1996, New York: Pocket Books. Copyright 1996 by Pocket Books.*

Environmental Influences

Environmental factors that may influence health are numerous, can be natural or man-made, and vary depending on geographic location and living conditions. Exposure to or ingestion of certain natural biological irritants can cause disease, such as results from exposure to poison ivy, and even death, such as results from ingestion of poisonous mushrooms. Exposure to chemicals such as asbestos in older buildings, lead paint in older houses, and mercury in polluted water sources also are health hazards. Radiation from the sun and some types of machinery can be harmful; extreme, prolonged exposure to solar radiation can even result in death. Natural disasters such as hurricanes, floods, volcanic eruptions, droughts, heat waves, blizzards, and other extreme weather conditions pose health risks, as do man-made environmental crises including wars, bombings, pollution, and overpopulation.

Personal Behavior

Personal behavior is the area with the most factors affecting health and wellness, and they are controlled entirely by the individual. It is the individual's decision to use or not to use these factors to promote health and wellness. Factors typically deemed to be under the individual's control include diet, exercise, personal care, sexual relationships, level of stress, tobacco and drug use, alcohol use, and safety.

Diet

Healthy eating habits and a proper diet greatly enhance an individual's overall state of health and well-being. Eating both fulfills the basic biological needs of sustenance, nutrition, and hydration and allows individuals to meet social and interpersonal needs (Figure 14-4). All of these factors contribute to overall wellness.

Exercise

Integrating physical activity into daily life is one of the best ways of promoting health. Exercise improves

Figure 14-4 *Sharing meals together is a wonderful means of meeting both physical and interpersonal needs.*

CULTURAL CONSIDERATIONS

Parents' Beliefs about Feeding Children
Many parents:

- Believe that milk alone will not satisfy their babies' hunger, so they begin feeding cereal and other solid foods earlier than recommended.
- Use food to console children.
- Believe a plump child is a healthier child.
- View a heavy infant or toddler as evidence of parental competence (Baughcum, 1998).

Nurses can work with these clients by respecting their cultural beliefs while enforcing the notion that a healthy child is a child who is satisfied following a meal and who shows a healthy, normal physical and emotional growth pattern. These factors, not plumpness, are indicators of wellness.

muscle strength, circulation, and emotional well-being; increases endurance; lowers blood pressure; and reduces the chances of heart attack, osteoporosis, and stroke. The individual who exercises regularly feels better and looks healthier.

Health clubs are used by many people in an effort to meet their need for exercise. Health clubs are a wonderful place for regular exercise, but also can be a source of disease. For example, perspiration on exercise machines is a prime source of impetigo. Clients should be made aware of such dangers so they can practice safety precautions, such as wearing thigh-length shorts and always keeping a towel between the body and the exercise equipment.

CLIENT TEACHING

Dietary Guidelines for Americans
Teach clients to develop nutritional wellness by:

Aim for Fitness
- Aiming for a healthy weight.
- Being physically active each day.

Build a Healthy Base
- Letting the Food Pyramid guide your meal choices.
- Choosing a variety of grains daily, especially whole grains.
- Choosing a variety of fruits and vegetables daily.
- Keeping food safe to eat.

Choose Sensibly
- Choosing a diet that is low in both saturated fat and cholesterol and moderate in total fat.
- Choosing beverages and foods to moderate your intake of sugars.
- Choosing and preparing foods with less salt.
- If you drink alcoholic beverages, doing so in moderation.

From *Home and Garden Bulletin No. 232* (5th ed.), by U.S. Department of Agriculture and U.S. Department of Health and Human Services, 2000.

Personal Care

The skin works with the immune system to defend the body against harmful allergens, bacteria, fungi, and viruses by protecting the body from outside elements. Regular skin, hair, and nail care will enhance wellness and foster self-esteem. Personal care also includes such wellness habits as proper posture, proper body mechanics, adequate sleep, and dental hygiene.

Sexual Relationships

Establishing intimacy and a sexual relationship with another person is a natural step in growth and development. To maintain health and wellness, the individual will use values, ethics, and morals to guide the development of the relationship. A healthy sexual relationship is based on mutual satisfaction of the parties, a consensual approach to pleasurable activities, and mutual respect for preferences and personal choices. One role of the nurse is to educate the client on ways to prevent sexually transmitted diseases.

Level of Stress

Not all stress is harmful. Limited stress raises one's energy level and makes one more alert. The way one responds to or copes with stressors dictates whether the situation is healthy or harmful. For instance one individual may enjoy the challenge of balancing work and family, while another may feel torn by these seemingly conflicting demands and will experience undue stress. Stress results not from an individual's life situation, but from that individual's reaction to and perception of the life situation.

Tobacco and Drug Use

Refraining from tobacco use is a strong step toward health promotion and maintenance. Even when a long-time smoker gives up the habit, the health risks begin to decrease at once, although it will take 10 to 15 years to eliminate all the effects of smoking from the lungs. The person who smokes exhales secondhand smoke, which presents a health risk to those who do not smoke.

Abuse of both illegal and prescription drugs is a serious medical and social problem in our society. Drugs prescribed by a physician are abused if they are not taken as directed, or if they are taken by anyone other than the client for whom they were prescribed. If not taken as directed, many prescribed drugs can be addictive. Health can be maintained when clients understand the effects, indications, side effects, and interactions of the prescription medications they are taking.

Alcohol Use

The decision to consume alcohol is a personal choice that can influence an individual's state of health. The amount of alcohol consumed will affect sobriety, decision-making ability, and, in many instances, safety. The use of alcohol can play a prominent role in drownings, suicides, traffic fatalities, adult fire deaths, and falling fatalities.

Safety

Personal choices concerning safety affect many areas of an individual's life and can be viewed collectively more as a lifestyle choice than individually as separate acts to promote safety. For example, individuals who embrace safety as a fundamental element of health and well-being will ensure safety in their homes by having smoke detectors, fire extinguishers, carbon monoxide detectors, practiced escape plans, locked medicine cabinets, and gates blocking dangerous stairways. These individuals will also most likely buckle their car seat belts, secure their children in child car seats, and obey speed limits when driving. All these elements of safety support a healthy lifestyle.

Health Care

Most people use the health care system to treat their illness or condition. However, health promotion and disease prevention are a more effective use of the health care system. Routine physical examinations with minimal testing are beneficial for preventing disease and maintaining health (Figure 14-5). Healthy adults should consider health care services based on family health history, personal habits, or personal health history. The presence of symptoms will alter the time frame for suggested health care services.

Figure 14-5 *Routine physical examinations are essential to maintaining health and preventing disease.*

Physical Exam

The physical examination begins with a review of family health history, personal health history, personal habits (sexual practices, tobacco, alcohol, and drug use), and concerns or questions the client may have. The client should write down questions and concerns before visiting the physician so none will be forgotten. Between the ages of 20 and 39 years, individuals should have a complete physical exam every 1 to 3 years; those 40 to 49 years of age, every 1 to 2 years; and those older than 50 years of age, every year. Women should have a breast exam with every physical exam before age 40 and yearly thereafter. Men should have a testicular exam and a rectal exam to check the prostate with every physical exam after age 40.

Immunizations

Adults who did not have the recommended immunizations as children should discuss this with their primary physicians. The physician may recommend having the immunizations as an adult based on the client's risk factors.

Every adult should have a tetanus booster every 10 years for life. Health care workers and college students; those with high risk of exposure; those with chronic heart, pulmonary, or kidney disease; those with diabetes; and those 65 years of age and older should have an influenza immunization every year and a pneumococcal pneumonia immunization every 6 years.

Tests

The following tests should be done with every physical exam: complete blood count, blood sugar, cholesterol, urinalysis, stool for blood, and, for women, a

Papanicolau (Pap) smear. An electrocardiogram (EKG or ECG) should be done at ages 20 and 40 and every 5 years thereafter (yearly if the client is at high risk). Women should have a baseline mammogram (Figure 14-6) at age 40 and yearly thereafter. Men should have a rectal exam of the prostate and testicular exam at each physical exam. A breast self-exam should be done by every

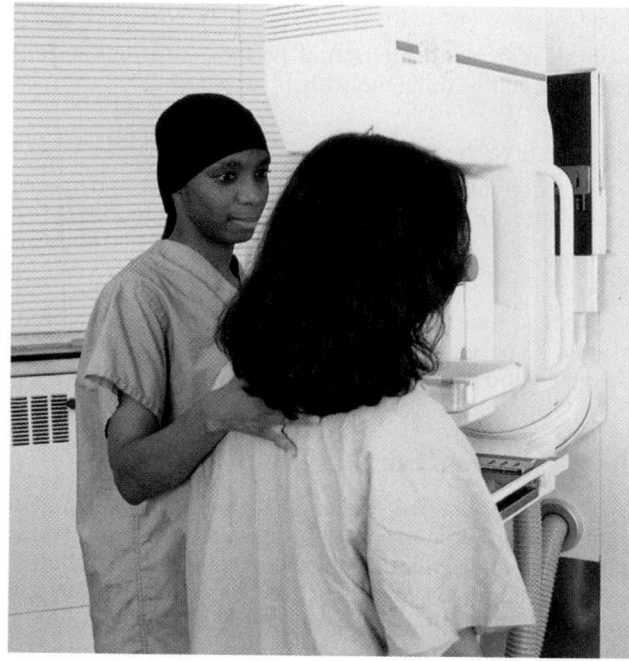

Figure 14-6 *Mammograms are a key element to wellness promotion for all women older than 40 years of age.*

CRITICAL THINKING

Wellness

How can you assist clients to assess their state of wellness? What preventive health care should be received by a person 20 years old, 42 years old, and 65 years old?

How does the nurse's state of wellness affect client care?

CLIENT TEACHING

Crucial Health Practices

Simon (1992) states that all the medical progress in the United States from 1900–1990 increased the life span of an average adult by 4 years; but that simple lifestyle changes increased the life span of an average adult by 11 years. He describes 10 crucial health practices:

- Use no tobacco or drugs.
- Consume no more than 2 ounces of alcohol per day.
- Eat a diet low in fat, cholesterol, and salt but high in fiber, fruits, vegetables, and fish.
- Exercise regularly—1 hour each week is helpful, 3 is ideal.
- Stay lean.
- Drive cars with air bags and wear seat belts; drive prudently, and never drink before driving.
- Avoid excessive stress.
- Minimize exposure to radiation, ultraviolet rays, chemical pollutants, and other environmental hazards.
- Protect self from sexually transmitted diseases.
- Obtain regular medical care including immunizations and screening tests.

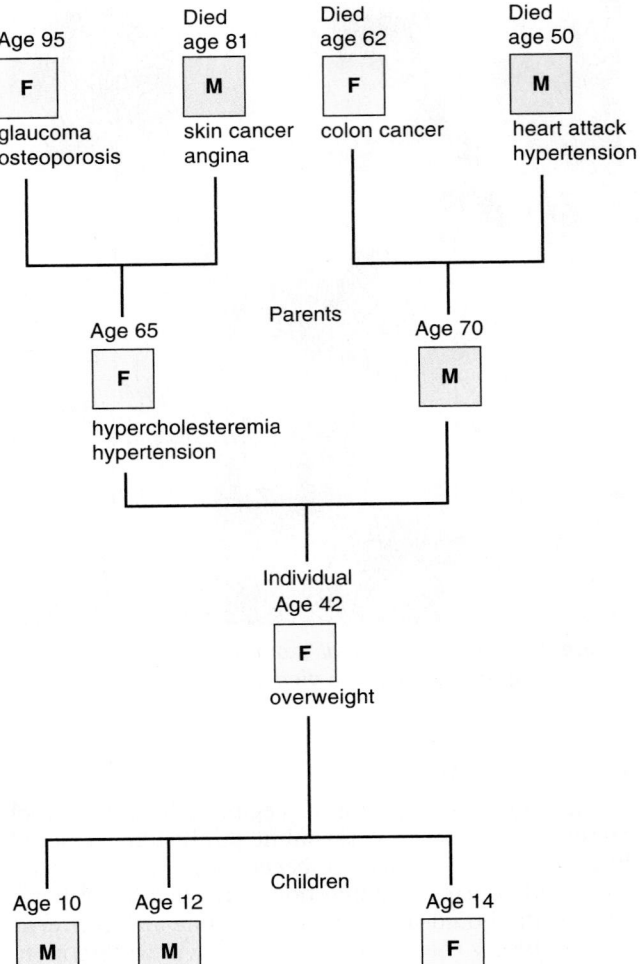

Figure 14-7 *Sample Genogram*

woman after each menstrual period. A testicular self-exam should be done monthly by every male.

Dental Exam

Throughout life, a dental exam, prophylaxis, and needed treatment should be performed every 6 to 12 months.

Eye Exam

An eye exam, including tonometry for glaucoma, should be performed every 2 to 3 years from ages 40 to 49 years and every 1 to 2 years after the age of 50.

MAKING A GENOGRAM

A **genogram** is a way to visualize family members, their birth and death dates or ages, and specific health problems. At least four generations should be included: the individual, the parents, the grandparents, and the children. Then it is easy to follow health problems through the generations. Health problems that may be encountered can be identified and steps taken to prevent them. Figure 14-7 shows a sample genogram.

GUIDELINES FOR HEALTHY LIVING

Because of their education and training, nurses are in a unique position to practice healthy living habits themselves and to promote such habits in their clients. Table 14-3 identifies the top 10 causes of death and the controllable factors that most contribute to these types of deaths. While it is important to remember that certain health variables such as gender and race cannot be controlled or changed, others such as diet and tobacco use result from individual choice. These lifestyle choices are based on individual preference, and nurses can help clients make the best choices to promote wellness and optimal functioning. Following is a list of select guidelines, for nurses and their clients, to promote healthy living and wellness in daily life.

Heart Disease:

- Eat a diet low in fat and cholesterol and high in fiber.
- Exercise regularly, 30 minutes three to five times a week (walking, swimming, cycling).
- Quit smoking or do not start to smoke.
- Reduce stress; use relaxation or meditation.
- Do not use caffeine or alcohol excessively.
- Maintain appropriate height-to-weight ratio.

CAUSE OF DEATH	CONTROLLABLE RISK FACTORS
Heart disease	Tobacco use, high blood pressure, high cholesterol, lack of exercise, excessive stress, diabetes, obesity
Cancer	Tobacco use, radiation, alcohol abuse, improper diet, environmental exposure
Stroke	Tobacco use, high blood pressure, high cholesterol, lack of exercise
Chronic lung disease	Tobacco use, environmental exposures
Accidents	Alcohol abuse, drug abuse, tobacco use, failure to use seat belts, fatigue, stress, recklessness
Diabetes	Obesity, improper diet, lack of exercise, excessive stress
Pneumonia and influenza	Chronic lung disease, environmental exposures, tobacco use, alcohol abuse, lack of immunization
Alzheimer's	None given
Kidney Disease	None given
Septicemia	

TABLE 14-3 CONTROLLABLE RISK FACTORS FOR TOP 10 CAUSES OF DEATH

Data from National Center for Health Statistics. (2001). *National Vital Statistics Report,* Vol. 51, No. 5. [Online]. Available: www.cdc.gov/nchs/fastats/deaths.htm

- Maintain normal blood pressure.
- Have a physical exam regularly.

Osteoporosis:
- Throughout life, eat a balanced diet and calcium-rich foods (milk and milk products).
- Get plenty of exercise.
- Discuss with the primary care physician the need for a calcium supplement and estrogen replacement therapy (females).
- Do not smoke.

Cancer:
- Do not smoke.
- Avoid unnecessary exposure to radiation.
- Protect skin from ultraviolet rays; use sunscreen.
- Avoid exposure to harmful chemicals.
- Minimize exposure to pesticides, herbicides, and poisons.
- Limit alcohol intake.
- Eat a well-balanced diet with adequate fiber.
- Exercise regularly.

- Practice safe sex.
- Have cancer screening tests—mammogram, Pap smear, rectal exam—fecal occult blood test with each physical exam.

Low-Back Pain:
- Exercise regularly.
- Practice good posture and proper body mechanics.

Colds and Flu:
- Wash hands frequently.
- Use paper tissues and dispose of properly.
- Have flu shots yearly.
- Eat a balanced diet.
- Drink plenty of fluids.

Breast Cancer:
- Eat a diet low in fat.
- Exercise regularly.
- Limit alcohol and caffeine intake.
- Perform monthly breast self-examinations.
- Have mammograms as recommended by the American Cancer Society.

Sexually Transmitted Diseases:
- Practice monogamous sex between noninfected individuals.
- Use latex condoms.

Tuberculosis (especially for health care workers):
- Take a Mantoux test.
- Receive isoniazid preventive therapy; any newly exposed and infected individual should take a full course of therapy.

Urinary Tract Infections:
- Drink plenty of water.
- Empty bladder frequently, especially before and after sexual intercourse.
- Wear cotton-crotch underwear.
- Wipe from front to back.
- Drink cranberry juice.
- Avoid bubble bath, douches, and colored or scented toilet paper.

Sickle-Cell Anemia and Thalassemia:
- Request genetic screening and counseling if a high-risk group.

Cataracts:
- Wear a brimmed hat and sunglasses.
- Eat a well-balanced diet.
- Do not smoke.

Glaucoma:
- Have tonometry performed.
- Have an optic nerve exam.

Sunburn:
- Always wear suncreen (with a minimum SPF of 15) when out in the sun.

Dental Caries and Periodontal Disease:
- Floss daily and brush after each meal.
- Use toothpaste with fluoride.
- Have a professional cleaning twice a year.
- Have a dental exam yearly.

Home Safety:

- Lock cupboards containing medicines and cleaning materials.
- Keep smoke alarms and fire extinguishers working.
- Use a carbon monoxide alarm in the presence of gas appliances and heaters.
- Plan escape routes in case of fire and have fire drills.
- Safety-proof home against falls.
- Know water safety rules.

Work Safety:

- Follow safety regulations at work.
- Report unsafe practices or equipment.

Travel Safety:

- Wear seat belts.
- Do not drive and drink.
- Drive defensively and safely.
- Use infant and child seats and restraints.
- Wear a helmet when riding a motorcycle or bicycle.
- Never swim alone.

Weight:

- Follow the Dietary Guidelines for Americans for a balanced diet.
- Exercise daily for 30 minutes.
- If overweight, eat the least number of servings recommended and use raw fruits or vegetables as snacks between meals.
- If underweight, eat the largest number of servings recommended and eat a nutritious snack between meals.

Stress:

- Identify sources of stress.
- Establish realistic expectations and goals.
- Try to be flexible.
- Express feelings and thoughts.
- Do not use alcohol or drugs for relaxation.
- Exercise regularly.
- Practice muscle relaxation and deep breathing.
- Get enough sleep.
- Have a sense of humor—laugh.
- Obtain professional help when needed.

Summary

- Wellness encompasses prevention, early detection, and treatment of health problems.
- The best way to maintain health is to follow the Dietary Guidelines for Americans, reduce stress, exercise regularly, prevent accidents, and receive routine health exams.
- Lifestyle changes can significantly reduce the leading causes of death.
- Physical, emotional, mental, social, and spiritual aspects all play key roles in the ability to resist disease and maintain health and wellness.

Review Questions

1. Health maintenance and disease prevention are the responsibility of the:

   a. nurse.
   b. physician.
   c. individual.
   d. nurse practitioner.

2. Primary prevention:

   a. is the nurse's job.
   b. is curing a disease in 5 days.
   c. occurs before a disease begins.
   d. includes all diseases or conditions.

3. Health can be improved by:

   a. not smoking.
   b. drinking alcohol.
   c. eating more pasta.
   d. sleeping 4 to 5 hours each night.

4. The nurse is aware that a genogram is used for:

   a. identifying a family tree.
   b. identifying potential health problems.
   c. preventing most diseases and illnesses.
   d. acknowledging the genes a person inherits.

5. Clients should be made aware that colds and flu can best be prevented by:

   a. smoking.
   b. staying warm and dry.
   c. washing hands frequently.
   d. having a flu shot every three years.

References/Suggested Readings

Baughcum, A. (1998). Mom's beliefs may cause child obesity. *Archives of Pediatric and Adolescent Medicine, 152,* 1010–1014.

Browder, S. (1998). *Attention, women over 50* [Online]. Available: www.seniornews.com/new-choices/article593.html

Centers for Disease Control and Prevention (CDC). (2000). *Mammography on the rise for women age 50 and over* [Online]. Available: www.od.nih.gov/ormh/press_rel/cdc_report.html

Cerrato, P. (1999). A radical approach to heart disease. *RN, 62*(4), 65–66.

Chopra, D., & Simon, D. (2001). *Grow younger, live longer.* New York: Harmony Books.

Edlin, G., Golanty, E., & McCormack-Brown, K. (1999). *Essentials for health and wellness.* Boston: Jones & Bartlett.

Floyd, P., Mimms, S., & Yelding-Howard, C. (1995). *Personal health: A multicultural approach.* Englewood, CO: Morton.

Hoeger, W., & Hoeger, S. (2000). *Lifetime physical fitness and wellness* (5th ed.). Belmont, CA: Wadsworth.

Hoeger, W., Turner, L., & Hafen, B. (2001). *Wellness: Guidelines for a healthy lifestyle* (3rd ed.). Belmont, CA: Wadsworth.

Hoffman, E. (1996). *Our health, our lives.* New York: Pocket.

Lee, I., & Paffenbarger, R. (1998). Exercise can cut stroke risk 50%. *Stroke, 29,* 2049–2054.

Lyon, B. (2000). Conquering stress. *Reflections on Nursing LEADERSHIP, 26*(1), 22–23, 43.

Malaty, H. (1998). Twin study: *H. pylori* tied to hygiene. *American Journal of Epidemiology, 148*, 793–797.

Matthews, K. (1998). Suppressed anger hard on women's hearts. *Psychosomatic Medicine, 60*, 633–638.

Maville, J., & Huerta, C. (2002). *Health promotion in nursing.* Clifton Park, NY: Thomson Delmar Learning.

National Center for Health Statistics. (1997). *Monthly vital statistics report, 45*(11S2), 23, 40–43 [Online]. Available: www.youfirst.com/risks.htm

National Center for Health Statistics. (2001). *National Vital Statistics Report*, Vol. 51, No. 5. [Online]. Available: www.cdc.gov/nchs/fastats/death.htm.

Oman, D., & Reed, D. (1998). Religious elderly tend to live longer. *American Journal of Public Health, 88*, 1469–1475.

Payne, W., & Hahn, D. (2000). *Understanding your health* (6th ed.). New York: McGraw-Hill.

Poliafico, F. (1999). Abstinence is not the only answer. *RN, 62*(1), 58–60.

Reed, D. (1998). Four factors predict "Healthy Aging." *American Journal of Public Health, 88*, 1463–1469.

Reichler, G., & Burke, N. (1999). *Active wellness: A personalized 10 step program for a healthy body, mind & spirit.* Richmond, VA: Time Life.

Seiger, L., Kanipe, D., Vanderpool, K., & Barnes, D. (2000). *Fitness and wellness strategies.* (2nd ed.). New York: McGraw-Hill.

Simmerman, J. M., & Mauzy, C. (2001). Finally! Babies can get this vaccine. *RN, 64*(7), 28–32.

Simon, H. (1992). *Staying well.* Boston: Houghton Mifflin.

Smith, C., & Maurer, F. (1999). *Community health nursing: Theory and practice.* (2nd ed.) Philadelphia: W. B. Saunders.

U.S. Department of Agriculture, U.S. Department of Health & Human Services (DHHS). (2000). *Home and Garden Bulletin No. 232* (5th ed.).

U.S. Department of Health & Human Services (DHHS). (1990). *Healthy People 2000: National health promotion and disease prevention objectives.* (DHHS Publication No. [PHS] 91-50212). Washington, DC.

U.S. Department of Health & Human Services (DHHS), Public Health Service. (1998). *Healthy People 2000: National health promotion and disease prevention objectives and first draft Healthy People 2010: National health promotion and disease prevention objectives* [Online]. Available: web.health.gov/healthypeople

U.S. Department of Health & Human Services (DHHS) Public Health Service. (2000a). *Healthy People 2010: National health promotion and disease prevention objectives* [Online]. Available: web.health.gov/healthypeople

U.S. Department of Health & Human Services (DHHS), Public Health Service. (2000b). *1998–1999 Progress Review* [Online]. Available: http://odphp.osophs.dhhs.gov/pubs/hp2000

Wash your hands (to help prevent colds). (1996, January). *Consumer Reports on Health, 2*(1).

Weil, A. (1998). *Natural health, natural medicine* (2nd ed.). Boston: Houghton Mifflin.

Weil, A. (2001). *Eating well for optimum health: The essential guide to bringing health and pleasure back to eating.* Camperdown, New South Wales, Australia: Quill.

Weil, A., & Daley, R. (2002). *The healthy kitchen: Recipes for a better body, life and spirit.* Westminster, MD: Knoph.

Resources

Aerobics and Fitness Association of America, 15250 Ventura Boulevard, Suite 200, Sherman Oaks, CA 91403-3297, 877-968-7263, www.aerobics.com

American Dietetic Association, 216 West Jackson Boulevard, Suite 800, Chicago, IL 60606-6995, 312-899-0040, www.eatright.org

American Health Care Association, 1201 L Street, NW, Washington, DC 20005, 202-842-4444, www.ahca.org

American Holistic Nurses' Association, P.O. Box 2130, Flagstaff, AZ 86003-2130, 800-278-2462, www.ahna.org

Center for Science in the Public Interest, 1875 Connecticut Avenue, NW, Suite 300, Washington, DC 20009-5728, 202-332-9110, www.cspinet.org

Centers for Disease Control and Prevention, *Morbidity and Mortality Weekly Report,* www.cdc.gov

Centers for Disease Control and Prevention, 1600 Clifton Road, NE, Atlanta, GA 30333, 404-639-3311, www.cdc.gov

Consumer Product Safety Commission, Washington, DC 20207, 800-638-2772, 800-638-8270 TDD, 800-492-8104 TTD in MD only

Dental Disease Prevention, Centers for Disease Control and Prevention (CDC), 1600 Clifton Road, NE, Atlanta, GA 30333

Environmental Protection Agency (EPA), Public Information Center, 401 M Street, SW, Washington, DC 20466, 800-424-9065, 202-260-2090, www.epa.gov

Food and Drug Administration, Office of Consumer Affairs, 5600 Fishers Lane, Rockville, MD 20857, 888-463-6332, www.fda.gov

Food and Nutrition Information Center, National Agricultural Library Building, Room 105, 10301 Baltimore Avenue, Beltsville, MD 20705-2351, 301-504-5719, www.nal.usda.gov

Healthy People 2010, Office of Disease Prevention and Health Promotion, 738-6 Humphrey Building, 200 Independence Avenue SW, Washington, DC 20201, 202-205-8583

Medic Alert Foundation International, P.O. Box 819008, Turlock, CA 95381-1009, 800-344-3226, 209-668-3333, www.medicalert.org

National Cholesterol Education Program Information Center, 4733 Bethesda Avenue, Room 530, Bethesda, MD 20814, 301-951-3260

National Council Against Health Fraud, 119 Foster Street, Building R, Second Floor, Peabody, MA 01960, 978-532-9383, www.ncahf.org

National Highway Traffic Safety Administration, NES-11 HL, U.S. Department of Transportation, 400 7th Street, SW, Washington, DC 20590, 888-327-4236, www.nhtsa.dot.gov

National Institute for Occupational Safety and Health, Clearinghouse for Occupational Safety and Health Information, Technical Information Branch, 4676 Columbia Parkway, Cincinnati, OH 45226, 800-356-4674

The National Institute on Aging, Building 31, Room 5C27, 31 Center Drive, MSC2292, Bethesda, MD 20892, 301-496-1752, www.nih.nia.gov

National Institutes of Health, Bethesda, MD 20892, 301-496-4000, www.nih.gov

National League for Nursing, 61 Broadway, #33 Floor, New York, NY 10006, 212-363-5555, 800-669-1656, Fax: 212-812-0393, www.nln.org

National Safety Council, 1121 Spring Lake Drive, Itasca, IL 60143-3201, 630-285-1121, www.nsc.org

National Wellness Institute, P.O. Box 827, Stevens Point, WI 54481-0827, 715-342-2969, www.nationalwellness.org

National Women's Health Network, 514 Tenth Street, NW, Washington, DC 20004, 202-347-1140

U.S. Department of Agriculture, 14th & Independence Avenue, SW, Washington, DC 20250, 800-535-4555, 202-720-2791, www.usda.gov

U.S. Department of Health and Human Services, Office of Disease Prevention and Health Promotion, 738-G Humphrey Building, 200 Independence Avenue, SW, Washington, DC 20201, 202-401-6295, www.odphp.osophs.dhhs.gov

World Health Organization, 525 23rd Street, NW, Washington, DC 20037, 202-974-3000, Headquarters, Avenue Appia 20, 1211 Geneva 27, Switzerland, www.who.int

COMPLEMENTARY/ ALTERNATIVE THERAPIES

MAKING THE CONNECTION

Refer to the following chapters to increase your understanding of complementary/alternative therapy:

Basic Nursing
- **Cultural Considerations**

- **Wellness Concepts**

LEARNING OBJECTIVES

Upon completion of this chapter, you should be able to:
- **Define key terms.**
- **Describe the influences of history on current complementary/alternative modalities.**
- **Discuss the connection between mind and body and how this affects a person's health.**
- **Explain the concept of the nurse as an instrument of healing.**
- **Identify the various mind-body, body-movement, energy healing, spiritual, nutritional, and other modalities that can be used as complementary therapies in client care.**
- **Discuss the use of complementary/alternative modalities.**

KEY TERMS

acupressure	hypnosis
acupuncture	imagery
alternative therapy	meditation
antioxidant	neuropeptide
aromatherapy	neurotransmitter
biofeedback	phytochemical
bodymind	psychoneuroimmunology
complementary therapy	shaman
curing	shamanism
energy therapy	therapeutic massage
free radical	therapeutic touch
healing	touch
healing touch	

INTRODUCTION

Our Western society generally equates health and healing with medicine, surgery, and other technological interventions. Many other cultures, however, promote healing through faith, ritual, magic, and other nonmedical approaches.

The use of **complementary therapies** (therapies used *in conjunction with* conventional medical therapies) and **alternative therapies** (therapies used *instead of* conventional or mainstream medical modalities) is becoming more prevalent among the general public (NCCAM, 2000).

This chapter addresses complementary/alternative (C/A) treatment methods that are currently being used in holistic nursing practice. Nurses must think critically before recommending or implementing any of these

therapies. Whether simply discussed with clients or performed, nurses should understand the ramifications. The abbreviation C/A will be used in this chapter.

LEGAL ASPECTS

Because more and more states are regulating C/A therapies, nurses must know the laws that govern these therapies in the states in which they work. Some states have outlawed certain therapies or consider them experimental procedures, whereas other states require licensure or certain educational standards before allowing practitioners to perform C/A therapies. Nurses who perform C/A therapies not in accordance with the laws of their respective states could have legal charges filed against them (Lorenzo, 2003).

Employer policy and the nurse's job description must also be checked to confirm that performing C/A therapies is within the nurse's scope of practice at that agency. Employer malpractice insurance policies typically do not cover situations where a client is injured as a result of a C/A therapy. The financial risk of any nurse who engages in C/A therapies will be lowered by having insurance that specifically covers those therapies.

HISTORIC FOUNDATION

People have tried to relieve pain and cure ills throughout history. Early cave drawings depict healers. Primitive healers believed that magic and superstition caused diseases, resulting in the intertwining of religious beliefs and health practices. Practices and remedies based in ancient traditions are being rediscovered and used. A brief look at ancient Greek, Far Eastern, Indian, and shamanistic practices will highlight their influences on modern C/A modalities.

Ancient Greece

In the ancient Greek culture, health was perceived as maintaining balance in all dimensions of life. In Greek mythology, Asclepius was the god of healing. Temples (called Ascleipions) were beautiful places for people (regardless of ability to pay) to worship, rest, and restore themselves. Their system of healing used symbols, myths, and rites administered by specially trained priest-healers. Illnesses were treated by restoring balance to a person's life through baths, massage, music, laughter, art, herbs, and simple surgery (Keegan, 1994). Many of our current therapies such as massage, art therapy, and herbal therapy have origins in ancient Greek traditions.

The Far East

Healing systems of the Far East have traditionally integrated body, mind, and spirit into a system balancing energy between the individual and the universe. The concept of a life force or life energy "has been recognized in many cultural traditions. . . . What is universally agreed on is that the more [life energy] you have, the more vital your mental and bodily processes" (Chopra, 1998). The origins of some energy therapies can be traced to the Far East.

Belief in the oneness of all things in nature is the basis of the traditional Chinese healing system. Life energy qi (pronounced "chee") flows through the universe and the person, creating a wholeness among all things and people. Qi provides vitality, warmth, and protection from illness. Qi flows along an invisible system of meridians (pathways), linking the organs together and connecting them to the external environment and to the universe. Illness and injury can alter the flow of this energy. The energy flow can be affected by stimulating points along the meridians.

Herbs are an important part of traditional Chinese healing practice. A discussion of the use of herbs in contemporary health practices appears later in this chapter.

Traditional Chinese healing techniques are being studied and used by contemporary Western health care providers. **Acupuncture,** one technique of traditional Chinese medicine, applies needles and heat to various points on the body to alter the energy flow (Figure 15-1).

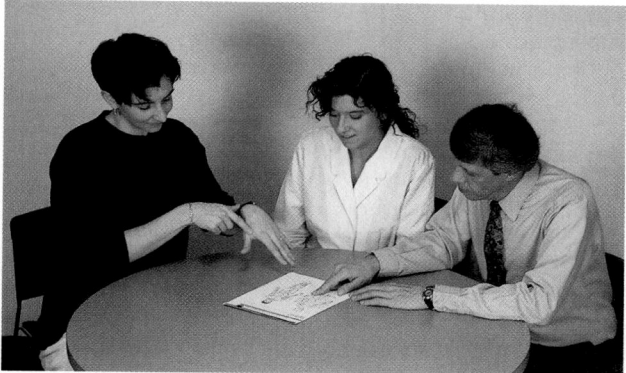

Figure 15-1 *Acupuncturist, Nurse, and Client*

The National Institutes of Health (NIH, 1997) acknowledged the efficacy of acupuncture in treating headaches, menstrual cramps, fibromyalgia, myofacial pain, osteoarthritis, low back pain, carpal tunnel syndrome, asthma, postoperative and chemotherapy-induced nausea and vomiting, and postoperative dental pain. They could not, however, determine a scientific basis for the circulation of qi.

India

For more than 4,000 years the people of India have practiced Ayurvedic medicine emphasizing prevention and a holistic approach to life (Keegan, 1994). The term *ayurveda* ("the science of life") refers to India's traditional medicine, which has an underlying spiritual basis. The life energy (prana) is moved through the body by a "wind" or Vata, which regulates every type of movement.

Vata, Kapha, and Pitta are the three metabolic principles (doshas) that provide life to all living things (Chopra, 1998). Kapha is the energy responsible for body structure. Pitta is the transformative process between Vata and Kapha. Each person is born with a unique balance of the three doshas. The dominant dosha determines temperament, body type, and susceptibility to certain illnesses.

The areas of energy concentration in the body are called chakras. Like the Chinese pathways (or meridians), these areas can become blocked and stagnant, causing illness. Ayurvedic healers try to activate chakra energy for self-healing.

The primary goals in the Ayurvedic system are preventing illness and restoring health by inner searching and spiritual growth. In contemporary practice, Ayurvedic intervention may consist of yoga, herbs, diet, and exercise; methods to cleanse the body, such as steam baths, cathartics, and detoxifying massage; and nasal purging.

Shamanistic Practices

Part of being human is a need to understand and explain life processes (i.e., birth, health, illness, and death). In many cultures, both modern and ancient, ritualized practices have been used to keep peace with the great spirits, to harness their power, to promote power, and to prevent death.

Shamanism refers to the practice of entering an altered state of consciousness with the intent to help others.

The **shaman** is a folk healer–priest who uses natural and supernatural forces to help others and who is skilled in many forms of healing, has an extensive knowledge of herbs, and serves as guardian of the spirits. Illness is believed to be the result of spirit loss. Shamans work with the spirits to encourage their full return to the individual. The shaman functions as both priest and healer and has access to the supernatural.

Seeking wisdom about the universe, establishing a relationship with the creator, and avoiding death are all feats accomplished through ritualized processes performed by the shaman. The shaman uses special objects such as power animals, fetishes, and totems, as well as dances, ritual songs, food, and clothing. Ritual chants, imagery, drumming, and hallucinogenic drugs may be used to create a trancelike state through which the shaman contacts the spirit world. The contemporary practices of hypnosis and guided imagery have roots in shamanistic traditions.

CURRENT TRENDS

The public perception of C/A treatment methods has been changing over the past few decades. In the late 1960s and early 1970s, the "natural," "new age," and "self-help" movements began to attract followers, first among consumers and later among health care practitioners. During that time period, there was a growing trend toward rejection of traditional medicine because of its perceived invasiveness, painfulness, cost, and ineffectiveness. A rekindled interest in Eastern religions, lifestyle, and medicine has fueled the development of contemporary holistic, C/A modalities. Clients are seeking out C/A therapies because most such therapies are noninvasive, holistic, and, in many instances, less expensive than going to a physician (Keegan, 1998).

In 1992, the U.S. government established the Office of Alternative Medicine (OAM) at the National Institutes of Health and allocated $2 million to disseminate information about complementary and alternative medicine to practitioners and the public. Congress increased the OAM's budget to $20 million for fiscal year 1998 (NCCAM, 2002).

Then in late 1998, Congress established the National Center for Complementary and Alternative Medicine (NCCAM), which replaced the OAM. Their budget for the fiscal year 2002 is $104.6 million (NCCAM, 2002). The NCCAM has the added responsibility of conducting and supporting basic and applied research and research training on C/A therapies. The NCCAM (2000) reports that as many as 42% of the U.S. population in 1997 used some type of C/A therapy, with a conservative estimate of spending $21.2 billion on these therapies.

Mind/Body Research

Traditional medicine is founded on the belief that the body, mind, and spirit are separate entities. A relatively new field of science, called **psychoneuroimmunology** (PNI), studies the complex relationship among the physical, cognitive, and affective aspects of humans. Psychoneuroimmunologists are studying how the brain sends signals along nerves to augment the body's normal immune functioning. This research supports the idea that the human mind can alter physiology.

All body cells have receptor sites for **neuropeptides,** amino acids produced in the brain and other sites in the body that act as chemical communicators. Neuropeptides are released when **neurotransmitters** (chemical substances produced by the body that facilitate nerve-impulse transmission) signal emotions in the brain. Pert, of the National Institutes of Health, wrote in 1986 that "the more we know about neuropeptides, the harder it is to think in the traditional terms of a mind and a body. It makes more sense to speak of a single integrated entity, a '*body*-mind'" (Pert, 1986).

Cells can be directly affected by emotions. This means that people can affect their health by what they feel and think. There are many examples of terminally ill persons hanging on to life until the occurrence of a specific event such as a child coming to visit or a grandchild's graduation or marriage.

This complex, intermeshed system of psyche and body chemistry is now called the **bodymind,** an inseparable connection and operation of thoughts, feelings, and physiological functions. This helps explain how some C/A therapies allow the calming influences of the parasympathetic system to take over during stress-inducing situations such as illness (Dossey, 1999b).

Holism and Nursing

The growing acceptance of the concept that body, mind, and spirit are interconnected is the basis for the expansion of the holistic health movement. The physiological, psychological, sociocultural, intellectual, and spiritual aspects of each individual are considered in holism. Holistic nursing is the art and science of caring for the whole person, knowing that each person is unique in all expressions of self. This means that the nursing assessment must include eliciting information regarding client use of C/A therapies (Hodge & Ullrich, 1999; Hatcher, 2001).

Nurses as holistic caregivers may use C/A techniques to promote clients' well-being. The focus of care in these practices is healing, as opposed to curing. The word **healing** comes from the Anglo-Saxon word *hael*, meaning "to make whole, to move toward, or to become whole." It is important to understand that healing is not **curing** (ridding one of disease), but is instead a process activating the individual's forces from within. The nurse as a healing facilitator enters into a relationship with the client to

CRITICAL THINKING

Alternative Methods

A close friend has AIDS and is experiencing a great deal of pain and discouragement. She wants to find alternative methods to ease the pain. She confides to you that she believes there may be a cure available at the holistic health center. How do you best help your friend in this situation? What do you advise?

assist the client by being a guide. The objective is to assist the client in releasing inner resources for healing.

COMPLEMENTARY/ALTERNATIVE THERAPIES

Many C/A therapies are used in holistic nursing practice. These interventions are categorized as mind/body, spiritual, manipulative and body-based, energy therapies, biologically based, and other methodologies.

Mind/Body Interventions

Mind/body interventions are methods by which an individual can, independently or with assistance, consciously control some sympathetic nervous system functions (e.g., heart rate, respiratory rate, and blood pressure). When the client is learning the way to perform these techniques, an assistant is involved; later, however, the client can perform them independently. Self-regulatory techniques include meditation, relaxation, imagery, biofeedback, and hypnosis.

Meditation

Meditation, a quieting of the mind by focusing attention on a sound or image or one's own breathing, is an ancient art. The person is no longer aware of worries or preoccupations, and stress is reduced. Health benefits from reduced stress include decreased respiration, heart rate, and oxygen consumption; improved mood; spiritual calm; and heightened awareness.

Nurses can assist clients with meditation by explaining what it is and answering any questions. When the client is in a comfortable position, instruct in a calm voice to concentrate on inhaling and exhaling. If the client's mind wanders, a refocus on breathing is needed. This should be practiced every day for 15 minutes.

Meditation has proved particularly beneficial for clients in labor.

Relaxation

Progressive muscle relaxation (PMR) is one method for achieving relaxation. It employs the alternate tensing and relaxing of muscles. Clients are instructed to con-

---

PROFESSIONAL TIP

Use of Complementary/Alternative Therapy

Nurses wanting to use C/A therapies should:

- Have a nonjudgmental attitude about these therapies.
- Ask clients whether they use any nontraditional therapies and, if so, which therapies, why, and the outcome.
- Discuss a therapy with the client *before* using it.
- Get adequate instruction in these therapies before trying to administer them.
- Try one or two basic therapies such as massage or guided imagery (Keegan, 1998).

CLIENT TEACHING

Progressive Muscle Relaxation

Explain the purpose and process of progressive muscle relaxation, then have the client:

- Assume a comfortable position in a quiet environment.
- Close eyes and keep them closed until the exercise is completed.
- Breathe in deeply to a count of 4.
- Hold breath for a count of 4.
- Breathe out to a count of 4.
- Continue to breathe slowly and deeply.
- Tense both feet until muscle tension is felt.
- Hold a gentle state of tension in both feet for a count of 5.

Tighten the muscles only until tense, but not painful.

- Slowly release the tension from the feet.
- Recognize the difference between tension and relaxation.
- Repeat the previous three steps.
- Gently tense the muscles of both lower legs.
- Continue the process with all muscle groups in a toe-to-head direction.
- After tensing and releasing all muscle groups, take in a few more deep relaxing breaths and scan your body for any areas that remain tense. Concentrate on tensing and relaxing the muscles in those areas.
- Breathe in deeply to a count of 4.
- Hold breath for a count of 4.
- Breathe out to a count of 4.
- Resume your usual breathing pattern.
- Slowly stretch and open your eyes.

This takes approximately 20 to 30 minutes and is most effective with repetition.

---

centrate on a certain body area (the jaw, for instance), tense the muscles for a count of five, then relax the muscles for a count of five. This process is repeated for muscle groups over the entire body until the client has achieved a state of overall relaxation. Nurses can use relaxation techniques to reduce pain and stress in clients.

Imagery

Imagery is a technique of using the imagination to visualize a pleasant, soothing image. The client is encouraged to use as many of the senses as possible to enhance the formation of vivid images. Table 15-1 presents examples of using all five senses in imagery.

Nurses can use guided imagery with clients capable of hearing and understanding the nurse's suggestions. For example, show and explain a chart of the stages of bone healing to a client who has suffered a fracture and ask the client to imagine this sequential activity in his body.

With guided imagery, the nurse can promote a sense of well-being in clients and help them change their perceptions about their disease, treatment, and healing ability (Dossey, 1999a). Studies have found that a combination of medication and guided imagery decreases physical tension, anxiety, and the adverse effects of chemotherapy

(Keegan, 1998). Helping clients use the power of the human imagination can be rewarding for the nurse.

Biofeedback

Biofeedback measures physiological responses, which assist individuals to improve their health by using

TABLE 15-1	USING ALL FIVE SENSES IN IMAGERY
SENSE	**IMAGERY**
Visual	See the white, fluffy clouds
Auditory	Hear the waves on the beach
Kinesthetic	Feel yourself floating in the water
Gustatory	Taste the tartness of the lemonade
Olfactory	Smell the hotdogs cooking on the grill

CLIENT TEACHING

Guided Imagery

Explain the purpose and process of guided imagery, then have the client:

- Assume a comfortable position in a quiet environment.
- Close their eyes and keep them closed until the exercise is completed.
- Breathe in deeply to a count of 4.
- Hold breath for a count of 4.
- Breathe out to a count of 4.
- Continue to breathe slowly and deeply.
- Think of your favorite place and prepare to take an imaginary journey there. Select a place in which you are relaxed and at peace.
- Picture in your mind's eye your favorite place. Look around you and see all the colors, the light and shadows, and all the pleasant sights.
- Listen to all the sounds. Pay attention to what you hear.
- Feel all the physical sensations . . . the temperature . . . the textures . . . the movement of the air.
- As you take in a deep breath, smell the aromas of your favorite place.
- Taste the foods and drinks you usually consume in your favorite place. Savor each taste fully.
- Focus all your attention totally on your favorite place.
- Breathe in deeply to a count of 4.
- Hold breath for a count of 4.
- Breathe out to a count of 4.
- Resume your usual breathing pattern.
- Slowly open your eyes and stretch, if desired.

This works best when all five senses are used, and becomes more effective with repetition.

signals from their own bodies. The biological functions commonly measured are muscle tension, skin temperature, heart rate, sweat gland activity, and brain wave activity. The individuals learn to alter their bodily responses after being "fed back" the information whether audibly or visually (AAPB, 2002a). Biofeedback is effective for migraine and tension headaches, urinary incontinence, hypertension, chronic pain, sleeping problems, enuresis, epilepsy, and Raynaud's disease (AAPB, 2002b).

Hypnosis

The practice of hypnosis was once overshadowed by mystery and misconception. Today, with the expanding knowledge of the human mind, hypnosis is being used more. Therapeutic **hypnosis** induces an altered state of consciousness or awareness resembling sleep and during which the person is more receptive to suggestion. Hypnosis does not magically cure anything.

Nurses desiring to use hypnosis in their practices must be aware of their scope of practice as defined by their respective state boards of nursing. They should also receive advanced training in hypnosis (Kolkmeier, 1999).

Spiritual Therapies

A state of health depends on one's relationship not only to the physical and interpersonal environments, but also to the spiritual part of self. The idea of a relationship between spirituality and health is not new. "From the earliest time of the shaman we have witnessed the mysterious spiritual element of healing . . . the connection of the healer with the divine" (Keegan, 1994).

Many cultures accept the inseparable link between the state of one's soul (life energy or spirit) and the state of one's health. Scientists (especially psychoneuroimmunologists) are beginning to validate that individuals have inner mechanisms of healing. Many religions have ideologies about health, illness, and healing.

Faith Healing At the heart of spiritual or faith healing is the belief that practitioners must purify themselves and reach a state of unity with God or a higher power before faith healing can occur. This process is usually accomplished through prayer. When preparing for healing, the practitioner adapts a passive and receptive mood to be a channel for divine power. The ill person's belief enhances, but is not necessary for healing.

Healing Prayer When praying, people believe they are communicating directly with God or a higher power. Prayer, an integral part of a person's spiritual life, can affect well-being. Florence Nightingale recognized that prayer helps connect individuals to nature and the environment (Nightingale, 1969). Medical research is currently investigating the effects of prayer on physical health (Dossey, 1999b).

Byrd and Sherrill (1995) investigated how prayer affected clients in critical care units. The results showed that clients receiving standard medical care plus intercessory prayers required less medication, had fewer complications, and improved faster than did clients in the control group, who received standard medical care and no prayers. Findings reported by Marwick (1995) showed that religious involvement may lead to improved physical health status.

Shamanism Shamanism was discussed earlier in this chapter.

Manipulative and Body-Based Methods

Body-based methods use techniques of manipulating or moving various body parts to achieve therapeutic outcomes. Movement/exercise, yoga, Tai-Chi, and chiropractic treatment are discussed in the following sections.

Movement/Exercise

The therapeutic intervention and health-promoting activity of movement is associated with athletic exercise, dance, celebration, and healing rituals. The primary goal of exercise is fitness (muscle strength, endurance, flexibility, and cardiovascular and respiratory health). There are many other positive outcomes of exercise, such as sleeping better and having more energy.

Nurses can help clients use movement as therapy through range-of-motion exercises, stretching exercises, and physical therapy. Movement is an effective method through which people of all ages can improve their level of functioning.

Yoga/Yoga Therapy

Yoga (meaning "union" in Sanskrit) integrates mental, physical, and spiritual energies to promote health and wellness. The basic elements of yoga are proper breathing, posture, and movement. The breathing is believed to promote relaxation and enhance the flow of prana (vital energy). Yoga develops proprioception (an awareness of where the body is in space and time) and an awareness of movement, weight distribution, and position (Davis, 2002).

Traditional yoga has always been primarily concerned with healthy individuals and promoting health by maintaining the balance and flow of life forces.

Yoga therapy is an effort to integrate traditional yogic concepts and techniques with Western medical and psychological knowledge (Feuerstein, 1998). The focus of yoga therapy is to holistically treat various psychological or somatic dysfunctions ranging from back problems to emotional distress.

Both yoga and yoga therapy are based on the understanding that the human being is an integrated body/mind system that best functions in a state of dynamic balance (Feuerstein, 1998). Studies regarding benefits of yoga practice have found that mentally challenged individuals become more aware of their bodies and enjoy improved coordination, while clients with os-

teoarthritis of the hands experience less pain (Keegan, 1998). Claims made by yoga authorities range from a beneficial effect on physical flexibility, muscle tone, and stamina to a reduction in obesity, back pain, hypertension, various respiratory diseases, anxiety, and memory loss (Feuerstein, 1998).

Tai Chi

The philosophy of looking for harmony with nature and the universe through complementary (yin and yang) balance is the basis for tai chi. When there is perfect harmony, everything functions spontaneously, effortlessly, perfectly, and according to the laws of nature. If one moves to the right, one must also move to the left. tai chi is a series of slow, continuously flowing movements. The movements, accompanied by deep breathing, improve flexibility, range of motion, muscle strength, and balance (Cerrato, 1999d).

Those who regularly practice tai chi believe that it enhances agility, stamina, and balance and that it boosts energy and bestows a sense of well-being. The entire tai chi form can take as little as 7 minutes or as long as an hour to practice. Tai chi has been shown to reduce blood pressure and the risk of falling in the elderly, and significantly reduced discomfort of clients with low back pain (Cerrato, 1999d).

Chiropractic Therapy

Chiropractic therapy is based on the principle that the brain sends vital energy to every organ in the body via the nerves originating in the spinal column. Disease, body disharmony, or malfunction results from vertebral subluxation complex (spinal nerve stress). The body is rebalanced and realigned using chiropractic "spinal adjustment" techniques.

The goal of chiropractic care is to awaken the client's own natural healing ability by correcting any areas of vertebral subluxation complex. Vitality, strength, and health are thus promoted. The Chiropractic Arts Center (2002) reports case histories of clients recovering from heart trouble, hyperactivity, fatigue, digestive problems, and many other conditions.

Stedman (1999) explains that chiropractic practitioners fall into one of two groups, the "straights" and the "mixers." The straights believe in the chiropractic therapy just described. The mixers use spinal adjustments mainly to relieve back pain, neck stiffness, and headaches, conditions that have sometimes been shown to be alleviated by chiropractic therapy. Most mixers are willing to work closely with a client's medical doctor.

LIFE CYCLE CONSIDERATIONS

Exercise and the Very Old

Positive results from regular exercise and weight lifting are achieved, including increased physical strength and flexibility and improved mental status in areas such as memory and depression in clients 95 years and older (Mills, 1994).

PROFESSIONAL TIP

Preparing for Chiropractic Therapy

Encourage clients considering the use of chiropractic services to first undergo a comprehensive health assessment to rule out any contraindications.

Chiropractic services have gained increasing acceptance in the United States. Chiropractors are licensed in all 50 states, and 41 states require insurance reimbursement for chiropractic services (Japsen, 1995).

Energy Therapies

One category of C/A therapies incorporated into nursing practice in the past 25 years is the **energy therapies,** use of the hands to direct or redirect the flow of the body's energy fields and enhance balance within those fields. These therapies are effective for many problems and can restore harmony in all aspects of health. These therapies can be used with persons of all ages and all stages of wellness and illness.

Energy therapies have their roots in traditional Chinese, ancient Eastern, and Native American philosophies. The fundamental concept is that individuals have a life force, energy not confined to physical skin boundaries. Figure 15-2 illustrates the energy field that extends beyond a person's physical body.

An individual's energy field consists of energy layers in constant flux. They can be reduced or otherwise adversely affected by any type of trauma, illness, or distress. The energy system can also be positively affected intentionally by the use of a practitioner's hands. The

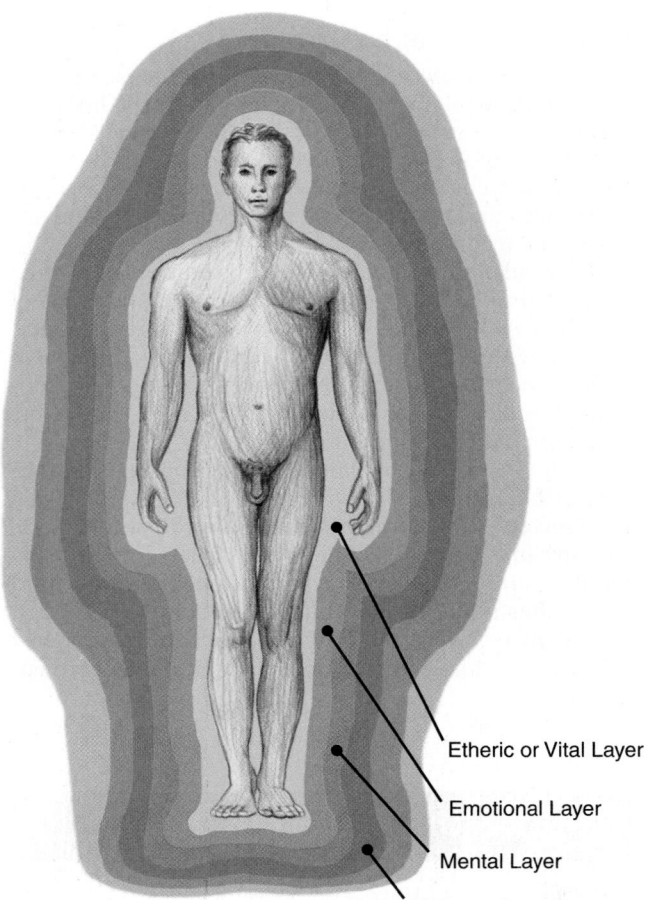

Figure 15-2 *Layers of the Human Energy Field Extending Beyond the Physical Boundaries*

Etheric or Vital Layer

Emotional Layer

Mental Layer

Intuitive or Spiritual Layer
(also called the astral body)

primary focus is to restore the optimal flow of life energy through the energy fields.

Many energy therapies are being used by nurses today, such as touch, therapeutic massage, therapeutic touch, and healing touch. Other therapies are acupressure and reflexology, which both involve deep-tissue body work and require advanced training for the practitioners.

Touch

The most universal C/A therapy is touch. **Touch** is the means of perceiving or experiencing through tactile sensation. Although it was used in all ancient cultures and shamanistic traditions for healing, the advent of scientific medicine and Puritanism led many healers away from the purposeful use of touch. It should be noted that touch carries with it taboos and prescriptions that are culturally dictated. Some cultures are very comfortable with physical touch; others specify that touch may be used only in certain situations and within specified parameters.

The nurse must be sure to convey positive intentions when touching. If in doubt, the nurse should not touch until establishing effective communication with the client. Touch is important in nursing practice, because it:

- Is an integral part of assessment.
- Promotes bonding between nurse and client (Figure 15-3).
- Is an important means of communication, especially when other senses are impaired.
- Assists in soothing, calming, and comforting.
- Helps keep the client oriented.

Therapeutic Massage

Therapeutic massage is the application of hand pressure and motion to improve the recipient's well-being. It involves rubbing, kneading, and using friction.

Figure 15-3 *Touch promotes bonding between nurse and client.*

Massage therapy is recognized as highly beneficial and is prescribed by many physicians. Many states now have licensing requirements for massage practitioners.

Traditionally, back rubs were given by nurses to provide comfort to hospitalized clients. Massage techniques can be used with all age groups and are especially beneficial to those who cannot move. A back rub or massage results in relaxation, increased circulation of the blood and lymph, and relief from musculoskeletal stiffness, spasm, and pain.

Safety: Precautions for Massage
- Increased circulation may be harmful in people with heart disease, diabetes, hypertension, or kidney disease.
- Never attempt massage in areas of circulatory abnormality, such as aneurysm, varicose veins, phlebitis, thrombus, or necrosis, or in areas of tissue injury, inflammation, open wounds, dermatitis, joint or bone injury, recent surgery, or sciatica.

Therapeutic Touch

Therapeutic touch, based on the ancient practice of the laying on of hands, consists of finding alterations in a person's energy field and using the hands to direct energy to achieve a balanced state. Therapeutic touch is based on four assumptions:

- A human being is an open energy system.
- Anatomically, a human being is bilaterally symmetrical.
- Illness is an imbalance in an individual's energy field.

Figure 15-4 *A nurse is administering therapeutic touch to a client.*

- Human beings have natural abilities to transform and transcend their conditions of living (Krieger, 1993).

Therapeutic touch is easily learned in workshops, can be done either with hands on or off the body, complements medical treatments, and has shown reasonably consistent and reliable results (Figure 15-4). The relaxation response may be seen in the client in 2 to 5 minutes after a treatment has begun, and some clients fall asleep or require less pain medication after a treatment.

Healing Touch

Healing touch is an energy therapy using the hands to clear, energize, and balance the energy field. Janet Mentgen, a nurse, developed it. The healing touch practitioner realigns the energy flow, which reactivates the mind/body/spirit connection to eliminate blockages to self-healing.

Healing touch can be administered in a few minutes or, ideally, in a one-hour session (Mentgen, 2002). The North American Nursing Diagnosis Association (NANDA, 2003) lists *Disturbed Energy Field,* defined as "a disruption of the flow of energy surrounding a person's being that results in disharmony of the body, mind, and/or spirit," as one of their approved nursing diagnoses. Implicit in this therapy is the need for follow-up or sequential treatments as well as discharge planning and referral to assist the client in adequately meeting goals.

Acupressure and Shiatsu

Both acupressure and shiatsu are based on the Chinese meridian theory, which states that the body is divided into meridian channels through which qi, or energy, flows. Cold, damp, fire, bacteria, or viruses may block the flow of qi, causing disease in the body. **Acupressure** is a technique of releasing blocked energy within an individual when specific points (Tsubas) along the meridians are pressed or massaged by the practitioner's fingers, thumbs, and heel of the hands. When the blocked energy is freed, the disease subsides. Shiatsu, a Japanese form of acupressure also uses the forearm, elbow, knee, and foot to activate the points. Both acupressure and Shiatsu relieve tension and many stress-related ailments. Contraindications

Reflexology

A client asks the nurse to rub his foot in a particular spot because that is where his reflexologist rubs to relieve his abdominal pain. How should the nurse handle this situation?

include venous stasis, phlebitis, and traumatic and deep-tissue injuries (Sutherland, 2000).

Shiatsu primarily focuses on health maintenance rather than on treatment of illness (Keegan, 1999b); that is, it is used to make sure the qi is able to flow freely so the individual does not become ill. Nurses must be self-aware when practicing shiatsu to enable them to concentrate completely on promoting the client's comfort.

Reflexology

Reflexology, rooted in ancient healing arts, is the art and science of enervating more than 7,000 nerves in the feet believed to correspond to every muscle system and organ in the body (Worden, 1999). The fundamental concept of reflexology divides the body into 10 equal, longitudinal zones running the length of the body, from the top of the head to the tip of the toes. These 10 zones correspond to the 10 fingers and toes. The foot is viewed as a microcosm of the entire body (Figure 15-5). Reflexology theory states that illness is evident as calcium deposits and acids in the corresponding part of the person's feet. Pressing certain points on the feet brings an autonomic nervous system response or reflex. Reflexology induces an optimal state of relaxation, which is conducive to healing. It promotes health by relieving pressures and accumulation of toxins in the corresponding body part.

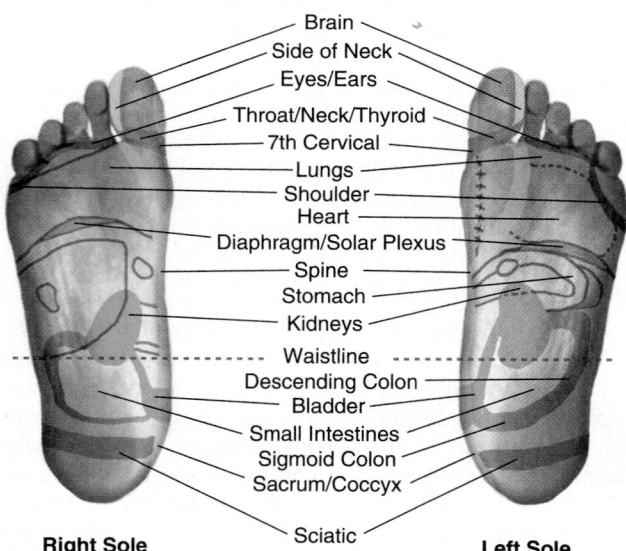

Figure 15-5 *Foot Reflexology Chart (Reproduced with permission from* Better Health with Foot Reflexology *[10th ed.]). Copyright 2001 by Dwight C. Byers, Ingham Publishing, Inc. POB 12642, St. Petersburg, FL 33733-2642.)*

Reflexology can be used as a complementary therapy for chronic conditions such as asthma, sinus infections, migraines, irritable bowel syndrome, constipation, and kidney stones.

Biologically Based Therapies

In the past 20 to 30 years, nutritional interventions for prevention and treatment of disease have generated increasing interest among consumers and health care providers. This section addresses the C/A nutritional and herbal approaches.

Phytochemicals

Currently, certain foods are being studied for their medicinal value. **Phytochemicals** are nonnutritive, physiologically active compounds present in plants in very small amounts (Simons, 1997). *Phyto* is the Greek word for "plant." Therefore, phytochemicals are plant chemicals. These chemicals have several functions, including storage of nutrients and provision of structure, aroma, flavor, and color. Phytochemicals protect against cancer and prevent heart disease, stroke, and cataracts. Phytochemicals are found in fruits and vegetables.

No single fruit or vegetable contains all phytochemicals. The consumption of a wide variety of fruits and vegetables provides the best supply. The major sources of phytochemicals are onions, garlic, leeks, chives, carrots, sweet potatoes, squash, pumpkin, cantaloupe, mango, papaya, tomatoes, citrus fruits, grapes, strawberries, raspberries, cherries, legumes, soybeans, tofu, and the cruciferous vegetables (broccoli, cauliflower, brussels sprouts, and cabbage). Nurses can use this information to encourage clients to eat more fruits and vegetables.

Antioxidants

Antioxidants are substances that prevent or inhibit oxidation, a chemical process whereby a substance is joined to oxygen. In the body, antioxidants prevent tissue damage related to **free radicals,** which are unstable molecules that alter genetic codes and trigger the development of cancer growth in cells. Vitamins C and E, beta-carotene (which is converted to vitamin A in the body), and selenium are antioxidants. Antioxidants may prevent heart disease, some forms of cancer, and cataracts. Antioxidants help repair eye tissue damaged from sunlight and thus prevent cataract formation (Simons, 1997). Other vitamins, minerals, trace elements, and enzymes are being investigated for their possible therapeutic value. Phytosterols (plant sterols) are

PROFESSIONAL TIP

Use of Medicinal Plants

Be cautious in the casual use of plants to treat self or others. "Natural" substances can be harmful if not processed properly, and many plants (including some herbs) can be poisonous.

LIFE CYCLE CONSIDERATIONS

Essential Oils

Essential oils should be used with caution in elderly persons. These clients are usually more sensitive to essential oils than are adults and teenagers and thus require smaller amounts and less-concentrated forms of the essence.

the active ingredients in the new lipid-lowering margarines. These inhibit absorption of dietary cholesterol and slow down the reabsorption of cholesterol secreted in bile (Cerrato, 1999a).

Herbs

Herbs and plants have been used for centuries in the care of the sick. Many of the drugs used today originally were plant remedies passed from one generation to the next.

Although herbs may have medicinal value (Table 15-2), some can cause potentially harmful herb–drug interactions when used with prescribed medications. It is important to ask during assessment specifically about the client's use of herbal and vitamin supplements. Feverfew, ginseng, and garlic prolong the clotting time. Encourage clients to reveal the use of herbs to their primary care provider.

Others

S-adenosylmethionine (SAMe) is a modified amino acid produced naturally by the body; however, the level decreases with age. Controlled research has shown that SAMe may work at least as well as certain antidepressants and may benefit clients with osteoarthritis by assisting in cartilage repair (Cerrato & Rowell, 1999).

Omega-3 fatty acids, found in salmon, trout, sardines, walnuts, canola oil, and flax seeds, help reduce the threat of cardiac arrhythmias. Research has also shown that the omega-3 fatty acids suppress inflammation of rheumatoid arthritis and may improve glucose control in Type 2 diabetes (Cerrato, 1999b).

Other Methodologies

Iridology, aromatherapy, humor, animal-assisted therapy, music therapy, and play therapy, are also used by holistic practitioners.

Iridology

According to Caradonna (2003), iridology began more than 100 years ago when two physicians began observing eyes and organizing their findings. Iridology is the study of the iris, or colored part, of the eye. It is theorized that the fibers and pigmentation of the iris reflects information about a person's physical and psychological makeup.

Aromatherapy

Aromatherapy is the therapeutic use of concentrated essences or essential oils extracted from plants and

flowers. Essential oils diluted in oil for massage or in warm water for inhalation may be stimulating, relaxing, or soothing. The following are some popular essential oils (Keville & Green, 1995):

- *Lavender* is said to have anti-inflammatory, antidepressant, and antibacterial effects.
- *Eucalyptus* is claimed to act as a decongestant, antimicrobial, and stimulant.
- *Chamomile* is believed to benefit the gastrointestinal tract, relieve allergies, and act as a sedative.
- *Marjoram* is purported to work as an antiseptic and anti-inflammatory agent and to relieve muscle spasms.
- *Peppermint* is believed to improve digestion and act as an antiseptic and decongestant.
- *Rosemary* is said to stimulate the circulation.
- *Geranium* is thought to balance the mind and body.

Aromatherapists use concentrated oils to treat specific ailments. The aromas cause physiological, psychological, and pharmacological reactions (Trevelyan, 1993). Some essential oils have antibacterial properties and are used in a wide variety of pharmaceutical preparations. These oils should be used intelligently and with caution.

A clinical study reported by Wilkinson (1995) concluded that massage oil with the essential oil Roman chamomile reduced anxiety and improved the quality of life of cancer clients to a greater extent than did unscented oil. Another study found that postcardiac surgery clients receiving foot massages with neroli oil (from orange flowers) experienced greater and more lasting psychological benefits than did those receiving massages without neroli oil (Stevenson, 1994). Weiss and James (1997), however, report clients with allergic contact dermatitis to essential oils.

Some contraindications for aromatherapy are listed in Table 15-3.

Safety: Aromatherapy
- Essential oils are very potent and should never be used in an undiluted form, be used near the eyes, or be ingested orally.
- Because some people are allergic to certain oils, a small skin-patch test should be done before generalized application.

Humor

Therapeutic humor includes any intervention that promotes health and wellness by stimulating a playful discovery, expression, or appreciation of the absurdity or incongruity of life's situations (AATH, 2001). It is probably the least understood, but the easiest to do.

To avoid giving offense, it is important to determine the client's perception of what is humorous. Whether a given situation is considered humorous or offensive will vary greatly from culture to culture and person to person. Good taste and common sense should serve as guides.

Nurses can promote humor in various ways. A humor cart (cart filled with cartoon and joke books, silly noses, and magic tricks) allows clients to select their own humor tools. A "humor room" may be made available, where clients can watch comedy videos or play fun games with visitors or other clients.

TABLE 15–2   MEDICINAL VALUE OF SELECTED HERBS

HERB	MEDICINAL VALUE	HERB	MEDICINAL VALUE
Aloe vera	• Improves wound healing • Soothes minor cuts, abrasions, and burns	Ginkgo biloba	• Increases cerebral blood flow • Helps lessen mild depression • Eases dementia • Combats impotence • Decreases peripheral vascular insufficiency • Relieves premenstrual syndrome symptoms • Decreases vascular fragility
Calendula	• Promotes healing of cuts, abrasions, minor burns, sunburn, acne, and athlete's foot • Soothes oral thrush (as a mouthwash) and vaginal thrush (as a douche)		
Celery	• Lowers cholesterol • Decreases dizziness • Relieves headache	Lavender	• Relieves headache • Reduces muscle spasms • Increases relaxation
Chamomile	• Induces a calming effect • Relieves nausea • Eases tension headache	Peppermint	• Relieves headache • Eases sinus congestion • Reduces muscle spasms
Echinacea	• Wound healing • Nonspecific immunostimulist for upper respiratory tract and urinary tract infections	Sage	• Acts as an antibacterial
		Saint John's Wort	• Relieves mild to moderate depression • Lessens severity of viral infections
Eucalyptus	• Acts as an antibacterial • Acts as a decongestant	Thyme	• Acts as an antimicrobial • Eases symptoms of common cold • Acts as an antispasmodic on bronchioles • Alleviates cystitis • Acts as an antifungal (especially when applied as a lotion for athlete's foot) • Used as a mouthwash for oral thrush
Garlic	• Acts as an antimicrobial remedy for intestinal worms • Guards against and treats respiratory infections • Used as expectorant in cases of bronchitis or a cold		
Ginger	• Relieves nausea (especially motion sickness and morning sickness) • Stimulates circulation in feet and hands • Acts as expectorant • Eases indigestion and flatulence • Relieves diarrhea		

NOTE: This information is not intended to serve as a guide for self-medication or the treatment of others. Consult a health care practitioner trained in the use of herbs before consuming or giving any herb for medicinal purposes.

From *Herbs for Health,* by S. Foster, 1995, The Herb Companion, 8(1), 63–86; *Down to Earth: An Ancient Herb for a Modern Garden,* by J. Long, 1995. The Herb Companion, 8(1), 22; *Eight Healing Herbs,* 1995, by M. Polunin and C. Robbins, 1995–1996, *Holistic Health Directory,* 30–34; *The Backyard Medicine Chest: An Herbal Primer,* by D. Schar, 1995, Washington, DC: Elliot & Clark; *Spontaneous Healing: How to Discover and Enhance Your Body's Natural Ability To Maintain and Heal Itself,* by A. Weil, 2000, New York: Ivy; *Herbal Medicines,* by C. O'Neil, J. Avila, & C. W. Fetrow, (1999), *Nursing99,* 29(4). Getting a handle on herbals, by M. Herbert-Ashton, 2002, *Travel Nursing Today* (supplement to *RN*) Sept., 16–24; and Understanding Echinacea (nontraditional choices), 2003, *Nursing 2003,* 3(1), 76.

TABLE 15-3 AROMATHERAPY CONTRAINDICATIONS

ESSENTIAL OIL	CONTRAINDICATION
Arnica, basil, celery, cypress, jasmine, juniper, marjoram, myrrh, sage, thyme	Pregnancy
Camomile, lavender	Use with care in pregnancies carrying the risk of bleeding or miscarriage
Peppermint, rose, rosemary	First trimester of pregnancy and only well-diluted later in pregnancy
Sweet fennel	Epilepsy
Rosemary, sage, thyme	Hypertension

Data from Aromatherapy by J. Trevelyan, 1993, *Nursing Times, 89*(25), 39.

Figure 15-6 *Pet therapy provides health benefits.*

Humor has many therapeutic outcomes. Norman Cousins, former chairperson of the Task Force in Psychoneuroimmunology at the School of Medicine at UCLA, tells how his recovery from an incurable connective tissue disorder, ankylosing spondylitis, was enhanced by watching films and movies that made him laugh daily (Cousins, 1979). Humor can effectively relieve anxiety, improve respiratory function, promote relaxation, enhance immunological function, and decrease pain by stimulating endorphin production.

Animal-Assisted Therapy

Animals were used in England in 1792 at York Retreat, where psychiatric clients cared for rabbits and poultry (McConnell, 2002). It was 1944 before animals were used in a therapeutic setting in the United States.

In animal-assisted therapy (AAT), a prepared handler and trained animal work one-on-one with a client toward identified short- and long-term goals.

Currently, AAT is used as a complementary therapy for people in both acute and long-term care settings (Figure 15-6).

Dogs are the animals most often used in AAT. Cats are less predictable, and many people are allergic to cat dan-

der (Miller & Connor, 2000). Animal-assisted therapy has many applications, including overcoming physical limitations, improving mood, lowering blood pressure, and improving socialization skills and self-esteem.

Music Therapy

Therapeutic use of music consists of playing music to elicit positive changes in behavior, emotions, or physiological response. Music encourages clients to actively participate in their health care and recovery and complements other treatment modalities.

Music is good to use with imagery, as it enhances the relaxation response and heightens images. All music stimulates the neurotransmitters evoking chemical changes in the bodymind, but different types of music elicit different responses (Achterberg, Dossey, & Kolkmeier, 1994). Music-thanatology is a holistic and palliative use of music with dying clients to help dissipate obstacles to peaceful transition to death (Schroeder-Shecker, 1994).

A tape or CD player with headphones playing music can be a useful tool for immobilized clients, those waiting for diagnostic tests, or those waiting for surgery (Figure 15-7). Some facilities allow clients to choose the type of music played while they undergo procedures such as cardiac catheterization. Pleasurable sound and music can reduce stress, perception of pain, anxiety, and feelings of isolation. Music can be very useful to help adolescents relax.

PROFESSIONAL TIP

Use of Humor

Never do or say anything that gives clients the idea that you are laughing *at* them as opposed to *with* them (McGhee, 1998).

CULTURAL CONSIDERATIONS

Music and Culture

- Each culture and each generation within each culture has its own preferred type of music.
- Music that is soothing to one client may be irritating to another.
- Either ask which type of music the client would prefer or allow the client to bring music.

Figure 15-7 *Music therapy helps client relax.*

Play Therapy

Play therapy is especially useful with children. Toys are used to allow children to learn about what will be happening to them and to express their emotions and their current situations. Drawing and artwork also provide a way for children to share their experiences. When language ability is reduced or not yet well developed, play therapy and drawings constitute a method for children to communicate their needs and feelings to care providers.

USE OF C/A APPROACHES

Western society labels some methods as C/A (e.g., acupuncture) when they have been validated by centuries of successful use. Biofeedback has been proven through research. Other C/A approaches such as therapeutic touch need further investigation and validation. Nurses have an important role to educate clients about nontraditional interventions appropriate throughout the life cycle (Table 15-4). The following terms are frequently used to describe approaches:

- *Proven:* have been scientifically tested in clinical trials
- *Experimental:* are undergoing Food and Drug Administration (FDA) investigations to ascertain safety and efficacy
- *Untested:* have not been investigated by the FDA with regard to safety and efficacy
- *Folklore:* have been passed from one generation to another as remedies, many of which have therapeutic value

TABLE 15-4 SUGGESTED COMPLEMENTARY THERAPIES THROUGH LIFE		
STAGE OF LIFE	**SUGGESTED COMPLEMENTARY THERAPIES**	
Infants	• Massage (modified) • Movement (rocking)	• Music
Young Children	• Massage • Music • Play	• Humor • Imagery • Art/drawing
School-age Children	• Massage • Music • Play • Humor • Animal-assisted therapy	• Imagery • Aromatherapy • Yoga • Tai chi
Adolescents	All therapies discussed in this chapter, as appropriate to the condition	
Adults	All therapies discussed in this chapter, as appropriate to the condition	
Older Adults	• Massage (lighter pressure and other modifications for body's status) • Animal-assisted therapy • Aromatherapy (with precautions) • Any other therapy discussed in this chapter, as appropriate to the condition and with precautions	
Terminally ill	• Massage • Reflexology • Energy therapies • Music	• Prayer • Any other therapies discussed in this chapter, as appropriate to the condition and with precautions

- *Quackery:* have not proven effective, may result in harm to consumers, and are usually marketed with numerous unfounded promises (e.g., as "cure-all" products or therapies) (Brown, Cassileth, Lewis, & Renner, 1994)

According to Keegan (1998), research has documented the effectiveness of specific C/A therapies:

- Meditation combined with guided imagery decreases physical tension, anxiety, and the adverse effects of chemotherapy.
- Nutrition, exercise, and meditation—without the use of medication or surgery—can reverse coronary heart disease.
- Yoga can help mentally challenged individuals become more aware of their bodies and improve coordination.
- Yoga can help reduce pain in clients with osteoarthritis of the hands.

The power of the nurse's presence with any client should never be underestimated. While many of the C/A approaches require further study and advanced training, nursing students are able to touch, listen, and care. Clients benefit from having another person present with them.

Summary

- More and more health care consumers are using nontraditional treatment modalities.
- Healing is not curing. It is regaining balance and finding harmony and wholeness as changes take place within the individual.
- No one can heal another, but a nurse can act as a guide and support system, for the client.
- Some of the mind/body modalities used by nurses are meditation, relaxation, imagery, biofeedback, and hypnosis.
- Body-movement modalities include movement and exercise and chiropractic therapy.
- Energy therapies can be used with clients of all ages and in various stages of illness and wellness.
- Nutritional/medicinal therapies include the use of antioxidants and herbal therapy.
- Other modalities such as aromatherapy, humor, animal-assisted therapy, music therapy, and play therapy are valuable adjuncts to conventional treatment.

Review Questions

1. Therapies that are used instead of mainstream medical practice are called:

   a. alternative therapies.
   b. contemporary therapies.
   c. complementary therapies.
   d. nontraditional therapies.

2. Therapies that are used in conjunction with conventional medical therapies are called:

   a. alternative therapies.
   b. contemporary therapies.
   c. complementary therapies.
   d. nontraditional therapies.

3. The National Center for Complementary and Alternative Medicine:

   a. investigates nontraditional treatment methods.
   b. refers persons to practitioners of nontraditional therapies.
   c. monitors the number of people using nontraditional therapies.
   d. grants a license to those who practice nontraditional therapies.

4. One of the most universal complementary/alternative modalities is:

   a. touch.
   b. massage.
   c. nutrition.
   d. faith healing.

5. The complementary therapy recommended for all ages in life is:

   a. massage.
   b. hypnosis.
   c. reflexology.
   d. aromatherapy.

References/Suggested Readings

Achterberg, J. (2002). *Imagery in healing: Shamanism and modern medicine*, Boston: Shambhala.

Achterberg, J., Dossey, B., & Kolkmeier, L. (1994). *Rituals of healing: Using imagery for health and wellness.* New York: Bantam.

American Association for Therapeutic Humor (AATH). (2001). *Purpose* [Online]. Available: aath.org/home_1.html

Association for Applied Psychophysiology & Biofeedback (AAPB). (2002a). *What is biofeedback?* [Online]. Available: www.aapb.org/public/articles/details.cfm?id=4

Association for Applied Psychophysiology & Biofeedback (AAPB). (2002b). *What kinds of problems can biofeedback help?* [Online]. Available: www.aapb.org/public/articles/details.cfm?id=7

Association of Psychophysiology and Biofeedback (AAPB). (2002). *What is biofeedback?* [Online]. Available: www.aapb.org

Astin, J. A. (1998). Why patients use alternative medicine: Results of a national study. *Journal of the American Medical Association, 279*(19), 1,248.

Avis, A. (1999). Aromatherapy in practice. *Nursing Standard, 13*(24), 14–15.

Benson, H. (1975). *The relaxation response.* New York: Morrow.

Brett, H. (1999). Aromatherapy in the care of older people. *Nursing Times, 95*(33), 56–57.

Brown, H., Cassileth, B. R., Lewis, J. P., & Renner, J. H. (1994, June 15). Alternative medicine—Or quackery? *Patient Care,* 80–98.

Byers, D. C. (2001). *Better health with foot reflexology.* (10th ed.). St. Petersburg, FL: Ingham.

Byrd, C., & Sherrill, J. (1995). The therapeutic effects of intercessory prayer. *Journal of Christian Nursing, 12*(1), 21–23.

Caradonna, B. (2003). *Iridology: An Introduction.* [Online]. Available: www.iridologyassn.org/index.php?page=2887

Carpenter, D. (2003). *Basic information.* [Online]. Available: www.iridologyassn.org/index.php?page=2889

Cerrato, P. (1998). Aromatherapy: Is it for real? *RN, 61*(6), 51–52.

Cerrato, P. (1999a). Using designer margarines to control lipid levels. *RN, 62*(10), 67–68.

Cerrato, P. (1999b). Omega-3 fatty acids: Nothing fishy here! *RN, 62*(8), 59–60.

Cerrato, P. (1999c). A radical approach to heart disease. *RN, 62*(4), 65–66.

Cerrato, P. (1999d). Tai chi: A martial art turns therapeutic. *RN, 62*(2), 59–60.

Cerrato, P. (2000). Diet and herbs for BPH? *RN, 63*(2), 63–64.

Cerrato, P. (2002). Complementary therapies update. *RN, 65*(9), 23.

Cerrato, P., & Rowell, N. (1999). SAMe: A dietary remedy for mind and body? *RN, 62*(12), 61–64.

Chiropractic Arts Center. (2002). *Frequently asked questions* [Online]. Available: www.chiroarts.com/faqs.htm

Chopra, D. (1998). *Ageless body, timeless mind.* New York: Harmony.

Cousins, N. (1979). *Anatomy of an illness.* New York: Norton.

Davis, J. (2002). *Yoga finds new twists in the U.S.* [Online]. Available: http://aolsvc.health.webmed.aol.com/content/article/1668.51358?SRC=aolkw&K W=yoga

Dossey, B. M. (Ed.). (1997). *Core curriculum for holistic nursing.* Gaithersburg, MD: Aspen.

Dossey, B. M. (1999a). Imagery: Awakening the inner healer. In B. M. Dossey, L. Keegan, C. E. Guzzetta, & L. G. Kolkmeier (Eds.), *Holistic nursing: A handbook for practice* (3rd ed.). Gaithersburg, MD: Aspen.

Dossey, B. M. (1999b). The psychophysiology of bodymind healing. In B. M. Dossey, L. Keegan, C. E. Guzzetta, & L. G. Kolkmeier (Eds.), *Holistic nursing: A handbook for practice* (3rd ed.). Gaithersburg, MD: Aspen.

Dossey, L. (1997). *Healing words: The power of prayer and the practice of medicine.* San Francisco: Harper.

Dossey, L. (1999). *Prayer, healing, and medicine: An evening with Larry Dossey.* Arvada, CO: Lutheran Medical Center Community Foundation, Arvada Center.

Dossey, L. (2003). *Healing beyond the body: Medicine and the infinite reach of the mind.* Boston, MA: Shambhala.

Dossey, L., Polkinghorne, J., & Benson, H. (2002). *Healing through prayer: Health practitioners tell the story.* Toronto, Ontario, Canada: Anglican Book Centre.

Evans, B. (1999). Complementary therapies & HIV infection. *AJN, 99*(2), 42–45.

Feuerstein, G. (1998). *Yoga and yoga therapy* [Online]. Available: members.aol.com/yogaresearch/yogatherapy.htm

Floyd, J., & Fernandes, J. (2003). Making a place for CAM in the ICU. *RN, 66*(7), 44–47.

Fonnesbeck, B. (1998). Are you kidding? *Nursing98, 28*(3), 64.

Frisch, N. (1997). Changing of the guard. *Beginnings, 17*(1), 1, 11.

Frisch, N., & Frisch, L. (2002). *Psychiatric mental health nursing.* (2nd ed.). Clifton Park, NY: Thomson Delmar Learning.

Gates, R. (1997). Legal issues in alternative medicine. *Alternative Therapies in Clinical Practice, 4*(4), 143.

Geiter, H. (2002). The spiritual side of nursing. *RN, 65*(5), 43–44.

Geller, U. (2002). *Mind medicine: The secret of powerful healing.* Boston: Element Books.

Guinness, A. (1993). *Family guide to natural medicine: How to stay healthy the natural way.* Pleasantville, NY: Reader's Digest.

Hatcher, T. (2001). The proverbial herb. *AJN, 101*(2), 36–43.

Herbert-Ashton, M. (2002). Getting a handle on herbals. *Travel Nursing Today* (Supplement to RN), Sept., 16–24.

Hodge, P., & Ullrich, S. (1999). Does your assessment include alternative therapies? *RN, 62*(6), 47–49.

Hover-Kramer, D. (2002). *Healing touch: A resource for health care professionals.* (2nd ed.). Clifton Park, NY: Thomson Delmar Learning.

Hutchison, C. (1999). Healing touch: An energetic approach. *AJN, 99*(4), 43–48.

Japsen, B. (1995, August 21). Cost-conscious providers take to holistic medicine. *Modern Healthcare,* 138–142.

Kane, J. (2001). *The healing companion: Simple and effective ways your presence can help people heal.* San Francisco, CA: Harper.

Keegan, L. (1994). *The nurse as healer.* Clifton Park, NY: Thomson Delmar Learning.

Keegan, L. (1998). Alternative & complementary therapies. *Nursing98, 28*(4), 50–53.

Keegan, L. (1999a). Nutrition, exercise, and movement. In B. M. Dossey, L. Keegan, C. E. Guzzetta, & L. G. Kolkmeier (Eds.), *Holistic nursing: A handbook for practice* (3rd ed., pp. 257–285). Gaithersburg, MD: Aspen.

Keegan, L. (1999b). Touch: Connecting with the healing power. In B. M. Dossey, L. Keegan, C. E. Guzzetta, & L. G. Kolkmeier (Eds.), *Holistic nursing: A handbook for practice* (3rd ed.). Gaithersburg, MD: Aspen.

Keegan, L. (2001). *Healing with complementary and alternative therapies.* Clifton Park, NY: Thomson Delmar Learning.

Keville, K., & Green, M. (1995). *Aromatherapy: A complete guide to healing art.* Freedom, CA: Crossing.

King, M. O., Pettigrew, A. C., & Reed, F. C. (1999). Complementary, alternative, integrative: Have nurses kept pace with their clients? *Medsurg Nursing, 8*(4), 249–56.

Klein, A. (2001). *How can you laugh at a time like this?* [Online]. Available: http://aath.org/art_klein.html

Kolkmeier, L. G. (1999). Relaxation: Opening the door to change. In B. M. Dossey, L. Keegan, C. E. Guzzetta, & L. G. Kolkmeier (Eds.), *Holistic nursing: A handbook for practice* (3rd ed.). Gaithersburg, MD: Aspen.

Krieger, D. (1993). *Accepting your power to heal: The personal practice of therapeutic touch.* Santa Fe, NM: Bear.

Levin, J. (2001). *God, faith and health: Exploring the spirituality-healing connection.* Hoboken, NJ: John Wiley & Sons.

Lorenzo, P. (2003). Complementary therapies—they're not without risk. *RN, 66*(1), 65–68.

Marwick, C. (1995). Should physicians prescribe prayer for health? Spiritual aspects of well-being considered. *Journal of the American Medical Association, 273*(20), 1561–1562.

Mason, J. (1999). Massage: The nursing touch. In Healing touch: An energetic approach by C. P. Hutchison. *AJN, 99*(4), 44.

Maxwell, J. (1997). The gentle power of acupressure. *RN, 60*(4), 53–56.

McConnell, E. (2002). Myths & facts about animal-assisted therapy. *Nursing2002, 32*(3), 76.

McGhee, P. (1998). Rx: Laughter. *RN, 69*(7), 50–53.

McGhee, P. (1999). *Health, healing, and the amuse system.* (3rd ed.). Dubuque, IA: Kendall/Hunt.

Mentgen, J. (2002). The clinical practice of healing touch. In D. Hover-Kramer (Ed.), *Healing touch: A resource for health care professionals* (2nd ed.). Clifton Park, NY: Thomson Delmar Learning.

Miller, J., & Connor, K. (2000). Going to the dogs . . . for help. *Nursing2000, 30*(11), 65–67.

Mills, E. M. (1994). The effect of low-intensity aerobic exercise on muscle strength, flexibility, and balance among sedentary elderly persons. *Nursing Research, 43*, 206–211.

Moyers, B. (1995). *Healing and the mind.* New York: Doubleday.

National Center for Complementary and Alternative Medicine (NCCAM). (2000a). *NCCAM Five-Year Strategic Plan.* [Online]. Available: http://nccam.nih.gov/about/plans/fiveyear

National Center for Complementary and Alternative Medicine (NCCAM). (2000b). *Untitled.* [Online]. Available: http://nccam.nih.gov/nccam/an/general/index.html

National Center for Complementary and Alternative Medicine (NCCAM). (2002). *Funding: Appropriations history.* [Online]. Available: http://nccam.nih.gov/about/appropriations/index.htm

National Institutes of Health (NIH). (1997). *Acupuncture: NIH consensus statement* [Online]. Available: http://odp.od.nih.gov/consensus/cons/107.107_intro.htm

Nightingale, F. (1969). *Nursing: What it is and what it is not.* New York: Dover.

Nontraditional Choices. (2001a). Discovering yoga. *Nursing2001, 31*(2), 20.

Nontraditional Choices. (2001b). Trying therapeutic massage. *Nursing2001, 31*(6), 26.

Nontraditional Choices. (2001c). Potentially dangerous herbs. *Nursing2001, 31*(10), 92.

Nontraditional Choices. (2001d). When patients ask about . . . reflexology. *Nursing2001, 31*(9), 68.

Nontraditional Choices. (2002a). Learning about acupuncture. *Nursing2002, 32*(1), 28–29.

Nontraditional Choices. (2002b). Learning about tai chi chuan. *Nursing2002, 32*(12), 86.

Nontraditional Choices. (2002c). Practicing meditation. *Nursing2002, 32*(4), 70.

Nontraditional Choices. (2002d). Understanding biofeedback. *Nursing2002, 32*(6), 88–90.

Nontraditional Choices. (2003a). Putting imagery to work for your patient. *Nursing2003, 33*(6), 73.

Nontraditional Choices. (2003b). Understanding echinacea. *Nursing2003, 33*(1), 76.

O'Neil, C., Avila, J., & Fetrow, C. W. (1999). Herbal medicines: Getting beyond the hype. *Nursing99, 29*(4), 58–61.

Payne, M. (2002). Power of touch. *Nursing2002, 32*(6), 102.

Pert, C. (1986). The wisdom of the receptors: Neuropeptides, the emotions, and bodymind. *Advances, 3*, 8–16.

Renner, J. H., Dillard, J. N., & Edelberg, D. (1999). Should the FDA regulate alternative medicines? *Hospital Health Network, 73*(10), 24.

Rosing, M. (2001). Warm hands, warm heart. *Nursing2001, 31*(12), 32.

Schroeder-Shecker, T. (1994). Music for the dying. *Journal of Holistic Nursing, 12*(1), 83–99.

Simons, S. (1997). *Vegetables and fruits: Natural "Phyters" against disease.* Paper presented at the Texas Agricultural Extension service conference.

Smith, M., Kemp, J., Hemphill, L., & Vojir, C. (2002). Outcomes of therapeutic massage for hospitalized cancer patients. *Journal of Nursing Scholarship, 34*(3), 257–262.

Snyder, J. R. (1999). Therapeutic touch in hospice care. In Healing touch: An energetic approach by C. P. Hutchison. *AJN, 99*(4), 46.

Spencer, J. W., & Jacobs, J. J. (Eds.) (1999). *Complementary/alternative medicine: An evidence-based approach.* St. Louis, MO: Mosby.

Stanley-Hermanns, M., & Miller, J. (2002). Animal-assisted therapy. *AJN, 102*(10), 69–76.

Stedman, M. (1999). Alternatives: You'd better shop around. *Health, 13*(1), 60–66.

Stevenson, C. (1994). The psychophysiological effects of aromatherapy massage following cardiac surgery. *Complementary Therapies in Medicine, 2*(1), 27.

Sutherland, J. A. (2000). Getting to the point. *AJN, 100*(9), 40–43.

Trevelyan, J. (1993). Aromatherapy. *Nursing Times, 89*(25), 38–40.

Vacca, V. (1998). Back to high touch. *RN, 69*(7), 88.

Weil, A. (1998). *Natural health, natural medicine: A comprehensive manual for wellness and self-care* (Rev. ed.). New York: Houghton Mifflin.

Weil, A. (2000). *Spontaneous healing: How to discover and enhance your body's natural ability to maintain and heal itself.* New York: Ivy Books.

Weiss, R. R., & James, W. D. (1997). Allergic contact dermatitis from aromatherapy. *American Journal of Contact Dermatology, 8*(4), 250.

Wilkinson, S. (1995). Aromatherapy and massage in palliative care. *International Journal of Palliative Nursing, 1*(1), 21.

Worden, J. (1999). *Overview of reflexology* [Online]. Available: www.aol.com/reflexology

Yoga Research and Education Center. (2000). *Frequently asked questions* [Online]. Available: www.yrec.org/faq.html

Resources

Acupressure Institute, 1533 Shattuck Avenue, Berkeley, CA 94709, 800-442-2232, www.acupressure.com

American Academy of Medical Acupuncture (AAMA), 4929 Wilshire Boulevard, Suite 428, Los Angeles, CA 90010, 323-937-5514, www.medicalacupuncture.org

The American Association for Applied and Therapeutic Humor, 1951 Camelback Road, Suite 445, Phoenix, AZ 85015, 602-995-1454, www.aath.org

American Holistic Nurses' Association, P.O. Box 2130, Flagstaff, AZ 86003-2130, 800-278-2462, www.ahna.org

American Massage Therapy Association (AMTA), 820 Davis Street, Suite 100, Evanston, IL 60201, 847-864-0123, www.amtamassage.org

Association for Applied Psychophysiology and Biofeedback, 10200 West 44th Avenue, Suite 304, Wheat Ridge, CO 80033-2840, 800-477-8892, 303-422-8436, www.aapb.org

Healing Touch International, Inc, 12477 West Cedar Drive, Suite 202, Lakewood, CO 80220, 303-989-7982, www.healingtouch.net

Holistic Alliance of Professional Practitioners Entrepreneurs Networkers, Inc. (HAPPEN), 1889 West Rose, Stockton, CA 95203, 888-8HAPPEN (42-7736), www.happen.org

International Iridology Practitioners Association, Attn: Ellen Tart, P. O. Box 3334, Escondido, CA 92033-3334, 888-682-2208, www.iridologyassn.org

The Laughter Remedy, 45 North Fullerton, Suite 402, Montclair, NJ 07042, 973-783-8383

National Center to Complementary and Alternative Medicine, NIH, P.O. Box 8218, Silver Spring, MD 20907-8218, 888-644-6226, www.nccam.nih.gov

Tai Chi Association, 4651 Roswell Road, Atlanta, GA 30342, 404-289-5652, www.tai-chi-association.com

Yoga Research and Education Center, 2400A County Center Drive, Santa Rosa, CA 95403, 707-566-9000, www.yrec.org

CHAPTER

16

BASIC NUTRITION

MAKING THE CONNECTION

Refer to the following chapters to increase your understanding of nutrition:

Basic Nursing
- **Life Cycle**
- **Cultural Considerations**
- **Diagnostic Tests**

Basic Procedures
- **Hand Hygiene**
- **Measuring Intake and Output**

Intermediate Procedures
- **Feeding and Medicating via Enteral Tube**

LEARNING OBJECTIVES

Upon completion of this chapter, you should be able to:
- Define key terms.
- Describe the role of the nurse in promoting proper nutrition.
- Explain how the body uses nutrients.
- Compare the six types of nutrients for functions, sources, digestion, absorption, storage, and signs of deficiency and excess.
- Describe factors affecting kilocalorie needs.
- Explain the food guide pyramid.
- Explain the purposes of the Dietary Guidelines for Americans and the recommended dietary allowances (RDAs).
- Discuss factors influencing nutrition.
- Explain the dietary needs and nutritional assessments for infancy, childhood, adolescence, older adulthood, pregnancy, and lactation.
- Explain the relationship between health and nutrition.
- Discuss weight management.
- Explain how to determine energy (kcal) needs.
- Describe three ways to promote food safety.
- Describe the standard hospital diets: regular, soft, liquid, mechanical, and pureed.
- Cite the proper procedure for serving a meal tray.
- List important points to follow when feeding a client.

KEY TERMS

absorption
anabolism
anthropometric
    measurements
atherosclerosis
basal metabolism
body mass index
calorie
catabolism
cholesterol
chyme
complete protein
deglutition
dehydration
diet therapy
dietary prescription/
    order
digestion
empty calories
enriched
enteral nutrition
euglycemia
excretion
extracellular fluid
fat-soluble vitamin
fortified
gluconeogenesis
glycogenesis
glycogenolysis
hyperglycemia
hypoglycemia

incomplete protein
ingestion
insensible water loss
insulin
interstitial fluid
intracellular fluid
ketosis
kilocalorie
kwashiorkor
lipid
marasmus
mastication
metabolic rate
metabolism
monounsaturated fatty
    acid
nutrition
obesity
oxidation
parenteral nutrition
peristalsis
phospholipid
polyunsaturated fatty
    acid
satiety
sensible water loss
triglyceride
villi
vitamin
water-soluble vitamin

INTRODUCTION

Nutrition encompasses all of the processes involved in consuming and utilizing food for energy, maintenance, and growth. These processes are ingestion, digestion, absorption, metabolism, and excretion. Much of the discussion throughout this chapter focuses on ingestion, because this is the process that the individual can control and with which the nurse can be of assistance to the client. Basic information is presented about proper nutrition and the role of the nurse in assisting clients to meet their nutritional needs. Topics covered include specific nutrients and their functions in the body; phytochemicals; promoting proper nutrition; factors influencing nutrition; nutritional needs during the life cycle; nutrition and health; weight management; food labeling, quality, and safety; food allergies; and nutrition and the nursing process.

PHYSIOLOGY OF NUTRITION

Five processes are involved in the body's use of nutrients: ingestion, digestion, absorption, metabolism, and excretion.

Ingestion

Nutrition begins with **ingestion,** taking food into the digestive tract, generally through the mouth. In special circumstances, ingestion occurs directly into the stomach, through a feeding tube; this situation is discussed later in the chapter.

Digestion

Digestion refers to the mechanical and chemical processes that convert nutrients into a physically absorbable state. Mechanical digestion includes **mastication** (chewing), breaking food into fine particles and mixing it with enzymes in saliva, and **deglutition** (swallowing food), the peristaltic waves and mucus secretions that move the food down the esophagus. Chemical diges-

tion is the process whereby enzymes, gastric and intestinal juices, bile, and pancreatic juices change food into the individual nutrients that can be used by the body.

Digestion begins in the stomach (except in the case of some starches, for which digestion begins in the mouth) and is completed in the intestines. **Peristalsis** (rhythmic, coordinated, serial contractions of the smooth muscles of the GI tract) forces **chyme** (an acidic, semifluid paste) through the small and large intestines. Only carbohydrates, proteins, and fats require chemical digestion to make the nutrients available for absorption. Figure 16-1 illustrates the basic elements and functions of the digestive system.

Absorption

Absorption is the process whereby the end products of digestion (i.e., individual nutrients) pass through the epithelial membranes in the small and large intestines and into the blood or lymph systems. The nutrients are absorbed and taken to the parts of the body that need them. Most nutrients are water soluble and can be absorbed directly through the **villi** (fingerlike projections that line the small intestine) and into the blood. Fats, which are not water soluble, are absorbed first into the lymph system and eventually enter the circulatory system.

Metabolism

The conversion of nutrients into energy by the body is called **metabolism;** this process is the sum total of all the biological and chemical processes in the body as they relate to the use of nutrients in every body cell. Metabolism involves two processes: anabolism and catabolism. **Anabolism** is the constructive process of metabolism, wherein new molecules are synthesized and new tissues are formed, as in growth and repair. This process requires energy. **Catabolism** is the destructive process of metabolism, wherein tissues or substances are broken into their component parts. This process releases energy. During metabolism, energy is also produced by the process of **oxidation,** which is the chemical process of combining nutrients with oxygen. The energy produced by the body is used in a number of ways: electrical energy for brain and nerve activities, chemical energy for metabolism, mechanical energy for muscle contractions, and thermal energy to keep the body warm.

Metabolic rate is the rate of energy utilization in the body; it is expressed in units called calories. One **calorie** is the amount of heat required to raise the temperature of one gram of water by 1° Celsius. Because of the large quantity of energy released during metabolism, the energy is expressed in **kilocalories** (kcal), each of which is equal to 1,000 calories.

Basal metabolism is the amount of energy needed to maintain essential physiologic functions, when a person is at *complete* rest. It is the lowest level of energy expenditure.

The major factor affecting basal metabolism is body composition. Lean muscle tissue has a higher metabolic rate and thus produces more energy than does fatty tissue. Generally, women have a lower metabolism than men because they have a higher percentage of fat tissue;

PROFESSIONAL TIP

Role of the LP/VN in Meeting Nutritional Needs

There are several aspects to the role of the licensed practical/vocational nurse (LP/VN) in meeting a client's nutritional needs. These are discussed throughout the chapter and are summarized as follows:

- Teach clients ways to meet their nutritional needs.
- Receive and implement physician's orders.
- Help clients understand their diets.
- Assist clients with eating their meals.
- Report and record observations about nutrient intake and the nutritional status of clients.
- Act as a communication link between the client, the physician, and the dietitian.

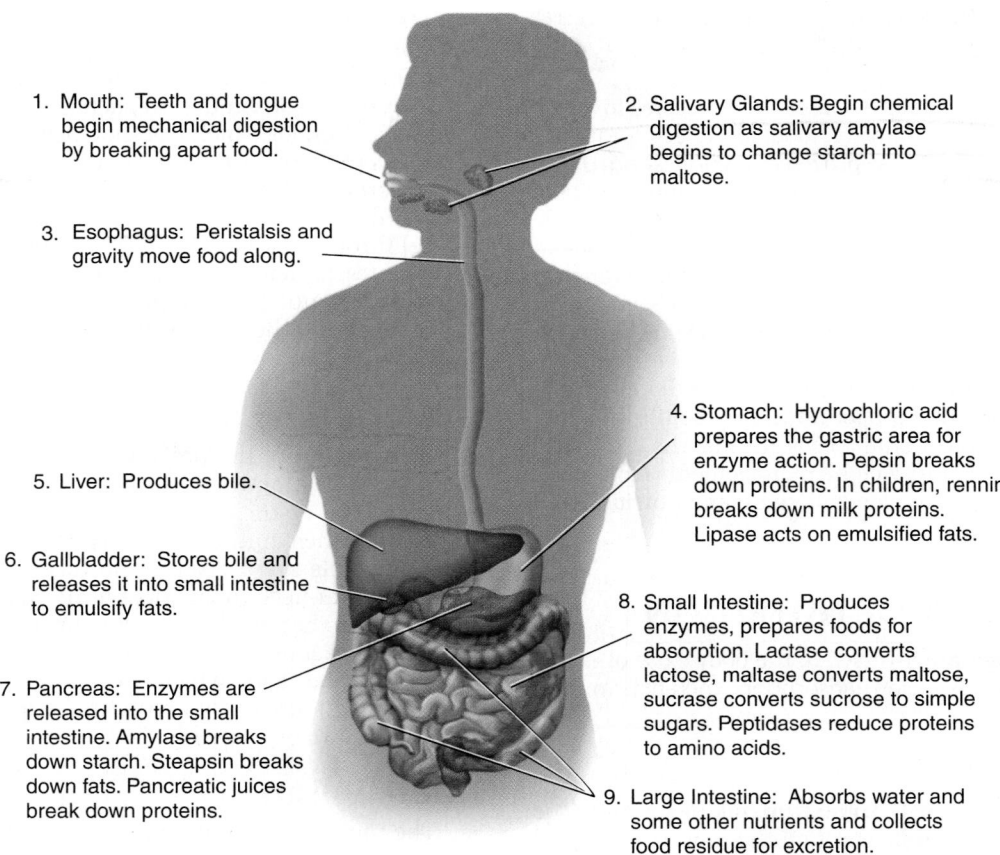

1. Mouth: Teeth and tongue begin mechanical digestion by breaking apart food.

2. Salivary Glands: Begin chemical digestion as salivary amylase begins to change starch into maltose.

3. Esophagus: Peristalsis and gravity move food along.

4. Stomach: Hydrochloric acid prepares the gastric area for enzyme action. Pepsin breaks down proteins. In children, rennin breaks down milk proteins. Lipase acts on emulsified fats.

5. Liver: Produces bile.

6. Gallbladder: Stores bile and releases it into small intestine to emulsify fats.

7. Pancreas: Enzymes are released into the small intestine. Amylase breaks down starch. Steapsin breaks down fats. Pancreatic juices break down proteins.

8. Small Intestine: Produces enzymes, prepares foods for absorption. Lactase converts lactose, maltase converts maltose, sucrase converts sucrose to simple sugars. Peptidases reduce proteins to amino acids.

9. Large Intestine: Absorbs water and some other nutrients and collects food residue for excretion.

Figure 16-1 *Functions of the Digestive System*

however, metabolism increases during menstruation, pregnancy, and lactation. Age is also an influence, because growth periods increase metabolism. Glandular activity, especially of the thyroid gland, affects metabolism. The rate of metabolism is governed primarily by the hormones triiodothyronine (T_3) and thyroxine (T_4). Hypothyroid activity, a decrease in the secretion of thyroid hormones, causes a lower rate of metabolism, whereas hyperthyroid activity, an increase in the secretion of thyroid hormones, causes a higher rate of metabolism.

Excretion

Excretion is the process of eliminating or removing waste products from the body. Dietary fiber and other indigestible materials, salts, and other products such as bile and water are formed into feces and excreted from the body as solid waste. Other excretory organs that aid the digestive system in the elimination of wastes include the kidneys, bladder, sweat glands, skin, and lungs. Most liquid waste is sent through the kidneys and bladder to be excreted as urine. Some liquid waste is removed through the sweat glands of the skin as perspiration. Gaseous waste is eliminated through the lungs.

NUTRIENTS

The body must have six types of nutrients to function efficiently and effectively. These are water, carbohydrates, fats, proteins, vitamins, and minerals. If a person eats a well-balanced diet, all the nutrients the body requires are provided by the food. Table 16-1 offers an overview of the first four nutrients in relation to their fuel value (the amount of energy they supply) and their daily requirements.

Nutrients are classified as energy nutrients, organic nutrients, and inorganic nutrients, as shown in Table 16-2.

Energy nutrients release energy for use by the body. Organic nutrients build and maintain body tissues and regulate body processes. Inorganic nutrients provide a medium for the body's chemical reactions, transport materials, maintain body temperature, promote bone formation, and conduct nerve impulses.

The functions of the nutrients are interrelated. Intake changes in one nutrient may lead to functional changes in another. Some examples of interrelated functions include: (1) Iron is better absorbed when vitamin C is present, and (2) calcium absorption depends on the presence of vitamin D.

Water

Water is the most important nutrient. It is more vital to life than is food. Virtually all body functions require water. An individual may live for weeks without food but for only approximately 10 days without water.

Water is the major constituent in every cell of the body. Approximately 55% to 65% of an adult's weight is

TABLE 16-1 NUTRIENTS, FUEL VALUES, AND DAILY REQUIREMENTS

NUTRIENT	FUEL VALUE	DAILY REQUIREMENTS
Water	0	1,000 mL/ 1,000 kcal eaten
Carbohydrates	1 g = 4 kcal	50% to 60% total kcal per day
Fats	1 g = 9 kcal	25% to 30% total kcal per day
Protein	1 g = 4 kcal	15% to 20% total kcal per day

TABLE 16-2 CLASSIFICATION OF NUTRIENTS

CLASSES	NUTRIENTS
Energy nutrients	Carbohydrates Fats (Lipids) Proteins
Organic nutrients	Carbohydrates Fats (Lipids) Proteins Vitamins
Inorganic nutrients	Water Minerals

Figure 16-2 *Body Water Balance (Approximate figures for a sedentary adult)*

water, and approximately 70% to 75% of an infant's weight is water. The body's water content decreases with age.

Approximately two-thirds of the water in the body is **intracellular fluid** (ICF), fluid within the cells. The other one-third is **extracellular fluid** (ECF), fluid outside the cells, including plasma fluid, lymph, cerebrospinal fluid, **interstitial fluid** (fluid in tissue spaces around each cell), and GI fluids.

Daily Requirements

The amount of water needed by the body varies based on environmental factors, such as temperature and humidity, and physical factors, such as activity level, metabolic need, functional losses (urine and feces), age, respiratory rate, and state of health. Higher environmental temperatures and vigorous physical activity cause more water loss as perspiration increases. Water lost must be replaced to maintain metabolism. Generally, 1,000 mL of water is needed to process every 1,000 kcal eaten.

A state of relative water balance exists when the body has adequate fluid distributed appropriately as ICF and ECF. A person's daily water intake and output should be equal (Figure 16-2). Excessive intake of fluids is not a problem in a healthy individual; more intake simply causes more output.

Functions

Water has many functions in the body:

- *Solvent:* Water is the liquid in which many substances are dissolved to form solutions.
- *Transporter:* Water carries nutrients, wastes, and other materials throughout the body and to and from each cell via blood, tissue fluids, and body secretions.
- *Regulator of body temperature:* Water is excreted as perspiration when the temperature goes up. Evaporation of perspiration cools the body.
- *Lubricant:* Water is a component of fluid within the joints, called synovial fluid, which provides smooth movement of the many joints in the body.
- *Component of all cells:* Water gives structure and form to the body.
- *Hydrolysis:* Water breaks apart substances, especially in metabolism.

Classification and Sources

There are three sources of water for the body:

- Liquids consumed, including water, coffee, juice, tea, milk, and soft drinks
- Foods consumed, especially vegetables and fruits
- Metabolism, which produces water when oxidization occurs

Digestion, Absorption, and Storage

Water is not digested but, rather, is absorbed and used by the body as we drink it. It is not stored by the body and is excreted daily. Water losses are classified as **sensible,** the person is aware of the loss, or **insensible,** the person is not generally aware of the loss. There are four ways the body normally loses water:

- *Urine:* accounts for the greatest amount of water lost from the body (sensible loss)

Dehydration

Infants, small children, and elderly persons are more susceptible to dehydration. For them, dehydration occurs more rapidly and is more severe.

- *Feces:* contains a small amount of water (insensible loss, except in cases of diarrhea)
- *Perspiration:* varies with temperature, but some fluid is always lost (insensible or sensible loss)
- *Respiration:* releases moisture with every breath (insensible loss)

Signs of Deficiency and Excess

Abnormal water losses from the body include profuse sweating, vomiting, diarrhea, hemorrhage, wound drainage (burns), fever, and edema. With edema, the water is still in the body, but is not usable.

A deficiency of water is called **dehydration**. Prolonged dehydration results in death.

Some conditions cause an excessive accumulation of fluid in the body. This condition is called *positive water balance.* It occurs when more water is taken in than is used and excreted, and edema results. Hypothyroidism, congestive heart failure, hypoproteinemia (low amounts of protein), some infections and cancers, and some renal conditions can cause such water retention because sodium is not being excreted normally.

Carbohydrates

Carbohydrates are made of the elements carbon, hydrogen, and oxygen. In nutrition, the first letters of these three elements are used as the abbreviation: CHO.

Carbohydrates constitute the chief source of energy for all body functions. They are also the major food source for all people, because they are the least expensive and the most abundant foods.

Daily Requirements

It is recommended that carbohydrates make up 50% to 60% of an individual's kcal intake per day. For example, if an individual's total energy requirement is 2,000 kcal, 50% of this number is 1,000; this number is then divided by 4 (the number of kcal in each gram of carbohydrate, Table 16-1), for an estimated carbohydrate requirement of 250 g/day. It is estimated that current U.S. diets contain only 45% of their kcal from carbohydrates (Townsend & Roth, 2000).

Functions

Carbohydrates constitute the primary source of energy for the body. The body must maintain a constant supply of energy; therefore, it stores approximately one-half a day's supply of carbohydrates in the liver and muscles for use as needed. A sufficient supply of carbohydrates spares proteins from being used for energy, thus allowing proteins to perform their primary function of building and repairing body tissues. Carbohydrates are needed to oxidize fats completely and for synthesis of fatty acids and amino acids. The central nervous system and erythrocytes rely solely on carbohydrates for energy.

Classification and Sources

Carbohydrates are classified as either simple or complex. Simple carbohydrates are single sugars (monosaccharides) such as glucose, fructose, and galactose found in fruits, honey, and corn syrup. Monosaccharides require no digestion, are quickly absorbed, and are either used for energy or stored as glycogen.

Double sugars (disaccharides), such as sucrose, maltose, and lactose, are two single sugars joined together. They are found in milk, sweeteners, sugar, and molasses. Before they can be absorbed by the body, disaccharides must be separated into monosaccharides through digestion.

Complex carbohydrates (polysaccharides) are composed of many single sugars joined together. Those important in nutrition are starch, glycogen, and dietary fiber (cellulose). The most significant of these in the diet is starch, which is found in grains, grain products, legumes, potatoes, and other vegetables. Complex carbohydrates are digested much more slowly than the simple carbohydrates, and they thus supply the body with energy for a longer period of time.

Glycogen is a form of carbohydrate made by the liver and stored in the liver and muscles. The body keeps a 12- to 48-hour store of glycogen. This reserve is used between meals and during sleep to maintain **euglycemia** (normal blood glucose level) for body functions. **Glycogenesis** is the process of converting glucose to glycogen. **Glycogenolysis** is the process of changing the glycogen back to glucose when it is needed by the body for energy. **Insulin** is a pancreatic hormone necessary for cells to produce energy and for the liver to produce and store glycogen. Glucose metabolism depends on the availability of insulin.

Dietary fiber has no nutritive value: The human body is unable to digest it. There are two types of dietary fiber: soluble and insoluble. Soluble dietary fiber slows gastric emptying and binds bile acids and cholesterol. This fiber provides **satiety** (a feeling of adequate fullness from food) and lowers the cholesterol level in the blood. Insoluble dietary fiber holds water, which increases fecal bulk and stimulates peristalsis for better elimination. Good sources of both kinds of dietary fiber are whole grains, whole-grain products, legumes, and fruits and vegetables with their skins.

Digestion, Absorption, and Storage

Digestion of cooked starches begins in the mouth, when the salivary enzyme ptyalin mixes with the starch in food during chewing. Little digestion takes place in the stomach. Carbohydrate digestion is completed in the small intestine by pancreatic and intestinal enzymes present there. Carbohydrates leave no waste for the kidneys to eliminate.

Glucose and other monosaccharides, the final products of carbohydrate digestion, are absorbed into the blood through the capillaries in the villi of the intestinal mucosa. Fructose and other monosaccharides are converted to glucose in the liver.

Glucose not needed for immediate energy is converted to glycogen by the liver and stored there and in the muscles. Any remaining glucose is then converted to fatty acids and stored as adipose tissue (fat). The body has no way to rid itself of excess carbohydrates; they are either used or stored.

Signs of Deficiency and Excess

A mild deficiency of carbohydrates can result in weight loss and fatigue. A diet seriously deficient in carbohydrates causes extra fat to be metabolized to meet the body's energy needs. Without carbohydrates, fat is incompletely oxidized, producing ketones, an acid by-product, which accumulates in the blood and urine causing **ketosis.** Ketosis can result from uncontrolled insulin-dependent diabetes mellitus, starvation, or diets extremely low in carbohydrates. It can lead to coma and even death.

Excess carbohydrate consumption is one of the most common causes of obesity. Although some of the surplus carbohydrate is changed to glycogen, the major part of any surplus becomes adipose tissue. Too many carbohydrates may cause tooth decay, irritate the lining of the stomach, or cause flatulence.

Fats

Fats constitute the most concentrated source of energy in the diet, providing 9 kcal per gram of fat. People in developed countries tend to eat diets relatively high in fat. Although fat is an essential nutrient, too much fat is a hazard to good health. The descriptive word for fats of all kinds is *lipids*. **Lipids** are organic compounds that are insoluble in water but soluble in organic solvents, such as ether and alcohol, and include true fats and fatlike compounds such as lipoids and sterols. Fats provide slightly more than twice the calorie content of carbohydrates. Like carbohydrates, fats are composed of carbon, hydrogen, and oxygen, but they have a substantially lower proportion of oxygen.

Daily Requirements

It is recommended that fats make up no more than 25% to 30% of an individual's caloric intake per day. For example, assuming that one's total energy requirement is 2,000 kcal/day, one-quarter (25%) of this would be 500 kcal. Dividing 500 kcal by 9 (the number of kcal in each gram of fat; Table 16-1) yields an estimated fat requirement of 55.5 g/day.

Functions

Fat has many functions in the body. It:

- Provides a concentrated source of energy (more than twice the kcal of carbohydrates).

- Assists in the absorption of fat-soluble vitamins.
- Is a major component of cell membranes and myelin sheaths.

- Improves the flavor of food and delays the stomach's emptying time, providing a feeling of satiety.
- Protects and helps hold organs in place.
- Insulates the body thus assisting in temperature maintenance.

Classification and Sources

Fat is formed by one molecule of glycerol being joined to one, two, or three fatty-acid molecules. The most important lipids are:

- **Triglycerides** (true fats), composed of one glycerol molecule attached to three fatty-acid molecules. Most dietary fat and body fat are triglycerides.
- **Phospholipids** (lipoids), composed of glycerol, fatty acids, and phosphorus. They are structural components of cells, for example, myelin (insulating covering of many nerves) and lecithin (a part of cell membranes).
- **Cholesterol** (a sterol), not essential in the diet because the liver manufactures approximately 1,000 mg every day. Cholesterol is found in all cell membranes, in brain and nerve tissue, and in blood, and it is excreted in bile. Cholesterol is required to produce several hormones, including estrogen, testosterone, adrenalin, and cortisone. The intake of dietary cholesterol from animal food products may affect the serum (blood) cholesterol level.

Fats can also be classified by source, visibility, and saturation. The source of fats can be either animal or plant (vegetable). Examples of animal fat are lard, butter, milk, cream, egg yolks, and the fat in meat, poultry, and fish. Examples of plant fat are oils (corn, safflower, olive, cottonseed, peanut, palm, and coconut), nuts, and avocado.

Fats are either visible or invisible. Visible fats are easy to identify, such as butter, oils, margarine, lard, shortening, bacon, salt pork, and the fat around beef. Examples of invisible fats are those in egg yolks, whole milk and whole-milk products, cheeses, nuts, seeds, olives, avocados, many desserts, and baked goods.

The saturation of a fat refers to its chemical composition. When fatty acids, the main building blocks of fats, contain all of the hydrogen ions possible in the molecule,

LIFE CYCLE CONSIDERATIONS

Children and Cholesterol

If children are not fed high-cholesterol foods on a regular basis, their chance of overusing these foods as adults lessens, as does their risk of heart attack and stroke.

they are said to be saturated. Saturated fats tend to be solid at room temperature. Generally, animal fats are saturated. Plant fats that are saturated are coconut, palm kernel, and palm oils. Unsaturated fats are missing a hydrogen ion at one or more places in the molecule. They tend to be soft or liquid at room temperature. Plant fats are generally unsaturated, with the exceptions already mentioned. Unsaturated fats are subdivided into monounsaturated and polyunsaturated fats. **Monounsaturated fatty acids** are those that form glycerol esters with one double or triple bond; foods in this category are nuts, fowl, and olive oil. **Polyunsaturated fatty acids** form glycerol esters that have many carbons unbonded to hydrogen atoms. Foods such as fish, corn, sunflower seeds, soybeans, cottonseeds, and safflower oil contain polyunsaturated fat.

There are three essential fatty acids (linoleic, linolenic, and arachidonic) necessary for growth, cholesterol metabolism, and heart action. They are found primarily in vegetable oils, egg yolks, and poultry.

Digestion, Absorption, and Storage

No chemical breakdown of fats occurs in the mouth, and very little fat digestion takes place in the stomach. When fat reaches the small intestine, digestion begins. The digestive agents for fat are bile, from the gallbladder, and enzymes, from the pancreas and the small intestine. The final products of fat digestion are fatty acids and glycerol. Approximately 95% of dietary fat is absorbed in the small intestine.

Fats not immediately needed by the body are stored as adipose tissue. Approximately 5 g of fat are excreted daily in the feces.

Signs of Deficiency and Excess

Deficiency symptoms occur when fats provide less than 10% of the total daily kcal requirement. Gross deficiency may result in eczema (inflamed and scaly skin condition), retarded growth, and weight loss.

Excess fat in the diet can lead to overweight and heart disease. In addition, studies point to an association between high-fat diets and cancers of the colon, breast, uterus, and prostate.

An elevated level of cholesterol in the blood is thought to be a contributing factor in heart disease, because hypercholesterolemia (high serum cholesterol) is common in clients with atherosclerosis. **Atherosclerosis** is a cardiovascular disease wherein plaque (fatty deposits containing cholesterol and other substances) forms on the inside of artery walls, reducing the space for blood flow.

Protein

Proteins are made of the elements carbon, hydrogen, oxygen, and nitrogen. In nutrition, the first letters of these four elements are used as the abbreviation: CHON.

Protein is the only nutrient that can build, repair, and maintain body tissues. An adequate supply of proteins in the daily diet is essential. All tissues and fluids in the body, with the exception of bile and urine, contain some protein. The basic building materials of protein are amino acids.

Daily Requirements

Daily protein requirement is determined by size, age, gender, and physical and emotional condition. A large person has more body cells to maintain than does a small person. A growing child, a pregnant woman, or a woman who is breastfeeding needs more protein for each pound of body weight than does the average adult. When digestion is inefficient, fewer amino acids are absorbed by the body; consequently, the protein requirement is higher. This is sometimes thought to be the case with elderly clients. Extra proteins are usually required after surgery or severe burns or during infections to replace lost tissue and manufacture antibodies. In addition, emotional trauma can cause the body to excrete more nitrogen than it normally does, thus increasing the need for protein-rich foods.

The National Research Council of the National Academy of Sciences considers the average adult's daily requirement to be 0.8 g of protein for each kilogram of body weight. Daily protein requirement is determined by multiplying body weight in kilograms (weight in pounds divided by 2.2) by 0.8. For instance:

$$130 \text{ lb. woman} \div 2.2 \text{ lb/kg} = 59.1 \text{ kg} \times 0.8 \text{ g/kg}$$
$$= 47.3 \text{ g protein/day}$$

Functions

The primary function of protein in the diet is to provide the amino acids necessary for the synthesis of body

proteins, which are used to build, repair, and maintain the body tissues. Protein composes most of the muscles, skin, hair, nails, brain, nerves, and internal organs.

Another function of protein is to assist in regulating fluid balance. Proteins are a vital part of enzymes, hormones, and blood plasma. Many body processes are regulated by enzymes and hormones. Plasma proteins help control water balance between the circulatory system and surrounding tissues. Protein is also used to build antibodies, which help defend the body against disease and foreign substances.

In the event of insufficient stores of carbohydrate and fat (the body's primary and secondary sources of energy), protein, in the form of amino acids, can be converted into glucose and used for energy. This process is called **gluconeogenesis**; however, when protein is used for energy, it is not available for its primary function. Using protein for energy also results in waste products that are difficult for the kidneys to excrete.

Classification and Sources

Protein is classified by source and completeness. Animal sources include meat, fish, poultry, eggs, milk, and dairy products. Plant sources are grains, legumes, nuts, and seeds.

The completeness of a protein refers to its quality. Of the 22 amino acids, 9 are called essential amino acids (i.e., they must be present in the diet because the body cannot synthesize them). **Complete proteins** contain all 9 essential amino acids. All animal proteins, with the exception of gelatin, are complete proteins; the only complete plant protein is soybeans.

Plant proteins (with the exception of soybeans) are **incomplete proteins** (i.e., one or more of the essential amino acids are missing). Because all plant proteins do not lack the same essential amino acids, they can be combined in various ways to provide all of the essential amino acids. When two plant protein foods are combined to provide the essential amino acids, they are said to be complementary. Some of the common complementary plant proteins are rice and beans (legumes); corn and beans; wheat bread and beans; toast and pea soup; and rice and lentils. Complementary proteins are a very important part of planning a healthy vegetarian diet.

Digestion, Absorption, and Storage

Chemical digestion of protein begins in the stomach, when hydrochloric acid activates the enzyme pepsin; however, most of the digestion takes place in the small intestine with the action of pancreatic and intestinal enzymes. The end product of protein digestion is amino acids. The body can then combine the amino acids to build, repair, and maintain body tissues.

The amino acids are absorbed into the blood by the capillaries in the villi of the intestinal mucosa. Amino acids not used to build proteins are converted to glucose, glycogen, or fat and are stored.

Signs of Deficiency and Excess

When people are unable to obtain an adequate supply of protein for an extended period, muscle wasting occurs, and arms and legs become very thin. At the same time, albumin (protein in blood plasma) deficiency causes edema, resulting in an extremely swollen appearance. The edema decreases when sufficient protein is eaten. Clients with edema become lethargic and depressed. These signs are seen in grossly neglected children or in the elderly poor or incapacitated. Children who lack sufficient protein do not grow to their potential size. Infants born to mothers eating insufficient protein during pregnancy can have permanently impaired mental capacities (Townsend & Roth, 2000).

Two deficiency diseases that affect children are caused by a grossly inadequate supply of protein, energy, or both. **Marasmus,** a condition resulting from severe malnutrition, afflicts very young children who lack both energy and protein foods as well as vitamins and minerals. The infant with marasmus appears emaciated but does not have edema; hair is dull and dry, and the skin is thin and wrinkled. **Kwashiorkor** results when there is a sudden or recent lack of protein-containing food (such as during a famine). This disease results in edema, painful skin lesions, and changes in the pigmentation of skin and hair (Townsend & Roth, 2000).

It is easy for people living in the developed parts of the world to ingest more protein than the body requires. This should be avoided because the saturated fats and cholesterol common to complete protein foods may contribute to heart disease and provide more kcal than needed. Some studies indicate a connection between long-term high-protein diets and colon cancer and high calcium excretion, which depletes the bones of calcium and may contribute to osteoporosis. People who eat excessive amounts of protein-rich foods may ignore essential fruits and vegetables, and excess protein intake may put more demands on the kidneys than they can handle (Townsend & Roth, 2000).

Vitamins

Vitamins are organic compounds essential to life and health. They regulate body processes and are needed in very small amounts. They have no fuel value

but are required for the metabolism of fats, carbohydrates, and proteins.

Daily Requirements

The Food and Nutrition Board of the National Academy of Sciences—National Research Council prepared a list of recommended dietary allowances for the 11 vitamins for which it considers current scientific research to be adequate for determining daily recommendations. Vitamin allowances are given by weight in milligrams (mg) or micrograms (mcg).

Vitamins taken in addition to the diet are called vitamin supplements. Lifestyle choices may affect the need for vitamin supplementation (Table 16-3).

Functions

The functions of vitamins are unique to each individual vitamin. Tables 16-4 and 16-5 list the functions of each type of vitamin.

Classification and Sources

Vitamins are commonly grouped according to solubility. Vitamins A, D, E, and K are fat soluble, and vitamin C and the B-complex vitamins are water soluble.

Fat-Soluble Vitamins The **fat-soluble vitamins** (A, D, E, and K) require the presence of fats for their absorption from the GI tract into the lymphatic system and for cellular metabolism. They must attach to protein carriers to be transported through the blood. The body's stored reserve makes daily intake unnecessary. In fact, the reserve can result in toxic levels if large supplemental doses are taken, especially in the case of vitamin A. Deficiencies can occur in conditions that interfere with fat absorption.

Water-Soluble Vitamins The **water-soluble vitamins** (C and the B-complex vitamins) require daily ingestion in normal quantities because they are not stored in the body. They are absorbed by the capillaries in the intestinal villi directly into the circulatory system. Deficiency symptoms develop quickly in response to inadequate intake. Foods should be cooked in the least amount of water possible, because the water-soluble vitamins are released into the cooking water: When the water is discarded, the vitamins are lost.

TABLE 16-3 SUPPLEMENTS FOR LIFESTYLE CHOICES	
LIFESTYLE CHOICE	**SUGGESTED SUPPLEMENT**
Restricted diets	B$_{12}$ (cobalamin)
Extensive exercise program	Riboflavin
Oral contraceptives	Pyridoxine, niacin, vitamin C
Smoking	Vitamin C
Alcohol	Thiamine, folate
Caffeine	B vitamins, vitamin C

TABLE 16-4   FAT-SOLUBLE VITAMINS

VITAMIN	FUNCTION	SOURCES	DEFICIENCY	TOXIC EFFECTS
A	• Aids in night vision • Promotes growth of bones and teeth • Maintains skin and mucous membranes	• Fish oils • Carrots • Sweet potatoes • Broccoli • Cantaloupe • Green leafy vegetables	• Night blindness • Dry, scaly skin • Diarrhea • Respiratory infections	• From supplementation: anorexia, diarrhea, hair loss, bone pain, liver damage
D	• Stimulates absorption of calcium and phosphorus for good bone mineralization	• Yeast • Fish liver oils • Fortified milk and cereals	• Rickets • Malformed teeth • Bone deformities	• Hypercalcemia • Kidney stones • Cardiovascular damage
E	• Acts as an antioxidant • Maintains cell membrane integrity • Protects red blood cells (RBCs) from hemolysis	• Vegetable oils • Leafy vegetables • Wheat germ	• Increased RBC hemolysis • Rare, except in cases of fat malabsorption	• Depression • Fatigue • Diarrhea • Cramps • Headaches
K	• Responsible for synthesis of prothrombin, needed for normal blood clotting	• Dark-green leafy vegetables • Made by intestinal bacteria	• Rare, except in newborns • Delayed blood clotting	• No toxic effects

TABLE 16-5   WATER-SOLUBLE VITAMINS

VITAMIN	FUNCTION	SOURCES	DEFICIENCY	TOXIC EFFECTS
C (asorbic acid)	• Builds and maintains strong tissues • Promotes wound healing • Aids in resisting infection • Enhances iron absorption	• Citrus fruits • Green and red peppers • Tomatoes • Melons • Cabbage • Broccoli • Strawberries	• Scurvy • Easy bruising • Delayed wound healing • Swollen, inflamed gums • Secondary infections	• Megadoses: excessive iron absorption • Nausea • Diarrhea
B_1 (thiamine)	• Promotes CHO metabolism • Ensures normal nervous system functioning	• Enriched grains and cereals • Pork • Legumes	• Beriberi • Mental confusion • Anorexia • Fatigue • Muscle weakness	• None known
B_2 (riboflavin)	• Promotes CHO, protein, and fat metabolism • Promotes deoxyribonucleic acid (DNA) synthesis • Aids in protein synthesis	• Milk and milk products • Meat, poultry, fish • Enriched grains and cereals	• Oral lesions • Dermatitis • Cheilosis • Red, swollen tongue • Reddening of cornea	• None known

continues

TABLE 16-5   continued

VITAMIN	FUNCTION	SOURCES	DEFICIENCY	TOXIC EFFECTS
Niacin (nicotinic acid)	• Aids in oxidation • Promotes CHO, protein, and fat metabolism • Aids tissue protein building	• Meat, poultry, fish • Legumes • Enriched grains • Peanuts	• Pellegra • Anorexia • Apathy • Weakness • Dermatitis • Diarrhea • Dementia	• Large doses: flushing, itching, hypotension, tachycardia
B_6 (pyridoxine)	• Is necessary for amino acid metabolism • Promotes blood formation • Maintains nervous tissue	• Chicken, fish, pork • Eggs • Whole grains	• Depression • Dermatitis • Abnormal brain wave patterns • Convulsions • Anemia	• Clumsiness • Nerve degeneration
B_{12} (cobolomin)	• Promotes normal function of all cells, especially those of the nervous system • Promotes blood formation • Promotes CHO, protein, and fat metabolism • Aids in synthesis of ribonucleic acid (RNA) and DNA • Is necessary for folate metabolism	• Fresh shrimp, oysters, meats, milk, eggs, and cheese	• Pernicious anemia • Anorexia • Indigestion • Paresthesia of hands and feet • Poor coordination • Depression	• None known
Folate (folic acid)	• Is necessary for synthesis of RNA and DNA • Promotes amino acid metabolism, RBC and white blood cell (WBC) formation • Prevents neural tube defects	• Green leafy vegetables • Milk • Eggs • Yeast	• Glossitis • Diarrhea • Macrocytic anemia	• None known
Pantothenic acid	• Promotes CHO, protein, and fat metabolism	• Animal tissues • Whole-grain cereals • Legumes • Milk	• Not observed in humans	• None known
Biotin	• Promotes CHO and fat metabolism • Is necessary for glycogen formation	• Egg yolk • Yeast • Milk • Soy flours • Cereals • Legumes • Made by intestinal bacteria	• Only induced with long-term total parenteral nutrition (TPN)	• None known

CLIENT TEACHING

Natural or Synthetic Vitamins

Some people believe that natural vitamins are superior in quality to synthetic vitamins. According to the U.S. Food and Drug Administration (FDA), however, the body cannot distinguish between a vitamin of plant or animal origin and one manufactured in a laboratory. The two types of the same vitamin are chemically identical.

CRITICAL THINKING

Vitamin Supplements

What recommendations should be made to a client regarding vitamin supplements?

Digestion, Absorption, and Storage

Vitamins do not require digestion. Fat-soluble vitamins are absorbed into the lymphatic system, whereas water-soluble vitamins are absorbed directly into the circulatory system. Excess amounts of fat-soluble vitamins cannot be excreted but are stored in the liver and adipose tissue. Water-soluble vitamins are excreted through urine, when excess amounts are taken into the body.

Signs of Deficiency or Excess

Vitamin deficiencies can occur and result in disease. Those persons inclined to vitamin deficiencies because they do not eat balanced diets include alcoholics; the poor; incapacitated elders; clients with serious diseases that affect appetite; mentally retarded persons; and young children who receive inadequate care. Deficiencies of fat-soluble vitamins occur in clients with chronic malabsorption diseases such as cystic fibrosis, celiac disease, and Crohn's disease.

Vitamins consumed in excess amounts can be toxic to the body (Tables 16-4 and 16-5).

Minerals

Minerals are inorganic elements that help regulate body processes and/or serve as structural components of the body. Like vitamins, they have no fuel value.

Chemical analysis shows that the human body is made up of specific chemical elements. Four of these elements—oxygen, carbon, hydrogen, and nitrogen—make up 96% of body weight. All the remaining elements are minerals, making up 4% of body weight. Nevertheless, these minerals are essential for good health.

Daily Requirements

Major minerals are required in amounts greater than 100 mg/day. Trace minerals are those required in amounts less than 100 mg/day.

Functions

The functions of minerals are unique to each individual mineral. Table 16-6 outlines the functions, sources, deficiencies, and toxic effects of each mineral.

Classification and Sources

Minerals are generally classified as major minerals and trace elements (Table 16-7). Minerals are found in

TABLE 16-6 MINERALS				
MINERAL	**FUNCTION**	**SOURCES**	**DEFICIENCY**	**TOXIC EFFECTS**
Calcium (Ca)	• Aids in bone and teeth formation • Promotes muscle contraction and relaxation • Aids blood clotting • Aids in nerve transmission • Promotes normal heart rhythm • Needs vitamin D for absorption	• Milk • Cheese • Sardines • Salmon • Green leafy vegetables • Whole grains	• Rickets • Osteoporosis • Tetany • Poor tooth formation	• Kidney stones • Deposits in joints and soft tissue • May inhibit iron and zinc absorption
Phosphorus (P)	• Aids in bone and teeth formation • Involved in energy metabolism • Regulates acid–base balance • Ensures structure of cell membranes • Is part of nucleic acids	• Fish, beef, pork, poultry • Cheese • Legumes • Milk • Carbonated beverages	• Rickets • Osteoporosis • Poor tooth formation • Disturbed acid base balance	• Low serum calcium • Kidney stones

continues

TABLE 16-6   continued

MINERAL	FUNCTION	SOURCES	DEFICIENCY	TOXIC EFFECTS
✓ Sodium (Na)	• Helps regulate fluid balance and acid–base balance • Regulates cell membrane irritability • Regulates nerve transmission	• Table salt • Milk • Meat • Processed foods • Carrots • Celery	• Hyponatremia • Nausea • Headache • Mental confusion • Hypotension • Anxiety • Muscle spasms	• Hypernatremia • Hypertension • Cardiovascular disturbance • Edema
✓ Potassium (K)	• Maintains fluid balance • Maintains acid–base balance • Regulates muscle activity • Aids in protein synthesis • Aids in CHO metabolism	• Fruits, especially oranges, bananas, and prunes • Red meats • Vegetables • Milk and milk products • Coffee	• Hypokalemia • Fluid and electrolyte imbalances • Tissue breakdown • Cardiac weakness • Muscle cramps	• Hyperkalemia • Muscle weakness • Severe dehydration • Mental confusion • Hypotension • Cardiac arrest
✓ Magnesium (Mg)	• Is necessary for muscle–nerve action • Regulates CHO, CHON, and fat metabolism • Activates enzymes • Aids in bone formation	• Green leafy vegetables • Whole grains • Legumes	• Hypomagnesemia • Tremors • Spasms • Convulsions	• Hypermagnesemia • Central nervous system (CNS) depression • Coma • Hypotension
✓ Chlorine (Cl)	• Helps regulate fluid balance and acid–base balance • Aids digestion as part of hydrochloric acid in stomach	• Table salt • Milk • Meat • Processed foods	• Rare	• Rare
Sulfur (S)	• Serves as component of amino acids • Aids vitamin, enzyme, and hormonal activity • Is part of skin, hair, nails, and soft tissue	• Cheese • Eggs • Poultry • Fish	• None specific	• None specific
Iron (Fe)	• Aids in formation of hemoglobin • Aids in antibody formation	• Meat • Whole grains • Egg yolk • Legumes • Prunes • Raisins • Apricots	• Iron deficiency • Anemia	• Hemochromatosis • GI cramping • Vomiting • Nausea • Shock • Convulsions • Coma
Iodine (I)	• Is a component of thyroid hormones	• Iodized salt • Seafood (salt water) • Milk	• Cretinism • Goiter	• Hyperthyroidism • Fatal in large amounts
Zinc (Zn)	• Is a component of DNA and RNA • Aids in physical and sexual development • Helps ensure normal taste and smell • Aids in wound healing	• Meats, oysters • Eggs • Milk • Whole grains	• Poor wound healing • Decreased taste and smell • Growth retardation	• Muscle incoordination • Vomiting • Diarrhea • Renal failure

continues

TABLE 16-6 continued

MINERAL	FUNCTION	SOURCES	DEFICIENCY	TOXIC EFFECTS
Selenium (Se)	• Acts as an antioxidant • Works with vitamin E	• Seafoods • Meats	• Muscle weakness • Cardiomyopathy	• Selenosis • Nausea • Peripheral neuropathy • Fatigue
Copper (Cu)	• Aids in bone and blood formation • Promotes iron absorption • Is part of myelin sheath	• Seafood • Nuts • Legumes	• Iron-deficiency anemia • Hypocholesterolemia	• None known
Manganese (Mn)	• Aids bone growth • Aids reproduction • Acts as enzyme activator	• Whole-grain cereals • Legumes • Tea	• Unknown	• Unlikely
Fluorine (Fl)	• Protects against dental caries • Contributes to bone formation and integrity	• Fluoridated water • Tea • Seafood	• Dental caries	• Mottled stains on teeth
Chromium (Cr)	• Associated with glucose metabolism	• Whole grains • Brewers yeast	• Insulin resistance • Impaired glucose tolerance	• Dietary: unlikely
Molybdenum (Mo)	• Helps ensure normal body metabolism	• Milk • Legumes • Whole grains	• Decreased production of uric acid	• Interferes with copper metabolism
Cobalt (Co)	• Is a component of vitamin B$_{12}$ • Aids in RBC formation	• Meat, as B$_{12}$	• Associated with vitamin B$_{12}$ deficiency	• Unknown

TABLE 16-7 MAJOR MINERALS AND TRACE ELEMENTS

MAJOR MINERALS	TRACE ELEMENTS	
	Essential	Questionable
Calcium (Ca)	Iron (Fe)	Arsenic (As)
Phosphorus (P)	Iodine (I)	Boron (B)
Sodium (Na)	Zinc (Zn)	Cadmium (Cd)
Potassium (K)	Selenium (Se)	Nickel (Ni)
Magnesium (Mg)	Copper (Cu)	Silicon (Si)
Chlorine (Cl)	Manganese (Mn)	Tin (Sn)
Sulfur (S)	Fluorine (Fl)	Vanadium (V)
	Chromium (Cr)	
	Molybdenum (Mo)	
	Cobalt (Co)	

water and in natural (unprocessed) foods, together with proteins, carbohydrates, fats, and vitamins. Minerals in the soil are absorbed by growing plants. Humans obtain minerals by eating plants grown in mineral-rich soil or by eating animals that have eaten such plants.

Highly processed or refined foods such as sugar and white flour contain almost no minerals. Iron, together with the vitamins thiamin, riboflavin, niacin, and folate is commonly added back to some flour and cereals, which are then labeled enriched.

Most minerals in food occur as salts, which are soluble in water. Therefore, the minerals leave the food and remain in the cooking water when foods are cooked in water. Foods should be cooked in as little water as possible or, preferably, steamed, and any cooking liquid should be saved to be used in soups, gravies, and white sauces. Using this liquid improves the flavor as well as the nutrient content of foods to which it is added.

Supplemental minerals may be required during growth periods and in some clinical situations. Individuals with iron-deficiency anemia require extra iron.

Persons taking potassium-losing diuretics need a potassium supplement.

Digestion, Absorption, and Storage

Minerals are absorbed in their ionic forms (i.e., carrying a positive or negative electrical charge). The amount of a mineral absorbed by the body is influenced by three factors:

- *Type of food:* Minerals in foods that come from animals are more readily absorbed than those in foods that come from plants.
- *Need of body:* If there is a deficiency of a mineral in the body, more will be absorbed.
- *Health of absorbing tissue:* If absorbing tissue (intestine) is affected by disease, less will be absorbed.

Signs of Deficiency and Excess

Because it is known that minerals are essential to good health, some people think "more is better." More can be hazardous to one's health when it comes to minerals. In a healthy individual eating a balanced diet, there will be some normal mineral loss through perspiration and saliva, and amounts in excess of body needs will be excreted in urine and feces. When concentrated forms of minerals are taken regularly over a period of time, however, they become more than the body can handle, and toxicity develops. An excessive amount of one mineral sometimes causes a deficiency of another mineral. Excessive amounts of minerals can cause hair loss and changes in the blood, hormones, bones, muscles, blood vessels, and nearly all tissues. Concentrated forms of minerals should be used only on the advice of a physician. Refer to Table 16-6 for specific signs of deficiency and toxicity of each mineral.

PROMOTING PROPER NUTRITION

Through the years, various ways to promote proper nutrition have been devised. The best known are the four food groups, the food guide pyramid, the *Dietary Guidelines for Americans*, the recommended daily allowances, and the dietary reference intakes.

Four Food Groups (Historical)

For many years, the four food groups assisted people in eating a well-balanced diet. Eating foods from the four groups—milk, meat, fruit/vegetable, and bread/cereal—provided most nutrients required in a daily diet. The minimum number of servings yielded approximately 1,200 kcal. Additional servings were to be added depending on the individual's age and activity level.

Food Guide Pyramid

In 1992, the U.S. Department of Agriculture introduced the food guide pyramid identifying the food groups from which additional servings should be obtained when calorie needs exceed the 1,200 kcal provided for by the minimum servings from the four food groups. The pyramid separates the fruit and vegetable groups and the suggested number of servings from each group. The food guide pyramid also identifies fat, because most American diets are too high in fat. Figure 16-3 shows the food guide pyramid.

Each food group of the food guide pyramid provides some, but not all, of the nutrients needed each day. Foods in one group cannot replace foods in another group. No one group is more important than another: All are needed.

Bread, Cereal, Rice, and Pasta Group

At the base of the pyramid is the bread, cereal, rice, and pasta group. The nutrients contributed by this

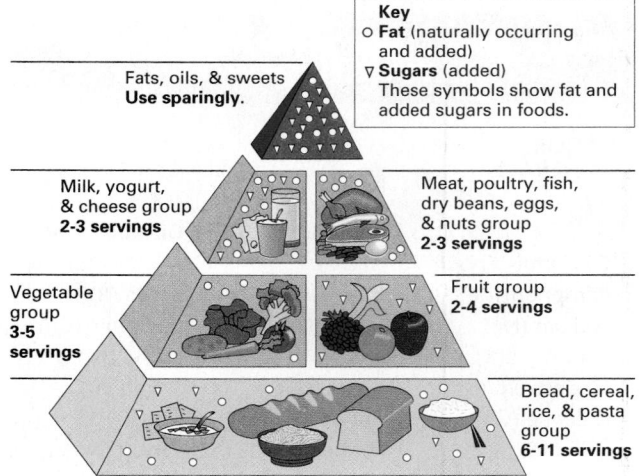

Figure 16-3 *Food Guide Pyramid [Courtesy of the U.S. Department of Agriculture, Center for Nutrition Policy and Promotion, 1996. Good Guide Pyramid (Home and Garden Bulletin, No. 252). Washington, DC: USDA.]*

group are complex carbohydrates, incomplete protein, the B vitamins, and iron, if the product is whole grain or **enriched** (nutrients that are removed during processing are added back) with iron. Six to eleven servings a day should come from this group. Examples of serving sizes from this group are one slice of bread, one tortilla, 1 ounce (1 cup) dry cereal, and $1/2$ cup cooked cereal, rice, or pasta.

Fruit and Vegetable Groups

On the second level of the pyramid are the fruits and vegetables. The nutritional contributions of fruits and vegetables are carbohydrates, vitamins, minerals, water, and very small amounts of proteins and fats. Dietary fiber, important for elimination, is found in the skin or pulp of many foods in this group.

Fruits Each person should have two to four servings of fruit every day. Citrus fruits, melons, and berries should be eaten regularly as they are high in vitamin C. Examples of serving sizes from the fruit group are one medium-size apple, pear, banana, or orange; $1/2$ cup of cooked, chopped, or canned fruit, or $3/4$ cup of fruit juice.

Vegetables Three to five servings a day from the vegetable group are suggested. Among the vegetables eaten daily, one should be a dark-green or deep-yellow vegetable to provide vitamin A. Sample serving sizes from the vegetable group include 1 cup of raw leafy vegetables, $1/2$ cup of cooked or chopped raw vegetables, or $3/4$ cup of vegetable juice.

Milk and Meat Groups

On the third level are the foods that come mostly from animals. These foods have significantly greater amounts of saturated fat or added sugar than do the foods on the first and second levels. Fewer servings should be eaten from this level each day.

Milk The nutritional contributions of the milk group are calcium, protein, riboflavin, fat, carbohydrates, phosphorus, sodium, vitamin B_{12}, and vitamin A. If skim milk or skim milk products are used, there is no fat and significantly fewer kcal. All commercial milk products are **fortified** (a nutrient not naturally occurring in a food is added to the food) with vitamin D. Vitamin D, not naturally found in milk, is added because the calcium provided by milk is better absorbed when vitamin D is present.

Two to three servings a day are suggested from the milk group. Eight ounces of milk is considered one serving. Other milk products and their serving sizes to provide the equivalent nutrients of 8 ounces of milk are $1^{1}/_{2}$ ounces of cheese, 1 cup of yogurt, $1^{1}/_{2}$ cups of cottage cheese, and $1^{1}/_{2}$ cups of ice cream. The kcal content of these foods varies, with ice cream containing more kcal than the other foods in the milk group.

Meat The meat group contributes complete protein, fats, iron, most other minerals, and the B vitamins. Cheese and bacon are not considered part of this group: cheese has too little iron and bacon has too much fat.

The suggested number of servings from the meat group is two to three each day. A serving size is 2 to 3 ounces of meat, fish, or poultry. Other foods that can be substituted for one serving of meat are two eggs, 4 table-spoons of peanut butter, or 1 cup cooked beans or peas (legumes). Legumes such as dried peas, beans, or lentils can be used instead of meat because of their high protein content. Peanuts as well as many other nuts are high in protein, but they are also high in fats and should be used sparingly.

Fats, Oils, and Sweets Group

Fats, oils, and sweets are placed at the very top of the pyramid because they do not fit into any of the other food groups. These other food items are considered **empty calories** (i.e., they generally provide many calories but very few nutrients). Items included are potato chips, cookies, cakes, pies, soft drinks, alcohol, jelly, syrup, fats, oils, salad dressings, pickles, olives, ketchup, and mustard. These foods are to be eaten in very small amounts and infrequently, as they have the most fat and added sugar and the least nutritional value of all the foods.

Number of Servings

The number of servings for an individual depends on the number of calories the individual needs. The number of calories needed by a person depends on age, gender, size, and activity. Almost everyone should have the minimum number of servings for each group. The serving recommendations for three general calorie levels are listed in Table 16-8.

The Vegetarian Diet

There are several vegetarian diets. The common factor among them is that they do not include red meat.

TABLE 16-8 SERVINGS FOR THREE CALORIE LEVELS

FOOD GROUP	TOTAL CALORIC INTAKE AND NUMBER OF SERVINGS PER GROUP		
	1,600 calories	2,200 calories	2,800 calories
Grain	6 servings	9 servings	11 servings
Vegetable	3 servings	4 servings	5 servings
Fruit	2 servings	3 servings	4 servings
Milk	2 to 3 servings	2 to 3 servings	2 to 3 servings
Meat	5 ounces	6 ounces	7 ounces

A 1,600-calorie diet is about right for sedentary women and older adults.

A 2,200 calorie diet is about right for most children, teenage girls, and active women and for many sedentary men. Pregnant and lactating women may need more calories.

A 2,800 calorie diet is about right for teenage boys, many active men, and some very active women.

From U.S. Department of Agriculture, Center for Nutrition Policy and Promotion, 1996. *Food Guide Pyramid* (Home and Garden Bulletin, No. 252). Washington, DC: USDA

When carefully planned, these diets can be nutritious. They can even contribute to a reduction in obesity, high blood pressure, heart disease, some cancers, and, possibly, diabetes (Townsend & Roth, 2000). They must be carefully planned so they include all the needed nutrients.

Lacto-ovo vegetarians use dairy products and eggs but no meat, poultry, or fish. Lacto vegetarians use dairy products but no meat, poultry, or eggs. Vegans avoid all animal foods. They use soybeans, chickpeas, meat analogues, and tofu. It is important that their meals be carefully planned to include appropriate combinations of the essential amino acids. For example, beans served with corn or rice, or peanuts eaten with wheat, are complementary proteins. Vegans can show deficiencies of calcium; vitamins A, D, and B_{12}; and, of course, proteins.

Dietary Guidelines

The *Dietary Guidelines* developed by the U.S. Department of Agriculture and the U.S. Department of Health & Human Services were last revised in 1990. They are now stated in positive terms (i.e., "eat . . ."; "consume . . .") instead of negative terms ("avoid . . ."). These guidelines attempt to prevent overnutrition by incorporating some of the concepts of the food guide pyramid (Table 16-9).

Recommended Dietary Allowances

Recommended dietary allowances (RDAs) of essential nutrients are the recommended intake levels judged adequate to meet the known nutrient needs of practically all healthy people. Recommendations are grouped according to infants, children, males, females, and pregnant/lactating women, and are subdivided within those groups according to age. The RDAs are compiled by the Food and Nutrition Board of the National Academy of Sciences and are periodically revised.

Dietary Reference Intakes

The dietary reference intakes (DRIs) are nutrient-based reference values for use in planning and assessing diets. They are intended to replace the old RDAs. The DRIs focus on decreasing the risk of chronic disease through nutrition, rather than on protecting against deficiency diseases, as do the RDAs.

The DRIs encompass four categories:

- *Estimated average requirement* (EAR) is the amount that meets the estimated nutrient need of 50% of the individuals in a specific group.
- *Recommended dietary allowance* (RDA) is the amount that meets the nutrient need of almost all (97% to 98%) healthy individuals in a specific age and gender group. It is the EAR plus an increase, based on scientific evidence, to account for variation within the specific group. The RDA should be used to achieve adequate nutrient intake aimed at decreasing the risk of chronic disease.
- *Adequate intake* (AI) is set when there is insufficient scientific evidence to estimate an average requirement. It is derived through experimental or observational data that show a mean intake that appears to sustain a desired indicator of health, such as calcium retention in bone.
- *Tolerable upper intake level* (UL) is the maximum intake by an individual that is unlikely to pose risks of adverse health effects in almost all healthy individuals in a specified group. It is not intended to be a recommended level of intake. There is no established benefit

TABLE 16-9 DIETARY GUIDELINES FOR AMERICANS

AIM FOR FITNESS	BUILD A HEALTHY BASE	CHOOSE SENSIBLY
• Aim for a healthy weight. • Be physically active each day. Following these two guidelines will help keep you and your family healthy and fit. Healthy eating and regular physical activity enable people of all ages to work productively, enjoy life, and feel their best. They also help children grow, develop, and do well in school.	• Use the food guide pyramid to make your food choices. • Choose a variety of grains daily, especially whole grains. • Choose a variety of fruits and vegetables daily. • Keep food safe to eat. Following these four guidelines builds a base for healthy eating. Let the food guide pyramid guide you so that you get the nutrients your body needs each day. Make grains, fruits, and vegetables the foundation of your meals. This forms a base for good nutrition and good health and may reduce your risk of certain chronic diseases. Be flexible and adventurous, try new choices from these three groups in place of some less nutritious foods or in place of higher calorie foods that you usually eat. Whatever you eat, always take steps to keep your food safe to eat.	• Choose a diet that is low in saturated fat and cholesterol and moderate in total fat. • Choose beverages and foods to moderate your intake of sugars. • Choose and prepare foods with less salt. • If you drink alcoholic beverages, do so in moderation. These four guidelines help you make sensible choices that promote health and reduce the risk of certain chronic diseases. You can enjoy all foods as part of a healthy diet as long as you don't overdo it on fat (especially saturated fat), sugars, salt, and alcohol. Read labels to identify foods that are higher in saturated fats, sugars, and salt (sodium).

From U.S. Department of Agriculture and U.S. Department of Health and Human Services, 2000. *Dietary Guidelines for Americans* (Home and Garden Bulletin, No. 232, 5th ed). Washington, D.C.: USDA.

for individuals to consume nutrients at levels above the RDA or AI.

FACTORS INFLUENCING NUTRITION

Many factors influence nutrition. Some of the major factors are culture, religion, socioeconomics, fads, and superstitions.

Culture

A person's culture encompasses a total way of life including values, attitudes, and practices. Food practices are a substantial part of a culture. These food habits are based on availability of foods, preparation techniques, methods of serving, and the personal meaning of food (Figure 16-4). American cuisine (cooking style) is a marvelous composite of countless national, regional, cultural, and religious food customs. Consequently, categorizing a client's food habits can be difficult. People who are ill commonly have little interest in food, and sometimes foods that were familiar to them during their childhood and youth are more tempting than other types. The following section briefly discusses some food patterns typical of various cultures, regions, and countries. Of course, there can be and usually are enormous variations within any one classification.

Native American

It is thought that approximately one-half of the edible plants commonly eaten in the United States today originated with the Native Americans. Examples are corn, potatoes, squash, cranberries, pumpkin, peppers, beans, wild rice, and cocoa beans. In addition, wild fruits, game, and fish were used. Foods were commonly prepared as soups and stews or were dried. The original Native American diets were probably more nutritionally adequate than current diets. Native American diets today may be deficient in calcium, vitamins A and C, and riboflavin (Townsend & Roth, 2000).

U.S. Southern

Hot breads such as corn bread and baking powder biscuits are common in the U.S. South because the wheat

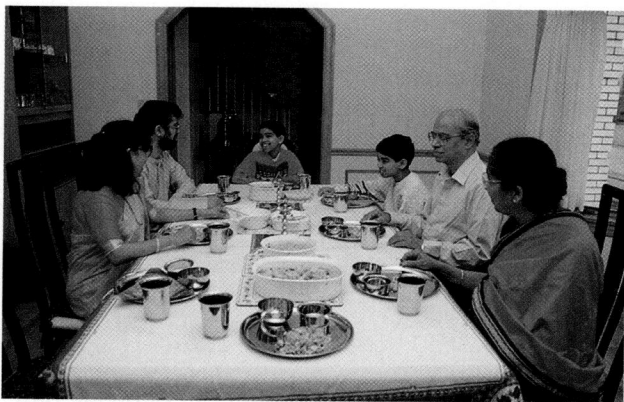

Figure 16-4 *Family and cultural values often affect diet.*

grown in this area does not make good-quality yeast breads. Grits and rice are also popular carbohydrate foods. Favorite vegetables include sweet potatoes, squash, green beans, and lima beans. Watermelon, oranges, and peaches are popular fruits. Fried fish is served often, as are barbecued and stewed meats and poultry. These diets have a great deal of carbohydrate and fat and limited amounts of protein in some cases. Iron, calcium, and vitamins A and C may be deficient (Townsend & Roth, 2000).

Mexican

Mexican food is a combination of Spanish and Native American foods. Beans, rice, chili peppers, tomatoes, and corn meal are favorites. Meat is often cooked with a vegetable, as in chili con carne. Cornmeal or flour is used to make tortillas, which are served as bread. The combination of beans and corn makes a complete protein. Corn tortillas filled with cheese (called enchiladas) provide some calcium, but the use of milk should be encouraged. Additional green and yellow vegetables and vitamin C–rich foods would also make these diets more well-balanced.

Puerto Rican

Rice is the basic carbohydrate food in Puerto Rican diets. Vegetables commonly used include beans, plantains, tomatoes, and peppers. Bananas, pineapple, mangoes, and papayas are popular fruits. Favorite meats are chicken, beef, and pork. Additional milk would make a more balanced diet (Townsend & Roth, 2000).

Italian

Pastas with various tomato or fish sauces and cheese are popular Italian foods. Fish and highly seasoned foods are common southern Italian cuisine; whereas meat and root vegetables are common northern cuisine. The eggs, cheese, tomatoes, green vegetables, and fruits in Italian diets provide excellent sources of many nutrients. Added fat-free milk and low-fat meat would make the diet more complete (Townsend & Roth, 2000).

Northern and Western European

Northern and Western European diets are similar to those of the U.S. Midwest, but with a greater use of dark breads, potatoes, and fish, and fewer green-vegetable salads. Beef and pork are popular, as are various cooked vegetables, breads, cakes, and dairy products. The addition of fresh vegetables and fruits would add vitamins, minerals, and fiber to these diets.

Central European

Citizens of Central Europe obtain the greatest portion of their calories from potatoes and grain, especially rye and buckwheat (Townsend & Roth, 2000). Pork is a popular meat. Cabbage cooked in many ways is a popular vegetable, as are carrots, onions, and turnips. Eggs and dairy products are used abundantly. Limiting the number of eggs consumed and using fat-free or low-fat dairy products would reduce the fat content in this diet.

Adding fresh vegetables and fruits would increase vitamins, minerals, and fiber.

Middle Eastern

Grains, wheat, and rice provide energy in Middle Eastern diets. Chickpeas in the form of hummus are popular. Lamb and yogurt are commonly used, as are cabbage, grape leaves, eggplant, tomatoes, dates, olives, and figs. Black, very sweet coffee is a popular beverage. There may be insufficient protein and calcium in this diet, depending on the amounts of meat and calcium-rich foods eaten. Fresh fruits and vegetables should be added to the diet to increase vitamins, minerals, and fiber.

Chinese

The Chinese diet is varied. Rice is the primary energy food and is used in place of bread. Vegetables are lightly cooked, and the cooking water is saved for future use. Soybeans are used in many ways, and eggs and pork are commonly served. Soy sauce is extensively used, but it is very salty and could present a problem for clients needing low-salt diets. Tea is a common beverage, but milk is not. This diet is typically low in fat (Townsend & Roth, 2000).

Japanese

Japanese diets include rice, soybean paste and curd, vegetables, fruits, and fish. Food is frequently served tempura style, which means fried. Soy sauce (shoyu) and tea are commonly used. Current Japanese diets have been greatly influenced by Western culture. Japanese diets may be deficient in calcium, given the near-total lack of milk in the diet (Townsend & Roth, 2000). Although fish is eaten with bones, this may not supply sufficient calcium to meet needs. Japanese diets may contain excessive amounts of salt.

Indian

Many Indians are vegetarians who use eggs and dairy products. Rice, peas, and beans are frequently served. Spices, especially curry, are popular. Indian meals are generally served as one course with many dishes.

Thai, Vietnamese, Laotian, and Cambodian

Rice, curries, vegetables, and fruit are popular in Thailand, Vietnam, Laos, and Cambodia. Meats and fish are used in small amounts. The wok (a deep, round fry pan) is used for sautéing many foods. A salty sauce made from fermented fish is commonly used. Thai, Vietnamese, Laotian, and Cambodian diets may be deficient in protein and calcium (Townsend & Roth, 2000).

Religion

Religious beliefs often influence nutrition by placing restrictions on the foods eaten and their preparation. A few examples follow.

Jewish

Interpretations of the Jewish dietary laws vary. Persons who adhere to the Orthodox view consider tradition important and always observe the dietary laws. Foods prepared according to these laws are called *kosher*. Conservative Jews are inclined to observe the rules only at home. Reform Jews consider their dietary laws to be essentially ceremonial and thus minimize their significance. Essentially the laws require the following (Townsend & Roth, 2000):

- Slaughtering must be done by a qualified person and in a prescribed manner.
- Meat and meat products may not be prepared with milk or milk products.
- The dishes used in the preparation and serving of meat products must be kept separate from those used for dairy foods.
- Dairy products and meat may not be eaten together. Six hours must elapse after eating meat before eating dairy products, and at least 30 minutes to 1 hour must elapse after eating dairy products before eating meat.
- The mouth must be rinsed after eating fish and before eating meat.
- The following may not be eaten: animals without cloven (split) hooves or animals that do not chew their cud; hindquarters of any animal; shellfish or fish without scales or fins; birds of prey; creeping things and insects; and leavened (containing ingredients that cause it to rise) bread during Passover.

There are prescribed fast days: Passover Week, Yom Kippur, and Feast of Purim. Chicken and fresh smoked and salted fish are popular, as are noodles, eggs, and flour dishes. These diets can be deficient in fresh vegetables and milk.

Roman Catholic

Although the dietary restrictions of the Roman Catholic religion have been liberalized, meat is not allowed on Ash Wednesday and Fridays during Lent.

Eastern Orthodox

The Eastern Orthodox religion includes Christians from the Middle East, Russia, and Greece. Although interpretations of the dietary laws vary, meat, poultry, fish, and dairy products are restricted on Wednesdays and Fridays and during Lent and Advent.

Seventh-day Adventists

In general, Seventh-day Adventists are lacto-ovo vegetarians, meaning that they use milk products and eggs, but no meat, fish, or poultry. Nuts, legumes, meat analogues (substitutes), and tofu (made from soybeans) may be used. Coffee, tea, and alcohol are considered to be harmful.

Mormon (Latter-day Saints)

The only dietary restriction observed by the Mormons is the prohibition of coffee, tea, and alcoholic beverages.

Islamic

Adherents of Islam are called Muslims. Dietary laws prohibit the use of pork and alcohol, and other meats must be slaughtered according to specific laws. During the month of Ramadan, Muslims do not eat or drink during daylight hours.

Hindu

To the Hindus, all life is sacred, and animals contain the souls of ancestors. Consequently, most Hindus are vegetarians and do not use eggs in food preparation because eggs represent life.

Socioeconomics

The amount of money available to purchase food certainly influences nutrition. More money, however, does not always mean better nutrition. Persons with less money often plan their meals and buy food more carefully than do those with higher incomes. Expensive food does not mean better nutrition. Many times, persons with no monetary worries eat what they want, when they want, without paying attention to nutritional value, thereby shortchanging themselves nutritionally.

Fads

Food fads are beliefs that persist for a period of time about certain foods and that generally have no scientific basis. Often, these fads are translated into diets that can be harmful if basic nutrients are missing or are in excess. One of the most popular diets some years ago was the grapefruit and egg diet. One of the more recent fads was the liquid-protein diet. This diet overloaded the body with protein, yet other nutrients were lacking. The excessive amount of protein damaged the kidneys of many people. Indeed, some people died from this fad diet (American Heart Association, 1999).

Superstitions

Superstitions are irrational beliefs about a food that are generally passed down from generation to generation. The nurse should be aware of the beliefs and the facts that contradict them so as to be knowledgeable and respectful. Examples of such superstitions are:

- *Superstition:* Toast is less fattening than bread.
  Fact: Only moisture is removed during toasting.
- *Superstition:* "Cravings" during pregnancy should be satisfied or the infant will be marked or deformed.
- *Fact:* Foods eaten or not eaten by the mother do not directly affect the infant; only the nutrients or lack thereof affect the unborn child.

NUTRITIONAL NEEDS DURING THE LIFE CYCLE

As a person grows and develops from birth to old age, nutritional needs change. These changes generally are based on growth needs, energy needs, and utilization of nutrients. A nutritional assessment should be conducted to ascertain the nutritional needs of the individual.

Infancy

Food and its presentation are extremely important during the baby's first year. Physical and mental development depend on the food itself, and psychosocial de-

---

PROFESSIONAL TIP

Nutritional Needs of Infants
It is important to remember that growth rates vary from child to child. Nutritional needs depend largely on a child's growth rate.

---

velopment is affected by the time and manner whereby the food is offered.

Although babies have been fed according to prescribed time schedules in the past, it is preferable to feed infants on demand. Feeding on demand prevents the frustrations that hunger can bring and helps the child develop trust in people. The newborn may require more frequent feedings, but, normally, the demand schedule averages approximately every 4 hours by the time the baby is 2 or 3 months old (Townsend & Roth, 2000).

Nutritional Requirements

The first year of life is a period of the most rapid growth in one's life. A baby doubles its birth weight by 6 months of age and triples it within the first year. This explains why the infant's energy, vitamin, mineral, and protein requirements are higher per unit of body weight than are those of older children or adults.

During the first year, the normal child needs approximately 100 kcal per kilogram of body weight each day. This is approximately two to three times the adult requirement. Infants who have suffered from low birth weight, malnutrition, or illness require more than the normal number of kcal per kilogram of body weight. The nutritional status of infants is reflected in many of the same characteristics as those of adults.

The American Academy of Pediatrics recommends breast milk for the first 12 months of life, although parents must decide on the method of feeding based on their lifestyle, values, and personal feelings.

Breast Milk Breastfeeding is nature's way of providing a good diet for the baby. It is, in fact, used as the guide by which nutritional requirements of infants are measured.

Mother's milk provides the infant with temporary immunity to many infectious diseases. It is sterile, easy to digest, and usually does not cause GI disturbances or allergic reactions. Breastfed infants grow more rapidly

---

CLIENT TEACHING

Breastfeeding

If the mother works and cannot be available for every feeding, breast milk can be expressed earlier, refrigerated or frozen, and used at the appropriate time, or a bottle of formula can be substituted. Never warm the breast milk in a microwave oven because the antibodies will be destroyed. Instead, warm a cup of water and place the bag of breast milk in the water to heat it.

CLIENT TEACHING

Cow's Milk

Infants younger than 1 year of age should not be given regular cow's milk. Its protein is more difficult and slower to digest than that of human milk and can cause GI blood loss. The kidneys are challenged by its high protein and mineral content, and dehydration and even damage to the CNS can result. In addition, the fat is less bioavailable, meaning it is not absorbed as efficiently as that in human milk (Townsend & Roth, 2000).

CLIENT TEACHING

Nursing Bottle Syndrome

Infants should not be put to bed with a bottle. Saliva, which normally cleanses the teeth, diminishes as the infant falls asleep. The milk then bathes the upper front teeth, causing tooth decay. Also, the bottle can cause the upper jaw to protrude and the lower to recede. The result is known as the baby bottle mouth, or nursing bottle syndrome. It is preferable to feed the infant the bedtime bottle, cleanse the teeth and gums with some water from another bottle or cup, and then put the infant to bed.

during the first few months of life than do formula-fed babies, and they typically have fewer infections (especially ear infections). Because breast milk contains less protein and minerals than infant formula, it reduces the load on the infant's kidneys. Breastfeeding also promotes oral motor development in infants because sucking requires more and different muscles than does bottle-feeding (Townsend & Roth, 2000).

One can be quite confident the infant is getting sufficient nutrients and kcal from breastfeeding if (1) there are six or more wet diapers per day; (2) there is normal growth; (3) there are one or two mustard-colored bowel movements per day; and (4) the breast becomes soft during nursing.

Formula If the baby is bottle-fed, the pediatrician provides information on commercial formulas and feeding instructions. Formulas are usually based on cow's milk because it is abundant and easily modified to resemble human milk in nutrient and kcal values.

When an infant is extremely sensitive or allergic to infant formulas, a synthetic formula made from soybeans may be given. Formulas with predigested proteins are used for infants unable to tolerate all other types of formulas (Townsend & Roth, 2000).

Formulas can be purchased in ready-to-feed, concentrated, or powdered forms. Sterile water must be mixed with the concentrated and powdered forms. The most convenient type is also the most expensive.

If the type purchased requires the addition of water, it is essential that the amount of water added be correctly measured. Too little water will create too heavy a protein and mineral load for the infant's kidneys; too much water will dilute the nutrient and kcal value such that the infant will not thrive.

Solid Foods Introducing solid foods before the age of 4 to 6 months is not recommended. The child's GI tract and kidneys are not sufficiently developed to handle solid

food before that age. Furthermore, it is thought that the early introduction of solid foods may increase the likelihood of overfeeding and the possibility of food allergies developing, particularly in children whose parents suffer from food allergies.

An infant's readiness for solid foods will be demonstrated by (1) the physical ability to pull food into the mouth rather than always pushing the tongue and food out of the mouth, (2) a willingness to participate in the process, (3) the ability to sit up with support, (4) having head and neck control, and (5) the need for additional nutrients. An infant drinking more than 32 ounces of formula or nursing 8 to 10 times in 24 hours should be started on solid food.

Solid foods must be introduced gradually and individually. One food is introduced and then no other new food for 4 or 5 days. If there is no allergic reaction, another food can be introduced, a waiting period allowed, then another, and so on. The typical order of introduction begins with cereal, usually iron-fortified rice, then oat, wheat, and mixed cereals. Cooked and pureed vegetables follow, then cooked and pureed fruits, egg yolk, and, finally, finely ground meats. Between 6 and 12 months, toast, zwieback, teething biscuits, custards, puddings, and ice cream can be added.

When the infant learns to drink from a cup, juice can be introduced. Juice should never be given from a bottle because babies will fill up on it and not get enough calories from other sources. Pasteurized apple juice is usually given first. It is recommended that only 100% juice products be given because they are nutrient dense (Townsend & Roth, 2000).

By the age of 1 year, most babies are eating foods from all the food guide pyramid's groups and may have most any food that is easily chewed and digested; however, precautions must be taken to avoid offering foods that might cause the child to choke. Examples include hot dogs, nuts, whole peas, grapes, popcorn, small candies, and small pieces of tough meat or raw vegetables. Foods should be selected according to the advice of the pediatrician.

Childhood

Although specific nutritional requirements change as children grow, nutrition always affects physical, mental, and emotional growth and development. Studies indi-

CLIENT TEACHING

Honey

Honey should never be given to an infant because it could be contaminated with *Clostridium botulinum* bacteria.

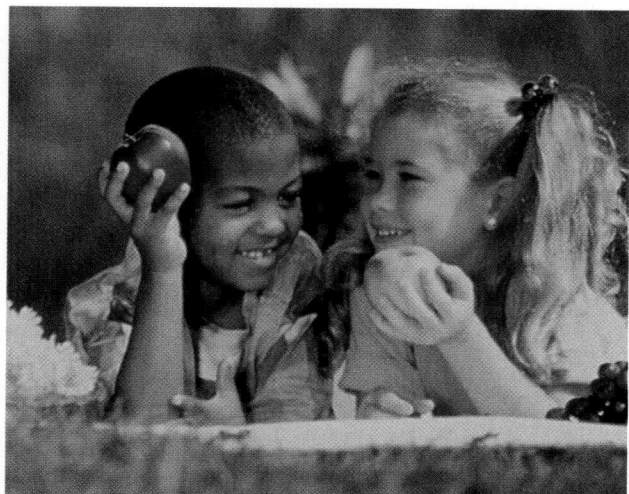

Figure 16-5 *Good health radiates from these two children. (Photo by Keith Weller, ARS/USDA.)*

cate that the mental ability and size of an individual are directly influenced by nutrition during the early years.

Eating habits develop during childhood. Once developed, poor eating habits are difficult to change. They can exacerbate emotional and physical problems such as irritability, depression, anxiety, fatigue, and illness. Good eating habits formed in early childhood will generally last a lifetime (Figure 16-5).

Parents should be aware that children's appetites vary. The rate of growth is not constant. As the child ages, the rate of growth actually slows. The approximate weight gain of a child during the second year of life is only 5 pounds. Children between the ages of 1 and 3 years learn to feed themselves.

As children continue to grow and develop, their likes and dislikes may change. New foods should be introduced gradually, in small amounts, and as attractively as possible.

Children should be offered nutrient-dense foods because the amount eaten will be small. Fats should not be limited before the age of 2 years, but meals and snacks should not be fat-laden either. Whole milk is recommended until the age of 2, but low-fat or fat-free should be served from 2 years on. The guideline for fat intake after the age of 2 is the same as that for adults. Children should not salt their food at the table or have foods prepared with a lot of salt (Townsend & Roth, 2000).

Children are especially sensitive to and reject hot (temperature) foods, but they like crisp textures, mild flavors, and familiar foods. They are wary of foods covered by sauce or gravy. Parents should set realistic goals and expectations as to the amount of food a child needs. A good rule of thumb for preschool children is one tablespoon of new food for each year of age. Table 16-10 details serving sizes according to age. Calorie needs depend on rate of growth, activity level, body size, metabolism, and health.

Nutritional Requirements

The rate of growth diminishes from the age of 1 year until about age 10, thus the kcal requirement per pound of body weight also diminishes during this period. For example, at 6 months, a girl needs approximately 54 kcal per pound of body weight, but by age 10, she will require only 35 kcal per pound of body weight.

Nutrient needs, however, do not diminish. From the age of 6 months to 10 years, nutrient needs actually increase because of the increased body size. Therefore, it is especially important that young children are given nutritious foods they will eat.

In general, the young child will need 2 to 3 cups of milk each day, or the equivalent in terms of calcium; however, excessive use of milk should be avoided because it can crowd out other iron-rich foods and possibly cause iron deficiency. The number of servings of the other food groups is the same as for adults, but the sizes will be smaller. The use of sweets should be minimized because children generally prefer them to nutrient-rich foods. Sweetened fruit juices should especially be avoided. Children also need water and fiber in their diets. They need to drink 1 mL of water for each kcal. If 1,200 kcal is eaten, five 8-ounce glasses of water are needed. Fiber needs are calculated according to age. After age 3 years a child's fiber needs are "age + 5g" and no more than

TABLE 16-10 FOOD PLAN FOR PRESCHOOL AND SCHOOL-AGE CHILDREN BASED ON THE FOOD GUIDE PYRAMID

FOOD GROUP	NUMBER OF SERVINGS	APPROXIMATE SERVING SIZE*			
		AGES 1–2	AGES 3–4	AGES 5–6	AGES 7–12
Milk, yogurt, and cheese	3	$\frac{1}{2}$ to $\frac{3}{4}$ cup or 1 oz	$\frac{3}{4}$ cup or $1\frac{1}{2}$ oz	1 cup or 2 oz	1 cup or 2 oz
Meat, poultry, fish, dry beans, eggs, and nuts	2 or more	1 oz or 1 to 2 Tbsp	$1\frac{1}{2}$ oz or 3 to 4 Tbsp	$1\frac{1}{2}$ oz or $\frac{1}{2}$ cup	2 oz or $\frac{1}{2}$ cup
Vegetables	3 or more	1 to 2 Tbsp	3 to 4 Tbsp	$\frac{1}{2}$ cup	$\frac{1}{2}$ cup
Fruits	2 or more	1 to 2 Tbsp or $\frac{1}{2}$ cup juice	3 to 4 Tbsp or $\frac{1}{2}$ cup juice	$\frac{1}{2}$ cup or $\frac{1}{2}$ cup juice	$\frac{1}{2}$ cup or $\frac{1}{2}$ cup juice
Bread, cereal, rice, and pasta	6 or more	$\frac{1}{2}$ slice or $\frac{1}{2}$ cup	1 slice or $\frac{1}{2}$ cup	1 slice or $\frac{3}{4}$ cup	1 slice or $\frac{3}{4}$ cup

*Use as a starting point. Increase serving size as energy yields dictate, but maintain variety in the diet by making sure all food groups are still appropriately represented.

Adapted from Food and Nutrition Services, U.S. Department of Agriculture: *Meal Plan Requirements and Offer versus Serve Manual*, FNS-265, 1990.

"age + 10g." A child eating more fiber than that might be too full to eat enough other foods providing the kcal needed for growth and development. Fiber should be added slowly, if not already in the diet, with fluids also increased. Childhood is a good time to develop the lifelong good habit of getting enough dietary fiber to prevent constipation and diseases such as colon cancer and diverticulitis (Townsend & Roth, 2000).

Adolescence

Adolescence is a period of rapid growth that causes major physiologic changes. The growth rate may be as much as 3 inches per year for girls and 4 inches for boys; nutrition plays a role in overall healthy adolescent development. Bones grow and gain density, muscle and fat tissue develop, and blood volume increases (Townsend & Roth, 2000).

Adolescents typically have enormous appetites. When good eating habits have been established during childhood and there is nutritious food available, the teenager's food habits should present no serious problem. Peer pressure is great at this time, and good eating habits may be forgotten. Many adolescents skip breakfast and/or lunch and then eat at fast-food places (Figure 16-6). Adolescents are concerned with body image and often compare their bodies to those of peers and popular media figures. They often restrict food intake, leading to inadequate nutrient intake.

Nutritional Requirements

Because of adolescents' rapid growth, kcal requirements naturally increase. Boys' kcal requirements tend to

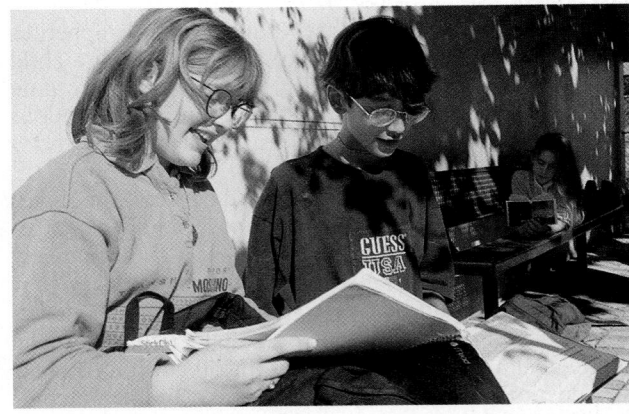

Figure 16-6 *Adolescents are vulnerable to peer pressure.*

be greater than girls', because boys are generally bigger, tend to be more physically active, and have more lean muscle mass than do girls (Townsend & Roth, 2000).

Except for vitamin D, nutrient needs increase dramatically at the onset of adolescence. Because of menstruation, girls have a greater need for iron than do boys. The RDAs for vitamin D, vitamin C, vitamin B_{12}, calcium, phosphorus, and iodine are the same for both sexes. The RDAs for the remaining nutrients are higher for boys than they are for girls (Townsend & Roth, 2000).

Young and Middle Adulthood

The period of young adulthood ranges from approximately 18 years to 40 years of age. They appear to have boundless energy for both social and professional activities, and are usually interested in exercise for its own sake, often participating in athletic events.

The middle adulthood period ranges from approximately 40 years to 65 years of age. This is a time when the physical activities of young adulthood typically begin to decrease, resulting in lowered kcal requirement for most individuals. During these years, people seldom have young children to supervise, and the strenuous physical labor of some occupations may be delegated to younger people. Middle-age people may tire more easily than they did when they were younger. They may not get as much exercise as they did in earlier years. Because appetite and food intake may not decrease, there is a common tendency toward weight gain during this period (Townsend & Roth, 2000).

Nutritional Requirements

Physical growth is usually complete by the age of 25 years. Consequently, except during pregnancy and lactation, the essential nutrients are needed only to maintain and repair body tissue and to produce energy. During these years, the nutrient requirements of healthy adults change very little.

Despite men's generally larger size, only 11 of the given RDAs are greater for men than for women. Six of the RDAs are the same for both sexes. The iron requirement for women throughout the childbearing years remains higher than that for men. Extra iron is needed to replace blood loss during menstruation and to help build both the infant's and the extra maternal blood needed during pregnancy. After menopause, this requirement for women matches that of men (Townsend & Roth, 2000).

The kcal requirement begins to diminish after the age of 25 years, as basal metabolism is reduced by approximately 2% to 3% per decade. This is a small amount each year, but, after 25 years, a person will gain weight if the total kcal value of the food eaten is not reduced accordingly. An individual's actual need, of course, will be determined primarily by activity and amount of lean muscle mass. Those who are more active will require more kcal than those with a high proportion of fat tissue.

A normal healthy adult should eat a variety of foods as shown on the food guide pyramid. This, along with following the *Dietary Guidelines for Americans*, should provide a healthy diet for the adult.

Older Adulthood

Physical changes of aging affect nutrition in several ways. The body's functions slow with age, and its ability to replace worn cells likewise diminishes. Metabolic rate slows; bones become less dense; lean muscle mass lessens; eyes do not focus on nearby objects as they once did and some grow cloudy from cataracts; poor dentition is common; the heart and kidneys become less efficient; and hearing, taste, and smell are less acute.

Digestion is affected because the secretion of hydrochloric acid and enzymes diminishes. This, in turn, decreases the intrinsic factor synthesis, which may lead to a vitamin B_{12} deficiency. The tone of the intestines is reduced, possibly resulting in constipation or, in some cases, diarrhea (Townsend & Roth, 2000).

Healthy eating habits throughout life, an exercise program suited to one's age, and enjoyable social activities can prevent or delay physical deterioration and depression during the senior years. They give purpose to the day, joy to the heart, and zest to the appetite. Nutrition and lifestyle should be carefully reviewed in any elderly client suspected of having depression.

Food–drug interactions must be monitored closely in the elderly client. Frequently, specific foods will prevent, decrease, or enhance the absorption of a particular drug.

Drug–drug interactions as well as food–drug interactions can contribute to decreased nutritional status. These interactions could affect both appetite and the absorption of nutrients from the food eaten. Careful monitoring is recommended.

Nutritional Requirements

In general, most elderly persons decrease their activity; thus their kcal needs also decrease.

The kcal requirement decreases approximately 2% to 3% per decade, because both metabolism and activity slow. If kcal intake is not reduced, weight will increase. Additional weight increases the work of the heart and puts increased stress on the skeletal system. An exercise

CLIENT TEACHING

Special Dietary Considerations for the Elderly

- Give special attention to water needs, regardless of physical activity, because the thirst mechanism is less responsive than in younger people.
- Decrease the kcal requirements in relation to activity: 10% for ages 51–75, and 20% to 25% for ages 75 and older. Bedridden and immobilized persons need a further reduction in kcal. Limit the quantities of empty-kcal foods (e.g., sugars, sweets, fats, oils, and alcohol).
- Maintain protein requirements, with 12% to 14% of kcal intake being derived from protein food (meat, eggs, poultry, milk, and cheese).
- Ensure adequate consumption of unsaturated fats, to provide a source of energy, provide the essential fatty acids, utilize the fat-soluble vitamins, and serve as a lubricating agent.
- Select carbohydrates as follows: limit concentrated sweets; use moderate amounts of simple sugars (candy, sugar, jams, jellies, preserves, and syrups); select most sources from complex carbohydrates (fruits, vegetables, cereals, and breads).
- Ensure adequate amounts of vitamin D, calcium, and phosphorus to maintain bone integrity (fortified milk is a good source).
- Consume high-fiber foods (dried fruits, whole-grain cereals, nuts, fresh fruit, and vegetables) to increase satiety and maintain intestinal motility and thereby prevent constipation.
- Maintain a safe, adequate intake of sodium, avoiding canned foods and salted or cured meats high in sodium content for those with cardiac problems and hypertension.
- Include foods from the food guide pyramid in the amounts that meet the RDAs for ages 51 and older.

plan appropriate to one's age and health can be helpful in burning excess kcal and in toning and strengthening the muscles.

Protein needs remain the same or may increase during illness. A well-balanced diet of a variety of foods should supply adequate amounts of vitamins and minerals. An increase in water and dietary fiber is often needed to maintain proper elimination.

Pregnancy and Lactation

Good nutrition during the 38 to 40 weeks of a normal pregnancy is essential for both mother and child. In addition to her normal nutritional requirements, the pregnant woman must provide nutrients and kcals for the fetus, the amniotic fluid, the placenta, and the increased blood volume and breast, uterine, and fat tissue.

The pregnant woman who follows a nutritionally adequate diet is more apt to feel better, retain her health, and bear a healthy infant than one who chooses her foods thoughtlessly (Townsend & Roth, 2000).

Studies have shown a relationship between the mother's diet and the health of the baby at birth. It is also thought that the woman who consumes a nutritious diet before pregnancy is more apt to bear a healthy infant than one who does not. Malnutrition of the mother is believed to cause growth and mental retardation in the fetus. Infants with low birth weight (less than 5.5 pounds) have a higher mortality (death) rate than those of normal birth weight.

Nutritional Requirements

Despite the saying, the pregnant woman is not "eating for two." No increase in kcal is required during the first 12 weeks of pregnancy. After that time, an extra 300 kcal/day is recommended. This increase can almost be accomplished by drinking two *extra* 8-ounce glasses of 2% milk each day, which supplies 240 kcal. Those two extra glasses of milk also supply the extra calcium, protein, and vitamin D required during pregnancy. The other nutrients that should be increased during pregnancy are folic acid and iron. Folic acid is necessary to prevent neural tube deformities in the fetus. Folic acid has been approved as a supplement for pregnant women. Good sources of folic acid are beef, legumes, wheat germ, and eggs. Good sources of iron are red meat, dried fruit, egg yolk, and whole-grain products.

To ensure that the nutritional requirements of pregnancy are met, vitamin supplements may be prescribed in addition to an iron supplement; however, it is *not* advisable for the mother to take any unprescribed nutrient supplement, as an excess of vitamins or minerals can be toxic to mother and infant. Excessive vitamin A, for example, can cause birth defects (Townsend & Roth, 2000).

The mother's kcal requirement increases during lactation. The kcal requirement depends on the amount of milk produced. Approximately 85 kcal are required to produce 100 mL ($3^1/_3$ oz) of milk. During the first 6 months, average daily milk production is 750 mL (25 oz), and for this, the mother requires approximately 640 extra kcal a day. During the second 6 months, when the baby begins to eat food in addition to breast milk, average daily milk production slows to 600 mL (20 oz), and the kcal requirement reduces to approximately 510 extra kcal a day.

NUTRITION AND HEALTH

An individual who embraces good nutrition is more likely to have good health than is someone who does not follow good nutritional practices. Of course, all situations of disease or ill health cannot be prevented by good nutrition.

The nutrients in the food we eat may be thought of as the building materials, fuel, and regulators necessary to keep the body functioning. When the body is supplied with nutrients in the proper amounts, it is most likely to function efficiently and effectively. The body is very adaptable and keeps functioning, although less effectively, even when not supplied with the proper amounts of nutrients. In this situation, however, the body is more susceptible to some diseases.

Primary Nutritional Disease

A primary nutritional disease occurs when nutrition is the cause of the disease. Usually, there is an inadequate intake of one or more nutrients. Some examples of such diseases are scurvy, from inadequate intake of vitamin C; rickets, from insufficient intake of vitamin D; and anemia, from a deficiency of iron in the diet.

Excesses of nutrients can also cause illness. These, however, occur when nutrient supplements are taken in excess, rather than from food intake. For instance, excess vitamin D may cause nausea, diarrhea, weight loss, and calcification of the renal tubules, blood vessels, and bronchi. Excess niacin may cause flushing, itching, and hypotension.

Secondary Nutritional Disease

Most nutritional diseases are secondary diseases; that is, they are a complication of another disease or condition. The original disease or condition interferes with digestion or absorption, or there is an increased need for one or more nutrients. For instance, in pregnancy, the body's need for iron increases. Not receiving the increased amount may cause anemia in the mother. In malabsorption disorders, the body is unable to absorb sufficient amounts of certain nutrients. The amount ingested may be adequate, but the body is unable to use it. Rapid excretion from the body, as in diarrhea, does not allow the nutrients to be absorbed and utilized. Uncontrolled diarrhea can lead to dehydration along with electrolyte and acid–base imbalance.

WEIGHT MANAGEMENT

Maintaining weight at a desired level can be very difficult for some people. Weight management is based on the relationship between the intake and use of kcal. When these two elements are balanced, weight is maintained at a steady level. A range of 10% over or under the desired weight is considered appropriate.

Determining Caloric Needs

The number of kcal needed to achieve or maintain a desired weight is based on two factors: basal energy needs and total energy requirements.

Basal Energy Needs

Basal energy need refers to the number of kcal required to keep an individual alive when at rest. There are two ways to determine basal energy (kcal) needs. One is based on the person's desired weight (Table 16-11), the other on the person's actual weight.
Calculation using desired weight is as follows:

Basal energy needs = desired weight × 10

Examples

Female: 5 ft 5 in tall
        5 ft = 100 lb
        5 in = 25 lb
           125 lb desired weight

TABLE 16-11	DETERMINING DESIRED WEIGHT	
BUILD	**WOMEN**	**MEN**
Medium	100 lb for 5 ft of height, plus 5 lb for each additional inch	106 lb for 5 ft of height, plus 6 lb for each additional inch
Small	Subtract 10%	Subtract 10%
Large	Add 10%	Add 10%

      125 × 10 = 1,250
      Basal energy needs = 1,250 kcal

Male: 5 ft 9 in tall
        5 ft = 106 lb
        9 in = 54 lb
           160 lb desired weight
      160 × 10 = 1,600
      Basal energy needs = 1,600 kcal

Calculation using actual weight is as follows:

Female weight in kg × 0.9 × 24 = basal kcal
Male weight in kg × 1 × 24 = basal kcal
(Weight in lb ÷ 2.2 = weight in kg)

Examples

Female weighs 130 lb

    130 ÷ 2.2 = 59.1 kg
    59.1 kg × 0.9 × 24 = 1,276.6
    Basal energy needs = 1,276.6 kcal

Male weighs 170 lb

    170 ÷ 2.2 = 77.3 kg
    77.3 kg × 1 × 24 = 1,855.2
    Basal energy needs = 1,855.2 kcal

Total Energy Requirements

People do not live their lives at rest. They are active! Kilocalories must be added to the basal metabolic requirement in order to meet the needs of activity. All activity is not equal in kcal needed, however. A person's overall activity level can be divided into sedentary (light, such as watching television), moderate (such as playing tennis), or strenuous (such as running a marathon). The following formulas can be used to determine the number of kcal to add given the activity level:

Sedentary: basal kcal × 1.3 = total kcal
Moderate: basal kcal × 1.5 = total kcal
Strenuous: basal kcal × 2.0 = total kcal

Example: The 125-lb woman in the preceding example who is planning on running a marathon would need the following:

1,250 (basal kcal) × 2 = 2,500 kcal

Factors in addition to activity that have an effect on the total kcal need are state of health and climate. A person who is ill needs more kcal to repair tissue. A cold climate requires a person to take in more kcal to provide more thermal energy to maintain body temperature.

Overweight

A person is considered to be overweight when 11% to 19% above the desired weight. **Obesity** is considered present in a person who is 20% or more above the desired weight. Overweight conditions can become serious health hazards by placing increased strain on the heart, lungs, muscles, bones, and joints. Overweight and obese people are more susceptible to diabetes and hypertension and tend to have a shorter life span.

According to the Centers for Disease Control and Prevention (1997), the Third National Health and Nutrition Examination Survey indicated that obesity is rising in the United States. Among children between the ages of 6 and 11 years, 13.7% are overweight; among adolescents ages 12 to 17, 11.5% are overweight. Among adults, 36.4% of men and 33.3% of women are overweight.

Causes

There is no single cause of obesity. Genetic, physiologic, biochemical, and psychological factors may all contribute to overweight conditions. Most often, the cause of being overweight or obese is an energy imbalance. That is, more kcal are being taken in than are being used. When this occurs, the body stores the excess kcal as adipose tissue. Hypothyroidism is a possible, but rare, cause of obesity. In this condition, basal metabolism is low, thereby reducing the number of kcal needed for energy. Unless corrected, this condition can result in excess weight (Townsend & Roth, 2000).

Treatment

Treatment for an overweight person involves two parts: revised eating habits and exercise. Revised eating habits include reducing daily kcal intake at mealtime, limiting between-meal snacks to fresh fruits or vegetables, and restricting or eliminating empty calories.

One pound of body weight equals 3,500 kcal. Therefore, to lose 1 pound per week, a person must reduce kcal intake by 500 kcal each day. Weight loss should be limited to 1 to 2 pounds per week, unless the client is under strict medical supervision. Diets should be planned according to the minimum servings of the food guide pyramid and should not be reduced to below 1,200 kcal/day in order for the dieter to receive adequate nutrients to sustain health.

Attention should also be given to food preparation. Frying adds many kcal from fat to a food item. Broiling, grilling, baking, roasting, boiling, and poaching are healthy ways to prepare foods. Vegetables should be eaten raw or steamed; the addition of butter, margarine, or sauces should be avoided. Eating habits may be adapted to decrease the amount eaten, and yet provide satisfaction: place food on a smaller plate; cut food into smaller bites; chew each bite at least 12 times; and place the fork on the plate between bites.

Exercise, particularly aerobic exercise, is an excellent adjunct to any weight-loss program. Aerobic exercise

CRITICAL THINKING

Weight Loss

What should the nurse know about nutrition in order to help an obese client lose weight?

uses energy from the body's fat reserves, as it increases the amount of oxygen the body takes in. Examples of aerobic exercise are dancing, jogging, bicycling, skiing, rowing, and power walking. Such exercise helps tone the muscles, burns kcal, increases the basal metabolism so that food is burned faster, and is fun for the participant. Any exercise program must begin slowly and increase over time so that no physical damage occurs.

Exercise alone can only rarely replace the need to be mindful of diet, however. The dieter should be made aware of the number of kcal burned by specific exercises to avoid overeating after the workout.

Underweight

Persons are considered to be underweight when their weight is 10% to 15% below the desired weight. An underweight person is more likely to have nutritional deficiencies because of the decreased intake of food. For women, this can cause complications during pregnancy. Being underweight may lower a person's resistance to infection. Being severely underweight may even cause death.

Causes

There are several possible causes of being underweight, such as an inadequate intake of food, excessive exercise, poor absorption of nutrients, or severe infection. Occasionally, hyperthyroidism may be the cause. After the adequacy of food intake and the appropriate activity level are ascertained, specific diagnostic tests must be done to determine whether poor absorption, infection, or hyperthyroidism are present.

Treatment

Dietary treatment for an inadequate intake of food is to gradually increase the amount of food eaten. Also, higher-kcal foods can be eaten. Between-meal snacks and a bedtime snack can help increase the intake of food.

If the individual is to gain 1 pound per week, 3,500 kcal in addition to the individual's basic normal weekly kcal requirement are prescribed. This means an extra 500 kcal must be taken in each day. If a weight gain of 2 pounds per week is required, an additional 7,000 kcal each week, or an additional 1,000 kcal per day, are necessary. This diet cannot be immediately accepted at full kcal value. Time will be needed to gradually increase the daily kcal value by increasing intake of foods rich in carbohydrates, some fats, and protein. Vitamins and minerals are supplied in adequate amounts. If there are deficiencies of some vitamins and minerals, supplements are prescribed (Townsend & Roth, 2000).

FOOD LABELING

In 1990, Congress passed the Nutrition, Labeling and Education Act (NLEA). This was the first legislation on labeling since the 1970s. Before this newest legislation, labeling was only required if a nutrient was added or a nutritional claim was made about the product. Now, labeling is required on virtually all retail food products, including bulk foods, fresh produce, and seafood. The nutrition information for fresh produce and seafood is to be displayed or made available at the point of purchase through counter cards, booklets, loose-leaf binders, signs, or tags.

The labels must follow the approved uniform format and use standard serving sizes and household measurements. Information on the label includes calories per serving; calories from fat; total fat, saturated fat, and cholesterol; total sodium; total carbohydrate, dietary fiber, and sugar; amount of protein; and percentages of vitamins A and C, calcium, and iron. A sample food label is shown in Figure 16-7.

Words used to describe nutrient content, such as *low*, *light*, *lean*, or *reduced*, now have specific, consistent definitions (Table 16-12).

The standardized label and word definitions make it easier for the consumer not only to know the amount of specific nutrients in a food or food product, but also to easily compare foods and food products.

TABLE 16-12 NUTRIENT CONTENT DESCRIPTORS

- **Free, without, no, zero:** The product contains only a tiny or insignificant amount of fat, cholesterol, sodium, sugar, and/or calories. For example, *fat-free* and *sugar-free* contain fewer than 0.5 g per serving. *Calorie-free* has fewer than 5 kcal per serving.
- **Low:** A food described as *low* in fat, saturated fat, cholesterol, sodium, and/or calories could be eaten fairly often without exceeding dietary guidelines. For instance, *low-fat* means no more than 3 g of fat per serving; *low-sodium* means no more than 140 mg of sodium per serving.
- **Lean:** *Lean* means that the product contains fewer than 10 g of fat, 4 g of saturated fat, and 95 mg of cholesterol per serving. *Lean* is not as lean as is *low*.
- **Extra lean:** *Extra lean* means that the product has fewer than 5 g of fat, 2 g of saturated fat, and 95 mg of cholesterol per serving. *Extra lean* is still not as lean as is *low*.
- **Reduced, less, fewer:** Means a diet product contains 25% less of a nutrient or calories. For example, hot dogs might be labeled *25% less fat than our regular hot dogs*.
- **Light/lite:** Means a diet product with $1/3$ fewer kcal or $1/2$ the fat of the original. *Light in sodium* means a product with $1/2$ the usual sodium.
- **More:** A food in which one serving has at least 10% more of the daily value of a vitamin, mineral, or fiber than usual.
- **Good source of:** One serving contains 10% to 19% of the daily value for a particular nutrient.
- **High:** One serving contains 20% or more of the daily value for a particular nutrient.

From U.S. Food & Drug Administration [FDA]. [1999]. The food label [Online]. Available: www.fda.gov/ opacom/ backgrounders/foodlabel/newlabel.html

Nutrition Facts

Serving Size 1/2 cup (114g)
Servings Per Container 4

Amount Per Serving

Calories 90	Calories from Fat 30

	% Daily Value
Total Fat 3g	5%
Saturated Fat 0g	0%
Cholesterol 0mg	0%
Sodium 300mg	13%
Total Carbohydrate 13g	4%
Dietary Fiber 3g	12%
Sugars 3g	
Protein 3g	

Vitamin A	80%	•	Vitamin C	60%
Calcium	4%	•	Iron	4%

• Percent Daily Values are based on a 2,000 calorie diet. Your daily values may be higher or lower depending on your calorie needs:

	Calories	2,000	2,500
Total Fat	Less than	65g	80g
Sat Fat	Less than	20g	25g
Cholesterol	Less than	300mg	300mg
Sodium	Less than	2,400mg	2,400mg
Total Carbohydrate		300g	375g
Fiber		25g	30g

Calories per gram:
Fat 9   •   Carbohydrate 4   •   Protein 4

Figure 16-7 *Sample Food Label*

FOOD QUALITY AND SAFETY

When planning an adequate diet, the quality and safety of the food must be considered in addition to the types of foods and serving sizes. To ensure the quality (nutrient content) and safety of food, proper storage, preparation, sanitation, and cooking are necessary; such measures will help prevent or reduce the risk of food-borne illnesses.

Quality of Food

Foods usually begin to lose nutrients when they are harvested, so they are best purchased when fresh in appearance and of bright color. Dates should be checked on all processed foods such as dairy products, lunch and other processed meats, crackers, and breads; all foods should be used before their expiration dates. All produce should be cooked until tender and thoroughly done, in the smallest amount of water possible to prevent loss of vitamins. Cooking meats via stewing increases mineral loss, so cooking methods that retain the most nutrients should be used instead; these include stir-frying, steaming, microwaving, or pressure cooking.

COMMUNITY/HOME HEALTH CARE

Resources for Meal Preparation

Ensure that the family has:

- Hot and cold running water
- A working refrigerator
- A working oven and range
- A clean, pest-free kitchen
- Fresh perishables stored in the refrigerator
- Adequate food supplies (including canned goods and staples, such as milk and bread), safely stored
- Appropriate adaptive equipment, if needed, such as low countertops that facilitate wheelchair access

Data from "Home Health Nutrition" by M. Costello, 1996, *MedSurg Nursing* 5(4), 229–238.

Safety of Food

There are three aspects to food safety: proper storage, proper sanitation, and proper cooking.

Proper Storage

Foods must be properly stored before and after purchase. Packages and jars should be tightly sealed, and cans should not leak or bulge. Any foods that look or smell unusual or show signs of mold or deterioration should be discarded. Hot foods should be kept hot—above 140°F—and cold foods should be kept below 40°F. Foods allowed to stand at temperatures between 40°F and 140°F provide an ideal breeding ground for pathogens. Leftovers must be refrigerated promptly and not allowed to cool before refrigerating.

Proper Sanitation

Proper sanitation means that all cooking utensils, pots, pans, and cutting boards, as well as the cook's hands, have been washed with soap and hot water before preparation begins. To prevent contamination of one food by another, cutting boards, utensils, and the cook's hands should be washed well with soap and hot water between preparation of different foods. A person who is ill should not prepare food. Good hand hygiene is a must before food preparation and following bathroom use.

Meat, fish, and poultry should be rinsed under cold running water and patted dry with several paper towels before preparing and cooking. A capful of chlorine bleach in a sink one-half full of water can be used to wash fruits and vegetables: leafy vegetables, cauliflower, broccoli, and other fruits and vegetables can be washed in the bleach water for a few minutes, rinsed, and then drained on paper towels.

Proper Cooking

Meats, fish, shellfish, and eggs should be cooked well done to ensure that harmful microorganisms are destroyed (Figure 16-8).

Figure 16-8 *Cook foods to a safe temperature. [From U.S. Department of Agriculture and U.S. Department of Health and Human Services, 2000. Dietary Guidelines for Americans (Home and Garden Bulletin, No. 232, 5th ed.). Washington, DC: USDA.]*

Food-Borne Illnesses

When proper storage, sanitation, or cooking are not maintained, food-borne illnesses often occur. These illnesses range in severity from fairly mild (such as staphylococcal food poisoning) to potentially fatal (such as botulism and *E. coli*). The important thing to remember is that food-borne illness is highly preventable with proper handling, preparation, and storage of food.

It is important to emphasize that nutrition involves the appropriate kinds and amounts of a variety of available foods so that a properly functioning body can digest and use the nutrients in the foods. If the foods are unsafe, they cannot adequately nourish the body.

NURSING PROCESS

Collection of subjective and objective data regarding the client's nutrition serves as the basis for determining the type of nutritional care the client requires.

Assessment

Proper assessment allows the health care team to determine the degree to which the client's nutritional needs are being met. Assessment must be performed logically and should include a nutritional history, physical examination, and the results of laboratory tests.

Age and pregnancy determine some specific items to be included in the nutritional assessment.

Nutritional assessment for an infant should include:

- Height and weight
- Sleeping habits
- Type of feeding (breast- or bottle-fed)
- If breastfeeding, the mother's nutritional status and use of alcohol, tobacco, caffeine, and drugs; infant's feeding schedule (how often fed and for how long)
- If formula feeding, type, frequency, and method of preparation and storage; feeding schedule; amount taken at each feeding
- Use of vitamin/mineral supplements
- If on solid foods, age at introduction, and any reactions or allergies
- Family attitudes about eating, food, and weight

The basic nutritional assessment for everyone over 1 year old should include:

- Nutritional status
- Height and weight
- Meal and snack pattern (food record or 24-hour recall)
- Adequacy of intake based on the food guide pyramid
- Food allergies
- Physical activity
- Cultural, ethnic, and family influences
- Use of vitamin/mineral supplements

In addition to the basic nutritional assessment, during childhood dental health should also be assessed.

In addition to the basic nutritional assessment, the following should be assessed for the adolescent client:

- Use of alcohol, tobacco, caffeine, and drugs
- Use of fad diets
- Family attitude toward thinness and the adolescent's weight

In addition to the basic nutritional assessment, the following should be assessed for the adult client:

- Use of alcohol, tobacco, caffeine, and drugs
- Use of fad diets
- Prescribed restricted diet

In addition to the basic nutritional assessment, the following should be assessed for elderly clients.

- Undesirable change in weight
- Dentition and swallowing
- Appetite
- Vision
- Hand–eye coordination
- Adequacy of daily intake of food
- Ability to self-feed
- Prescribed restricted diet
- Use of alcohol, tobacco, caffeine, and drugs

In addition to the basic nutritional assessment, the following should be assessed for the pregnant client:

- Weight and rate of weight gain
- Diet changes in response to pregnancy
- Cravings for foods or nonfoods (pica)
- Intake of supplemental vitamins/minerals
- Feeding plans (breast or formula)
- Use of alcohol, caffeine, tobacco, or drugs

Subjective Data

Subjective data can be obtained through a nutritional history by asking clients questions. Several methods can be used in collecting these subjective data: 24-hour recall, food-frequency questionnaire, food record, and diet history. Although the history data may indicate adequate nutrition, clients must be reassessed periodically to prevent nutritional problems.

24-Hour Recall The 24-hour recall requires client identification of everything consumed in the previous 24 hours. It is performed easily and quickly by asking pertinent questions; however, clients may be unable to accurately recall their intake or anything atypical in the diet. Family members can often assist with these data, if necessary.

Food-Frequency Questionnaire The food-frequency method gathers data relative to the number of times per day, week, or month that the client eats particular foods. The nurse can tailor the questions to particular nutrients, such as cholesterol and saturated fat. This method helps to validate the accuracy of the 24-hour recall and provides a more complete picture of foods consumed.

Food Record The food record provides quantitative information regarding all foods consumed, with portions weighed and measured for three consecutive days. This method requires full client or family member cooperation.

PROFESSIONAL TIP

Nutritional History

Food preferences are an expression of an individual's likes and dislikes. They may be related to the texture of food, how it is prepared, or what was served to the individual during childhood; however, preferences can also be an expression of the person's economic, ecological, ethical, or religious beliefs.

Peer pressure often dictates what teenagers eat. Stress, depression, and alcohol abuse alter the appetite. Medications can alter food absorption and excretion and affect the taste of food. Gastrointestinal disorders can cause anorexia, nausea, vomiting, diarrhea, constipation, discomfort, and pain, all of which may alter eating habits and food preferences.

TABLE 16-13	PHYSICAL INDICATORS OF NUTRITIONAL STATUS	
BODY AREA	**GOOD NUTRITION**	**INADEQUATE NUTRITION**
General	Alert, responsive, sleeps well, energetic, seldom ill	Apathetic, easily fatigued, looks tired, often ill
Weight	Appropriate for age, height, body build	Overweight, underweight
Skeleton	Good posture, no malformations	Poor posture
Skin	Good color, no rashes or swelling, smooth, moist, good turgor	Rough, dry, pale, poor turgor
Muscles	Firm, good tone	Flaccid, poor tone
Nails	Pink, firm	Pale, brittle
Eyes	Clear, bright, moist	Dull, pale, dry
Hair	Shiny, smooth	Dull, dry, brittle
Elimination	Regular, soft	Diarrhea or constipation

Diet History The diet history elicits detailed information regarding the client's nutritional status, general health pattern, socioeconomic status, and cultural factors. This method incorporates information similar to that collected by the 24-hour recall and food-frequency questionnaire. The history may require more than one interview because of the amount of data to be collected.

Objective Data

A physical examination may elicit findings that suggest nutritional imbalance. Table 16-13 lists physical indicators of nutritional status.

The measurement of a client's intake and output and daily weight are critical assessments, especially for hospitalized clients. **Anthropometric measurements** (measurement of the size, weight, and proportions of the body) are indicative of the client's calorie–energy expenditure balance, muscle mass, body fat, and protein reserves. The measurements used are body mass index (calculated using weight and height), skinfolds, and limb and girth circumferences.

Body Mass Index Body mass index (BMI) is a measurement used to determine whether a person's weight (in kilograms) is appropriate for height (in meters). It is calculated using a simple formula:

$$BMI = \frac{weight\ (kg)}{[height\ (m)]^2}$$

A BMI of 27 or greater indicates obesity. For example, a person who weighs 65 kilograms and is 1.6 meters tall would have a BMI of 65 kg/(1.6)^2, or 25.4. Go to the CDC's website for a body mass index calculator at www.cdc.gov.

Skinfold Measurement Skinfold measurement indicates the amount of body fat. The skinfold is measured by grasping the subcutaneous tissue and taking a reading using a special caliper. Measurements can be taken of the tricep, subscapular, bicep, and suprailiac skinfolds.

Other Measurements Mid–upper-arm circumference serves as an index of skeletal muscle mass and protein reserve. Abdominal-girth measurement serves as

an index as to whether the abdomen is increasing, decreasing, or remaining the same. Both of these measurements should be made repeatedly over a span of time, for best assessment.

Laboratory Tests Several laboratory tests provide information about a client's nutritional status. These include the protein indices of serum albumin, pre-albumin, and serum transferrin; hemoglobin; total lymphocyte count; blood urea nitrogen (BUN); and urine creatinine. The serum albumin blood test is used to measure prolonged protein depletion that occurs in chronic malnutrition, liver disease, and nephrosis. The pre-albumin test indicates protein depletion in acute conditions such as trauma and inflammation. Serum transferrin also measures the protein level as indicated by iron stores. Hemoglobin is a measurement of the oxygen- and iron-carrying capacity of the blood. Total lymphocyte count may reflect protein-calorie malnutrition, which inhibits lymphocyte synthesis. Blood urea nitrogen is a nitrogen balance study that indicates the degree to which protein is being depleted or replaced, and urine creatinine excretion indicates the amount of creatinine eliminated by the kidneys.

Nursing Diagnosis

Nursing diagnoses (NANDA, 2003) related specifically to nutrition include:

*Imbalanced **N**utrition: Less than Body Requirements*
*Imbalanced **N**utrition: More than Body Requirements*
*Risk for Imbalanced **N**utrition: More than Body Requirements*

PROFESSIONAL TIP

Creatinine Excretion
Record the client's height and gender on the laboratory request for a creatinine excretion test because the normal values are standardized on the basis of these variables.

Other possible nursing diagnoses related to nutritional problems include the following:

Disturbed **B**ody Image
Ineffective **B**reastfeeding
Impaired **D**entition
Deficient **K**nowledge (specify)
Impaired **O**ral Mucous Membrane
Acute **P**ain, Chronic **P**ain
Feeding **S**elf-Care Deficit
Chronic Low **S**elf-Esteem
Risk for Impaired **S**kin Integrity

Planning/Outcome Identification

A plan should be formulated by the nurse and client to achieve mutually agreed-upon goals. The plan is individualized to meet the client's specific needs. These needs may include achieving desired weight, correcting nutritional deficiencies, maintaining a special diet, preventing nutritional disorders secondary to a particular therapy, or improving nutrition to promote health and prevent disease.

Goals for clients with nutritional alterations might be as follows:

Client will maintain intake and output balance.
Client will comply with diet therapy, avoiding high-sodium foods.
Client will gain 2 pounds in 4 weeks.

Implementation

The nurse and client actually carry out the plan through specific actions. Interventions to accomplish the goals may include diet therapy, assistance with meals, weight and intake monitoring, and nutritional support.

 ### Diet Therapy

Diet therapy is the treatment of a disease or disorder with a special diet. A **dietary prescription/order** is an order written by the physician for food, including liquids. This is similar to a medication prescription written for medications a client receives. A client must not be given anything to eat or drink without an order. The dietary prescription is written for one or more of the following purposes:

• Provide the client with nutrients needed for maintenance or growth.
• Prepare a client for diagnostic tests.
• Treat the client with a disease or condition.

When the dietary prescription has been received, the dietary department must be notified so the proper food will be sent to the client.

Many times a client needs some help in understanding changes in the diet and the reasons the changes are necessary. A basic knowledge of nutrition and diet therapy contributes to the nurse's ability to competently answer the client's questions about nutrition and diet. It is important, however, for the nurse to recognize when to refer questions to the dietitian.

The dietary prescription may be for nothing by mouth, a standard diet, or a special diet.

Nothing by Mouth Nothing by mouth (nil per os, NPO) status is a type of diet modification as well as a fluid restriction. This is often prescribed before surgery and certain diagnostic procedures, to rest the GI tract, or when the client's nutritional problem has not been identified.

Standard Diets Each health care agency has standard or house diets. The standard diets include general (sometimes called regular), soft, clear liquid, full liquid, mechanical soft, and pureed.

General or Regular Diet The general or regular diet is planned according to the food guide pyramid. There are no restrictions of any kind. It is an adequate diet providing approximately 2,000 kcal a day.

Soft Diet A soft diet provides foods that are easy to chew and swallow, thus promoting mechanical digestion of foods. Foods to be avoided include nuts, seeds (tomatoes and berries with seeds), raw fruits and vegetables, fried foods, and whole grains. The food guide pyramid is the basis for this diet, although fewer kcal, usually approximately 1,800, are provided.

Clear-Liquid Diet The clear-liquid diet, also called the surgical liquid diet, is ordered as preparation for diagnostic tests or as the first meal or two after surgery. It consists mostly of water and carbohydrates, providing approximately 500 kcal/day. This is a very nutritionally inadequate diet but does relieve thirst, aids in hydration, and mildly stimulates peristalsis. Liquids included are water; clear, fat-free broth; tea; coffee; clear and strained fruit juices; jello; popsicles; and carbonated drinks such as lemon-lime soda.

Full-Liquid Diet A full-liquid diet provides approximately 800 to 1,000 kcal per day. It includes all foods that are liquid at room temperature. In addition to the liquids on a clear-liquid diet, milk; milk drinks; cream soups; strained, cooked cereals; ice cream; puddings; all fruit and vegetable juices; and custard are included.

Mechanical Soft or Edentulous Diet A mechanical soft or edentulous diet consists of food fixed especially for a person who has no teeth or has difficulty chewing. The food is either ground or chopped into very small pieces and cooked very soft, to ease the work of chewing.

Pureed Diet A pureed diet uses foods that have been blended to a smooth consistency. It is prescribed for clients who have difficulty swallowing.

Special Diets A special diet restores or maintains a client's nutritional status. These diets are variations of the general diet; however, they still must provide all the nutrients of the general diets. Special diets may provide specific amounts of nutrients or may increase or restrict certain foods. Low-residue, high-fiber, liberal bland, fat-controlled, and sodium-restricted are types of special diets.

Low-Residue Diet The low-residue diet of 5 to 10 g of fiber a day reduces the normal work of the intestines by reducing food residue. Some low-residue diets limit tough or coarse meats, milk, and milk products. The low-residue diet is prescribed to decrease GI mucosal irritation in clients with diverticulitis, ulcerative colitis, and Crohn's disease. Foods to be avoided include raw fruits (except bananas), vegetables, seeds, plant fiber, and whole grains. Dairy products are limited to two servings per day.

High-Fiber Diet A high-fiber diet contains 25 to 35 g or more of dietary fiber. A high-fiber diet is an integral part of the treatment regimen for diverticulosis because it increases the forward motion of the indigestible wastes through the colon. This diet is believed to help prevent constipation, hemorrhoids, and colon cancer, along with helping to treat diabetes mellitus and atherosclerosis.

The recommended foods for this diet include coarse and whole-grain breads and cereals, bran, all fruits, vegetables (especially raw), and legumes. This nutritionally adequate diet must be introduced gradually to prevent the formation of gas and the discomfort that accompanies it. Eight 8-oz glasses of water also must be consumed along with the increased fiber.

Liberal Bland Diet A liberal bland diet eliminates chemical and mechanical food irritants such as fried foods, alcohol, and caffeine. This diet is prescribed for clients with gastritis and ulcers because it reduces GI irritation.

Fat-Controlled Diet The fat-controlled diet reduces the total fat ingested by replacing saturated fats with monounsaturated and polyunsaturated fats and restricting cholesterol. This diet is prescribed for clients with atherosclerosis, heart disease, and obesity. Saturated-fat foods to be avoided include animal fats, gravies, sauces, chocolate, and whole-milk products.

Sodium-Restricted Diet Sodium-restricted diets tailor the level of sodium to mild (2 to 3 g); moderate (1,000 mg); strict (500 mg); or severe (250 mg). This diet is prescribed for clients with fluid volume excess, hypertension, heart failure, myocardial infarction, or renal failure.

Assistance with Meals

Assisting with meals consists of preparing the client, preparing the environment, serving the tray, and assisting with eating.

Preparing the Client Before taking a meal tray into a client's room, the nurse must ensure that the client is ready to eat: face and hands are washed, oral hygiene completed, and if necessary, the bladder emptied. The nurse should help the client into a comfortable eating position; this must be individualized to each client, as not everyone is allowed or able to sit up to eat a meal.

Preparing the Environment The nurse should make every effort to see that the physical environment is as conducive to a pleasant mealtime atmosphere as possible. This may necessitate cleaning and clearing the overbed table so the tray can be placed on it, tidying the room to remove offensive sights and smells, and brightening the room.

Serving the Tray The nurse should check that the tray contains the diet ordered, that everything on the tray is appropriate for the diet, and that nothing has spilled. For example, if a low-sodium diet tray has a salt packet, the packet should be removed. The nurse should then check the client's ID band against the name on the tray; it is very important that the correct meal is served to each client. The nurse should prepare the food by opening cartons or cutting food, if necessary.

Assisting with Eating The client who needs assistance in eating should be served last. This way, the nurse will have ample time and not have to hurry the client through the meal (Figure 16-9).

Weight and Intake Monitoring

Measuring weight daily or weekly and measuring the amount of food and fluid intake monitors therapy effectiveness.

Recording and Reporting

After the client has finished eating, the tray should be promptly removed. The amount of food eaten should be recorded, usually as the percentage of the meal eaten. When a client with diabetes does not eat all the food on the tray, both the charge nurse and the dietitian must be notified so that a supplemental feeding can be sent later. If the client is on intake and output (I & O), the amount of fluids consumed during the meal must be recorded.

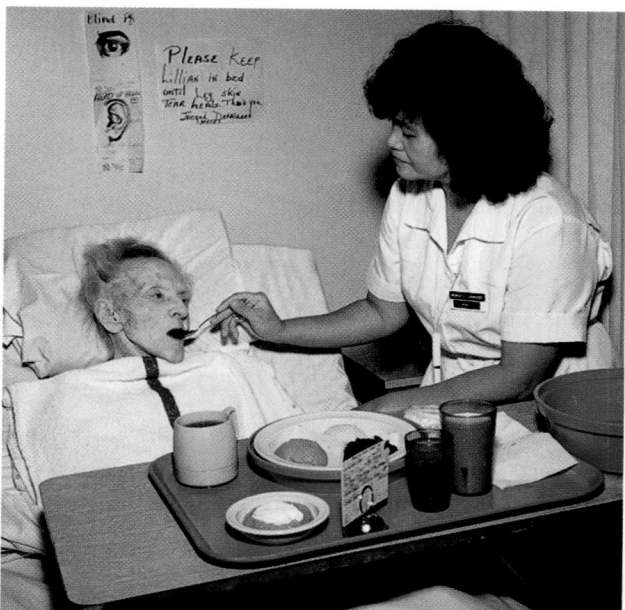

Figure 16-9 *Older adults may have health problems that affect their ability to self-feed.*

Any problems or difficulty in eating as well as likes and dislikes should be reported and documented on the client's medical record.

Nutritional Support

There are two ways nutritional support for adult clients are delivered: enteral nutrition and parenteral nutrition. **Enteral nutrition** includes both the ingestion of food orally and the delivery of nutrients through a GI tube, but is generally used to mean the latter. **Parenteral nutrition** refers to nutrients bypassing the GI system and entering the blood directly.

Enteral Nutrition When clients cannot or will not take food by mouth, but their GI tracts are working, they are given tube feedings (TF). Sometimes, this may be necessary because of unconsciousness, surgery, stroke, severe malnutrition, or extensive burns. Tube feedings maintain the structural and functional integrity of the GI tract, enhance the utilization of nutrients, and are a safe, economical way to provide nutrients.

Usually, for periods that do not exceed 6 weeks, tube feeding is administered through a nasogastric (NG) tube inserted through the nose and into the stomach or small intestine. When the tube cannot be placed in the nose or when tube feedings will be required for more than 6 weeks, an opening called an ostomy is surgically created into the esophagus (esophagostomy), the stomach (gastrostomy), or the intestine (jejunostomy) (Figure 16-10). The physician selects the route and type of feeding tube. The tubes used for these feedings are soft, flexible, and as small as they can be and still allow the feeding to pass through. Numerous commercial formulas are available, with varying types and amounts of nutrients.

There are three methods for administering tube feedings: intermittent, bolus, and continuous. Usually, tube feedings are administered by the continuous infusion

Nasogastric Route   Nasoduodenal Route

Nasojejunal Route   Esophagostomy Route

Gastrostomy Route   Jejunostomy Route

Figure 16-10 *Enteral Feeding Routes*

method, preferably with a pump. This means the feeding is continuous over a 16- to 24-hour period. Sometimes, the formula is given at half strength at a rate of 30 to 50 mL per hour. This rate may be increased by approximately 25 mL every 4 hours until tolerance has been established. As soon as the client tolerates the half-strength formula, a full-strength formula is initiated at the appropriate rate. When clients are ready to return to oral feedings, the transfer must be done gradually.

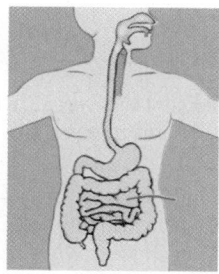 **Parenteral Nutrition** Parenteral nutrition is the infusion of a solution of nutrients directly into a vein to meet the client's daily requirements. It is used if the GI tract is not functional or if normal feeding is not adequate for the client's needs. Formerly called hyperalimentation, it is now generally referred to as total parenteral nutrition (TPN). The solution used in this intravenous infusion contains dextrose, amino acids, fats, essential fatty acids, vitamins, and minerals. Administration of TPN is generally a function of the registered nurse.

Evaluation

The effectiveness of the plan is evaluated in relation to attaining the desired goals. The nurse must assess whether the goals were met. The plan is continued or modified based on the evaluation.

SAMPLE NURSING CARE PLAN

THE CLIENT WITH ALTERED NUTRITION

Mrs. Vincent, age 58 years, is seen in the clinic for her yearly physical examination. She says, "I hardly have the energy to get up and dressed in the morning. Cleaning the house and doing the laundry make me exhausted." She does not work and is not involved in community activities. Her daily routine involves cooking for her husband, reading, and watching TV for 6 to 8 hours. She loves to bake fresh breads and pastry. She has a history of being overweight and does not exercise. She says, "I eat because I have nothing else to do." Assessment reveals: height, 5'3"; weight, 166 pounds; weight gain, 14 pounds in the past year; sedentary lifestyle; eats in response to having nothing to do.

Nursing Diagnosis   *Imbalanced Nutrition: More than Body Requirements*, related to excess intake of high-calorie foods, eating in response to boredom, and sedentary lifestyle as evidenced by height–weight relationship and weight gain

Nursing Outcomes Classification (NOC)	Nursing Interventions Classification (NIC)
Nutritional Status	*Nutrition Management*
Weight Control	*Exercise Promotion*
	Weight Reduction Assistance

PLANNING/GOALS	NURSING INTERVENTIONS	RATIONALE
Mrs. Vincent will verbalize factors contributing to excess weight.	Conduct a dietary history, using open-ended questions to assist Mrs. Vincent in exploring factors that may contribute to excess eating.	Encourages client trust and honesty.
Mrs. Vincent will lose 1 to 2 pounds each week while eating well-balanced meals.	Assess Mrs. Vincent's motivation to lose weight.	Will influence success.
	Suggest methods to adapt eating habits to decrease amount of intake (smaller servings, taking small bites and chewing each bite 12 times, placing the fork on the plate between bites, drinking water with meals, eating only at mealtime, chewing sugar-free gum when watching TV).	Helps the client eat to satisfy hunger, not boredom.
	Ask Mrs. Vincent to maintain a daily dietary intake log: time, food, and amount.	Helps the client recognize her eating patterns and note healthy and unhealthy behaviors.
	Provide and review the food guide pyramid and *Dietary Guidelines*; plan with Mrs. Vincent a diet for 1 week, taking into consideration food preferences.	Ensures that the client has information necessary to plan healthy meals within recommended guidelines.
Mrs. Vincent will engage in 20 to 30 minutes of exercise three times a week.	Review with Mrs. Vincent age-appropriate exercises; emphasize the need for walking.	Increases self-esteem, burns calories, increases energy level, and decreases boredom.
Mrs. Vincent will explore outside interests to decrease boredom and increase feelings of self-worth.	Review with Mrs. Vincent community interests outside the home, unrelated to cooking and eating.	Helps the client focus on activities not involving food, thereby decreasing boredom and increasing self-esteem.

EVALUATION   Mrs. Vincent verbalized boredom as the main reason for eating. Mrs. Vincent is drinking water with meals, chewing her food slowly, and chewing gum while watching TV. She has lost 1.5 pounds in 1 week. Mrs. Vincent now walks 30 minutes 4 days a week. Mrs. Vincent will begin volunteering 2 hours three times a week at the church's child care center.

Summary

- The LP/VN plays an important role in promoting proper nutrition.
- The six types of nutrients are water, carbohydrates, fats, protein, vitamins, and minerals.
- Water is the most vital nutrient.
- There must always be a balance between water intake and output to maintain health.
- Nutrients build, repair, and maintain body tissue; provide energy; and regulate body processes.
- The food guide pyramid identifies the five food groups for a well-balanced diet along with a range of servings to meet varying kcal needs.
- Nutritional needs vary as an individual moves through the life cycle.
- Nutrition is influenced by culture, religion, socioeconomics, fads, superstitions, age, and health.
- The kcal needs of an individual are based on basal energy needs plus activity.
- Weight management is based on the relationship between the intake and the use of kcal.
- Food safety is based on proper storage, proper sanitation, and proper cooking.
- Food-borne illnesses can be fairly mild or fatal.

Review Questions

1. The role of the LP/VN in meeting the nutritional needs of the client includes:
   a. writing the diet order.
   b. preparing food for clients.
   c. preparing a complete diet plan.
   d. answering questions about nutrition.

2. Which of the following would most likely be on a clear liquid diet?
   a. milkshake
   b. tomato soup
   c. orange juice
   d. cranberry juice

3. Which of the following is the best source of dietary fiber?
   a. popcorn
   b. chicken
   c. tomato juice
   d. macaroni and cheese

4. Cholesterol:
   a. is made in the body.
   b. has no function in the body.
   c. is not important in any disease.
   d. should not be included in the diet.

5. Why should the nurse advise a client to take an iron supplement with orange juice?
   a. to prevent heartburn
   b. to prevent constipation
   c. to improve absorption of the iron
   d. to improve digestion of the orange juice

References/Suggested Readings

Abarzanek, E., Kimm, S. Y. S., et al. (2001). Long-term safety and efficacy of a cholesterol-lowering diet in children with elevated low-density lipoprotein cholesterol: Seven-year results of the Dietary Intervention Study in Children (DISC). *Pediatrics, 107*(2), 256.

American Heart Association. (2002). *Delicious Decisions.* [Online]. Available: www.deliciousdecisions.org/

Centers for Disease Control and Prevention. (1997). Update: Prevalence of overweight among children, adolescents, and adults—United States, 1988–1994. *MMWR, 46*(9), 199.

Centers for Disease Control and Prevention (CDC). (2002). *Body Mass Index Web Calculator.* [Online]. Available: www.cdc.gov/nccdphp/dnpa/bmi/calc-bmi.htm

Cerrato, P. (1999). When food is the culprit. *RN, 62*(6), 52–56.

Cobb, M. (1997). Improving your patient's nutritional status. *Nursing97, 27*(6), 32hhr, 32hh6.

Collins, J. (2002). Helping an older patient eat well to stay well. *Nursing2002, 32*(11), 32hn6–32hn8.

Costello, M. (1996). Home health nutrition. *MedSurg Nursing, 5*(4), 229–238.

Craig, W. (1997). Phytochemicals: Guardians of our health. *Journal of the American Dietetic Association, 97*(10 Suppl. 2), S199–S204.

Dochterman, J., & Bulechek, G. (2004). *Nursing Interventions Classification (NIC)* (4th ed.). St. Louis, MO: Mosby.

Dudek, S. G. (2000). Malnutrition in hospitals: Who's assessing what patients eat? *AJN, 100*(4), 36–42.

Dudek, S. (2001). *Nutrition essentials for nursing practice* (4th ed). Philadelphia: Lippincott Williams & Wilkins.

Estes, M. E. Z. (2002). *Health assessment & physical examination* (2nd ed.). Clifton Park, NY: Thomson Delmar Learning.

Gartner, L., & Greer, F. (2003). Prevention of rickets and vitamin D deficiency: New guidelines for vitamin D intake. *Pediatrics, 111*(4 Pt 1), 908.

Goldrick, B. (2003). Foodborne diseases. *AJN, 103*(3), 105–106.

Institute of Medicine (IOM) and Food and Nutrition Board (FNB). (1997). *Dietary reference intakes for calcium, phosphorus, magnesium, vitamin D, and fluoride.* Washington, DC: National Academy Press. Also [Online]. Available: www.nap.edu/books/0309063507/html/index.html

Institute of Medicine (IOM) and Food and Nutrition Board (FNB). (2000a). *Dietary reference intakes for thiamin, riboflavin, niacin, vitamin B_6, folate, vitamin B_{12}, pantothenic acid, biotin, and choline.* Washington, DC: National Academy Press. Also [Online]. Available: www.nap.edu/books/0309065542/html/index.html

Institute of Medicine (IOM) and Food and Nutrition Board (FNB). (2000b). *Dietary reference intakes for vitamin C, vitamin E, selenium, and carotinoids.* Washington, DC: National Academy Press. Also [Online]. Available: www.nap.edu/books/0309069351/html/

Institute of Medicine (IOM) and Food and Nutrition Board (FNB). (2002). *Dietary reference intakes for vitamin A, vitamin K, arsenic, boron, chromium, copper, iodine, iron, manganese, molybdenum, nickel, silicon, vanadium, and zinc.* Washington, DC: National Academy Press. Also [Online]. Available: www.nap.edu/books/0309072694/html/

Kohn-Keeth, C. (2000). How to keep feeding tubes flowing freely. *Nursing2000, 30*(3), 58–59.

Kurtzwell, P. (1998). Staking a claim to good health [Online]. Available: www.fda.gov/fdca/features/1998/698_labl.html

Loan, T., Magnuson, B., & Williams, S. (1998). Debunking six myths about enteral feeding. *Nursing98, 28*(8), 43–48.

McConnell, E. (1998). Administering parenteral nutrition. *Nursing98, 28*(7), 18.

McConnell, E. (2001). Administering total parenteral nutrition. *Nursing2001, 31*(11), 17.

McConnell, E. (2002). Measuring fluid intake and output. *Nursing2002, 32*(7), 17.

Metheny, N., & Titler, M. (2001). Assessing placement of feeding tubes. *AJN, 101*(5), 36–45.

Moorhead, S., Johnson, M., & Maas, M. (2004). *Nursing Outcomes Classification (NOC)* (3rd ed.). St. Louis, MO: Mosby.

National Academy of Sciences. (1989). *Recommended dietary allowances: 10th edition.* Washington, DC: National Academy Press. Also [Online]. Available: http://bob.nap.edu.books/0309046335/html

North American Nursing Diagnosis Association (NANDA). (2003). *Nursing diagnoses: Definitions and classification, 2003–2004.* Philadelphia: Author.

Sheff, B. (2002). Salmonella. *Nursing2002, 32*(7), 81.

Simons, S. (1997). *Vegetables and fruits: Natural "phyters" against disease.* Texas Agriculture Extension Service.

Stanfield, P. (1997). *Nutrition and diet therapy* (3rd ed.). Boston: Jones & Bartlett.

Townsend, C., & Roth, R. (2000). *Nutrition & diet therapy.* (7th ed.). Clifton Park, NY: Thomson Delmar Learning.

USDA. (1996). *The food guide pyramid* (Home and Garden Bulletin, No. 252). Washington, DC: U.S. Department of Agriculture, Center for Nutrition Policy and Promotion. Also [Online]. Available: www.usda.gov/cnpp/pyrabklt.pdf

USDA. (2000). *Nutrition and your health: Dietary guidelines for Americans* (5th ed., Home and Garden Bulletin, No. 232). Washington, DC: U.S. Department of Agriculture and U.S. Department of Health and Human Services. Also [Online]. Available: www.health.gov/dietaryguidelines/dga2000/document/contents.htm

U.S. Food & Drug Administration (FDA). (1999). The food label. [Online]. Available: www.fda.gov/opacom/backgrounders/foolaabel/newlabel.html

Washington, H. (1998). The vitamin revolution. *Health, 12*(6), 104–110.

Wilkes, G. (2000). Nutrition: The forgotten ingredient in cancer care. *AJN, 100*(4), 46–51.

Williams, S. (2001). *Basic nutrition and diet therapy* (11th ed.). St. Louis, MO: Mosby.

Resources

American Dietetic Association, 216 West Jackson Blvd., Chicago, IL 60606-6995, 312-899-0040, 800-877-1600, www.eatright.org

Food and Nutrition Board, Institute of Medicine, 2101 Constitution Avenue, NW, Washington, DC 20418, 202-334-2169, www.iom.edu

Food and Nutrition Information Center, USDA/National Agricultural Library, 10301 Baltimore Boulevard, Room 105, Beltsville, MD 20705-2351, 301-504-5719, www.nal.usda.gov

REST AND SLEEP

LEARNING OBJECTIVES

Upon completion of this chapter, you should be able to:
- **Define key terms.**
- **Describe the phases and stages of sleep.**
- **Discuss age-related sleep variations.**
- **State the outcomes of sleep deprivation.**
- **Delineate nursing interventions that promote rest and sleep.**

KEY TERMS

biological clock ✓	REM movement disorder
bruxism	rest ✓
cataplexy	restless leg syndrome
chronobiology	sleep ✓
circadian rhythm ✓	sleep apnea
hypersomnia	sleep cycle
insomnia	sleep deprivation
narcolepsy	somnambulism
parasomnia	

INTRODUCTION

The quality of rest and sleep can have a significant impact on a person's health, including physical well-being, mental status, and coping effectiveness. This chapter discusses the importance of rest and sleep and nursing care to assist clients maintain optimal health when disturbances in rest and sleep occur.

REST AND SLEEP

Rest and sleep are basic to health well-being. In the past century, the average time asleep has been reduced by 20% (NSF, 2001e). Age, developmental level, health status, activity level, and cultural norms influence the need for rest and sleep.

Rest is a state of mental and physical relaxation and calmness. Rest can take place when lying down, reading a book, or taking a quiet walk. The nurse should try to ascertain which activities and places the client finds restful (Figure 17-1).

Sleep is a state of altered consciousness during which a person has minimal physical activity; changes in level of consciousness; and a slowing of physiologic processes. Sleep is cyclical, usually lasting for several hours. Disruptions in the usual sleep routine can be distressing to clients and often prevent further sleep. Sleep is a restorative function needed for physiologic and psychological healing. It is important that health care providers, clients, and their significant others understand the normal sleep–wake cycle and how sleep affects healing and mood.

Physiology of Sleep

Centers in the brain control the cycles of wakefulness and sleep, which are influenced by environmental factors and routines. An individual's biological clock helps determine the specific cycles of wakefulness and sleep.

Phases and Stages of Sleep

The stages of sleep are identified by electroencephalograph (EEG) patterns, eye movements, and

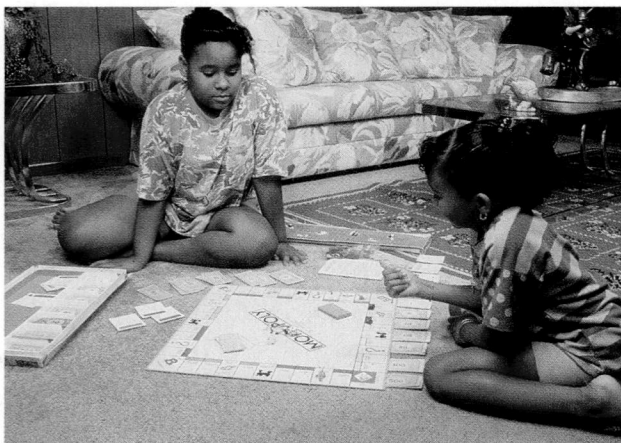

Figure 17-1 *Playing a quiet board game can be a relaxing activity for children.*

muscle activity. Sleep phases are classified as non–rapid eye movement (NREM) and rapid eye movement (REM) sleep.

NREM Sleep The first phase of sleep is called non–rapid eye movement, or NREM, sleep and consists of four stages. *Stage 1 sleep* is a light sleep, in which muscles relax and brain waves are rapid and irregular (NSF, 2001e). In adults with normal sleep patterns, stage 1 sleep usually lasts 10 minutes or so. During this stage, it is easy to awaken a sleeper.

Stage 2 sleep is still fairly light sleep. Brain waves become larger with bursts of electrical activity. Half of normal adult sleep may be spent in stage 2. After 20 minutes or so in stage 2 sleep, a deep sleep is entered.

Stage 3 and *stage 4 sleep* are usually discussed together because they are difficult to identify and separate. Stage 3 is a medium-deep sleep, and stage 4 is the deepest sleep. Each stage lasts 15 to 30 minutes. During these stages large, slow waves are seen on the EEG. Vital signs are significantly lower than when awake. It is difficult to awaken a person in this stage of sleep.

Stages 3 and 4 sleep are thought to have restorative value, needed for physical recovery. Human growth hormone is secreted mainly at night, especially during stages 3 and 4 sleep, near the beginning of a sleep period. Growth hormone is necessary for growth and also for normal tissue repair in individuals of all ages. About 75% of sleep is NREM sleep.

LIFE CYCLE CONSIDERATIONS

REM Sleep

- Rapid eye movement sleep accounts for 50% of sleep in the newborn. This percentage gradually declines to about 25% of sleep by early childhood and remains fairly constant throughout the remainder of the life span.
- An adult typically has four to six REM-sleep periods during the night.

REM Sleep After the first 60 to 90 minutes of NREM sleep in adults, the individual enters rapid eye movement, or REM, sleep. The brain waves are almost the same as when awake. This is a highly active time with rapid eye movements, heart rate, respiratory rate, and blood pressure similar to when awake; and muscles are flaccid, making the body paralyzed. This is the time when dreams occur. Dreams are ways for individuals to consolidate memories, solve problems, adapt behaviors, and clarify thoughts and emotions. About 25% of sleep is REM sleep, with REM-sleep periods becoming longer as the night goes on.

Sleep Cycle

The **sleep cycle** is the sequence of sleep beginning with the four stages of NREM sleep, a return to stage 3 and then stage 2 (the first phase), followed by the first REM sleep (Figure 17-2). The duration of a sleep cycle is usually 60 to 90 minutes, and the sleeper will generally go through four to six sleep cycles during a sleep period of 7 to 8 hours.

The length of the NREM and REM periods of sleep change as the sleep period progresses, and dreams during REM sleep may become more vivid and intense. Whenever the sleep cycle is broken, a new sleep cycle starts, beginning again at NREM sleep stage 1.

Biological Clock

The **biological clock** is an internal mechanism in a living organism capable of measuring time. It controls the daily variations in hundreds of physiologic processes, including body temperature, respiratory rate, alertness, performance, and the level of several hormones. According to Coleman (1986), the major characteristics of biological clocks are:

- They are internal physiologic systems that measure the passage of time.
- They have their own daily cycle length, which is close to, but not exactly, 24 hours.

Figure 17-2 *The Two Phases and Four Stages of the Sleep Cycle*

Biorhythms

Chronobiology is a relatively new branch of science that studies the rhythms controlled by our biological clocks, or biorhythms. The **circadian rhythms,** those that cycle on a daily basis, such as the sleep–wake cycle, are the most widely studied. Other biological rhythms include:

- *Ultradian:* those lasting much shorter than a day, such as the milliseconds it takes for a neuron to fire
- *Infradian:* those lasting a month or more, such as the monthly menstrual cycle
- *Circannual:* those requiring approximately 1 year to complete, such as seasonal affective disorder, which causes depression in susceptible people during the short days of winter

Jet Lag

When traveling by plane through several time zones, a person must allow several days for his biological clock to adjust to the new time. This is known as **jet lag.** The body wants to go to sleep in daylight and wake up during the night. Suggestions to minimize jet lag include the following:

- Get up earlier and go to bed earlier for several days before a trip eastward and later for a trip westward.
- During the flight, change your watch to the time at the destination.
- Avoid caffeine and alcohol for 4 hours before bedtime.
- Avoid strenuous exercise for 2 hours before bedtime.
- Wear earplugs and a blindfold while sleeping.
- Stay out in the sunlight as much as possible.

(NSF, 2001i)

- When exposed to normal environmental cues, such as the day–night cycle, they adapt to a 24-hour day.
- When free of environmental cues, such as the day–night cycle, the organism's internal cycle length determines its behavior.

When external time cues such as day–night, mealtimes, and sleep–wake are inconsistent, a desynchronization of the circadian biological rhythms occurs. This internal desynchronization disrupts the timing of physiologic and behavioral activity, which, in turn, causes disrupted sleep patterns, chronic fatigue, and decreased performance and coping abilities. An example of desynchronization is shift workers who try to sleep in the daytime when activities around them and their own biological clock tells them to be awake.

Factors Affecting Rest and Sleep

Several factors can influence the quality and quantity of both rest and sleep. Often, sleep problems result from a combination of many factors.

Physical Factors

Comfort is a very subjective experience. The nurse must make sure the client's physical and psychological needs are met. When basic needs are not met, the person encounters discomfort, which leads to physiologic tension and anxiety and, possibly, disturbed rest and sleep. For example, a client experiencing hunger or pain may become restless and irritable and will focus on getting these needs met instead of getting restful sleep.

Some physical problems can interfere with the ability to fall asleep or stay asleep. Conditions that cause discomfort or pain, such as arthritis, make it difficult to sleep well, as can breathing disorders such as sleep apnea and asthma. Hormonal changes that cause premenstrual syndrome (PMS) or menopause with its hot flashes can disrupt sleep. Even pregnancy, especially during the last few weeks, may make sleeping difficult.

Psychological Factors

An active mind and restless body interfere with the ability to sleep. Many individuals have intrusive thoughts or muscle tension, which interferes with rest and sleep. Anxiety related to family demands, work pressures, and other stressors does not necessarily cease when an individual tries to go to sleep, and often results in difficulty falling or staying asleep. Usually, sleep problems disappear when the stressful situation is resolved.

Environment

Temperature, lighting, ventilation, odors, and noise level can interrupt sleep when different from the person's usual sleep environment. The comfort and size of the bed, firmness of the pillow, and habits (snoring or movements) of a sleep partner may all interfere with sleep.

Sleep is especially disrupted when a person is hospitalized. Some factors associated with hospitalization that lead to sleep impairment include:

- Physical or emotional pain
- Unfamiliar surroundings
- Change in routine
- Fear of the unknown
- Timing of assessments, procedures, and treatments
- Intrusive lighting or equipment
- Noise level (especially unfamiliar noises)
- Lack of privacy

Lifestyle Stressors

A fast-paced life with many stressors may result in a person being unable to relax easily or fall asleep quickly. Relaxation precedes healthy sleep. Vigorously exercising within an hour of going to bed or performing mentally intense activities just before or after getting into bed often work against getting a good night's sleep.

A work schedule that does not fit with an individual's biological clock (e.g., working at times other than

CLIENT TEACHING

Methods to Reduce Anxiety

Teach clients the following methods to relieve anxiety:

- Progressive muscle relaxation
- Guided imagery
- Deep breathing
- Thought stopping
- Meditation
- Therapeutic massage

PROFESSIONAL TIP

Providing Environmental Comfort

A firm pillow is suggested for side-sleepers, a medium pillow for back-sleepers, and a soft pillow for stomach sleepers (*Pillow Firmness Key*, 1998).

the day shift) may interfere with sleep. Approximately 20% of employees in the United States are shift workers (NSF, 2001a). Individuals who frequently change work shifts or travel across several times zones face a real challenge in trying to stabilize their biological rhythms and rest comfortably.

Diet

Foods high in caffeine, such as coffee, colas, and chocolate, are stimulants and often delay sleep. Consuming a large, spicy, or heavy meal just before bedtime may cause indigestion, which often interferes with sleep. Going to bed when hungry can also delay sleep because the individual will be focused on food and hunger pangs instead of on sleep.

Medications and Other Substances

Many medications, both prescription and over the counter, list fatigue, restlessness, sleepiness, agitation, or insomnia as side effects. A small amount of alcohol may help some people fall asleep; however, alcohol may interrupt sleep later in the night. Nicotine, a stimulant, also delays sleep.

CRITICAL THINKING

Caffeine

Which foods and beverages have the most and least caffeine? Check out the National Sleep Foundation's (NSF) Caffeine Calculator on their website at www.sleepfoundation.org.

CULTURAL CONSIDERATIONS

Expectations Affecting Sleep

Some people perceive sleep as a luxury to be indulged in when they are not too busy with "important" activities. Others view sleep as an absolute necessity. The amount of sleep that a person considers necessary is partially determined by the attitudes of family and culture.

 Safety: Medications and Sleep

Some medications used to treat high blood pressure, asthma, or depression may cause sleeping difficulties. For instance, captopril (Capoten) and theophylline (Theomar), used to treat high blood pressure and asthma, respectively, may cause insomnia, whereas trazodone (Desyrel), an antidepressant, can either induce drowsiness or cause insomnia.

Age/Aging

Some sleep variations are based on age.

The neonate (birth–1 month) sleeps 16 to 20 hours per day in 3- to 4-hour intervals. The newborn usually sleeps very soundly and with little activity occurring during sleep ("sleeping like a baby"). There is often no difference in day and night sleep patterns.

As the infant gets older, the amount of sleep needed decreases. When infants begin to sleep through the night, they will usually have two or three naps during the day.

Toddlers typically sleep 10 to 12 hours at night with one or two daytime naps (Figure 17-3). Bedtime rituals such as a bath, brushing teeth, and reading books help establish expectations and provide nighttime security.

During preschool years, daytime napping decreases or ceases, and vivid dreams and nightmares may occur at night. These often awaken the child several times during the night.

School-age children need 10 to 12 hours of sleep daily but may resist bedtime as they struggle for inde-

Figure 17-3 *Young children require naps and rest periods throughout the day.*

CRITICAL THINKING

Age-Related Sleep Variations

What age-related sleep variations should be considered when assessing the sleep habits of neonates, infants, toddlers, school-age children, adolescents, and elders?

LIFE CYCLE CONSIDERATIONS

Sleep and Aging

- Sleep needs do not decline with age, but stay fairly constant at 7 to 9 hours per day.
- Middle-aged and elderly clients are more likely to experience sleep apnea, restless leg syndrome, and periodic limb movement disorder (NSF, 2001f).

pendence. They may develop a fear of the dark and need reassurance and a system to cope with this fear.

Adolescents need 8 to 10 hours of sleep per day. Irregular sleeping habits often become the norm as their high activity level often interferes with regular sleep patterns.

The young adult requires about 8 hours of sleep per day. Sleep may be interrupted by their young children or by work responsibilities. Lifestyle stressors cause difficulties in falling or staying asleep.

Most middle-age adults sleep 6 to 8 hours each day. Daily stressors may result in insomnia and the use of sleep-inducing medications.

Most older adults sleep less at one time than do those who are younger, although overall sleep needs remain constant at 7 to 9 hours (NSF, 2001e). They may go to sleep earlier, wake up more often, get less deep sleep, and rise earlier (NSF, 2001a). Often, a daytime nap is taken. The quality of sleep may diminish due to frequent waking and physical discomfort. The percentage of REM sleep remains fairly constant.

Sleep Pattern Alterations

Sleep disturbances are varied and are quite common. It is estimated that 30 to 40 million Americans have a serious sleep disorder (NSF, 2001e). Sleep pattern alterations are either primary sleep disorders (those where the fundamental problem is the sleep alteration) or secondary sleep disorders (those where a medical or clinical cause results in or contributes to the sleep alteration). The most common sleep alterations include insomnia, hypersomnia, narcolepsy, sleep apnea/snoring, sleep deprivation, parasomnias, restless leg syndrome, and periodic limb movement disorder.

Insomnia

Insomnia refers to difficulty falling asleep or staying asleep (AASM, 2000). According to NSF (2002) 56% of

American adults experience insomnia a few nights per week. Insomnia is not a disease, but it may be a manifestation of many illnesses. Causes may include stress, depression, medical problems, caffeine, alcohol, pain, poor sleep habits, or changes in sleep patterns related to travel or shift work. The person experiencing insomnia often gets caught up in a vicious cycle of not being able to sleep, trying harder to fall asleep, and experiencing increasing anxiety about not sleeping, which, in turn, increases the inability to fall asleep.

Symptoms of insomnia include difficulty falling asleep, waking frequently during the night, waking very early and not being able to go back to sleep, feeling unrested in the morning and/or tired during the day, and becoming anxious and restless as bedtime arrives. Many who have insomnia actually sleep significantly more than they think they do.

Often, insomnia may occur only for a night or two. If it continues or is viewed as very disturbing or disruptive by the individual, a health care provider should be consulted for relief. Treatment is best focused on modifying the factors or behaviors causing it.

Hypersomnia

Hypersomnia is characterized by excessive sleep, especially in the daytime. Persons with hypersomnia often feel they do not sleep enough at night, so they sleep late into the morning and nap several times during the day. Causes of hypersomnia can be physical (such as a disease or medication) or psychological (such as a self-imposed short sleep time); treatment must address the underlying cause.

Narcolepsy

Narcolepsy is a sudden, irresistible urge to fall asleep during the daytime. Approximately 1 in 2,000 people have narcolepsy (NSF, 2001e). These "sleep attacks" can occur during a conversation or while driving, and last from a few seconds to more than 30 minutes. The hallmark symptom of narcolepsy is **cataplexy,** a sudden loss of muscle tone without loss of consciousness, which may cause the person to fall (Stansberry, 2001).

Individuals with narcolepsy often sleep adequately at night. There is no cure, but symptoms may be controlled by taking scheduled daytime naps, waking at the same time each morning, and avoiding caffeine, food, and alcohol after 8 P.M. (Stansberry, 2001).

Sleep Apnea/Snoring

Apnea is a Greek word meaning "without breath." **Sleep apnea** is a period, during sleep, of not breathing following a period of loud snoring. People with untreated sleep apnea may stop breathing hundreds of times for up to 60 seconds or more. Sleep apnea affects 12 million people in the United States and is most common in men older than 40 (ASAA, 2002).

There are three types of apnea: obstructive, caused by relaxation of muscles in the back of the throat that block the airway; central, caused by a failure of the brain to signal the muscles to breathe; and mixed, a combination of the two (ASAA, 2002; NSF, 2001g).

PROFESSIONAL TIP

Sleep Apnea

Sleep apnea and snoring are more common in obese persons, although the obesity connection is much weaker among older people. Among middle-aged people, 4% of men and 2% of women have sleep apnea. After the age of 65, the rate increases to 28% for men and 24% for women (NSF, 2001g).

The unaware sleeper wakes up several hundred times per night for 5 to 10 seconds, takes a deep breath, rolls over, and goes back to sleep, only to start another cycle of apnea. Usually, those with sleep apnea have no idea they are not breathing or that they are continually waking up (NSF, 2001g).

Sleep apnea results in REM-sleep deprivation, manifesting as excessive daytime sleepiness. Persons with sleep apnea have a three to seven times greater risk of falling asleep while driving (NSF, 2001e). Sleep apnea can cause hypertension and an increased risk of heart attack or stroke. A nasal continuous positive airway pressure (CPAP) device, which maintains airflow with a small compressor, may give relief. Dental appliances that reposition the tongue may also help (NSF, 2001e). With some individuals, surgical intervention is required to correct the cause of the apnea.

Sleep Deprivation

Sleep deprivation is a term used to describe prolonged inadequate quality and quantity of sleep, either of the REM or the NREM type. Sleep deprivation can result from age, prolonged hospitalization, drug and substance use, illness, and frequent changes in lifestyle patterns. Sleep and dreaming have a restorative value necessary for mental and emotional recovery, and they

PROFESSIONAL TIP

Sleep Deprivation

Sleep deprivation can be deadly, and the price tag is staggering. According to the National Sleep Foundation (NSF, 2001b), the costs of drowsy drivers are estimated to be $12.5 billion per year. Drowsy drivers are blamed for 100,000 police-reported crashes and 4% of all traffic fatalities each year in the United States, and 30% to 40% of heavy truck crashes.

The person who is deprived of restful sleep is less alert, less attentive, less able to perform even simple tasks, more irritable, and has poorer concentration and judgment and mood problems that make relationships with family, friends, and coworkers difficult. No matter the cause of sleep deprivation, inadequate sleep reduces the quality of life and is harmful to health.

appear to enhance the ability to cope with emotional problems. Therefore, sleep deprivation can cause symptoms ranging from irritability, hypersensitivity, and confusion to apathy, sleepiness, and diminished reflexes. Treating or minimizing the factors that cause the sleep deprivation is the most effective intervention.

Parasomnia

Parasomnia refers to disorders that intrude on sleep in very active ways. **Somnambulism** (sleepwalking), sleeptalking, night terrors, REM movement disorder, bed wetting, and **bruxism** (teeth grinding) are the most common parasomnias; the first four are discussed in more detail following. Treatment for parasomnias varies, and the client and family should be helped to understand the disorder and its potential safety problems.

Somnambulism Sleepwalking, mostly done by children, is typically not remembered by the individual the next morning. The sleepwalker usually moves around furniture very safely. Doors and windows must be kept locked at night to protect the sleepwalker from harm. Sleepwalkers are difficult to rouse during an episode, and if awakened are often confused and without any specific recall of events that led to their behavior. Sleepwalking tends to run in families and usually stops at puberty (NSF, 2001e).

Sleeptalking Sleeptalking can occur at any age. It may be a word or two or a long speech, sometimes understandable and sometimes gibberish. The person has no memory of talking, but the sleep partner may have been awakened.

Sleep Terrors Sleep terrors are more common in children and seldom continue into adulthood. The child suddenly appears to awaken, thrashes about, sweats, and may even cry. This can last anywhere from 1 minute to approximately 15 minutes. The child remembers nothing in the morning (NSF, 2001e). Reassurance by the parents during the episode is the only treatment; the child will eventually outgrow the behavior.

REM Movement Disorder **REM movement disorder** results when the normal paralysis of REM sleep is absent or incomplete and the sleeper acts out the dream. It is most common among older men. Violent behavior and injuries may result. The person *can* remember the dream in the morning. Medication usually is effective in controlling the physical movements.

Restless Leg Syndrome

Restless leg syndrome (RLS) is the uncomfortable sensations of tingling or crawling in the muscles and twitching, burning, prickling, or deep aching in the foot, calf, or upper leg when at rest that is only relieved by walking, standing, or moving or rubbing the legs (NSF, 2001d). The sensations return in seconds or minutes. The legs frequently jump involuntarily if they are not moved. Symptoms worsen at night. If sleep does come, the leg movements awaken the person frequently.

Although the cause is unknown, some cases of RLS have been linked to iron deficiency, dialysis treatment, peripheral neuropathy, pregnancy, excessive caffeine intake, alcohol dependence, smoking, and rheumatoid arthritis (NSF, 2001d). The disorder is more common among women who have passed middle age. Avoiding or reducing smoking, caffeine, and alcohol intake may help. Symptoms may be relieved by opiates, benzodiazepines, or L-dopa.

Periodic Limb Movements in Sleep

Periodic limb movements in sleep (PLMS) is a condition of repetitive leg movements every 20 to 40 seconds throughout the night (NSF, 2001c). It is typically not uncomfortable for the affected person, but may be distressing to the sleep partner. Multiple sleep interruptions occur, leading to daytime sleepiness and nighttime insomnia.

The disorder is quite common in persons older than age 65 years. Approximately 35% of elders have at least a mild form of PLMS, which occurs only during sleep and is not as uncomfortable as RLS (NSF, 2001c).

Nocturnal Sleep-Related Eating Disorder

Nocturnal sleep-related eating disorder (NSRED) is rapid and chaotic eating when partially or fully awake with variable recall of the episode. An estimated 4 million people have this disorder, with two-thirds being women (Montgomery, Haynes, & Garner, 2002). This combination sleep and eating disorder may be misdiagnosed as anorexia, bulimia, or depression.

Clients gain weight with only moderate daytime eating, are not hungry in the morning, and are chronically tired. They typically eat food high in calories and fat at night, often foods they do not eat in the daytime. A spouse, partner, or family member may be able to shed light on the situation.

NURSING PROCESS

All standardized nursing history tools include questions related to a client's rest and sleep patterns. Care of the client who is diagnosed with a sleep disorder is collaborative, with the nurse participating in an interdisciplinary team providing treatment.

Assessment

Discussion of sleep habits is part of the regular health history. The client with a sleep disturbance should be thoroughly assessed to determine sleep routines, types of disturbance, sleep alterations, and impact of sleep problems. Usually, the client is a reliable source for this information, but a spouse or partner sharing sleeping arrangements may add valuable information to the client's report. Questions regarding the client's usual sleep patterns should focus on the following:

- Nature of sleep (restful, uninterrupted)
- Quality of sleep (feeling on waking)
- Sleep environment (description of room, temperature, noise level)
- Associated factors (bedtime routines, use of sleep medications or any other sleep inducers)
- Opinion of sleep (adequate, inadequate, problematic)

PROFESSIONAL TIP

Sleep History

To help detect a sleep disorder, ask the client:

- What time do you usually go to bed?
- How long does it take to fall asleep?
- What wakes you up in the morning?
- What time do you wake up in the morning?
- Do you take a nap during the day? When? How long?
- How much food do you eat in the evening?
- Do you drink caffeinated beverages? How much? In the evening?
- Do you drink alcohol? How much? In the evening?
- Do you take medications or herbal supplements to help you sleep?

To discover information about altered sleep patterns, ask questions about:

- Type of problem (inability to fall asleep, difficulty remaining asleep, inability to fall asleep after awakening, restless sleep, daytime sleepiness)
- Quality of the problem (number of hours of sleep versus number of hours spent trying to sleep, duration and frequency of naps, number of awakenings per sleep period)
- Environmental factors (lighting, bed, noise level, surrounding stimulation, sleep partner)
- Other factors (relation to meals eaten, activity before retiring, life stressors, work stressors, anxiety level, pain, recent illness or surgery)
- Alleviating factors (mild diet, warm drink before retiring, reading, listening to quiet music, taking a hot bath)
- Effect of problem (fatigue, irritability, confusion)

A daily journal of their sleep patterns may be helpful for clients whose sleep problems are not well defined. Other factors such as age, medical diagnosis, occupation, allergies, and psychiatric disorders must also be considered when assessing sleep problems.

Nursing Diagnosis

After information about the sleep impairment has been collected, the data must be analyzed to formulate appropriate nursing diagnoses. Alterations in sleep can manifest as verbal complaints on the part of the client, physical signs such as yawning or dark circles under the eyes, or alterations in mood, such as apathy or irritability. The primary diagnosis for individuals experiencing sleep problems is *Disturbed Sleep Pattern*. According to the North American Nursing Diagnosis Association (NANDA, 2003), *Disturbed Sleep Pattern* is defined as "time-limited disruption of sleep (natural, periodic suspension of consciousness) amount and quality."

Another diagnosis related to rest and sleep is *Sleep Deprivation* (NANDA, 2003). This diagnosis is defined as "prolonged periods of time without sleep (sustained natural, periodic suspension of relative unconsciousness)."

If the client has problems in addition to a sleep disturbance, think about the possibility that the sleep disturbance is the *cause* (not the effect) of another problem. For example, a client may be experiencing **A***ctivity Intolerance* related to lack of sleep as evidenced by verbal complaint, extreme fatigue, disorientation, confusion, and lack of energy.

Planning/Outcome Identification

Client input should be incorporated into the plan and goals. The plan of care and the goals must focus on the true cause of the alteration or sleep disturbance. For example, if the client is experiencing *Disturbed Sleep Pattern* because of bedwetting, the bedwetting should be the focus of intervention.

Many sleep disturbances require long periods of time (weeks or months as opposed to days) to correct. Sleep is by nature habitual and part of the person's lifestyle patterns. When planning care, the nurse should time procedures and treatments so they do not disturb sleep time.

Implementation

Several interventions can promote rest and sleep in clients; these are discussed following.

Trusting Nurse–Client Relationship

The client's ability to rest and sleep can be enhanced by the quality of the nurse–client relationship. Knowing that the nurse is trustworthy and genuinely cares about the client allows the client to relax and feel secure. Anxiety can be minimized by the nurse's use of therapeutic communication skills. The therapeutic use of self helps allay client anxiety.

Relaxing Environment

A place to sleep should be inviting. The immediate surroundings should be arranged to promote sleep for the sleep-impaired client. The nurse should ascertain what environment the client finds relaxing, then try to provide this environment in the inpatient setting or help the client establish this type of environment in the home setting.

Relaxation Techniques

The client's mood before sleep is very important. Believing that one can and will sleep affects both sleep quality and quantity. The calm, relaxed client is likely to fall asleep quickly and stay asleep all night. Relaxation techniques are useful sleep aids (Figure 17-4). Progressive muscle relaxation may be helpful for the person who has tense muscles. A warm bath may be relaxing.

Nutritional Considerations

Some foods enhance sleep. Tryptophan, an amino acid in milk, promotes sleep by stimulating the brain's production of serotonin. Scientific data supports the old wives' tale that drinking warm milk promotes sleep. Other ways to promote sleep are to avoid caffeine after noon, avoid

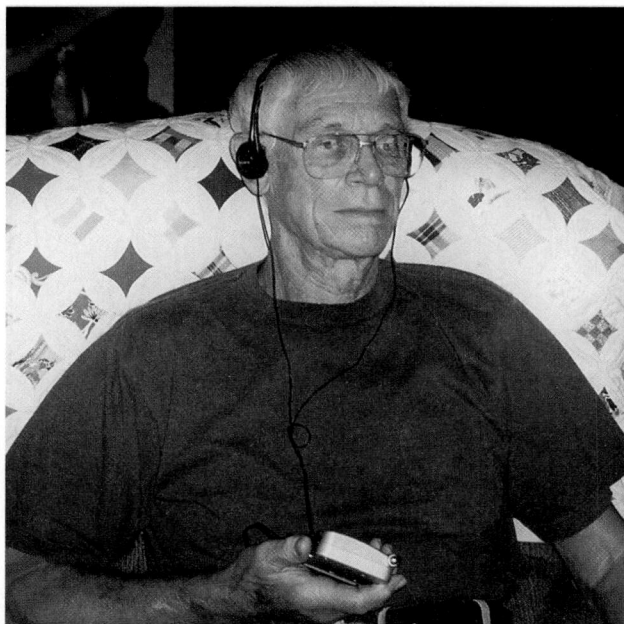

Figure 17-4 *Listening to favorite music can be very relaxing before going to bed.*

PROFESSIONAL TIP

Variables to Consider in Evaluation

When evaluating the care of the client experiencing a sleep disorder, consider the following questions:

- Were the client's basic needs met?
- Did client education include the family or significant others?
- Was an environment conducive to rest maintained?
- Were therapeutic activities balanced with the client's need for rest and sleep?
- Were the client's bedtime rituals followed as closely as possible?
- Were anxiety-reduction techniques used appropriately?

large or heavy meals close to bedtime, and refrain from eating foods that cause gastrointestinal distress.

Pharmacologic Interventions

If pain is a reason for sleep disturbance, interventions should first focus on pain management. Some nonpharmacologic relaxation and imagery interventions may be effective.

Pharmacologic agents such as tricyclic antidepressants, antihistamines, and short-acting hypnotics may be helpful for clients with sleep disturbances (McCaffery & Pasero, 1999). The tricyclic antidepressant amitriptyline (Elavil) improves the client's ability to fall asleep and stay asleep by causing sedation when given 1 to 3 hours before bedtime; doses are significantly less than those given for depression.

If given at bedtime, antihistamines such as hydroxyzine (Vistaril, Atarax) and diphenhydramine (Benadryl) have mild sedative effects that can promote sleep.

The last group are the short-acting hypnotics. These are *not* recommended for long-term or routine use, as they may cause insomnia; however, for short-term treatment they may be effective. When used, a hypnotic with a short half-life is recommended.

Client Education

Educating the client about sleep-promoting activities is a good investment of the nurse's time. By providing clients with ways of promoting good sleep habits, the nurse helps them gain a sense of control over their sleep disturbances and boosts their confidence so that they can successfully meet their sleep and rest needs.

Evaluation

The plan of care must be updated on a regular basis with additional interventions used as needed.

SAMPLE NURSING CARE PLAN

THE CLIENT WITH TROUBLE SLEEPING

Six-year-old Jacques Porcheron is brought to your clinic by his father, who states that Jacques has trouble sleeping at night. In the evenings after a dinner of hot dogs, corn or baked beans, and chocolate milk, Jacques reads some books, then watches his favorite superhero video. Afterward, he runs and plays, mimics the actions he sees in the video, and refuses to take a bath or cooperate when getting ready for bed. After being put to bed at 9 P.M., he is up several times for any number of reasons and often is not asleep until midnight. When his father wakes him at 7 A.M. for school, Jacques is disagreeable, tired, and difficult to get moving.

Nursing Diagnosis *Disturbed Sleep Pattern (less than age-normal total sleep time)* related to environmental factors (excessive stimulation) and parental lack of knowledge of sleep-promoting behaviors as evidenced by parental complaint, ineffective bedtime rituals, and insufficient hours of sleep for developmental age

continues

SAMPLE NURSING CARE PLAN

Nursing Outcomes Classification (NOC)
Rest
Sleep

Nursing Interventions Classification (NIC)
Sleep Enhancement
Energy Management

PLANNING/GOALS	NURSING INTERVENTIONS	RATIONALE
Jacques and his family will determine those sleeping behaviors they would like to achieve.	Explain that the normal sleep requirement for a child of Jacques' age is 10 to 12 hours each day.	Helps family understand Jacques' sleep requirements.
Jacques and his family will develop bedtime rituals to help Jacques wind down from the day.	Teach the family about the effect that certain foods can have on digestion and sleep habits, and identify with them those foods that are good choices for dinner.	Informs family about potential adverse effects of certain foods and allows them to plan meals more appropriately.
	Discuss those bedtime activities that can be detrimental to sleep induction.	Assists the family in modifying pre-bedtime behaviors.
	Suggest appropriate bedtime rituals such as taking a bath, brushing the teeth, reading a book, or listening to calming music.	Helps the body and mind prepare for bedtime.
Jacques and his family will identify behaviors that are helpful before bedtime.	Explain that overstimulation close to bedtime, such as watching superhero movies and engaging in rowdy play, prevents the body and mind from slowing down and preparing for sleep.	Helps the family in choosing more appropriate bedtime activities.
	Emphasize the importance of establishing a calming bedtime routine that is followed every night, especially for the school-age child.	Helps Jacques know what is expected of him by practicing appropriate bedtime routines.
	Describe an appropriate sleep environment for Jacques, such as a calm room kept at a comfortable temperature and lit only by a night light.	Such an environment promotes sleep and does not interfere with falling back asleep once awake.

EVALUATION   Jacques and his family have decided they would like Jacques to cooperate in getting ready for bed and to be asleep in 30 minutes. Together they have established a bedtime ritual that begins with playing quietly, followed by taking a warm bath, reading two books, brushing teeth, and then going to bed. The behaviors identified as helpful include no watching of stimulating videos after 7 P.M. and engaging in quiet play such as reading, arts and crafts, or writing. Some modification to Jacques' diet is planned for the next few weeks.

Summary

- Sleep has two phases: non–rapid eye movement (NREM) and rapid eye movement (REM).
- The biological clock controls the daily variations of many physiologic processes.
- Nonpharmacologic interventions should be used in promoting rest and sleep.
- The amount of sleep required differs according to developmental stage.
- Pharmacologic agents can be therapeutic for clients experiencing sleep pattern disturbances. However, the medications should not be the only interventions used.

Review Questions

1. A new sleep cycle for a client who is awakened during stage 4 NREM sleep will begin in:

   a. REM sleep.

   b. stage 1 sleep.

   c. stage 2 sleep.

   d. stage 3 sleep.

2. Individuals have several rhythms controlled by their biological clocks. The circadian rhythm cycle occurs:

   a. daily.

   b. every year.

   c. every month or so.

   d. several times a day.

3. The older adult:

   a. needs less sleep.

   b. often takes a nap.

   c. experiences less REM sleep.

   d. experiences good-quality sleep.

4. Sleep apnea occurs mostly in:

   a. adolescents.

   b. young adults.

   c. middle-age adults.

   d. elders (those over age 65).

5. REM-sleep deprivation results from:

   a. sleep apnea.

   b. somnambulism.

   c. restless leg syndrome.

   d. periodic limb movements in sleep.

References/Suggested Readings

American Academy of Sleep Medicine (AASM). (2000). *Insomnia* [Online]. Available: www.aasmnet.org

American Sleep Apnea Association (ASAA). (2002). *Information about sleep apnea.* [Online]. Available: www.sleepapnea.org/geninfo.html

Coleman, R. M. (1986). *Wide awake at 3:00 AM: By choice or by chance?* New York: Freeman.

Coren, S. (1997). *Sleep thieves: An eye-opening exploration into the science and mysteries of sleep.* New York: Free Press.

Dochterman, J., & Bulechek, G. (2004). *Nursing Interventions Classification (NIC)* (4th ed.). St. Louis, MO: Mosby.

Hogstel, M. O. (2001). *Gerontology: Nursing care of the older adult* (4th ed.). Clifton Park, NY: Thomson Delmar Learning.

McCaffery, M., & Pasero, C. (1999). *Pain: Clinical manual* (2nd ed.). St. Louis, MO: Mosby.

Merritt, S. L. (2000). Putting sleep disorders to rest. *RN, 63*(7), 26–30.

Montgomery, L., Haynes, L., & Garner, L. (2002). An unusual sleep disorder. *RN, 65*(4), 41–43.

Moorhead, S., Johnson, M., & Maas, M. (2004). *Nursing Outcomes Classification (NOC)* (3rd ed.). St. Louis, MO: Mosby.

National Sleep Foundation (NSF). (1998). *Why Target Sleep?* [Online]. Available: www.sleepfoundation.org

National Sleep Foundation (NSF). (2001). *New insomnia treatment approved.* [Online]. Available: www.sleepfoundation.org/PressArchives/sonata_pr.html

National Sleep Foundation (NSF). (2001a). *ABCs of ZZZs.* [Online]. Available: www.sleepfoundation.org/publications/ZZZs.html

National Sleep Foundation (NSF). (2001b). *Drowsy driving.* [Online]. Available: www.sleepfoundation.org/activities/daaamain.html

National Sleep Foundation (NSF). (2001c). *Facts about PLMS.* [Online]. Available: www.sleepfoundation.org/publications/fact_plms.html

National Sleep Foundation (NSF). (2001d). *Facts about restless legs.* [Online]. Available: www.sleepfoundation.org/publications/fact_rls.html

National Sleep Foundation (NSF). (2001e). *The nature of sleep.* [Online]. Available: www.sleepfoundation.org/publications/nos.html

National Sleep Foundation (NSF). (2001f). *Sleep & aging.* [Online]. Available: www.sleepfoundation.org/publications/sleepage.html

National Sleep Foundation (NSF). (2001g). *Sleep apnea.* [Online]. Available: www.sleepfoundation.org/publications/sleepap.html

National Sleep Foundation (NSF). (2001h). *Sleep strategies for shift workers.* [Online]. Available: www.sleepfoundation.org/publications/shiftworker.html

National Sleep Foundation (NSF). (2001i). *Sleep and the traveler.* [Online]. Available: www.sleepfoundation.org/publications/travel.html

North American Nursing Diagnosis Association. (2003). *Nursing diagnoses: Definitions and classification, 2003–2004.* Philadelphia: Author.

Pillow Firmness Key to Sleeping Well. (1998). [Online]. Available: www.thirdage.com Sorrell, J. (1999). Taking steps to calm restless legs syndrome. *Nursing99, 29*(9), 60–61.

Sorrell, J (1999). Taking steps to calm restless legs syndrome. *Nursing99, 29*(9), 60–61.

Stansberry, T. (2001). Narcolepsy: Unveiling a mystery. *AJN, 101*(8), 50–53.

Tate, J., & Tasota, F. (2002). More than a snore: Recognizing the danger of sleep apnea. *Nursing2002, 32*(8), 46–49.

Resources

American Sleep Apnea Association, 1424 K Street NW, Suite 802, Washington, DC 20005, 202-293-3650, www.sleepapnea.org

American Academy of Sleep Medicine, One Westbrook NW, Suite 300, Rochester, MN 55901, www.aasmnet.org

Narcolepsy Network, 10921 Reed Hartman Highway, Cincinnati, OH 45242, 513-891-3522, www.websciences.org

National Sleep Foundation, 1522 K Street, NW, Suite 510, Washington, DC 20005, 202-347-3471, www.sleep-foundation.org

Restless Leg Syndrome Foundation, Inc., 819 Second Street SW, Rochester, MN 55902-2985, www.rls.org

CHAPTER

18

SAFETY/HYGIENE

MAKING THE CONNECTION

Refer to the following chapters to increase your understanding of safety/hygiene:

Basic Nursing
- **Holistic Care**
- **Legal and Ethical Responsibilities**
- **Communication**
- **Nursing Process/Documentation**
- **Cultural Considerations**
- **Stress, Adaptation, and Anxiety**
- **Wellness Concepts**
- **Complementary/Alternative Therapies**
- **Infection Control/Asepsis**
- **Standard Precautions and Isolation**
- **Assessment**
- **Diagnostic Tests**

Adult Health Nursing
- **The Older Adult**

Basic Procedures
- **Hand Hygiene**
- **Bedmaking: Unoccupied Bed**
- **Bedmaking: Occupied Bed**
- **Bathing a Client in Bed**
- **Perineal Care**
- **Oral Care**
- **Eye Care**
- **Giving a Back Rub**
- **Shaving a Client**
- **Application of Restraints**

Intermediate Procedures
- **Assisting with Crutches, Cane, or Walker**

LEARNING OBJECTIVES

Upon completion of this chapter, you should be able to:
- Define key terms.
- Describe the kinds of accidents that can occur in health care settings.
- Describe the importance of and procedure for correctly identifying clients.
- Identify safety factors to be considered before using equipment.
- Recount safety measures related to the use of protective restraints.
- Detail safety measures related to preventing fire when oxygen is in use.
- Discuss the factors influencing a client's personal hygiene practices.
- Explain how assessment maintains a safe environment.
- Describe the modifications that can be used to resolve environmental hazards in institutional and home settings.

KEY TERMS

body image	physical restraint
chemical restraints	poison
client behavior accident	pyorrhea
dental caries	restraint
equipment accident	self-care deficit
gingivitis	sensory overload
halitosis	stomatitis
hygiene	therapeutic procedure
perineal care	accident

INTRODUCTION

Safety is basic to the care of all clients. Nurses are responsible for providing professional, quality nursing care to the client in a safe environment. This involves both safety precautions and hygiene assistance. The nurse's role in these areas is described in this chapter.

SAFETY

Safety is the number-one priority when providing client care. The first step is to raise nurses' awareness regarding risk factors because prevention is the key to safety. Nurses must be aware of those factors that have the potential to endanger a client's safety. Constant attention to these factors enables the nurse to maintain a safe environment for the client.

A safety committee is required in all health care facilities, with the purpose of maintaining an overall safe facility for clients, employees, and visitors. The committee is composed of representatives from all departments of the facility. Responsibilities range from analyzing environmental safety in the facility to researching illness rates.

Safety is associated with health promotion and illness prevention. A safe environment reduces the risk of accidents and subsequent alterations in health and lifestyle; it also helps contain the cost of health care services

(Figure 18-1). Many factors in the environment can threaten safety.

FACTORS AFFECTING SAFETY

Client safety and health are influenced by several factors including age, lifestyle/occupation, mobility, sensory and perceptual alterations, and emotional state.

Age

Injury risk varies with chronological age and developmental stage. Education about preventive measures can prevent injury among clients of various ages.

The potential for injury increases as infants mature. Most accidents occur as infants, toddlers, and preschoolers explore the environment. These can be prevented with careful adult supervision.

Figure 18-1 *Use of stair gates, life vests, seat belts, and hand rails minimizes safety risks.*

PROFESSIONAL TIP

Workplace Safety

Employee Right-to-Know Laws

Under the authority of the Occupational Safety and Health Administration (OSHA) of the Department of Labor and Industry, several states have passed employee right-to-know laws, which state that employees are legally entitled to information regarding hazardous substances or harmful agents in the workplace. Such substances include skin and eye irritants, flammables, poisons, carcinogens, pathogens, and harmful rays (radiation).

Regulations Relating to Hazardous Materials

OSHA also outlines and enforces regulations that all health care facilities must follow with regard to employees' exposure to and handling of potentially infectious materials.

Material Safety Data Sheet

As part of conforming to OSHA regulations, all facilities must have a material safety data sheet (MSDS) for each hazardous substance. The MSDS describes the substance in question, including the associated dangers. Protective equipment, safe handling techniques, and first-aid information are also given. The MSDSs for toxic materials must be kept on site for no fewer than 30 years. All employees must know how to use the MSDS.

The risk for injury increases when school-age children explore the environment outside the home. During this stage, preventive measures should focus on stranger awareness; traffic safety rules; bicycle, skating, and swimming safety; protective equipment; and avoidance of substance abuse.

While good physical health is usually enjoyed by adolescents and young adults, their lifestyle may put them at risk for injury. Because this age group spends much time away from home, educational efforts of parents, schools, and community health care providers must focus on environmental safety. High-risk factors for injury and death are automobile accidents, substance abuse, violence, unwanted pregnancies, and sexually transmitted diseases.

The injury risk for adults is usually related to lifestyle, behaviors, and work practices. Preventive measures for adults emphasize exercise, nutrition, and occupational safety. High-risk factors for this age group include anxiety, fatigue, caregiver role strain, sleep pattern disturbances, and altered health maintenance.

The older adult is prone to falls, especially in the bathroom, bedroom, and kitchen because of poor vision and mobility; loss of muscle strength and flexibility; changes in the inner ear that upset the sense of balance; effects of medications; and chronic diseases such as osteoarthritis, Parkinson's disease, and Alzheimer's disease (Walker, 1998). Preventive measures for older adults include good lighting, using hand rails, changing position slowly, skidproof mats in bathtub or shower, and removing throw rugs and loose carpets.

According to the CDC (2002b), one in three adults older than age 65 falls each year. Of those who fall, 20% to 30% have mobility and independence permanently reduced and the risk of premature death is increased.

Lifestyle/Occupation

Lifestyle practices, reflecting an individual's personal choices about activities or habits to pursue, can increase a person's risk for injury and potential for disease. For instance, individuals who operate machinery; experience excessive stress, anxiety, and fatigue; use alcohol and drugs (prescription and nonprescription); and live in high-crime neighborhoods are at increased risk for injury and alterations to health. Risk-taking behaviors, such as participating in daredevil activities, driving vehicles at high speeds, and not wearing seat belts, are factors that pose a threat to an individual's safety and well-being. Unlike other factors such as age, however, lifestyle/occupation practices are modifiable.

NIOSH (2002) reports that an average of 9,000 U.S. workers sustain disabling injuries each day, costing $145 billion each year. Compare this cost to $33 billion for AIDS and $170.7 billion for cancer.

Sensory/Perceptual Changes

Sensory functions are essential for environmental safety. Clients having visual, hearing, smell, taste, communication, or touch impairments have an increased risk for injury, because they may not be able to perceive a potential danger.

PROFESSIONAL TIP

Accidents in the Health Care Setting

In the health care setting, accidents are categorized by their causative agent: client behaviors, therapeutic procedures, or equipment:

- **Client behavior accidents** result from the client's behavior or actions. Examples include poisonings, burns, and self-inflicted cuts and bruises.

- **Therapeutic procedure accidents** result from the delivery of medical or nursing interventions. Examples include medication errors, client falls during transfers, contamination of sterile instruments or wounds, and improper performance of nursing activities.

- **Equipment accidents** result from the malfunction or improper use of medical equipment such as electrocution and fire. National and institutional policies establish safety standards with regard to equipment. For example, a facility may attempt to minimize the risk of equipment accidents by requiring the biomedical engineering department to check equipment before use.

All accidents and incident reports must be fully documented according to institutional protocol.

Mobility

A client with impaired mobility has an increased risk for injury, especially from falls. Impaired mobility may result from poor balance or coordination, muscle weakness, or paralysis. Immobility may lead to physiologic and emotional complications such as pressure ulcers and depression.

Emotional State

Emotional states such as depression and anger affect the perception of environmental hazards and the degree of risk associated with certain behaviors. These emotional states alter a person's thinking patterns and reaction time. During periods of emotional stress, usual safety precautions may be forgotten.

HYGIENE

Hygiene is the study of health and ways of preserving health. Hygiene provides comfort and relaxation, improves self-image, and promotes cleanliness and healthy skin. Client hygiene is part of client safety in that proper hygiene protects the client against disease. The body's first line of defense, the skin and mucous membranes, is kept healthy by proper hygiene. Nurses are responsible for ensuring that client hygiene needs are met. The care provided depends on the client's needs, ability, and practices.

Factors Influencing Hygiene Practices

Hygiene practices are unique to each client. Nurses provide individualized care based on needs and these practices. Hygiene practices are influenced by body image, personal preferences, social and cultural practices, knowledge, and socioeconomic status.

Body Image

Body image is the individual's perception of physical self including appearance, function, and ability. Body image is linked to the person's attitude, mood, emotions, and values. Body image directly affects the practice of personal hygiene, which may change if the client's body

---

CULTURAL CONSIDERATIONS

Hygiene

- Some cultures do not permit women to submerge their bodies in water during menstruation because of a fear that the woman may drown.
- In North America, people typically bathe daily and use deodorant products.
- In Europe, many people do not bathe daily, nor do they use deodorant products. They do not consider the smell of human perspiration offensive.

---

image is altered because of surgical procedures or illness. At these times, the nurse should assist the client to maintain the client's pre-illness level of hygiene and personal preferences.

Personal Preferences

Personal preferences include the timing of bathing, products used for bathing, and how bathing is performed. For example, some men shave before bathing, whereas others shave after bathing; some people bathe in the morning, whereas others bathe at bedtime to encourage relaxation and sleep. The client should be permitted to practice usual routines and to use preferred hygiene products unless the client's health is adversely affected. Individualized nursing care incorporates the client's personal hygiene preferences.

Social and Cultural Practices

Social and cultural practices and beliefs come from family, religious, and personal values developed during maturation. Clients learn hygiene practices in early childhood. Later, hygiene practices are influenced by socialization outside the family. For example, teenagers often follow the trends in personal hygiene accepted by their peers.

Clients from various cultural backgrounds have differing hygiene practices. A nonjudgmental attitude must be maintained when assessing or providing hygiene care to clients from different social or cultural backgrounds.

Knowledge

The client's understanding of the hygiene and health relationship is influenced by knowledge. For clients to practice basic hygiene, however, they must have more than knowledge; they must be motivated and believe that they are capable of self-care.

An illness or surgical procedure frequently results in a knowledge deficit about the correct hygiene procedure or type of hygiene that can be used. Providing the necessary education about hygiene during an illness is the nurse's responsibility. The nurse may have to perform all hygiene care for a client during an illness until the client is able to do so again.

Socioeconomic Status

A client's hygiene practices may also be influenced by socioeconomic status. Limited economic resources may affect the frequency, extent, and type of hygiene practiced. Some clients may not be able to afford soap, shampoo, toothpaste, and deodorants. The nurse can advocate for the client by contacting social services for referrals to community agencies providing assistance to needy persons.

NURSING PROCESS

The nursing process facilitates providing nursing care to clients at risk for injury or a self-care deficit.

Assessment

Assessment data are the basis for prioritizing the client's problems and the nursing diagnoses. Clients at risk for injury require frequent reassessment, so appropriate changes can be made in the plan of care and expected outcomes.

The health history and physical examination data correlated with laboratory data identify those clients at risk for problems relating to safety or hygiene. Appropriate risk appraisals may be incorporated into the nursing health history interview.

Subjective Data

The nursing health history interview provides the client's subjective account of specific health data. It is important for the nurse to gather complete, pertinent, and relevant information at this point.

Health History Key elements of relevant data regarding the client at risk for injury and infection are obtained in the health history. A health history questionnaire may be used, but depending on the client's status, the nurse may have to perform an interview to obtain these data. When the client cannot provide the subjective data, the nurse must specify, either on the questionnaire or in the nursing progress notes, who provided the information.

During the nursing health history interview, the client's general health perception and management status should be assessed to ascertain how the client manages self-care. This information will provide data regarding the client's routine self-care and health-promotion needs.

Objective Data

Objective data are gathered through the physical examination and the diagnostic and laboratory findings.

Physical Examination When assessing the client specifically for the level of risk for injury and hygiene deficits, the nurse should focus on the following areas and signs:

- Level of consciousness: The Glasgow Coma Scale (GCS) is an objective measurement tool (Neurological System chapter).

- Range of motion: Immobilization of an extremity and/or limited mobility are risk factors for developing skin breakdown, joint contractures, and muscle atrophy.
- Secretions or exudate of the skin or mucous membranes
- Condition of the skin: Skin condition provides data about a client's nutritional and hydration status, skin integrity, hygiene practices, and overall physical abilities.

Risk Appraisals Specifically developed risk assessment tools appraise the client for potential risks. The client's self-care abilities are appraised during the health history. An analysis of relevant risk factors identifies actual or possible risks. For instance, the risk of impaired skin integrity increases when a person is placed on bed rest. A skin integrity risk appraisal (Table 18-1) should be completed to assist with planning care.

Client in an Inpatient Setting Inpatient clients should be assessed for skin and fall risk factors. The client's

---

TABLE 18-1　SKIN BREAKDOWN POTENTIAL CHECKLIST

_____ (1) Fair:　Major underlying disease, controlled
_____ (2) Poor:　Uncontrolled underlying disease

Mental Status
_____ (1) Lethargic:　Listless
_____ (2) Confused:　Inappropriate communication
_____ (4) Comatose:　Unresponsive

Mobility/Activity
_____ (2) Minor Deficit:　Some limitation in movement Needs assistance w/ADLs
_____ (4) Major Deficit:　Movement requires assistance
_____ (6) Immobile:　No voluntary movement

Incontinence
_____ (1) Mild:　Stress incontinence, 1 BM/day
_____ (4) Frequent:　No bladder control, BMs > 2-4/day
_____ (6) Total:　No bladder control, frequent/continuous BM

Nutrition
_____ (2) Fair:　Intake < body requirements, eats 75% or less
_____ (3) Poor:　Eats 50% or less, started on TPN or tube feeding
_____ (4) Compromised:　No intake, dehydrated

Skin Integrity
_____ (2) Fair:　Single stage I or II
_____ (4) Poor:　More than one break in skin integrity
_____ TOTAL SCORE OF 8 OR ABOVE, ENTER SKIN INTEGRITY POTENTIAL ON
PCP PROBLEM LIST, INITIATE PREVENTATIVE ADLs

Excerpt from Patient Admission Data Base, Courtesy of CHRISTUS Spohn Health System, Corpus Christi, TX.

TABLE 18-2 SAFETY ASSESSMENT

☐ (5) Age greater than 60		**Medications**
☐ (5) History of previous falls		☐ (5) Diuretics
☐ (3) From nursing home		☐ (5) Laxatives/G.I. preps
☐ (3) Has had sitter/companion at home		☐ (3) Antihypertensives
		☐ (3) Antiseizures
Status: Mental/Physical		☐ (5) Sedative/hypnotics
☐ (5) Confused/Judgement Impaired		☐ (3) Analgesics
☐ (5) Sensory impairment		☐ (3) Antipsychotics/antidepressants
☐ (5) Combative/Aggressive		
☐ (5) "Sundowners" Syndrome		
☐ (5) Noncompliance/uncooperativeness		
☐ (5) Paralysis/amputee		☐ LEVEL 1 (0–17)
☐ (5) Weakness/debilitation		☐ LEVEL 2 (18–24)
☐ (5) Urgent/frequent elimination needs		☐ LEVEL 3 (25 or greater)
_____ TOTAL		
☐ Safety precautions implemented		☐ Patient/family instructed
☐ Restraints per protocol		☐ Color coded band on

Excerpt from Patient Admission Data Base, Courtesy of CHRISTUS Spohn Health System, Corpus Christi, TX.

risk of falling is identified after gathering specific assessment data, as shown in Table 18-2. Each of these indicators carries a specific weight to determine the client's risk. Special safety measures are implemented as required.

The client should be assessed for safety risks every shift or according to institutional policy. Nurses ensure a safe environment by leaving the bed in low position, side rails up, nurse call light and personal belongings within easy reach, and assistive devices (e.g., a walker) nearby, as shown in Figure 18-2.

Client in the Home Injuries in the home primarily result from falls, poisonings, fires, suffocation, and malfunctioning household equipment (Stanhope & Knollmueller, 2000). Home health nurses may use a safety risk appraisal to determine the client's level of safety knowledge.

The safety risk data assessed in the home direct the nurse's planning for the client's and caregiver's education. Assessment, teaching, and outcome evaluation of the safety hazards can take several home visits.

Diagnostic and Laboratory Data Appraising the client's risk for injury also involves evaluating laboratory findings related to an abnormal blood profile (e.g., anemia, infection). Malnourished clients are at risk for injury.

Nursing Diagnosis

Following data collection and analysis, the nurse formulates a nursing diagnosis. The main nursing diagnoses that relate to safety and hygiene deficits are *Risk for Injury* and the *Self-Care Deficit* diagnoses.

Risk for Injury

The primary nursing diagnosis *Risk for Injury* exists when the client is "at risk of injury as a result of environmental conditions interacting with the individual's adaptive and defensive resources" (NANDA, 2003). Although this diagnostic label has no defining charac-

Figure 18-2 *This client's safety risk has been assessed and responded to through the measures shown here.*

teristics set forth by NANDA, it is categorized as having either internal or external risk factors. An internal biochemical risk factor for a client with impaired vision would be stated as *Risk for Injury* related to the risk factor of sensory dysfunction (visual). In contrast, medications on a nightstand in a home with a toddler present should be identified by a home health nurse as creating an external chemical risk factor for the toddler; the nursing diagnosis would be stated as *Risk for Injury* related to the risk factor of medications in the environment.

Examples of the other risk nursing diagnoses that may be a risk factor for *Risk for Injury* are:

Risk for Aspiration: risk for entry of gastrointestinal secretions, oropharyngeal secretions, or solids or fluids into the tracheobronchial passages

Risk for Disuse Syndrome: at risk for deterioration of body systems as the result of prescribed or unavoidable musculoskeletal inactivity

Risk for Falls: increased susceptibility to falling that may cause physical harm

Risk for Latex Allergy Response: at risk for allergic response to natural latex rubber products

Risk for Poisoning: at accentuated risk of accidental exposure to, or ingestion of, drugs or dangerous products in doses sufficient to cause poisoning

Risk for Suffocation: accentuated risk of accidental suffocation (inadequate air available for inhalation)

Risk for Suicide: at risk for self-inflicted, life threatening injury.

Risk for Trauma: accentuated risk of accidental tissue injury (e.g., wound, burn, fracture)

These eight nursing diagnoses allow specific nursing interventions to be related to the diagnosed problem. For example, the specific nursing diagnosis for the toddler encountering medications on a nightstand in the home would be *Risk for Poisoning*, related to the risk factor of medications accessible to children. The level of risk would be higher if the medications were in open containers or if the closed containers did not have childproof caps. This diagnosis points to specific nursing interventions directed toward the need for client teaching.

Self-Care Deficits

A **self-care deficit** exists when an individual is not able to perform one or more activities of daily living (ADLs). Three self-care deficits related to hygiene practices are identified by NANDA (2003). These nursing diagnoses, definitions, defining characteristics, and related factors are presented in Table 18-3.

Other Nursing Diagnoses

The client at risk for injury or having a self-care deficit may have other associated physiologic or psychological problems. The following nursing diagnoses may also be appropriate:

Imbalanced Nutrition: less than body requirements
Imbalanced Nutrition: more than body requirements
Ineffective Protection
Impaired Tissue Integrity
Impaired Skin Integrity
Social Isolation
Risk for Loneliness
Ineffective Coping
Impaired Bed Mobility

TABLE 18-3   SELF-CARE DEFICITS RELATED TO HYGIENE PRACTICES

NURSING DIAGNOSIS AND DEFINITION	DEFINING CHARACTERISTICS	RELATED FACTORS
Bathing/Hygiene Self-Care Deficit: Impaired ability to perform or complete bathing/hygiene activities for oneself	Inability to get bath supplies, wash body or body parts, obtain or get to water source, regulate the temperature or flow of bath water, get in and out of bathroom, dry body	Decreased or lack of motivation; weakness and tiredness; severe anxiety; inability to perceive body part or spatial relationship; perceptual or cognitive impairment; pain; neuromuscular impairment; musculoskeletal impairment; environmental barriers
Dressing/Grooming Self-Care Deficit: Impaired ability to perform or complete dressing and grooming activities for oneself	Inability to choose clothing, use assistive devices, use zippers, remove clothes, put on socks, put clothing on upper body, maintain appearance at a satisfactory level, put clothing on lower body, pick up clothing; put on shoes, impaired ability to put on or take off necessary items of clothing, obtain or replace articles of clothing, fasten clothing	Decreased or lack of motivation; pain; severe anxiety; perceptual or cognitive impairment; neuromuscular impairment; musculoskeletal impairment; discomfort; environmental barriers; weakness or tiredness
Toileting Self-Care Deficit: Impaired ability to perform or complete own toileting activities	Inability to manipulate clothing, carry out proper toilet hygiene, sit on or rise from toilet or commode, get to toilet or commode, flush toilet or commode	Environmental barriers; weakness or tiredness; decreased or lack of motivation; severe anxiety; impaired mobility status; impaired transfer ability; musculoskeletal impairment; neuromuscular impairment; pain; perceptual or cognitive impairment

From *Nursing Diagnoses: Definitions and Classification 2003–2004,* by North American Nursing Diagnosis Association, 2003, Philadelphia: Author.

*Impaired Physical **M**obility*

*Impaired Wheelchair **M**obility*

***H**opelessness*

***P**owerlessness*

*Deficient **K**nowledge (specify)*

*Acute **P**ain*

***A**nxiety*

***F**ear*

Planning/Outcome Identification

The primary nursing goal is to provide safe care by identifying actual or potential risks and implementating safety measures. The nurse reviews assessment data with the client and records what the client indicates are needs for change and health teaching. These findings, when incorporated into the plan of care, reflect the individualized needs of each client. Identified outcomes provide direction for nursing care implemented to reduce the risk of injury.

Another important part of the care plan is client/caregiver education related to identifying potential risks and health-promotion practices. The nursing care plan should include educating the client about preventive actions and changes for an unsafe environment.

Implementation

Implementation involves continual assessment of client health risks and prioritization of nursing interventions aimed at risk reduction, such as:

- Promoting adequate rest and exercise
- Teaching client about health risks
- Administering prescribed medications
- Providing balanced nutritional intake

Implementation of safety measures may require an alteration in the physical environment, as identified by agency fall prevention protocol.

Identify Client

In order to provide safe care, it is essential that nurses correctly match clients with the activity, medication, diet, or treatment ordered for them. The client's well-being is placed in jeopardy by administering unordered care.

The identification (ID) band or bracelet is the primary means of correctly identifying a client. It lists the client's name, room number, bed number, hospital number, and doctor and may include other information such as age, sex, and religion.

This band is placed on the client's wrist upon admission to the hospital. Each time care is given, the band must be checked against the assignment sheet, order sheet, diet card, and medication and treatment sheet or card (Figure 18-3). The client's identity should always be further verified by one other method, such as stating the client's name, asking the client to state his name, or obtaining a positive identification from another person. None of these methods is safe when used alone, but when used with the ID band, can help the nurse verify identity.

If a client is discovered without an ID band, care should be withheld until positive identification is made.

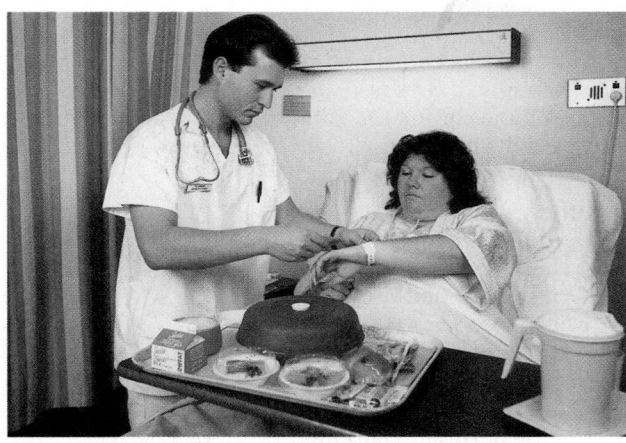

Figure 18-3 *Checking the client's ID band ensures that the correct person receives care.*

A new ID band should be placed on the client's wrist as soon as identity is verified.

Most nursing home residents also wear ID bands. Some, however, do not, and other methods of identification, such as photographs, are used. Nurses working in such long-term care facilities must learn to safely use the identification system. Whatever the system, client identification is essential before rendering any care.

Increase Safety Awareness

In all settings, nurses must show an awareness of safety hazards and teach clients accordingly. Clients must be made aware of safety precautions such as specific information about the use of heating devices, oxygen, intravenous equipment, and automatic bed controls.

A 1996 Food and Drug Administration (FDA) safety alert discussed entrapment hazards related to side rails on hospital beds. The FDA received 102 reports of head and body entrapment incidents resulting in 68 deaths, 22 injuries, and 12 entrapments without injury (FDA, 1996). These incidents occurred in private homes, hospitals, and long-term care facilities. All reported methods of entrapment are illustrated in Figure 18-4.

Figure 18-4 *Entrapment Hazards Associated with Hospital Bed Side Rails:* **A,** *Between the bars of the side rail;* **B,** *Between two side rails;* **C,** *Between the side rail and mattress;* **D,** *Between the headboard or footboard, side rail, and mattress (Source: Food and Drug Administration, Safety Alert, August 1996)*

Prevent Falls

Most falls occur when clients are weak, uncoordinated, fatigued, confused, paralyzed, or disoriented. The data obtained from the safety risk appraisal identifies those clients requiring special measures to prevent falls. The risk for falls can be reduced by:

- Properly supervising clients
- Orienting clients to the environment and the call system
- Providing ambulatory aids (e.g., a wheelchair or walker)
- Keeping personal items and call light in easy reach
- Keeping beds in lowest position and side rails up
- Using rubber mats in shower and tub
- Having adequate lighting

Specific nursing interventions aimed at preventing falls include wiping up spills; use of side rails; applying restraints; encouraging use of assistive devices for walking; using proper body mechanics; ensuring adequate lighting; and removing obstacles. These are discussed following.

Wipe Up Spills Floors must be kept clean and free of spills. Although the housekeeping department usually does the actual washing of floors, it is the nurse's responsibility to either wipe up a spill when it occurs or mark the area as a safety hazard and notify the appropriate person for immediate cleanup. Wet or sticky floors can easily cause a weak, unsteady client to slip or trip. Even those unimpaired by illness, such as visitors and hospital personnel, are at risk.

Use Side Rails Side rails have been used to prevent falls from hospital beds for more than 50 years. Since the 1970s, health care facilities have had side rails on virtually all beds and written policies for the routine use of side rails with all clients. Side rails may be full-length, half-length, or one-third-length.

Clients use side rails to help turn from side to side in bed, sit up on the edge of the bed, and as a support when standing (Figure 18-5). Some clients feel more secure in a strange bed and environment with the side rails up.

Injuries and deaths have occurred with side rail use when clients try to get out of bed by climbing over the rails or when the client becomes entrapped in the rail or between the rail, mattress, and bed frame (refer to Figure 18-4). Many cognitively impaired or older clients feel they are "in jail" or being "treated like a child" and resist the use of side rails.

The Centers for Medicare and Medicaid Services (CMS) have identified that if the client cannot easily remove or release a side rail, it is considered a restraint and must meet the requirements for restraints (discussed in next section) (CMS, 2002).

Talerico & Capezuti (2001) suggest safe alternatives to side rail use, including low-height beds, motion sensors, hip pads, floor mats alongside the bed, full-length body pillows, adequate nighttime pain control, individualized nighttime toileting rounds, bed alarms, treating depression and sleep disorders, and individualized sleep regimens. Choosing the appropriate alternative to restrictive side rails (restraint) requires a thorough client assessment. *Clients at risk for falls must always be closely monitored.*

Use Restraints **Restraints** are devices used to limit the physical activity of a client or to immobilize a client or extremity. Restraints are used to protect the client from falls, protect a body part, keep the client from interfering with therapies (e.g., pulling out tubes, disconnecting intravenous setups, or removing wound coverings), and reduce the risk of injury to self and others. Restraints should *never* be used as a substitute for close observation and supervision by nursing personnel.

Before using restraints, find the cause of the problem and then intervene appropriately. Alternatives to restraints may include assessing for pain or other discomfort, using diversional activities, reducing stimuli, coordinating care to minimize sleep interruptions, adjusting room temperature, providing extra pillows and blankets, lowering bed to lowest level, placing call bell within client's reach, having a clock with large numbers and a calendar with large print at the bedside, reintroducing yourself each time you enter the room, providing bathroom breaks every 2 hours, and keeping fluids available and within reach (unless contraindicated) (Sweeney-Calciano, Solimene, & Forrester, 2003; Napierkowski, 2002).

Restraint use is very controversial because of client injuries related to these devices. The Omnibus Budget Reconciliation Act (OBRA) of 1987 defines clients'

Figure 18-5 *The use of side rails* can *contribute to a safe and secure environment.*

PROFESSIONAL TIP

Key Elements of Restraint Documentation

- Reason for using a restraint
- Type of restraint
- Explanation given to client and family
- Date and time of and client's response to application
- Length of time restraint used
- Frequency of monitoring and client's response
- Safety (release from the restraint along with periodic, routine exercise and assessment for circulation and skin integrity)
- Assessment for continued need of restraint
- Outcome of restraint use

Figure 18-6 *Types of Restraints: **A**, Jacket or vest restraint; **B**, Belt restraint for chair; **C**, Mitten or hand restraint; **D**, Limb or extremity restraint; **E**, Elbow restraint; **F**, Mummy restraint. (Parts A and B courtesy of J. T. Posey Co., Inc.)*

rights and choices and gives the following as acceptable reasons for using physical restraints:

- Restraints are part of the medical treatment.
- All other interventions have been tried first.
- Other disciplines have been consulted for assistance with the problem.
- Supporting documentation has been provided.

The Joint Commission on Accreditation of Healthcare Organizations (JCAHO) has also updated its guidelines on physical restraints. Citing studies, JCAHO stated that the use of restraints may violate clients' rights and cause "physical and psychological harm, loss of dignity . . . and even death" (JCAHO, 2001).

Since 1999, the Centers for Medicare and Medicaid Services (CMS) have had regulations regarding the use of restraints. Physicians must do a face-to-face assessment of the client before writing a restraint order. Each order has a maximum limit of 4 hours for adults, 2 hours for children ages 9 to 17, and 1 hour for clients younger than age 9. They can be written for a shorter time frame. Nurses must continually assess, monitor, and reevaluate the client so the restraint can be removed at the earliest possible time. The physician may be telephoned for an order renewal based on the nurse's most recent assessment. The physician must perform another face-to-face assessment every 24 hours if the restraint is still used (CMS, 2002).

Once restrained, clients are rendered less able to care for their own basic needs; thus, the nurse's responsibility in meeting these needs increases. Facility policy regarding use of restraints, care of the client in restraints, and method of documentation must be followed precisely.

Restraints can be physical or chemical. **Physical restraints** reduce the client's movement through the application of a device (Figure 18-6). **Chemical restraints** are medications used to control the client's behavior. Anxiolytics and sedatives are commonly used chemical restraints.

The nursing plan of care should include safety measures to reduce the potential for injury from restraints. Additional safety measures to observe when using restraint devices are as follows:

- Restraints should never interfere with a treatment (e.g., intravenous therapy) or intensify the client's health problem.
- At least once every 2 hours, the nurse must assess the color, temperature, sensation, motion, and capillary refill in the area distal to the restraint and perform range-of-motion exercises.
- The client and significant others should be provided psychological support, as needed.

Safety: Restraints
- Placing a jacket or belt restraint too tightly on the diaphragm will inhibit lung expansion.
- To avoid accidental injury in the event that the side rail is released, the restraint strap should be secured to the bed frame, *not* to the side rail.

Use Assistive Devices for Walking Devices used to assist walking include canes, crutches, walkers, and wheelchairs.

Canes Canes are curved walking devices that provide support to the weak side of the body. Three common types of canes are the single stick, the tripod (three-footed), and the quad (four-footed). All types should have a sturdy grip and rubber tips. The tips should be checked frequently for signs of wear.

Canes should be held on the strong side of the body (Figure 18-7). The affected side and the cane should move simultaneously while the weight is supported on the strong side. The strong side is moved while the weight is supported on the cane and the weaker side.

Crutches Crutches are wooden or metal staffs used either temporarily or permanently to increase mobility. There are two types of crutches: the axillary crutch and the Lofstrand, or forearm, crutch. The axillary crutch, the type most commonly used, fits under the axilla, with the weight being placed on the handgrips. The Lofstrand crutch has a handgrip and a metal cuff that fits around the arm. This type of crutch is more convenient but not as stable as the axillary crutch.

To prevent slipping, crutches have rubber tips, which must be kept dry. The tips should also be inspected regularly. If tips become loose or worn, they must be replaced immediately. The structure of the crutch must also be inspected regularly. The person's weight will not be properly dispersed if there are cracks or bends in the crutch.

CRITICAL THINKING

Restraints

An 83-year-old widow fractured her hip when she fell in the bathtub. She had hip replacement surgery yesterday. Tonight she is very confused and is trying to dislodge the bandage and stitches. She is now being restrained for her protection. What other nursing activities could have been implemented before use of restraints? Do you think restraints will affect her mental status? If so, in what way(s)? What are some other effects she may experience as a result of being restrained?

Figure 18-7 *A nurse ensures the safety of a client using a quad cane.*

Walkers A walker is a waist-high metal tubular device with a handgrip and four legs. Some walkers have wheels on the front two legs, whereas other walkers have rubber tips on all four legs. Walkers give a sense of security and extra support, as well as independence, to clients. The client first moves the walker forward and then takes a step while balancing weight on the walker.

Wheelchairs A wheelchair is a means of ambulation for clients who are unable to support their weight while standing. The nurse should instruct the client in the safe use of a wheelchair by reminding the client to keep the wheelchair locked when not moving and to lift the footrests out of the way when getting in or out of the wheelchair. The wheelchair should be pushed slowly from behind and should be backed into doorways and into and out of elevators.

Use Proper Body Mechanics The human body is able to move in many different ways, some more efficient than others. The most effective, safest way of lifting and moving things is by using the principles of body mechanics, including center of gravity, base of support, and body alignment.

Center of Gravity The center of gravity is located in the center of the body, in the pelvic area. Body weight is approximately equal above and below this area. All movement should pivot around this central point. This keeps the weight over the base of support, making it easier to stay balanced. Keeping the back straight and bending at the knees and hips helps maintain the center of gravity in the pelvic area. If the center of gravity shifts, the body tends to fall.

Base of Support Feet are the base of support. The feet should be kept wide apart when lifting heavy items because it is easier to stay balanced with a wide base of support. Furthermore, one foot should be kept a little forward of the other to give stability from front to back. Keeping the knees slightly bent allows for quick movement and for jolts to the body to be absorbed. When turning, the feet rather than the body should be moved, in order to prevent injury to the back.

Body Alignment Proper body alignment requires that the various parts of the body be kept in proper anatomic relationship to each other.

Safety: Body Mechanics

- Stoop to lift objects from the floor: bend at the hips and the knees, keeping the back straight and base of support wide. The large muscles of the legs can then be used to straighten the body and lift the object.
- Avoid bending from the waist because doing so strains the lower back muscles.
- To prevent undue stress and strain on the back when caring for clients, adjust the height of the bed to one of comfort and ease.
- Carry objects close to the midline of the body.
- Avoid stretching to reach objects.

Ensure Adequate Lighting Adequate lighting helps people see environmental hazards. Rooms should have adequate light so the client can safely perform ADLs and health care providers can perform procedures.

Remove Obstacles Obstacles in heavily traveled areas represent a risk to the client's safety. Older adults and persons unfamiliar with the environment have the greatest risk of injury from obstacles.

Reduce Bathroom Hazards

Bathrooms pose a threat to the client because of the presence of water. Accidents common to the bathroom are falls, scalds, or burns. Accidents can be reduced by using grab bars near the tub, shower, and toilet; nonslip mats in the tub and shower; a secured bathroom rug near the tub or shower; and always check the temperature of the water before entering the tub or shower. Medications should be stored in a locked cabinet, out of reach of children and disoriented or confused adults.

Prevent Fire

Fire is a potential danger in institutional and home environments. Fire requires the interaction of three elements: sufficient *heat* to ignite the fire, combustible material *(fuel)*, and *oxygen* to support the fire.

Immobilized or incapacitated clients are at great risk during a fire. Common causes of fire are smoking in bed, discarding cigarette butts in trash cans, and faulty electrical equipment. Because smoking is a health hazard, most health care facilities are now smoke free.

COMMUNITY/HOME HEALTH CARE

Preventing Fires and Burns

- Turn handles of pots and pans toward the center of the stove to prevent children from pulling them down and burning themselves.
- Keep matches in a metal can and in a place where children cannot reach them.
- Be aware of loose, flowing clothing when cooking, especially over an open flame.
- Avoid using candles for light or heat and never leave a burning candle unattended.
- Install smoke alarms near bedrooms and check batteries twice a year.
- Do not place portable heaters near curtains, which can easily catch on fire.
- Allow only certified electricians to work on wiring in the home.
- Do not place electrical cords under carpeting.
- Do not use multiple-plug outlets.
- Do not stick anything into appliances that are plugged in (e.g., a fork in the toaster).
- Teach family members routes of escape from the house, pick a place to meet outside to verify that everyone is safe, and conduct practice fire drills.
- Teach *stop, drop, and roll* to extinguish fire on clothing.

Goals regarding fire are twofold: fire prevention and client protection during a fire. Interventions to prevent or reduce the risk of fire are:

- Make sure fire exits are clearly marked.
- Identify the locations and demonstrate the operation of fire extinguishers.
- Practice fire evacuation procedures.
- Post emergency phone numbers near all telephones.
- Keep open spaces and hallways clear of obstacles.
- Check electrical cords for exposed or damaged wires.
- Teach clients about fire hazards.

When there is a fire, follow institutional policy and procedures for fire containment and evacuation (Figure 18-8). During a fire, nursing interventions are focused on protecting the client from injury and containing the fire. When a fire occurs, nurses should ensure client safety, immediately report the exact location and type of fire, and evacuate if necessary. Nurses should know the locations and operation of fire extinguishers (Figure 18-9). The four types of fire extinguishers are water, carbon dioxide, dry chemical, and Halon. Each type of fire extinguisher is used for a specific class of fire, as outlined in Table 18-4.

Ensure Equipment Safety

Checking all equipment and supplies carefully before use and refusing to use any damaged goods or equipment can prevent many accidents. A good rule to follow is *never use any piece of equipment that is damaged in any way or not working properly.* If a wheel comes off an overbed table, do not attempt to prop the table up, but

Figure 18-8 *All personnel should be familiar with the evacuation plan and emergency exits.*

Figure 18-9 *Know the location and use of fire extinguishers.*

remove it from the room and send it to the appropriate area for repair. The same holds true for smaller supplies given to or used on clients. The safety of clients must always come first.

Glass and Plastic Glass and plastic equipment and supplies should be inspected for cracks and chips before use. The nurse should also check that there are no rough edges that may injure clients.

Disposable Sterile Supplies When using disposable sterile supplies, the nurse should first always check that the package is intact. Any break in or wetness of the wrapper renders it unsterile. Expiration dates should also be verified before use.

Electrical Equipment The hospital environment has a variety of electrical equipment such as bed controls and intravenous and patient-controlled analgesia (PCA) pumps. Each piece of electrical equipment should have a three-pronged, grounded electrical plug. A grounded plug transmits any stray electrical current from equipment to ground. To protect the client from electrical injury, the nurse should read the warning labels on all equipment, check for frayed electrical cords, use only grounded electrical equipment, avoid overloading circuits, and report any shocks received from equipment to the biomedical department (Figure 18-10).

Personal electrical appliances that the client is allowed to keep at the bedside, such as shavers, hair dryers, or curling irons, should be safety checked by the biomedical department before being used.

If a client receives an electrical shock, the electricity should be turned off before touching the client. Then, the client's pulse should be checked; if no pulse, CPR should be initiated. The nurse should assess vital signs, mental status, and skin integrity for burns on the client with a pulse. The physician should be notified of the event, and an incident report filled out.

Reduce Exposure to Radiation

Injury from radiation can occur to clients during diagnostic testing and therapeutic interventions if overex-

posure or exposure to untargeted tissues occurs. Dislodged radiation implants can result in exposure to untargeted tissues. Time, distance, and shielding are the basis of radiation exposure and protection. Protection from radiation therapy involves the following:

- Minimize the time spent in contact with the radiation source (implant or client).
- Maximize the distance from the radiation source (implant or client).
- Use appropriate radiation shields.
- Monitor radiation exposure with a film badge.
- Label all potentially radioactive material.
- Never touch dislodged implants or the body fluids of a client receiving radiation therapy.

The client's risk for injury can be reduced by following all instructions and precautions. The nurse's risk for injury can be reduced by observing all radioactive labels, wearing gloves when handling radioactive body discharges, wearing a lead apron, washing hands, disposing of radioactive substances in special containers, reducing the length of client contact, and wearing a badge that measures the amount of radiation exposure.

Prevent Poisoning

A **poison** is any substance that, when taken into the body, interferes with normal physiologic functioning. Poisons may be inhaled, injected, ingested, or absorbed into the body. Many substances can be poisonous if taken in sufficient quantity.

 Safety: Aspirin
Aspirin can be poisonous when taken in sufficient quantity.

TABLE 18-4 FIRE EXTINGUISHERS

NEW LABEL   **OLD LABEL**

 Class A: Puts out ordinary combustibles such as wood, paper, and cloth.
Ordinary Combustibles

 Class B: Used on fires of flammable liquids such as grease, gasoline, and oil.
Flammable Liquids

Class C: Suitable for electrical fires.
Electrical Equipment

NONE Class D: For flammable metals, specific for the type of metal.
Combustible Metals

Extinguishing Agents	Use
Water	Class A
Carbon Dioxide	Class B & C
Dry Chemical	Class A, B & C
Halon (leaves no residue on valuable electrical equipment)	Class C

Data from *HFD: All you ever wanted to know about fire extinguishers*, 2001, U.S. Department of Energy. [Online]. Available: www.hanford.gov/fire/safety/extingrs.htm

Figure 18-10 *Heed warning labels on electrical equipment.*

Dangerous chemicals may be found in any workplace, but some are specific to the health care industry, such as radioactive isotopes, laboratory dyes, antiseptics, irrigating solutions, disinfectants, and therapeutic drugs. The nurse must ensure that potentially dangerous materials are never left unattended in clients' rooms. Alcohol and other antiseptics or medications used for dressing changes or other procedures must be removed from the client's room after use.

Safety: Medication and Cleaning Carts

- Medication carts and cleaning and supply carts should never be left unattended.
- Confused, visually impaired, or very young clients may help themselves to something harmful or something they may use in a harmful way.
- Medication cupboards and carts must be kept locked when not in use.

On admission, clients are asked whether they have brought any medications to the facility. If so, these medications must be either removed to a safe place or sent home with the client's family. Family members sometimes bring in remedies that the client used at home. The nurse should be observant for potentially harmful substances in client rooms.

When poisoning is suspected, the poison control center should be notified. The number can generally be found on the inside cover or first few pages of the telephone book. The person reporting the poisoning should know the amount and type of poison inhaled, ingested, or injected and the client's age and symptoms. Anyone ingesting poison should be turned on the side to prevent aspiration while awaiting further treatment (Stanhope & Knollmueller, 2000).

Prevent Choking

To prevent choking on food, special techniques are used when feeding clients in at-risk categories. Nothing should ever be given by mouth to an unconscious client, because the epiglottis does not function, and choking and suffocation are likely. Likewise, to prevent aspiration of vomitus, food and drink are usually withheld before the induction of general anesthesia. After some tests, such as a bronchoscopy, food and drink are withheld until the gag reflex returns.

Prevent Suffocation

Smothering can be prevented by proper nursing observation of at-risk clients such as infants, those who are impaired with regard to ADLs, and paralyzed or unconscious clients. Such clients should be repositioned frequently and checked for a patent (open) airway. Soft pillows, mattresses, and comforters, in which they might bury their faces, should not be used. In the presence of oral secretions, the client's head should be turned to the side to prevent choking. Monitors that beep if breathing ceases should be used for at-risk clients.

Prevent Drowning

Infants, young children, and weak or confused clients are most at risk for drowning. These clients should never be left alone in the bathtub. If the nurse must leave for any reason, either the client must be removed from the tub or another member of the health care team must stay with the client until the nurse returns or the bath is completed.

Clients should be instructed in the use of call systems installed in tub and shower rooms. Clients should also be instructed to first pull the plug in the tub and then call the nurse, should they feel weak or faint.

Reduce Noise Pollution

Noise pollution, an uncomfortable noise level, often occurs in health care facilities from visitor traffic, personnel, and medical equipment. It can result in sensory overload and a disorganized environment. **Sensory overload** is an increased rate and intensity of auditory and visual stimuli. Sensory overload can alter a client's recovery by increasing or causing anxiety, paranoia, hallucinations, and depression.

Safety: Noise Pollution
- Maintain a quiet environment.
- Control traffic.
- Provide earplugs.

Provide for Client's Bathing Needs

An essential component of nursing care is bathing clients. The nurse is responsible for ensuring that the hygiene needs of the client are met whether the nurse performs the bath or delegates the activity to another health care provider. The purpose of the bath and the client's self-care abilities determine the type of bath provided. The two general types of baths are cleansing and therapeutic.

Cleansing Baths Cleansing baths are routine client care for personal hygiene. The five types of cleansing baths are shower, tub bath, self-help, bed bath, complete bed bath, and partial bath.

Shower Most ambulatory clients are capable of taking a shower. Clients with physical limitations can use a waterproof chair in the shower. The nurse may provide some assistance with the shower.

Tub Bath Some clients may prefer and enjoy a tub bath. Tub baths can also be therapeutic. Clients with physical limitations should be assisted when entering and exiting the tub.

Safety: Tub Bath
Water temperature must be checked in the bathtub before allowing the client to enter.

Self-Help Bath A self-help bed bath provides hygiene care to clients confined to bed. The nurse prepares the bath equipment and assists in washing difficult-to-reach body areas such as the back, legs, feet, and perineal area.

Complete Bed Bath A complete bed bath is provided for dependent clients who are confined to bed. The nurse washes the client's entire body.

PROFESSIONAL TIP

Bathing
- Baths are an excellent time to assess the skin.
- Bathing provides time to meet the client's psychosocial needs through assessment and counseling and to educate the client on basic and special hygiene needs.

Partial Bath In a partial bath, only those body areas that would cause discomfort or odor are cleansed. These areas are the face, hands, axillae, and perineal area. The client or nurse may perform a partial bath, depending on the client's self-care abilities. Partial baths may be performed with the client in bed or standing at the sink.

Therapeutic Baths A physician's order is required for therapeutic baths, stating the type of bath, body surface to be treated, temperature of the water, and type of medicated solutions to be used. A therapeutic bath is usually taken in a tub and lasts approximately 20 to 30 minutes. They are classified as hot, warm, tepid, or cool; soak or sitz; and oatmeal (Aveeno), cornstarch, or sodium bicarbonate.

Hot- or warm-water tub baths reduce muscle spasms, soreness, and tension, but can cause skin burns. Cool or tepid baths relieve tension and lower body temperature. To prevent chilling and rapid temperature fluctuations during a tepid or cool bath, the nurse must not leave the client in the tub too long.

A soak is usually limited to a body part but can involve the entire body. Water, with or without a medicated solution, is applied to reduce irritation, pain, or swelling, or to soften or remove dead tissue.

Sitz baths reduce inflammation and cleanse the perineal and anal areas. Sitz baths are usually used for hemorrhoids or anal fissures and after perineal or rectal surgery.

Skin irritations can be soothed with oatmeal (Aveeno), cornstarch, or sodium bicarbonate baths.

Provide Clean Bed Linens

Clean linens are placed on the bed to promote comfort after a bath. Clients able to be out of bed can sit in a chair while the nurse makes the bed.

If the client cannot be out of bed, the nurse will make an occupied bed. If the client cannot be turned or is in traction, assistance will be needed. Care must be taken to avoid disturbing any traction weights.

Provide Perineal Care

Perineal care is the cleansing of the external genitalia, the perineum, and surrounding area. Perineal care may be called *peri-care*. Perineal care prevents or eliminates infection and odor, promotes healing, removes secretions, and provides comfort. Perineal care can be provided as part of the bath or separately.

PROFESSIONAL TIP

Perineal Care
Perineal care may be embarrassing for both the client and the nurse, especially if the client is of the opposite sex. In this situation, the nurse may provide the client with warm water, a moistened washcloth, soap, a dry towel, and privacy. The nurse is responsible for providing perineal care in a professional and private manner if the client is unable to do so.

Offer Back Rubs

Back rubs and massages stimulate the client's circulation, relieve muscle tension, and relax muscles, and give the nurse an opportunity to assess the skin. Cream and lotion facilitate the rubbing and skin lubrication during a back rub or massage.

The client lies either on the side or prone. The nurse uses friction and pressure when rubbing the hands on the client's skin. Friction creates heat, which dilates the peripheral blood vessels and increases the blood supply to the skin. Pressure stimulates the muscle fibers, which relaxes the muscles. The nurse must check for contraindications before giving a back rub or massage. Be cautious when massaging limbs, especially the lower limbs. A thrombus (blood clot) might be dislodged, resulting in an embolus (circulating blood clot). Bony prominences should be massaged lightly to prevent damage to underlying tissue.

Provide Foot and Toenail Care

Proper foot and toenail care are necessary for standing and ambulation. Often, foot and toenail care are ignored until problems arise. Foot and toenail problems may result from poorly fitted shoes, inadequate foot and toenail hygiene, incorrect nail trimming, and exposure to harsh chemicals. These problems may cause a loss of skin integrity and potential for infection.

Pain or tenderness is usually the first sign of foot and toenail problems. These symptoms may result in limping, causing strain to certain muscle groups. Clients with diabetes mellitus have changes in circulation predisposing them to foot problems requiring special foot and toenail care.

Foot and toenail care prevents infection and soft tissue trauma from ingrown or jagged nails and eliminates odor. Hygiene care of feet and toenails includes regular cleansing, rinsing, and drying the feet and toenails; trimming the toenails; cleaning under the toenails; and wearing properly fitted shoes.

Soaking facilitates cleansing dirty or thickened toenails. Use an orangewood stick to clean under the toenails, because a metal instrument roughens the nail and causes harboring of dirt. The nail clipper is the safest instrument to trim the toenails; however, some people think that cutting the nails makes them brittle. The client who chooses not to cut the nails should file them straight across with an emery board. The areas between the toes should be carefully dried. An emollient, such as cold cream, helps keep toenails and cuticles soft.

Callused areas should never be cut. Lotion applied to the feet maintains moisture and softens callused areas. Soaking also facilitates callus removal. If the client's feet

are excessively moist (sweat), water-absorbent powder can be applied between the toes.

Everyone should wear clean, properly fitted shoes. Shoes should not be too tight but should be snug enough to provide support to the feet and have arch supports. Shoes should be $1/2$ inch longer than the longest toe.

Provide Oral Care

The oral cavity takes in food, chews it, secretes mucus to moisten and lubricate the food, and secretes a digestive enzyme. Common problems occurring in the oral cavity include:

- Bad breath **(halitosis)**
- Cavities **(dental caries)**
- Inflammation of the gums **(gingivitis)**
- Inflammation of the oral mucosa **(stomatitis)**
- Periodontal disease **(pyorrhea)**
- Plaque

Poor oral hygiene and loss of teeth affects a person's social interaction, body image, and nutritional intake. Daily oral care is vital to maintain the integrity of the mucous membranes, gums, teeth, and lips. Preventive measures can preserve the oral cavity and teeth. Preventive oral care consists of flossing, brushing, and rinsing with fluoride.

Fluoride Research has determined that fluoride can prevent dental caries so communities add fluoride to their water supplies. Fluoride is common in toothpastes and mouthwashes, but persons with very dry or irritated mucous membranes should not use commercial mouthwashes because the alcohol content further dries the mucous membranes.

Infants can be given fluoride drops as early as 2 weeks of age to prevent dental caries. Nurses should inform

PROFESSIONAL TIP

Oral Care for the Unconscious Client

Special care should be taken when doing oral care for the unconscious client to prevent both client aspiration and injury to the nurse (from the client biting because of the gag reflex).

- Never use your fingers to hold a client's mouth open; use a bite block or padded tongue blade.
- Assess for gag reflex.
- Turn the client's head to one side with a basin under the mouth.
- Use only a small amount of liquid and oral suctioning to facilitate removal of secretions.
- Brush the teeth and tongue in the usual manner. Exercise caution to prevent aspiration.

clients that excessive fluoride can darken the color of tooth enamel. Fluoride should be administered with a dropper directed toward the back of the throat to prevent discoloration of the tooth enamel.

Flossing Flossing should be done daily before brushing the teeth. Flossing prevents the formation of plaque and removes plaque and food debris between the teeth. Regular flossing can prevent dental caries and periodontal disease.

Brushing Brushing promotes blood circulation in the gums and removes plaque and food debris. Tooth brushing should follow flossing. Brush teeth after each meal using a dentifrice (toothpaste) containing fluoride. Brush the tongue to remove bacteria and prevent halitosis. Dentures are brushed the same way as teeth. The oral cavity of a client who wears dentures must also be cleansed. Dentures should be kept moist by putting back in the mouth or immersing in water after cleansing.

Provide Hair Care

Hair affects a person's appearance and body image. Hair maintains body temperature and is a receptor for the sense of touch. Hair texture, growth, and distribution provides information on a person's general health status. Common hair problems include hair loss, dandruff, tangled or matted hair, and infestations such as lice and pediculosis. Daily hair care can reduce hair problems and promote hair growth; prevent hair loss, infections, or infestations; promote circulation to the scalp, evenly distribute oils along hair shafts, and maintain the client's physical appearance. Hair care consists of brushing and combing, shampooing, shaving, and mustache and beard care.

Brushing and Combing Hair should be brushed or combed daily in the client's preferred manner. A clean brush or comb should be used to brush from the scalp toward the hair ends. Be gentle when brushing or combing sensitive scalps.

Some clients may have tangled or matted hair. Prevent pain when combing tangled or matted hair by holding the tangled hair near the scalp while combing.

The hair can be loosely braided to prevent tangling or matting if the client permits. Tight braids may cause pain and hair loss. Written informed consent must be received before cutting a client's hair.

Shampooing Hair should be shampooed according to the client's usual routine. Shampooing removes soil from the hair, stimulates scalp circulation, and facilitates brushing and combing. Depending on the client's abilities and preferences, hair can be shampooed in the tub, in the shower, at the sink, or in the bed.

Hair can be shampooed with water or with shampoos not requiring water. Use the fingertip pads to gently massage the scalp. Thoroughly rinse and dry with an absorbent towel, comb and style as the client desires.

Shaving Shaving is the removal of hair from the skin surface. Males often shave to remove facial hair, and women may shave to remove leg and/or axillary hair. Operative procedures may also require shaving an area of the body.

Shaving may be performed before, during, or after the bath. The area should be washed with soap and warm water to soften the hair before shaving. Apply shaving cream or mild soap to the area to ease hair removal. Pull the skin taut, hold the razor at a 45-degree angle, and move the razor over the skin in firm, short strokes in the direction of hair growth. Care should be taken to avoid cutting the skin. Wash, rinse, and pat the skin dry following shaving.

Safety: Shaving
- Review the client's medical record and the facility's policy regarding the use of razors for shaving.
- Clients prone to bleeding should use only electrical razors for shaving.
- The nurse should wear gloves unless using an electric razor.

Mustache and Beard Care Mustaches and beards need daily care to keep the hair clean, trimmed, and combed. They can be washed with soap or shampoo but often require only gentle wiping with a moist washcloth. A mustache or beard should never be shaved off by the nurse without written informed consent from the client.

Provide Eye, Ear, and Nose Care

Eye, ear, and nose care should be included in routine hygiene care.

Eye Care Eyes are continually cleansed by tears and the movement of the eyelids over the eyes. Eyelids should be washed daily with a warm washcloth and from the inner to the outer canthus.

Infection Control: Eye Care
In order to prevent the transfer of pathogens, a new, clean corner of the washcloth should be used for each eye and with each stroke.

Eyelashes prevent foreign material from entering the eyes and conjunctival sacs. Eyelashes and eyebrows should be washed with the face.

Although some artificial eyes (prosthetics) are permanently implanted, others may require daily removal and cleaning: The eye is removed from the eye socket and washed.

Comatose clients lack a blink reflex and need special eye care. Lubricants or eyedrops should be frequently instilled to prevent corneal abrasions.

Clients who can insert, remove, and manage the care of their contact lenses require little assistance from the nurse. The client who also has corrective eyeglasses may wish to wear eyeglasses during hospitalization. There are hard and soft types of contact lenses. Each type requires different cleansing and care. The lenses should be removed during emergency situations and placed in the appropriate solution.

Ear Care Foreign material or wax in the external ear canal can affect hearing. Cleansing the ears involves cleansing the external ear canal and auricles. No objects should be inserted into the ear canal. Excess wax or foreign material may be removed with a warm washcloth while pulling the ear downward in the adult client. The ear is pulled up and back in children. Irrigation of the ear may be necessary to remove dried wax; this will require a physician's order.

Hearing aids amplify sound. Hearing aids should be cleansed regularly to ensure proper functioning.

If the hearing aid is not functioning properly, the nurse should check the on–off switch and volume control; the battery (and replace as necessary); the plastic tubing, for cracks and loose connections; and the telephone switch, which should be in the off position unless the client is using the phone. Hearing aids should be handled carefully because bumping or dropping them can damage their delicate mechanisms. The hearing aid should be stored in a container when not in use because dust and dirt can damage the mechanism.

Nose Care The nose is the organ of smell, which humidifies inhaled air, facilitates breathing, and prevents entrance of foreign material into the respiratory tract. Excessive or dried secretions may impair nasal function. If the client cannot blow the nose, insert a cotton-tip applicator moistened with water or saline into the nostrils but not beyond the cotton tip. A suction bulb can remove excessive nasal secretions in infants. The client with a nasogastric tube should receive meticulous skin care to the nose area to prevent skin breakdown.

Evaluation

Evaluation looks for achievement of goals and expected outcomes.

The client should not only be kept free of injury during hospitalization, but also helped to develop an awareness of the factors increasing the risk for injury. In the home, modifications to ensure a safe environment serve as evidence for the home health nurse that learning has taken place.

The therapeutic value of hygiene is greatest when the client participates and is free from infection and changes in skin integrity. Evaluation identifies the client's level of functioning in self-care activities. At the time of discharge, appropriate referrals can be made to home health care agencies to assist the client in safety and hygiene practices.

SAMPLE NURSING CARE PLAN

THE CLIENT AT RISK FOR INJURY

Mr. Simon, age 75 years, presents with coronary heart disease (CHD) upon being admitted to the hospital. He has a family history of CHD. He smokes two packs of cigarettes per day, has diabetes mellitus, and is obese. He has gained 7 pounds in the past month and exhibits diminished visual acuity, decreased bladder tone, weakness, and syncope. His blood cholesterol is 320 mg/dL, and his high-density lipoprotein (HDL) level is 28 mg/dL. On the Glasgow Coma Scale (GCS), he received a score of 12 (15 is fully oriented; 7 is comatose). His blood pressure is 186/116.

Nursing Diagnosis *Risk for Injury* related to failure to adapt to sensory dysfunctions as evidenced by diminished visual acuity and a GCS score of 12

Nursing Outcomes Classification (NOC)
Risk Control: Cardiovascular Health
Neurological Status

Nursing Interventions Classification (NIC)
Surveillance
Surveillance: Safety

continues

SAMPLE NURSING CARE PLAN

PLANNING/GOALS	NURSING INTERVENTIONS	RATIONALE
Mr. Simon will be protected from injury during hospitalization.	Initiate fall-prevention protocol.	Identifies and reduces the risk for injury.
	Place Mr. Simon in a room as close as possible to the nurses' station.	Facilitates faster response time to the client's needs.
	Place fall-alert signs on Mr. Simon's door and head of bed.	Alerts other health care workers to the client's risk status.
	Turn the bed alarm on.	Helps monitor client status and facilitates prompt response if the client tries to get out of bed unassisted.
	Monitor Mr. Simon and the environment every 2 hours and whenever a caregiver passes by his room.	Provides information on status, progress, and needs of the client; encourages team approach to client care.
	Reassess Mr. Simon's status every 4 hours.	Identifies changes and, thus, the need to modify the plan of care.
	Instruct all caregivers to respond promptly to the call light.	Ensures rapid response to the client's needs.
	Teach Mr. Simon to use the call light; reinforce teaching each time before leaving him alone.	Ensures that the client has the means and knowledge to call for assistance if necessary.

EVALUATION   The fall prevention protocol was implemented. When discharged on the third day of hospitalization, Mr. Simon was free of injury.

Summary

- Maintaining a safe environment for clients must be the highest priority for nurses.
- The best way to ensure safety is to recognize hazards and eliminate them. Prevention is the best safety measure.
- Clients having a high risk factor for injury must be provided extra protection measures.
- Factors influencing client safety are age, lifestyle, sensory and perceptual alterations, mobility, and emotional state.
- Accidents occurring in health care settings are related to client behavior, therapeutic procedures, and equipment.

- A safety risk appraisal is part of an assessment of a safe environment.
- Nurses can help clients maintain a safe environment by eliminating hazards related to falls, lighting, obstacles, the bathroom, fire, electricity, radiation, poisoning, and noise pollution.
- Safety precautions should be explained thoroughly to clients and/or families.
- Hygiene practices are influenced by personal preference, social and cultural practices, body image, socioeconomic status, and knowledge.
- Basic hygiene practices include bathing, skin care, perineal care, back rubs, foot and nail care, oral care, hair care, and eye, ear, and nose care.

Review Questions

1. Mingo, a 60-year-old diabetic, had his left leg amputated. He is in a semiprivate room with another client who is receiving oxygen. What sign should be posted on the door?

    a. "Amputee"
    b. "No Visitors"
    c. "No Smoking"
    d. "Regular Diet"

2. Felicita, just admitted to the hospital, is overweight, unsteady on her feet, and visually impaired. Her two daughters enter the room as the nurse puts the side rails up on the bed. Felicita begins to cry. The daughters accuse her of being a baby. The best nursing intervention would be to:

    a. tell the daughters to leave until Felicita has calmed down.
    b. explain to the daughters that they are making their mother feel worse.
    c. explain to Felicita that side rails must be used to protect her from falling out of bed.
    d. explain to Felicita and her daughters both the purpose of the side rails and the facility's alternate policy.

3. The priority for nursing care is:

    a. safety.
    b. timeliness.
    c. one-to-one care.
    d. the execution of procedures exactly as written.

4. The use of side rails:

    a. is only needed at night.
    b. is required for all clients.
    c. has caused injury to clients.
    d. relieves the nurse from checking on the client as frequently.

5. Hygiene is considered a safety measure because:

    a. it changes a person's self-image.
    b. the same thing is done for all clients.
    c. it rids the body of all microorganisms.
    d. it promotes the health of the body's first line of defense.

References/Suggested Readings

Association for Professionals in Infection Control and Epidemiology, Inc. (2003). *The use of hand sanitizers in the healthcare setting.* [Online]. Available: www.apic.org/pdf/FINALHandSanitizers.pdf

Carpenito, L. (2002). *Handbook of nursing diagnosis* (9th ed). Philadelphia: Lippincott Williams & Wilkins.

Carroll, P. (1998). Preventing nosocomial pneumonia. *RN, 61*(6), 44–47.

Centers for Disease Control and Prevention (CDC), National Center for Injury Prevention and Control (NCIPC). (2002a). *Preventing falls.* [Online]. Available: www.cdc.gov/ncipc/duip/spotlite/falls.htm

Centers for Disease Control and Prevention (CDC), National Center for Injury Prevention and Control (NCIPC). (2002b). *The costs of fall injuries among older adults.* [Online]. Available: www.cdc.gov/ncipc/factsheets/fallcost.htm

Centers for Medicare & Medicaid Services (CMS). (2002). *Questions and answers for hospital conditions of participation for patients' rights.* [Online]. Available: www.cms.gov/cop/2b.asp

Continuing Education Offering (2001). Oral care: The inside story. *Nursing2001, 31*(5), between pages 32 and 33.

Dochterman, J., & Bulechek, G. (2004). *Nursing Interventions Classification (NIC)* (4th ed.). St. Louis, MO: Mosby.

Food and Drug Administration. (1996). *FDA safety alert: Entrapment hazards with hospital bed side rails.* [Online]. Available: www.fda.gov/cdrh/bedrails.html

Guyton, A. C., & Hall, J. (2000). *Textbook of medical physiology* (10th ed.). Philadelphia: W. B. Saunders.

Joint Commission on Accreditation of Healthcare Organizations. (2001). *Comprehensive accreditation manual for hospitals.* Oakbrook Terrace, IL: Author.

Kimbell, S. (2001). Before the fall: Keeping your patient on his feet. *Nursing2001, 31*(8), 44–45.

Larson, E. (2002). The "hygiene hypothesis": How clean should we be? *AJN, 102*(1), 81–89.

Moorhead, S., Johnson, M., & Maas, M. (2004). *Nursing Outcomes Classification (NOC)* (3rd ed.). St. Louis, MO: Mosby.

Napierkowski, D. (2002). Using restraints with restraint. *Nursing2002, 32*(11), 58–62.

National Institute for Occupational Safety & Health (NIOSH). (2002). *About NIOSH research and services* [Online]. Available: www.cdc.gov/niosh/about.html

North American Nursing Diagnosis Association. (2003). *Nursing diagnoses: Definitions and classification 2003-2004.* Philadelphia: Author.

Parini, S., & Myers, F. (2003). Keeping up with hand hygiene recommendations. *Nursing2003, 33*(92), 17.

Parker, K., & Miles, S. H. (1997). Deaths caused by bedrails. *Journal of the American Geriatric Society, 45*(7), 797–802.

Ramponi, D. (2001). Eye on contact lens removal. *Nursing2001, 31*(8), 56–57.

Richman, D. (1998). To restrain or not to restrain? *RN, 61*(7), 55–60.

Salladay, S. (1998). Severing the ties that bind. *Nursing98, 28*(5), 30.

Schweon, S., & Novatnack, E. (2003). Don't underestimate Group A strep. *RN, 66*(8), 28–32.

Stanhope, M., & Knollmueller, R. (2000). *Handbook of community-based and home health nursing practice: Tools for assessment, intervention, and education* (3rd ed.). St. Louis, MO: Mosby.

Swauger, K., & Tomlin, C. (2002). Moving toward restraint free patient care. *Journal of Nursing Administration, 30*(6), 325–329.

Sweeney-Calciano, J., Solimene, A., & Forrester, D. (2003). Finding a way to avoid restraints. *Nursing2003, 33*(5), 32hn1–32hn4.

Talerico, K., & Capezuti, E. (2001). Myths and facts about side rails. *AJN, 101*(7), 43–48.

U.S. Department of Energy (Hanford Fire Department). (2001). *HFD: All you ever wanted to know about fire extinguishers.* [Online]. Available: www.hanford.gov/fire/safety/extingrs.htm

U.S. Department of Labor. (2002). *Workplace fire safety.* [Online]. Available: www.cdc.gov/nasd/docs/d000701-0000800/d000737/d000737.html

Walker, B. (1998). *Injury prevention for the elderly: Preventing falls.* Gaithersberg, MD: Aspen.

Walker, B. (1998). Preventing falls. *RN, 61*(5), 40–42.

Yoneyama, T. et al. (2002). Oral care reduces pneumonia in older patients in nursing homes. *Journal of the American Geriatric Society, 50*(3).

Resources

Association for Professionals in Infection Control and Epidemiology, Inc., 1275 K Street NW, suite 1000, Washington, DC 20005-4006, 202-789-1890, www.apic.org

Centers for Medicare & Medicaid Services, 7500 Security Boulevard, Baltimore, MD 21244-1850, 410-786-3000, www.cms.hhs.gov

Consumer Product Safety Commission, Washington, DC 20207, 800-638-2772, www.cpsc.gov

Environmental Protection Agency, Public Information Center, 401 M Street SW, Washington, DC 20460, 202-260-2090, www.epa.gov

Food and Drug Administration, Office of Consumer Affairs, 5600 Fishers Lane, Rockville, MD 20857, 888-463-6332, www.fda.gov

Joint Commission on Accreditation of Healthcare Organizations (JCAHO), One Renaissance Boulevard, Oakbrook Terrace, IL 60181, 630-792-5000, www.jcaho.org

National Institute for Occupational Safety and Health, Clearinghouse for Occupational Safety and Health Information, Technical Information Branch, 4676 Columbia Parkway, Cincinnati, OH 45226, 800-356-4674, www.cdc.gov

UNIT

6

Infection Control

INFECTION CONTROL/ASEPSIS

MAKING THE CONNECTION

Refer to the following chapters to increase your understanding of infection control/asepsis:

Basic Nursing
- **Basic Nutrition**
- **Safety/Hygiene**
- **Standard Precautions and Isolation**
- **Fluid, Electrolyte, and Acid–Base Balance**

Basic Procedures
- **Hand Hygiene**
- **Use of Protective Equipment**

Intermediate Procedures
- **Surgical Asepsis: Preparing and Maintaining a Sterile Field**
- **Performing Open Gloving**
- **Applying a Dry Dressing**

LEARNING OBJECTIVES

Upon completion of this chapter, you should be able to:
- **Define key terms.**
- **Describe the chain of infection.**
- **Discuss the body's nonspecific and specific immune defenses.**
- **Describe the stages of the inflammatory process.**
- **Discuss the stages of the infectious process.**
- **Identify the signs and symptoms of inflammation and infection.**
- **Explain the principles of medical and surgical asepsis.**
- **Provide client care maintaining the principles of medical and/or surgical asepsis.**

INTRODUCTION

Nurses are responsible for providing quality care that incorporates infection-control principles. These principles are a major component of a safe environment. This chapter discusses infection-control principles including naturally occurring microorganisms, pathogens, infection and colonization, chain of infection, body defenses, stages of the infectious process, and nosocomial infections. Discussion of the nurse's role in controlling infections is emphasized.

KEY TERMS

acquired immunity
agent
airborne transmission
antibody
antigen
asepsis
aseptic technique
bactericide
biological agent
carrier
chain of infection
chemical agent
clean object
cleansing
colonization
communicable agent
communicable disease
compromised host
contact transmission
convalescent stage
dirty object
disinfectant
disinfection
edema
erythema
flora
fomite

germicide
hand hygiene
host
humoral immunity
illness stage
immunization
incubation period
infection
infectious agent
inflammation
localized infection
lymphokine
medical asepsis
mode of transmission
nosocomial infection
pathogen
pathogenicity
physical agent
portal of entry
portal of exit
prodromal stage
purulent exudate
reservoir
resident flora
sebum
spore
sterilization

FLORA

Flora are microorganisms that occur or have adapted to live in a specific environment, such as intestinal, skin, vaginal, or oral flora. There are two types of flora: resident and transient. **Resident (normal) flora** are microorganisms that are always present, usually without altering the client's health; an example would be *proprionibacterium* on the skin. Resident flora prevent the overgrowth of harmful microorganisms; only when the balance is upset does disease result. **Transient flora** are microorganisms that are episodic (of limited duration); an example would be *staphylococcus aureus.* They attach to the skin for a brief period of time but do not continually live on the skin. Transient flora are usually acquired from direct contact with the microorganisms on environmental surfaces.

PATHOGENICITY AND VIRULENCE

Although most microorganisms found in the environment do not cause disease and infection, some do. Disease-producing microorganisms are called **pathogens; pathogenicity** refers to the ability of a microorganism to produce disease. **Virulence** refers to the frequency with which a pathogen causes disease. The factors affecting virulence are the strength of the pathogen to adhere to healthy cells; the ability of a pathogen to damage cells or interfere with the body's normal regulating systems; and the ability of a pathogen to evade the attack of white blood cells (WBCs).

Five types of microorganisms can be pathogenic: bacteria, viruses, fungi, protozoa, and *Rickettsia.*

Bacteria

Bacteria are small, one-celled microorganisms that lack a true nucleus or mechanism to provide metabolism. Therefore, bacteria need an environment that will provide food for survival. Bacteria can be spherical, rodlike, spiral, or curving in shape, usually appearing as single cells, pairs, chains, or groups. Although most bacteria multiply by simple cell division, some forms of bacteria produce **spores,** a resistant stage that withstands unfavorable environments. When proper environmental conditions return, spores germinate and form new cells. Spores are difficult to kill because of their resistance to heat, drying, and disinfectants. The growth rate of bacteria is affected by environmental factors such as changes in temperature and nutrition. The optimal temperature for pathogenic bacteria is 98.6°F.

Bacteria can be found in all environments, yet not all bacteria are harmful or cause disease. Only a small percentage of bacteria are actually pathogenic. Common bacterial infections include diarrhea, pneumonia, sinusitis, urinary tract infections, cellulitis, meningitis, gonorrhea, otitis media, and impetigo.

Viruses

Viruses are organisms that can live only inside cells. They cannot get nourishment or reproduce outside cells. Viruses contain a core of deoxyribonucleic acid (DNA) or ribonucleic acid (RNA) surrounded by a protein coating. Some viruses have the ability to create an additional coating called an envelope, which helps protect the cell from attack by the immune system. Viruses damage the cells they inhabit by blocking the normal protein synthesis of the cells and by using the cell's mechanism for metabolism to reproduce.

The same viral infection may cause different symptoms in different individuals, based on the individual's immune response to the invading virus. Some viruses will immediately trigger a disease response, whereas others may remain latent for many years. Common viral infections include influenza, measles, common cold, chickenpox, hepatitis B, genital herpes, and HIV.

Fungi

Fungi grow in single cells, as in yeast, or in colonies, as in molds. Fungi obtain food from dead organic matter or from living organisms. Most fungi are not pathogenic and make up many of the body's normal flora. Disease from fungi is found mainly in individuals who are immunologically impaired. Fungi can cause infections of the hair, skin, nails, and mucous membranes.

Protozoa

Protozoa are single-celled parasitic organisms with the ability to move (Figure 19-1). Most protozoa obtain their nourishment from dead or decaying organic matter. Infection is spread through ingestion of contaminated food or water or through insect bites. Common protozoan infections include malaria, gastroenteritis, and vaginal infections.

Rickettsia

Rickettsia are intracellular parasites that need to be in living cells to reproduce. Infection from *rickettsia* is spread through fleas, ticks, mites, and lice. Common *rickettsia* infections include typhus, Rocky Mountain spotted fever, and Lyme disease.

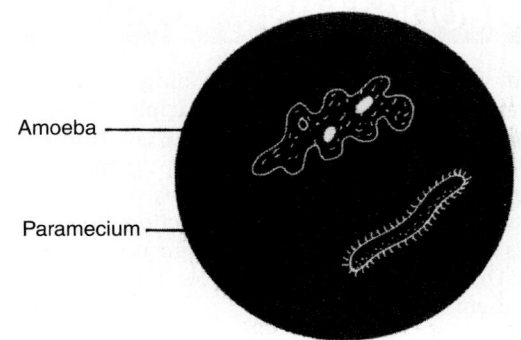

Figure 19-1 *Protozoa*

COLONIZATION AND INFECTION

Colonization is the multiplication of microorganisms on or within a host that does not result in cellular injury; an example of colonization is the normal flora (microorganisms) in the intestines. However, if host susceptibility increases or the microorganism's virulence increases, colonized microorganisms on a host may be a potential source of infection.

Infection is the invasion and multiplication of pathogenic microorganisms in body tissue that results in cellular injury; an example is strep throat. These microorganisms are called **infectious agents**. Infectious agents capable of being transmitted to a client by direct or indirect contact, through a vehicle (or vector) or airborne route are called **communicable agents**. Diseases produced by these agents are referred to as **communicable diseases**.

CHAIN OF INFECTION

Neither a susceptible host nor the presence of a pathogen means that an infectious process will occur. The **chain of infection** describes the development of an infectious process. An interactive process involving an agent, host, and environment is required. This interactive process involves several essential elements, or "links in the chain," for transmission of microorganisms to occur. Figure 19-2 identifies the six essential links (elements) in the chain of infection. An infectious process cannot occur without the transmission of microorganisms.

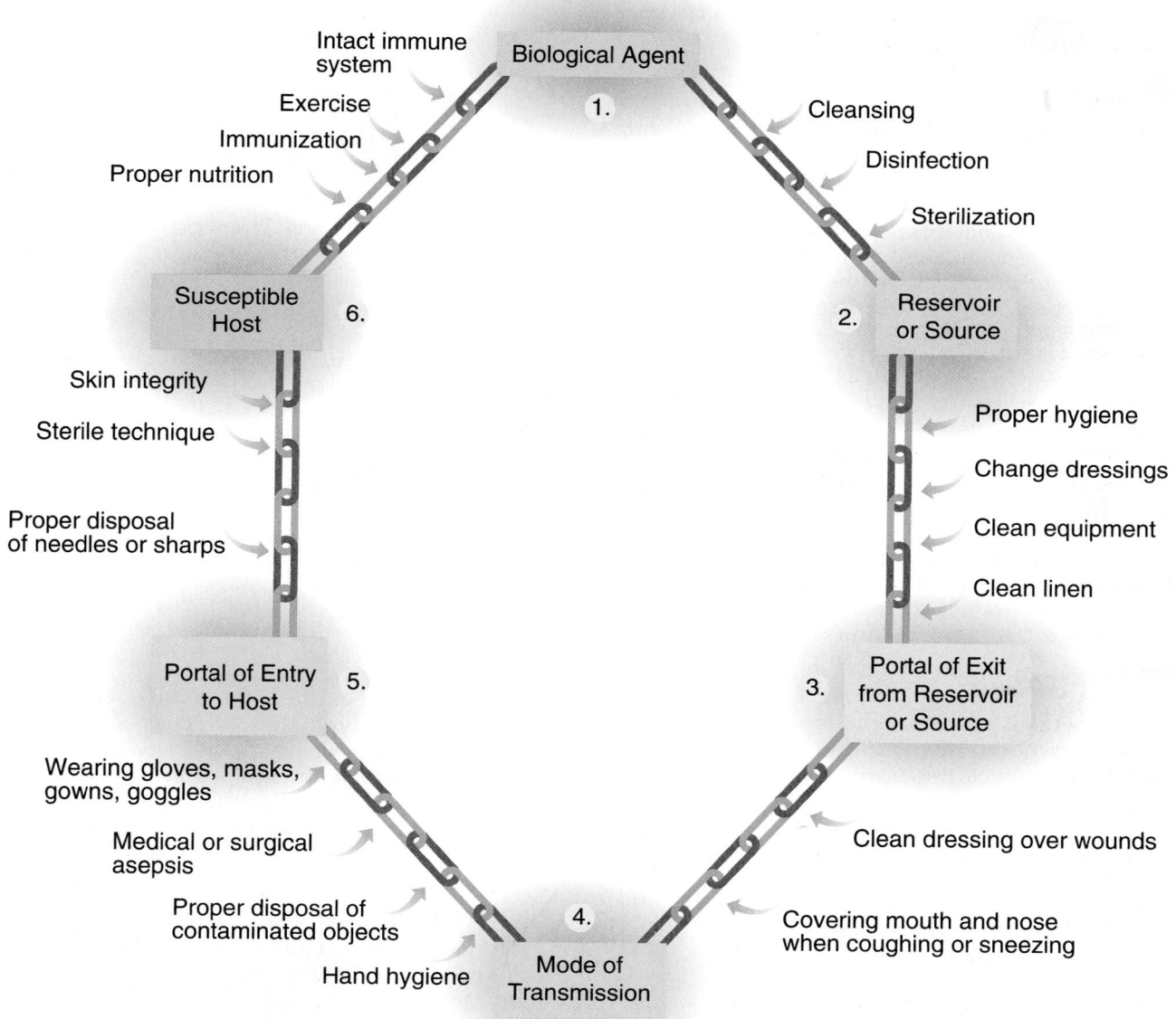

Figure 19-2 *The Chain of Infection: Preventive Measures Follow Each Link of the Chain*

Therefore, knowledge about the chain of infection facilitates control or elimination of microorganism transmission by breaking the links in the chain. Breaking the chain of infection is achieved by altering the interactive process of the agent, host, and environment. Each of the six links in the chain of infection is discussed following.

Agent

An **agent** is an entity that is capable of causing disease. Agents that cause disease may be as follows:

- **Biological agents.** Living organisms that invade the host, causing disease, such as bacteria, viruses, fungi, protozoa, and *rickettsia*
- **Chemical agents.** Substances that can interact with the body, causing disease, such as food additives, medications, pesticides, and industrial chemicals
- **Physical agents.** Factors in the environment that are capable of causing disease, such as heat, light, noise, and radiation.

In the chain of infection, the main concern is biological agents and their effect on the host.

Reservoir

The **reservoir** is a place where the agent can survive. Colonization and reproduction take place while the agent is in the reservoir. A reservoir that promotes growth of pathogens must contain the proper nutrients (such as oxygen and organic matter), maintain proper temperature, contain moisture, maintain a compatible pH level (neither too acidic nor too alkaline), and maintain the proper amount of light exposure. The most common reservoirs are:

- Humans
- Animals
- Environment
- **Fomites** (objects contaminated with an infectious agent, such as bedpans, urinals, bed linens, instruments, dressings, specimen containers, and other equipment)

Humans and animals can have symptoms of the infectious agents or can be strictly carriers of the agent. **Carriers** have the infectious agent but are symptom free. The agent can be spread to others in both instances.

Portal of Exit

The **portal of exit** is the route by which an infectious agent leaves the reservoir to be transferred to a susceptible host. The agent leaves the reservoir through body secretions including:

- Sputum, from the respiratory tract
- Semen, vaginal secretions, or urine, from the genitourinary tract
- Saliva and feces, from the gastrointestinal tract
- Blood
- Draining wounds
- Tears

Modes of Transmission

The **mode of transmission** is the process of the infectious agent moving from the reservoir or source

TABLE 19-1   MODES OF TRANSMISSION

MODE	EXAMPLES
Contact	Direct contact of health care provider with client: • Touching • Bathing • Rubbing • Toileting (urine and feces) • Secretions from client Indirect contact with fomites: • Clothing • Bed linens • Dressings • Health care equipment • Instruments used in treatments • Specimen containers used for laboratory analysis • Personal belongings • Personal care equipment • Diagnostic equipment
Airborne	Inhaling microorganisms carried by moisture or dust particles in air: • Coughing • Talking • Sneezing
Vehicle	Contact with contaminated inanimate objects: • Water • Blood • Drugs • Food • Urine
Vectorborne	Contact with contaminated animate hosts: • Animals • Insects

through the portal of exit to the portal of entry of the susceptible "new" host. Most infectious agents have a usual or primary mode of transmission; but some microorganisms may be transmitted by more than one mode (Table 19-1). Depending on the agent, almost anything in the environment can become a potential mode of transmission.

Contact Transmission

The most important and frequent mode of transmission is **contact transmission**. This involves the transfer of an agent from an infected person to a host by direct contact with the infected person, indirect contact with the infected person through a fomite, or close contact with contaminated secretions (Figure 19-3). Sexually transmitted diseases are spread by direct contact.

Figure 19-3 *Care must be taken in handling bodily fluids to prevent the transfer of infectious agents through contact.*

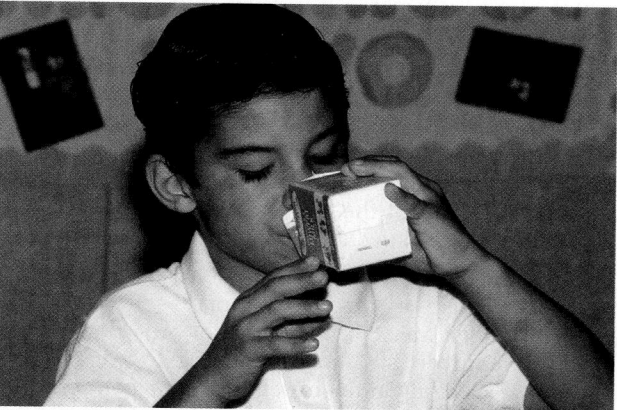

Figure 19-4 *Vehicle transmission occurs through contamination of inanimate objects, such as milk.*

Common viral infections (cold, measles, flu) are spread by close contact with contaminated secretions.

Airborne Transmission

Airborne transmission occurs when a susceptible host contacts droplet nuclei or dust particles that are suspended in the air. Particle size influences the length of time that the organism can remain airborne. The longer the particle is suspended, the greater the chance it will find an available port of entry to the human host. A disease that relies on airborne transmission is measles. Contaminated droplets containing the measles virus are in the spray from sneezing. The droplet can find a portal of entry through the mucous membranes or conjunctiva. Droplets that do not remain airborne or settle out are excluded from this category (Chin, 2000).

Vehicle Transmission

Vehicle transmission occurs when an agent is transferred to a susceptible host by contaminated inanimate objects such as water, food, milk (Figure 19-4), drugs, and blood. Cholera is transmitted through contaminated drinking water, and salmonellosis is transmitted through contaminated meat.

Vectorborne transmission

Vectorborne transmission occurs when an agent is transferred to a susceptible host by animate means such as mosquitoes, fleas, ticks, lice, and other animals (Figure 19-5). Lyme disease, malaria, and West Nile virus are examples of diseases spread by vectors.

Deer tick

Figure 19-5 *Lyme disease and other infections are caused by the bite of a tick.*

Portal of Entry

A **portal of entry** is the route by which an infectious agent enters the host. Portals of entry include the following:

- *Integumentary system*, through a break in the integrity of the skin or mucous membranes (e.g., infections of surgical wounds)
- *Respiratory tract*, by inhaling contaminated droplets (such as cold, influenza, measles)
- *Genitourinary tract*, through contact with infected vaginal secretions or semen (as in sexually transmitted diseases)
- *Gastrointestinal tract*, by ingesting contaminated food or water (e.g., typhoid, hepatitis A)
- *Circulatory system*, through the bite of insects (such as mosquito bites resulting in malaria)
- *Transplacental*, through transfer of microorganisms from mother to fetus via the placenta and umbilical cord (including HIV, hepatitis B)

Host

A **host** is an organism that can be affected by an agent. A human being is usually considered a host. A **susceptible host** is a person who has no resistance to an agent and thus is vulnerable to disease. For example, an individual who has not received the measles vaccine is more likely to contract the infection because of the lack of immunity to the infectious agent. A **compromised host** is a person whose normal body defenses are impaired and is therefore susceptible to infection. For example, a person with a common cold or superficial burns is at greater risk for infection because of the impaired state of the body system mechanisms.

Characteristics of the host influence the susceptibility to and severity of infections. These include:

- *Age.* As a person ages, immunity declines, thus increasing susceptibility to infection.
- *Concurrent diseases.* The existence of comorbid diseases indicates an environment susceptible to infection.
- *Stress.* An individual experiencing a compromised emotional state may have altered or decreased immune system response.
- *Immunization/vaccination status.* Individuals who are not fully immunized are at greater risk for infection.
- *Lifestyle.* Lifestyle practices such as having multiple sex partners or sharing intravenous drug needles increase an individual's potential for illness.
- *Occupation.* Forms of employment that involve an increased exposure to pathogens might include dealing with chemical agents (such as asbestos) or handling sharp instruments (such as scalpels).
- *Nutritional status.* Individuals who maintain targeted weight for height and body frame are less prone to illness.
- *Heredity.* Some individuals are naturally more susceptible to infection than others (Black & Matassarin-Jacobs, 1999).

Interaction between agent and host occurs in the environment, which is everything other than the agent and host. Many of the conditions promoting transmission of microorganisms reflect changes in the relationship between humans and their environments.

BREAKING THE CHAIN OF INFECTION

Nurses focus on breaking the chain of infection by applying proper infection-control practices to interrupt the transmission of microorganisms. Specific strategies can be directed at breaking or blocking the transmission of infection from one link in the chain to the next. A discussion regarding each of the six links follows (refer back to Figure 19-2).

 Infection Control: First Line of Defense
Hand hygiene is the first line of defense against infection and is the single most important practice in preventing the spread of infection.

CRITICAL THINKING

Chain of Infection
How is the chain of infection applicable in everyday life in a person's home?

PROFESSIONAL TIP

Infectious Diseases
Berlinguer (1992) notes that the causes of most emerging infectious diseases are the same today as throughout recorded history: the transfer and dissemination of existing agents to new host populations (a process called "global microbial traffic"). For instance, cholera probably originated in Asia in ancient times; in the 19th century, it spread to Europe and the New World because of increased global travel. Cholera entered South America for the first time in 1992, through the possible contaminated bilge water released from a Chinese freighter. West Nile virus was unknown in the United States until 1999 (APIC, 2002c). The causes of emerging infectious diseases and outbreaks require careful consideration of changes in relationship between humans and their environments.

Between Agent and Reservoir

The first link in the chain of infection is between the agent and the reservoir. The keys to eliminating infection at this point in the chain are cleansing, disinfection, and sterilization. These practices prevent the formation of a reservoir where infectious agents can live and multiply.

Cleansing

Cleansing is the removal of soil or organic material from instruments and equipment used in providing client care. Nurses often cleanse instruments after assisting or performing invasive procedures. To reduce the amount of contamination and loosen the material on reusable objects, the objects are cleansed before sterilization or disinfection. Cleansing involves the use of water, mechanical action, and, sometimes, a detergent. Contaminated objects are cleansed using a soft-bristled brush to scrub the surface. The steps for proper cleansing are:

1. Wet the object with *cold* water; warm water coagulates the proteins in organic material and makes them stick.
2. Apply detergent and scrub the object under running water using a soft-bristled brush.
3. Rinse the object under warm running water.
4. Dry the object before sterilization or disinfection.

 Infection Control: Cleansing
Cleansing is a potential hazard to the nurse from the splashing of contaminated material onto the body. Nurses should wear gloves, masks, and goggles during cleansing.

Disinfection

Disinfection is the elimination of pathogens, except spores, from inanimate objects. **Disinfectants** are chemical solutions used to clean inanimate objects. Bedpans, linens, thermometers, and some types of endoscopes are disinfected. The U.S. Environmental Protection Agency (EPA) licenses intermediate and low-level disinfectants.

The Food and Drug Administration (FDA) regulates high-level disinfectants (NICOD, 2002). Common disinfectants are alcohol, sodium hypochlorite, quaternary ammonium, phenolic solutions, and glutaraldehyde.

A **germicide** is a chemical that can be applied to both animate (living) and inanimate objects to eliminate pathogens. Antiseptic preparations such as alcohol and silver sulfadiazine are germicides.

Sterilization

Sterilization is destroying all microorganisms including spores. Equipment that enters normally sterile tissue or blood vessels must be sterilized. Methods of achieving sterilization are moist heat (steam), dry heat, and ethylene oxide gas. The method of sterilization depends on the object to be sterilized and the kind and amount of contamination.

Autoclaving sterilization, which uses moist heat or steam, is the most common sterilization technique used in the hospital setting (Figure 19-6). Boiling water is not an effective sterilization measure, because some viruses and spores can survive boiling water. Objects that have been boiled in water for 15 to 20 minutes at 121°C (249.8°F) are considered clean but not sterile (Department of Labor, 1991).

Between Reservoir and Portal of Exit

Promoting proper hygiene, changing dressings and linens, and ensuring that clean equipment is used in client care are ways to break the chain of infection between the reservoir and the portal of exit. The goal is to eliminate the reservoir for the microorganism before a pathogen can escape to a susceptible host.

Proper Hygiene

Educate clients on the importance of maintaining the cleanliness and integrity of the skin and the mucous membranes. Clean skin, hair, and nails maintain the body's normal flora and eliminate transient flora from the client's system. Bathing and hand hygiene are important ways to eliminate the potential for infection.

Figure 19-6 *Sterilized Packages. The strips below each package show the way they looked before sterilization. The strips on the packages have changed color because they have been sterilized.*

Clients should be encouraged to practice daily bathing and teeth brushing. Clients who are unable to perform these activities independently should be assisted.

Change Dressings

Any open injury or other break in skin integrity represents a potential reservoir for infectious agents and portal of exit for a pathogen to be transferred to another individual. Dressings on open or oozing wounds must be changed regularly. To protect both yourself and the client from infection, follow proper aseptic technique when changing dressings. This technique is discussed in detail later in this chapter.

Clean Linens

Bed linens, gowns, and towels are catch-alls for bodily secretions. Infectious agents can be easily transferred from one individual to the next through contact with a client's linens. Linens must be changed regularly, and soiled linens must be properly disposed. When changing linens, take care to keep the soiled articles from contact with your uniform. This will prevent being infected from the soiled linens or passing the infection on to other clients.

Clean Equipment

All equipment used in the care of a client must be cleansed and disinfected after each use. Although many items such as disposable gowns can be discarded after use, items such as beds must be thoroughly cleansed after each use. Clients should be instructed never to share care items. Any nondisposable equipment used in an invasive procedure (such as equipment used in the operating room [OR]) must be sterilized before being used again. Wear gloves and masks when cleansing equipment to avoid being splashed with contaminated waste products or secretions.

Between Portal of Exit and Mode of Transmission

The goal in breaking the chain of infection between the portal of exit and the mode of transmission is to prevent the exit of the infectious agents. Clean dressings must be maintained on all wounds. Clients should be encouraged to cover their mouths and noses when sneezing or coughing, and the nurse must do so as well. Gloves must be worn when caring for a client who may have infectious secretions, and care must be taken to properly dispose of any contaminated article.

Between Mode of Transmission and Portal of Entry

To break the chain of infection between the mode of transmission and the portal of entry, asepsis must be ensured and barrier protection worn when the care of clients involves contact with body secretions. Gloves, masks, gowns, and goggles are barrier protection that can be used. Proper hand hygiene and proper disposal of contaminated equipment and linens are ways to prevent transmission of microorganisms to other clients and health care workers. A thorough discussion of asepsis and disposal of contaminated items is included later in this chapter.

Between Portal of Entry and Host

Maintaining skin integrity and using sterile technique for client contacts are methods of breaking the chain of infection between portal of entry and host. Avoiding needle sticks by properly disposing of sharps also reduces the potential for infection by denying a portal of entry. The goal at this point in the chain is to prevent the transmission of infection to a client or health care worker who is not infected.

Between Host and Agent

Breaking the chain of infection between host and agent means eliminating infection before it begins. There are many ways to reduce the risk of acquiring infection: Proper nutrition, exercise, and immunizations allow an individual to maintain an intact immune system, thus preventing infection.

Proper Nutrition

Proper nutrition assists the body's immune system to function properly. Clients need adequate amounts of protein in their diets to maintain and repair tissue as well as to produce the antibodies needed to fight infection. A balanced diet also allows the body to maintain appropriate acid–base balance.

Exercise

Exercise maintains the body's metabolic rate and, therefore, allows the body to maintain the antibodies and energy necessary to ward off infection.

Immunization

Immunization is the process of creating immunity, or resistance to infection, in an individual. Many immunizations are given in early childhood (e.g., measles, mumps, and rubella). Immunization for the flu must be given every year, and for tetanus every 10 years.

BODY DEFENSES

A host's immune system is a defense against infectious agents. The immune system is able to recognize "self" and "nonself"; that is, the immune system recognizes what is not consistent with the genetic composition of the host (self). These agents are called **antigens** (nonself). An immune response against an antigen protects the body from infection. Immune defenses are identified as nonspecific and specific and work together to defend the host from pathogens (Bouman, 1999; Porche, 1998).

Nonspecific Immune Defense

The nonspecific immune defense protects the host from all microorganisms; it does not depend on prior exposure to an antigen. Nonspecific immune defenses are skin and normal flora; mucous membranes; coughing, sneezing, and tearing reflexes; elimination and acidic environment; and inflammation.

Skin and Normal Flora

The skin, the first line of defense against infection, serves as a physical barrier to infectious agents. Skin cells, shed daily, remove potentially harmful microorganisms. **Sebum,** a substance produced by the skin, contains fatty acids that kill some bacteria. The normal flora residing on the skin and in the body compete with pathogenic flora for food and inhibit pathogen multiplication. The balance of normal flora may become disrupted, al-

CLIENT TEACHING

Inappropriate Use of Antibiotics

- Do not pressure the physician or nurse practitioner to prescribe antibiotics for every illness. Antibiotics are not always appropriate. They are not effective against viruses.
- When antibiotics are prescribed, the client should take *all* of the medication as directed.
- Antibiotics taken only until the client feels better allow the microorganisms to become resistant to the antibiotic, and the antibiotic will no longer be effective.
- Antibiotics also destroy normal flora microorganisms, and other illnesses may ensue.

lowing pathogenic organisms to proliferate, causing infection or superinfection.

Mucous Membranes

Mucous membranes also are a physical barrier to infectious agents. Mucus produced by these membranes entraps infectious agents and inhibits bacterial growth. For example, the cilia of the respiratory tract trap and propel mucus and microorganisms away from the lungs, thereby reducing the potential for infection.

Coughing, Sneezing, and Tearing Reflexes

The cough and sneeze reflexes forcibly expel mucus and microorganisms from the respiratory tract. Tears protect the eyes by continually flushing away microorganisms. Tears also contain **bactericides,** which are bacteria-killing chemicals.

Elimination and Acidic Environment

Elimination and an acidic environment usually prevent growth of pathogenic organisms. Resident flora of the large intestines prevent the growth of pathogens. The mechanical process of defecation removes microorganisms with the feces. Urine acidity prevents microbial growth. Urination flushes and cleans the bladder neck and urethra of microorganisms and prevents microorganisms from ascending into the urinary tract.

Normal vaginal flora prevent growth of several pathogens. At puberty, lactobacilli ferment and produce sugars in the vagina that lower the pH to an acidic range. The acidic environment of the vagina prevents pathogenic growth.

Inflammation

Inflammation is a nonspecific cellular response to tissue injury. Tissue injury caused by bacteria, trauma, chemicals, heat, or any other occurrence releases substances, producing dramatic secondary changes in the injured tissue. This entire complex of tissue changes in response to injury is called the *inflammatory process* (Table 19-2). The body's response to injury produces characteristic local and systemic signs of inflammation.

Inflammation, while not necessarily the result of invading microorganisms, does have signs and symptoms similar to those of an infection. The primary signs of inflammation and infection are as follows:

- Redness **(erythema),** results from increased blood flow to the area
- Heat results from increased blood flow and metabolism in the area
- Pain results from increased pressure on pain sensors in the area
- Swelling **(edema,** a detectable accumulation of increased interstitial fluid) results from fluid and leukocytes entering the tissues from the circulatory system
- Loss of function results from both pain and swelling, is the body's way of resting the injured part
- Pus **(purulent exudate),** resulting from infection, a secretion made up of white blood cells, dead cells, bacteria, and other debris

The inflammatory process intensity is usually in proportion to the degree of tissue injury.

Specific Immune Defense

The specific immune defense is a response specific to the invading antigen. It is activated when phagocytes fail to completely destroy the antigen. This causes production of T lymphocytes (T cells), which regulate the immune response by activating other cells. The T cells move to the injured area and release chemical substances called **lymphokines.** Lymphokines attract other phagocytes and lymphocytes to the injured area and assist in antigen destruction.

STAGE	DESCRIPTION	RESULT
	TABLE 19-2 STAGES OF THE INFLAMMATORY PROCESS	
1	Initial injury causes release of chemicals: histamine, bradykinin, serotonin, prostaglandins, and lymphokines.	Initiates the inflammation process
2	Blood flow increases to the injured area.	Produces characteristic redness and warmth
3	Increased capillary permeability leaks large amounts of plasma into the damaged tissue; tissue spaces and lymphatics are blocked by fibrinogen clots.	"Walls off" infection; results in nonpitting edema
4	Leukocytes infiltrate damaged tissue and engulf the bacteria and necrotic tissue. After several days, these leukocytes die and form a cavity of necrotic tissue and dead leukocytes.	Produces purulent exudate (pus)
5	Destroyed tissue cells are replaced by identical or similar structural and functioning cells and/or fibrous tissue.	Promotes tissue healing or the formation of fibrous (scar) tissue, which may reduce the functional capacity of the tissue.

The T cells also stimulate the production of B cells, which become plasma cells, producing antibodies specific to the antigen. **Antibodies** are protein substances that destroy the antigen. The stimulation of B cells and the production of antibodies are collectively known as **humoral immunity.**

Memory B cells are formed to remember the antigen and prepare the host for future antigen invasion. When the antigen enters the body again, the immune response occurs faster by rapidly producing antibodies. The formation of these antibodies is referred to as **acquired immunity,** which protects the individual against future invasions of already experienced antigens such as lethal bacteria, viruses, toxins, and even foreign tissues.

The process of **vaccination** (inoculation with a vaccine to produce immunity against specific diseases) provides acquired immunity. There are three types of vaccines:

1. Dead organisms that are no longer capable of causing disease but still have their chemical antigens, such as typhoid, whooping cough, and diphtheria
2. Toxins that have been chemically treated so their toxic nature is destroyed but their antigens are still intact, such as for tetanus and botulism
3. Live organisms that have been attenuated (rendered incapable of causing the disease yet still have the specific antigen), such as for poliomyelitis, yellow fever, measles, smallpox, and many other viral diseases (Guyton & Hall, 2000)

TYPES AND STAGES OF INFECTIONS

Infection is the result of tissue invasion and damage by an infectious agent. There are two types of infections:

1. **Localized infections** are limited to a defined area or single organ with symptoms that resemble inflammation (redness, tenderness, and swelling), such as a cold sore.
2. **Systemic infections** affect the entire body and involve multiple organs, such as AIDS.

All infections progress through four stages: incubation, prodromal, illness, and convalescence.

Incubation Stage

The **incubation period** is the time between entry of an infectious agent in the host and the onset of symptoms. During this time, the infectious agent invades the tissue and multiplies to produce an infection. The client is typically infectious to others during the latter part of this stage. For example, the incubation period for varicella (chickenpox) is 2 to 3 weeks; the infected person is contagious from 5 days before any skin eruptions to no more than 6 days after the skin eruptions appear.

 Safety: Incubation Period
Always verify the incubation period of a suspected infection. Remember that a client may be able to transmit the infection to another person before the onset of symptoms.

Prodromal Stage

The **prodromal stage** is the time from the onset of nonspecific symptoms until specific symptoms begin to manifest. The infectious agent continues to invade and multiply in the host. A client may also be infectious to other persons during this time period. In the client with chickenpox, a slight elevation in temperature will occur during this stage, followed within 24 hours by eruptions on the skin.

Illness Stage

The **illness stage** is the time when the client has specific signs and symptoms of an infectious process. The client with chickenpox will experience a further rise in temperature and continued outbreaks of skin eruptions for at least 2 to 3 more days.

Convalescent Stage

The **convalescent stage** is from the beginning of the disappearance of acute symptoms until the client returns to the previous state of health. The client with chickenpox will see the skin eruptions and irritation begin to resolve during this stage.

NOSOCOMIAL INFECTIONS

A **nosocomial infection** is an infection acquired in a hospital or other health care facility that was not present or incubating at the time of the client's admission. They also include those infections that become symptomatic after the client is discharged and infections passed among medical personnel. Nosocomial infections are also called *hospital-acquired infections.* These types of infections typically fall into four categories: urinary tract, surgical wounds, pneumonia, and septicemia.

Most nosocomial infections are transmitted by health care personnel who fail to practice proper hand hygiene or who fail to change gloves between client contacts.

The hospital environment provides exposure to a variety of organisms to which the client has not typically been exposed in the past. Therefore, the client has no resistance to these organisms. Illness impairs the body's defenses.

NURSING PROCESS

Quality nursing care requires the reduction of microorganism transmission in the health care environment. Infection-control practices are directed at controlling or eliminating sources of infection in the health care agency or home. Nurses are responsible for protecting clients and themselves by using infection-control practices.

Assessment

Assessment data guides the prioritization of the client's problem and identification of appropriate nursing diagnoses. Clients at risk for infection require frequent reassessment followed by appropriate changes in the plan of care, goals, and nursing interventions.

The health history and physical examination data correlated with the laboratory results identify those clients at risk for infection. Appropriate risk appraisals may be incorporated into the nursing health history interview.

Subjective Data

Relevant data regarding the client at risk for infection are obtained in the health history. A comprehensive assessment also involves appraising the client's environment to detect potential hazards and the client's self-care abilities. Reviewing such factors as work environment, immunization status, and other health-related issues may help identify actual or possible infection risks.

Objective Data

Objective data are gathered through the physical examination and the diagnostic and laboratory findings.

Physical Examination A complete health assessment includes a systematic physical examination, generally conducted from head to toe, to obtain objective data relative to the client's health status and presenting problems. When assessing the client to determine the level of risk for infection, focus the physical examination on:

- Range of motion and mobility (A client with limited mobility is at risk for developing joint contractures, skin breakdown, and muscle atrophy.)
- Localized redness, warmth, swelling, pain, and loss of use in a specific body part
- Fever with an increase in pulse and respirations; weakness; anorexia, nausea, vomiting, and/or diarrhea; enlarged and/or tender lymph nodes
- Secretions or exudate of the skin or mucous membranes; hydration status
- Auscultation of the lungs for crackles or wheezes

Diagnostic and Laboratory Data The laboratory indicators for an infection are:

- An elevated leukocyte (white blood cell [WBC]) and WBC differential:

Neutrophils. Increased in acute, severe inflammation

Lymphocytes. Increased in chronic bacterial and viral infections

Monocytes. Increased in some protozoan and rickettsial infections and TB

Eosinophils and basophils. Unaltered in an infectious process
- An elevated erythrocyte sedimentation rate (ESR): increased in the presence of inflammation
- An elevated pH of involved body fluids (gastric, urine, or vaginal secretions): indicative of microorganism presence
- Positive cultures of involved body fluids (blood, sputum, urine, or other drainage): indicative of microorganism growth (Guyton & Hall, 2001)

Nursing Diagnosis

After data collection and analysis, identify a nursing diagnosis. The North American Nursing Diagnosis Association (NANDA) identifies one nursing diagnosis related to infection: *Risk for Infection.*

Risk for infection is an increased risk for being invaded by pathogenic organisms (NANDA, 2003). The risk factors that increase a client's susceptibility to infections are as follows:

- Inadequate primary defenses (broken skin, traumatized tissue, decrease in ciliary action, stasis of body fluids, change in pH of secretions, and altered peristalsis)
- Inadequate secondary defenses (decreased hemoglobin, leukopenia, suppressed inflammatory response)
- Inadequate acquired immunity
- Immunosuppression
- Tissue destruction and increased environmental exposure
- Chronic disease
- Malnutrition
- Invasive procedures
- Pharmaceutical agents
- Trauma
- Rupture of amniotic membranes
- Insufficient knowledge to avoid exposure to pathogens (NANDA, 2003)

Clients who are at risk for infection may have other associated physiologic and psychological concerns. The common nursing diagnoses that often accompany *Risk for Infection* include:

- *Imbalanced Nutrition: Less than Body Requirements* or *More than Body Requirements*
- *Ineffective Protection*
- *Impaired Tissue Integrity*
- *Impaired Oral Mucous Membrane*
- *Impaired Skin Integrity*
- *Deficient Knowledge* (specify)

This list indicates several related problems that must be considered when planning care for the client at risk for infection.

Planning/Outcome Identification

The nurse collaborates with the client and other health care providers to determine goals, outcomes, and interventions to reduce the risk of infection. Outcomes provide direction for nursing care to reduce the risk of infection. Client and caregiver education about identifying potential hazards and health-promotion practices is another critical element of the care plan.

Implementation

Nurses are responsible for providing the client with a safe environment, including prevention of nosocomial infections. Nursing interventions to reduce the risk of infection center around ensuring asepsis and properly disposing of infectious materials to reduce or eliminate infectious agents. **Asepsis** refers to the absence of microorganisms. **Aseptic technique** is the infection-control practice used to prevent the transmission of pathogens. The use of aseptic technique decreases the risk and spread of nosocomial infections. There are two types of asepsis: medical and surgical.

Medical Asepsis

The term **medical asepsis** refers to those practices used to reduce the number, growth, and spread of microorganisms. It is also called *clean technique.* In medical asepsis, objects are generally referred to as "clean" or "dirty." **Clean objects** are considered to have the presence of some microorganisms that are usually not pathogenic. **Dirty** (soiled) **objects** are considered to have a high number of microorganisms, some being potentially pathogenic. Common medical aseptic measures used for clean or dirty objects are hand hygiene, daily changing of linens, and daily cleansing of floors and hospital furniture.

Hand Hygiene Hand hygiene is a general term that includes *handwashing* (using plain soap and water), *antiseptic handwash* (using antimicrobial substances and water), *antiseptic hand rub* (using alcohol-based hand rub), and *surgical hand antisepsis* (using antiseptic handwash or antiseptic hand rub preoperatively by surgical personnel to eliminate transient and reduce resident hand flora) (CDC, 2002). Perform hand hygiene after arriving at work, before leaving work, before and after each client contact, after removing gloves, when hands are visibly soiled, before eating, after excretion of body waste (urination and defecation), after contact with body fluids, and after handling contaminated equipment. *When hands are visibly dirty, wash hands with soap (plain or antimicrobial) and water. If hands are not visibly soiled, an alcohol-based hand rub may be used* (CDC, 2002).

Handwashing is the rubbing together of all surfaces and crevices of the hands using plain soap and water, followed by rinsing in a flowing stream of water. Friction physically removes soil and transient flora, and a flowing stream of water rinses it all away. To remove transient flora from the hands, a washing time of 15 seconds is recommended. High-risk areas such as nurseries usually require a handwash of approximately 2 minutes duration. Soiled hands usually require more time (APIC, 2002b; CDC, 2002; Department of Labor, 1991). Handwashing is the most basic and effective infection-control measure to prevent and control the transmission of infectious agents. It is the single most important procedure for preventing nosocomial infections (APIC, 2002b).

Infection Control: Hand Hygiene
- Cleanse hands before and after every client contact.
- The most common cause of nosocomial infections is contaminated hands of health care providers.
- When in doubt, *cleanse your hands.*

Antiseptic hand rub uses an alcohol-containing preparation designed to reduce the number of viable microorganisms on the hands. In the United States, these preparations usually contain 60% to 95% ethanol or isopropanol. Apply product to palm of one hand and rub hands together, covering all surfaces of hands and fingers, until hands are dry. Follow the manufacturer's recommendation for the amount of product to use (CDC, 2002).

Surgical Asepsis

Surgical asepsis, or sterile technique, consists of those practices that eliminate all microorganisms and spores from an object or area. Surgical asepsis relates to surgical handwashing, establishing and maintaining sterile fields, donning surgical attire (caps, masks, and eyewear), and sterile gloves, gowning, with closed gloving.

Surgical asepsis is practiced in the OR, in labor and delivery, and for many therapeutic and diagnostic interventions at the client's bedside. Common nursing procedures requiring sterile technique are:

- All invasive procedures, either entry into a bodily orifice (tracheobronchial suctioning, insertion of a urinary catheter) or intentional perforation of the skin (injections, insertion of intravenous needles or catheters)

- Nursing interventions when there is a disruption of skin surfaces (changing a surgical wound or intravenous site dressing) or destruction of skin layers (trauma and burns)

Surgical Hand Antisepsis Surgical hand antisepsis scrub removes soil and microorganisms from the skin. Workers in the OR do surgical hand antisepsis to minimize the client's risk for infection. The skin on the hands and arms should be intact (free of lesions). Agency policy determines the method and timing for the scrub.

Sterile Field and Equipment Establish and maintain a sterile field when performing procedures that require sterile technique, such as inserting a urinary catheter or changing wound dressings. Before preparing the sterile field, review the agency's policy and gather all the necessary supplies.

Donning Surgical Attire Surgical nurses are required to wear a surgical mask (Figure 19-7) and a clean cap covering all of the hair. Protective eyewear (glasses or goggles) is worn during all procedures posing a threat of body fluids splashing into the eyes. Masks, caps, eyewear, gowns, and gloves are considered barrier precautions because they are a physical impediment to the spread of microorganisms.

Donning Sterile Gloves There are two methods of applying sterile gloves: open and closed. The open method is used when performing procedures requiring sterile technique, such as dressing changes. The closed method is used when the nurse wears a sterile gown, as in the OR.

Gowning with Closed Gloving When donning a sterile gown, nurses in the OR and special procedure areas such as cardiac cath labs use the closed gloved method. After the surgical scrub, don the sterile gown and gloves using the closed method. The sterile gown serves as a barrier to decrease the risk of wound contamination and also allows the nurse to move freely in the environment of sterile fields.

Disposal of Infectious Materials All health care facilities must have guidelines for the disposal of infectious-waste materials as required by the OSHA Act of 1991. The types of materials included are:

- Laboratory wastes
- All body fluids including blood, blood products

Figure 19-7 *Putting on a Surgical Mask*

CRITICAL THINKING

Medical and Surgical Asepsis

How are medical asepsis and surgical asepsis the same? How are they different?

- Client care items (soiled bed linen and protection pads, urinals, and bedpans)
- Disposable instruments
- Medication and soiled treatment items
- Surgical wastes

All health care workers must be diligent in observing the biological hazard symbol and handling all infectious materials as hazardous.

When disposing of infectious waste, all personnel must be sure to:

- Wear gloves.
- Use the proper containers (red or one labeled with the biological hazard symbol as required by the facility), sharps containers for needles, scalpels, and other sharp instruments or devices; and leakproof plastic bags for waste from client areas (soiled dressings, gloves, linen).
- Ensure that all infectious waste is properly labeled.
- Carefully handle plastic bags to avoid punctures and tearing.
- Disinfect carts used to carry infectious waste.
- Dispose of waste only in designated areas
- Wash hands after disposing of hazardous materials.

Containers for contaminated sharps should be readily accessible to personnel and maintained in an upright position.

 Infection Control: Needle Disposal
- Used needles should not be recapped, bent, or broken.
- Needles should be placed in a puncture-resistant, marked or color-coded container close to the work site.
- Correct disposal decreases the risk of needle punctures to caregivers.

Finkelstein and Mendelson (1998) report that results from multicenter studies estimate the transmission rate for HIV as being 0.36% after percutaneous exposure and for hepatitis C virus (HCV) as being 1.8% when injured by hollow-bore needles. Most health care workers acutely infected with HBV will eventually clear the virus, but 5% to 10% may develop chronic infection.

Evaluation

Evaluation of the effectiveness of nursing care is based on the achievement of goals and expected outcomes. Keeping the client free from infection requires frequent reassessment followed by timely adjustments made in the plan of care in order for nursing interventions to be effective. It is important for the client to remain free of infection during hospitalization as well as develop a true awareness of the factors that increase the risk for infection.

SAMPLE NURSING CARE PLAN

THE CLIENT AT RISK FOR INFECTION

Mr. Filar, a 38-year-old homeless person, was struck and dragged by a speeding car as he crossed the street. He was taken to the hospital by ambulance. His left leg is broken, and there are lacerations and abrasions on his right side, arm, and leg. The left leg is in a cast and the lacerations have been sutured. Mr. Filar grimaces when he tries to move his legs, but he does not verbalize pain. Mr. Filar is very thin and says that he has not eaten for 2 days.

Nursing Diagnosis 1   *Risk for **I**nfection* related to inadequate primary defenses as evidenced by lacerations and abrasions

Nursing Outcomes Classification (NOC)	**Nursing Interventions Classification (NIC)**
Tissue Integrity: Skin & Mucous Membranes	*Wound Care*
Nutritional Status	*Nutrition Management*

PLANNING/GOALS	NURSING INTERVENTIONS	RATIONALE
Mr. Filar will not have developed an infection in the lacerations and abrasions at discharge.	Use proper hand hygiene before and after caring for Mr. Filar.	Reduces microorganisms on hands.
	Use sterile technique when caring for lacerations and abrasions.	Prevents introduction of microorganisms into lacerations and abrasions.
	Apply antibiotic ointment on abrasions, as ordered.	Promotes healing of abrasions.
	Keep bed linens clean and dry.	Removes any drainage that may harbor microorganisms.
	Administer oral antibiotics, as ordered.	Prevents or cures infection.

EVALUATION   Mr. Filar has some redness around one laceration.

Nursing Diagnosis 2   *Acute **P**ain* related to physical injury as evidenced by facial grimacing

Nursing Outcomes Classification (NOC)	**Nursing Interventions Classification (NIC)**
Pain Control	*Pain Management*
Symptom Severity	*Analgesic Administration*
	Hope Instillation

PLANNING/GOALS	NURSING INTERVENTIONS	RATIONALE
Mr. Filar will experience increased comfort and will verbalize that pain is under control within 24 hours.	Use pain scale to determine level of discomfort.	Provides objective measure of pain.
	Assist client to a position of comfort and elevate extremities.	Reduces pain and swelling by increasing blood return to the heart.
	Administer analgesics, as ordered.	Provides comfort.

EVALUATION   Mr. Filar states that he is experiencing less discomfort by 16 hours but that he still desires pain medication.

continues

SAMPLE NURSING CARE PLAN

Nursing Diagnosis 3 *Imbalanced Nutrition: Less than Body Requirements* related to economic factors as evidenced by extreme thinness and not having eaten for 2 days

Nursing Outcomes Classification (NOC)
Nutritional Status: Nutrient Intake

Nursing Interventions Classification (NIC)
Nutrition Management

PLANNING/GOALS	NURSING INTERVENTIONS	RATIONALE
Mr. Filar will eat balanced meals while hospitalized.	Assist Mr. Filar to select foods high in protein, vitamins A and C, calcium, zinc, and copper.	Wound healing depends on the availability of protein, vitamins, and minerals.
	Provide between-meal snacks, especially milk or milk products.	Snacks will increase overall caloric intake; increased protein will promote wound healing; increased calcium will promote bone healing.

EVALUATION   Mr. Filar eats everything on his meal trays and the between-meal snacks.

Summary

- Flora are microorganisms that occur or have adapted to live in a specific environment.
- Pathogens are microorganisms that cause disease; they include bacteria, viruses, fungi, protozoa, and *rickettsia.*
- The elements of the chain of infection include the agent, the reservoir, the portal of exit, the modes of transmission, the portal of entry, and the host.
- The body has two primary defenses: the nonspecific immune defense, protecting the host from all microorganisms regardless of previous exposure, and the specific immune defense, reacting to a specific antigen that the body has previously experienced.
- Infections progress through four stages: incubation, prodromal, illness, and convalescence.
- Hand hygiene must be done before and after every client contact and after removing gloves. It is the most important procedure for preventing nosocomial infections.
- Other means of preventing the spread of infection include cleansing equipment, cleansing soiled linen, changing dressings over wounds, practicing barrier precautions, maintaining skin integrity, and receiving all appropriate immunizations.
- The OSHA regulations mandate that sharps be properly disposed of immediately after use.

Review Questions

1. With regard to the chain of infection, the main focus of attention in infection control in a health care facility is the:
   a. portal of exit.
   b. infectious agent.
   c. susceptible host.
   d. mode of transmission.

2. The most important procedure for preventing nosocomial infection is:
   a. sterilizing.
   b. hand hygiene.
   c. disinfecting.
   d. the use of bactericides.

3. Living organisms that invade a host are called:
   a. animated agents.
   b. physical agents.
   c. chemical agents.
   d. biological agents.

4. The redness noted during the inflammation process is the result of:
   a. fluid entering the tissues.
   b. increased pressure in the area.
   c. increased blood flow to the area.
   d. increased metabolism in the area.

5. A client is infectious to other persons during the:

    a. illness stage.
    b. prodromal stage.
    c. incubation period.
    d. convalescent stage.

References/Suggested Readings

Association for Professionals in Infection Control and Epidemiology (APIC). (2002a). *Infection control—A few ounces of prevention.* [Online]. Available: www.apic.org/cons/icdesc.cfm

Association for Professionals in Infection Control and Epidemiology, Inc. (APIC). (2002b). *Infection control tips on handwashing* [Online]. Available: www.apic.org/cons/washtips.cfm

Association for Professionals in Infection Control and Epidemiology, Inc. (APIC). (2002c). *West Nile Virus: Consumer Information.* [Online]. Available: www.apic.org/cons/westnile.cfm

Beaumont, E. (1997). Technology scoreboard: Focus on infection control. *AJN, 97*(12), 51–54.

Bender, K., & Thompson, F. (2003). West Nile Virus: A growing challenge. *AJN, 103*(6), 32–39.

Benner, J. (1998). Combating infection: Help from the web. *Nursing98, 28*(11), 71-72.

Berlinguer, G. (1992). The interchange of disease and health between the old and new worlds. *American Journal of Public Health, 82*(10), 1407-1414.

Black, J. M., & Matassarin-Jacobs, E. (1999). *Medical–surgical nursing: Clinical management for continuity of care* (5th ed.). Philadelphia: W. B. Saunders.

Bouman, C. C. (1999). Functions of the immune system. In P. Beare, & J. Myers (Eds.), *Adult health nursing* (3rd ed.). St. Louis, MO: Mosby.

Centers for Disease Control and Prevention (CDC). (1991). *Recommendations for preventing transmission of human immunodeficiency virus, hepatitis B virus to patients during exposure-prone invasive procedures.* Washington, DC: U.S. Government Printing Office.

Centers for Disease Control and Prevention. (1992). *Principles of epidemiology: Agent, host, environment* (2nd ed.). Atlanta, GA: Public Health Practice Program Office.

Centers for Disease Control and Prevention. (2000). Hospital-acquired infections hit fewer ICU patients. *Morbidity and Mortality Weekly Report, 49*(8), 149.

Centers for Disease Control and Prevention (CDC). (2002). *Guideline for hand hygiene in health care settings.* [Online]. Available: www.cdc.gov/mmwr/preview/mmwrhtml/rr5116a1.htm

Chin, J. (Ed.). (2000). *Control of communicable diseases manual* (17th ed.). Washington, DC: American Public Health Association.

Combating Infection. (1997). Tackling disease transmission. *Nursing97, 27*(7), 65.

Combating Infection. (2001). Handwashing: First defense against infection. *Nursing2001, 31*(9), 20.

Department of Labor. (1991). Bloodborne pathogens rules and regulations. *Federal Register, 58,* 64175-64182.

Dochterman, J., & Bulechek, G. (2004). *Nursing Interventions Classification (NIC),* (4th ed.). St. Louis, MO: Mosby.

Finkelstein, L., & Mendelson, M., with Bailey, E. (1998). Exposure to bloodborne pathogens. *AJN, 98*(3), 67-68.

Goldrick, B., & Goetz, A. (2003). Keeping West Nile Virus at bay. *Nursing2003, 33*(8), 44-47.

Guyton, A. C., & Hall, J. (2001). *Textbook of medical physiology* (10th ed.). Philadelphia: W. B. Saunders.

Hegner, B., Caldwell, E., & Needham, J. (1999). *Nursing assistant: A nursing process approach* (8th ed.). Clifton Park, NY: Thomson Delmar Learning.

Infection Control Update 1997. (1997). How to prevent IV catheter contamination. *Nursing97, 27*(6), 60.

Infection Control. (2002). "Hand hygiene" news. *Nursing2002, 32*(5), 32hn6.

Infectious Disease. (2000). Blood contamination in 50% of reusable tourniquets. *AJN, 100*(4), 17.

Inman, W. B. (2000). Combating infection: Pathogens invade 21st century. *Nursing2000, 30*(8), 22-24.

Moorhead, S., Johnson, M., & Maas, M. (2004). *Nursing Outcomes Classification (NOC),* (3rd ed.). St. Louis, MO: Mosby.

National Center for Infectious Disease (NCID). (2002). *Sterilization or disinfection of medical devices: General principles* [Online]. Available: www.cdc.gov/ncidod/hip/sterile/sterilgp.htm

North American Nursing Diagnosis Association (NANDA). (2003). *Nursing diagnoses: Definitions & classification 2003-2004.* Philadelphia: Author.

OSHA Regulations (1996). *Bloodborne pathogens 1910.1.3.(d)(4)(111)(A)(1).* [Online]. Available: www.osha.gov/oshstd_data/1910_1030html

Pittet, D. (2001). Improving adherence to hand hygiene practice: A multidisciplinary approach. *Emerging Infectious Diseases, 7*(2). [Online]. Available: www.cdc.gov/ncidod/eid/vol7no2/pittet.htm

Porche, D. J. (1999). Nursing management of adults with immune disorders. In P. Beare & J. Myers (Eds.), *Adult health nursing* (3rd ed.). St. Louis, MO: Mosby.

Schweon, S. (2003). West Nile Virus: Get ready for its return. *RN, 66*(4), 56–60.

Weltman, A. C., Short, L. J., & Mendelson, M. H. (1995). Disposal-related sharps injuries at a New York City teaching hospital. *Infection Control and Hospital Epidemiology, 16*(5), 268-274.

Resources

American Public Health Association, 800 I Street NW, Washington, DC 20001, 202-777-2742, www.apha.org

Association for Professionals in Infection Control and Epidemiology, Inc. (APIC), 1275 K Street, NW, Suite 1000, Washington, DC 20005-4006, 202-789-1890, www.apic.org

Centers for Disease Control and Prevention, 1600 Clifton Road, Atlanta, GA 30333, 800-311-3435, www.cdc.gov

Environmental Protection Agency (EPA), Disinfectant Hotline, 401 M Street, SW, Washington, DC 20460-0003, 800-447-6349, Antimicrobial Program Branch, 703-308-0127

Hospital Infection Program (HIP), Office of the Director, HIP Mailstop A07, National Center for Infectious Diseases, Centers for Disease Control and Prevention, 1600 Clifton Rd., Atlanta, GA 30333, www.cdc.gov

National Foundation for Infectious Diseases, 4733 Bethesda Ave., Suite 750, Bethesda, MD 20814, 301-656-0003, www.nfid.org

Society for Healthcare Epidemiology of America (SHEA), 19 Mantua Road, Mt. Royal, NJ 08061, 856-423-0087, www.shea-online.org

STANDARD PRECAUTIONS AND ISOLATION

MAKING THE CONNECTION

Refer to the following chapter to increase your understanding of Standard Precautions and isolation:

Basic Nursing
- **Infection Control/Asepsis**

Adult Health Nursing
- **Surgery**

Basic Procedures
- **Hand Hygiene**

Intermediate Procedures
- **Performing Open Gloving**

Advanced Procedures
- **Initiating Strict Isolation Precautions**

LEARNING OBJECTIVES

Upon completion of this chapter, you should be able to:
- **Define key terms.**
- **Describe each of the eleven aspects of Standard Precautions.**
- **Identify the three transmission-based precautions and when each is to be used.**
- **Apply Standard Precautions in providing appropriate client care.**

KEY TERMS

airborne precautions	isolation
aseptic technique	nosocomial infection
barrier precautions	reverse isolation
contact precautions	Standard Precautions
droplet precautions	Transmission-Based
endemic	Precautions
epidemic	

INTRODUCTION

For more than 120 years, health care facilities and their personnel have struggled to prevent the spread of infections among their clients. This chapter reviews some of the historical methods as well as the current methods used to prevent the spread of infection.

HISTORICAL PERSPECTIVE

A hospital handbook published in 1877 recommended placing clients with infectious diseases in a separate facility (Lynch, 1949). These facilities became known as infectious-disease hospitals. Yet, **nosocomial infections** (infections acquired in the hospital that were not present or incubating at the time of the client's admission) continued in these facilities because the infected clients were not separated according to disease, and **aseptic technique** (infection-control practices used to

prevent the transmission of pathogens) was seldom, if ever, practiced. To combat the continuing problem of nosocomial infections in the infectious-disease hospitals, personnel began to set aside a floor or ward for clients with similar diseases (Gage, Landon, & Sider, 1959).

Nursing has always been at the forefront of preventing the spread of infections among clients and personnel. Infectious-disease hospital personnel began practicing aseptic technique as recommended in nursing textbooks published from 1890 to 1900 (Lynch, 1949). Isolation practices and the use of infectious-disease hospitals were altered in 1910 when the cubicle system of isolation was introduced in U.S. hospitals (Gage et al., 1959). The cubicle system of **isolation** (separation from other persons, especially those with infectious diseases) placed clients in multiple-bed wards, with hospital personnel using a separate gown when caring for each client, washing their hands in an antiseptic solution after contact with each client, and disinfecting objects contaminated by any client. These nursing procedures were known as *barrier nursing*. Barrier nursing was aimed at preventing transmission of pathogenic organisms to other clients and to health care personnel. The cubicle system of isolation, including the barrier nursing procedures, gave the clients the alternative of receiving care in general hospitals instead of the infectious-disease hospitals (Centers for Disease Control and Prevention [CDC]/Hospital Infection Control Practices Advisory Committee [HICPAC], 1997a).

During the 1950s, infectious-disease hospitals closed, with the exception of the tuberculosis (TB) hospitals, which closed in the 1960s. Thus, by the end of the 1960s, clients with infectious diseases were cared for in general hospitals.

In 1970, the CDC published *Isolation Technique for Use in Hospitals* (National Communicable Disease Center, 1970), a revised edition of which was released in 1975 (CDC, 1975). This manual introduced and recommended seven categories of isolation: Strict Isolation, Respiratory Isolation, Protective Isolation, Enteric Precautions, Wound and Skin Precautions, Discharge Precautions, and Blood Precautions. By the mid-1970s, 93% of U.S. hospitals had adopted the recommendations of this book (Haley & Schactman, 1980).

By 1980, **endemic** (occurring continuously in a particular population and having low mortality) and **epidemic** (infecting many people at the same time, in the same geographic area) nosocomial infections were surfacing. Some of these infections were caused by multidrug-resistant (MDR) microorganisms, others by newly identified pathogens. Both types required isolation precautions different from those specified in any of the seven isolation categories. As Schaffner (1980) describes, isolation precautions needed to be directed more specifically at nosocomial transmission in special-care units rather than at community-acquired infectious diseases being spread within the hospital.

In 1983, the CDC replaced the 1975 isolation manual with the *Guideline for Isolation Precautions in Hospitals* (Garner & Simmons, 1983). One of the most important changes was the emphasis on decision making by the users as to which guideline was appropriate in a particular situation (Garner, 1984; Haley, Garner, & Simmons, 1985).

Another change was to rename Blood Precautions, primarily used for clients who were chronic carriers of hepatitis B virus (HBV), to Blood and Body Fluid Precautions, which now were to apply to clients with acquired immunodeficiency syndrome (AIDS); body fluids other than blood, such as semen and vaginal secretions; amniotic, cerebrospinal, pericardial, peritoneal, pleural, and synovial fluids; and any other body fluid visibly contaminated with blood. It did not apply to feces, nasal secretions, sputum, sweat, tears, urine, or vomitus unless blood was visible in them.

Until 1985, clients placed in isolation either had a confirmed diagnosis or were suspected of having an infectious disease. Mainly because of the human immunodeficiency virus (HIV) epidemic and those other blood-borne infections often yet unrecognized in a client, it was decided that Blood and Body Fluid Precautions were to be applied universally to all clients, regardless of their presumed infection status (CDC, 1985). Thus, the new name became Universal Precautions.

A new system of isolation called Body Substance Isolation (BSI) was proposed in 1987 as an alternative to the diagnosis-driven isolation system of the 1983 *Guideline for Isolation Precautions in Hospitals*. Body Substance Isolation focused on isolating all moist and potentially infectious body substances (blood, feces, urine, sputum, saliva, wound drainage, and other body fluids) from *all* clients. The use of gloves was the primary method of isolating infectious agents; however, BSI did not contain adequate provisions to prevent droplet transmission, direct or indirect contact transmission, or true airborne transmission of infections. Also, BSI recommended handwashing after removal of gloves only if the hands were soiled (Lynch, Jackson, Cummings, & Stamm, 1987), whereas Universal Precautions recommended handwashing after every removal of gloves (CDC, 1987; CDC, 1988).

In 1991, the Hospital Infection Control Practices Advisory Committee (HICPAC) was established to provide advice and guidance to the Secretary and Assistant Secretary of the U.S. Department of Health and Human Services (USDHHS), the Director of the CDC, and the Director of the National Center for Infectious Diseases (CDC/HICPAC, 1997a). The committee also provides advice to the CDC about updating guidelines and other policy statements related to the prevention of nosocomial infections.

The CDC, with the assistance of HICPAC, revised the *Guideline for Isolation Precautions in Hospitals* in 1996. The new guideline combined the major features of Universal Precautions and Body Substance Isolation into a single set of Standard Precautions, and the specific isolation categories into three Transmission-Based Precautions (CDC/HICPAC, 1997b).

The CDC recommendations are not subject to legal enforcement; however, regulations of the Occupational Safety and Health Administration (OSHA) must be followed by all health care facilities. These regulations, laws enforced through the Department of Labor (OSHA, 1991), ensure that Standard Precautions and Transmission-Based Precautions are followed. According to OSHA regulations, all health care facilities must:

- Determine which employees have occupational exposure.
- Provide hepatitis B vaccine free of charge to all employees with occupational exposure.
- Provide personal protective equipment (e.g., gowns, gloves, masks, goggles) for all employees with occupational exposure.
- Provide adequate handwashing facilities and supplies.
- Provide training regarding these rules to all employees with occupational exposure, both at hire and, then, annually.
- Provide evaluation and follow-up for any employee who experiences an exposure incident.
- Provide appropriate, properly labeled containers for contaminated sharps.
- Provide and prominently display an exposure control plan for staff to follow.

STANDARD PRECAUTIONS

Standard Precautions, listed on the inside back cover of this book, are preventive practices to be used in the care of all clients in hospitals regardless of diagnosis or presumed infection status. These guidelines are designed to reduce the risk of microorganism transmission from both recognized and unrecognized sources of infection in hospitals (CDC/HICPAC, 1997b).

Standard Precautions apply to:

- Blood
- All body fluids, secretions, and excretions *except* sweat, regardless of whether those fluids contain visible blood
- Nonintact skin
- Mucous membranes

Infection Control: Standard Precautions
- Standard Precautions must be practiced with all clients.
- Standard Precautions represent the most effective means of decreasing the risk of infection among clients and caregivers.

Barrier precautions, used to minimize the risk of exposure to blood and body fluids, involve the use of personal protective equipment, such as masks, gowns, and gloves, to create a barrier between the person and the microorganism and thus prevent transmission of the microorganism. *Hand hygiene, however, is the most basic aspect of Standard Precautions.* The other aspects of Standard Precautions are gloves; mask, eye protection, face shield; gown; client-care equipment; environmental control; linen; occupational health and blood-borne pathogens; and client placement.

Hand Hygiene

Refer to hand hygiene in the Infection Control chapter. To prevent cross-contamination of different body sites on one client, hand hygiene may be necessary between tasks and procedures on that client.

Gloves

Clean, nonsterile gloves are to be worn when touching blood, body fluids, secretions, excretions, and contaminated items. Clean gloves should be put on just before touching mucous membranes and nonintact skin. Gloves must be changed between tasks and procedures being performed on one client if material that may contain microorganisms in high concentrations is touched. Gloves must be removed promptly after use, and hands must be cleansed immediately before touching uncontaminated items or providing care to another client.

Safety: Latex Allergies
- Standard Precautions include the use of gloves when there is a possibility of contact with client body fluids.
- Be alert that health care personnel or the client may be allergic to the latex gloves. Reactions range from an eczematous contact dermatitis to anaphylactic shock.
- Before touching clients when wearing latex gloves, ask whether they have a known allergy to latex products. If they do, use nonlatex gloves for those clients.

Mask, Eye Protection, Face Shield

A mask and eye protection or a face shield should be worn to protect the mucous membranes of the eyes, nose, and mouth when procedures and client-care activities are likely to generate splashes or sprays of blood, body fluids, secretions, or excretions.

Gown

A clean, nonsterile gown should be worn to protect the skin and prevent soiling of clothing during procedures and client-care activities that are likely to generate splashes or sprays of blood, body fluids, secretions, or excretions. A gown that is appropriate for the activity and potential amount of fluids should be selected. A soiled gown should be removed as promptly as possible, and the hands cleansed to prevent transfer of microorganisms to other clients or environments.

Client-Care Equipment

Client-care equipment soiled with blood, body fluids, secretions, or excretions must be handled in a manner to prevent skin and mucous membrane exposure, clothing contamination, and microorganism transfer to other clients or environments. Reusable equipment must not be used in the care of another client until it has been cleansed and sterilized appropriately. All single-use items must be properly discarded.

Environmental Control

The hospital must have adequate procedures for the routine care, cleansing, and disinfection of environmental surfaces, beds, bed rails, bedside equipment, and other frequently touched surfaces. All personnel must ensure that these procedures are followed.

Linen

Linen that is soiled with blood, body fluids, secretions, or excretions must be handled, transported, and processed in a manner to prevent skin and mucous membrane exposure, clothing contamination, and microorganism transfer to other clients and environments. Follow agency policy.

Occupational Health and Blood-Borne Pathogens

Care must be taken to prevent injury when using needles, scalpels, and other sharp instruments and when handling, cleansing, and disposing of such items after use. The OSHA regulations state that "contaminated (used) sharps shall be discarded immediately or as soon as feasible in containers that are closable, puncture-resistant, leakproof on the sides and bottom and are labeled or color coded" (OSHA, 1991) (Figure 20-1).

Used needles should never be recapped by using both hands. A one-handed "scoop" method is acceptable. Used needles should never be removed from disposable syringes by hand, nor should they be bent, broken, or otherwise manipulated by hand. Disposable syringes and needles, scalpel blades, and other sharp items should be placed in designated puncture-resistant containers. Reusable syringes and needles should be placed in a separate puncture-resistant container and transported to the appropriate area for cleansing and sterilizing.

In areas where the need for resuscitation is predictable, mouth pieces, resuscitation bags, or other ventilation devices should be used instead of the direct mouth-to-mouth resuscitation method.

Figure 20-1 *Sharps-Disposal Container*

Client Placement

Any client who contaminates the environment or who does not or cannot be expected to assist with maintaining appropriate hygiene or environment control should be placed in a private room. When a private room is unavailable, infection-control professionals must be consulted.

ISOLATION

The 1996 CDC guideline eliminated the previous category-specific isolation precautions and condensed the former disease-specific precautions into three sets of precautions based on the route of transmission: airborne (Figure 20-2), contact (Figure 20-3), or droplet (Figure 20-4). These new, Transmission-Based Precautions are to be used *in addition to* the Standard Precautions. **Transmission-Based Precautions** are practices designed for clients documented as or suspected of being infected with highly transmissible or epidemiologically important pathogens for which additional precautions beyond the Standard Precautions are required to interrupt transmission in hospitals (CDC/HICPAC, 1997b) (Table 20-1).

The Transmission-Based Precautions are also to be used in addition to the Standard Precautions in the event of suspicious infections and with clients who are im-

AIRBORNE PRECAUTIONS
(In addition to Standard Precautions)

VISITORS: Report to nurse before entering

 Patient Placement
Private room that has:
Monitored negative air pressure,
6 to12 air changes per hour,
Discharge of air outdoors or HEPA filtration if recirculated.
Keep room door closed and patient in room.

 Respiratory Protection
Wear an **N95 respirator** when entering the room of a patient with known or suspected infectious pulmonary **tuberculosis**.
Susceptible persons should not enter the room of patients known or suspected to have **measles** (rubeola) or **varicella** (chickenpox) if other immune caregivers are available. If susceptible persons must enter, they should wear an **N95 respirator**.(Respirator or surgical mask not required if immune to measles and varicella.)

 Patient Transport
Limit transport of patient from room to essential purposes only.
Use **surgical mask** on patient during transport.

Figure 20-2 *Transmission-Based Precautions: Airborne Precautions (From Brevis Corporation, 3310 S. 2700, Salt Lake City, UT 84109. Copyright 1996 by Brevis Corporation. Reprinted with permission.)*

CONTACT PRECAUTIONS
(In addition to Standard Precautions)

VISITORS: Report to nurse before entering

Patient Placement
Private room, if possible. Cohort if private room is not available.

Gloves
Wear gloves when entering patient room.
Change gloves after having contact with infective material that may contain high concentrations of microorganisms (**fecal** material and **wound drainage**).
Remove gloves before leaving patient room.

Wash
Wash hands with an **antimicrobial** agent immediately after glove removal. After glove removal and handwashing, ensure that hands do not touch potentially contaminated environmental surfaces or items in the patient's room to avoid transfer of microorganisms to other patients or environments.

Gown
Wear gown when **entering** patient room if you anticipate that your clothing will have substantial contact with the patient, environmental surfaces, or items in the patient's room, or if the patient is **incontinent**, or has **diarrhea**, an **ileostomy**, a **colostomy**, or **wound drainage** not contained by a dressing. **Remove** gown before leaving the patient's environment and ensure that clothing does not contact potentially contaminated environmental surfaces to avoid transfer of microorganisms to other patients or environments.

Patient Transport
Limit transport of patient to essential purposes only. During transport, ensure that precautions are maintained to minimize the risk of transmission of microorganisms to other patients and contamination of environmental surfaces and equipment.

Patient-Care Equipment
Dedicate the use of noncritical patient-care equipment to a single patient. If common equipment is used, clean and disinfect between patients.

Figure 20-3 *Transmission-Based Precautions: Contact Precautions (From Brevis Corporation, 3310 S. 2700, Salt Lake City, UT 84109. Copyright 1996 by Brevis Corporation. Reprinted with permission.)*

DROPLET PRECAUTIONS
(In addition to Standard Precautions)

VISITORS: Report to nurse before entering

Patient Placement
Private room, if possible. Cohort or maintain spatial separation of **3 feet** from other patients or visitors if private room is not available.

Mask
Wear mask when working within **3 feet** of patient (or upon entering room).

Patient Transport
Limit transport of patient to essential purposes only.
Use **surgical mask** on patient during transport.

Figure 20-4 *Transmission-Based Precautions: Droplet Precautions (From Brevis Corporation, 3310 S. 2700, Salt Lake City, UT 84109. Copyright 1996 by Brevis Corporation. Reprinted with permission.)*

munosuppressed either from disease or chemotherapy. More than one of the transmission-based precautions is used at the same time for clients with certain infections or conditions.

CRITICAL THINKING

Transmission-Based Precautions

How are the three Transmission-Based Precautions the same? How are they different?

Isolation precautions are usually ordered by the physician; however, nurses may initiate these precautions whenever a nursing diagnosis related to the infectious process is identified, for example, *Risk for Infection* related to decreased resistance of immune system. Most agencies require nurses to obtain a culture from a draining body area and to initiate isolation precautions when positive cultures are reported. After isolation precautions have been instituted, visitors and all personnel should comply with the agency's policy regarding isolation precautions. Signs should be posted in a prominent location outside the client's room. The signs should indicate the type of isolation precautions and preparation required before entering the room (Figure 20-5). The necessary supplies should be readily available.

Clients requiring isolation should be placed in a private room with adequate ventilation and should have their own supplies. Personal belongings should be kept to a minimum, and health care providers should use disposable supplies and equipment whenever possible. All articles leaving the room, such as soiled linen and collected specimens, should be labeled and either placed in impermeable bags or double bagged.

Reverse isolation, also known as protective isolation, is a barrier protection designed to prevent infection

COMMUNITY/HOME HEALTH CARE

Isolation

- Provide the client and family with appropriate written isolation instructions relative to the specific precautions.
- Provide necessary supplies or suggest a list of those things to buy and places to purchase the supplies.

PROFESSIONAL TIP

Psychological Interventions for Clients in Isolation

- Explain the pertinent isolation procedures and rationales.
- Discuss the client's feelings about the isolation procedures.
- Convey a sense of empathy and understanding.
- Permit visitors in accordance with isolation precautions.
- Support existing coping mechanisms.
- Visit the client.

TABLE 20-1   PRECAUTIONS RELATED TO TYPE OF DISEASE

PRECAUTION	TYPE OF DISEASE
Standard Precautions	All clients, regardless of disease or condition
Airborne Precautions	In addition to Standard Precautions, used for clients known to have or suspected of having serious illnesses spread by airborne droplet nuclei, including: • Measles • Varicella • Tuberculosis

Contact Precautions	In addition to Standard Precautions, used for clients known to have or suspected of having serious illnesses easily spread by direct client contact or contact with fomites, including:
	• Wound infections
	• Gastrointestinal infections
	• Respiratory infections
	• Skin infections including:
	  Herpes simplex
	  Impetigo
	  Major abscesses, cellulitis, or pressure ulcers
	  Pediculosis
	  Scabies
	  Varicella (Zoster)
	• Viral hemorrhagic infections (Ebola)

Droplet Precautions	In addition to Standard Precautions, used for clients known to have or suspected of having illnesses spread by large particle droplets, including: • Meningitis • Adenovirus • Pneumonia • Influenza • Diphtheria • Mumps • Pertussis • Rubella • Scarlet fever • Parvovirus B19

From *Table I: Synopsis of Types of Precautions and Patients Requiring Precautions,* by Centers for Disease Control and Prevention (CDC)/Hospital Infection Control Practices Advisory Committee (HICPAC), 2002. [Online]. Available: www.cdc.gov/ncidod/hip/isolat/isotab_1.htm

Figure 20-5 *The sign on the door to the client's room indicates the type of isolation precaution and preparation needed before entering the room.*

in clients who are severely compromised and highly susceptible to infection. This includes clients who:

• are taking immunosuppressive medications
• are receiving chemotherapy or radiation therapy
• have diseases such as leukemia, which depress resistance to infectious organisms
• have extensive burns, dermatitis, or other skin impairments that prevent adequate coverage with dressings

These clients are at increased risk for infection from their own microorganisms, contact with health care workers whose hands have not been properly cleansed, and exposure to improperly disinfected and nonsterile items such as air, food, water, and equipment. Nursing responsibilities toward these clients include ensuring that everyone entering the client's room has completed a meticulous hand hygiene and is properly attired in gown, gloves, and mask; ensuring that the client's environment is as clear of pathogens as possible; and knowing the institutional policy regarding caring for clients requiring reverse isolation.

Figure 20-6 *Nurse Interacting with Client Requiring Isolation Precautions*

CLIENT RESPONSES TO ISOLATION

Isolation precautions are for the client's protection; however, clients who are placed on isolation precautions may experience psychological discomfort (Figure 20-6). Symptoms of anxiety, depression, rejection, guilt, or loneliness may be found in isolated clients. Clients should be educated on those isolation precautions that will be practiced and their purposes. Clients should be encouraged to verbalize their feelings regarding the isolation precautions and should be provided with intellectual stimulation and diversional activities such as paperback books, crossword puzzles, music, radio, or television. Visitors should be encouraged as a method to alleviate the client's feelings of isolation and loneliness. Wearing appropriate barrier precautions, visitors can safely enter an isolated client's room.

Summary

- Standard Precautions are to be used when caring for *every* client.
- Airborne Precautions are to be used when caring for clients who have or may have serious illnesses spread by airborne droplet nuclei.
- Droplet Precautions are to be used when caring for clients who have or may have serious illnesses spread by large-particle droplets.
- Contact Precautions are to be used when caring for clients who have or may have serious illnesses spread by direct client contact or fomite contact.

Review Questions

1. In 1996, the revised *Guideline for Isolation Precautions in Hospitals* combined Universal Precautions and Body Substance Isolation into:
   a. Barrier Precautions.
   b. Contact Precautions.
   c. Standard Precautions.
   d. Transmission-Based Precautions.

2. The use of masks, gowns, and gloves is termed:
   a. Droplet Precautions.
   b. Barrier Precautions.
   c. Contact Precautions.
   d. Standard Precautions.

3. The nursing action most basic to Standard Precautions is:
   a. gloving.
   b. gowning.
   c. hand hygiene.
   d. wearing a face mask.

4. Airborne Precautions require:
   a. paper masks.
   b. a private room.
   c. the wearing of gloves.
   d. the wearing of a gown.

5. Those precautions to be used in the care of all clients in hospitals regardless of diagnosis or presumed infection status are called:
   a. Standard Precautions.
   b. Airborne Precautions.
   c. Universal Precautions.
   d. Body Substance Isolation.

References/Suggested Readings

Borton, D. (1997). Isolation precautions: Clearing up the confusion. *Nursing97, 27*(1), 49.

Centers for Disease Control and Prevention (CDC). (1975). *Isolation techniques for use in hospitals* (2nd ed.), (HHS [CDC] Publication No. 80-8314). Washington, DC: U.S. Government Printing Office.

Centers for Disease Control and Prevention (CDC). (1985). Recommendations for preventing transmission of infection with human T-lymphotropic virus type III/lymphadenopathy-associated virus in the workplace. *Morbidity and Mortality Weekly Report (MMWR), 34,* 681–686, 691–695.

Centers for Disease Control and Prevention (CDC). (1987). Recommendations for prevention of HIV transmission in health-care settings. *MMWR, 36*(2S), 1S–18S.

Centers for Disease Control and Prevention (CDC). (1988). Update: Universal precautions for prevention of transmission of human immunodeficiency virus, hepatitis B virus, and other blood borne pathogens in health-care settings. *MMWR, 37*(24), 377–382, 387–388. [Online]. Available: www.cdc.gov/mmwr/preview/mmwrhtml/00000039.htm

Centers for Disease Control and Prevention (CDC). (1996). Guideline for isolation precautions in hospitals. In *Guidelines for the prevention and control of nosocomial infections*. Atlanta, GA: Author.

Centers for Disease Control and Prevention (CDC). (Updated 1999). *Universal precautions for prevention of transmission of HIV and other bloodborne infections.* [Online]. Available: www.cdc.gov/ncidod/hip/Blood/UNIVERSA.HTM

Centers for Disease Control and Prevention (CDC). (2002). *Guideline for hand hygiene in health care settings.* [Online]. Available: www.cdc.gov/mmwr/preview/mmwrhtml/rr5116a1.htm

Centers for Disease Control and Prevention (CDC)/Hospital Infection Control Practices Advisory Committee (HICPAC). (1997a). *Part I: Evolution of isolation practices.* [Online]. Available: www.cdc.gov/ncidod/hip/isolat/isopart1.htm

Centers for Disease Control and Prevention (CDC)/Hospital Infection Control Practices Advisory Committee (HICPAC). (1997b). *Part II. Recommendations for isolation precautions in hospitals.* [Online]. Available: www.cdc.gov/ncidod/hip/isolat/isopart2.htm

Centers for Disease Control and Prevention (CDC)/Hospital Infection Control Practices Advisory Committee (HICPAC). (1997c). *Table II. Clinical syndromes warranting additional emperic precautions to prevent transmission of epidemiologically important pathogens pending confirmation of diagnosis.* [Online]. Available: www.cdc.gov/ncidod/hip/isolat/isotab_2.htm

Centers for Disease Control and Prevention (CDC)/Hospital Infection Control Practices Advisory Committee (HICPAC). (1997d). *Appendix A: Type and duration of precautions needed for selected infections and conditions.* [Online]. Available: www.cdc.gov/ncidod/hip/isolat/isoapp_a.htm

Centers for Disease Control and Prevention (CDC)/Hospital Infection Control Practices Advisory Committee (HICPAC). (2002). *Table I. Synopsis of types of precautions and patients requiring precautions.* [Online]. Available: www.cdc.gov/ncidod/hip/isolat/isotab_1.htm

Department of Labor. (1991). Bloodborne pathogens rules and regulations. *Federal Register, 58,* 64175–64182.

Gage, N. D., Landon, J. F., & Sider, M. T. (1959). *Communicable disease.* Philadelphia, PA: F. A. Davis.

Garner, J. S. (1984). Comments on CDC guideline for isolation precautions in hospitals, 1984. *American Journal of Infection Control, 12,* 163.

Garner, J. S., & Simmons, B. P. (1983). *CDC Guideline for Isolation Precautions in Hospitals* (HHS [CDC] Publication No. 83-8314). Atlanta, GA: U.S. Department of Health and Human Services, Public Health Service, Centers for Disease Control. *Infection Control* (1983) 4:245–325; and *American Journal of Infection Control* (1984) 12:103–163.

Haley, R. W., & Shachtman, R. H. (1980). The emergence of infection surveillance and control programs in U.S. hospitals: An assessment, 1976. *American Journal of Epidemiology, 111,* 574–591.

Haley, R. W., Garner, J. S. & Simmons, B. P. (1985). A new approach to the isolation of patients with infectious diseases: Alternative systems. *Journal of Hospital Infection, 6,* 128–138.

Hospital Infection Control Practices Advisory Committee (HICPAC). (1995). Recommendations for preventing the spread of Vancomycin resistance. *Infection Control and Hospital Epidemiology, 16*(2), 105–113.

Infection Control. (2002). "Hand hygiene" news. *Nursing2002, 32*(5), 32hn6.

Jagger, J. (2002). Avoiding blood and body fluid exposures. *Nursing2002, 32*(8), 68.

Jarvis, W. (2001). Infection control and changing health-care delivery systems. *Emerging Infectious Diseases, 7*(2). [Online]. Available: www.cdc.gov/ncidod/eid/vol7no2/jarvis.htm

Lynch, P., Jackson, M. M., Cummings, J., & Stamm, W. E. (1987). Rethinking the role of isolation practices in the prevention of nosocomial infections. *Annals of Internal Medicine, 107,* 243–246.

Lynch, T. (1949). *Communicable disease nursing.* St. Louis, MO: Mosby.

Occupational Safety and Health Administration (OSHA). (1991). Occupational exposure to bloodborne pathogens: Final rule, 29CRF 1919;1030. *Federal Register, 56,* 64175.

Perry, J. (2001). The bloodborne pathogens standard, 2001. *Nursing2001, 31*(6), 32hn16.

Porche, D. J. (1998). Nursing management of adults with immune disorders. In P. Beare & J. Myers (Eds.), *Adult health nursing* (3rd ed.). St. Louis, MO: Mosby.

Schaffner, W. (1980). Infection control: Old myths and new realities. *Infection Control, 1,* 330–334.

Resources

Association for Professionals in Infection Control and Epidemiology (APIC), 1275 K Street NW, Suite 1000, Washington, DC 20005-4006, 202-789-1890, www.apic.org

Centers for Disease Control and Prevention, 1600 Clifton Road, Atlanta, GA 30333, 404-639-3311, www.cdc.gov

Occupational Safety and Health Administration, 200 Constitution Avenue NW, Washington, DC 20210, www.osha.gov

FLUID, ELECTRO YTE
AND ACID-BASE
BALANCE

UNIT
7

Fundamental Nursing Care

21

FLUID, ELECTROLYTE, AND ACID–BASE BALANCE

MAKING THE CONNECTION

Refer to the following chapters to increase your understanding of fluid, electrolyte, and acid–base balance:

Basic Nursing
- Assessment
- Diagnostic Tests

Adult Health Nursing
- Respiratory System

- **Cardiovascular System**

Basic Procedures
- **Measuring Intake and Output**

LEARNING OBJECTIVES

Upon completion of this chapter, you should be able to:
- Define key terms.
- Discuss the importance of pH regulation in the body.
- Describe the three buffer systems of the body.
- Describe and give examples in the body of diffusion, osmosis, and filtration.
- Name the fluid compartments, the fluids contained in them, and the function of those fluids.
- Describe the way the kidneys work to maintain fluid and electrolyte balance.
- Describe the way the lungs work to maintain pH in the body.
- Detail causes, assessment data, nursing interventions, and criteria for evaluating effectiveness of care for clients with a nursing diagnosis of *Deficient Fluid Volume* or *Excess Fluid Volume.*
- Detail causes, assessment data, nursing diagnoses, nursing interventions, and criteria for evaluating the effectiveness of nursing care for clients with sodium, potassium, calcium, and magnesium imbalances.
- Relate principles of nursing management for clients receiving fluids and electrolytes via oral supplements, intravenous solutions, enteral feedings, and total parenteral nutrition.
- Differentiate the causes, assessment data, and nursing management of metabolic and respiratory acidosis and alkalosis.
- Use the nursing process to plan care for a client experiencing a fluid, electrolyte, and/or acid–base imbalance.

KEY TERMS

acid	hypotonic solution
acidosis	hypoxemia
alkalosis	infiltration
anion	interstitial fluid
arterial blood gases	intracellular fluid
atom	intravascular fluid
base	intravenous therapy
buffer	ion
cation	isotonic solution
compound	isotope
crenation	matter
decomposition	mixture
dehydration	molecule
dialysis	osmolality
diffusion	osmolarity
edema	osmosis
electrolyte	osmotic pressure
element	oxidized
extracellular fluid	permeability
filtration	salt
hemolysis	semipermeable
homeostasis	membrane
hydrostatic pressure	synthesis
hypertonic solution	turgor

INTRODUCTION

The external environment within which we live undergoes continual changes, both small and large. For example, the daily and seasonal temperatures may fluctuate over a wide range. The light intensity is bright on sunny days and less so on cloudy days. The humidity may be either high or low. These are just a few of the many factors that constantly change in the external environment. Our bodies must continually adjust to such changes in the external environment. In order for life to continue, however, our internal environment—the one inside our bodies—must remain relatively constant, varying only slightly within narrow ranges. This internal environment consists of the various body fluids such as the fluid inside cells, the blood, tissue fluids that bathe the cells, and other fluids. Maintenence of the internal environment within very narrow limits is termed **homeostasis** (equilibrium).

✳ HOMEOSTASIS

Homeostasis is an ongoing process; that is, the body simply does not reach a state of equilibrium and remain there. Small changes constantly occur in response to physiologic processes. The body must therefore continuously make subtle adjustments to maintain the constancy of the internal environment within a normal range.

Homeostasis is accomplished by various physiologic processes and the coordinated activities of the organ systems. Some examples are as follows:

- The gastrointestinal (GI) system changes large, complex molecules of ingested food to simpler, less-complex molecules that can be utilized by the cells of the body to produce the energy necessary for life.
- The respiratory system supplies the cells with the constant source of oxygen required to release the energy from the products of digestion. It also eliminates carbon dioxide, the waste product produced by the cells as a result of energy production.
- The blood acts as a transport mechanism, carrying the products of digestion along with hormones and oxygen to the cells, where these substances are utilized.
- It also transports carbon dioxide from the energy-releasing processes of the cells to the lungs, where it will be eliminated.
- All of the activities of the various organ systems are integrated and coordinated through the nervous system and the endocrine system.

When the body loses the ability to maintain homeostasis and the internal environment changes, the physiologic processes can be interrupted or changed, leading to disease, disorder, or death. In essence, then, maintaining homeostasis is essential to life. Because the processes of homeostasis involve many chemical and physical processes, it is necessary to examine some of these before studying homeostasis in more detail.

CHEMICAL ORGANIZATION

The human body is highly organized. This organization exists in increasing levels of complexity. Most basic is the chemical level. To understand the higher levels of organization, it is necessary to know something about basic chemical and physical principles.

Elements

The cell consists of living matter. **Matter** is anything that occupies space and possesses mass. All matter has certain physical properties such as color, odor, hardness, and density. Matter also has extensive properties such as size, shape, and weight. Matter is composed of basic substances called **elements.** Elements are made of tiny units called atoms. Atoms of each element are alike. Different elements have different kinds of atoms. Presently, 108 elements are recognized. Some examples are iron, gold, carbon, hydrogen, oxygen, nitrogen, and copper. Many of the elements occur in the human body in varying amounts. Some are present in large amounts, and others are found in only trace amounts. The four elements oxygen, carbon, hydrogen, and nitrogen constitute more than 95% of the total body weight of the elements. Some of the elements and their function in the body are presented in Table 21-1.

Atoms

An **atom** is the smallest unit of chemical structure, and no chemical change can alter it. Atoms are made up of three basic particles: protons, neutrons, and electrons. Protons and neutrons are similar in size, but whereas protons have a positive electrical charge, neutrons have no charge. Together, they form the nucleus of the atom. Because the protons have a positive charge and the neutrons are neutral, the nucleus of an atom has a positive charge. The electrons have a negative charge and move in an orbit around the nucleus. There are as many electrons as protons, rendering the overall atom neutral. The number of protons in an atom is called its atomic number. The simplest element is hydrogen. It has an atomic number of 1. One proton with a positive charge forms the nucleus, and one electron moves in an orbit around the nucleus. Hydrogen atoms may or may not have a neutron. A hydrogen atom is illustrated in Figure 21-1.

Depending on the element, other atoms may have more than one proton and one electron and may have neutrons. The number of protons and neutrons in the nucleus is approximately equal to the atomic weight. Thus hydrogen has an atomic weight of 1.

Isotopes

The number of protons in the nucleus is the same for all atoms of a given element, but the number of neutrons may vary in atoms of the same element. For instance, all hydrogen atoms have one proton and one electron; however, some hydrogen atoms have one neutron in the nucleus, while others have two (Figure 21-2). Atoms of the same element that have different atomic weights (i.e., have a different number of neutrons) are called **isotopes.** All of the isotopes of a given element react the same way chemically.

Some isotopes, called radioactive isotopes, have an unstable nucleus, which decomposes and gives off energy in the form of radiation. This radiation can be in the form of alpha, beta, or gamma rays. All are damaging to cells. Alpha radiation is the least harmful, and gamma

TABLE 21-1 ELEMENTS OCCURRING IN THE HUMAN BODY

ELEMENT	APPROXIMATE % OF BODY WEIGHT	FUNCTION
Major Elements		
Oxygen (O)	65.0	Found in both organic and inorganic compounds; as a gas, is necessary in metabolizing glucose and other chemical compounds into energy
Carbon (C)	18.5	Found in all organic compounds such as carbohydrates, protein, lipids, and nucleic acids; necessary for cellular respiration
Hydrogen (H)	9.5	Found in many organic and inorganic compounds; in ionic form, involved in pH; component of water; necessary for life
Nitrogen (N)	3.2	Important in proteins, which are the body's building blocks, an energy source, and a component of hormones
Calcium (Ca)	1.5	Important element in bone and tooth composition; involved in nerve conduction, muscle contraction, and blood clotting
Phosphorus (P)	1.0	Found in bones, teeth, the high-energy carrying compound adenosine triphosphatase (ATP), some proteins, and nucleic acid
Potassium (K)	0.4	Major electrolyte in intracellular fluid; important in muscle contraction and transmission of nerve impulses; activates enzymes; influences cellular osmotic pressure; involved in kidney function and acid–base balance
Sulfur (S)	0.3	Found in some proteins, nucleic acids, and some vitamins and hormones
Sodium (Na)	0.2	Constitutes major electrolyte in extracellular fluid; important in osmoregulation and acid–base balance; necessary for nerve transmission and muscle contraction
Chlorine (Cl)	0.2	Found in extracellular fluid; important in water balance, acid–base balance, and production of hydrochloric acid in the stomach
Magnesium (Mg)	0.1	Important to muscle and nerve function and bone formation and in some coenzymes
Essential Trace Elements		
Present in the human body in minimal amounts, constituting approximately 0.1% of body weight; have known functions		
Cobalt (Co)		Important component of vitamin B_{12}
Copper (Cu)		Necessary for formation of hemoglobin and for bone development
Chromium (Cr)		A cofactor involved with enzymes for fat, cholesterol, and glucose metabolism
Fluorine (F)		Gives hardness to teeth and bones
Iodine (I)		Necessary for synthesis of thyroid hormone
Iron (Fe)		Necessary for transportation of oxygen by hemoglobin
Manganese (Mn)		Necessary in activating some enzymes
Selenium (Se)		Acts with vitamin E as an antioxidant; component of teeth
Zinc (Zn)		Found in some enzymes; needed for protein metabolism and carbon dioxide transport
Other Trace Elements		
Have probable, but as yet undetected, functions		
Aluminum (Al) Nickel (Ni) Arsenic (As) Tin (Sn) Boron (B) Silicon (Si) Cadmium (Cd) Vanadium (V)		

radiation is the most harmful. Iodine, oxygen, and cobalt are examples of elements having radioactive isotopes. Some of the radioactive isotopes are useful as biological markers and can be used to track metabolic pathways of food. Others such as iodine[131] can be injected into the body and used to track the circulation of blood. Still others such as cobalt[60] are used in cancer treatment.

Molecules and Compounds

Atoms of the same element can unite with each other to form a **molecule.** For example, atoms of hydrogen unite to form a hydrogen molecule. This can be expressed in a chemical equation using the chemical symbol for hydrogen:

$$H + H \rightarrow H_2$$

In this reaction, the atoms on the left are the reactants; the arrow is read as "yield"; and the last symbol is the product—a molecule of hydrogen. A chemical equation uses the chemical symbols of elements and shows the ratios by which they combine. Because atoms of elements always combine in the same ratio under similar conditions, it is possible to predict the nature of a chemical change.

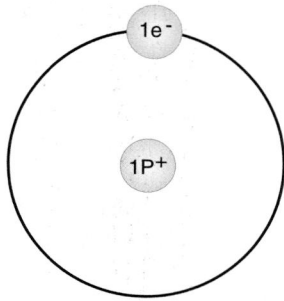

Figure 21-1 *Hydrogen Atom Showing Positively Charged Proton in the Nucleus and Negatively Charged Electron in Orbit*

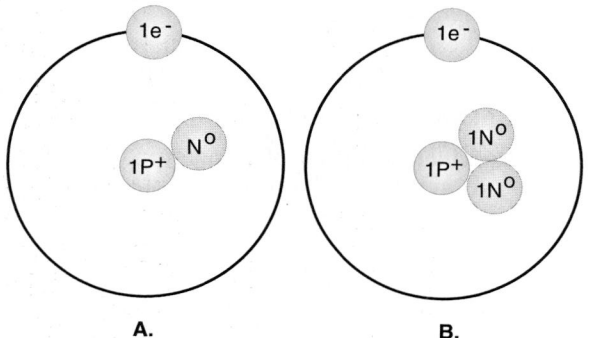

Figure 21-2 *Isotopes of Hydrogen:* **A,** *Deuteridium has one positively charged proton and one neutron in the nucleus and one electron in orbit;* **B,** *Tritium has one positively charged proton and two neutrons in the nucleus and one electron in orbit.*

When atoms of two or more different elements combine (react), they form a **compound.** For example, if one atom of sodium (Na) and one atom of chlorine (Cl) react, they form a molecule of the compound called sodium chloride. This is expressed in the following equation:

$$Na + Cl \rightarrow NaCl$$

Compounds can be divided into two groups. Those without carbon are inorganic compounds, and those with carbon are organic compounds. By using chemical equations, chemical changes, called reactions, can be shown. Sometimes, different substances are combined in no specific way, and the components do not have a definite ratio every time. For instance, water, sugar, and table salt mixed without being measured will yield different results depending on the ratio of each substance. Such a combination is called a **mixture.** Its composition may vary each time the components are mixed.

Chemical reactions occur whenever atoms join together or separate. They join together by forming bonds, and they separate by breaking bonds. Either way, new combinations result. When two or more atoms (reactants) bond and form a more complex molecular product, the reaction is called **synthesis.** A sample equation would be as follows:

$$2H^- + O \rightarrow H_2O$$
hydrogen and oxygen yields water

When the bonding between the atoms in a molecule is broken and simpler products are formed, the reaction is called **decomposition.** If a molecule of sodium chloride is decomposed, it forms sodium and chlorine. This can be expressed as follows:

$$NaCl \rightarrow Na + Cl$$
sodium chloride yields sodium and chloride
(decomposition)

It is important to understand that when synthesis occurs, energy is tied up in the bonds formed during the reaction. When decomposition occurs, energy is released. In the cells of the body, these kinds of chemical reactions are repeatedly occurring: Molecules form and decompose. Body cells can utilize these reactions to form energy sources and to free energy to drive the various metabolic processes of the cells.

Ions

When some compounds are placed in water, they decompose, or ionize. The result is an **ion,** an atom bearing an electrical charge. An ion with a positive charge is called a **cation;** an ion with a negative charge is termed an **anion.** For example, sodium chloride in water dissociates to form sodium ions bearing a positive charge and chloride ions bearing a negative charge (Figure 21-3). Because the atoms in this combination are charged, they will conduct electricity. The reaction can be shown as follows:

$$NaCl \rightarrow Na^+ + Cl^-$$
sodium chloride yields sodium and chloride
(cation)   (anion)

A compound that dissociates into ions in water is called an **electrolyte.** Many electrolytes are extremely important in body chemistry.

WATER

Water constitutes approximately 60% of the total body weight of an adult and is involved in many of the physical and physiological processes of the body. Because water is so integral to the body's processes, fluctuations in

Figure 21-3 *Dissociation of Electrolytes*

the amount of water in the body can have harmful or even fatal consequences.

Water is the major component of blood. Approximately 92% of the body's organic and inorganic compounds dissolve in this water into less-complex molecules and atoms and then are transported throughout the body. Necessary substances such as oxygen and nutrients from the GI system are carried to the cells, where they are utilized. Cellular waste products such as carbon dioxide, urea, and excessive minerals are carried by water to sites of elimination: carbon dioxide to the lungs, urea and minerals to the kidneys.

Water also absorbs heat resulting from muscle contractions and distributes this heat over the body. Water in the form of perspiration released from sweat glands in the skin can cool the body by evaporation. Water also can break apart the bonds in large molecules such as starches to form smaller molecules in the digestive process. This type of reaction is called *hydration*.

GASES

Two important gases in the body are oxygen (O_2) and carbon dioxide (CO_2). Because these elements are gases, their molecules are free and can move swiftly in all directions. Oxygen enters the body through the lungs and is transported by the red blood cells throughout the body to the cells. The cells use oxygen in the release of energy from glucose and other molecules. This energy is needed by the cells to carry out their activities. As a result of the energy-releasing processes, carbon dioxide is produced by the cells and transported in the blood to the lungs, where it is eliminated.

ACIDS, BASES, SALTS, AND PH

Other chemical substances important for life are acids, bases, and salts; pH is the measure of acid and base strength.

Acids

An **acid** is any substance that in solution yields hydrogen ions bearing a positive charge. As an example,

hydrochloric acid (HCl) in water dissociates as shown following:

$$HCl \rightarrow H^+ + Cl^-$$
hydrochloric acid yields hydrogen and chlorine

The hydrogen ion characterizes this as an acid. Important acids in the body are hydrochloric acid, produced in the stomach, and carbonic acid, formed when the carbon dioxide released from cells reacts with some of the water in the extracellular fluid (all body fluids except for those contained within the cells).

Bases

A **base** is a substance that when dissociated produces ions that will combine with hydrogen ions. For example, when sodium hydroxide dissociates in water, it forms a sodium ion bearing a positive charge and a hydroxyl ion bearing a negative charge as shown following:

$$NaOH \rightarrow Na^+ + OH^-$$
sodium hydroxide yields sodium and hydroxyl

The hydroxyl ion is capable of combining with a hydrogen ion to form water. Sodium bicarbonate is an example of a base found in the body.

Salts

A **salt** is formed when an acid and a base react with each other. Salts result from the neutralization of an acid by a base, as illustrated by the following reaction:

$$HCl + NaOH \rightarrow H_2O + NaCl$$
hydrochloric and sodium yields water and sodium
acid   hydroxide   chloride

The hydrochloric acid reacts with the sodium hydroxide to form a molecule of water and a molecule of a salt—sodium chloride. When salts are placed in water, they dissociate into a cation and an anion. For instance, in water, the sodium chloride would dissociate into Na^+ and Cl^-. One reason salts are of great biological importance is that many of the compounds that dissociate into ions in living cells are salts. For example, sodium and chlorine ions are present in great amounts in body fluids. Many other salts occur in lesser amounts.

pH

Acid and bases are classified as either strong or weak by the number of hydrogen ions or hydroxyl ions they produce when they dissociate. Strong acids release many hydrogen ions; weak acids release relatively few. The same is true of hydroxyl ions in strong and weak bases. The acidity or alkalinity of a solution is determined by the concentration of hydrogen ions in the solution. Potential hydrogen (pH) indicates the hydrogen ion concentration in a solution, expressed as a number from 0 to 14. A solution with a pH of 7 is neutral (i.e., it is neither an acid or a base). A solution with a pH greater than 7 is a base, or alkaline. A solution with a pH less than 7 is an acid. The higher above 7 the pH, the more alkaline the solution; the lower below 7 the pH, the more acid the solution. pH is of great biological importance. The human body can tolerate only very slight changes in pH. For example, the pH of human blood ranges from 7.35 to 7.45. Blood pH above or below this range can cause severe or even fatal physiological problems.

Although small amounts of acids may enter the body through food intake, the greatest source of acids—and thus H^+ ions—is cellular metabolism, resulting in products including lactic acid, phosphoric acid, pyruvic acid, and many fatty acids. When blood pH falls below 7.35 as a result of an elevated concentration of H^+ ions, **acidosis** occurs. Rarely does blood pH fall to 7 or become acidic, because death will usually occur first. As acidosis increases, the central nervous system (CNS) becomes involved, and the client may become unconscious. The heartbeat may become weak and irregular, and blood pressure may decrease or even disappear.

When blood pH increases above 7.45, **alkalosis** occurs. Alkalosis is a condition characterized by an excessive loss of hydrogen ions. This happens less often than does acidosis. Symptoms of alkalosis include a heightened state of nervous system activity, resulting in spasmodic muscle contractions, convulsions, and even death.

BUFFERS

Buffers are substances that attempt to maintain pH range, or H^+ ion concentration, in the presence of added acids or bases. Buffers usually occur in pairs in the body fluids. They act to keep the pH of body fluids within normal range. If body fluids become acidic, buffers in the body fluids combine with the excess hydrogen ions and restore normal pH. Likewise, if the body fluids become alkaline, other buffers in the blood combine with the strong bases, converting them to weak bases and restoring normal pH.

Three important buffer systems occur in body fluids: the bicarbonate buffer system, the phosphate buffer system, and the protein buffer system. Because a change in pH of one fluid may bring corresponding changes in the pH of other fluids, an interplay between buffer systems acts to maintain the body's pH. The buffer systems react quickly to prevent excessive changes in the hydrogen ion concentration.

Bicarbonate Buffer System

The bicarbonate buffer system is found in both the extracellular and intracellular fluids and is the body's primary buffer system. It has two components: carbonic acid (H_2CO_3) and sodium bicarbonate ($NaHCO_3$). When a strong acid such as hydrochloric acid is added to this buffer system, the acid will react with the sodium bicarbonate and form a weaker acid (carbonic acid) and a salt (sodium chloride).

$$HCl + NaHCO_3 \rightarrow H_2CO_3 + NaCl$$

hydrochloric and sodium yields carbonic and sodium
acid   bicarbonate   acid   chloride

The strong acid is converted into a weak acid, and the pH is raised toward normal.

If a strong base such as sodium hydroxide is added to this buffer system, the carbonic acid will react with it to form a weak base (sodium bicarbonate) and water.

$$NaOH + H_2CO_3 \rightarrow NaHCO_3 + H_2O$$

sodium   and carbonic yields sodium   and water
hydroxide   acid   bicarbonate

The strong base, which initially raised the pH, is converted to a weak base, which will lower the pH toward normal. It is vital to note that hydrochloric acid and sodium hydroxide are substances not normally added to the blood. They are used here only as good examples of the way buffers work. This buffer system normally buffers organic acids found in body fluids.

In the body, bicarbonate helps stabilize pH by combining reversibly with hydrogen ions. Most of the body's bicarbonate is produced in red blood cells, where the enzyme carbonic anhydrase accelerates the conversion of carbon dioxide to carbonic acid. The production of bicarbonate is illustrated in the following reversible equation:

$$CO_2 + H_2O \leftrightarrow H_2CO_3 \leftrightarrow H^+ + HCO_3^-$$

carbon   water carbonic   hydrogen bicarbonate
dioxide   acid

When the hydrogen ion concentration increases in the extracellular (outside of the cell) space, the reaction shifts toward the left. A decreased concentration of hydrogen ions drives the reaction to the right.

Phosphate Buffer System

The phosphate buffer system is involved in regulating the pH of intracellular fluid and the fluid of the kidney tubules. It has two phosphate compounds: sodium monohydrogen phosphate ($NaHPO_4$) and sodium dihydrogen phosphate (NaH_2PO_4). In the presence of a strong acid such as hydrochloric acid, the sodium monohydrogen phosphate reacts with the acid to form a weak acid (sodium dihydrogen phosphate) and a salt (sodium chloride), thus raising the pH.

$$HCl + NaHPO_4 \rightarrow NaH_2PO_4 + NaCl$$

hydro-   and sodium   yields sodium   and sodium
chloric   monohydrogen   dihydrogen   chloride
acid   phosphate   phosphate

When sodium dihydrogen phosphate encounters a strong base such as sodium hydroxide, a weak base (sodium monohydrogen phosphate) and water are formed.

$$NaOH + NaH_2PO_4 \rightarrow NaHPO_4 + H_2O$$

sodium   and sodium   yields sodium   and water
hydroxide   dihydrogen   monohydrogen
             phosphate   phosphate

Protein Buffers

Proteins are complex substances formed when amino acids bond. Each amino acid contains a carboxyl group (COOH) and an amino group (NH_2). The carboxyl group can ionize and release hydrogen, thus acting as an acid. The amino group can accept hydrogen, thus acting as a base. This ability allows proteins to act as a buffer system. The protein buffer system is found inside cells, especially in the hemoglobin of red blood cells, where the proteins can act to maintain the pH inside the cell. They are also found in the plasma.

SUBSTANCE MOVEMENT

Substances must be able to both enter and leave cells. For example, oxygen and various end products of digestion must enter a cell through the cell membrane for use by the cell. Waste products from cellular processes must be eliminated from the cell. Various ions must also both enter and leave cells. Everything that enters and leaves the cell must pass through the cell membrane. Thus the cell membrane serves not only as an envelope around the cell, but also as a gatekeeper, regulating which substances can enter and leave the cell. The cell membrane is a very thin and delicate, but complex and living, elastic covering around each cell. It consists of an inner and outer layer of phospholipids in which protein molecules are embedded. Many small channels pass through the membrane. These channels allow some water molecules and some water-soluble substances to pass through the membrane. The ability of a membrane to permit substances to pass through it is called **permeability.** Because a cell membrane allows passage of only certain substances, it is called a selective permeable membrane, or **semipermeable membrane.**

Some substances can pass through the cell membrane without energy expenditure on the part of the cell. This is called passive transport. The passage of other substances requires an expenditure of energy by the cell. This is called active transport.

Passive Transport

There are several types of passive transport: diffusion, osmosis, and filtration.

Diffusion

Diffusion is the tendency of molecules of either gases, liquids, or solids to move from a region of higher molecular concentration to a region of lower molecular concentration until an equilibrium is reached. This movement is caused by the kinetic energy in molecules. Kinetic energy causes the molecules to move constantly, colliding with one another and knocking each other about, thus causing them to move farther apart. An example is a drop of black ink placed in a glass of water; over time, the glass of water will turn a uniform black color because of diffusion, as shown in Figure 21-4.

In the body, oxygen moves by diffusion from the lungs to the bloodstream because the oxygen concentration is higher in the lungs and lower in the blood. Carbon dioxide moves by diffusion from the bloodstream, where the concentration of carbon dioxide is higher, to the lungs, for elimination. The size of the channels in the cell membrane can prevent large molecules from passing through the membrane. Some substances, such as glucose molecules, combine with carrier molecules, which carry them into the interior of the cell, where they are released.

The term **dialysis** is used when diffusion is employed to separate molecules out of a solution by passing them through a semipermeable membrane. Dialysis is the process used in the artificial kidney. As blood from a client circulates through a machine, small, toxic waste molecules such as urea leave the blood and pass through the semipermeable membrane by diffusion and out into the surrounding fluid. The blood, thus cleaned, is then returned to the body.

Osmosis

Osmosis is the diffusion of water through a semipermeable membrane from a region of higher water concentration to a region of lower water concentration. In a solution undergoing osmosis, only the water (solvent) molecules move through the membrane; the dissolved molecules do not (Figure 21-5).

If a cell, having both a membrane that will not allow sodium chloride to pass through and a molecular concentration of 10% sodium chloride, were placed in a container with a 5% sodium chloride solution, the cell would contain 10% sodium chloride and 90% water, and the 5% solution in which it was placed would contain 5% dissolved sodium chloride and 95% water. There would be more water outside than inside the cell; thus water would pass through the membrane into the cell. Because the cell membrane is elastic, the cell would increase in size as a result of the water accumulation within it facilitated by the process of osmosis. The pressure exerted against the cell membrane by the water inside the cell is called **osmotic pressure.**

A solution that has the same molecular concentration as the cell is called an **isotonic solution.** It neither increases nor decreases the size of the cell. A solution that has a lower molecular concentration than the cell is

Figure 21-4 *Diffusion is the spreading of particles from an area of greater concentration to an area of lesser concentration. Dye put into a beaker of water gradually spreads throughout the water.*

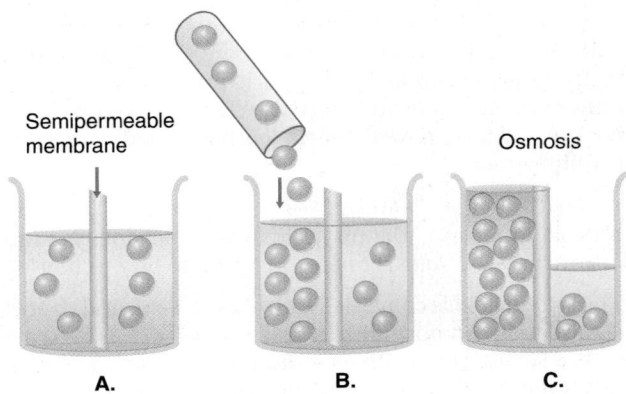

Semipermeable membrane

Osmosis

A.   B.   C.

Figure 21-5 *The Process of Osmosis*

called a **hypotonic solution.** Placing cells in a hypotonic solution causes them to swell, possibly to the point of eventual rupture. The rupture of red blood cells due to osmosis is called **hemolysis.** As red blood cells swell, the hemoglobin contained within passes to the outside of the cell and into the solution surrounding the cell, rendering the blood cells no longer capable of carrying oxygen. A solution that has a higher molecular concentration than the cell is called a **hypertonic solution.** When placed in such a solution, water leaves the cell, and the cell decreases in size. In the case of red blood cells, they shrivel and become wrinkled. This shrinkage, called **crenation,** leaves the cells incapable of functioning.

In persons who have lost large volumes of blood, it is sometimes necessary to administer additional fluids to maintain blood pressure. Generally, normal saline can be used. This 0.9% sodium chloride solution has approximately the same osmotic concentration as blood. Because it is isotonic, it will not damage the cells. Figure 21-6 shows osmosis in cells with different solution concentrations.

Filtration

In **filtration,** fluids and the substances dissolved in them are forced through cell membranes by **hydrosta-**

Figure 21-6 *Osmosis is the movement of water through a membrane from an area of lower concentration to one of higher concentration.* **A,** *In a hypotonic solution, the water moves into the cells, causing them to swell and burst.* **B,** *In an isotonic solution, cells are normal in size and shape because the same amount of water is entering and leaving the cells.* **C,** *In a hypertonic solution, cells are losing water because water moves from an area of lower concentration (inside the cell) to an area of higher concentration (outside the cell).*

tic pressure—the pressure the fluid exerts against the membrane. The molecules passing through the membrane are determined by the size of the pores in the membrane. Tissue fluids are formed by filtration. As blood passes through the capillaries, hydrostatic pressure exerted by the pumping action of the heart causes some of the liquid fraction of the blood (but not the cells) to pass out of the capillaries, resulting in formation of the tissue fluid (Figure 21-7). As the blood circulates through the capillaries of the kidneys, the hydrostatic pressure of the blood causes many materials to leave the blood through the filtration process. These materials pass into the tubules of the kidneys, where the toxic waste products are removed to form urine. The urine is then eliminated from the body.

Active Transport

In the processes discussed thus far, the movement of molecules depends on the concentration of molecules or on pressure. In other words, the cells do not have to expend energy to move the molecules in or out of the cell. In active transport, the cell must use energy to move the molecules. For instance, in the body, sodium ions are in higher concentration in the fluids surrounding the cell than inside the cell. Although some sodium ions can diffuse into the cell, the cell actively transports them through the membrane to the outside. Active transport is accomplished by means of carrier molecules, which can latch onto specific molecules and transport them in or out of the cell. This process requires an expenditure of cellular energy (Figure 21-8). Examples of important ions transported by this process are calcium, sodium, potassium, and magnesium.

FLUID AND ELECTROLYTE BALANCE

Human life is suspended in a saline solution having a salt concentration of 0.9%. This solution, which both surrounds the cells and is contained within them, constitutes the body fluids. The water and electrolytes composing these body fluids come from ingested water and nutrients, and from the water that results from metabolism.

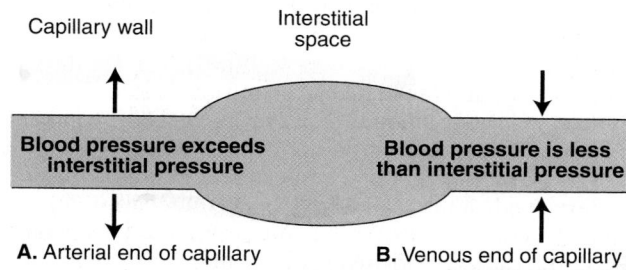

Figure 21-7 *Filtration:* **A,** *Pressure in the arteriole is greater then interstitial (between the cells) pressure, causing fluid with dissolved substances to move out of capillaries.* **B,** *Pressure in venules is less than interstitial fluid pressure, causing fluid and waste products to move back into the capillaries.*

Figure 21-8 *Active Transport of Molecules from an Area of Lesser Concentration to an Area of Greater Concentration*

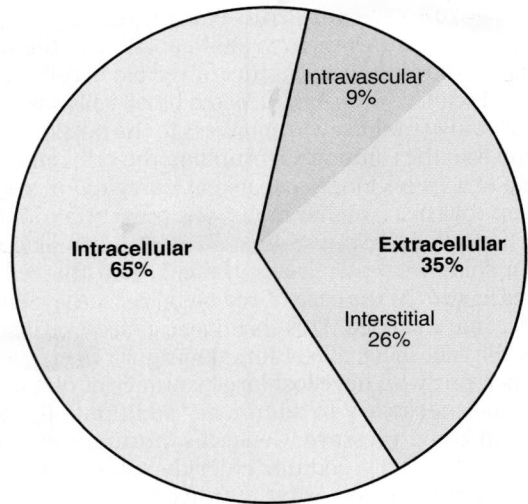

Figure 21-9 *Body Fluid Compartments of an Adult*

For life to continue and the cells to function properly, the body fluids must remain fairly constant with regard to the amount of water and the specific electrolytes of which they are composed. Water is essential because it is the basic component of all the body fluids. Water is involved in many of the metabolic processes in the body and is a by-product of some of these reactions. The various electrolytes all have essential roles in cellular physiological processes. If some of either is lost, it must be replaced, and if either water or an electrolyte is in excess, it must be removed. Maintaining the consistency of this fluid environment is homeostasis.

For cells to survive and carry out their multitude of physiologic functions, they need both a continuing source of water, nutrients, and oxygen and a mechanism to remove cellular wastes. These physiologic processes affect the amount of water, the pH, and the ions both inside and outside the cells. A balance must be maintained between the components of the fluids inside and outside the cell. Because the ions are dissolved in water, these two components are tied together: Anything affecting the amount of water in the body will affect the ion concentration.

Body Fluids

Much of the body weight of an average adult is due to the water in the body fluids surrounding the cells and contained within them. The fluid around the cells cushions them and serves as the medium of exchange. Everything that enters or leaves the cells must pass through this fluid layer.

There are two kinds of body fluids. They can be thought of as being contained within two separate containers, called compartments. The **intracellular fluid** (ICF) compartment contains all of the water and ions inside the cells. By far the largest amount of water in the body, approximately 65%, is found within this compartment.

The extracellular fluid compartment contains the remaining body fluids, called **extracellular fluid** (ECF), or fluid outside the cells. These can be further subdivided into interstitial, intravascular, and other fluids. **Interstitial fluid** is the fluid in the tissue spaces around each cell. The **intravascular fluid** is the plasma in the blood vessels and the lymph in the lymphatic system (Figure 21-9). There are also small amounts of other specialized body fluids such as synovial fluid, cerebrospinal

fluid, serous fluid, aqueous and vitreous humor, and the endolymph and perilymph. The proportions of extracellular fluid and intracellular fluid vary with age.

Generally speaking, the major ions in the extracellular fluid are sodium (Na^+), chloride (Cl^-), and bicarbonate (HCO_3^-), although other ions do occur. In the intracellular fluid, the major ions are potassium (K^+), phosphate (PO_4^{--}), and magnesium (Mg^{++}), with lesser amounts of other ions present. There are also large numbers of protein molecules bearing a negative charge.

Exchange between the Extracellular and Intracellular Fluids

Water and ions moving between the extracellular and intracellular fluids must first pass through the selectively permeable cell membrane. This movement is governed primarily by osmosis. Diffusion and active transport also play a role.

The difference in the ion concentration inside the cell and outside the cell is primarily due to the cell's ability to pump some ions inside and pump others out. If the intracellular fluid becomes hypertonic to the extracellular fluid, water from the extracellular fluid will move by osmosis into the cell to restore the balance, and vice versa.

A fluid balance also occurs between the interstitial fluid and the plasma. This balance is regulated primarily by hydrostatic pressure (blood pressure) and osmotic pressure. When the circulating blood passes from the arterioles into the capillaries, the pressure in the capillaries is higher than that in the interstitial fluid. This forces some of the water from the plasma out of the capillaries and into the interstitial fluid. Because of osmotic pressure, some of the water in the interstitial fluid is forced back into the capillaries in the area where they join the venules. Some water is also returned to the bloodstream through the lymphatic system. If the amount of interstitial fluid returned to the circulatory system lessens and the fluid accumulates in the tissue spaces, the tissues become swollen. This condition is called **edema.** Several conditions can cause edema, including kidney or liver disease and heart disorders. Many of these conditions can have serious consequences.

When more water is lost from the body than is replaced, **dehydration** occurs. Among the various causes of dehydration are water deprivation, excessive urine production, profuse sweating, diarrhea, and extended periods of vomiting. As water is lost, the amount of water in the interstitial fluid decreases. Water then moves from the cells to the tissue spaces by osmosis, causing an electrolyte imbalance. Circulatory impairment occurs, which in turn affects the kidney's ability to function normally. This condition is corrected by supplying water and the appropriate electrolytes.

Regulators of Fluid and Electrolyte Balance

There must be a balance in the amounts of fluids and electrolytes consumed and lost daily. Under typical conditions, the average adult loses some water through the skin, lungs, and GI tract and loses the largest amount of water through urine production. This can amount to a per-day fluid loss of approximately 2,500 mL, depending on conditions.

Skin

In the average adult, an estimated water loss of 300 to 400 mL per day occurs by diffusion through the skin. Because the person is not aware of this water loss, it is called *insensible loss.* Water is also lost through the skin by perspiration. The total amount of water lost through perspiration varies depending on environmental factors and body temperature.

Lungs

In the average adult, an estimated insensible water loss of 300 to 400 mL per day occurs with expired air, which is saturated with water vapor. This amount varies with the rate and depth of respirations.

Gastrointestinal Tract

Although a large amount of fluid—approximately 8,000 mL per day in the average adult—is secreted into the gastrointestinal tract, almost all of this fluid is reabsorbed by the body. In adults, approximately 200 mL of water is lost per day in feces. Severe diarrhea can cause a fluid and electrolyte deficit because the GI fluids contain a large amount of electrolytes.

Kidneys

The kidneys play a major role in maintaining fluid balance by excreting 1,200 to 1,500 mL of water per day in the average adult. The excretion of water by healthy kidneys is proportional to the fluid ingested and the amount of waste or solutes excreted.

When an extracellular fluid volume deficit occurs, hormones play a key role in restoring the extracellular fluid volume. Release of the following hormones into circulation causes the kidneys to conserve water:

- *Antidiuretic hormone (ADH).* Released by the posterior pituitary gland; acts on the distal tubules of the kidneys to reabsorb water
- *Aldosterone.* Produced in the adrenal cortex; causes the reabsorption of sodium from the renal tubules, leading to water retention in the extracellular fluid, thereby increasing its volume
- *Renin.* Released by the juxtaglomerular cells of the kidneys; promotes vasoconstriction and the release of aldosterone

The interaction of these hormones with regard to renal functions serves as the body's compensatory mechanism to maintain homeostasis.

Sodium is the main electrolyte that promotes the retention of water. An intravascular water deficit causes the renal tubules to reabsorb more sodium into circulation. Because water molecules go with the sodium ions, the intravascular water deficit is corrected by this action of the renal tubules.

Fluid and Food Intake

Fluids must be replaced in the amounts lost. The primary source of fluid replacement is water consumption. Approximately 60% may be obtained in this way, with an additional 30% being obtained from foods and 8% to 10% being a product of metabolism (metabolic water), for a total of 2,500 mL. Figure 21-10 illustrates fluid balance.

Figure 21-10 *Water Balance*

Thirst

Water consumption usually occurs in response to the sensation of thirst. This mechanism is poorly understood. It is generally believed to be brought about by the loss of body fluids, which in turn causes a dryness in the mouth and the thirst sensation. Replacing the lost fluids by water consumption causes the sensation to diminish. The thirst mechanism appears to be regulated by the hypothalamus in the brain.

Dehydration is one of the most common and most serious fluid imbalances that can result from poor monitoring of fluid intake. One nursing goal is to ensure that all clients understand both the role that water plays in health and the way to maintain adequate hydration.

DISTURBANCES IN ELECTROLYTE BALANCE

In health, normal homeostatic mechanisms function to maintain electrolyte balance. In illness, one or more of the regulating mechanisms may be affected, or an imbalance may become too great for the body to correct without treatment. Electrolytes are measured by laboratory analysis of a blood sample.

Sodium

Sodium (Na^+) is the major electrolyte in extracellular fluid. It regulates fluid balance through osmotic pressure that results from water following sodium in the body. Sodium stimulates conduction of nerve impulses and helps maintain neuromuscular activity. Excretion occurs primarily via the kidneys. The normal serum sodium for an adult is 136 to 145 mEq/L. Critical values are <130 or >160 mEq/L (Daniels, 2002).

Hyponatremia

A subnormal serum sodium value indicates hyponatremia. The cause is either a sodium deficit or a water excess. A hypo-osmotic state exists: The water moves out of the vascular space, into the interstitial space, and then into the intracellular space, causing edema. Hyponatremia may be caused by prolonged vomiting, diarrhea, or gastric or intestinal suctioning. This can be life threatening.

Hypernatremia

An elevated serum sodium level indicates hypernatremia. Excess sodium or a loss of water causes a rise in the extracellular osmotic pressure and pulls water out of the cells and into the extracellular space.

Potassium

Potassium (K^+) is the major electrolyte in intracellular fluid. Its concentration inside cells is approximately 150 mEq/L. The normal value range of extracellular (serum) potassium is narrow: 3.5 to 5.5 mEq/L. Critical values are <2.5 or >6.5 mEq/L (Daniels, 2002). Consequently, the slightest changes can dramatically affect physiological functions. Potassium maintains normal nerve and muscle activity, especially of the heart,

---

and osmotic pressure within the cells. It also assists in the cellular metabolism of carbohydrates and proteins. The kidneys prefer to retain sodium and excrete potassium, even when both electrolytes are depleted. When potassium is lost from cells, sodium and hydrogen move into the cells. This aids in regulating acid–base balance. Intracellular potassium deficit may coexist with an excess of extracellular potassium.

Hypokalemia

A low serum potassium level indicates hypokalemia. Excessive loss of gastric fluids and the use of diuretics can place the client at risk for hypokalemia and an acid–base imbalance (metabolic alkalosis). Potassium-wasting diuretics, such as furosemide (Lasix) or chlorothiazide (Diuril) can cause hypokalemia.

 Safety: Potassium Chloride
- Use IV route only when hypokalemia is life threatening or when oral replacement is not feasible.
- Always dilute potassium chloride in a large amount of IV solution.
- Never administer more than 10 mEq/L of IV potassium chloride (KCl) per hour; the normal dose of IV KCl is 20 to 40 mEq/L infused over an 8-hour period.
- Never give KCl intramuscularly (IM) or as an IV bolus; potentially fatal hyperkalemia may result.
- Monitor the IV site frequently for early signs of infiltration, as potassium is caustic to the tissues.

Hyperkalemia

An elevated serum potassium level indicates hyperkalemia. Clients with renal disease develop hyperkalemia because potassium cannot be excreted adequately by the kidneys. Extensive trauma causes potassium to be released from the cells and enter the bloodstream, leading to hyperkalemia. Hyperkalemia inhibits the action of digitalis. This condition is much more critical than is hypokalemia.

Calcium

Calcium (Ca^{++}) plays an essential role in bone and teeth integrity, blood clotting, muscle functioning, and nerve impulse transmission. Vitamin D is required for absorption of calcium from the GI tract. Only 1% of the body's calcium is found in the blood plasma (serum).

Normally, 50% of the serum calcium is ionized (physiologically active), with the remaining 50% being bound to protein. Free, ionized calcium is needed for cell membrane permeability. The calcium that is bound to plasma protein cannot pass through the capillary wall and, therefore, cannot leave the intravascular compartment. Total serum calcium concentration measures both the ionized calcium and the calcium bound to albumin. The normal value range of total serum calcium concentration for an adult is 8.5 to 10.5 mg/dL. Critical values are <7.0 or >12 mg/dL. Values for the older adult are slightly lower (Daniels, 2002).

Hypocalcemia

Hypocalcemia is indicated by a low serum calcium level. Alkalosis, elevated serum albumin, and the rapid administration of citrated blood increase the activity of calcium binders, thereby decreasing the amount of free calcium.

Hypercalcemia

An elevated total serum calcium level indicates hypercalcemia. Generally, three separate evaluations of either total serum calcium or ionized serum calcium are performed before a diagnosis of hypercalcemia is made. Hypercalcemia is often a symptom of an underlying disease such as metastatic bone tumors, Paget's disease, acromegaly, and hyperparathyroidism, which all increase bone reabsorption and, thereby, foster the release of calcium into circulating blood. Calcium-containing antacids and excess calcium from the diet may also cause hypercalcemia.

Magnesium

Most magnesium (Mg^{++}) is found in intracellular fluid and in combination with calcium and phosphorus

in bone, muscle, and soft tissue. Blood serum contains only approximately 1%. Magnesium plays an important role as a coenzyme, in the metabolism of carbohydrates and proteins, and as a mediator, in neuromuscular activity. It is the only cation that is found in higher concentration in cerebrospinal fluid than in extracellular fluid. When a magnesium deficiency develops, the body conserves magnesium at the expense of excreting potassium. A close relationship exists between magnesium, calcium, and potassium in the intracellular fluid: A low level of one results in low levels of the other two. The normal serum magnesium level for an adult is 1.6 to 2.6 mEq/L (Daniels, 2002).

Hypomagnesemia

A serum magnesium level of <1.0 mEq/L indicates hypomagnesemia (Daniels, 2002), which most commonly results from chronic alcoholism. Increased renal excretion is associated with prolonged diuretic therapy or use of gentamicin (Garamycin), cyclosporin (Sandimmune), or cisplatin (Platinol).

Hypermagnesemia

A serum magnesium level of >5.0 mEq/L indicates hypermagnesemia (Daniels, 2002). This condition rarely occurs if kidney function is normal. An increased magnesium level is associated with uncontrolled diabetes (ketoacidosis), renal failure, and ingestion of magnesium antacids (Maalox, Mylanta) or laxatives (milk of magnesia [MOM], magnesium citrate [Citromal]).

 Safety: Magnesium Level
When the serum magnesium level reaches 10 to 15 mEq/L, respiratory paralysis may occur.

Phosphate

Phosphate (PO_4^{--}) is the main intracellular anion. It appears as phosphorus in the serum, where the normal value range is 3.0 to 4.5 mg/dL (Daniels, 2002). Phosphorus is critical for normal cell functioning. Most phosphorus is found combined with calcium in teeth and bones. Phosphate and calcium exist in an inverse relationship (i.e., as one increases the other decreases).

Hypophosphatemia

A client with a low serum phosphorus level has hypophosphatemia. Rarely does this condition result from decreased dietary intake. More commonly, it stems from respiratory alkalosis. Intense, prolonged hyperventilation can cause severe hypophosphatemia.

Hyperphosphatemia

A client with an elevated serum phosphorus level has hyperphosphatemia. This condition most commonly results from renal failure with resultant decreased renal phosphorus excretion. Excessive use of phosphate-containing laxatives or phosphate enemas may cause hyperphosphatemia.

Chloride

Chloride (Cl^-) is the major anion in extracellular fluid. Chloride functions in combination with sodium to maintain osmotic pressure. It also assists in maintaining acid–base balance. When the carbon dioxide level increases, bicarbonate shifts from the intracellular compartment to the extracellular compartment. Chloride, in an effort to maintain homeostasis, then moves into the intracellular compartment. The kidneys selectively excrete chloride or bicarbonate ions depending on the acid–base balance. The normal serum chloride range is 98 to 106 mmol/L. Critical values are <70 or >120 mmol/L (Daniels, 2002).

Hypochloremia

A low serum chloride level indicates hypochloremia. Excess losses of chloride may result from prolonged diarrhea or diaphoresis. Loss of hydrochloric acid related to vomiting, gastric suctioning, or gastric surgery may cause hypochloremia.

Hyperchloremia

An elevated serum chloride level indicates hyperchloremia, which usually occurs in conjunction with dehydration, hypernatremia, or metabolic acidosis.

ACID–BASE BALANCE

As described earlier, the body maintains a normal pH within the relatively narrow range of 7.35 to 7.45. Body

pH is maintained by the buffer systems, the respiratory system, and the kidneys. A pH below 7.35 is termed acidosis, and a pH above 7.45 is termed alkalosis. Either of these conditions can be brought about by respiratory or metabolic changes.

Regulators of Acid–Base Balance

The body has three main control systems that regulate acid–base balance to counter acidosis or alkalosis: the buffer systems, respirations, and renal control of hydrogen ion concentration. These systems vary in their reaction times in regulating and restoring balance to the hydrogen ion concentration.

Buffer Systems

The buffer systems—bicarbonate, phosphate, and protein—were previously discussed. They react quickly to prevent excessive changes in the hydrogen ion concentration.

Respiratory Regulation of Acid–Base Balance

The respiratory system helps maintain acid–base balance by controlling the content of carbon dioxide in extracellular fluid. The *rate of metabolism* determines the formation of carbon dioxide. Various intracellular metabolic processes continuously form carbon dioxide in the body. The carbon in foods is **oxidized** (joined with oxygen) to form carbon dioxide.

It takes the respiratory regulatory mechanism several minutes to respond to changes in the carbon dioxide concentration of extracellular fluid. With the increase of carbon dioxide in extracellular fluid, respiration increases in rate and depth so that more carbon dioxide is exhaled. As the respiratory system removes carbon dioxide, less carbon dioxide is present in the blood to combine with water to form carbonic acid. Likewise, if the blood level of carbon dioxide is low, respirations decrease to maintain a normal ratio between carbonic acid and basic bicarbonate.

Renal Control of Hydrogen Ion Concentration

The kidneys control extracellular fluid pH by eliminating either hydrogen ions or bicarbonate ions from body fluids. If the bicarbonate concentration in the extracellular fluid is greater than normal, the kidneys excrete more bicarbonate ions, making the urine more alkaline. Conversely, if more hydrogen ions are excreted in the urine, the urine becomes more acidic. The renal mechanism for regulating acid–base balance cannot readjust the pH within seconds, as can the extracellular fluid buffer system, nor within minutes, as can the respiratory compensatory mechanism; but it can function over a period of several hours or days to correct acid–base imbalance.

Diagnostic and Laboratory Data

The biochemical indicators of acid–base balance are assessed by measuring the **arterial blood gases** (ABGs). The arterial blood gas test measures the levels of oxygen and carbon dioxide in arterial blood. The test assesses pH, partial pressure of oxygen (PO_2 or PaO_2), partial pressure of carbon dioxide (PCO_2 or $PaCO_2$), saturation of oxygen (SaO_2), and bicarbonate (HCO_3). pH has already been discussed.

The PO_2 or PaO_2 expresses the amount of oxygen that can combine with hemoglobin to form oxyhemoglobin, the form in which oxygen is transported through the body. At sea level, the normal range is 80 to 100 millimeters of mercury (mm Hg). The rate at which the oxygen/hemoglobin reaction occurs is influenced by pH. The rate decreases as the pH value decreases.

The PCO_2 or $PaCO_2$ in the blood is a reflection of the efficiency of gaseous exchange in the lungs. At sea level, the normal range is 35 to 45 mm Hg. If the alveoli are obstructed or damaged by disease, carbon dioxide cannot be eliminated and will combine with water to form carbonic acid, which in turn causes acidosis. Conversely, in a person who is hyperventilating, too much carbon dioxide is eliminated, which may trigger alkalosis.

The SaO_2 is the percentage of oxygen that combines with hemoglobin in the blood. The normal range is 95% to 100% saturation. This value, along with the PO_2 and hemoglobin levels, indicates the degree to which the tissues are receiving oxygen. Oxygen saturation can also be measured with a pulse oximeter, a noninvasive technique.

Determining the amount of bicarbonate (HCO_3) in the blood is important because, along with carbonic acid, bicarbonate is a major buffer in the blood. The two substances occur in a ratio of 20 parts bicarbonate to 1 part carbonic acid. Regardless of the carbonic acid and bicarbonate values, the pH of the blood will remain in the normal range as long as the ratio remains 20:1. The normal range for HCO_3 at sea level is 24 to 28 mEq/L. The carbonic acid level is always 3% of the PCO_2 level.

DISTURBANCES IN ACID–BASE BALANCE

The acid–base imbalances are respiratory acidosis and alkalosis and metabolic acidosis and alkalosis. In determining whether the acid–base imbalance is caused by a respiratory or a metabolic alteration, the key indicators are bicarbonate and carbonic acid levels (Figure 21-11). Table 21-2 lists those changes in laboratory values that indicate the various acid–base imbalances.

Respiratory Acidosis

When carbon dioxide is not eliminated by the lungs as fast as it is produced by cellular metabolism, the amount of carbon dioxide increases in the blood. It then reacts

Figure 21-11 *Acid–Base Balance and Imbalance*

with water and forms excess hydrogen ions, as shown in the following reaction:

$$CO_2 + H_2O \rightarrow H^+ + HCO_3$$

In respiratory acidosis there is an increased concentration of hydrogen ions (a blood pH below 7.35), an increased PCO_2 level (greater than 45 mm Hg), and an excess of carbonic acid. It is caused by hypoventilation or any condition that depresses ventilation. Hypoventilation can be caused by brain injury, chest injuries, emphysema, and chronic obstructive pulmonary disease (COPD). When the respiratory rate and the amount of oxygen supplied to the lungs suddenly lessen, acute respiratory acidosis can occur. This condition can be life threatening, and it must be recognized and corrected quickly. Chronic respiratory acidosis occurs when the respiratory rate is continually depressed.

Clients with respiratory acidosis experience neurological changes as a result of the cerebrospinal fluid and brain cells acidity. Hypoventilation causes **hypoxemia** (decreased oxygen in the blood), which in turn causes further neurological impairment. Hyperkalemia may accompany acidosis.

Respiratory Alkalosis

In respiratory alkalosis there is a decreased concentration of hydrogen ions (a blood pH above 7.45) and

SITUATION	PH	PCO₂	HCO₃
TABLE 21-2 — LABORATORY VALUES IN ACID–BASE IMBALANCES			
Normal parameters	7.35 to 7.45	35 to 45 mm Hg	24 to 28 mEq/L
Respiratory acidosis			
Acute	<7.35	>45 mm Hg	Normal
Chronic	<7.35	>45 mm Hg	>28 mEq/L
Respiratory alkalosis	>7.45	<35 mm Hg	Normal
Metabolic acidosis	<7.35	Normal	<24 mEq/L
Metabolic alkalosis	>7.45	Normal	>28 mEq/L

PROFESSIONAL TIP

Metabolic Alkalosis

The following clinical conditions can place clients at risk for metabolic alkalosis:

- Vomiting and nasogastric suctioning or lavage cause a loss of hydrochloric acid and chloride. With the loss of the hydrogen and chloride ions, bicarbonate ions are absorbed, unneutralized, into the bloodstream, and the pH of the extracellular fluid rises (alkalosis).
- Diarrhea and steroid or diuretic therapy can cause excessive loss of potassium, chloride, and other electrolytes. The potassium deficit causes the kidneys to exchange hydrogen ions (instead of potassium ions) for sodium ions, which promotes the loss of hydrogen, thereby increasing bicarbonate level.

acids. The kidneys try to increase the pH and the excretion of hydrogen by exchanging sodium ions for hydrogen ions. Metabolic acidosis is most common in individuals with kidney disease or diabetes mellitus.

Metabolic Alkalosis

In metabolic alkalosis there is a loss of acid from the body or a gain in base (increased level of bicarbonate). Blood pH is above 7.45. Excessive ingestion of antacids and milk may cause a gain in base. These substances neutralize acids, resulting in alkalosis and hypercalcemia. Excessive oral or parenteral intake of sodium bicarbonate or other alkaline salts (e.g., sodium or potassium acetate, lactate, or citrate) increases the amount of base in extracellular fluid. Loss of gastric fluids from vomiting or suctioning may result in metabolic alkalosis.

The renal and respiratory compensatory mechanisms respond to an increased bicarbonate/carbonic acid ratio. In an effort to retain carbon dioxide, the rate and depth of respirations decreases. To counter the pH imbalance of metabolic alkalosis, the arterial carbon dioxide concentration rises, creating respiratory acidosis.

A normal serum potassium level is necessary for renal compensation. When potassium ions enter the cells in exchange for hydrogen ions, in alkalosis hypokalemia results. The kidneys cannot function as a compensatory mechanism when hypokalemia is present; they continue to excrete hydrogen, and bicarbonate excess continues.

NURSING PROCESS

The nursing process assists the nurse in planning client care.

Assessment

Assessment data are used to identify clients who have potential or actual alterations in fluid volume. Electrolyte and acid–base imbalances are identified primarily with laboratory data, while fluid balances are identified primarily with the health history and physical examination.

PROFESSIONAL TIP

Electrolyte Shift

An electrolyte shift occurs in metabolic acidosis. Hydrogen and sodium ions move into the cells, and potassium moves into the extracellular fluid. Hyperkalemia may cause ventricular fibrillation and death.

a below-normal PCO₂ level (lower than 35 mm Hg). It is caused by hyperventilation (excessive exhalation of carbon dioxide) resulting in hypocapnia (decreased arterial carbon dioxide concentration). As the breathing rate increases, the amount of carbon dioxide in the blood decreases, which in turn increases the pH of the blood.

Hyperventilation can be triggered by anxiety, fear, fever, pain, rapid mechanical ventilation, and hypoxia at high altitudes. This condition is usually self-correcting. As the breathing returns to normal, the carbon dioxide level in the blood increases, and the normal pH is restored. Other causes of hyperventilation, which involves overstimulation of the respiratory center, include salicylate poisoning, brain tumors, meningitis, encephalitis, and pulmonary embolus.

Metabolic Acidosis

In metabolic acidosis there is an increased concentration of hydrogen ions (blood pH below 7.35) or a decrease in bicarbonate concentration. Such a change may be brought about by kidney disease when the mechanism to excrete excess hydrogen ions is compromised. Diarrhea, diabetes mellitus, and, sometimes, diuretics may also be responsible. The lungs eliminate more carbon dioxide but are usually ineffective in decreasing

Health History

The nursing history should elicit data in the following areas:

- Lifestyle (sociocultural and economic factors, stress, exercise)
- Dietary intake (recent changes in the amount and types of fluid and food, increased thirst)
- Weight (sudden gain or loss)
- Fluid output (recent changes in the frequency or amount of urine output)
- Gastrointestinal disturbances (prolonged vomiting, diarrhea, anorexia, ulcer, hemorrhage)
- Fever and diaphoresis
- Burns, trauma, draining wounds
- Disease conditions that can upset homeostasis (renal disease, endocrine disorders, neural malfunction, pulmonary disease)
- Therapeutic programs that can produce imbalances (special diets, medications, chemotherapy, IV fluid or total parenteral nutrition [TPN] administration, gastric or intestinal suction)

Physical Examination

Because fluid alterations may affect any body system, the nurse performs a complete physical examination and identifies all abnormalities.

Daily Weight Changes in the body's total fluid volume are reflected in body weight. For instance, each liter (1,000 mL) of fluid gained or lost is equivalent to 1 kilogram (2.2 lb) of weight.

Vital Signs The client with an elevated temperature is at risk for dehydration related to an increased loss of body fluid. Changes in the pulse rate, strength, and rhythm may indicate fluid alterations. Fluid volume changes may cause the following pulse changes:

- *Fluid volume deficit.* Increased pulse rate and weak pulse strength
- *Fluid volume excess.* Increased pulse strength and third heart sound

Inspect chest wall movement, count the respiratory rate, and auscultate the lungs to assess respiratory changes. Rate and depth changes may cause respiratory acid–base imbalances or may indicate a compensatory response to metabolic acidosis or alkalosis.

The degree of fluid volume deficit can be assessed by blood pressure measurements. Fluid volume deficit can lower the blood pressure. A narrow pulse pressure (lower than 20 mm Hg) may indicate severe hypovolemia (fluid volume deficit).

Intake and Output The client's I&O should be measured and recorded for a 24-hour period to assess for an actual or potential imbalance. A minimum intake of 1,500 mL is essential to balance urinary output and the body's insensible water loss. All liquids taken by mouth (e.g., soup, ice cream, gelatin, juice, and water) and liquids administered through tube feedings (nasogastric or jejunostomy) and parenterally (IV fluids and blood or its components) are included. Output includes urine, vomitus, diarrhea, and drainage from tubes such as gastric suction or surgical drains.

Safety: Fluid Measurements
To protect both the nurse and the client from transfer of microorganisms, Standard Precautions are always followed during fluid administration and output measurement.

Thirst Thirst is the most common indicator of fluid volume deficit. The hypothalamus triggers a thirst response when there is a decrease in extracellular fluid volume or an increase in plasma osmolality.

Food Intake Ingested food also helps maintain extracellular fluid volume. One-third of the body's fluid needs are met with ingested food. Electrolytes are also provided by food.

Skin Edema and skin turgor are two important indicators of fluid, electrolyte, and acid–base balances.

Edema The main symptom of fluid volume excess is edema. It may be confined to a specific area (localized) or occur throughout the body (generalized). The skin is taut, shiny, smooth, and pale in localized edema. Before edema is noticeable, the body may retain 5 to 10 pounds of fluid (Bulechek & McCloskey, 1999). The dependent body parts—sacrum, back, and legs—should be assessed for peripheral edema. Pitting edema is rated on a four-point scale, as follows:

+0: no pitting
+1: 0 to $^1/_4$ inch pitting (mild)
+2: $^1/_4$ to $^1/_2$ inch pitting (moderate)
+3: $^1/_2$ to 1 inch pitting (severe)
+4: greater than 1 inch pitting (severe)

Turgor Skin **turgor** refers to the normal resiliency of the skin, a reflection of hydration status. When skin is pinched and released, it springs back to a normal position because the cells and interstitial fluid exert outward pressure. To measure the client's skin turgor, use the thumb and forefinger to grasp and raise and then release a small section of skin. Dehydration is the main cause of decreased skin turgor, which manifests as lax skin that returns slowly to the normal position. Increased skin turgor, which occurs in conjunction with edema, manifests as smooth, taut, shiny skin that cannot be grasped and raised.

Buccal (Oral) Cavity The nurse should inspect the buccal cavity. With fluid volume deficit, saliva decreases, causing sticky, dry mucous membranes and dry, cracked lips. The tongue has longitudinal furrows.

Eyes The eyes should be inspected for sunkenness, dry conjunctiva, and decreased or absent tearing, all signs of fluid volume deficit. Puffy eyelids (periorbital edema or papilledema) are signs of fluid volume excess. The client may have a history of blurred vision.

LIFE CYCLE CONSIDERATIONS

Skin Turgor in Elderly Clients

The skin loses elasticity with aging, causing reduced skin turgor. In elderly clients, assess the tongue for creases or furrows to monitor dehydration (Hogstel, 2001).

Figure 21-12 *Client Position When Assessing Jugular Vein Distention*

Jugular and Hand Veins Circulatory volume is assessed by measuring venous filling of the jugular and hand veins. With the client in a low Fowler's position:

1. Palpate the jugular (neck) veins. Fluid volume excess causes a distention in the jugular veins (Figure 21-12).
2. Place the client's hand below heart level and palpate the hand veins. Fluid volume deficit causes decreased venous filling (flat hand veins).

Neuromuscular System Fluid and electrolyte imbalances may cause neuromuscular alterations. The muscles lose tone, becoming soft and flabby, and reflexes diminish. Calcium and magnesium imbalances cause an increase in neuromuscular irritability. To assess for neuromuscular irritability, the tests for Chvostek's sign and Trousseau's sign are performed. Other neurological signs of fluid, electrolyte, and acid–base imbalances include inability to concentrate, confusion, and emotional lability.

Diagnostic and Laboratory Data

Laboratory tests can reveal imbalances before clinical symptoms are evident in the client; however, unless clients are having the tests for some other reason, symptoms are detected first.

Hemoglobin and Hematocrit Indices The hemoglobin (Hgb) level decreases in the event of severe hemorrhage. Hematocrit (Hct) is affected by changes in plasma volume. For instance, with severe dehydration and hypovolemic shock, hematocrit increases. Conversely, overhydration decreases hematocrit.

Osmolality **Osmolality** is a measurement of the total concentration of dissolved particles (solutes) per kilogram of water. Osmolality measurements are performed on both serum and urine samples to identify changes in fluid and electrolyte balance.

Serum Osmolality Serum osmolality is a measurement of the total concentration of dissolved particles per kilogram of water in serum, recorded in milliosmoles per kilogram (mOsm/kg). The particles measured in serum osmolality include electrolyte ions (i.e., sodium and potassium), and electrically inactive substances (i.e., glucose and urea). Water and sodium are the main entities controlling the osmolality of body fluids. Serum sodium is responsible for 90% of the serum osmolality (Daniels,

2002). The normal range of serum osmolality is 280 to 295 mOsm/Kg (Daniels, 2002). The value increases with dehydration and decreases with water excess.

In clinical practice, the terms *osmolality* and **osmolarity** (the concentration of solutes per liter of cellular fluid) are often used interchangeably to refer to the concentration of body fluid; however, these terms actually have different meanings, in that *osmolality* refers to the concentration of solutes in the total body water rather than in cellular fluid. The appropriate term to use in conjunction with IV fluid therapy is *osmolarity* (Bulechek & McCloskey, 1999).

Urine Osmolality Urine osmolality measures the number of solute particles in a defined amount of solution. The particles measured are nitrogenous waste (creatinine, urea, and uric acid), with urea being predominant. Urine osmolality varies greatly with diet and fluid intake and reflects the kidney's ability to concentrate urine. The normal range of urine osmolality is 500 to 800 mOsm/kg (Daniels, 2002).

Urine pH The measurement of urine pH reveals the hydrogen ion concentration in the urine, indicating the urine's acidity or alkalinity. The pH of the urine should be within normal range (4.5 to 8.0) when the kidney buffering system is compensating for either metabolic acidosis or alkalosis. This is considered a sign of normal function; however, when the renal compensatory function fails to respond to the blood pH, the urine pH will either increase, with acidosis, or decrease, with alkalosis.

Nursing Diagnosis

NANDA (2003) identifies the primary nursing diagnoses for clients with fluid imbalances as *Deficient Fluid Volume, Excess Fluid Volume, Risk for Deficient Fluid Volume,* and *Risk for Imbalanced Fluid Volume.* Numerous secondary nursing diagnoses may also apply.

Deficient Fluid Volume

Deficient Fluid Volume is defined as "decreased intravascular, interstitial, and/or intracellular fluid. This refers to dehydration, water loss alone without change in sodium" (NANDA, 2003). The many causes of fluid volume deficit include:

- Excessive fluid loss resulting from diaphoresis, vomiting, diarrhea, hemorrhage, burns, ascites, wound drainage, indwelling tubes, or suction
- Diabetes insipidus
- Diabetes mellitus

- Addison's disease (adrenal insufficiency)
- Gastrointestinal fistula or draining abscess
- Intestinal obstruction

Assessment findings in the client with fluid volume deficit include thirst and weight loss of an amount consistent with the degree of dehydration. Marked dehydration manifests as dry mucous membranes and skin; poor skin turgor; low-grade temperature elevation; tachycardia; respirations of 28 or greater; decreased (10 to 15 mm Hg) systolic blood pressure; slowed venous filling; decreased urine output (less than 25 mL/hr); concentrated urine; elevated Hct, Hgb, and BUN; and acidic blood pH (less than 7.4).

Severe dehydration is characterized by the symptoms of marked dehydration plus a flushing of the skin. Systolic blood pressure continues to drop (60 mm Hg or below), and behavioral changes (restlessness, irritability, disorientation, and delirium) occur. The signs of fatal dehydration are anuria and coma, leading to death.

Excess Fluid Volume

Excess Fluid Volume is defined as "increased isotonic fluid retention" (NANDA, 2003). Fluid volume excess is related to excess fluid in either the tissues or the extremities (peripheral edema) or the lung tissues (pulmonary edema). The several causes of excess fluid volume include:

- Excessive fluid intake (e.g., IV therapy, sodium)
- Excessive loss or decreased intake of protein (chronic diarrhea, burns, kidney disease, malnutrition)
- Compromised regulatory mechanisms (kidney failure)
- Decreased intravascular movement (impaired myocardial contractility)
- Lymphatic obstruction (cancer, surgical removal of lymph nodes, obesity)
- Medications (steroid excess)
- Allergic reactions

The client with fluid volume excess will exhibit acute weight gain; decreased serum osmolality (lower than 275 mOsm/Kg), Hgb, Hct; protein and albumin, blood urea nitrogen (BUN); increased central venous pressure (greater than 12 to 15 cm H_2O); and signs and symptoms of edema. The clinical expressions of edema are relative to the area of involvement, either pulmonary or peripheral (Table 21-3).

Risk for Deficient Fluid Volume

Risk for Deficient Fluid Volume is defined as "at risk for experiencing vascular, cellular, or intracellular dehydra-

PROFESSIONAL TIP

Loss of Gastric Juices

Clients who lose excessive amounts of gastric juices, either through vomiting or suctioning, are prone to not only fluid volume deficit but also metabolic alkalosis, hypokalemia, and hyponatremia. Gastric juices contain hydrochloric acid, pepsinogen, potassium, and sodium.

TABLE 21-3 CLINICAL MANIFESTATIONS OF EDEMA

PULMONARY EDEMA	PERIPHERAL EDEMA
Cough	Pitting edema in extremities
Pink, frothy sputum	Edematous area: tight, smooth, dry
Dyspnea	
Cold, clammy skin	Shiny, pale, cool skin
Engorged neck and hand veins	Puffy eyelids
	Weight gain
Crackles and wheezes in lungs	
Tachypnea	
Tachycardia	

tion" (NANDA, 2003). The many factors that place a client at risk for fluid volume deficit were listed previously.

Risk for Imbalanced Fluid Volume

Risk for Imbalanced Fluid Volume is defined as "at risk for a decrease, increase, or rapid shift from one to the other of intravascular, interstitial, and/or intracellular fluid. This refers to body fluid loss, gain, or both" (NANDA, 2003). The greatest risk factor is a client undergoing a major invasive procedure.

Other Nursing Diagnoses

In clients with a fluid imbalance, the relationship between the primary nursing diagnoses previously discussed and the secondary nursing diagnoses is reciprocal: The primary nursing diagnoses influence and are influenced by the secondary nursing diagnoses. Some commonly identified secondary nursing diagnoses include:

- *Impaired **G**as Exchange*
- *Decreased **C**ardiac Output*
- *Ineffective **B**reathing Pattern*
- ***A**nxiety*
- *Disturbed **T**hought Processes*
- *Risk for **I**njury*
- *Risk for **I**nfection*
- *Impaired **O**ral Mucous Membrane*
- *Deficient **K**nowledge (specify)*

Planning/Outcome Identification

Holistic nursing care requires collaborating with each client to identify goals for each nursing diagnosis. These individualized goals should reflect the client's abilities and limitations.

Nursing interventions are selected and prioritized to support the client's achievement of expected outcomes based on the goals. For example, if vomiting and diarrhea along with dry mucous membranes and a 5% weight loss led to a nursing diagnosis of *Deficient Fluid Volume*, the goals might include to relieve vomiting and diarrhea and achieve the proper balance of intake and output.

Implementation

The nurse has a responsibility to collaborate with and advocate for clients to ensure they receive appropriate and ethical care based on practice standards. The data obtained from the history serve as the basis for formulating expected outcomes and selecting nursing interventions appropriate to the client's natural patterns as revealed in their history.

Interventions related to changes in fluid, electrolyte, or acid–base balance are based on the goal of maintaining homeostasis and regulating and maintaining essential fluids and nutrients. Clients' adaptive capabilities are kept in mind when selecting interventions based on the clients' perceptions of their support systems, strengths, and options.

The nurse is responsible for performing frequent assessments and monitoring for adverse effects of fluid and electrolyte therapy to prevent complications.

Nursing activities related to assessment and implementation often involve the same measurements (e.g., weight and vital signs). Common interventions that promote reaching expected outcomes for restoring and maintaining homeostasis are discussed following.

Monitor Daily Weight

One of the main indicators of fluid and electrolyte balance is weight. The accurate measuring and recording of the client's daily weight is a vital responsibility. This information along with other clinical findings determine fluid therapy requirements for the client.

Measure Vital Signs

The client's acuity level and clinical situation determine the frequency of vital sign measurement. For example, vital signs are taken every 15 minutes until stable on the typical postoperative client, whereas vital signs should be monitored continuously on the client in shock or hemorrhaging. Vital signs and other clinical data are used to determine the amount and type of fluid therapy.

Measure Intake and Output

Intake and output measurements monitor the client's fluid status over a 24-hour period. Agency policy for I&O may vary regarding:

- Times for charting (e.g., every 8 hours versus every 12 hours)
- Time when 24-hour totals are calculated
- Definition of "strict" I&O

COMMUNITY/HOME HEALTH CARE

Considerations for Measuring I&O

- Ask for client and family input to select household items for intake measurement.
- Provide containers for measuring output, adapting the urinary container to home facilities, and teach client and family about proper washing and storage of the containers.
- Teach proper hand hygiene.
- Provide written instructions on what is to be measured.
- Leave sufficient I&O forms to last until the nurse's next visit.
- Identify the parameters for evaluating a discrepancy between the intake and the output and for notifying the nurse or physician.

 Safety: Remove Gloves Before Charting
To prevent the transfer of microorganisms when the I&O form is removed from the client's room, remove gloves and wash hands before recording the amount of drainage on the form.

Review the client's 24-hour I&O calculations to evaluate fluid status. Intake should exceed output by 500 mL to offset insensible fluid loss. Intake and output and daily weight are critical interventions because they are used to evaluate the effectiveness of rehydration or diuretic therapy.

Having an accurate I&O requires the efforts of the client and family. The client and family must be taught how to measure and record the I&O.

Provide Oral Hygiene

Providing oral hygiene that promotes both client comfort and the integrity of the buccal cavity is an important responsibility. The condition of the client's buccal cavity and the type of fluid imbalance dictates the frequency of oral hygiene.

Initiate Oral Fluid Therapy

Depending on the client's clinical situation, oral fluids may be totally restricted, commonly referred to as *nothing by mouth* (NPO, which is from the Latin *non per os*), or they may be restricted or forced.

Nothing by Mouth Clients are designated NPO as prescribed by the physician. Based on agency policy and

---

PROFESSIONAL TIP

"Strict" I&O

- "Strict" I&O measurement usually involves accounting for incontinent urine, emesis, and diaphoresis and might require weighing soiled bed linens.
- *Gloves should always be worn when handling soiled linen.*

PROFESSIONAL TIP

Mouthwashes

Mouthwashes with alcohol or glycerin and swabs with lemon or glycerin may feel refreshing, but these ingredients dry the mucous membranes.

clarification from the physician, the client may be allowed small amounts of ice chips when designated NPO. The NPO status may be required to:

- Avoid aspiration in unconscious, perioperative, and preprocedural clients who will receive anesthesia or conscious sedation.
- Rest and heal the GI tract when there is severe vomiting or diarrhea or a GI disorder (inflammation or obstruction).
- Prevent more loss of gastric juices in clients on nasogastric suctioning.

Clients who are NPO should receive oral hygiene every 1 to 2 hours or as needed to prevent alterations of the mucous membranes and for comfort.

Restricted Fluids Fluid intake is commonly restricted when treating fluid volume excess related to heart and renal failure. Intake may be restricted to 200 mL in a 24-hour period.

The way fluids are limited should be determined in collaboration with the client. For example:

- Half of the allowed fluid might be divided between breakfast and lunch, and
- The remaining half might be divided between the evening meal and before bedtime, unless the client must be awakened during the night for medication.

Forced Fluids "Forcing" or encouraging the intake of oral fluids, mainly water, is sometimes done when treating clients who are at risk for dehydration or who have renal and urinary problems (kidney stones). Compliance is obtained through client education and honoring client preferences of timing and type of liquids. A client might, for example, be requested to consume 2,000 mL over a 24-hour period. Explain that this is only eight glasses or one glass every 2 hours. Also tell the client that ice, gelatin, soups, and ice cream all count as liquid.

Maintain Tube Feeding

The client who cannot ingest oral fluids but has a normal GI tract can have fluids and nutrients administered through a feeding tube as prescribed by a physician.

Monitor Intravenous Therapy

Fluid volume is replaced parenterally when fluid loss is severe or the client cannot tolerate oral or tube feedings. **Intravenous** (IV) **therapy** is the administration of fluids, electrolytes, nutrients, or medications by the venous route. The physician prescribes IV therapy to prevent or treat fluid, electrolyte, or nutritional imbalances. There are specific nursing responsibilities during IV therapy. Specifically, the nurse must:

- Know why the IV fluid is prescribed.
- Document client understanding.
- Select, according to agency policy, the appropriate equipment.
- Obtain the correct prescribed solution.
- Assess the client for allergies to iodine, tape, ointment, or antibiotic preparations used for skin preparation of the venipuncture site.
- Administer the fluid at the prescribed rate.
- Observe for signs of **infiltration** (seepage of the fluid into the interstitial tissue as a result of accidental dislodgement of the needle from the vein) and other complications that are fluid specific.
- Document in the client's medical record the implementation of the prescribed IV therapy.

Evaluation

Evaluation is an ongoing process. When evaluating whether the time frames and expected outcomes are realistic (such as whether the intake and output are within 200 to 300 mL of each other), the focus should be on the client's responses such as vital signs within normal limits, the IV infusion rate maintains the client's hydration, and the IV site remains free from erythema, edema, and purulent drainage. The nursing care plan should be modified as necessary to support the client's expected outcomes.

SAMPLE NURSING CARE PLAN

THE CLIENT WITH EXCESS FLUID VOLUME

When brought to the emergency department by his granddaughter, Mr. Gomez, a 68-year-old widower, stated, "I can't breathe." Mr. Gomez has a history of hypertension and heart disease, and he is obese. The practitioner ordered a stat chest x-ray, CBC, and electrolytes, which revealed pulmonary congestion (x-ray), decreased Hct, and decreased Hgb. The physical assessment results were as follows: Wt 162; TPR 97.6, 98, 30 (labored); BP 186/114; shortness of breath, crackles; constant cough; pitting edema (ankles); and engorged neck veins. Mr. Gomez stated, "I thought I could stop taking the heart medication and eat what I wanted when I felt good again."

Nursing Diagnosis 1   *Excess Fluid Volume* related to a compromised regulatory mechanism as evidenced by edema, shortness of breath, crackles, decreased Hgb and Hct, and jugular vein distention

Nursing Outcomes Classification (NOC)
Cardiac Pump Effectivenss
Respiratory Status: Ventilation

Nursing Interventions Classification (NIC)
Fluid Management
Medication Management

PLANNING/GOALS	NURSING INTERVENTIONS	RATIONALE
Mr. Gomez will have a balanced I&O for 2 days.	Measure and document hourly I&O; restrict fluids as ordered	Monitors fluid status
	Administer diuretics as ordered and document response	Increases excretion of fluids and electrolytes
Mr. Gomez will identify a specific amount of weight to lose over the next 6 months.	Weigh daily at the same time, with the same scale, and with Mr. Gomez wearing the same clothing	Allows weight to be compared from one day to another
	Discuss with Mr. Gomez the need for weight loss	Allows Mr. Gomez to voice his thoughts about weight loss and provides an avenue to determine number of pounds to be lost
Mr. Gomez will show normal hydration status before discharge.	Measure and document vital signs every hour until shortness of breath subsides, then every 2 hours	Monitors Mr. Gomez's response to therapy
	Hourly assess heart sounds; breath sounds; rate, rhythm, and depth of respirations; and the position Mr. Gomez takes to relieve the shortness of breath	Provides information for use in modifying the plan of care

EVALUATION   Output for the first 3 hours was 2,020 mL; on day two, I&O indicated fluid balance. Mr. Gomez identified the need to lose 30 pounds over the next 6 months. Mr. Gomez demonstrated normal hydration status, as shown by normal levels of Hct and Hgb; BP 156/92; normal breath sounds; and absence of shortness of breath, jugular engorgement, and peripheral edema.

Nursing Diagnosis 2   *Deficient Knowledge* related to information misinterpretation as evidenced by Mr. Gomez's statement "I thought I could stop taking the heart medication and eat what I wanted when I felt good again."

Nursing Outcomes Classification (NOC)
Knowledge: Disease Process
Communication: Receptive Ability
Memory

Nursing Interventions Classification (NIC)
Teaching: Disease Process
Teaching: Prescribed Medication
Medication Management

continues

SAMPLE NURSING CARE PLAN

PLANNING/GOALS	NURSING INTERVENTIONS	RATIONALE
Mr. Gomez will demonstrate an understanding of the causes of fluid excess and the role of heart medications, foods, and exercise in assisting with weight reduction.	Assess Mr. Gomez's knowledge of hypertension; decreased cardiac output; digitalis; the effects of a large abdominal girth on breathing; and foods low in sodium, fats, and carbohydrates	Provides a basis for educating Mr. Gomez about causes, aggravating and alleviating factors, and effects of fluid excess

EVALUATION Mr. Gomez was unable to verbalize understanding of how weight, high-sodium diet, and failure to take his heart medications caused the fluid excess. He was referred to home health for client teaching.

Summary

- Homeostasis is the maintenance of the body's internal environment within a narrow range of normal values. It is an ongoing process, with changes constantly occurring in the body.
- Compounds that ionize in water are called electrolytes.
- The normal range of blood pH is 7.35 to 7.45. A decrease or increase beyond this range can cause severe or even fatal physiologic problems.
- The bicarbonate buffer system works to regulate pH in both intracellular and extracellular fluids.
- The phosphate buffer system works to regulate the pH of intracellular fluid and fluid in kidney tubules.
- Protein buffers work to regulate pH inside cells, especially red blood cells.
- Substances move in and out of cells by the passive transport methods of diffusion, osmosis, and filtration and by active transport.
- The kidneys regulate fluid and electrolyte balance.
- Sodium is the main electrolyte that promotes the retention of water.
- The slightest decrease or increase in electrolyte levels can cause serious, adverse, or life-threatening effects on physiologic functions.
- Hospitalized clients, especially elderly clients, are at risk for developing dehydration.
- Clients receiving IV therapy require constant monitoring for complications.

Review Questions

1. The phosphate buffer system is involved in regulating the pH of the:
   a. carbonic acid in the lungs.
   b. carbon dioxide in the lungs.
   c. bicarbonate ions in the lungs.
   d. intracellular fluid and the fluid in the kidney tubules.

2. Diffusion is:
   a. the movement of molecules from a region of high concentration to a region of low concentration.
   b. the movement of molecules from a region of low concentration to a region of high concentration.
   c. the movement of a liquid from a region of high concentration through a membrane to a region of low concentration.
   d. the movement of a liquid from a region of low concentration through a membrane to a region of high concentration.

3. When gas is exchanged in the lungs:
   a. carbon dioxide concentration is equal in the alveoli and lungs.
   b. oxygen concentration is higher in the alveoli than in the blood.
   c. oxygen concentration is higher in the blood than in the alveoli.
   d. carbon dioxide has a higher concentration in the alveoli than in the blood.

4. Acidosis and alkalosis are identified by changes in the pH. Which of the following statements is true?

   a. A pH above 7.45 is called acidosis.

   b. A pH above 7.45 is called alkalosis.

   c. A pH increase caused by an increase of bicarbonate in the blood is metabolic acidosis.

   d. A pH decrease caused by an accumulation of carbonic acid results in respiratory alkalosis.

5. The maximum amount of IV potassium chloride that can be infused per hour is:

   a. 5 mEq.

   b. 10 mEq.

   c. 15 mEq.

   d. 20 mEq.

References/Suggested Readings

Bulechek, G., & McCloskey, J. (1999). *Nursing interventions: Effective nursing treatments* (3rd ed). Philadelphia: W. B. Saunders.

Castiglione, V. (2000). Hyperkalemia. *AJN, 100*(1), 55–56.

Chernecky, C., Macklin, D., & Murphy-Ende, K. (2001). *Fluids & Electrolytes.* Philadelphia: W. B. Saunders.

Cook, L. (1999). The value of lab values. *AJN, 99*(5), 66–75.

Daniels, R. (2002). *Delmar's Guide to Laboratory and Diagnostic Tests.* Clifton Park, NY: Thomson Delmar Learning.

Estes, M. E. Z. (2002). *Health assessment & physical examination* (2nd ed.). Clifton Park, NY: Thomson Delmar Learning.

Hadaway, L. (2002). I.V. infiltration: Not just a peripheral problem. *Nursing2002, 32*(8), 36–42.

Hamilton, S. (2001). Detecting dehydration & malnutrition in the elderly. *Nursing2001, 31*(12), 56–57.

Hogstel, M. (2001). *Nursing care of the older adult* (4th ed.). Clifton Park, NY: Thomson Delmar Learning.

I.V. therapy: Update97. (1997). *Nursing97, 27*(11), 60–61.

Incredibly Easy! (2002). Understanding hypokalemia. *Nursing2002, 32*(3), 56.

Incredibly Easy! Understanding hypokalemia. *Nursing2000, 30*(11), 74–76.

Josephson, D. L. (1999). *Intravenous infusion therapy for nurses: Principles and practice.* Clifton Park, NY: Thomson Delmar Learning.

Kee, J., & Paulanka, B. (1999). *Fluids and electrolytes with clinical applications* (6th ed.). Clifton Park, NY: Thomson Delmar Learning.

Krueger, D., & Tasota, F. (2003). Keeping an eye on calcium levels. *Nursing2003, 33*(6), 68.

Mader, S. (2001). *Understanding human anatomy & physiology* (4th ed.). Boston: McGraw Hill College Division.

Marieb, E. (2002). *Essentials of human anatomy & physiology* (7th ed.). Redwood City, CA: Cummings.

Martini, F., & Welch, K. (2001). *Fundamentals of anatomy and physiology* (5th ed.). Englewood Cliffs, NJ: Prentice-Hall.

McConnell, E. (1999). Performing pulse oximetry. *Nursing99, 29*(11), 17.

McConnell, E. (2002). Measuring fluid intake and output. *Nursing2002, 32*(7), 17.

North American Nursing Diagnosis Association (NANDA). (2003). *Nursing diagnoses: Definitions & classification 2003-2004.* Philadelphia: Author.

Scanlon, V., & Sanders, T. (2003). *Essentials of anatomy and physiology* (4th ed.). Philadelphia: F. A. Davis.

Schmidt, T. C., & Williams-Evans, S. A. (2000). How to recognize hypokalemia. *Nursing2000, 30*(2), 22.

Sensi-Scott, A., & Fong, E. (1998). *Body structures and functions* (9th ed.). Clifton Park, NY: Thomson Delmar Learning.

Tasota, F., & Wesmiller, S. (1998). Balancing act: Keeping blood pH in equilibrium. *Nursing98, 28*(12), 34–40.

Thibodeau, G., & Patton, K. (2000). *Structure & function of the body* (11th ed.). St. Louis, MO: Mosby.

White, V. (1997). Hyperkalemia. *AJN, 97*(6), 35.

Wong, F. (1999). A new approach to ABG interpretation. *AJN, 99*(8), 34–36.

Resources

Infusion Nurses Society, 220 Norwood Park South, Norwood, MA 02062, 781-440-9408, www.ins1.org

MEDICATION ADMINISTRATION AND IV THERAPY

MAKING THE CONNECTION

Refer to the following chapters to increase your understanding of medication administration and IV therapy:

Basic Nursing
- Legal and Ethical Responsibilities
- Nursing Process/Documentation
- Basic Nutrition
- Infection Control/Asepsis
- Standard Precautions and Isolation
- Diagnostic Tests

Basic Procedures
- Administering an Enema
- Measuring Intake and Output

Intermediate Procedures
- Administering an Oral, Sublingual and Buccal Medication
- Withdrawing Medication from an Ampule

- Withdrawing Medication from a Vial
- Administering an Intradermal Injection
- Administering a Subcutaneous Injection
- Administering an Intramuscular Injection
- Administering an Eye and Ear Medication

Advanced Procedures
- Performing Venipuncture (Blood Drawing)
- Preparing an IV Solution and Starting an IV
- Setting the IV Flow Rate
- Administering Medications via IV Piggyback
- Assessing and Maintaining an IV Insertion Site

LEARNING OBJECTIVES

Upon completion of this chapter, you should be able to:
- Define key terms.
- Describe how drug standards and legislation influence medication administration.
- Explain pharmacokinetics, including absorption, distribution, metabolism, and excretion of drugs.
- Describe factors that can affect a drug's action.
- Explain the different types of medication orders, when each is used, and the nurse's responsibilities for each type.
- Identify principles of safe medication administration.
- Discuss potential liabilities for the nurse administering medications.
- Develop teaching guidelines for clients regarding medication administration in the home.
- Explain procedures for the various methods of medication administration, including the choice of route and site.

KEY TERMS

absorption	infiltration
angiocatheter	intracath
aspiration	intradermal (ID)
bioavailability	intramuscular (IM)
butterfly needle	intravenous (IV)
chemical name	IV push (bolus)
distribution	metabolism
drug allergy	onset of action
drug incompatibility	parenteral
drug interaction	patency
drug tolerance	peak plasma level
enteral instillation	pharmacokinetics
excretion	phlebitis
extravasation	piggyback
flashback	plateau
flow rate	stock supply
generic name	subcutaneous (SC/SQ)
half-life	toxic effect
hypervolemia	trade (brand) name
idiosyncratic reaction	unit dose
implantable port	vesicant

INTRODUCTION

Managing medications requires collaboration of many health care providers. Medications are prescribed by a physician, dentist, or other authorized prescriber such as advanced practice registered nurses as determined by individual state licensing boards. Medications are prepared and dispensed by pharmacists. Nurses are responsible for administering medications. Dietitians may be involved in identifying possible food–drug interactions.

Medication administration requires specialized knowledge, judgment, and nursing skills based on the principles of pharmacology. This chapter focuses on assisting students to apply knowledge of pharmacology and to acquire safe administration of medications skills. The nursing process directs nursing decisions about safe drug administration and ensures compliance with standards of practice.

DRUG STANDARDS AND LEGISLATION

A drug is a chemical substance intended to have a specific effect. Nurses assume, before administering any medication, that the drug will be safe for the client if the dose, route, and frequency are within the therapeutic range for that drug. This assumption is implied by standards ensuring drug uniformity in strength, purity, efficacy, safety, and **bioavailability** (readiness to produce a drug effect).

Standards

Standards ensure drug uniformity for predictable effects. The *United States Pharmacopeia* and the *National Formulary* (USP and NF) are books of drug standards used in the United States. The USP and NF list drugs recognized for compliance with legal standards of purity, quality, and strength.

The USP has been providing standards for pharmaceutical preparations since its first edition was published in 1851. The American Pharmaceutical Association first published the NF in 1898 to provide a list of drugs complying with established standards.

Legislation

The USP and the NF were designated by the Pure Food and Drug Act of 1906 as the official bodies to establish drug standards. The authority to enforce these standards was given to the federal government. The federal Food, Drug, and Cosmetic Act of 1938 authorized the Food and Drug Administration (FDA) to test all new drugs for toxicity before giving approval to market a drug. In 1952, the federal Food, Drug, and Cosmetic Act of 1938 was amended to differentiate prescription (legend) drugs from nonprescription (over-the-counter) drugs and to regulate prescription dispensing. Drug effectiveness testing came with the Kefauver-Harris Act of 1962 (Lehne, 2004).

In 1914, the Harrison Narcotic Act classified habit-forming drugs as narcotics and began regulating them.

TABLE 22-1   CONTROLLED SUBSTANCES

Schedule (C-I): Includes substances for which there is a high abuse potential and no current approved medical use (e.g., heroin, marijuana, LSD, other hallucinogens, certain opiates and opium derivatives).

Schedule (C-II): Includes drugs that have a high abuse potential and a high ability to produce physical and/or psychological dependence and for which there is a current approved or acceptable medical use.

Schedule (C-III): Includes drugs for which there is less potential for abuse than drugs in Schedule II and for which there is a current approved medical use. Certain drugs in this category are preparations containing limited quantities of codeine. Also, anabolic steroids are classified in Schedule III.

Schedule (C-IV): Includes drugs for which there is a relatively low abuse potential and for which there is a current approved medical use. Examples include diazepam and lorazepam.

Schedule (C-V): Drugs in this category consist mainly of preparations containing limited amounts of certain narcotic drugs for use as antitussives and antidiarrheals. Federal law provides that limited quantities of these drugs (e.g., codeine) may be bought without a prescription by an individual at least 18 years of age. The product must be purchased from a pharmacist, who must keep appropriate records. However, state laws vary, and in many states such products require a prescription.

From PDR Nurse's Handbook 2004 by G. Spratto & A. Woods, 2004, Clifton Park, NY: Thomson Delmar Learning. Copyright 2004 by Thomson Delmar Learning. Reprinted with permission.

This law and other drug abuse laws were replaced with the Comprehensive Drug Abuse Prevention and Control Act (Controlled Substance Act) in 1970. This act defines a *drug-dependent person* in terms of physical and psychological dependence and provides for strict regulation of narcotics and other controlled drugs such as barbiturates with the five categories of scheduled drugs (Table 22-1). Records must be kept by the dispensing pharmacist for all controlled substances. Pharmacists employed by the Drug Enforcement Agency (DEA) inspect records and prescriptions to discover illicit distribution of these substances.

All states must adhere to the schedule of controlled substances as minimum standards; however, individual states can pass stricter controls of these substances. For example, the Controlled Substance Act has antitussives with codeine as a schedule V drug, but an individual state may place this drug in the more restrictive schedule II category.

DRUG NOMENCLATURE

The terms *medication, medicine,* and *drug* are used interchangeably by laypersons and health care providers.

Drugs are identified by a chemical, generic, official, or trade name. The **chemical name** is a precise description of the drug's chemical formula. The **generic name** *(nonproprietary)* in the United States is the name assigned by the U.S. Adopted Names Council to the manufacturer who first develops the drug. When a drug is approved, it is given an *official name,* which may be the same as the nonproprietary name (Lehne, 2004). Drugs with proven therapeutic value are listed by their official name in the USP and NF. Pharmaceutical companies assign a *proprietary name,* also called a **trade (brand) name,** when they market a drug. One generic drug may have several trade names depending on how many companies market the drug. For example, ibuprofen is a generic name; trade names for this drug include Advil, Motrin, Excedrin IB, and Nuprin. *Generic names are not capitalized, but trade names are always capitalized.*

DRUG ACTION

Drug action refers to a drug's ability to combine with a cellular receptor. Depending on the location of cellular receptors affected by a given drug, a drug can have a local effect, a systemic effect, or both. For example, when diphenhydramine hydrochloride (Benadryl) cream is applied to the skin, it has only a local effect; however, when administered in a tablet or injectable form, it has both a systemic and local effect.

Pharmacology

The study of drug effects on living organisms is called pharmacology. This section discusses the pharmacological activities of drug action as related to medication management, drug classification, and routes of administration.

Medication Management

Medication management is to produce the desired drug action by maintaining a constant drug level. Drug action is based on the half-life of a drug. A drug's **half-life** is the time it takes the body to eliminate half of the blood concentration level of the original drug dose. For example, if a drug has a half-life of 8 hours, 50% of the drug's original dose is present in the blood 8 hours after administration, and 25% of the drug is present 16 hours after administration. Because of a drug's half-life, repeated doses are given to maintain the drug level over a 24-hour interval.

Other terms describing drug action include onset, peak plasma level, and plateau. **Onset of action** is the time for the body to respond to a drug after administration. **Peak plasma level** is the highest blood concentration of a single drug dose before the elimination rate equals the rate of absorption. The blood concentration level will decrease steadily once the peak plasma level is reached, unless another dose is given. When a series of scheduled drug doses is administered, the blood concentration level is maintained, called a **plateau.**

Classification

Drugs are generally classified by the body system with which they interact (e.g., cardiovascular) or by the drug's approved therapeutic usage (e.g., antihypertensive). Drugs with several therapeutic uses are usually classified by their most common use.

Routes

Drugs are prepared in many forms for administration by a specific route (Table 22-2). The route is how the drug is absorbed: oral, buccal, sublingual, parenteral, topical, and respiratory.

 Safety: Do Not Substitute Drug Forms
Drugs prepared for administration by one route cannot be substituted by the drug prepared for another route. For example, when a client has difficulty swallowing a large tablet or capsule, an oral solution or elixir of the same drug cannot be administered without first consulting the physician. A liquid may be more easily and completely absorbed, producing a higher blood level than a tablet.

Oral Route Most drugs are administered by the oral route because it is the most convenient, least expensive, and safest method, but it acts more slowly than the other routes. Drugs are not given orally to clients with GI intolerance, those on NPO (nothing by mouth) status, or those in a coma.

The buccal or sublingual route is used when small amounts of drugs are required. Buccal and sublingual drugs act quickly because of the oral mucosa's thin epithelium and large vascular system, allowing the drug to be quickly absorbed.

Buccal drugs are to be placed in the buccal pocket (superior-posterior aspect of the internal cheek next to the molars) for absorption by the mucous membrane. Sublingual medications are made to dissolve quickly when placed under the tongue. For example, nitroglycerin (Nitrostat), an antianginal drug, can be given either sublingually or buccally as prescribed, whereas isoproterenol hydrochloride (Isuprel), a bronchodilator, is only given sublingually and methyltesterone (Testred), an androgen, is only given buccally.

Parenteral Route Parenteral drugs are administered by injection using sterile technique. By definition, **parenteral** route refers to any route other than the oral-gastrointestinal tract; however, the medical usage of the term excludes topical and respiratory routes. The four routes that nurses use to administer medications parenterally are:

- **Intradermal** (ID), an injection into the dermis
- **Subcutaneous** (SC or SQ), an injection into the subcutaneous tissue

---

PROFESSIONAL TIP

Special Considerations for Oral Route

- Chewable tablets are to be chewed before swallowing; chewing enhances gastric absorption.
- Buccal and sublingual medications must dissolve completely before the client drinks or eats.
- Suspensions and emulsions should be administered immediately after shaking and pouring from the bottle.

TABLE 22-2   TYPES OF DRUG PREPARATIONS

TYPE DESCRIPTION

Oral Solids	• Tablets: compressed or molded substances, to be swallowed whole, chewed before swallowing, or placed in the buccal pocket or under the tongue (sublingual) • Capsules: substances encased in a hard or a soft soluble cover or gelatin shell that dissolves in the stomach • Caplets: gelatin-coated tablets that dissolve in the stomach • Powders and granules: finely ground substances • Troches, lozenges, and pastilles: designed to dissolve in the mouth • Enteric-coated tablets: coated tablets that dissolve in the intestines • Time-release capsules: encased substances that are further enclosed in smaller casings that deliver a drug dose over an extended period • Sustained-release: compounded substances that release a drug slowly to maintain a steady plasma level
Topicals	• Liniments: substances mixed with an alcohol, oil, or soapy emollient; applied to the skin • Ointments: semisolid substances for topical use • Pastes: semisolid substances, thicker than ointments, absorbed slowly through the skin • Suppositories: gelatin substances designed to dissolve when inserted in the rectum, urethra, or vagina
Inhalants	• Inhalations: drugs or dilutions of drugs administered by the nasal or oral respiratory route for a local or systemic effect
Solutions	• Solutions: contain one or more soluble chemical substances dissolved in water • Enemas: aqueous solutions for rectal instillation • Douches: aqueous solutions that function as a cleansing or antiseptic agent that may be dispensed in the form of a powder with directions for dissolving in a specific quantity of warm water • Suspensions: particles or powder substances that must be mixed with, not dissolved in, a liquid by shaking vigorously before administration • Emulsions: two-phase systems in which one liquid is dispersed in the form of small droplets throughout another liquid • Syrups: substances dissolved in a sugar liquid • Gargles: aqueous solutions • Mouthwashes: aqueous solutions that may contain alcohol, glycerin, and synthetic sweeteners • Nasal solutions: aqueous solutions instilled as drops or sprays • Optic (eye) and otic (ear) solutions: aqueous solutions instilled as drops • Elixirs: solutions that contain water, varying amounts of alcohol, and sweeteners

• **Intramuscular** (IM), an injection into the muscle
• **Intravenous** (IV), an injection into a vein

Other parenteral routes, such as intrathecal or intraspinal, intrapleural, intracardiac, intra-arterial, and intra-articular, are used by physicians and sometimes by advanced-practice registered nurses.

Topical Route Most topical drugs are given to deliver a drug at, or immediately beneath, the point of application. Many topical drugs are applied to the skin, but other topical drugs include eye, nose and throat, ear, rectal, and vaginal preparations. Drugs directly applied to the skin are absorbed into the dermis, where they have a local effect or are absorbed into the bloodstream. The vascularity of the skin varies the drug action. Usually several applications over a 24-hour period are required for the desired therapeutic effect.

Transdermal patches are used to deliver medications such as nitroglycerin (Transdermal-NTG), an antianginal, and some supplemental hormone replacements for

absorption to produce systemic effects. Some topical drugs, such as eye and nasal drops and vaginal and rectal suppositories, applied directly to the mucous membranes, are absorbed quickly and, depending on the drug's dose (strength and quantity), may cause systemic effects.

Respiratory Route Inhalants such as oxygen and most general anesthetics deliver gaseous or volatile substances that are almost immediately absorbed into systemic circulation. The inhalants, delivered into the alveoli of the lungs, promote fast absorption due to:

• Permeability of the alveolar and vascular epithelium
• Abundant blood flow
• Very large surface area for absorption

Oropharyngeal handheld inhalers deliver topical drugs to the respiratory tract to create local and systemic effects. The three types of inhalers—the metered-dose inhaler, or nebulizer; the turbo-inhaler; and the nasal inhaler—are explained later in this chapter.

Pharmacokinetics

Pharmacokinetics is the study of the absorption, distribution, metabolism, and excretion of drugs to determine the relationship between the dose of a drug and the drug's concentration in biological fluids. This knowledge is used by health care providers in medication management.

The physician is concerned mainly with the dose and route that will produce the most therapeutic effects. Pharmacists, physicians, and nurses work together to identify appropriate times for drug administration and to avoid interactions with other substances that might alter the drug's actions. Nurses and physicians monitor the client's response to the drug's action. Drug actions are dependent on four properties: absorption, distribution, metabolism, and excretion.

Absorption

The degree and rate of **absorption,** or movement of a drug from administration site into the bloodstream, depend on several factors: the drug's physicochemical effects, its dosage, its route of administration, its interactions with other substances, and various client characteristics such as age (Blanchard & Loeb, 2003). Oral preparations, such as tablets and capsules, must first disintegrate into smaller particles for gastric juices to dissolve and prepare the drug for absorption in the small intestines.

Intramuscularly administered drugs are absorbed through the muscle into the bloodstream. Suppositories are absorbed through the mucous membranes into the blood. Intravenous drugs are immediately bioavailable because they are directly injected into the blood.

Distribution

Distribution is the movement of drugs from the blood into various body tissues and fluids. Drug distribution in the body is limited by the degree of binding between blood proteins and chemical substances. The amount of drug distributed can be altered by the client's health condition.

Metabolism

Metabolism is the physical and chemical processing of a drug by the body. Most drugs are metabolized in the liver. The presence of enzymes in the liver that detoxify the drugs determine the rate of metabolism. Some drugs can increase the rate of metabolism.

Excretion

Excretion is the elimination of drugs from the body. This occurs mainly through hepatic metabolism and renal excretion, but the lungs, exocrine glands, skin, and intestinal tract can eliminate some drugs.

Drug Interaction

Drug interaction is the effect one drug can have on another drug. Drug interactions may occur when two drugs are administered at the same time or within a short time interval. Drugs can be purposely combined for a positive effect; for example, hydrochlorothiazide (HydroDIURIL), a potassium-depleting diuretic, and spironolactone (Aldactone), a potassium-sparing diuretic, when combined maintain a normal blood level of potassium. When one drug is purposely given to potentiate the action of another drug, as in preoperative medications, a positive drug interaction occurs.

Not all drug interactions are therapeutic. Some interactions can interfere with the absorption, effect, or excretion of other drugs. For example, calcium products and magnesium-containing antacids can cause inadequate absorption of tetracycline (Tetracyn), an antibiotic, in the digestive tract.

Side Effects and Adverse Reactions

Drug effects other than those therapeutically intended and expected are called *adverse reactions*. A nontherapeutic effect may be mild and predictable (side effect) or unexpected and potentially dangerous (adverse reaction). There are several types of adverse reactions: drug allergy, drug tolerance, toxic effect, and idiosyncratic reactions.

A **drug allergy** (hypersensitivity to a drug) is an antigen–antibody immune reaction occurring when an individual previously exposed to a drug has developed antibodies against the drug. The type of reaction may be mild (skin rash, urticaria, headache, nausea, or vomiting) or severe (anaphylaxis). Drug reactions are often seen on the skin because of its abundant blood supply.

Anaphylaxis is an immediate, life-threatening reaction to a drug, such as penicillin, marked by respiratory distress, sudden severe bronchospasm, and cardiovascular collapse. Anaphylaxis can be fatal if emergency measures are not begun immediately (administration of epinephrine, bronchodilators, and antihistamines).

Drug tolerance occurs when the body is so accustomed to a specific drug that larger doses are needed to produce the desired therapeutic effect. For example, clients with cancer experiencing severe pain may require larger and larger doses of morphine (a narcotic analgesic) to control the pain.

A **toxic effect** occurs when the body cannot metabolize a drug and the drug accumulates in the blood. Digoxin, a cardiac drug, has a narrow margin of safety between an effective therapeutic dose and a toxic dose (Spratto & Woods, 2004).

An **idiosyncratic reaction** is a very unpredictable response that may be an overresponse, an underresponse, or an atypical response. For example, 1 of 40,000 clients will develop aplastic anemia after receiving chloramphenicol (an antibiotic) (Blanchard & Loeb, 2003).

Food–Drug Interactions

Medication management works to avoid possible food–drug interactions. There are three main types of food–drug interactions:

1. Some drugs interfere with the absorption, excretion, or use in the body of one or more nutrients.
2. Some foods increase or decrease the absorption of a drug into the body.

3. Some foods alter the chemical actions of drugs, preventing the therapeutic effect on the body.

Most interaction problems occur with the use of oral antibiotics, diuretics, anticoagulant, and antihypertensive drugs. Clients on sodium-restricted diets should consult with a pharmacist about the sodium content of prescription and over-the-counter drugs. Some drugs contain almost half the total daily allowance of sodium. Alcohol interacts with many drugs, such as antihistamines, antibiotics, anticoagulants, and sleeping pills. Food–drug interactions vary depending on the dose and the form of the drug taken and the client's age, gender, nutritional status, body weight, and specific medical condition.

Many herbals interact with drugs to change their effect, such as with digoxin, a cardiac drug. Herbal teas such as Woodruff, tonka bean, and melitot contain natural coumarins that can potentiate the effects of Coumadin, a blood thinner (Spratto & Woods, 2004).

FACTORS INFLUENCING DRUG ACTION

Individual client characteristics such as genetic factors, age, height, weight, and physical and mental conditions can influence drug actions on the body. Genetic factors can interfere with drug metabolism, producing an abnormal sensitivity to certain drugs.

The physician often correlates the client's age, height, and weight to determine the dosage for many drugs. This information must be accurately recorded in the client's medical record. The amount of body fat may also alter drug distribution.

The client's physical condition can also alter the effects of drugs. For example, in an edematous client, the drug must be distributed to a larger volume of body fluids than in a nonedematous client; therefore, the edematous client may require a larger dose to produce the desired action, whereas a dehydrated client may require a smaller dosage. Diseases affecting liver and renal functioning can alter the metabolism and elimination of most drugs.

MEDICATION ORDERS

In health care facilities, medication orders are written on a physician's order form in each client's medical record.

LIFE CYCLE CONSIDERATIONS

Age-Related Factors Influence Drug Action and Dosing

- Neonates and infants have underdeveloped gastrointestinal systems, muscle mass, and metabolic enzyme systems and inadequate renal function.
- Elderly clients often experience decreased hepatic or renal function and diminished muscle mass.

All orders must be written clearly and legibly. A drug order should contain seven parts:

1. Client's name
2. Date and time when the order is written
3. Name of the drug to be administered
4. Dosage
5. Route for administration and special directives about its administration
6. Time of administration and frequency
7. Signature of the person writing the order, such as the physician or advanced practice registered nurse

Drug prescriptions outside acute care facilities may also specify whether the generic or trade name drug is to be used, the quantity to be given, and how many times the prescription can be refilled.

If, in the nurse's judgment, a drug order is in error, the nurse is responsible and held accountable for questioning that order. The error may be in any part of the drug order, and the nurse should clarify the order with the prescriber. The conversation must be documented in the client's medical record (Smith, 2003). A drug error has serious legal implications if the nurse involved could have been expected, on the basis of experience and knowledge, to have noted the error.

Most agencies have policies relative to medication administration, such as stop dates for certain types of drugs, regularly scheduled times to administer medications as specified in the drug order, and a listing of abbreviations officially accepted for use in the agency. The agency's medical records department maintains the official listing of abbreviations adopted by the medical staff of that agency. Only abbreviations from the official list can be used in any part of the client's medical record at that agency (see appendices).

Types of Orders

Medications are prescribed differently, depending on their purpose. Medications can be prescribed as stat, single-dose, scheduled, and prn orders.

Stat Orders

Stat medication orders are those that should be administered immediately, not an hour or two later. Stat orders are often encountered in emergency situations, such as a stat dose of nitroglycerin for a client experiencing chest pain. The client's response to all stat medications must be assessed and documented.

Single-Dose Orders

Single-dose orders are one-time medications. They should be administered either at a time specified by the prescriber or at the earliest convenient time. These orders are often used in preparation for a diagnostic or therapeutic procedure; for example, a laxative may be ordered to prepare for a lower GI x-ray.

Scheduled Orders

Scheduled orders are administered as specified until the order is changed or canceled by another order or until the specified number of days have elapsed as set by agency policy. Scheduled orders are used to maintain the desired blood level of the medication.

Agency policy sets the actual times for administering medications over a 24-hour time interval. For example, t.i.d. drugs may be administered at 0800, 1400, and 2000 or at 0900, 1500, and 2100. Medications ordered qd may have a time specified in the order, such as Isophane (NPH) Insulin 10 U SC qd at 0630, or they will be given at the agency's designated time; for example, Lanoxin 0.25 mg po qd would be given at 0900.

An order specifying the number of days or dosages the client is to receive has an automatic stop date for the drug. For example, an order for tetracycline 250 mg po q6h for 5 days would provide tetracycline 250 mg orally every 6 hours for 5 days, a total of 20 doses. Day one begins with the administration of the first dose.

PRN Orders

A PRN (as needed) drug is administered when, in the nurse's judgment, the client's condition requires it. This type of order is generally written for laxatives, analgesics, and antiemetics. For example, a client may have an order for morphine, a narcotic analgesic, gr $^1/_4$ IM q3–4h PRN. The pain medication is given based on the assessment of the client's pain and as specified in the order.

SYSTEMS OF WEIGHT AND MEASURE

Medication administration requires a knowledge of weight and volume measurement systems. In the United States three different systems of measurement are used in medication management: metric, apothecary, and household.

Metric System

In 1890, the USP adopted the metric system of weights and measures exclusively except for equivalent dosages. In 1944, the Council on Pharmacy and Chemistry of the American Medical Association adopted the metric system exclusively. The metric system is used in every major country of the world except the United States but is used almost exclusively in U.S. health care facilities.

The metric (decimal system) is a simple system based on units of 10. Move the decimal point to the right to change from a larger unit to a smaller unit, and move the decimal point to the left to change from a smaller unit to a larger unit. For example:

5 g = 5,000 mg	0.5 mg = 500 mcg
5 mcg = 0.005 mg	1.25 L = 1,250 mL
0.25 g = 250 mg	2.45 kg = 2,450 g

The basic measurement units are the meter (linear), the liter (volume), and the gram (mass, or weight). Important abbreviations and equivalents to remember are:

- Volume (liquid)
1 milliliter (mL)	= 1 cubic centimeter (cc)
1,000 milliliters	= 1 liter (L)

TABLE 22-3	METRIC SYSTEM PREFIXES
PREFIX	**EXAMPLE**
Latin Prefixes— subdivisions of the basic unit	deci (1/10, or 0.1) centi (1/100, or 0.01) milli (1/1,000, or 0.001) micro (1/1,000,000, or 0.000001)
Greek Prefixes— multiples of the basic unit	deka (10) hecto (100) kilo (1,000)

- Weight
1,000 micrograms (mcg)	= 1 milligram (mg)
1,000 milligrams	= 1 gram (g)
1,000 grams	= 1 kilogram (kg)

The metric system uses Latin prefixes to designate subdivisions of the basic units and Greek prefixes to designate multiples of the basic units (Table 22-3).

 Safety: Metric System
A zero is *always* placed in front of the decimal for values less than 1 (0.5) to prevent error.

Apothecary System

The apothecary system originated in England and is based on the weight of one grain of wheat. The grain (gr) is the basic unit of weight and the minim (the approximate volume of water that weighs a grain) is the basic unit of volume. Important equivalents and abbreviations are:

- Volume (liquid)
60 minums (♏)	= 1 fluid dram (fl dr, or ℨ)
8 fluid drams	= 1 fluid ounce (fl oz, or ℥)
16 fluid ounces	= 1 pint (pt)
- Weight
60 grains (gr)	= 1 dram (dr, or ℨ)
8 drams	= 1 ounce (oz, or ℥)
12 ounces	= 1 pound (lb)

Household System

The household system of measurement is the least accurate of the three systems. It is not ordinarily used to calculate dosage, but only as a reference to help the client. The units of liquid measure are drop (gtt), teaspoon (tsp), tablespoon (Tbsp), ounce (oz), and cup (Figure 22-1). The 16-ounce pound of the household system *is* used to calculate dosage, with 2.2 lb equal to 1 kg.

The USP recognizes the teaspoon for household medication administration and states that the teaspoon may be regarded as representing 5 mL (American Hospital Formulary Service, 2002). Household spoons are not accurate (varying sizes) for measuring a liquid medication; therefore, the USP recommends using a calibrated oral syringe or dropper for accurate measurement of liquid drug doses.

Household units are generally used in calculating a client's intake and output. Important household equivalents and abbreviations to remember are:

Figure 22-1 *Relationship between Household Measures*

- Volume (liquid)

60 drops (gtt)	= 1 teaspoon (tsp)
3 tsp	= 1 tablespoon (Tbsp)
2 Tbsp	= 1 ounce (oz)
8 oz	= 1 cup (c)
2 cup	= 1 pint (pt)
2 pints	= 1 quart (qt)

- Weight

16 ounces	= 1 pound (lb)

APPROXIMATE EQUIVALENTS

The conversion of metric with the apothecary and household systems are *approximate equivalents* (Table 22-4). The approximate equivalents represent quantities usually ordered by physicians using either the metric or apothecary system of weights and volumes for drug doses (American Hospital Formulary Service, 2002). When a dosage is prescribed in the metric system, the pharmacist may dispense the corresponding approximate equivalent in the apothecary system and vice versa. For example, if the physician prescribes morphine 15 mg, the pharmacist may dispense morphine gr $^1/_4$. The USP and NF reference *exact equivalents* that must be used to calculate quantities in pharmaceutical formularies and prescription compounding.

Converting Units of Weight and Volume

Knowledge of measurement systems and their conversions must be applied when a drug dosage is prescribed in one system and the pharmacy dispenses the equivalent dose in another. The conversions may be accomplished with either a proportion or a ratio. For example:

Proportion

Means

2 : 4 = 6 : 12

└─ Extremes ─┘

Ratio

$$\frac{2}{4} = \frac{6}{12}$$

In a proportion, the product (multiplication) of the means equals the product of the extremes. In a ratio, the products of cross-multiplication are equal.

$$4 \times 6 = 24 \qquad 2 \times 12 = 24$$
$$2 \times 12 = 24 \qquad 4 \times 6 = 24$$

If one of the terms is unknown, it can be determined by substituting x for the number. The term with the x (unknown) is always put on the left.

$$2 : x = 6 : 12 \qquad \frac{2}{x} = \frac{6}{12}$$
$$6x = 24 \qquad 6x = 24$$
$$x = 4 \qquad x = 24$$

Proof that the answer is correct can be determined by substituting the answer for the x and multiplying.

TABLE 22-4	APPROXIMATE EQUIVALENTS TO THE METRIC SYSTEM					
METRIC		**APOTHECARY**		**HOUSEHOLD**		
Liquid (Volume)					**Weight**	
Liquid	*Weight*	*Liquid*	*Weight*			
0.06 mL	= 60 mg	= 1 ♍	= 1 gr	= 1 gtt	0.4 mg (400 mcg)	= 1/150 gr
1 mL	= 1 g	= 15–16 ♍	= 15 gr	= 15 gtt	1 mg (1,000 mcg)	= 1/60 gr
5 mL	= 5 g	= 1 fl dr	= 1 dr	= 1 tsp	4 mg	= 1/15 gr
15 mL	= 15 g	= 4 fl dr	= 4 dr	= 1 Tbsp	10 mg	= 1/6 gr
30 mL	= 30 g	= 1 fl oz	= 1 oz	= 1 oz	15 mg	= 1/4 gr
240 mL	= 240 g	= 8 fl oz	= 8 oz	= 8 oz	30 mg	= 1/2 gr
380 mL	= 380 g	= 12 fl oz	= 1 lb	= 16 oz	1000 g (1 kg)	= 2.2 lb
500 mL	= 500 g	= 1 pt	= 16 oz	= 1 pt		
1,000 mL	= 1,000 g	= 1 qt	= 32 oz	= 1 qt		

Proportion can be used when converting units of weight and volume, conversions within the metric system, conversions between systems, and in drug dosage calculations. When the physician orders morphine gr $^{1}/_{4}$ and the pharmacist dispenses morphine 15 mg, the nurse is responsible for ensuring the correct dose. The nurse knows that 1 grain equals 60 milligrams; to convert the ordered dose to milligrams, the nurse should use the following calculation:

$$1 \text{ gr} : 60 \text{ mg} = 1/4 \text{ gr} : x$$
(the grains cancel out)
$$1 \ x = (60 \text{ mg})(1/4)$$
(divide 60 by 4)
$$x = 15 \text{ mg}$$

Safety: Know What Is Being Calculated
All terms must be labeled (gr, mg, mL, and so on) to avoid errors.

Conversions within the Metric System

Dose equivalents within the metric system are computed by either dividing or multiplying. For example, to change milligrams to grams (1,000 mg equals 1 g) or milliliters to liters (1,000 mL equals 1 L), divide the number by 1,000:

$$250 \text{ mg} = x \text{ g}$$
(move the decimal point three places to the left)
$$x = 0.25 \text{ g}$$
or
$$500 \text{ mL} = x \text{ L}$$
(move the decimal point three places to the left)
$$x = 0.5 \text{ L}$$

To convert grams to milligrams or liters to milliliters, multiply the number by 1000:

$$0.005 \text{ g} = x \text{ mg}$$
(move the decimal point three places to the right)
$$x = 5 \text{ mg}$$
or
$$0.725 \text{ L} = x \text{ mL}$$
(move the decimal point three places to the right)
$$x = 725 \text{ mL}$$

Converting the volume of liters and milliliters may be necessary for enemas and irrigating solutions for bladder and wound irrigations. Intravenous solutions are prepackaged, sterile solutions dispensed in volumes as ordered by the physician, such as 50 mL, 100 mL, 250 mL, 500 mL, or 1,000 mL (1 liter).

Conversions between Systems

Converting between systems is necessary when the physician orders nitroglycerin (an antianginal drug) gr 1/150 po for chest pain and the dispensed dose is 0.4 mg:

$$1 \text{ gr} : 60 \text{ mg} = 1/150 \text{ gr} : x$$
$$1 \text{ gr} \ x = (60 \text{ mg})(1/150 \text{ gr})$$
(the grains cancel out)
$$1 \ x = 60/150 \text{ mg}$$
(divide 60 by 150)
$$x = 0.4 \text{ mg}$$

The nurse can use proportion when converting pounds to kilograms (2.2 lb = 1 kg). For example, if the client weighs 154 lb, what is the weight in kilograms?

$$2.2 \text{ lb} : 1 \text{ kg} = 154 \text{ lb} : x$$
(the pounds cancel out)
$$2.2 \ x = 154$$
(divide 154 by 2.2)
$$x = 70 \text{ kg}$$

Dosage Calculations

Several formulas may be used by the nurse when calculating drug doses. One formula uses ratios based on the *desired dose* and the *dose on hand*. For example, cephalexin hydrochloride (Keftab), an anti-infective cephalosporin, 500 mg po q.i.d. (dose desired) is ordered by the physician; the dose on hand is 250 mg/5 mL. The formula is as follows:

$$\frac{500 \text{ mg (desired dose)}}{250 \text{ mg (dose on hand)}} \times \frac{x \text{ (quantity desired)}}{5 \text{ mL (quantity on hand)}}$$
(cross-multiply)
(milligrams cancel out)
$$250 \ x = 500 \times 5$$
$$\frac{500 \times 5}{250}$$
$$x = 10 \text{ mL}$$

In another example, the physician orders heparin (an anticoagulant) 10,000 units SC; the dose on hand is 40,000 units/mL:

$$\frac{10,000 \text{ units}}{40,000 \text{ units}} \times \frac{x}{1 \text{ mL}}$$
(cross-multiply)
(units cancel out)
$$40,000 \ x = 10,000$$
(zeros cancel out)
$$x = {}^{1}/_{4} \text{ mL}$$

Because $^{1}/_{4}$ mL would be difficult to measure, it is best converted to minums. It is known that 1 mL = 15–16℩. It will be best to use 16 so it will come out with a whole number for the answer.

$$1 \text{ mL} : 16℩ = {}^{1}/_{4} \text{ mL} : x$$
(mL cancel out)
$$1 \ x = (16)({}^{1}/_{4})$$
$$x = 4℩$$

Pediatric Dosages

There are several rules to calculate infants' and childrens' dosages, such as *Young's Rule*, *Clark's Rule*, and *Fried's Rule*. Another method, body surface area (BSA), is considered to be one of the most accurate methods of

PROFESSIONAL TIP

Reasonable Answer

- *The final step in figuring dosage is to ask whether the answer is reasonable.*
- Seldom are more than 2 or 3 tablets or capsules given of one medication or more than 2 or 3 ounces of a liquid medication.
- Seldom is a parenteral injection, except for IV, given of more than 3 mL.
- If your calculations are outside these parameters, recheck your calculations and have a colleague check the calculations too.

Directions for use: (1) Determine client height. (2) Determine client weight. (3) Draw a straight line to connect the height and weight. Where the line intersects on the SA line is the derived body surface area (M²).

Figure 22-2 *Nomogram for Estimating Body Surface Area (From Nelson Textbook of Pediatrics [17th ed.] by R. E. Behrman, R. Kliegman, & H. B. Jenson, 2004, Philadelphia: Saunders. Copyright 2000 by Saunders. Reprinted with permission.)*

calculating medication dosages for infants and children up to 12 years of age (Rice, 2001). No matter which method is used in calculating pediatric drug dosages, the dosages are approximate and, depending on the child's response, may need adjustment.

Body surface area refers to the square meter surface area method of relating the surface area of individuals to drug dosage. The BSA based on height and weight gives an approximate dose using the following formula:

$$\frac{\text{Body surface area of child}}{\text{Body surface area of adult}} \times \frac{\text{Usual adult dose}}{} = \frac{\text{Child's dose}}{}$$

The BSA of an adult is 1.73 square meters (m²); the 1.73 m² is based on an adult weighing 150 pounds.

A nomogram is used to compute the child's BSA (Figure 22-2). Draw a straight line from the child's height in the left column to the child's weight in the right column. The point where this line intersects the body surface area column (designated SA) is the child's BSA. For example: A 3-year-old child is 38 inches tall and weighs 36 pounds. The physician orders meperidine (Demerol) for pain. The average adult dose is 50 mg. How much Demerol should the child receive? From the nomogram the child's BSA is 0.66 m².

$$\frac{0.66\ (m^2)}{1.73\ (m^2)} \times 50\ mg$$

(square meters cancel out)

$$\frac{33}{1.73}$$

(divide 33 by 1.73)

$$= 19.07\ mg = 19\ mg$$

Now use the desired dose/dose on hand formula to determine how much to give.

$$\frac{19\ mg}{50\ mg} = \frac{x}{1\ mL}$$

(milligrams cancel out)
(cross-multiply)
$$50x = 19\ mL$$
$$x = 0.32\ mL$$

This will have to be given in a tuberculin syringe. Nomograms are used primarily in calculating pediatric drug dosages; however, they are also used when calculating some adult drug dosages such as aminoglycosides and antineoplastic agents.

DRUG ADMINISTRATION SAFETY

Many drugs must be administered in an efficient and safe manner according to nursing standards of practice and agency policy. Other responsibilities of the nurse include safe storage and maintaining an adequate supply of drugs.

The nurse should document the actual administration of medications on the MAR. The medication administration record (MAR) contains the drug's name, dose, route, and frequency of administration. Drug data are entered either by the pharmacist when dispensing the order (computer-generated form; Figure 22-3) or by the nurse when transcribing the order (handwritten onto the form).

PHARMACY MAR

START	STOP	MEDICATION	SCHEDULED TIMES	OK'D BY	0001 HRS. to 1200 HRS.	1201 HRS. to 2400 HRS.
08/31/xx 1800 SCH		PROCAN SR 500 MG TAB-SR [500 MG] [Q6H] [PO]	0600 1200 1800 2400	JD	0600 LW 1200 LW	1800 MS 2400 JD
09/03/xx 0900 SCH		DIGOXIN (LANOXIN) 0.125 MG TAB [1 TAB] [QOD] [PO] ODD DAYS-SEPT.	0900	JD	0900 LW	
09/03/xx 0900 SCH		FUROSEMIDE (LASIX) 40 MG TAB [1 TAB] [QD] [PO]	0900	JD	0900 LW	
09/03/xx 0845 SCH		REGLAN 10 MG TAB [10 MG] [AC&HS] [PO] GIVE ONE NOW!	0730 1130 1630 2100	JD	0730 LW 1130 LW	1630 MS 2100 MS
09/04/xx 0900 SCH		K-LYTE 25 MEQ EFFERVESCENT TAB [1 EFF. TAB] [BID] [PO] DISSOLVE AS DIR. START 9-4	0900 1700	JD	0900 LW	1700 MS
09/03/xx 1500 PRN		NITROGLYCERIN 1/50 GR 0.4 MG TAB-SL [1 TABLET] [PRN*] [SL] PRN CHEST PAIN		JD		
09/03/xx 1700 PRN		DARVOCET-N 100* [1 TAB] [Q4-6H] [PO] PRN MILD-MODERATE PAIN		JD		
09/03/xx 2100 PRN		MEPERIDINE*(DEMEROL) INJ [50 MG] [Q4H] [IM] PRN SEVERE PAIN W PHENERGAN		JD		2200 Ⓗ MS
09/03/xx 2100 PRN		PROMETHAZINE (PHENERGAN) INJ [50 MG] [Q4H] [IM] PRN SEVERE PAIN W DEMEROL		JD		2200 Ⓗ MS

Gluteus	Thigh	Nurse's Signature	Initial	Allergies: NKA	Patient: Patient, John D.
A. Right	H. Right				Patient #: 3-81512-3
B. Left	I. Left	7-3 L. White, R.N.	LW		Admitted: 08/31/xx
Ventro Gluteal		3-11 M. Smith, R.N.	MS	Diagnosis: CHF	Physician: J. Physician, MD
C. Right	J. Right	11-7 J. Doe, R.N.	JD		Room: PCU-14 PCU
D. Left	K. Left				
E. Abdomen 1|2 3|4					

Figure 22-3 *Computerized Medication Administration Record*

Guidelines for Medication Administration

Nurses have traditionally used the "five rights" of drug administration as a guideline to protect clients from medication errors.

1. Right drug
2. Right dose
3. Right client
4. Right route
5. Right time

The nurse is legally responsible for knowing the usual dose, the expected action, the side effects, the adverse reactions, and any interactions with other drugs or food of every drug administered. Without this knowledge, the nurse should not administer any medication.

Right Drug

The medications listed on the MAR or, less frequently, on a medication card are checked against the physician's order before any medication is administered. When procuring a medication, check the label on the container against the MAR at least three times.

1. When removing the drug container from the client's medication drawer
2. When removing the drug from the container
3. Before returning it to the client's medication drawer

Right Dose

Know how to correctly calculate dosages and have them checked before administration. Policy in some facilities requires two nurses to check insulin dosages to ensure accuracy.

Scored tablets are seldom broken, but if they are, make sure the tablets are broken evenly. This prevents overdosage or underdosage. After crushing pills with a mortar and pestle, thoroughly cleanse the mortar and pestle to avoid mixing different medications.

Right Client

Correctly identify the client by checking the client's identification band and asking the client to state his or her full name. Never identify a client by calling the person's name because confused clients will answer to any name.

Right Route

The route for giving the medication is specified in the written order. If a route is not identified in the order, the route ordered differs from the recommended one, or the route prescribed is questioned, the prescriber should be consulted. For example, the nurse should never substitute an oral medication for an intramuscular medication simply because the oral medication is available.

Right Time

Medications have to be given in a timely manner to maintain their effects. They are generally ordered on a schedule and should not be given more than an hour before or after the scheduled time, or as per agency policy, without first checking with the physician.

Safety: Medication Administration
- *Never administer medications prepared by another nurse.* You are responsible for a medication error if you administer a medication that was inaccurately prepared by another nurse.
- Listen carefully to the client questioning the addition or deletion of a medication and recheck the order.
- When circumstances prevent giving prescribed medications to the client, the exact reason must be documented in the client's record.
- *Do not leave medications at the client's bedside.*
- Initial the MAR only for those medications you actually have administered.
- Advise clients not to offer their medications to others and not to take medications belonging to others.

In the home health and community care settings, such as a retirement home, the nurse has different responsibilities regarding drug safety (Figure 22-4).

Documentation of Drug Administration

Documentation is a critical element of drug administration. The standard is *"if it was not documented, it was not done."* Appropriate documentation can prevent many drug errors. The nurse administering a medication must initial the medication on the MAR for the time the drug was given. Usually space is available for a full signature

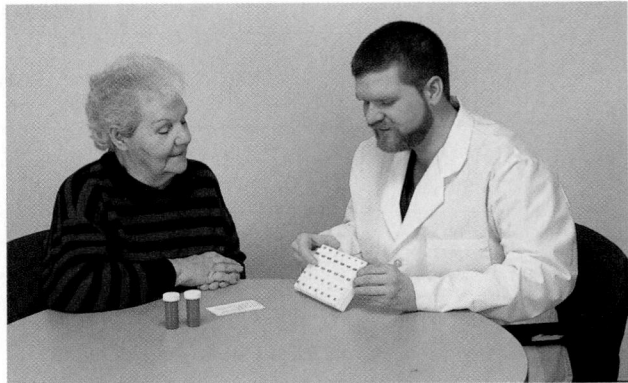

Figure 22-4 *Assisting Client at Home with a Pillbox Correlated to the Days of the Month*

on the record. Documentation should be done *after* the client has received the drug.

If a client refuses to take a medication, document that a dose was missed, why the dose was missed, and notify the physician. Clients do have the right to refuse a medication, but most will be willing to take it if they understand the actions of the medication. Medication times must be rescheduled for clients having various diagnostic tests or treatments at the time the medication is to be administered and the change documented.

Drug Supply and Storage

Drugs are dispensed by the pharmacy to nursing units by various methods, accommodating the facility's medication system. After the pharmacy delivers drugs to a nursing unit, the nurse is responsible for their safe storage.

Scheduled drugs are usually dispensed in a unit dose form for each client. **Unit dose** is a system of packaging and labeling each dose of medication by the pharmacy, usually to supply the scheduled drugs for a 24-hour time period. Unit dose drugs are usually stored in a medication cart containing individual drawers for each client's medications or in a medication room in separate containers for each client. The unit dose system makes it easy to administer the correct dose, thereby minimizing the number of medication errors.

COMMUNITY/HOME HEALTH CARE

Considerations for Drug Safety

- Encourage and assist the client in removing outdated prescriptions and over-the-counter drugs from medication cabinets.
- Encourage the client or caregivers to maintain drug refills to decrease the risk of missing scheduled medications.
- Use a pillbox or reminder calendar (Figure 22-4) to help the client or caregiver remember to take or administer medications as scheduled.

At the beginning of each shift, the nurse usually checks the medications in each client's drawer. Some medication carts are locked and the nurse keeps the key. When the nurse is preparing medications for administration, the medication drawers should be removed one at a time from the cart. A drawer should never be left on top of the cart unattended. Drugs should not be used from one client's supply for another client.

Certain drugs may be **stock supplied** (dispensed and labeled in large quantities) and are kept together in a secured area. Some medications and intravenous fluids must be stored in a designated medication refrigerator to preserve the integrity of the drug. *Only drugs can be stored in the medication refrigerator.*

Narcotics and Controlled Substances

Health care facilities have special forms to record the supply on hand and the administration of narcotics and controlled substances according to federal regulations. These forms usually require the following information for each drug administered:

- Name of the client receiving the drug
- Amount of the drug used
- Time the drug was administered
- Name of the prescribing physician
- Name of the nurse administering the drug

Nurses are required to count the narcotics and controlled substances at specified times, usually at the change of shifts. One nurse going off duty counts the drugs with a nurse coming on duty. Each drug dose must be accounted for on the narcotic record. When the narcotic count does not check, the discrepancy must be reported immediately. Narcotics and controlled substances are kept in a double-locked drawer, box, room, or medication-dispensing cart, such as a computer-controlled dispensing system as shown in Figure 22-5. The law requires these safety precautions for narcotics and controlled substances.

MEDICATION COMPLIANCE

When clients do not take their prescribed medications consistently or when they adjust the scheduling or dose of the medication, they are *noncompliant.*

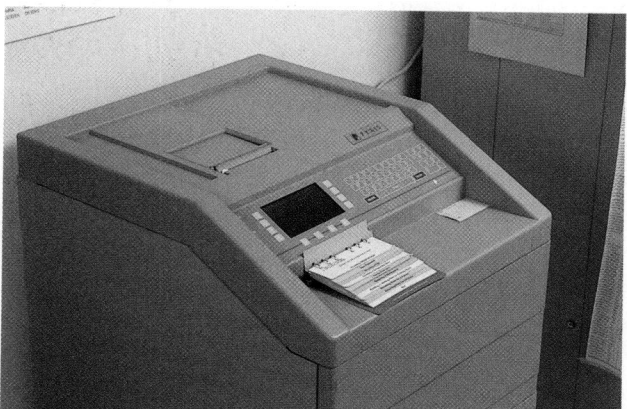

Figure 22-5 *Computer-Controlled Dispensing System*

Clients may have several reasons why they choose not to take ordered medications. They may not understand the need to take prescribed medications, medications may cost too much for the client on a fixed income, the medication may not provide prompt relief, or the medication may cause undesirable side effects.

Compliance can be enhanced by giving the client information on the medications to take at home. Large print or illustrations should be used if the client is elderly. When educating the client, include the caregiver. Compliance may be enhanced by giving the client a telephone number to call if questions arise.

LEGAL ASPECTS OF MEDICATION ADMINISTRATION

Remember the "five rights" for safe administration of medications. Giving the wrong medicine to the client is an error; giving the right medicine but wrong dose or wrong route is an error; giving a medication at the wrong time is an error. The physician must be informed of all errors and needs accurate information to make appropriate decisions. Medications given in error must be documented on the MAR.

Medication errors must be reported in a timely manner. Incident reports are generally required for medication errors. The report must include the name of the medication, dose given, route, time administered, specific error, time the physician was contacted about the error, what countermeasures were taken, and the client's response.

Sometimes nurses discover errors made by other nurses. These must also be reported and documented.

NURSING PROCESS

The nursing process is vital in planning client care and in ensuring safe and accurate medication administration.

Assessment

The subjective data include medication history and medical history. Objective data include a physical examination and diagnostic and laboratory data.

Medication History

A medication history obtained when a client is admitted to a health care facility should contain information about the client's medication background, including allergies, and use of prescription and over-the-counter drugs.

CRITICAL THINKING

Incorrect Drug

You discover that a similar but incorrect drug (not the drug ordered) is being given IV to a client. What is the first thing you should do? What is your next course of action? How do you feel about the nurse who made the medication error and did not recognize it?

Allergies Inquire about all medication and food allergies. The client who has had an allergic reaction to a drug should describe the details of the reaction: name of the drug; dosage, route, and number of times the drug was taken before the reaction; onset of the reaction; and evidences of the reaction. Ask about possible contributing factors to the allergic reaction, such as concurrent use of stimulants or depressants (tobacco, alcohol, or illegal drugs) or significant changes in nutritional status.

Allergies to foods should also be discussed because drugs may contain the same substances that cause allergic reactions to some foods. For example, clients who are allergic to shellfish may have a reaction to drugs containing iodine. Vaccines are commonly derived from chick embryos and would be contraindicated for clients with allergies to eggs.

Prescription Drugs The client should identify all current prescription drugs and describe the following:

- Why the drug was prescribed and by whom
- The drug's dosage, route, and frequency
- The client's knowledge of the drug's action: side and adverse effects, when to notify the physician, and special administration considerations such as with or without foods

Over-the-Counter Drugs Ask specifically about nonprescription drugs taken by the client. For example, determine if the client takes aspirin, laxatives, or antacids routinely, along with the dosage, route, and frequency of these drugs. Also ask about the use of creams, ointments, patches, or sprays.

Medical History

Gather information about chronic diseases and disorders and correlate these data with the prescription drugs.

Sensory and Cognitive Status Assess for and inquire about sensory deficits such as vision or hearing impairments. Assess the client's cognitive abilities during the history interview by noting if the client is alert and oriented and interacts appropriately.

Physical Examination

The client's condition is assessed before administering any drug to establish the client's baseline, or normal, health status. For example, the nurse assesses the client's apical pulse before administering digoxin (Lanoxin), an inotropic, so that the heart rate after receiving the drug can be compared with the baseline measurement.

Diagnostic and Laboratory Data

Common laboratory values, such as electrolytes, blood urea nitrogen, creatinine, glucose, complete blood count, and a white blood cell count, are usually monitored over a period to identify trends and to measure the body's response to medications.

Nursing Diagnosis

Once the actual or potential problems are identified, relevant nursing diagnoses can be identified. The NANDA (2003) nursing diagnoses commonly related to medication administration include:

- Ineffective **H**ealth Maintenance
- Deficient **K**nowledge (specify)
- Ineffective **T**herapeutic Regimen Management
- Impaired Physical **M**obility
- Disturbed **S**ensory Perception
- Impaired **S**wallowing

Planning/Outcome Identification

The care plan and goals are developed based on the nursing diagnoses. For example, the client with a knowledge deficit related to a newly prescribed drug may have the following expected outcomes:
Before discharge the client will:

- Correctly state the actions of the drug in the body.
- Prepare the correct dose of the drug.
- List the possible side effects of and possible adverse reactions to the drug.
- Correctly identify special considerations (i.e., take with food, no alcohol).

Implementation

The main nursing interventions related to medication management are assessment, administration, and teaching. Use the time spent when administering medications to assess the client's knowledge of and response to the drug.

Medication administration requires implementing safety guidelines, following the "five rights." Medications are administered according to set procedures based on the prescribed route. This section presents information for medication administration by the following routes: oral, including sublingual and buccal; parenteral; site-specific topical applications; and inhalation.

Drug teaching usually takes place in two phases. The first phase is usually a formal teaching session, when the drug's action, route, side and adverse effects, and the specific signs of a drug reaction that require physician notification are explained. Clients may need assistance developing a drug schedule that fits their lifestyle. Teaching the client and/or support person specific procedural techniques, such as subcutaneous injection, may be necessary.

The second phase of client teaching occurs whenever a drug is administered. At each interaction, assess and reinforce the client's knowledge of drugs. When a client is

---

CLIENT TEACHING

Written Medication Information

Written medication information for clients should be accurate, specific, comprehensive, and presented in a legible and understandable format. It should:

- Include generic and trade names.
- State indications for use, contraindications, precautions, adverse reactions, risks, and storage.
- Provide straightforward instructions.
- Have conspicuous drug warnings.
- Have print size appropriate to client's visual abilities.
- Be appropriate for client literacy level.

taught self-administration, the teaching plan should identify dates for teaching and a date for achievement of goals.

Oral Drugs

Oral administration of drugs is the most common
route; however, potential risk factors must be considered. Assess the client's ability to take the medication before administering oral drugs by assessing the client's
state of consciousness, gag reflex, and presence of nausea and vomiting. These assessments assist in protecting
the client from aspiration. **Aspiration** is the inhalation
of secretions or fluids into the pulmonary system.

Liquid medications are measured out in a calibrated
medicine cup. Doses smaller than 1 dr, 1 tsp, or 5 mL are
measured in a syringe for accuracy. Solid oral medications are put into a medicine cup or small paper (soufflé)
cup, depending on agency policy. Individually wrapped
medications should be opened at the bedside.

Remain with the client when administering oral
drugs, until all medications have been swallowed. When
in doubt that the client has swallowed a pill, don a nonsterile glove and visually inspect the client's mouth using
a tongue depressor (Figure 22-6).

Sublingual and Buccal Assess the integrity of the
mucous membranes by inspecting under the client's
tongue and in the buccal cavity before administering
sublingual and buccal drugs. When oral membranes are
excoriated or painful, withhold the medication and notify the physician. For buccal drugs that irritate the mucosa, alternate sides of the mouth. Drugs given by these
routes are quickly absorbed by the mucosa's abundant
blood supply and the thin epithelium.

Enteral **Enteral installation** is the delivery of drugs
through a gastrointestinal tube. Enteral tubes provide a
way to directly instill medications into the gastrointestinal system of clients who cannot take them orally.

There are several types of enteral tubes. A nasogastric
tube (NG) is a soft rubber or plastic tube inserted through a
nostril and into the stomach. The gastrostomy tube is surgically inserted into the stomach through the abdomen.

Check the tube for **patency** and placement and assess
the client for the presence of bowel sounds before administering a medication. Patency is being freely open.

Figure 22-6 *Check the client's mouth if unsure that medications have been swallowed.*

When the tube is obstructed or improperly placed, the
client is vomiting, or bowel sounds are absent, the instillation of drugs is contraindicated.

Once the patency and placement of the tube have
been determined, prepare the medication for instillation
as prescribed by the physician. When the physician orders a drug in tablet form, crush the tablet into minute
particles and dissolve the crushed tablet in 15 to 30 mL
of warm water before instillation. Cold water may cause
abdominal cramps when instilled. Open capsules and
empty the contents into a liquid.

Parenteral Drugs

Parenteral medications are given through a route other than the alimentary canal; these routes are intradermal, subcutaneous, intramuscular, or intravenous. The insertion angle of the needle and the depth of penetration indicate the type of injection (Figure 22-7).

Equipment To administer parenteral medications, special equipment such as syringes, needles, ampules, and vials are used.

Syringes A syringe has three basic parts: the hub, which connects with the needle; the barrel, or outside part, which has measurement calibrations; and the plunger, which fits inside the barrel and has a rubber tip (Figure 22-8). The hub, the inside of the barrel, and the shaft and rubber plunger tip must be kept sterile. When handling a syringe, touch only the outside of the barrel and the plunger's handle.

Most syringes are disposable, made of plastic, and individually packaged. There are hypodermic, insulin, and tuberculin syringes (Figure 22-9). When a medication is incompatible with plastic, it is usually prefilled into a single-dose glass syringe. Syringes are often packaged with the size and gauge needle commonly used.

The *hypodermic syringe* comes in 2-, 2.5-, and 3-mL sizes. The measurement calibrations are usually in cubic centimeters (cc) and minims. Most syringes are marked in cubic centimeters, while most drugs are ordered in milliliters; these are equivalent measurements (1 cc = 1 mL). The hypodermic syringe is used most often when a medication is ordered in milliliters. When the order is written in minims, it is safer to use a tuberculin syringe.

The *insulin syringe* is designed especially for use with insulin. For example, if the physician writes the order for 30 units of U-100 insulin, use an insulin syringe calibrated on the 100-unit scale. Always compare the size of

Figure 22-9 *Type of Syringes:* **A,** *Hypodermic;* **B,** *Standard U-100 insulin (Courtesy of Becton Dickinson Consumer Products);* **C,** *1-mL tuberculin (Courtesy of Becton Dickinson and Company)*

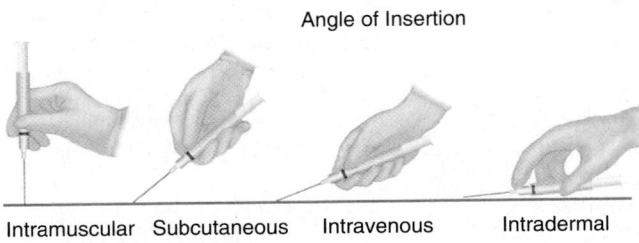

Figure 22-7 *Angle of Insertion for Parenteral Injections*

Figure 22-8 *The Parts of a Syringe*

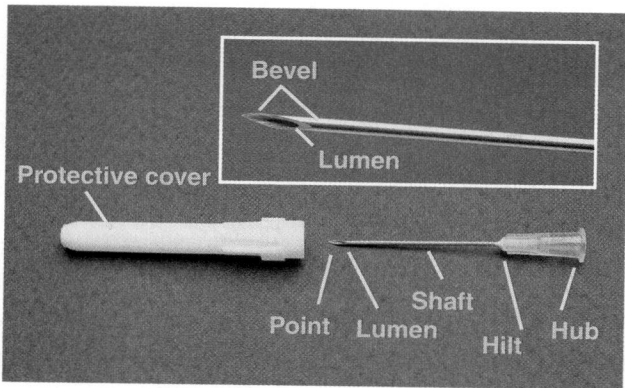

Figure 22-10 *Parts of a Needle*

Figure 22-11 *A*, *Ampules;* ***B*,** *Vials*

the insulin syringe and the strength indicated on the insulin bottle with the physician's order; all three units must be the same.

The *tuberculin syringe* is a narrow syringe, calibrated in tenths and hundredths of a milliliter (up to 1 mL) on one scale and in sixteenths of a minim (up to 1 minim) on the other scale. This syringe is generally used to administer small or precise doses (i.e., pediatric dosages). The tuberculin syringe should be used for doses 0.5 mL or less.

Prefilled single-dose syringes should not be confused with a unit dose. The prescribed dose must be checked against that in the prefilled syringe and the excess discarded. For example, if the physician orders diazepam (Valium) 5 mg IM as a preoperative sedative and the prefilled single-dose contains 10 mg/2 mL, the dosage must be calculated (5 mg/1 mL) and 1 mL discarded from the syringe before administration.

Needles Most needles are made of stainless steel, disposable, and individually packaged. Reusable needles are seldom used today, except in surgery and special procedure rooms. These needles require frequent inspection to ensure that the needle is sharp, and resterilization is necessary between uses.

A needle has three aspects: the hub, which fits onto the syringe hub; the cannula, or shaft; and the bevel, which is the slanted part at the tip of the shaft (Figure 22-10). Needles come in many sizes, from $1/4$ to 5 inches long, with gauges from 28 to 14. The *gauge* refers to the diameter of the shaft; the larger the number, the smaller the diameter of the shaft. Smaller needles (larger gauge) produce less trauma to the body's tissue; however, the viscosity of a solution must be considered when selecting the gauge.

The *shaft* of the needle indicates its length. The length of the needle is selected based on the client's muscle development and weight and the type of injection, such as intravenous versus intramuscular.

Needles may have a short or a long *bevel*. The bevel length is selected based on the type of injection. Long bevels are sharp and produce less pain when inserted into the subcutaneous or muscle tissues. A short bevel is used for intradermal and intravenous injections to prevent the tissue or blood vessel wall from occluding the bevel.

The hub of the needle should be immediately attached to the hub of the syringe when removed from its sterile wrapper to prevent contamination. The protective cover should remain on the needle until it is ready to be used.

Used needles must be disposed of in the proper receptacles, such as a sharps container, to prevent needlesticks. All client care areas have sharps containers in most facilities. Discussion of the needleless system is found under IV therapy later in this chapter.

Ampules and Vials Drugs for parenteral injections must be sterile. Those that deteriorate in solution are dispensed as tablets or powders to be dissolved in a solution immediately before injection. Drugs remaining stable in solution are dispensed in ampules and vials in an aqueous or an oily solution or suspension.

Ampules are glass containers of single-dose drugs (Figure 22-11A). The glass container has a constriction in the stem to facilitate opening the ampule. Drugs may be irritating to the subcutaneous tissue, so the needle should be changed after withdrawing a drug from an ampule.

Glass, single- or multiple-dose rubber-capped drug containers are called vials (Figure 22-11B). A vial usually has an easily removed soft metal cap. The needle should be changed after withdrawing a drug from a vial.

PROFESSIONAL TIP

Expiration Date

- Laws require manufacturers to put expiration dates on all drugs.
- To ensure a drug is current, check the expiration date.
- Return outdated drugs to the pharmacy for proper disposal.

Intradermal Injection Intradermal (ID) or intracutaneous injections are used to administer local anesthetics, identify allergens, and diagnose tuberculosis. Below the epidermis is the location for administering ID injections; drugs are absorbed slowly from this site. Commonly used sites for ID injection are the inner aspect of the forearm, upper back, and upper chest.

The drug's dosage for an ID injection is usually a small amount of solution (0.01 to 0.1 mL). To provide accurate measurement, use a 1-mL tuberculin syringe with a short bevel, 25 to 27 gauge, $^3/_8$- to $^1/_2$-inch needle. For repeated doses the site should be rotated. Intradermal injections are administered into the epidermis by angling the needle 10 to 15 degrees to the skin.

Subcutaneous Injection Subcutaneous (SC or SQ) injections are used to administer insulin and heparin because they are absorbed slowly, creating a sustained effect. Subcutaneous injections put the medication between the dermis and the muscle into the subcutaneous tissue. The amount of medication given varies but seldom exceeds 1.5 mL. For repeated doses the site should be rotated.

Common sites for SC injections include the abdomen, the lateral aspect of the upper arm or the anterior aspect of the upper thigh, the scapular area on the back, and the upper ventrodorsal gluteal area. Select a sterile 0.5- to 3-mL syringe with a 23 to 25 gauge and a $^3/_8$- to $^3/_4$- inch needle. The medication is administered by angling the needle 45 degrees to the skin.

Intramuscular Injection Intramuscular (IM) injections promote rapid drug absorption and provide another route for drugs that are irritating to subcutaneous tissue. The absorption rate is greater because there are more blood vessels in the muscles than in subcutaneous tissue; however, the client's circulatory status may affect the absorption rate.

The four common sites for administering IM injections are the dorsogluteal and ventrogluteal (gluteus maximus muscle); the anterolateral aspect of the thigh (vastus lateralis muscle); and the upper arm (deltoid muscle). These sites are identified by using appropriate anatomic landmarks. An IM injection is administered at a 90-degree angle to the skin.

Z-Track Injection A Z-track (zig-zag) injection is a method for administering IM injections, most commonly in the ventrogluteal and dorsogluteal muscles.

For administration of a Z-track injection, the client is placed in the prone position; the skin is pulled to one side, the needle is inserted at a 90-degree angle, and the medication is administered. After 10 seconds the needle is withdrawn and then the skin is released. Do not massage the site; it may cause tissue irritation. Never inject more than 5 mL in a single site (Giving Z-track Injections, 2002).

Intravenous Therapy Intravenous (IV) therapy requires parenteral fluids (solutions) and special equipment: administration set, IV pole, filter, regulators to control IV flow rate, and an established venous route.

Parenteral Fluids Read the physician's order in the client's medical record to confirm the type and amount of IV solution. Intravenous solutions are sterile and usually packaged in plastic bags. Solutions incompatible with plastic are in glass containers.

Plastic IV solution bags collapse under atmospheric pressure, allowing the solution to enter the infusion set. Plastic solution bags are packaged with an outer plastic bag, which should remain intact until the solution is prepared for administration. The solution bag should be dry when removed from its outer wrapper. If it is wet, the solution should not be used. Moisture on the bag shows that the integrity of the bag has been compromised, and the solution cannot be considered sterile. Return the bag to the department that issued the solution. Glass containers are discussed in the section on equipment.

Parenteral fluids are classified based on their relationship to normal blood plasma. Solutions may be hypotonic, isotonic, or hypertonic. The solution prescribed is based on the client's diagnosis and the goal of therapy. The solution's effect is:

- *Hypotonic fluid.* Lowers osmotic pressure and makes fluid move into the cells. Water intoxication may result if fluid is infused beyond the client's tolerance.
- *Isotonic fluid.* Increases only extracellular fluid volume. Cardiac overload may result if fluid is infused beyond the client's tolerance.
- *Hypertonic fluid.* Increases osmotic pressure and draws fluid from the cells. Cellular dehydration may result if fluid is infused beyond the client's tolerance (Bulechek & McCloskey, 2000).

Common intravenous solutions are shown in Table 22-5.

TABLE 22-5 COMMON INTRAVENOUS SOLUTIONS

TONICITY	SOLUTION	CONTENTS (MEQ/L)	CLINICAL IMPLICATIONS
Hypotonic	Sodium chloride 0.45%	77 Na$^+$, 77 Cl$^-$	Daily maintenance of body fluid and establishment of renal function.
Isotonic	Dextrose 2.5% in 0.45% saline	77 Na$^+$, 77 Cl$^-$	Promotes renal function and urine output.
	Dextrose 5% in 0.2% saline	77 Na$^+$, 77 Cl$^-$	Daily maintenance of body fluids when less Na$^+$ and Cl$^-$ are required.
	Dextrose 5% in water (D$_5$W)	38 Na$^+$, 38 Cl$^-$	Promotes rehydration and elimination; may cause urinary Na$^+$ loss; good vehicle for K$^+$.
	Ringer's lactate	130 Na$^+$, 4 K$^+$, Ca^{2+}, 109 Cl$^-$, 28 lactate	Resembles the normal composition of blood serum and plasma; K$^+$ level below body's daily requirement.
	Normal saline (NS), 0.9%	154 Na$^+$, 154 Cl$^-$	Restores sodium chloride deficit and extracellular fluid volume.
	Dextran 40 10% in NS (0.9%) or D$_5$W		A colloidal solution used to increase plasma volume of clients in early shock; *it should not be given to* severely dehydrated clients and clients with renal disease, thrombocytopenia, or active hemorrhaging.
	Dextran 70% in NS		A long-lived (20 hours) plasma volume expander; used to treat shock or impending shock caused by hemorrhage, surgery, or burns. *It can prolong bleeding and coats the RBCs (draw type and crossmatch before administering).*
Hypertonic	Dextrose 5% in 0.45% saline	77 Na$^+$, 77 Cl$^-$	Daily maintenance of body fluid and nutrition; treatment of FVD.
	Dextrose 5% in saline 0.9%	154 Na$^+$, 154 Cl$^-$	Fluid replacement of sodium, chloride, and calories (170).
	Dextrose 10% in saline 0.9%	154 Na$^+$, 154 Cl$^-$	Fluid replacement of sodium, chloride, and calories (340).
	Dextrose 5% in lactated Ringer's	130 Na$^+$, 4 K$^+$, 3 Ca^{2+}, 109 Cl$^-$, 28 lactate	Resembles the normal composition of blood serum and plasma; K$^+$ level below body's daily requirement; caloric value 180.
	Hyperosmolar saline 3% and 5% NaCl	856 Na$^+$, 865 Cl$^-$	Treatment of hyponatremia; raises the Na osmolarity of the blood, and reduces intracellular fluid excess.
	Ionosol B with dextrose 5%	57 Na$^+$, 25 K$^+$, 49 Cl$^-$, 25 lact., 5 Mg^{2+}, 7 PO^{4-}	Treatment of polyionic parenteral replacement caused by vomiting-induced alkalosis, diabetic acidosis, fluid loss from burns, and postoperative FVD.

From *Fluids and Electrolytes with Clinical Applications* (7th ed.), by J. L. Kee & B. J. Paulanka, 2004, Clifton Park, NY: Thomson Delmar Learning. Copyright 2004 by Thomson Delmar Learning. Reprinted with permission.

Equipment Intravenous equipment is disposable, sterile, and prepackaged with user instructions. The user instructions, including a schematic labeling the parts, are usually placed on the outside of the package, which allows the user to read the package before opening. IV equipment requires sterile technique when handling because it is in direct contact with fluids to be infused into the bloodstream.

The administration (infusion) set includes an insertion spike with a protective cap, a drip chamber, tubing with a slide clamp and regulating (roller) clamp, a rubber injection port, and a protective cap over the needle adapter (Figure 22-12). Protective caps keep both ends of the set sterile and are removed only when used. The insertion spike is inserted into the port of the IV solution container.

Infusion sets are vented or nonvented. The nonvented type is used with plastic bags and vented bottles. The vented set is used for nonvented glass containers (Figure 22-13).

There are two types of drip chambers: a macrodrip, which releases 10 to 20 drops per milliliter of solution, and a microdrip, which releases 60 drops per milliliter. The drop rate, which varies with the manufacturer, is indicated on the package.

The roller clamp compresses the plastic tubing to control the flow rate. At the end of the IV tubing is a needle

Figure 22-12 *Sample Basic Administration Set*

Figure 22-13 *Sample Vented-Administration Set*

adapter that connects to a sterile injection device inserted into the client's vein. Extension tubing may be used to lengthen the primary tubing or provide additional Y-injection ports for administering additional solutions.

Intravenous Filters Intravenous filters remove particulate matter that may cause irritation and **phlebitis** (inflammation of a vein) from the solution. Intravenous filters come in various sizes. An in-line filter is found in many IV catheters. Then, it is not necessary to add a filter to the tubing.

Needles and Catheters Needles and catheters provide access to the venous system. A variety of devices of different sizes to accommodate the age of the client and the type and duration of therapy are available (Figure 22-14). The larger the number, the smaller the lumen of the needle or catheter; a 20 is larger than a 28.

Butterfly (scalp vein or wing-tipped) **needles** are short, beveled needles with plastic wings attached to the shaft. The wings (which are flexible) are held tightly together to facilitate needle insertion and then are flattened against the skin and taped to prevent dislodgment. These are generally used for short-term or intermittent therapy and for infants and children.

Several types of catheters are used to access peripheral veins. Some of these catheters are threaded over a needle, and others are threaded inside a needle during insertion. **Intracath** refers to a plastic tube inserted into a vein. An **angiocatheter** (angiocath, for short) is a type of intracath with a metal stylet to pierce the skin and vein; then the plastic catheter is threaded into the vein and the metal stylet is removed.

Needle-Free System Safety is a concern with IV therapy. Accidental needlestick injuries and puncture wounds with contaminated devices increase the employee's risk for infectious diseases such as AIDS, hepatitis (B and C), and other viral, rickettsial, bacterial, fungal, and parasitic infections. Many health care facilities use totally needle-free IV systems to increase employee safety.

Vascular Access Devices Vascular access devices (VADs) include various cannulas, catheters, and infusion ports that allow long-term IV therapy or repeated access to the central venous system. The client's diagnosis and the type and length of treatment determine the kind of VAD used. Central venous catheters (CVCs) are inserted by a physician.

The **implantable port** (a device made of a radiopaque silicone catheter and a plastic or stainless steel injection port with a self-sealing silicone-rubber septum) is another type of VAD. *Only nurses who have been specially trained are allowed to access an implanted port because of the risk of infiltration into the tissue if needle placement is incorrect.*

Preparing an Intravenous Solution Before preparing an IV solution, first read the physician's order and the agency's protocol, then gather necessary equipment. Because IV solutions and equipment are sterile, the

Figure 22-14 *Peripheral IV Devices:* **A,** *Butterfly;* **B,** *Angiocatheter*

Selecting Needle Gauge

Consider the client's age and body size and the type of solution to be administered when selecting the gauge of the needle or catheter.

- Infants and small children, 24 gauge
- Preschool through preteen, 24 or 22 gauge
- Teenagers and adults, 22 or 20 gauge
- Elderly, 24 or 22 gauge

package expiration date should be checked before use. The IV can be prepared in the client's room or in a nurses' work area.

Prepare a time strip and apply it to the IV solution bag to easily monitor the infusion rate prescribed by the physician (Figure 22-15). Tag the IV tubing with the date and time to notify when the tubing needs to be replaced. Intravenous tubing is changed every 24 to 48 hours according to agency policy. The time strip and the IV tubing tag should be initiated by the nurse.

 Safety: Marking an IV Bag
The ink from a felt-tip pen can leak through the plastic and contaminate the solution. Do not use such a pen.

Initiating IV Therapy Before starting IV therapy, consider the type of fluid to be infused, calculate the flow rate, and assess for a venipuncture site. Ellenberger

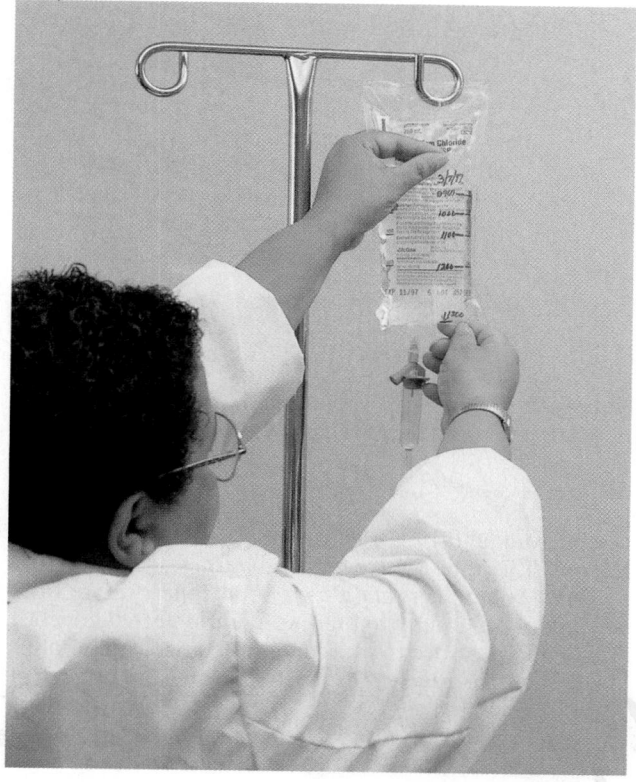

Figure 22-15 *Applying a Time Strip to the IV Container*

PROFESSIONAL TIP

Inserting a CVC

When assisting with the insertion of a long-line central catheter, observe the client for symptoms of a pneumothorax: sudden shortness of breath or sharp chest pain; increased anxiety; a weak, rapid pulse; hypotension; pallor or cyanosis. These symptoms indicate accidental puncture of the pleural membrane.

LIFE CYCLE CONSIDERATIONS

Locating a Vein

For clients who are elderly or have fragile veins, eliminate the tourniquet or apply it very loosely if a vein can be palpated.

(1999) suggests that the smallest gauge and shortest needle appropriate be selected (22 gauge for maintenance fluids and routine antibiotics, 20 gauge or larger for blood products).

Calculating Flow Rate The physician prescribes the **flow rate,** the volume of fluid to infuse over a set period. For example, 125 mL per hour or 1,000 mL over an 8-hour period. The hourly infusion rate is calculated as follows:

$$\frac{\text{Total volume}}{\text{Number of hours to infuse}} = \text{mL/hour infusion rate}$$

For example, if 1,000 mL is to be infused over 8 hours:

$$\frac{1,000}{8} = 125 \text{ mL/hour}$$

Calculate the actual infusion rate (drops per minute) as follows:

$$\frac{\text{Total fluid volume}}{\text{Total time (minutes)}} \times \text{Drop factor} = \text{Drops per minute}$$

For example, if 1,000 mL is to be infused over 8 hours with a tubing drop factor of 10 drops per milliliter:

$$\frac{1,000 \text{ mL}}{8(60)\text{min}} \times 10 \text{ drops/mL} = \frac{10,000 \text{ drops}}{480 \text{ min}} = 20.8, \text{ or } 21, \text{ drops/min}$$

Another way to calculate the actual infusion rate is to use the hourly infusion rate; for the first example:

$$\frac{125 \text{ mL} \times 10 \text{ drops/mL}}{60 \text{ min}} = 20.8 \text{ or } 21 \text{ drops/min}$$

Consider body size, age, skin condition, clinical status, and impairments when assessing for a potential IV site. Venipuncture site, contraindications are as follows:

- Any signs of infection, infiltration, or thrombosis
- Affected arm of a postmastectomy client
- Arm with a functioning arteriovenous fistula (dialysis)
- A paralyzed arm
- Arm with circulatory or neurological impairments

Because venous blood flows upward toward the heart, select a vein for an IV at its most distal end to maintain the integrity of the vein. When a vein is punctured with a needle, fluids can infiltrate (leak from the vein into the tissue at the site of puncture). When IV therapy is discontinued for infiltration, it can only be restarted above the initial puncture site. Generally, it is best to begin with the hand and advance up the arm if new sites are needed. Figure 22-16 illustrates common peripheral sites for initiating IV therapy.

Locating a Vein With the client's arm extended on a firm surface, place a tourniquet on the arm, tight enough to impede venous flow yet loose enough that a radial pulse can still be palpated. Next, the index and middle fingers of the nondominant hand are used to palpate a vein. It should feel soft and resilient and not have a pulse. If no vein can be seen or felt, a warm, moist compress may be applied for 10 to 20 minutes, the area may be massaged toward the heart, or the client may open and close the fist (Ellenberger, 1999).

Placing the Needle After hand hygiene and gloving is completed, prepare the selected site according to agency policy. Without touching the prepared site, stabilize the vein by placing your thumb beside the vein and pulling down. Hold the needle at a 10- to 30-degree angle, bevel up to puncture the skin, then lessen the angle to prevent puncturing the back of the vein (Ellenberger, 1999). Secure the needle in place according to agency policy.

Infection Control: Venipuncture

Standard Precautions must be followed when performing a venipuncture.

Administering IV Therapy When the solution has been prepared and the rate calculated, explain the procedure to the client. Administration may be continuous over a 24-hour period, or intermittent, 1,000 mL once in a 24-hour period. Although fluids may be continuous, the type of fluids can change over a 24-hour period. For example, an order might read: *Add 40 mEq of KCl to first bag of 1,000 mL of normal saline.*

Intravenous medications may be **piggybacked**, connected to an existing IV to infuse concurrently. Refrigerated solutions and medications should be warmed to room temperature before administration (usually for 30 minutes) for client comfort.

Regulating IV Solution Flow Rate The flow rate for IV solutions can be regulated by calculating the drops per

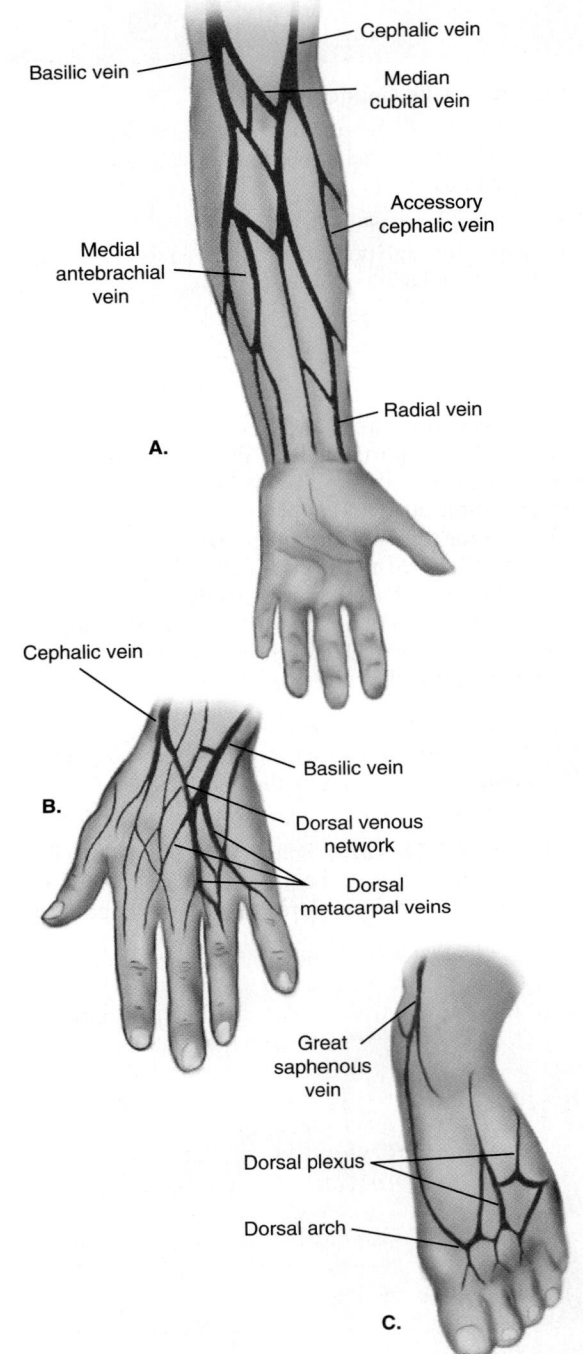

Figure 22-16 *Peripheral Veins Used in Intravenous Therapy: A, Forearm; B, Dorsum of the hand; C, Dorsal plexus of the foot*

minute and adjusting the drip rate to that number or by the use of volume controllers and pumps.

Volume Controllers and Pumps Controllers are devices dependent on gravity to maintain a preselected flow but do not add pressure to overcome resistance (e.g., Dial-a-Flo or Buretrol). Resistance may develop from the use of a large catheter in a small vein, high venous pressure, infusing a viscous solution, or a decrease in the height of the container from the IV site. Resistance causing a de-

IV-Related Sepsis

If a client has chills and fever, check how long the IV solution has been hanging and the needle or catheter has been in place. Assess the client's vital signs and for other symptoms of pyrogenic reactions, such as backache, malaise, headache, nausea, and vomiting. If IV-related sepsis occurs, the pulse rate increases, and temperature is usually above 100°F. Stop the infusion, notify the physician, and obtain blood specimens if ordered.

crease in the flow will sound the controller alarm. Volumetric controllers permit flow rates to be set in milliliters per hour.

Pumps maintain a preselected volume delivery by adding pressure when needed. Pumps may be used when large volumes must be delivered in a short period and for viscous fluids. Pumps have maximum pressure limits that sound an alarm when reached. When a drug or solution is administered under high pressure, clients have a greater risk for complications.

Managing IV Therapy Intravenous therapy requires frequent client monitoring to ensure an accurate flow rate. Other nursing actions are to ensure client comfort and position; check the IV solution to ensure that the solution, amount, and timing are correct; monitor expiration dates of the IV system (tubing, venipuncture site, dressing) and change as necessary; and be aware of safety factors.

Client care must be coordinated with the maintenance of IV lines. Changing the gown and IV tubing when doing site care decreases the number of times the access device is manipulated, thereby decreasing the risk for infiltration and phlebitis. Peripherally inserted devices are changed every 72 hours as directed by the Centers for Disease Control and Prevention (CDC) guidelines.

Hypervolemia **Hypervolemia** (increased circulating fluid volume) may result from rapid IV infusion of solutions, causing cardiac overload, which can lead to pulmonary edema and cardiac failure. The infusion rate must be monitored hourly to prevent this.

When a solution infuses at a rate greater than prescribed, decrease the rate to *keep vein open* (KVO) and immediately notify the physician. Report the amount and type of solution that was infused over the exact time period and the client's response.

Infiltration **Infiltration** (inadvertent administration of a nonvesicant solution into surrounding tissue) may result from dislodging the device from the vein, inserting the wrong type of device, or using the wrong-gauge needle. Using a high pressure pump may also cause infiltration or vein irritation. The client usually complains of discomfort at the IV site. Inspect the site by palpating for swelling and feeling the temperature of the skin (coolness and paleness of skin are indications of infiltration).

Confirm that the needle is still in the vein by pinching the IV tubing. This action should cause **flashback** (blood will rush into the tubing if the needle is still in the vein).

If flashback does not occur, the injection port nearest the device should be aspirated. The needle or catheter should be removed from the vein if it cannot be aspirated and a sterile dressing applied to the puncture site.

The puncture site may ooze or bleed after the IV has been removed (especially in clients receiving anticoagulants). If oozing or bleeding occurs, apply pressure until it stops and reapply a sterile dressing. Accurately assess and document the degree of edema.

Injury may occur from infiltration. If an IV site is grossly infiltrated, the soft tissue edema may cause nerve compression with permanent loss of function to the extremity. **Extravasation** is the inadvertent administration of a **vesicant** (medication that causes blistering and tissue injury when it escapes into surrounding tissue) into surrounding tissue. This may cause significant tissue loss with permanent disfigurement and loss of function (Hadaway, 2002a).

Phlebitis Phlebitis may result from either mechanical or chemical trauma. Inserting a device with too large a gauge, using a vein that is too small or fragile, or leaving the device in place for too long may cause mechanical trauma. Chemical trauma may result from infusing too rapidly or from an acidic solution, hypertonic solution, a solution containing electrolytes (especially potassium and magnesium) or other medications.

Phlebitis may be a precursor of sepsis. Client descriptions of tenderness are usually the first indication of an inflammation. The IV site must be inspected for changes in skin color and temperature (a reddened area or a pink or red stripe along the vein, warmth, and swelling are indications of phlebitis).

If phlebitis is present, the IV infusion must be discontinued. Before removing and discarding the venous device, check the facility's protocol to see whether the tip of the device is to be cultured. If so, it must be sent to the laboratory for a culture and sensitivity test. After removing the device, apply a sterile dressing to the site and wet, warm compresses to the affected area. Document the time, symptoms, and nursing interventions.

Intravenous Dressing Change Standard Precautions and aseptic technique are followed for intravenous dressing changes. The frequency of care is determined by institutional protocol and the type of intravenous access device and dressing. Persistent drainage at the IV site may require more frequent dressing changes or may necessitate changing the IV site.

Intravenous Drug Therapy When a rapid drug effect is desired or a medication is irritating to tissue, the intravenous (IV) route is used. Intravenous administration immediately releases medication into the bloodstream; therefore, it can be dangerous. Intravenous medications are administered by one of the following modes:

- Intravenous fluid container
- Volume-control administration set
- Intermittent infusion by piggyback or partial fill
- Intravenous push (IVP or bolus)

Adding Drugs to an Intravenous Fluid Container Before administering IV medications, assess the patency of the infusion system and the condition of the injection site for signs of infiltration and phlebitis. Some IV medications or solutions with high or low pH or high osmolarity are irritating to veins and can cause phlebitis. Also note the client's allergies, drug or solution incompatibilities, the amount and type of diluent needed to mix the medication, and the client's general condition to establish a baseline before administering medication. **Drug incompatibilities** are an undesired chemical or physical reaction between a drug and a solution, between a drug and the container or tubing, or between two drugs. For example, diazepam (Valium) and chlordiazepoxide hydrochloride (Librium) are not compatible with a saline solution; insulin sticks to the inside of the solution bag, so use glass bottles.

Adding Drugs to a Volume-Control Administration Set
A volume-control set is used to administer small volumes of IV solution. They have various names, such as Soluset, Metriset, VoluTrol, or Buretrol. To use this method, do the following:

- Withdraw the prescribed amount of medication into a syringe.
- Cleanse the injection port of a partially filled volume-control set with an alcohol swab.
- Inject the prepared medication through the port of the volume-control set.
- Gently mix the solution in the volume-control chamber.
- Check the infusion rate and adjust as necessary.

Administering Medications by Intermittent Infusion A common method of administering IV medications is by using a secondary, or partial-fill additive bag, often called IV piggyback (IVPB). The secondary line is a complete IV set (fluid container and tubing with either a microdrip or a macrodrip system) connected to a Y-port of a primary line. The primary line maintains venous access. The IVPB is used for medication administration. When the IVPB medication is incompatible with the primary IV solution, flush the primary IV tubing with normal saline before and after administering the medication.

Intermittent Infusion Devices When the client requires only IV medications without a quantity of solution, an intermittent infusion device is attached to a peripheral needle or catheter in the client's vein. This device is commonly referred to as a heparin or saline lock, depending on the facility's policy of heparin or saline maintenance. A lock provides continuous venous access, eliminating the need for a continuous IV and increasing the client's mobility.

The device can be used to infuse intermittent IVPB or IV push (also called bolus) medications, or it can be converted to a primary IV. An **IV push (bolus)** is the administration of a large dose of medication in a relatively short time, usually 1 to 30 minutes. A heparin lock device provides venous access in case of an emergency and is routinely used with cardiac clients.

Administering IV Push Medications An IV push medication can be injected into a saline or a heparin lock (Figure 22-17A) or into a continuous infusion line. When giving an IV push medication into a continuous infusion line, stop the fluids in the primary line by pinching the IV tubing closed while injecting the drug (Figure 22-17B). This technique is safe and prevents having to recalculate the drip rate of the primary infusion line.

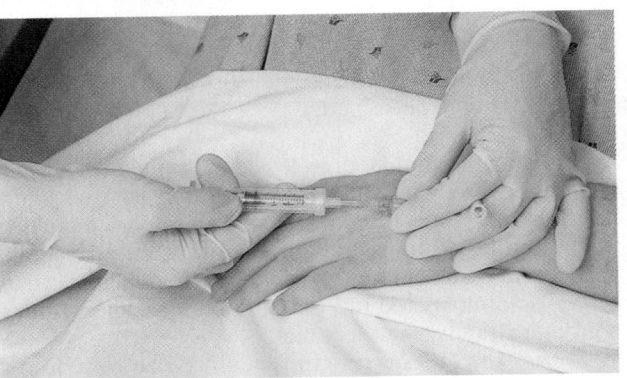

Figure 22-17 *Injecting an IV Push (Bolus) Medication:* **A,** *into a Peripheral Saline Lock;* **B,** *into a Primary Infusion Line. The IV tubing must be pinched closed first.*

Documentation

When IV therapy is begun, the date, time, venipuncture site, number of attempts made, amount and type of fluid, and equipment used must be documented. Each time the insertion site, venipuncture device, or IV tubing is changed, the reason for the change must be documented (e.g., routine, infiltration). The condition of the insertion site and the fluid type, amount, and flow rate are documented each shift and at intervals specified by agency policy. Any complications are precisely documented along with the nurse's actions.

Blood Transfusion

A blood transfusion is given to replace blood loss (deficit) with whole blood or blood components. Based

---

COMMUNITY/HOME HEALTH CARE

Blood Temperature

Blood is transported to the client in a container that maintains proper storage temperature for 6 hours. Because the container does not have thermometers and alarms, it is not considered "monitored" storage, and the blood cannot be returned to inventory if the transfusion is canceled (Fitzpatrick & Fitzpatrick, 1997).

on the client's unique needs, the physician determines the type of transfusion, either whole blood or a component of whole blood.

Whole Blood and Blood Products Whole blood contains red blood cells (RBCs) and plasma components of blood. It is used when all the components of blood are needed to restore blood volume, and to restore the oxygen-carrying capacity of the blood.

When the physician prescribes whole blood or a blood product, the client's blood is typed and crossmatched. If time and the client's condition permit, the family may arrange for donors. The blood is stored in the blood bank after typing and crossmatching.

Whole blood has a refrigerated shelf life of 35 days, but platelets must be administered within 3 days after extracted from whole blood. If the RBCs and plasma are frozen, their shelf life is up to 3 years (Kee & Paulanka, 2004).

Initial Assessment and Preparation Before administering blood, perform an initial assessment, including the following:

- Verify that the client has signed a blood administration consent form and that this consent matches what the physician has prescribed.
- Identify the gauge of needle or catheter used if IV in place. The viscosity of whole blood usually requires an 18-gauge needle or catheter to prevent red blood cell damage. If blood is to be infused quickly, a 14- or 15-gauge device must be used.
- Ensure patency of the existing IV site.
- Establish vital signs baseline data, especially temperature, and assess skin for eruptions or rashes.
- Verify label on the whole blood or blood component with the client's blood type before administration, to ensure compatibility.
- Assess the client's age and state of nutrition.

Scheduled IV medications should be infused before blood administration to prevent a medication reaction while blood is infusing. If a reaction were to occur, it would not be known whether the medication or the blood was causing the reaction.

Administering Whole Blood or a Blood Component A facility's blood protocol may require that a licensed person sign a release for blood from the blood bank and that two licensed personnel check blood products before infusion. Information that must be on the blood bag label and verified for accuracy includes the client's name and identification number, ABO group and Rh factor, donor number, type of product ordered and expiration date.

To maintain RBC integrity and decrease the chance of infection, blood administration should begin within 30 minutes after it was received from the bank. Whole blood should not be unrefrigerated for more than 4 hours. Room temperature causes RBC lysis, releasing potassium and causing hyperkalemia.

Safety Measures Observe the client for the initial 15 minutes for a transfusion reaction. Take vital signs every 15 minutes for the first hour, then every hour while the blood is infusing.

Safety: Blood Transfusion Incompatibilities
Only normal saline can be used with a blood product. Blood transfusions are incompatible with dextrose and with Ringer's solution.

The three basic types of transfusion reactions are allergic, febrile, and hemolytic and may be mild or severe, depending on the cause. Hemolytic reactions may be immediate or delayed up to 96 hours, depending on the cause of the reaction. Other complications include sepsis, hypervolemia, and hypothermia. The classic symptoms of a reaction and sepsis are fever and chills.

The nursing actions for all types of reactions and complications are given in Table 22-6.

Topical Medications

Topical medications may be administered to the skin, eyes, ears, nose, throat, rectum, and vagina. The

---

LIFE CYCLE CONSIDERATIONS

Initial Assessment

If pediatric, elderly, or malnourished clients are at risk for circulatory overload, notify the blood bank to divide the 500-mL bag of blood into two 250-mL bags or discuss with the physician other alternatives, such as packed RBCs rather than whole blood.

PROFESSIONAL TIP

Transfusion Reaction

Transfusion reaction severity is related to the time of onset. Severe reactions usually occur shortly after the blood begins to infuse. At the first sign of a reaction, stop the blood infusion immediately.

TABLE 22-6	NURSING ACTIONS FOR BLOOD REACTIONS	
IMMEDIATE NURSING ACTION	**OTHER MEASURES**
• Stop transfusion. • Keep vein open with normal saline. • Notify the physician.	• Monitor client's vital signs every 15 minutes for 4 hours or until stable. • Monitor I&O. • Send IV tubing and bag of blood back to the blood bank. • Obtain a blood and urine specimen. • Label specimen "Blood Transfusion Reaction." • Process a transfusion reaction report.

medication provides a local effect but may also have systemic effects. Drugs applied directly to the skin for a local effect include lotions, pastes, creams, ointments, powders, and aerosol sprays. The vascularity of the area determines the rate and degree of the drug's absorption.

Topical drugs provide continuous absorption to produce various effects: to relieve pruritus (itching), to prevent or treat an infection, to provide local anesthesia, to protect the skin, or to create a systemic effect. Topical medications are usually applied two or three times a day to achieve their therapeutic effect.

Before applying a topical preparation, the condition of the skin must be assessed for any rashes, open lesions, or areas of erythema and skin breakdown. The nurse should check with the client and the medical record for any known allergies.

Cleanse the area by washing it with soap and warm water, unless contraindicated by a specific order. Allow the skin to thoroughly dry before applying a topical medication. Open wounds require the use of aseptic technique.

When the skin is dry, the medication can be applied. To apply a paste, cream, or an ointment, follow Standard Precautions. To prevent cross-contamination, use a sterile tongue depressor for removing the medication from the container. Transfer the medication from the tongue blade to a gloved hand for application. Apply the medication in long, smooth strokes in the direction of the hair follicles to prevent the medication from entering the hair follicles. When more medication is removed from the container, a new sterile tongue depressor must be used. Assess the area for signs of an allergic reaction 2 to 4 hours after the application.

Eye Medications Eye medications can be drops, ointments, or disks. These drugs are used for diagnostic and therapeutic purposes, to lubricate the eye or socket for a prosthetic eye, and to treat or prevent eye conditions such as glaucoma (elevated pressure within the eye) and infection. Diagnostically, eyedrops are used to dilate the pupil, anesthetize the eye, or stain the cornea to identify abrasions and scars.

 Safety: Prevent Cross-Contamination
- Never share a bottle of eyedrops between clients.
- After instillation, discard any solution remaining in the dropper.
- Discard the dropper if the tip is accidentally contaminated (i.e., touching the bottle or any part of the client's eye).

Medication disks are inserted at bedtime because they usually cause blurred vision. Follow Standard Precautions when administering eye care and medications; there is a potential for contact with bodily secretions.

Ear Medications Solutions ordered for the ear are often called *otic* (pertaining to the ear) drops or irrigations.

Eardrops may be instilled to soften ear wax, treat infection or inflammation, produce anesthesia, or facilitate removal of a foreign body. External auditory canal irrigations are usually performed for cleansing purposes.

Inspect the ear for signs of drainage (an indication of a perforated tympanic membrane) before instilling a solution into the ear. Eardrops are usually contraindicated with a perforated tympanic membrane. Aseptic technique must be used if the tympanic membrane is damaged. Otherwise, medical asepsis is used for ear medications.

Nasal Instillations Nasal instillations can be either drops or nebulizers (atomizer or aerosol). Nasal drugs produce one or more of the following effects: shrink swollen mucous membranes, loosen secretions and facilitate drainage, or treat infections of the nasal cavity or sinuses. Because the nose is connected with the sinuses, medical asepsis is used when performing nasal instillations.

Many of these products are nonprescription drugs, so clients should be taught their correct usage. Nasal decongestants are common over-the-counter drugs to shrink swollen mucous membranes; however, they may have a reverse or rebound effect by increasing nasal congestion when used in excess.

Nebulizers (inhalers) deliver a fine mist containing medication droplets. The client who is discharged with a nasal inhaler must be taught how to store and use the device. Assist clients in the use of atomizers and aerosols:

- Have the client clear the nostrils by blowing the nose.
- Client should be in an upright position with head tilted back slightly.

For atomizers:
- Occlude one nostril to prevent air from entering the nasal cavity and allow the medication to flow freely into the open nostril.
- Insert the atomizer tip into the open nostril and ask the client to inhale, while the atomizer is squeezed once, then ask the client to exhale.

For aerosols:
- Shake the aerosol well before each use.
- Grasp between thumb and index finger and insert the adapter tip into one nostril while occluding the other nostril with a finger, then press the adapter cartridge firmly to release one measured dose of medication.
- Repeat the above steps for the other nostril.
- Have the client keep the head tilted backward for 2 to 3 minutes and breathe through the nose while the medication is being absorbed.

Respiratory Inhalants Respiratory inhalants are delivered by devices that produce fine droplets to be inhaled deep into the respiratory tract. They are absorbed very quickly through the alveolar epithelium into the bloodstream. This section discusses only oropharyngeal handheld inhalers.

Oropharyngeal handheld inhalers deliver medications, such as bronchodilators and mucolytics, that produce both local and systemic effects. Bronchodilators (drugs that dilate the bronchi) improve airway patency and prevent or treat asthma, bronchospasms, and allergic reactions. Mucolytics liquify tenacious (thick) bronchial secretions.

Clients must be able to assemble the turbo-inhaler and form an airtight seal around the inhaling devices. This requirement prevents some clients from using these devices. Bronchodilators are contraindicated for clients having a history of tachycardia.

Rectal Instillations Rectal instillations can be in the form of suppositories, ointments, or enemas. Rectal ointments are used to treat local conditions and hemorrhoid symptoms of pain, inflammation, and itching. Rectal suppositories are cone-shaped medications designed to melt at body temperature and be absorbed at a slow and steady rate.

Suppositories are a convenient and safe route for administering drugs that interact poorly with digestive enzymes or have a bad taste or odor. They are used to provide temporary relief for clients who cannot tolerate oral preparations (e.g., to relieve nausea and vomiting). They

CLIENT TEACHING

Tampon Use
Clients should not use tampons after the insertion of vaginal medications because the tampon can absorb the medication and decrease the drug's effect.

are also used to reduce fever, relieve pain and local irritation, and stimulate peristalsis and defecation in clients who are constipated.

The rectum should be assessed for irritation or bleeding and sphincter control checked. Some clients may have a problem retaining the suppository. Ask those clients to remain in Sims' position for at least 15 minutes or have the client lie on the abdomen, if allowed, and hold the buttocks closed. When the client is unable to retain a suppository, notify the physician so that another route can be ordered.

Vaginal Instillations Medications inserted into the vagina may be suppositories, creams, ointments, gels, foams, or douches. They are used to treat infections, inflammation, and discomfort or as a contraceptive measure.

Vaginal creams, gels, ointments, and foams usually come with a disposable applicator with a plunger to insert the drug. Suppositories are usually inserted with the index finger of a gloved hand; however, small suppositories may come with an applicator. After insertion of these preparations, the client may notice drainage and should be told to expect this. To prevent soiling of the underpants, the client should be told to wear a perineal pad.

Agency policy usually requires sterile technique when administering a vaginal douche (irrigation). Check that the client does not have an allergy to iodine because many vaginal preparations contain povidone-iodine.

Evaluation

Administering medications according to the five "rights" requires the nurse to verify that safe nursing care was provided. Evaluation includes that each client knows the effects, side effects, adverse reactions, special considerations, and when to call the physician for each drug.

A nurse identifying a potential medication risk and initiating actions to prevent client injury is performing another form of evaluation.

PROFESSIONAL TIP

Contraindications for Rectal Suppositories
- Cardiac clients because insertion may stimulate the vagus nerve, causing cardiac dysrhythmias (abnormal heart patterns).
- Clients recovering from rectal or prostate surgery because suppositories may cause pain on insertion and trauma to the tissues.

Summary

- The *United States Pharmacopeia* and the *National Formulary* list drug standards for use in the United States.
- The Food and Drug Administration tests all drugs before granting a company the right to market a drug.
- Drugs are usually referred to by their generic name (not capitalized) or by their trade name (always capitalized).
- The safest and least expensive administration route is the oral route, although it is also the slowest to act.

SAMPLE NURSING CARE PLAN

THE CLIENT WITH DEEP VEIN THROMBOSIS

Mrs. Landry, a 45-year-old, was admitted to your floor with a diagnosis of deep vein thrombosis. She noticed swelling of her left leg about a week ago but decided to treat it at home. Four days later the lower leg was very edematous, warm, and painful to move. After an office visit, Mrs. Landry was admitted to the hospital. This is her first hospitalization. On examination the left leg is warmer than the right. The left thigh circumference is 3 inches larger than the right. The physician ordered a heparin IV drip after a loading dose bolus was given. The drip contained 10,000 units heparin in 500 mL of D_5W at 10 mL/h (200 units/h). The physician anticipates that Mrs. Landry will be weaned off of the heparin drip and started on subcutaneous heparin within 5 days. At the time of discharge she will be given Coumadin.

Nursing Diagnosis 1 *Ineffective Tissue Perfusion (peripheral)* related to the development of venous thrombi in the deep femoral vein as evidenced by left leg being warmer than right leg and left thigh circumference being 3 inches larger than right thigh circumference

Nursing Outcomes Classification (NOC)	**Nursing Interventions Classification (NIC)**
Tissue Perfusion: Peripheral	*Embolus Care: Peripheral*
Circulation Status	*Circulatory Care: Venous Insufficiency*

PLANNING/GOALS	NURSING INTERVENTIONS	RATIONALE
Mrs. Landry will:	Maintain on bedrest.	Reduces the possibility of embolus; may decrease the pain and swelling.
Report an absence of pain.	Apply moist heat to the affected extremity.	Provides an analgesic effect; it decreases venospasms and pain.
Have a decrease of edema.	Elevate the legs above the heart.	Facilitates venous return and decreases the edema.
	Measure the circumference of the left thigh and compare with that of the right thigh.	Provides a quantitative reference point that can be used to evaluate the swelling.
Experience the same degree of skin temperature in both legs.	Administer the heparin drip at 200 units/h.	Prevents the conversion of fibrinogen to fibrin and prothrombin to thrombin, thereby limiting the extension of the thrombus.
	Monitor the partial thromboplastin time (PTT).	Monitors heparin therapy because heparin, a short-acting anticoagulant, increases the PTT.

EVALUATION   Mrs. Landry is able to ambulate without difficulty or pain. Mrs. Landry's left thigh is only $1/2$ inch larger than her right thigh. Mrs. Landry has no temperature difference between her legs.

Nursing Diagnosis 2   *Risk for Injury (bleeding)* related to the administration of an anticoagulant.

Nursing Outcomes Classification (NOC)	**Nursing Interventions Classification (NIC)**
Risk Detection	*Teaching: Disease Process*
	Medication Management

continues

SAMPLE NURSING CARE PLAN

PLANNING/GOALS	NURSING INTERVENTIONS	RATIONALE
Mrs. Landry will:	Withhold the medication in the event that bleeding occurs and to notify the physician immediately.	The dose may need to be adjusted.
Not demonstrate evidence of bleeding from gums or nose, in urine or stool, or under the skin.	Encourage the client to discontinue smoking.	May increase the metabolism of the medication, necessitating an increase in the dose.
Maintain her prothrombin time (PT) or international normalized ratio (INR) within therapeutic range.	Advise the client to watch food intake.	Foods high in fat and foods rich in vitamin K can interfere with the PT.
	Warn against taking oral contraceptive medication.	Decreases anticoagulant effect.
	Warn against taking aspirin and other over-the-counter medications.	May increase the risk of bleeding; it inhibits platelet formation.

EVALUATION   Mrs. Landry has had no bleeding episodes. Mrs. Landry still has many questions about taking the oral anticoagulant on discharge. Discharge follow-up will be needed to monitor the client's progress on the oral anticoagulant.

- Parenteral drugs are injected through intradermal (ID), subcutaneous (SC or SQ), intramuscular (IM), or intravenous (IV) routes and are typically fast-acting.
- The pharmacokinetics of drugs includes absorption, distribution, metabolism, and excretion.
- The five "rights" of safe drug administration are right drug, right dose, right client, right route, and right time.
- Nurses are legally and morally responsible for correct administration of medications.
- Oral liquid medications are poured and measured at eye level to ensure accuracy.
- Although the physician determines the dose and route of a parenteral drug, the nurse chooses the correct gauge and length of the needle to be used.
- Always monitor client reactions to medications and ensure that clients know the actions, side effects, and contraindications of all medications they take.
- Clients receiving intravenous therapy or blood transfusions require constant monitoring for complications.

Review Questions

1. A client is unable to swallow the pills ordered by the physician. The best action for the nurse is to:
   a. tell the client to chew the pills.
   b. crush the pills and give them to the client.
   c. call the physician for a change in the orders.
   d. ask the pharmacy to send the medications in liquid form.

2. The client is in the bathroom when the nurse brings the medications. The best action for the nurse is to:
   a. return with the medications when the client is finished in the bathroom.
   b. leave the medications for the client to take when finished in the bathroom.
   c. knock on the bathroom door and give the medications to the client at this time.
   d. ask the nursing assistant to see that the client takes the medications when finished in the bathroom.

3. The best time for the nurse to document medication administration is:
   a. whenever the nurse has time.
   b. before the client receives the medication.
   c. only after the client has received the medication.
   d. toward the end of the shift so all medications can be charted at one time.

4. Standard Precautions are required with:
   a. venipuncture.
   b. IM injections.
   c. oral medications.
   d. nasal instillation.

5. A client receiving a blood transfusion tells the nurse, who is taking the first set of 15-minute vital signs, that she is cold (chills) and her chest hurts. The first thing the nurse should do is:

   a. stop the transfusion.

   b. get a warm blanket for the client.

   c. call the blood bank to come and check the blood.

   d. stay with the client and talk quietly to her to help her relax.

References/Suggested Readings

American Hospital Formulary Service, McEvoy, G. (ed.). (2002). *AHFS drug information 2002*. Bethesda, MD: American Society of Health System Pharmacists.

Behrman, R. E., Kliegman, R., & Jenson, H. B. (Eds.). (2004). *Nelson textbook of pediatrics* (17th ed.). Philadelphia: W. B. Saunders.

Blanchard & Loeb. (2003). Nurse's Drug Handbook 2003. Philadelphia: Blanchard & Loeb Publishers, LLC.

Bulechek, G.M., & McCloskey, J.C. (2000). *Nursing interventions: Effective nursing treatments* (3rd ed.). Philadelphia: W. B. Saunders.

Carroll, P. (2003). Medication errors: The bigger picture. *RN, 66*(1), 52–57.

Charting Tips. (2000). Documenting IV therapy, part I. *Nursing2000, 30*(2), 73.

Charting Tips. (2000). Documenting IV therapy, part II. *Nursing2000, 30*(3), 83.

Daniels, J., & Smith, L. (1999). *Clinical calculations* (4th ed.). Clifton Park, NY: Thomson Delmar Learning.

Dochterman, J., & Bulechek, G. (2004). *Nursing Interventions Classification (NIC)*, (4th ed.). St. Louis, MO: Mosby.

Ellenberger, A. (1999). Starting an IV line. *Nursing99, 29*(3), 56–59.

Fitzpatrick, L., & Fitzpatrick, T. (1997). Blood transfusion: Keeping your patient safe. *Nursing97, 27*(8), 34–41

Giving Z-track injections. (2002). *Nursing2002, 32*(9), 81.

Goldy, D. (1998). Circulatory overload secondary to blood transfusion. *AJN, 98*(7), 33.

Hadaway, L. C. (1999a). Choosing the right vascular access device, part I. *Nursing99, 29*(2), 18.

Hadaway, L. C. (1999b). Choosing the right vascular access device, part II. *Nursing99, 29*(7), 28–29.

Hadaway, L. (2002a). IV infiltration: Not just a peripheral problem. *Nursing2002, 32*(8), 36–42.

Hadaway, L. (2002b). What you can do to decrease catheter-related infections. *Nursing2002, 32*(9), 46–48.

Hadaway, L. (2003). Infusing without infecting. *Nursing2003, 33*(10), 58–63.

Hrouda, B. S. (2002). Warming up to IV infusion. *Nursing2002, 32*(3), 54–55.

Josephson, D. L. (1999). *Intravenous infusion therapy for nurses: Principles and practice*. Clifton Park, NY: Thomson Delmar Learning.

Karch, A., & Karch, F. (2002). Double dosing. *AJN, 102*(10), 23.

Karch, A., & Karch, F. (2003). Not so fast. *AJN, 103*(8), 71.

Kee, J., & Paulanka, B. (2004). *Fluids and electrolytes with clinical applications* (7th ed.). Clifton Park, NY: Thomson Delmar Learning.

Larouere, E. (1999). Deaccessing an implanted port. *Nursing99, 29*(6), 60–61.

Lehne, R. (2004). *Pharmacology for nursing care* (5th ed.). Philadelphia: W. B. Saunders.

Macklin, D. (2000). Removing a PICC. *AJN, 100*(1), 52–54.

Masoorli, S. (2002). How to accurately document IV insertion. *Nursing2002, 32*(6), 65.

Matheny, N., Wehrle, M. A., Wiersema, L., & Clark, J. (1998). Testing feeding tube placement: Auscultation vs. pH method. *AJN, 98*(5), 37–42.

McConnell, E. (1998). Giving medications through an enteral feeding tube. *Nursing98, 28*(3), 6.

McConnell, E. (1999). Administering a Z-track IM injection. *Nursing99, 29*(1), 26.

McConnell, E. (2001). Instilling ear drops. *Nursing2001, 31*(4), 17.

McConnell, E. (2002). Administering medication through a gastrostomy tube. *Nursing2002, 32*(12), 22.

Metheny, N., & Titler, M. (2001). Assessing placement of feeding tubes, *AJN, 101*(5), 36–45.

Millam, D. (original manuscript), Hadaway, L. (revised manuscript). (2003). On the road to successful I.V. starts. A supplement to *Nursing2003, 33*(5 Supp1), between pages 64 and 65.

Moorhead, S., Johnson, M., & Maas, M. (2004). *Nursing Outcomes Classification (NOC)*, (3rd ed.). St. Louis, MO: Mosby.

North American Nursing Diagnosis Association. (2003). *Nursing diagnoses: Definitions and classification 2003-2004.* Philadelphia: NANDA.

Obenour, P. (1998). Administering an S.C. medication continuously. *Nursing98, 28*(6), 20.

Pickar, G. (2004). *Dosage calculation* (7th ed.). Clifton Park, NY: Thomson Delmar Learning.

Pope, B. (2002). How to administer subcutaneous and intramuscular injections. *Nursing2002, 32*(1), 50–51.

Przybylek, C. (2002). Two ways to avoid a "sticky" IV situation. *Nursing2002, 32*(11), 47–49.

Rice, J. (2001). *Medications & mathematics for the nurse* (9th ed.). Clifton Park, NY: Thomson Delmar Learning.

Royer, T. (2001). Looking for a vein? Stick with venous ultrasound. *Nursing2001, 31*(11), 72–73.

Saxton, D., & O'Neill, N. (1998). *Math and meds for nurses*. Clifton Park, NY: Thomson Delmar Learning.

Schatzlein, K. (2003). Hold tight: Keeping catheters secure. *Nursing2003, 33*(3), 20–21.

Smetzer, J. (2001). Take 10 giant steps to medication safety. *Nursing2001, 31*(11), 49–53.

Smith, L. (2003). Clarifying a medication order. *Nursing2003, 33*(5), 26.

Spratto, G., & Woods, A. (2004). *PDR nurse's drug handbook 2004.* (8th ed.). Clifton Park, NY: Thomson Delmar Learning.

Togger, D., & Brenner, P. (2001). Metered dose inhalers. *AJN, 101*(10), 26–32.

Trimble, T. (2003a). Peripheral IV starts: Insertion tips. *Nursing2003, 33*(8), 17.

Trimble, T. (2003b). Starting peripheral IVs: Tips for planning ahead. *Nursing2003, 33*(4), 30.

Resources

Infusion Nurses Society, Fresh Pond Square, 10 Fawcett Street, Cambridge, MA 02138, 616-441-3008, www.ins1.org

Institute for Safe Medication Practices, 1800 Baberry Road, Suite 810, Huntingdon Valley, PA 19006, 215-947-7797, www.ismp.org

National Coordinating Council for Medication Error Reporting and Prevention, www.nccmerp.org

U.S. Pharmacopeia, 12601 Twinbrook Parkway, Rockville, MD 20852, 800-822-8772, www.usp.gov

ASSESSMENT

MAKING THE CONNECTION

Refer to the following chapters to increase your understanding of health assessment:

Basic Nursing
- **Communication**
- **Cultural Considerations**
- **Loss, Grief, and Death**
- **Complementary/Alternative Therapies**
- **Fluid, Electrolyte, and Acid–Base Balance**
- **Pain Management**

Adult Health Nursing
- **The Older Adult**

Basic Procedures
- **Hand Hygiene**
- **Taking a Temperature**
- **Taking a Pulse**
- **Counting Respirations**
- **Taking Blood Pressure**
- **Weighing Client, Mobile and Immobile**

LEARNING OBJECTIVES

Upon completion of this chapter, you should be able to:
- **Define key terms.**
- **Identify the components of functional health patterns.**
- **Utilize the framework of functional health to facilitate a holistic assessment process.**
- **Analyze the components of the head-to-toe assessment.**
- **Incorporate the four assessment techniques within the head-to-toe assessment.**
- **Utilize the head-to-toe assessment in clinical situations.**

KEY TERMS

adventitious breath sound	orthostatic hypotension
affect	palpation
auscultation	percussion
borborygmi	pleural friction rub
bradycardia	pulse amplitude
bradypnea	pulse deficit
bronchial sound	pulse rate
bronchovesicular sound	pulse rhythm
crackle	review of systems
cyanosis	sibilant wheeze
dyspnea	Snellen chart
eupnea	sonorous wheeze
health history	stridor
hyperventilation	tachycardia
hypoventilation	tachypnea
inspection	vesicular sound

INTRODUCTION

Within the scope of the nursing profession, a complete nursing assessment is necessary to analyze each client's needs in a holistic manner. Nursing assessment includes both physical and psychosocial aspects to evaluate a client's condition. Caring, respect, and concern are demonstrated for each client when doing a nursing assessment.

A thorough nursing assessment includes both a health history and a physical examination. For a health history, the client is interviewed to identify how the client adjusts to or lives within the environment. This is subjective data, or information based on client self-report. The physical examination, objective data, includes observations made by the nurse while utilizing the assessment techniques of inspection, palpation, percussion, and auscultation. Other sources of objective data are laboratory tests, x-rays, and measurements of the client's vital signs, height, and weight.

The initial nursing assessment generally occurs within 8 hours of a client's admission to a health care facility and continues throughout the stay. In a physician's office or health care clinic, the nursing assessment would be completed immediately. Most institutions have a standard assessment form (Figure 23-1).

Usually a health history is completed before the physical examination, but in emergency situations or when performing care in a health care facility after the initial admitting assessment, it will be necessary to incorporate history-taking into the physical examination. When incorporating a health history into the head-to-toe assessment, the nurse must remember to incorporate questions about the client's habits or usual patterns along with the physical data collected in the head-to-toe assessment. Functional assessment is best done within the framework of the physical assessment because the environment in which each client resides and participates becomes a part of the physical assessment. The functional assessment brings the environment in which the client lives and the physical needs of that client together to establish a holistic picture.

HEALTH HISTORY

A primary focus of the data collection interview is the health history. The **health history** is a review of the client's functional health patterns before the current contact with a health care agency. Whereas the medical history concentrates on symptoms and the progression of disease, the nursing health history focuses on the client's functional health patterns, responses to changes in health status, and alterations in lifestyle. The health history is also used in developing the plan of care.

Demographic Information

Personal data including name, address, date of birth, gender, religion, race/ethnic origin, occupation, and type of health plan/insurance should be included. This information may be useful in understanding a client's perspective.

Reason for Seeking Health Care

The client's reason for seeking health care should be described in the client's own words. For example, the statement "fell off four-foot ladder and landed on right shoulder; unable to move right arm" is the client's actual report of the event that precipitated a need for health care. The client's perspective is important because it explains what is significant about the event from the client's point of view. It is also important to know the time of the onset of symptoms.

Perception of Health Status

Perception of health status refers to the client's opinion of his or her general health. It may be useful to ask clients to rate their health on a scale of 1 to 10 (with 10 being ideal and 1 being poor), along with the client's rationale for the rating score. For example, the nurse may record a statement such as the following to represent the client's perception of health: "Rates health a 7 on a scale of 1 (poor) to 10 (ideal) because he must take medication regularly to maintain mobility, but the medication sometimes upsets his stomach."

Previous Illnesses, Hospitalizations, and Surgeries

The history and timing of any previous experiences with illness, surgery, or hospitalization are helpful in order to assess recurrent conditions and to anticipate responses to illness because prior experiences often affect current responses.

Client/Family Medical History

Ascertain any family history (blood relative) of acute and chronic illnesses that tend to be familial. Health history forms often include checklists of various illnesses that can be used as the basis for questions. It is also helpful to indicate the relative's relationship to the client (e.g., mother, father, sister).

Immunizations/Exposure to Communicable Diseases

A record of current immunizations should be obtained. This is particularly important with children; however, records of immunizations for tetanus, influenza, pneumonia, and hepatitis B are important for adults. A history of childhood or other communicable diseases should be noted. If the client has traveled out of the country, the time frame should be noted in order to determine incubation periods for relevant diseases. Also ask about potential exposure to communicable diseases such as tuberculosis or human immunodeficiency virus (HIV).

Allergies

Any drug, food, or environmental allergies should be noted in the health history, along with the type of reaction to the substance. For example, a client may report that a rash or shortness of breath developed after taking penicillin. This reaction should be recorded. Clients may report an "allergy" to a medication because their stomach was upset after ingesting it. This is a side effect that would not preclude administration of the drug in the future.

 Safety: Assessment for Allergies
It is essential to explore possible allergies before administering any medications. Allergic reactions can be life-threatening and can occur with very low dosages of medications. A client's sensitivity to a drug can also change over time, resulting in severe reactions even though the client has successfully taken the drug during prior illnesses or experienced only mild reactions to the drug in the past.

Current Medications

All medications currently taken, both prescription and over-the-counter, should be recorded by name, frequency, and dosage. Ask about birth control pills, lax-

FUNCTIONAL SCREENING (ADULT)

*Physical Therapy:
0 pts = complete independence
1 pt = recent onset of neurological problem
1 pt = recent onset of orthopedic problem
1 pt = recent onset of problem with impaired mobility (ambulation, stair climbing, bed mobility, transferring)
2 pts = open wound or an acute burn
TOTAL POINTS
* A Score of 2 or More Points Requires a Physical Therapy Screening.
Physical Therapy Screening Requested
☐ Yes ☐ No

*Occupational Therapy
0 pts = complete independence
1 pt = acute decline in upper extremity function
1 pt = recent onset of a neurological or orthopedic problem
1 pt = recent onset of a problem causing a decrease in ADL function (Bathing, Dressing, Feeding Toileting)
TOTAL POINTS
* A Score of 2 or More Points Requires an Occupational Therapy Screen.
Occupational Therapy Screening Requested
☐ Yes ☐ No

*Speech Therapy
0 pts = no identified problems
2 pt = recent onset of swallowing problems
1 pt = recent onset of speech difficulty
1 pt = recent neurological problem affecting ability to follow commands
2 pt = radical ENT surgery
TOTAL POINTS
* A Score of 2 or More Points Requires a Speech Therapy Screen.
Speech Therapy Screening Requested
☐ Yes ☐ No

PASTORAL CARE SCREEN

[ ] Would you like a special request sent for a visit from our chaplain?
[ ] Yes [ ] No
[ ] If Yes, Send Request to Pastoral Care

PATIENT INSTRUCTION CHECKLIST

☐ Signal Light   ☐ Telephone   ☐ Shower   ☐ Dentures/Hearing Aid
☐ Bed Controls   ☐ Brochure   ☐ T.V.
☐ Light Controls   ☐ Visiting Privileges   ☐ I.D./Allergy Band On
☐ Bathroom   ☐ Safety Precautions   ☐ Pillow Speaker Placement

PSYCHOSOCIAL/DISCHARGE PLANNING SCREEN

PSYCHOSOCIAL STATUS (circle all that apply)
History of non-compliance impacting medical treatment   1
History alcohol/chemical abuse needing treatment   1
Suspected neglect/abuse   4
Unsafe home environment (domestic violence/self-neglect)   4
Prolonged confusion/disorientation   1
Illness related anxiety impacting care   1
Ineffective family coping patterns   1
Recent loss of body limb   4
Terminal illness   1
Suicide attempt/Ideation   1
Significant Grief impacting care/treatment   1
Teen Pregnancy (with high risk social factors)   2
Birth Anomalies or retardation   4
Loss of Infant (fetal demise)   4
Adoption   4
Other:

LIVING ARRANGEMENT:
Family Unable to help/no known friends   2
Age > 70 years lives alone   1
Patient admitted from other institution: 1
SNF _____ NH _____
_____ Rehab _____ Other Hospital
Patient is disabled   1
Homeless or no address available   3

ADMISSION STATUS:
Readmitted within 1 -30 days   1
Admitted through ER   1
TOTAL OF ALL. _____

Low Risk = 0-2
Moderate Risk = 3 pts
High Risk = 4 or > pts
*HIGH RISK requires Social Services consult. Social Services notified ☐ Yes ☐ No

Current Resource Being Utilized: Yes No
Home Health   ☐ ☐
Provider   ☐ ☐
Private Sitter   ☐ ☐
Meals on wheels   ☐ ☐
Hospice   ☐ ☐
MHMR   ☐ ☐
Adult Day Program   ☐ ☐
WIC Program   ☐ ☐

DME AT HOME
☐ Oxygen   ☐ Walker
☐ Wheelchair   ☐ Trapeze
☐ Hospital Bed
☐ Bedside commode
Living with _____

VALUABLES BROUGHT WITH PATIENT TO HOSPITAL   (SECURITY TAG)

☐ Cane/Walker   ☐ Bridgework no. of pieces   Date:
☐ Clocks   ☐ Eyeglasses   ☐ Prothesis type   ☐ Money (purse)   ☐ Electric Razor
☐ Dentures U/L   ☐ Contact Lens   ☐ Hearing Aids L/R   ☐ Wheelchair   ☐ Clothing
☐ Partial U/L   ☐ Watches   ☐ Jewelry   ☐ Radio   ☐ Other
☐ Money (billfold)   ☐ T.V.

I take entire responsibility for keeping in my possession the articles listed above. I am holding nothing in my possession which I have not declared here. I understand and agree that Christus Spohn Health System shall not be liable for the loss or damage to any money, jewelry, eyeglasses, dentures, hearing aids or other articles of value left in the care, custody and control of the patient or family/significant other. It is understood and agreed that Christus Spohn Health System maintains a locked safe for money and valuables. The hospital shall not be liable for any of the patient's personal property that is not secured in the valuables storage envelope or in the hospital locked safe.

SIGNATURE OF PATIENT
I have fully explained to this patient that Christus Spohn Health System takes no responsibility for articles retained by the patient.
SIGNATURE OF EMPLOYEE RECORDING ARTICLES

Valuables given to:
VALUABLES STORAGE ENVELOPE: When valuables storage envelope is used, record the following information:
Valuables Storage Envelope Number   Date property received
Employee taking envelope to cashier   2705318-2.F10 02/25/99

DATE: _____
TIME: _____

REASON FOR HOSPITALIZATION (E.R. TRIAGE/DIAGNOSIS)

MODE OF ARRIVAL
Ambulance ☐
Wheelchair ☐
Stretcher ☐
Ambulatory ☐

ONSET OF SYMPTOMS (E.R. TRIAGE)

PAST HISTORY: (Past Surgeries / Hospitalization) (E.R. TRIAGE)

COMMENTS:

VITAL SIGNS
TEMP
PULSE
RESP
BP   STATED
HEIGHT   ACTUAL
STATED
WEIGHT   ACTUAL

HEALTH HISTORY
✓ Only those conditions that patient has history or current condition
GLAUCOMA ☐   GASTRIC ULCERS ☐
CANCER ☐   HEPATITIS ☐
LUNG DISEASE ☐   HIV DISEASE ☐
ASTHMA ☐   DIABETIC # OF YRS ☐
KIDNEY DISEASE ☐   ANESTHESIA REACTION ☐
HEART DISEASE ☐   STROKE ☐

ALLERGIES
PACEMAKER ☐   SEIZURE ☐
HYPERTENSION ☐   TUBERCULOSIS ☐
FOOD ☐   ALCOHOL ☐   PSYCHIATRIC DX ☐
LATEX ☐   SMOKING ☐   BLOOD TRANSFUSION ☐
OTHER ☐   DRUGS ☐   IN PAST 10 YEARS ☐

PERSON TO NOTIFY IN CASE OF EMERGENCY
NAME
RELATIONSHIP
HAS POWER OF ATTORNEY FOR HEALTH CARE?
☐ YES ☐ NO
TELEPHONE #

DRUG ALLERGIES   REACTION   DATE
1.
2.
3.
4.
5.

MEDICATIONS (E.R. MEDS)

Name	Dose	Freq	Reason	Last Dose

ORGAN DONATION
Do you want information on organ donation?
YES ☐   NO ☐
Referred to: ☐ Organ Transplant Alliance   887-6189

PATIENT RIGHTS
☐ Received copy of Patient Rights
☐ Verbalizes understanding and ability to implement
SIGNATURES:
Completed by: _____
Entered by: _____

CHRISTUS SPOHN HEALTH SYSTEM
PATIENT ADMISSION DATA BASE
Meds Sent Home: YES ☐   NO ☐   N/A ☐

2705318   NEW: 06/95
REVISED: 02/99.F10

4013

Figure 23-1 Patient Admission Database (Courtesy of CHRISTUS Spohn Health System, Corpus Christi, TX)   (continues)

RN ASSESSMENT: DATE: _____ TIME: _____ SIGNATURE: _____, RN

INSTRUCTION:
1. Complete physical assessment
2. Identify problems/nursing diagnosis for each system as appropriate
3. Prioritize Problems
4. Enter problems for problem list in computer

SYSTEMS

SYSTEMS	YES	NO	COMMENTS	PROBLEM

NEUROLOGICAL

L.O.C.
- Alert
- Drowsy
- Comatose
- Disoriented
- Cooperative
- Agitated

☐ Thought processes, alteration in
☐ Coping, ineffective
☐ Communication, impaired
☐ Tissue perfusion alterations in

EYES
- Pearl
- Vision Normal
- Prosthesis

☐ Injury potential
☐ Vision, impaired
☐ Comfort, alterations in pain:

MOUTH
- Moist
- Lesions
- Teeth
- Other

☐ Sensory, perception
☐ Other

EARS
- Responds to normal voice tone

SPEECH
- Clear
- Slurred
- Hoarse / raspy
- Aphasic

ACUTE ☐
CHRONIC ☐

CARDIOVASCULAR
Apical Rate
Rhythm (circle one)   Regular   Irregular

On Cardiac Monitor:
If Yes: Rhythm

Peripheral Pulses: Right   Left
- Carotid
- Radial
- Popliteal
- Femoral
- Pedal

Pacemaker
Peripheral Edema
Chest Pain
Jugular Vein Distention
Extremity Discoloration
Rt. Arm/Hand
Lt. Arm/Hand

	YES	NO	COMMENTS

ACUTE ☐
CHRONIC ☐
Post Operative ☐
Other ☐

RESPIRATORY

RESPIRATIONS
- Rate
- Labored

BREATH SOUNDS
- Clear
- Wheezes
- Rales / Rhonchi

COUGH
- Present
- Sputum

☐ Airway clearance, ineffective
☐ Breathing pattern ineffective
☐ Gas exchange, impaired
☐ IF PROBLEM IDENTIFIED SEND RESPIRATORY CONSULT
☐ Other

MUSCLE / SKELETAL

EXTREMITIES
- Moves all on command

WEAKNESS (specify)
RA ___ LA ___
RL ___ LL ___
- Edema
- Normal ambulation
- Prosthesis (specify)

☐ Self Care deficit
☐ Mobility impaired, physical
☐ Activity intolerance comfort, alterations in

ACUTE ☐
CHRONIC ☐
☐ Tissue perfusion; alterations in

GENITOURINARY

VOIDING
- Normal
- Frequency
- Burning

Decreased Force of urinary stream
INCONTINENCE:
- Stress
- Nocturia

UROSTOMY
DIALYSIS
If Yes: Hemo   Peritoneal
Routine schedule
Date of last Dialysis
Catheter insertion
Date of last menstrual period

☐ Urinary Elimination, alterations in pattern
☐ Urinary Retention
☐ Incontinence, Total
☐ Incontinence, Stress
☐ Comfort, alterations in

ACUTE ☐
CHRONIC ☐

27055183.F10.02/1299

GASTROINTESTINAL

ABDOMEN	YES	NO	COMMENT	PROBLEM

- Soft
- Distended
- Tenderness

ELIMINATION
- Bowel Sounds
- Diarrhea
- Constipation
- Incontinence
- Ostomy
Last B.M. Date:

Bowel elimination alterations in
☐ Diarrhea
☐ Constipation
☐ Incontinence,
☐ Comfort altered pain
ACUTE ☐
CHRONIC ☐

SAFETY ASSESSMENT

	MEDICATIONS	
☐ (5) Age greater than 60	☐ (5) Diuretics	
☐ (5) History of previous falls	☐ (5) Laxatives / G.I. preps	
☐ (5) From nursing home	☐ (5) Antihypertensives	
☐ (5) Has had sitter / companion at home	☐ (3) Antiseizures	
STATUS: MENTAL/PHYSICAL	☐ (3) Sedative / hypnotics	
☐ (5) Confused / Judgement Impaired	☐ (3) Analgesics	
☐ (5) Sensory impairment	☐ (3) Antipsychotics / antidepressants	
☐ (5) Combative/Aggressive		
☐ (5) "Sundowners" Syndrome		
☐ (5) Noncompliance/uncooperativeness		
☐ (5) Paralysis / amputee	☐ LEVEL 1 (0-17)	
☐ (5) Weakness / debilitation	☐ LEVEL 2 (18-24)	
☐ (5) Urgent/frequent elimination needs	☐ LEVEL 3 (25 or greater)	

TOTAL _____

☐ Safety precautions implemented   ☐ Patient/family instructed
☐ Restraints per protocol   ☐ Color coded band on

NUTRITIONAL SCREENING

Indicate as appropriate for patient   Previous diet
☐ (8) TPN/Parenteral Nutrition
☐ (8) Tube Feeding
☐ (2) Unplanned weight loss or gain > 20 lbs in 3 months
☐ Referral to S.S. screen for neglect/abuse?
☐ (1) Loss of appetite/Eats less than 50% of meal
☐ (1) Nausea, vomiting or diarrhea
☐ (1) Difficulty chewing
☐ (1) Difficulty swallowing
☐ *Diagnosis of:
☐ (2) Heart disease, hypertension, CHF, gestational diabetic, hepatic or renal failure, diabetic, anemia, cancer other than ENT, geriatric surgery
☐ (5) AIDS, malnutrition, DKA, decubitus ulcer, septic condition requiring ICU, burn patient, ENT cancer
☐ (1) modified diet; NPO for 48 hrs.
☐ (1) age > 65 years

*LAB VALUES: Albumin   Glucose   Hgb
☐ (1) 2.5 - 3.0   ☐ (1) <60 or   ☐ (1) male < 13
☐ (2) < 2.5   ☐ (2) > 300   ☐ (1) female < 11

TOTAL SCORE _____   SEND NUTRITION SCREEN
High Risk - 8 pts or >   CONSULT WITH TOTAL SCORE
Moderate Risk - 5-7 pts   OF 5 OR ABOVE AND IDENTIFY
Low Risk - 0-4 pts   SCORE OF PATIENT IN ORDER

PATIENT / SIGNIFICANT OTHER PARTICIPATION IN ADMISSION PROCESS

1. Answered question   Yes _____   No _____   3. Family/significant other present   Yes _____   No _____
2. Volunteered information   Yes _____   No _____   4. Plan of care reviewed with: Patient _____   Family / Significant other _____
5. Comments:

INTEGUMENTARY

	YES	NO	COMMENT	PROBLEM

SKIN
- Color Normal
- Warm, dry
- Turgor good
- Bruises
- abrasions, lacerations   Color, Size, Location
- Poor hygiene
- Rash, lesions
- Scars
- Dressing
- Pressure points intact
  - coccyx
  - heels
  - elbows
  - hips
  - ankles
  - cast edges
- Other _____
E-Z graph
- Vascular access

Type: _____   Insertion Date: _____
Site: _____   Purpose: _____

☐ Referral to Social Service (screen for neglect / abuse)

☐ Other: _____
☐ Tissue perfusion, alterations in
☐ Skin integrity impairment of: actual
☐ Skin integrity impairment of: potential
☐ Tissue integrity, comfort, alterations in pain
ACUTE ☐
CHRONIC ☐
WOUND CARE ☐

SKIN BREAKDOWN POTENTIAL CHECKLIST

_____ (1) Fair: Major underlying disease, controlled
_____ (2) Poor: Uncontrolled underlying disease

MENTAL STATUS
_____ (1) Lethargic: Listless
_____ (2) Confused: Inappropriate communication
_____ (4) Comatose: Unresponsive

MOBILITY / ACTIVITY
_____ (2) Minor Deficit: Some limitation in movement
_____ (4) Needs assistance w / ADL's
_____ (4) Major Deficit: Movement requires assistance
_____ (6) Immobile: No voluntary movement

INCONTINENCE
_____ (1) Mild: Stress incontinence, 1 BM / day
_____ (4) Frequent: No bladder control, BMs > 2-4 /day
_____ (6) Total: No bladder control, frequent / continuous BM

NUTRITION
_____ (2) Fair: Intake < body requirements, eats 75% or less
_____ (3) Poor: Eats 50% or less, started on TPN or tube feeding
_____ (4) Compromised: No intake, dehydrated

SKIN INTEGRITY
_____ (2) Fair: Single stage I or II
_____ (4) Poor: More than one break in skin integrity

TOTAL SCORE OF 8 OR ABOVE, ENTER SKIN INTEGRITY POTENTIAL ON PCP PROBLEM LIST, INITIATE PREVENTATIVE ADL's

270318-4.F10

Figure 23-1 *(continued)*

atives, nonprescription pain relief medications, herbal remedies, and vitamin and mineral supplements.

Developmental Level

Knowledge of developmental level is essential for considering appropriate norms of behavior and for appraising the achievement of relevant developmental tasks. Any recognized theory of growth and development can be applied in order to determine if clients are functioning within the parameters expected for their age group. For example, if Erikson's stages of psychosocial development are used, validation of an adult client's attainment of the developmental task of generativity versus stagnation can be made by a statement such as "client prefers to spend time with his family; very involved in children's school activities."

Psychosocial History

Psychosocial history refers to assessment of self-concept and self-esteem as well as usual sources of stress and the client's ability to cope. Sources of support for clients in crisis, such as family, significant others, religion, or support groups, should be explored.

Sociocultural History

The client's sociocultural history includes the home environment, family situation, and client's role in the family. For example, the client could be the parent of three children and the sole provider in a single-parent family. The responsibilities of the client are important data through which the impact of changes in health status and the most beneficial care plan for the client are determined. Caffeine and alcohol intake and use of tobacco or recreational drugs should also be explored.

Complementary/ Alternative Therapy Use

The University of Maryland Medicine (2002) reports that nearly 70% of U.S. citizens have used at least one complementary/alternative therapy in their lifetime. The question is: How many tell their health care providers? Simple open-ended questions such as "Do you do anything to improve your health?" may provide important information. If a complementary/alternative therapy is mentioned, the nurse might ask if this is something the client would consider using (Hodge & Ullrich, 1999).

Activities of Daily Living

The activities of daily living (ADL) is a description of the client's lifestyle and capacity for self-care and is use-

ful both as baseline information and as a source of insight into usual health behaviors. This baseline should include information on nutritional intake and eating habits, elimination patterns, rest/sleep patterns, and activity/exercise.

Review of Systems

The **review of systems** (ROS) is a brief account from the client of any recent signs or symptoms associated with any of the body systems. This can most effectively be obtained as the physical examination is being performed. The ROS relies on subjective information provided by the client rather than on the physical examination. When a symptom is encountered, either while eliciting the health history or during the physical examination of the client, as much information as possible about the symptom should be obtained. Relevant data include:

- *Location.* The area of the body in which the symptom (such as pain) is felt.
- *Character.* The quality of the feeling or sensation (e.g., sharp, dull, stabbing).
- *Intensity.* The severity or quantity of the feeling or sensation and its interference with functional abilities. The sensation can be rated on a scale of 1 (very little) to 10 (very intense).
- *Timing.* The onset, duration, frequency, and precipitating factors of the symptom.
- *Aggravating/alleviating factors.* The activities or actions that make the symptom worse or better.

PHYSICAL EXAMINATION

A physical examination is performed for all age groups in all health care settings (home, outpatient facilities, extended care institutions, and acute care facilities) to gather comprehensive, pertinent client data. The physical examination, a picture of the client's physiological functioning, combined with a health and psychosocial assessment, forms a database for decision making. The examination should be performed according to the agency's policy, which may vary from one agency to another.

To ensure a thorough assessment of each system, the physical examination is done in a sequential, head-to-toe fashion. This method decreases the number of times the nurse and the client have to change positions and prevents forgetting to examine an area,

The physical or the head-to-toe assessment is performed by using the specific assessment techniques of inspection, palpation, percussion, and auscultation.

Inspection

Inspection consists of a thorough visual observation of the client, providing a picture of the body's outward response to its internal functioning. Inspection of the skin, for example, can assist in identifying signs of a fever by the client's flushed face. The skin can also be an indicator of a decreased oxygen supply when **cyanosis,** a bluish or dark purple coloration, is noted in the client's lips, skin, or nail beds. Sharing observations with the client during inspection enhances the holistic data collected. For example, when mentioning the observation of visible scars, the client may discuss previous surgeries or hospitalizations. Instruments such as a penlight and otoscope are often used to enhance visualization.

Effective inspection requires adequate lighting and exposure of the body parts being observed. Show sensitivity to the client's feelings of embarrassment by discussing the technique with the client and using appropriate draping.

Palpation

Palpation uses the sense of touch to assess texture, temperature, moisture, organ location and size, vibrations, pulsations, swelling, masses, and tenderness. The finger pads are placed flat against the client's skin, exerting slight pressure for light palpation, as seen in Figure 23-2. Assessment of the kidneys, liver, spleen, bowel, and fundal height may be accomplished through deep palpation, in which more pressure is exerted. Pulses are also palpated. The abdomen is palpated for distention, softness, firmness, rigidity, or tenderness.

Palpation requires a calm, gentle approach and is used systematically, with light palpation preceding deep palpation and palpation of tender areas performed last.

Safety: Palpation
Deep palpation is a technique requiring significant expertise and should not be employed by beginning nursing students without supervision.

Percussion

Percussion uses short, tapping strokes on the surface of the skin to create vibrations of underlying organs. It is used to assess the density of structures or determine the location and size of organs. The fingertips are used to tap the client's body to produce sounds and vibrations. Place the middle finger of the nondominant hand on the client's skin in the area to be percussed, then tap lightly with the middle finger of the dominant hand on the distal phalanx of the middle finger positioned on the body surface (Figure 23-3). Tap twice in one place before moving to a new area.

Percussion should not be painful to the client. If it is painful, the percussion should be discontinued and the response documented.

Percussion requires much practice to master, and it is important to be familiar with the sounds produced when percussion is used. Table 23-1 describes the various percussion tones.

Auscultation

Auscultation involves listening to sounds in the body that are created by movement of air or fluid. Areas most often auscultated include the lungs, heart, abdomen, and blood vessels. A stethoscope is used to channel the sound (Figure 23-4).

HEAD-TO-TOE ASSESSMENT

Some important concepts should be kept in mind and utilized throughout the examination. The client's privacy should be respected by pulling the curtain, closing the door, and providing appropriate draping. When possible, distracting noises such as radio or television and people talking should be eliminated. Assessment should be performed under natural light because fluorescent light can change the color tones of the skin. All procedures should be explained to the client and confidentiality of data acquired during the examination maintained.

Infection Control: Standard Precautions
Remember to utilize Standard Precautions when in contact with any body fluids by using gloves, gown, or mask as appropriate.

The client should be positioned to ensure accessibility to the body part being assessed. Figure 23-5 illustrates positions used in conducting a physical examination.

Figure 23-2 *Light Palpation*

Figure 23-3 *Percussion*

TABLE 23-1	DESCRIPTION OF PERCUSSION TONES				
TONE	INTENSITY	PITCH	DURATION	QUALITY	NORMAL LOCATION
Dullness	Medium	High	Medium	Thudlike	Liver
Flatness	Soft	High	Short	Extreme dullness	Muscle
Hyperresonance	Very loud	Very low	Long	Booming	Child's lung
Resonance	Loud	Low	Long	Hollow	Peripheral lung
Tympany	Loud	High	Medium	Drumlike	Stomach

Draping the client prevents unnecessary exposure during the examination. Embarrassment causes tension and restlessness and decreases the client's ability to cooperate. Draping also prevents the client from being chilled.

General Survey

During the introductory time, use inspection to make a general assessment of the client. This overview is the first impression of the client and is the beginning point of the head-to-toe assessment. Such aspects as the general state of health and any signs of distress, such as pain or breathing difficulties, the client's awareness of the surroundings, body type and posture, facial expressions, and mood are noted.

Document the general survey data to portray an overall picture of the client. The elderly, disabled, and abused clients will require special consideration during the physical examination.

Elderly

Before assessing elderly clients, it is important to know the normal changes of aging. Aging may reduce the body's tolerance of stress, resistance to illness, and ability to recuperate from illness. Be sure the client understands and can follow instructions, and allow extra time for the client having difficulty changing positions.

CRITICAL THINKING

Performing a Physical Assessment

What are your feelings about performing a complete physical assessment on a client? What is the best way to handle the situation?

LIFE CYCLE CONSIDERATIONS

The Older Client

- All senses are less acute.
- Endorphin level rises with age, which decreases awareness of painful events.
- Temperature normal range is 96°F to 98.9°F.
- Strength and endurance decline.
- Height decreases.
- Digestive and urinary functions slow down.
- Older clients are prone to constipation and nocturia.
- Respirations are slowed.
- Older clients are prone to fatigue, dizziness, and falls (Andresen, 1998).

CULTURAL CONSIDERATIONS

Cultural Values and Assessment

Although cleanliness is highly valued by mainstream American society, in some cultures, a daily bath is not believed necessary or desirable. In fact, some cultures do not interpret natural body odors as offensive. Consider the client in the context of cultural beliefs. The terms *dirty, unkempt,* or *foul-smelling* are value-laden and can cloud the assessment process and care provided to a client.

Figure 23-4 *Auscultation*

Sitting
To examine head, neck, back, posterior thorax and lungs, anterior thorax and lungs, breast, axillae, heart, extremities.

Client can expand lungs; nurse can inspect symmetry. *Institute risk precautions for elderly and debilitated clients.*

Dorsal recumbent
To examine head, neck, anterior thorax and lungs, breast, axillae, heart.

Client comfortable; increases abdominal muscle tension. *Contraindicated in abdominal assessment.*

Prone
To examine posterior thorax and lungs, hip

Assessment of hip extension. *Contraindicated in clients with cardiopulmonary alterations.*

Supine
To examine head, neck, anterior thorax and lungs, breasts, axillae, heart, abdomen, extremities.

Client relaxed; decreases abdominal muscle tension; nurse can palpate all peripheral pulses. *Contraindicated in clients with cardiopulmonary alterations.*

Sims'
To examine rectum and vagina.

Relaxes rectal muscles. Painful for clients with joint deformities.

Knee-chest
To examine rectum

Maximal rectal exposure. *Contraindicated in clients with respiratory alterations.*

Lithotomy
To examine female genitalia, rectum, genital tract.

Maximal genitalia exposure; embarrassing and uncomfortable for client. *Contraindicated in clients with joint disorders.*

Figure 23-5 *Various Positions for Physical Examination*

Disabled Clients

When assessing disabled clients, adapt the process to the client's ability; for example, a hearing-impaired client should be given a written questionnaire. Simple, direct sentences and questions or pictures might be required for an intellectually impaired client. It is best to determine the client's ability to participate before conducting the examination. To allay the disabled client's fears and anxiety, a family member may be allowed to remain with the client during the examination. The client's level of independence and feelings about the disability should be noted.

Abused Clients

Observe for signs of abuse, especially in children and the elderly. Symptoms may be psychological as well as physical; for example, refusal to be touched, inability to maintain eye contact, or unwillingness to talk about bruises, burns, or other injuries may indicate abuse. Bruises or lacerations most typically appear on breasts, buttocks, thighs, or genitalia. Inspect for healed scarring or burns and know state laws and agency policies for reporting possible abuse.

Vital Signs

After establishing rapport with the client through introductions, measurement of vital signs is the next step in an assessment. Vital signs are the "signs of life," providing a way of connecting the external inspection with the internal functioning of the client's organs. When checking vital signs, obtain the temperature (T), pulse

TABLE 23-2   VITAL SIGNS AND VARIATIONS

VITAL SIGN	NORMAL READING		VARIATIONS
Temperature	Axillary	36.5°C or 97.6°F	<36°C or 96.8°F Hypothermia
	Tympanic	37°C or 98.6°F	>38°C or 100.4°F Pyrexia
	Oral	37°C or 98.6°F	
	Rectal	37.5°C or 99.6°F	
Pulse	60–100 beats/min.		<60 Bradycardia
			<100 Tachycardia
Respirations	16–20 resp./min.		<16 Bradypnea
			>20 Tachypnea
Blood Pressure	90/60–140/90		<90/60 Hypotension
			>140/90 Hypertension

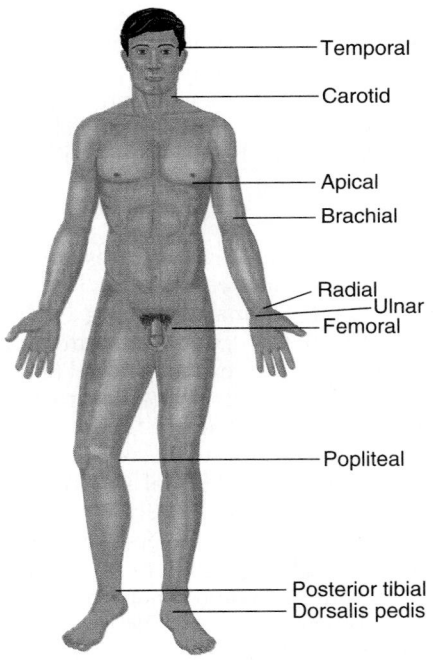

Figure 23-6 *Pulse Points*

(P), respirations (R), blood pressure (BP), and pain assessment of the client. See Table 23-2 for normal values and variations.

Temperature

When assessing the client's temperature (T), an electronic, chemical, or mercury thermometer can be used. Body temperature can be taken by five routes: oral, rectal, axillary, skin, or tympanic membrane. The route chosen depends on the client's age and physical condition. Factors such as age, gender, physical activity, and environment can affect a person's temperature. Craig et al. (2002) found ear temperatures in children to be inac-

Temperature Conversion

To convert Fahrenheit to Celsius (centigrade):

$$(\text{Temperature } °F - 32) \times {}^5/_9 = °C$$

Example:

$$98.6°F - 32 = 66.6 \times {}^5/_9 = 37°C$$

To convert Celsius to Fahrenheit:

$${}^9/_5 \times \text{temperature}°C + 32 = °F$$

Example:

$${}^9/_5 \times 40°C = 72 + 32 = 104°F$$

curate. Consumption of hot or cold food or beverage and smoking 15 to 30 minutes before taking an oral temperature can affect the results.

Pulse

Pulse assessment measures a pressure pulsation created when the heart contracts and ejects blood into the aorta. Assessment of pulse characteristics provides clinical data regarding the heart's pumping action and the adequacy of peripheral artery blood flow.

There are many pulse points (Figure 23-6). The most accessible are the radial and carotid sites. The body diverts blood to the brain when a cardiovascular emergency such as hemorrhage occurs, so in these situations the carotid site should always be used to assess the pulse. Pulse point assessments are described in Table 23-3.

Assessment of the client's pulse (P) includes the rate, rhythm, and amplitude.

Pulse rate is an indirect measurement of cardiac output obtained by counting the number of peripheral

TABLE 23-3   PULSE POINT USES

PULSE POINT	USE
Temporal: over temporal bone, lateral and superior to eye	For infants and when radial is inaccessible
Carotid: under lower jaw in neck along medial edge of sternocleidomastoid muscle	For infants and during shock or cardiac arrest when other peripheral pulses are too weak to palpate; also to assess cranial circulation
Apical: left midclavicular line at fourth to fifth inter-costal space	To auscultate heart sounds and assess api-cal-radial deficit
Brachial: between groove of biceps and triceps muscles at antecubital fossa	In cardiac arrest for in-fants, to assess lower arm circulation, and to auscultate blood pressure
Radial: inner aspect of fore-arm on thumb side of wrist	To routinely assess pulse
Ulnar: outer aspect of fore-arm on finger side of wrist	To assess circulation to ulnar side of hand and to perform the Allen's test
Femoral: in groin, below in-guinal ligament (midpoint between symphysis pubis and anterosuperior iliac spine)	To assess circulation to legs and during cardiac arrest
Popliteal: behind knee, at center in popliteal fossa	To assess circulation to legs and to auscultate leg blood pressure
Posterior tibial: inner aspect of ankle between Achilles tendon and tibia	To assess circulation to feet
Dorsalis pedis: over instep, midway between extension tendons of great and sec-ond toe	To assess circulation to feet

PROFESSIONAL TIP

Carotid Pulse Assessment
When assessing a carotid pulse, apply light pressure to only one carotid artery to avoid disruption of cerebral blood flow. Then assess the other one.

Pulse amplitude is a measurement of the strength or force exerted by the blood against the arterial wall with each heart contraction. It is described as normal (full, easily palpable), weak (thready and usually rapid), or strong (bounding).

Usual assessment of the radial pulse occurs for 30 seconds, and the number of beats is doubled for documentation. If the pulse rhythm is irregular, assessment must occur for 60 seconds. In addition, the nurse must assess for a **pulse deficit** (condition in which the apical pulse rate is greater than the radial pulse rate). A pulse deficit results from the ejection of a volume of blood that is too small to initiate a peripheral pulse wave.

During the pulse assessment, integrate questions about endurance, fatigue, and any possible episodes of palpitations, "feeling the heart beating," over the chest area.

Respirations

Respiratory assessment measures the breathing pattern. This provides clinical data regarding the pH of arterial blood. Normal breathing is slightly observable, quiet, effortless, regular, and automatic. Assess by observing chest wall expansion and bilateral symmetrical movement of the thorax. Another way to assess breathing is to place the back of the hand next to the client's nose and mouth to feel the expired air.

Assessment of external respirations (R) should include specific characteristics of respirations as well as the use of any type of oxygen equipment, the route, and flow rate. Each respiration includes one complete inhalation (breathing in) and exhalation (breathing out) by the client. When identifying the characteristics of respirations, the rate, depth, and rhythm of each breath should be determined.

Eupnea refers to easy respirations with a rate that is age-appropriate. **Bradypnea** is a respiratory rate of

pulse waves over a pulse point. A normal pulse rate for adults is between 60 and 100 beats per minute. **Bradycardia** is a heart rate less than 60 beats per minute in an adult. **Tachycardia** is a heart rate greater than 100 beats per minute in an adult.

Pulse rhythm is the regularity of the heartbeat. It indicates how evenly the heart is beating: regular (the beats are evenly spaced) or irregular (the beats are not evenly spaced); also called dysrhythmia or arrhythmia.

PROFESSIONAL TIP

Positioning for Dyspneic Clients
Dyspneic clients should be maintained in a semi-Fowler's or Fowler's position, never flat in bed. For maximal lung expansion, have the client leaning forward over a padded, raised overbed table with head and arms resting on the table.

10 or fewer breaths per minute. **Hypoventilation** is characterized by shallow respirations. **Tachypnea** is a respiratory rate greater than 24 breaths per minute. **Hyperventilation** is characterized by deep, rapid respirations. **Dyspnea** refers to difficulty breathing as observed by labored or forced respirations by using accessory muscles in the chest and neck. Dyspneic clients are very aware of their respirations and feel short of breath.

Also observe for nasal flaring and the use of accessory muscles for breathing as evidenced by sternal, costal, and subclavicular retractions. Children and males typically utilize abdominal muscles to breathe, but women use thoracic muscles (Fuller & Schaller-Ayers, 2000).

During respiration assessment, determine functional ability by asking about any shortness of breath, difficulty in breathing with increased exercise, or problems completing activities of daily living.

Blood Pressure

After checking a client's respirations, assess the client's blood pressure (BP). The most common site for indirect blood pressure measurement is the client's arm over the brachial artery.

When pressure measurements in the upper extremities are not accessible, the popliteal artery, located behind the knee, is the site of choice. Blood pressure can also be assessed in other sites, such as the radial artery in the forearm and the posterior tibial or dorsalis pedis artery in the lower leg. The extremity should be at the level of the heart when blood pressure is measured. Because it is difficult to auscultate sounds over the radial, tibial, and dorsalis pedis arteries, these sites are usually palpated to obtain a systolic reading.

A person's blood pressure is the result of the interaction of cardiac output and peripheral resistance, and depends on the speed with which the arterial blood flows, the volume of blood supplied, and the elasticity of the walls of the artery. The force exerted by the blood against the wall of the artery as the heart contracts and relaxes is called the *arterial pressure.* When the ventricles contract and blood is forced into the aorta and pulmonary arteries, the *systolic pressure* is measured. This is the first sound heard. When the heart is in the filling or relaxed stage, the force is described as the *diastolic pressure.* This is when the last sound is heard. The difference between the systolic and diastolic blood pressures is called the *pulse pressure.* A pulse pressure is usually between 30 and 40 mm Hg.

An accurate reading requires the correct width of blood pressure cuff, determined by the circumference of the client's extremity. According to the American Heart Association (1987), the bladder width should be approximately 40% of the circumference of the extremity. To measure the width of the bladder, place the cuff lengthwise on the client's extremity and extend the width to cover 40% of the extremity's circumference (Figure 23-7). Table 23-4 recommends bladder sizes based on different arm circumferences. A falsely elevated reading results if the bladder is too narrow, and a falsely low reading results if it is too wide.

Figure 23-7 *Measure width of arm by holding cuff against client's upper arm.*

TABLE 23-4	GUIDELINES FOR BLOOD PRESSURE CUFF SELECTION	
MIDPOINT* ARM CIRCUMFERENCE	**BLADDER CUFF WIDTH**	**LENGTH**
13–20 cm (child)	8 cm	13 cm
24–32 cm (average adult)	13 cm	24 cm
32–42 cm (large adult)	17 cm	32 cm

*Distance between the acromion and olecranon processes.

This is an appropriate time to ask if the client ever becomes lightheaded or dizzy when moving from a reclining position to a sitting or standing position. This may occur as a result of an abnormally low blood pressure caused by the inability of the peripheral blood vessels to compensate quickly for the change in position and is referred to as **orthostatic hypotension.**

Pain

According to the Joint Commission on Accreditation of Healthcare Organizations (JCAHO) standards for ambulatory care, behavioral health care, home care, hospital, health care network, long-term care, and long-term care pharmacy, pain is considered the fifth vital sign. Pain is to be assessed and recorded along with the client's temperature, pulse, respirations, and blood pressure (JCAHO, 2000a; JCAHO, 2000b). The pain assessment is to include pain intensity and quality (character, frequency, location, and duration). Regular assessment and follow-up are according to agency policy. This statement on pain management, "All patients have a right to pain relief," is to be posted in all client care areas (e.g., client rooms, clinic rooms, waiting rooms) (JCAHO, 2000a).

Height and Weight Measurement

Height and weight measurements are as important as the client's vital signs. Routine measurement provides data about growth and development in infants and children. Alterations may indicate illness at any age. Height and weight are routinely taken on visits to physicians' offices, clinics, on admission to acute care facilities, and in other health care settings.

Height

A height-measuring rod, calibrated in either inches or centimeters, is usually found on a standing weight scale. The client should stand erect on the scale's platform. The metal arm attached to the back of the scale is extended to gently rest on the top of the client's head. The measurement is read at eye level.

Weight

When a client has an order for "daily weight," the weight should be obtained at the same time of day on the same scale, with the client wearing the same type of clothing. The scale should be balanced before each client is weighed.

 Infection Control: Measuring Weight
When standing on a scale, the client should wear some type of light foot covering, such as socks or disposable operating room slippers, to prevent the transmission of infection and to enhance comfort.

Head and Neck Assessment

Assessment of the head and neck determines the client's mental and neurological status and the client's overall **affect** (outward expression of mood or emotion).

Hair and Scalp

The hair and scalp of a client should be inspected. Note hair distribution, quantity, texture, and color. The scalp should be smooth and free of any debris or infestations.

Eyes

Examine the eyes to determine if they are symmetrical. Look at the eyebrows and eyelids to see if there is any drooping, which may be a sign of muscle weakness or neurological impairment. Note the color of the sclera and conjunctiva, as well as the presence of any drainage.

Assess the pupils to determine their size, shape, and reaction to light. This is accomplished by darkening the room and asking the client to gaze into the distance. Move a light in from the side and notice if the pupil constricts; this is called the *direct light reflex*. Note the pupil size in millimeters both before and after the light response (Figure 23-8). Accommodation is tested by asking the client to focus on an object in the distance; this will dilate the pupils. The client is then asked to move his or her gaze to a near object such as a pen or finger held approximately 3 inches from the nose. The pupils should constrict as they focus on the near object, and the eyes will converge or move in toward midline. This normal response is documented as Pupils Equal, Round, Reactive to Light and Accommodation (PERRLA).

Ask if the client wears glasses and for what reason, if any eye problems such as blurry vision, diplopia (double vision), or difficulty seeing at night are experienced.

Visual acuity is assessed by a simple, noninvasive procedure using a **Snellen chart** (a chart that contains various-sized letters with standardized numbers at the end of each line of letters). The standardized numbers (called the denominator) indicate the degree of visual acuity when the client is able to read that line of letters at a distance of 20 feet.

Nose

The nose should be symmetrical, midline, and in proportion to other features. Note any deformity, inflammation, or prior trauma. The patency of the nostrils can be tested by asking the client to sniff inward while closing off each nostril. Ask the client if the following are ever experienced: nosebleeds, dryness, or decrease in sense of smell.

Lips and Mouth

The lips and mucous membranes of the mouth are observed for color, symmetry, moisture, or lesions. Ask the client with dentures or partial plates to remove them

Figure 23-8 *Scale Used to Measure Pupil Size, in Millimeters*

Common Abnormal Breath Odors
- Acetone breath ("fruity" smell) is common in malnourished or diabetic clients with ketoacidosis.
- Musty smell is caused by the breakdown of nitrogen and presence of liver disease.
- Ammonia smell occurs during the end stage of renal failure from a buildup of urea.

for a more thorough inspection of the mouth. Unusual breath odors should be noted. Inspect the oral mucosa by inserting a tongue depressor between the teeth and the cheek. The mucous membranes and gums should be pink, moist, smooth, and free of lesions. Inspection of the tongue assists in determining the client's hydration. The tongue should be pink with a slightly rough texture. During the examination, determine if the client is able to enunciate words appropriately and if there are any voice changes such as hoarseness. Usual dental hygiene practices should be discussed and the client's history of tobacco usage obtained.

Neck

The neck is assessed for full range of motion. The accessory neck muscles should be symmetrical. As the client moves the head, note any enlargement of the lymph nodes or thyroid gland. Observe for any pulsations in the neck. The carotid pulsation, seen just below the angle of the jaw, normally is the only visible pulsation while the client is in the sitting position.

Mental and Neurological Status and Affect

A head-to-toe assessment incorporates an assessment of the client's mental and neurological status and affect. A client's mental status includes the level of orientation to person, place, and time and the client's responsiveness to the environment. When assessing, observe for responsiveness, the client's ability to follow directions and to respond appropriately to comments and to his or her name when called.

Neurological assessment of the client focuses on the level of consciousness (LOC), pupil response, hand grasps, and foot pushes. Each of these assessments is discussed in the area of the head-to-toe assessment in which it is observed. The LOC is the client's degree of wakefulness. For example, a client who is alert is fully awake with eyes open and responds to environmental stimuli. The client who is less awake will be drowsy and slow responding to environmental stimuli.

When documenting the client's affect, judgmental words such as *pleasant, happy, cooperative, uncooperative, angry, depressed,* or *hostile* should not be used. Focus specifically on the behaviors exhibited by the client, such as facial expression and verbal and nonverbal behaviors. In doing this, the accuracy of the conversation or the be-

haviors observed is maintained as well as the legal appropriateness of the assessment.

Skin Assessment

Skin assessment should be performed as each area of the body is assessed. Note the color of the skin as well as its moisture or dryness. Inspect and palpate the client's skin, assessing temperature, turgor, edema, and integrity. Palpation of the skin with the dorsal aspect of the hand on the right and left sides of the body provides a comparison of the client's skin temperature. Ask the client if any pain or discomfort in relation to the skin and/or mucous membranes has occurred. Identification of the skin's turgor is best accomplished by gently pinching the skin of the anterior chest and observing the speed of skin return to its previous position. If the skin stays pinched, it may indicate dehydration, and further assessment is needed.

Palpate dependent areas (sacrum, legs, ankles, feet) for edema. Firmly apply pressure with a finger for 5 seconds. The degree of edema is based on the depth of indentation and how long it remains (Gehring, 2002):

1+ indentation of 1 cm or less, disappears rapidly
2+ indentation of 1.5 cm, disappears in 10-15 seconds
3+ indentation of 2 cm, last more than 1 minute
4+ indentation of 2.5 cm, lasts 2 to 5 minutes

Note the location, size, distribution, and appearance of skin lesions throughout the body. Document any breaks or changes in the skin integrity, such as scratches, bruises, skin tears, cuts, and scars from previous injuries or surgeries. Note the general hygiene of the skin and ask the client about usual skin care routines.

CULTURAL CONSIDERATIONS

Skin Color
- The darker the client's skin, the more difficult it is to assess changes in color.
- Establish a baseline skin color by observing the least pigmented skin surfaces, which include the volar surfaces of the forearms, the palms of the hands, the soles of the feet, the abdomen, and the buttocks. There should be an underlying red tone in these areas. Absence of this red tone may indicate pallor.
- Oral hyperpigmentation often is found in dark-skinned persons. If the hard palate is not hyperpigmented, it has a yellow discoloration in the presence of jaundice.
- The lips may be used to assess jaundice and cyanosis, and the sclera may be used to assess jaundice if a baseline color has been established for each.
- The conjunctiva reflect color changes of cyanosis or pallor.
- Nail beds can be used to note how quickly the color returns after pressure has been released from the free edge of the nail, regardless of the nail bed color.

Thoracic Assessment

During thoracic assessment, the condition of the client's cardiovascular and respiratory systems along with assessment of the breasts are determined.

Cardiovascular Status

Assessment of the client's cardiovascular status by the LP/VN focuses specifically on listening to the apical pulse, identifying heart tones, and checking the nail beds. The apical pulse is determined by using auscultation and palpation. To assess the apical pulse, palpate over the apex of the heart at the fifth left intercostal space at the midclavicular line. A slight, short duration tap against the fingers will be felt, and this is where the apical pulse is auscultated (Figure 23-9). Listening to the apical pulse is the most accurate assessment of the heart rate and should occur for 60 seconds. The apical pulse is assessed first with the diaphragm of the stethoscope for the regularity or irregularity of its rhythm. Second, the bell of the stethoscope is used to differentiate the loudness or tones of the heart. Along with the apical pulse, the other pulse points may be assessed now or when the extremities are assessed.

To assess blood perfusion of peripheral vessels and skin, note changes in skin temperature, color, and sensation; changes in the pulses; and feel the toes for warmth and color. Because the position of the extremities can affect the skin temperature and appearance, extremities must always be assessed at heart level and at normal room and body temperature. Compare peripheral pulses bilaterally, and note changes in strength and quality.

The focus of the functional assessment includes personal habits contributing to or preventing cardiovascu-lar disease. Ask about the client's personal exercise habits and elicit information regarding past chest pain or shortness of breath. The client should describe any pain, its location, duration, precipitating factors, and what is done to alleviate the pain. Also ask if the client has ever fainted or felt dizzy. Any lower leg swelling and its cause should also be noted.

Respiratory Status

Breath sound assessment is performed after assessing the apical pulse rate. The presence of normal and abnormal breath sounds is revealed by respiratory auscultation. The client should be asked to breathe only through the mouth during auscultation, because mouth breathing decreases air turbulence, which interferes with an accurate assessment.

There are three types of normal breath sounds, each having a unique pitch, quality, intensity, location, and duration in the inspiratory and expiratory phases of respiration:

- **Bronchial sounds.** Loud, high-pitched sounds with a hollow quality heard longer on expiration than inspiration from air moving through the trachea
- **Bronchovesicular sounds.** Medium-pitched, blowing sounds heard equally on inspiration and expiration from air moving through the large airways, posteriorly between the scapula and anteriorly over bronchioles lateral to the sternum at the first and second intercostal spaces
- **Vesicular sounds.** Soft, breezy, low-pitched sounds heard longer on inspiration than expiration resulting from air moving through the smaller airways over the lung's periphery, with the exception of the scapular area

Non-normal breath sounds are described as either abnormal or **adventitious breath sounds.** Adventitious breath sounds include sibilant wheeze (formerly wheeze), sonorous wheeze (formerly rhonchi), fine and coarse crackle (formerly rales), pleural friction rub, and stridor. **Sibilant wheezes** are high-pitched, whistling sounds heard during inhalation and exhalation. A **sonorous wheeze** is a low-pitched snoring sound that is louder on exhalation. Coughing may alter the sound if caused by mucus. **Crackles** are popping sounds heard on inhalation or exhalation, not cleared by coughing. A **pleural friction rub** is a low-pitched grating sound on inhalation and exhalation. **Stridor** is a high-pitched, harsh sound heard on inspiration when the trachea or larynx is obstructed. Assess breath sounds of the anterior, posterior, and lateral chest wall for normal as well as adventitious breath sounds. Monitor adventitious breath sounds consistently. The lungs are assessed from side to side so the two sides can be compared, as shown in Figure 23-10.

The functional assessment information to be obtained when assessing the respiratory status includes any difficulty breathing or the presence of a cough. Ask the client if the cough is nonproductive or productive and to describe the secretions produced. Terms used to describe secretions expectorated would be *thick, thin, yellow, green.*

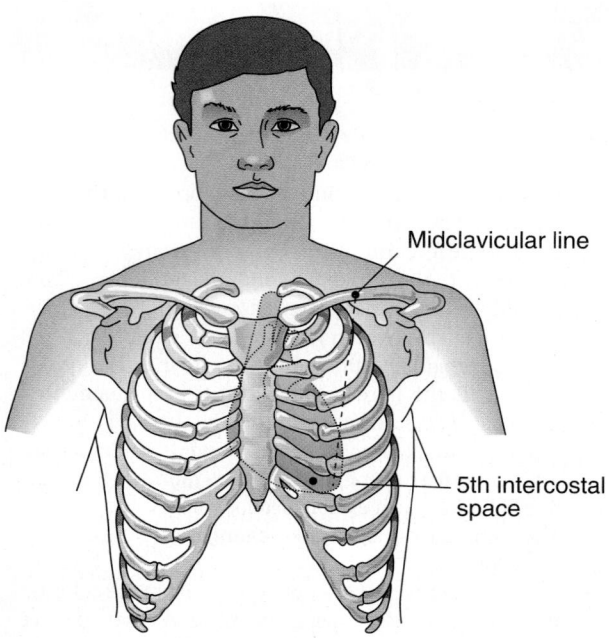

Midclavicular line

5th intercostal space

Figure 23-9 *Assessing the Apical Pulse*

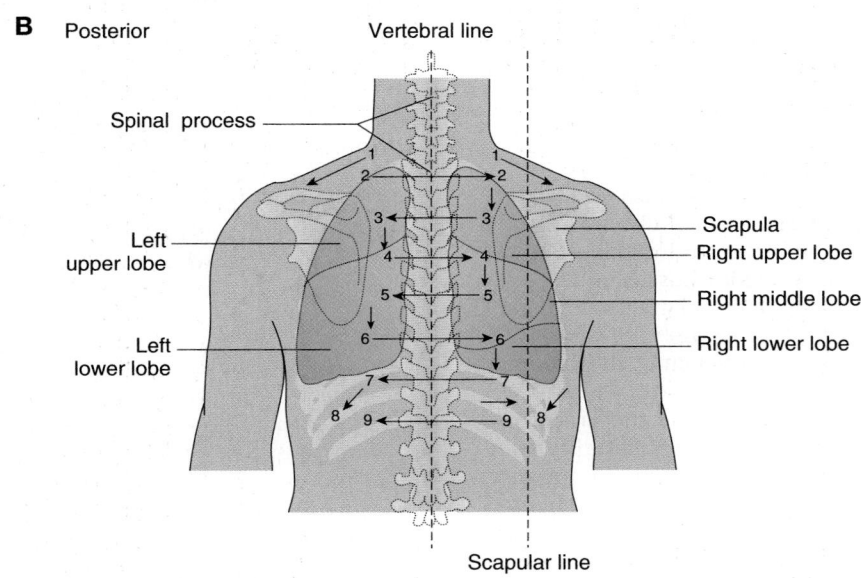

Figure 23-10 *Symmetrical Assessment of Breath Sounds:* **A,** *Anterior;* **B,** *Posterior*

The client's occupational or home environment may affect breathing patterns; exposure to dust, chemicals, vapors, tobacco, smoke, or paint fumes, and irritants such as asbestos should be noted.

Wounds, Scars, Drains, Tubes, Dressings

When assessing the thorax, note any type of wounds, scars, drains, tubes, or dressings. Documentation of these must include the location, size, and amount of drainage or discharge, and if present, signs of inflammation.

Breasts

Assessment of the breasts should be done for both male and female clients. Begin by inspecting the breasts for size and symmetry. It is common to have a slight difference in size of breasts. Note any obvious masses, dimpling (a depression in the surface skin), or inflammation. The skin normally is smooth and even in color. Determine if the nipples and areola are symmetrical in size, shape, and color, and note any discharge from the nipples.

Any abnormal area should be palpated for size, consistency, mobility, tenderness, and location of the lesion. Another area to include in breast assessment is the axillary lymph nodes that drain the breasts. Palpate the axilla for enlarged or inflamed lymph nodes, ask if there is any tenderness, and determine if and when the client performs breast self-exams. Note if the client has had a mammogram and when the last one was taken.

Figure 23-11 *The Four Quadrants of the Abdomen*

Abdominal Assessment

Abdominal assessment determines the status of the client's gastrointestinal and genitourinary systems. Note any type of wounds, scars, drains, tubes, dressings, or ostomies. Documentation of these must include the location, size, and amount of drainage or discharge, and if present, signs of inflammation.

Gastrointestinal Status

The abdomen is first inspected for rashes and scars. Assess if the abdomen is flat, rounded, or distended, and observe the abdomen for symmetry and visible signs of peristalsis or pulsations. If the abdomen is distended, ask the client questions pertaining to bowel movements and urinary status.

Auscultation is the second component of the abdominal assessment of a client's bowel status. A "bubbly-gurgly" sound, caused by peristalsis and movement of the intestinal contents, can be heard by placing the stethoscope on each quadrant of the abdomen and listening for approximately 1 minute. These sounds should be present in all four quadrants of the abdomen, beginning in the right lower quadrant (RLQ) and moving clockwise around the four quadrants, as shown in Figure 23-11. When approximately 5 to 20 bowel sounds are heard per minute, or one at least every 5 to 15 seconds, the bowel sounds are considered active.

The absence of bowel sounds during 1 minute of auscultation in each quadrant is documented as absent bowel sounds. Bowel sounds of less than five per minute are described as hypoactive, while an excess of 20 or more bowel sounds per minute is defined as hyperactive. High-pitched, loud, rushing sounds heard with or without a stethoscope are termed **borborygmi.** This is caused by the passage of gas through the liquid contents of the intestine.

Percussion of the abdomen is done in all four quadrants. The predominant abdominal percussion sound is tympany caused by percussing over the air-filled stomach and intestines.

Light palpation of the abdomen is done to assess for muscle tone, masses, pulsations, or any signs of ten-derness or discomfort. Abdominal muscles may be palpated and should feel relaxed on light palpation, not tightly contracted or spastic. If the client is anxious, muscle contraction may be evident. Palpation of a separation of the rectus abdominous muscle may be felt, especially in clients who are obese or pregnant. The rectus abdominous muscle includes two large, midline muscles that extend from the xiphoid process to the symphysis pubis and can be palpated midline as the client raises his or her head. Rebound tenderness, indicating possible inflammation of the appendix, may be elicited by depressing the abdomen and quickly withdrawing the fingers. This examination is done at the end of the abdominal assessment because of the possibility of increasing the client's level of pain. If any of the abdominal organs can be felt with light palpation, this is abnormal and should be reported to the nursing supervisor. After assessment of bowel sounds, question the client about diet, usual bowel patterns, appetite, weight changes, indigestion, heartburn, nausea, pain, and use of enemas or laxatives.

Genitourinary Status

Assessment of the client's urinary and reproductive status is accomplished mainly by inspection and use of interview skills. Genitourinary assessment includes examination of the abdomen, urinary meatus and genitalia, and assessment of the client's urine.

Inspect the abdomen for any enlargement or fullness. In the normal adult, the abdomen is smooth, flat, and symmetrical. The urinary meatus should be inspected for any abnormalities such as inflammation and discharge, which may signal a urethral infection.

In females, observe the appearance of the genitalia (labia, clitoris, vaginal opening). Questions to ask the client that focus on the reproductive history include pregnancies, use of birth control, menstrual cycle history, present sexual activity, use of protection during intercourse, date of the last Pap test, and determination of how any present illness has or will affect sexual activity.

In males, inspect the penis, urethral meatus, foreskin (if uncircumcised), and scrotum. Questions to ask the client that focus on the reproductive history include present sexual activity, use of protection during intercourse, and how the present illness has or will affect sexual activity. Ask if the client performs testicular self-examinations.

Note any lesions or ulcerations that may indicate sexually transmitted disease. The usual voiding pattern and any recent changes should be determined if the client has had any history of urinary tract infections, kidney stones, change in the urinary stream, or painful urination or nocturia.

Musculoskeletal and Extremity Assessment

Assess symmetry and strength of major muscle groups throughout the head-to-toe assessment. Any time during the assessment when the client is repositioned, observe the range of movement the client utilizes to make that position change. Ask the client to walk across the room and observe the client's movements and posture when sitting up in bed to assess gross motor movement and posture. Assessment of the client's handshake gives an estimate of muscle strength. Palpating muscles lightly identifies swelling, tone, or any specific changes in the shape of the muscles.

Hand grasps and foot pushes assess the strength and equality of the client's extremities. Upper extremity strength is assessed by having the client grasp the nurse's index and middle fingers of each hand. The grasp should be equal in both hands. Foot pushes assess the lower extremities. The nurse's hands should be placed on the soles of the client's feet. The client is asked to push both feet against the nurse's hands. The push should be equal in both feet. Ask the client to touch the tip of her nose with a finger and then the tip of the nurse's finger as it is moved to different locations to test the client's coordination skills.

Assess strength and symmetry of some of the major muscle groups by watching gait and postural movements. Note any aids to ambulation. Examine muscles, first in one extremity and then the other; note equality of size, contour, tone, and strength.

Carefully assess the skin of the lower extremities to determine color changes, loss of feeling or hair, change in temperature within the extremity and from one extrem-

ity to the other, and presence of varicose veins, ulcers, and edema. Ask if the client experiences any leg pain or cramps or if muscle weakness is experienced or if difficulty or pain when walking or performing routine daily activities occurs. The functional assessment includes asking the client about routine activities such as cooking, shopping, exercise, yard work, and hobbies. Tolerance limitations can be identified by observing for stiffness, crepitus, or fatigue during ambulation. Determine if the client can safely and appropriately perform functions essential for home life and activities of daily living.

Summary

- Psychosocial needs of clients are identified within the scope of a functional assessment.
- The health history and the physical examination used together present a holistic view of client needs.
- Collection of vital signs is the foundation of each head-to-toe assessment and includes temperature, pulse, respirations, blood pressure, and pain.
- Assessment of a client's mental and neurological status is determined by obtaining information about the client's level of consciousness, pupil response, as well as hand grip and foot push capabilities.
- When describing a client's affect, utilize terms that are descriptive of the specific behavior observed, not a judgment about the behavior.
- Assessing the cardiovascular status of each client includes palpation of specific pulse points.
- Auscultation of lung fields assists in collection of data regarding the breath sounds of the client.
- An abdominal assessment includes use of inspection, auscultation, percussion, and palpation within the four quadrants of the abdomen to establish bowel status and function.
- Through observation of client gait and overall range of movement, some knowledge of the symmetry and strength of muscles is obtained.
- During the assessment of wounds, drains, dressings, and other external devices, maintain accurate documentation of the amount of drainage, color, or other changes.

Review Questions

1. Mrs. Jones is 54 years old. While performing the assessment overview, Mrs. Jones states, "I just get so lightheaded when I first get up in the morning." Mrs. Jones most likely has:

   a. cyanosis.

   b. hypertension.

   c. orthostatic hypertension.

   d. orthostatic hypotension.

2. During the physical head-to-toe assessment of the client, the nurse checks the pulse and blood pressure. Which of the four assessment techniques did the nurse utilize?

   a. auscultation, palpation, and inspection
   b. auscultation, percussion, and inspection
   c. auscultation and palpation
   d. palpation and inspection

3. Upon admission to your unit, the client verbalizes increased pain in her left leg. What would be the pertinent assessment information to collect about this client?

   a. Listen to the client's bowel sounds.
   b. Check circulation in the right leg.
   c. Assess both of the client's legs.
   d. Ask the client about her current diet.

4. How often a nurse assesses a client's vital signs depends on the:

   a. availability of personnel.
   b. doctor's orders.
   c. nurse's discretion.
   d. client's condition.

5. The nurse checks the radial pulse for 30 seconds and multiplies by 2. She notices an irregularity in the beat. What is the next action the nurse should take?

   a. Check the radial pulse for 60 seconds.
   b. Listen to the apical pulse for 60 seconds.
   c. Listen to the apical for 30 seconds and multiply by 2.
   d. Continue with the rest of the assessment.

References/Suggested Readings

American Heart Association (AHA). (1987). *Recommendations for human blood pressure determination.* (AHA Publication No. 701005). Dallas, TX: Author.

Andresen, G. (1998). Assessing the older patient. *RN, 61*(3), 46–55.

Barkauskas, V. H., Bauman, L. C., & Darling-Fisher, C. S. (2002). *Health and physical assessment* (3rd ed.). St. Louis: Mosby.

Bickley, L. S. & Sailagyi, P. (2002). *Bates' guide to physical examination and history taking* (8th ed.). Philadelphia: Lippincott Williams & Wilkins.

Craig, J. V. et al. (2002). Now, hear this: Ear temps in children found to be inaccurate. *Lancet, 360*(9333), 603–609.

Crow, S. (1997). Your guide to gloves. *Nursing97, 27*(3), 26–28.

Estes, M. E. Z. (2002). *Health assessment & physical examination* (2nd ed.). Clifton Park, NY: Thomson Delmar Learning.

Finesilver, C. A. (2001). Perfecting your skills: Respiratory assessment. *RN's Travel Nursing Today,* April 2001, 16–26.

Fuller, J., & Schaller-Ayers, J. (2000). *Health assessment: A nursing approach.* (3rd ed.). Philadelphia: Lippincott Williams & Wilkins.

Gallauresi, B. A. (1998). Pulse oximeters. *Nursing98, 28*(9), 31.

Gehring, P. E. (2002). Perfecting your skills: Vascular assessment. *RN's Travel Nursing Today,* April 2002, 16–24.

Heery, K. (2000). Straight talk about the patient interview. *Nursing 2000, 30*(6), 66–67.

Hodge, P., & Ullrich, S. (1999). Does your assessment include alternative therapies? *RN, 62*(6), 47–49.

Husain, M., & Coleman, R. (2002). Should you treat a fever? *Nursing2002, 32*(10), 66–70.

Joint Commission on Accreditation of Healthcare Organizations (JCAHO). (2000a). *Comprehensive accreditation manual for hospitals (CAMH) revised pain management standards* [Online]. Available: www.jcaho.org/standard/pm_hap.html

Joint Commission on Accreditation of Healthcare Organizations (JCAHO). (2000b). *Pain assessment and management standards* [Online]. Available: www.jcaho.org/standard/pm_coll.html

Karch, A. M., & Karch, F. E. (2000). When a blood pressure isn't routine. *AJN, 100*(3), 23.

Kirton, C. A. (1997). Assessing bowel sounds. *Nursing97, 27*(3), 64.

Klingman, L. (1999). Assessing the female reproductive system. *AJN, 99*(8), 37–43.

Klingman, L. (1999). Assessing the male genitalia. *AJN, 99*(7), 47–50.

Lower, J. (2002). Facing neuro assessment fearlessly. *Nursing2002, 32*(2), 58–64.

Mehta, M. (2003a). Assessing the abdomen. *Nursing2003, 33*(5), 54–55.

Mehta, M. (2003b). Assessing cardiovascular status. *Nursing2003, 33*(2), 56–58.

Mehta, M. (2003c). Assessing respiratory status. *Nursing2003, 33*(2), 54–56.

Murray, R. B., & Zentner, J. P. (2001). *Health promotion strategies through the lifespan* (7th ed.). Norwalk: Prentice Hall.

O'Hanlon-Nichols, T. (1997). Basic assessment series: The adult cardiovascular system. *AJN, 97*(12), 34–40.

O'Hanlon-Nichols, T. (1998). Basic assessment series: Gastrointestinal system. *AJN, 98*(4), 48–53.

O'Hanlon-Nichols, T. (1998). Basic assessment series: Musculoskeletal system. *AJN, 98*(6), 48–52.

O'Hanlon-Nichols, T. (1998). Basic assessment series: The adult pulmonary system. *AJN, 98*(2), 39–45.

O'Hanlon-Nichols, T. (1999). Neurologic assessment. *AJN, 99*(6), 44–50.

Owen, A. (1998). Respiratory assessment revisited. *Nursing98, 28*(4), 48–49.

Pullen, R. (2003). Using an ear thermometer. *Nursing2003, 33*(5), 24.

Rice, K. L. (1998). Sounding out blood flow with a Doppler device. *Nursing98, 28*(9), 56–57.

Rice, K. L. (1999). Measuring thigh BP. *Nursing99, 29*(8), 58–59.

Stanley, W. (2003). Nailing a key assessment. *Nursing2003, 33*(8), 50–51.

Taylor, C., Lillis, C., & LeMone, P. (2001). *Fundamentals of nursing: The art and science of nursing care* (4th ed.). Philadelphia: Lippincott Williams & Wilkins.

Thomas, J., & Feliciano, C. (2003). Measuring BP with a doppler device. *Nursing2003, 33*(7), 52–53.

University of Maryland Medicine. (2002). *An introduction to CAM.* [Online]. Available: www.umm.edu/altmed/ConsModalities/AnIntroductionToCAMcm.html

Warner, P., Rowe, T., & Whipple, B. (1999). Shedding light on the sexual history. *AJN, 99*(6), 34–40.

Weber, J., & Kelley, J. (2002). *Health assessment in nursing.* (2nd ed.). Philadelphia: Lippincott Williams & Wilkins.

PAIN MANAGEMENT

MAKING THE CONNECTION

Refer to the following chapters to increase your understanding of pain management:

Basic Nursing
- **Communication**
- **Cultural Considerations**
- **Loss, Grief, and Death**
- **Complementary/Alternative Therapies**

Intermediate Procedures
- **Administering Oral, Sublingual, and Buccal Medication**
- **Withdrawing Medication from an Ampule**
- **Withdrawing Medication from a Vial**
- **Administering an Intradermal Injection**
- **Administering a Subcutaneous Injection**
- **Administering an Intramuscular Injection**

LEARNING OBJECTIVES

Upon completion of this chapter, you should be able to:
- **Define key terms.**
- **Identify the four components of pain conduction.**
- **Discuss the gate control theory of pain.**
- **Describe the types of pain.**
- **List three guidelines that should be included in a thorough pain assessment.**
- **Identify three general principles of pain management.**
- **List the nurse's responsibilities in administration of analgesics.**
- **Identify site of action of both nonopioid and opioid analgesics.**
- **Describe three examples of nonpharmacological measures for pain relief.**
- **Discuss nursing interventions that promote comfort.**

KEY TERMS

acupuncture
acute pain
adjuvant medication
afferent pain pathway
analgesia
analgesic
ceiling effect
chronic acute pain
chronic nonmalignant
 pain
chronic pain
colic
cryotherapy
cutaneous pain
distraction
efferent pain pathway
endorphin
epidural analgesia
gate control pain theory
hypnosis
intrathecal analgesia
ischemic pain
mixed agonist-
 antagonist
modulation

myofascial pain
 syndromes
neuralgia
nociceptor
noxious stimulus
pain
pain threshold
pain tolerance
patient-controlled
 analgesia
perception
phantom limb pain
progressive muscle re-
 laxation
recurrent acute pain
referred pain
reframing
relaxation technique
somatic pain
tolerance
transcutaneous electrical
 nerve stimulation
transduction
transmission
visceral pain

INTRODUCTION

Pain is a phenomenon found in all specialties of nursing. No matter the setting, including neonatal intensive care, intraoperative, home care, or clinics, there are challenges in pain management. While other health care team members address pain management with clients, the nurse spends the most time with the client experiencing pain. For example, in an acute care setting, the physician orders the **analgesics** (substances that relieve pain) for the client, but may only spend 10 to 15 minutes a day with that client. Nurses are present 24 hours a day, administer the medications, assess the client's response, and report the response to the physician. The nurse's role can be pivotal in relieving the client's pain.

The experience of pain can have a significant impact on a client's health. It is a personal experience affecting all aspects of an individual's health, including physical well-being, mental status, and effectiveness of coping mechanisms. This chapter provides an overview of the complex phenomenon of pain, including pain definitions, pain physiology, and pain assessment. Strategies to control pain are also discussed, including pharmacological, noninvasive, and invasive techniques.

DEFINITIONS OF PAIN

The phenomenon of pain is referenced as far back as the Babylonian clay tablets. Aristotle (4th century B.C.) described pain as an emotion, being the opposite of pleasure. Although emotions certainly play an important role in pain perception, there is much more to the experience than the feelings involved.

In the Middle Ages, pain had religious connotations. Pain was seen as God's punishment for sins, or as evidence that an individual was possessed by demons. This definition of pain is still embraced by some clients, who might tell the nurse that the suffering is their "cross to bear." Pain relief may not be the goal for those individuals who believe in this definition of pain. Spiritual counseling may need to be implemented before this person is willing to work toward relief.

The most widely accepted definition of **pain** is one developed by the International Association for the Study of Pain (IASP). This organization defines pain as "an unpleasant sensory and emotional experience associated with actual or potential tissue damage or described in terms of such damage" (Merskey & Bogduk, 1994). This definition incorporates both the sensory and emotional components of pain. It also acknowledges that evidence of actual tissue damage is not required in order for the pain to be considered real.

Many pain experts emphasize the subjective nature of pain. Unlike a blood pressure or a blood glucose measurement, the intensity of discomfort the client is feeling cannot be measured with an instrument. McCaffery and Pasero (1999) say it best by defining pain as "whatever the person experiencing it says it is, existing whenever [he or she] says it does." This philosophy is emphasized in professional pain management guidelines. For example, the 1994 Agency for Health Care Policy and Research (AHCPR)—now called Agency for Healthcare Research and Quality (AHRQ)—from the guideline for cancer pain states, "Health professionals should ask about pain, and the patient's self-report should be the primary source of assessment." Guidelines are still published under the old name. The American Pain Society (APS) also stresses the importance of self-report: "Pain is always subjective. . . . The clinician must accept the patient's report of pain" (1999).

Although pain has had many definitions throughout history, research in pain physiology shows that pain is a complex phenomenon. Pain is often difficult for clients to describe and nurses to understand; yet it is among the most common complaints leading individuals to seek health care. Until recently, pain was viewed as a symptom that required diagnosis and treatment of the underlying cause. It is now clear that pain itself can be detrimental to the health and healing of clients. McCaffery and Pasero (1999) write that pain control, not just relief from pain once it occurs, must be recognized as a priority in the care of clients in all settings.

NATURE OF PAIN

Pain experience is a signal of tissue damage, as in the pain of cancer and chronic illness. Pain can also be a protective mechanism to prevent further injury, as when a client guards or protects an injured body part. Pain, as a warning of potential tissue damage, may be absent in people with hereditary sensory neuropathies, congenital nerve or spinal cord abnormalities, multiple sclerosis, diabetic neuropathy, alcoholism, leprosy, and nerve or spinal cord injury.

COMMON MYTHS ABOUT PAIN

Pain is often misunderstood and misjudged because it is subjective (depends on the client's perception) and cannot be objectively measured through a laboratory test or diagnostic data. A client's report of the level of pain varies based on cultural and experiential background. The nurse's interpretation of a client's pain is filtered through the nurse's biases and expectations. Some common myths related to pain are discussed in Table 24-1.

TYPES OF PAIN

Pain can be described by its origin or cause and by its nature or description. Pain categorized by its origin is either cutaneous, somatic, or visceral; by its nature is either acute or chronic.

Pain Categorized by Origin

Cutaneous pain is caused by stimulating the cutaneous nerve endings in the skin and results in a well-localized "burning" or "prickling" sensation; tangled hair that is pulled during combing causes cutaneous pain. **Somatic pain** is nonlocalized and originates in support structures such as tendons, ligaments, and nerves; twisting an ankle results in somatic pain. **Visceral pain** is discomfort in the internal organs, is less localized, and more slowly transmitted than cutaneous pain. Pain originating from the abdominal organs is often called **referred pain** because pain is not felt in the organ but instead is perceived at the spot where the organs were located during fetal development, making it difficult to assess (Figure 24-1).

Pain Categorized by Nature

It is important to understand the difference between acute and chronic pain because they each present a different clinical picture.

TABLE 24-1 COMMON MYTHS ABOUT PAIN

MYTH	FACT
• The nurse is the best judge of a client's pain.	• Pain is a subjective experience; only the client can judge the level and severity of pain.
• If pain is ignored, it will go away.	• Pain is a real experience that is appropriately treated with nursing and medical intervention.
• Clients should not take any measures to relieve their pain until the pain is unbearable.	• Pain control and relief measures are effective in lowering the pain level, which will help clients function more normally and comfortably.
• Most complaints of pain are purely psychological (e.g., "it's all in your head"); only "real" pain manifests in obvious physical signs such as moaning or grimacing.	• Most clients honestly report their perception of pain, both physical and emotional, and need effective intervention and teaching; physical responses vary greatly depending on experience and cultural norms, and visible expressions of pain are not always reliable indicators of its severity.
• Clients taking pain medications will become addicted to the drug.	• Addiction is unlikely when analgesics are carefully administered and closely monitored.
• Clients with severe tissue damage will experience significant pain; those with lesser damage will feel less pain.	• Individuals' perceptions of pain are subjective; the extent of tissue damage is not necessarily proportional to the extent of pain experienced.
• Clients ask for pain medication when they need it.	• Many clients do not ask for medication because they are afraid of side effects, do not want to bother the nurse, have cultural norms and beliefs against it, or believe pain is inevitable and untreatable.

Acute Pain

Acute pain has a sudden onset, relatively short duration, mild to severe intensity, with a steady decrease in intensity over a period of days to weeks. Once the **noxious stimulus** (underlying pathology) is resolved, the pain usually disappears (Table 24-2). It is usually associated with a specific condition, injury, or tissue damage caused by disease. As healing occurs, acute pain should diminish. Everyone has experienced acute pain (e.g., toothaches, headaches, needlesticks, skinned knees, burns, muscle pain, childbirth, postoperative pain, a sprained ankle, and fractures). The client is usually able to pinpoint the hurt. Acute pain is often described as sharp, although deep pain may be described as dull and aching. The client will exhibit elevated heart rate, respiratory rate, and blood pressure; and may become diaphoretic and have dilated pupils. These signs resemble those of anxiety, which often accompanies acute pain. Behaviors may include crying and moaning, rubbing the site of pain, guarding, frowning, grimacing, and verbal complaints of the discomfort.

Recurrent acute pain is repetitive painful episodes that recur over a prolonged period or throughout the client's lifetime. Pain-free intervals alternate with painful episodes. Examples of recurrent pain seen in children include recurrent abdominal, chest, limb pain, and headaches. In adults, recurrent pain experience includes migraine headaches, sickle cell crises pain, and angina pain.

Chronic Pain

Chronic pain is usually defined as long-term (lasting 6 months or longer), persistent, nearly constant, or recurrent pain producing significant negative changes in the client's life. Chronic pain may last long after the pathology is resolved. Although some infants, children, and adolescents experience chronic pain, it is more common in adults. In the United States, one in four live with chronic pain. Chronic pain is the reason for more than 80% of all physician visits (NPF, 2002).

Chronic acute pain occurs almost daily over a long period, months or years, and may never stop. Cancer and severe burns are examples of pathophysiology leading to chronic acute pain. Sometimes the pain ends only at the time of death, as in terminal cancer clients (McCaffery & Pasero, 1999). This type of pain is also called *progressive pain*.

Chronic nonmalignant pain, also called *chronic benign pain*, occurs almost daily and lasts for at least 6 months, ranging from mild to severe intensity. Three critical characteristics of chronic nonmalignant pain are identified by McCaffery and Pasero (1999):

- Caused by non–life-threatening causes
- Not responsive to currently available pain relief methods.
- May continue for the rest of the client's life

Examples of pathophysiology leading to chronic nonmalignant pain include the following:

Figure 24-1 *Areas of Referred Pain:* **A,** *Anterior View;* **B,** *Posterior View*

- Many forms of **neuralgia** (paroxysmal pain that extends along the course of one or more nerves)
- Low-back pain
- Rheumatoid arthritis
- Ankylosing spondylitis
- **Phantom limb pain** (a form of neuropathic pain that occurs after amputation with pain sensations referred to an area in the missing portion of the limb)
- **Myofascial pain syndromes** (a group of muscle disorders characterized by pain, muscle spasm, tenderness, stiffness, and limited motion)

When chronic nonmalignant pain is severe enough to disable the client, it is identified as *chronic intractable nonmalignant pain syndrome.*

Signs and Symptoms The signs and symptoms of chronic pain can look very different from those of acute pain. The body cannot tolerate the sympathetic nervous system signs for a long period and, therefore, adapts. Vital signs will often be normal, with no accompanying pupil dilatation or perspiration. Lack of these signs may prompt some health care workers to question the client's description of pain.

The hopelessness, listlessness, and loss of libido and weight of chronic pain are similar to those of depression. The client often describes exhaustion and fatigue. Behaviors include no complaint of pain unless asked and physical inactivity or immobility leading to functional disability. The crying, moaning, guarding, and grimacing that most clinicians associate with pain are absent. Treatment of chronic pain is more complex than that of acute pain. Chronic pain is viewed by pain experts as a disease state, rather than a symptom. Management includes identifying the cause of pain, recognizing emotional and environmental factors contributing to the pain, and rehabilitation to improve the client's functional abilities.

TABLE 24-2	ACUTE VERSUS CHRONIC PAIN	
	ACUTE	**CHRONIC**
Time Span	Less than 6 months	More than 6 months
Location	Localized, associated with a specific injury, condition, or disease	Difficult to pinpoint
Characteristics	Often described as sharp, diminishes as healing occurs	Often described as dull, diffuse, and aching
Physiologic Signs	• Elevated heart rate • Elevated BP • Elevated respirations • May be diaphoretic • Dilated pupils	• Normal vital signs • Normal pupils • No diaphoresis • May have loss of weight
Behavioral Signs	• Crying and moaning • Rubbing site • Guarding • Frowning • Grimacing • Complains of pain	• Physical immobility • Hopelessness • Listlessness • Loss of libido • Exhaustion and fatigue • Complains of pain only when asked

PURPOSE OF PAIN

Pain serves as a protective mechanism. If a person touches a hot stove, the pain signal causes the person to pull the hand away immediately. The skin would be seriously burned if this did not happen.

Pain can be a diagnostic tool. The quality and duration of the pain give important clues in determining a client's medical diagnosis. For example, in acute appendicitis, the clinician looks for rebound tenderness (the pain increases when pressure is released) when palpating the abdomen. This particular type of pain helps confirm the diagnosis of appendicitis rather than other gastrointestinal disorders.

PHYSIOLOGY OF PAIN

The opioid system and the nonopioid system are the two known endogenous (developing within) analgesia systems in humans. The best known is the opioid system. It is mediated by **endorphins** (endogenous opiate-like substances). The nonopioid system is mediated by monoamine substances such as norepinephrine and serotonin.

When pain occurs, sensory input from injured tissue causes peripheral **nociceptors** (receptive neurons for painful sensations) and central nervous system (CNS) pain pathways to enhance future responses to pain stimuli. Long-lasting changes in cells within the spinal cord **afferent** (ascending) and **efferent** (descending) **pain pathways** may thus occur after a brief noxious stimulus.

Physiological responses (such as elevated blood pressure, respiratory rate, and pulse rate; dilated pupils; perspiration; and pallor) to even a brief acute pain episode will show adaptation within minutes to a few hours. The body cannot sustain the extreme stress response physiologically for more than short periods. The body conserves its resources by physiological adaptation: a return to normal or near normal blood pressure, respiratory rate, and pulse rate; pupil size; and dry skin with little evidence of poor perfusion, *even with continuing pain of the same intensity.*

Stimulation of Pain

The specific action of pain depends on the type of pain. Cutaneous pain rapidly travels through a simple reflex arc from the nerve ending (point of pain) to the spinal cord at approximately 300 feet per second, with a reflex response evoking an almost immediate reaction. This is why, when a hot stove is touched, the person's hand jerks back *before* there is conscious awareness of damage (Figure 24-2). After a hot stove is touched, a sensory nerve ending in the finger skin initiates nerve transmission that travels through the dorsal root ganglion to the dorsal horn in the gray matter of the spinal cord. The impulse then travels though an interneuron that synapses with a motor neuron at the same level in the spinal cord. This motor neuron stimulating the muscle is responsible for the swift movement of the hand away from the hot stove.

In the case of the hot stove, the sensory neuron also synapses with an afferent sensory neuron. The impulse travels up the spinal cord to the thalamus, where a

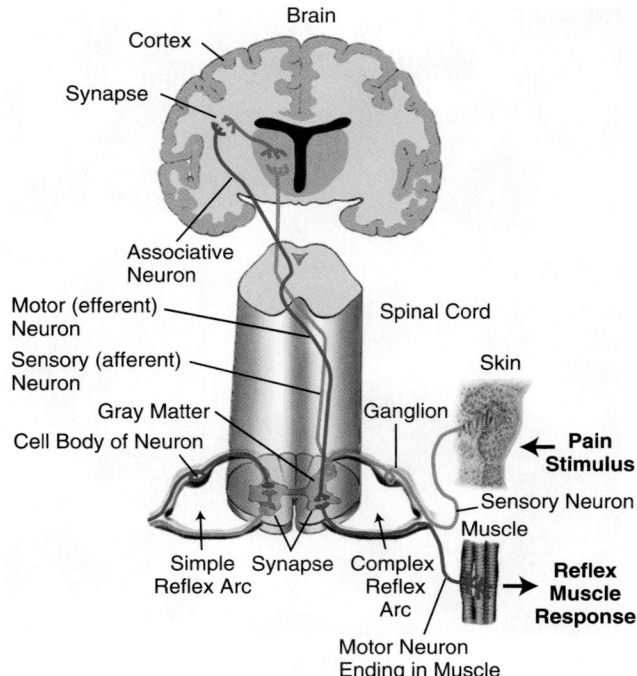

Figure 24-2 *Reflex Arcs*

synapse sends the impulse to the brain cortex. Once the impulse is interpreted, the information is consciously available. Then the person is aware of the location, intensity, and quality of pain. Previous experience adds the affective feature to the pain experience. Descending or efferent motor neuron response moves from the brain through the spinal cord, synapsing with a motor neuron in the spinal cord, and innervates the muscle.

The transmission of visceral pain impulses is slower and less localized than cutaneous pain. Internal organs (including the gastrointestinal tract) have few nociceptors, which is why visceral pain is poorly localized and is felt as a throbbing sensation or dull ache; however, internal organs are very sensitive to distension. The cramping pain of **colic** (acute abdominal pain) results when:

- Constipation or flatus distends the stomach or intestines.
- There is hyperperistalsis, as in gastroenteritis.
- Something tries to pass through an opening that is too small.

The physiology of **ischemic pain,** or pain occurring when the blood supply to an area is restricted or cut off completely, also differs. Blood flow restriction causes in-

---

PROFESSIONAL TIP

Sensation of Pain

To feel pain in the cornea of the eye, it takes 0.2 grams of pressure per square millimeter, on the forearm 20 grams, on the sole of the foot 200 grams, and on the fingertips 300 grams (Brand & Yancey, 1993).

adequate oxygenation of the tissue supplied by those vessels and inadequate removal of metabolic wastes. The onset of ischemic pain is most rapid in an active muscle and much slower in a passive muscle. Examples of ischemic pain are muscle cramps, myocardial infarction, angina pectoris, and sickle cell crisis. When ischemic pain occurs in a muscle that continues to work, a muscle spasm (cramp) occurs. If the blood supply to the heart is completely cut off or severely restricted and not restored quickly, a myocardial infarction occurs.

 Safety: Ischemic Pain
Administer supplemental oxygen and pain medication quickly to clients with ischemic pain to minimize oxygen deprivation and prevent infarction (tissue death).

Substances released from injured tissue in acute pain episodes lead to stress hormone responses. There is an increase in metabolic rate, enhanced breakdown of body tissue, increased blood clotting, impaired immune function, and water retention. The fight-or-flight reaction is triggered, leading to tachycardia and negative emotions.

The Gate Control Theory

Pain transmission and interpretation theories try to describe and explain the pain experience. Early pain theorists focused on the neuroanatomical and neurophysiological mechanisms.

In 1965, Melzack and Wall proposed the **gate control pain theory,** which was the first one recognizing that psychological aspects of pain are as important as physiological aspects. The gate control theory combined cognitive, sensory, and emotional components—in addition to the physiological aspects—and proposed that they can act on a gate control system to block the individual's perception of pain. The basic premise is that transmission of potentially painful nerve impulses to the cortex is modulated by a spinal cord gating mechanism and by CNS activity. As a result, the level of conscious awareness of painful sensation is altered.

The theory suggests that nerve fibers that contribute to pain transmission converge at a site in the dorsal horn of the spinal cord. This site is thought to act as a gating mechanism that determines which impulses will be blocked and which will be transmitted to the thalamus. The image of a gate is useful in teaching clients and their families about pain relief measures. If the "gate" is closed, the signal is stopped before it reaches the brain, where **perception** (being aware of) of pain occurs. If the gate is open, the signal will continue on through the spinothalamic tract to the cortex, and the client will feel the pain. Whether the gate is opened or closed is influ-

enced by impulses from peripheral nerves (the sensory components) and nerve signals that descend from the brain (motivational-affective and cognitive components). For example, stimulation of some types of peripheral nerves by cutaneous stimulation such as massage can close the gate, whereas stimulation of the nociceptors will open the gate.

If a person is anxious, the gate can be opened by signals sent from the brain down to the mechanism in the dorsal horn of the spinal cord. On the other hand, if the person has had positive experiences with pain control in the past, the cognitive influence can send signals down to the gating mechanism and close it. The gate theory offered a great benefit by suggesting new approaches to relieving both acute and chronic pain. Pain could be relieved by blocking the transmission of pain impulses to the brain by both physical modalities and by altering the individual's thought processes, emotions, or other behaviors.

Conduction of Pain Impulses

Conduction of pain impulses refers to the physiologic processes that occur from the initiation of the pain signal to the realization of pain by the individual. Four processes are involved in the conduction of this signal. The first, **transduction,** is when a noxious stimulus triggers electrical activity in the endings of afferent nerve fibers (nociceptors). Once the signal is triggered, **transmission** occurs. The impulse travels from the receiving nociceptors to the spinal cord. Projection neurons then carry the message to the thalamus, and the message continues to the somatosensory cortex. Then the third step, perception of pain, occurs. Here neural messages are converted into the subjective experience. The fourth process, **modulation,** is a CNS pathway that selectively inhibits pain transmission by sending blocking signals back down to the dorsal horn of the spinal cord.

FACTORS AFFECTING THE PAIN EXPERIENCE

According to McCaffery and Pasero (1999), *the client is the only authority about the existence and nature of his or her pain.* Age, previous experience with pain, drug abuse, and cultural norms account for the differences in clients' individual responses to pain.

Age

Age can greatly influence clients' perception of pain. They may continue pain behaviors learned as children and may be reluctant to admit pain or seek medical care because they fear the unknown or fear how treatment may impact their lifestyle. Older adults may ignore their pain, believing it is a consequence of aging. Family and health care members may thoughtlessly support this idea and be less responsive to an older client's complaints of pain.

Previous Pain Experiences

Previous experience with pain often influences clients' reactions. Past coping mechanisms may affect

LIFE CYCLE CONSIDERATIONS

Elders and Pain

Older clients often live with pain, believing that nothing can be done. Pain often is not reported by older clients for fear of being labeled a "bother" or "complainer." Encourage the client to request pain relief as needed.

clients' judgments about how pain will affect their lives and which measures they can use to successfully manage the pain on their own. Teaching clients about pain expectations and management methods can often allay their fears and lead to successful pain management.

Drug Abuse

According to Compton (1999), a drug abuser is likely to be *less* tolerant of pain than someone who does not use drugs. Drug abuse may cause changes in the central nervous system, resulting in an exaggerated neurophysiologic response to painful stimuli. To keep a drug abuser comfortable, withdrawal must be prevented.

Cultural Norms

Cultural differences in pain responses can lead to pain management problems. Studies on subjects of various cultures found no significant difference among the groups in the intensity level at which pain becomes perceptible. The same studies showed that the intensity level or duration of pain the client was willing to endure differed significantly. Cultural values guide the expression of pain. Some cultures tolerate pain and "suffering in silence," whereas others fully express pain, including physical and emotional responses. Be careful not to equate the level of pain expression with the level of actual pain experienced, but consider cultural and other influences that affect the expression of pain.

JCAHO STANDARDS

Pain management standards were included in the 2000–2001 standards of the Joint Commission on Accreditation of Healthcare Organizations (JCAHO). They were first scored for compliance in 2001.

The health care organizations are expected to:

- Recognize the right of patients to appropriate assessment and management of pain.
- Assess the existence and, if so, the nature and intensity of pain in all patients.
- Record the results of the assessment in a way that facilitates regular reassessment and follow-up.
- Determine and assure staff competency in pain assessment and management and address pain assessment and management in the orientation of all new staff.
- Establish policies and procedures that support the appropriate prescription or ordering of effective pain medications.

- Educate patients and their families about effective pain management.
- Address patient needs for symptom management in the discharge planning process (JCAHO, 1999).

NURSING PROCESS

The nursing process provides the framework for managing a client's pain.

Assessment

Assessment of the client's pain is a crucial nursing function. During the assessment process, be aware of your own values and expectations about pain behaviors. Just as the client's experience and cultural background help determine how pain is demonstrated, nurses' cultures and experiences help determine which pain behaviors are viewed as acceptable. Be aware of these values and avoid biases when assessing client pain and planning client care. Once a self-assessment about pain has been conducted, the nurse is ready to assess the client.

Pain assessment tools are the most effective method to identify the presence and intensity of pain in clients. *These tools must be used, and the results must be accepted* (Figure 24-3).

The JCAHO (2000a) now considers pain as the fifth vital sign. It is to be assessed and recorded along with the client's temperature, pulse, respiration, and blood pressure.

Subjective Data

The first step in pain assessment is gathering subjective information regarding the client's pain. A client's pain threshold and pain tolerance level should be determined. **Pain threshold** is the intensity level where a person feels pain. It varies with each individual and with each type of pain. **Pain tolerance** is the intensity level or duration of pain the client is able or willing to endure.

The client's description of the pain should cover several qualifiers, including its location, onset and duration, quality, intensity, aggravating factors (variables that worsen the pain, such as exercise, certain foods, or stress), alleviating factors (measures the client can take that lessen the effect of the pain, such as lying down, avoiding certain foods, or taking medication), associated manifestations (factors that often accompany the pain, such as nausea, constipation, or dizziness), and what pain means to the client.

Whenever subjective and objective data conflict, the subjective reports of pain are to be considered the primary source.

Location The client can point to the location of the pain on the client's own body or locate it on a body diagram on a pain assessment tool. The client should be asked if there is more than one site of pain; if the pain radiates, and if so to where; and ask if the pain is deep or superficial.

Onset and Duration Ask the client how long the pain has existed; what, if anything, triggers its onset; and if there are any patterns to the pain (e.g., whether it is worse at certain times of the day or night).

Quality Ask the client what the pain feels like, and record the words used to describe the pain. Clients may

COMPLETE WITH 1ST DOSE OF PAIN MEDICATION	INITIALS	SIGNATURE

1. Onset and frequency (When did it start?) (How often)_____
2. Provokes (What makes it worse?)_____
_____
3. Radiates?_____
4. Severity/Intensity (What is an acceptable level of pain [0–10])_____
5. Timing/Duration (How long does it last?)_____
6. Past & Current analgesic/alternative modalities that make it better._____
_____

7. Does your pain affect: sleep__ appetite__ physical activity__ emotions__
social relationships__

COMMENTS:

Pediatrics/Noncommunicative Clients (0–10)

A. Verbal/Vocal
0=positive
1=other complaint, whimper
2=pain, crying
3=screaming

B. Body Movements
0=moves easily
1=neutral shifting
2=tense, flailing arms & legs

C. Facial
0=smiling
1=neutral
2=frown, grimace
3=clenched teeth

D. Touching (localizing pain)
0=no touching
1=reaching, patting
2=grabbing

Source of Information
1=Patient
2=Child
3=Parent
4=Nurse
5=Family
6=Other

Side Effects:
1=Nausa/Vomiting
2=Resp. Depression
3=Pruritis
4=Urinary Retention
5=Altered Mental Status
6=None

Safety:
1=Bed low
2=Call bell in reach
3=Side rails ×2
4=Side rails ×4
5=Bed alert
6=Family/Sitter

Nonpharmacological Interventions
1=Cold   7=Massage
2=Distractions   8=Music
3=Environmental Control   9=Positioning
4=Exercises   10=Relaxation
5=Heat   11=TENS
6=Imagery   12=Spiritual Care

Pediatrics
13=Holding
14=Rocking
15=Pacifier
16=Security object

Mode of Administration
PCA   SQ   Rectal (R)
IV   PO   Nasal (N)
IM   SL
Epidural (EP)
Transdermal (TD)

LEVEL OF CONSCIOUSNESS KEY (LOC)*
1. Alert, engages in conversation; puposefully travels with eyes, if mute
2. Lethargic, drowsy, sedate—focuses on personal interchange—but unable to maintain focus
3. Responds only to maximal stimulation (shaking). Response only a grunt or moan—not a clear sentence.
4. Coma—unable to respond at all.

Date/ Time	Location of Pain	Character: Dull, Stabbing, Pressure, Sharp, Throbbing	Severity Rating 0–10	Pharmacologic// (Med Name)/ Nonpharmacologic	Mode of Adminis- tration	Source of Information	B	P	R	Side Effects / LOC	Safety	Time of Evaluation	Evaluation of Interventions/ Frequency Rating 0–10 Response/ Comments	Initails

CHRISTUS SPOHN HEALTH SYSTEM

PAIN MANAGEMENT FLOW SHEET
PATIENT CARE SERVICES

2006

2763751

NEW: 07/99
REVISED: 05/30/2001
FM15

Figure 24-3 *Pain Assessment and Management (Courtesy of CHRISTUS Spohn Health System, Corpus Christi, TX)* use sensory-type words, such as "pricking," "radiating," "burning," or "throbbing." Other clients use words that have an affective connotation, such as "fearful," "sickening," or "punishing." Other words used may be evaluative, such as "miserable" or "unbearable." The quality of pain provides information that may be useful in diagnosing the cause of the pain. For example, pain described as "burning" or "freezing" is usually neuropathic in origin.

Intensity The client may have difficulty in judging the intensity of pain; however, it is important to obtain an estimate of the severity of the pain. This information allows the clinician to evaluate the effectiveness of pain relief measures tried by comparing intensity before and after the interventions.

Pain intensity scales are an effective method for clients to rate the intensity of their pain (Figure 24-4). The simple descriptive pain-intensity scale and the visual analog scale (VAS) are best used by showing the scale to the client and asking the client to point to the spot on the scale that corresponds to the present pain. The pain scale most frequently used with adolescent and adult clients is the verbal 0 to 10 scale. It needs no equipment or supplies and requires only one question: "On a scale of 0 to 10, with 0 being no pain at all and 10 being the worst pain possible, how much do you hurt right now?" If there are multiple painful areas, this question can be asked regarding each area. Twycross et al. (1996) report that pain ratings higher than 3 on a 0 to 10 scale interfered with client activities, and scores of 6 and 7 greatly interfered with client quality of life.

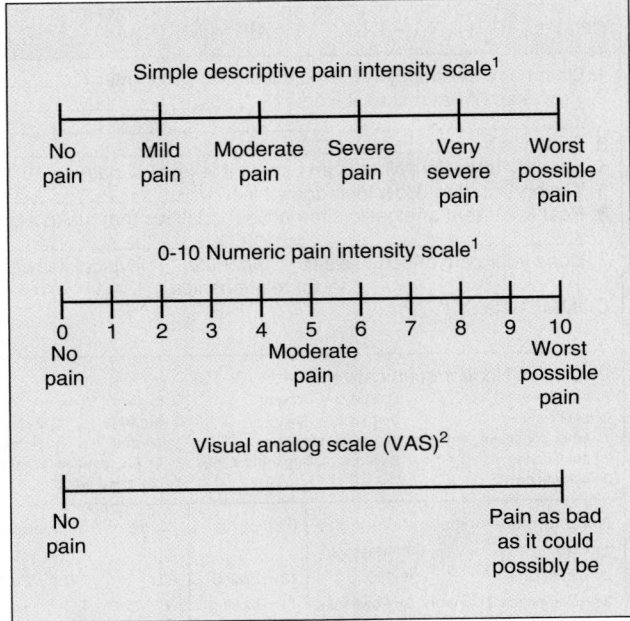

[1] If used as a graphic rating scale, a 10-cm baseline is recommended.
[2] A 10-cm baseline is recommended for VAS scales.

Figure 24-4 *Pain Intensity Scales: Three Commonly Used Self-Report Intensity Scales (Courtesy of Agency for Health Care Policy and Research, 1992)*

Clients must be taught how to correctly use the pain intensity scale (McCaffery, 2001).

Although developed for use with children, the FACES Pain Rating Scale (Figure 24-5) can be used effectively with clients when a language barrier exists. A translator should be used initially to explain what the faces represent.

A new pain assessment tool is the "Painometer" developed by Dr. Gaston-Johansson (Mattson, 2000). The client positions a pointer between "no pain" and "worst possible pain." Quantifying numbers are on the back. The client also indicates the quality of pain by selecting sensory and affective descriptors from a list.

Aggravating and Alleviating Factors Ask the client about what makes the pain worse and what makes the pain better, including behaviors or activities that influence the pain. This information helps in developing the plan of care for the client in pain. If specific activities relieve the pain, incorporate them into the care plan. Being aware of activities that increase the pain can allow for interventions that may prevent the pain. For example, if physical therapy exercises trigger an increase in pain, an analgesic can be administered as ordered before treatment.

Associated Manifestations The initial pain assessment should include the impact of pain on the activities of daily living. Pain may cause changes in sleep patterns or the ability to work and carry out the many roles in a client's life. Pain may affect appetite, mood, sexual functioning, or the ability to participate in recreational activities. If pain is interfering with daily life, the client's quality of life can be greatly affected.

0 No hurt | 1 Hurts little bit | 2 Hurts little more | 3 Hurts even more | 4 Hurts whole lot | 5 Hurts worst

Figure 24-5 *Wong/Baker FACES Pain Rating Scale (From Wong's Nursing Care of Infants and Children [7th ed.] by M. Hockenberry-Eaton, D. Wilson, & M. L. Winkelstein, 2003, New York: Elsevier Science. Copyright 2003 by Elsevier Science. Reprinted with permission.)*

Pain is fatiguing. It requires a significant amount of energy to deal with pain. The longer a person has pain, the greater the level of fatigue. Although there is no conscious awareness of pain during sleep, there may be a dream-state awareness (McCaffery & Pasero, 1999). The stress response (which can be seen even in clients under general anesthesia) continues, and the body physiologically pays the price. Clients also wake up with more pain than they had going to sleep, thereby requiring even more intervention (pharmacologic and nonpharmacologic) to reduce the pain.

Meaning of Pain Because of the motivational-affective components of the pain experience, the meaning of pain can have a great impact on how the client perceives the pain. A frequently cited classic study on this phenomenon was conducted by Beecher (1956), who compared the pain perceived by soldiers wounded in battle to pain perceived by civilians with similar surgical wounds. He found that only 32% of the soldiers required narcotics for pain relief, whereas 85% of the civilians needed the narcotics. This was interpreted that for the soldiers, the wound represented a ticket away from the battlefield, while for the civilians, the surgical wound was a depressing event.

Explore with the client what implications the pain may have for the individual. Does it mean that the client's cancer is metastasizing? Or that the client's con-

dition is worsening? All of these interpretations may influence the pain experience for the client.

Objective Data
As discussed when addressing acute versus chronic pain, the objective data often presents a different picture depending on the type of pain the client is experiencing.

Physiologic Acute pain activates the sympathetic nervous system, and the client may exhibit elevated heart rate, elevated respiratory rate, elevated blood pressure, diaphoresis, pallor, muscle tension, and dilated pupils. These signs resemble those of anxiety, which often accompanies acute pain. The signs and symptoms of chronic pain show adaption and, therefore, are different from those of acute pain, with vital signs being normal and no accompanying pupil dilation or perspiration.

Behavioral Acute pain behaviors may include crying and moaning, rubbing the site of pain, restlessness, a distorted posture, clenched fists, guarding the painful area, frowning, and grimacing. The client usually speaks of the discomfort and may be restless or afraid to move.

The client in chronic pain may demonstrate behaviors similar to those of depression, such as hopelessness, listlessness, and loss of libido and weight. Chronic pain often leads to physical inactivity or immobility, which can lead to functional disability. **Distraction** (focusing attention on stimuli other than pain) may also be used by clients. According to McCaffery and Pasero (1999), clients often minimize the pain behaviors they are able to control for several reasons, including:

• To be a "good" client and avoid making demands
• To maintain a positive self-image by not being a "sissy"
• Distraction makes pain more bearable (young children are particularly adept at this)
• Exhaustion

Client pain behaviors (AHCPR, 1992) include splinting of the painful area, distorted posture, impaired mobility, anxiety, insomnia, attention seeking, and depression. Occasionally, a discrepancy exists between pain behaviors observed by the nurse (objective data) and the client's self-report of pain. Discrepancies between behaviors and the client's self-report can result from good coping skills (e.g., relaxation techniques or distraction), anxiety, stoicism, or cultural differences in pain behaviors. Whenever these discrepancies occur, they should be addressed with the client and the pain management plan renegotiated accordingly.

Ongoing Assessment
The initial assessment obtains a baseline of information about the client's pain, while subsequent assessments

http://www.oucher.org

THE OUCHER: A SUMMARY

What is the OUCHER?

The OUCHER is a poster developed for children to help them communicate how much pain or hurt they feel. There are two scales on the OUCHER: A number scale for older children and a picture scale for younger children.

Which scale should be used?

Children who are able to count to 100 by ones or tens and who understand, for example, that 71 is greater than 43, can use the numerical scale. Children who do not understand numbers should use the picture scale. Some children who are able to use the number scale might prefer to use the picture scale. Ask the child which scale he or she would prefer.

How do I use the OUCHER?

Picture scale: The following is an example of how to explain the picture scale to a younger child. The words can be changed when using the picture scale with an older child.

This is a poster called the OUCHER. It helps children tell others how much hurt they have. (For younger children, it might be useful to ask: Do you know what I mean by hurt? If the child is not sure, then an explanation should be provided.) Here's how this works. This picture shows not hurt (point to the bottom picture), this picture shows just a little bit of hurt (point to the 2nd picture), this picture shows a little more hurt (point to the 3rd picture), this picture shows even more hurt (point to the 4th picture), this picture shows a lot of hurt (point to the 5th picture), and this picture shows the biggest hurt you could ever have (point to the 6th picture). Can you point to the picture that shows how much hurt you are having right now?

Once a child selects a picture, their picture selection is changed to a number score from 0-10.

10 – Picture at the top of the scale
8 – Second picture from the top
6 – Third picture from the top
4 – Fourth picture from the top
2 – Fifth picture from the top
0 – Picture at the bottom of the scale

Number scale: The following is an example of how to explain the number scale.

This is a poster called the OUCHER. It helps children tell others how much hurt they have. Here's how it works. 0 means no hurt. Here (point to the lower third of the scale, about 1 to 3), this means you have little hurts; here (point to the middle third of the scale, about 3 to 6) it means you have middle hurts. If your hurt is about here (point to the upper third of the scale, about 6 to 9), it means you have big hurts. But if you point to 10, it means you have the biggest hurt you could ever have. Can you point to the number (or tell me which number) that is like the hurt you are having right now?

The pain score for the number scale is the exact number from 0 to 10 that the child gives you.

What does the score mean? How should it be used?

The person who has pain is the expert or the one who knows best how the pain feels. The OUCHER score gives parents, teachers, nurses, and doctors some idea of how much pain the child is feeling. OUCHER scores can be used as a means to see if certain actions used to relieve pain, such as rest, applying heat or cold, eating or drinking, and medicine make a difference in how much pain the child feels. OUCHER scores can be recorded over a period of hours or days and would be useful information to share with nurses and doctors.

Remember, OUCHER scores only communicate how much pain the child is feeling. Other observations, such as changes in activity, location of the pain, what it feels like, and how long it lasts, are important. If you, as a parent or teacher, are concerned about the child's pain, you should contact your health care provider.

© The Caucasian version of the OUCHER was developed and copyrighted by Judith E. Beyer, PhD, RN, (University of Missouri-Kansas City),1983. The African-American version was developed and copyrighted by Mary J. Denyes, PhD, RN, (Wayne State University), and Antonia M. Villarruel, PhD, RN, (University of Michigan) at Children's Hospital of Michigan, 1990. Cornelia P. Porter, PhD, RN, and Charlotta Marshall, RN, MSN, contributed to the development of the scale. The Hispanic version was developed and copyrighted by Antonia M. Villarruel, PhD, RN, and Mary J. Denyes, PhD, RN, 1990.

For information about the Oucher, write to: Dr. Judith E. Beyer, P.O. Box 411714, Kansas City, MO 64141 or go to the www.OUCHER.com website.

Figure 24-6 *The Oucher Pain Assessment Tool: For Use with Children 3–12 Years of Age. Caucasian, Hispanic, and African American versions are available. (The Caucasian version of the Oucher, developed and copyrighted by Judith E. Beyer, RN, PhD, 1983.)*

provide information regarding the effectiveness of the interventions. Physiologic and behavioral signs, and most important, the client's subjective pain ratings of the intensity, all help the health care team determine whether the interventions should be continued or changed. Pain assessments should be performed when the intervention should be providing the most relief. For example, the onset of intravenous morphine is rapid, peaking approximately 20 minutes after administration. If the client has not obtained relief by 20 minutes, the intravenous morphine was ineffective, and the plan of care would need to be changed.

Recording Pain Assessment Findings

Pain assessment is of little value unless the information is recorded in a manner easily understood by the health care team. A flow sheet provides one place to document most of the information used to make pain management decisions, including pain rating, vital signs, analgesic administered, and level of arousal. The client's report of pain must be accepted and recorded, with pain management decisions based on that report (Pasero & McCaffery, 2001).

Nursing Diagnoses

The two primary nursing diagnoses used to describe pain are *Acute Pain* and *Chronic Pain.* According to the

North American Nursing Diagnosis Association (NANDA, 2003), *Acute Pain* is defined as "an unpleasant sensory and emotional experience arising from actual or potential tissue damage or described in terms of such damage . . . [with] sudden or slow onset of any intensity from mild to severe, with an anticipated or predictable end and a duration of less than 6 months." *Chronic Pain* is defined the same as *Acute Pain*, with the last phrase replaced by "constant or recurring without an anticipated or predictable end and a duration of greater than 6 months."

Pain may be the etiology (cause) of other problems (e.g., *Impaired Physical Mobility*, related to arthritic hip pain). Whether the pain is addressed in the problem statement or the etiology is determined by the client's primary problem. Many diagnoses can be related to the client in pain depending on the effects of the pain:

- *Activity Intolerance*
- *Anxiety*
- *Constipation*
- *Deficient Knowledge (specify)*
- *Disturbed Body Image*
- *Disturbed Sleep Pattern*
- *Disturbed Thought Processes*
- *Fatigue*
- *Fear*
- *Hopelessness*
- *Impaired Social Interaction*
- *Ineffective Breathing Pattern*
- *Ineffective Individual Coping*
- *Ineffective Role Performance*
- *Ineffective Therapeutic Regimen Management*
- *Powerlessness*

Planning/Outcome Identification

When planning care, mutual goal setting with the client experiencing pain is of utmost importance. The nurse and client work together to develop realistic outcomes. Consider both nonpharmacologic and pharmacologic interventions.

Often, several approaches must be combined for adequate relief to be obtained. No matter which type of intervention is being utilized, general principles apply: individualization, prevention, and utilization of a multidisciplinary approach.

Individualize the Approach

A variety of pain relief measures can be tried in many combinations until the goal of pain relief is reached. This often means some trial-and-error of interventions until the right combination is found. It is important to include measures that the client believes will be effective. The cognitive component of pain perception can have a powerful influence on the effectiveness of interventions. This may mean including folk remedies or nonscientific relief measures. It is important to keep an open mind. This comes with the caution to avoid those remedies that may harm the client.

Use a Preventive Approach

Pain is much easier to control if it is treated before it gets severe. Interventions should be implemented when pain is mild or when it is anticipated. For example, medicate a client before a painful dressing change or treatment rather than waiting for the pain to occur.

Use a Multidisciplinary Approach

Pain relief is a complex phenomenon requiring input from various members of the health care team. The nurse's role is pivotal in managing a client's pain. The physician also plays a key role, diagnosing and treating the medical cause of the pain, which includes prescribing appropriate medications. In complex cases, other professionals, such as physical therapists, psychologists, social workers, or chaplains, may be needed. The multidisciplinary team approach is the most successful way to manage chronic pain and improve the quality of a client's life.

Implementation

Pharmacologic and nonpharmacologic interventions can both be effective in caring for clients in pain. Nonpharmacologic techniques may be the primary intervention in some cases of mild pain, with medication available as "backup." Cases of moderate to severe pain may use nonpharmacologic techniques as effective adjunctive, or complementary, treatment.

There are three categories of pain control interventions: pharmacological, noninvasive, and invasive. Each category is discussed separately, but these methods are often used in combination.

Pharmacological Interventions

Drug therapy is the mainstay of treatment for pain control. The American Pain Society (1999) and AHCPR (1992, 1994) have published guidelines that provide specific recommendations for the use of drug therapy in pain control. These guidelines were developed by panels of experts who analyzed current research available on pain control and represent concise information that can help nurses, physicians, and other health care workers to effectively administer medications for pain relief.

The World Health Organization (WHO) has made worldwide relief of cancer pain one of their primary goals (1990). In order to help meet this goal, it developed an analgesic ladder to help the clinician determine which analgesic to prescribe (Figure 24-7). Combining analgesics and the use of adjuvant medication provides effective pharmacologic intervention for clients with pain. **Adjuvant medications** are those drugs used to enhance the analgesic efficacy of opioids, to treat concurrent symptoms that exacerbate pain, and to provide independent analgesia for specific types of pain. The ladder recommends that the analgesic, plus or minus an adjuvant, is chosen based on the level of pain the client is experiencing. For mild pain, the ladder recommends a nonopioid. If the pain persists or if the client has moderate pain to begin with, WHO recommends a weak opioid, plus or minus the nonopioid, plus or minus an adjuvant. If pain persists, a strong opioid is used. The *nonopioid should be continued,* and an adjuvant medication should be considered (AHCPR, 1994). This ladder gives health care workers guidelines in determining if the drug regimen is appropriate for the client with cancer pain.

Figure 24-7 *WHO Analgesic Ladder gives guidelines for choosing analgesic therapy for cancer pain based on the level of pain the client is experiencing. (Courtesy of World Health Organization, 1990. Used with permission.)*

Nurses' Role in Administration of Analgesics

The nurse spends the most time with the client in pain and is the team member who most often assesses the effectiveness of pain control interventions. When analgesics are prescribed, the nurse often has choices of drug, route, and interval. For example, the postoperative client may have the following orders:

- Morphine 10–15 mg IM or IV q2–4h prn severe pain
- Vicodin i–ii tabs q3–4h prn moderate pain

When this client complains of pain, which analgesic should the nurse administer? Which route? Which dose? How frequently? The nurse has a large responsibility in making these decisions but also has autonomy in making these decisions. Each nurse may make a different decision, often based on the nurse's own biases.

McCaffery and Pasero (1999) identify the following as the responsibilities of the nurse in administering analgesics:

- Determine whether to give the analgesic, and if more than one is ordered, which one.
- Assess the client's response to the analgesic, including assessing the effectiveness in pain relief and occurrence of any side effects.
- Report to the physician when a change is needed, including making suggestions for changes based on the nurse's knowledge of the client and pharmacology.
- Teach the client and family regarding the use of analgesics.

Principles of Administering Analgesics "How an analgesic is used is probably more important than which one is used" (McCaffery & Pasero, 1999). Principles should be applied in the administration of analgesics, no matter which one is given.

Establishing and maintaining a therapeutic serum level is important. Peaks and valleys often occur when analgesics are administered in the traditional PRN (as needed) manner. When the dose is administered on an intermittent schedule, a larger dose is often required, causing the client to have a peak serum drug level in the sedation range. The client must wait for the return of pain before requesting the next dose of analgesic. Depending on the length of time it takes to obtain the medication and, once taken, to reestablish an adequate blood level, there could be a period of up to an hour or so without adequate pain control.

Preventive Approach Pain is much easier to control if treated when it is anticipated or at a mild intensity. Once pain becomes severe, the analgesics ordered may not be effective enough to relieve it. Many clinicians still teach their clients to wait to take medication until they are sure they really need it. This practice leads to uncontrolled pain. There are two ways the preventive approach may be implemented:

- ATC (around the clock). When pain is predictable, for example, the first few days following surgery or with chronic cancer pain, the medication is administered on a scheduled basis. This prevents the peaks and valleys of serum drug level that can lead to oversedation or toxicity and recurrence of pain, respectively. If the analgesics are ordered by the physician to be given PRN, it can still be a nursing measure to administer the drugs ATC, as long as they are given within the time constraints of the order.
- PRN (Latin for *pro re nata*, which means "as required"). Pain is not always predictable; therefore

PRN dosing may be required. For some clients this may be used in addition to scheduled dosing for "breakthrough" pain (pain that surpasses the level of **analgesia,** or pain relief without anesthesia, that the steady level of analgesics is providing). Examples of this include a cancer client on prolonged-release morphine who needs extra analgesics to participate in activities such as shopping or receiving visitors. Another example would be the orthopedic client who is receiving regularly scheduled analgesics for postoperative pain who needs additional pain relief for therapy sessions. In order to implement the preventive approach with PRN dosing, the medications should be given as soon as the pain appears, or when it is anticipated to begin.

Titrate to Effect Because of the unique nature of the pain experience, the analgesic regimen needs to be titrated until the desired effect is achieved. This involves adjusting the following:

- *Dosage.* Some clients may require more or less than the standard dose. Many factors may influence the pharmacokinetics in an individual client. The individual's response is assessed, and the dosage of the analgesic is regulated accordingly. In clients with chronic cancer pain, opioid analgesics are recommended to be increased until pain relief is obtained or unacceptable side effects occur. This may be done because of the lack of a **ceiling effect** (the dosage beyond which no further analgesia occurs) in pure opioids. The lack of a ceiling effect means there is no limit to the dose that can be given. For example, cancer clients have been known to receive more than 1 gram per hour intravenously. Because the dosage is gradually increased, the client develops a **tolerance** (requiring larger and larger doses of an analgesic to achieve the same level of pain relief) to the side effects of the opioid.
- *Interval.* Some clients metabolize the analgesics faster than others. For example, young adults tend to metabolize opioids faster; therefore, they may need more frequent doses. Older clients tend to metabolize them slower, so they require a longer interval between doses.
- *Route.* The appropriate route is chosen depending on how rapidly pain relief is required, the client's ability to take medications orally, the client's diagnosis, and assessment of the client's response to the current route. Intravenous administration provides the most rapid onset of pain relief. All other routes require a lag time for absorption of the analgesic into the circulation. In postoperative pain, IV is the preferred route for opioids when the oral route is not appropriate. If IV access is not available, sublingual, rectal, or transdermal routes should be considered (AHCPR, 1992).

With cancer pain, the oral route is preferred. If the client is unable to take oral medications, rectal and transdermal routes are preferred because they are less invasive than other routes (AHCPR, 1994). In addition, tolerance develops at a slower rate with the oral route compared to the more invasive routes.

- *Choice of drug.* If one drug is not providing relief or has unacceptable side effects, another analgesic may be tried.

The key to administering an analgesic is to monitor the client's response to it. This includes assessing the effectiveness of pain relief and the occurrence of side effects.

Classes of Analgesics Three classes of drugs are used for pain relief: (1) nonopioid analgesics; (2) opioid analgesics; and (3) analgesic adjuvants already discussed (WHO, 1986).

Nonopioids The medications in this category are useful for a variety of painful conditions, including surgery, trauma, and cancer (American Pain Society, 1999). The indications include mild to moderate pain, and they are used in conjunction with opioids. These drugs differ from opioids in several ways in that they:

- Are subject to the ceiling effect.
- Do not produce the effect of tolerance or physical dependence.
- Are antipyretic and should not be given in cases where they may mask an infection.

Ketorolac is the only nonsteroidal anti-inflammatory drug (NSAID) available in parenteral form and has proven useful in clients on NPO status who would benefit from a NSAID. Even when administered intramuscularly or intravenously, ketorolac produces significant gastric irritation and the potential for gastric bleeding. The most frequent use of ketorolac is orally or intramuscularly in adults, but some pediatric centers have used it intravenously under strict supervision for a limited course (less than 5 days) in children and adolescents with great success.

Action Action of these drugs is thought to inhibit prostaglandin formation. If prostaglandins are inhibited, the sensory neurons are less likely to receive the pain signal. Thus this class of analgesics works in the peripheral nervous system.

Opioids The opioid analgesics fall into three classes: pure opioid agonists, partial agonists, and **mixed agonist-antagonists** (a compound that blocks opioid effects on one receptor type while producing opioid effects on a second receptor type). Pure agonists produce a maximal response from cells when they bind to the cells' opioid receptor sites. Morphine (the gold standard against which all other opioids are measured), fentanyl, methadone (Dolophine), hydromorphone hydrochloride (Dilaudid), and codeine are pure agonists. Meperidine (Demerol), although classified as a pure agonist, is not recommended except in clients with a true allergy to all other narcotics, because of its neurotoxicity. Meperidine produces clinical analgesia for only 2.5 to 3.5 hours when given intramuscularly in adults.

Unlike the NSAIDs, pure agonist opioids are not subject to the ceiling effect. As the dosage is increased, pain relief increases.

PROFESSIONAL TIP

Ketorolac

Ketorolac should not be given to a client with any history of renal dysfunction, gastric irritation, bleeding problems, low platelet count, or allergy to aspirin or other NSAIDs.

PROFESSIONAL TIP

Types of Nonopioid Drugs

- *Salicylates.* These include aspirin and other salicylate salts. Common side effects of aspirin include gastric disturbances and bleeding caused by the antiplatelet effect. Some of the salicylate salts, such as choline magnesium trisalicylate (Trilisate) and salsalate (Salgesic) have fewer gastrointestinal and bleeding effects than aspirin.
- *Acetaminophen.* This nonsalicylate is similar to aspirin in its analgesic action but has no anti-inflammatory effect. Its mechanism of action for pain relief is not known.
- *NSAIDs.* The effectiveness of these drugs varies, with some being close to the effectiveness of aspirin and acetaminophen, whereas others are much stronger. Clients tend to vary in response, so once the maximum recommended dose has been tried with ineffective results, it would be worth trying another NSAID. The drugs in this group inhibit platelet aggregation and are contraindicated in clients with coagulation disorders or on anticoagulation therapy.

Action Opioids act in the CNS by binding to opiate receptor sites on afferent neurons. The pain signal is stopped at the spinal cord level and does not reach the cortex where pain is perceived.

Side Effects The only limiting factor in the use of pure agonist opioids is the degree of side effects, particularly respiratory depression and constipation. Other side effects include pruritus and nausea, but the degree to which they are present from each medication varies among individuals. Clients must be instructed regarding these normal responses to opioids and informed that it does not mean that they are allergic to them. A true allergy to opioids would be indicated by a rash or hives that starts after receiving the opioid, a local histamine release at the site of infusion, or anaphylaxis. Clients also need to know that the pruritus and nausea generally subside after 4 to 5 days of opioid therapy. In the meantime, an antihistamine such as diphenhydramine hydrochloride (Benadryl) or hydroxyzine hydrochloride (Atarax, Vistaril) may be used for pruritus, and an antiemetic such as metoclopromide hydrochloride (Clopra) or trimethobenzamide hydrochloride (Tigan) can be used to treat the nausea.

Almost all medications used to treat side effects have their own side effect of sedation. Thus there is the possibility of a cumulative effect of severe sedation. These medications must be used with caution and appropriate monitoring until the client's response is determined. Ondansetron hydrochloride (Zofran) is one antiemetic on the market with little, if any, sedative effect. It has recently received Food and Drug Administration (FDA) approval for use with postoperative nausea and has been effective in clients with refractory nausea and vomiting unresponsive to other antiemetics. The current cost per dose, close to $100 in many hospitals, limits its use to the extreme nausea associated with cancer chemotherapy or to clients with refractory nausea and vomiting.

LIFE CYCLE CONSIDERATIONS

Effects of Meperidine (Demerol)

- In the elderly, most of whom show decreased glomerular filtration rates, there is generally a higher peak and longer duration of action because it takes longer to excrete the opioid as well as its toxic metabolite, normeperidine.
- In pediatric clients receiving intravenous meperidine, analgesia may last for only 1.5 to 2 hours.

LIFE CYCLE CONSIDERATIONS

Opioid Analgesia in the Elderly

- Cheyne-Stokes respiratory patterns are not unusual during sleep in the elderly and should not be used as a reason to restrict appropriate opioid pain relief unless accompanied by unacceptable degrees of arterial desaturation (less than 85%).
- The elderly are more sensitive to sedation and respiratory depressant effects and experience a higher peak and longer duration of effect from opioid medications.
- Opioid dose titration must be based on analgesic effects and degree of side effects, such as sedation, urinary retention, constipation, respiratory depression, or exacerbation of Parkinson's disease (AHCPR, 1992).

Mixed agonist-antagonist opioids are believed to be subject to the ceiling effect for pain relief, as well as a ceiling effect for respiratory depression. Mixed agonist-antagonist opioids activate one opioid receptor type while simultaneously blocking another type. Butorphanol tartrate (Stadol), pentazocine hydrochloride (Talwin), and nalbuphine hydrochloride (Nubain) are the most frequently used in pain management.

Opioid antagonists include naloxone (Narcan) and naltrexone (Trexal), with the most commonly used being naloxone (Narcan). They work by blocking opioid stimulation of receptor sites. Naloxone effectively reverses opioid side effects of sedation, respiratory depression, and nausea *and it completely reverses any pain control.*

Alternative Delivery Systems Opioids are administered in more than just the traditional oral, subcutaneous, intramuscular, intravenous, and rectal routes.

Patient-Controlled Analgesia **Patient-controlled analgesia** (PCA) is most often delivered by a device that allows the client to control the delivery of intravenous, epidural, or subcutaneous pain medication in a safe, effective manner through a programmable pump (Figure 24-8). This system helps eliminate the time required for the nurse to draw up the medication and allows the client to feel some control over the pain. The pump has the safety feature of locking out once a maximum dose has been reached. This prevents the client from overdosing. Requirements for the use of PCA are the cognitive ability to understand how to use the pump and the physical ability to push the button. The PCA has been successfully used with many types of pain and in many settings, including pediatrics and home health.

Oral PCA is relatively new in hospitals and, according to Pasero (2000a), is becoming increasingly popu-

Figure 24-8 *Client on IV Patient-Controlled Analgesia (PCA)*

lar. Client teaching is the key for success. The client must understand how pain, pain medication, and pain relief are related and how to maintain a pain-relief diary. A Velcro®-sealed wrist pouch is applied to the client with one or two doses of the prescribed oral analgesic, even controlled substances, in the pouch. The client notifies the nurse when a dose is taken, so it can be replaced. If the client does not comply with the oral PCA policy, it is discontinued.

Epidural/Intrathecal Analgesia **Epidural analgesia** refers to administering the opioid via a catheter that terminates in the epidural space, the space outside the dura mater that protects the spinal cord. **Intrathecal analgesia** refers to administering the drug directly into the subarachnoid space. These may be administered as a one-time injection by the anesthesiologist or via a catheter that has been placed. Both of these routes are occasionally referred to as *intraspinal anesthesia.* Because the opioid is delivered close to the site of action, these routes require much lower doses of opioid (usually morphine [Duramorph] or fentanyl [Sublimaze] are used) for pain relief. The incidence of systemic side effects is also much lower with these routes. Duration is longer than

PROFESSIONAL TIP

Constipation and Opioids

Clients who are expected to require opioid analgesics for more than 1 or 2 days should be administered a stool softener as soon as they are taking fluids orally. While they are still NPO, a glycerin or bisacodyl (Dulcolax) suppository should be administered if the client has not had a bowel movement in 1 or 2 days.

systemic routes (e.g., the duration of one dose of intrathecal morphine can last 24 hours).

Transdermal Analgesia Another route of opioid administration is the transdermal patch. The only opioid drug currently available via this route is fentanyl (Duragesic). This medication is on an adhesive patch that attaches to the skin. It is available in 25, 50, 75, and 100 mcg/hour dosages. The fentanyl transdermal patch allows slow infusion of the drug through the skin. The fentanyl patch is indicated for continuous pain with high dosage requirements. The advantage of this route is that it is simple to apply and effective for 72 hours. The disadvantage is that dosage adjustments are difficult to make because of the slow infusion rate. In addition, side effects may not be reversed as rapidly as when opiates are administered via the oral route.

Local Anesthesia Local anesthetics are effective for pain management in a variety of settings. Topical anesthetics are available for teething, sore throats, denture pain, laceration repair, and intravenous catheter insertions. One topical anesthetic, EMLA cream, is a mixture of local anesthetics, combining prilocaine and lidocaine (Xylocaine). It produces complete anesthesia for at least 60 minutes when topically applied on intact skin. Another topical anesthetic, TAC, is available for anesthesia during closure of lacerations. It is a combination of tetracaine hydrochloride (Pontocaine) 0.5%, adrenaline (epinephrine) 1:2000, and cocaine 11.8% in a normal saline solution that can be applied directly to the open wound surface in place of local anesthetic infiltration with a needle. This allows pain-free cleansing of the laceration as well as suturing. Because both adrenaline (epinephrine) and cocaine cause vasoconstriction, TAC cannot be used in areas supplied by end-arteriolar blood supply such as digits, the ear, or the nose. It also is contraindicated on burned or abraded skin because this could lead to increased systemic absorption of cocaine and tetracaine, thus placing the client at risk for seizures.

Noninvasive Interventions

Noninvasive relief measures consist of cognitive-behavioral strategies and physical modalities that use cutaneous stimulation. These treatments can be used to supplement pharmacological therapy and other modalities to control pain. Clients and their families can also be instructed to utilize these treatments at home and in inpatient settings.

Cognitive-Behavioral Interventions The cognitive-behavioral interventions influence the cognitive and the motivational-affective components of pain perception. These methods can not only help influence the level of pain, but also help the client gain a sense of self-control.

Trusting Nurse–Client Relationship Establishing a therapeutic relationship is the foundation for effective nursing care. The clients most likely to be comfortable are those who trust their nurses to be there, to listen, and to act.

Relaxation Relaxation techniques (a variety of methods used to decrease anxiety and muscle tension) result in decreased heart rate and respiratory rate, and decreased muscle tension. The body's response to pain is almost "tricked" into reversing itself when relaxation exercises are implemented.

Relaxation exercises help reduce pain by decreasing anxiety and decreasing reflex muscular contraction. There are a wide variety of relaxation techniques, including focused breathing, progressive muscle relaxation, and meditation. Simple techniques should be used during episodes of brief pain (e.g., during procedures) or when pain is so severe that the client is unable to concentrate on complicated instructions.

To teach simple relaxation techniques, the nurse can instruct the client to (1) take a deep breath and hold it; (2) exhale slowly and concentrate on going limp; and (3) start yawning (McCaffery & Pasero, 1999). The yawning triggers a conditioned response in the client (i.e., the body associates yawning with relaxation and will relax when the client yawns). The technique can be enhanced if the nurse starts yawning. It is so contagious that even the client compromised by severe pain will usually start yawning with the nurse.

A more complex technique is **progressive muscle relaxation,** a strategy in which muscles are alternately tensed and relaxed. This type of technique is especially useful for clients who do not know what muscle relaxation feels like. By purposely contracting and releasing the muscle groups, the client is able to compare the difference and identify feelings of relaxation. Meditative relaxation techniques are also available, including audiotapes sold in most bookstores.

Relaxation is a learned response. The more frequently the client practices these techniques, the more skilled the body will be in learning to relax. Ideally, the best time to teach the client these methods is when pain is controlled or before the pain occurs (e.g., in the preoperative period).

Reframing Reframing is a technique that teaches clients to monitor their negative thoughts and replace them with more positive ones. For example, teach a client to replace an expression such as, "I can't stand this pain, it's never going away," with one such as, "I've had similar pain before, and it's gotten better."

Distraction Distraction focuses one's attention on something other than the pain, therefore placing pain on the periphery of awareness (McCaffery & Pasero,

---

LIFE CYCLE CONSIDERATIONS

Injections and Children
Children lack the cognitive ability to weigh the pain of injection against the pain relief from the medication, so oral and rectal routes are preferred over injections.

PROFESSIONAL TIP

Using Distraction
Distraction should never be the *only* pain management intervention used, but it can be very helpful while waiting for other techniques to take effect.

1999). Successful use of distraction does not eliminate the pain; it makes it less troublesome. The main disadvantage of distraction is that as soon as the distractive stimuli stop, the pain returns in full force. For this reason, the most appropriate use of distraction techniques is for the relief of brief, episodic pain. It can be effective for procedural pain or the period between administration of an analgesic and the onset of the drug. Examples of distraction include the following:

- Active listening to recorded music (have the client tap fingers in rhythm to the beat)
- Reciting a poem or rhyme (children do this well)
- Describe a plot of a novel or movie
- Describe a series of pictures

Guided Imagery Guided imagery uses one's imagination to provide a pleasant substitute for the pain. It incorporates features of both relaxation and distraction. The client imagines a pleasant experience, such as going to the beach or the mountains. The experience should use all five senses to fully involve the client in the image.

The images chosen need to be ones that are pleasant for the client. Describing an ocean cruise would not be appropriate for a person who becomes seasick.

Humor The old saying, "Laughter is the best medicine," carries some truth to it. Although there is nothing very funny about pain, laughing has been shown to provide pain relief. The act of laughing can cause distraction from the pain, induce relaxation by taking deep breaths and releasing tension, release endorphins, and provide a pleasant substitute for pain. Norman Cousins (1991) relates obtaining 2 hours of pain relief from watching episodes of the Candid Camera television show and Marx Brothers films. This technique can be implemented by encouraging the client to watch humorous movies, read funny books, or listen to comedy routines. Because different people see humor in different types of situations, be sensitive to what the client views as funny.

Biofeedback Biofeedback is a method that may help the client in pain to relax and relieve tension. Individuals learn to influence their physiological responses to stimuli and thus alter their pain experience.

Cutaneous Stimulation The technique of cutaneous stimulation involves stimulating the skin to control pain. It is theorized that this technique provides relief by stimulating nerve fibers that send signals to the dorsal horn of the spinal cord to "close the gate." The main advantage of these therapies is that many techniques are easy for the nurse to implement and easy to teach the client and family to perform. They are not usually meant to replace analgesic therapy, but to complement it.

Hot and Cold Application In addition to stimulating nerves that can block pain transmission, superficial heat application increases circulation to the area, which promotes oxygenation and nutrient delivery to the injured tissues. It also decreases joint and muscle stiffness. Heat is contraindicated in cases of acute injury because it can increase the initial response of edema. It is also contraindicated in rheumatoid arthritis flare-ups and over topical applications of mentholated ointments. Heat treatments should be limited to 20- to 30-minute intervals because maximum vasodilatation occurs in that time.

CLIENT TEACHING

Hot or Cold Applications
Teach the client or family that hot or cold applications:

- Must have at least one layer of towel between the heating or cooling device and the skin.
- Should be placed on the skin only for short periods.
- Should not be applied to tissue that has been exposed to radiation therapy (AHCPR, 1994).

Cryotherapy (cold applications) induces local vasoconstriction and numbness, therefore altering the pain sensations. It is contraindicated in any condition where vasoconstriction might increase symptoms (e.g., peripheral vascular disease). For best results, cold therapy should be limited to 20- to 30-minute intervals. Either heat or cold can be used as cutaneous stimulation unless one is specifically contraindicated. Cold often provides faster relief (McCaffery & Pasero, 1999). If the client has used heat or cold before, incorporate the modality that the client believes will be the most effective. Combining the two might provide better relief. An example of this would be to apply a hot pack for 4 minutes, followed by an ice pack for 2 minutes, repeated four times. In a hospital setting, a physician order is required for this therapy.

Acupressure and Massage One of the first responses to pain is to rub the painful part. People seem to instinctively understand the pain-relieving aspects of this intervention. In addition to blocking the pain transmission through nerve stimulation, massage can also promote relaxation. Acupressure is a type of massage that consists of continuous pressure on or the rubbing of acupuncture points. It is based on the same principles as acupuncture, but needles are not used. Massage also provides a form of nonverbal communication that can be therapeutic on its own.

Mentholated Rubs Ointments or lotions containing menthol are thought to provide relief by providing a counterirritation to the skin. The menthol gives the client the perception that the temperature of the skin has changed (becoming either warmer or cooler). This alters the sensation of pain or provides a distraction from the pain. Client response varies to mentholated rubs; some gain effective relief, but others have poor results. Their use is contraindicated on broken skin, on mucous membranes, or if pain increases.

Transcutaneous Electrical Nerve Stimulation Transcutaneous electrical nerve stimulation (TENS) is the process of applying a low-voltage electrical current to the skin through cutaneous electrodes. This modulates pain transmission, as do other cutaneous stimulation methods, but also distracts the client from pain. Research supports the effectiveness of using TENS for the relief of postoperative pain (AHCPR, 1992). It has also been used successfully in many pain syndromes (e.g., chronic low-back pain, menstrual cramps, temporomandibular joint [TMJ] syndrome, phantom limb pain, and others). It is administered by specially trained health professionals, usually a physical therapist. Other modalities of pain management should *not* be abandoned while a trial of TENS occurs.

 Safety: TENS Contraindications
- No electrodes should be placed in the area over or surrounding demand cardiac pacemakers.
- No electrodes can be placed over the uterus of a pregnant woman.

Exercise Exercise is an important treatment for chronic pain because it helps mobilize joints, strengthens weak muscles, and helps restore balance and coordination. Do not use passive range of motion if it increases discomfort or pain. Immobilization is frequently used to stabilize fractures or for clients with episodes of acute pain. Prolonged immobilization can lead to muscle atrophy and cardiovascular deconditioning.

Psychotherapy Psychotherapy may be beneficial to some clients, particularly those:

- Who are clinically depressed
- Who have a history of psychiatric problems
- Whose pain is difficult to control

Some psychotherapists use **hypnosis** (altered state of consciousness when a person is more receptive to suggestion) to help clients alter pain perception. Hypnosis can be effective but should be used only by specially trained professionals.

Positioning The final noninvasive technique is proper positioning and body alignment. Moving the client with the least possible stress on joints and skin will minimize exposure to painful stimuli. This includes supporting joints appropriately and maintaining wrinkle-free sheets.

Invasive Interventions

Invasive interventions are meant to complement behavioral, physical, and pharmacological therapies in those clients who do not obtain relief from those measures alone (AHCPR, 1994). Invasive measures are indicated primarily for chronic cancer pain and in some cases of chronic benign pain. These procedures are usually tried only when noninvasive measures have been attempted first with poor results.

Nerve Block Neural blockade is the process of injecting a local anesthetic or neurolytic agent into the nerve. An anesthetic agent may be injected to act as a diagnostic tool in order to identify the nerves involved in a pain syndrome. A neurolytic agent is a chemical agent that causes destruction of the nerve and, therefore, creates an interruption in the pain signal.

Neurosurgery Neurosurgical measures for pain control include neurostimulation procedures and destructive or ablative procedures. Neurostimulation procedures involve the implantation of electrical stimulation devices that send impulses to different parts of the nervous system. Some of these devices stimulate areas of the brain; others stimulate the spinal cord. Relief is thought to be provided by blocking the afferent fiber input at the spinal cord level or by stimulating release of endorphins using the body's ability to modulate pain.

Destructive or ablative procedures are used to destroy part of the nervous system that conducts pain. By interrupting the pain signal, it is prevented from reaching the cortex where realization of pain occurs. These procedures are reserved for clients with terminal illness.

Radiation Therapy Radiation can be used as a palliative measure for pain relief in clients with cancer. It can relieve both metastatic pain and pain caused by tumors at the primary cancer site. It enhances other pain management strategies, such as analgesic therapy, because it is aimed specifically at the cause of the client's pain. When administered for pain relief, the smallest dose of radiation is utilized to minimize side effects.

Acupuncture **Acupuncture** is the insertion of small needles into the skin at specific (hoku) sites. The sites are chosen after the practitioner takes a detailed history and uses traditional Asian diagnostic techniques. The needles used for acupuncture have rounded ends that enter the skin without cutting the tissue. The practitioner may twirl or vibrate the needles manually or electrically. It is important that the nurse keep an open mind when the client chooses this therapy, or the client may be reluctant to discuss its use.

Evaluation

Evaluating pain management interventions is ongoing, focusing primarily on the client's subjective reports. Objective data to evaluate pain management include the following:

- Continuing use of pain assessment tools
- Client's facial expression and posture
- Presence (or absence) of restlessness
- Vital sign monitoring

Summary

- *Pain* may be defined as "an unpleasant sensory and emotional experience associated with actual or potential tissue damage," and "whatever the client says it is, existing whenever the client says it does."
- The gate control theory proposes that several processes (sensory, motivational-affective, and cognitive) combine to determine how a person perceives pain.
- Assessment of pain helps establish a baseline of data and helps evaluate the effectiveness of interventions.
- Factors influencing pain perception include age, previous experience with pain, and cultural norms.
- The subjective data to gather include location of pain, onset and duration, quality, intensity (on a scale of 0 to 10), aggravating and relieving factors, and how pain affects the activities of daily living.

CRITICAL THINKING

Noninvasive Intervention
How would you decide which noninvasive intervention to use with a client?

SAMPLE NURSING CARE PLAN

THE CLIENT WITH CHRONIC PAIN

Sally Jeffries, a 48-year-old woman, injured her back 3 years ago while lifting some boxes of paper at work. Since that time, she has had four epidural steroidal injections for the pain associated with two ruptured discs. Her pain has been intermittent, with some alleviation from the epidural injections. Her last epidural was 3 months ago. She arrives at the clinic stating, "I just don't know how I can go on like this. The pain has been tolerable until last night. I'm hurting so bad!" She is tearful and pacing, saying, "It hurts too much when I sit down." Verbalizes pain is "9" on a 1 to 10 pain intensity scale. Blood pressure is 148/90. Pulse is strong and regular at 92. She has guarded movements.

Nursing Diagnosis 1   *Chronic Pain,* related to muscle spasm and ruptured discs as evidenced by back injury 3 years ago and client statement "I just don't know how I can go on like this. The pain has been tolerable until last night. I'm hurting so bad!"

Nursing Outcomes Classification (NOC)
Pain Level
Well-Being

Nursing Interventions Classification (NIC)
Pain Management

PLANNING/GOALS	NURSING INTERVENTIONS	RATIONALE
Ms. Jeffries will verbalize a decrease in pain.	Assess Ms. Jeffries's level of pain, determining the intensity at its best and worst.	Determines a baseline for future assessment.
	Listen to Ms. Jeffries while she discusses the pain; acknowledge the presence of pain.	Decreases anxiety by communicating acceptance and validating her perceptions.
	Discuss reasons why pain may be increased or decreased.	Helps Ms. Jeffries understand her pain.
Ms. Jeffries will practice selected noninvasive pain relief measures.	Teach relaxation techniques such as deep breathing, progressive muscle relaxation, and imagery.	Reduces skeletal muscle tension and anxiety, which potentiates the perception of pain.
	Teach Ms. Jeffries about the use of medication for pain relief. Provide accurate information to reduce fear of addiction.	Lack of knowledge and fear may prohibit Ms. Jeffries from taking analgesic medications as prescribed.
	Encourage Ms. Jeffries to rest during the day.	Fatigue increases the perception of pain.

EVALUATION   After practicing relaxation techniques, Ms. Jeffries rates her pain as a 2 to 3 on the pain intensity scale. Ms. Jeffries demonstrates the use of deep breathing and progressive muscle relaxation.

Nursing Diagnosis 2   *Anxiety* related to chronic pain as evidenced by pacing and tears

Nursing Outcomes Classification (NOC)
Coping
Acceptance: Health Status

Nursing Interventions Classification (NIC)
Coping Enhancement
Progressive Muscle Relaxation

continues

SAMPLE NURSING CARE PLAN

PLANNING/GOALS	NURSING INTERVENTIONS	RATIONALE
Ms. Jeffries will verbalize an increase in psychological and physiological comfort level.	Assess Ms. Jeffries's level of anxiety.	Determines baseline for future assessment.
	Encourage Ms. Jeffries to verbalize angry feeling.	Provides an outlet for her anger.
Ms. Jeffries will demonstrate ability to cope with anxiety as evidenced by normal vital signs and a verbalized reduction in pain intensity.	Speak slowly and calmly.	Avoids escalating Ms. Jeffries's anxiety level and increases the likelihood of her comprehension.

EVALUATION   After practicing relaxation techniques, Ms. Jeffries rates her pain as a 2 to 3 on the pain intensity scale. She voices concern that the pain will soon come back. After a relaxation session, her vital signs returned to normal. Ms. Jeffries denies feeling angry.

- The three general principles to follow with pain relief measures are (1) individualize the approach; (2) use a preventive approach; and (3) use a multidisciplinary approach.
- The nurse carries a great deal of autonomy in administering analgesics, which leads to specific responsibilities for which the nurse is accountable.
- Pharmacologic agents can be therapeutic for clients experiencing pain; however, the medications should not be the only interventions used.
- Noninvasive treatments for pain relief are measures that can supplement pharmacological and invasive treatments for pain relief.
- Invasive techniques are interventions used when the noninvasive and pharmacological measures do not provide adequate relief. Methods include nerve blocks, neurosurgery, radiation therapy, and acupuncture.

Review Questions

1. According to McCaffery and Pasero, pain may be defined as:
   a. discomfort resulting from identifiable physiologic or iatrogenic sources.
   b. a syndrome of behavioral and physical manifestations that can be objectively identified by the nurse.
   c. whatever the patient says it is, existing whenever and wherever the patient says it does.
   d. a sensory response to noxious stimuli.

2. Which of the following is a useful tool for assessing the intensity of pain that is easy to use?
   a. the gate control scale
   b. acute pain monitor
   c. numeric pain scale
   d. pressure pain monitor

3. Mr. Levy, 45, has experienced chronic low-back pain since a fall 8 years ago. He describes his pain as "a gnawing, constant dull pain" that makes him feel tired. The nurse caring for him recognizes that one of the differences between acute and chronic pain characteristics is:
   a. acute pain is more severe.
   b. chronic pain is often described as dull and is difficult to localize.
   c. chronic back pain is often not real.
   d. acute pain is more diffuse and difficult to describe.

4. Nancy Johnson, 84 years old, is recuperating from a total hip replacement. Morphine, 8 mg IV q4h PRN, is prescribed for Ms. Johnson. Her respiratory rate is 18, her pulse rate is 96 beats per minute, and her blood pressure is elevated slightly above her normal level. She is complaining of severe pain, 8 on a scale of 0 to 10. The most appropriate initial nursing intervention is:
   a. question the physician regarding the dosage amount for a client this age.
   b. turn her and then reevaluate her need for opioid analgesia.
   c. administer the medication as ordered.
   d. advise Ms. Johnson to cough and breathe deeply since you are unable to give her anything for pain until her respiratory rate is 20.

5. Ms. Redgrave, 55 years old, is hospitalized with an exacerbation of rheumatoid arthritis. She has a favorite television show she watches every afternoon. She reports feeling comfortable during this show and seldom requests pain medication when she is watching it. The nurse's assessment of this phenomenon is that:

a. the assessment of pain that prompted hospitalization is inaccurate.

b. Ms. Redgrave is bored and the boredom usually makes her pain seem worse.

c. inactivity is the best approach to Ms. Redgrave's pain.

d. distraction is an effective modifier of the pain experience for Ms. Redgrave.

References/Suggested Readings

Acello, B. (2000a). Meeting JCAHO standards for pain control. *Nursing2000, 30*(3), 52–54.

Acello, B. (2000b). Facing fears about opioid addiction. *Nursing2000, 30*(5), 72.

Adler, P., Good, M., Roberts, B., & Snyder, S. (2000). The effects of tai chi on older adults with chronic arthritis pain. *Journal of Nursing Scholarship, 32*(4), 377.

Agency for Health Care Policy and Research. (1992). *Clinical practice guideline: Acute pain management: Operative or medical procedures and trauma.* (AHCPR Publication No. 92-0032). Rockville, MD: U.S. Department of Health and Human Services.

Agency for Health Care Policy and Research. (1994). *Clinical practice guideline: Management of cancer pain.* (AHCPR Publication No. 94-0592). Rockville, MD: U.S. Department of Health and Human Services.

American Pain Society. (1995). *Pain: The fifth vital sign.* [Online]. Available: www.ampainsoc.org/advocacy/fifth.htm

American Pain Society. (1999). *Principles of analgesic use in the treatment of acute pain and cancer pain* (4th ed.). Glenview, IL: Author.

Beecher, H. K. (1956). Relationship of significance of wound to pain experienced. *JAMA, 161,* 1609–1613.

Brand, P., & Yancey, P. (1993). *Pain: The gift nobody wants.* New York: HarperCollins.

Brown, J., Horn, J., Calbert, J., & Nolan-Goslin, K. (1999). A question of pain. *Nursing99, 29*(10), 48–51.

Chapman, G. F. (1999). Documenting a pain assessment. *Nursing99, 29*(11), 25.

Choiniére, M. (2001). Burn Pain: A unique challenge. *Pain: Clinical Updates, 9*(1). [Online]. Available: http://iasp-pain.org/PCU01-1.html

Collins, P. M., Auclair, M., Butler, E., Hush, M., Bernstein, B. J., Aguirre, F., & Huston, M. (2000). Educating staff about pain management. *AJN, 100*(1), 59.

Compton, P. (1999). Managing a drug abuser's pain. *Nursing99, 29*(5), 26–28.

Controlling Pain. (2001). Taming pain with TENS. *Nursing2001, 31*(11), 84.

Cousins, N. (1991). *Anatomy of an illness as perceived by the patient.* Toronto: Bantam.

D'Arcy, Y. (2002). How to treat arthritis pain. *Nursing2002, 32*(7), 30–31.

Derby, S. A. (1999). Opioid conversion guidelines for managing adult cancer pain. *AJN, 99*(10), 62–65.

Dillard, J., & Hirschman, L. (2002). *The chronic pain solution: The comprehensive, step-by-step guide to choosing the best alternative and conventional medicine.* Philadelphia: Bantam Doubleday Dell.

Dochterman, J. M., & Bulechek, G. (2004). *Nursing Interventions Classification (NIC)* (4th ed.). St. Louis, MO: Mosby.

Faries, J. (1998a). Easing your patient's postoperative pain. *Nursing98, 28*(6), 58–60.

Faries, J. (1998b). Making a smooth switch from IV analgesia. *Nursing98, 28*(7), 26.

Feinberg, S. D. (2000). Complex regional pain syndrome. *AJN, 100*(12), 23–24.

Flor, H. Birbaumer, N., & Sherman, R. (2000). Phantom limb pain. *Pain: Clinical Updates, 8*(3). [Online]. Available: http://iasp-pain.org/PCU00-3.html

Haddad, A. (2000). Ethics in action: Treating pain in substance abusers. *RN, 63*(1), 21–24.

Hockenberry-Eaton, M., Wilson, D., & Winkelstein, M. L. (2003). *Wong's nursing care of infants and children* (7th ed.). New York: Elsevier Science.

Joint Commission on Accreditation of Healthcare Organizations (JCAHO). (1999). *Joint Commission focuses on pain management* [Online]. Available: www.jcaho.org/news/nb207.html

Joint Commission on Accreditation of Healthcare Organizations (JCAHO). (2000a). *Comprehensive accreditation manual for hospitals (CAMH) revised pain management standards* [Online]. Available: www.jcaho.org/standard/pm_hap.html

Joint Commission on Accreditation of Healthcare Organizations (JCAHO). (2000b). *Pain assessment and management standards* [Online]. Available: www.jcaho.org/standard/pm_coll.html

Juarez, G. (1995). When culture clashes with pain control. *Nursing95, 25*(5), 90.

Kedziera, P. (1998). The two faces of pain. *RN, 61*(2), 45-46.

Loeb, J. L. (1999). Pain management in long-term care. *AJN, 99*(2), 48–52.

Mattson, J. E. (2000). The language of pain. *Reflections on Nursing LEADERSHIP, 26*(4), 10–14.

Mayer, D., Torma, L., Byoch, I., & Norris, K. (2001). Speaking the language of pain. *AJN, 101*(2). 44–49.

McCaffery, M. (1979). *Nursing management of the patient with pain* (2nd ed.). Philadelphia: Lippincott Williams & Wilkins.

McCaffery, M. (1999a). Pain control. *AJN, 99*(8), 18.

McCaffery, M. (1999b). Understanding your patient's pain tolerance. *Nursing99, 29*(12), 17.

McCaffery, M. (2001). Using the 0-to-1 pain rating scale. *AJN, 101*(10), 81–82.

McCaffery, M. (2002). Choosing a faces pain scale. *Nursing2002, 32*(5), 68.

McCaffery, M. (2003). Switching from IV to PO: Maintaining pain relief in the transition. *AJN, 103*(5), 62–63.

McCaffery, M. & Ferrell, B. R. (1999). Opioids and pain management. *Nursing99, 29*(3), 48–52.

McCaffery, M., & Pasero, C. (1999). *Pain: Clinical manual* (2nd ed.). St. Louis, MO: Mosby.

McCaffery, M., & Robinson, E. (2002). Your patient is in pain: Here's how you respond. *Nursing2002, 32*(10), 36–45.

McDevitt, M. J. (1995). A(TENS)tion! *Nursing95, 25*(12), 46–47.

Melzack, R., & Wall, P. D. (1965). Pain mechanisms: A new theory. *Science, 150,* 971–979.

Merskey, J., & Bogduk, N. (Eds.). (1994). *Classification of chronic pain* (2nd ed., pp. 209–214). Task Force on Taxonomy. Seattle, WA: IASP.

Moorhead, S., Johnson, M., & Maas, M. (2004). *Nursing Outcomes Classification (NOC)* (3rd ed.). St. Louis, MO: Mosby.

Morris, D. B. (2001). Ethnicity and pain. *Pain: Clinical Updates.* [Online]. Available: http://iasp-pain.org/PCU01-4.html

Morrison, C. (2000). Fear of addiction: Balancing the facts and concerns about opioid use. *AJN, 100*(7), 81.

Nichols, R. (2003). Pain management in patients with addictive disease, *AJN, 103*(3), 87–90.

North American Nursing Diagnosis Association. (2003). *Nursing diagnoses: Definitions & classification, 2003–2004.* Philadelphia: Author.

Pace, J. (2002). Understanding nociceptive pain. *Nursing2002, 32*(3), 74–75.

Panke, J. (2002). Difficulties in managing pain at the end of life. *AJN, 102*(7), 26.

Pasero, C. (1999). Using superficial cooling for pain relief. *AJN, 99*(3), 48–52.

Pasero, C. (2000a). Oral patient-controlled analgesia. *AJN, 100*(3), 24.

Pasero, C. (2000b). Continuous local anesthetics. *AJN, 100*(8), 22–23.

Pasero, C., & McCaffery, M. (2000a). Reversing respiratory depression with naloxone. *AJN, 100*(2), 26.

Pasero, C., & McCaffery, M. (2000b). When patients can't report pain. *AJN, 100*(9), 22–23.

Pasero, C., & McCaffery, M. (2001). The patient's report of pain. *AJN, 101*(12), 73–74.

Pasero, C., & Montgomery, R. (2002). Intravenous fentanyl. *AJN, 102*(4), 73–76.

Perkins, E. (2002). Less morphine, or more? *RN, 65*(11), 51–54.

Portenoy, R. K., Payne, R. et al. (1999). Oral transmucosal fentanyl citrate (OTFC) for the treatment of breakthrough pain in cancer patients: A controlled dose titration study. *Pain, 79*, 303.

Poulain, P., Langlade, A., & Goldberg, J. (1997). Cancer pain management in the home. *Pain Clinical Updates, 5*(1). [Online]. Available: www.iasp-pain.org/PCU97a.html.

Reiff, P., & Niziolek, M. (2001). Troubleshooting TIPS for PCA. *RN, 64*(4), 33–37.

Scholz, M. (2000). Managing constipation that's opioid-induced. *RN, 63*(6), 103.

Slaughter, A., & Pasero, C. (2002). Unacceptable pain levels. *AJN, 102*(5), 75–76.

Smith-Stoner, M. (2003). How Buddhism influences pain control choices. *Nursing2003, 33*(4), 17.

Spratto, G., & Woods, A. (2004). *2004 PDR® Nurse's Drug Handbook™.* Clifton Park, NY: Thomson Delmar Learning.

Strevy, S. (1998). Myths and facts about pain. *RN, 61*(2), 42–45.

The National Pain Foundation (NPF). (2002). *The need for the National Pain Foundation.* [Online]. Available: www.painconnection.com/AboutUs/default.asp

Thomas, M., & Lundeberg, T. (1996). Does acupuncture work? *Pain Clinical Updates, 4*(3). [Online]. Available: www.iasp-pain.org/PCU96c.html.

Travell, J. G., & Simons, D. G. (1983, 1999). *Travell & Simon's myofascial pain and dysfunction: The trigger point manual* (2nd ed.), (Vols. 1 & 2). Baltimore: Lippincott Williams & Wilkins.

Twycross, R. et al. (1996). A survey of pain in patients with advanced cancer. *Journal of Pain Symptom Management, 12*(5), 273–282.

Vasudevan, S. V. (1993). *Pain: A four letter word you can live with.* Milwaukee, WI: Montgomery Media.

Victor, K. (2001). Properly assessing pain in the elderly. *RN, 64*(5), 45–49.

Wentz, J. (2003). Understanding neuropathic pain. *Nursing2003, 33*(1), 22.

Wong, D. (2003). Topical local anesthetics. *AJN, 103*(6), 42–45.

World Health Organization. (1986). *Cancer pain relief.* Geneva, Switzerland: Author.

World Health Organization. (1990). Cancer pain relief and palliative care. *Report of a WHO expert committee [World Health Organization Technical Report Series, 804].* Geneva, Switzerland: Author.

Young, D., Mentes, J. C., & Titler, M. G. (1999). Acute pain management protocol. *Journal of Gerontological Nursing, 26*(5), 10.

Resources

Agency for Healthcare Research and Quality (AHRQ), Office of Health Care Information, Executive Office Center, Suite 501, 2101 East Jefferson St., Rockville, MD 20852, www.ahcpr.gov

American Chronic Pain Association, P.O. Box 850, Rocklin, CA 95677-0850, 916-632-0922, www.theacpa.org

American Pain Society (APS), 4700 W. Lake Avenue, Glenview, IL 60025, 847-375-4715, www.ampainsoc.org

American Society of Pain Management Nurses, 7794 Grow Drive, Pensacola, FL 32514, 888-342-7766, www.aspmn.org

International Association for the Study of Pain (IASP), 909 Forty-third Street NE, Suite 306, Seattle, WA 98105-6020, 206-547-6409, www.iasp-pain.org

Joint Commission on Accreditation of Healthcare Organizations (JCAHO), One Renaissance Boulevard, Oakbrook Terrace, IL 60181-4294, 630-792-5000, www.jcaho.org

National Chronic Pain Outreach Association, P.O. Box 274, Millboro, VA 24460-0274, 540-862-9437, www.medhelp.org

National Committee on Treatment of Intractable Pain, 1920 N Street NW, Suite 300, Washington, DC 20036, 202-452-4886

National Guidelines Clearinghouse, www.guideline.gov

- Clinical Practice Guideline for managing acute pain. Available in three formats: (1) The clinical practice guideline (Publication No. 92-0032); (2) Quick reference guides (Adults—No. 92-0019 and Pediatric—No. 92-0020); and (3) Pain Control after Surgery: A Patient's Guide (No. 92-0021)

- Clinical Practice Guideline for managing cancer pain. Available in three formats: (1) The clinical practice guideline (Publication No. 94-0592); (2) Quick reference guides (Adults—No. 94-0593 and Pediatric—No. 92-0594); and (3) Patient's Guide (No. 94-0595)

National Headache Foundation, 428 W. St. James Place, 2nd Floor, Chicago, IL 60614-2750, 888-843-5552, www.headaches.org

National Hospice and Palliative Care Organization, 1700 Diagonal Road, Suite 300, Alexandria, VA 22304, 703-837-1500, www.nhpco.org

Nursing Research and Education/City of Hope Pain Resource Center, 1500 East Duarte Road, Duarte, CA 91010, 626-359-8111 ext. 3829, http://mayday.coh.org

The National Pain Foundation, P.O. Box 102605, Denver, CO 80250-2605, www.painconnection.org

DIAGNOSTIC TESTS

CHAPTER

25

MAKING THE CONNECTION

Refer to the following chapters to increase your understanding of diagnostic tests:

Basic Nursing
- **Complementary/Alternative Therapies**
- **Assessment**

Basic Procedures
- **Urine Collection: Closed Drainage System**
- **Urine Collection: Clean Catch Female/Male**

Intermediate Procedures
- **Performing Urinary Catheterization: Female/Male**
- **Performing a Skin Puncture**

Advanced Procedures
- **Performing Venipuncture (Blood Drawing)**

LEARNING OBJECTIVES

Upon completion of this chapter, you should be able to:
- **Define key terms.**
- **Discuss the care of the client before, during, and after diagnostic testing.**
- **Describe the methods of specimen collection.**
- **Describe common noninvasive and invasive diagnostic procedures.**
- **Demonstrate the nursing responsibilities for common diagnostic procedures.**

KEY TERMS

agglutination	ketone
agglutinin	lipoprotein
agglutinogen	lumbar puncture
analyte	magnetic resonance
aneurysm	imaging
angiography	necrosis
antibody	noninvasive
antigen	occult blood
arteriography	oliguria
ascites	Papanicolaou test
aspiration	paracentesis
bacteremia	phlebotomist
barium	pneumothorax
biopsy	port-a-cath
central line	procedural sedation
computed tomography	radiography
contrast medium	sensitivity
culture	stable
cytology	stress test
electrocardiogram	thoracentesis
electroencephalogram	transducer
electrolyte	trocar
endoscopy	type and crossmatch
enzyme	ultrasound
fluoroscopy	urobilinogen
hematuria	venipuncture
invasive	void

INTRODUCTION

Information from a thorough history and physical examination determines the need for diagnostic testing. Results of diagnostic procedures are used to formulate a medical diagnosis and plan a course of treatment. The challenge of cost-effective health care encourages practitioners to rely on basic assessment and to be selective about expensive diagnostic tests. The emphasis on cost containment has changed the nurse's role from doing for the client to teaching clients to do for themselves. The nurse teaches the client, family, and significant others about the diagnostic testing, how to prepare for the specific test(s), and the care required after the test. Although the primary focus is on teaching, the nurse may assist in performing various diagnostic tests. To deliver appropriate care to the client, nurses must know the implications of diagnostic tests and must know anatomy and physiology to understand the nature of diagnostic tests. Nurses can then relate diagnostic tests to specific disease processes and understand the test results.

This chapter discusses common diagnostic tests. The terms *test* and *procedure* are used interchangeably. The term *practitioner* is used to refer to either the physician or an advanced-practice registered nurse. Most state boards of nursing allow advanced-practice registered nurses to order and perform certain diagnostic tests.

DIAGNOSTIC TESTING

Diagnostic tests are either noninvasive or invasive. **Noninvasive** means that the body is not entered with any type of instrument; the skin and other body tissues, organs, and cavities remain intact. **Invasive** means that the body's tissues, organs, or cavities are accessed through some type of instrument.

Client Care

Diagnostic testing is a critical element of assessment. In collaboration with the client, assessment data are used to formulate nursing diagnoses, outcome measures, and a plan of care. Evaluation of the client's expected outcomes requires the incorporation of diagnostic findings.

Safety: Diagnostic Testing
To protect your health and safety, as well as that of other health care providers and the client, use Standard Precautions whenever performing invasive or noninvasive procedures.

Preparing the Client for Diagnostic Testing

The nurse plays a key role in scheduling and preparing the client for diagnostic testing. Tests not scheduled correctly inconvenience the client and delay interventions, which may place the client's health at risk. The institution is also at risk to lose money. Table 25-1 outlines a sample protocol of nursing care to prepare a client for diagnostic testing.

Ensure that the client is wearing an identification band and understands those things to be done. Also see that needed consent forms have been signed (Figure 25-1).

Nursing measures to ensure client safety are establish baseline vital signs, identify known allergies, and assess teaching effectiveness. In ambulatory and outpatient centers, there might be only one opportunity to assess and record vital signs. It is important to confirm that the vital signs are normal values *for the client.* Compare the vital signs taken during and after the procedure to those obtained before as baseline data to accurately assess the client's response to anesthetic agents and the procedure performed.

Advise the client of those things to expect during the procedure. Such teaching can both increase the level of cooperation and decrease the degree of anxiety. The client's family should also be informed of what will happen during the procedure and approximately how long the procedure

Figure 25-1 *Preparing a Client for Diagnostic Testing*

should last. Know the facility's specific protocols and procedures, because these are not standardized.

Care of the Client during Diagnostic Testing

Although client care must be individualized according to the specific procedure, general guidelines for client care during a procedure are outlined in Table 25-2. Protocols are used to assist with client care.

Standard Precautions are used when possible exposure to body fluids may occur. Protective barriers, such as gown, gloves, and goggles, should be used during invasive procedures.

Label all specimens with the client's name and room number (for hospitalized clients) and the date, time, and specimen source. Some specimens may need to be taken immediately to the laboratory or placed on ice (e.g., arterial blood gases [ABGs]).

Ongoing assessment of the client is required during any procedure. The patency of the client's airway should be continuously assessed, because it may be compromised by the client's position, by anesthesia, or by the procedure itself. During an invasive procedure, monitor for signs and symptoms of accidental perforation of an organ (e.g., sudden changes in vital signs).

The nurse has the following additional responsibilities:

- Prepare the procedure room (e.g., ensure adequate lighting).
- Gather and charge for supplies to be used during the procedure.
- Test the equipment to ensure it is functional and safe.
- Secure proper containers for specimen collection.

Practitioners usually have preference cards within the diagnostic testing area that specify the type of equipment to be used, the position in which to place the client, and the type of sedative or anesthetic agent to be used.

Some diagnostic tests are performed with the RN administering IV sedation, also called procedural sedation. **Procedural sedation** is a minimally depressed level of consciousness during which the client retains the ability to maintain a continuously patent airway and respond appropriately to physical stimulation or verbal commands. The nurse managing procedural sedation functions in an

TABLE 25-1	**PROTOCOL: PREPARING THE CLIENT FOR DIAGNOSTIC TESTING**
Purpose	To increase the reliability of the test by providing client teaching on the reason the test is being performed, those things the client can expect during the test, and the outcomes and side effects of the test
	To decrease the client's anxiety about the test and the associated risks
Supportive Data	Increase the client's knowledge, thereby promoting cooperation and enhancing the quality of the testing
	Decrease the time required to perform the tests, thereby increasing cost effectiveness
	Prevent delays by ensuring proper physical preparation
Assessment	Ensure that the client is wearing an identification band
	Review the medical record for allergies and previous adverse reactions to dyes and other contrast media; a signed consent form; and the recorded findings of diagnostic tests relative to the procedure
	Assess for the presence, location, and characteristics of physical and communicative limitations or pre-existing conditions
	Monitor the client's knowledge of the reasons for the test and things to expect during and after testing
	Monitor vital signs, including pain, of the client scheduled for invasive testing, to establish baseline data
	Assess client outcome measures relative to the practitioner's preferences for preprocedure preparations
	Monitor level of hydration and weakness for clients who are designated nothing by mouth (NPO)
Report to Practitioner	Notify practitioner of allergy, previous adverse reaction, or suspected adverse reaction following the administration of drugs
	Notify practitioner of any client or family concerns not alleviated by discussions with nurse
Interventions	Clarify with practitioner whether regularly scheduled medications are to be administered
	Implement NPO status, as determined by the type of test
	Administer cathartics or laxatives as noted on the test's protocol; instruct clients who are weak to call for assistance to the bathroom
	Teach relaxation techniques, such as deep breathing and imagery
	Establish intravenous (IV) access if necessary for the procedure
Evaluation	Evaluate the client's knowledge of those things to expect
	Evaluate the client's anxiety level
	Evaluate the client's level of safety and comfort
Client Teaching	Discuss the following with the client and family, as appropriate to the specific test:
	• The reason for the test and those things to expect
	• An estimate of how long the test will take
	• Specifics of NPO status, including amount of water to drink if oral medication is to be taken
	• Cathartics or laxative: amount, frequency
	• Sputum: cough deeply, do not clear throat
	• Urine: voided, clean-catch specimen; timing of collection
	• Removal of objects (e.g., jewelry or hair clips) that will obscure x-ray film
	• Contrast medium:
	Barium: taste, consistency, after-effects (lightly colored stools for 24 to 72 hours; possibly, obstruction/impaction)
	Iodine: metallic taste, delayed allergic reaction (itching, rashes, hives, wheezing and breathing difficulties)
	• Positioning during the test
	• Positioning posttest (e.g., immobilize limb after angiography)
	• Posttest (encourage fluid intake if not contraindicated)
Documentation	Record in the client's medical record:
	• Practitioner notification of allergies or suspected adverse reaction to contrast media
	• Presence, location, and characteristics of symptoms
	• Teaching and the client's response to teaching
	• Responses to interventions (client outcomes)

TABLE 25-2   PROTOCOL: CARE OF THE CLIENT DURING DIAGNOSTIC TESTING

Purpose	To increase cooperation and participation by allaying the client's anxiety
	To provide the maximum level of safety and comfort during a procedure
Supportive Data	Encourage relaxation of the muscles and thus facilitate instrumentation by increasing the client's participation and comfort
	Ensure efficient use of time during the test and reliable results from the test with proper client preparation
Assessment	Check the client's identification band to ensure the correct client
	Review the medical record for allergies
	Assess the client's reaction to the preprocedure sedatives administered prior to the induction of anesthesia during the procedure
	Assess airway maintenance and gag reflex, if a local anesthetic is sprayed into the client's throat
	Assess vital signs, including pain, throughout the procedure and compare to baseline data
	Assess the client's ability to maintain and tolerate the prescribed position
	Assess the client's comfort level (pain) to ensure the effectiveness of the anesthetic agent
	Assess for related symptoms indicating complications specific to the procedure (e.g., accidental perforation of an organ)
Report to Practitioner	Notify the practitioner of any client concerns or questions not answered in discussions with the nurse
	Notify the practitioner of any family members present and their location during the procedure
	Notify the practitioner when the client is positioned properly and the anesthetic agent has been administered to the client
Interventions	Institute Standard Precautions or appropriate aseptic technique for the specific test
	Report to all personnel involved in the test any known client allergies
	Place the client in the correct position, drape, and monitor to ensure that breathing is not compromised
	Remain with the client during induction and maintenance of anesthesia
	If the procedure requires the administration of a dye, ensure that the client is not allergic to the dye; if the client has not received the dye before, perform the skin allergy test according to the manufacturer's instructions that accompany the medication
	Monitor the client's airway and keep resuscitative equipment available
	Assist the client to relax during insertion of the instrument by telling the client to breathe through the mouth and to concentrate on relaxing the involved muscles
	Explain what the practitioner is doing so that the client knows what to expect
	Label and handle the specimen according to the type of materials obtained and the testing to be done
	Report to the practitioner any symptoms of complications
	Secure client transport from the diagnostic area
	Posttest in the diagnostic area:
	• Assist the client to a comfortable, safe position
	• Provide oral hygiene and water to clients who were designated NPO for the test, if they are alert and able to swallow
	• Remain with the client awaiting transport to another area
Evaluation	Evaluate the client's ventilatory status and tolerance to the procedure
	Evaluate the client's need for assistance
	Evaluate the client's understanding of what was performed during the procedure
	Evaluate the client's understanding of findings identified during the procedure
	Evaluate the client's knowledge of what to expect after the procedure
Client Teaching	Discuss the following with the client and family, as appropriate to the specific test:
	• Those things that occurred during the procedure
	• Questions and concerns of the client or family member
	• Those things to expect during the immediate recovery phase
	• Those things to report to the nurse during the immediate recovery phase

continues

TABLE 25-2 continued	
Documentation	Record in the client's medical record: • Person who performed the procedure • Reason for the procedure • Type of anesthestic, dye, or other medications administered • Type of specimen obtained and where it was sent • Vital signs and other assessment data such as client's tolerance of the procedure or pain/discomfort level • Any symptoms of complications • Person who transported the client to another area (designate the names of persons who provided transport and the destination)

expanded role that requires additional education and demonstrated ability beyond the basic education.

Care of the Client after Diagnostic Testing

Postprocedure nursing care is directed toward restoring the client's prediagnostic level of functioning (Table 25-3). Nursing assessment and interventions are based mainly on the nature of the test and whether the client received anesthesia.

The client is closely monitored for signs of respiratory distress and bleeding. Some diagnostic tests require vital signs measurement every 15 minutes for the first hour, and then at gradually longer intervals until the client is **stable** (alert and with vital signs within the client's normal range).

Some diagnostic tests use medications that are excreted through the kidneys. The client's intake and output (I&O) is monitored for 24 hours. The client is taught to monitor I&O and to report **hematuria** (presence of blood in the urine).

 Safety: Radioactive Iodine and Urine Collection
Clients receiving radioactive iodine must have their urine collected and properly discarded in a special container, according to agency policy for handling radioactive medical wastes.

Clients should receive written instructions when discharged after diagnostic testing. Most agencies have discharge forms on which teaching regarding medications, dietary and activity restrictions, and signs and symptoms to be reported immediately to the practitioner are documented.

LABORATORY TESTS

Common laboratory studies are usually simple measurements to determine the amount or number of **analytes** (i.e., measured substances) present in a specimen. Laboratory tests are ordered by the practitioner to:

- Detect and quantify future disease risk.
- Establish or exclude diagnoses.
- Assess the disease process severity and formulate a prognosis.
- Guide intervention selection.

- Monitor the progress of the disorder.
- Monitor treatment effectiveness.

Specimen Collection

The scheduling and sequencing of laboratory tests are important. All tests requiring **venipuncture** (the use of a needle to puncture a vein to aspirate blood) should be grouped together so the client has only one venipuncture. Fasting laboratory and radiological studies should be scheduled on the same day so that the client is only required to fast for 1 day. The client's comfort level and satisfaction increases with appropriate scheduling.

Accuracy in laboratory testing requires that:

- The correct requisition form is used.
- All requested information is written on the form (e.g., the client's full name and medical number).
- Pertinent data that could influence the test's results, such as medications taken, is included.
- Specimen collection from the correct client is confirmed by checking the identification band.
- Laboratory results are placed in the correct medical record.

Venipuncture

Various members of the health care team can perform venipuncture. Although laboratories employ **phlebotomists** (individuals who perform venipuncture) to collect blood specimens, nurses must know how to perform venipuncture, because they routinely perform venipuncture in hospital critical care units, the home, and long-term care settings.

PROFESSIONAL TIP

Documentation of Specimen-Collection Difficulties
Document on the laboratory requisition slip and in the nurses' notes any difficulty experienced during collection. Such problems may indicate adverse effects related to the nature of the test and thus must be reported and treated immediately.

TABLE 25-3	PROTOCOL: CARE OF THE CLIENT AFTER DIAGNOSTIC TESTING
Purpose	To restore the client's prediagnostic level of functioning by providing care and teaching relative to both those things the client can expect after a test and the outcomes or side effects of the test
Supportive Data	Decrease client anxiety by increasing the client's participation and knowledge of expected outcome measures after a diagnostic test
	Through proper postprocedure care and client teaching, alert the client to those signs and symptoms that must be reported to the practitioner
Assessment	Check the identification band and call the client by name
	Assess the client closely for signs of airway distress, adverse reactions to anesthestic or other medications, and other signs that may indicate accidental perforation of an organ
	Assess for bleeding in those areas where a biopsy was performed
	Assess the client's vital signs, including pain
	Assess vascular access lines or other invasive monitoring devices
	Assess the client's ability to expel air, if air was instilled during a gastrointestinal test
	Assess the client's knowledge of those things to expect during the recovery phase
Report to Practitioner	Notify the practitioner of any signs of respiratory distress, bleeding, or changes in vital signs; adverse reactions to anesthetic, sedative, or dye; and other signs of complications
	Notify the practitioner of client or family concerns or questions not answered in discussions with the nurse
	Notify the practitioner when any results are obtained from the diagnostic test
	Notify the practitioner when the client is fully alert and recovered (for an order to discharge)
Interventions	Implement the practitioner's orders regarding the postprocedure care of the client
	Institute Standard Precautions or surgical asepsis as appropriate to the client's care needs
	Position the client for comfort and accessibility so as to facilitate performance of nursing measures
	Monitor vital signs according to the frequency required for the specific test
	Observe the insertion site for hematoma or blood loss; replace pressure dressing, as needed
	Monitor the client's urinary output and drainage from other devices
	Enforce activity restrictions appropriate to the test
	Schedule client appointments as directed by the practitioner
Evaluation	Evaluate the client's respiratory status, especially if an anesthetic agent was used
	Evaluate the client's tolerance of oral liquids
	Evaluate the client's understanding of the procedural findings of when the practitioner expects to receive written results
	Evaluate the client's knowledge of those things to expect after discharge
Client Teaching	Based on client assessment and evaluation of knowledge, teach the client or family about the following:
	• Dietary or activity restrictions
	• Signs and symptoms that should be reported immediately to the practitioner
	• Medications
Documentation	Record in the client's medical record on the appropriate forms:
	• Assessment data, nursing interventions, and achievement of expected outcomes
	• Client or family teaching and demonstrated level of understanding
	• Written instructions given to the client or family members

Venipuncture can be performed by using either a sterile needle and syringe or a vacuum tube holder with a sterile two-ended needle. Test tubes with different colored stoppers are used to collect blood specimens. The stoppers indicate the type of additive in the test tube. The tubes are universally color coded as follows:

- Red: no additive
- Lavender: ethylenediaminotetraacetic acid (EDTA)
- Light blue: sodium citrate
- Green: sodium heparin
- Gray: potassium oxalate
- Black: sodium oxalate

Puncture site

Figure 25-2 *Capillary Puncture of Fingertip*

Arterial Puncture

Arterial blood gases reveal the lung's ability to exchange gases by measuring the partial pressures of oxygen (PaO_2) and carbon dioxide ($PaCO_2$) and evaluates the potential of hydrogen (pH) of arterial blood. Blood gases are ordered to evaluate:

- Oxygenation
- Ventilation and the effectiveness of respiratory therapy
- Acid–base balance in the blood

Arterial blood is drawn from a peripheral artery (e.g., radial or femoral) or from an arterial line. The blood is collected in a 5-mL heparinized syringe. The syringe is then rotated to mix the blood with the heparin to prevent clotting and then placed on ice.

In some agencies, it is within the scope of nursing practice to perform radial artery puncture, but femoral artery puncture is usually performed only by an advanced practitioner because of the associated increased risk of hemorrhage. It is not common practice for student nurses to draw ABG samples, but students often assist with the procedure and care for the client afterward.

The nurse is responsible for assessing the client for symptoms of postpuncture bleeding or occlusion. Apply direct pressure to the puncture site until all bleeding has stopped (a minimum of 5 minutes). Symptoms of impaired circulation include:

- Numbness and tingling
- Bluish color (cyanosis)
- Absence of a peripheral pulse

Capillary Puncture

When small quantities of capillary blood are needed for analysis or when the client has poor veins, a capillary puncture is performed. They are also used for blood glucose analysis. Figure 25-2 illustrates a capillary puncture of a fingertip.

Central Lines

A blood sample can also be collected from a **central line** (a venous catheter inserted into the superior vena cava through the subclavian or internal or external jugular vein). Central lines are used to treat fluid or electrolyte imbalances, such as severe dehydration caused by vomiting. Central lines are inserted when a peripheral route cannot be obtained, can be used for treatment, and to withdraw blood for analysis.

The first blood sample drawn from a central line cannot be used for diagnostic testing. It must be discarded, with the volume of discard being the same as the dead space (catheter size). Agency protocol should specify the volume to discard relative to the type and size of catheter.

Central line care requires strict sterile technique. The practitioner must write an order for a blood sample to be obtained from a central line.

Implanted Port

Some clients have a **port-a-cath** (a port that has been implanted under the skin) over the third or fourth rib. The port's catheter is inserted into the superior vena cava or right atrium through the subclavian or internal jugular vein. This implanted port is used for the same purpose as a central line. Using strict sterile technique, blood can be withdrawn for analysis by accessing the port. This should be performed only by a nurse who has the education to properly do so. Students are not usually taught how to access an implanted port.

Urine Collection

Urine can be collected for various studies. The type of testing determines the method of collection. The different methods of urine collection are as follows:

- Random collection (routine analysis)
- Timed collection (24-hour urine)
- Collection from a closed urinary drainage system
- Sterile specimen (catheterized)
- Clean-voided specimen

The client's age and the method of collection determine client teaching. The collection method should be written on the laboratory requisition.

Safety: Standard Precautions and Urine Collection
All urine collection requires the use of Standard Precautions to prevent transmission of microorganisms among nurses, clients, and other health care providers. All specimen containers should be sealed in a biohazard bag prior to transport to the laboratory.

Random Collection The practitioner writes the order for a UA (routine urine analysis), also called a random collection. The specimen can be collected at any time using a clean, not sterile, cup. The specimen should be taken immediately to the laboratory to prevent bacterial growth and changes in the urine's analytes.

Timed Collection Timed collection is done over a 24-hour period. The urine is collected in a plastic gallon container that contains preservative(s), some of which are caustic.

For a timed collection, the client is told to **void** (eliminate urine) and discard the specimen at the beginning of the collection. Timing for a 24-hour urine collection begins after the first voiding has been discarded. For example, if the client voids at 1000 hours (24-hour [military] time), that urine should be discarded, but all urine is saved until 1000 hours the following day, when the last urine is saved. The client can void into a clean container and pour the urine into the collection bottle. Toilet tissue should not be dropped into the container used to catch the urine. The collection container should be refriger-

ated or kept on ice the entire 24 hours to stabilize the analytes and retard bacterial growth.

Collection from a Closed-Drainage System A sterile specimen can be collected from a client with an indwelling Foley catheter and closed-drainage system. A sterile specimen is used for urine culture. The urine specimen should *not* be obtained from the drainage bag because the analytes in the urine drainage bag change, leading to inaccurate results, and bacteria grows quickly in the drainage bag. The closed-drainage tubing has an aspiration port for sterile specimen collection.

Sterile Specimen When a sterile urine specimen is required and the client does not have an indwelling catheter and closed-drainage system, the client is catheterized. A small amount of urine is allowed to run out of the catheter into a basin, then the urine is allowed to flow into a sterile specimen bottle.

Clean-Voided Specimen Clean-voided (clean-catch, or midstream) specimen collection is done to have a specimen uncontaminated by skin flora. The collection technique is different for women and men. The female client is instructed to cleanse from the front to the back and then void into the specimen bottle; the male client is instructed to cleanse from the tip of the penis downward and then void into the specimen bottle.

Stool Collection

The reason for collecting a stool specimen should be explained to the client. The client is then instructed to defecate into a clean bedpan or container, and discard used tissue in the toilet. Stools can be collected one time or over 24, 48, or 72 hours. Stools to be collected over a prolonged period must be placed into a container and refrigerated. Once all stools have been collected, the container should be labeled with the client's name, the date and time, and the test to be performed. All stool specimens are placed in a biohazard bag before being transported to the laboratory.

Safety: Collecting Stool from a Client with Hepatitis
Write on the requisition form that the client has hepatitis. Doing so alerts laboratory personnel to be especially careful when handling the specimen.

Blood Tests

Many tests can be performed on the blood. Tests specific to the hematologic system are described in Table 25-4.

Type and Crossmatch

A **type and crossmatch** identifies the client's blood type and determines compatibility of blood between a potential donor and recipient (client). There are four basic blood types: A, B, AB, and O. The blood types are determined by the presence or absence of A or B antigens. **Antigens** are substances, usually proteins, that cause the formation of and react specifically with antibodies. **Antibodies** are immunoglobulins produced by the body in response to bacteria, viruses, or other antigenic substances. Type A and type B are antigens that are classified as **agglutinogens,** or substances that cause

TABLE 25-4 TESTS SPECIFIC TO THE HEMATOLOGIC SYSTEM

TEST	EXPLANATION/NORMAL VALUES	NURSING RESPONSIBILITIES
Red blood cells (RBCs)	Number of RBCs per mm³ of blood. May be low in clients with rheumatoid arthritis. Clients living in high altitudes may have an elevated RBC level. Normal: Male: 4.6–6.2 million/mm³ Female: 4.2–5.5 million/mm³	The client is not required to fast for the test.
White blood cells (WBCs)	Number of WBCs per mm³ of blood. Elevation is associated with infectious processes. Normal: 4100–10,800 mm³	The client is not required to fast for the test. Exercise, stress, last month of pregnancy, labor, previous splenectomy, and eating may increase level and alter differential values. Note medications taken that may affect test; aspirin, heparin, and steroids may increase WBC level, whereas antibiotics and diuretics may decrease WBC level.
Differential count Neutrophils	Percentage of types of WBCs in 1 mm of blood. Increase in bacterial infections and trauma. Normal:	The client is not required to fast for the test.
Segs (mature neutrophils)	Segs: 50%–65%	
Bands (immature neutrophils)	Bands: 0%–5%	
Eosinophils	Increased in allergic reactions or parasitic infestation. Normal: 1%–3%	Corticosteroid therapy causes a decreased level.
Basophils	Increased in allergic reactions and during healing periods. Normal: 0.4%–1.0%	Steroids cause a decreased level.
Lymphocytes	Increased in viral infections and other diseases, such as pertussis and tuberculosis (TB). Decreased in acquired immunodeficiency syndrome (AIDS). Normal: 25%–35%	Steroids cause a decreased level.
Monocytes	Increased in chronic diseases, such as malaria, TB, Rocky Mountain spotted fever. May be low in clients with rheumatoid arthritis. Normal: 4%–6%	
Hemoglobin (Hgb)	Measures the oxygen-carrying compound in RBCs. Normal: Male: 14–18 g/dL Female: 12–16 g/dL Critical value: <5 g/dL	The client is not required to fast for the test. Sample may be drawn from a finger of a child or the heel of an infant.
Hemoglobin electrophoresis	Detects abnormal forms of hemoglobin. Performed after positive sickle cell test. If the hemoglobin electrophoresis is negative, the client has the sickle cell trait. If the hemoglobin electrophoresis is positive, the client has sickle cell anemia. Normal: Hgb S: 0% Hgb F: <2% Hgb Ca: 0%	If the client has had a blood transfusion within the last 12 weeks, the results of the test may be altered.

continues

TABLE 25-4   continued

TEST	EXPLANATION/NORMAL VALUES	NURSING RESPONSIBILITIES

Hematocrit (Hct)	Measures the percentage of blood cells in a volume of blood. Clients living in high altitudes may have an increased level.
	
	Normal:
	
	  Male: 40%–54%
	  Female: 38%–47%
	
	Critical value: <15% or >60%
		The client is not required to fast for the test.

Platelet count	Measures the number of platelets per cubic milliliter of blood. Normal: 150,000–450,000/mm^3 Critical level: <50,000 and >1 million/mm^3	Instruct the client that strenuous exercise and oral contraceptives increase platelet level. Instruct the client that aspirin, acetaminophen, and sulfonamides decrease platelet level. If the client has a low platelet count, maintain digital pressure to the puncture site.
Bleeding time	Measures the length of time for a platelet plug to occlude a small puncture wound. Normal: 1–9 minutes (Ivy method) Critical value: >15 minutes	Notify the laboratory if the client is taking aspirin, anticoagulants, or other medications that may affect the clotting process.
Prothrombin time (PT, protime)	Measures the effectiveness of several bloodclotting factors. Normal: 10–13.4 seconds INR: 2.0–3.0 In the presence of anticoagulant therapy, the values should be 1$^1/_2$–2 times the normal value. Critical value: >20 seconds In the presence of anticoagulant therapy, the critical value should be >3 times the normal critical value.	Ensure that the blood specimen is drawn before the daily dose of warfarin (Coumadin) is administered. Instruct the client that alcohol intake may increase PT and that a diet high in fat may decrease PT. Note those medications taken that may affect results; salicylates, sulfonamides, and methyldopa (Aldomet), as these may increase PT, whereas digitalis and oral contraceptives decrease the level. Instruct the client not to take any medication without notifying the physician, as medications may affect the PT level.
International normalized ratio (INR)	Normal: 2–3 (2.5–3.5 for the client with a mechanical prosthetic heart valve). The INR is more accurate than PT in monitoring warfarin (Coumadin) therapy.	The daily warfarin (Coumadin) dose should be given after blood has been drawn for the INR.

Partial thromboplastin time (PTT), also called activated partial thromboplastin time (APTT)	Normal:
	
	  PTT: 60–70 sec
	  APTT: 21–35 sec
	
	In the presence of anticoagulant therapy, the normal value is 1.5–2.5 times the control value.
	
	Critical value:
	
	  APTT: >70 seconds
	  PTT: >100 seconds
		If the client is receiving intermittent heparin doses, schedule the APTT to be drawn 30–60 minutes before the next heparin dose.
		If heparin is given continuously, the blood specimen can be drawn at any time.
		If PTT is greater than 100 seconds, the client is at risk for bleeding, and the physician is notified.
		The antidote for heparin is protamine sulfate.
		Note whether the client is taking antihistamines, vitamin C, or salicylates, as these prolong PTT time.

D dimer test (fragment D dimer, fibrin degradation fragment)	Measures a fibrin split product that is released when a clot breaks. Confirms the diagnosis of disseminated intravascular coagulation (DIC). Normal: <10 mg/mL	Note whether the client is on thrombolytic therapy, as the results of this test would be increased from negative to positive.

CRITICAL THINKING

Type and Rh

If a client's blood type is AB positive, what are the possible blood types of the client's parents? Can the client receive Rh-negative blood? Explain your answer.

agglutination (clumping of RBCs). **Agglutinins** are specific kinds of antibodies whose interaction with antigens manifests as agglutination.

Blood types are also identified as positive or negative, depending on the presence or absence of the Rh factor. The Rh factor is an antigen that may be found on the RBC. The designation *Rh positive* means the antigen is present; *Rh negative* means the antigen is absent. An individual's blood type and Rh are determined genetically.

Crossmatch identifies the compatibility of the donor's blood with that of the recipient. A sample of the recipi-

ent's blood is mixed with the blood of a possible donor in the laboratory. If the mixed sample does not agglutinate, it is compatible.

Blood Chemistry

Blood chemistry tests are often grouped together, requiring one requisition and one venous specimen. Tests performed include glucose, electrolytes, enzymes, lipids, creatinine, and protein values. Other tests that may be performed on a blood specimen are listed in Table 25-5.

Blood Glucose Blood for measuring glucose is obtained by either skin puncture or venipuncture and is either fasting (FBS) or nonfasting (usually 2 hours postprandial) blood sugar. If the results of this screening test for diabetes mellitus are abnormal, the practitioner may order a glucose tolerance test, the most accurate test for diagnosing hypoglycemia and hyperglycemia (diabetes mellitus).

Serum Electrolytes An **electrolyte** is a substance that, when in solution, separates into ions and conducts electricity. Some electrolytes act on the cell membrane

Text continues on p. 499

TABLE 25-5 ADDITIONAL TESTS PERFORMED ON BLOOD SPECIMEN

TEST	EXPLANATION/NORMAL VALUES	NURSING RESPONSIBILITIES
Acid phosphatase	Acid phosphatase is an enzyme found in the prostate gland, seminal fluid, and RBCs. An elevated level is seen in clients with prostatic cancer and hemolytic anemias. If tumors are treated successfully, the level will decrease. A rising level may indicate a poor prognosis. Normal: 0–0.80 U/L	Tell the client that no food or drink restrictions are associated with this test. Apply pressure to the venipuncture site. Observe the site for bleeding. Used in rape investigations.
Adrenocorticotropic hormone (ACTH), corticotropin	Determines the function of the anterior pituitary. Because of diurnal variation, specimens should be drawn in both morning and evening. Normal: 4–22 pmol/L	Emotional or physical stress or recent radioisotope scans can interfere with test results. Drugs that may increase ACTH level include corticosteroids, estrogens, ethanol, and spironolactone. Explain the procedure to the client. This is especially important to decrease the client's stress level. Evaluate the client for increased stress level. Initiate NPO status 12 hours before test. The blood specimen must be drawn with a heparinized syringe, chilled by placing the specimen on ice, and immediately transported to the lab.
ACTH stimulation test, cortisol stimulation test, cosyntropin test	Monitors plasma cortisol level to indicate adrenal gland response to ACTH. Normal: 1 hour: ↑ 20 μg/dL at least above baseline	Note those medications taken that may affect results: cortisone, estrogens, hydrocortisone, and spironolactone may increase plasma cortisol level. Explain the procedure to the client. Initiate NPO status after midnight. For all tests, obtain baseline serum cortisol level. Administer injection of cosyntropin IM or IV. Draw blood specimen 30 to 60 minutes after injection. *continues*

TABLE 25-5   continued

TEST	EXPLANATION/NORMAL VALUES	NURSING RESPONSIBILITIES
Alanine aminotransferase (ALT, formerly serum glutamic pyruvic transaminase [SGPT])	ALT is an enzyme released in response to liver injury. Normal: varies with testing methods	Note those medications taken that affect results: many medications may increase level, including antibiotics, narcotics, oral contraceptives, and many others.
Alkaline phosphatase (ALP)	Alkaline phosphatase is an enzyme found primarily in the liver, biliary tract, and bone. Detection is important for determining possible liver and bone disease. Normal: varies widely depending on method	Fasting may be required. Apply pressure to the venipuncture site. Observe the site for bleeding.
Alpha-fetoprotein (AFP)	Test for tumor marker; elevated in nonseminomatous testicular cancer. Performed between 16 and 18 weeks of pregnancy. A high level is suggestive of neural tube defects. Normal: 0.9 ng/mL 16–18 weeks gestation: 30–43 µg/mL	Apply pressure to site and watch for bleeding or hematoma. Sample must be drawn between 15–20 weeks of gestation.
Amylase (AMS)	Amylase is an enzyme secreted by the pancreas. Elevation indicates pancreatitis. Normal: 25–125 IU/L	Note those medications taken that affect test results; steroids, aspirin, alcohol, some narcotics, some diuretics, and other drugs may increase level, whereas citrate, glucose, and oxalates may decrease level.
Antidiuretic hormone (ADH), vasopressin	Determines the production of ADH by the posterior pituitary. Normal: <1.5 pg/L	Explain the procedure to the client. Note those medications taken that may interfere with test results. Drugs that elevate ADH level include acetaminophen, barbiturates, cholinergic agents, estrogen, nicotine, oral hypoglycemic agents, some diuretics such as thiazides, and tricyclic antidepressants. Drugs that decrease ADH level include alcohol, beta-adrenergic agents, morphine antagonists, and phenytoin (Dilantin). Client should fast for 12 hours before the test. Evaluate the client for high level of physical or emotional stress.
Antinuclear antibodies (ANAs)	ANAs attack cell nuclei. The result is positive in 95% of clients with systemic lupus erythematosus. Levels are low in clients with mononucleosis, rheumatic fever, and liver diseases. Normal: negative at 1:20 dilution	Fasting is not required. Hydralazine (Apresoline) and procainamide (Pronestyl) may increase level. A radioactive scan in the past week may alter results; inform the lab, if applicable.
Antistreptolysin O (ASO)	High titer indicates presence of *beta-hemolytic streptococcus*, which may cause rheumatic fever or acute glomerulonephritis. Upper limit of normal varies with age, season, and geographic area. Normal: Adult: <1:100 12–19 years: <1:200 2–5 years: <1:100	There are no food or fluid restrictions. Antibiotics decrease ASO level. Check urine output if ASO is elevated. Urine output of less than 600 mL/24 h is associated with acute glomerulonephritis.

continues

TABLE 25-5 continued

TEST	EXPLANATION/NORMAL VALUES	NURSING RESPONSIBILITIES
Antithyroid microsomal antibody, antimicrosomal antibody, microsomal antibody, thyroid autoantibody, thyroid antimicrosomal antibody	Used to detect thyroid microsomal antibodies found in clients with Hashimoto's thyroiditis. Normal: titer <1:100	Explain the procedure to the client.
Aspartate aminotransferase (AST, formerly serum glutamic oxaloacetic transaminase [SGOT])	AST is an enzyme that indicates inflammation of heart, liver, skeletal muscle, pancreas, or kidneys. Normal: Male: 8–46 U/L Female: 7–31 U/L	Avoid intramuscular (IM) injections; record date and time of any injections. Avoid hemolysis. Withhold medications that affect results, for 12 hours if possible; several medications, such as antihypertensives, cholinergic agents, anticoagulants, digitalis, and others, may increase level, as may exercise.
Arterial blood gases (ABGs)	Direct measurement of the pH, PaO_2, and $PaCO_2$, and calculated measurement of HCO_3^- and SaO_2 from samples of arterial blood. pH = expresses the acidity or alkalinity of the blood. PaO_2 = partial pressure of oxygen in the blood. $PaCO_2$ = partial pressure of carbon dioxide in the blood. SaO_2 = arterial oxygen saturation. HCO_3^- = bicarbonate ion concentration in the blood. The oxygen content of the blood expressed as a percentage of the oxygen carrying capacity of the blood. Normal: Critical level: pH: 7.35–7.45 <7.2 or >7.6 PaO_2: 75–100 mm Hg <40 mm Hg $PaCO_2$: 35–45 mm Hg <20 or >70 HCO_3^-: 22–26 mEq <10 or >40 SaO_2: >95% (at sea level) <60%	Explain that an arterial sample of blood is required. Arterial punctures cause more discomfort than venous. Instruct the client not to move. Assess the adequacy of collateral circulation. The blood sample is drawn in a syringe containing heparin. After the specimen has been obtained, rotate the syringe to mix the blood and heparin. The blood sample is placed on ice and taken immediately to the lab. Apply pressure to the arterial site for 3 to 5 minutes or 15 minutes if client is on an anticoagulant. Assess site for bleeding.
Bilirubin	Measures bilirubin in the blood. Indicates how well the liver is functioning. Normal: Total: 0.1–1.3 mg/dL Direct: 0.0–0.3 mg/dL Indirect: 0.1–1.0 mg/dL	Note those medications taken that affect results; steroids, antibiotics, oral hypoglycemics, narcotics, as well as others may cause increased level, whereas barbiturates, caffeine, penicillins, and salicylates may cause decreased level. Fasting may be required. Do not shake the tube; protect the tube from light.
Blood glucose, fasting blood sugar (FBS)	Measures blood level of glucose (serum values). Results depend on method used by laboratory. Normal: 70–110 mg/dL Diabetic: ≥126 mg/dL Critical values: >400 mg/dL <50 mg/dL	Client must fast (except for water) for 12 hours before test. Withhold insulin or oral antidiabetic medications until blood is drawn. Be certain client receives medications and meal after fasting specimen drawn. Cortisone, thiazide, and loop diuretics cause increase.
2 hour post prandial glucose (2h PPG) or 2 hour post prandial blood sugar (2h PPBS)	Measures blood glucose 2 hours after a meal. Normal: 70–140 mg/dL Diabetic: >140 mg/dL	Instruct the client to eat entire meal and then to not eat anything else until blood is drawn. Notify the laboratory of the time meal was completed.

continues

TABLE 25-5 continued

TEST	EXPLANATION/NORMAL VALUES	NURSING RESPONSIBILITIES
Blood urea nitrogen (BUN)	Measures urea, end product of protein metabolism. Normal: 5–20 mg/dL	Initiate NPO status 8 hours prior to test, if possible. Note the client's hydration status. Note those medications taken that may affect results, including phenothiazines, nephrotoxic drugs, diuretics (hydrochlorothiazide [Hydro-Diuril], ethacrynic acid [Edecrin], furosemide [Lasix]); antibiotics (bacitracin, gentamicin, kanamycin, methicillin, neomycin); antihypertensives (methyldopa [Aldomet], guanethidine [Ismelin]), sulfonamides, propranolol, morphine, lithium, salicylates.
CA-15-3	CA-15-3 (cancer antigen) is a tumor marker for monitoring breast cancer. Because benign breast or ovarian disease can also cause elevations, it has limited use in diagnosis. Normal: <22 U/mL	Fasting is not required. Apply pressure to the venipuncture site. Observe the site for bleeding.
CA-19-9	CA-19-9 (cancer antigen) is a tumor marker used primarily in the diagnosis of pancreatic carcinoma. Normal: <37 U/mL	Fasting is not required. Apply pressure to the venipuncture site. Observe the site for bleeding.
CA-125	CA-125 (cancer antigen) is a tumor marker especially helpful in making the diagnosis of ovarian cancer. Normal: 0–35 U/mL	Fasting is not required. Apply pressure to the venipuncture site. Observe the site for bleeding.
Calcitonin, HCT, thyrocalcitonin	Determines thyroid and parathyroid activity. Also used as a tumor marker to detect thyroid cancer and several other cancers. Normal: basal <151 pg/mL	Note those medications taken that may increase calcitonin level, including calcium, cholecystokinin, epinephrine, glucagon, pentagastrin, and oral contraceptives. Explain the procedure to the client. The client should fast 8 hours but may have water.
Carcinoembryonic antigen (CEA)	CEA is found in clients with cancer, especially colorectal cancer. It is especially useful in monitoring treatment response and is occasionally the first sign of tumor recurrence. Normal: <5 ng/mL Smoker <2.5 ng/mL Nonsmoker	Fasting is not required. Apply pressure to the venipuncture site. Observe the site for bleeding. Note whether the client smokes or has a disease that will alter results, such as hepatitis, cirrhosis, or colitis.

Cardiac enzymes
  Serum AST
	Indicates possible tissue damage if elevated.
	Normal:
	  Male: 7–21 U/L
	  Female: 6–18 U/L
		Neither fasting nor NPO status is necessary.
		Pattern of elevated levels of AST, CPK, and LDH is indicative of myocardial infarction (MI).

Creatine kinase CPK (CK)	Normal:
	  Male: 55–170 U/L
	  Female: 30–135 U/L
		CPK is the first enzyme elevated after MI, and peaks within the first 24 hours.

CK isoenzymes	Present in skeletal muscle, brain, lungs, and heart muscle. Normal:	Elevation of an isoenzyme indicates damage to tissue in a specific organ; CK-MB is specific for myocardial cells. Level increases 3–6 hours following myocardial infarction, peaks in 12–24 hours and returns to normal in 18–24 hours.
CK-MM (muscle)	100%	
CK-BB (brain)	0%	
CK-MB (heart)	0%	
Lactic dehydrogenase (LDH)	Normal: 45–90 U/L Critical Level: 300–800 U/L following myocardial infarction	LDH_1 value greater than LDH_2 value is indicative of an acute MI. LDH_5 is elevated with congestive heart failure (CHF).

continues

TABLE 25-5 continued

TEST	EXPLANATION/NORMAL VALUES	NURSING RESPONSIBILITIES
Cardiac enzymes (continued)		
LDH isoenzymes LDH$_1$ (heart and erythrocytes) LDH$_2$ (reticuloendothelial system) LDH$_3$ (lungs and other tissues) LDH$_4$ (kidney, placenta, pancreas) LDH$_5$ (liver and striated muscles)	*17.5%–28.3% *30.4%–36.4% *18.8%–26.0% *9.2%–16.5% *5.3%–13.4%	
Cardiac troponin I and T	Proteins found in cardiac muscle. Protein is released when the muscle is injured or dead. Troponin I elevated level in 4–6 hours Normal: <1.5 ng/mL Troponin T elevated level in 1–3 hours Normal: <0.6 ng/mL	Explain to client that blood sample is needed. Test very expensive. Often used in the ED.
CD4 T-cell count	Predictor of HIV progression; baseline taken after positive HIV test. Normal: 500–1000/mm³ Critical value: <200/mm³	Explain the meaning of the test. Provide follow-up explanation of test results.
Cholesterol (lipid profile)	Lipid necessary for steroid, bile, and cell membrane production. Normal: <200 mg/dL (total)	Have client fast 12–14 hours prior to test. No alcohol 24 hours prior to test. Diet intake 2 weeks prior to test will affect results. Note those medications taken that may affect results; steroids, phenytoin, diuretics, and others may elevate level, whereas MAO inhibitors, some antibiotics, lovastatin, and others may decrease level. If elevated, increased risk of coronary artery disease (CAD), hypertension, and MI.
High density lipoprotein (HDL) Low density lipoprotein (LDL) Very low density lipoprotein (VLDL) Triglycerides	Normal: 30–70 mg/dL Normal: 60–160 mg/dL Normal: 25%–50% Normal: 40–150 mg/dL	Elevated level in CAD; level increases when LDL level increases.
Complement assay (total complement, C3 and C4)	Decreased levels in autoimmune diseases due to depletion of complement by antibody–antigen complexes. Normal: C3: Male: 80–180 mg/dL Female: 76–120 mg/dL C4: 15–45 mg/dL	Fasting is not required.
Coombs' test (direct antiglobulin test)	Detects whether immunoglobulins are attached to RBCs. Normal: negative	Note whether the client is taking ampicillin (Unasyn), captopril (Capoten), indomethacin (Indocin), or insulin, as these cause false-positive results.
Cortisol, hydrocortisone	Determines adrenal cortex function. There is normally a diurnal variation, with higher level around 6 to 8 A.M. and lowest levels around midnight.	Note whether the client has been under physical or emotional stress as either can artificially elevate plasma cortisol level. Likewise, recent use of radioisotopes can interfere with test results.

*% of total LDH

continues

TABLE 25-5 continued

TEST	EXPLANATION/NORMAL VALUES	NURSING RESPONSIBILITIES
Cortisol, hydrocortisone (continued)	Normal: 8 A.M.: 6–28 μg/dL, or 170–625 nmol/L 4 P.M.: 2–12 μg/dL, or 80–413 nmol/L	Note those medications taken that may affect results. Drugs that may increase plasma cortisol level include estrogen, oral contraceptives, and spironolactone (Aldactone). Drugs that may decrease plasma cortisol level include androgens and phenytoin (Dilantin) Explain the procedure to the client. Two specimens are drawn—one at 8 A.M. and another at 4 P.M. Assess the client for physical or emotional stress and report to the physician. Indicate times of collection on laboratory requisitions.
C-reactive protein test (CRP)	An abnormal protein appears in the blood of clients with an acute inflammatory process. Used to monitor the progress of clients with autoimmune disorders such as rheumatoid arthritis. More sensitive than erythrocyte sedimentation rate (ESR). Normal: less than 6 mg/L	Fast, except for water, for 8 hours. Note those medications that may affect results: nonsteroidal antiinflammatory drugs (NSAIDs), steroids, and salicylates may decrease level; oral contraceptives and intrauterine devices (IUDs) may increase level. Inform laboratory, if applicable.
Culture	Identifies pathogens in blood. Normal: None	There are no food or fluid restrictions.
Dexamethasone suppression test (DST), prolonged/rapid DST, cortisol suppression test (ACTH suppression test)	Monitors plasma cortisol level to measure adrenal gland function. Normal: <5 mg/dL	Stress can interfere with test results. Note those medications taken that may affect results, including barbiturates, estrogens, oral contraceptives, phenytoin (Dilantin) spironolactone, steroids, and tetracyclines. Explain the procedure to the client. Weigh the client for baseline weight. Rapid test: Administer dexamethasone 1 mg orally at 11 P.M. with milk or antacid. Administer sedative, if ordered. At 8 A.M., before client rises, draw plasma cortisol level. Overnight 8-mg dexamethasone suppression test: If no cortisol suppression occurs, repeat test using 8 mg dexamethasone. If there is still no cortisol suppression, a prolonged test over 6 days involving six 24-hour urine collections should be done.
Electrolytes	Determines blood electrolyte levels. First four are the most commonly measured.	Sodium and potassium are necessary for cardiac electrical conduction.
Sodium (Na⁺)	Measures level of serum sodium. Function in the body: Major electrolyte in extracellular fluid, regulates fluid balance, stimulates conduction of nerve impulses, helps maintain neuromuscular activity. Normal: 135–145 mEq/L	There are no food or fluid restrictions.
Potassium (K⁺)	Measures level of serum potassium. Function in the body: Major electrolyte in intracellular fluid, maintains normal nerve and muscle activity, assists in cellular metabolism of carbohydrates and proteins. Normal: 3.5–5.5 mEq/L	There are no food or fluid restrictions. If the client has hypokalemia or hyperkalemia, evaluate the client for cardiac dysrhythmias.

TABLE 25-5 continued

TEST	EXPLANATION/NORMAL VALUES	NURSING RESPONSIBILITIES
Electrolytes (continued)		
Chloride (Cl⁻)	Measures level of serum chloride Function in the body: 　Major electrolyte in extracellular fluid, functions in combination with sodium to maintain osmotic pressure, assists in maintaining acid–base balance Normal: 100–110 mEq/L	There are no food or fluid restrictions.
Calcium, total/ionized Ca⁺⁺	Indicates parathyroid gland function and calcium metabolism. Because ionized calcium is unaffected by serum albumin, it can give more accurate results; however, most laboratories do not have the equipment to perform the test. Normal: 　Total: 8.5–10.5 mg/dL, or 2.25–2.75 nmol/L 　Ionized: 4.5–5.6 ng/dL, or 1.05–1.30 nmol/L	Note those medications taken that may affect results. Drugs that may increase serum calcium level include calcium salts, hydralazine, lithium, thiazide diuretics, parathyroid hormone (PTH), thyroid hormone, and vitamin D. Drugs that may decrease serum calcium level include acetazolamide, anticonvulsants, asparaginase, aspirin, calcitonin, cisplatin, corticosteroids, heparin, laxatives, loop diuretics, magnesium salts, and oral contraceptives. Vitamin D and excessive milk ingestion can also interfere with test results. Explain the procedure to the client. Fasting is not required for serum calcium, but might be required if other blood chemistry tests are to be drawn.
Magnesium (Mg⁺⁺)	Measures level of serum magnesium Function in the body: 　Combines with calcium and phosphorous in intracellular bone tissue, essential for neuromuscular contraction, synthesis of protein, and body temperature regulation Normal: 1.6–2.6 mEq/L	There are no food or fluid restrictions.
Phosphate (PO₄⁻⁻)	Measures level of serum phosphate Function in the body: 　An essential intracellular electrolyte, exists in an inverse relationship with calcium Normal: 3–4.5 mg/dL	Initiate NPO status after midnight. Intravenous fluids containing glucose are sometimes discontinued several hours before the test.
Bicarbonate (HCO₃⁻) (total carbon dioxide content or carbon dioxide capacity)	Always in a 20:1 ratio with carbonic acid. Normal: venous 22–29 mEq/L 　　　arterial 21–28 mEq/L	There are no food or fluid restrictions. Loss of gastric contents is the most common reason for increased level.
ELISA	Screening test used to indicate the presence of HIV Normal: negative	Inform the client that if the first ELISA test is positive, a second ELISA will be drawn before confirmation is done with Western blot. Provide pretest counseling. Obtain informed consent. Provide or arrange for post-test counseling.
Erythrocyte sedimentation rate (ESR or sed rate test)	Measures, in mm, RBC descent in a normal saline solution after 1 hour. Level is increased in inflammatory, infectious, necrotic, or cancerous conditions, due to increased protein content in plasma. Used to monitor the course of therapy for clients with autoimmune diseases, such as rheumatoid arthritis. Normal: 　Male: 0–13 mm/hr 　Female: 0–20 mm/hr	The test should be performed within 3 hours after the blood is drawn. Menstruation or pregnancy may increase level. Ethanbutal, quinine, aspirin, cortisone, and prednisone may alter results.

continues

TABLE 25-5 continued

TEST	EXPLANATION/NORMAL VALUES	NURSING RESPONSIBILITIES
Folic acid (Folate level)	Measures folic acid level in the blood. Normal: 5–20 ug/mL, or 14–34 mmol/L	Fasting is not required. Instruct the client not to drink any alcoholic beverages before the test. The test is drawn before folic acid medications are administered. Note whether the client is taking phenytoin (Dilantin), primidone (Mysoline), methotrexate, antimalarial agents, or oral contraceptives, as these cause decreased level.

Follicle-stimulating hormone (FSH)	Determines anterior pituitary function. Usually measured with luteinizing hormone level.
	Normal: varies with phase of menstrual cycle
	  Follicular: 5–20 mU/mL
	  Midcycle peak: 15–30 mU/mL
	  Luteal: 5–15 mU/mL
	  Postmenopause: 50–100 mU/mL
	  Male: 5–20 mU/mL
		Note whether client is taking estrogen or progesterone, as these may decrease FSH level. Recent use of radioisotopes can also interfere with test results.
		Explain the procedure to the client.
		Indicate on the laboratory requisition the date of the last menstrual period (LMP) or that the client is postmenopausal. Indicate use of estrogen or progesterone on laboratory requisition.
		The client should be relaxed and recumbent for 30 minutes before the test.

Gamma-glutamyl transpeptidase (GGT or GGTP)	Enzyme that detects liver cell dysfunction. Normal: 5–38 IU/L	The client must fast for 8 hours prior to test. Note alcohol, Dilantin, and phenobarbital may elevate results, whereas oral contraceptives and clofibrate may decrease results.
Globulin	Key for antibody production. Indicates how well the liver is functioning. Normal: 2.3–3.5 g/dL	Note those medications taken that affect results (see albumin).

Glucose tolerance test (GTT)	Evaluates blood and urine glucose 30 minutes before, and 1, 2, and 3 hours after a standard glucose load.
	Normal: fasting 70–110 mg/dL
	  1 hr 160 mg/dL
	  2 hr 115 mg/dL
	  3 hr 70–110 mg/dL
		The client must fast (except for water) for 6–8 hours prior to the test.
		Withhold drugs that interfere with results.
		After administration of glucose load, withhold all food. The client should drink water, however.
		Collect urine specimens at hourly periods.
		Administer meal and medications after test is completed.

Glycosylated hemoglobin (GHB)	Measures glycohemoglobin, evaluating average blood glucose level over 120 days.
	Normal: nondiabetic 3.5%–6%
	  Good control: 7.5% or less
	  Fair control: 7.6%–8.9%
	  Poor control: >9% or more
		Fasting is not required.
		Blood can be drawn at any time.

Hepatitis B surface antigen (HB$_s$AG)	A positive result indicates presence of hepatitis or that the person is a carrier. Normal: negative	

Human chorionic gonadotropin (hCG)	Test for tumor marker; elevated in germ cell testicular cancer.
	Normal: negative
	  Female, pregnant: positive, peaks at 8–12 weeks then falls
	  Female, abnormal pregnancy or choriocarcinoma: remains high or increases
		Apply pressure to the site and observe for bleeding or hematoma.

continues

TABLE 25-5 continued

TEST	EXPLANATION/NORMAL VALUES	NURSING RESPONSIBILITIES
Human leukocyte antigen DW4 (HLA-DW4)	Positive (present in 50% of clients with rheumatoid arthritis). Normal: negative	Fasting is not required.
Lupus erythematosus test (LE prep)	Positive in 70%–80% of clients with systemic lupus erythematosus. May be positive in clients with rheumatoid arthritis. Used to diagnose and monitor the course of treatment for clients with systemic lupus erythematosus. Normal: negative	Fasting is not required. May be ordered daily for 3 days. Note whether the client is taking Apresoline, Pronestyl, oral contraceptives, quinidine, penicillin, Aldomet, tetracycline, isoniazid, or reserpine, as these may cause false-positive results.
Luteinizing hormone (LH) assay	Determines anterior pituitary function. It can be used to determine whether ovulation has occurred. Can also determine whether gonadal insufficiency is primary or secondary. Normal: 　Males: 7–24 mU/mL 　Females: 6–30 mU/mL	Note whether the client is taking estrogen or progesterone, as these may decrease LH level. Recent use of radioisotopes can also interfere with test results. Explain the procedure to the client. Indicate on the laboratory requisition the date of the LMP or that the client is postmenopausal.
Parathyroid hormone (PTH), parathormone	Measures the quantity of PTH to determine hyperparathyroidism or whether hypercalcemia is caused by parathyroid glands. Normal: 10–60 pg/mL	Recent use of radioisotope can interfere with test results. Explain the procedure to the client. Initiate NPO status after midnight, except for water. Obtain morning blood specimen and indicate time of collection.
Phosphorus	Determines the level of phosphorus in the blood. Normal: 3.0–4.5 mg/dL, or 0.97–1.45 nmol/L	Laxatives or enemas containing sodium phosphate can increase serum phosphorus level. Note those medications taken that may affect results. Drugs that may increase serum phosphorus level include methicillin and excessive vitamin D. Recent carbohydrate ingestion including IV administration causes decreased serum phosphorus level, as do antacids and mannitol. Explain the procedure to the client. Initiate NPO status 12–14 hours before test. Discontinue IV fluids containing glucose for several hours before test, if possible.
Polymerase chain reaction (PCR)	Detects HIV-specific DNA (virus). Normal: negative	Explain the meaning of the test. Provide follow-up explanation of test results.
Progesterone assay	Determines ovulation and function of corpus luteum. Adrenal tumors can elevate level. Normal: 　Male: <100 ng/dL 　Female: midcycle: 300–2,400 ng/dL 　　Pregnancy 7–13 weeks 1,500–5,000 ng/dL 　　　　14+ weeks 6,500–20,000 ng/dL	Recent use of radioisotopes or hemolysis resulting from rough handling of blood specimen can interfere with test results. Note those medications taken that may interfere with test results, including estrogen and progesterone. Explain the procedure to the client. Indicate the date of LMP on the laboratory requisition. *continues*

TABLE 25-5 continued

TEST	EXPLANATION/NORMAL VALUES	NURSING RESPONSIBILITIES
Prolactin level (PRL)	Determines anterior pituitary secretion. Among the problems indicated by an elevated level are pituitary tumors or primary hypothyroidism. Normal: Female, or male: 0–20 ng/mL Pregnant: 20–400 ng/mL	Note those medications taken that may affect results. Drugs that may increase prolactin level include phenothiazines, oral contraceptives, reserpine, opiates, verapamil, histamine antagonists, monoamine oxidase (MAO) inhibitors, and antihistamines. Drugs that may decrease prolactin level include ergot alkaloid derivatives, clonidine, levodopa, and dopamine. Explain the procedure to the client. The blood specimen should be obtained in the morning and placed on ice if not taken immediately to the laboratory.
Prostate-specific antigen (PSA)	PSA is an antigen detected in all males; level increases with prostatic cancer. It is more sensitive and specific than the acid phosphatase. Normal: <4 ng/mL	Fasting is not required. Apply pressure to the venipuncture site. Observe the site for bleeding.
Protein	Measures total protein in the blood. Normal: 6–8 g/dL	Note those medications taken that may affect results; steroids and hormones such as insulin, and growth hormones may increase level, whereas oral contraceptives and liver toxic drugs may decrease level.
Renin assay, plasma renin activity (PRA)	Measures the amount of renin and is used as a screening procedure to detect essential or renal hypertension. When combined with plasma aldosterone level, determines adrenal cortex activity. Normal: Upright position, sodium depleted or restricted diet: 20–39 years: 2.9–24 ng/mL/h >40 years: 2.9–10.8 ng/mL/h Upright position, sodium repleted or normal diet: 20–39 years: 0.1–4.3 ng/mL/h >40 years: 0.1-3.0 ng/mL/h	Pregnancy, salt intake, or licorice ingestion can interfere with test results. Time of day (early in the day), a low-salt diet, or an upright position increases renin value. Note those medications taken that may interfere with test results, including antihypertensives, diuretics, estrogens, oral contraceptives, and vasodilators. Explain the procedure to the client. The client should maintain a normal diet with sodium restricted to 3 grams per day for 3 days before the test. Drugs and licorice should be discontinued for 2 to 4 weeks before the test. The client should stand or sit upright for 2 hours before blood is drawn. Client position, dietary status, time of day, and drugs should be recorded on the laboratory requisition. Blood specimen should be placed in ice and taken immediately to the laboratory. After blood specimen is obtained, the client may resume a normal diet and restart medications.
Rheumatoid factor (RF)	Abnormal protein in serum of approximately 80% of clients with rheumatoid arthritis. Formed as a result of the reaction of IgM to an abnormal IgG. Also elevated in clients with other autoimmune diseases such as systemic lupus erythematosus. Normal: negative	Fasting is preferred.
Serum acid phosphatase (prostatic) (ACP)	Serum measurement of prostatic acid phosphatase, elevated in malignancy; because it detects cancer in the later stages, no longer commonly used. Normal: 0.0–0.8 U/L	Apply pressure to the site. Observe the site for bleeding or hematoma.
Serum alkaline phosphatase (ALP)	Serum measurement of alkaline phosphates, elevated in malignancy. Normal: 30–120 U/L	Apply pressure to the site. Observe the site for bleeding or hematoma.

continues

TABLE 25-5 continued

TEST	EXPLANATION/NORMAL VALUES	NURSING RESPONSIBILITIES
Serum creatinine	Specific indicator of renal disease. Normal: 0.4–1.5 mg/dL	Note those medications taken that may affect results, including amphotericin B, cephalosporins (cepfazolin [Ancef], cephalothin [Keflin]), methicillin, ascorbic acid, barbiturates, lithium carbonate, methyldopa (Aldomet), triamterene (Dyrenium).
Sickledex (sickle-cell test)	Screening test to determine the presence of Hgb S. Normal: no Hgb S If results are positive, a hemoglobin electrophoresis test is done.	There are no food or fluid restrictions. Note on the laboratory requisition whether the client had a blood transfusion in the past 3 to 4 months.
Thyroid-stimulating hormone (TSH), thyrotropin	Determines thyroid function as well as monitors exogenous thyroid replacement. Normal: 2–10 µU/mL, or 2–10 mU/L	Recent use of radioisotopes may affect test results. Severe illness may decrease TSH level. Drugs that may increase TSH level include antithyroid drugs, lithium, potassium iodide, and TSH injection. Drugs that may decrease TSH level include aspirin, dopamine, heparin, steroids, and T_3. Explain the procedure to the client. The client should be relaxed and recumbent for 30 minutes before the test.
TSH stimulation test	Differentiates between primary and secondary hypothyroidism. Normal: none given	Explain the procedure to the client. Obtain baseline level of radioactive iodine intake or serum T_4. Administer 5–10 units of TSH intramuscularly for 3 days. Repeat radioactive iodine intake or T_4 as indicated for comparison studies.
Thyrotropin-releasing hormone (TRH) test, thyrotropin-releasing factor (TRF) test	Assesses the responsiveness of the anterior pituitary by its secretion of TSH in response to an IV injection of TRH. Also tests the function of the thyroid gland. Normal: undetectable to 15 µU/mL	Pregnancy may increase TSH response to TRH. Note those medications taken that may modify TSH response, including antithyroid drugs, aspirin, corticosteroids, estrogens, levodopa, and T_4. Explain the procedure to the client. Any thyroid preparations should be discontinued for 3–4 weeks before the test.
Thyroxine (T_4) Screen	Directly measures the amount of T_4 present. Normal: radioimmunoassay: 5–12 µg/dL, or 65–155 nmol/L	X-ray iodinated contrast studies may increase T_4 levels. Pregnancy will increase T_4 level. Note those medications taken that may affect results. Drugs that may increase T_4 level include clofibrate, estrogens, heroin, methadone, and oral contraceptives. Drugs that may decrease T_4 level include anabolic steroids, androgens, antithyroid drugs, lithium, phenytoin (Dilantin), and propranolol (Inderal). Explain the procedure to the client. Evaluate the client's drug history. If needed, instruct the client to stop exogenous T_4 medications for 1 month prior to test. *continues*

TABLE 25-5 continued

TEST	EXPLANATION/NORMAL VALUES	NURSING RESPONSIBILITIES
Thyroxine free, FTI, FT₄	Measures the amount of free T₄ that actually enters the cells and is active in metabolism. A true indicator of thyroid activity. Can be used to diagnose thyroid status in pregnant females or clients on drugs that can interfere with results of other tests. Normal: 280–480 pg/dL	Recent radionuclear scans can interfere with test results. Explain the procedure to the client. Blood specimens for T₄ and T₃ uptake must be obtained to calculate T₄.
Total iron-binding capacity (TIBC)	Determines the ability of iron to bind to a protein called transferrin. Normal: 300–360 mg/dL	NPO 12 hours prior to the test. A recent blood transfusion or a diet high in iron may affect test results. Note whether the client is taking oral contraceptives, as these increase TIBC level.
Triglycerides	Form of fat produced in the liver. Normal: 30–150 mg/dL	Client to fast 12–14 hours prior to the test, and have no alcohol for 24 hours before. Diet of prior 2 weeks affects results.
Triiodothyronine (T₃) radioimmunoassay (T₃ by RIA)	Determines thyroid gland function Normal: 110–230 ng/dL, or 1.2–1.5 nmol/L	Radioisotope administration may interfere with test results. Pregnancy increases T₃ results. Note those medications taken that may affect results. Drugs that may increase T₃ level include: estrogen, methadone, and oral contraceptives. Drugs that may decrease T₄ level include anabolic steroids, androgens, phenytoin (Dilantin), propranolol (Inderal), reserpine, and salicylates (high dose). Explain the procedure to the client. Determine whether exogenous T₃ is being taken. With physician's approval, withhold those drugs that would interfere with test results.
Triiodothyronine (T₃) serum free	Measures the amount of free T₃ that actually enters the cells and is active in metabolism. A true indicator of thyroid activity. Can be used to diagnose thyroid status in pregnant females or clients on drugs that can interfere with results of other tests. Normal: 0.2–0.6 ng/dL	Explain the procedure to the client. Blood specimens for T₃ and T₄ uptake must be obtained to calculate T₃.
Uric acid	Elevated in gout. Normal: Male: 2.1–8.5 mg/dL Female: 2.0–8.0 mg/dL	There are no food or drink restrictions. Note those medications and other substances taken that may affect results, including ascorbic acid, diuretics, levadopa, allopurinol, and Coumadin.
VDRL (Venereal Disease Research Laboratory), RPR (rapid plasma reagin), FTA-ABS (fluorescent treponemal antibody-absorption test), Reiter test, fluorescent antibody Treponema pallidum immobilization (TPI) test (performed only at Centers for Disease Control [CDC] in Atlanta)	Blood tests for presence of syphilis. Normal: negative or nonreactive	Explain the test to the client, including amount of blood to be drawn.
Western blot	Confirmatory test for the presence of antibodies to HIV. Normal: negative	Provide pretest counseling. Obtain informed consent. Provide or arrange post-test counseling.

to allow the transmission of electrochemical impulses in nerve and muscle fibers, whereas others determine the activity of cellular metabolism (Guyton & Hall, 2000).

Cations are ions that have a positive charge, such as sodium (Na^+), potassium (K^+), calcium (Ca^{++}), and magnesium (Mg^{++}). Anions are ions that have a negative charge, including chloride (Cl^-), bicarbonate (HCO_3^-), and phosphate (HPO_4^{--}).

Blood Enzymes Enzymes are globular proteins produced in the body that catalyze chemical reactions within the cells. Enzyme tests are key to diagnosing tissue damage, mainly to the myocardium and, to a lesser degree, to the brain.

Plasma levels of intracellular enzymes elevate in the presence of myocardial **necrosis** (tissue death as the result of disease or injury). Enzymes in the blood are directly proportional to the degree of cellular damage. The enzymes are not used alone in determining a diagnosis but, rather, are reviewed with other diagnostic studies.

Blood Lipids An elevated serum lipid level is one of the controllable contributing risk factors to congestive heart disease (CHD). **Lipoproteins** (blood lipids bound to protein) are measured along with cholesterol.

PROFESSIONAL TIP

Drugs and Laboratory Tests
Note drugs the client is taking when those drugs may influence the results of laboratory tests.

Urine Tests

Urinalysis assists in the diagnosis of various conditions. Substances not normally found in the urine include RBCs, white blood cells (WBCs), protein, glucose, ketones, and casts. Tests often performed on a urine specimen are found in Table 25-6.

Urine pH

The hydrogen ion concentration in the urine determines the pH. Diabetes mellitus, diarrhea, dehydration, emphysema, and starvation make the urine acidic. Urinary tract infections, chronic renal failure, renal tubular acidosis, and salicylate poisoning make the urine alkaline.

TABLE 25-6 TESTS PERFORMED ON URINE

TEST	EXPLANATION/NORMAL VALUES	NURSING RESPONSIBILITIES
Urinalysis		Explain the procedure and purpose to the client and assist with specimen collection, if needed.
Color	Clear amber	Ensure that specimen is taken to the laboratory in a timely manner.
Odor	Pleasantly aromatic until left standing; offensive and unpleasant in kidney infection.	
pH	4.6–8.0	
Specific gravity	1.015–1.030	
Glucose	Negative	
Acetone (ketone)	Negative	
Casts	Rare	
Albumin (protein)	Negative	
RBCs	2–3/HPF	
WBCs	4–5/HPF	
Bilirubin	Negative	
Bacteria	Negative	
Aldosterone Assay	A blood test or 24-hour urine collection to evaluate the adrenal cortex, especially for tumors. The 24-hour urine is more reliable, but the blood specimen is more convenient. Normal, blood: Male: 6–22 ng/dL, or 0.17–0.61 nmol/L Female: 5–30 ng/dL, or 0.14–0.80 nmol/L Normal, urine: 2–80 μg/24 h, or 5.5–72.0 nmol/24 h	Strenuous exercise and stress can increase aldosterone level. Excessive licorice ingestion can decrease aldosterone level. Client should be upright (sitting or standing) for 4 hours before test. Explain the procedure to the client. The client should follow a normal diet with 3 grams of sodium/day and no licorice for at least 2 weeks before the test. Medications should be stopped for at least 2 weeks before the test, if possible. Initiate 24-hour urine collection. Send collection to laboratory immediately upon conclusion.

continues

TABLE 25-6 continued

TEST	EXPLANATION/NORMAL VALUES	NURSING RESPONSIBILITIES
Bence Jones Protein	Bence Jones proteins are immunoglobulins typically found in the urine of clients with multiple myeloma. They may also be associated with tumor metastases to the bone and chronic lymphocytic leukemia. Normal: negative	Instruct the client for a clean catch or 24-hour urine specimen. Instruct the client not to contaminate specimen with toilet paper or stool.
Creatinine clearance	Normal: Male: 95–135 mL/min Female: 85–125 mL/min Minimum: 10 mL/min to maintain life	Instruct the client about the 24-hour urine test. Encourage hourly water intake. Keep urine on ice or in special refrigerator. Cephalosporins and vigorous exercise affect results.
17-hydroxycorticosteroids (17-OHCS)	24-hour urine test that measures adrenal cortex function. Normal: Male: 3–10 mg/24 h Female: 2–6 mg/24 h	Emotional or physical stress or licorice ingestion may increase adrenal activity. Note those medications taken that may affect results. Drugs that may increase 17-OHCS level include acetazolamide, chloral hydrate, ascorbic acid, and erythromycin. Drugs that may decrease 17-OHCS level include estrogens, oral contraceptives, phenothiazines, and reserpine. Explain the procedure to the client. Initiate 24-hour urine collection. Send collection to laboratory immediately upon conclusion.
17-ketosteroids (17-KS)	24-hour urine test that measures adrenal cortex function. Normal: Male: 5–23 mg/24 h, or 24–88 μmol/24 h Female: 2–15 mg/24 h, or 14–52 μmol/24 h	Stress may increase adrenal activity. Note medications taken that may affect results. Drugs that increase 17-KS level include antibiotics and dexamethasone. Drugs that may decrease 17-KS level include estrogen and oral contraceptives. Explain the procedure to the client. With physician's approval, withhold all drugs for several days before test. Monitor client for stress and report to physician. Initiate 24-hour urine collection. Send collection to laboratory immediately upon conclusion.
Schilling test	Determines vitamin B_{12} absorption by the intestine. Differentiates between pernicious anemia and gastrointestinal malabsorption problems. Normal: 8%–40% of the radioactive vitamin B_{12} is excreted in the urine within 24 hours.	Collect the urine for a 24- to 48-hour period. Laxatives are not given during the test, as they decrease the absorption of vitamin B_{12}.
Urine cortisol, hydrocortisone	24-hour urine test that measures adrenal cortex function. Normal: 22–69 μmol/24 h, or 8–25 mg/24 h	Pregnancy or stress increases cortisol level. Recent radioisotope scans can interfere with test result. Note medications taken that may interfere with test result, including oral contraceptives and spironolactone. Explain the procedure to the client. Assess for stress and report to physician. Initiate 24-hour urine collection. Send collection to laboratory immediately upon conclusion.

continues

TABLE 25-6 continued

TEST	EXPLANATION/NORMAL VALUES	NURSING RESPONSIBILITIES
Vanillylmandelic acid (VMA) and catecholamines (epinephrine, norepinephrine, metanephrine, normetanephrine, dopamine)	24-hour urine test that diagnoses pheochromocytoma and other adrenal tumors. Normal: VMA: 2–7 mg/24 h, or 10–35 µmol/24 h Epinephrine: 0.5–20.0 µg/24 h, or <275 nmol/24 h Norepinephrine: 15–80 µg/24 h Metanephrine: 24–96 µg/24 h Normetanephrine: 75–375 µg/24 h Dopamine: 65–400 µg/24 h	Certain foods (e.g., tea, coffee, cocoa, vanilla, chocolate), vigorous exercise, stress, or starvation may increase VMA level. Uremia, alkaline urine, or iodinated contrast dyes may falsely decrease VMA level. Note those medications taken that may affect results. Drugs that may increase VMA level include caffeine, epinephrine, levodopa, lithium, and nitroglycerine. Drugs that may decrease VMA level include clonidine, disulfiram (Antabuse), guanethidine, imipramine, MAO inhibitors, phenothiazines, and reserpine. Drugs that may increase catecholamine level include ethyl alcohol, aminophylline, caffeine, chloral hydrate, clonidine (chronic therapy), contrast media (iodine containing), disulfiram (Antabuse), epinephrine, erythromycin, insulin, methenamine, methyldopa, nicotinic acid (large doses), nitroglycerin, quinidine, riboflavin, and tetracyclines. Drugs that may decrease catecholamine level include guanethidine, reserpine, and salicylates. Explain the procedure to the client. The client should be on a VMA-restricted diet for 2–3 days before the test. Items restricted include coffee, tea, bananas, chocolate, cocoa, licorice, citrus fruit, anything with vanilla, and aspirin. Client should not take antihypertensive drugs before the test. Initiate 24-hour urine collection.

Specific Gravity

Specific gravity measures the number of solutes in a solution. Urea and uric acid, by-products of nitrogen metabolism, are the greatest influence on urine specific gravity.

Specific gravity increases with excess fluid loss from the body. Renal disease decreases specific gravity.

Urine Glucose

Glucose spills into the urine when the blood level of glucose exceeds the renal threshold (180 mg/dL). Measuring urine glucose is not as accurate as measuring the blood glucose level.

PROFESSIONAL TIP

Testing for Blood Lipid Level
To allow for the proper balance between the vascular and extravascular compartment and ensure valid test results, the blood should always be drawn after the client has been sitting quietly for 5 minutes.

Urine Ketones

Ketones, products of incomplete fat metabolism, are completely metabolized by the liver under normal conditions. The most common cause of ketonuria (excessive ketones in the urine) is diabetes.

Urine Cells and Casts

The urine is normally free of blood cells and casts. In cases of nephritis, renal damage or failure, and urinary stones or infections, the following can occur:

- Bleeding, resulting in RBCs in the urine
- Accumulation of epithelial cells accompanied by cast formation
- WBCs in the urine, indicating infection

Stool Tests

Stool specimens are examined for normal substances (such as urobilinogen) and blood, bacteria, and parasites (Table 25-7).

Urobilinogen

Urobilinogen, a colorless derivative of bilirubin, is formed by the normal action of intestinal flora on bilirubin. It increases in situations of severe hemolysis and decreases with most biliary obstructions.

TABLE 25-7	TESTS PERFORMED ON STOOL	
TEST	**EXPLANATION/NORMAL VALUES**	**NURSING RESPONSIBILITIES**
Stool occult blood (guaiac) Fecal occult blood test (FOBT) Hemoccult	Fecal occult blood screening studies may be utilized as possible indicators of colorectal cancer. Normal: negative for blood	Place a smear of stool on a card. Medications such as anticoagulants, aspirin, iron preparations, NSAIDs, and steroids may cause a false-positive result, whereas vitamin C may cause a false negative. Red meat should not be ingested for 3 days prior to the test. For premenopausal women, wait at least 4 days after menstrual period. Wear gloves when obtaining and handling the specimen.
Stool O & P (ova & parasite)	A positive result indicates infection. Normal: negative	Place the stool specimen in a container and take warm to the laboratory. Usually done 3 times.

Occult Blood

Occult blood is invisible blood in the stool that can be detected only by chemical means or with a microscope. The digestive process in the GI tract acts on blood, making it occult. Random sampling for occult blood is done to diagnose gastrointestinal bleeding, ulcers, and malignant tumors.

To decrease the possibility of a false-positive result when occult blood is to be used to confirm suspicions of a gastrointestinal disorder, the client is placed on a 3-day diet free of meat, poultry, and fish. Drugs causing a false-positive test for occult blood are salicylate, steroids, and indomethacin.

Parasites

The gastrointestinal tract can harbor parasites and their eggs (ova). Whereas some of these parasites are harmless, others cause clinical symptoms. Most common parasites except pinworms (which can enter the body through both the oral and anal routes) enter the body through the mouth when contaminated water or food is ingested.

Culture and Sensitivity Tests

Culture is the growing of microorganisms to identify the pathogen. Culture and **sensitivity** (C&S) tests are performed to identify both the pathogen and its susceptibility to commonly used antibiotics. Sensitivity allows the selection of appropriate antibiotic therapy. All C&S specimens should be immediately taken to the laboratory.

Blood Culture

Bacteremia is bacteria in the blood. A blood culture should be procured while the client is having chills and fever. A series of three collections are performed using strict sterile technique. The needle should be changed after the specimen is collected and before injecting the blood sample into the test tube.

Throat (Swab) Culture

The throat normally hosts many organisms. Throat cultures identify such pathogens as beta-hemolytic streptococci, *Staphylococcus aureus*, meningococci, gonococci, *Bordetella pertussis,* and *Corynebacterium diphtheria*. A throat swab is commonly done to identify streptococcal infections, which can cause rheumatic fever or glomerulonephritis if left untreated.

To obtain a throat swab, use a wooden blade to depress the tongue and swab the white patches, exudate, or ulcerations of the throat with a sterile applicator. The applicator should not touch any other parts of the mouth. The applicator is then placed in a sterile container.

Sputum Culture

Sputum tests include culture, smear, and cytology. Sputum, created by the mucous glands and goblet cells of the tracheobronchial tree, is sterile until it reaches the throat and mouth, where it comes in contact with normal flora. For a more accurate identification of pulmonary organisms, sputum can be obtained by tracheobronchial suctioning and transtracheal aspiration.

In addition to the organism(s) found in a culture, a sputum smear identifies eosinophils, epithelial cells, and other substances. Smears help diagnose asthma (eosinophils) and fungal infections. The specimen must be refrigerated if it cannot be taken immediately to the laboratory.

PROFESSIONAL TIP

Cultures

All culture tests should be performed before initiating antibiotic therapy so as to identify the type of pathogen and its sensitivity to specific antibiotics.

Sputum **cytology** (the study of cells) is performed to diagnose cancer of the lungs. The specimen should be collected early in the morning and after a deep cough.

Urine Culture

Urinary C&S tests are performed whenever a urinary tract infection is suspected.

Stool Culture

Stool C&S is performed to identify bacterial infections. If the client has diarrhea, a rectal swab can be taken and used as a specimen, but fecal material must be visible on the swab for the laboratory to perform the test.

Papanicolaou Test

The **Papanicolaou test** (a smear method of examining stained exfoliative cells), commonly called a Pap smear,

evaluates the metabolic activity, cellular maturity, and morphological variations of cervical tissue. Papanicolaou testing can also be done on specimens from other organs, such as gastric secretions and bronchial aspirations.

RADIOLOGICAL STUDIES

Radiography (the study of film exposed to x-rays or gamma rays through the action of ionizing radiation) is used by the practitioner to study internal organ structure. When used in conjunction with a **contrast medium** (a radiopaque substance that facilitates roentgen imaging of the body's internal structures), **fluoroscopy** (immediate, serial images of the body's structure and function) reveals the motion of organs. X-rays are valuable in formulating a diagnosis and helping to determine if other studies (e.g., a lung lesion requiring biopsy to differentiate between a benign or malignant tumor) are necessary.

Some radiological tests require a contrast medium such as barium and iodine that often interferes with other diagnostic studies. Draw a blood sample for thyroid function before beginning an intravenous pyelogram (IVP), where radioactive iodine dye is administered. If a client needs both an IVP and a barium enema, perform the IVP first because the barium is likely to decrease kidney visualization. Commonly performed radiological studies are described in Table 25-8.

Text continues on p. 507

TABLE 25-8 RADIOLOGIC STUDIES

TEST	EXPLANATION/NORMAL VALUES	NURSING RESPONSIBILITIES
Radiograph (x-ray)	Most common diagnostic study. Identifies traumatic disorders, i.e., fractures, dislocations, tumors, bone disorders, joint deformities, bone density, and changes in bone relationships. Performed by a technician.	Explain the procedure to the client. Prepare the client as ordered. No specific post procedure care is required. Administer an analgesic, especially for the arthritic client.
Abdominal x-rays	Determines diaphragm position and gas and fluid distribution in the abdomen.	No preparation is required.
Adrenal angiography, Adrenal arteriogram	Study of adrenal glands and arterial system after injection of radiopaque dye to detect benign or malignant tumors or hyperplasia of the adrenal glands. Normal: no growth or enlargement	Assess for allergy to shellfish or iodine; arteriosclerosis; pregnancy; or blood disorders, as they preclude the test. Explain the procedure to the client. Assess for allergies. Informed and written consent must be obtained before the procedure. Note whether client has been taking anticoagulants. *continues*

TABLE 25-8   continued

TEST	EXPLANATION/NORMAL VALUES	NURSING RESPONSIBILITIES
Adrenal angiography, Adrenal arteriogram (continued)		Initiate NPO status after midnight. Mark peripheral pulses with a pen before the procedure. Inform the client that a warm flush may be felt when the dye is injected. Observe the puncture site. Monitor vital signs. Monitor peripheral pulses, color, and temperature of extremities. Institute bed rest for 12–24 hours. Apply cold compresses to puncture site, if needed. Force fluids to prevent possible dehydration from the dye.
Adrenal venography	Involves insertion of a catheter through the femoral vein and into the adrenal vein to withdraw a blood specimen to detect the function of each adrenal gland. A contrast dye is injected to visualize size and position of the adrenal glands. Normal: no growth or enlargement	Explain the procedure to the client. Assess for allergies. Obtain informed and written consent. Inform the client that a burning sensation may be experienced when the dye is injected. Although this study involves the venous system, monitor vital signs and injection site as well as pulses, temperature, and color of extremities.
Arthrogram (-graphy)	Visualization of a joint. Radiopaque dye or air is injected into the joint cavity to outline soft tissue, usually on knee/shoulder joints. Local anesthetic and sterile technique are used. Performed by a physician; takes approximately 30 minutes. Normal: absence of lesions, fractures, or tears	Explain the procedure to the client. Obtain informed consent. Client wears an elastic bandage for several days; check for edema. Administer a mild analgesic for pain. Monitor for increased pain. Neither fasting nor sedation is required.
Barium enema	An enema of barium is given while x-rays are taken of the large intestine.	Initiate NPO status the night before. Administer the ordered medication to clean the bowel. Observe the results of the laxatives, and inform the x-ray department if there have been no results. After the test, force oral fluids and administer a cleansing enema, as ordered. Document status of abdomen and stools.
Barium swallow	The client drinks a glass of barium while x-rays are taken of the esophagus and cardiac sphincter.	Initiate NPO status the evening before. Explain the procedure and the time frame for results. Encourage the client to drink fluids and eat fiber after the test. A laxative is sometimes given after the test. The client should be instructed that bowel movements will be white for 1–2 days. During the test, the client will be tilted on the x-ray table in various positions. There may be repeated pictures taken at $^1/_2$-hour intervals as the barium moves through the bowel. Document the client's tolerance of the procedure and passage of the barium. Because the procedure can be lengthy, encourage the client to take reading material.
Cardiac catheterization (cardiac angiogram, coronary arteriogram)	A catheter is passed into the right and/or left side of the heart to determine oxygen level, cardiac output, and pressure within the heart chambers.	Assess the client for allergy to iodine or shellfish. The client is to fast for 6 hours prior to the test, but medications can be taken with sips of water. Inform the client of the possibility of feeling warm or flushed during the test. After the procedure, assess the peripheral pulses every 15 minutes for 2–4 hours, or according to physician's orders. Assess color, temperature, and pulse in the extremity below the catheter insertion site. Instruct the client to keep the involved extremity straight for 6–8 hours. *continues*

TABLE 25-8 continued

TEST	EXPLANATION/NORMAL VALUES	NURSING RESPONSIBILITIES
Chest x-ray	Provides a two-dimensional image of the lungs without using contrast media. Used to detect the presence of fluid within the interstitial lung tissue or the alveoli; tumors or foreign bodies; and the presence and size of a pneumothorax. The size of the heart can also be determined by chest x-ray.	Explain the test to the client. If appropriate, inquire whether the client may be pregnant, to prevent exposure of the fetus to x-ray. The client is generally required to stand for various views; if the client is unable to stand, views may be obtained with the client in a sitting position, or a portable x-ray may be obtained. Instruct the client to inspire deeply and hold the breath. Instruct the client to remove all metal objects from the chest and neck area and to don a hospital gown that does not have snap closures.
Conduitogram	Radiopaque dye is injected through a catheter into either the conduit or a piece of ileum to assess by means of x-ray the length and emptying ability of the conduit as well as the presence of stricture or obstruction.	A conduit is a connection between the bladder or pouch and the outside of the body. Explain the procedure to the client. Assess the client for allergies to iodine-based dye.
Fistula gram	Radiopaque dye or barium is given to drink, and x-rays are taken as the dye or barium passes through the gastrointestinal tract. The dye shows the location of the fistula and how it is connected to the gastrointestinal tract.	Initiate NPO status as ordered. Explain the procedure and the time frame for the results and identify the person who will give the client the results.
Fluoresce in angiography	Following IV injection of sodium fluorescein, rapid-sequence photographs of the fundus are taken with a special camera. Visualization of microvascular structures of the retina and choroid are enhanced, allowing evaluation of the entire retinal vascular bed.	Instill eye drops to dilate the pupils. Start an IV so the sodium fluorescein can be injected. Remove the IV following completion of the test. Inform the client that skin and urine may be yellow for 24–48 hours.
Gallbladder series	X-ray visualization of the gallbladder.	Administer dye tablets the evening before the test. Provide a low-fat or fat-free meal the evening before. Initiate NPO status except for water after taking the dye.
Hysterosalpingogram	Radiopaque dye is instilled through the cervix. Used to diagnose uterine cavity and tubal abnormalities. Performed as a part of an infertility workup.	Explain the procedure and prepare the client in the lithotomy position. The test is done in the radiology department. Inquire about allergies to iodine or other dyes. Assist the physician.
Intravenous pyelogram (IVP)	Infusion of radiopaque dye into a vein, allowing visualization of the urinary system. The renal pelvis, ureters, and bladder can be seen. If BUN is over 40 mg/dL, the test may not be performed.	Explain the procedure to the client. Explain that client will experience a warm feeling during dye injection. Ask the client about allergy to iodine or shellfish. Serve a light supper, then initiate NPO status overnight. Administer a laxative or enema. Schedule test before barium studies. Post-test, observe for untoward reaction to dye. Encourage fluids for 24 hours to eliminate dye.
Kidney-ureter-bladder x-ray (KUB)	Shows abnormalities such as calculi, tumors, or changes in anatomic position.	Explain the procedure to the client. No preparation is required.
Long bone x-rays	Serial x-rays of the long bones to determine bone growth.	Explain the procedure to the client. Instruct the client to keep extremities still while the x-ray is being taken. Shield ovaries, testes, or pregnant uterus. Remove all metallic objects from area being x-rayed. *continues*

TABLE 25-8 continued

TEST	EXPLANATION/NORMAL VALUES	NURSING RESPONSIBILITIES
Lymphangiogram	A contrast dye is injected into the lymph vessels in the hands or feet to examine the lymph vessels and nodes. Used to stage lymphomas and evaluate the effectiveness of chemotherapy and radiation therapy. Normal: Normal-sized lymph nodes with no malignant cells	The dye remains in the lymph nodes for 6 months to 1 year, so disease progress can be evaluated with an x-ray. Obtain informed consent. Inform the client that if a blue-colored dye is used, the skin and urine may have a bluish discoloration. Assess the client's breath sounds after the procedure, as lipoid pneumonia is a possible complication if the dye gets into the thoracic duct.
Mammography	Used to diagnose benign and malignant disorders of the breast.	Explain the procedure to the client. The breast will be compressed, possibly causing discomfort for several seconds. Explain that it is important to have a baseline mammogram done between the ages of 35 and 40 and a breast examination done by a physician or nurse practitioner every 3–4 years. For women ages 40–49, a mammogram should be performed every 1–2 years; for those over 50, an annual mammogram is recommended along with an annual breast examination by physician or nurse practitioner.
Myelogram	X-ray of spinal subarachnoid space following injection of an opaque medium.	Follow nursing responsibilities for lumbar puncture in Table 25-14. Inform the client that the table may be tilted during the procedure. Obtain informed consent according to facility guidelines. Withhold the meal prior to procedure. Administer a light sedative, if ordered. Postprocedure care is determined by the type of medium used; follow physician's orders for activity and fluids.
Pouchogram	Installation of radiopaque dye into the Kock or Indiana pouch. Done with the continent ostomies to determine the state of healing and size of the pouch created.	Assess the client for allergy to iodine. Explain the procedure to the client.
Pulmonary angiography	Assesses the arterial circulation of the lungs. Most often used to detect pulmonary emboli.	Explain the procedure to the client. Assess for allergy to iodine or shellfish. Inform the client that an arterial puncture is required, usually of the femoral artery, and that injection of the dye may cause a flushing or warm sensation due to vasodilation. After the study, assess the arterial puncture site frequently for evidence of bleeding. Assess vital signs and respiratory status. The client may be required to lie flat for up to 6 hours if the femoral artery is used for access. Obtain informed consent per facility policy.
Renal angiography	A catheter is inserted into the femoral artery and threaded into the renal artery. Dye is injected to show blood vessels in the kidney.	Initiate NPO status; administer enema. Assess client for allergy to iodine or shellfish. Check vital signs and peripheral pulses. Institute post-test bedrest, with leg straight. Monitor vital signs, peripheral pulses, urine output, and puncture site. *continues*

TABLE 25-8 continued

TEST	EXPLANATION/NORMAL VALUES	NURSING RESPONSIBILITIES
Voiding cystourethrography	The bladder is filled with dye, and x-rays are taken to observe bladder filling and emptying. Detects structural abnormalities of the bladder and urethra and reflux into the ureters.	Administer enema. Insert a Foley catheter and inject dye into bladder while x-rays are taken. Remove catheter and ask the client to void while more x-rays are taken. Allow the client to express feelings, as this test may be embarrassing.
Computed tomography (CT) scan	Provides a three-dimensional cross-sectional view of tissues. Computer-constructed picture interprets densities of various tissues. Most useful for viewing tumors in the chest, abdominal cavity, and brain.	Explain the procedure to the client. Obtain informed consent. Remove wigs and hairpins and clips for head CT. Initiate NPO status 8 hours prior to scan. Assess for iodine allergy. Observe for signs of anaphylaxis, if dye is used. Check for claustrophobia. Inform the client that the test will take approximately 45 minutes to 1 hour. The client must lie still on a hard, flat table and will be put through a large machine. Because barium will interfere with the test, schedule tests using barium either after or 4 or more days before the scan.
Cardiac positron emission tomography (PET) scan	Radioactive tracers are injected intravenously prior to the test. Nuclear imaging is used to confirm tissue that has adequate blood supply and tissue that has become impaired due to a lack of blood.	Instruct the client not to have caffeine, alcohol, or smoke for 24 hours prior to the test. Initiate NPO status from 10 P.M. the evening before the test, except for medications and water. Obtain informed written consent. Encourage the client to drink fluids after the procedure to facilitate faster excretion of the radioactive material.
Orbital CT scan	Allows visualization of abnormalities not readily seen on standard x-rays, delineating size, position, and relationship to adjoining structures. The orbital CT is a series of images reconstructed by a computer and displayed as anatomic slices on an oscilloscope. It identifies space-occupying lesions earlier and more accurately than do other x-ray techniques. It also provides three-dimensional images of orbital structures, especially the ocular muscles and optic nerve. the Enhancement with a contrast agent may help define ocular tissue and circulation abnormalities.	Explain the test and the procedure to the client: that the client is positioned on an x-ray table; that the head of the table is moved into the scanner; that the scanner rotates during the test and may make loud, crackling sounds; that if an IV contrast agent is required, the client may feel flushed and warm or experience a transient headache; and that salty taste, nausea, and vomiting may occur following injection of the IV contrast dye. Reassure the client that the reaction is common and she may signal the technician if she is unable to tolerate the test.

CRITICAL THINKING

Test Scheduling

The physician orders gallbladder x-rays, a barium swallow, and a barium enema for a client. In which order should these tests be scheduled? Why?

 Safety: X-rays
- Question the client about the possibility of pregnancy, asthma, and allergic reactions to contrast media (iodine), as well as to other foods and drugs, before scheduling x-rays.
- If the client has not previously received iodine, note this on the requisition to indicate that allergic status is unknown.

Chest X-Ray

The chest x-ray is the most common radiological study. Chest x-rays are taken from various views (Figure 25-3), because multiple views of the chest are needed to assess the entire lung field. To prepare for a chest x-ray, the client should remove all clothing from the waist up and don a gown. The client should also remove all metal objects (jewelry) because metal will appear on the x-ray film, thereby obscuring visualization of parts of the chest. Pregnant women are advised against x-rays; however, if x-ray is absolutely necessary, the woman should be draped with a lead apron to protect the fetus.

Computed Tomography

Computed tomography (CT) is the radiological scanning of the body. X-ray beams and radiation detectors transmit data to a computer that transcribes the data into quantitative measurement and multidimensional

Figure 25-3 *Radiographic Projection Positions*

Figure 25-4 *Computed Tomography*

images of the internal structures. Figure 25-4 illustrates the sagittal, transverse, and coronal planes used in CT scanning.

The procedure requires the client's informed consent. The client's cooperation is essential during CT scanning because the client will be positioned and asked to remain motionless. Prepare the client by providing an explanation and pictures of what to expect.

Safety: Contrast Media
If a contrast medium is used, observe the client for indicators of allergic reaction to the dye, such as respiratory distress, urticaria, hives, nausea, vomiting, decreased production of urine (**oliguria**), and decreased blood pressure.

Barium Studies

Barium (a chalky white contrast medium) is a preparation that permits roentgenographic visualization of the internal structures of the digestive tract. Barium studies can reveal congenital abnormalities, reflux, spasm, stricture, obstruction, inflammation, ulceration, lesions, varices, and fistula.

Angiography

Angiography allows visualization of vascular structures by using fluoroscopy and a contrast medium. It

---

PROFESSIONAL TIP

Computed Tomography
Assess the client's ability to relax, and review imagery relaxation. Sedation can be administered with an order from the practitioner.

shows blood flow to the heart, lungs, brain, kidneys, lower extremities, and is useful in diagnosing an **aneurysm** (weakness in the wall of a blood vessel).

Arteriography

Arteriography is the radiographic study of the vascular system after radiopaque dye is injected through a catheter. Using fluoroscopy, the catheter is threaded through a peripheral artery into the area to be studied, such as the aorta or the cerebral, coronary, pulmonary, renal, iliac, femoral, or popliteal artery. With the client on a cardiac monitor, dye is injected through the vascular catheter, and a rapid sequence of films is taken.

Dye Injection Studies

Iodine, a common dye used in radiographic studies, might cause the client to experience the following temporary symptoms: shortness of breath, nausea, and a warm to hot flushed sensation. Most dye injection studies are invasive and thus require written informed consent.

ULTRASONOGRAPHY

An **ultrasound,** also called an echogram or sonogram, is a noninvasive procedure using high-frequency sound waves to visualize deep body structures. To ensure accuracy, this procedure should be scheduled before studies using a contrast medium or air, because the contrast medium would reflect the sound waves differently than body structures do. The client must lie still during the procedure.

Ultrasound is used to evaluate the brain, thyroid gland, heart, abdominal aorta, vascular structures, liver, gallbladder, pancreas, spleen, and pelvis. During pregnancy, an ultrasound is commonly done to evaluate the size of the fetus and placenta. A full bladder is needed to ensure visualization.

To increase the contact between the skin and the **transducer** (instrument that converts electrical energy to sound waves), a coupling agent (lubricant) is placed on the surface of the body area to be studied. The transducer sends sound waves through the body tissue, which are reflected back and recorded. The varying density of body tissues deflects the waves into a differentiated pattern on an oscilloscope. Photographs are taken of the sound wave pattern on the oscilloscope. Table 25-9 describes some ultrasound tests.

MAGNETIC RESONANCE IMAGING

Magnetic resonance imaging (MRI) uses radiowaves and a strong magnetic field to make continuous cross-sectional images of the body. During the study, a noniodine IV paramagnetic contrast agent may be used. The study reveals lesions and changes in the body's organs, tissues, and vascular and skeletal structures (Table 25-10).

TABLE 25-9   ULTRASOUND TESTS

TEST	EXPLANATION/NORMAL VALUES	NURSING RESPONSIBILITIES
Ultrasound	High-frequency ultrasound waves are sent into the body, and echoes are recorded as they strike tissues of different densities, producing an image or photograph. Useful in distinguishing between cystic and solid masses. Most often used to assess the pelvis, heart, and abdomen. Diagnostic for cysts, tumors, pregnancy, fetal gestational age, and multiple gestation.	Explain the procedure to the client. Most ultrasound tests require no special preparation: Pelvic sonogram: Instruct the client to have a full bladder. Abdominal sonogram: Initiate NPO status at bedtime; prepare bowel as directed. Gallbladder sonogram: Initiate NPO status for 12 hours and institute a fat-free diet the evening before the test. Vaginal sonogram: Client does not need to have a full bladder.
Doppler ultrasound	Determines patency of veins and arteries in conditions such as arterial occlusive disease, arteriosclerotic disease, or Raynaud's disease. Normal: audible "swishing" sound of the Doppler when placed over vessel. A Doppler unit with blood pressure cuffs can measure the pulse volume of arteries and veins. An AB index is obtained by dividing the blood pressure reading in the ankle by the blood pressure reading in the arm (brachial artery). This is known as the ankle-to-brachial arterial blood pressure. There should be a less than 20 mm Hg difference between the pressure in the lower extremity as compared to the pressure in the upper extremity. Normal, AB index: 0.85 or greater	Inform the client that the procedure is painless. Remove clothing from the extremity being evaluated. Instruct the client not to smoke for 30 minutes prior to the test, because nicotine causes vasoconstriction of the vessels. Remove conductive or acoustic gel from the skin after the test is completed.

continues

TABLE 25-9   continued

TEST	EXPLANATION/NORMAL VALUES	NURSING RESPONSIBILITIES
Echocardiogram	An ultrasound of the heart to determine hypertrophies, cardiomyopathies, or congenital defects. Very helpful in diagnosing valve abnormalities and pericardial effusion.	Explain the procedure to the client and assure the client that there is no discomfort during the procedure, although some pressure may be felt on the chest wall from the transducer.
Thyroid ultrasound	Detects the size, shape, and position of the thyroid gland.	Explain the procedure to the client: that the client will lie supine, with the neck hyperextended; that breathing or swallowing will not be affected by the sound transducer; that a liberal amount of lubricating gel will be placed on the neck for the transducer; and that a series of photos will be taken over a 15-minute period. Assist the client in removing the lubricant.
Transrectal bladder ultrasound	Produces an image of the prostate or bladder and surrounding tissue.	Explain the procedure to the client.

TABLE 25-10   MAGNETIC RESONANCE IMAGING

TEST	EXPLANATION/NORMAL VALUES	NURSING RESPONSIBILITIES
Magnetic resonance imaging (MRI)	Uses magnetic field and radio waves to detect edema, hemorrhage, blood flow, infarcts, tumors, infections, aneurysms, demyelinating disease, muscular disease, skeletal abnormalities, intervertebral disk problems, and causes of spinal cord compression. Provides greater tissue discrimination than do chest x-ray or CT scans. Performed by qualified technologist. Takes approximately 1 hour.	Assess the client for the presence of metal objects within the body (i.e., shrapnel, cochlear implants, pacemakers). Explain the procedure to the client: the client will be required to lie still for up to 20 minutes at a time; the client will be placed within a scanning tunnel; sedation may be required if the client has claustrophobic tendencies; the magnet will make a loud thumping noise as images are obtained (provide earplugs as necessary). As the test may require up to 2 hours to perform, have the client void prior to entering the scanning tunnel. Obtain informed written consent, per facility policy.

NUCLEAR SCANS

Radionuclide imaging (nuclear scanning) uses radionuclides (or radiopharmaceuticals) to show morphological and functional changes in the body's structure. A scintigraphic scanner, placed over the area of study, detects emitted radiation and produces a visual image. The results reveal congenital abnormalities, skeletal changes, infections, lesions, and glandular and organ enlargement (Table 25-11). For all nuclear scans, written informed consent is required. The client must remove all jewelry and metal objects.

ELECTRODIAGNOSTIC STUDIES

Electrodiagnostic tests measure electrical activity of the brain, heart, and skeletal muscles. Electrical sensors (electrodes) are placed at certain points to measure the velocity, tone, and direction of the impulses. The impulses are then transmitted to an oscilloscope or printed on graphic paper. Table 25-12 describes the various electrodiagnostic studies.

Electroencephalography

An **electroencephalogram** (EEG) is the graphic recording of the brain's electrical activity. During the procedure, electrodes are placed on the client's scalp. The electrodes transmit impulses from the brain to an EEG machine. The machine amplifies the brain's impulses and records the waves on strips of paper. An EEG can reveal not only the presence of a seizure disorder or intracranial lesion but also the type. The absence of the brain's electrical activity is used to confirm death.

Electrocardiography

An **electrocardiogram** (EKG or ECG) is a graphic, noninvasive recording of the heart's electrical activity.

TABLE 25-11   NUCLEAR SCANS

TEST	EXPLANATION/NORMAL VALUES	NURSING RESPONSIBILITIES
Scan (radioisotope test)	A radioactive substance or isotope is taken up by the part of the body being examined. Organ sites most frequently studied are the liver, spleen, lungs, heart, urinary tract, thyroid, and brain. The radioactive substance is given orally or intravenously by nuclear medicine personnel.	Explain the procedure to the client: that the client must lie still for 30–60 minutes and that the machine makes clicking noise at times. For liver, spleen, lung, thyroid, and brain scans, no special preparation is required. For a heart scan, initiate NPO status the evening before. For a kidney scan, hydrate as ordered.
Radioactive iodine uptake (RAIU), iodine uptake test, ^{131}I uptake	Uses oral radioactive iodine to determine thyroid function by the thyroid's ability to trap and retain iodine. Normal: 2 hours: 4%–12% absorbed 6 hours: 6%–15% absorbed 24 hours: 8%–30% absorbed	The client who is allergic to iodine or shellfish or is pregnant should not have the test. Client should fast overnight. Drugs that decrease RAIU level include ACTH, antihistamines, saturated solution of potassium iodine, thyroid drugs, antithyroid drugs, and tolbutamide.
Radionuclide angiography (multiplegated radioisotope scan, multigated acquisition scanning, MUGA)	A radioisotope is injected to evaluate the function of the left ventricle. The ejection fraction (a comparison of the volume of blood pumped by the left ventricle to the total volume of blood left in the ventricle) is measured.	
Technetium pyrophosphate scanning	Important in diagnosing acute MIs, with the best accuracy obtained at 48 hours after the client experiences symptoms suggestive of an infarct. A tracer or radioisotope, which is injected intravenously, accumulates in the damaged or infarcted tissue areas, called "hot spots."	Instruct the client not to smoke or consume caffeine or alcohol for 3 hours before the test. Inform the client that the test will take 45–60 minutes.
Ventilation-perfusion scan (lung scan)	Assesses ventilation and perfusion of the lungs. Most often used to detect the presence of pulmonary emboli.	Assess for allergy to iodine and shellfish. Explain the procedure to the client: that a radioactive contrast media will be introduced via an IV access and inhalation of radioactive gas and that the client will be required to hold the breath for short periods as images are obtained.

TABLE 25-12   ELECTRODIAGNOSTIC STUDIES

TEST	EXPLANATION/NORMAL VALUES	NURSING RESPONSIBILITIES
Electrocardiogram (EKG or ECG)	Electrodes are placed on the skin to record wave patterns of the electrical conduction of the heart. Detects myocardial damage, rhythmic disturbances, and hyperkalemia.	Explain the procedure to the client. Inform the client that the test is painless.
Electroencephalogram (EEG)	Record of electrical activity generated in the brain and obtained through electrodes applied to the scalp or microelectrodes placed in brain tissue during surgery.	Withhold caffeine due to stimulant effect. Serve meal so that blood sugar will not be altered. Shampoo hair night before test. Explain the procedure to the client: that the test takes approximately 45 minutes to 2 hours; the procedure is painless; the client may be asked to open and close the eyes during the test and that there may be flashing lights or small electrical stimulations.

continues

TABLE 25-12   continued

TEST	EXPLANATION/NORMAL VALUES	NURSING RESPONSIBILITIES
Electromyography (EMG)	Detects primary muscular disorders. A needle electrode is inserted into the muscle being examined. Measures electrical activity of skeletal muscle at rest and during voluntary muscle contraction.	Explain the procedure to the client. Obtain informed written consent. Instruct the client to refrain from consuming caffeine and smoking for 3 hours before the test. Assure client that the needle will not cause electrocution. Inform the client that there will be temporary discomfort when the needle electrode is inserted. Observe the site for hematoma or inflammation after the test. The procedure takes approximately 1 hour.
Electroretinogram (ERG)	A record of the changes in the retina's electric potential following stimulation by light. Clinically useful in some clients with retinal disease. Performed by placing a contact lens electrode on the anesthetized cornea. The electrical potential recorded on the cornea is identical to the response that would be obtained if the electrodes were placed directly on the surface of the retina.	Explain the test and procedure to the client.
Esophageal motility studies (manometry)	Evaluates muscle contractions and coordination by using a tube with transducers. Used as a diagnostic tool for disorders of the esophagus and lower esophageal sphincter (LES).	Initiate NPO status 6–8 hours prior to the test.
Holter monitor	A portable EKG monitors and records the electrical conduction of the heart for a period of 24 hours. The heart rhythm is compared to client activities.	Instruct the client to engage in normal daily activities and to keep a journal of symptoms experienced in performing these activities.
Stress test	An EKG taken as the client exercises. Evaluates the effects of exercise on the heart. Often, the client is asked to walk on a treadmill, the incline of which is elevated at various times throughout the test. Used frequently on clients who have CAD.	Explain the procedure to the client. Encourage the client to wear good walking shoes during the test.
Thallium test (myocardial perfusion scan)	A radioactive tracer (Thallium^{201}) is injected and accumulates in myocardial tissue that is well perfused. Accumulation is lessened in areas of myocardial tissue that are not well perfused, areas called "cold spots." The client may be asked to perform exercise, such as riding a bike, during the test to evaluate the perfusion of myocardial tissue during exercise.	Instruct the client to refrain from eating and drinking for 3 hours prior to the test.

Lubricated electrodes are applied to the chest wall and extremities. The client is asked to lie still during the test. The pain-free test can reveal abnormal transmission of impulses and electrical position of the heart's axis.

A portable cardiac monitor (Holter monitor) records the heart's electrical activity, producing a continuous recording over a specified time (e.g., 24 hours) (Figure 25-5). It allows the client to ambulate and perform regular activities. Clients keep a log of activities resulting in the heart beating faster or irregularly. The EKG tracing is reviewed in relation to the client's log to determine if certain activities, such as walking, are associated with abnormal transmission of impulses.

Stress Test

A **stress test** measures the client's cardiovascular fitness. It shows the myocardium's ability to respond to increased oxygen requirements (the result of exercise) by increasing the blood flow to the coronary arteries.

Figure 25-5 *Holter Monitor*

The client walks on a treadmill while connected to an EKG machine. Continuous EKG recordings are made during frequent changes in the treadmill's slope and speed. If the client experiences any symptoms of decreased cardiac output (chest pain, dyspnea, fatigue, or ischemic changes revealed by the EKG monitor), the test is stopped immediately.

Thallium Test

Thallium[201] is a radioactive isotope that emits gamma rays and closely resembles potassium. Although a radioactive study, the thallium test is discussed here because it is often performed in conjunction with an EKG. Thallium is rapidly absorbed by normal myocardial tissue but is slowly absorbed by areas with poor blood flow and damaged cells. During the test, thallium is administered intravenously and the scanner detects the radiation and makes a visual image. The light areas on the image represent heavy isotope uptake (normal myocardial tissue), whereas the dark areas represent poor isotope uptake (poor blood flow and damaged cells).

There are two types of thallium test: resting imaging and stress imaging. Resting imaging can detect a myocardial infarction within its first few hours. Stress imaging (thallium stress test) is performed while the client is on a treadmill and being monitored with an EKG. At peak stress, the IV thallium is injected. Scanning is performed in 3 to 5 minutes and again in 2 to 3 hours. The test is stopped immediately if the client becomes symptomatic for ischemia.

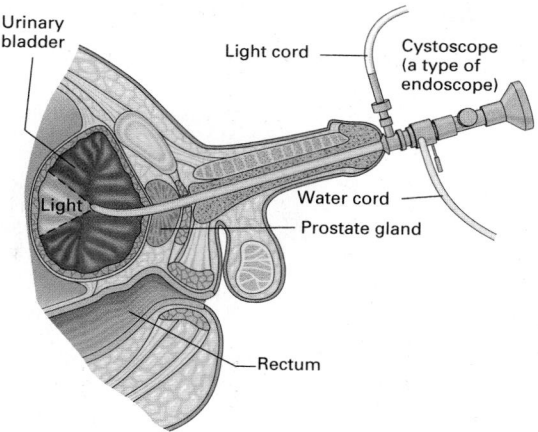

Figure 25-6 *Cystoscope*

ENDOSCOPY

Endoscopy is the visualization of a body organ or cavity through a scope. An endoscope (a metal or fiberoptic tube) is inserted directly into the body structure to be studied (Figure 25-6). A light and, in some studies, a camera at the end of the scope allow the practitioner to assess, via direct visualization or television picture, for lesions and structural problems. The endoscope has an opening at the distant tip that allows the practitioner to administer an anesthetic agent and to lavage, suction, and biopsy tissue. Common endoscopic procedures are listed in Table 25-13.

After the procedure, monitor vital signs, observe for bleeding, and assess for procedural risks (e.g., return of the gag and swallowing reflexes following a bronchoscopy performed under local anesthesia).

ASPIRATION/BIOPSY

Aspiration is performed to withdraw fluid that has abnormally collected or to obtain a specimen. To minimize client discomfort when the skin is pierced by the needle, a local anesthetic is administered in the area to be studied.

A hollow-bore needle with stylet is used to pierce the skin. The stylet is withdrawn once the needle is in place, leaving only the outer needle to aspirate the fluid. A **biopsy** (excision of a small amount of tissue) can be obtained during aspiration or in conjunction with other diagnostic tests (e.g., bronchoscopy). Table 25-14 outlines various aspiration/biopsy procedures.

Bone Marrow Aspiration/Biopsy

The iliac crest and sternum are common sites for bone marrow puncture. A fluid specimen (aspiration) or a core of marrow cells (biopsy) can be obtained. Both tests are often done to obtain the best possible marrow specimen. The test identifies anemias; cancers such as multiple myeloma, leukemia, or Hodgkin's disease; or the client's response to chemotherapy.

TABLE 25-13 ENDOSCOPIC PROCEDURES

TEST	EXPLANATION/NORMAL VALUES	NURSING RESPONSIBILITIES
Endoscopy	Permits visual examination of internal structures of the body using specially designed instruments. The observation may be done through a natural body opening or through a small incision. A biopsy of suspicious areas may then be done for further study.	Explain the procedure to the client. Initiate NPO status 8–10 hours before test, except for sigmoidoscopy, before which a liquid diet should be followed for several days prior to the examination. Administer a laxative and then a cleansing enema.
Arthroscopy	Endoscopic procedure for direct visualization of a joint. Done in an operating room under sterile conditions and local or general anesthesia.	Perform frequent neurovascular checks. Elevate the client's leg. Apply compression dressing. Administer analgesic for discomfort.
Bronchoscopy	Direct visual examination of the bronchi through a fiber optic scope. Used to remove foreign bodies, for aggressive pulmonary cleansing, and to obtain sputum and tissue specimens.	Obtain written informed consent per facility policy. Explain the procedure to the client: that the client must be NPO for at least 6 hours prior to the test; that, if ordered, preprocedure sedation is administered; that an IV access will be obtained and sedation given during the procedure via this route. Following the procedure, frequently assess vital signs and respiratory status. Assess the client for unusual amounts of bleeding. Inform the client that sputum may be blood tinged initially following the procedure. Maintain the client in a side-lying position until the gag reflex returns. Withhold all food and fluids until the client is fully awake and has a gag reflex.
Colonoscopy	Examination of the rectum, colon, cecum, and ileocecal valve.	Initiate sedation. Cleanse the bowel. Offer only clear liquids after cleansing. Initiate NPO status for 6–8 hours prior to the test. Inform the client that flatulence and cramping will be experienced after the test.
Cystoscopy	A cystoscope is passed through the urethra and into the bladder to examine the interior of the bladder for inflammation, stones, tumors, or congenital abnormalities. A biopsy may be performed, and small stones may be removed. Ureteral catheters may be inserted to obtain urine from each kidney. May require topical, spinal or general anaesthesia.	Explain the procedure to the client. Obtain informed written consent. Check vital signs. Instruct in deep breathing, if general anesthesia is to be used. Allow a full liquid diet if topical anesthetic is to be used. Monitor I&O.
Endoscopic retrograde cholangiopancreatogram (ERCP)	Examination of the common bile duct (CBD) and biliary and pancreatic systems following injection of dye. Sphincterotomy, stone crushing, and stone removal can be done.	Initiate sedation. X-ray is used in conjunction. Initiate NPO status 6–8 hours prior to examination. Inform the client that the test can last up to 2 hours.
Esophagogastro-duodenoscopy (EGD)	Examination of the esophagus, stomach, and duodenum. Biopsies can be taken, and dilations done.	Initiate sedation. Initiate NPO status 6–8 hours prior to the examination. Remove dentures and eye wear.
Flexible sigmoidoscopy	Examination of the sigmoid colon and rectum.	Sedation is optional. Administer enemas prior to examination. Inform the client to expect some flatulence and cramping after the examination.
Laparoscopy	Examination of the internal pelvic structures by direct visualization with a laparoscope. Usually performed under general anesthesia. Diagnostic for pelvic disorders and infertility problems.	Explain the procedure to the client. Prepare the client, conduct pre- and postoperative assessment, and institute interventions. Provide discharge instructions on activity and follow-up.

TABLE 25-14 ASPIRATION/BIOPSY PROCEDURES

TEST	EXPLANATION/NORMAL VALUES	NURSING RESPONSIBILITIES
Aspiration Procedures		
Arthrocentesis	Procedure to obtain fluid from a joint using strict sterile technique. The knee is anesthetized, the sterile needle is inserted into joint space, and synovial fluid is aspirated. Used to diagnose infections, crystal-induced arthritis, and synovitis, and to inject anti-inflammatory medications. Normal: RBCs, O; WBCs, 0-150/mm³, neutrophils >25%	Explain the procedure to the client. Obtain written informed consent. Assess site for edema, pain. The client should fast if possible. Apply pressure dressing and ice.
Bone marrow aspiration	Evaluates how well the bone marrow is producing RBCs, WBCs, and platelets. Normal: adequate numbers of RBCs, WBCs, and platelets.	Obtain written informed consent. Inform the client that pressure will be felt when the physician aspirates the bone marrow. Assess the site for bleeding after the procedure is completed. Bed rest for 30 minutes.
Gastric acid stimulation	Determines the amount of hydrochloric (HCl) acid in the stomach. If no HCl acid is present, that indicates parietal cells are malfunctioning. Parietal cells secrete the intrinsic factor that is essential for vitamin B_{12} absorption. Used to diagnose pernicious anemia. Normal tube test: 　Basal acid output: 2–6 mEq/h 　Maximal acid output: 16–26 mEq/h Normal, tubeless test: presence of dye in urine (usually blue or blue-green in color)	If the client is having the tube test, initiate NPO status after midnight and instruct the client not to smoke prior to the test. Inform the client that a nasogastric tube is inserted prior to the test so that gastric contents can be aspirated after the administration of pentagastrin. If the client is having the tubeless test, inform the client of the possibility of a blue or blue-green discoloration of urine. Note any medications taken that affect results; antacids, anticholinergics, and cimetidine (Tagamet) decrease HCl level, whereas adrenergic-blocking agents, cholinergics, steroids, and alcohol elevate HCl level.
Lumbar puncture (LP) (spinal tap)	A needle is inserted into the subarachnoid space to measure CSF pressure and/or to obtain a specimen. Normal pressure: 60–180 mm water pressure Normal specific gravity: 1.007 Normal glucose: 45–100 mg/100 mL Normal complete blood count (CBC): 0 Normal WBC: 0–5 cells/mm³	Obtain informed written consent. Have the client empty the bowel and bladder prior to procedure. Assist in setting up a sterile field and pouring solutions, if not included in the tray. Assist the client to maintain the position. Postprocedure, deliver the specimen to the lab for testing, keep the client flat in bed for 3–24 hours or as ordered by physician; encourage fluid intake to replace fluids lost; and monitor vital and neurological signs.
Paracentesis	Fluid is withdrawn from the abdominal cavity by inserting a needle into the abdomen. The specimen is analyzed for infection or bleeding.	Have the client empty the bladder prior to the procedure. Prepare the abdomen by scrubbing it with a surgical prep solution and draping it with a sterile drape. Postprocedure, dress the site with a sterile dressing and monitor the site for further drainage. Assess vital signs one time postprocedure.
Pericardiocentesis	Fluid is removed from the pericardial sac for analysis or to relieve pressure.	Obtain written informed consent. Position the client in the semi-Fowler's position during the procedure and attach to an EKG monitor. Postprocedure, take vital signs every 15 minutes and monitor EKG rhythm.

continues

TABLE 25-14   continued

TEST	EXPLANATION/NORMAL VALUES	NURSING RESPONSIBILITIES
Thoracentesis	Removal of fluid for diagnostic purposes. May also obtain biopsy, instill medications, and remove fluid for client comfort and safety.	Explain the procedure to the client. Obtain written informed consent. Position the client in an upright sitting position, leaning forward. Have client rest the arms on an overbed table to facilitate this position. Explain to the client that the area will be anesthetized prior to the procedure. Instruct the client to hold as still as possible during the insertion of the thoracentesis needle. Assist the physician during the procedure. Deliver the specimen to the laboratory as soon as possible. Observe the thoracentesis site for bleeding following the procedure. Assess breath sounds before and after the procedure. Report absent breath sounds immediately.
Biopsy procedures	Removal of sample tissue for microscopic study. Tissue may be quickly frozen or placed in formalin before it is chemically stained and thinly sliced for analysis. Frozen section analysis takes only a few minutes and is often completed while a client is still in surgery. The full biopsy analysis takes 24–48 hours to complete but is the most accurate means of establishing a cancer diagnosis. Tissue biopsy is essential to confirming the type of cancer, the amount of lymph node involvement, and whether the cancer was successfully removed.	Explain the procedure to the client. Follow the physician's orders and/or agency protocol for client preparation. Obtain informed written consent.
Breast biopsy	Performed with or without local or general anesthesia and by aspiration, needle biopsy, excision, or incision. Tissue or fluid is obtained and sent to pathology for examination and identification of abnormal cells. New method of obtaining breast biopsies may be done with the stereotactic mammography studies.	Explain the procedure to the client. Have the client undress down to the waist. Cleanse the biopsy region and shave the area, if needed. Drape the breast and adjacent skin. Provide emotional support prior to, during, and following the procedure. Monitor vital signs. Apply a sterile dressing or bandage. Instruct the client in postbiopsy wound care.
Cardiac biopsy	Done during a cardiac catheterization. The tissue sample is taken from the apex or septum to determine toxicity related to drugs; inflammation; or rejection of a transplanted heart.	Preparation is the same as for Cardiac Catheterization (see Table 25-8). After the procedure, observe the client for symptoms of a perforation, such as chest pain, decreased blood pressure, or dyspnea.
Endometrial biopsy	Obtained with special biopsy instruments and used to diagnose endometrial tissue abnormalities.	Explain the procedure to the client. Prepare the tissue preservation agent and label and send the sample to pathology. Assist the client in relaxing during the procedure, to offset the discomfort/cramping she may experience.
Liver biopsy	Obtained by inserting a needle into the liver. May be done with ultrasound or CT scan to guide needle placement. Evaluates cirrhosis, cancer, and hepatitis.	Schedule H&H, PT, PTT, and platelet tests prior to the procedure. Instruct the client to refrain from using NSAIDs including aspirin for 1 week prior to the procedure. Prepare the site by scrubbing it with a surgical prep solution and draping with a sterile towel. Monitor for signs of hemorrhage post procedure by frequently monitoring vital signs and pain. Have the client lie on the right side. Support the biopsy site with a towel or bath blanket for 2 hours. Monitor the site for ecchymosis.
Prostatic biopsy	Removal of a small piece of tissue for microscopic examination.	Monitor for and educate the client about signs and symptoms of hemorrhage, infection, and postprocedure pain.
Testicular biopsy	Determines presence of sperm and rules out vas deferens obstruction.	Monitor for and educate the client about signs and symptoms of infection or hemorrhage.

continues

TABLE 25-14 continued		
TEST	**EXPLANATION/NORMAL VALUES**	**NURSING RESPONSIBILITIES**
Thyroid biopsy	Excision of thyroid tissue for histological examination after noninvasive tests prove abnormal or inconclusive. Can be obtained through needle biopsy or open surgical biopsy under general anesthesia.	Explain the procedure to the client. Obtain informed written consent. Assess for allergies. Have coagulation blood studies done. Assess for bleeding and respiratory and swallowing difficulties after the test. To prevent undue strain on the biopsy site, instruct the client to put both hands behind the neck when sitting up. Warn the client that a sore throat is possible after the biopsy.

Client positioning is determined by the site used: supine for the sternum and side lying for the iliac crest. The site is prepped to decrease the skin's normal flora. Explain to the client that pressure may be experienced as the specimen is withdrawn. The client should hold still because a sudden movement may dislodge the needle.

After the procedure, the client should be kept on bed rest for 1 hour. Monitor vital signs to assess for bleeding (rapid pulse rate, low blood pressure). Instruct client to report to the practitioner any bleeding or signs of inflammation.

Paracentesis

Paracentesis is the aspiration of fluid from the abdominal cavity. It can be diagnostic, therapeutic, or both. With end-stage liver or renal disease, for instance, **ascites** (an accumulation of fluid in the abdomen) occurs. Pressure from ascites can interfere with breathing and gastrointestinal functioning. In this instance, aspiration is therapeutic. If a specimen for culture is taken, it is also diagnostic.

The client should void and be weighed before the procedure. The client should be placed in a high-Fowler's position in a chair or sitting on the side of the bed. The skin is prepped, anesthetized, and punctured with a **trocar** (a sharply pointed surgical instrument contained in a cannula). The trocar is held perpendicular to the abdominal wall and advanced into the peritoneal cavity. The trocar is removed when fluid appears, leaving the inner catheter in place to drain the fluid. The client is observed for changes resulting from the rapid removal of fluid.

After the procedure, a sterile dressing is applied to the puncture site, and the client is monitored for changes in vital signs and electrolytes. Instruct the client to record the color, amount, and consistency of drainage on the dressing after discharge.

Thoracentesis

Thoracentesis is the aspiration of fluids from the pleural cavity. The pleural cavity normally has a small amount of fluid to lubricate the lining between the lungs and pleura. Inflammation, infection, and trauma may cause increased fluid production, which can impair ventilation.

To facilitate access to the rib cage, position the client with the arms crossed and resting on a bedside table (Figure 25-7). The client should not cough during insertion of the trocar. The practitioner selects, preps, and anesthetizes the puncture site. The trocar is usually inserted into the intercostal space at the place of maximum dullness to percussion. This should be above the seventh rib laterally and above the ninth rib posteriorly.

During the procedure, the client must be carefully monitored for symptoms of a **pneumothorax** (collection of air or gas in the pleural space, causing the lungs to collapse), such as dyspnea, pallor, tachycardia, vertigo, and chest pain. After the procedure, assess for signs of cardiopulmonary changes and a mediastinum shift, as indicated by bloody sputum and changes in vital signs.

Cerebrospinal Fluid Aspiration

Lumbar puncture (LP, "spinal tap") is the aspiration of cerebrospinal fluid (CSF) from the subarachnoid space. The specimen is examined for organisms, blood, and tumor cells. A spinal tap is also performed:

Figure 25-7 *Client Position for Thoracentesis*

- To obtain a pressure measurement when blockage is suspected
- During a myelogram
- To instill medications (anesthetics, antibiotics, or chemotherapeutic agents)

The client assumes a lateral recumbent position, with the craniospinal axis parallel to the floor, the flat of the back perpendicular to the procedure table. The client should assume a flexed knee-chest position to bow the back, thereby separating the vertebrae. Most clients require assistance in maintaining this position throughout the procedure. Face the client and place one hand across the client's shoulder blades and the other hand over the client's buttocks.

The practitioner selects, preps, and anesthetizes the puncture site (usually interspace L3–L4, L4–L5, or L5–S1). The needle and stylet are inserted into the midsagittal space and advanced through the longitudinal subarachnoid space (Figure 25-8).

When positioned, the stylet is removed, leaving the needle in place. An initial CSF pressure reading is taken. If the pressure reading is greater than 200 mm H_2O or falls quickly, only 1 or 2 mL of CSF is withdrawn for analysis. If the pressure is less than 200 mm H_2O, an adequate specimen is withdrawn slowly.

After the pressure reading is taken, the stopcock is turned so the CSF slowly flows into a sterile test tube. A sterile cap is placed on the test tube, and the sample is taken to the laboratory. Rapid withdrawal of CSF can cause a transient postural headache. The client's cardiorespiratory status is monitored throughout the procedure.

OTHER TESTS

Other diagnostic tests are described in Table 25-15.

Figure 25-8 *Lumbar puncture: Position of client and insertion of the needle into the subarachnoid space are shown.*

TABLE 25-15 OTHER TESTS		
TEST	**EXPLANATION/NORMAL VALUES**	**NURSING RESPONSIBILITIES**
Arterial plethysmography (pulse volume recorder)	Determines arteriosclerotic disease in the upper extremities and occlusive disease in the lower extremities. Done by applying three blood pressure cuffs to an extremity. The cuffs are connected to a pulse volume recorder, which records the amplitude of each pulse wave. If there is a decrease in the amplitude of the pulse wave, an occlusion is in the artery proximal to the cuff. A decrease of 20 mm Hg of pressure indicates arterial occlusion. The test is not as reliable as arteriography but also does not have the risks associated with an arteriogram. Normal: normal arterial pulse waves	Explain to the client that the test is painless. Instruct the client to lie still during the test. Instruct the client not to smoke for 30 minutes prior to the test. Instruct the client to remove clothing from the extremity on which the test is to be done.

continues

TABLE 25-15 continued

TEST	EXPLANATION/NORMAL VALUES	NURSING RESPONSIBILITIES
Audiometric testing	Evaluates both bone and air conduction and determines the degree of hearing loss. The client wears headphones, through which a series of tones is delivered at different frequencies. The client signals to the audiologist when the tones are audible. The results are recorded on an audiogram. The client is kept in a soundproof booth during the test.	Explain the procedure and its purpose to the client. Ensure that the client is not claustrophobic.
Brainstem auditory-evoked response (ErA and BAER)	Detects hearing dysfunctions of the central nervous system and cochlear nerve (cranial nerve VII). Valuable for testing comatose clients, clients with neurological damage, and children. An altered appearance of the brainstem waveforms or a delay or loss of a waveform indicates an abnormality including a possible cochlear lesion or acoustic neuroma.	Explain the procedure and its purpose to the client particularly that the client will be in a darkened room and will have both electrodes attached to the head and earphones in place.
Caloric test	Assesses alteration in vestibular function. The client is placed in a supine or Fowler's position and each ear is irrigated with cold and then warm water. Cold water causes rotary nystagmus away from injected ear and back to midline; warm water toward injected ear. Most commonly done on comatose clients. A punctured eardrum or Ménière's disease may contraindicate the test.	Explain the procedure and its purpose to the client. Tell the client that nystagmus, vertigo, nausea, vomiting, and an unsteady gait represent a normal response. Stay with the client and have an emesis basin and tissues available.
Color vision tests	Most common color vision tests use pseudoisochromatic (seemingly the same color) plates comprising patterns of dots of the primary colors superimposed on backgrounds of randomly mixed colors. A client with normal vision can identify the patterns; a client with a color deficiency cannot distinguish between pattern and background.	Explain the test and procedure to the client.
Colposcopy	Direct visualization of the vagina and cervix through a high-powered microscope. Acetic acid is applied to the tissue to dehydrate the cells for improved visualization. Used to diagnose cervical dysplasia or carcinoma in situ of the cervix. Biopsies may be obtained as needed.	Explain the procedure and prepare the client in the dorsal lithotomy position. Assist with the procedure. Prepare biopsy specimens for pathological examination.
Culture and sensitivity (C&S)	Determines presence of microorganism and identifies the antibiotic that will kill or inhibit growth of microorganism. Drainage from infected lesions is obtained with a sterile swab and is incubated in order to identify the causative organism and to determine antibiotic sensitivity. Normal: negative for microorganism growth.	Ensure that the specimen has been obtained before initiating antibiotic therapy. Specimens should be taken to the laboratory within 30 minutes of being obtained.

continues

TABLE 25-15   continued

TEST	EXPLANATION/NORMAL VALUES	NURSING RESPONSIBILITIES
Cytology	The study of cells and fluids obtained from various organs by scrapings, brushings, or needle aspiration. Cytologic smears, such as the Pap smear, are routinely done to study cells from the female genital tract. A cytological smear showing evidence of malignancy is followed by a biopsy to facilitate a more comprehensive diagnosis.	Explain the procedure to be used for obtaining cells and fluids for study. Follow agency protocol for client preparation.
Dark field examination of wart scrapings	Microscopic examination to differentiate genital warts from syphilis condylomata.	Take a careful client history. Examine the genital area carefully and provide scalpel and slide, if specimen is to be obtained. Explain the procedure thoroughly to the client.
Dilatation and curettage (D&C)	Surgical scraping of the endometrial lining, performed under general, epidural, or paracervical anesthesia and on an outpatient basis. Diagnostic or therapeutic for uterine bleeding disorders.	Explain the procedure to the client. Perform pre- and postoperative assessment and provide care. Provide discharge instructions related to activities and follow-up appointments.
Dynamic infusion cavernosometry and cavernosography (DICC)	Group of diagnostic tests that measure neurovascular events of penile erection.	Perform baseline assessment, monitor during the procedure, and assess for postoperative complications; advise the client of possible discomfort related to the injection. Explain the procedure to the client. Assess for allergies. If preferred by the laboratory, initiate NPO status after midnight. Restrict iodine and thyroid preparations a week before test. Inform the client that radioactive iodine may be given orally or intravenously. Withhold food for 45–60 minutes after the iodine is given. Provide the client with a list of times to report to radiology. Tell the client that he will lie supine for test, which takes about 30 minutes, and that neither isolation nor specific urine precautions are necessary.
Huhner test (post-coital test)	Performed in the office. The couple has intercourse 2 hours before the appointment. A sample of secretions is removed from the vagina and placed on a microscopic slide. The sperm are observed for number and motility in the cervical mucous. Normal: a minimum of 20 sperm per field that demonstrate good motility	Explain the procedure to the client and schedule it near client's normal ovulation. Prepare the client in the lithotomy position. Assist the physician or nurse practitioner with the procedure. Perform microscopic observations as directed.
Nocturnal tumescence penile monitoring	Various devices are attached to the penis at night to monitor swelling (tumescence).	Explain to the client that the test will require application of a device to the penis and that the device is to be worn while sleeping. Show the client the device and explain how to apply it.
Papanicolaou (Pap) smear	Cells are obtained from the external and internal cervical canal. Screening tool for premalignant and malignant cervical changes.	Explain the procedure. Have client empty bladder and undress. Position client in dorsal lithotomy position. Help client relax during procedure. Prepare microscopic slides for pathology. Instruct the client on the importance of having an annual Pap smear.

continues

TABLE 25-15 continued

TEST	EXPLANATION/NORMAL VALUES	NURSING RESPONSIBILITIES
Past-point testing	Measures the ability or inability to accurately place a finger on some part of the body, usually the client's or examiner's face and fingers. For example, the examiner will instruct the client to close her eyes and touch her nose, then, with eyes open, touch the examiner's nose or the examiner's index finger.	Explain the test and procedure to the client. Explain that it is painless and represents a helpful measure of vestibular function (coordination).
Patch testing	Allergens within occlusive patches are applied to normal skin (usually the upper back) for 48 hours. If the client is allergic to a specific allergen, an erythematous skin reaction will occur.	Clean and dry the skin where the patches are to be applied. Tell the client that the patches must be left in place for the full 48 hours.
Pelvic examination (recommended annually for women over 18 through menopause)	Performed by a physician or nurse practitioner. The external and internal pelvic structures are visualized, the pelvic organs are palpated via bi-manual examination, and the cervix is examined via a speculum. A Pap smear and rectovaginal exam are also performed, and cultures and wet smears may be obtained.	Explain the procedures to the client; prepare the client by having her void and undress; position the client on the examination table in a dorsal lithotomy position; help the client to relax during the examination, prepare slides and culture medium; obtain other supplies; and assist with the procedure.
Prostatic smears	Microscopic examination of prostatic secretions obtained via rectal massage performed by a physician.	Explain to the client that to obtain the specimen, the prostate must be massaged via the rectum and that this will cause some discomfort.
Pulmonary function tests (PFTs)	A group of studies used to evaluate ventilatory function. Measurements are obtained directly via spirometer or calculated from the results of spirometer measurements. Bronchodilators may be used during the study. Measurements included are: Tidal volume: the amount of air inhaled and exhaled in one breath: 500 mL at rest. Inspiratory reserve volume: the amount of air inspired at the end of a normal inspiration. Expiratory reserve volume: the amount of air expired following a normal expiration. Residual volume: the amount of air left in lungs after maximal expiration. Vital capacity: the total volume of air that can be expired after maximal inspiration. Total lung capacity: the total volume of air in the lungs when maximally inflated. Inspiratory capacity: the maximum amount of air that can be inspired after normal expiration. Forced vital capacity: the capacity of air exhaled forcefully and rapidly following maximal inspiration. Minute volume: the amount of air breathed per minute.	Explain the procedure to the client, PFTs should not be done within 1–2 hours after a meal. After the test, monitor respiratory status. Advise the client to avoid activity and to rest following the test, as fatigue may result.

continues

TABLE 25-15 continued

TEST	EXPLANATION/NORMAL VALUES	NURSING RESPONSIBILITIES
Pulse oximetry	A noninvasive procedure. A transdermal clip is placed on a finger or earlobe to detect the arterial oxygen saturation (SaO_2). Normal: >95% (at sea level)	Explain the procedure to the client. Assess peripheral circulation, as this may alter results. Place the sensor on the earlobe, fingertip, or pinna of the ear. Keep the sensor intact until a consistent reading is obtained. Observe and record readings. Report to the physician measurements below 95%.
Rinne test (tuning fork)	Detects loss of hearing in one or both ears. Tuning fork is struck and placed against the mastoid bone to measure the sound conduction through the bone. The tuning fork is then placed beside and parallel to the ear to test conduction through the air. If the sound is louder when the tines are placed beside the ear, hearing is normal or the hearing loss is sensorineural. If the sound is louder when conducted through the bone, the hearing loss is conductive.	Explain the procedure and its purpose to the client.
Romberg test	Assesses vestibular (balance) function. The client stands with the eyes closed, arms extended in front, and feet together. Normal: slight swaying.	Explain the procedure and its purpose to the client. Stand close and reassure the client that someone will catch him if he begins to fall.
Schiller test	Performed during colposcopy. An iodine solution is applied to the cells of the cervix. Abnormal cells turn white or yellow. Aids in visualization of abnormal tissue and indicates areas for biopsy. Normal: cells turn brown	Explain the reason for the application of the solution. Assist with the biopsy procedure as necessary. Label tissue specimens and send to histology.
Segmented bacteriologic localization cultures	The first 5–10 mL of urine is collected, the next 200 mL is discarded, then 5–10 mL is collected midstream. The prostate is then massaged until prostatic secretions can be collected. Finally, 5–10 mL urine is collected before the bladder is emptied. Four samples are needed in sterile culture tubes.	Ensure that the client is well hydrated and has a full bladder.
Semen analysis	Determines the presence, number, and motility of sperm.	Teach the client about proper collection of sperm.
Skin scrapings	A lesion is scraped with an oiled scalpel blade. The cells are then examined under a microscope. Used to diagnose fungal lesions.	Explain the procedure and its purpose to the client.
Speech audiometry (Spondee threshold)	Evaluates ability to hear and understand the spoken word. A series of two-syllable words commonly recognized by their vowel sounds (like *toothbrush* and *baseball*) are delivered through earphones. When the client correctly repeats the word, the sound intensity is recorded in decibels. The test is normally conducted in a soundproof booth.	Explain the procedure and its purpose to the client. Ensure that the client is not claustrophobic.

continues

TABLE 25-15 continued

TEST	EXPLANATION/NORMAL VALUES	NURSING RESPONSIBILITIES
Sputum analysis	Sputum samples are examined for the presence of bacteria, fungi, molds, yeasts, and malignant cells. Appropriate antibiotic therapy is determined via C&S studies.	Explain the procedure and its purpose to the client. Obtain specimens early in the morning to prevent contamination via ingested food or fluids. Instruct the client to breathe deeply and cough, so as to facilitate collection of a specimen originating from the lower respiratory tract. If necessary, pulmonary suctioning may be used to induce such a specimen. Instruct the client to expectorate sputum into the appropriate container. Deliver specimens to the laboratory as soon as possible.
Tonometry	Used to measure intraocular pressure and to aid in the diagnosis and follow-up evaluation of glaucoma. Two types of tonometric devices are used for assessment: applanation and indentation. An applanation tonometer is the most accurate and commonly used device and measures the force (delineated by the reading on the tension dial on the tonometer) required to flatten a small, standard area of the cornea. An indentation tonometer measures the deformation of the globe in response to a standard weight placed on the cornea. Before use of either apparatus, the eyes are anesthetized with a local ophthalmic solution, such as benoxinate with fluorescein or tetracaine, so that the pressure from the tonometer will not be felt. Normal: 20 mm Hg or lower	Explain the procedure and its purpose to the client. Explain to the client that this test measures the pressure within the eyes and that although the test requires the client's eyes to be anesthetized, the anesthesia will wear off shortly after the examination is complete. Reassure the client that the procedure is painless.
Typanometry	Measures the movement of the eardrum in response to air pressure in the ear canal. Evaluates the presence of fluid in the middle ear and is commonly used to evaluate otitis media in children or adults.	Explain the procedure and its purpose to the client. Inform the client a small burst of air is introduced through the otoscope, which may produce an uncomfortable sensation.
Tzanck smear	Fluid from the base of a vesicle is applied to a glass slide, stained, and examined under a microscope. Used to diagnose herpes zoster, herpes simplex, varicella, or pemphigus. Normal: negative	Describe to the client how the laboratory technician will obtain the specimen and that although the procedure will likely not be painful, the client must remain still to prevent injury. Provide scalpel blade, glass slide, and stain for collection.
Urethra pressure profile (UPP)	Assesses functional urethral length and general competency of the urethra and sphincter, either at rest or during coughing, straining, or voiding. Functional profile length is the length from bladder outlet to the point in the urethra where urethral pressure equals intravesical pressure. Used to diagnose stress or overflow incontinence or urethral obstruction. Normal: 　Male: bladder outlet through membranous urethra 　Female: bladder outlet through mid-urethra	Explain the procedure and its purpose to the client: that it is often performed when the bladder is empty and the client is at rest; that it may be performed simultaneously with CMG; and that the client may be asked to cough or void. Provide privacy, as the test can be embarrassing.
Uroflowmetry	Noninvasive assessment of urination. An electronic device connected to a funneled commode calculates the rate of urine flow, volume voided, and time taken to void.	Explain the procedure and its purpose to the client. Instruct the client to void as usual, leaving client alone to do so, if possible.

continues

TABLE 25-15 continued

TEST	EXPLANATION/NORMAL VALUES	NURSING RESPONSIBILITIES
Weber test (tuning fork)	Detects loss of hearing in one or both ears. Tuning fork is struck and the handle is placed in the middle of the forehead. Clients with normal hearing or bilateral deafness will hear or not hear the sound equally in both ears. Clients with unilateral hearing loss will hear the sound only in the unaffected ear.	Explain the procedure and its purpose to the client.
Wood's light examination	Skin and hair are examined under ultraviolet light (black light) in a darkened room. Used to diagnose fungal infections (tinea) of hair and skin.	Explain the procedure and its purpose to the client. Reassure the client that the rays are not harmful.

Summary

- Most invasive procedures require that the client give written informed consent.
- Prepare clients for diagnostic testing by ensuring client understanding and compliance with preprocedural requirements.
- Clients, families, and significant others must be involved in the testing process; advise them of the estimated procedure time.
- To help offset the discomfort and anxiety experienced during procedures, teach the client how to perform relaxation techniques such as imagery.
- After a diagnostic test, provide care and teach the client those things to expect, including the outcomes or side effects of the test.
- The nurse facilitates the scheduling of diagnostic tests, performs client teaching, performs or assists with procedures, and assesses clients for adverse responses.
- Schedule diagnostic procedures to promote client comfort and cost containment.
- Standard Precautions are used when obtaining a specimen or assisting with an invasive procedure.
- Before a procedure, obtain baseline vital signs and assess the client's preparation for testing.
- After a procedure, assess the client for secondary procedural complications and perform any necessary nursing interventions.

Review Questions

1. Scheduling and sequencing of laboratory tests are important functions of the:
   a. nurse.
   b. physician.
   c. phlebotomist.
   d. laboratory supervisor.

2. When collecting a 24-hour urine specimen, the nurse knows:
   a. to put a large bottle at the client's bedside.
   b. the collection begins at the time of the first discarded voiding.
   c. that the client must urinate at a specific start time.
   d. to teach the client how to void in the large collection bottle.

3. The nurse knows that glucose spills into the urine when the blood glucose level exceeds the renal threshold of:
   a. 120 mg/mL.
   b. 140 mg/mL.
   c. 160 mg/mL.
   d. 180 mg/mL.

4. When scheduling a series of tests, the nurse knows to schedule:
   a. a barium enema before an upper GI.
   b. an ultrasound after all other tests.
   c. an upper GI before a gallbladder x-ray.
   d. a gallbladder x-ray before any barium studies.

5. A test that combines a radioactive scan with an electrodiagnostic study is a:
   a. MUGA.
   b. brain scan.
   c. thallium stress test.
   d. radioactive iodine uptake test.

References/Suggested Readings

Ahmed, D. S. (2000). Hidden factors in occult blood testing. *AJN, 100*(12), 25.

Beattie, S. (1999). Cut the risks for cardiac cath patients. *RN, 62*(1), 50–54.

Carr, M., & Grey, M. (2002). Magnetic resonance imaging. *AJN, 102*(12), 26–33.

Clinical Rounds. (2002). Quick blood test identifies heart failure. *Nursing2002, 32*(6), 34.

Connolly, M. (2001). Chest X-rays: Completing the picture, *RN*, *64*(6), 56–62.

Cook, L. (1999). The value of lab values: Incorporate lab results into the nursing diagnosis. *AJN, 99*(5), 66–75.

Daniels, R. (2002). *Delmar's guide to laboratory and diagnostic tests.* Clifton Park, NY: Thomson Delmar Learning.

Darty, S., Thomas, M., Neagle, C., Link, H., Wesley-Farrington, D., & Hundley, G. (2002). Cardiovascular magnetic resonance imaging. *AJN, 102*(12), 34–38.

Ernst, D. (1999). Collecting blood culture specimens. *Nursing99, 29*(7), 56–58.

Gallauresi, B. (1998). Pulse oximeters. *Nursing98, 28*(9), 31.

Guyton, A. C., & Hall, J., (2000). *Textbook of medical physiology* (10th ed.). Philadelphia: W. B. Saunders.

Hill, J., & Newton, J. (1998). Contrast echo: Your role at the bedside. *RN, 61*(10), 32–35.

Kee, J. L. (1998). *Laboratory and diagnostic tests with nursing implications* (5th ed.). Upper Saddle River, NJ: Prentice Hall.

Lawrence, B., & Tasota, F. (2003). Detecting neuromuscular problems with electromyography. *Nursing2003, 33*(4), 82.

McEnroe-Ayers, D. (2002a). EBCT: Beaming in on coronary artery disease. *Nursing2002, 32*(4), 81.

McEnroe-Ayers, D. (2002b). Preparing a patient for cardiac catheterization. *Nursing2002, 32*(9), 82.

Montes, P. (1997). Managing outpatient cardiac catheterization. *AJN, 97*(8), 34–37.

Nursing2002. (2002). Teaching your patient about cardiovascular tests. *Nursing2002, 32*(1), 62–64.

Ryan, D. (2000). Is it an MI?: A lab primer. *RN, 63*(2), 26–30.

Shortall, S. P., & Perkins, L. A. (1999). Interpreting the ins and outs of pulmonary function tests. *Nursing99, 29*(12), 41–46.

Tasota, F. (2002). Full-body scans: Screening for problems. *Nursing2002, 32*(7), 22.

Tasota, F., & Tate, J. (2001a). Assessing thyroid function with serum tests. *Nursing2001, 31*(1), 22.

Tasota, F., & Tate, J. (2001b). Diagnosing pulmonary embolism with spiral CT. *Nursing2001, 31*(5), 75.

Tasota, F., & Tate, J. (2001c). Digital mammography: Enhanced imaging in real time. *Nursing2001, 31*(4), 70.

Tasota, F., & Tate, J. (2001d). Interpreting the highs and lows of platelet counts. *Nursing2001, 31*(2), 25.

Tasota, F., & Tate, J. (2001e). Teaching patients about lipid levels. *Nursing2001, 31*(3), 68.

Tasota, F., & Tate, J. (2001f). Using PET to detect abnormalities. *Nursing2001, 31*(11), 24.

Wong, F. W. H. (1999). A new approach to ABG interpretation. *AJN, 99*(8), 34–36.

Resources

National Library of Medicine, www.nlm.nih.gov (then click on "Search MEDLINE")

National Network of Libraries of Medicine (NN/LM) Regional Medical Libraries, 800-338-7657

Nursing Procedures

BASIC PROCEDURES

PROCEDURE 26-1   Hand Hygiene

OVERVIEW

Hand hygiene is a general term that includes *handwashing* (using plain soap and water), *antiseptic handwash* (using antimicrobial substances and water), *antiseptic hand rub* (using alcohol-based hand rub), and *surgical hand antisepsis* (using antiseptic handwash or antiseptic hand rub preoperatively by surgical personnel to eliminate transient and reduce resident hand flora) (CDC, 2002). *When hands are visibly dirty, wash hands with soap (plain or antimicrobial) and water. If hands are not visibly soiled, an alcohol-based hand rub may be used* (CDC, 2002).

Handwashing is the rubbing together of all surfaces and crevices of the hands using a soap or chemical and water. Handwashing is a component of all types of isolation precautions and is the most basic and effective infection-control measure to prevent and control the transmission of infectious agents.

The three essential elements of handwashing are soap or chemical, water, and friction. Soaps that contain antimicrobial agents are frequently used in high-risk areas such as emergency departments and nurseries. Friction is the most important element of the trio because it physically removes soil and transient flora.

Handwashing should be performed after arriving at work, before leaving work, between client contacts, after removing gloves, when hands are visibly soiled, before eating, after excretion of body waste (urination and defecation), after contact with body fluids, before and after performing invasive procedures, and after handling contaminated equipment. The exact duration of time required for handwashing depends on the circumstances. A washing time of 10 to 15 seconds is recommended to remove transient flora from the hands. High-risk areas, such as nurseries, usually require about a minimum 2-minute handwash. Soiled hands usually require more time (CDC, 2002).

ASSESSMENT

1. Assess the environment **to establish if facilities are adequate for cleansing the hands.** Is the water clean? Is soap available? Is there a clean towel to dry hands?
2. Assess your hands **to determine if they have open cuts, hangnails, broken skin, or heavily soiled areas.**

POSSIBLE NURSING DIAGNOSIS

Risk for Infection

PLANNING

Expected Outcomes

1. The caregiver's hands will be cleansed adequately to remove microorganisms, transient flora, and soiling from the skin.

Equipment Needed

- Soap
- Paper or cloth towels
- Sink
- Running water

DELEGATION TIPS

All hospital personnel are expected to maintain proper hand hygiene technique and routinely practice Standard Precautions.

continues

IMPLEMENTATION—ACTION/RATIONALE

ACTION

Handwashing

1. Remove jewelry. Wristwatch may be pushed up above the wrist (midforearm). Push sleeves of uniform or shirt up above the wrist at midforearm level.
2. Assess hands for hangnails, cuts, or breaks in the skin, and areas that are heavily soiled.

3. Turn on the water. Adjust the flow and temperature. Temperature of the water should be warm.
4. Wet hands and lower forearms thoroughly by holding under running water. Keep hands and forearms in the down position with elbows straight. Avoid splashing water and touching the sides of the sink.

5. Apply about 5 mL (1 teaspoon) of liquid soap. Lather thoroughly.
6. Thoroughly rub hands together for about 10 to 15 seconds. Interlace fingers and thumbs and move back and forth to wash between digits. Rub palms and back of hands with circular motion (Figure 26-1-1). Special attention should be provided to areas such as the knuckles and fingernails, which are known to harbor organisms (Figure 26-1-2).

RATIONALE

1. Provides access to skin surfaces for cleaning. Facilitates cleaning of fingers, hands, and forearms.

2. Intact skin acts as a barrier to microorganisms. Breaks in skin integrity facilitate development of infection and should receive extra attention during cleaning.
3. Running water removes microorganisms. Warm water removes less of the natural skin oils.
4. Water should flow from the least contaminated to the most contaminated areas of the skin. Hands are considered more contaminated than arms. Splashing of water facilitates transfer of microorganisms. Touching of any surface during cleaning contaminates the skin.
5. Lather facilitates removal of microorganisms. Liquid soap harbors less bacteria than bar soap.
6. Friction mechanically removes microorganisms from the skin surface. Friction loosens dirt from soiled areas.

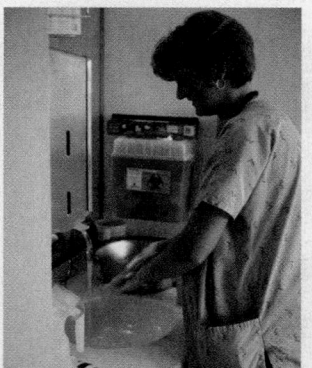

Figure 26-1-1   Lather thoroughly and rub hands together.

Figure 26-1-2   Give special attention to fingernails and knuckles.

7. Rinse with hands in the down position, elbows straight. Rinse in the direction of forearm to wrist to fingers.
8. Blot hands and forearms to dry thoroughly. Dry in the direction of fingers to wrist and forearms. Discard the paper towels in the proper receptacle.
9. Turn off the water faucet with a clean, dry paper towel.

7. Flow of water rinses away dirt and microorganisms.

8. Blotting reduces chapping of skin. Drying from cleanest (hand) to least clean area (forearms) prevents transfer of microorganisms to cleanest area.
9. Prevents contamination of clean hands by a less clean faucet.

continues

Alcohol-based Hand Rub

10. Apply the recommended amount of product to one hand.
11. Rub hands together, covering hands and fingers on all sides.
12. Continue rubbing until hands are dry.

10. Amount of rub required varies by product.

11. Spreads rub to cover all aspects of hands and fingers.

12. Allows the rub to work.

EVALUATION

- The hand hygiene was adequate to control topical flora and infectious agents on the hands.
- The hands were not recontaminated during or shortly after the hand hygiene.

DOCUMENTATION

No documentation is needed for routine hand hygiene by the nurse.

PROCEDURE 26-2   Use of Protective Equipment

OVERVIEW

Infection control is an essential area of concern for the nurse in any setting. Effective implementation prevents or reduces the incidence of nosocomial infections. The hospitalized client is at increased risk for infection because of added exposure to pathogens, compromised immunologic state, and potential invasive procedures. Development of infection can delay healing, prolong hospital stay, or cause permanent disability, or even loss of life.

Medical asepsis is the process of reducing microorganisms and preventing their spread. Hand hygiene is the single most important technique for infection control. Surgical asepsis takes this further with procedures implemented to eliminate any microorganisms. This is practiced in the surgical arena to reduce the risk of infection for the client.

Standard Precautions consider all clients and their bodily fluids (except sweat) to be potentially infectious, thereby replacing the term Universal Precautions, which applied only to blood and visibly bloody fluids (CDC, 2002).

- Gloves are required when hand contact with any body fluids is anticipated. This includes touching mucous membranes and nonintact skin. Latex- and powder-free gloves are recommended. Hands should be cleansed after the gloves are removed.
- Impervious gowns must be worn by health care workers to prevent soiling of clothing by splashes of blood or body fluids, and masks, along with eye protection, are mandated if splashes toward the face are anticipated.
- Masks are worn when caring for clients on airborne and/or droplet precautions and immunocompromised clients.
- Hair should be covered by a cap when in the semirestricted and restricted areas of the surgical suite and in areas of the hospital where special procedures are done (i.e., bone marrow transplant).
- Eye protection (goggles) or face shields should be worn during care activities that may be associated with splashes or sprays of blood or body fluids.
- Soiled protective items should be removed promptly after use and disposed of as appropriate. Handle and process soiled gowns to the laundry according to facility protocol.

ASSESSMENT

1. Assess if Standard Precautions are being followed or if specific isolation precautions are needed for the client's condition. **The type of microorganism and mode of transmission determine the degree of precautions.**
2. Assess the client's laboratory results **to learn which organism the client is infected with and the client's immune responses.**
3. Assess what nursing measures are required before entering the room **to have all the necessary equipment ready.**
4. Assess the client's knowledge for the need to wear a cap, gown, and mask during care **to direct client teaching.**
5. Assess whether the isolation is airborne, droplet, or contact and which isolation attire is necessary.

continues

POSSIBLE NURSING DIAGNOSES

Ineffective Protection
Social Isolation
Situational Low Self-Esteem

PLANNING

Expected Outcomes

1. The client and staff will remain free of nosocomial infection.
2. The health care provider will be protected from infection when caring for the client.
3. The staff will avoid transmitting microorganisms to others.
4. The client will interact on a social level with nurse, family members, and other visitors.

Equipment Needed

- Gloves, clean—sterile if necessary
- Gown, sterile or clean
- Cap
- Mask
- Goggles
- Face mask

DELEGATION TIPS

Donning and removing gloves, caps, and masks is a skill that is required of all personnel, including ancillary personnel. Proper technique should be monitored by the nursing staff.

IMPLEMENTATION—ACTION/RATIONALE

ACTION

✢ Check client's identification band ✢ Explain procedure before beginning ✢

1. Cleanse hands.
2. The first item of apparel donned should be the cap or surgical hat/hood. Hair should be tucked in a manner so that all hair is covered (Figure 26-2-1).

RATIONALE

1. Reduces the transmission of microorganisms.
2. Because hair acts as a filter when left uncovered, it collects bacteria in proportion to its length, curliness, and oiliness. Loose hair may fall in the surgical area. Shedding hair may lead to surgical wound infection.

Figure 26-2-1 Caps and surgical caps should cover the head, and hair should be tucked in.

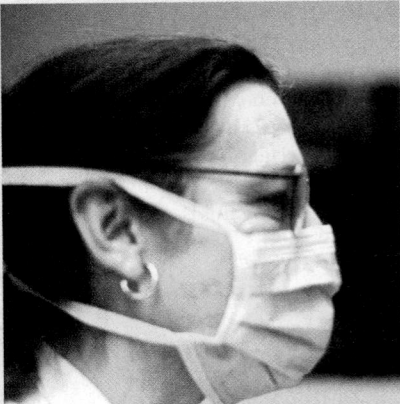

Figure 26-2-2 Bottom of the mask should fit snugly under chin.

continues

3. Apply a mask around mouth and nose and secure in a manner that prevents venting. For masks with strings:
   a. Hold mask by top and pinch center (metal strip) over bridge of nose.
   b. Pull top two strings over ears and secure at top, back of head.
   c. Tie two lower ties around back or nape of neck so bottom of mask fits snugly under chin (Figure 26-2-2).
4. Open gown, slip arms into sleeves, and secure at neck and side (Figure 26-2-3 A&B).

Figure 26-2-3A Put on the gown before putting on gloves.

5. Protective eyewear should be worn whenever health care provider or client are at risk for splash and contamination. These are applied as goggles/glasses or face shields, which have elastic ties for around the ears.
6. Don clean gloves. If sterile gloves are required for a procedure, use open or closed method.

7. The open glove technique:
   a. Slide the hands into the gown all the way through the cuffs on the gown.
   b. Pick up the cuff of the left glove using the thumb and index finger of the right hand.
   c. Pull the glove onto the left hand, leaving the cuff of the glove turned down.
   d. Take the gloved left hand and slide the fingers under the cuff of the right glove, keeping the gloved fingers under the folded cuff.
   e. Pull the glove onto the right hand.
   f. Rotate the arm as the cuff of the glove is pulled over the gown.
8. The closed glove technique:
   a. Slide the hands into the gown all the way through the cuffs on the gown.
   b. Use right hand to pick up left glove.

3. Masks are worn to contain and filter droplets of microorganisms that are expelled when talking, sneezing, or coughing. Masks prevent the transmission of oral and nasopharyngeal organisms between the nurse and client.

4. Gowns act as a protective barrier and should be worn to reduce exposure to blood, body fluid, or other potentially infectious liquids.

Figure 26-2-3B Tie the gown at the neck and waist.

5. Protective eyewear reduces the incidence of contamination to the eyes. If eyewear or face shields become contaminated, they should be discarded immediately and replaced with a clean barrier.
6. Gloves are worn to prevent gross contamination of the hands. They should be changed between clients and hands cleansed. The open method is used when performing procedures that require sterile technique but do not require donning a sterile gown or when both gloves need to be changed without assistance during a surgical procedure (Procedure 27-2). The closed method is used by scrubbed personnel in the operating room.
7. The open glove method is commonly used for sterile procedures or when both gloves need to be changed without assistance during a surgical procedure.

8. The closed glove technique is used by the scrubbed personnel in the operating room. This is preferred because the possibility of the glove touching the skin is eliminated.

continues

c. Place the glove on the upward-turned left hand—palm side down thumb to thumb with the fingers extending along the forearm pointing toward the elbow.

d. Hold the glove cuff and sleeve cuff together with the thumb of the left hand.

e. The right hand stretches the cuff of the left glove over the opened end of the sleeve.

f. Work the fingers into the glove as the cuff is pulled onto the wrist.

g. The right glove is done in the same manner.

9. Enter the client's room and explain the rationale for wearing the attire.

10. After performing necessary tasks, remove gown, gloves, mask, and cap before leaving the room.

11. Removal of gown: Untie gown and remove from shoulders. Fold and roll gown down in front into a ball, so contaminated area is rolled onto center of gown. Dispose in approved receptacle.

12. Removal of gloves:

a. Grasp outside cuff of one glove and pull off, turning inside out. Hold it with the remaining gloved hand (Figure 26-2-4).

b. Pull the second glove off without touching the outside of the second glove. Turn the second glove as it is removed (Figure 26-2-5). Dispose into receptacle with first glove.

9. Minimizes anxiety and feelings of isolation.

10. Reduces transmission of organisms.

11. Reduces transmission of organisms.

12.

a. Reduces risk of contamination.

b. Reduces risk of contamination.

Figure 26-2-4   Grasp the outside cuff and turn the glove inside out.

Figure 26-2-5   Turn the second glove over the first glove.

13. Removal of mask: Untie bottom strings of mask first, then top strings, and lift off face. Hold mask by strings and discard.

14. Removal of cap: Grasp top surface of cap and lift from head.

15. Cleanse hands.

13. Prevents contaminated surface of mask from contacting uniform.

14. Minimizes contact of hands to hair.

15. Reduces transmission of microorganisms.

continues

EVALUATION

- The client remains free of any nosocomial infection.
- The health care provider and staff are protected from infection and microorganisms are contained without cross-contamination.
- The client interacts on a social level with nurse, family members, and other visitors.

DOCUMENTATION

Nurses' Notes

- Type of protective barriers used and any breaks in isolation technique
- Client's compliance with and verbalization of understanding and adjustment to isolation
- Family members' compliance of isolation procedures

PROCEDURE 26-3 Taking a Temperature

OVERVIEW

Monitoring body temperature is a basic skill necessary in nursing and medical decision making. When heat production exceeds heat loss, and body temperature rises above the normal range, pyrexia (fever) occurs. Pyrexia can accompany any inflammatory response, loss of body fluid, or prolonged exposure to high temperatures. When the body is exposed to temperatures lower than normal for a prolonged length of time, hypothermia occurs. Hospitalized clients are at particular risk for infection and accompanying fever. Clients are stressed by their presenting conditions, and their bodies are further stressed by the hospital environment; thus they are more susceptible to the infectious agents found there. Hypothermia generally occurs in response to prolonged exposure to cold weather or as a result of being immersed in cold water. Accurate monitoring and recording of a client's temperature is essential for diagnosis, treatment, and monitoring of the client.

ASSESSMENT

1. Assess body temperature for changes when exposed to pyrogens (endogenous or exogenous substances that cause fever) or to extreme hot or cold external environments **because such environments may indicate the cause of an infection.**
2. Assess the client for the most appropriate site to check temperature **to obtain an accurate reading.**
3. Confirm that the client has not consumed hot or cold food or beverage nor smoked for 15 to 30 minutes before the measurement **because these activities may alter the oral reading.**
4. Assess for mouth breathing and tachypnea **because both can cause an inaccurate oral reading.**
5. Assess for oral lesion, especially herpetic lesions, **because herpes viruses are extremely contagious and require implementation of Standard Precautions of the Centers for Disease Control and Prevention. Clients with herpetic lesions should have their own glass thermometer or disposable thermometer to prevent transmission to others.**

POSSIBLE NURSING DIAGNOSES

*Ineffective **H**ealth Maintenance*
*Risk for **I**nfection*

Hypothermia
Hyperthermia
Ineffective Thermoregulation
Deficient Fluid Volume
Risk for Imbalanced Body Temperature

PLANNING

Expected Outcomes

1. An accurate temperature reading will be obtained.
2. The client will verbalize understanding of the reason for the procedure.

Equipment Needed

- Thermometer (one of the following)
  — Electronic thermometer with disposable protective sheath
  — Tympanic membrane thermometer with probe cover
  — Disposable, single-use chemical strip thermometer
  — Glass (mercury free): oral or rectal at client's bedside, usually color coded to avoid cross use
- Lubricant for rectal and glass thermometer
- Two pairs of nonsterile gloves
- Tissues

continues

DELEGATION TIPS

The skill of temperature measurement is often delegated to ancillary personnel; however, the nurse retains responsibility for knowledge of the client's temperature and appropriate actions. The expectation is that ancillary personnel will have documented instruction and competency validation of their ability to:
- *Select the correct route for measurement of the temperature.*
- *Correctly position the client for measurement.*
- *Correctly perform the measurement according to established guidelines and record on the appropriate flow sheet (clinical record).*
- *Recognize and report abnormal findings to the nurse.*

IMPLEMENTATION—ACTION/RATIONALE

ACTION

RATIONALE

❋ Check client's identification band ❋ Explain procedure before beginning ❋

1. Review medical record for baseline data and factors that influence vital signs.

2. Explain to the client that vital signs will be assessed. Encourage the client to remain still and refrain from drinking, eating, and smoking, and to avoid mouth breathing, if possible.
3. Assess client's toileting needs and proceed as appropriate.

4. Gather equipment.
5. Provide for privacy.
6. Cleanse hands and apply gloves when appropriate.

1. Establishes parameters for client's normal measurements, provides direction in device selection, and helps determine site to use for measurement. Vital signs are measured in the order of temperature, pulse, and respiration (TPR) and blood pressure (BP), usually without interruptions, to provide the nurse with an objective clinical database to direct decision making.
2. Encourages participation, allays anxiety, and ensures accurate measurements. Cold or hot liquids and smoking alter circulation and body temperature. Mouth breathing can alter temperature.
3. Prevents interruptions during measurements, communicates caring, and promotes client comfort.
4. Facilitates organization.
5. Decreases embarrassment.
6. Hands are cleansed before and after every contact with a client to reduce the transmission of microorganisms. Gloves are worn to avoid contact with bodily secretions and to reduce transmission of microorganisms.

Oral Temperature—Electronic Thermometer

7. Repeat Actions 1 to 6.
8. Place disposable protective sheath over probe.
9. Grasp top of the probe's stem. Avoid placing pressure on the ejection button.
10. Place tip of thermometer under the client's tongue and along the gumline to the posterior sublingual pocket lateral to center of lower jaw (Figure 26-3-1).
11. Instruct client to keep mouth closed around thermometer.
12. Thermometer will signal (beep) when a constant temperature registers (Figure 26-3-2).
13. Read measurement on digital display of electronic thermometer. Push ejection button to discard disposable sheath into receptacle and return probe to storage well.
14. Inform client of temperature reading.
15. Remove gloves and cleanse hands.

7. See Rationales 1 to 6.
8. Reduces transmission of microorganisms.
9. Pressure on the ejection button releases the sheath from the probe.
10. Sublingual pocket contains superficial blood vessels.

11. Maintains thermometer in proper place and decreases amount of time required for an accurate reading.
12. Signal indicates final temperature reading.
13. Reduces transmission of microorganisms. Ensures that the electronic system is ready for next use.

14. Promotes client's participation in care.
15. Reduces transmission of microorganisms.

continues

Figure 26-3-1   Place probe tip in the posterior sublingual pocket.

Figure 26-3-2   Listen for audible beep signal when temperature registers.

16. Record reading according to institution policies.

17. Return electronic thermometer unit to charging base, checking that it is plugged in.
18. Cleanse hands.

Tympanic Temperature: Infrared Thermometer

19. Repeat Actions 1 to 6.
20. Position client in Sims' or sitting position.
21. Remove probe from container and attach probe cover to tympanic thermometer unit (Figure 26-3-3).
22. Turn client's head to one side. For an adult, pull pinna upward and back; for a child, pull down and back. Gently insert probe with firm pressure into ear canal (Figure 26-3-4).
23. Remove probe after the reading is displayed on digital unit (usually 2 seconds).
24. Discard probe cover into receptacle and replace probe in storage container.
25. Return tympanic thermometer to storage unit.

16. Accurate documentation by site allows for comparison of data.
17. Ensures charging base is plugged into electrical outlet and thermometer is ready for next use.
18. Reduces transmission of microorganisms.

19. See Rationales 1 to 6.
20. Promotes access to ear.
21. Prevents contamination.

22. Provides access to ear canal. Gentle insertion prevents trauma to external canal. Firm pressure is needed to ensure probe will record an accurate temperature.

23. Reading is displayed within seconds.

24. Reduces transmission of microorganisms. Protects reusable probe from damage.
25. Recharges batteries of unit for future use.

Figure 26-3-3   Attach disposable probe cover to unit.

Figure 26-3-4   Insert temperature probe into ear canal.

continues

26. Record reading according to institution policy.
27. Cleanse hands.

26. Promotes accurate documentation for data comparison.
27. Reduces transmission of microorganisms.

Using a "Tempa-Dot"

28. Repeat Actions 1 to 6.
29. Position the client in a sitting or lying position.

28. See Rationales 1 to 6.
29. Promotes client's comfort, and promotes site access for all measurement.

Figure 26-3-5 "Tempa-Dot" Single-Use Disposable Thermometer

Figure 26-3-6 Oral (blue tip) and Rectal (red tip) Glass Thermometers

30. Prepare Tempa-Dot according to directions (Figure 26-3-5).
    • Oral measurement: Place Tempa-Dot under tongue as far back as possible. Have client press tongue down on thermometer and keep mouth closed for 60 seconds. Remove thermometer, read the last blue dot; ignore any skipped dot.
    • Axillary measurement: Place thermometer high in the armpit, vertical to the body, with dots against the torso. Lower client's arm to hold thermometer in place. Remove thermometer after 3 minutes.
31. Record temperature, indicate the method, and discard the thermometer.
32. Cleanse hands.

30. Promotes accurate measurement and client safety.

31. Nursing documentation, practice clean technique.

32. Reduces transmission of microorganisms.

Oral Temperature: Glass Thermometer

33. Repeat Actions 1 to 6.
34. Select correct color tip of thermometer from client's bedside container (Figure 26-3-6).
35. Remove thermometer from storage container, hold at end away from bulb and cleanse under cool water.

36. Use a tissue to dry thermometer from bulb's end toward fingertips.
37. Read thermometer by locating colored solution or mercury level. It should read 35.5°C (96°F).
38. If thermometer is not below normal body temperature reading, grasp thermometer with thumb and forefinger and shake vigorously by snapping the wrist in a downward motion to move mercury to a level below normal.

33. See Rationales 1 to 6.
34. Identifies correct device; a blue tip usually denotes an oral thermometer.
35. Cleansing removes disinfectant, which can irritate oral mucosa. Cool water prevents expansion of the colored solution/mercury. Touching the bulb will heat the solution and cause an inaccurate reading.
36. Wipe from area of least contamination to most contaminated area.
37. Thermometer must be below normal body temperature to ensure an accurate reading.
38. Shaking briskly lowers level of mercury in column. Because glass thermometers break easily, make sure that nothing in the environment comes in contact with the thermometer when shaking it.

continues

Figure 26-3-7   Place bulb of thermometer in the posterior sublingual pocket. Have client close lips around thermometer.

Figure 26-3-8   Wipe the thermometer with a tissue from fingertips to bulb end.

39. Place thermometer in client's mouth under the tongue and along the gumline to the posterior sublingual pocket. Instruct client to hold lips closed (Figure 26-3-7).

40. Leave in place as specified by institution policy, usually 3 to 5 minutes.

41. Remove thermometer and wipe with a tissue away from fingers toward the bulb's end (Figure 26-3-8).

42. Read at eye level and rotate slowly until mercury level is visualized.

43. Shake thermometer down, cleanse glass thermometer with soapy water, rinse under cold water, and return to storage container.

44. Remove and dispose of gloves in receptacle. Cleanse hands.

45. Record reading according to institution policy.

46. Cleanse hands.

39. Ensures contact with large blood vessels under the tongue. Prevents environmental air from coming in contact with the bulb.

40. Thermometer must stay in place long enough to ensure an accurate reading.

41. Mucus on thermometer may interfere with the effectiveness of the disinfectant solution. Wipe from area of least contamination to most contaminated area.

42. Ensures an accurate reading.

43. Mechanical cleansing removes secretions that promote growth of microorganisms. Hot water may cause coagulation of secretions and cause expansion of mercury in the thermometer.

44. Reduces transmission of microorganisms.

45. Accurate documentation by site allows for comparison of data.

46. Reduces transmission of microorganisms.

Rectal Temperature

47. Repeat Actions 1 to 6.

48. Place client in the Sims' position with upper knee flexed. Adjust sheet to expose only anal area.

49. Place tissues in easy reach. Apply gloves.

50. Prepare the thermometer.

51. Lubricate tip of rectal thermometer or probe (a rectal thermometer usually has a red tip or cap).

52. With dominant hand, grasp thermometer. With other hand, separate buttocks to expose anus (Figure 26-3-9).

53. Instruct the client to take a deep breath. Insert the thermometer or probe gently into anus: infant, 1.2 cm (0.5 inches); adult, 3.5 cm (1.5 inches). If resistance is felt, do not force insertion.

54. Hold in place for 2 minutes.

55. Wipe off secretions on the glass thermometer with a tissue. Dispose of tissue in a receptacle.

47. See Rationales 1 to 6.

48. Proper positioning ensures visualization of anus. Flexing knee relaxes muscles for ease of insertion.

49. Tissue is needed to wipe anus after device is removed.

50. Ensures a smooth procedure and an accurate reading.

51. Promotes ease of insertion of thermometer or probe.

52. Aids in visualization of anus.

53. Relaxes anal sphincter. Gentle insertion decreases discomfort to client and prevents trauma to mucous membranes.

54. Prevents trauma to mucosa and breakage of glass thermometer.

55. Removes secretions and fecal material for visualization of mercury level. Prevents transmission of microorganisms.

continues

Figure 26-3-9 Preparation for the Insertion of a Rectal Thermometer

56. Read measurement and inform the client of the temperature reading.
57. While holding glass thermometer in one hand, use other hand to wipe anal area with tissue to remove lubricant or feces. Dispose of soiled tissue. Cover client.
58. Cleanse thermometer.
59. Remove and dispose of gloves in receptacle. Cleanse hands.
60. Record reading according to institution policy.

56. Promotes client's participation in care.
57. Prevents contamination of clean objects with soiled thermometer, decreases skin irritation, and promotes client comfort. Prevents embarrassment.
58. Reduces transmission of microorganisms.
59. Reduces transmission of microorganisms.
60. Accurate documentation by site allows for comparison of data.

Axillary Temperature

61. Repeat Actions 1 to 6.
62. Remove client's arm and shoulder from one sleeve of gown. Avoid exposing chest.
63. Make sure axillary skin is dry; if necessary, pat dry.
64. Prepare thermometer.
65. Place thermometer or probe into center of axilla. Fold the client's upper arm straight down, and place arm across the client's chest.
66. Leave glass thermometer in place as specified by institution policy (usually 6 to 8 minutes). Leave an electronic thermometer in place until signal is heard.
67. Remove and read thermometer.
68. Inform client of temperature reading.
69. Shake down thermometer, cleanse glass thermometer with soapy water, rinse under cold water, and return to storage container.
70. Assist the client with replacing the gown.
71. Record reading according to institution policy.
72. Cleanse hands.

61. See Rationales 1 to 6.
62. Exposes axillary area.
63. Removes moisture and prevents a false low reading.
64. Ensures accurate use of thermometer.
65. Puts device in contact with axillary blood supply. Maintains the device in proper position.
66. Device must stay in place long enough to ensure an accurate reading. Signal indicates final temperature reading.
67. Allows accurate reading of temperature.
68. Promotes client's participation in care.
69. Prevents breakage of glass thermometer and transmission of microorganisms.
70. Promotes comfort.
71. Promotes accurate documentation for data comparison.
72. Reduces transmission of microorganisms.

Disposable (Chemical Strip) Thermometer

73. Repeat Actions 1 to 6.
74. Apply tape to appropriate skin area, usually forehead.
75. Observe tape for color changes.

76. Record reading and indicate method.
77. Cleanse hands.

73. See Rationales 1 to 6.
74. Tape must be in direct contact with the client's skin.
75. Color indicates temperature reading (refer to the manufacturer's instructions).
76. Promotes accurate documentation for data comparison.
77. Reduces transmission of microorganisms.

continues

EVALUATION

- Establish client's baseline temperature.
- Compare temperature with the client's baseline temperature.
- Evaluate the client's condition for trauma caused by the instrument.

DOCUMENTATION

Vital Signs Flow Sheet

- Temperature measurement and site
- Plot the temperature on a graph to identify patterns, or sudden elevations and drops (a condition known as spiking).

Medication Administration Record

- Antipyretic (fever-reducing) medications and temperature reading

Nurses' Notes

- Response to antipyretic medications

PROCEDURE 26-4   Taking a Pulse

OVERVIEW

Pulse assessment is the measurement of a pressure pulsation created when the heart contracts and ejects blood into the aorta. The amplitude of the pulse reflects the stroke volume with each ejection. Assessment of pulse characteristics provides clinical data regarding the heart's pumping action and the adequacy of peripheral artery blood flow. The radial pulse is most often used for basic assessment; however, other site areas are used in total assessment and when specific areas of circulation are to be determined.

PULSE-TAKING TECHNIQUES

Palpation

- Palpation of a pulse involves the index and middle fingers of one hand. Start with gentle pressure to locate the strongest pulsation, and then use firmer palpation for the counting. When counting, also assess the rhythm and quality of the pulse. Measure the pulse for 30 and 60 seconds, and then multiply the counts if need be to obtain the one-minute reading.

Auscultation

- Auscultation is usually used to assess the apical pulse. The apical pulse is the most accurate pulse, especially when the peripheral pulse is difficult to locate. Auscultation requires the stethoscope. The stethoscope should be equipped with a bell and a diaphragm. The diaphragm side is normally used for low-pitch sound, such as normal heart sound, bowel sound, or breath sound; the bell side is used for high-pitch sound, such as murmur and abnormal heart sound.

Doppler

- An ultrasonic Doppler device is usually used when the pulse cannot be detected by palpation. The Doppler can detect the peripheral pulses in situations such as cardiopulmonary collapse in obese clients, infants with small arms, or clients with edema in which palpation of the pulse is difficult.
- A vendor-recommended conductive gel should be applied to the skin as a coupling medium for ultrasound transmission. The transmitting device (probe) is then placed over the artery to be assessed. The Doppler usually is equipped with both high- and low-frequency probes. A high-frequency (8 to 10 Hz) probe is usually used on the surface vessel sites. A low-frequency (2 to 3 Hz) probe often is used for deeper sites, such as obstetric assessment.
- The sounds can be amplified and heard through an earpiece or speaker attached to the device, assessing with low volume initially. Tilt the back of the probe toward the hand at an angle of about 45 degrees. Search the area of the assessed artery and tilt the probe for best Doppler sounds. Adjust the sound volume control to a comfort level for counting.

continues

ASSESSMENT

1. Assess client for need to monitor pulse **because certain diseases or conditions, such as history of heart disease or cardiac dysrhythmias, chest pain, invasive cardiovascular diagnostic tests, infusion of large volume of IV fluids, or hemorrhage, can cause an increased risk for alterations in pulse.**
2. Assess the pulse for rate, amplitude, contour, and regularity.
3. Assess for signs and symptoms of cardiovascular alterations, such as dyspnea, chest pain, orthopnea, syncope, palpitations, edema of extremities, cyanosis, or fatigue, **because these signs may indicate deficient cardiac or vascular function.**
4. Assess client for factors that may affect the character of the pulse, such as age, medications, exercise, change in position, or fever. **This enables the nurse to accu-** rately assess for the significance of an alteration in pulse.
5. Assess for the appropriate site for measuring pulse **so the pulse will be accurate.**
6. Assess the baseline heart rate and rhythm in the client's chart **to compare it with the current measurement.**
7. Assess circulatory status by using appropriate site (Table 26-4-1) **because pulses may be affected by surgery, medical condition, arterial blood draws, or poor circulation.**

POSSIBLE NURSING DIAGNOSES

Decreased **C**ardiac Output
Ineffective **T**issue Perfusion (Cardiopulmonary)

TABLE 26-4-1   PULSE POINT ASSESSMENT

PULSE POINT	LOCATION	ASSESSMENT CRITERIA
1. Temporal	Over the temporal bone, lateral to the eye, upper to the ear	Accessible; used routinely for infants and when radial is inaccessible
2. Carotid	Bilateral, under the lower jaw, beneath the sternomastoid muscles. Carotid pulse best represents the aortic pulse for its close location to the central circulation. Palpation of the carotid artery on the neck may cause stimulation of the carotid sinus and result in decrease of the pulse rate	Accessible; used routinely for infants and during shock or cardiac arrest when other peripheral pulses are too weak to palpate; also used to assess cranial circulation Take a carotid pulse on only one side of the neck at a time
3. Apical	Left ventricle, fourth to fifth intercostal space, on the midclavicular line	Used to auscultate heart sounds and assess apical-radial deficit
4. Brachial	Inner side between the groove of bicep and tricep muscles at the antecubital fossa	Used in cardiac arrest for infants, to assess lower arm circulation, and to auscultate blood pressure
5. Radial	On the thumb side, inner aspect of the wrist	Accessible; used routinely in adults to assess character of peripheral pulse
6. Ulnar	On the little finger side, outer aspect of the wrist	Used to assess circulation to ulnar side of hand and to perform the Allen test
7. Femoral	Below the inguinal ligament, in the anterior medial aspect of the thigh, midway to the anterior-superior iliac spine and symphysis pubis	Used to assess circulation to legs and during cardiac arrest
8. Popliteal	Behind the knee. Medial or lateral to the popliteal fossa	Used to assess circulation to legs and to auscultate leg blood pressure
9. Posterior Tibial	Inner side of the ankle, between the Achilles tendon and tibia	Used to assess circulation to feet
10. Pedal/Dorsal Pedal	Lateral to the extension tendon, from the great toe toward the ankle	Used to assess circulation to feet

continues

PLANNING

Expected Outcomes

1. Pulse rate, quality, rhythm, and volume will be within normal range for the client's age group.
2. The client will be comfortable with the procedure and demonstrate an understanding regarding its importance.

Equipment Needed

- Watch with a second hand
- Stethoscope
- Alcohol swab
- Gloves

DELEGATION TIPS

The radial pulse assessment is often delegated to trained ancillary personnel; however, the nurse is responsible for knowing the results. Assessment of the apical pulse may be delegated to specially prepared staff. The assessment of peripheral circulation is delegated after proper training in the monitoring of peripheral sites for the presence of abnormal color, motion, or sensation in the extremity. The absence of pulses must be immediately reported for further assessment by the nurse, and the nurse is responsible for reviewing the data collected in a timely manner and revalidating the results, if indicated. The institution's policy should clearly indicate the training and validation requirements before the nurse delegates the monitoring of apical pulses and peripheral vascular assessments on stable clients. These tasks should not be delegated if the client is unstable.

IMPLEMENTATION—ACTION/RATIONALE

ACTION	RATIONALE

❖ Check client's identification band ❖ Explain procedure before beginning ❖

Taking a Radial (Wrist) Pulse

ACTION

1. Cleanse hands.
2. Inform client of the site(s) at which you will measure pulse.
3. Flex client's elbow and place lower part of arm across chest.

4. Support client's wrist by grasping outer aspect with thumb.
5. Place your index and middle fingers on inner aspect of client's wrist over the radial artery and apply light but firm pressure until pulse is palpated (Figure 26-4-1).

RATIONALE

1. Reduces transmission of microorganisms.
2. Encourages participation and allays anxiety.

3. Maintains wrist in full extension and exposes artery for palpation. Placing client's hand over chest will facilitate later respiratory assessment without undue attention to your action. (It is difficult for any person to maintain a normal breathing pattern when someone is observing and measuring.)
4. Stabilizes wrist and allows for pressure to be exerted.

5. Fingertips are sensitive, facilitating palpation of pulsating pulse. The nurse may feel his or her own pulse if palpating with thumb. Applying light pressure prevents occlusion of blood flow and pulsation.

Figure 26-4-1 Place index and middle fingers over radial artery.

continues

6. Identify pulse rhythm.

7. Determine pulse volume.

8. Count pulse rate by using second hand on watch.
   For a regular rhythm, count number of beats for 30 seconds and multiply by 2.
   For an irregular rhythm, count number of beats for a full minute, noting number of irregular beats.

Taking an Apical Pulse

9. Cleanse hands.
10. Raise client's gown to expose sternum and left side of chest.
11. Cleanse earpiece and diaphragm of stethoscope with an alcohol swab.

12. Put stethoscope around your neck.
13. Locate apex of heart:
    • With client lying on left side, locate suprasternal notch.
    • Palpate second intercostal space to left of sternum.
    • Place index finger in intercostal space, counting downward until fifth intercostal space is located.
    • Move index finger along fourth intercostal space left of the sternal border and to the fifth intercostal space, left of the midclavicular line to palpate the point of maximal impulse (PMI) (Figure 26-4-2).
    • Keep index finger of nondominant hand on the PMI.
14. Inform client that you are going to listen to his or her heart. Instruct client to remain silent.
15. With dominant hand, put earpiece of the stethoscope in your ears and grasp diaphragm of the stethoscope in palm of your hand for 5 to 10 seconds.
16. Place diaphragm of stethoscope over the PMI and auscultate for sounds S_1 and S_2 to hear lub-dub sound (Figure 26-4-3).
17. Note regularity of rhythm.

6. Palpate pulse until rhythm is determined. Describe as regular or irregular.
7. Quality of pulse strength is an indication of stroke volume. Describe as normal, weak, strong, or bounding.
8. An irregular rhythm requires a full minute of assessment to identify the number of inefficient cardiac contractions that fail to transmit a pulsation, referred to as a "skipped" or irregular beat.

9. Reduces transmission of microorganisms.
10. Allows access to client's chest for proper placement of stethoscope.
11. Decreases transmission of microorganisms from one health care practitioner to another (earpiece) and from one client to another (diaphragm).
12. Ensures stethoscope is nearby for frequent use.
13. Identification of landmarks facilitates correct placement of the stethoscope at the fifth intercostal space in order to hear point of maximal impulse.
    • Ensures correct placement of stethoscope.

14. Elicits client support. Stethoscope amplifies noise.

15. Dominant hand facilitates psychomotor dexterity for placement of earpiece with one hand. Heat warms metal or plastic diaphragm and prevents startling client.
16. Movement of blood through the heart valves creates S_1 and S_2 sounds. Listen for a regular rhythm (heartbeats are evenly spaced) before counting.
17. Establishment of a rhythmic pattern determines length of time to count the heartbeats to ensure accurate measurement.

Figure 26-4-2 Palpating the Apical Pulse

Figure 26-4-3 Place diaphragm of stethoscope over the PMI to hear the heart rate.

continues

18. Start to count while looking at second hand of watch. Count lub-dub sound as one beat:
   • For a regular rhythm, count rate for 30 seconds and multiply by 2.
   • For an irregular rhythm, count rate for a full minute, noting number of irregular beats.
19. Share your findings with client.
20. Record by site the rate, rhythm, and, if applicable, number of irregular beats.
21. Cleanse hands.

18. Ensures sufficient time to count irregular beats.

19. Promotes client participation in care.
20. Record rate and characteristics at bedside to ensure accurate documentation.
21. Reduces transmission of microorganisms.

EVALUATION

• Compare client's pulse with baseline rate, amplitude, and rhythm to detect any changes.
• If pulse is irregular or abnormal, ask another nurse to check the pulse and then report to health care provider.
• Evaluate pulse site as required by client's condition and compare bilateral pulses. Example: For clients with poor peripheral circulation in the lower extremities, compare both pedal/dorsal or both posterior tibial pulses.

DOCUMENTATION

Nurses' Notes and/or Flow Sheet

• Pulse rate
• Observations regarding regularity, volume, or rate
• New irregularities in pulse reported to the client's health care provider

---

PROCEDURE 26-5   Counting Respirations

OVERVIEW

Respiratory assessment is the measurement of the breathing pattern. Assessment of respirations provides clinical data regarding the pH of arterial blood.

Normal breathing is slightly observable, effortless, quiet, automatic, and regular. It can be assessed by observing chest wall expansion and bilateral symmetric movement of the thorax or by placing the back of the hand next to the client's nose and mouth to feel the expired air.

When assessing respiration, ascertain the rate, depth, and rhythm of ventilatory movement. Assess the rate by counting the number of breaths taken per minute. Note the depth and rhythm of ventilatory movements by observing for the normal thoracic and abdominal movements and symmetry in chest wall movement. Normal respirations are characterized by a rate ranging from 12 to 20 breaths per minute.

One inspiration and expiration cycle is counted as one breath. The nurse can observe the rise and fall of the chest wall and count the rate by placing the hand lightly on the chest to feel it rise and fall. Count the number of respirations for a 30-second interval and multiply by 2 if respirations are regular and even. If the client is experiencing any respiratory difficulty, count the rate for a full minute.

Also observe alterations in the movement of the chest wall: Costal (thoracic) breathing occurs when the external intercostal muscles and the other accessory muscles are used to move the chest upward and outward; diaphragmatic (abdominal) breathing occurs when the diaphragm contracts and relaxes as observed by movement of the abdomen. Dyspnea refers to difficulty in breathing as observed by labored or forced respirations through the use of accessory muscles in the chest and neck to breathe. Dyspneic clients are acutely aware of their respirations and complain of shortness of breath.

Respiratory alterations may cause changes in skin color as observed by a bluish appearance of the nail beds, lips, and skin. The bluish color (cyanosis) results from reduced oxygen level in the arterial blood. Changes in the level of consciousness (restlessness, anxiety, and dyspnea) may also occur with decreased oxygen level. Clients assume a forward-leaning position or may have to stand to increase the expansion capacity of the lungs.

Metabolic alterations such as diabetic ketoacidosis can cause Kussmaul's respirations, which are abnormally deep but regular.

continues

Apnea is the cessation of breathing for several seconds. Persistent apnea is called respiratory arrest. Irregular rhythm with alternating periods of apnea and hyperventilation is called Cheyne-Stokes respirations. The cycle begins with slow, shallow breaths that gradually increase to abnormally deep and rapid respirations, which then gradually slow and return to shallow breathing followed by apnea. This is common in clients who are dying (see Figure 26-5-2).

ASSESSMENT

1. Assess the movement of client's chest wall **to see if it is equal bilaterally, if the movement is labored, or if the client is using accessory muscles to breathe.**
2. Assess the rate of respirations **to identify slow, rapid, or irregular respirations or even periods of apnea.**
3. Assess the depth of the client's breaths **to monitor shallow, deep, or uneven respirations. Think if there might be something influencing the client's respirations. Is the client in pain, frightened, talking, or smoking?**
4. Assess for risk factors such as fever, pain, anxiety, diseases, or trauma to the chest wall **that may alter the respirations because certain conditions may cause increased risk of alterations in respirations.**
5. Assess for factors that normally influence respirations such as age, exercise, anxiety, pain, smoking, medications, or postural changes **so that an accurate assessment can be made.**

POSSIBLE NURSING DIAGNOSES

*Impaired **G**as Exchange*
*Impaired Spontaneous **V**entilation*
*Ineffective **A**irway Clearance*
*Ineffective **B**reathing Pattern*

PLANNING

Expected Outcomes

1. An accurate evaluation of a client's respiratory rate and character will be obtained.
2. The respiratory rate and character will be normal.

Equipment Needed

- Watch with a second hand
- Stethoscope if needed

DELEGATION TIPS

The skill of respiratory rate measurement is often delegated to properly trained ancillary personnel; however, the nurse is responsible for this information and appropriate action. Respiration counts over 30 (adult) or 60 (child) should be immediately reported to the nurse for further assessment.

IMPLEMENTATION—ACTION/RATIONALE

ACTION	RATIONALE
❋ Check client's identification band ❋ Explain procedure before beginning ❋	
1. Cleanse hands.	1. Reduces transmission of microorganisms.
2. Be sure chest movement is visible. Client may need to remove heavy clothing.	2. Facilitates observation of chest wall and abdominal movements.
3. Observe one complete respiratory cycle. If it is easier, place the client's hand across the abdomen and your hand over the client's wrist.	3. Helps determine what constitutes a breath. Helps to determine what to count. Hand rises and falls with inspiration and expiration.
4. Start counting with first inspiration while looking at the second hand of a watch (Figure 26-5-1).	4. Respiratory rate is one complete cycle (inspiration and expiration).
• Infants and children: Count a full minute.	• Infants and children usually have an irregular rate.
• Adults: Count for 30 seconds and multiply by 2. If an irregular rate or rhythm is present, count for one full minute.	

continues

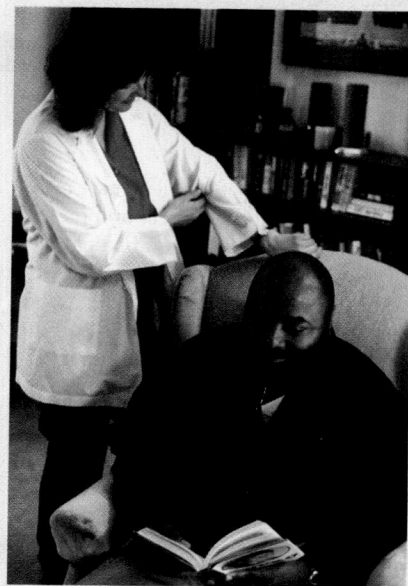

Figure 26-5-1   Count inspirations for a full 30 seconds.

Figure 26-5-2   When assessing respirations, observe skin color and level of consciousness as well as respiratory rate and rhythm.

5. Observe character of respirations:
   • Depth of respirations by degree of chest wall movement (shallow, normal, or deep)
   • Rhythm of cycle (regular or interrupted)
6. Observe skin color and level of consciousness (Figure 26-5-2).
7. Replace client's gown if needed.
8. Record rate and character of respirations.

9. Cleanse hands.

5. Reveals volume of air movement into and out of the lungs.

6. Reveals reduced oxygen level in arterial blood.

7. Prevents embarrassment and chilling.
8. Record rate and characteristics at bedside to ensure accurate documentation.
9. Reduces transmission of microorganisms.

EVALUATION

• Evaluate client's respirations as a baseline value.
• Compare respirations with baseline to detect any alterations.

DOCUMENTATION

Vital Signs Flow Sheet

•   Respiratory rate

Nurses' Notes

•   Depth, rhythm, and character of respirations
•   Respiratory rate outside the normal age range, an irregular rhythm, inadequate depth, or any abnormal characteristics such as dyspnea

PROCEDURE 26-6   Taking Blood Pressure

OVERVIEW

Blood pressure measurement is performed during a physical examination, at initial assessment, and as part of routine vital signs assessment. Depending on the client's condition, the blood pressure is measured by either a direct or indirect technique.

The indirect method requires use of the sphygmomanometer and stethoscope for auscultation and palpation as needed. The most common site for indirect blood pressure measurement is the client's arm over the brachial artery. When the client's condition prevents auscultation of the brachial artery, assess the blood pressure in the forearm or leg sites. When pressure measurements in the upper extremities are not accessible, the popliteal artery, located behind the knee, is the site of choice. Blood pressure can also be assessed in other sites, such as the radial artery in the forearm and the posterior tibial or dorsalis pedis artery in the lower leg. Because it is difficult to auscultate sounds over the radial, tibial, and dorsalis pedis arteries, these sites are usually palpated to obtain a systolic reading.

The direct method requires an invasive procedure in which an intravenous catheter with an electronic sensor is inserted into an artery and the artery-transmitted pressure on an electronic display unit is read.

ASSESSMENT

1. Assess the condition of the potential blood pressure (BP) site **so that a site with an injury or surgery proximal to the site can be avoided.**
2. Assess the artery for any compromise to it **so that compressing the artery briefly will not cause decrease in circulation.**
3. Assess the distal pulse **to check if it is intact and palpable.**
4. Assess the circumference of the extremity for the right size cuff to be used **so an accurate reading can be obtained.**
5. Assess for factors that affect blood pressure, such as age, anxiety, fear, medications, smoking, eating, or exercising within 30 minutes before BP assessment, and postural changes **so an accurate reading can be obtained.**
6. Determine client's baseline blood pressure by reading the medical record **so a comparison can be made with each BP reading.**

POSSIBLE NURSING DIAGNOSES

*Ineffective **T**issue Perfusion (Cardiopulmonary)*
*Decreased **C**ardiac Output*
***D**eficient Knowledge (blood pressure control)*

PLANNING

Expected Outcomes

1. An accurate estimate of the arterial pressure at diastole and systole will be obtained.
2. Blood pressure is within normal range for the client.
3. Client will be able to understand why the blood pressure is taken and what it means.

Equipment Needed

- Stethoscope
- Sphygmomanometer/bladder with mercury column or aneroid dial
- Gloves, if required
- Alcohol swabs

DELEGATION TIPS

The measurement of blood pressure is often delegated to ancillary personnel who have been properly educated to use both manual and electronic equipment; however, the nurse is responsible for carefully monitoring this information for significant changes and taking appropriate action. The delegation of blood pressure measurement would be reserved for a client in stable physical condition and measured at sites without intravenous solutions infusing, dialysis shunt or fistula, painful extremity, or recent mastectomy.

continues

IMPLEMENTATION—ACTION/RATIONALE

ACTION

RATIONALE

* Check client's identification band * Explain procedure before beginning *

Auscultation Method Using Brachial Artery

1. Cleanse hands.
2. Determine which extremity is most appropriate for reading. Do not take a pressure reading on an injured or painful extremity or one in which an intravenous line is running.
3. Select a cuff size appropriate for the client. Estimate by inspection, or measure with a tape, the circumference of the bare upper arm at the midpoint between the shoulder (acromion) and the elbow (olecranon process) (Figure 26-6-1).

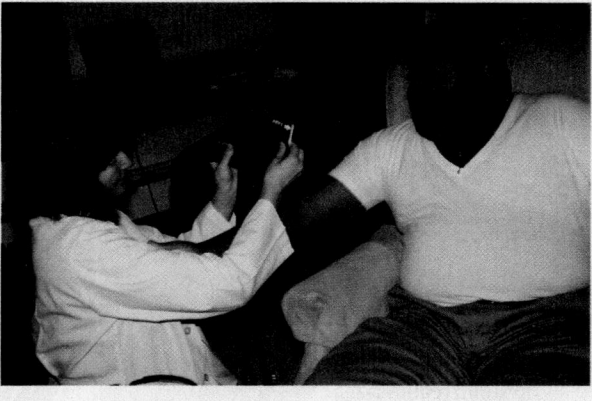

1. Reduces transmission of microorganisms.
2. Cuff inflation can temporarily interrupt blood flow and compromise circulation in an extremity already impaired or a vein receiving intravenous fluid.
3. The bladder inside the cuff should encircle 80% of the arm in adults and 100% of the arm of children less than 13 years old. If in doubt, use a larger cuff to ensure equalization of pressure on the artery and accurate measurement.

Figure 26-6-1 Select proper cuff size. An obese client may need a larger cuff size to obtain an accurate reading.

4. Have the client's bared arm resting on a support so the midpoint of the upper arm is at the level of the heart. Extend the elbow with palm turned upward.
5. Make sure the bladder cuff is fully deflated and the pump valve moves freely. Place the manometer so the center of the mercury column or aneroid dial is at eye level and easily visible to the observer.
6. Palpate the brachial artery, in the antecubital space, and place the cuff so that the midline of the bladder is over the arterial pulsation. Next, wrap and secure the cuff snugly around the client's bare upper arm. The lower edge of the cuff should be 1 inch (2 cm) above the antecubital fossa (bend of the elbow), where the head of the stethoscope is to be placed (Figures 26-6-2 and 26-6-3).
7. Inflate the cuff rapidly to 70 mm Hg and increase by 10-mm increments while palpating the radial pulse. Note the level of pressure at which the pulse disappears and subsequently reappears during deflation.

8. Insert the earpieces of the stethoscope into the ear canals with a forward tilt to fit snugly.

4. Blood pressure increases when the arm is below the level of the heart and decreases when the arm is above the level of the heart.
5. Equipment must be visible and function properly to obtain an accurate reading.

6. Ensures even pressure distribution over the brachial artery. Rolling up the sleeve may form a tourniquet around the upper arm. Always use a bare arm.

7. The palpatory method provides the necessary preliminary approximation of systolic blood pressure to ensure an accurate reading. When frequent measurements are required, such as every 15 minutes, the palpatory method is generally not incorporated with each pressure check.
8. The bell, the low-frequency position of the stethoscope, enhances sound transmission from chest piece to ears.

continues

Figure 26-6-2   Palpate the brachial artery to determine placement of the stethoscope.

Figure 26-6-3   Center the blood pressure cuff over the brachial artery.

9. Relocate the brachial artery with your nondominant hand, and place the bell of the stethoscope over the brachial artery pulsation. The bell should be held firmly in place, ensuring that the head is in direct contact with the skin and not touching the cuff (Figure 26-6-4).
10. With the dominant hand, turn the valve clockwise to close. Compress the pump to inflate the cuff rapidly and steadily until the manometer registers 20 to 30 mm Hg above the level previously determined by the palpation.
11. Partially unscrew (open) the valve counterclockwise to deflate the bladder at 2 mm/sec while listening for the appearance of the five phases of the Korotkoff sounds. Note the manometer reading for these sounds.
    I   A faint, clear tapping sound that increases in intensity
    II   Swishing sound
    III   Intense sound
    IV   Abrupt, distinctive muffled sound
    V   No sound

9. Sound is heard best directly over the artery. Wedging the head of the stethoscope under the edge of the cuff results in considerable extraneous noise and may cause an inaccurate reading.
10. Prevents air leaks during inflation. Ensures the cuff is inflated to a pressure greater than the client's systolic pressure.
11. Maintains constant release of pressure to ensure hearing first systolic sound. Identify manometer readings for each of the five phases.
    • Identify two consecutive tapping sounds to confirm systolic reading.
    • The American Heart Association (2002) recommends using Phase IV as the diastolic level in children less than 13 years old. Even though 5 phases of Korotkoff sounds have been identified, most clients have only 2 clearly distinct sounds (phase I and V), identified as the systolic and diastolic sounds.

Figure 26-6-4   The stethoscope chestpiece should not touch the blood pressure cuff.

continues

12. After the last Korotkoff sound is heard, deflate the cuff slowly for at least another 10 mm Hg to ensure that no other sounds are audible; then, deflate rapidly and completely.

13. Allow the client to rest for at least 30 seconds and re- move cuff. (A measurement should be repeated after 30 seconds and the two readings averaged. It may be done in the same or opposite arm) (American Heart Association, 2002).

14. Inform the client of the reading.

15. The systolic (Phase I) and diastolic (Phase V) pressure should be immediately recorded, rounded off (upward) to the nearest 2 mm Hg. (In children and when sounds are heard nearly to the level of 0 mm Hg, the Phase IV pressure should also be recorded.)

16. If appropriate, lower bed, raise side rails, and place call light in easy reach.

17. Put all equipment in proper place.

18. Cleanse hands.

12. Prevents arterial occlusion and client discomfort from numbness or tingling.

13. Releases trapped blood in the vessels. Ensures accurate measurement.

14. Promotes client's participation in health care.

15. Ensures accuracy.

16. Promotes client's safety.

17. Fosters maintenance of equipment.

18. Reduces transmission of microorganisms.

EVALUATION

- Evaluate the blood pressure reading for accuracy by comparing with the medical record.
- Evaluate the client's blood pressure for being within the normal range.
- Identify variations in the client's blood pressure of more than 5 to 10 mm Hg from one arm to the other.
- Evaluate if the client's blood pressure changes signifi- cantly when he or she stands up.
- Report abnormal measurements to charge nurse or health care provider.

DOCUMENTATION

Vital Signs Flow Sheet

- Blood pressure measurement
- Site where recording was done
- Method of obtaining the pressure—auscultation or palpation

PROCEDURE 26-7   Weighing a Client, Mobile and Immobile

OVERVIEW

A client's weight is an essential piece of data used in monitoring his or her response to a variety of therapies. Changes in a client's weight could necessitate an alteration in the assessment and intervention plans. An accurate weight is important, therefore, to ensure appropriate care.

ASSESSMENT

1. Assess the client's ability to stand independently and safely on a scale. **Consider factors requiring the use of a sling scale: The client is somnolent or comatose; paralyzed; too weak to stand; or un- steady when standing.**

2. Determine if clothing is similar to that worn during previous weight measurement **to help determine ac- curacy of the new weight.**

continues

POSSIBLE NURSING DIAGNOSES

*Imbalanced **N**utrition: More than Body Requirements*
*Imbalanced **N**utrition: Less than Body Requirements*
*Excess **F**luid Volume*
*Deficient **F**luid Volume*

PLANNING

Expected Outcomes

1. Health care provider obtains accurate weight.
2. Client incurs no injuries.
3. Client maintains privacy.

Equipment Needed

- Scale: standing electronic or balance scale (see Figure 26-7-1) or sling scale (Figure 26-7-2)
- Recommended disinfectant
- 1 to 3 other staff members to assist when using sling scale
- Plastic cover for sling scale
- Gloves (when applicable)

DELEGATION TIPS

The skill of weighing the mobile and immobile client is routinely delegated to trained ancillary personnel. The personnel should be instructed to do the following:

- *Select the correct scale for measurement.*
- *Properly and safely position the client for measurement.*
- *Correctly and safely perform the measurement according to established guidelines and record on the appropriate flow sheet (clinical record).*
- *Recognize and report abnormal findings promptly to the nurse.*

Figure 26-7-1   The standing balance scale is used to weigh ambulatory clients.

Figure 26-7-2   The sling scale is used to weigh clients in bed.

continues

IMPLEMENTATION—ACTION/RATIONALE

ACTION

RATIONALE

✻ Check client's identification band ✻ Explain procedure before beginning ✻

Standing Scale

1. Cleanse hands.
2. Place the scale near the client.
3. Turn on the scale and calibrate it to zero.
4. Ask client to remove shoes if necessary, step up on the scale, and stand still.
   Electronic scale: Read weight after digital numbers have stopped fluctuating.
   Balance scale: Slide the larger weight into the notch most closely approximating the client's weight. Slide the smaller weight into the notch so the balance rests in the middle. Add the two numbers for the client's weight.
5. Ask the client to step down. Assist the client back to the bed or chair, if necessary.
6. Wipe the scale with appropriate disinfectant.
7. Cleanse hands.

1. Reduces transmission of microorganisms.
2. Reduces risk of fall or injury.
3. Ensures accurate reading.
4. Obtains weight.

   Reading is not accurate when the numbers are still fluctuating.
   Weights on scale must be balanced to obtain accurate reading.

5. Reduces risk of injury if client needs assistance.

6. Reduces risk of spread of infection.
7. Reduces transmission of microorganisms.

Sling Scale

8. Cleanse hands and put on gloves if needed.
9. Place plastic covering on sling if available (can usually be ordered in bulk from the manufacturer).
10. Remove pillows. Turn the client to one side and place half of sling on bed next to the client, with remaining half rolled up against the client's back (Figure 26-7-3).
11. Turn the client to the other side, and unroll the rest of the sling so it lays flat beneath the client.
12. Roll the scale over the bed such that the legs of the scale are underneath the bed (Figure 26-7-4). Open and lock the legs of the scale.
13. Turn on scale and calibrate to zero.

8. Reduces risk of nosocomial infection.
9. Reduces risk of spreading infection between clients.
10. Most accurate weight will be obtained by leaving no other bedding between the client and sling.
11. Turning in this manner maximizes client comfort.
12. Ensures equipment is being used safely to reduce risk of injury.
13. Ensures accurate reading.

Figure 26-7-3 Turn client on one side and place sling on the bed.

Figure 26-7-4 After unrolling the rest of the sling under the client, move the scale into position over the bed.

continues

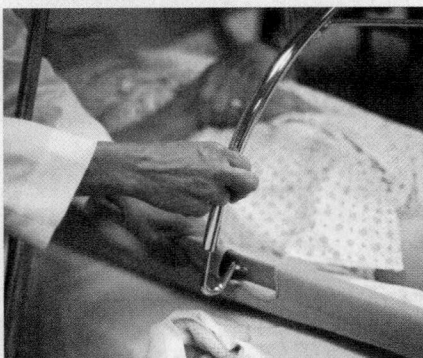

Figure 26-7-5   Attach the hooks through the holes in the sling.

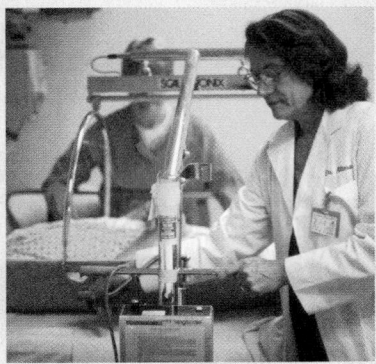

Figure 26-7-6   Pump the scale until the sling lifts completely off the bed.

14. Lower arms of the scale and slip hooks through holes in sling (Figure 26-7-5).
15. Pump scale until sling rests completely off the bed (Figure 26-7-6).
16. Remind the client to remain still. Read weight after digital numbers have stopped fluctuating (Figure 26-7-7).
17. Lower the client back to bed and remove arms of the scale from sling (Figure 26-7-8).
18. Unlock scale legs, return to their original position, and remove scale from bed.
19. Turn the client on his or her side, roll up sling, turn client to the other side.
20. Realign the client with pillows and covers.
21. Remove plastic covering from the sling and discard as per hospital policy.
22. Remove gloves and cleanse hands.

14. Attaches sling to scale to obtain weight.

15. Ensures accurate weight.

16. Reading is not accurate when the numbers are still fluctuating.

17. Prepares for removal of sling.

18. Allows for removal of equipment that obstructs proximity to the client, thereby facilitating removal of the sling.
19. Facilitates removal of the sling.

20. Ensures comfort and privacy.
21. Reduces risk of spread of infection and nosocomial infection.
22. Reduces transmission of microorganisms.

Figure 26-7-7   Read the weight after the numbers have stopped fluctuating.

Figure 26-7-8   Lower the client back to the bed and remove the sling.

EVALUATION

• Compare weight obtained to previously recorded weight. Repeat weight if large discrepancy is noted.
• If large discrepancy still remains, notify appropriate health care team members.

DOCUMENTATION

Vital Signs Flow Sheet

• Date, time of day, and the weight of the client on the appropriate flow sheet

PROCEDURE 26-8   Proper Body Mechanics

OVERVIEW

Skills needed to care for clients often require physical strength to provide individuals with assistance required to remain mobile. Nurses/caregivers may need to carry, pull, push, or lift clients and/or equipment to accomplish daily care. It is imperative to know and use proper lifting techniques and seek assistance as needed to avoid injury to self and clients. Body mechanics is the term used when referring to lifting techniques. Correct body mechanics are essential to avoid work-related musculoskeletal injuries, diminish excessive strain and fatigue, and minimize the potential for injury (Figure 26-8-1).

Body mechanics involve pushing, pulling, stooping, carrying, and lifting correctly. Knowledge of various client transfer techniques, the use of a team as needed, and the use of proper supportive equipment are included in this skill. Proper techniques of body mechanics, specialized lifting skills of transfer from bed to stretcher and from bed to chair or wheelchair, and the use of the bed transfer board and a hydraulic lift are reviewed. Specific tips for client and staff safety are highlighted. Promotion of client independence and self-help behavior as an intervention to reduce the risk of client and nurse injury is discussed.

ASSESSMENT

1. Assess the need and degree to which the client requires assistance to achieve physical movement. **Identifies client's ability to attain maximum level of self-help before initiating intervention.**
2. Identify the type of physical movement required **to ensure the use of proper body mechanics such as pushing, pulling, or lifting.**
3. Identify the potential need for assistive equipment to accomplish the goal of safe lifting **to minimize the risk of client/nurse injury.**

4. Identify any unusual risks to safe lifting, such as an extra-heavy client or a home care setting. **Allows nurse to plan modifications to ensure good body mechanics and reduce the risk of injury.**
5. Assess the client's vital signs, pain status, and need for pain medications before ambulating. Assess incisional areas and/or areas of injury.
6. Check equipment to ensure that it is in working order to facilitate a safe and uninterrupted transfer. Especially check locks on wheelchair.
7. Identify all equipment and tubes connected to the client and take appropriate preventive measures.

Figure 26-8-1 Always follow these eight rules for lifting. (Reprinted with permission from Ergodyne Corporation, St. Paul, MN.)

continues

Frequently, clients that require lifting or transfer have intravenous tubing, other tubing, and/or orthopedic equipment.

8. Assess the client's understanding of the steps required to achieve the goal of a safe transfer and the ability to assist. Explanation of the steps in a clear, concise fashion will decrease anxiety, secure cooperation, and ease physical requirements for both the client and the nurse/caregiver.

POSSIBLE NURSING DIAGNOSES

Risk for **I**njury
Impaired Physical **M**obility

PLANNING

Expected Outcomes

1. Clients will be safely lifted/transferred by staff utilizing appropriate equipment and correct body mechanics.

2. Accidents during lifting of clients will be avoided by using proper body alignment and mechanics.
3. Heavy lifting will be facilitated by mechanical devices and a team effort.
4. Clients and families will be taught safe lifting/transfer techniques to facilitate this process in home and extended-care environments.
5. The nurse will practice safe lifting and proper body mechanics when performing nursing care that requires bending or lifting.

Equipment Needed

- Transfer or gait belts
- Wheelchair equipped with working locks
- Transfer board
- Draw or lift sheet
- Nonslip shoes or slippers
- Safety or gait belt
- Stretcher equipped with working locks
- Hydraulic lift

DELEGATION TIPS

Delegation to ancillary personnel of the moving, transferring, and lifting of clients is an expectation of their role after proper instruction and/or certification. Ancillary personnel are routinely expected to place the bed at proper height, use a wide base of support, properly position the client, and safely use assistive devices. After repositioning the client, ancillary personnel are expected to evaluate the client's level of comfort. The client who requires complex turning or lifting devices needs the supervision of the professional nurse.

IMPLEMENTATION—ACTION/RATIONALE

ACTION	RATIONALE

* Check client's identification band * Explain procedure before beginning *

ACTION	RATIONALE
1. Cleanse hands.	1. Reduces the transmission of microorganisms.
2. Assess the situation for obstacles, heavy clients, poor handholds, or equipment or objects in the way. Reduce or remove safety hazards prior to lifting the client or object. Assess for any tubing or equipment connected to the client.	2. Good planning helps prevent accidental injury.
3. Assess the situation for slippery surfaces, including wet floors; slippery shoes on client, helper, or nurse; and towels, linen, or paper on the floor. Resolve the slippery surface before lifting the client or object.	3. Removes the cause of many falls and slips.
4. Assess the situation for hidden risks, including client confusion, combativeness, orthostatic hypotension, drug effects, pain, or fear.	4. Allows the nurse to anticipate and plan for unexpected events.
5. Maintain low center of gravity by bending at the hips and knees, not the waist. Squat down rather than bend over to lift and lower (Figure 26-8-2).	5. Provides for the equal distribution of body weight and assists in maintaining safe balance.
6. Establish a wide support base with feet spread apart (Figure 26-8-3).	6. Provides stability and lowers the center of gravity.

continues

Figure 26-8-2 Squat, rather than bend, to maintain good posture.

Figure 26-8-3 Spread feet apart to establish a wide base of support.

7. Use feet to move, not a twisting or bending motion from the waist.
8. When pushing or pulling, stand near the object and stagger one foot partially ahead of the other.
9. When pushing a client or an object, lean into the client or object and apply continuous light pressure. When pulling a client or an object, lean away and grasp with light pressure. Never jerk or twist your body to force a weight to move.
10. When stooping to move an object, maintain a wide base of support with feet, flex knees to lower body, and maintain straight upper body.
11. When lifting or carrying an object, squat in front of the object, take a firm hold, and assume a standing position by using the leg muscles and keeping the back straight.
12. When rising up from a squatting position, arch your back slightly. Keep the buttocks and abdomen tucked in and rise up with your head first.
13. When lifting or carrying heavy objects, keep the weight as close to your center of gravity as possible.
14. When reaching for a client or an object, keep the back straight. If the client or object is heavy, do not try to lift the client or object without repositioning yourself closer to the weight (Figure 26-8-4).

7. Assists in maintaining correct body alignment, which increases strength to lift, push, pull, and carry.
8. Provides a safety net for avoiding potential back injuries.
9. Firm pressure will provide continuous movement of the object and will avoid abrupt movements that require the expenditure of increased energy.

10. Provides the appropriate mechanics for the strength and endurance to achieve the task and to stand up straight upon completion.
11. This stance will avoid the use of the back, diminish the potential for spinal twisting, and provide the lifter with a firm center of gravity and strength to lift the required weight.
12. Keeps the back from bowing and increasing the strain on the back muscles.

13. Reduces the strain on arm, leg, and back muscles.

14. Avoids straining the back and arm muscles.

Figure 26-8-4 Keep your back straight when reaching.

continues

Figure 26-8-5   Use gait belts for better grip and control.

Figure 26-8-6   Use lifts to carry the weight of the client. Monitor equipment, lines, tubes, and drains and adjust as needed to prevent them from being dislodged.

Figure 26-8-7   Use transfer boards to reduce shearing forces and to reduce the effort needed to slide the client.

15. Use safety aids and equipment. Use gait belts (Figure 26-8-5), lifts (Figure 26-8-6), drawsheets, and other transfer assistance devices (Figure 26-8-7). Encourage clients to use handrails and grab bars. Wheelchair, cart, and stretcher wheels should be locked when they are not actually being moved.

15. Reduces the strain on the nurse and improves the safety for the client.

EVALUATION

- The client or object is lifted and/or moved without sustaining injury or damage.
- The nurse who is lifting and moving clients or objects is not injured.

DOCUMENTATION

Nurses' Notes

- Type of lift or transfer in the progress notes
- Client's tolerance of the lift or move

PROCEDURE 26-9

Performing Passive Range-of-Motion (ROM) Exercises

OVERVIEW

Passive range-of-motion (ROM or PROM) exercises seek to maintain or improve the current level of functional mobility of a client's extremities. The nurse provides, assists with, and teaches the client functional movements in all available planes and directions of involved joints. ROM exercises prevent contractures and shortening of muscles and tendons, increase circulation to extremities, decrease vascular complications of immobility, and facilitate comfort for the client.

ASSESSMENT

1. Be aware of the client's medical diagnosis. **Understand the expected functional limits of a client with this diagnosis.**
2. Familiarize yourself with the client's current range of motion. Note any joint pain, stiffness, or inflammation that might limit the client's motion. **Understanding the client's current ROM will help you assess the functional limits of movement of each joint.**
3. Assess client consciousness and cognitive function. **Client should be encouraged to participate in ROM as actively as possible.**

POSSIBLE NURSING DIAGNOSES

Impaired Physical Mobility
Risk for Activity Intolerance

PLANNING

Expected Outcomes

1. Client will maintain or improve current functional mobility in all involved joints and extremities.
2. Client will regain or improve strength and/or voluntary movement in involved joints and extremities.
3. Client will avoid complications of immobility, including pressure ulcers, contractures, decreased peristalsis, constipation, fecal impaction, orthostatic hypotension, pulmonary embolism, and thrombophlebitis.

Equipment Needed

- No special equipment is needed, except gloves when contact with body fluids is possible.

DELEGATION TIPS

Administering passive range-of-motion exercises may be delegated to properly trained ancillary personnel. Outcomes must be reported to the nurse.

IMPLEMENTATION—ACTION/RATIONALE

ACTION

❋ **Check client's identification band** ❋ **Explain procedure before beginning** ❋

1. Cleanse hands, wear gloves if contact with body fluids is possible.
2. Provide for privacy, including exposing only the extremity to be exercised.
3. Adjust bed to comfortable height for performing ROM.
4. Lower bed rail only on the side you are working.
5. Describe the passive ROM exercises you are performing, or verbally cue client to perform ROM exercises with your assistance.
6. Start at the client's head and perform ROM exercises down each side of the body.

RATIONALE

1. Reduces the transmission of microorganisms.
2. Decreases embarrassment.
3. Prevents muscle strain and discomfort for nurse.
4. Prevents falls.
5. Exercises all joint areas.
6. Provides a systematic method to ensure that all body parts are exercised.

continues

7. Repeat each ROM exercise as the client tolerates, to a maximum of 5 times. Perform each motion in a slow, firm manner. Encourage full joint movement, but do not go beyond the point of pain, resistance, or fatigue.

8. Head
   Perform these movements with the client in a sitting position, if possible.
   • Rotation: Turn the head from side to side.
   • Flexion and extension: Tilt the head toward the chest and then tilt slightly upward.
   • Lateral flexion: Tilt the head on each side so as to almost touch the ear to the shoulder.

9. Neck
   Perform these movements with the client in a sitting position, if possible.
   • Rotation: Rotate the neck in a semicircle while supporting the head.

10. Trunk
    Perform these movements with the client in a sitting position, if possible.
    • Flexion and extension: Bend the trunk forward, straighten the trunk, and then extend slightly backward.
    • Rotation: Turn the shoulders forward and return to normal position.
    • Lateral flexion: Tip trunk to the left side, straighten trunk, tip to the right side.

11. Arm
    • Flexion and extension: Extend the arm in a straight position upward above the head, then downward along the side and back.
    • Adduction and abduction: Extend the arm in a straight position toward the midline (adduction) and away from the midline (abduction).

12. Shoulder
    • Internal and external rotation: Bend the elbow at a 90-degree angle with the upper arm parallel to the shoulder; rotate the shoulder by moving the lower arm upward and downward.

13. Elbow
    • Flexion and extension: Supporting the arm, flex and extend the elbow.
    • Pronation and supination: Flex elbow, move the hand in palm-up and palm-down position.

14. Wrist
    • Flexion and extension: Supporting the wrist, flex and extend the wrist (Figure 26-9-1).
    • Adduction and abduction: Supporting the lower arm, turn wrist right to left, left to right, then rotate the wrist in a circular motion.

15. Hand
    • Flexion and extension: Supporting the wrist, flex and extend the fingers (Figure 26-9-2).
    • Adduction and abduction: Supporting the wrist, spread fingers apart and then bring them close together.
    • Opposition: Supporting the wrist, touch each finger with the tip of the thumb.
    • Thumb rotation: Supporting the wrist, rotate the thumb in a circular manner.

7. Provides exercise to the client's tolerance or to a level that will maintain the joint function.

8. Optimizes the performance of the movements, to preserve muscle tone and joint flexibility.

9. Optimizes the performance of the movements, to preserve muscle tone and joint flexibility.

10. Optimizes the performance of the movements, to preserve muscle tone and joint flexibility.

11. Optimizes the performance of the movements, to preserve muscle tone and joint flexibility.

12. Optimizes the performance of the movements, to preserve muscle tone and joint flexibility.

13. Optimizes the performance of the movements, to preserve muscle tone and joint flexibility.

14. Optimizes the performance of the movements, to preserve muscle tone and joint flexibility.

15. Optimizes the performance of the movements, to preserve muscle tone and joint flexibility.

continues

Figure 26-9-1 Flex and extend the wrist.

Figure 26-9-2 Flex and extend the fingers.

16. Hip and leg
    Perform these movements with the client in a supine position, if possible.
    - Flexion and extension: Supporting the lower leg, flex the leg toward the chest and then extend the leg.
    - Internal and external rotation: Supporting the lower leg, angle the foot inward and outward.
    - Adduction and abduction: Slide the leg away from the client's midline and then back to the midline (Figure 26-9-3).
17. Knee
    - Flexion and extension: Supporting the lower leg, flex and extend the knee (Figure 26-9-4).
18. Ankle
    - Flexion and extension: Supporting the lower leg, flex and extend the ankle.

16. Optimizes the performance of the movements, to preserve muscle tone and joint flexibility.

17. Optimizes the performance of the movements, to preserve muscle tone and joint flexibility.

18. Optimizes the performance of the movements, to preserve muscle tone and joint flexibility.

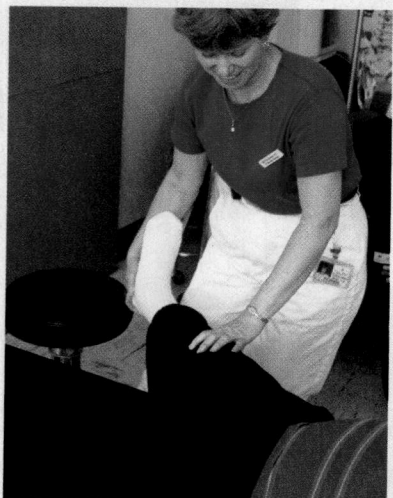

Figure 26-9-3 Slide the leg away from the client's midline, then return.

Figure 26-9-4 Flex and extend the knee.

continues

19. Foot
   • Adduction and abduction: Supporting the ankle, spread the toes apart and then bring them close together.
   • Flexion and extension: Supporting the ankle, extend the toes upward and then flex the toes downward.
20. Observe client's joints and face for signs of exertion, pain, or fatigue during movement.
21. Replace covers and position client in proper body alignment.
22. Place side rails in original position.
23. Place call light within reach.
24. Cleanse hands.

19. Optimizes the performance of the movements, to preserve muscle tone and joint flexibility.

20. Alerts nurse to discontinue exercise.

21. Promotes comfort.

22. Prevents falls.
23. Facilitates communication.
24. Reduces the transmission of microorganisms.

EVALUATION

- Client has maintained or improved current functional mobility in all involved joints and extremities.
- Client has regained or improved strength and/or voluntary movement in involved joints and extremities.
- Client has avoided complications of immobility, including pressure ulcers, contractures, decreased peristalsis, constipation, fecal impaction, orthostatic hypotension, pulmonary embolism, and thrombophlebitis.

DOCUMENTATION

Nurses' Notes

- Performance of ROM exercises. Include joints and extremities on which ROM was performed, the types and degrees of limitation observed, the extent of the client's active involvement in exercises, any reports of pain or discomfort, and any observations of intolerance to exercise.
- Unusual findings

PROCEDURE 26-10   Ambulation Safety and Assisting from Bed to Walking

OVERVIEW

Client ambulation (assisted or unassisted walking) is encouraged soon after the onset of illness or surgery to prevent the complications of immobility. First, assess the strength, endurance, mobility, and orientation of the client. Assist with client ambulation, especially if equipment (IV infusions, urinary catheters, closed chest drainage systems, drainage tubes) is present. Evaluate client ambulation to plan the progression of activity.

Clients at high risk for falls include those with prolonged hospitalization, those taking sedatives or tranquilizers, confused clients, or those with a history of physical restraint use. A great majority of falls:
- Occur in the evening
- Occur in the client's room
- Involve wheelchairs
- Involve confused clients
- Involve unattended clients
- Involve clients with poor footwear
- Occur with poor lighting
- Involve clients with poor vision
- Occur with clients experiencing neuromuscular impairment

Awareness of risk factors for falls allows many client injuries to be prevented. When the client is comfortably able to tolerate sitting on the side of the bed and then standing at the side of the bed, progressive ambulation activities can be initiated.

continues

Disturbances in balance, coordination, proprioception, as well as weakness, low endurance, and deconditioning often occur as consequences of medical/surgical procedures. These clients need assistance with ambulation.

Continually evaluate the client's strength and endurance during the entire ambulation process.

ASSESSMENT

1. Determine the client's most recent activity level and tolerance **to evaluate the client's current ambulatory ability.**
2. Assess the client's current status, including vital signs, fatigue, pain, and medications **to identify conditions that might adversely affect ambulation.**
3. **To evaluate the client's environment for safety:** Check for handrails to help the client stand and to hold onto while walking. Check that the floor is level, clean, and not slippery or wet. Make sure there is adequate lighting so the client can see where he or she is going.
4. Assess the client's ambulation equipment, including the use of a walker, cane, or other assistive device **to determine whether the equipment is in safe condition.**
5. Check the client's clothing **to determine that the client's shoes or slippers are safe to walk in and that he or she has adequate covering for warmth and privacy.**
6. While the client is ambulating, assess his or her gait and bearing. **Determines how well he or she is tolerating the activity and allows detection of hypotension, diaphoresis, breathlessness, or weakness.**
7. After ambulation, assess the client's ability to recover from the activity, including exhaustion, energy, and recovery times. **Determine if modifications need to be made in the distance, type of assistance, or length of time the client is ambulating.**

POSSIBLE NURSING DIAGNOSES

*Risk for **I**njury*
*Impaired Physical **M**obility*
***A**ctivity Intolerance*

PLANNING

Expected Outcomes

1. The client will be able to walk a predetermined distance, with assistance as needed, and return to the starting point.
2. While walking, the client will not suffer any injury.
3. The client will be able to increase the distance he or she can walk and/or will require less assistance to accomplish the distance on a regular basis.

Equipment Needed

- Gait belt (transfer) as needed (PRN)
- Assistive devices
- Shoes or nonslip footwear

DELEGATION TIPS

The ambulation and safe movement of clients is routinely delegated after proper instruction regarding planning the move, arranging for adequate help, if necessary, and positioning oneself close to the client to prevent injury.

IMPLEMENTATION—ACTION/RATIONALE

ACTION	RATIONALE

* Cleanse hands * Check client's identification band * Explain procedure before beginning *

Ambulation Safety

1. When assisting a client with an intravenous (IV) infusion, place the IV pole with wheels at the head of the bed before having the client dangle the legs, so there is room to swing the legs from the bed to the floor. If orders allow, place a saline lock on the IV.	1. Prevents the client's legs from becoming tangled in the IV pole or tubing, causing a fall or causing the tubing to become dislodged. Provides more freedom of movement.

Figure 26-10-1   Ambulating Client with an IV

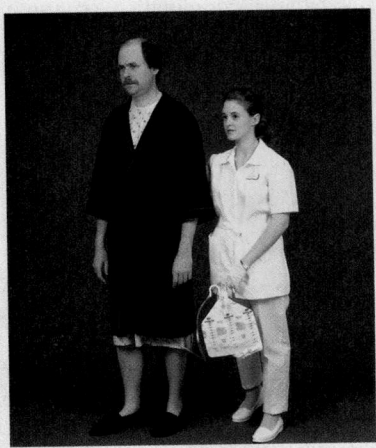

Figure 26-10-2   Ambulating Client with a Urinary Drainage Bag

2. Transfer the IV infusion from the bed IV pole to the portable IV pole. The client or the nurse can guide the portable IV pole ahead during ambulation (Figure 26-10-1).

3. When assisting the client with a urinary drainage bag, empty the drainage bag before ambulation. Have the client sit on the side of the bed with legs dangling.

   Remove the urinary drainage bag from the bed. The nurse or client can hold the urinary drainage bag during ambulation. Make sure the drainage bag remains below the level of the bladder (Figure 26-10-2).

4. When the client has a drainage tube such as a T-tube, hemovac, or Jackson–Pratt drainage system, be sure to secure the drainage tube and bag before ambulation. Place a rubber band around the drainage tube near the drainage bag. Secure the drainage tube and bag with a safety pin through the rubber band. Allow slack. The safety pin can be secured to the client's gown or robe (Figure 26-10-3).

2. Supports the IV while the client ambulates.

3. Emptying the bag reduces the weight of the bag. An empty bag kept below the level of the bladder reduces the risk of urine flowing back into the bladder, and, hence, reduces risk of contamination.

   Having the nurse hold the drainage bag allows the client to concentrate on safe ambulation.

4. Prevents the tubing from becoming dislodged or tangled in clothing or other tubes.

Figure 26-10-3   Secure tubes and drainage bags prior to ambulation, so they do not become dislodged.

continues

Figure 26-10-4   Ambulating the Client Using a Gait Belt for Better Grip and Control

5. Ambulating the client with a closed chest tube drainage system often requires two nurses, one assisting the client and one nurse managing the closed chest tube drainage system. While the client is sitting on the edge of the bed with feet dangling, remove the hangers from the drainage system. Hold the closed chest tube drainage system upright at all times to maintain the water seal. Do not pull or tug on the chest tubes; they may not be sutured into place.

6. Use a transfer belt or gait belt when ambulating a client who is weak (Figure 26-10-4). For additional safety, a wheelchair can be pushed alongside the client for ready access if the client feels weak, tired, or faint.

7. If a client feels faint or dizzy during dangling, return the client to a supine position in bed and lower the head of the bed. Monitor the client's blood pressure and pulse.

8. If the client feels faint or dizzy during ambulation, allow the client to sit in a chair. Stay with the client for safety. Request another nurse to secure a wheelchair if not already available to return the client to bed.

9. If the client feels faint or dizzy during ambulation and starts to fall, ease the client to the floor while supporting and protecting the client's head. Position yourself next to and slightly behind the ambulating client, thus being able to step behind the client and safely ease the client to the floor. Ask other personnel to assist you in returning the client to bed. Assess orthostatic blood pressures.

10. Encourage the client to void before ambulating, especially with elderly clients.

Bed to Walking

1. Inform client of the purposes and distance of the walking exercise.
2. Elevate the head of the bed and wait several minutes.
3. Lower the bed height.

5. Two nurses allow one to focus on the client's safety and ambulation while the other focuses on maintaining the chest drainage system and keeping tubes from becoming dislodged.

6. The transfer belt is a 2-inch-wide webbed belt worn by the client for stabilization during transfers and ambulation. It provides more support for the client by having the nurse hold the back of the belt.

7. Keeps the client from falling from the bed. Lowering the head of the bed will allow gravity to support blood flow to the brain in the hypotensive client.

8. May stop the client from progressing to full syncope.

9. Easing the client to the floor prevents injury to the client.

10. Prevents need to interrupt ambulation. Restroom may not be readily available.

1. Reduces client anxiety and increases cooperation.

2. Prevents orthostatic hypotension.

3. Reduces distance client has to step down, thus decreasing risk of injury.

continues

4. Encourage client to actively move legs, or this may be done passively.

4. Stimulates flow of blood, especially elevation of systolic blood pressure to prevent possible orthostatic hypotension.

5. With one arm on the client's back and one arm under the client's upper legs, move the client into the dangling position.

5. Provides client support and reduces risk of falling.

6. Encourage client to dangle at side of bed for several minutes.

6. Prevents orthostatic hypotension. Allows for assessing tolerance for the sitting position.

7. Place gait belt around client's waist; secure the buckle in front. Place ambulation device such as a walker within reach of the client, if necessary (Figure 26-10-5). Assist client into standing position. Make sure bed is locked and floor is not slippery. Client shoes should have nonslip soles.

7. Provides handholds for the caregiver to support the client. Provides for client and caregiver safety.

8. Stand in front of client with your knees touching client's knees.

8. Prevents client from sliding forward if dizziness or faintness occurs.

9. Place arms under client's axilla.

9. Supports client's trunk.

10. Assist client to a standing position, allowing client time to balance.

10. Reduces risk of fall.

11. If client is able to proceed with ambulating, assume a position beside the client and assist the client as necessary using the gait belt. Place yourself in a guarding position so as to assist client quickly and safely, if necessary. Use additional assistance, as necessary (Figure 26-10-6).

11. Provides for client and caregiver safety.

12. Following ambulation, return client to bed, remove gait belt, and monitor vital signs, as necessary. Make the client comfortable, and make sure all lines and tubes are secure.

12. Promotes safety and comfort.

13. Place the call light within reach of the client.

13. Provides for client safety.

14. Move the bedside table close to the bed and place items of frequent use within reach of the client.

14. Provides for client safety.

15. Cleanse hands.

15. Reduces the transmission of microorganisms.

Figure 26-10-5 Place the walker in front of the client.

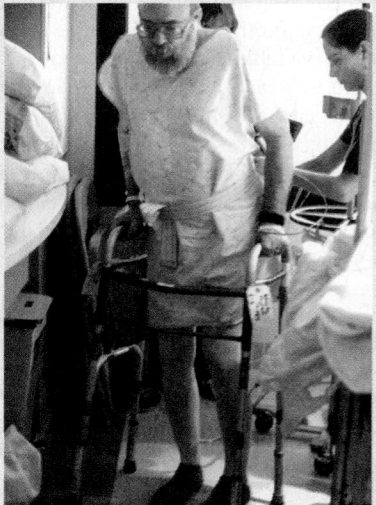

Figure 26-10-6 Assist the client to maintain the standing position if needed.

continues

EVALUATION

- The client was able to walk a predetermined distance, with assistance as needed, and return to the starting point.
- While walking, the client did not suffer any injury.
- The client was able to increase the distance walked and/or required less assistance to accomplish the distance on a regular basis.

DOCUMENTATION

Nurses' Notes

- Distance the client was able to ambulate and how the client tolerated the ambulation
- Assistive devices the client required and teaching done regarding using the device
- Special concerns or unusual findings observed while ambulating the client

PROCEDURE 26-11   Turning and Positioning a Client

OVERVIEW

Clients are not always able to independently move and position themselves in bed. Proper turning and positioning allows the health care provider to make clients as comfortable as possible, prevent contractures and pressure sores, make portions of the client's body available for treatment or procedures, and allows clients greater access to their environment. There are three key concepts to remember when positioning a client: pressure, friction, and skin shear.

Any area that contacts the surface the client is lying on is a pressure site. Because of circulatory compromise, the pressure sites over bony prominences are at the highest risk of skin breakdown and ulceration. Always assess the blood flow to skin and tissue areas put under increased pressure when placing a client in a given position. When repositioning a client, be sure the sheets under the client are smooth. This helps prevent areas of increased pressure that could contribute to pressure sores.

Skin shear is caused when the skin is dragged across a hard surface. The deep layers of skin are torn by the resistance of being dragged. This damage to the skin can lead to skin breakdown and ulceration. To prevent skin shear, or friction burn from the sheets, do not drag a client across the bed. Lift the client into proper position or use a turning sheet.

Friction is caused when the skin is dragged across a rough surface, thereby causing heat and damaging the skin's surface. Any damage to the skin's integrity can lead to infection and skin breakdown.

Clients who cannot reposition themselves must be repositioned at least every two hours and more frequently if they are uncomfortable, incontinent, or have poor circulation, fragile skin, decreased cognition, decreased sensation, or poor nutritional status. When repositioning a client, assess the skin for redness and integrity. Areas of redness should be resolved before the client is repositioned on that area. Areas of redness that do not resolve within 30 minutes after pressure relief should be documented. A plan to reposition the client more frequently may need to be instituted. Areas of prolonged redness are more likely to sustain tissue damage, as are tissue areas covering bony prominences. Hip, back, neck, or head conditions may require that a client be turned keeping the body in alignment, turning as one unit, as a log. This is called log rolling. Remember that proper body mechanics are essential to protect the caregiver's back and to ensure client safety.

ASSESSMENT

1. Assess the client's ability to move independently. **Determine if the client can assist with turning and repositioning.**
2. Assess the client's flexibility. **If clients have contractures or other flexibility limitations, their positions may need to be modified to allow for the restrictions.**
3. Assess the client's age, medical diagnosis, cognitive status, skin integrity, nutritional status, continence, altered sensation, as well as the overall condition of the musculoskeletal system. **Helps determine the client's potential for pressure sore development.**
4. Assess the physician's or qualified practitioner's orders for specific restrictions regarding client positioning **to ensure the correct positioning is implemented.**

continues

POSSIBLE NURSING DIAGNOSES

Risk for Impaired Skin Integrity
Impaired Physical Mobility
Activity Intolerance
Acute Pain

PLANNING

Expected Outcomes

1. The client will maintain skin integrity without skin burns, pressure areas, or pressure ulcers.

2. The client will be comfortable as evident by verbal and nonverbal cues.

Equipment Needed

- Pillows
- Rolled blankets or towels
- Footboard
- Heel protectors
- Hand rolls
- Gloves (if chance of exposure to body fluids)

DELEGATION TIPS

Turning and positioning are routinely delegated to ancillary personnel who have received the appropriate training. The caregiver must protect him or herself and the client from injury and report the client's response to the activity to the nurse.

IMPLEMENTATION—ACTION/RATIONALE

ACTION	RATIONALE
✴ Check client's identification band ✴ Explain procedure before beginning ✴	
1. Cleanse hands.	1. Reduces the transmission of microorganisms.
2. Gather all necessary equipment. Provide for client privacy.	2. Ensures client dignity and allows for a smooth procedure.
3. Secure adequate assistance to safely complete task.	3. Prevents caregiver back and muscle strain as well as provides for client safety.
4. Adjust bed to comfortable working height. Lower side rail on side of bed from which you are assisting client.	4. Prevents caregiver back and muscle strain.
5. Follow proper body mechanics guidelines: When moving a client in bed, position the bed so that your legs are slightly bent at the knees and hips. Maintain the natural curves in your back while lifting. Position one foot slightly in front of the other and spread feet apart to create a wide base for balance. When your arms are placed under the client, slowly lean backward onto your back leg using your body weight to help you lift the client to one side of the bed. Do not extend or rotate your back to move a client in bed. If you cannot move the client easily, always ask for and obtain assistance for both your and the client's safety (Figure 26-11-1). Be sure the floor is not slippery and that the bed is locked. Always use a turning sheet when rolling a client because this gives you better support and control of the client (Figure 26-11-2).	5. Prevents caregiver back injury and muscle strain and promotes client safety. Spreading feet to create a wide base helps prevent loss of balance.
6. Position drains, tubes, and IVs to accommodate for new client position.	6. Prevents accidental dislodgment and/or discomfort from movement by reduced mechanical tension.
7. Place or assist client into appropriate starting position. Monitor client status, and provide adequate rest breaks or support as necessary.	7. Prevents client injury.

continues

Figure 26-11-1 If the client is heavy or hard to move, always obtain assistance for both the client's and your safety.

Figure 26-11-2 When rolling a client, use a turning sheet for better support and control.

Moving from Supine to Side-Lying Position

8. Slide your hands underneath the client. Move the client to one side of the bed by lifting the client's body toward you in stages—first the upper trunk, then the lower trunk, and finally the legs. Lift the client's body; do not drag the client across the sheets. Move to other side of bed.

   Roll the client to side-lying position by placing the client's inside arm next to the client's body with the palm of the hand against the hip. Cross the client's outside arm and leg toward midline and log roll the client toward you using the client's outside shoulder and hip for leverage while maintaining stability and control of top arm and leg.

8. Prevents shearing of skin tissue. Maintains client body alignment. Protects caregiver's back and prevents muscle strain. Prevents client injury and shearing of skin tissue.

Maintaining Side-Lying Position

9. Repeat Actions 1–8.
10. Pillows may be placed to support the client's head and arms (Figure 26-11-3). An additional pillow may be used to support the topside leg, and fully and equally support the thigh, knee, ankle, and foot (Figure 26-11-4). Move the lower arm forward slightly at the shoulder and bend the elbow for comfort. If the client is unstable, a pillow placed against the back will provide additional support and keep the client from rolling supine.

9. See Rationales 1–8.
10. Provides support and comfort.

Figure 26-11-3 Place pillows to support the head and arms.

Figure 26-11-4 Place pillows to support the leg, ankle, and foot.

continues

Moving from Side-Lying to Prone Position

11. Repeat Actions 1–8.
12. Remove positioning towels, pillows, or other support devices. Assess whether the client's position in bed needs to be adjusted to accommodate the continued movement into prone. Move the client's inside arm next to the client's body with palm against hip. Roll the client onto the stomach using the shoulder and hip as key points of control. The head must be placed in a comfortable position to one side without excessive pressure to sensitive areas. Pillows under the trunk are placed as needed to relieve pressure and increase comfort. The client's arms are placed comfortably at the client's side and the legs are uncrossed with the feet approximately a foot apart.

11. See Rationales 1–8.
12. Ensures comfort and safety in movement.

Maintaining Prone Position

13. A shallow pillow or a folded towel may be used to support the client's head comfortably as well as a pillow placed under the abdomen to support the back. An additional pillow may be placed under the lower leg to reduce the pressure of the toes and forefoot against the bed.

13. Provides support and comfort.

Moving from Prone to Supine Position

14. Repeat Actions 1–8.
15. Remove positioning towels, pillows, or other supporting devices. Slide your hands underneath the client. Move the client segmentally to one side of the bed to accommodate the new position. Position the inside arm next to the client's body with the client's palm next to the hip. Roll the client to supine by log rolling the client toward you using the client's outside shoulder and hip for leverage. Have the client's face positioned away from the direction of the roll to prevent undue pressure to the face or neck. When the client reaches supine, uncross the client's arms and legs and place them comfortably into anatomic positions.

14. See Rationales 1–8.
15. Provides support and comfort.

Maintaining Supine Position

16. A footboard may be used to support the foot as well as heel protectors or a pillow placed between the heel and gastrocnemius muscle to reduce the pressure on the heels. Assess and compare warmth, sensation, color, and movement of feet. To prevent excessive external rotation of the lower extremity, a trochanter roll may be used. For comfort, additional pillows may be used to support the client's head, arms, or lower back.

16. Provides support and comfort. Heel protectors and routine assessment of the feet help to prevent pressure sores. Trochanter rolls and pillows help to prevent displacement of the acetabulum (hip joint).

Log Rolling

17. Repeat Actions 1–8.
18. Use three nurses. Place a turning/draw sheet under client's head, back, and buttocks (if not already present).
19. Place pillow between client's legs.
20. Have client fold arms across chest.

17. See Rationales 1–8.
18. Provides for client safety. Reduces shearing force.
19. Keeps legs in alignment with body.
20. Prevents getting the client's arms trapped or injured.

continues

21. Roll up draw sheet on the far side until it is next to the client.

21. Provides support under the heavy parts of the client and places the nurses' hands close to the weight to be turned.

22. One nurse places hands under the client's far leg, another holds rolled draw sheet at client's buttocks, and third nurse holds rolled draw sheet at chest and shoulder level.

22. Ensures client is turned like a log, as a unit.

23. Nurse nearest the client's head gives the signal to turn: 1-2-3 turn.

23. Ensures a smooth, coordinated turn.

24. Tuck pillows at client's back and abdomen.

24. Helps maintain side-lying position.

25. Assess the client for comfort and proper alignment.

25. Comfort is subjective. Ensures alignment.

26. Procedure can be reversed to reposition client on back or opposite side.

26. Reduces pressure ulcer development.

27. Be sure to replace side rails to upright position as well as to lower bed to beginning position.

27. Provides for client safety.

28. Place call light within reach of the client.

28. Provides for client safety.

29. Move bedside table close to bed and place items of frequent use within reach of the client.

29. Provides for client safety.

30. Cleanse hands.

30. Reduces the transmission of microorganisms.

EVALUATION

- Safe and proper body alignment and movement were achieved for both client and caregiver.
- The client is comfortable in the new position as evident by verbal and nonverbal cues.
- The client's skin and underlying organs and tissues were protected from pressure, friction, and shear.

DOCUMENTATION

Nurses' Notes

- Client's new position and time of the position change
- Report or observation of pain, discomfort, or dyspnea
- Integumentary assessment, including color and integrity of skin and length of time redness persists over bony prominences

PROCEDURE 26-12   Moving a Client in Bed

OVERVIEW

Prolonged immobility is uncomfortable and presents an increased risk of many complications. Muscle wasting, clot formation, and skin breakdown are the most common risks associated with immobility. Clients who are unable to move themselves in bed or are only able to assist with moving in bed are at risk for discomfort and complications related to immobility. Often, clients' restlessness in bed will cause them to slide down toward the foot of the bed. This is especially true in beds where the head raises up to a Fowler's or semi-Fowler's position. If the client slides down toward the foot of the bed while the head is elevated, it can lead to reduced respiratory effort, reduced lung capacity, and skin breakdown, thus impairing the client's recovery.

The nurse is often called on to move a client to a more comfortable position. Repositioning a client can sometimes be done by a single staff member, but often it requires two or more people to do this procedure safely.

continues

ASSESSMENT

1. Assess the client's ability to assist with repositioning. Determine if the client can move with the aid of an overhead trapeze or the side rail. Judge how much assistance will be needed. **Determines safety for the client and the nurse and good body mechanics for the nurse.**
2. Assess the client's ability to understand and follow directions and assist and cooperate with the move. **Affects how the procedure will be carried out. Affects client teaching.**
3. Assess the client's environment. Check the bed for cleanliness. Has the client been restless, sweaty, or incontinent? Check to see if the sheets have been turned or twisted. Tubes, lines, wires, traction, casts, or splints must be moved carefully. **Affects how the procedure will be carried out. Affects what additional procedures will be performed. Prepares the caregivers to keep tubes and equipment from becoming dislodged or tipping or pulling.**

POSSIBLE NURSING DIAGNOSES

*Impaired Physical **M**obility*
***A**ctivity Intolerance*
*Risk for Impaired **S**kin Integrity*

PLANNING

Expected Outcomes

1. The client will be moved in bed without injury to self.
2. The client will be moved in bed without injury to the staff.
3. The client will report an increase in comfort following the move.
4. All tubes, lines, and drains will remain patent and intact.

Equipment Needed

- Hospital bed with side rails
- Trapeze if required
- Turn sheet or draw sheet

DELEGATION TIPS

Turning and positioning is routinely delegated to ancillary personnel who have received appropriate training. The caregiver must protect him or herself and the client from injury and report the client's response to the activity to the nurse.

IMPLEMENTATION—ACTION/RATIONALE

ACTION

RATIONALE

❋ Check client's identification band ❋ Explain procedure before beginning ❋

Moving a Client Up in Bed with One Nurse

1. Cleanse hands.
2. Elevate bed to just below waist height. Lower head of bed if tolerated by client. Lower side rails on the side where you are standing.
3. Remove the pillow and place it against the headboard.

4. Have client hold on to the overhead trapeze, if available (Figure 26-12-1).
5. Have the client bend the knees and place the feet flat on the bed if able (Figure 26-12-2).
6. Stand at an angle to the head of the bed, feet apart, knees bent, feet toward the head of the bed.
7. Slide one hand and arm under the client's shoulder, the other under the client's thigh.
8. Rock forward toward the head of the bed, lifting the client with you. Simultaneously have the client push with the legs.

1. Reduces the transmission of microorganisms.
2. Lessens strain on nurse's back muscles.

3. Prevents having to move against the pillow. Provides padding of the headboard if the client should be moved too high in the bed.
4. Promotes client autonomy by allowing the client to assist with the move.
5. Allows the client to assist in the move; promotes client autonomy.
6. Promotes good body mechanics.

7. Distributes the client's weight more evenly. Promotes good lifting technique.
8. Allows a smooth motion to lift the client. Client assistance lessens strain on nurse's back muscles; promotes client autonomy.

continues

Figure 26-12-1 Have client hold onto the overhead trapeze, if one is available, to assist in the move.

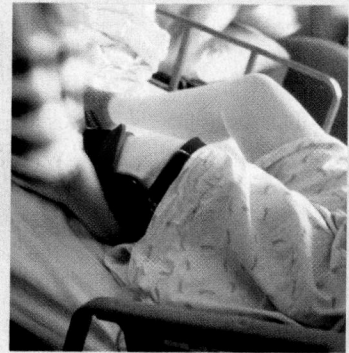

Figure 26-12-2 Have the client bend the knees and place feet flat on the bed.

9. If the client has a trapeze, have the client pull up holding onto the trapeze as you move the client upward in bed.
10. Repeat these steps until the client is moved up high enough in bed.
11. Return the client's pillow under the head.
12. Elevate head of bed, if tolerated by client.

13. Assess client for comfort.
14. Adjust the client's bedclothes as needed for comfort.
15. Lower bed and elevate side rails.
16. Cleanse hands.

Moving a Client Up in Bed with Two or More Nurses

17. Cleanse hands and apply gloves if needed.
18. Elevate bed to just below waist height. Lower head of bed if tolerated by client. Lower side rails.
19. With two nurses, place turn/draw sheet under client's back and head.
20. Roll up the draw sheet on each side until it is next to the client (Figure 26-12-3).

21. Follow Actions 3–5.
22. The nurses stand on either side of the bed, at an angle to the head of the bed, with knees flexed, feet apart in a wide stance.

9. Client assistance lessens strain on nurse's back muscles; promotes client autonomy.

10. Large or very immobile clients are often not moved far enough in one step.
11. Promotes client comfort.
12. Promotes comfort; facilitates eating and drinking; facilitates communication.
13. Comfort is subjective.
14. Promotes comfort.
15. Promotes client safety.
16. Reduces the transmission of microorganisms.

17. Reduces the transmission of microorganisms.
18. Lessens strain on nurses' back muscles.

19. Reduces shearing force, which can precipitate skin breakdown.
20. Provides support under the heavy parts of the body and places the nurse's hands close to the weight to be moved.
21. See Rationales 3–5.
22. Promotes good body mechanics.

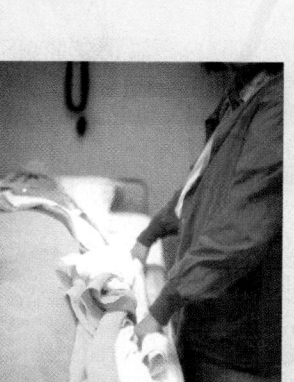

Figure 26-12-3 Rolling the draw sheet up tightly next to the client places the nurse's hands close to the weight of the client.

continues

Figure 26-12-4   At the signal from the lead nurse, lift and pull in one smooth motion.

23. The nurses hold their elbows as close as possible to their bodies.
24. The lead nurse gives the signal to move: 1-2-3 go. The nurses will lift up (off the bed) on the turn/draw sheet and forward (toward the head of the bed) in one smooth motion (Figure 26-12-4). The move is coordinated to transfer the client toward the head of the bed. Simultaneously, have the client push with the legs or pull using the trapeze.
25. Repeat until the client is moved up high enough in bed to be comfortable.
26. Return the client's pillow under the head.
27. Elevate head of bed, if tolerated by client.

28. Assess client for comfort.
29. Adjust the client's bedclothes for comfort.
30. Lower bed and elevate side rails.
31. Cleanse hands.

23. Allows the muscles of the torso to assist the arm muscles in bearing and moving the weight of the client.
24. Allows a smooth motion to lift the client. Client assistance lessens strain on the nurses' back muscles; promotes client autonomy.

25. Large or very immobile clients are often not moved far enough in one step.
26. Promotes client comfort.
27. Promotes comfort; facilitates eating and drinking; facilitates communication.
28. Promotes comfort.
29. Promotes comfort.
30. Promotes client safety.
31. Reduces the transmission of microorganisms.

EVALUATION

- The client was moved without injury to self or staff.
- The client reported an increase in comfort following the move.
- All tubes, lines, and drains remained intact.

DOCUMENTATION

Nurses' Notes

- Time and position the client was moved
- Unusual findings

PROCEDURE 26-13   Transferring from Bed to Wheelchair, Commode, or Chair

OVERVIEW

Client activity is an important part of the healing process. Activity improves muscle tone, increases venous return to the heart, and stimulates peristalsis. Moving a client from the bed to a chair is an important part of client activity.

Moving a client from the bed to a chair, wheelchair, commode, or stretcher is called a transfer. Transferring a client requires good planning to avoid injury to the client and the nurse. When transferring a client, consider the client's ability to assist with

continues

the transfer. If the client is unable to provide any assistance or is large, one or more staff members may be needed to help perform the transfer safely.

The most frequent complication in transferring a client is falling during the transfer. If a client does start to fall while being transferred, lower him or her gently to the floor, making sure the head does not strike anything. If a client does fall, obtain assistance and perform a thorough assessment of the client before moving him or her.

Another possible hazard in client transfers is pulling on or dislodging indwelling tubes or catheters. Think ahead about ways tubes will move with the transfer and try to avoid snagging them. Take care to appropriately anchor all tubes and catheters before transferring a client.

Clients are also at risk of damage to their skin during a transfer. Sliding across the sheets, side rails, and wheelchair armrest can bruise or injure the client. Use a transfer board or pad any sharp exposed areas to help prevent injury to the client.

Be sure the client is wearing shoes or slippers with firm, nonslip soles when transferring a client. Even if the client will be standing only briefly, the feet need to be protected from potential injury and contamination from the floor and the client from slipping.

When transferring a client with weakness on one side of the body, use the "Good to go" maxim. This means that the client needs to lead off with the "good" or strong side of the body. Perform the transfer in the direction of the good side, so the client pivots and supports the weight on the good side. This allows maximum strength and stability on the client's part.

ASSESSMENT

1. Assess the client's current level of mobility. Determine how much the client is able to assist with the transfer. Assess for pain or confusion, which might impair ability to assist. Check for a "weak" side. **Affects how the procedure will be carried out.**
2. Assess for any impediments to mobility, including casts, drainage tubes, catheters, IVs, or intubation. **Affects how the procedure will be carried out. Prepares caregivers to keep tubes and equipment from becoming dislodged, tipping, or pulling.**
3. Assess the client's level of understanding and anxiety regarding the procedure. **Affects how the procedure will be carried out. Affects client teaching.**
4. Assess the client's environment. Assess the available space for maneuvering the wheelchair to the bed. **Affects how the procedure will be carried out. Affects safety and good body mechanics for caregivers.**
5. Assess the equipment. Check the bed and chair height. See whether they are adjustable. Check for chair footings and wheelchair brakes. **Affects safety for client and caregivers.**

POSSIBLE NURSING DIAGNOSES

Impaired Physical Mobility
Activity Intolerance
Risk for Injury

PLANNING

Expected Outcomes

1. The client will be transferred from the bed to the wheelchair, commode, or chair without pain or injury.
2. Drainage tubes, IVs, or other devices will be intact.
3. The client's skin will be intact and undamaged.

Equipment Needed

- Bed
- Wheelchair, chair, or commode
- Any splints, braces, or supportive equipment specific to the client
- Shoes or slippers with nonskid soles
- Gait belt
- Transfer board (if necessary)

DELEGATION TIPS

Assisting a client from a bed to a wheelchair, commode, or chair is a skill routinely delegated to properly trained ancillary personnel.

IMPLEMENTATION—ACTION/RATIONALE

ACTION	RATIONALE
* Check client's identification band * Explain procedure before beginning *	
1. Cleanse hands.	1. Reduces transmission of microorganisms.
2. Assess client for ability to assist with the transfer and for presence of cognitive or sensory deficits.	2. Allows planning regarding the amount of assistance and cooperation to expect from the client.

continues

3. Lock the bed in position.
4. Place any splints, braces, or other devices on the client.
5. Place the client's shoes or slippers on the client's feet.
6. Lower the height of the bed to lowest possible position.

7. Slowly raise the head of the bed if this is not contraindicated by the client's condition.
8. Place one arm under the client's legs and one arm behind the client's back. Slowly pivot the client so the client's legs are dangling over the edge of the bed and the client is in a sitting position on the edge of the bed (Figure 26-13-1).
9. Allow client to dangle for 2 to 5 minutes. Help support client if necessary (Figure 26-13-2).
10. Bring the chair or wheelchair close to the side of the bed. Place it at a 45-degree angle to the bed. If the client has a weaker side, place the chair or wheelchair on the client's strong side.
11. Lock wheelchair brakes and elevate the foot pedals. For chairs, lock brakes if available.
12. If using a gait belt to assist the client, place it around the client's waist.
13. Assist client to side of bed until feet are firmly on the floor and slightly apart.
14. Grasp the sides of the gait belt or place your hands just below the client's axilla. Using a wide stance, bend your knees and assist the client to a standing position.

15. Standing close to the client, pivot until the client's back is toward the chair.
16. Instruct the client to place hands on the arm supports, or place the client's hands on the arm supports of the chair.
17. Bend at the knees and ease the client into a sitting position.
18. Assist client to maintain proper posture. Support weak side with pillow if needed.

3. Prevents the bed from rolling during the procedure.
4. Provides support and prevents injury to the client.
5. Provides a nonslip surface for stability.
6. Reduces distance client has to step down, thus decreasing risk of injury.
7. Minimizes lifting.

8. Supports the client while sitting him or her upright.

9. Allows time for assessing client's response to sitting; reduces possibility of orthostatic hypotension.
10. Minimizes transfer distance. Allows the client to pivot on the stronger leg.

11. Provides stability.

12. Provides a secure handhold for the nurse during the transfer.
13. Moves client into proper position for transfer. Provides stable footing for client.
14. Wide stance increases nurse stability and minimizes strain on the back. Avoids putting pressure directly on the axilla, and risking nerve damage or shoulder subluxation.
15. Moves client into proper position to be seated.

16. Allows client to gain balance and judge distance to seat.

17. Increases stability and minimizes strain on back.

18. Increases client comfort.

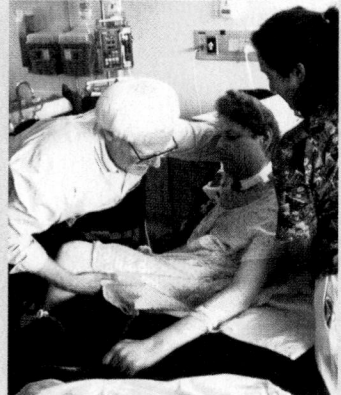

Figure 26-13-1 Pivot the client to a sitting position on the edge of the bed.

Figure 26-13-2 Support the client, if needed, while the client adjusts to the sitting position.

continues

Figure 26-13-3 Once the client is moved, make sure skin, tubing, or equipment is not pinched between the client and the chair.

Figure 26-13-4 Position the wheelchair footrests or use a footstool if the client is sitting in a chair.

19. Secure the safety belt, place client's feet on feet pedals, and release brakes if you will be moving the client immediately. Make sure tubes and lines, arms, and hands are not pinched or caught between the client and the chair (Figure 26-13-3). If the client is sitting in a chair, offer a footstool if available (Figure 26-13-4).
20. Cleanse hands.

19. Ensures client safety; prepares client for movement.

20. Reduces the transmission of microorganisms.

EVALUATION

- Client was transferred from the bed to the wheelchair without pain or injury.
- Drainage tubes, IVs, or other devices remain intact.
- Client's skin is intact and undamaged.

DOCUMENTATION

Nurses' Notes

- Client's tolerance of the activity, any aids that were required, how much assistance was required, and the client's ability to assist
- Unusual events during the transfer

PROCEDURE 26-14 — Transferring from Bed to Stretcher

OVERVIEW

Some clients are not strong enough to sit erect in a wheelchair or have some injury that prevents them from sitting, so they must be moved while lying flat. The most commonly used equipment for transferring a client is a stretcher (gurney). A stretcher is a narrow, cartlike bed that rolls on wheels. For client safety, stretchers are equipped with side rails or safety straps to prevent accidental falls during transport. The wheels on a stretcher lock to prevent accidental movement during client transfers.

ASSESSMENT

1. Assess the client's current level of mobility. **Knowing whether a client is able to assist with the transfer will affect how the transfer is performed.**

2. Assess for injury. **Caregivers may need to keep the client in the same alignment as much as possible.**
3. Assess for any impediments to mobility such as a cast, drainage tubes, IVs, or intubation. **This will affect how the transfer is performed.**

continues

4. Assess the client's level of understanding of the procedure. **This will affect client comfort, anxiety, and cooperation.**
5. Assess the client's environment. Assess how close the stretcher will move to the bed. Assess the height of the bed. **This allows for a safe transfer. Plan for good body mechanics.**
6. Make sure the stretcher is safe to use. Check for working brakes, side rails, safety straps that are intact and usable, and an IV pole attachment if needed. **This allows for a safe transfer. Plan for good body mechanics.**

POSSIBLE NURSING DIAGNOSES

Impaired Physical Mobility
Activity Intolerance

PLANNING

Expected Outcomes

1. The client will be transferred from the bed to the stretcher without pain or injury.
2. Drainage tubes, IVs, or other devices will remain intact.
3. The client's skin will be intact and undamaged.

Equipment Needed

Transferring a Client with Minimum Assistance
• Bed
• Stretcher

Transferring a Client with Maximum Assistance
• Bed
• Stretcher
• Pillows
• Transfer/slider boards
• Lift sheet
• Other qualified personnel to assist

DELEGATION TIPS

Assisting a client from a bed to a stretcher is a skill routinely delegated to properly trained ancillary personnel.

IMPLEMENTATION—ACTION/RATIONALE

ACTION	RATIONALE
* Check client's identification band * Explain procedure before beginning *	

Minimum Assistance

ACTION	RATIONALE
1. Cleanse hands.	1. Reduces the transmission of microorganisms.
2. Raise the height of bed to 1 inch higher than the stretcher and lock brakes of bed.	2. Reduces distance nurse must bend, thus preventing back strain; prevents bed from moving.
3. Instruct client to move to side of bed close to stretcher. Lower side rails of bed and stretcher. Leave side rails on opposite side up.	3. Decreases risk of client falling.
4. Stand at outer side of stretcher and push it toward bed.	4. Diminishes the gap between bed and stretcher; secures the stretcher position.
5. Instruct client to move onto stretcher with assistance as needed.	5. Promotes client independence.
6. Cover client with sheet or bath blanket.	6. Promotes comfort; protects privacy.
7. Elevate side rails on stretcher and secure safety belts about client. Release brakes of stretcher.	7. Prevents falls.
8. Stand at head of stretcher to guide it when pushing.	8. Pushing, not pulling, ensures proper body mechanics.
9. Cleanse hands.	9. Reduces the transmission of microorganisms.

Maximum Assistance

ACTION	RATIONALE
10. Repeat Actions 1 and 2.	10. See Rationales 1 and 2.
11. Assess amount of assistance required for transfer. Usually 2 to 4 staff members are required for the maximum-assisted transfer.	11. Promotes client independence; ensures that enough staff are present before beginning transfer.

continues

12. Lock wheels of bed and stretcher.
13. Have one nurse stand close to client's head.
14. Log roll the client (keep in straight alignment) and place a lift sheet under the client's back, trunk, and upper legs. The lift sheet can extend under the head if client lacks head control abilities.
15. Empty all drainage bags (e.g., T-tube, Hemo Vac, Jackson–Pratt). Record amounts. Secure drainage system to client's gown before transfer.
16. Move client to edge of bed near stretcher. Lift up and over to avoid dragging.
17. Because the client is now on the side of the bed, without the side rail up, the nurse on nonstretcher side of bed holds the stretcher side of the lift sheet up (by reaching across the client's chest) to prevent the client from falling onto the stretcher or off the bed.
18. Place pillow and slider board overlapping the bed and stretcher (Figure 26-14-1).
19. Have staff members grasp edges of lift sheet. Be sure to use good body mechanics (Figure 26-14-2).
20. On the count of three, have staff members pull lift sheet and the client onto the stretcher.
21. Position client on stretcher, place pillow under head, and cover with a sheet or bath blanket (Figure 26-14-3).
22. Secure safety belts and elevate side rails of stretcher.
23. If IV is present, move it from bed IV pole to stretcher IV pole after client transfer.
24. Cleanse hands.

12. Prevents falls.
13. Supports client's head during the move.
14. Prevents flexion and rotation of client's hips and spine; maintains correct body alignment.

15. Decreases possibility of spills; prevents dislodging of tubes.

16. Prevents dragging, which causes shearing force.

17. Protects the client from falling.

18. Protects head from injury. Slider board eases movement of the client.
19. Provides surface for client to slide on. Prevents dragging and shearing.
20. Working in unison makes the overall job easier and prevents staff injury.
21. Promotes comfort and provides for privacy.

22. Prevents falls.
23. Prevents tubing from being pulled and IV from being dislodged.
24. Reduces the transmission of microorganisms.

Figure 26-14-1 Place pillow and slider board overlapping the bed and stretcher.

Figure 26-14-2 Firmly grasp edges of lift sheet.

Figure 26-14-3 Place pillow under head and cover client with blanket.

continues

EVALUATION

- The client was transferred from the bed to the stretcher without pain or injury.
- All drainage tubes, IVs, or other devices remain intact.
- Assess whether the client's skin is intact and undamaged.

DOCUMENTATION

Kardex

- Amount of assistance the transfer required and amount the client was able to assist

Nurses' Notes

- Time, date, reason for transfer, type of transfer, and how the client tolerated the activity

---

PROCEDURE 26-15   Bedmaking: Unoccupied Bed

OVERVIEW

After the client takes a bath, clean linens are placed on the bed to promote comfort and decrease transmission of microorganisms. If the client is able to get out of bed, assist the client to a chair and proceed with making the bed. After surgery, the client should be returned to a clean bed with the linens folded to the foot of the bed to promote easy client transfer.

ASSESSMENT

1. Assess your equipment. Check for all linens necessary to change the bed. Check for a dirty linen hamper. **Facilitates a smooth procedure.**
2. Assess whether the bed needs cleaning before placing clean sheets on it. **Reduces the transmission of microorganisms.**
3. Assess the client's needs in the bed. Check for profuse drainage, incontinence, or special needs for comfort or skin integrity. **Determines how the procedure will be performed.**
4. Assess the client's ability to be out of bed in a safe place while changing linens.

POSSIBLE NURSING DIAGNOSIS

Risk for Impaired Skin Integrity

PLANNING

Expected Outcomes

1. The client will have clean linens on the bed.
2. The clean linens will be appropriate to the client's needs and condition.

Equipment Needed

- Bottom sheet (fitted, if available)
- Top sheet
- Draw sheet (regular top sheet may be used)
- Pillowcase (each pillow on the bed)
- Mattress pad
- Antiseptic solution, washcloth, and towel
- Linen bag hamper outside the room
- Nonsterile gloves

DELEGATION TIPS

Bed making is usually delegated to ancillary personnel. Their instruction should include safety precautions for themselves and the client, and understanding the appropriate use of Standard Precautions.

continues

IMPLEMENTATION—ACTION/RATIONALE

ACTION

*Cleanse hands * Check client's identification band * Explain procedure before beginning*

1. Place hamper by client's door if linen bags are not available. Assess condition of blanket and/or bedspread.
2. Gather linens and gloves. Place linens on a clean, dry surface in reverse order of usage at the client's bedside (pillowcases, top sheet, draw sheet, bottom sheet).
3. Inquire about the client's toileting needs and attend as necessary.
4. Assist client to a safe, comfortable chair.
5. Apply gloves.

6. Position bed: flat, side rails down, adjust height to waist level.
7. Remove and fold blanket and/or bedspread. If clean and reusable, place on clean work area.
8. Remove soiled pillowcases by grasping the closed end with one hand and slipping the pillow out with the other. Place the soiled cases on top of the soiled sheet, and place the pillows on clean work area.
9. Remove soiled linens: Start on the side of the bed closest to you; free the bottom sheet and mattress pad (if used) by lifting the mattress and rolling soiled linens to the middle of the bed. Go to the other side of the bed, repeat action.
10. Fold (do not fan or flap) soiled linens: head of bed to middle, foot of bed to middle. Place in linen bag or hamper, keeping soiled linens away from uniform.
11. Check mattress. If the mattress is soiled, clean it with an antiseptic solution and dry it thoroughly.
12. Remove gloves, cleanse hands, and apply a second pair of clean gloves (when appropriate).
13. Open the clean mattress pad lengthwise onto the bed. Unfold half the pad's width to the center crease and smooth the pad flat. If there are elastic bands to hold the pad in place, slide them under the corners of the mattress.
14. Proceed with placing the bottom sheet onto the mattress. Linens differ from facility to facility. Bottom sheets may be fitted or they may be flat. Proceed to the appropriate action for the linen available.

Fitted Bottom Sheet

15. Position yourself diagonally toward the head of the bed.
16. Start at the head with seamed side of the fitted sheet toward the mattress.
17. Lift the mattress corner with your hand closest to the bed; with your other hand, pull and tuck the fitted sheet over the mattress corner; secure at the head of the bed.
18. Pull and tuck the fitted sheet over the mattress corners at the foot of the bed.

RATIONALE

1. Provides for proper disposal of soiled linens. Allows for organization of supplies.

2. Provides easy access to items.

3. Provides for client comfort and prevents interruptions during bed making.
4. Increases client's comfort and decreases risk of falls.
5. Reduces risk of infection from soiled, contaminated linens.
6. Promotes good body mechanics and decreases back strain.
7. Keeps reusable bed linens clean.

8. Allows easy removal of the pillowcases without contamination of uniform by soiled linens and keeps pillows clean.

9. Prevents tearing and fanning of linens. Linens are folded from cleanest area to most soiled to prevent contamination.

10. Fanning or flapping linens increases the number of microorganisms in the air. Folding linens reduces the risk of transmission of infection to others.
11. Reduces the transmission of microorganisms.

12. Reduces the transmission of microorganisms to clean linens.
13. Facilitates making bed in an organized, time-saving manner by not having to go from one side of the bed to the other.

14. Use linen available at the facility.

15. Ensures good body mechanics and efficient procedure.
16. Placement of seamed side toward mattress prevents irritation to the client's skin.
17. Prevents straining of back muscles; decreases the chance that the sheet will pull out from under the mattress.

18. Prevents straining of back muscles; decreases the chance that the sheet will pull out from under the mattress.

continues

Flat Regular Sheet

19. Unfold the bottom sheet with the seamed side toward the mattress. Align the bottom edge of the sheet with the edge of the mattress at the foot of the bed.

20. Allow the sheet to hang 10 inches (25 cm) over the mattress on the side and at the top of the bed.

21. Position yourself diagonally toward the head of the bed. Lift the top of the mattress corner with the hand closest to the bed and smoothly tuck the sheet under the mattress.

22. Miter the corner at the head of the bed using the following technique.

23. Face the side of bed and lift and lay the edge of the sheet onto the bed to form a triangular fold.

24. With your palms down, tuck the lower edge of sheet (hanging free at the side of the mattress) under the mattress.

25. Grasp the triangular fold, bring it down over the side of the mattress. Allow the sheet to hang free at the side of the mattress.

26. Place the draw sheet on the bottom sheet and unfold it to the middle crease.

27. Face the side of the bed, palms of hands down. Tuck both the bottom and draw sheets under the mattress. Ensure that the bottom sheet is tucked smoothly under the mattress all the way to the foot of the bed.

28. Go to the other side of the bed, unfold the bottom sheet, and repeat the actions used to apply the mattress pad and bottom sheet.

29. Unfold the draw sheet, if used, and grasp the free-hanging sides of both the bottom and draw sheets. Pull toward you, keeping your back straight, and with a firm grasp (sheets taut) tuck both sheets under the mattress. Use your arms and open palms to extend the linen under the mattress. Place the protective pad on the bottom sheet.

30. Place the top sheet on the bed and unfold lengthwise, placing the center crease (width) of the sheet in the middle of the bed. Place the top edge of the sheet (seam up) even with the top of the mattress at the head of the bed. Pull the remaining length toward the bottom of the bed.

31. Unfold and apply the blanket or spread. Follow the same technique as used in applying the top sheet (Figure 26-15-1).

32. Miter the bottom corners. With your palms down, tuck the lower edge of the sheet under the mattress. Grasp the triangular fold and bring it down over the side of the mattress. Allow the sheet to hang free at the side of the mattress (Figures 26-15-2 and 26-15-3).

33. Face the head of the bed and fold the top sheet and blanket over 6 inches (15 cm). Fanfold the sheet and blanket (from the foot to the middle of the bed).

19. Placement of the seamed side toward the mattress prevents irritation to the client's skin. Ensure proper placement of the sheet so that it can be tightly secured at the top and on both sides of the bed.

20. Proper placement of linens ensures adequate sheeting for all sides of the bed.

21. Prevents straining of back muscles; decreases the chance that the sheet will pull out from under the mattress.

22. Secures sheet tightly to the mattress, with the triangular fold providing a smooth tuck to keep the linen in place.

23. Forms the base for the tuck.

24. Forms the first half of the tuck.

25. Will form the final portion of the mitered corner when tucked in.

26. Provides a sheet to lift and move the client in bed without having to use the bottom sheet and remake the bed. Helps to keep the bottom sheet clean.

27. Keeps sheet taut, in place, and wrinkle-free, thereby decreasing the risk of skin irritation.

28. Unfolding decreases air current; air currents can spread microorganisms.

29. Uses your body's weight in pulling the sheet taut and prevents strain on your back muscles.

30. Saves time and movement, making one side of the bed at a time. Seam will be folded down to prevent contact with the client's skin, which can result in irritation.

31. Provides warmth.

32. Secures linen at the foot of the bed.

33. Allows the client easy access to the bed.

continues

Figure 26-15-1 Place the blanket or spread over the top sheet.

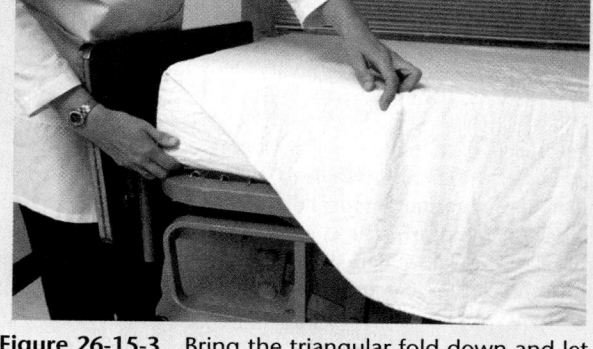

Figure 26-15-3 Bring the triangular fold down and let it hang freely at the side of the mattress.

Figure 26-15-2 Lift and lay the edge of the sheet and blanket on the bed to form a triangular fold.

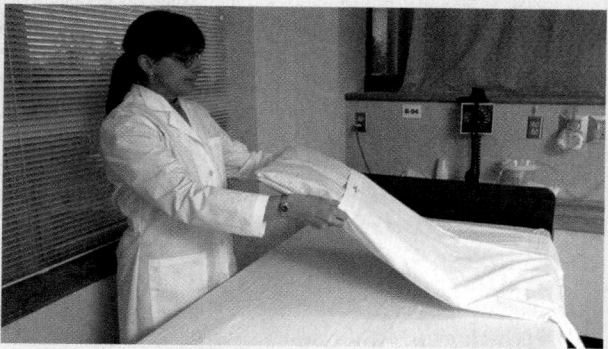

Figure 26-15-4 Place a clean pillowcase on each pillow while keeping the clean pillowcase away from your uniform.

34. Apply a clean pillowcase on each pillow (Figure 26-15-4). With one hand, grasp the closed end of the pillowcase. Gather the pillowcase and turn it inside out over hand. With same hand, grasp the middle of one end of the pillow. With the other hand, pull the case over the length of the pillow. The corners of the pillow should fit snugly into the corners of the case.
35. Return the bed to the lowest position and elevate the head of the bed 30 to 45 degrees. Put side rails up on side, farthest from client.
36. Inquire about toileting needs of the client; assist as necessary.
37. Assist the client back into the bed and pull up the side rails; place call light in reach; take vital signs.

38. Remove gloves and cleanse hands.

34. Keeps clean pillowcase away from your uniform.

35. Provides for client safety.

36. Saves client energy and provides time to care for the client's needs.
37. Promotes client safety and a means to call for assistance. Sitting up in a chair and movement may cause changes in the client's vital signs.
38. Reduces the transmission of microorganisms.

EVALUATION

- Confirm that fresh linens were placed on the bed in a manner appropriate to the client's needs.

DOCUMENTATION

Nurses' Notes

- Client's tolerance to being out of bed. (Linen changes are not generally documented.)

PROCEDURE 26-16   Bedmaking: Occupied Bed

OVERVIEW

After the client takes a bath, clean linens are placed on the bed to promote comfort and decrease the transmission of microorganisms. If the client is unable to get out of bed, change the linens around the client. Assistance will be needed if the client is in traction or cannot be turned. Care must be taken to avoid disturbing the traction weights. If the client cannot be turned, change the linens from head to toe. Place a waterproof draw sheet on the beds of clients who are incontinent or have profuse drainage. The type and amount of linens placed on the bed will vary based on the type of bed the client is using. Air beds and Clinitron beds, for example, use only minimal linens under the client.

ASSESSMENT

1. Assess your equipment. Check for all the linens necessary to change the bed. Check for a dirty linen hamper. **Facilitates a smooth procedure.**
2. Assess whether the bed needs cleaning before placing clean sheets on it. **Reduces the transmission of microorganisms.**
3. Assess the client's needs in the bed. Check for profuse drainage, incontinence, or special needs for comfort or skin integrity. **Determines how the procedure will be performed.**
4. Assess the client's ability to assist with the procedure, including mobility, mental status, and muscle strength. **Determines whether assistance will be needed to change the client's linens.**
5. Assess for the presence of dressings, IV lines, tubes, or any equipment that may be attached to the client.

POSSIBLE NURSING DIAGNOSIS

Risk for Impaired Skin Integrity

PLANNING

Expected Outcomes

1. The client will have clean linens on the bed.
2. The clean linens will be appropriate to the client's needs and condition.
3. The linens will be changed with a minimum of trauma to the client.

Equipment Needed

- Linen hamper
- Top sheet, draw sheet, bottom sheet
- Pillowcase
- Blanket
- Bath blanket
- Gloves (if needed)

DELEGATION TIPS

Bed making is usually delegated to ancillary personnel. Their instruction should include the appropriate use of Standard Precautions and safety precautions for themselves and the client, such as the proper movement of the client in bed, how to manage drains and dressings, and the use of proper body mechanics. In certain situations where the client is in critical condition and multiple tubes, especially chest tubes, are present, the nurse should assist.

IMPLEMENTATION—ACTION/RATIONALE

ACTION	RATIONALE
❖ Cleanse hands ❖ Check client's identification band ❖	
1. Explain procedure to client.	1. Promotes client cooperation.
2. Bring equipment to the bedside.	2. Facilitates procedure organization.

continues

3. Cover client with a bath blanket (Figure 26-16-1). Remove top sheet and blanket. Loosen bottom sheet at foot and sides of bed. Lower side rail nearest the nurse, if necessary for access.

3. Bath blanket prevents exposure and chills. Facilitates easy removal of linens. Lowering only side rail close to nurse reduces client's risk of falls.

4. Position client on side, facing away from you. Reposition pillow under head.

4. Provides space to place clean linens.

5. Fanfold or roll bottom linens close to client toward the center of the bed.

5. Keeps soiled linen together. Promotes comfort when client later rolls to other side.

6. Place clean bottom linens with the center fold nearest the client. Fanfold or roll clean bottom linens nearest client and tuck under soiled linen (Figure 26-16-2). Maintain an adequate amount of sheet at head of bed for tucking. Have sheet even with bottom of mattress.

6. Provides for maximum fit of sheets and decreases chance of wrinkles.

7. Miter bottom sheet at head of bed. To miter, lift the mattress and tuck the sheet over the edge of the mattress, lift edge of sheet that is hanging to form a triangle, and lay upper part of sheet back onto bed; tuck the lower hanging section under the mattress. Repeat for each corner. Tuck the sides of the sheet under the mattress.

7. Holds linens firmly in place.

8. Fold the draw sheet in half. Identify the center of the draw sheet and place it close to the client. Fanfold or roll draw sheet closest to client and tuck under soiled linen. Smooth linen. Add protective padding if needed. Tuck draw sheet under mattress, working from the center to the edges. Draw sheet should be positioned under the lower back and buttocks.

8. Draw sheet facilitates moving and lifting clients while in bed.

9. Roll client over onto side facing you. Raise side rail.

9. Positions client off soiled linen. Protects client from falling.

10. Move to other side of bed. Remove soiled linens by rolling into a bundle and place in linen hamper without touching uniform.

10. Prevents cross-contamination.

11. Unfold/unroll bottom sheet, then draw sheet. Look for objects left in the bed. Grasp each sheet with knuckles up and over the sheet and pull tightly while leaning back with your body weight. Client may be positioned supine.

11. Tight sheets keep linens wrinkle-free and decrease the risk of skin irritation. Leaning back uses body weight for good body mechanics.

12. Place top sheet over client with center of sheet in middle of bed. Unfold top of sheet over client. Remove bath blankets left on client. Place top blanket over client, same as the top sheet.

12. Provides client with top sheet and blanket to prevent chilling.

Figure 26-16-1 Cover client with a bath blanket for warmth and modesty while top sheet and blanket are removed.

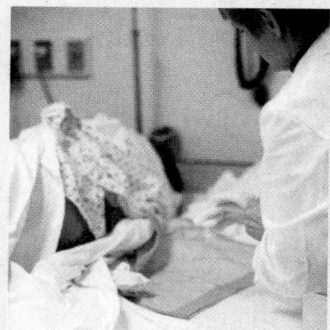

Figure 26-16-2 Place clean linens and protective pad on mattress. Tuck clean linen nearest client under soiled linen. Change gloves, if soiled, before handling clean linen.

continues

13. Raise foot of mattress and tuck the corner of the top sheet and blanket under. Miter the corner. Repeat with other side of mattress. Bend knees and not the back for proper mechanics.

13. Secures top sheet and blanket in place.

14. Grasp top sheet and blanket over client's toes and pull upward, then make a small fanfold in the sheet.

14. Provides room under the tight top sheet and blanket for client to move feet. Prevents toe decubitus and sheet burns from pressure.

15. Remove soiled pillowcase. Grasp center of clean pillowcase and invert pillowcase over hand/arm. Maintain grasp of pillowcase while grasping center of pillow. Use other hand to pull pillowcase down over pillow. Place pillow under client's head.

15. Provides clean pillowcase without shaking pillow or pillowcase. Promotes comfort.

16. Cleanse hands.

16. Reduces the transmission of microorganisms.

EVALUATION

- The client has clean, unwrinkled linen.
- The linen placed on the bed is suitable for the client's special needs.
- The linen was changed with a minimum of pain and trauma to the client.

DOCUMENTATION

Nurses' Notes

- How the client tolerated the bed change, and any unusual findings. (Bed change is not generally documented.)

PROCEDURE 26-17   Bathing a Client in Bed

OVERVIEW

Bathing clients is an essential component of nursing care and a critical time to assess the client. Whether the nurse performs the bath or delegates the activity to another health care provider, the nurse is responsible for ensuring that the hygienic needs of the client are met. The type of bath provided depends on the purpose of the bath and the client's self-care ability. The two categories of baths are cleansing and therapeutic. Cleansing baths are provided as routine client care. The purpose of a cleansing bath is personal hygiene. Following are the five types of cleansing baths:

1. Shower
2. Tub
3. Self-help, or assisted bed bath
4. Complete bed bath
5. Partial bath

For clients confined to bed, the bed bath is used to provide hygienic care. There are several variations of bed bath depending on the client's ability to assist with care. The complete bed bath is provided to dependent clients confined to bed. The nurse washes the client's entire body during a complete bed bath. A partial bed bath and a self-help bed bath are variations of the complete bed bath.

ASSESSMENT

1. Assess the client's level of ability to assist with the bath. **Determine if the client is able to follow directions. Check the client's ability to assist with cleaning any portion of the body.**

2. Assess the client's level of comfort with the procedure. Check into potential cultural, sexual, or generational issues. **Determine whether the client is uncomfortable, tense, or nervous about being bathed by someone else.**

continues

3. Assess the environment. Verify that the equipment needed is available. Assess if the client has skin intact or dressings, IV lines, or drainage tubes in place. Check whether clean, warm water is available. **Determine whether the need for modesty and privacy can be met. The environment should be conducive to a clean, safe, and comfortable procedure.**

POSSIBLE NURSING DIAGNOSES

*Risk for Impaired **S**kin Integrity*
*Bathing/Hygiene **S**elf-care Deficit*

PLANNING

Expected Outcomes

1. Clients will be cleaned without damage to their skin.
2. Clients' privacy will be maintained throughout the procedure.

3. Clients will participate in their own hygiene as much as possible.
4. Clients will not become overly tired or experience increased pain, cold, or discomfort as a result of the bath.

Equipment Needed

- Bath towels
- Washcloths
- Bath blanket
- Washbasin
- Soap
- Soap dish
- Lotion
- Deodorant
- Clean gown
- Clean linen
- Disposable, latex-free gloves

DELEGATION TIPS

This skill is routinely delegated to ancillary personnel who should allow the client to perform as much of the bath as possible or permitted. The caregiver employs Standard Precautions, properly positions the client, and observes and reports the client's skin condition and color to the nurse. The nurse retains the responsibility to assess the client.

IMPLEMENTATION—ACTION/RATIONALE

ACTION	RATIONALE
✽ **Check client's identification band** ✽ **Explain procedure before beginning** ✽	
1. Assess the client's preferences about bathing.	1. Provides client opportunity to participate in care.
2. Prepare environment. Close doors and windows, adjust temperature, provide time for elimination needs, and provide privacy.	2. Protects from chills during bath and increases sense of privacy.
3. Cleanse hands. Apply gloves. Gloves should be changed when emptying water basin.	3. Reduces the transmission of microorganisms.
4. Lower side rail on the side close to you. Position client in a comfortable position close to the side near you.	4. Prevents unnecessary reaching. Facilitates use of good body mechanics.
5. If bath blankets are available, place bath blanket over top sheet. Remove top sheet from under bath blanket. Remove client's gown. Bath blanket should be folded to expose only the area being cleaned at that time. (Top sheets or towels may also be used for bath blankets.)	5. Prevents exposure of client. Promotes privacy. Protects from chills.
6. Fill washbasin two-thirds full. Permit client to test temperature of water with hand. Water should be changed when a soap film develops or water becomes soiled.	6. Prevents accidental burns or chills.
7. Wet the washcloth and wring it out.	7. Prevents unnecessarily wetting of client.

continues

8. Make a bath mitten with the washcloth. To make a mitten, grasp the edge of the washcloth with the thumb; fold a third over the palm of the hand; wrap remainder of cloth around hand and across palm, and grasp the second edge under the thumb; fold the extended end of the washcloth onto the palm and tuck under the palmar surface of the cloth.

8. Prevents ends of washcloth from dragging across skin. Promotes friction during bath.

9. Wash the face (Figure 26-17-1). Ask the client about preference for using soap on the face. Use a separate corner of the washcloth for each eye, wiping from inner to outer canthus. Wash neck and ears. Rinse and pat dry. Male clients may want to shave at this time. Provide assistance with shaving as needed.

9. Some clients may not use soap on the face. Using separate corners of washcloth reduces risk of transmitting microorganisms. Patting dry reduces skin irritation and drying.

10. Wash arms, forearms, and hands. Wash forearms and arms using long, firm strokes in the direction of distal to proximal. Arm may need to be supported while being washed. Wash axilla. Rinse and pat dry. Apply deodorant or powder if desired. Immerse client's hand into basin of water. Allow hand to soak about 3 to 5 minutes. Wash hands, interdigit area, fingers, and fingernails. Rinse and pat dry.

10. Long strokes promote circulation. Soaking hands softens nails and loosens soil from skin and nails. Strokes directed distal to proximal promote venous return.

11. Wash chest and abdomen. Fold bath blanket down to umbilicus. Wash chest using long, firm strokes. Wash skin fold under the female client's breast by lifting each breast. Rinse and pat dry. Fold bath blanket down to suprapubic area. Use another towel to cover chest area. Wash abdomen using long, firm strokes. Rinse and pat dry. Replace bath blanket over chest and abdomen. Cover chest or abdomen area in between washing, rinsing, and drying to prevent chilling.

11. Promotes privacy and prevents chills. Long strokes promote circulation. Perspiration and soil collect within skin folds.

12. Wash legs and feet. Expose leg farthest from you by folding bath blanket to midline. Bend the leg at the knee. Grasp the heel, elevate the leg from the bed, and cover bed with bath towel. Place washbasin on towel. Place client's foot into washbasin (Figure 26-17-2). Allow foot to soak while washing the leg with long, firm strokes in the direction of distal to proximal. Rinse and pat dry. Clean soles, interdigits, and toes. Rinse and pat dry. Perform same procedure with the other leg and foot.

12. Supports joints to prevent strain and fatigue. Soaking foot loosens dirt, softens nails, and promotes comfort.

Figure 26-17-1   Wash the client's face first.

Figure 26-17-2   Place feet in basin. Clean interdigits and soles of feet.

continues

13. Wash back. Assist client into prone or side-lying position facing away from you. Wash the back and buttocks using long, firm strokes. Rinse and pat dry. Give back rub and apply lotion.
14. Perineal care: Assist client to supine position. Perform perineal care (see Procedure 26-18).
15. Apply lotion as desired or needed. Apply clean gown.
16. Cleanse hands.

13. Exposes back and buttocks for washing. Back rub promotes relaxation and circulation.

14. Removes genital secretions and soil.

15. Lotion lubricates skin.
16. Reduces the transmission of microorganisms.

EVALUATION

• The client was cleaned adequately without skin damage.
• The client's modesty was maintained throughout the procedure.
• The client participated in the procedure as much as possible.
• The client remained comfortable during the procedure.

DOCUMENTATION

Nurses' Notes

• Client was bathed. Indicate how much of the bath the client assisted with and how well the client tolerated the activity.
• Unusual findings including rashes, open sores, poor turgor, and so on

PROCEDURE 26-18   Perineal Care

OVERVIEW

The perineum is the external structure of the pelvic floor. It is composed of the skin and muscle surrounding the genitalia; it is the area between the scrotum and anus in the male and between the vulva and anus in the female. Care of the perineum and genitalia is directed toward maintaining a hygienic perineal environment. Perineal and genital care is usually self-care; however, alterations in the client's ability to perform self-care or alterations in the perineum and genitalia are reasons for nurses or other care providers to perform this skill. Perineal and genital care is an emotionally and culturally difficult subject. Many cultures have specific beliefs and taboos regarding the perineal/genital area. Many people are embarrassed by the idea of anyone else seeing or touching their genitals, particularly a stranger. Be aware of these possibilities when approaching genital/perineal care. In general, a professional, nonjudgmental approach will put the client more at ease with the procedure. Ask the client or the client's caregiver, if possible, about any preferences the client may have in this area.

ASSESSMENT

1. Evaluate client status: level of consciousness, ability to ambulate, ability to perform self-care, frequency of urination and defecation, skin condition. **This allows the nurse to decide who, where, how, and when to perform perineal care.**
2. Identify cultural preferences for perineal care. **Perineal care is strongly associated with cultural practices, for example, who may touch the perineal area and how, and the proper way to "wipe." To the extent possible, these preferences should be identified and incorporated into the client's care.**
3. Assess the client's perineal health. Ask the male client if he has any perineal/genital itching or discomfort.

Ask the female client if she has any urethral, vaginal, or anal discharge. **Determines the presence of signs and symptoms that may need additional assessment and intervention.**
4. Determine if the client is incontinent of urine or stool. **Affects how the procedure will be done and what additional procedures may be necessary.**
5. Assess whether the client has recently had perineal/genital surgery. **Affects how the procedure will be done and what additional procedures may be necessary.**

POSSIBLE NURSING DIAGNOSES

Risk for Impaired Skin Integrity
Bathing/Hygiene Self-Care Deficit

continues

PLANNING

Expected Outcomes

1. Perineum and genitalia will be dry, clean, and free of secretions and unpleasant odors.
2. The client will report feeling comfortable and clean in the perineal area.
3. The client will not experience discomfort or undue embarrassment during the procedure.
4. The perineum will be free of skin breakdown or irritation.

Equipment Needed

- Personal protective equipment (gloves, gown)
- Toilet paper/washcloths
- Waterproof pads
- Cleansing solution if needed
- Perineal wash bottle (fill with plain, warm water).
- Water receptacle (bedpan or toilet if client is ambulatory)
- Dry towels
- Perineal treatment (i.e., ointment or lotions) if necessary
- Linen receptacle
- Room deodorizer

DELEGATION TIPS

This skill is routinely delegated to ancillary personnel who should be trained in Standard Precautions and proper client positioning, and to report color, odor, and amount of any discharge, if present, to the nurse.

IMPLEMENTATION—ACTION/RATIONALE

ACTION

* Check client's identification band * Explain procedure before beginning *

1. Cleanse hands and wear gloves. If appropriate and splashing is likely, wear gown, mask, and goggles.
2. Close privacy curtain or door.
3. Position client.

4. Place waterproof pads under the client in the bed or under bedpan if used.
5. Remove fecal debris with toilet paper and dispose in toilet.

6. Spray perineum with washing solution if indicated. Alternatively, plain water may be used.

7. Cleanse perineum with wet washcloths (front to back on females), changing to clean area on washcloth with each wipe. Cleanse the penis on the male (Figure 26-18-1).
8. Carefully examine gluteal folds and scrotal folds for debris. Gently visualize vulva for debris.
9. If soap is used, spray area with clean water from the peri-bottle.
10. Change gloves.
11. Dry perineum carefully with towel.

12. If indicated, apply barrier lotion or ointment.

13. Reposition or dress client as appropriate.

RATIONALE

1. Reduces the transmission of microorganisms.

2. Provides privacy.
3. If client is ambulatory, perineal care may be done either with client on or standing at the toilet. If perineal care is to be performed in the bed, place the client on the side or over a deep bedpan.
4. Protects bed linen.

5. May require several attempts. If performing at the bedside, may collect paper in disposable pad or linens until end of procedure.
6. Several perineal solutions are available, which may or may not require rinsing. Carefully evaluate this requirement. Solutions that require rinsing may cause skin breakdown if left on the skin.
7. Maximizes cleaning; prevents spread of rectal flora to vagina.

8. Fecal material causes irritation and skin breakdown rapidly when left in contact with skin.
9. Rinses soap, which can irritate the skin, from the area.

10. Reduces the transmission of microorganisms.
11. Residual moisture provides an ideal environment for the growth of microorganisms.
12. Barrier ointments may be used if client is incontinent or skin folds tend to harbor moisture.
13. Promotes client comfort.

continues

Figure 26-18-1 Cleanse the penis with a warm, wet washcloth.

14. Dispose of linens and garbage according to hospital policy.
15. Cleanse hands.
16. Deodorize room if appropriate.

14. Prevents spread of disease or bacteria.
15. Reduces the transmission of microorganisms.
16. Promotes client comfort. This may also be done at the beginning of the procedure.

EVALUATION

- The perineum and genitalia are dry, clean, and free of secretions and unpleasant odors.
- The client reports feeling comfortable and clean in the perineal area.
- The client did not experience discomfort or undue embarrassment during the procedure.

DOCUMENTATION

Nurses' Notes
- Time and type of perineal care provided
- Unusual findings such as skin breakdown, infection, or unusual drainage
- Client special preferences or cultural considerations

Kardex
- Special preferences or cultural considerations

PROCEDURE 26-19   Routine Catheter Care

OVERVIEW

An indwelling catheter is used to provide continuous drainage of urine from the bladder. The catheter, which is attached to a drainage bag, may be used for episodic or long-term urinary drainage. Because the catheter is in the bladder through the urethra, bacteria may enter the urinary system; therefore, care must be taken to ensure that the surrounding area is clean to decrease contamination of the catheter by bacterial flora. Clients may be embarrassed or frightened by the catheter and related care and, therefore, require emotional support.

ASSESSMENT

1. Assess catheter patency and urine color, consistency, and amount while performing the care **to determine if catheter and drainage system are functioning correctly.**

2. Determine the condition of the urinary meatus and perineal area **to monitor for redness, swelling, or drainage, stool, or vaginal discharge, as indicators of infection. External infections may migrate up the catheter and lead to urinary tract infection.**

continues

3. Determine the client's emotional reaction and feelings related to the catheter. **This may prevent untoward reactions to the care and allow the nurse to help the client deal with some deeper emotional issues.**

POSSIBLE NURSING DIAGNOSES

Risk for Infection
Risk for Impaired Skin Integrity

PLANNING

Expected Outcomes

1. The client will be free of signs and symptoms of urinary tract infection.

2. The client will understand the reason for the catheter and related cares.
3. The meatus and surrounding area will be clean and free of drainage.

Equipment Needed

- Clean latex-free gloves
- Washcloth, soap, and water
- Waterproof pad
- Antiseptic solution
- Sterile swabs

DELEGATION TIPS

Routine catheter care is a procedure ancillary personnel are able to perform after proper instruction and supervision. Instruction should include notifying the nurse regarding the appearance of catheter drainage and any problems with catheter tubing, such as leaks.

IMPLEMENTATION—ACTION/RATIONALE

ACTION

RATIONALE

* Check client's identification band * Explain procedure before beginning *

1. Cleanse hands.
2. Check institutional protocol or care plan.
3. Provide privacy.
4. Place client in supine position and expose perineal area and catheter.

5. Place waterproof pad under client.
6. Put on clean gloves.
7. After performing perineal care (Procedure 26-18), cleanse meatus if there is excessive purulent drainage with nonirritating antiseptic solutions on cotton balls.
8. Cleanse catheter from meatus out to end of catheter, taking care not to pull on catheter.
9. Be sure to repeat catheter care any time it becomes soiled with stool or other drainage.
10. Place linen or cotton balls in proper receptacle for laundry or disposal.
11. Cleanse hands.

1. Reduces the transmission of microorganisms.
2. Ensures proper procedure.
3. Protects client dignity.
4. Allows for visualization of field. If unable to visualize the perineal area with the client supine, try placing the client in a side-lying position.
5. Protects bed linens.
6. Reduces transmission of microorganisms.
7. Moving from the most clean area out decreases risk of recontamination.

8. Moving from most clean area out does not traumatize urethra or bladder.
9. Reduces chance of infection.

10. Reduces transmission of infection to other clients.

11. Reduces transmission of microorganisms.

EVALUATION

- The client is free of signs and symptoms of urinary tract infection.
- The client understands the reason for the catheter and related care.
- The meatus and surrounding area are clean, intact, and free of drainage.

DOCUMENTATION

Nurses' Notes

- Time the procedure was performed and condition of area surrounding the catheter

PROCEDURE 26-20   Oral Care

OVERVIEW

The oral cavity functions in mastication, secretion of mucus to moisten and lubricate the digestive system, secretion of digestive enzymes, and absorption of essential nutrients. Common problems occurring in the oral cavity include the following:

- Bad breath (halitosis)
- Dental cavities (caries)
- Plaque
- Periodontal disease
- Inflammation of the gums (gingivitis)
- Inflammation of the oral mucosa (stomatitis)

Poor oral hygiene and loss of teeth may affect a client's social interaction and body image as well as nutritional intake. Daily oral care is essential to maintain the integrity of the mucous membranes, teeth, gums, and lips. Through preventive measures, the oral cavity and teeth can be preserved. Preventive oral care consists of fluoride rinsing, flossing, and brushing.

Fluoride

Researchers determined that fluoride can prevent dental caries. Fluoride is a common component of many mouthwashes and toothpastes; however, people with excessive dryness or irritated mucous membranes should avoid commercial mouthwashes because of the alcohol content, which causes drying of mucous membranes. Educate clients about fluoride being an excellent preventive measure against dental caries, but excessive fluoride exposure can affect the color of tooth enamel.

Flossing

Floss daily in conjunction with brushing of teeth. Flossing prevents the formation of plaque, removes plaque between the teeth, and removes food debris. Dental caries and periodontal disease can be prevented by regular flossing. Many floss holders are available to facilitate flossing.

Brushing

Teeth should be brushed after each meal. Brushing should be performed using a dentifrice (toothpaste) that contains fluoride to aid in preventing dental caries. An effective homemade dentifrice is the combination of two parts salt with one part baking soda. Brushing removes plaque and food debris and promotes blood circulation of the gums. Dentures should be brushed using the same brushing motion as that used for brushing teeth.

ASSESSMENT

1. Assess whether the client is able to assist with oral care and to what extent. **Promotes independence where possible.**
2. Evaluate whether the client has an understanding of proper oral hygiene. **Promotes self-care and teaching.**
3. Check whether the client has dentures. **Determines how oral care will be performed.**
4. Assess the condition of the client's mouth. **Determines how oral care will be performed.**
5. Assess whether inflammation, bleeding, infection, or ulceration is present. **Determines how oral care will be performed. Determines the need for additional assessment and intervention.**
6. Assess what cultural practices must be taken into consideration. **Determines how oral care will be performed.**
7. Assess whether there are any appliances or devices present in the client's mouth such as braces, endotracheal tube, or bridgework. **Determines how oral care will be performed.**
8. Check that the proper equipment is available to perform oral care. **Ensures a smooth procedure.**

POSSIBLE NURSING DIAGNOSES

*Risk for **I**nfection*
*Impaired **O**ral Mucous Membrane*
*Bathing/Hygiene **S**elf-Care Deficit*
*Deficient **K**nowledge-Oral Hygiene*

continues

PLANNING

Expected Outcomes

1. Client's mouth, teeth, gums, and lips will be clean and free of food particles.
2. Any inflammation, bleeding, infection, or ulceration present will be noted and treated.
3. The oral mucosa will be clean, intact, and well hydrated.

Equipment Needed

Brushing and Flossing
- Toothbrush
- Toothpaste with fluoride
- Emesis basin
- Towel
- Cup of water
- Nonsterile gloves
- Dental floss, floss holder
- Mirror
- Lip moisturizer

Denture Care
- Denture brush
- Denture cleaner
- Emesis basin
- Towel
- Cup of water
- Nonsterile gloves
- Tissue
- Denture cup

Special Care Items for Clients with Impaired Physical Mobility or Who Are Unconscious (comatose)
- Soft toothbrush or toothette
- Tongue blade
- 3 × 3 gauze sponges
- Cotton-tip applicators
- Prescribed solution
- Plastic Asepto syringe
- Suction machine and catheter

DELEGATION TIPS

Oral care is routinely delegated to ancillary personnel, who should allow the client to perform as much of the oral care as possible or permitted. The caregiver should be trained to employ Standard Precautions, to properly position the client, and to observe and report the client's mucous membrane condition and color to the nurse.

IMPLEMENTATION—ACTION/RATIONALE

ACTION   RATIONALE

❋ Check client's identification band ❋ Explain procedure before beginning ❋

Self-Care Client: Flossing and Brushing

1. Assemble articles for flossing and brushing.
2. Provide privacy.
3. Place client in a high Fowler's position.
4. Cleanse hands and apply gloves.
5. Arrange articles within client's reach.
6. Assist client with flossing and brushing as necessary. Position mirror, emesis basin, water with straw near the client, and a towel across the chest (Figure 26-20-1).
7. Assist client with rinsing mouth.
8. Reposition client, raise side rails, and place call button within reach.
9. Rinse, dry, and return articles to proper place.
10. Remove gloves, cleanse hands, and document care.

1. Promotes efficiency.
2. Relaxes the client.
3. Decreases risk of aspiration.
4. Reduces the transmission of microorganisms.
5. Facilitates self-care.
6. Flossing and brushing decrease microorganism growth in the mouth. Use of mirror permits cleaning back and sides of teeth.
7. Removes toothpaste and oral secretions.
8. Promotes comfort, safety, and communication.

9. Promotes a clean environment.
10. Reduces the transmission of microorganisms and documents nursing care.

Self-Care Client: Denture Care

11. Assemble articles for denture cleaning.
12. Provide privacy.

11. Promotes efficiency.
12. Relaxes the client.

continues

Figure 26-20-1 Promote independence, but assist with flossing or brushing as necessary.

Figure 26-20-2 Dentures may include full upper or lower plates, or partial plates.

13. Assist client to a high Fowler's position.
14. Cleanse hands and apply gloves.

15. Assist client with denture removal:
   a. Top denture:
      • With tissue, grasp the denture with thumb and forefinger and pull downward.
      • Place in denture cup.
   b. Bottom denture:
      • Place thumbs on the gums and release the denture. Grasp denture with thumb and forefinger and pull upward.
      • Place in denture cup.
16. Apply toothpaste to brush, and brush dentures either with cool water in the emesis basin or under running water in the sink. Pad sink with towel to protect dentures in case they are dropped.
17. Rinse thoroughly.
18. Assist client with rinsing mouth and replacing dentures.
19. Reposition client, with side rails up and call button within reach.
20. Rinse, dry, and return articles to proper place.
21. Remove gloves and cleanse hands.

Full-Care Client: Brushing and Flossing

22. Assemble articles for flossing and brushing.
23. Provide privacy.
24. Cleanse hands and apply gloves.

25. Position client as condition allows: high Fowler's, semi-Fowler's, or lateral position, head turned toward side (Figure 26-20-3).
26. Place towel across client's chest or under face and mouth if head is turned to one side.
27. Moisten toothbrush or toothette, apply small amount of toothpaste, and brush teeth and gums.

13. Facilitates removal of dentures.
14. Reduces the transmission of microorganisms and exposure to body fluids.
15. Breaks seal created with dentures without causing pressure and injury to oral membranes. Prevents breaking of dentures (Figure 26-20-2).

16. Facilitates removal of microorganisms.

17. Removes toothpaste.
18. Freshens mouth and facilitates intake of solid food.

19. Promotes comfort, safety, and communication.

20. Maintains a clean environment.
21. Reduces the transmission of microorganisms.

22. Promotes efficiency.
23. Relaxes client.
24. Reduces the transmission of microorganisms and exposure to body fluids.
25. Decreases risk of aspiration.

26. Catches secretions.

27. Moistens mouth and facilitates plaque removal.

continues

Figure 26-20-3   If client is unable to sit up, turn head to the side.

28. Grasp the dental floss in both hands or use a floss holder and floss between all teeth; hold floss against tooth while moving floss up and down sides of teeth.
29. Assist the client in rinsing mouth.
30. Reapply toothpaste and brush the teeth and gums using friction in a vertical or circular motion. On inner and outer surfaces of teeth, hold brush at 45-degree angle against teeth and brush from sulcus to crowns of teeth. On biting surfaces, move brush back and forth in short strokes. All surfaces of teeth should be brushed from every angle.
31. Assist the client in rinsing and drying mouth.
32. Apply lip moisturizer, if appropriate.
33. Reposition client, raise side rails, and place call button within reach.
34. Rinse, dry, and return articles to proper place.
35. Remove gloves and cleanse hands.

Clients at Risk for or with an Alteration of the Oral Cavity

36. Follow Actions 22–24.
37. Bleeding:
    a. Assess oral cavity with a padded tongue blade and flashlight for signs of bleeding.
    b. Proceed with the actions for oral care for a full-care client except:
       • Do not floss.
       • Use a soft toothbrush, toothette, or a tongue blade padded with 3 × 3 gauze sponges to gently swab teeth and gums.
       • Dispose of padded tongue blade into a biohazard bag according to institutional policy.
       • Rinse with tepid water.
38. Infection:
    a. Assess oral cavity with a tongue blade and flashlight for signs of infection.
    b. Culture lesions as ordered.
    c. Proceed with the actions for oral care for a full-care client except:
       • Do not floss.
       • Use prescribed antiseptic solution.

28. Removes plaque and prevents gum disease.

29. Removes toothpaste and oral secretions.
30. Permits cleaning of back and sides of teeth and decreases microorganism growth in mouth.

31. Removes toothpaste and oral secretions.
32. Maintains skin integrity of lips.
33. Promotes comfort, safety, and communication.

34. Provides an orderly environment.
35. Reduces the transmission of microorganisms.

36. See Rationales 22–24.
37.
    a. Determines whether bleeding is present, amount, and specific areas.
    b.

       • Decreases risk of bleeding and trauma to gums.
       • Decreases risk of bleeding and trauma to gums.

       • Promotes proper disposal of contaminated waste.

       • Cleanses mouth.
38.
    a. Determines appearance, integrity, and general condition.
    b. Identifies growth of specific microorganisms.
    c.

       • Prevents irritation, pain, and bleeding.
       • Antiseptic solutions decrease growth of microorganisms.

continues

- Use a tongue blade padded with 3×3 gauze sponges to gently swab the teeth and gums.
- Dispose of padded tongue blade into a biohazard bag according to institutional policy.
- Rinse mouth with tepid water.
- Apply additional solution as prescribed.

39. Ulceration:
  a. Assess oral cavity with a tongue blade and flashlight for signs of ulceration.
  b. Culture lesions as ordered.
  c. Proceed with actions for oral care for a full-care client except:
    - Do not floss.
    - Use prescribed antiseptic solution.
    - Use a tongue blade padded with 3×3 gauze sponges to gently swab the teeth and gums.
    - Dispose of padded tongue blade into a biohazard bag according to institutional policy.
    - Rinse mouth with tepid water.
    - Apply additional solution as prescribed.

- Promotes proper disposal of contaminated materials.
- Cleanses mouth.
- Provides a coating that promotes healing of the tissue.

39.
  a. Determines appearance, integrity, and general condition.
  b. Identifies growth of specific microorganisms.
  c.

  - Prevents irritation, pain, and bleeding.
  - Antiseptic solutions decrease growth of microorganisms.

  - Promotes proper disposal of contaminated materials.
  - Cleanses mouth.
  - Provides a coating that promotes healing of the tissue.

Unconscious (Comatose) Client

40. Follow Actions 22–24.
41. Place the client in a lateral position, with the head turned toward the side.
42. Use a floss holder and floss between all teeth.
43. Moisten toothbrush or toothette, and brush the teeth and gums using friction in a vertical or circular motion. Do not use toothpaste. On inner and outer surfaces of teeth, hold brush at 45-degree angle against teeth and brush from sulcus to crowns of teeth. On biting surfaces, move brush back and forth in short strokes. All surfaces of teeth should be brushed from every angle.
44. After flossing and brushing, rinse mouth with an Asepto syringe (do not force water into the mouth) and perform oral suction.
45. Dry the client's mouth.
46. Apply lip moisturizer.
47. Leave the client in a lateral position with head turned toward side for 30 to 60 minutes after oral hygiene care. Suction one more time. Remove the towel from under the client's mouth and face.
48. Dispose of any contaminated items in a biohazard bag and clean, dry, and return all articles to the appropriate place.
49. Remove gloves and cleanse hands.

40. See Rationales 22–24.
41. Prevents aspiration.

42. Prevents transfer of microorganisms from a client bite.
43. Permits cleaning of back and sides of teeth and decreases microorganism growth in mouth. Toothpaste may foam and cause aspiration.

44. Promotes cleansing and removal of secretions and prevents aspiration.

45. Prevents skin irritation.
46. Maintains skin integrity of lips.
47. Prevents pooling of secretions and aspiration.

48. Promotes proper disposal of contaminated materials.

49. Reduces the transmission of microorganisms.

EVALUATION

- The client's mouth, teeth, gums, and lips are clean and free of food particles.
- Inflammation, bleeding, infection, or ulceration are noted and cared for.
- The oral mucosa is clean, intact, and well hydrated.
- The oral care was performed with a minimum of trauma to the client.

DOCUMENTATION

Nurses' Notes

- Unusual findings

PROCEDURE 26-21   Eye Care

OVERVIEW

Generally, the eye needs little daily care. Normally, eyes are continually cleansed by the production of tears and movement of eyelids over the eyes. Some clients, however, do have special eye care needs.

Contact Lenses

Self-care is the best method of care for a client with contact lenses; however, accidents or illness may render a client unable to remove or care for the lenses. Some lenses may be left on the cornea for up to a week without damage. Most must be removed daily for cleaning and to prevent hypoxia of the cornea. It is a nursing responsibility to determine whether the client is wearing contact lenses and to properly care for the lenses and the client's eyes. In acute care situations, encourage the client to wear glasses if possible and send the contact lenses home with a family member.

Prosthetic Eyes

Some clients have an artificial eye (ocular prosthesis) in place. Artificial eyes are created to look identical to the client's biologic eye. They are generally made from glass or plastic. Some artificial eyes are permanently implanted in the eye socket, but others must be removed daily for cleaning. The eye socket should also be gently cleansed to remove crusts and mucus, and the prosthesis replaced in the eye socket.

ASSESSMENT

1. Determine if the client is wearing contact lenses or has an ocular prosthesis. If the client is unable to answer questions, you will need to find out another way. Does it indicate in the client's chart if the client wears contact lenses or has a prosthesis? Are there family members present to ask? **This will affect how eye care is given.**
2. Are the eye care supplies needed available? If the client can tell you what kind of eye care products he or she normally uses, ask or have a family member bring these products from home. **This will affect how eye care is given.**
3. Assess whether the client can do his or her own eye care. If not, evaluate what kind of assistance the client will need. **This promotes maximum independence in the client.**

POSSIBLE NURSING DIAGNOSES

Ineffective **H**ealth Maintenance
Bathing/Hygiene **S**elf-Care Deficit
Disturbed **S**ensory Perception (Visual)

PLANNING

Expected Outcomes

1. The client's contact lenses will be safely removed and stored.

2. The client's ocular prosthesis will be safely removed, cleaned, and either stored or returned to the client's eye socket.
3. The client's contacts or prosthesis will be cared for with a minimum of trauma to the client's eyes.
4. The client's eyes will be free of crusts and exudate.

Equipment Needed

Artificial Eye
- Storage container
- Mild soap
- 3 × 3 gauze sponges
- Cotton balls
- Towel
- Emesis basins
- Eye irrigation syringe (optional)
- Running water
- Sterile gloves
- Biohazard bag
- Saline solution
- Protector pad

Contact Lenses
- Lens container
- Soaking solution—type used by client
- Towel
- Suction cup (optional)
- Scotch tape (optional)
- Nonsterile gloves

continues

DELEGATION TIPS

Eye care requires the assessment and intervention of the nurse and delegation to ancillary personnel is inappropriate.

IMPLEMENTATION—ACTION/RATIONALE

ACTION

RATIONALE

* Check client's identification band * Explain procedure before beginning *

Artificial Eye Removal

1. Inquire about client's care regimen and gather equipment accordingly.
2. Provide privacy.
3. Cleanse hands; apply gloves.
4. Place client in a semi-Fowler's position.
5. Place the cotton balls in an emesis basin filled halfway with warm tap water.
6. Place 3 × 3 gauze sponges in bottom of second emesis basin and fill halfway with mild soap and tepid water.
7. Grasp and squeeze excess water from a cotton ball. Cleanse the eyelid with the moistened cotton ball, starting at the inner canthus and moving outward toward the outer canthus. After each use, dispose of cotton ball in biohazard bag. Repeat procedure until eyelid is clean (without dried secretions).
8. Remove the artificial eye:
   a. Using dominant hand, raise the client's upper eyelid with index finger and depress the lower eyelid with thumb.
   b. Cup nondominant hand under the client's lower eyelid.
   c. Apply slight pressure with index finger between the brow and the artificial eye and remove it. Place it in an emesis basin filled with warm, soapy water.
9. Grasp a moistened cotton ball and cleanse around the edge of the eye socket. Dispose of the soiled cotton ball into biohazard bag.
10. Inspect the eye socket for any signs of irritation, drainage, or crusting.
    Note: If the client's usual care regimen or physician order requires irrigation of the socket, proceed with Action 11; otherwise, go to Action 12.
11. Eye socket irrigation:
    a. Lower the head of the bed and place the client in a supine position. Place protector pad on bed; turn head toward socket side and slightly extend neck.
    b. Fill the irrigation syringe with the prescribed amount and type of irrigating solution (warm tap water or normal saline).
    c. With nondominant hand, separate the eyelids with your forefinger and thumb while resting fingers on the brow and cheekbone.

1. Promotes continuity of care.
2. Relaxes the client.
3. Reduces the transmission of microorganisms.
4. Facilitates procedure and client participation.
5. Dry cotton balls could cause irritation.
6. Gauze serves as padding to prevent breakage of the prosthesis.
7. Eliminating the excess water prevents water from running down the client's face. Cleansing the eyelid prevents contamination of the lacrimal system (inner canthus area). Disposal of cotton balls reduces transmission of microorganisms to other health care workers.
8. Cleanses the artificial eye.
   a. Promotes removal of artificial eye.

   b. Cupping reduces dropping and possible breaking of the eye.
   c. Applying pressure will help the prosthesis to slip out.

9. Cleanses the eye socket. Disposal of cotton ball reduces transmission of microorganisms to other health care workers.
10. Indicates an infection.

11. Cleanses the eye socket and removes secretions.
    a. Positioning of client facilitates ease in performing the procedure and client comfort.
    b. Ensures compliance with client's regimen or prescribed orders.
    c. Keeps the eyelid open and the socket visible.

continues

d. Hold the irrigating syringe in dominant hand several inches above the inner canthus; with thumb, gently apply pressure on the plunger, directing the flow of solution from the inner canthus along the conjunctival sac.

e. Irrigate until the prescribed amount of solution has been used.

f. Wipe the eyelids with a moistened cotton ball after irrigating. Dispose of soiled cotton ball in biohazard bag.

g. Pat the skin dry with the towel.

h. Return the client to a semi-Fowler's position.

i. Remove gloves, cleanse hands, and apply clean gloves.

12. Rub the artificial eye between index finger and thumb in the basin of warm, soapy water.

13. Rinse the prosthesis under running water or place in the clean basin of tepid water. Do not dry the prosthesis.
    Note: Either reinsert the prosthesis (Action 14) or store in a container (Action 15).

14. Reinsert the prosthesis:
    a. With the thumb of the nondominant hand, raise and hold the upper eyelid open.
    b. With the dominant hand, grasp the artificial eye so that the indented part is facing toward the client's nose and slide it under the upper eyelid as far as possible.
    c. Depress the lower lid.
    d. Pull the lower lid forward to cover the edge of the prosthesis.

15. Place the cleaned artificial eye in a labeled container with saline or tap water solution.

16. Grasp a moistened cotton ball and squeeze out excessive moisture. Wipe the eyelid from the inner to the outer canthus. Dispose of the soiled cotton ball in a biohazard bag.

17. Clean, dry, and replace equipment.

18. Reposition the client, raise side rails, and place call light in reach.

19. Dispose of biohazard bag according to institutional policy.

20. Remove gloves and cleanse hands.

Contact Lens Removal

21. Assess level of assistance needed and provide privacy.

22. Cleanse hands.

23. Assist the client to a semi-Fowler's position if needed.

24. Drape a clean towel over the client's chest.

25. Prepare the lens storage case with the prescribed solution.

26. Instruct the client to look straight ahead. Assess the location of the lens. If it is not on the cornea, either you or the client should gently move the lens toward the cornea with pad of index finger (Figure 26-21-1).

d. Prevents injury to the client.

e. Ensures compliance with client's regimen of prescribed orders.

f. Reduces the transmission of microorganisms to prosthesis.

g. Prevents maceration of the skin.

h. Promotes client comfort.

i. Reduces the transmission of microorganisms.

12. Creates cleaning with friction and prevents breakage of the prosthesis.

13. Removes soap and secretions. Keeping the artificial eye wet prevents irritation from lint or other particles that might adhere to it and facilitates reinsertion.

14. Allows for client comfort.
    a. Facilitates reinsertion of the prosthesis without discomfort to the client.
    b. Positions the prosthesis for insertion.

    c. Allows the prosthesis to slide into place.
    d. Holds the prosthesis in place.

15. Protects the prosthesis from scratches and keeps it clean.

16. Squeezing the cotton ball removes moisture. Cleansing the eyelid prevents contamination of lacrimal system. Disposal of cotton ball reduces the transmission of microorganisms to other health care workers.

17. Promotes a clean environment.

18. Promotes client's comfort, safety, and communication.

19. Reduces the transmission of microorganisms to other health care workers.

20. Same as Rationale 19.

21. Level of assistance determines level of intervention. Privacy reduces anxiety.

22. Reduces the transmission of microorganisms.

23. Facilitates removal of lens.

24. Provides a clean surface and facilitates the location of a lens if it falls during removal.

25. Hard lenses can be stored dry or in a special soaking solution. Soft lenses are stored in sterile normal saline without a preservative.

26. Client's position promotes easy removal of lens. Positioning lens on the cornea aids removal. Use of the finger pad of the index finger prevents damage to cornea and lens.

continues

Figure 26-21-1 If the lens is not on the cornea, gently move it toward the cornea with the pad of the index finger.

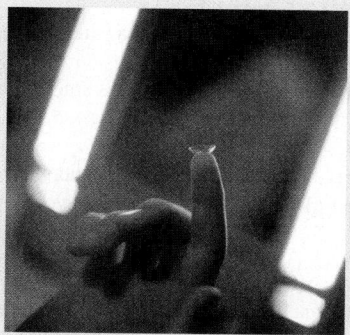

Figure 26-21-2 Be careful with the lens when it is out of the client's eye. It may be easily dropped or lost.

27. Remove the lens.
   a. Hard lens:
   - Cup nondominant hand under the eye.

   - Gently place index finger on the outside corner of the eye and pull toward the temple and ask client to blink. Catch the lens in your nondominant hand.
   b. Soft lens:
   - With nondominant hand, separate the eyelid with your thumb and middle finger.
   - With the index finger of the dominant hand gently placed on the lower edge of the lens, slide the lens downward onto the sclera and gently squeeze the lens.
   - Release the top eyelid (continue holding the lower lid down) and remove the lens with your index finger and thumb (Figure 26-21-2).
      Note: If Action 27 is unsuccessful, secure a suction cup to remove the contact lens. If you are unable to remove the lens, notify the physician or qualified practitioner.
28. Store the lens in the correct compartment of the case ("right" or "left"). Label with the client's name.
29. Remove and store the other lens by repeating Actions 27 and 28.
30. Assess eyes for irritation or redness.
31. Store the lens case in a safe place.
32. Dispose of soiled articles and clean and return reusable articles to proper location.
33. Reposition the client, raise side rails, and place call light in reach.
34. Remove gloves and cleanse hands.

27. Provides for cleaning and storage of the lens.
   a.
   - Cupping the hand under eye helps catch the lens and prevent breakage.
   - Pulling the corner of the eye tightens the eyelid against the eyeball. Pressure on the upper edge of lens causes the lens to tip forward.

   b.
   - Separating the eyelid exposes the lower edge of lens.
   - Positions lens for easy grasping with the pad of the index finger, which prevents injury to the cornea and lens. Squeezing the lens allows air to enter and release the suction.
   - Ensures control of the lens.

   - Suction cup is used to remove a lens from an unconscious or dependent client.

28. Storage prevents damage to the lenses and ensures that each lens will be reinserted into the correct eye.
29. Refer to Rationales 27 and 28.

30. Signs of corneal irritation.
31. Prevents damage or loss.
32. Reduces the transmission of infection.

33. Promotes client comfort, safety, and communication.

34. Reduces the transmission of infection.

continues

EVALUATION

- The client's contact lenses were safely removed and stored.
- The client's ocular prosthesis was safely removed, cleaned, and either stored or returned to the client's eye socket.
- The client's contacts or prosthesis were cared for with a minimum of trauma to the client's eyes.
- The client's eyes are free of crusts and exudate.
- The client is comfortable.

DOCUMENTATION

Nurses' Notes

- Whether the client wears contact lenses
- Location and condition of the lenses
- Whether the client requires assistance to place and remove the contact lenses
- Whether the client has an ocular prosthesis and which eye.
- Condition of the prosthesis and the condition of the eye socket
- Care performed on the prosthesis and the socket and how the client tolerated the activity
- Client teaching

Kardex

- Whether the client wears contact lenses or glasses or has an ocular prosthesis
- Special care requirements

PROCEDURE 26-22   Giving a Back Rub

OVERVIEW

Giving a back rub is a basic nursing skill. Back massage can be an effective means of building a sense of trust and increased rapport between the nurse and client. Clients are often touch-deprived in the busy health care industry of today. The small amount of time that it takes to do a simple back massage can often soothe and relax a "difficult" client and increase the effectiveness of the nurse–client relationship.

Massage can be performed in many different ways, from light strokes to heavy kneading. Various forms include effleurage, deep or gentle stroking, and petrissage, a kneading performed with the tips of the fingers and thumbs or palm of the hand. Massage stimulates circulation and promotes lymphatic drainage, thereby helping to rid the body of metabolic wastes, speed healing, and provide gentle relaxation. Massage can open lines of communication and improve the therapeutic relationship between a nurse and client.

ASSESSMENT

1. Assess the client's willingness to have a massage. **The client may not want a massage or may not enjoy the tactile experience of a massage.**
2. Assess the client for contraindications of a back rub. Conditions include open sores or lesions, vertebral fractures, burns, and signs of pressure ulcers. **To prevent injuring the client.**
3. Assess any limitations the client has in positioning **to determine if the client has any conditions that prohibit a side-lying or prone position.**
4. Assess the client for fatigue, stiffness, or soreness in the back and shoulders. **Knowing areas of particular**

concern allows you to focus your energies toward "trouble areas."
5. Assess the client for anxiety or emotional disturbances. **Massage can help reduce anxiety and calm people in distress.**
6. If possible, have the client quantify the degree of discomfort using a 1 to 10 rating scale. **Quantifying the results can provide more validity to the intervention.**

POSSIBLE NURSING DIAGNOSES

*A*nxiety (mild, severe, panic)
Impaired Physical Mobility

continues

PLANNING

Expected Outcomes

1. The client will experience a reduction in tension, anxiety, pain, and fatigue.
2. The nurse will establish a better rapport with the client.

Equipment Needed

- Quiet environment, free of interruptions, with a comfortable room temperature
- Comfortable bed or massage table that allows a client to lie in a side-lying or prone position
- Bath blanket
- Bath towel, to absorb excess moisture, oils
- Lotion, baby powder, or massage oil
- Gloves if necessary

DELEGATION TIPS

Giving a back rub to a client is routinely delegated to properly trained ancillary personnel, who should communicate the client's response to a back rub to the nurse.

IMPLEMENTATION—ACTION/RATIONALE

ACTION	RATIONALE

❋ Check client's identification band ❋ Explain procedure before beginning ❋

ACTION	RATIONALE
1. Cleanse your hands and apply gloves if necessary.	1. Reduces the transmission of microorganisms.
2. Help client to a prone or side-lying position (Figure 26-22-1).	2. Allows exposure of back and shoulder area.
3. Drape the bath blanket, and undo the client's gown, exposing the back, shoulder, and sacral area, but keeping the remainder of the body covered.	3. Prevents chilling and excess exposure.
4. Pour a small amount of lotion in your hand and warm between your palms for a few moments. The lotion bottle can also be submerged in a bowl of warm water for a few minutes to warm the lotion. Baby powder may be substituted for oils or lotions (Figure 26-22-2).	4. Prevents the shock of cold lotion being applied to the body. Some clients may be sensitive to oils or lotions.
5. Begin in the sacral area with smooth, circular strokes, moving upward toward the shoulders. Gradually lengthen the strokes to the upper back, scapulae, and upper arms. Apply firm, continuous pressure without breaking contact with the client (Figures 26-22-3).	5. Applying firm, continuous pressure increases circulation and relaxation.

Figure 26-22-1 Position client in a prone or side-lying position.

Figure 26-22-2 Pour lotion on your hand and warm between your palms.

continues

Figure 26-22-3 Apply firm, continuous pressure without breaking contact between your hands and the client's skin.

Figure 26-22-4 Finish the massage with light brush strokes, using the fingertips.

6. Assess client's back as you are massaging for areas of redness and signs of decreased circulation.
7. Provide a firm, kneading massage to areas of increased tension if desired, in areas such as the shoulders and gluteal muscles.
8. Complete the massage with long, very light brush strokes, using the tips of the fingers (Figure 26-22-4).
9. Gently pat or wipe excess lubricant off the client and cover the client.
10. Cleanse hands.

6. Monitors for signs of early skin breakdown.

7. Firm, kneading strokes can decrease muscle tension, reducing pain and increasing relaxation.

8. This is a very relaxing stroke and signals an end to the massage.
9. Prevents soiling of the bed with excess lotions and keeps the client warm.
10. Reduces the transmission of microorganisms.

EVALUATION

- The client experienced a reduction in tension, anxiety, pain, and fatigue.
- The nurse established better rapport with the client.

DOCUMENTATION

Nurses' Notes

- Time and date the back rub was performed
- Client's response to the back rub
- Complaints of pain or tension the client reported
- Unusual findings

PROCEDURE 26-23   Shaving a Client

OVERVIEW

Shaving the male client is done to remove facial hair if the client is unable to complete this self-care. It is usually done after a bath or shower and as often as required to remove unwanted facial hair. Most men shave every day, although the facial hair of older clients does not grow as rapidly. If a beard or mustache is present, it should be groomed daily and trimmed as appropriate. Do not shave off beards or mustaches without the client's permission.

continues

ASSESSMENT

1. Assess whether the client is able to perform self-care. **Promote independence when possible.**
2. Assess the client's skin for areas of redness, skin breakdown, moles, or skin lesions. **Shaving could irritate the skin further.**
3. Assess whether the client has a bleeding tendency or is on anticoagulants. **If there is an increased risk of bleeding, an electric razor should be used.**
4. If the client prefers to shave himself, assess the client's ability to manipulate the razor. **The client must be able to shave safely.**
5. Assess the client's preference for the type of shaving, type of equipment, and type of lotion (if there are options). **This promotes independence.**

POSSIBLE NURSING DIAGNOSES

Dressing/Grooming **S***elf-Care Deficit*
Risk for **I***njury*
Risk for Situational Low **S***elf-Esteem*

PLANNING

Expected Outcomes

1. The client will be neat and well-groomed.
2. The client's skin integrity will remain intact.
3. If the client is able to shave or able to assist, the client will attain a sense of independence.
4. The client will be comfortable following the procedure.

Equipment Needed

* Electric razor or disposable razor
* Shaving cream or soap
* Warm water
* Washcloth and bath towel
* Washbasin
* Aftershave lotion (if the client has no skin irritation and prefers lotion)
* Mirror
* Sharp scissors and comb if mustache care required
* Gloves

DELEGATION TIPS

Shaving the adult male client is routinely delegated. Caution must be exercised with intubated clients to maintain the integrity of their tubes.

IMPLEMENTATION—ACTION/RATIONALE

ACTION

❋ **Check client's identification band** ❋ **Explain procedure before beginning** ❋

1. Cleanse hands and apply gloves.
2. Assist the client to a comfortable position. If the client can shave himself, set up the equipment and supplies, including warm water, and watch the client for safety. Adjust lighting as needed.
3. Place a towel over the client's chest and shoulder.
4. Raise the bed to a comfortable height.
5. Fill a washbasin with water at approximately 44°C (110°F). Check temperature for comfort.
6. Place the washcloth in the basin and wring out thoroughly. Apply the cloth over the client's entire face.
7. Apply shaving cream.
8. Take the razor in the dominant hand and hold it at a 45-degree angle to the client's skin. Start shaving across one side of the client's face. Use the nondominant hand to gently pull the skin taut while shaving. Use short, firm strokes in the direction hair grows. Use short, downward strokes over the upper lip area (Figure 26-23-1).
9. Rinse the razor in water as cream accumulates.

RATIONALE

1. Reduces transmission of microorganisms.
2. Facilitates comfort and ease of shaving. Encourages sense of self-control and independence.

3. Protects the client and gown from soil.
4. Facilitates comfort of staff.
5. Warm water helps soften the skin and beard. Warmth can be relaxing.
6. Warm water helps soften the skin and beard. Warmth can be relaxing.
7. Helps soften the whiskers.
8. Holding the skin taut prevents razor cuts and discomfort during shaving.

9. Keeps the cutting edge of the razor clean.

continues

Figure 26-23-1   Shave with short, firm strokes in the direction the hair grows.

Figure 26-23-2   When finished shaving, rinse the face thoroughly with a warm washcloth.

10. Check the face to see if all the facial hair is removed.
11. After all the facial hair is removed, rinse the face thoroughly with a moistened washcloth (Figure 26-23-2).
12. Dry the face thoroughly and apply aftershave lotion if desired.
13. Assist the client to a comfortable position and allow him to inspect the results of the shave.
14. Dispose of equipment in proper receptacle.

15. Cleanse hands.

10. Ensures a neat appearance.
11. Promotes comfort and cleanliness.

12. Stimulates and lubricates the skin.

13. Facilitates comfort and a sense of control.

14. Equipment should not be shared between clients in accordance with Standard Precautions because disruption of skin and bleeding may occur. The client may, however, keep his own razor. Clean and store it at the bedside.
15. Reduces the transmission of microorganisms.

EVALUATION

- The client is neat and well-groomed.
- The client's skin integrity remained intact.
- If the client was able to shave or able to assist, the client attained a sense of independence.
- The client is comfortable following the procedure.

DOCUMENTATION

Nurses' Notes

- Procedure, if the client was able to assist, and how the client tolerated the activity
- Unusual findings or injury that may have occurred

PROCEDURE 26-24   Applying Antiembolic Stockings

OVERVIEW

Antiembolic hose, also called TED® hose or elastic stockings, are used to promote circulation by compression and are useful to prevent thrombophlebitis. They are used on the legs of a client after surgery, on clients who are immobile, and on clients who have vascular disorders such as thrombophlebitis, varicose veins, and other conditions of impaired circulation of the lower extremities.

continues

ASSESSMENT

1. Assess the condition of the client's lower extremities, noting edema, color, temperature, intact skin, ulcers, or infections. **Establishes a baseline for comparison.**
2. Assess the quality and equality of peripheral pulses in the legs (either dorsalis pedis or posterior tibial pulses) **to determine circulatory status.**
3. Assess the client's understanding of the reasons for, and the use of, the antiembolic stockings **to determine the amount of client teaching required.**
4. Assess the client for signs and symptoms of deep vein thrombosis, such as increased calf size or color change, **to determine the appropriateness of the TED® hose placement.**

POSSIBLE NURSING DIAGNOSES

Risk for Impaired **S**kin Integrity
Decreased **C**ardiac Output
Ineffective **T**issue Perfusion

PLANNING

Expected Outcomes

1. The client will experience no signs or symptoms of deep venous thrombosis or thrombophlebitis.
2. The client's venous return will be improved.
3. The client's popliteal, posterior tibial, and dorsalis pedis pulses will remain intact while stockings are in place.
4. The client will have good circulation while stockings are in place, as evident by warm skin temperature, capillary return within normal limits, sensation present, and no edema present in both extremities.

Equipment Needed

- Antiembolic stockings and package directions (latex-free, if necessary)
- Tape measure

DELEGATION TIPS

Ancillary personnel routinely remove and reapply antiembolic stockings. Instruction should be given to staff to apply stockings while client is supine in bed and to inspect and report any skin breakdown, impaired circulation, or excessive edema to the nurse.

IMPLEMENTATION—ACTION/RATIONALE

ACTION

* Check client's identification band * Explain procedure before beginning *

1. Cleanse hands.
2. Review the orders with the client, including the reason for the stockings and the type of stockings ordered (e.g., knee or thigh high).
3. With the client in a supine position in bed, measure the client's leg for the correct size:
   - Thigh-high stockings: from Achilles tendon to the gluteal fold, circumference of the midthigh
   - Below-the-knee stockings: from the Achilles tendon to the popliteal fold, circumference of the midcalf
4. Compare the obtained measurements with the package insert to ascertain proper size.

5. Apply stockings. The best time to apply stockings is early in the morning, before the client gets out of bed or immediately after surgery. Keep client in supine position until stockings are applied.

6. Open the package and turn stockings inside out over hand and arm. Place hand deep enough inside a stocking to grasp the stocking toe.

RATIONALE

1. Reduces transmission of microorganisms.
2. Facilitates compliance.

3. Supine position encourages venous return and decreases swelling, thereby allowing accurate measurement for size of stockings.

4. Correct size is essential for stockings to apply the appropriate pressure for adequate venous return without compromise to circulation.
5. Feet are less swollen in the morning because the feet have been in a nondependent position during the night and most venous return has occurred. This, of course, is not the case in a client who has been up frequently during the night.
6. Because stockings contain strong elastic, application can be difficult if not initiated from the bottom up and if stockings are not turned inside out. Wrinkles in stockings can also occur if a systematic approach is not used for application.

continues

Figure 26-24-1   Place the stocking over the client's toes and foot.

Figure 26-24-2   Pull the stocking smoothly and evenly up the client's leg.

Figure 26-24-3   Smooth out any wrinkles and make sure the toes are comfortable.

7. Using the hand inside the stocking, hold onto the client's toes. Invert the stocking with the other hand and pull it over the hand and the client's toes. Release toes.

8. Hold each side of the stocking and pull it from the client's toes to the heel in one motion (Figure 26-24-1).

9. Continuing to hold each side of the stockings, firmly pull the stocking up by using the thumbs to guide the stockings upward over the ankles and up the client's leg (Figure 26-24-2).

10. Repeat with the other leg, if necessary.

11. Smooth and remove any wrinkles in the stockings (Figure 26-24-3).

12. Assess circulatory and neurostatus of feet. (CMS: circulatory, movement, sensation)

13. Cleanse hands.

7. See Rationale 6.

8. See Rationale 6.

9. See Rationale 6.

10. See Rationale 6.

11. Wrinkles can create skin breakdown and can cause a tourniquet effect on the leg.

12. Establishes baseline assessment.

13. Reduces transmission of microorganisms.

EVALUATION

- The client has not experienced any signs or symptoms of deep venous thrombosis or thrombophlebitis.
- The client's venous return is improved.
- The client's popliteal, posterior tibial, and dorsalis pedis pulses remain intact while stockings are in place.
- The client has good circulation while stockings are in place, as evident by warm skin temperature, capillary return within normal limits, sensation within normal limits, and no edema in either extremities.

DOCUMENTATION

Nurses' Notes

- Use of stockings
- Skin integrity, any presence of venous problems, and circulatory status of extremities
- Equality of pedal pulses
- Size and length of stockings

PROCEDURE 26-25   Assisting with a Bedpan or Urinal

OVERVIEW

Voiding and bowel elimination for the client confined to bed require a bedpan and/or a urinal. Reduced mobility, pain, privacy issues, the need for assistance, delays in getting assistance when needed, and the fear of interruption can all alter normal elimination patterns. Fear of creating embarrassing noises, sights, or odors may compel the client to reduce fluid intake or avoid the urge to eliminate while in the hospital. This can lead to an increased risk of urinary tract infection. Sensitivity and proper technique by caregivers support the client on bed rest.

ASSESSMENT

1. Assess your equipment. Do you have the necessary items within reach? **Prevents having to stop the procedure and leave the client's bedside.**
2. Assess how much the client can assist in positioning and removing the bedpan. **Determines how the procedure will be done and whether assistance will be required.**
3. Check whether the client is confused, combative, in traction, or immobile. **Determines how the procedure will be done and whether assistance will be required.**
4. Check for casts, braces, or dressings, which need to be protected from accidental contamination with waste products. **Determines how much preparation will need to be done before toileting.**
5. Check for privacy and unexpected interruptions. **Determines if extra steps need to be taken to ensure privacy before toileting.**
6. Assess if client has orders to record intake and output. **Determines need to take steps for measurement and may require containers with measurement markings.**

POSSIBLE NURSING DIAGNOSES

Constipation
Bowel Incontinence

Stress Urinary Incontinence
Urge Urinary Incontinence
Urinary Retention
Toileting Self-Care Deficit
Situational Low Self-Esteem
Powerlessness

PLANNING

Expected Outcomes

1. Clients will be able to void and defecate when necessary.
2. Clients will have as much privacy and comfort as allowable, given their physical condition.
3. Intake and output will be accurately measured as needed.
4. The urinal or bedpan will be placed without skin damage.
5. The bedpan will be removed and emptied without spillage.

Equipment Needed

- Bedpan (regular or fracture) or urinal
- Disposable gloves
- Bedpan cover
- Toilet paper
- Washcloth and towel

DELEGATION TIPS

This skill is routinely delegated to ancillary personnel who have been trained in Standard Precautions and proper body positioning, and to report color, odor, and amount of output to the nurse.

continues

IMPLEMENTATION—ACTION/RATIONALE

ACTION

RATIONALE

* Check client's identification band * Explain procedure before beginning *

Positioning a Bedpan

ACTION	RATIONALE
1. Close curtain or door.	1. Provides for privacy.
2. Cleanse hands; apply gloves.	2. Reduces transmission of microorganisms.
3. Lower head of bed so client is in supine position.	3. The supine position will increase ability of client to move to side-lying position.
4. Elevate bed.	4. Ensures proper body mechanics.
5. Assist client to side-lying position using side rail for support.	5. Provides for best position for proper placement of bedpan.
6. Warm bedpan under warm water if needed; powder bedpan if necessary (Figure 26-25-1).	6. For comfort; prevents bedpan from sticking to the skin.
7. While holding the bedpan with one hand, help the client roll onto his or her back, while pushing against the bedpan (toward the center of the bed) to hold it in place.	7. Prevents dislocation or alignment of bedpan.
8. Alternate: Help the client raise the hips using the overbed trapeze, and slide the pan in place. Alternate: If the client is unable to turn or raise hips, use a fracture pan instead of a bedpan. With a fracture pan, the flat side is placed toward the client's head (Figure 26-25-2).	8. Provides an alternate way to position the pan. Fracture pan reduces the amount of movement and lift required to place the pan.
9. Check placement of bedpan by looking between client's legs.	9. May prevent spillage from misalignment of bedpan.
10. If indicated, elevate head of bed to 45-degree angle or higher for comfort.	10. Check order of physician or qualified practitioner; bed remains flat if client has a spinal cord injury or spinal surgery. Elevating the head of bed creates a more normal elimination position.
11. Place call light within reach of client; place side rails in upright position, lower bed, and provide privacy.	11. Privacy allows for a more comfortable elimination environment; elevated side rails provide for safety.
12. Remove gloves; cleanse hands.	12. Reduces transmission of microorganisms.

Figure 26-25-1   Applying powder to the bedpan prevents it from sticking to the skin.

Figure 26-25-2   A fracture pan is used when the client is unable to turn or raise hips.

continues

Figure 26-25-3 Lift the covers and place the urinal. Allow the client to adjust the position.

Figure 26-25-4 If the client is unable to assist, place the penis into the opening of the urinal.

Positioning a Urinal

13. Repeat Actions 1 and 2.
14. Lift the covers and place the urinal so the client may grasp the handle and position it. If the client cannot do this, you must position the urinal and place the penis into the opening (Figures 26-25-3 and 26-25-4).
15. Remove gloves; cleanse hands.

Removing a Bedpan

16. Cleanse hands; apply gloves.
17. Gather toilet paper and washing supplies.

18. Lower head of bed to supine position.
19. While holding bedpan with one hand, roll client to side and remove the pan, being careful not to pull or shear skin sticking to the pan and being careful not to spill contents.
20. Assist with cleaning or wiping; always wipe from front to back.

21. Empty bedpan (observe and measure urine output and check for occult blood if ordered), clean bedpan, and store it in proper place; if bedpan is to be emptied outside client's room, cover it during transport.
22. Remove soiled gloves. Cleanse hands.
23. Allow client to cleanse hands.
24. Place call light within reach; recheck that side rails are in the upright position.
25. Cleanse hands.

Removing a Urinal

26. Cleanse hands and apply gloves.
27. Empty the urinal, measuring urine output if ordered, rinse the urinal and replace it within the client's reach. Observe odor and color of urine before discarding.

28. Remove soiled gloves. Cleanse hands.
29. Allow client to cleanse hands.
30. Place call light within reach; recheck that side rails are in the upright position.
31. Cleanse hands.

13. See Rationales 1 and 2.
14. Ensures proper placement of the urinal and reduces the risk of spillage.

15. Reduces transmission of microorganisms.

16. Reduces transmission of microorganisms.
17. Having supplies at the bedside allows smooth and safe completion of the procedure.
18. Increases client's ability to move to side-lying position.
19. Prevents possible spillage of bedpan contents.

20. Client may not be able to clean self; wiping from front to back decreases chances of cross-contamination from anus to urethra.
21. Promotes privacy and decreases the chance of spilling contents. Assessment of types of stool evaluates for constipation and diarrhea.

22. Reduces transmission of microorganisms.
23. Provides for physical hygiene and comfort.
24. Ensures client safety and comfort.

25. Reduces transmission of microorganisms.

26. Reduces transmission of microorganisms.
27. Provides a way to measure the client's output. Keeping the urinal within reach promotes client autonomy. Helps evaluate for concentrated urine, infection, and renal problems.
28. Reduces transmission of microorganisms.
29. Provides for physical hygiene and comfort.
30. Ensures client safety and comfort.

31. Reduces transmission of microorganisms.

continues

EVALUATION

- The client was able to void or defecate as needed.
- The client's request for assistance was answered promptly.
- The bedpan or urinal was removed and emptied without spillage.
- Ordered tests were performed and samples were collected.
- The client's skin integrity was maintained without skin shear or tearing.
- The client was provided with as much privacy and comfort as possible.

DOCUMENTATION

Nurses' Notes

- Elimination and voiding. Include color, odor, consistency, and any unusual findings such as blood or mucus.
- Client complaints such as constipation or burning with urination
- Condition of the client's skin

Intake and Output Record

- Time the client voided and the amount of urine voided

PROCEDURE 26-26   Applying a Condom Catheter

OVERVIEW

The condom catheter is an external drainage system to collect urine from male clients who have incontinence. It is less invasive than a retention catheter and allows less contact of the skin with urine than a diaper or blue pad. Condom catheters require an order from an appropriate health care provider.

ASSESSMENT

1. Assess skin integrity around the penis and perineal area **to look for signs of irritation and skin breakdown.**
2. Assess the client for ability to cooperate with the application and retention of the condom catheter **to determine what type of teaching will be necessary.**
3. Assess the amount and pattern of urinary incontinence **to determine if the condom catheter is the best continence method for the client.**
4. Assess for latex allergy.

POSSIBLE NURSING DIAGNOSES

*Impaired **U**rinary Elimination*
*Risk for Impaired **S**kin Integrity*
*Toileting **S**elf-Care Deficit*

PLANNING

Expected Outcomes

1. The client will have a condom catheter in place without leakage or discomfort.
2. The client will have no skin irritation from the condom catheter.
3. The client will understand the reason for, and cooperate with, the placement and retention of the condom catheter.

Equipment Needed

- Condom catheter kit with adhesive strip
- Urinary drainage bag
- Clean gloves
- Basin with warm water and soap
- Towel and washcloth

DELEGATION TIPS

Application of a condom catheter may be delegated to properly trained ancillary personnel. The need for condom drainage and the ongoing assessment of the client's skin condition should be followed up by the nurse.

continues

IMPLEMENTATION—ACTION/RATIONALE

ACTION

RATIONALE

* Check client's identification band * Explain procedure before beginning *

1. Cleanse hands.
2. Protect the client's privacy by closing the door and pulling curtains around the bed.
3. Position the client in a comfortable position, preferably a supine position, if tolerated by the client. Raise the bed to a comfortable height for the nurse.
4. Apply latex-free gloves.
5. Fold the client's gown across the abdomen and the sheet just below pubic area.
6. Assess the client's penis for any signs of redness, irritation, or skin breakdown.

7. Clean the client's penis with warm soapy water. Retract the foreskin on the uncircumcised male and clean thoroughly in folds.
8. Return the client's foreskin to its normal position.

9. Shave any excess hair around the base of the penis if required by institutional policy.
10. Rinse and dry the area.

11. If a condom kit is used, open the package containing the skin preparation (Figure 26-26-1). Wipe and apply skin preparation solution to the shaft of the penis. If the client has an erection, wait for termination of erection before applying the catheter.
12. Apply the double-sided adhesive strip around the base of the client's penis in a spiral fashion. The strip is applied 1 inch from the proximal end of the penis. Do not completely encircle the penis or tightly encompass penis.
13. Position the rolled condom at the distal portion of the penis and unroll it, covering the penis and the double-sided strip of adhesive. Leave a 1- to 2-inch space between the tip of the penis and the end of the condom (Figure 26-26-2).

1. Reduces transmission of microorganisms.
2. Allows privacy for the client.

3. Facilitates the cleaning and application of the catheter. Raising the bed to a comfortable height promotes good body mechanics.
4. Prevents possible transmission of microorganisms.
5. Provides minimal exposure of the client, thereby reducing the client's embarrassment.
6. A significant amount of skin breakdown may require an indwelling catheter. Provides baseline data for comparison with future assessments.
7. Removes microorganisms that could enter the urinary meatus and cause a urinary tract infection. Avoids trapping microorganisms in folds around the meatus.
8. Failure to return the foreskin to a normal position can lead to swelling of the penis and possible constriction.
9. Prevents discomfort from the adhesive strip when the condom catheter is removed.
10. Moist warm environment can lead to the growth of microorganisms.
11. Preparation solution protects the client's skin from irritation. An erection may occur from manipulation of the penis while cleaning the area. This is a normal reaction and will terminate in a few minutes.

12. Applying the adhesive in a spiral fashion does not compromise circulation of the penis. Encircling the penis can constrict the penis, impair circulation, and cause edema.
13. The condom sticks to the adhesive and remains in place. The extra spacing prevents pressure and erosion of the tip of the penis.

Figure 26-26-1 After preparing the penis, open the condom kit. Apply the skin preparation solution.

Figure 26-26-2 Unroll the condom from the distal portion of the penis upward to the base.

continues

Figure 26-26-3 Make sure the drainage bag tubing lies over the client's leg.

14. Gently press the condom to the adhesive strip.

15. Attach the drainage bag tubing to the catheter tubing. Make sure the tubing lays over the client's legs, not under. Secure the drainage bag to the side of the bed below the level of the client's bladder or to the drainage bag attached to the leg (Figure 26-26-3).

16. Determine that the condom and tubing are not twisted.

17. Cover the client.

18. Dispose of the used equipment in appropriate receptacle.

19. Empty the bag, measure the client's urinary output, and record every 4 hours. Remove gloves and cleanse hands after procedure.

20. Return the client's bed to the lowest position and reposition client to comfortable or appropriate position.

21. Remove the condom once a day to clean the area and assess the skin for signs of impaired skin integrity.

14. Enables the condom to adhere evenly to the adhesive strip.

15. Promotes urine flow away from the client. Constant exposure to urine and moisture can irritate the penis. Prevents reflux of the urine onto the penis and microorganisms from entering the penis.

16. If the condom or tubing is twisted, the urine cannot flow out and the condom will leak or fall off.

17. Maintains privacy of the client.

18. Reduces transmission of microorganisms.

19. Records output and prevents bag from becoming overly full and/or too heavy. Reduces transmission of microorganisms.

20. Reduces potential injury from falls.

21. Promotes hygiene and reduces the possibility of skin breakdown.

EVALUATION

- The client's condom catheter is in place without leakage or discomfort.
- The client does not have any skin irritation from the condom catheter.
- The client understands the reason for, and cooperates with, the placement and retention of the condom catheter.

DOCUMENTATION

Nurses' Notes

- Time the procedure was performed
- Condition of the client's skin, recording any irritation, rashes, or open areas
- Client teaching performed

Intake and Output Record

- Amount of urine emptied from the urine drainage bag

PROCEDURE 26-27 Administering an Enema

OVERVIEW

An enema is a solution inserted into the rectum and sigmoid colon to remove feces and/or flatus. Enemas can also be used to instill medications or nutrition. A cleansing enema is probably the most common type of enema. This type of enema stimulates peristalsis via irritation of the colon/rectum and by causing intestinal distention with fluid. There are two general types of cleansing enemas: the large-volume enema and the small-volume enema.

A large-volume enema is designed to clean the colon of as much feces as possible. In a large-volume enema, between 500 and 1,000 cc of fluid are instilled into the rectum/colon, and the client is asked to retain the fluid as long as possible.

Small-volume enemas are designed to clear the rectum and the sigmoid colon of fecal matter. Small-volume enemas can be delivered with the traditional enema kit using 50 to 200 cc of solution, but most frequently they are administered using a prepackaged disposable kit. Prepackaged enemas are easily administered and available over-the-counter in most drugstores. This makes them ideal for home care use.

An oil retention enema is a small-volume enema that instills oil into the rectum, retained for up to an hour to soften very hard stool. It is often followed by a large-volume cleansing enema. A small-volume enema can deliver a medicated solution directly to the rectal mucosa. This method is useful when the rectum is the area to be medicated, if the client is unable to take oral medications, or if rapid absorption of the medication is required. The return-flow enema, used to remove flatus and stimulate peristalsis, is frequently given following abdominal surgery to reduce intestinal distention and to stimulate the resumption of bowel function.

Many different solutions are used for enemas, including tap water, normal saline, hypertonic solutions, soap solutions, oil, and carminative solutions. Tap water is a hypotonic solution. Because it is a less concentrated solution than the body's cells, it is drawn into the body and may cause water toxicity, electrolyte imbalance, or circulatory overload. Normal saline is an isotonic solution. It is the same concentration as the body's own fluids and is considered a safe enema solution. It is important that children and infants be given only normal saline enemas because their small size predisposes them to fluid imbalances. Prepackaged small-volume enemas use hypertonic solutions to draw fluid from the body to lubricate the stool and distend the rectum. Hypertonic solutions are contraindicated in dehydrated clients and small children. Carminative solutions are used to prevent gas from forming.

Enemas are contraindicated in clients with bowel obstruction, inflammation, or infection of the abdomen or if the client has had recent rectal or anal surgery. If there is any question regarding the advisability of administering an enema, consult the client's health care provider.

ASSESSMENT

1. Identify the type of enema ordered as well as the rationale for the enema. **Allows the nurse to verify the appropriateness of the type of enema ordered.**
2. Assess the physical condition of the client. Determine if the client has bowel sounds. Assess for a history of constipation, hemorrhoids, or diverticulitis. Determine if the client will be able to hold a side-lying or knee-chest position or be able to retain the enema solution. **Allows the nurse to plan the procedure with the client's limitations in mind.**
3. Assess the client's mental state, including ability to understand and cooperate with the procedure, the client's knowledge level regarding the procedure, and any pre-existing fears the client may have regarding the procedure. Knowing if the client can comprehend and cooperate with the procedure will help the nurse plan ahead. **Many clients have preexisting fears and beliefs regarding enemas and their administration.**

POSSIBLE NURSING DIAGNOSES

Constipation
Risk for Deficient Fluid Volume
Risk for Situational Low Self-Esteem

PLANNING

Expected Outcomes

1. The client's rectum will be free of feces and flatus.
2. The client will experience a minimum of trauma and embarrassment from the procedure.

continues

Equipment Needed

Large-Volume Cleansing Enema
- Absorbent pad for the bed
- Disposable gloves
- Bedside commode or bedpan if client will not be able to ambulate to bathroom
- Lubricant
- Enema container
- Tubing with clamp and nozzle
- Thermometer for enema solution
- Toilet tissue
- IV pole
- Washcloth, towel, and basin

Small-Volume Prepackaged Enema
- Prescribed prepackaged enema
- Lubricant if the tip is not prelubricated

- Toilet tissue
- Bedpan or commode if the client cannot use the bathroom
- Absorbent pad for bed
- Gloves

Return-Flow Enema
- Absorbent pad for the bed
- Disposable gloves
- Bedside commode or bedpan if client will not be able to ambulate to bathroom
- Prescribed solution
- Lubricant
- Enema container
- Tubing with clamp and nozzle
- Thermometer
- Toilet tissue

DELEGATION TIPS

Administering an enema is a procedure that ancillary personnel are able to perform after proper instruction and supervision. Instruct ancillary personnel to notify the nurse if any difficulty in administering or negative reactions such as severe cramping or inability to retain the enema occur. Results should be documented and reported to the nurse.

IMPLEMENTATION—ACTION/RATIONALE

ACTION	RATIONALE

❖ Check client's identification band ❖ Explain procedure before beginning ❖

Large-Volume Cleansing Enema

ACTION	RATIONALE
1. Cleanse hands.	1. Reduces transmission of microorganisms.
2. Assess client's understanding of procedure and provide privacy.	2. Prepares client for procedure.
3. Apply gloves.	3. Prevents contact with feces.
4. Prepare equipment (Figure 26-27-1).	4. Ensures a smooth procedure.
5. Place absorbent pad on bed under client. Assist client in attaining left lateral position with right leg flexed as sharply as possible. If there is a question regarding the client's ability to hold the solution, place a bedpan on the bed nearby (Figure 26-27-2).	5. Facilitates flow of solution into the rectum and colon. The flexed leg provides the best exposure of the anus.

Figure 26-27-1   Assemble equipment at the bedside.

Figure 26-27-2   Position the client in the left lateral position with the right leg sharply flexed.

continues

Figure 26-27-3 Lubricate 2 inches of the rectal tube with lubricant.

Figure 26-27-4 Gently and smoothly insert the rectal tube into the rectum.

6. If specified, heat solution to desired temperature using thermometer to measure. Enemas administered to adults are usually given at 105° to 110°F (40.5° to 43°C), and those administered to children are usually administered at 100°F (37.7°C). Solution should be at least body temperature to prevent cramping and discomfort.

6. Enemas work best when solution is warm. If enemas are too hot, damage can be done to the bowel mucosa. If enemas are too cold, spasms may occur.

7. Pour solution into the bag or bucket; add water if needed. Open clamp and allow solution to prime tubing. Clamp tubing when primed.

7. Expels air from the tubing, which could cause intestinal distention and discomfort.

8. Lubricate 5 cm (2 inches) of the rectal tube unless the tube is part of a prelubricated enema set (Figure 26-27-3).

8. Minimizes trauma to the anal sphincter during insertion of the rectal tube.

9. Hold the enema container level with the rectum. Ask the client to take a deep breath. Simultaneously, slowly and smoothly insert rectal tube into rectum approximately 7 to 10 cm in an adult. The rectum of an adult is usually 10 to 20 cm (4 to 6 inches). The tube should be inserted beyond the internal sphincter. Aim the rectal tube toward the client's umbilicus (Figure 26-27-4).

9. A deep breath helps relax the sphincter. Insertion of rectal tube toward the umbilicus guides tube along rectum.

10. Raise the solution container and open clamp. (If using an enema set, squeeze the container holding solution). The solution should be 30 to 45 cm (12 to 18 inches) above the rectum for an adult and 7.5 cm (3 inches) above the rectum for an infant. The solution may be placed on an IV pole at the proper height.

10. Solution should be at a height above rectum that allows gravity flow of solution into the rectum, but does not cause damage to the rectal lining because of a too-rapid increase in rectal pressure.

11. Slowly administer the fluid.

11. Decreases the incidence of intestinal spasms and cramps.

12. When solution has been completely administered or when the client cannot hold any more fluid, clamp the tubing, remove the rectal tube, and dispose of it properly.

12. The urge to defecate indicates that a sufficient amount of fluid has been administered.

13. Clean lubricant, any solution, and any feces from the anus with toilet tissue.

13. Minimizes skin irritation.

14. Have the client continue to lie on the left side for the prescribed length of time.

14. Certain types of enemas are more effective when retained for a specified amount of time. It is easier for the client to retain the enema in a lying position, where gravity can be resisted.

15. When the client has retained the enema for the prescribed amount of time, assist to the bedside commode or toilet or onto the bedpan. If the client is using the bathroom, instruct not to flush the toilet when finished.

15. Client will be prepared to expel fluid and feces. Caregiver can see results of the enema.

continues

16. When the client is finished expelling the enema, assist to clean the perineal area if needed.
17. Return the client to a comfortable position. Place a clean, dry protective pad under the client to catch any solution or feces that may continue to be expelled.
18. Remove gloves and cleanse hands.

Small-Volume Prepackaged Enema

19. Cleanse hands.
20. Remove prepackaged enema from packaging (Figure 26-27-5). Be familiar with any special instructions included with the enema. The packaged enema may be stood in a basin of warm water to warm the fluid before use.
21. Apply gloves.
22. Place absorbent pad on bed under client. Assist client in attaining left lateral position with right leg flexed as sharply as possible, or you may use the knee-chest position (Figure 26-27-6). If there is a question regarding the client's ability to hold the solution, place a bedpan on the bed nearby.
23. Remove the protective cap from the nozzle and inspect the nozzle for lubrication. If the lubrication is not adequate, add more.
24. Squeeze the container gently to remove any air and prime the nozzle.
25. Have the client take a deep breath. Simultaneously, gently insert the enema nozzle into the anus, pointing the nozzle toward the umbilicus.
26. Squeeze the container until all the solution is instilled.
27. Remove the nozzle from the anus and dispose of the empty container in a trash receptacle.
28. Clean lubricant, any solution, and any feces from the anus with toilet tissue.
29. Have the client continue to lie on the left side for the prescribed length of time.

30. When the client has retained the enema for the prescribed amount of time, assist to the bedside commode or toilet or onto the bedpan. If the client is using the bathroom, instruct not to flush the toilet when finished.

16. Prevents skin breakdown and excoriation.
17. Provides comfort for the client and protects the linen from potential soiling.
18. Reduces transmission of microorganisms.

19. Reduces transmission of microorganisms.
20. Prepares the enema for use.

21. Protects hands from exposure to feces.
22. Facilitates flow of solution into the rectum and colon. The flexed leg provides the best exposure of the anus. The knee-chest position provides good exposure and allows gravity to aid in retention of the enema.

23. Prevents trauma to the rectal mucosa.

24. Reduces introduction of air into the rectum.

25. Relaxes the rectal sphincter. Pointing the nozzle toward the umbilicus positions the nozzle away from the rectal walls.
26. Allows the client to get the full benefit of the solution.
27. Prevents the spread of microorganisms.

28. Minimizes skin irritation.

29. Certain types of enemas are more effective when retained for a specified amount of time. It is easier for the client to retain the enema in a lying position, where gravity can be resisted.
30. Client will be prepared to expel fluid and feces.

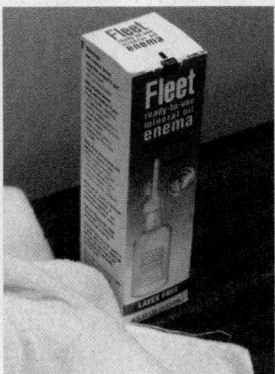

Figure 26-27-5 A Commercial Enema

Figure 26-27-6 Alternately, you may position the client in the knee-chest position.

continues

Figure 26-27-7 Raise the container 12 to 18 inches above the rectum and instill 200 cc of solution.

Figure 26-27-8 Lower the container 12 to 18 inches below the client's rectum. Observe for air bubbles as the solution returns.

31. When the client is finished expelling the enema, assist to clean the perineal area if needed.
32. Return the client to a comfortable position. Place a clean, dry protective pad under the client to catch any solution or feces that may continue to be expelled.
33. Remove gloves and cleanse hands.

Return-Flow Enema

34. Follow Actions 1–9.
35. Raise the solution container and open clamp. The solution should be 30 to 45 cm (12 to 18 inches) above the rectum for an adult and 7.5 cm (3 inches) above the rectum for an infant (Figure 26-27-7).
36. Slowly administer approximately 200 cc of solution.

37. Clamp the tubing and lower the enema container 12 to 18 inches below the client's rectum. Open the clamp (Figure 26-27-8).
38. Observe the solution container for air bubbles as the solution returns. Note any fecal particles that may be returned.
39. When no further solution is returned to the container, clamp the tubing and raise the enema container 12 to 18 inches above the client's rectum. Open the clamp and instill approximately 200 cc of fluid.
40. Repeat raising and lowering the solution container until no further flatus is seen. Most institutions have guidelines regarding the number of returns to perform. A good rule of thumb is not more than 3 times.
41. After the final return of fluid, clamp the tubing and gently remove it from the client's anus. Clean the anus with tissue to remove any lubricant or solution.
42. If the client feels the need to empty his or her rectum, assist onto the bedpan or up to the bathroom or commode.
43. When the client is finished expelling any retained solution, assist to clean the perineal area if needed.
44. Return the client to a comfortable position. Place a clean, dry protective pad under the client to catch any solution or feces that may continue to be expelled.
45. Remove gloves and cleanse hands.

31. Prevents skin breakdown and excoriation.

32. Provides comfort for the client and protects the linen from potential soiling.

33. Reduces transmission of microorganisms.

34. See Rationales 1–9.
35. Solution should be at a height that allows gravity flow of solution into the rectum, but does not cause damage to the rectal lining because of a too rapid increase in rectal pressure.
36. Momentary pauses decrease the incidence of intestinal spasms and cramps.
37. Allows the solution to flow back out of the rectum.

38. Assesses the effectiveness of the procedure. Air bubbles in the container indicate flatus being passed from the rectum.
39. Continues to stimulate peristalsis and remove flatus.

40. Limiting the number of returns prevents unduly tiring or stressing the client.

41. Prevents skin irritation.

42. Allows any retained solution to be expelled. Stimulates peristalsis.

43. Prevents skin breakdown and excoriation.

44. Provides comfort for the client and protects the linen from potential soiling.

45. Reduces transmission of microorganisms.

continues

EVALUATION

- The client's rectum is free of feces or flatus.
- The client experienced a minimum of trauma and embarrassment from the procedure.

DOCUMENTATION

Nurses' Notes

- Time and date of the procedure
- Type of enema given, amount of fluid infused and returned, and amount and description of the feces expelled

- Client's tolerance for the procedure and any complaints or unusual findings

Medication Administration Record (MAR)

- If this is a medicated enema, be sure to note it on the MAR.

Intake and Output Record

- If the amount of fluid returned is significantly less than the amount infused, note this on the I&O record.

PROCEDURE 26-28   Measuring Intake and Output

OVERVIEW

One of the most basic methods of monitoring a client's health is measuring intake and output, commonly called "I&O." By monitoring the amount of fluids a client takes in and comparing this to the amount of fluid a client puts out, the health care team gains valuable insights into the client's general health as well as monitors specific disease conditions.

To maintain good health, fluid intake should approximately equal fluid output. Intake that exceeds output can indicate medical conditions ranging from renal failure to congestive heart failure. Output that exceeds intake can be caused by things as serious as life-threatening diarrhea or as benign as diuretic medications. An accurate record of a client's fluid balance is an important nursing function.

I&O monitoring is often ordered by the health care provider but can also be initiated by the nurse. Ideally, I&O should be monitored over several days to obtain an accurate record of the client's status. In critical situations, however, this may not be possible, and the client's I&O may be monitored and reported on an hourly basis. A urine output of less than 30 cc per hour should be reported.

A daily weight is often done in conjunction with I&O because it can indicate fluid retention or loss. One gallon of water weighs 8 pounds. An 8-pound weight gain over a 24- to 48-hour period could indicate a life-threatening condition for the client. A significant change in a client's weight or a significant difference in a client's total I&O should be reported to the client's health care provider.

Intake is considered to be any fluid consumed or infused. This includes water, juice, coffee, milk, ice cream, soup broth, and Jell-O. Be sure to calculate the amount of water the client has consumed from the bedside water pitcher. Any fluids infused through IV lines, central lines, feeding tubes, or irrigant that is not returned is considered intake. Blood and blood products as well as the saline used to flush IV lines before and after the transfusion are also included in this count. IV piggybacks, fluids used to measure cardiac output, central line flushes, and *TKO* (to keep open) fluids are also considered in the intake total.

Urine is the largest component of output fluid volume, but several other fluid loss avenues must be considered. Diarrhea, diaphoresis, wound drainage, gastric or other fluids removed by suction, and bleeding are all fluid losses as well. These losses should be measured or estimated and recorded in the total output.

Clients who are able to understand and cooperate with the I&O measurement should be encouraged to keep track of their fluid balance. Particularly in clients who are on a fluid restriction, client understanding and participation can greatly increase cooperation.

ASSESSMENT

1. Assess the client's risk factors for fluid overload, such as congestive heart failure, renal failure, or ascites **because edema can result from excess volume in extracellular fluid spaces and transferring of fluid into tissues.**

2. Determine if the client is receiving fluids or medications that would predispose to fluid overload, such as large amounts of IV fluids or steroid therapy, **because steroids cause sodium and water retention and excretion of potassium.**

3. Assess the client's risk factors for fluid loss, such as diaphoresis, rapid respirations, diarrhea, gastric suction,

continues

blood loss, or wound drainage, **because dehydration can result from reduction of fluid within the tissues and circulatory system.**

4. Determine if the client's urine output is in excess of fluid intake **because the kidneys excrete excess fluid during periods of overhydration and conserve body water during periods of dehydration.**

5. Assess the client's ability to understand and cooperate with intake and output measurement **because cooperation in these measurements will help ensure accuracy.**

POSSIBLE NURSING DIAGNOSES

Excess **F***luid Volume*
Deficient **F***luid Volume*
Risk for Deficient **F***luid Volume*

PLANNING

Expected Outcomes

1. The client's fluid intake and output will be accurately measured and recorded.
2. The client will participate in the recording of fluid intake and output if possible.

Equipment Needed

- I&O form at bedside
- I&O graphic record in chart
- Glass or cup
- Bedpan, urinal, or bedside commode
- Graduated container for output
- Nonsterile gloves
- Sign at bedside stating client is on I&O

DELEGATION TIPS

Intake and output measurement may be delegated to ancillary personnel, who should be knowledgeable regarding the following:
- *Obtaining accurate measurements and reporting incontinence*
- *Observing the amount, color, and any odor from the output*
- *Protecting themselves from contamination from a body fluid and storing collection containers in designated areas*
- *Recording measurements on proper clinical records*

IMPLEMENTATION—ACTION/RATIONALE

ACTION

Check client's identification band * *Explain procedure before beginning* *

1. Cleanse hands.
2. Explain the rules of I&O record. All fluids taken orally must be recorded on the client's intake and output form (sometimes called a fluid balance flow sheet).
   - Client must void into bedpan, urinal, or "hat" in toilet for collecting urine, not into toilet.
   - Toilet tissue should be disposed of in plastic-lined container, not in bedpan.

Intake

3. Measure all oral fluids in accord with agency policy (e.g., cup = 150 mL, glass = 240 mL). Record all IV fluids as they are infused.
4. Record time and amount of all fluid intake in the designated space on bedside form (e.g., oral, tube feedings, IV fluids).
5. Transfer 8-hour total fluid intake from bedside I&O record to graphic sheet or 24-hour I&O record on client's chart.
6. Record all fluid intake in the appropriate column of the 24-hour record.
7. Complete 24-hour intake record by adding all 8-hour totals.

RATIONALE

1. Reduces transmission of microorganisms.
2. Elicits client support.

   - Fluid voided into the toilet cannot be measured.

   - Liquids absorbed into toilet tissue cannot be measured by volume.

3. Provides for consistency of measurement.

4. Documents fluids.

5. Provides for data analysis of the client's fluid status.

6. Documents intake by type and amount.

7. Provides consistent data for analysis of the client's fluid status over a 24-hour period.

continues

Figure 26-28-1 Urine in Foley drainage bag must be measured.

Figure 26-28-2 Empty urine into a graduated container or commode "hat."

Output

8. Cleanse hands and apply nonsterile gloves.
9. Empty urinal, bedpan, or Foley drainage bag (Figure 26-28-1) into graduated container or commode "hat" (Figure 26-28-2).
10. Remove gloves and cleanse hands.
11. Record time and amount of output (e.g., urine, drainage from nasogastric tube, drainage tube) on I&O record.
12. Transfer 8-hour output totals to graphic sheet or 24-hour I&O record on the client's chart.
13. Complete 24-hour output record by totaling all 8-hour totals.
14. Cleanse hands.

8. Reduces potential for transmission of pathogens.
9. Provides accurate measurement of urine.

10. Prevents cross-contamination.
11. Documents output.

12. Provides for data analysis of the client's fluid status.
13. Provides consistent data for analysis of the client's fluid status over a 24-hour period.
14. Reduces transmission of microorganisms.

EVALUATION

• The client's fluid intake and output was accurately measured and recorded.
• Note if the client was able to participate in the recording of fluid intake and output to the best of his or her ability.
• Note and report any abnormal findings to the client's health care provider.

DOCUMENTATION

Intake and Output Record

• All fluid I&O
• Totals at the end of every shift
• Totals for 24 hours

Nurses' Notes

• Unusual findings, excessive intake, excessive output, or serious imbalance of intake and output and report to the client's health care provider

PROCEDURE 26-29 Urine Collection—Closed Drainage System

OVERVIEW

Indwelling catheters are used frequently in acute care settings for episodic or continuous drainage of urine. Specimens may be required to evaluate urine content, such as electrolytes, dilution, hormones, glucose, or abnormal factors, or renal function. Bacteria can be identified in urine specimens to determine if the catheter needs to be removed or if antibiotic therapy is indicated. Catheter tubing is generally designed to allow for easy access to obtain specimens without disconnecting the catheter from the tubing. Careful technique should prevent contamination of the system and, hence, risk for infection.

ASSESSMENT

1. Identify the purpose of the urine test **to determine the amount of urine needed and the proper container to collect it in.**
2. Assess the client's understanding of the test **to determine the amount of instruction needed.**
3. Identify the type of collecting tubing attached to the indwelling catheter **to determine if you need to disconnect the catheter from the system or can obtain the specimen from a closed system.**

POSSIBLE NURSING DIAGNOSIS

Risk for Infection

PLANNING

Expected Outcomes

1. Client understands the reason for the specimen.
2. Specimen is obtained in the proper container in a timely manner.
3. Specimen will remain uncontaminated.

Equipment Needed

- Nonserrated clamp or rubber band
- Nonsterile gloves
- 10-cc syringe with needle (1-inch)
- Specimen container, plastic bag, and labels
- Povidone-iodine swabs

DELEGATION TIPS

Obtaining a urine specimen from an indwelling catheter requires the skill and problem-solving ability of a nurse. This task cannot be delegated to ancillary personnel.

IMPLEMENTATION—ACTION/RATIONALE

ACTION	RATIONALE

＊ Check client's identification band ＊ Explain procedure before beginning ＊

ACTION	RATIONALE
1. Cleanse hands.	1. Reduces transmission of microorganisms.
2. Check health care provider's order.	2. Determines test and container needed for the specimen.
3. Provide privacy.	3. Maintains client dignity.
4. Check for urine in the tubing.	4. Determines if there is sufficient urine in the collecting tubing for a specimen. *Urine from the collection bag should not be used for sterile specimens.*
5. If more urine is needed, clamp the tubing using a nonserrated clamp or a rubber band for 10 to 15 minutes (Figure 26-29-1).	5. Collects 10 mL of urine, which is needed for most urinalyses.
6. Put on clean gloves.	6. Practices Standard Precautions.
7. Clean sample port with a povidone-iodine swab.	7. Prevents entrance of microorganisms into the system.
8. Insert sterile needle of syringe into the sample port of catheter at a 45-degree angle and withdraw 10 mL of urine (Figure 26-29-2).	8. Obtains specimen with sufficient volume for most urine tests.

continues

Figure 26-29-1 Clamp the tubing by folding it over and securing it with a rubber band to collect an adequate sample.

Figure 26-29-2 Cleanse the sample port and insert a sterile needle and syringe into the sample port.

9. Put urine into sterile container and close tightly, taking care not to contaminate the lid of the container.
10. Place needle and syringe into sharps container; *never recap a contaminated needle.*
11. Remove clamp and rearrange tubing avoiding dependent loops.
12. Label specimen container, put it in a plastic bag, and transport to the laboratory.
13. Cleanse hands.

9. Prevents contamination of specimen and spill of urine.
10. Prevents accidental needlesticks.
11. Reestablishes urine flow and drainage into the system.
12. Ensures right test and controls transfer of pathogens.
13. Reduces transmission of microorganisms.

EVALUATION

- Client understands the reason for the specimen.
- Specimen was obtained in the proper container in a timely manner.
- Specimen remained uncontaminated.

DOCUMENTATION

Nurses' Notes

- Date and time the specimen was sent to the laboratory
- Date, time, client name and room number, and test(s) ordered

Intake and Output Record

- Amount of urine collected for the specimen

PROCEDURE 26-30   Urine Collection—Clean Catch, Female/Male

OVERVIEW

A clean urine specimen to be used for culture and sensitivity can be collected without using an invasive method such as catheterization. This procedure is referred to as a clean-voided, clean-catch, or midstream urine specimen in that it is not a sterile procedure such as catheterization but, rather, a method of obtaining a clean specimen. This procedure is best accomplished with the client on the toilet because the use of a urinal or bedpan increases the risk of contamination. The client is asked to clean him or herself and initiate urination. After the client starts voiding, a sterile collection cup is placed under the stream of urine and a specimen collected. Hence it is called midstream collection. The initial urine is not collected because this portion of the stream flushes the urethral opening and meatus of any bacteria. The end urine is not collected because as the urine stream slows, and increased dripping and contact with the meatus occurs, the chance of contamination increases. The clean-catch specimen is sent to a laboratory for analysis.

continues

ASSESSMENT

1. Evaluate the client's ability to obtain a clean-catch specimen to **determine if the client is able to clean him or herself appropriately and understands the need to obtain a midstream specimen.**
2. Assess the presence of signs and symptoms of urinary tract infections or other abnormalities **because burning or the inability to control urination may hamper the client's ability to obtain a clean specimen.**

POSSIBLE NURSING DIAGNOSES

Impaired **U***rinary Elimination*
Acute **P***ain*
Deficient **K***nowledge* (collecting clean-catch urine specimen)

PLANNING

Expected Outcomes

1. Client will be able to obtain a clean, midstream specimen.
2. Client will have absence of urinary abnormalities, such as burning, tingling, pain upon urination, or inability to control stream.
3. Client will understand procedure.

Equipment Needed

- Sterile collection container with lid and label
- Sterile midstream kit, antiseptic towelettes, or cotton balls with antiseptic solution
- Toilet paper
- Nonsterile latex-free gloves
- Sterile gauze (optional)

DELEGATION TIPS

Collection of a clean-catch specimen may be delegated to ancillary personnel properly trained in the technique of cleaning the client and obtaining the voided specimen.

IMPLEMENTATION—ACTION/RATIONALE

ACTION
RATIONALE

＊ Check client's identification band ＊ Explain procedure before beginning ＊

1. Check orders and assess need for the procedure.
2. Gather equipment.
3. Assess the client's ability to complete the procedure, including understanding, mobility, and balance.
4. If the nurse is to perform the procedure: Cleanse hands and apply gloves. If the client is to perform the procedure, instruct the client to cleanse hands before and after the procedure. If the client wishes, provide a pair of gloves.
5. Provide privacy.
6. Using sterile procedure, open kit or towelettes (Figure 26-30-1). Open sterile container, placing the lid with sterile side up on a firm surface (Figure 26-30-2).
7. Female client: Sit with legs separated on the toilet. Use the thumb and forefinger to separate the labia, or have the client separate the labia with fingers (Figure 26-30-3).

   With the labia separated, use a downward stroke (from the top of the labia down toward the rectal area), and cleanse one side of the labia with the towelette (Figure 26-30-4).

   Discard the towelette and repeat the procedure on the other side with another towelette, keeping the labia separated at all times. With a third towelette, use a downward stroke from the top of the urethral opening to the bottom. Discard the towelette.

1. Provides understanding of the purpose of the procedure.
2. Provides for organization.
3. Improves compliance and likelihood of obtaining clean specimen.
4. Decreases transmission of microorganisms.

5. Decreases embarrassment.
6. Prevents contamination of the specimen.

7. Provides access for cleaning the labia. Cleanses area and prevents contamination of clean area. Prevents contamination by feces. Keeping labia separated avoids contamination and decreases microorganisms in specimen.

continues

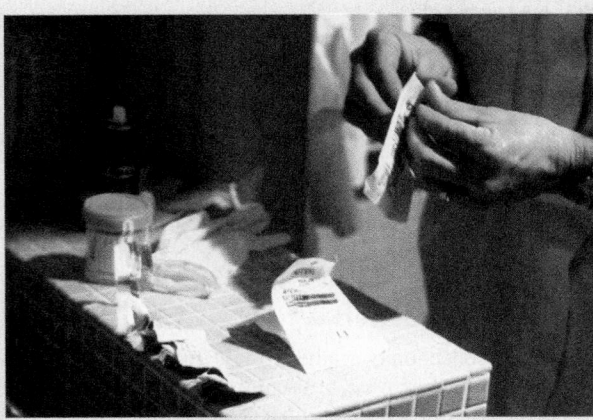

Figure 26-30-1   Open specimen cup and kit or cleansing towel packages prior to beginning the procedure.

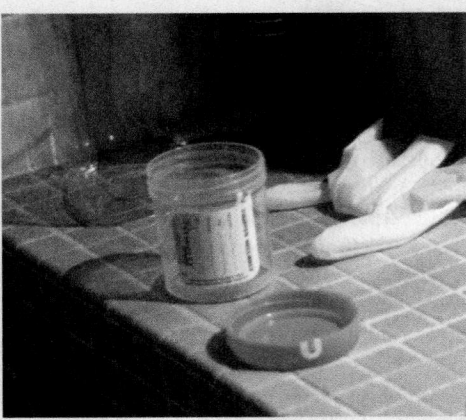

Figure 26-30-2   Place the lid on a firm surface, sterile side up. Do not touch the inside of the lid.

Figure 26-30-3   Separate the labia with the fingers of the nondominant hand.

Figure 26-30-4   Cleanse each side and down the middle using a single downward stroke for each towelette. Keep the labia separated.

8. Male client: Stand in front of toilet. Pull back the foreskin (if present in uncircumcised male) and clean with a single stroke around meatus and glans. Use a circular motion, starting with the head of the penis at the urethral opening, moving down the glans shaft. Discard the towelette and repeat the procedure with another towelette, keeping the foreskin retracted. Cleanse the head of the penis three times using a circular motion. Use a new towelette each time.

9. Ask the client to begin to urinate into the toilet. After the stream starts with good flow, place the collection cup under the stream of urine. Avoid touching the skin with the container. Fill the container with 30 to 60 cc of urine and remove the container before urination ceases. Wipe with toilet paper.

10. Place the sterile lid back onto the container and close tightly.
    Clean and dry the outside of the container with a towelette. Cleanse hands. Label and enclose in a plastic biohazard bag, and follow facility policy for transporting specimen to the laboratory.

11. Remove and dispose of gloves and cleanse hands.

8. Prevents contamination of microorganisms from foreskin. Single strokes and moving away from opening prevents contamination of the urethral opening.

9. The specimen is collected midstream to avoid contamination of urine that touches the labia. The initial urine flushes bacteria from the orifice and the end urine may have contact with the meatus or labia and, hence, be contaminated.

10. Prevents contamination of clean specimen, prevents spillage, and ensures accuracy.

11. Decreases transmission of microorganisms.

continues

EVALUATION

- Clean midstream specimen obtained.
- Client understood procedure.
- Client had no complaints associated with urination, such as burning, pain, or inability to initiate urination.

DOCUMENTATION

Nurses' Notes

- Procedure
- Characteristics of urine
- Client's signs and symptoms associated with urination

PROCEDURE 26-31   Collecting Nose, Throat, and Sputum Specimens

OVERVIEW

A nose, throat, or sputum specimen is a simple diagnostic tool for clients with signs or symptoms of upper respiratory or sinus infections. Nose and throat specimens are collected from the client using a sterile swab. Sputum specimens are collected in a sterile cup. Sputum specimens can also be obtained via a specimen trap connected to suction. Specimens are sent to the laboratory and placed in a culture medium to allow pathogenic organisms to grow. The type of organism can be identified, thereby enabling diagnosis and appropriate antimicrobial therapy.

ASSESSMENT

1. Assess the client's understanding of the purpose of the procedure **so the client will be able to cooperate.**
2. Assess the type of nasal or sinus drainage **to determine what kind of collection equipment will be needed.**
3. Review the health care provider's orders for the cultures requested **so repeat cultures are not done.**
4. Assess the client for postnasal drip, sinus headache or tenderness, nasal congestion, or sore throat **to know why the procedure is being done.**
5. Identify whether the client has received recent antimicrobials and obtain a specimen before treatment, if possible.

POSSIBLE NURSING DIAGNOSES

*Risk for **I**nfection*
Anxiety
*Risk for **I**njury*
*Deficient **K**nowledge* (regarding the procedure)

PLANNING

Expected Outcomes

1. An adequate specimen will be obtained and sent to the laboratory.
2. The procedure will be performed with a minimum of trauma to the client.

Equipment Needed

- Two sterile swabs in sterile culture tubes or a flexible wire sterile swab with cotton tip for nose or throat cultures
- Tongue blades
- Penlight
- Facial tissues
- Clean, disposable latex-free gloves
- Nasal speculum (optional)
- Emesis basin or clean container
- Sterile specimen cup, or sputum specimen collector

DELEGATION TIPS

Sputum specimens may be obtained by ancillary personnel. Avoiding specimen collection immediately after meals is important, as is the use of Standard Precautions when handling the specimen. Obtaining nose and throat cultures requires the problem-solving skills and techniques of a nurse, so obtaining these specimens may not be delegated.

continues

IMPLEMENTATION—ACTION/RATIONALE

ACTION

RATIONALE

* Check client's identification band * Explain procedure before beginning *

ACTION	RATIONALE
1. Cleanse hands and put on clean gloves.	1. Reduces transmission of microorganisms.
2. Ask the client to sit erect in the bed or on a chair facing the nurse.	2. Provides easy access to the nose or throat.
3. Prepare a sterile swab for use by loosening the top of the container.	3. Prevents contamination of the swab.

Collecting Throat Culture

4. Ask the client to tilt the head backward, open the mouth, and say "ah."	4. Promotes visualization of the pharynx, relaxes the throat muscles, and minimizes the gag reflex.
5. Depress the anterior one-third of the tongue with a tongue blade for better visualization.	5. Promotes visualization of the pharynx, but may induce the gag reflex.
6. Insert the swab without touching the cheek, lips, teeth, or tongue.	6. Prevents contamination of the specimen with oral flora.
7. Swab the tonsillar area from side to side in a quick, gentle motion (Figure 26-31-1).	7. Ensures collection of microorganisms. Retains microorganisms in the culture tube and ensures the life of bacteria for testing.
8. Withdraw the swab without touching adjacent structures and place in the culture tube. Crush ampule at bottom of tube and push swab into liquid medium (Figure 26-31-2).	8. Prevents contamination from outside microorganisms and erroneous culture results.
9. Secure the top to the culture tube and label with the client's name.	9. Prevents identification mistakes.
10. Discard the tongue depressor. Remove gloves and discard. Cleanse hands.	10. Reduces transmission of microorganisms.

Collecting Nose Culture

11. Instruct the client to blow nose and check nostrils for patency with penlight.	11. Clears nasal passages of mucus containing resident bacteria.
12. Ask the client to occlude one nostril, then the other, and exhale.	12. Determines the optimal nasal passage from which to obtain the specimen.
13. Ask the client to tilt the head back.	13. Promotes visualization of the sinuses.
14. Insert the swab into the nostril until it reaches the inflamed mucosa and rotate the swab.	14. Ensures the swab will be covered with the appropriate exudate.

Figure 26-31-1 Swab the sample area using a quick, gentle motion.

Figure 26-31-2 Crush ampule to release the culture medium.

continues

15. Withdraw the swab without touching adjacent structures and place in culture tube. Crush ampule at bottom of tube and push swab into liquid medium.
16. Secure the top to the culture tube and label with the client's name.
17. Remove gloves and discard. Cleanse hands.

15. Prevents contamination from normal nasal flora and erroneous culture results.
16. Prevents identification mistakes.
17. Reduces transmission of microorganisms.

Collecting of Nasopharyngeal Culture

18. Follow Actions 11 to 17, except use a swab on a flexible wire that can reach the nasopharynx via the nose.

18. Allows for access to the nasopharyngeal area.

Collecting a Sputum Culture

19. Explain to the client that the specimen must be sputum, coughed up from the lungs.
20. Have a sterile specimen cup ready for the sample and some tissues at hand.
21. Have the client take several deep breaths and then cough deeply.
22. Have the client expectorate the sputum into the sterile cup without touching the inside of the cup.
23. Place the lid on the specimen container without touching the inside of the lid or the container.
24. Provide the client with tissues and make him or her comfortable.

19. Promotes client cooperation.
20. The specimen must be collected in a sterile cup to prevent contamination.
21. Helps loosen secretions so the client will be able to provide a specimen.
22. Prevents contamination of the specimen.
23. Prevents contamination of the specimen.
24. Promotes client comfort.

Alternative Sputum Collection Method

Generally used if the client is unable to expectorate an adequate sample.
25. Obtain a sterile suction catheter and an in-line sputum collection container.
26. Provide the client with warm humidified air for about 20 minutes if it is not contraindicated by the client's condition.
27. Hook up the sputum collector to the suction tubing and a suction device (Figure 26-31-3). Hook up the suction catheter to the sputum collector.

25. Prevents contamination of the specimen.
26. Helps loosen secretions in the lungs.
27. Prepare the equipment before having the client cough.

Figure 26-31-3 Sputum Collector for Use with Suction

continues

28. If the client is able to cooperate, have him or her take several deep breaths and cough.
29. As the client is coughing up sputum, carefully insert the catheter either orally or nasopharyngeally into the back of the throat and suction the sputum into the specimen container.
30. Safely dispose of the suction catheter.
31. Close the specimen container.
32. Provide tissues or other measures for client comfort.
33. Cleanse hands.
34. Label each specimen with the client's name and send to the laboratory.

28. Loosens the secretions and brings them up to the back of the throat.
29. Obtains a sterile specimen that is not contaminated with saliva.

30. Prevents spread of microorganisms.
31. Prevents contamination of the specimen.
32. Promotes client comfort.
33. Reduces transmission of microorganisms.
34. Promotes the correct diagnosis for the client.

EVALUATION

- An adequate specimen was obtained.
- The procedure was performed with a minimum of trauma to the client.

DOCUMENTATION

Nurses' Notes

- Date, time, and site from which the specimen was obtained
- Bleeding or obvious trauma as a result of the procedure
- Description and time the specimen was collected and if the specimen is the first morning specimen, not pooled secretions

---

PROCEDURE 26-32   Collecting a Stool Specimen

OVERVIEW

Stool specimens are not collected as frequently as urine or blood specimens, but they are extremely valuable in evaluating and diagnosing a variety of gastrointestinal diseases. The most common tests on a stool specimen are occult blood, culture, fecal fat, fecal leukocyte, and OVA and parasite (parasite screen). A stool specimen can help identify GI bleeding; screen for carcinomas, polyps, diverticulitis, and colitis; diagnose and monitor various pathogenic microorganisms; diagnose inflammatory bowel disorders, pancreatitis, and malabsorption syndrome; and identify parasitic infestations. A single specimen is often not diagnostic, and at least three stool cultures are required for a pathogenic diagnosis (Daniels, 2002).

ASSESSMENT

1. Assess the client's or family member's understanding of the need for the test **so the nurse can provide needed teaching.**
2. Assess the client's ability to cooperate with the procedure to collect the specimen **to maintain privacy while a sample is obtained.**
3. Assess the client's medical history for bleeding or GI disorders. **The nurse can initiate screening tests.**
4. Assess any medications the client receives that can cause GI bleeding, such as anticoagulants, steroids, or acetylsalicylic acid, **to help determine the need for testing and/or the possible source of bleeding.**

POSSIBLE NURSING DIAGNOSES

Constipation
Diarrhea
*Deficient **K**nowledge* (need and test procedure)

PLANNING

Expected Outcomes

1. The client will understand the purpose of the test.
2. The client will be able to collect the specimen, or allow the specimen to be collected.
3. The test will be conducted properly and results recorded.

continues

Equipment Needed

- Paper towel
- Disposable gloves
- Wooden applicator
- Specimen container
- Gloves
- Clean, dry bedpan, bedside commode, or toilet "hat"

DELEGATION TIPS

The collection of stool may be delegated. Ancillary personnel should be instructed to report the presence of red blood in the stool immediately to the nurse.

IMPLEMENTATION—ACTION/RATIONALE

ACTION	RATIONALE

* Check client's identification band * Explain procedure before beginning *

ACTION	RATIONALE
1. Cleanse hands and apply clean gloves.	1. Reduces transmission of microorganisms from fecal specimen to nurse.
2. Depending on agency policy, assist client as needed to bedside commode or toilet. Have client void before moving bowels. Then, prepare for specimen collection. If client is not ambulatory, use a bedpan. For the toilet, use "hat" (Figure 26-32-1).	2. Allows client privacy and the ability to move bowels in a more normal physiological position.
3. Instruct the client not to contaminate the specimen with urine, vaginal discharge, or toilet paper.	3. Minimizes risk of skewed laboratory results.
4. Ask the client to notify you as soon as the specimen is available.	4. Reduces the risk of contamination of specimen, allows the nurse to collect a fresh specimen, and reduces embarrassment to client.
5. Assist the client with hygiene, help the client back to bed (as required), and ensure client comfort before turning attention to specimen.	5. Promotes client cleanliness and dignity.
6. Apply gloves and wear gown if client is on isolation or at risk for infectious stool, such as vancomycin-resistant enterococcus (VRE).	6. Reduces the risk of transmission of microorganisms.
7. Assess the stool for color, consistency, and odor, and presence or absence of visible blood or mucus.	7. Facilitates comprehensive client assessment.

Figure 26-32-1 Use a toilet (commode) "hat" to collect a stool sample.

continues

8. Using one or two tongue blades (depending on how much specimen is needed and for which test), transfer a representative sample of stool to the specimen card or container, taking care not to contaminate the outside of the container (or the inside of a sterile specimen cup). If using a culture swab, swab in a representative area of stool, particularly if any purulent material is visible. Check with laboratory regarding the volume of stool needed for a particular test.

8. Provides a high-quality sample for optimal results.

9. Close the card, place the lid on the container, or place the swab in the culture tube (according to agency policy) as soon as specimen is collected.

9. Reduces the risk of spread of microorganisms and reduces odor.

10. Place the specimen container in a biohazard bag for transport to the lab after proper labeling is done according to agency policy. Be careful not to contaminate the outside of bag. Provide requisition for test according to agency policy.

10. Properly identifies specimen to client; makes transport of specimen to lab more aesthetic for personnel. Provides client privacy. Reduces spread of microorganisms.

11. Dispose of rest of stool according to agency policy.

11. Reduces spread of microorganisms.

12. Remove gloves and cleanse hands.

12. Reduces spread of microorganisms.

13. Send specimen to laboratory immediately.

13. Maximizes quality of specimen for testing.

EVALUATION

- Note presence or absence of color change in the guaiac paper.
- Note color, character, and consistency of stool.
- Ask the client to explain the rationale and procedure for the stool test.

DOCUMENTATION

Nurses' Notes

- Date and time the collection was obtained
- Color, character, and consistency of the stool
- When the results of the test were reported to the health care provider

---

PROCEDURE 26-33   Applying Abdominal, T-, Breast, and Scultetus Binders

OVERVIEW

In the past, abdominal binders were primarily used to provide support and comfort for an incision following abdominal surgical procedures. Today binders are most often used to hold dressings in place, to support soft tissue, or to suppress lactation. Single and double T-binders hold rectal or perineal dressings in place. Abdominal binders support the abdomen and hold abdominal dressings in place. Stretch net binders are not designed for support, but simply to hold dressings in place.

A breast binder or a tight bra is used as a nonpharmacologic device to aid in lactation suppression. In addition, a breast binder may be used after breast reduction surgery, a mastectomy, or breast reconstruction surgery. The binder is placed over the breast to prevent breast and nipple stimulation. Ice packs are used in conjunction with breast binders to relieve discomfort associated with breast engorgement.

Proper placement of any binder is essential for optimum comfort and effect. The binder must be smooth, the right size for the client, not interfere with circulation, or put too much pressure on the bound area.

ASSESSMENT

1. Assess the reason the binder is needed **to determine the correct binder and correct placement.**

2. Assess the client's skin condition for rashes, inflammation, open areas, or dressings **to provide a baseline for future assessments.**

continues

3. Assess and measure the client **to determine what size binder will be needed.**

4. Assess for any special circumstances that may affect the placement of the binder, such as dressings, tubing, catheters or IV lines **to determine a plan for binder placement.**

5. Assess the client's understanding of the reasons for the binder and the method of placing the binder **to determine what types of client teaching will be needed.**

POSSIBLE NURSING DIAGNOSES

Interrupted **B**reastfeeding
Impaired Physical **M**obility

PLANNING

Expected Outcomes

1. For breast binder, lactation will be suppressed.
2. Binder will provide support for dressings or soft tissue.
3. Binder will not be too tight or compress the skin.
4. T-binder in a male client will not compress the testicles.
5. Client will assist in placement of the binder as much as possible.

Equipment Needed

- Correct binder for intended purpose (latex-free if indicated)
- Safety pins or fasteners

DELEGATION TIPS

Abdominal binder application may be performed by ancillary personnel after the nurse has assessed the client's tolerance of the binder. The client should be able to breathe effectively and move adequately. In addition, ancillary personnel should be instructed to ensure that the client's skin is intact and to report any breakdown for nurse evaluation.

IMPLEMENTATION—ACTION/RATIONALE

ACTION	RATIONALE

❋ **Check client's identification band** ❋ **Explain procedure before beginning** ❋

Abdominal Binders

1. Cleanse hands.
2. Choose correct binder. If a stretch net binder is being used, select the correct circumference and cut length to fit.
3. Help the client into the proper position to place the binder.
   - For abdominal binders, the client should lie supine and lift the hips, or, alternatively, position the client on one side, and roll the client onto the binder. For stretch net binders, slide the net over the head and neck, or slide the net up from the feet, depending on which is easier for the client.
   - Place the scultetus binder (Figure 26-33-1) with the upper border no higher than the waist.
4. Wrap the straight abdominal binder, starting from the lower abdomen and working upward.
   - Stretch net binders should be adjusted to cover the dressings they will be holding in place.
   - Bring the tails of the scultetus binder across the center of the abdomen, one at a time, alternating sides, starting at the bottom. (For a postpartum client, work from the top down.) Each tail should overlap the next lower one by about half the width of tail for maximal support. Secure only the last tail.

1. Reduces transmission of microorganisms.
2. Select the correct binder for the job. The correct size will make the binder most effective.

3. Applying binders can be awkward if the client is not positioned correctly. If binders are too high, they interfere with breathing.

4. Supports the abdomen and, if needed, secures dressings.

continues

5. Secure binders with fasteners. If the binder does not have Velcro fasteners, secure with safety pins. Stretch net binders cling and stretch over the body part and do not need additional fastening. Check for snug fit.
6. Adjust if necessary. Be sure that binders are not restricting breathing or circulation. Be sure that sterile dressings are in place between the binder and any wound.
7. Cleanse hands.

T-Binders

8. Cleanse hands.
9. Select a single-tail binder for a female, a double-tail binder for a male. Have the client lift the hips or, alternatively, position the client on one side and roll the client onto the binder. Place the waistband at the waist, with the single or double tails pointing downward along the spine.
10. Wrap waistband around the waist and secure.
    • Bring the tail(s) of the T-binder up between the client's legs. For the male, one tail should be placed on each side of the testicles. Join tails to the waistband and secure.
11. Cleanse hands.

Breast Binders

12. Cleanse hands.
13. Assist the client to a sitting position.

14. Apply binder, adjusting for a snug fit.

15. Adjust if necessary. Be sure that breast binder is not restricting breathing or causing skin irritation.

16. Add use of adjunctive treatments (e.g., ice packs, analgesics) for additional comfort, if needed.
17. Cleanse hands.

5. Fasteners will keep binder in place. Be sure that all fasteners are closed securely to prevent possible client injury.

6. Binders that are too tight may make breathing difficult and may contribute to skin irritation or breakdown. Binders are generally not sterile.
7. Reduces transmission of microorganisms.

8. Reduces transmission of microorganisms.
9. Proper binder keeps dressing in place.

10. Secures dressing and promotes client comfort.

11. Reduces transmission of microorganisms.

12. Reduces transmission of microorganisms.
13. Sitting will allow ease in placement of the binder. If not possible, turn client side-to-side while applying binder.
14. The tightness of the binder will be instrumental in adequate lactation suppression.
15. Breast binders that are too tight may make breathing difficult and/or may contribute to skin irritation or breakdown.
16. If breasts are engorged, adjunctive treatment may be required to increase client's level of comfort.
17. Reduces transmission of microorganisms.

EVALUATION

• For breast binder, lactation is suppressed.
• Binder provides support for dressings or soft tissue.
• Binder is not too tight and does not compress the skin.
• T-binder on a male client does not compress the testicles.
• Client assists in placement of the binder as much as possible.

DOCUMENTATION

Nurses' Notes

• Time, date, and type of binder
• Difficulty the client experienced with the procedure

Figure 26-33-1 Scultetus Binder

PROCEDURE 26-34   Application of Restraints

OVERVIEW

A restraint is a physical or mechanical method of involuntarily restricting movement and physical activity so that the confused, agitated, or disoriented client is protected from causing harm to self and/or to others. Restraints may be used to prevent movement during a procedure. If a client is restless or confused, a restraint may be used to prevent the client from damaging therapeutic equipment.

The procedure to restrain a client is fairly simple, but legal, emotional, and ethical considerations accompanying this procedure are complex. State and federal laws as well as hospital policies govern the use of restraints. Nurses or caregivers may not restrain or confine clients without documented necessity; however, the nurse or caregiver can be liable if a confused client sustains injury without appropriate protection, which may include restraints. Many people see the use of restraints as demeaning and dehumanizing. Others feel that restraints are used to replace nursing contact in understaffed environments. Confused clients often feel they are being imprisoned. While trying to balance these considerations, the nurse has a legal and ethical duty to keep clients safe. The decision to restrain a client and how much is a delicate balancing act of nursing judgment.

Restraints range from a simple armboard to prevent movement of a wrist or elbow to more complex locked restraints. The restraints most commonly used are soft restraints made of mesh or soft canvas. They are designed to gently restrain the client without damaging the skin. Chest restraints, cloth wrist restraints, mitten restraints, and "posey" restraints fall into this category. Other types of restraints include locked web belt restraints, locked leather restraints, and full-body restraints. These are more often used in settings where clients are extremely agitated and belligerent.

ASSESSMENT

1. Assess the client's level of consciousness. **This will help you determine the client's ability to protect him or herself from potential harm.**
2. Assess the client's degree of orientation. **A client who is confused regarding time, place, or person is more likely to be at risk of injuring him or herself. A client who is agitated or angry may be at risk of injuring others.**
3. Assess the client's physical condition. **A client who has weakness, paralysis, or impaired balance or mobility is at increased risk of injury. Impaired vision or hearing also increases the client's risk of injury.**
4. Assess the client's history for falls, accidents, confusion, agitation, or self-inflicted injury. **A client who has a history of this type is at increased risk for injury.**
5. Assess the client's intent. **A client who is verbalizing threats to harm self or others is at increased risk of injury.**
6. Assess the need for restraints. Determine if the client's treatment plan requires and allows restraints, if orders are in place, and hospital policies and laws are specified. **This will prevent the inappropriate use of restraints and is necessary for legal protection in the event of an injury.**
7. Assess client and family knowledge regarding the use of and rationale for restraints or protective devices. **The more the client and family understand regarding the reason for restraints, the more cooperative and understanding they will be.**

POSSIBLE NURSING DIAGNOSES

*Risk for **I**njury*
*Low **S**elf-Esteem*
***P**owerlessness*
*Deficient **K**nowledge* (need for restraints)
*Impaired Physical **M**obility*

PLANNING

Expected Outcomes

1. The client will remain uninjured.
2. The client will not suffer injury or impairment from the restraints.
3. The client's therapeutic equipment will remain intact and functional.
4. Others will not be harmed by the client.
5. The client will be restrained just enough to prevent injury.

Equipment Needed

- Restraints appropriate to the client's condition and type of restraint required
- Cotton batting or foam padding

continues

IMPLEMENTATION—ACTION/RATIONALE

ACTION	RATIONALE

※ Cleanse hands ※ Check client's identification band ※

Chest Restraint

ACTION	RATIONALE
1. Explain that the client will be wearing a jacket attached to the bed. Explain that this is for safety.	1. Promotes client cooperation.
2. Place the restraint over the client's hospital gown or clothing.	2. Provides for client privacy and prevents the restraint from rubbing the client's skin.
3. Place the restraint on the client with the opening in the front.	3. Allows movement but restricts freedom.
4. Overlap the front pieces, threading the ties through the slot/loop on the front of the vest.	4. Secures the restraint.
5. If the client is in bed, secure the ties to the movable part of the mattress frame with a half-knot (Figure 26-34-1).	5. Allows the restraint to move with the bed if the head of the bed is raised or lowered.
6. If the client is in a chair, cross the straps behind the back of the chair and secure the straps to the chair's lower legs, out of the client's reach (Figure 26-34-2). If it is a wheelchair, be sure the straps will not get caught in the wheels.	6. Provides support for the client to sit up while restricting freedom.
7. Step back and assess the client's overall safety. Be sure the restraint is loose enough not to be a hazard to the client but tight enough to restrict the client from getting up and harming him or herself.	7. Looking at the overall picture can allow you to see dangers you might have missed.
8. Cleanse your hands.	8. Prevents spread of microorganisms.

Figure 26-34-1 Secure ties to the movable part of the frame.

Figure 26-34-2 Secure restraining straps out of the client's reach.

continues

Applying Wrist or Ankle Restraints

1. Explain to the client that you will be placing a wrist or ankle band that will restrict movement.
2. Place padding around the client's wrist/ankle.
3. Wrap the restraint around the client's wrist/ankle, pulling the tie through the loop in the restraint and tie a square knot.
4. Secure the restraint to the movable portion of the mattress frame.
5. Slip two fingers under the restraint to check for tightness. Be sure the restraint is tight enough that the client cannot slip it off but loose enough that the neurovascular status of the client's extremity is not impaired.
6. Step back and assess the client's overall safety. Be sure the restraint is loose enough not to be a hazard to the client but tight enough to restrict the client from getting up and harming him or herself.
7. Place the call light within the client's reach.

8. Check on the client every half hour while restrained. Assess the safety of the restraint placement and the client's neurovascular status.

9. Cleanse your hands.

1. Promotes client cooperation.

2. Prevents restraint from chafing the skin.
3. Secures the restraint, and prevents the restraint from overtightening at the wrist.

4. When the head or foot of the client's bed is moved, the restraint will move with it.
5. If the restraint is too tight, the client's neurovascular status may be impaired, causing injury to the client.

6. Looking at the overall picture can allow you to see dangers you might have missed.

7. Allows the client to contact the nurse to have any needs met. Provides the client with an increased sense of safety.
8. Assures that the client remains safe. Clients may try to escape from restraint and injure themselves in the attempt. States and institutions may have regulations outlining the frequency of client checks if the client is in restraints. Be aware of regulations that apply.
9. Prevents spread of microorganisms.

EVALUATION

- The client remains uninjured.
- The client has not suffered injury or impairment from the restraints.
- The client's therapeutic equipment has remained intact and functional.
- Others have not been harmed by the client.
- The client is restrained just enough to prevent injury.

DOCUMENTATION

Nurses' Notes

- Use of restraints including reason the client was restrained, type of restraint placed, time the restraints

were placed, condition of the client's skin at the site of restraint at the time of placement, and any unusual findings at the time the client was restrained
- Nurses' notes should be made at least every 2 hours even if a flow sheet is used.
- Ongoing need for restraints
- If the client's status changes, restraints may no longer be necessary.

Flow Sheet

- Some institutions have flow sheets that are used when a client is restrained. These flow sheets document the frequency of client checks, the client's condition, and how often the restraints are released.

PROCEDURE 26-35   Performing the Heimlich Maneuver

OVERVIEW

Foreign body obstruction of the breathing passages has consistently ranked as one of the top ten causes of accidental deaths in the United States. Complete or partial airway obstruction by a foreign body can occur in numerous settings. In adults, large, poorly chewed pieces of food are most frequently the cause of airway obstruction. Pediatric clients are at risk for choking, especially the infant and young child, and in this population, food (e.g., grapes, hot dogs, raisins, and peanuts) as well as foreign bodies (e.g., coins, beads, marbles, thumbtacks, and paper clips) often cause airway obstruction. The Heimlich maneuver or subdiaphragmatic abdominal thrusts can assist a health care provider in successfully treating airway obstruction. It is important in the pediatric population to differentiate airway obstruction as a result of infection (e.g., epiglottitis) versus a foreign body aspiration.

Health professionals frequently teach the Heimlich maneuver to the general public because most food/foreign body obstructions occur outside the hospital/clinic settings. It is important to have a good comfort level with this skill as well as the ability to disseminate this information in an easily understood manner to the public.

ASSESSMENT

1. Assess air exchange. A foreign body obstruction can be complete or partial. Partial airway obstruction will have some air exchange. If the client can cough, this should be encouraged, and do not interfere with the client's efforts. In the event of partial airway obstruction, the client will usually be able to cough but may wheeze between coughs. **If the client has complete airway obstruction as indicated by a weak, ineffective cough, high-pitched inspiratory noises (stridor), and signs of respiratory distress (cyanosis, loss of consciousness), intervention is necessary.**
2. Establish airway obstruction. The universal sign of airway obstruction is clutching the neck with hands. In addition, the inability to talk or breathe as well as cyanosis and the progression to an unconscious state indicate airway obstruction. **Determine the problem.**
3. In the pediatric client, differentiate between infection and airway obstruction. Fevers, gradually increasing respiratory distress, retractions, stridor, and drooling are all signs of infection. **In this situation, it is important to maintain an upright position, keep the child as calm as possible, and seek immediate medical attention.** The Heimlich maneuver is not appropriate in these cases.

POSSIBLE NURSING DIAGNOSES

Impaired **G**as Exchange
Ineffective **A**irway Clearance
Ineffective **B**reathing Pattern
Risk for **S**uffocation
Risk for **A**spiration
Fear

PLANNING

Expected Outcomes

1. The client will demonstrate improved clinical status as evident by airway clearance or establishment of a patent airway.
2. The client will demonstrate improved gas exchange as evident by absence of signs and symptoms of partial or complete airway obstruction (e.g., cough, wheezing, stridor, loss of consciousness, cyanosis).
3. The client will experience minimal discomfort during the Heimlich maneuver or other method of airway clearance.
4. The client will not experience complications related to airway obstruction/hypoxia.

Equipment Needed

- An individual with the training to perform this procedure

DELEGATION TIPS

The Heimlich maneuver may be performed by any trained individual. A technique adjustment may need to be demonstrated in pregnant women.

continues

IMPLEMENTATION—ACTION/RATIONALE

ACTION

RATIONALE

Foreign Body Obstruction—All Clients

1. Assess airway for complete or partial blockage.

2. Encourage attempts to cough and breathe.

3. Activate emergency response assistance if respiratory distress or complete blockage; for example, ask bystander to call 911.

1. If there is good air exchange and the client is able to forcefully cough, do not intervene or interfere with the client's attempts to expel the foreign body.
2. Attempts to cough will provide a more forceful effort. If complete airway obstruction is apparent, the Heimlich maneuver or alternative method of subdiaphragmatic thrust should be performed immediately.
3. Provides follow-up care by professionally trained personnel.

Conscious Adult Client—Sitting or Standing (Heimlich Maneuver)

4. Stand behind the client and wrap your arms around the client's waist (Figure 26-35-1).
5. Make a fist with one hand and grasp the fist with your other hand, placing the thumb side of the fist against the client's abdomen. The fist should be placed midline, below the xiphoid process and lower margins of the rib cage and above the navel (Figure 26-35-2).
6. Perform a quick upward thrust into the client's abdomen; each thrust should be separate and distinct.
7. Repeat this process six to ten times until the client either expels the foreign body or loses consciousness.

4. Proper positioning is necessary to provide an effective subdiaphragmatic thrust.
5. Correct hand placement is important to prevent internal organ damage.

6. This subdiaphragmatic thrust can produce an artificial cough by forcing air from the lungs.
7. Attempts to dislodge food or a foreign body to relieve airway obstruction should be continued as long as necessary because of the serious consequences of hypoxia.

Unconscious Adult Client or Adult Client Who Becomes Unconscious

8. Repeat Actions 1 to 3.

9. Position the client supine; kneel astride the client's abdomen.

8. Determines the need for intervention and summons essential help.
9. Proper positioning is necessary to provide an effective subdiaphragmatic thrust.

Figure 26-35-1 Wrap both arms around the client's waist.

Figure 26-35-2 Make a fist. Place the fist below the xiphoid process, above the client's navel.

continues

10. Place the heel of one hand midline, below the xiphoid process and lower margin of the rib cage and above the navel. Place the second hand directly on top of the first hand.
11. Perform a quick upward thrust into the diaphragm, repeating six to ten times.
12. Perform a finger sweep:

   a. Use one hand to grasp the lower jaw and tongue between your thumb and fingers and lift. This will open the mouth and pull the tongue away from the back of the throat.
   b. Using the index finger of the other hand, insert the finger into the client's mouth next to the cheek and dislodge any foreign body using a hooking motion. Caution must be used to prevent pushing the foreign body farther down into the airway.
13. Open the client's airway and attempt ventilation.

14. Continue sequence of Heimlich maneuver, finger sweep, and rescue breathing as long as necessary.

Airway Obstruction—Infants and Small Children

15. Differentiate between infection and airway obstruction.

Infant Airway Obstruction

16. Straddle infant over your forearm in the prone position with the head lower than the trunk. Support the infant's head, positioning a hand around the jaws and chest.
17. Deliver five back blows between the infant's shoulder blades.
18. Keeping the infant's head down, place the free hand on the infant's back and turn the infant over, supporting the back of the child with your hand and thigh.
19. With your free hand, deliver five thrusts in the same manner as infant external cardiac compressions.
20. Assess for a foreign body in the mouth of an unconscious infant and utilize the finger sweep *only* if a foreign body is visualized.
21. Open airway and assess for respiration. If respirations are absent, attempt rescue breathing. Assess for the rise and fall of the chest; if not seen, reposition infant and attempt rescue breathing again.
22. Repeat the entire sequence again: five back blows, five chest thrusts, assessment for foreign body in oral cavity, and rescue breathing as long as necessary.

10. Proper positioning is necessary to provide an effective subdiaphragmatic thrust.

11. A client who becomes unconscious may become more relaxed so that the previously unsuccessful Heimlich maneuver may be successful.
12. Should only be used on the unconscious client, who will not fight the action.
   a. Draw the tongue away from any foreign body lodged in the back of the throat.

13. The brain can suffer irreversible damage if it is without oxygen for more than 4 to 6 minutes.
14. Life-saving efforts must continue until they are successful, or until the rescuer becomes exhausted and cannot go on.

15. Infectious complications that lead to airway obstruction require immediate medical attention, establishment of a patent airway (intubation or emergency tracheotomy), and treatment of the underlying infection. Food/foreign body airway obstruction also needs immediate attention; however, airway management differs for each scenario.

16. Proper positioning is essential for success of the maneuver and prevention of other organ damage.

17. Provides correct technique for dislodging the obstruction.

18. Safely rotates the infant's position to continue life-saving procedures.

19. Technique for dislodging the obstruction.

20. A blind finger sweep is avoided in infants and children because a foreign object can be pushed back farther into the airway, increasing obstruction.
21. Many times some air can get around the foreign body causing the airway obstruction. This allows for some oxygenation of the client. Without oxygen, irreversible brain damage can occur within 4 to 6 minutes.
22. Life-saving efforts must continue until they are successful or until the rescuer becomes exhausted and cannot go on.

continues

Small Child—Airway Obstruction (Conscious, Standing or Sitting)

23. Assess air exchange and encourage coughing and breathing. Provide reassurance to the child that you are there to help.

24. Ask the child if he or she is choking. If the response is affirmative, follow the steps outlined below. In addition, if the child has poor air exchange (and infection has been ruled out), initiate the following steps:
    a. Stand behind the child with your arms wrapped around his or her waist and administer six to ten subdiaphragmatic abdominal thrusts.
    b. Continue until foreign object is expelled or the child becomes unconscious.

Small Child—Airway Obstruction (Unconscious)

25. Position the child supine and kneel at the child's feet and gently deliver five subdiaphragmatic abdominal thrusts in the same manner as for an adult but more gently.
26. Open airway by lifting the lower jaw and tongue forward. Perform a finger sweep only if a foreign body is visualized.

27. If breathing is absent, begin rescue breathing. If the chest does not rise, reposition the child and attempt rescue breathing again.

28. Repeat this sequence as long as necessary.

29. Cleanse hands.

23. Inability to breathe is a distressing event for anyone, especially a small child who may not fully understand the circumstance. Reassurance is important to gain the child's trust and cooperation with the maneuvers necessary to help him or her, especially if the child is conscious.

24. Many small children are capable of responding to simple questions such as "Are you choking?"

    a. Proper positioning is essential for success of the maneuver and prevention of other organ damage.

    b. Life-saving efforts must continue until they are successful or until the rescuer becomes exhausted and cannot go on.

25. This is the recommended position for small children; the astride position may be used for larger children. Proper positioning is essential for success of the maneuver and prevention of other organ damage.
26. Opens the airway and allows visualization of the oral cavity. A blind finger sweep can cause increased obstruction by pushing a foreign object farther back into the airway.
27. Many times some air can get around the foreign body causing the airway obstruction. This allows for some oxygenation of the client. Without oxygen, irreversible brain damage can occur within 4 to 6 minutes.
28. Life-saving efforts must continue until they are successful or until the rescuer becomes exhausted and cannot go on.
29. Reduces transmission of microorganisms.

EVALUATION

- The client demonstrates improved clinical status as evident by airway clearance or establishment of a patent airway.
- The client demonstrates improved gas exchange as evident by absence of signs and symptoms of partial or complete airway obstruction (e.g., cough, wheezing, stridor, loss of consciousness, cyanosis).
- The client experienced minimal discomfort during the Heimlich maneuver or other method of airway clearance.
- The client did not experience complications related to airway obstruction/hypoxia.

DOCUMENTATION

- If the airway obstruction occurs in the health care setting, document the following in the narrative notes and in the emergency procedure notes if needed:

— Time and date of onset of symptoms
— Presentation, including onset and type of symptoms
— Type (complete or partial) and cause of obstruction, if known
— Interventions utilized to alleviate obstruction
— Results of interventions
— Other emergency support needed (e.g., emergency tracheotomy)

- If the airway obstruction occurs in an alternate setting (e.g., restaurant, home), provide the following information to the responding health care providers for documentation:

— Presentation, including onset and type of symptoms
— Type (complete or partial) and cause of obstruction, if known
— Interventions utilized to alleviate obstruction
— Length of time with airway obstruction
— Results of interventions

PROCEDURE 26-36   Performing Cardiopulmonary Resuscitation (CPR)

OVERVIEW

Cardiac or respiratory arrest can occur at any time to individuals of all ages. It is a crisis event that can be the result of an accident (e.g., foreign body aspiration, motor vehicle accident, drowning) or a disease process (e.g., cardiac arrhythmia, epiglottitis). Cardiopulmonary resuscitation (CPR) is the basic life-saving skill utilized in the event of cardiac, respiratory, or cardiopulmonary arrest to maintain tissue oxygenation by providing external cardiac compressions and/or artificial respiration.

This life-saving skill is initiated in the event that an individual is found with or develops the absence of a pulse or respiration or both. The basic goals of CPR, which are often referred to as the ABCD of emergency resuscitation, are as follows:

A: Establish **A**irway
B: Initiate **B**reathing
C: Maintain **C**irculation
D: **D**efibrillate

Cardiopulmonary resuscitation must be initiated immediately once it is determined that a cardiac or pulmonary arrest has occurred. Lack of oxygen to the tissues can result in permanent cardiac and brain damage within 4 to 6 minutes.

Cardiopulmonary resuscitation is a basic life-saving skill that nurses are expected to be able to perform not only in the hospital and other clinical settings but in the outside environments as well. It is expected that nurses maintain certification in the administration of CPR to individuals of all ages and participate in annual review or recertification courses. In addition, this skill is frequently taught to the lay public and caregivers of medically fragile individuals.

ASSESSMENT

1. Assess responsiveness and level of consciousness by gently shaking or tapping the client while shouting, "Are you OK?" **It is important to differentiate an unconscious individual from someone who is intoxicated, hypoglycemic, sleeping, or in shock. In addition, it is important to touch clients in case they are hearing impaired.**
2. Assess the amount and abilities of any available assistance. **CPR cannot be performed indefinitely by a single individual. If in the hospital or a clinical setting, activate the appropriate "code" to signify there is an emergency situation. If outside the hospital, call for help to activate emergency assistance (e.g., call 911 or the local emergency medical service).**
3. Assess the client's position. **Proper positioning, in a supine position (flat) on a hard surface, is essential to assess respiratory and cardiac status and to adequately perform cardiopulmonary resuscitation. Care must be taken when positioning the client with a suspected neck injury.**
4. Assess respiratory status by looking for chest rise and fall, listening for air exchange, and feeling for the presence of air movement. **Presence of respirations contraindicates the initiation of artificial respiration. In addition, assessment of the respiratory status will uncover complicating factors, including foreign body obstruction and vomit or other excessive airway secretions. These complicating factors will need to be resolved in order to open the airway before the initiation of artificial respirations.**

5. Assess circulatory status by using the carotid or brachial pulse points. **Presence of pulse contraindicates the initiation of external chest compressions.**

POSSIBLE NURSING DIAGNOSES

*Ineffective **A**irway Clearance*
*Ineffective **B**reathing Pattern*
*Impaired **G**as Exchange*
*Impaired Spontaneous **V**entilation*
*Decreased **C**ardiac Output*

PLANNING

Expected Outcomes

1. Client will experience improved clinical status, as evident by:
   • Patent airway with spontaneous respirations
   • Return of cardiac circulation
2. Client does not experience negative sequela related to hypoxic event.
3. Client does not have damage inflicted by incorrect positioning for CPR (e.g., paralysis from manipulation of neck injury, cracked ribs or sternum).
4. Cardiopulmonary resuscitation will be terminated only in the following situations:
   • Cardiopulmonary resuscitation was successful in reestablishing respirations and circulation.
   • The client is placed on advanced life support (e.g., intubated and transferred to the intensive care unit).
   • The rescuer is unassisted, fatigued, and unable to continue.

continues

- The physician or qualified practitioner pronounces the client dead and orders CPR to be discontinued.

- Ambu®-bag
- Oral airway
- Emergency resuscitation cart (including defibrillator)
- Documentation forms

Equipment Needed

Hospital or Clinical Setting
- Hard, flat surface (e.g., chest compression board)
- Body substance isolation items
  — Gloves
  — Face shield
  — Mask/CPR oral barrier device

Outside: Public Environment
- Hard, flat surface (e.g., floor)
- Body substance isolation items, if available
  — Gloves
  — Face shield
  — Mask/CPR oral barrier device

DELEGATION TIPS

The administration of CPR to adults and children is a skill that may be delegated to ancillary personnel and caregivers after proper instruction and CPR certification.

IMPLEMENTATION—ACTION/RATIONALE

ACTION

CPR: One Rescuer—Adult, Adolescent

1. Assess responsiveness by tapping or gently shaking client while shouting, "Are you OK?"

2. Activate emergency medical system (EMS). In the hospital or clinical setting, follow institutional protocol. In the community or home environment, activate the local emergency response system (e.g., 911).

3. Position client in a supine position on a hard, flat surface (e.g., floor or cardiac board). Use caution when positioning a client with a possible head or neck injury.

4. Apply appropriate body substance isolation items (e.g., gloves, face shield) if available.

5. Position self. Face the client on your knees parallel to the client, next to the head, to begin to assess the airway and breathing status.

6. Open airway. The most commonly used method is the head-tilt/chin-lift method. This is accomplished by placing one hand on the client's forehead and applying a steady backward pressure to tilt the head back while placing the fingers of the other hand below the jaw at the location of the chin and lifting the chin (Figure 26-36-1). In the event of a suspected head or neck injury, this lift is modified and the jaw thrust is used. To perform the jaw thrust, place hands at the angles of the lower jaw and lift, displacing the mandible forward while tilting the head backward (Figure 26-36-2). Additionally, if available, insert oral airway.

RATIONALE

1. Prevents injury to a client who is not experiencing cardiac or respiratory arrest. Also assists in assessing level of consciousness and possible etiology of crisis.

2. Activates assistance from personnel trained in advanced life support. *Note:* According to the new CPR guideline, September 2000 (American Heart Association), rescuers should notify the EMS or phone 911 for unresponsive adults before beginning CPR.

3. Proper positioning facilitates assessment of the cardiac and respiratory status and successful external cardiac massage. Prevents further damage to a potential head or neck injury.

4. Prevents transmission of disease.

5. Proper positioning prevents rescuer fatigue and facilitates CPR by allowing the rescuer to move from chest compressions to artificial breathing with minimal movement.

6. A patent airway is essential for successful artificial respirations. The head-tilt/chin-lift assists in preventing the tongue from obstructing the airway. The jaw thrust is used when a head or neck injury is suspected because it prevents extension of the neck and decreases the potential of further injury.

continues

Figure 26-36-1 Use the head-tilt/chin-lift method to open airway.

Figure 26-36-2 The jaw-thrust method is used to open the airway if a neck injury is suspected.

7. Assess for respirations. Look, listen, and feel for air movement (3 to 5 seconds).

8. If respirations are absent:
   • Occlude nostrils with the thumb and index finger of the hand on the forehead that is tilting the head back (Figure 26-36-3).
   • Form a seal over the client's mouth using either your mouth or the appropriate respiratory assist device (e.g., Ambu®-bag and mask) and give two full breaths of approximately 0.5 to 2 seconds, allowing time for both inspiration and expiration (Figure 26-36-4).
   • In the event of a serious mouth or jaw injury that prevents mouth-to-mouth ventilation, mouth-to-nose ventilation may be used by tilting the head as described earlier with one hand and using the other hand to lift the jaw and close the mouth.

9. Assess for the rise and fall of the chest:
   • If the chest rises and falls, continue to Action 10.
   • If the chest does not move, assess for excessive oral secretions, vomit, airway obstruction, or improper positioning.

7. Cardiopulmonary resuscitation should not be administered to a client with spontaneous respirations or pulse because of the potential risk of injury.

8. Occluding the nostrils and forming a seal over the client's mouth will prevent air leakage and provide full inflation of the lungs. Excessive air volume and rapid inspiratory flow rates can create pharyngeal pressures that are greater than esophageal opening pressures. This will allow air into the stomach, resulting in gastric distention and increased risk of vomiting.

9. Visual assessment of chest movement helps confirm an open airway. A volume of 800–1200 mL is usually sufficient to make the chest rise in most adults.

Figure 26-36-3 Occlude both nostrils with fingers.

Figure 26-36-4 Give two full breaths.

continues

Figure 26-36-5   Palpate for a carotid pulse.

Figure 26-36-6   Place the heel of one hand next to the index finger on the client's sternum.

10. Palpate the carotid pulse (5 to 10 seconds) (Figure 26-36-5):
    • If present, continue rescue breathing, at the rate of 12 breaths per minute.
    • If absent, begin external cardiac compressions.

11. Cardiac compressions are performed as follows:
    • Maintain a position on knees parallel to sternum.
    • Position the hands for compressions:
      a. Using the hand nearest to the legs, use the index finger to locate the lower rib margin and quickly move the fingers up to the location where the ribs connect to the sternum.
      b. Place the middle finger of this hand on the notch where the ribs meet the sternum and the index finger next to it.
      c. Place the heel of the opposite hand next to the index finger on the sternum (Figure 26-36-6).
      d. Remove the first hand from the notch and place it on top of the hand that is on the sternum so they are on top of each other.
      e. Extend or interlace fingers and do not allow them to touch the chest (Figure 26-36-7).
      f. Keep arms straight with shoulders directly over hands on sternum and lock elbows (Figure 26-36-8).

10. Performing chest compressions on an individual with a pulse could result in injury. Additionally, the carotid pulse may persist when peripheral pulses are no longer palpable. Hyperventilation assists in maintaining blood oxygen levels. Additionally, a pulse may be present for approximately 6 minutes after respirations have ceased.

11. Irreversible brain and tissue damage can occur if a client is hypoxic for more than 4 to 6 minutes. Proper positioning is essential for the following reasons:
    • Allows for maximum compression of the heart between the sternum and vertebrae.
    • Compressions over the xiphoid process can lacerate the liver.
    • Keeping fingers off the chest during compressions reduces the risk of rib fracture.

Figure 26-36-7   Extend or interlace the fingers.

Figure 26-36-8   Proper position of rescuer. Keep arms straight and lock elbows.

continues

g. Compress the adult chest 3.8–5.0 cm (1$\frac{1}{2}$–2 inches) at the rate of approximately 100 compressions per minute.

h. The heel of the hand must completely release the pressure between compressions, but it should remain in constant contact with the client's skin.

i. Use the mnemonic "one and, two and, three and . . . " to keep rhythm and timing.

j. Ventilate client as described in Action 8.

12. Maintain the compression rate for approximately 100 times per minute, interjecting 2 ventilations after every 15 compressions. (compression:ventilation rate at 15:2)

13. Reassess the client after four cycles.

CPR: Two Rescuers—Adult, Adolescent

14. Follow the steps above with the following changes:
- One rescuer is positioned facing the client parallel to the head while the other rescuer is positioned on the opposite side facing the client parallel to the sternum next to the trunk (Figure 26-36-9).
- The rescuer positioned at the client's trunk is responsible for performing cardiac compressions and maintaining the verbal mnemonic count. This is rescuer 1.
- The rescuer positioned at the client's head is responsible for monitoring respirations, assessing the carotid pulse, establishing an open airway, and performing rescue breathing. This is rescuer 2.
- Maintain the compression rate for approximately 100 times per minute, interjecting two ventilations after every 15 compressions. (compression:ventilation rate at 15:2)
- Rescuer 2 palpates the carotid pulse with each chest compression during the first full minute.
- Rescuer 2 is responsible for calling for a change when fatigued, following this protocol:
- Rescuer 1 calls for a change and completes the 15 chest compressions.
- Rescuer 2 administers two breaths and then moves to a position parallel to the client's sternum and assumes the proper hand position.
- Rescuer 1 moves to the rescue breathing position and checks the carotid pulse for 5 seconds. If cardiac arrest persists, rescuer 1 says, "continue CPR" and delivers one breath. Rescuer 2 resumes cardiac compressions immediately after the breath.

CPR: One Rescuer—Child (1–7 years)

15. Assess responsiveness, position the child, apply appropriate body substance isolation, position self, open airway, and assess for respirations as described in Actions 1, 3–7. Remember respiratory arrest is more common in the pediatric population.

12. Faster rate increases blood flow to key organ tissues.

13. Determines return of spontaneous pulse and respirations and need to continue CPR.

14. Proper positioning allows one rescuer to perform artificial respirations while the other administers chest compressions without getting in each other's way. In addition, this facilitates ease in changing positions when one of the rescuers becomes fatigued. Palpating the carotid pulse with each chest compression during the first full minute assures that adequate stroke volume is being delivered with each compression.

Two rescuers are needed because one person cannot maintain CPR indefinitely. When a rescuer becomes fatigued, chest compressions can become ineffective, decreasing the volume of oxygenated blood circulated to key organs and tissue.

Figure 26-36-9 Two-rescuer positioning. One person kneels on each side of the client.

15. See Rationales 1, 3–7.

continues

16. If respirations are absent, begin rescue breathing:
- Give two slow breaths (1–1¹/₂ sec/breath), pausing to take a breath in between.
- Use only the amount of air needed to make the chest rise. When you see the chest rise and fall, you are using the right volume of air.

17. Palpate the carotid pulse (5 to 10 seconds). If present, ventilate at a rate of once every 4 seconds or 15 times per minute. If absent, begin cardiac compressions.

18. Cardiac compressions (child 1–7 years):
- Maintain a position on knees parallel to child's sternum.
- Position the hands for compressions:
  a. Locate the lower margin of the rib cage using the hand closest to the feet and find the notch where the ribs and sternum meet.
  b. Place the middle finger of this hand on the notch and then place the index finger next to the middle finger.
  c. Place the heel of the other hand next to the index finger of the first hand on the sternum with the heel parallel to the sternum (1 cm above the xiphoid process).
  d. Keeping the elbows locked and the shoulders over the child, compress the sternum 2.5–3.8 cm (1–1¹/₂ inches) at the approximate rate of 100 times per minute.
  e. Keep the other hand on the child's forehead.
  f. At the end of every fifth compression administer a ventilation (1–1¹/₂ seconds).
  g. Reevaluate the child after 20 cycles. If respirations are still absent, call 911.

CPR: One Rescuer—Infant (1–12 months)

19. Assess responsiveness, activate emergency medical system, position the child, apply appropriate body substance isolation, position self, open airway, and assess for respirations as described in Actions 1, 3–7. Remember, respiratory arrest is more common in the pediatric population.

20. If respirations are absent, begin rescue breathing:
- Avoid overextension of the infant's neck.
- Place a small towel or diaper under the infant's shoulders or use a hand to support the neck.
- Make a tight seal over both the infant's nose and mouth and gently administer artificial respirations.
- Give two slow breaths (1–1¹/₂ seconds per breath), pausing to take a breath in between.

16. Hypoxia can cause irreversible brain and tissue damage after 4 to 6 minutes.
- The volume of air in a small child's lungs is less than an adult's. Excessive air volume and rapid inspiratory rates can increase pharyngeal pressures that exceed esophageal opening pressures. This allows air to enter the stomach, causing gastric distention, increasing the risk of vomiting, and further compromising the client's respiratory status.

17. Performing chest compressions on a child with a pulse could result in injury. Additionally, the carotid pulse may persist when peripheral pulses are no longer palpable. Hyperventilation assists in maintaining blood oxygen levels. Additionally, a pulse may be present for approximately 6 minutes after respirations have ceased.

18. Irreversible brain and tissue damage can occur if a client is hypoxic for more than 4 to 6 minutes. Proper positioning is essential for the following reasons:
- Allows for maximum compression of the heart between the sternum and vertebrae.
- The backward tilt of the head lifts the back of small children.
- Compressions over the xiphoid process can lacerate the liver.
- Keeping fingers off the chest during compressions reduces the risk of rib fracture.
- Keeping one hand on the child's forehead helps maintain an open airway.

g. Guidelines published by the American Heart Association recommend that a 1-minute CPR be performed for infants and children up to age 8 before calling 911. In institutions, follow hospital protocol.

19. See Rationales 1, 3–7.

20. Irreversible brain and tissue damage can occur if a client is hypoxic for more than 4 to 6 minutes. Proper positioning is essential for the following reasons:
- It is believed that overextension of an infant's head can cause a closing or narrowing of the airway.
- Proper positioning with support allows maximum compression of the heart between the sternum and vertebrae.

continues

• Use only the amount of air needed to make the chest rise.

• Making a complete seal over the infant's mouth and nose prevents air leakage.
• The volume of air in a small child's lungs is less than an adult's. Excessive air volume and rapid inspiratory rates can increase pharyngeal pressures that exceed esophageal opening pressures. This allows air to enter the stomach, causing gastric distention, increasing the risk of vomiting, and further compromising the client's respiratory status.

21. Assess circulatory status using the brachial pulse:
• Locate the brachial pulse on the inside of the upper arm between the elbow and shoulder by placing your thumb on the outside of the arm and palpating the proximal side of the arm with the index finger and middle fingers.
• If a pulse is palpated, continue rescue breathing 20 times per minute or once every 3 seconds.
• If a pulse is absent, begin cardiac compressions.

21. The carotid pulse is often difficult to locate in the infant; therefore the brachial artery is the recommended site.

22. Cardiac compressions (infant 1–12 months):
• Maintain a position parallel to the infant. Infants can easily be placed on a table or other hard surface.
• Place a small towel or other support under the infant's shoulders/neck.
• Position the hands for compressions:
   a. Using the hand closest to the infant's feet, locate the intermammary line where it intersects the sternum.
   b. Place the index finger 1 cm below this location on the sternum and place the middle finger next to the index finger.
   c. Using these two fingers, compress in a downward motion 1.3–2.5 cm ($^1/_2$–1 inch) at the rate of 100 times per minute.
   d. Keep the other hand on the infant's forehead.
   e. At the end of every fifth compression, administer a ventilation (1–1$^1/_2$ seconds).
   f. Reevaluate infant after 20 cycles. If respirations are still absent, call 911.

22. Irreversible brain and tissue damage can occur if a client is hypoxic for more than 4 to 6 minutes. Proper positioning is essential for the following reasons:
• Allows for maximum compression of the heart between the sternum and vertebrae.
• A small towel, diaper roll, or some other type of support is necessary for effective cardiac compressions.
• Compressions over the xiphoid process can lacerate the liver.
• Keeping other fingers and hands off the chest during compressions reduces risk of rib fracture.
• Keeping one hand on the infant's forehead helps maintain an open airway.

   f. New guidelines published by the American Heart Association recommend that a 1-minute CPR be performed for infants and children up to age 8 before calling 911. In institutions, follow hospital protocol (American Heart Association, 2000).

CPR: Two Rescuers—Child (1–7 years) and Infant (1–12 months)

23. Follow Action 14 for two-rescuer CPR for adults with the following changes:
• Utilize the child or infant procedure for chest compressions.
• Change the ratio of compressions to ventilation to 5 : 1 (five chest compressions to one ventilation).
• Deliver the ventilation on the upstroke of the third compression.

23. Improper hand placement can cause internal organ damage or other medical complications in infants or children. Increased rate of ventilation allows for maximum oxygen delivery to prevent tissue hypoxia. Delivering ventilation during the upstroke phase allows for full lung expansion during inspiration.

CPR—Neonate or Premature Infant

24. Follow the infant guidelines with the following changes for chest compressions:
• Encircle the chest with both hands.
• Position thumbs over the midsternum.

24. Improper hand placement can cause internal organ damage or other medical complications in infants or children.

continues

- Compress the midsternum with both thumbs.
- Compress 1.3–1.8 cm ($^{1}/_{2}$–$^{3}/_{4}$ inch) at a rate of 100–120 times per minute.

25. If properly trained use an automated external defibrillator (AED). AEDs are not recommended for children younger than 8 years of age.

    In hospital setting, use defibrillator as specified by institution protocol. Defibrillator should be placed only by properly trained personnel.

25. The use of an AED can increase the client's chances for survival by restoring rhythm and circulation. AEDs have been adequately tested in children, and excessive joules may cause injury.

    Protocol in hospital setting include the use of defibrillator with codes and can increase survival. Injury to self, staff, or the client may occur with untrained personnel.

EVALUATION

- There should be a constant evaluation for the return of spontaneous pulse and respirations.
- Successful intervention with CPR is illustrated as follows:
  — An open airway is maintained, as evident by the chest rise and fall.
  — The resistance and compliance of the client's lungs is felt.
  — Airway movement during expiration is felt and heard.
  — Circulation indicators, such as color, improve.
  — The client has return of spontaneous pulse and respirations, as evidenced by a palpable carotid or brachial pulse and the presence of respiratory effort.
- Assist with transfer to hospital/advanced life-support unit.
- If CPR was unsuccessful, assist in notifying next of kin and providing psychosocial support.

DOCUMENTATION

Nurses' Notes/Code Record

- Time and condition in which the client was found
- Interventions that were implemented, including accurate times, results of the implementations, orders received from the physicians, vital signs of the client, timing of the incident, and status of the client afterward

Medication Administration Record

- Medications the client received, including time and route, during the procedure
- If the incident occurs in a noninstitutional setting, report findings and interventions to aid personnel when they arrive.

PROCEDURE 26-37   Admitting a Client

OVERVIEW

The procedure for admitting a client to a health care facility is extremely important. First impressions of the facility and caregivers are lasting ones. A calm, caring approach instills confidence in the client and the belief that the client's needs are important. Orienting the client to the room, nursing unit, and facility will help the client to be comfortable in the health care environment.

ASSESSMENT

1. Assess the client's comfort level about being in a health care facility. **Identifies needed nurse–client interactions.**

2. Assess client's physical and mental state. **Provides basis for nursing care. Shows caring and concern for the client.**

3. Assess client's knowledge of reason for admission. **Provides basis for nurse–client interaction and client teaching.**

continues

POSSIBLE NURSING DIAGNOSES

Fear
Anxiety
Deficient Knowledge (health care facility)

PLANNING

Expected Outcomes

1. Client will be comfortable in health care facility.
2. Client will understand how to use call bell system, bed controls, television, and telephone.
3. The client will adjust to facility routine.

Equipment Needed

- Admission kit: wash basin, emesis basin, pitcher, glass, etc.
- Client orientation materials
- Valuables envelope (if needed)
- Belongings checklist
- Admission Nursing Assessment form
- Sphygmomanometer, stethoscope, thermometer

DELEGATION TIPS

Admitting a client may be delegated to ancillary personnel after proper instruction. The nursing assessment must be performed by the nurse and may not be delegated.

IMPLEMENTATION—ACTION/RATIONALE

ACTION

❋ Cleanse hands ❋

1. Welcome client to unit. Introduce yourself by name and title. Ask client to state his or her name.
2. Orient client to room and nursing unit. Describe items such as nurse call bell system, location of bathroom, place for clothing, bed controls, television, telephone, visiting hours, meal times, Standard Precautions, and review items in client education materials such as client rights and other written information about the facility.
3. Provide privacy for client to change into pajamas or hospital gown, if not already done.
4. Show client ID bracelet to double-check proper identification. Attach bracelet to wrist. (This may have been done in Admitting Department.) Review drug allergies and attach allergy bracelet to same wrist, according to agency policy.
5. Document and store client's belongings and valuables according to agency policy.
6. Begin nursing assessment, according to agency policy.
7. Perform any other actions, as directed by agency policy.

RATIONALE

1. Verifies identification.

2. Reduces client anxiety; allows fuller participation in care.

3. Respects client privacy.

4. Confirms client identification; promotes client safety.

5. Reduces the risk of loss.

6. Starts development of client database.
7. Different facilities have different needs, regulations, and guidelines for client admission.

EVALUATION

- The client is comfortable in the health care facility.
- The client uses call bell system, bed controls, television, and telephone.
- The client has adjusted to facility routing.

DOCUMENTATION

- Complete admitting nursing assessment record
- Time and condition of client on admission
- All valuables sent to the safe
- Client's belongings
- Client's comfort level

PROCEDURE 26-38   Transferring a Client

OVERVIEW

Transferring a client to a different unit in a health care facility can be very stressful to the client. It may mean that the client's condition has deteriorated (transferring to ICU) or improved (transferring to a rehabilitation unit after a hip replacement), thus requiring different treatments.

However short the stay before a transfer, the client has a sense of knowing the environment and the health care personnel on that unit. Explaining the reason for transfer to the client and family, as well as gathering all equipment, medications, and client's personal belongings, help ease the stress of a transfer.

Introducing the client and family to health care personnel working on the new unit and sharing some of the client's personal preferences in the client's presence (i.e., prefers one pillow and an extra blanket) shows caring and concern for the client and helps ensure continuity of care.

ASSESSMENT

1. Assess client's knowledge and feelings about the transfer. **Allows for explanations and discussion about the situation.**
2. Assess which equipment is to be transferred with the client and that those medications and client's personal belongings are ready to move. **Provides organization to the transfer and encourages completeness.**
3. Assess readiness of new unit to accept client. **Allows transfer to proceed smoothly with no waiting.**

POSSIBLE NURSING DIAGNOSES

Anxiety
Fear
Hopelessness

PLANNING

Expected Outcomes

1. Client will understand reason for transfer.
2. Client will be safely moved with needed equipment and medications and all personal belongings.
3. Client's move will be communicated to appropriate department for continuity of care (i.e., Dietary, Pharmacy).

Equipment Needed

- Client's medical record (if not electronic)
- Client's imprint card
- Client's medications
- Stretcher or wheelchair
- Cart to carry client's belongings

DELEGATION TIPS

Transferring a client is a skill that ancillary personnel may assist with. The nurse is responsible for transferring the client's medical record and medications and for giving a thorough report to the accepting nurse on the new unit.

IMPLEMENTATION—ACTION/RATIONALE

ACTION

RATIONALE

∗ Cleanse hands ∗ Check client's identification band ∗

ACTION	RATIONALE
1. Check to see if order is needed to initiate transfer according to agency policy.	1. Policies differ among facilities.
2. Call nursing unit of new location to see if bed is ready and to give report.	2. Provides continuity of care.
3. Explain the transfer to the client (and family, if appropriate). Answer any questions. Allay anxieties about moving.	3. Keeps client informed and promotes cooperation.
4. Review the valuables and belongings checklist completed on admission. Compare with belongings.	4. Ensures all of client's belongings are transferred with the client. Prevents loss.

continues

5. Gather records and any other equipment that will be transferred with the client, according to agency policy, such as eyedrops, other medications, IV pump, respiratory therapy equipment, and so on.
6. Transfer client by appropriate vehicle (wheelchair, stretcher). Accompany client to new unit. Transfer care to another staff member in person. Ensure that call bell is within reach or staff member is in room before leaving client.
7. Document time of transfer and any other information required by agency policy.
8. Upon return to unit, notify appropriate personnel according to agency policy that client has left the unit. Arrange for personnel to clean the bed and surroundings the client has left.

5. Helps make transfer more efficient and reduces multiple trips to new area.

6. Enhances continuity of care. Promotes safety.

7. Promotes communication among members of the health care team.
8. Prepares bed for new admission. Reduces transfer of microorganisms.

EVALUATION

- The client understands the reason for transferring to a new unit.
- The client is safely moved with needed equipment and medications and all personal belongings.
- The client's move was communicated to appropriate departments for continuity of care.

DOCUMENTATION

- Client's condition when leaving unit
- Equipment and medications transferred with the client
- Personal belongings sent with client.
- Report on client given to receiving nurse
- Departments notified of client's transfer

PROCEDURE 26-39   Discharging a Client

OVERVIEW

A client may be discharged from a health care facility to another facility or to home. This can be a frightening experience depending on the level of recuperation the client has achieved, the amount and type of medications prescribed, dietary needs or restrictions, and other treatments to be conducted. Being transferred from one facility to another may be seen either as improvement or as a lack of progress in recovery.

Discuss with the client and family the discharge process. Complete all paperwork and all discharge teaching. Collect the client's belongings and valuables (as documented on admission) so they can accompany the client. These things will help make the discharge process pleasant and effective.

ASSESSMENT

1. Assess client's feelings about being discharged. **Opens communication about the discharge.**
2. Assess that family and home or the other facility is prepared to receive the client. **Provides a smooth process with less stress for the client.**
3. Assess client's or family's knowledge of care at home. **Ensures continuity of care.**

POSSIBLE NURSING DIAGNOSES

Anxiety
Readiness for Enhanced Therapeutic Regimen Management

continues

PLANNING

Expected Outcomes

1. Client will complete discharge to another facility with no problems.
2. Client will feel confident about care at home.

Equipment Needed

- Required facility paperwork
- Stretcher or wheelchair
- Cart for client's belongings

For discharge to home

- Prescriptions
- Instructions—care, diet, medications, follow-up appointment

DELEGATION TIPS

The physical movement of the client for discharge may be done by ancillary personnel. The nurse must review with the client prescriptions and instructions on care, diet, medications, and making a follow-up appointment.

IMPLEMENTATION—ACTION/RATIONALE

ACTION	RATIONALE
* Cleanse hands * Check client's identification band *	
1. Check order for discharge.	1. Most agency policies require order for discharge.
Discharge to Another Facility	
2. Explain discharge to client, and family, if appropriate.	2. Includes client in care. Promotes cooperation.
3. Complete intra-agency transfer form, according to policy. Be sure to note last time of medication doses. Complete nursing discharge summary. Prepare transfer paperwork, according to policy.	3. Facilitates continuity of care. Promotes client safety.
4. Notify receiving agency of impending transfer. Provide report and confirm ability to receive client.	4. Facilitates continuity of care. Ensures that new facility will accept client before client leaves current facility.
5. Arrange for transportation to new facility. Call transportation company according to agency policy.	5. Reduces waiting time; facilitates continuity of care.
6. Review the valuables and belongings checklist completed on admission. Compare with belongings.	6. Ensures all of client's belongings leave with the client. Prevents loss.
7. When personnel from transportation company arrive, assist client transfer to stretcher or wheelchair. Provide transportation personnel with required information, such as client's DNR status, for transfer. See that client's belongings accompany client, along with any required paperwork or equipment.	7. Provides continuity of care.
Discharge to Home	
8. Discuss discharge with client, and family, if appropriate. Confirm that discharge teaching has been done. Ask client if there are any questions about self-care at home. If so, follow up with appropriate personnel (typically, RN).	8. Promotes client cooperation. Allays anxiety.

continues

9. LP/VN or RN (according to agency policy) reviews with client: prescriptions to be filled, including telling client when next dose is due based on medications administered in the facility; food and drug interactions and any other essential medication information; care of incision or dressings, if indicated; dietary needs or restrictions or other pertinent information; and when client should make appointment for follow-up with private physician.

10. Have client/family provide return demonstration of skills required for self-care at home.

11. Check that transportation to home is available. Check client room area for any personal belongings.

12. Complete any paperwork with client, as required by agency policy.

13. Escort client to transportation vehicle.

For Any Discharge

14. Notify appropriate personnel according to agency policy that client has left the unit. Arrange for personnel to clean the bed and surroundings the client has left.

9. Promotes continuity of care.

10. Demonstrates that learning has occurred.

11. Reduces waiting time.

12. Meets regulatory requirements.

13. Promotes client safety.

14. Prepares bed for new admission. Reduces transfer of microorganisms.

EVALUATION

- The client encountered no problems in discharge to another facility.
- The client, with the assistance of family, is confident about care at home.

DOCUMENTATION

- Date and time of discharge
- Belongings and valuables with client

Discharge to another facility

- Person receiving report on client
- Company transporting client

Discharge to home

- Mode of taking client to transportation vehicle
- Person taking client home
- Prescriptions and instructions given to client

References/Suggested Readings

Centers for Disease Control and Prevention (CDC). (2002). *Guideline for hand hygiene in health-care settings.* [Online]. Available: www.cdc.gov/mmwr/preview/mmwrhtml/rr5116a1.htm

Daniels, R. (2002). *Delmar's Guide to Laboratory and Diagnostic Tests.* Clifton Park, NY: Thomson Delmar Learning.

Infection Control. (2002). "Hand hygiene" news. *Nursing2002, 32*(5), 32hn6.

Martin, P. (2003). CPR when the patient's pregnant. *RN, 66*(8), 34–39.

Nelson, A., Owen, B., Lloyd, J., Fragala, G., Matz, M., Amato, M., Bowers, J., Moss-Cureton, S., Ramsey, G., & Lentz, K. (2003). Safe patient handling and movement. *AJN, 103*(3), 32–43.

North American Nursing Diagnosis Association. (2003). *Nursing Diagnoses: Definitions & Classification 2003–2004.* Philadelphia, PA: Author.

Parini, S., & Myers, F. (2003). Keeping up with hand hygiene recommendations. *Nursing2003, 33*(2), 17.

Pullen, R. (2003). Caring for a patient on pulse oximetry. *Nursing2003, 33*(9), 30.

Ramponi, D. (2001). Eye on contact lens removal. *Nursing2001, 31*(8), 56–57.

INTERMEDIATE PROCEDURES

PROCEDURE 27-1 — Surgical Asepsis: Preparing and Maintaining a Sterile Field

OVERVIEW

Preparing and maintaining a sterile field is basic to many nursing procedures, such as inserting a urinary catheter and changing surgical dressings. It takes practice to develop a "sterile conscience," a consistent awareness of what is sterile, and to maintain the sterility.

ASSESSMENT

1. Assess all packages to determine that they are dry and intact. **Assesses the sterility of packages.**
2. Assess the local environment for a dry, horizontal, stable area. **A dry, flat workspace is best for a sterile field.**

POSSIBLE NURSING DIAGNOSIS

Risk for Infection

PLANNING

Expected Outcomes

1. Sterility of the field and all packages, while being opened, will be maintained.
2. Sterility of the procedure will be maintained.

Equipment Needed

- Sterile kit as needed for procedure
- Sterile gloves (if not in kit)
- Sterile drape (if needed)
- Sterile solution (if needed)
- Other sterile items as required

DELEGATION TIPS

Only nurses should prepare and maintain a sterile field, with the exception of surgical technicians in the OR.

IMPLEMENTATION—ACTION/RATIONALE

ACTION	RATIONALE
* Cleanse hands * Check client's identification band *	
1. Gather equipment for the type of procedure: a. Select only clean, dry packages marked sterile, and read listing of contents. b. Check the package for integrity and expiration date.	1. Prevents break in technique during procedure. If the package is moist or outdated, it is considered contaminated and cannot be used.

continues

2. Select a clean area in the client's environment to establish the sterile field.
3. Explain procedure to the client; provide specific instructions if client assistance is required during the procedure.
4. Inquire about and attend to the client's toileting needs.
5. Hospital environment: If the procedure is to be performed at the client's bedside, the client should be in a private room or moved to a clean treatment room if available.
6. Home environment: Secure privacy and remove pets from the room.
7. Position client and attend to comfort measures; the client's position should provide easy access to the area and facilitate good body mechanics during the procedure.
8. Cleanse hands.
9. Place sterile package (drape or tray) in the center of the clean, dry work area.

2. Promotes access to the sterile field during the procedure.
3. Gains client's understanding and cooperation during the procedure.
4. Prevents break in technique during the procedure.
5. Minimizes microorganisms in the environment.

6. Puts the client at ease and promotes a clean environment.
7. Helps the client relax and prevents movement during the procedure; prevents reaching, decreasing the risk of contamination and back strain.
8. Prevents transmission of microorganisms.
9. Prevents reaching over exposed sterile items when wrapper is removed.

Drape

10. Open the wrapper, pulling away from the body first.
11. Grasp the top edge of drape with fingertips of one hand.
12. Remove the drape by lifting up and away from all objects while it unfolds; discard the outer wrapper with other hand.
13. With free hand, grasp the other drape corner, keeping it away from all objects.
14. Lay the drape on the surface, with the drape bottom first touching the surface farthest from you; step back and allow the drape to cover the surface.

10. Prevents contamination.
11. Edges are considered unsterile.
12. If the drape touches an unsterile object, it is contaminated and must be discarded.
13. Avoids contamination.
14. Prevents you from reaching over the sterile field; stepping back decreases risk that drape will touch your uniform.

Tray

15. Remove outer wrapping and place the tray on the work surface so that the top flap of the sterile wrapper opens away from you.
16. Reach around the tray, not over it. With thumb and index fingertips grasping the wrapper's top flap, gently pull up, then down to open over the surface.
17. Repeat the same steps to open the side flaps.
18. Grasp the corner of the bottom flap with fingertips, step back, and pull flap down (Figure 27-1-1).

15. Prevents reaching over the sterile items.

16. Only the edges of the field can be contaminated, pulling up frees the top folded flap.

17. Keeps the arm from reaching over the sterile field.
18. Creates a sterile work surface.

Figure 27-1-1 Grasp the corner of the bottom flap with fingertips, step back, and pull flap down (gloves not required for this procedure).

continues

Figure 27-1-2 Grasp the flaps of the wrapped supply and pull downward.

Figure 27-1-3 Add contents to the sterile field by holding the package 6 inches (15 cm) above the field and allowing the contents to drop onto the field.

Adding Additional Sterile Items to Sterile Field

19. While facing the sterile field, step back, remove the outer wrapper, and grasp the item in your nondominant hand so that the top flap will open away from you.
20. With your dominant hand, open the flaps as previously described.
21. With your dominant hand, pull the wrapper back and away from the sterile field (toward your nondominant arm holding the item) and place the item onto the field.
22. When adding additional gauze or dressings to the sterile field, open the package as directed, grasp the top flaps of the wrapper and pull downward (Figure 27-1-2), then drop the contents onto the center of the field (Figure 27-1-3).

19. Keeps your dominant hand free, item remains sterile.

20. Prevents reaching over the sterile item.

21. Prevents the wrapper from touching the sterile field.

22. Prevents contamination of item and sterile field.

Adding Solutions to Sterile Field

23. Read the labels and strengths of all solutions three times before pouring.
24. Remove the lid from the bottle of solution and invert the lid onto a clean surface.
25. Hold the bottle, label facing ceiling, 4 to 6 inches (10 to 15 cm) over the container on the sterile field; slowly pour the solution into the container to avoid splashing. Pour from the side of the sterile field. Do not reach over it.

26. Replace the lid on the container, label the container with the date and time, and initial the container.

23. Ensures proper solution and strength.

24. Inverting the lid prevents contamination of the inner surface.

25. Prevents the label from getting wet. If the solution splashes onto the label, the field is contaminated because moisture conducts microorganisms from the nonsterile surface. Prevents contamination. If the solution splashes out of the container and the drape becomes wet, the field is contaminated.

26. Sterility of the solution will be lost if exposed to air for an extended period.

Using Sterile Gloves

27. Cleanse hands and perform open gloving (see Procedure 27-2).
28. Continue with procedure, keeping gloved hands above waist level at all times, touching only items on the sterile field.
29. If using a solution to cleanse a site, use the sterile forceps to prevent contamination of gloves; dispose of forceps after use or process instruments according to agency policy.

27. Prevents transmission of microorganisms.

28. Decreases chance of contamination.

29. Prevents field contamination.

continues

30. Postprocedure, dispose of all contaminated items in colored plastic bag.	30. Decreases risk of transmission of microorganisms to all health care workers.
31. Remove gloves as shown in Procedure 27-2.	31. Minimizes risk of contact with infectious wastes on the gloves.
32. Reposition the client.	32. Promotes client comfort.
33. Clean the environment; cleanse hands.	33. Prevents transmission of microorganisms.

EVALUATION

- Sterility of field was maintained.
- Sterility of procedure was maintained.

DOCUMENTATION

- Procedure completed following sterile technique.

PROCEDURE 27-2   Performing Open Gloving

OVERVIEW

Asepsis, or sterile technique, consists of those practices that eliminate all microorganisms and spores from an object or area. The use of sterile gloves is at the heart of aseptic technique. The ability to manipulate sterile items without contaminating them is critical to many diagnostic and therapeutic interventions. Common nursing procedures that require sterile technique are:

- All invasive procedures, either intentional perforation of the skin (injection, insertion of IV needles or catheters) or entry into a body orifice (tracheobronchial suctioning, insertion of a urinary catheter)
- Nursing measures for clients with disruption of skin surfaces (changing a surgical wound or IV site dressing) or destruction of skin layers (trauma and burns)

There are two methods for applying sterile gloves: open and closed. The open method is used most frequently when performing procedures that require the sterile technique, such as dressing changes, but that do not require donning a sterile gown.

ASSESSMENT

1. Assess the glove package. Is it intact? Is it wet or otherwise contaminated? **Assesses the sterility of the glove.**
2. Assess the local environment. Is there an area suitable for opening the package and applying the gloves? Is it dry? Is it reasonably stable and horizontal? Are there obvious airborne contaminants? **A flat, clear workspace is necessary to successfully carry out the procedure.**
3. Assess the correct glove size for proper fit. **Gloves come in many sizes, and proper fit is conducive to maintaining asepsis.**

POSSIBLE NURSING DIAGNOSIS

Risk for Infection

PLANNING

Expected Outcomes

1. Sterility of the gloves will be maintained while they are being applied.
2. Sterility of the procedure will be maintained.

Equipment Needed

- Package of proper-sized sterile gloves

DELEGATION TIPS

Sterile gloving is only delegated if the personnel are specifically trained, such as in a surgical suite or a testing laboratory setting.

continues

IMPLEMENTATION—ACTION/RATIONALE

ACTION

1. Cleanse hands.
2. Read the manufacturer's instructions on the package of sterile gloves; proceed as directed in removing the outer wrapper from the package (Figure 27-2-1), placing the inner wrapper onto a clean, dry surface. Open inner wrapper to expose gloves (Figure 27-2-2).

Figure 27-2-1 Remove the outer wrapper of the sterile glove package.

3. Identify right and left hand; glove dominant hand first.

4. Grasp the 2-inch- (5-cm-) wide cuff with the thumb and first two fingers of the nondominant hand, touching only the inside of the cuff (Figure 27-2-3).
5. Gently pull the glove over the dominant hand, making sure the thumb and fingers fit into the proper spaces of the glove.
6. With the gloved dominant hand, slip your fingers under the cuff of the other glove, gloved thumb abducted, making sure it does not touch any part on your nondominant hand (Figure 27-2-4).
7. Gently slip the glove onto your nondominant hand, making sure the fingers slip into the proper spaces (Figures 27-2-5 and 27-2-6).

Figure 27-2-3 Grasp first cuff with the nondominant hand.

RATIONALE

1. Prevents transmission of microorganisms.
2. Different manufacturers package gloves differently; the instructions will tell you how to open properly to avoid contamination of the inner wrapper; any moisture on the surface will contaminate the gloves.

Figure 27-2-2 Open the inner wrapper to expose glove.

3. Dominant hand should facilitate motor dexterity during gloving.
4. Maintains sterility of the outer surfaces of the sterile glove.

5. Prevents tearing the glove material; guiding the fingers into proper places facilitates gloving.

6. Cuff protects gloved fingers, maintaining sterility.

7. Contact is made with two sterile gloves.

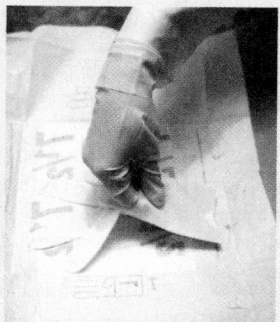

Figure 27-2-4 Slip fingers under the cuff of the second glove.

continues

Figure 27-2-5   Pull on the second glove.

Figure 27-2-6   Make sure all fingers are in the proper spaces.

8. With gloved hands, interlock fingers to fit the gloves onto each finger. If the gloves are soiled, remove by turning inside out as follows:

8. Promotes proper fit over the fingers.

Removing Gloves

9. Slip gloved fingers of the dominant hand under the cuff of the opposite hand or grasp the outer part of the glove at the wrist if there is no cuff.

9. Contact is made with two sterile gloves.

10. Pull the glove down to the fingers, exposing the thumb (Figure 27-2-7).

10. Frees the thumb for the next step.

11. Slip the uncovered thumb into the opposite glove at the wrist allowing only the glove-covered fingers of the hand to touch the soiled glove (Figure 27-2-8).

11. Contact is made with two sterile gloves.

Figure 27-2-7   Peel glove down to fingers, exposing one thumb.

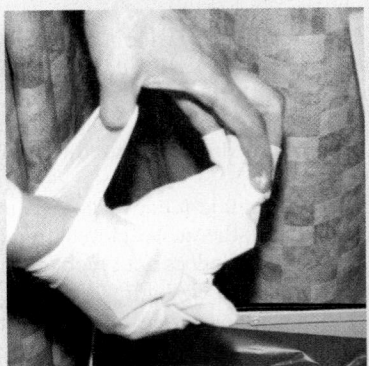

Figure 27-2-8   Slip uncovered thumb into the opposite glove.

12. Pull the glove down over the dominant hand almost to the fingertips and slip the glove over the first glove (Figure 27-2-9).

12. Removes glove without contact with soiled surfaces.

13. With the dominant hand touching only the inside of the other glove, pull the glove over the dominant hand so that only the inside (clean surface) is exposed.

13. Exposes only the clean surface of the gloves.

14. Dispose of soiled gloves according to institutional policy and cleanse hands (Figure 27-2-10).

14. Prevents transfer of microorganisms.

continues

Figure 27-2-9 When soiled gloves are removed correctly, only the inside, clean surface of one glove is exposed.

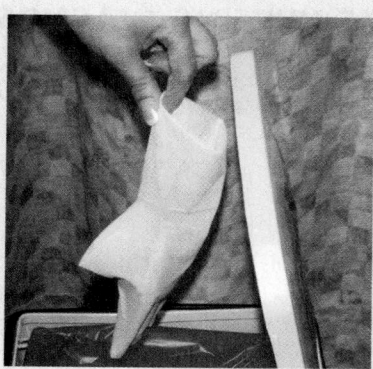

Figure 27-2-10 Dispose of gloves in appropriate receptacle.

EVALUATION

- Sterility of the gloves and sterile field was maintained without breaks.

DOCUMENTATION

Nurses' Notes

- Procedure was performed using sterile technique.

PROCEDURE 27-3   Performing Urinary Catheterization: Female/Male

OVERVIEW

Catheterization involves passing a rubber or plastic tube into the bladder via the urethra to drain urine from the bladder or to obtain a urine specimen. Intermittent catheterization may be used to obtain a sample or to relieve bladder distention. Indwelling catheters may be used short-term to keep the bladder empty, prevent urinary retention, or allow precise measurement of urine. Long-term indwelling, or retention, catheters are used to control incontinence, prevent retention, or prevent the leakage of urine. Catheterization is a sterile procedure.

ASSESSMENT

1. Assess the need for catheterization and the type of catheterization ordered **to ensure the proper procedure is carried out.**
2. Assess for the need for perineal care before catheterization **to reduce the transmission of microorganisms.**
3. Assess the urinary meatus for signs of infection or inflammation. Ask the client for any history of latex allergy, difficulty with prior catheterizations, anxiety, or urinary strictures. **Allows detection of potential complications.**
4. Assess the client's ability to assist with the procedure. Can she maintain the proper position while you perform the procedure? Is the client agitated, and could she contaminate the sterile field? Will you need assistance to hold her legs in position? **Determines how the procedure is to be carried out.**
5. Assess the light. Will you be able to see well enough to place the catheter, or do you need a secondary light source? **Determines what preparation needs to be done to ensure a successful procedure.**
6. Assess for an allergy to povidone-iodine and/or latex **to avoid an allergic reaction.**
7. Watch for indications of distress or embarrassment, especially if the nurse is of the opposite gender, **to determine what teaching and support are needed.** Explore further if indicated.

continues

POSSIBLE NURSING DIAGNOSES

*Risk for **I**nfection*
*Risk for **I**mpaired Skin Integrity*
*Deficient **K**nowledge* (insertion of a catheter)

PLANNING

Expected Outcomes

1. A catheter will be inserted without pain, trauma, or injury to the client.
2. The client's bladder will be emptied without complication.
3. The nurse will maintain the sterility of the catheter during insertion.

Equipment Needed

- Straight or indwelling catheter with drainage system (Figure 27-3-1)
- Sterile catheterization kit (Figure 27-3-2)
- Adequate lighting source
- Disposable clean gloves
- Blanket or drape
- Soap and washcloth
- Warm water
- Towel

Figure 27-3-1 Indwelling and Straight Catheters

Figure 27-3-2 Catheterization Kit

DELEGATION TIPS

Insertion of an indwelling catheter in a female client is generally not delegated to ancillary personnel. The delegation of this skill depends on institution policy and the availability of licensed staff versus properly trained ancillary personnel. Male urinary catheterization may be delegated to properly trained ancillary personnel depending on institution policies. The nurse is responsible to evaluate the client for contraindications to delegating this procedure, such as the risk for a difficult or traumatic insertion. The nurse may then decide to perform the procedure or to defer to the health care practitioner.

IMPLEMENTATION—ACTION/RATIONALE

ACTION

RATIONALE

❋ **Check client's identification band** ❋ **Explain procedure before beginning** ❋

Performing Urinary Catheterization

1. Gather the equipment needed. Read the label on the catheterization kit. Note if the catheter is included in the kit and, if so, what type it is. Gather any supplies you will need that are not in the prepackaged kit.

2. Provide for privacy. Assess for allergy to povidone-iodine.

1. Promotes efficiency in the procedure. Kits from various manufacturers come with different equipment. The catheter may or may not be packaged in the kit. Sterile gloves and the urine drainage bag may also need to be gathered separately.

2. Promotes client dignity. Prevents known allergic reactions.

continues

Figure 27-3-3 Position the client supine with legs spread.

Figure 27-3-4 Open the catheterization kit, using the wrapper to establish a sterile field between the client's legs.

3. Set the bed to a comfortable height to work, and raise the side rail on the side opposite you.
4. Assist the client to a supine position with legs spread and feet together (Figure 27-3-3).
5. Drape the client's abdomen and thighs for warmth if needed.
6. Ensure adequate lighting of the perineal area.
7. Cleanse hands and apply disposable gloves.
8. Wash perineal area.
9. Remove gloves and cleanse hands.
10. Open the catheterization kit, using aseptic technique. Use the wrapper to establish a sterile field (Figure 27-3-4).

11. If the catheter is not included in the kit, drop the sterile catheter onto the field using aseptic technique. Add any other items needed.
12. Apply sterile gloves. These may be included in the kit.

13. If inserting a retention catheter, attach the syringe filled with sterile water to the Luerlock tail of the catheter. Inflate and deflate the retention balloon. Detach the water-filled syringe (Figure 27-3-5).
14. Attach the catheter to the urine drainage bag if it is not preconnected.

15. Generously coat the distal portion of the catheter with water-soluble, sterile lubricant and place it nearby on the sterile field (Figure 27-3-6).

3. Promotes proper body mechanics and ensures client safety.
4. Relaxes muscles and allows visualization of the area to facilitate insertion of the catheter.
5. Promotes client comfort and warmth.

6. Facilitates proper execution of technique.
7. Reduces transfer of microorganisms.
8. Reduces transfer of microorganisms.
9. Reduces transfer of microorganisms.
10. Provides an area for the sterile equipment to be laid out and assembled. Establish the sterile field close to the client. If the client is able to cooperate, the sterile field can sometimes be established in the open area between the client's legs.
11. Prevents contamination of the sterile equipment and the sterile field.

12. Prevents contamination of the sterile equipment and the sterile field.
13. Tests the patency of the retention balloon. Detaching the syringe prevents accidental inflation during catheter insertion.

14. The catheter and drainage system may be preconnected; otherwise connect it before catheterization to avoid exposing the client to ascending infection from an open-ended catheter.
15. Facilitates catheter insertion.

Figure 27-3-5 Inflate and deflate the retention balloon to test its patency.

Figure 27-3-6 Open the lubrication package and squeeze lubricant onto the sterile field where it will be used to lubricate the catheter.

continues

Figure 27-3-7 Spread the labia minora and visualize the urinary meatus.

Figure 27-3-8 Using forceps, pick up a cotton ball soaked in povidone-iodine. Cleanse the periurethral mucosa.

Female Client

16. Place the fenestrated drape from the catheterization kit over the client's perineal area with the labia visible through the opening.

17. Gently spread the labia minora with the fingers of your nondominant hand and visualize the urinary meatus (Figure 27-3-7).

18. Holding the labia apart with your nondominant hand, use the forceps to pick up a cotton ball soaked in povidone-iodine, and cleanse the periurethral mucosa. Use one downward stroke for each cotton ball and dispose. Keep the labia separated with your nondominant hand until you insert the catheter (Figure 27-3-8).

19. Holding the catheter in the dominant hand, steadily insert the catheter into the meatus until urine is noted in the drainage bag or tubing (Figure 27-3-9).

20. If the catheter will be removed as soon as the client's bladder is empty, insert the catheter another inch and hold the catheter in place as the bladder drains.

21. If the catheter will be indwelling with a retention balloon, continue inserting another 1 to 3 inches.

16. Provides a sterile field at the procedural site. Prevents accidental contamination from adjacent areas.

17. Helps locate the meatus, so the catheter can be placed in the correct spot.

18. Cleans the area and minimizes the risk of urinary tract infection by removing surface pathogens.

19. Provides a visual confirmation that the catheter tip is in the bladder.

20. The catheter needs to be inserted far enough to allow complete bladder drainage, but not so far as to possibly irritate the bladder, causing spasms.

21. Ensures adequate catheter insertion before retention balloon is inflated.

Figure 27-3-9 Steadily insert the catheter into the meatus.

continues

Male Client

22. Place the fenestrated drape from the catheterization kit over the client's perineal area with the penis extending through the opening.

23. If inserting a retention catheter, attach the syringe filled with sterile water to the Luerlock tail of the catheter. Inflate and deflate the retention balloon. Detach the water-filled syringe.

24. Attach the catheter to the urine drainage bag if it is not preconnected.

25. Generously coat the distal portion of the catheter with water-soluble, sterile lubricant and place it nearby on the sterile field.

26. With your nondominant hand, gently grasp the penis and retract the foreskin (if present). With your dominant hand, cleanse the glans penis with a povidone-iodine solution or other antimicrobial cleanser (Figure 27-3-10).

27. Hold the penis perpendicular to the body and pull up gently.

28. Inject 10 mL sterile, water-soluble lubricant (use a 2% Xylocaine lubricant whenever feasible) into the urethra.

29. Holding the catheter in the dominant hand, steadily insert the catheter about 8 inches, until urine is noted in the drainage bag or tubing (Figure 27-3-11).

30. If the catheter will be removed as soon as the client's bladder is empty, insert the catheter another inch, place the penis in a comfortable position, and hold the catheter in place as the bladder drains.

31. If the catheter will be indwelling with a retention balloon, continue inserting until the hub of the catheter (bifurcation between drainage port and retention balloon arm) is met.

32. Reattach the water-filled syringe to the inflation port.

33. Inflate the retention balloon using manufacturer's recommendations or according to the health care provider's orders (Figure 27-3-12).

22. Provides a sterile field at the procedural site. Prevents accidental contamination from adjacent areas.

23. Tests the patency of the retention balloon. Detaching the syringe prevents accidental inflation during catheter insertion.

24. The catheter and drainage system may be preconnected; otherwise it is connected before catheterization to avoid exposing the client to ascending infection from an open-ended catheter.

25. Facilitates catheter insertion.

26. Removes dirt and minimizes the risk of urinary tract infection by removing surface pathogens.

27. Facilitates catheter insertion by straightening urethra.

28. Avoids urethral trauma and discomfort during catheter insertion and facilitates insertion.

29. Provides a visual confirmation that the catheter tip is in the bladder.

30. The catheter needs to be inserted far enough to allow complete bladder drainage, but not so far as to possibly irritate the bladder, causing spasms.

31. Ensures adequate catheter insertion before retention balloon is inflated.

32. Provides a sterile method of inflating the retention balloon.

33. Ensures retention of the balloon. Retention catheters are available with a variety of balloon sizes. Use a catheter with the appropriate size balloon.

Figure 27-3-10   Cleanse the glans penis with a povidone-iodine solution.

Figure 27-3-11   Steadily insert the catheter.

continues

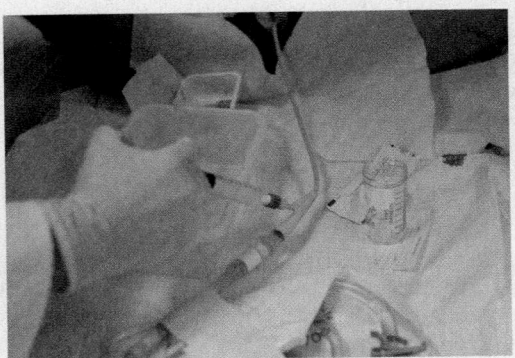

Figure 27-3-12   Inflate the retention balloon.

Figure 27-3-13   Tape the catheter to the client's thigh.

34. Instruct the client to immediately report discomfort or pressure during balloon inflation; if pain occurs, discontinue the procedure, deflate the balloon, and insert the catheter farther into the bladder. If the client continues to complain of pain with balloon inflation, remove the catheter and notify the client's health care provider.

35. Once the balloon has been inflated, gently pull the catheter until the retention balloon is resting snugly against the bladder neck (resistance will be felt when the balloon is properly seated).

36. Tape the catheter to the thigh with enough slack so it will not pull on the bladder (Figure 27-3-13).

37. Place the drainage bag below the level of the bladder. Do not let it rest on the floor. Make sure the tubing lies over, not under, the leg (Figures 27-3-14 and 27-3-15).

38. Remove gloves, dispose of equipment, and cleanse hands.

39. Help client adjust position. Lower the bed.

40. Assess and document the amount, color, odor, and quality of urine (Figure 27-3-16).

41. Cleanse hands.

34. Pain or pressure indicates inflation of the balloon in the urethra; further insertion will prevent misplacement and further pain or bleeding.

35. Maximizes continuous bladder drainage and prevents urine leakage around the catheter.

36. Prevents excessive traction from the balloon rubbing against the bladder neck, inadvertent catheter removal, or urethral erosion.

37. Maximizes continuous drainage of urine from the bladder (drainage is prevented when the drainage bag is placed above the abdomen).

38. Prevents transfer of microorganisms.

39. Promotes client comfort and safety.

40. Monitors urinary status.

41. Reduces transmission of microorganisms.

Figure 27-3-14   Place the drainage bag tubing over the leg.

Figure 27-3-15   Place the drainage bag below the level of the bladder, but do not rest it on the floor.

continues

Figure 27-3-16 Monitor the urinary status. Assess and document the amount, color, and quality of urine.

EVALUATION

- The catheter was inserted without pain, trauma, or injury to the client.
- The client's bladder was emptied without complication.
- The nurse maintained the sterility of the catheter during insertion.

DOCUMENTATION

Nurses' Notes

- Time and date the catheter was inserted
- Size and type of catheter used, including the size of the retention balloon and the amount of sterile water used to inflate the balloon
- Client's response to the procedure and the amount, color, and quality of urine returned

Intake and Output Record

- Amount of urine returned

PROCEDURE 27-4   Irrigating a Urinary Catheter

OVERVIEW

Open intermittent irrigation of a urinary catheter is generally done for one of two reasons: either to instill medication into the bladder or to irrigate the catheter itself, which may be blocked by either blood clots or urinary sediment. This irrigation is referred to as "open" because the closed bladder drainage system is opened where the drainage tubing inserts into the urinary catheter; the catheter is generally indwelling. Maintaining sterility of the system is paramount in this type of irrigation.

ASSESSMENT

1. Identify the following items in the health care provider's orders: type of irrigation (bladder or catheter); purpose of the irrigation; type and amount of solution to irrigate with; any premedication ordered; and any other details of the order. **Allows the nurse to anticipate responses to the procedure and assess pertinent features of the client's condition.**

2. Assess the condition of the client as it relates to the procedure: patency of the catheter, characteristics of urinary drainage, and total intake and output status of the client. **Establishes a baseline of the client's condition as it relates to elimination and in the case of PRN catheterization, which may indicate whether there is a need for the procedure.**

3. Assess for current pain or bladder spasms. **Even when medication is not specifically ordered, medicating**

continues

for pain before the procedure can increase client comfort, and if irrigation does not relieve spasms, the client may need medication afterward.

4. Assess client's knowledge about the procedure **to determine need for education and reduce anxiety about the procedure.**

5. If this is a repeat of the procedure, read the charting from previous times. **Provides a history of how this client tolerates the procedure and of any teaching done.**

POSSIBLE NURSING DIAGNOSES

*Risk for **I**nfection*
*Impaired **U**rinary Elimination*
*Risk for Deficient **F**luid Volume*
*Acute **P**ain*

PLANNING

Expected Outcomes

1. Urinary catheter will be patent.
2. Sediment/blood clots will be passed through the catheter.
3. Bladder will be free of sources of local irritation.
4. Urinary pH will be lowered to a more acidic state.

Equipment Needed

- Sterile gloves
- Sterile cover for the end of the drainage tubing
- Disposable, water-resistant drape or towel
- Sterile asepto or Toomey syringe with container for irrigant
- Sterile antiseptic swabs
- Sterile irrigating solution (labeled with date and time of opening, if opened)

DELEGATION TIPS

The procedure of irrigating a urinary catheter cannot be delegated because it requires the skills and problem-solving abilities of a nurse.

IMPLEMENTATION—ACTION/RATIONALE

ACTION

* Check client's identification band * Explain procedure before beginning *

1. Verify the need for bladder or catheter irrigation.

2. Assemble all supplies.

3. Provide for client privacy with a closed door or curtain.
4. Assist the client to a dorsal recumbent position.
5. Cleanse your hands.
6. Empty the collection bag of urine.

7. Expose the indwelling catheter and place the water-resistant drape underneath it.
8. Open the sterile syringe and container. Stand it up carefully in or on the wrapper and add 100 to 200 mL sterile diluent without touching or contaminating the tip of the syringe or the inside of the receptacle.
9. Open the end of the antiseptic swab package, exposing the swab sticks, and the sterile cover for drainage tube.
10. Apply the sterile gloves.
11. Disinfect the connection between the catheter and the drainage tubing.
12. After the disinfectant dries, loosen the ends of the connection.

RATIONALE

1. Ensures that procedure is being applied correctly, to reduce unnecessary opening of the system and risk of infection.
2. Having all supplies in room enables the nurse to maintain sterility of supplies once they are opened and laid out.
3. Decreases client anxiety.

4. Facilitates the flow of irrigant into the bladder.
5. Decreases transmission of microorganisms.
6. Starting with an empty collection bag makes it easier to identify clots or sediment passed as a result of irrigation.
7. Protects the bedclothes and client from urine and body fluids.
8. Enables nurse to maintain sterility of gloves once they are applied.

9. Enables nurse to maintain sterility of gloves once they are applied.
10. Maintains sterility of the procedure.
11. Minimizes risk of contaminating the system.

12. Enables the nurse to open the connection without accidentally contaminating either end.

continues

Figure 27-4-1 Separate the catheter and tube.

Figure 27-4-2 Insert the tip of the syringe into the catheter and gently instill the solution.

13. Grasp the catheter and tubing 1 to 2 inches from their ends, with catheter in the nondominant hand.

14. Fold the catheter to pinch it closed between the palm and last three fingers; use the thumb and first finger to hold the sterile cap for the drainage tube.

15. Separate the catheter and tube, covering the tube tightly with the sterile cap.

16. Fill the syringe with 30 mL for catheter irrigation, 60 mL for bladder irrigation. Insert the tip of the syringe into the catheter and gently instill the solution into the catheter (Figures 27-4-1 and 27-4-2).

17. Clamp catheter if ordered (medicated solution). If not clamped, irrigant may be released into a collection container or aspirated back into the syringe (Figure 27-4-3).

18. If the bladder or catheter is being irrigated to clear solid material, repeat irrigation until return is clear.

19. Reconnect system and remove sterile gloves. Cleanse your hands (Figure 27-4-4).

20. Monitor client for pain, urine color and clarity, any solid material passed, and total intake and output.

21. Cleanse hands.

13. Maintains sterility of the procedure and allows the nurse to be positioned to use the dominant hand for the syringe.

14. Allows for one nurse to handle all equipment simultaneously, thus maintaining sterility.

15. Maintains sterility of equipment.

16. Catheter can be irrigated with 30 mL of solution, minimizing bladder discomfort, while irrigating a bladder takes 60 mL.

17. Fine sediment or clear irrigant with medication can run freely; material with more solids (sediment or clots) may need gentle aspiration.

18. Clearing the catheter completely in this irrigation means a lower total number of irrigations and less opening of the system, thus decreasing the risk of infection.

19. Maintains sterility of system and reduces transmission of microorganisms.

20. Monitoring output after irrigation evaluates the efficacy of the treatment.

21. Reduces transmission of microorganisms.

Figure 27-4-3 Irrigant is released into a collection container.

Figure 27-4-4 Reconnect the tubing to the catheter.

EVALUATION

- Urinary catheter remains patent.
- Any sediment/blood clots were passed through the catheter.
- Bladder is free of local irritation.
- Urinary pH was more acidic.

DOCUMENTATION

Nurses' Notes

- Assessment indicating need for irrigation, such as decreased output, increased sediment, clots, bladder spasms/pain, or palpation of a full bladder
- Type of irrigant and amount in each instillation
- Amount and quality of returns (returns often include urine trapped in the bladder)

- Medication given before or after the procedure and response to same
- Urine output, color, and clarity and any solids passed 30 to 60 minutes after procedure
- Client response, especially changes in pain, spasms, or discomfort

Medication Administration Record

- Type of irrigant, if medicated, and amount in each instillation
- Any medication given before or after the procedure

Intake and Output Record

- Amount of urine emptied from the drainage bag prior to and following the procedure
- Amount of irrigant instilled

PROCEDURE 27-5 — Irrigating the Bladder Using a Closed-System Catheter

OVERVIEW

Surgical procedures such as prostate resections and bladder surgery or traumatic injury may require frequent or continuous bladder irrigation. To prevent the potential introduction of infectious organisms and as a practical matter, open bladder irrigation is not used in these cases. A closed bladder irrigation system is preferable under these circumstances. Closed bladder irrigation may be used to instill medication, encourage hemostasis, or flush clots and debris out of the catheter and bladder.

A three-way catheter is used for closed bladder irrigation. If the client will require closed irrigation following surgery, the surgeon often places the three-way catheter during the operation. If a standard indwelling catheter has been placed, a Y adapter can be used for intermittent irrigation. A three-way catheter has three ports: one for inflation of the retention balloon, one for urine drainage, and one for instilling irrigant.

As with open bladder irrigation, closed bladder irrigation is a sterile procedure. The irrigant, tubing, and drainage systems must be maintained as a closed sterile system to decrease the risk of infection. Because of the risk of blockage from clots and debris, the system must also be monitored closely for equal amounts of irrigant instilled and irrigant returned.

ASSESSMENT

1. Assess the client for bladder distention or complaints of fullness or discomfort **to assess the patency of the drainage system.**
2. Assess the drainage system for equal or larger amounts of drainage versus infused irrigant **to assess the patency of the system.**
3. Assess the color, consistency, and clarity of the bladder drainage as well as noting any clots or debris present **to assess the effectiveness of the irrigation.**

POSSIBLE NURSING DIAGNOSES

Risk for Infection
Impaired Urinary Elimination

PLANNING

Expected Outcomes

1. The client will not exhibit signs or symptoms of bladder or urinary tract infection.
2. The client will not experience pain or discomfort as a result of the bladder irrigation.

continues

3. The catheter will remain patent, and the client's bladder will not be distended.

Equipment Needed

• Three-way indwelling catheter or Y adapter
• IV pole

• Ordered irrigation solution
• Sterile gloves
• Closed-irrigation tubing
• Large urine collection bag
• Antiseptic swabs

DELEGATION TIPS

This procedure cannot be delegated. Bladder irrigation using a closed-system catheter requires the skills of a nurse.

IMPLEMENTATION—ACTION/RATIONALE

ACTION   RATIONALE

❋ **Check client's identification band** ❋ **Explain procedure before beginning** ❋

Intermittent Bladder Irrigation Using a Standard Indwelling Catheter and a Y Adapter

ACTION	RATIONALE
1. Cleanse hands.	1. Prevents spread of microorganisms.
2. Close privacy curtain or door.	2. Provides privacy.
3. Hang the prescribed irrigation solution from an IV pole.	3. Different solutions may be ordered depending on the results the health care provider desires. Bladder irrigant is generally packaged in 2,000- to 4,000-mL bottles.
4. Insert the clamped irrigation tubing into the bottle of irrigant and prime the tubing with fluid, expel all air and reclamp the tube (Figure 27-5-1).	4. Prevents introduction of air into the bladder.
5. Prepare sterile antiseptic swabs and sterile Y connector.	5. Prevents contamination of sterile gloves and field.
6. Clamp the urinary catheter.	6. Prevents urine leakage onto the bed linens.
7. Apply sterile gloves.	7. Minimizes the client's risk of infection.
8. Unhook the drainage bag from the indwelling catheter.	8. Allows the Y adapter to be inserted into the system.
9. While holding the drainage tubing and the drainage port of the catheter in your nondominant hand, cleanse both the tubing and the port with antiseptic swabs.	9. Reduces risk of contamination and infection.
10. Connect one port of the Y connector to the drainage port of the catheter.	10. Provides a bifurcation for irrigant to instill as well as urine to drain.

Figure 27-5-1   Insert the clamped irrigation tubing into the bottle of irrigant.

continues

11. Connect another port of the Y adapter to the drainage tubing.

11. Collects the urine and drained irrigant. This may be the established urine collection bag or a new, sterile bag that is large enough to hold the increased volume of drainage.

12. Attach the third port of the Y adapter to the irrigant tubing.

12. Instills the irrigant into the closed system.

13. Unclamp the urinary catheter and establish that urine is draining through the catheter into the drainage bag.

13. If the urine does not flow freely after unclamping, the catheter may have become clogged with a clot or debris. Notify the client's health care provider of the lack of urine drainage.

14. To irrigate the catheter and bladder, clamp the drainage tubing distal to the Y adapter.

14. Prevents the irrigant from bypassing the bladder and flowing directly into the drainage bag.

15. Unclamp irrigation tubing and instill the prescribed amount of irrigant.

15. The bladder normally feels full when it contains approximately 300 mL of urine. If a prescribed amount of irrigant was not ordered, do not instill more than 150 mL of irrigant. If the client has undergone bladder surgery, do not instill irrigant without knowing the specific amount ordered.

16. Clamp the irrigant tubing (Figure 27-5-2).

16. Prevents further instillation of irrigant.

17. If the health care provider has ordered the irrigant to remain in the bladder for a measured length of time, wait the prescribed length of time.

17. Some irrigation solutions contain medication and are meant to remain in contact with the bladder wall for a prescribed length of time.

18. Unclamp the drainage tubing and monitor the drainage as it flows into the drainage bag.

18. Assess the drainage for volume, color, clarity, and the presence of any clots or debris.

Closed Bladder Irrigation Using a Three-Way Catheter

19. Follow Actions 1–4.

19. See Rationales 1–4.

20. Prepare sterile antiseptic swabs and any other sterile equipment needed.

20. Prevents contamination of sterile gloves and field.

21. Clamp the urinary catheter.

21. Prevents leakage of urine onto the bedclothes.

22. Apply sterile gloves.

22. Minimizes the client's risk of infection when connecting the irrigant to the catheter and drainage system.

23. Remove the cap from the irrigation port of the three-way catheter (Figure 27-5-3).

23. Allows access for the irrigant tubing.

24. Cleanse the irrigation port with the sterile antiseptic swabs.

24. Minimizes the risk of infection.

25. Attach the irrigation tubing to the irrigation port of the three-way catheter.

25. Connects irrigant to the system.

26. Remove the clamp from the catheter and observe for urine drainage (Figure 27-5-4).

26. Ensures catheter remains patent after being clamped. Some surgical procedures can cause bleeding and clotting of the catheter.

Figure 27-5-2 Clamp the irrigant tubing.

Figure 27-5-3 Remove the cap from the irrigation port of the three-way catheter.

continues

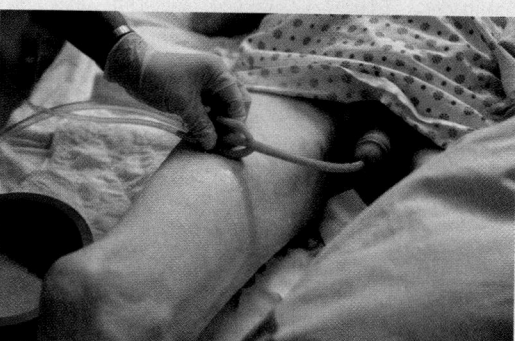

Figure 27-5-4 Attach the irrigation tubing, remove the clamp from the catheter, and observe for urine drainage. Carefully observe the drainage for color, clarity, and the presence of debris.

If intermittent irrigation has been ordered:
27. Follow Actions 15–16.
28. If the health care provider has ordered the irrigant to remain in the bladder for a measured length of time, clamp the drainage tube before instilling the irrigant and wait the prescribed length of time.
29. Monitor the drainage as it flows into the drainage bag.

If continuous bladder irrigation has been ordered:
30. Adjust the clamp on the irrigation tubing to allow the prescribed rate of irrigant to flow into the catheter and bladder.
31. Monitor the drainage for color, clarity, debris, and volume as it flows back into the drainage bag.
32. Tape the catheter securely to the thigh.
33. Cleanse hands.

27. See Rationales 15–16.
28. Some irrigation solutions contain medication and are meant to remain in contact with the bladder wall for a prescribed length of time.

29. Assesses the drainage for volume, color, clarity, and the presence of any clots or debris.

30. Regulates the amount of irrigant flowing in and out of the bladder to prevent distention or damage to any surgical site.
31. Assesses for bleeding, clotting, and blockage of urine drainage or other complications.
32. Prevents the catheter from becoming dislodged.
33. Reduces transmission of microorganisms.

EVALUATION

- The client does not exhibit signs or symptoms of bladder or urinary tract infection.
- The client has not experienced pain or discomfort as a result of the bladder irrigation.
- The catheter remains patent, and the client's bladder is not distended.

DOCUMENTATION

Intake and Output Record

- Amount of irrigant instilled and amount of drainage measured. Subtracting the used irrigant from the drainage total will leave the amount of the client's urine output.

Nurses' Notes

- Client's tolerance for the procedure
- Color, clarity, volume, and debris in the drainage

PROCEDURE 27-6   Pouching a Stoma

OVERVIEW

A colostomy is an opening surgically created from the ascending, transverse, or descending colon to the abdominal wall. An ileostomy is an opening from the ileum to the abdominal wall. Colostomies and ileostomies function to discharge waste (liquids, solids, and gases) to the outside of the body. Pouching a fecal diversion ensures that the client's peristomal skin remains intact and provides the client with artificial continence.

The purpose of creating ileostomies and colostomies is to improve survival and the quality of life. Anger, grief, body image disturbances, socialization disturbances, depression, and helplessness often accompany these procedures.

ASSESSMENT

1. Inspect the stoma for color and texture. **Allows the nurse to determine the viability and turgor of the stoma.**
2. Inspect the condition of the skin surrounding the stoma. **Alterations in skin integrity prohibit a closed drainage system from adhering to the skin.**
3. Measure the dimensions of the stoma before obtaining an ostomy appliance system from central supply. **Alleviates the problem of obtaining the wrong size equipment.**

POSSIBLE NURSING DIAGNOSES

*Risk for Impaired **S**kin Integrity*
*Impaired **S**kin Integrity*
*Disturbed **B**ody Image*

PLANNING

Expected Outcomes

1. Peristomal skin integrity will remain intact.
2. Irritated or denuded peristomal skin will heal.
3. Client will acknowledge the change in body image.
4. Client will express positive feelings about self.
5. Client will maintain fluid balance.

Equipment Needed

- Clean washcloth or 4 × 4 gauze pads
- Warm tap water
- Appropriate drainable ostomy appliance (Figures 27-6-1 and 27-6-2)
- Scissors
- Pen or pencil
- Clean gloves

Figure 27-6-1   Ostomy Skin Barriers (also called wafers)

Figure 27-6-2   Ostomy Drainage Bags

DELEGATION TIPS

This procedure cannot be delegated to ancillary personnel. Changing an ostomy appliance requires the skills and problem-solving ability of a nurse.

continues

IMPLEMENTATION—ACTION/RATIONALE

ACTION

*Check client's identification band * Explain procedure before beginning*

1. Cleanse hands.
2. Assemble drainable pouch and wafer.
3. Apply clean gloves.
4. Remove current ostomy appliance after emptying pouch of stool, if present.

5. Dispose of appliance in appropriate waste container.
6. Remove gloves and cleanse hands.
7. Apply clean gloves.
8. Cleanse stoma and skin with warm tap water. Pat dry.

9. Measure stoma using a measuring guide for appropriate length and width of stoma at base (where skin meets stoma).
10. Place gauze pad over orifice of stoma to wick stool while you are preparing the wafer and pouch for application.
11. Trace pattern onto paper backing of wafer.

12. Cut wafer as traced.
13. Attach clean pouch to wafer. Make sure port closure is closed.

14. Remove gauze pad from orifice of stoma.
15. Remove paper backing from wafer and place on skin with stoma centered in cutout opening of wafer (Figures 27-6-3 and 27-6-4).
16. Tape the wafer edges down with hypoallergenic tape (optional).
17. Cleanse hands.

RATIONALE

1. Prevents spread of microorganisms.
2. Ensures that all equipment is ready to use.
3. Prevents spread of microorganisms.
4. Prevents contamination of surrounding environment if stool accidentally leaks from appliance when removed from client's skin.
5. Practices infection control.
6. Prevents spread of microorganisms.
7. Follows Standard Precautions.
8. Gentle care of the stoma prevents injury to the mucosa, which has no nerve endings and is very friable.
9. Correct measurement of the stoma's dimensions ensures a good fit of the ostomy appliance without excess skin at the base of the stoma exposed to stool.
10. Ensures a good seal of the wafer to the client's skin.

11. Inaccurate pattern size results in either laceration of the stoma by the wafer or maceration of peristomal skin from constant contact with stool.
12. Ensures a snug fit.
13. Preattaching the pouch to the wafer saves time and prevents stool from leaking underneath the wafer during application process.
14. It is easier to visualize the stoma.
15. Paper backing needs to be removed from wafer in order for wafer to adhere to skin.

16. Ensures that the edges of the wafer will not adhere to client's clothing.
17. Reduces transmission of microorganisms.

Figure 27-6-3 Place the wafer and pouch with the stoma centered in the cutout opening of the wafer.

Figure 27-6-4 Check to make sure the stoma fits the hole so a minimum of the surrounding skin is exposed to contact with stool.

continues

EVALUATION

- Peristomal skin integrity remains intact.
- Irritated or denuded peristomal skin integrity is healed.
- Client acknowledges the change in body image.
- Client expresses positive feelings about self.
- Client maintains fluid balance.

DOCUMENTATION

Nurses' Notes

- Assessment of peristomal skin
- Assessment of stoma
- Stoma measurements (length, width, height)
- Color and amount of drainage
- Peristomal skin care if alteration in skin integrity was noted
- Type of ostomy pouch applied

PROCEDURE 27-7 — Application of Heat and Cold

OVERVIEW

Heat application is used to promote vasodilatation, increase capillary permeability, decrease blood viscosity, increase tissue metabolism, and reduce muscle tension. Moist heat can be in the form of immersion of a body part in a warmed solution or water. It can also be accomplished by wrapping body parts in dressings that are saturated with warmed solution.

Dry heat can be used to enhance circulation, promote healing, reduce swelling and inflammation, reduce pain, reduce muscle spasms, and increase systemic temperature.

Cold therapy is used to decrease blood flow to an area by promoting vasoconstriction and increased blood viscosity. These changes facilitate clotting and control bleeding. Cold decreases tissue metabolism, reduces oxygen consumption, and decreases inflammation and edema formation. Cold therapy has a local anesthetic effect by raising the threshold of pain receptors. It causes a decrease in muscle tension. Cold is used to reduce fever.

ASSESSMENT

1. Assess the area to receive heat or cold treatment for circulation. **Heat increases circulation; adequate vasculature must be present to be effective. Cold decreases circulation; adequate circulation must be present to prevent further tissue damage.**
2. Assess the skin sensation and integrity around the area to be treated. **Heat treatment cannot be used over areas of blisters, burns, or redness indicative of burning.**
3. Assess for open wounds that may be affected by the treatment. **Moist heat provides an ideal climate for the growth of microorganisms. Moist heat should be applied to open wounds only with orders from a physician or qualified practitioner. Dry heat is frequently used on open wounds.**
4. Check the client's systemic temperature. **If large areas are exposed to heat or cold, the total body temperature may be increased or decreased.**
5. Assess age. **Tolerance to heat and cold varies with individuals and is related to age, thinner layers of skin, or general sensitivity to heat and cold.**

POSSIBLE NURSING DIAGNOSES

*Ineffective **T**issue Perfusion*
*Acute **P**ain*
*Risk for Impaired **S**kin Integrity*
*Risk for Imbalanced **B**ody Temperature*
*Ineffective **T**hermoregulation*
*Risk for **I**njury*

PLANNING

Expected Outcomes

1. The client will derive the intended benefits of the heat or cold treatment.
2. The client will not experience any injury to skin integrity.

continues

Equipment Needed

- Aquathermia pad
- Commercial heat or cold pack
- Solution for heat or cold treatment
- 4 × 4 gauze and waterproof pads
- Examination gloves
- Sterile gloves if open wounds
- Towel
- Heat cradle
- Pain for hot or cold soak
- Portable sitz bath

DELEGATION TIPS

These procedures are routinely delegated to properly trained ancillary personnel. Reassessment of the client after application to maintain proper temperature and to evaluate the client response is essential.

IMPLEMENTATION—ACTION/RATIONALE

ACTION
RATIONALE

* Check client's identification band * Explain procedure before beginning *

Moist Heat

ACTION	RATIONALE
1. Check the physician's order and the reason for warm compress.	1. A physician's or nurse practitioner's order is generally required.
2. Cleanse hands.	2. Reduces transmission of microorganisms.
3. Assess the client's skin for areas of redness, breakdown, or scar tissue. If open wounds are involved, carefully assess the open wounds.	3. Provides baseline information for comparison assessments. Because scar tissue may be heat sensitive or insensitive, this area should be avoided, if possible, when the compress is applied. Any open wounds should be avoided unless the treatment is specific for these areas.
4. Review the client's condition, medical diagnosis, and any history of diabetes mellitus or impairments in sensation.	4. Sensation is often impaired in peripheral vascular disease, diabetes, and especially in peripheral neuropathy. People with impairments in sensation may not be able to identify when the compresses are too hot. The risk of burns is greater with moist heat than with dry heat. The client's history and medical diagnosis may alert you to other problems.
5. Warm the container of sterile saline or tap water by placing it in a bath basin filled with hot tap water. Sterile saline should be warmed to 105°–113°F. If you are using a commercial compress, follow the manufacturer's directions for heating the compress.	5. Sterile saline is used to prevent any contamination of the wound. A temperature above 113°F will cause further injury.
6. Place a waterproof pad under the body area that needs the warm compress.	6. Protects the client's bed and clothing.
7. A thin layer of petroleum jelly may be placed on the client's skin in the area to be treated. Do not put petroleum jelly on an open wound or use with oxygen therapy.	7. Helps protect the client's skin.
8. Pour the sterile saline into the sterile basin. Soak an appropriate-size piece of gauze or a towel, wring out the excess saline, and place it on the affected area. Wear gloves if there is any drainage of the client's body fluids. Wear sterile gloves if there is an open wound.	8. A sterile basin is used to prevent further contamination. Excess saline may increase the chance of burns.

continues

Figure 27-7-1   Wrap the hot, moist towel with a waterproof pad and secure the pad.

9. Wrap the area with a waterproof pad or apply a disposable heat or aquathermia pad (Figure 27-7-1).
10. Check the client's skin periodically for signs of heat intolerance. Tell the client to report any signs of discomfort immediately.
11. If it is tolerated, leave the compress in place for approximately 30 minutes and then remove it.

12. Dry the affected area with sterile towels if there is an open wound and with clean towels if there is no open wound.
13. Properly dispose of all single-use equipment according to hospital protocol.

14. Clean the bath basin and thermometer. Return the sterile basin to the appropriate place for resterilization.
15. Remove gloves if they were worn and cleanse hands.
16. Reassess the condition of the client's skin.

Sitz Bath

17. Cleanse hands and assemble equipment.

18. Run tap water to preferred temperature (between 100°F and 110°F). Have client test the temperature on the dorsal surface of the wrist.
19. For toilet insert model, raise the seat of the toilet. Set the basin on the rim of the toilet bowel.
    Fill water bag and prime tubing. Close the clamp.
    Hang the water bag above the toilet. Thread the tubing through the front of the basin. Secure the tubing in the notch in the bottom of the basin.
20. For stand-alone model, fill basin with water (Figure 27-7-2).
21. Pad the seat with a towel (Figure 27-7-3).
22. Always use Standard Precautions when assisting with perineal care treatments.
    Have client remove and dispose of peri-pad using Standard Precautions.
23. Ensure that the floor is dry. Assist client to the bathroom if necessary.

9. Maintains or holds in the heat.
10. Signs of intolerance may include redness or further swelling.

11. A longer period of time may damage the client's skin and predispose the client to edema formation from circulatory congestion.
12. The client may feel chilled when the warm compress is removed. Dry the area completely to prevent chilling.
13. The basins and thermometer can be used again. Proper disposal of all other equipment reduces transmission of microorganisms.
14. Reduces transmission of microorganisms and gets the equipment ready for use again.
15. Reduces transmission of microorganisms.
16. The condition of the client's skin and any signs of heat sensitivity should be assessed and documented.

17. Reduces transmission of microorganisms and organizes time.
18. Prevents burn injury.

19. Basin will rest on the bowl.
    Water bag will create a gentle swirling of water. The higher the bag, the more forceful the flow and the faster the water will run out.

20. Allows client to sit in the water.

21. Provides client comfort.
22. Prevents infection.

23. Prevents injury from falling.

continues

Figure 27-7-2   Fill the sitz bath basin with warm water.

Figure 27-7-3   Pad the seat of the sitz bath with a towel for comfort.

24. Have client sit in the basin. For toilet insert model, demonstrate how to unclamp the tubing to start the water flow.
25. Cover client's lap for warmth and modesty.
26. Ensure that the client can reach the call button. Instruct the client to call before standing up.
27. After 20 minutes (or sooner if client is finished), help the client dry the area by gently patting with clean towels.
28. Assist client to bed. Encourage client to lie flat or elevate hips for 20 minutes.
29. For toilet insert model, empty remaining water into toilet. Rinse basin and bag and allow to air dry. Then clean according to institutional policy. For stand-alone model, empty water from drain trap into basin. Clean according to institutional policy.

Dry Heat

30. Check the physician's or qualified practitioner's order and the purpose of the heat treatment.

31. Determine if there are any underlying problems that may affect the use of heat treatment such as decreased sensation; decreased mentation; or a history of diabetes mellitus, bleeding disorders, peripheral vascular disease, or peripheral neuropathy.
    Heat should not be used over areas of scarring.
32. Cleanse hands.
33. Check the skin for lotions or ointments and remove if present.
34. Gather equipment and complete as follows:
    For a disposable heat pack:
    • Activate the pack according to the manufacturer's directions. Some packs must be heated in boiling water, others can be heated by microwave, and some require bending and chemical activation.
    • Wrap the pack in a towel or protective covering (some manufacturers include cover). Do not use pins. Use tape if needed to secure the towel.

24. Water flow is soothing and helps cleanse the area.

25. Provides client comfort and privacy.
26. Water may splash over the floor, creating a slipping hazard.
27. Warm soaks should last no longer than 20 minutes to prevent rebound vasoconstriction.

28. Prevents congestion and decreases swelling.

29. Prepares equipment for the next use.

30. An order is required. Because there are many purposes of heat treatment, it is helpful to know what outcomes are expected and the site/sites to be treated.
31. If the client has decreased sensation or mental status, heat treatment should be used only if the client can be observed closely.
    Heat should not be applied over areas where the client cannot alert the nurse about the sensation of burning.
32. Reduces transmission of microorganisms.
33. Lotions and ointments retain heat and can lead to an increased risk of burning.
34.

    • Manufacturer's directions should be followed because activation differs. If a microwave is used to heat a pack that should be heated in boiling water, the bag might break.
    • A barrier between the client's skin and the heat source is necessary to avoid burns.

continues

• Discard after use.

For an aquathermia pad:
• Follow manufacturer's directions.

• Fill the control unit with distilled water or as indicated by manufacturer's directions.
• Check the control unit and tubing for leaks. Turn on the unit and check the temperature of the water with a thermometer after several minutes.
   The proper temperature of the water is 105°F. Some units require that the control unit is level with the pad to function because overcoming gravity can put undue strain on the motor.

For a heat lamp with a 60-watt or infrared bulb:
• Position client so that the area to be treated is exposed, and drape the client to protect privacy. If the buttock or perineum is to be treated, it may be necessary to tape the buttock to hold apart and keep the area to be treated exposed (Figure 27-7-4).
• Place the lamp 18–24 inches from the client and ensure that the lamp does not touch the client (Figure 27-7-5). Instruct the client not to touch the lamp or move to avoid contact with the lamp.
• Check the area after 5 minutes of heat. Remove the lamp after 20 minutes and check the area for burning, redness, rash, or any adverse reaction. Reposition the client in a comfortable position.
• Clean equipment

For a heat cradle:
• Use a 25-watt bulb. Place the cradle over the affected area, positioned 18–24 inches from the client. Cover the cradle and client with a bath blanket.
• Check the client in 5 minutes and remove the cradle after 10–15 minutes.
   Assess the skin for burning, redness, or any adverse reaction. Reposition the client for comfort. Clean the equipment.

35. Cleanse hands.

• Chemically activated packs will not reactivate once activated. In medical facilities, gel packs cannot be reheated in common areas without causing the transmission of microorganisms. In the home setting, packs activated by boiling or the microwave can be used on the same client again.

• There are various brands of aquathermia pads and each one may have slight differences in operating instructions.
• Distilled water prevents the accumulation of mineral deposits that will damage equipment.
• This will ensure that the control unit is properly functioning. If there is a leak in the tubing, another pad should be obtained because this presents an electrical danger to the client and the staff.

• Because the client will be positioned to expose the area to be treated, which many times includes the perineum, further draping is necessary to ensure privacy.

• The lamp should be not closer than 18 inches to protect the client from burning. Check the area shortly after the treatment is started because client's sensitivity to heat will vary.
• Do not use beyond 20 minutes or the client may have adverse reactions. Reposition the client because many times clients are placed in unnatural positions to expose the area to be treated.
• Reduces transmission of microorganisms.

• A 25-watt bulb ensures that the temperature inside the cradle does not exceed 125°F and burn the client or alter systemic temperature.
• If the client is checked frequently, adverse reactions can be prevented.

35. Reduces transmission of microorganisms.

Figure 27-7-4 Tape the skin up if needed to expose the area being treated.

Figure 27-7-5 Place the heat lamp 18–24 inches from the client.

continues

Application of Cold

36. Cleanse hands.
37. Assess the client's sensation and skin color at the site of planned application. Determine if any tissue damage is present. Assess for bleeding or wound drainage.
38. Review whether the client has a history of circulatory impairment or neuropathy.

39. Check the physician's or qualified practitioner's order and the reason for the application of cold.
40. If using an ice bag with moist gauze or towels, fill the bag three-fourths full with ice and remove the remaining air from the bag. Close the bag. Check for leaks. Wrap the bag in a towel or protective cover and place it on the affected area. If cold soaks are being applied, use the appropriate-size basin for the body part to be soaked.
41. If an ice collar is used, fill the collar three-fourths full with ice and remove the remaining air from the collar before closing the collar. Check for leaks. Place the collar in a protective cover and around the client's neck.

42. If a disposable cold pack is used, activate the pack according to the manufacturer's directions, wrap the pack in a towel, and place it on the affected area. Some packs come with covers. Secure pack in place with tape, elastic wrap, or bandage. Dispose of the pack after the treatment.
43. Assess the client's skin periodically for signs of cold intolerance or tissue damage.
44. If the client can tolerate the cold, leave the cold application in place for approximately 20–30 minutes at approximately 15°C (59°F).

45. Dispose of equipment according to agency policy.
46. Reassess the condition of the client's skin or exposed tissue.
47. Cleanse hands.

36. Reduces transmission of microorganisms.
37. Provides baseline data for post-treatment comparison.

38. Cold causes vasoconstriction and decreased metabolism and can cause tissue damage in people with impaired circulation and sensation.
39. A physician's or qualified practitioner's order is needed in most situations of cold treatment.
40. If air is removed from the bag, the bag will be easier to mold to the client's body. The bag is wrapped to prevent injury to the client's skin or exposed tissue because direct cold can cause damage.

41. Easier to mold to the client's body. The collar is wrapped to prevent injury to the client's skin.

42. When the pack is squeezed or kneaded, an alcohol-based solution is released, creating the cold temperature. The pack cannot be used again.

43. Signs of intolerance to cold are pallor, blanching, mottling, or numbness of the skin.
44. Longer application can cause tissue damage, especially because the client's pain sensation is decreased in the presence of cold. A reflex vasodilation occurs after 20–30 minutes, thereby negating the therapeutic effect of the cold treatment.
45. Reduces transmission of microorganisms.
46. The client's skin should be assessed, and any signs of cold changes and intolerance should be documented.
47. Reduces transmission of microorganisms.

EVALUATION

- The client derived the intended benefits of the heat or cold treatment.
- The client had no injury to skin integrity.

DOCUMENTATION

Nurses' Notes

- Procedure and the client's response to the procedure
- Equipment used
- Length of time of application
- Client's skin condition after the procedure

PROCEDURE 27-8

Administering Oral, Sublingual, and Buccal Medications

OVERVIEW

The easiest and most common method of administering a medication is usually by mouth. Clients may be taught to administer the medication by themselves at home, or a nurse can prepare the medications and dispense to clients. Oral medications are contraindicated for clients with gastrointestinal alterations, using nasogastric tube or gastrostomy tube, or who have a poor gag reflex. Clients with an inability to swallow because of neuromuscular disorder, esophageal stricture, or lesion of the mouth or those who are unresponsive or comatose are also ineligible to receive oral administration of medication.

Nurses need to know the action, normal dosage, side effects, and nursing implications for each drug they administer. In some settings, medications for several clients may be prepared at one time in the medication room or medication cart by carefully identifying each client's doses. Most hospitals use a computerized limited-access medication system.

ASSESSMENT

1. Assess the five rights: right client, right medication, right route, right dose, and right time. **Prevents errors in medication administration.**
2. Review the action, purpose, normal dosage and route, common side effects, time of onset and peak action, and nursing implications of each drug **so the client's response to the medication may be monitored.**
3. Assess the client's condition to be sure the order of the health care provider is appropriate **because the client's condition may have changed since the order was written.**
4. Assess the client's ability to swallow food and fluid **because an alternate route for medication may be needed if unable to swallow a pill.**
5. Assess for any contraindications for administering an oral medication such as nausea and vomiting, gastric suction, or gastric surgery resulting in decreased peristalsis **because alterations in gastrointestinal function may interfere with drug absorption and excretion.**
6. Assess the client's medical record for a history of allergies to food or medications **so these medications can be avoided.**
7. Assess the client's knowledge about the use of medications **so client teaching can be tailored to client's needs. This may also assess compliance for taking the drugs at home or reveal drug dependence or abuse.**
8. Assess the client's age **because pediatric or geriatric clients may have special needs according to their ability to swallow a pill.**
9. Assess the client's need for fluids **because swallowing a pill is usually easier with fluid and promotes fluid intake; however, fluid restrictions are sometimes necessary.**
10. Assess the client's ability to sit or turn to the side. **The client must be able to swallow the pill without aspiration.**

POSSIBLE NURSING DIAGNOSES

Noncompliance
Impaired Swallowing
Deficient Knowledge (medication regimen)

PLANNING

Expected Outcomes

1. The client will swallow the prescribed medication.
2. The client will be able to explain the purpose and schedule for taking the medication.
3. The client will have no gastrointestinal discomfort or alterations in function.
4. The client will show the desired response to the medication such as pain relief, regular heart rate, or stable blood pressure.

Equipment Needed

- Health care provider's order for the medication
- Medication administration record (MAR)
- Medication cart or dispensing computer
- Medication tray
- Disposable medication cups
- Glass of water, juice, or other liquid
- Drinking straw
- Mortar and pestle, if needed
- Paper towels

continues

DELEGATION TIPS

The procedure of medication administration and assessment of effects is not delegated to ancillary personnel in acute care settings. This may vary in state or federal institutions. Ancillary personnel are generally informed about the medications the client is receiving if adverse effects are anticipated or are being monitored.

IMPLEMENTATION—ACTION/RATIONALE

ACTION	RATIONALE
1. Cleanse hands.	1. Reduces the number of microorganisms.
2. Arrange the medication tray and cups in the medication room or on the medication cart outside the client's room. Most hospitals use a computerized limited-access medication cart. Follow institutional protocol.	2. Organizing medications and equipment saves time and reduces the possibility of error.
3. Unlock the medication cart or log on to the computer.	3. Medications need to be safeguarded.
4. Prepare the medication for one client at a time following the five rights. Select the correct drug from the medication drawer according to the MAR. Calculate the drug dosage if needed.	4. The five rights are right client, right time, right medication, right dose, and right route. Comparing the MAR with the label reduces error. Double-checking reduces error in calculation.
5. To prepare a tablet or capsule: Pour the required number of tablets or capsules into the bottle cap and transfer the medication to a medication cup without touching them.	5. Avoids wasting expensive medications and avoids contamination of medication.
• Scored tablets may be broken, if necessary, using gloved hands or with a pill-cutting device (Figure 27-8-1).	• Tablets that are not scored are not meant to be broken. The medication's effectiveness would be diminished if the tablet were broken or crushed.
• A unit-dose tablet should be placed directly into the medicine cup *without* opening it until it is administered to the client.	• The wrapper maintains cleanliness and identification until it is administered.
• For clients with difficulty in swallowing, some tablets may be crushed into a powder using a mortar and pestle or by being placed between two paper medication cups and ground with a blunt object, then mixed in a small amount of applesauce or custard. *Time-released or specially coated medications must not be crushed.* Check with the pharmacy if you are uncertain (Figure 27-8-2).	• A large tablet is usually easier to swallow if it is ground and mixed with soft food.

Figure 27-8-1 Scored tablets may be broken, if necessary.

Figure 27-8-2 Some medications may be crushed and mixed with a soft food, such as applesauce, for clients who have difficulty in swallowing.

continues

Figure 27-8-3   Measure liquid medications at eye level.

Figure 27-8-4   Identify the client by reading the client's name bracelet and asking his or her name before administering medication.

6. To prepare a liquid medication: Remove the bottle cap from the container and place cap upside down on the cart. Hold the bottle with the label up and the medication cup at eye level while pouring (Figure 27-8-3). Fill the cup to the desired level using the surface or base of the meniscus as the scale, not the edge of the liquid on the cup. Wipe lip of bottle with paper towel.

7. To prepare a narcotic, obtain the key to the narcotic drawer and check the narcotic record for the drug count when signing out the dose. If the drug count does not agree with records, report to charge nurse.

8. Check expiration date on all medications.
   • Double-check the MAR with the prepared drugs.
   • Return stock medications to their shelf or drawer.
   • Place MARs with the client's medications.
   • Do not leave drugs unattended.

9. Administer medications to client: Observe the correct time to give the medication.
   • Identify the client by reading the client's name bracelet, repeating the name, and/or asking the client to state his or her name (Figure 27-8-4). Additionally, check the hospital number if name alert or client is not reliable.
   • Check the drug packaging if it is present to ensure the medication type and dosage.
   • Assess the client's condition and the form of the medication.
   • Perform any assessment required for specific medications such as a pulse or blood pressure.
   • Explain the purpose of the drug and ask if the client has any questions.
   • Assist the client to a sitting or lateral position.
   • Allow client to hold the tablet or medication cup.
   • Give a glass of water or other liquid, and straw if needed, to help the client swallow the medication.
   • For *sublingual* medications, instruct client to place medication under the tongue and allow it to dissolve completely.

6. Placing the bottle cap upside down on the cart prevents contamination of the inside of the container. Holding the bottle with the label up keeps spilled liquid from obliterating the label. Holding the medication cup at eye level ensures an accurate dose. Wiping the lip of the bottle prevents the bottle cap from sticking.

7. Controlled substance laws require records of each dose dispensed. Early identification of errors assists in corrective action. Facility may require an incident report be filed.

8. Expired medications may lose their effectiveness.
   • Reduces risk of error.
   • Ensures safety of stock medications.
   • Ensures identification of medications.
   • Drugs are safeguarded by nurse.

9. Ensures the therapeutic effect of the drug when given within 30 minutes of the prescribed time. *(Right time.)*
   • Identification bracelets made at the time of admission are the most reliable source of identification even if the client is unable to state his or her name. *(Right client.)*

   • Prevents giving the wrong medication or wrong dose. *(Right medication, right dose.)*
   • Allows you to assess the route of the medication and if this route is appropriate. *(Right route.)*
   • Determines whether the medication should be given at that time or not.
   • Improves compliance with drug therapy.

   • Prevents aspiration during swallowing.
   • Client becomes familiar with medications.
   • Promotes client comfort in swallowing and can improve fluid intake.
   • Drug is absorbed through the mucous membranes into the blood vessels. If swallowed, the drug may be destroyed by gastric juices or detoxified in the liver too quickly so that its intended effects will not occur.

continues

- For *buccal* administration of drugs, instruct the client to place the medication in the mouth against the cheek until it dissolves completely.
- For oral medications given through a *nasogastric tube,* crush tablets or open capsules and dissolve powder with 20 to 30 mL of warm water in a cup. Be sure medication will still be properly absorbed if crushed and dissolved. Check placement of the feeding tube or nasogastric tube before instilling anything but air into the tube.
- Remain with the client until each medication has been swallowed or dissolved.
- Assist the client into a comfortable position.

10. Dispose of soiled supplies and cleanse hands.
11. Return the cart to the medicine room; restock the supplies as needed. Clean the work area.

- Promotes local activity on mucous membranes.

- Allows medication administration via NG or feeding tube. Ensures that the medication is absorbed and utilized correctly.

- Ensures that the client receives the dose and does not save it or discard it.
- Maintains client's comfort.

10. Reduces transmission of microorganisms.
11. Assists other staff in completing duties efficiently.

EVALUATION

- Evaluate the client's response to the drug within 30 minutes of administration or sooner if an allergic reaction is anticipated.
- Ask client or caregiver to discuss the purpose, action, dosage schedule, and side effects of the drug.

DOCUMENTATION

Medication Administration Record

- Date and time each drug was administered, including initials and signature
- If drug is withheld, circle the time the drug was scheduled on the MAR.

Nurses' Notes

- Date, time, and reason a drug was withheld
- Response to drug administered

PROCEDURE 27-9   Withdrawing Medication from an Ampule

OVERVIEW

Ampules are containers that hold a single dose of medication. The ampules are made of clear glass and have a distinctive shape with a constricted neck. The head of the ampule is broken off at the neck, and the medication is withdrawn with a needle and syringe.

The neck of the ampule is often colored and usually scored. This scoring allows the neck to be broken off easily from the body to obtain the medication. Place a sterile piece of gauze around the neck of the ampule and break the neck in an outward motion. The gauze protects the nurse's fingers from the glass.

Medication can become trapped in the uppermost portion of the ampule. Before opening the ampule, flick the upper portion of the ampule with a fingernail to drop the medication from the upper segment down into the body of the ampule. This step may need to be repeated several times.

ASSESSMENT

1. Identify the correct ampule, including medication, dosage strength, dosage volume, dosage route, and expiration date **to avoid medication errors.**

2. Assess the syringe, filter needle, and injection needle for expiration date and package intactness **to evaluate the sterility of the equipment.**

continues

3. Assess the fluid in the ampule for cloudiness, particulate matter, or color changes **to evaluate for usability of the medication.**
4. Identify the medication's intended action, purpose, normal dosage range, time of action, common side effects, and nursing implications **to avoid medication errors.**

POSSIBLE NURSING DIAGNOSES

Risk for Impaired Skin Integrity
Risk for Infection

PLANNING

Expected Outcomes

1. The correct medication ampule will be selected.
2. The medication will be drawn into an appropriate syringe.

DELEGATION TIPS

The procedure of medication administration is not delegated to ancillary personnel in acute care settings. This may vary in state or federal institutions. Ancillary personnel are generally informed about the medications the client is receiving if adverse effects are anticipated or are being monitored.

3. Microorganisms will not be introduced into the sterile system.
4. Foreign objects will not be introduced into the sterile system.

Equipment Needed

• Medication ampule
• Sterile gauze pad or alcohol pad
• Syringe with filter needle
• Replacement needle
• Clean work space
• Medication administration record (MAR)
• Gloves (optional)

IMPLEMENTATION—ACTION/RATIONALE

ACTION

1. Cleanse hands. Apply gloves (optional).
2. Select appropriate ampule (Figure 27-9-1).
3. Select syringe with filter needle.
4. Obtain a sterile gauze pad.

5. Select and set aside the appropriate length of safety needle for planned injection.

RATIONALE

1. Decreases transmission of microorganisms.
2. Ensures client receives correct medication.
3. Filter needle entraps any glass fragments.
4. Using a gauze pad prevents cuts on the jagged edge of the broken ampule.
5. Accurate needle length ensures the medication is administered where it is intended.

Figure 27-9-1 Medication Ampules

continues

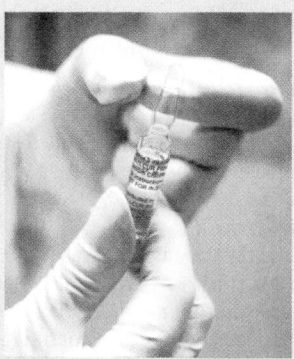

Figure 27-9-2   Flick the neck of the upright ampule to dislodge medication from the top of the vial.

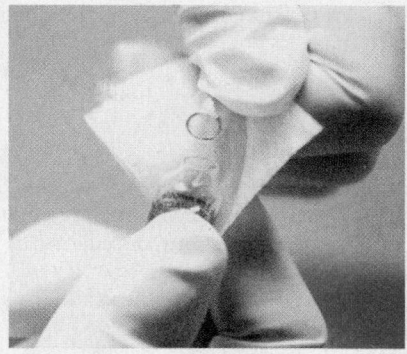

Figure 27-9-3   Wrap gauze or alcohol pad around the neck to protect fingers. Snap off the top in a quick outward motion.

6. Clear a work space.

7. Observe ampule for location of the medication.

8. If the medication is trapped in the top, flick the neck of the ampule repeatedly with your fingernail while holding the ampule upright (Figure 27-9-2).

9. Wrap the sterile gauze pad around the neck and snap off the top in an outward motion directed away from self (Figure 27-9-3).

10. Invert ampule and place the needle into the liquid. Gently withdraw medication into the syringe (Figure 27-9-4).

11. Alternately, place the ampule on the counter, hold and tilt slightly with the nondominant hand. Insert the needle below the level of liquid and gently draw liquid into the syringe, tilting the ampule as needed to reach all the liquid.

12. Remove the filter needle and replace with the safety injection needle.

13. Dispose of filter needle and glass ampule (including lid) in appropriate sharps container (Figure 27-9-5).

6. Prevents contamination with microdroplets that may spill when the ampule is broken.

7. The medication frequently becomes trapped in the top of the ampule.

8. Flicking the neck and top of the ampule moves the medication into the body of the ampule.

9. The gauze prevents the nurse from being cut by the jagged edge of the broken ampule. The outward motion provides added safety for the nurse.

10. Inverting the ampule allows all of the medication to be withdrawn into the syringe. Surface tension will hold the medication in the ampule until the negative pressure of the syringe barrel draws it into the syringe.

11. While it is more difficult to read the syringe calibrations, it is easier to hold the ampule steady. Choose the method most comfortable for you.

12. The filter needle is designed to trap glass particles and must not be used for client injections.

13. Needles or sharp glass objects must always be disposed of in puncture and leak-proof containers to provide safety for clients and health care workers.

Figure 27-9-4   Invert ampule and gently draw the liquid into the syringe.

Figure 27-9-5   Dispose of the filter needle, ampule, and ampule top in a sharps container.

continues

14. Label the syringe with drug, dose, date, and time.
15. Cleanse hands.

14. Prevents medication errors from taking place.
15. Decreases transmission of microorganisms.

EVALUATION

- The correct medication ampule was selected.
- The medication was drawn into an appropriate syringe.
- Microorganisms were not introduced into the sterile system.
- Foreign objects were not introduced into the sterile system.

DOCUMENTATION

Medication Administration Record

- Name of the medication
- Dosage drawn up
- Date and time the medication was drawn up

If the medication drawn up is a controlled substance, document in the Controlled Substances Record Book:
- Name of the medication
- Dosage drawn up
- Date and time the medication was drawn up
- Any controlled substance that was wasted
- Name of nurse drawing up the controlled substance

Controlled substances must be documented at the time they are removed from the locked cabinet. Documentation on the MAR is done after the medication is administered.

PROCEDURE 27-10   Withdrawing Medication from a Vial

OVERVIEW

Vials are often used to package multidose or single-dose parenteral medication. A vial is a small glass bottle with a rubber seal at the top. Glass vials come with a protective plastic or metal cap that prevents the rubber from being punctured before use. The rubber top must be cleaned with 70% alcohol with every usage of the medication. In order to aspirate the medication from the vial, an equal amount of air must be injected into the vial before attempting to withdraw any medication. In order to draw the medication out of the vial, the entire vial should be turned upside down. The syringe should be held at eye level to ensure an accurate amount of medication is drawn into the syringe.

ASSESSMENT

1. Assess the expiration date on the vial to be sure it is current **to avoid administering outdated medications.**
2. Assess the contents of the medication vial you are about to use for the correct medication in the correct dosage strength **to avoid medication error.**
3. Assess the contents of the vial for color, consistency, and debris **to avoid administering contaminated medication.**
4. Assess the integrity of the vial and its stopper **to avoid using a vial that may be contaminated.**
5. Assess the integrity of the syringe and needle that will be used to withdraw the medication **to avoid using equipment that may be contaminated.**

POSSIBLE NURSING DIAGNOSES

*Risk for **I**nfection*
*Risk for **I**njury*

PLANNING

Expected Outcomes

1. The correct medication will be drawn from the vial using sterile technique.
2. The correct dose will be drawn from the vial.
3. The remaining contents of multiuse vials will not be contaminated.
4. The date will be marked on the vial after opening using an ink pen.

continues

Equipment Needed

- Medication vial
- Syringe with needle
- Alcohol sponge pad
- Gloves (optional)
- Clean work space
- Medication administration record (MAR)

DELEGATION TIPS

The procedure of medication administration is not delegated to ancillary personnel in acute care settings. This may vary in state or federal institutions. Ancillary personnel are generally informed about the medications the client is receiving if adverse effects are anticipated or are being monitored.

IMPLEMENTATION—ACTION/RATIONALE

ACTION

1. Cleanse hands. Apply gloves (optional).
2. Select the appropriate vial (Figure 27-10-1).

Figure 27-10-1 Carefully select the ordered medication.

3. Verify health care provider's orders.
4. Check expiration date on vial.

5. Determine the route of medication delivery and select the appropriate size syringe and needle.
6. While holding the syringe at eye level, withdraw the plunger to the desired volume of medication.
7. Clean the rubber top of the vial with a 70% alcohol pad. Use a circular motion starting at the center and working out.
8. Using sterile technique, uncap the needle and lay the needle cap on a clean surface.
9. Placing the needle in the center of the vial, inject the air slowly. Do not cause turbulence.

10. Invert the vial and slowly, using gentle negative pressure, withdraw the medication. Keep the needle tip in the liquid.
11. With the syringe at eye level, determine that the appropriate dose has been reached by volume (Figure 27-10-2).
12. Slowly withdraw the needle from the vial. Follow the institution's policy regarding recapping and changing needles (Figure 27-10-3).
13. Using ink, mark the current date and time and initials on the vial.
14. Label the syringe with drug, dose, date, and time.
15. Cleanse hands.

RATIONALE

1. Decreases transmission of microorganisms.
2. Prevents medication errors.

3. Prevents medication errors.
4. Avoids giving expired medication, which may have altered potency.
5. The route of medication delivery is essential to selecting the appropriate size syringe and needle.
6. Holding the syringe at eye level makes it easier to read the syringe calibrations and increases accuracy.
7. Ensures that the center of the rubber top is the cleanest area for needle entry. Reduces potential contamination with microorganisms.
8. Prevents spread of microorganisms.
9. Adding air prevents the buildup of negative pressure in the vial. Turbulence, which can result in air bubbles forming within the vial, can affect the accuracy of the volume of liquid being withdrawn.
10. Decreases the number of air bubbles that tend to form with unsteady, fast, jerky motions. Keeping the needle tip in the liquid prevents drawing in air.
11. Ensures client receives the ordered dose of medication.

12. Avoids splatter of medication and potential contamination of nearby supplies. Keeps the needle sterile.

13. Prevents using a medication that has been opened too long per institutional protocol.
14. Prevents medication errors.
15. Decreases transmission of microorganisms.

continues

Figure 27-10-2 Invert the vial and slowly withdraw the medication until the appropriate dosage has been reached.

Figure 27-10-3 Follow the institutional policy regarding recapping needles.

EVALUATION

- The correct medication ampule was selected.
- The vial was current and the rubber seal intact.
- The correct amount of medication was withdrawn.
- The needle did not become contaminated or damaged.

DOCUMENTATION

Medication Administration Record

- Name of the medication
- Dosage drawn up
- Date and time the medication was drawn up

If the medication drawn up is a controlled substance, document in the Controlled Substances Record Book:
- Name of the medication
- Dosage drawn up
- Date and time the medication was drawn up
- Any controlled substance that was wasted
- Name of nurse drawing up the controlled substance

Controlled substances must be documented at the time they are removed from the locked cabinet. Documentation on the MAR is done after the medication is administered.

PROCEDURE 27-11   Administering an Intradermal Injection

OVERVIEW

An intradermal injection is a method used to administer medications just below the skin. Potent medications that should be absorbed slowly are given intradermally because of the less richly supplied blood vessels of this layer; however, the client may respond rapidly and should be monitored for allergic reactions.

The most common reason for an intradermal injection is skin testing such as tuberculin screening or allergy testing. Only small amounts (0.01 to 0.10 mL) of fluid are given intradermally.

The most common sites for injections are forearms and upper back. The site should be lightly pigmented, free of lesions, and hairless. Because these areas are easily accessible, the nurse can monitor the reaction (Figure 27-11-1).

A tuberculin or small hypodermic syringe is used with a short ($^1/_4$ to $^1/_2$ inch), fine (26 to 27) gauge needle.

continues

As of April 2001, a Federal Needle Stick Safety and Prevention Law requires safe medical devices. The position of the Occupational and Safety Health Act (OSHA) provides that whenever exposure to blood-borne pathogens is anticipated, controls to eliminate employee exposure should be used, hence, safe devices. Examples of such devices are needle-protected or needleless systems. In the case of intradermal injections, safety syringes or needles should be used. These can be safety-glide needles or safety-retraction or slide syringes. Instruction should be provided appropriate to manufacturers' specifications.

Figure 27-11-1 Common intradermal injection sites: A. Inner aspect of the forearm; B. Upper chest; C. Upper back

ASSESSMENT

1. Assess the five rights: right client, right medication, right route, right dose, and right time. **Prevents errors in medication administration.**
2. Review health care provider's order **so the drug is administered safely and correctly.**
3. Review information regarding the expected reaction to the allergen **to anticipate the type of reaction a client may have.**
4. Assess for the indications for intradermal injection, including the client's allergy history, **so the nurse will not administer a substance to which the client is known to be sensitive.**
5. Check the expiration date of the medication vial **because the drug loses its potency over time.**
6. Assess client's knowledge regarding the medication to be received **so client education may be tailored according to need.**
7. Assess the client's response to discussion about an injection **because some clients may express anticipatory anxiety, which may increase pain.**

Figure 27-11-2 Syringes come in many sizes. Select a 1-mL tuberculin safety-syringe for intradermal injections.

POSSIBLE NURSING DIAGNOSES

Risk for Infection
Impaired Skin Integrity
Deficient Knowledge (procedure)
Anxiety

PLANNING

Expected Outcomes

1. The client will experience only minimal pain or burning at the injection site.
2. The client will experience no allergic reaction or other side effects from the injection.
3. The client will be able to explain the significance of the presence or absence of a skin reaction.
4. The client will keep follow-up appointments within the recommended time frame to have responses to the medication evaluated.

Equipment Needed

- Tuberculin syringe, 1 ml (Figure 27-11-2)
- Needle (25- to 27-gauge, $1/4$- to $5/8$-inch)
- Antiseptic or alcohol swabs
- Medication ampule or vial
- Medication card or medication administration record
- Gloves

DELEGATION TIPS

The procedure of medication administration is not delegated to ancillary personnel in acute care settings. This may vary in state or federal institutions. Ancillary personnel are generally informed about the medications the client is receiving if adverse effects are anticipated or are being monitored.

continues

IMPLEMENTATION—ACTION/RATIONALE

ACTION

RATIONALE

* Check client's identification band * Explain procedure before beginning *

1. Cleanse hands and put on clean gloves.
2. In the inpatient setting, close door or curtains around bed and keep gown or sheet draped over body. In the outpatient setting, close door to exam or treatment room. Identify client.
3. Select 1 mL tuberculin syringe and $^1/_4$- to $^5/_8$-inch 25- to 27-gauge needle.
4. Assist client into a comfortable position. Forearm site: Relax the arm with elbow and forearm extended on a flat surface. Distract client by talking about an interesting subject.
5. Select injection site.
   • Inspect skin for bruises, inflammation, edema, masses, tenderness, and sites of previous injections.
   • Forearm site should be 3 to 4 finger widths below antecubital space and one hand width above wrists on inner aspect of forearm.
6. Use antiseptic swab in a circular motion to clean skin at site.
7. While holding the swab between fingers of nondominant hand, pull cap from needle.
8. Administer injection:
   • With nondominant hand, stretch skin over site with forefinger and thumb.
   • Insert needle slowly at a 5- to 15-degree angle, bevel up, until resistance is felt; then advance to no more than $^1/_8$ inch below the skin. The needle tip should be seen through the skin.
   • Slowly inject the medication. Resistance will be felt.

   • Note a small bleb, like a mosquito bite, forming under the skin surface (Figure 27-11-3).
9. Withdraw the needle while applying gentle pressure with the antiseptic swab.
10. Do not massage the site.

1. Reduces transmission of microorganisms.
2. Provides privacy. Ensures medication is given to right client.

3. Ensures that needle will be inserted into the dermis.

4. Relaxation minimizes discomfort. Distraction reduces anxiety.

5. Injection site should be free of lesions. Repeated daily injections should be rotated. Ensures a clear site for interpreting results.

6. Circular motion and mechanical action of swab remove secretions containing microorganisms.
7. Swab remains accessible during procedure. Prevents contamination of needle.
8.
   • Needle penetrates tight skin easier than loose skin.

   • Ensures needle tip is in the dermis.

   • Dermal layer is tight and does not expand easily when fluid is injected.
   • Indicates the medication was deposited in the dermis.
9. Supporting tissue around injection site minimizes discomfort.
10. Prevents medication from being dispersed into the tissue and altering test results.

Figure 27-11-3 Note a small bleb, like a mosquito bite, forming under the skin surface as the medication is injected.

continues

11. Assist the client to a comfortable position.
12. Discard the uncapped needle and syringe in a sharps container.
13. Remove gloves and cleanse hands.

11. Promotes comfort.
12. Decreases risk of needlestick.

13. Reduces transmission of microorganisms.

EVALUATION

- The client experienced only minimal pain or burning at the injection site.
- The client experienced no allergic reaction or other side effects from the injection.
- The client was able to explain the significance of the presence or absence of a skin reaction.
- The client kept all follow-up appointments within the recommended time frame to have responses to the medication evaluated.

DOCUMENTATION

Medication Administration Record

- Date, time, medication, dose, route, site, and signature or initials

Nurses' Notes

- Date and time of skin reaction
- Date and time of any systemic side effects of the medication. Report to health care provider.

PROCEDURE 27-12   Administering a Subcutaneous Injection

OVERVIEW

A subcutaneous injection is a method used to administer medications into the loose connective tissues just below the dermis of the skin. Medications that do not need to be absorbed as quickly as those given intramuscularly are given subcutaneously because of the less richly supplied blood vessels in the subcutaneous tissue; however, the client may respond more rapidly to a subcutaneous injection than to oral medication and should be monitored for potential side effects, allergic reactions, the risk of infection, or bleeding.

Only small (0.5- to 1-mL) doses of isotonic, nonirritating, nonviscous, and water-soluble medications should be given subcutaneously, such as insulin, tetanus toxoid, allergy medications, epinephrine, and vitamin B_{12}. If larger volumes of medications remain in these sensitive tissues, a sterile abscess could form, causing a hard, painful lump.

The most common sites for subcutaneous injections are the vascular areas around the outer aspect of the upper arms, the abdomen, and the anterior aspect of the thighs (Figure 27-12-1). Because these areas are easily accessible, the client may learn how to self-administer medications. Rotation of sites of injections should be observed so that no site is used more often than every 6 to 7 weeks.

For a subcutaneous injection, a 2- to 3-mL syringe or a 1-mL syringe is recommended. U-100 insulin syringes in 30-, 50-, and 100-unit sizes are used for subcutaneous insulin injections. The most commonly used needle for a subcutaneous injection is a $^5/_8$-inch 25-gauge needle. Adjustments need to be made for pediatric, obese, or cachectic clients.

As of April 2001, a Federal Needle Stick Safety and Prevention Law requires safe medical devices. The position of the Occupational and Safety Health Act (OSHA) pro-

Figure 27-12-1 Subcutaneous injection sites: **A,** Abdomen; **B,** Lateral and anterior aspects of upper arm and thigh; **C,** Scapular area or back; **D,** Upper ventrodorsal gluteal area.

continues

vides that whenever exposure to blood-borne pathogens is anticipated, controls to eliminate employee exposure should be used, hence, safe devices. Failure to comply with using safe devices and safe disposal can result in fines. Examples of safe devices are needle-protected or needleless systems with proper disposal in clearly marked sharps containers. In the case of subcutaneous injections, safety syringes or needles should be used. These can be safety-glide or retraction needles or slide syringes. Instruction should be provided appropriate to manufacturers' specifications.

ASSESSMENT

1. Assess the five rights: right client, right medication, right route, right dose, and right time. **Prevents errors in medication administration.**
2. Review health care provider's order **so the drug is administered safely and correctly.**
3. Review information regarding the drug ordered, such as action, purpose, time of onset and peak action, normal dosage, common side effects, and nursing implications **to anticipate the drug's effects and anticipate a reaction.**
4. Assess client for factors that may influence an injection such as circulatory shock or reduced local tissue perfusion **because reduced tissue perfusion will interfere with the absorption and distribution of the drug.**
5. Assess for previous subcutaneous injections **in order to rotate sites and avoid repeating a dose in the same site.**
6. Assess for the indications for subcutaneous injection **because an injection is preferred for clients who are confused or unconscious, are unable to swallow a tablet, or have a gastrointestinal disturbance, including the use of nasogastric suction.**
7. Assess the client's age **because older clients or pediatric clients have special needs based on their physiologic status.**
8. Assess client's knowledge regarding the medication to be received **so client education may be tailored according to need.**

9. Assess the client's response to discussion about an injection **because some clients may express anticipatory anxiety, which may increase pain.**

POSSIBLE NURSING DIAGNOSES

Risk for Infection
Impaired Skin Integrity
Anxiety
Deficient Knowledge (procedure)

PLANNING

Expected Outcomes

1. The client will experience only minimal pain or burning at the injection site.
2. The client will experience no allergic reaction or other side effects from the injection.
3. The client will be able to explain the action, side effects, dosage and schedule of the medication, and rationale for rotation of sites.

Equipment Needed

• Syringe appropriate for the medication being given
• Needle (25- to 27-gauge, $^3/_8$- to $^5/_8$-inch)
• Antiseptic or alcohol swabs
• Medication ampule or vial
• Medication record
• Gloves

DELEGATION TIPS

The procedure of medication administration is not delegated to ancillary personnel in acute care settings. This may vary in state or federal institutions. Ancillary personnel are generally informed about the medications the client is receiving if adverse effects are anticipated or are being monitored.

IMPLEMENTATION—ACTION/RATIONALE

ACTION	RATIONALE
✴ Check client's identification band ✴ Explain procedure before beginning ✴	
1. Cleanse hands and put on clean gloves.	1. Reduces the number of microorganisms.
2. Close door or curtains around bed and keep gown or sheet draped over client.	2. Provides privacy.

continues

3. Select injection site.
   - Inspect skin for bruises, inflammation, edema, masses, tenderness, and sites of previous injections and avoid these areas.
   - Use subcutaneous tissue around the abdomen, lateral aspects of upper arm or thigh, or scapular area.
4. Select needle size:
   - Measure skinfold by grasping skin between thumb and forefinger.
   - Be sure needle is one-half the length of the skinfold from top to bottom.
5. Assist client into a comfortable position:
   - Relax the arm, leg, or abdomen.
   - Distract client by talking about an interesting subject or explaining what you are doing step by step.
6. Use antiseptic swab to clean skin at site.

7. While holding swab between fingers of nondominant hand, pull cap from needle.
8. Administer injection:
   - Hold syringe between thumb and forefinger of dominant hand like a dart.
   - Pinch skin with nondominant hand (Figure 27-12-2).

   - Inject needle quickly and firmly (like a dart) at a 45- to 90-degree angle (Figure 27-12-3).

   - Release the skin.

   - Grasp the lower end of the syringe with nondominant hand and position dominant hand to the end of the plunger. Do not move the syringe.
   - Pull back on the plunger to ascertain that the needle is not in a vein. If no blood appears, slowly inject the medication. (Aspiration is contraindicated with some medications; check with the pharmacy if you are unclear.)
9. Remove hand from injection site and quickly withdraw the needle. Apply pressure with the antiseptic swab. Do not push down on the needle with the swab while withdrawing it, because this will cause more pain.

3. Injection site should be free of lesions.
   - Repeated daily injections should be rotated.

   - Avoids injury to underlying nerves, bone, or blood vessels.
4. Ensures that needle will be inserted into subcutaneous tissue.

5. Relaxation minimizes discomfort. Distraction reduces anxiety.

6. Circular motion and mechanical action of swab remove microorganisms.
7. Swab remains accessible during procedure. Prevents contamination of needle.
8.
   - Quick, smooth injection is easier with proper position of syringe.
   - Needle penetrates tight skin easier than loose skin. Pinching skin elevates subcutaneous tissue.
   - Quick, firm injection minimizes discomfort. Angle depends on amount of subcutaneous tissue present and the site used.

   - Injection requires smooth manipulation of syringe parts. Movement of syringe may cause discomfort.

   - Aspiration of blood indicates intravenous placement of needle so procedure may have to be abandoned.

9. Supporting tissue around injection site minimizes discomfort. Removing hand before withdrawing needle reduces chance of needlestick.

Figure 27-12-2 Pinch the skin with the nondominant hand.

Figure 27-12-3 When injecting at a 90° angle, hold the syringe like a dart and pierce the skin quickly and firmly.

continues

10. Apply pressure. Some medications should not be massaged. Ask the pharmacy if you are unclear.
11. Assist the client to a comfortable position.
12. Discard the uncapped needle and syringe in a disposable needle receptacle.
13. Remove gloves and cleanse hands.

10. Stimulates circulation and improves drug distribution and absorption.
11. Promotes comfort and encourages client to remain still.
12. Decreases risk of needlestick.
13. Reduces transmission of microorganisms.

EVALUATION

• Ask the client about pain, burning, numbness, or tingling at the injection site.
• Assess the client's response to the medication 30 minutes later.
• Ask the client to discuss the purpose, action, schedule, and side effects of the medication.

DOCUMENTATION

Medication Administration Record

• Date, time, medication, dose, route, site of injection, and signature or initials

Nurses' Notes

• Date and time of response to the medication
• Date and time of any side effects of the medication

PROCEDURE 27-13   Administering an Intramuscular Injection

OVERVIEW

An intramuscular injection is a method used to administer medications into the deep muscle tissue. Medications will be absorbed quickly because of the richly supplied blood vessels in the muscle. Most aqueous medications are absorbed in 10 to 30 minutes. Average-sized adults can tolerate up to 3 mL of medication injected into a large muscle because muscle is less sensitive to irritating and viscous drugs than subcutaneous tissue.

The most common sites for intramuscular injections are the vastus lateralis, the ventrogluteal, the dorsogluteal, and the deltoid muscles (Figure 27-13-1). The *vastus lateralis* muscle is located on the anterior lateral aspect of the thigh. This easily accessible site is the preferred site for clients of all ages because it has no major blood vessels or nerves nearby. The *ventrogluteal* site is the preferred site in adults because it is located deep and away from major blood vessels and nerves. It is preferred over the dorsogluteal for the following reasons: There is less risk of damage to the sciatic nerve and blood vessels; this site is less painful because the muscle is most often not tense even in an anxious client. The *dorsogluteal* muscle in the upper outer quadrant of the buttock poses greater risk of damage to the sciatic nerve, major blood vessels, and the greater trochanter bone. It should not be used in children younger than 5 years of age because this muscle is not developed. The *deltoid* muscle is found on the upper arm about 1 to 2 inches below the acromion process. Major nerves and blood vessels are beneath this site, and only small volumes of medication should be injected.

Originally the Z-track method of intramuscular injections was used as a special procedure for only certain medications. Medications such as iron dextran and hydralazine hydrochloride can be irritating to the tissues and stain the skin. Using the Z-track method prevents potentially irritating medications from being tracked up through the tissues by interrupting the injection tract. This method can help reduce pain also with nonstaining or irritating substances.

There are many different types and sizes of syringes. Prefilled syringes that consist of a prefilled barrel and needle assembly placed in a reusable plunger are often used (Figure 27-13-2). For an intramuscular injection, a 2- to 3-mL syringe is recommended with a $1^1/_4$- to $1^1/_2$-inch, 19- to 23-gauge needle. Adjustments need to be made for pediatric, obese, or cachectic clients.

As of April 2001, a Federal Needle Stick Safety and Prevention Law requires safe medical devices. The position of the Occupational and Safety Health Act (OSHA) provides that whenever exposure to blood-borne pathogens is anticipated, controls to eliminate employee exposure should be used, hence, safe devices. Failure to comply with using safe devices and safe disposal

continues

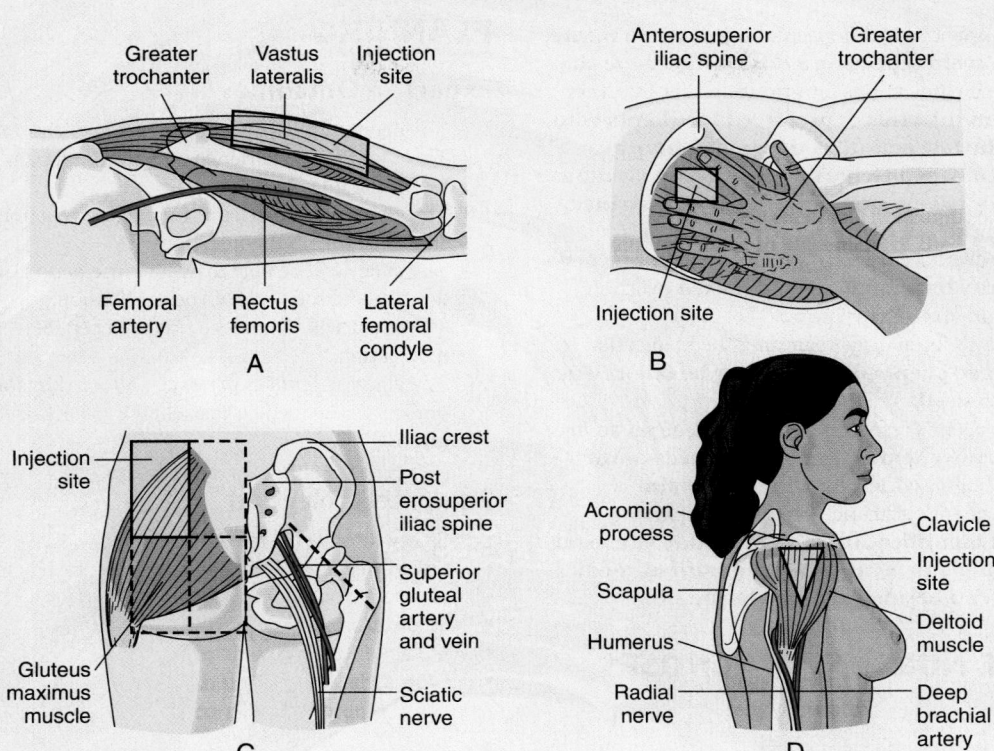

Figure 27-13-1 Intramuscular injection sites. **A,** Vastus lateralis: Identify greater trochanter; place hand at lateral femoral condyle; injection site is middle third of anterior lateral aspect. **B,** Ventrogluteal: Place palm of left hand on right greater trochanter so that index finger points toward anterosuperior iliac spine; spread first and middle fingers to form a V; injection site is the middle of the V angle. **C,** Dorsogluteal: Place hand on iliac crest and locate the posterosuperior iliac spine. Draw an imaginary line between the trochanter and the iliac spine; the injection site is the outer quadrant. **D,** Deltoid: Locate the lateral side of the humerus from two to three finger widths below the acromion process in adults or one finger width below the acromion process in children.

Figure 27-13-2 A prefilled syringe consists of a prefilled barrel and needle assembly placed in a reusable plunger.

can result in fines. Examples of safe devices are needle-protected or needleless systems with proper disposal in sharps containers clearly marked. With intramuscular injections, safety syringes or needles should be used. These can be safety-glide or retraction needles or slide syringes. Instruction should be provided appropriate to manufacturers' specifications.

ASSESSMENT

1. Assess the five rights: right client, right medication, right route, right dose, and right time. **Prevents errors in medication administration.**
2. Review health care provider's order **so the drug is administered safely and correctly.**
3. Review information regarding the drug ordered, such as action, purpose, time of onset and peak action, normal dosage, common side effects, and nursing implications **to anticipate the drug's effects and anticipate a reaction.**
4. Assess client for factors that may influence an injection, such as circulatory shock, reduced local tissue perfusion, or muscle atrophy **because reduced tissue perfusion will interfere with the absorption and distribution of the drug.**

continues

5. Assess for previous intramuscular injections **to rotate sites and avoid repeating a dose in the same site.**
6. Assess for the indications for intramuscular injection **because an injection is preferred for clients who require the fast action of the medication, are confused or unconscious, are unable to swallow a tablet, or have a gastrointestinal disturbance, including the use of nasogastric suction.**
7. Assess the client's age **because older clients or pediatric clients have special needs based on their physiologic status.**
8. Assess client's knowledge regarding the medication to be received **so client education may be tailored according to need.**
9. Assess the client's response to discussion about an injection **because some clients may express anticipatory anxiety, which may increase pain.**
10. Assess the client's size and muscle development. **Assists in identification of appropriate site, needle size, angle to be used, and amount of medication that can be administered in the site.**

POSSIBLE NURSING DIAGNOSES

Risk for Infection
Impaired Skin Integrity
Anxiety
Deficient Knowledge (injection)

PLANNING

Expected Outcomes

1. The client will receive the correct medication.
2. The client will experience only minimal pain or burning at the injection site.
3. The client will experience no allergic reaction or other side effects from the injection.
4. The client will be able to explain the action, side effects, dosage, and schedule of the medication.
5. The client will obtain the expected benefit from the medication.
6. The client will not experience pain or skin staining secondary to the medication when Z-track injection is given.

Equipment Needed

- Safety-syringe (1- to 3-mL)
- Safety-needle (19- to 23-gauge, $1^1/_4$ to $1^1/_2$ inches)
- Antiseptic or alcohol swabs
- Medication ampule or vial
- Medication record
- Gloves

DELEGATION TIPS

The procedure of medication administration is not delegated to ancillary personnel in acute care settings. This may vary in state or federal institutions. Ancillary personnel are generally informed about the medications the client is receiving if adverse affects are anticipated or are being monitored.

IMPLEMENTATION—ACTION/RATIONALE

ACTION

* Check client's identification band * Explain procedure before beginning *

1. Cleanse hands and put on clean gloves.
2. Close door or curtains around bed and keep gown or sheet draped over client.
3. Select injection site (Figure 27-13-1).
   - Inspect skin for bruises, inflammation, edema, masses, tenderness, and sites of previous injections.
   - Use anatomic landmarks.

4. Select needle size: Assess size and weight of client and site to be used.

RATIONALE

1. Reduces the number of microorganisms.
2. Provides privacy.

3. Injection site should be free of lesions.
   - Repeated daily injections should be rotated.

   - Avoids injury to underlying nerves, bone, or blood vessels. Site should be selected based on muscle development, type, and amount of medication, and comfortable access to site.
4. Ensures that needle will be inserted into the muscle.

continues

Figure 27-13-3 Have the client stand or sit with arm relaxed at side.

Figure 27-13-4 Inject needle quickly and firmly at a 90° angle.

5. Assist client into a comfortable position:
   - For vastus lateralis, lying flat or supine with knee slightly flexed
   - For ventrogluteal, lying on side or back with knee and hip slightly flexed
   - For dorsogluteal, lying prone with feet turned inward or on side with upper knee and hip flexed and placed in front of lower leg
   - For deltoid, standing with arm relaxed at side or sitting with lower arm relaxed on lap or lying flat with lower arm relaxed across abdomen (Figure 27-13-3).
   - Distract client by talking about an interesting subject.
6. Use antiseptic swab to clean skin at site.

7. While holding swab between fingers of nondominant hand, pull cap from needle.
8. Administer injection:
   - Hold syringe between thumb and forefinger of dominant hand like a dart.
   - Spread skin tightly or pinch a generous section of tissue firmly—for cachectic clients.
   - Inject needle quickly and firmly (like a dart) at a 90-degree angle (Figure 27-13-4).
   - Release the skin.
   - Grasp the lower end of the syringe with nondominant hand and position dominant hand to the end of the plunger. Do not move the syringe.
   - Pull back on the plunger and aspirate to ascertain if needle is in a vein. If no blood appears, slowly inject the medication.
9. Remove nondominant hand and quickly withdraw the needle. Apply pressure with the antiseptic swab.

10. Apply pressure. Certain protocols suggest gentle massage action.

Z-track Injection

11. Create an air lock. Add 0.1 to 0.2 mL of air to the dose in the syringe. The air will push the medication out of the needle when the last of the medication has been injected.

5. Relaxation minimizes discomfort. Distraction reduces anxiety.

6. Circular motion and mechanical action of swab remove secretions containing microorganisms.
7. Swab remains accessible during procedure. Prevents contamination of needle.
8.
   - Quick, smooth injection is easier with proper position of syringe.
   - Needle penetrates tight skin more easily than loose skin.
   - Quick, firm injection minimizes discomfort.

   - Injection requires smooth manipulation of syringe parts. Movement of syringe may cause discomfort.

   - Aspiration of blood indicates intravenous placement of needle so procedure may have to be abandoned.
9. Supporting tissue around injection site minimizes discomfort. Removing hand before withdrawing needle prevents needlestick.
10. Pressure prevents medication from leaking out of site. Gentle massage stimulates circulation and improves drug distribution and absorption.

11. The injected medication is followed by air to clear the medication from the needle.

continues

Skin pulled taut   Skin released

Figure 27-13-5 Administering intramuscular injection using Z-track technique.

12. Using your nondominant hand, pull the skin and sub-cutaneous tissue to the side or downward about an inch, out of alignment with the underlying muscle (Figure 27-13-5). (Do not use this technique in the deltoid; dorsogluteal is the preferred site).

13. Using sterile technique, remove the needle guard using your nondominant hand.

14. While maintaining traction on the skin, using your dominant hand, dart the needle into the skin at a 90-degree angle.

15. Aspirate for a minimum of 5 seconds. Observe for a blood return.

16. If no blood return is present, slowly (at a rate of 1 mL/10 seconds) inject the medication.

17. Allow the needle to stay in place for 10 seconds after the medication is injected.

18. While still maintaining traction on the skin with the nondominant hand, smoothly remove the needle and allow the skin to return to its normal position.

19. Do not rub or wipe the skin after removal of the needle.

20. Assist the client to a comfortable position.

21. Discard the uncapped needle and syringe in a specified biohazard sharps container.

22. Remove gloves and cleanse hands.

12. Pulling the tissue to the side or downward prior to the injection will break the injection track after removing the needle and not allow the medication to track back up to the surface of the skin. Also, by pulling the tissue tight, the skin becomes firm and facilitates entry of the needle.

13. Ensures the needle is not contaminated with microorganisms.

14. Darting the needle is more comfortable for the client. A 90-degree angle will ensure the needle reaches muscle tissue and is not trapped in the subcutaneous or adipose tissue.

15. Blood from small vessels can take up to 5 seconds to appear in the syringe.

16. Allows the medication to diffuse, causing less stretch on the muscle fibers and thus is better tolerated by the client.

17. Allows the medication to diffuse before the needle is removed, which decreases the chance that any medication will be tracked back up through the skin.

18. Holding traction on the tissue prevents any irritation caused by the needle being removed. Allowing the tissue to slide over the track seals the track.

19. This can cause seepage of the medication back to the surface and result in irritation.

20. Promotes comfort.

21. Decreases risk of needlestick.

22. Reduces transmission of microorganisms.

EVALUATION

- The client received the correct medication.
- Ask the client about any pain, burning, numbness, or tingling at the injection site.
- Assess the client's response to the medication 10 to 30 minutes later.
- Ask the client to explain the purpose, action, schedule, and side effects of the medication.
- The client obtains the expected benefit.

DOCUMENTATION

Medication Administration Record

- Name of medication
- Dosage
- Route of administration
- Location of injection
- Time administered
- Initials and signature of nurse administering medication

Nurses' Notes

- Time and type of client complaint
- Medication administered
- Outcome of treatment (patient response)
- Nurse's signature

PROCEDURE 27-14   Administering Eye and Ear Medications

OVERVIEW

Eye Medications

Eye medications refer to drops, ointment, and disks. These drugs are used for diagnostic and therapeutic purposes—to lubricate the eye or socket for a prosthetic eye and to prevent or treat eye conditions such as glaucoma (elevated pressure within the eye) and infection. Diagnostically, eyedrops can be used to anesthetize the eye, dilate the pupil, and stain the cornea to identify abrasions and scars.

Review the abbreviations used in medication orders to ensure that the medication is instilled in the correct eye. Cross-contamination is a potential problem with eyedrops. Adhere to the following safety measures to prevent cross-contamination:

- Each client should have his or her own bottle of eyedrops.
- Discard any solution remaining in the dropper after instillation.
- Discard the dropper if the tip is accidentally contaminated by touching the bottle or any part of the client's eye.

Ear Medications

Solutions ordered to treat the ear are often referred to as otic (pertaining to the ear) drops or irrigation. Eardrops may be instilled to soften ear wax, to produce anesthesia, to treat infection or inflammation, or to facilitate removal of a foreign body, such as an insect. External auditory canal irrigations are usually performed for cleaning purposes and less frequently for applying heat and antiseptic solutions.

Before instilling a solution into the ear, inspect the ear for signs of drainage, which is an indication of a perforated tympanic membrane. Eardrops are usually contraindicated when the tympanic membrane is perforated. If the tympanic membrane is damaged, all procedures must be performed using sterile technique; otherwise, medical asepsis is used when instilling medication into the ear.

Certain conditions have contraindications for specific drugs (e.g., hydrocortisone eardrops are contraindicated in clients with a fungal infection or a viral infection such as herpes).

ASSESSMENT

1. Assess the five rights: right client, right medication, right route, right dose, and right time. **Prevents errors in medication administration.**
2. Assess the condition of the client's eyes and/or ears. Are there any contraindications to administering this medication present? Is there drainage from the ear indicating a possible tympanic rupture? If so, the medication administration must be done using sterile technique. **Reassessing the client before every medication dose prevents possibly injuring the client.**
3. Assess the medication order. Is the medication for only one eye/ear or both? With eye medications be sure to understand the abbreviations used for right eye (OD), left eye (OS), and both eyes (OU). **Prevents errors in medication administration.**

POSSIBLE NURSING DIAGNOSES

*Risk for **I**njury*
*Deficient **K**nowledge* (medication regime)
*Disturbed **S**ensory Perception* (visual or auditory)

PLANNING

Expected Outcomes

1. The client will receive the right dose of the right medication via the right route at the right time.
2. The client will encounter minimum discomfort during the medication administration procedure.
3. The client will receive maximum benefit from the medication.

Equipment Needed

Eye Medication

- Medication administration record (MAR)
- Eye medication
- Tissue or cotton ball
- Nonsterile latex-free gloves (if needed)

Ear Medication

- Medication administration record (MAR)
- Medication
- Nonsterile latex-free gloves
- Cotton-tipped applicator
- Tissue

continues

DELEGATION TIPS

The procedure of medication administration is not delegated to ancillary personnel in acute care settings. This may vary in state or federal institutions. Ancillary personnel are generally informed about the medications the client is receiving if adverse effects are anticipated or are being monitored.

IMPLEMENTATION—ACTION/RATIONALE

ACTION

* Check client's identification band * Explain procedure before beginning *

RATIONALE

Eye Medication

1. Check with the client and the chart for any known allergies or medical conditions that would contraindicate use of the drug.
2. Gather the necessary equipment.
3. Follow the five rights of drug administration.
4. Take the medication to the client's room and place on a clean surface.
5. Inquire if the client wants to instill medication. If so, assess the client's ability to do so.
6. Cleanse hands, and don nonsterile latex-free gloves if needed.
7. Place client in a supine position with the head slightly hyperextended.

1. Prevents occurrence of adverse reactions.

2. Promotes efficiency.
3. Promotes safety.
4. Decreases risk of contamination of bottle cap.

5. Some clients are used to instilling their own medication.

6. Reduces transmission of microorganisms. Decreases contact with bodily fluids.
7. Minimizes drainage of medication through the tear duct.

Instilling Eyedrops

8. Remove cap from eye bottle and place cap on its side.
9. Place a tissue below the lower lid.
10. With dominant hand, hold eyedropper $^1/_2$–$^3/_4$ inch above the eyeball; rest hand on client's forehead to stabilize.
11. Place hand on cheekbone and expose lower conjunctival sac by pulling down on cheek.
12. Instruct the client to look up and drop prescribed number of drops into center of conjunctival sac (Figure 27-14-1).

8. Prevents contamination of the bottle cap.
9. Absorbs the medication that flows from the eye.
10. Reduces risk of dropper touching eye structure, and prevents injury to the eye.
11. Stabilizes hand and prevents systemic absorption of eye medication.
12. Reduces stimulation of the blink reflex; prevents injury to the cornea.

Figure 27-14-1 To administer eye medication, gently press the lower lid down and have the client look upward while instilling drops into the lower conjunctival sac.

Figure 27-14-2 Placing the fingers on the sides of the client's nose closes the tear ducts and prevents the medication from draining out of the eye.

continues

13. Instruct client to gently close eyes and move eyes. Briefly place fingers on either side of the client's nose to close the tear ducts and prevent the medication from draining out of the eye (Figure 27-14-2).
14. Remove gloves; cleanse hands.

Eye Ointment Application

15. Repeat Actions 1–7.
16. Lower lid:
    • With nondominant hand, gently separate client's eyelids with thumb and finger and grasp lower lid near margin immediately below the lashes; exert pressure downward over the bony prominence of the cheek.
    • Instruct the client to look up.

    • Apply eye ointment along inside edge of the entire lower eyelid, from inner to outer canthus.
17. Upper lid:
    • Instruct client to look down.
    • With nondominant hand, gently grasp client's lashes near center of upper lid with thumb and index finger, and draw lid up and away from eyeball.
    • Squeeze ointment along upper lid starting at inner canthus.
18. Remove gloves; cleanse hands.

Medication Disk

19. Repeat Actions 1–7.
20. Open sterile package and press dominant, sterile gloved finger against the oval disk so that it lies lengthwise across fingertip.
21. Instruct the client to look up.

22. With nondominant hand, gently pull the client's lower eyelid down and place the disk horizontally in the conjunctival sac.
    • Then pull the lower eyelid out, up, and over the disk.
    • Instruct the client to blink several times.
    • If disk is still visible, repeat steps.
    • Once the disk is in place, instruct the client to gently press the fingers against the closed lids; do not rub eyes or move the disk across the cornea.
    • If the disk falls out, pick it up, rinse under cool water, and reinsert.
23. If the disk is prescribed for both eyes (OU), repeat Actions 20–22.
24. Remove gloves; cleanse hands.

Removing an Eye Medication Disk

25. Repeat Actions 6–7.
26. Remove the disk:
    • With nondominant hand, invert the lower eyelid and identify the disk.

13. Distributes solution over conjunctival surface and anterior eyeball.

14. Reduces transmission of microorganisms.

15. See Rationales 1–7.
16.
    • Provides access to the lower lid.

    • Reduces stimulation of the blink reflex and keeps cornea out of the way of the medication.
    • Ensures drug is applied to entire lid.
17.
    • Keeps cornea out of the way of the medication.

    • Ensures medication is applied to entire length of lid.
18. Reduces transmission of microorganisms.

19. See Rationales 1–7.
20. Promotes sticking of disk to fingertip.

21. Reduces stimulation of the blink reflex and keeps cornea out of the way of the medication.
22. Allows the disk to automatically adhere to the eye.

    • Secures the disk in the conjunctival sac.
    • Allows the disk to settle into place.
    • Ensures correct placement of the disk.
    • Secures disk placement. Prevents corneal scratches.

    • Preserves medication. This is not a sterile procedure. Health care provider must wear gloves to pick up disk.
23. Ensures both eyes are treated at the same time.

24. Reduces transmission of microorganisms.

25. See Rationales 6–7.
26.
    • Exposes the disk for removal.

continues

- If the disk is located in the upper eye, instruct the client to close the eye, and place your finger on the closed eyelid. Apply gentle, long, circular strokes; instruct client to open the eye. Disk should be located in corner of eye. With your fingertip, slide the disk to the lower lid, then proceed.
  - With dominant hand, use the forefinger to slide the disk onto the lid and out of the client's eye.

- Safely moves the disk to the lower conjunctival sac.

- Safely removes the disk without scratching the cornea.

27. Remove gloves; cleanse hands.
28. Record on the MAR the removal of the disk.

27. Reduces transmission of microorganisms.
28. Provides documentation that the disk was removed.

Ear Medication

1. Check with client and chart for any known allergies.
2. Check the MAR against the health care provider's written orders.
3. Cleanse hands.
4. Place the client in a side-lying position with the affected ear facing up.
5. Straighten the ear canal by pulling the pinna down and back for children less than 3 years of age or upward and outward in adults and older children.
6. Instill the drops into the ear canal by holding the dropper at least $1/2$ inch above the ear canal (Figure 27-14-3).

1. Prevents the occurrence of hypersensitivity reactions.
2. Ensures accuracy in identification of the medication.
3. Reduces transfer of microorganisms.
4. Facilitates the administration of the medication.
5. Opens the canal and facilitates introduction of the medication.
6. Prevents injury to the ear canal.

Figure 27-14-3 Slowly instill the drops, holding the dropper at least $1/2$ inch above the ear canal.

7. Ask the client to maintain the position for 2 to 3 minutes.
8. Place a cotton ball on the outermost part of the canal.
9. Cleanse hands.

7. Allows for distribution of the medication.
8. Prevents the medication from escaping when the client changes to a sitting or standing position.
9. Reduces the transmission of microorganisms.

EVALUATION

- The client received the right dose of the right medication via the right route at the right time.
- The procedure was performed with minimum trauma and/or discomfort to the client.
- The client received maximum benefit from the medication.
- All the prescribed medication went into the eye or ear and none was spilled.

DOCUMENTATION

Medication Administration Record (MAR)

- Date, time, medication, location, and dosage administered
- If an ordered medication was not given, note this, usually by circling the time of the missed medication.

Nurses' Notes

- If an ordered medication was not given, record the reason.
- If an as-needed medication was given, note the reason for giving the medication and the client's response.

PROCEDURE 27-15   Administering Skin/Topical Medications

OVERVIEW

Topical medications are directly applied to the skin or mucous membranes. These types of medications are used for their local effect or to produce systemic effects by absorption from percutaneous routes. Topical medications include creams, ointments, and lotions. Topical medications applied to the skin are commonly used to relieve itching, prevent local infections, moisten the skin, or for vasodilation. Most topical medications are used for local effects; however, certain medications can be absorbed percutaneously to provide systemic effects, such as topical nitroglycerin, nicotine patches, or certain estrogen products.

ASSESSMENT

1. Assess the five rights: right client, right medication, right route, right dose, and right time. **Prevents errors in medication administration.**
2. Assess the area where treatment will be applied **to establish a baseline condition of the skin for future comparison.**
3. If drug is being used for systemic effect, assess for area free of scars, moles, or other skin aberrations **to facilitate selection of a site with no barriers to absorption.**

POSSIBLE NURSING DIAGNOSIS

Risk for Impaired Skin Integrity

PLANNING

Expected Outcomes

1. Good skin integrity
2. Relief of itching, irritation, or pain
3. Improved circulation

Equipment Needed

- Correct medication
- Correct applicator (cotton balls, sterile gauze pad, tongue blades, or cotton applicator)
- Gloves (sterile if broken skin integrity)
- Basin with warm water
- Mild soap (if appropriate and not contraindicated by skin condition or interaction with medication)
- Washcloth and towel
- Gauze dressing, tape as indicated
- Disposable waterproof pad
- Chart or medication sheet for medication verification
- Latex-free gloves

DELEGATION TIPS

The application of some creams, lotions, and ointments may be delegated to properly trained ancillary personnel, but these are generally over-the-counter preparations and not prescription medications.

IMPLEMENTATION—ACTION/RATIONALE

ACTION	RATIONALE
❋ Check client's identification band ❋ Explain procedure before beginning ❋	
1. Cleanse hands.	1. Reduces transmission of microorganisms.
2. Ascertain client's allergic status.	2. Avoids allergic reactions. Nurses are responsible for medication errors including reactions. Charts may not always be current regarding allergies or an oversight might have occurred.
3. If unfamiliar with medication, read label and insert or seek appropriate information.	3. Prevents inappropriate medication administration and errors. Medications should never be administered without knowledge about the medication.

continues

4. In some facilities, topical medications used for skin irritations are kept in the client's room, so verification must be done at the bedside.

5. Position the client appropriately for administration of medication. Keep client draped for privacy.

6. Put on gloves. If dressing is over area to be treated, remove, discard, and change gloves.

7. If an open wound, clean area to be treated with mild soap (if no allergies or reactions to soap) and water. If skin is irritated, use only warm water. If administering a systemically absorbed topical medication, clean the skin surface thoroughly and pat skin dry, leaving no residues of soap. Do not rub vigorously because absorption can be altered.

8. Assess the client's skin condition, making notation of circulation, drainage, color, temperature, or any altered skin integrity.

9. Change gloves.

10. Apply medication according to label. If lotion or ointment, apply a thin layer and smooth into skin as indicated.

11. If an aerosol spray is used, shake the container and administer according to direction. Spray evenly over affected area and avoid spraying close to client's or caregiver's face.

12. If gels or pastes are used, applicators may be needed. Apply evenly. If applying over an area with hair growth, follow direction of hair.

13. If powders are used, dust lightly and avoid inhalation by client and caregiver.

14. If nitroglycerin ointment or paste are used, follow instructions and orders carefully to administer correct dosage.

   • Remove the old ointment strip and clean the old site thoroughly. New ointment will be applied in different area.
   • Cleanse the new site with the appropriate cleaner.
   • Squeeze the dose out onto the enclosed medication measuring strip (Figure 27-15-1). Nitroglycerin paste dosages are measured in inches and applied to the paper measuring strip before being applied to the client.
   • Flatten the roll of nitroglycerin so the ointment will be spread over a wider area when applied to the client.
   • Apply the measuring paper, ointment side down, to a portion of the client's body without hair.
   • Tape the paper in place.

15. If a transdermal patch is used, follow the manufacturer's directions and apply the patch to a smooth, cleaned skin surface.
   • Remove the old patch and wash the site of the old patch.

4. Identifies appropriate medication with right client.

5. Keeps the client in a comfortable position for medication administration. Protects privacy.

6. Decreases contact with microorganisms.

7. Soap can irritate an open wound. If skin is already irritated, soap may cause more irritation. Systemically absorbed medication can be effected by residue on the skin or rubbing, which causes vasodilation.

8. Information can be compared with future assessment and effect of medication.

9. Prevents spread of microorganisms and avoids absorption of medication by caregivers. (This is especially important with systemically absorbed medication.)

10. Medication dosages have been studied and are recommended according to certain standards.

11. Aerosol may need to be mixed to be effective. Avoid inhalation because it may have adverse effects on the mucous membranes and lungs.

12. Apply evenly to affected areas. Excess gel or paste will be wasted because absorption can only occur at skin level. The client will experience less discomfort if hair growth pattern is followed.

13. Excess powder will be wasted because absorption can only occur at skin level. Inhalation can cause untoward effects on the lungs and mucous membranes.

14. Nitroglycerin is systemically absorbed and accurate dosing is essential. If thick lines of ointment are applied, the dose will be different; therefore, the manufacturer's suggestions must be followed carefully for safe use of this drug.
   • If areas of ointment from previous doses are not removed, the client will be receiving more than one dose at a time.
   • Ensures proper absorption of the medication.
   • Use care not to over or undermedicate by squeezing out a line of ointment that is too thick or too thin.

   • The wider area of contact and thinner coating of ointment increases absorption.

   • Using a nonhairy area increases the absorption of the medication.
   • Keeps the medication in place.

15. Patches offer a more reliable means of controlling dosage; however, patches are generally more expensive than ointments.
   • Prevents overdose.

continues

Figure 27-15-1 Squeeze the correct dose out onto the enclosed medication measuring strip.

Figure 27-15-2 When applying a transdermal patch, remove the protective covering and apply the patch.

- Wash and prepare the skin at a new site.
- Remove the protective covering over the transdermal portion of the patch and apply the new patch (Figure 27-15-2).

16. Remove gloves; cleanse hands.

- Allows for maximal medication absorption.
- Removing the protective covering allows the medication to be absorbed.

16. Reduces transmission of microorganisms.

EVALUATION

- The client's skin integrity was maintained.
- The client experienced relief of itching, irritation, or pain if this was the intent of the medication.
- The client experienced maximum effect from the topical medication.

DOCUMENTATION

Medication Administration Record

- Date, time, and site of application of the topical medication

Nurses' Notes

- Changes in the client's skin integrity, coloration, or sensation
- If medication was for irritation, itching, or rash, document any improvement or change.
- Unusual findings or client complaints

PROCEDURE 27-16   Administering Nasal Medications

OVERVIEW

Nasal medications may be administered by drops or sprays. Sprays may be packaged as pump sprays, sprays in aerosolized containers (pressurized containers, sometimes called nasal nebulizers), or powdered turbo inhalers. Prescribed medications are generally available in pump sprays or aerosolized sprays, whereby sprays and nasal drops are available in over-the-counter medications. Nasal medications may be used to achieve local effects on the nasal mucosa, indirect effects on the sinuses, or a systemic effect. Examples of medications that have systemic effects and are available in nasal sprays are insulin, agents to suppress nicotine use, and agents to treat migraine headaches. The four groups of sinuses (frontal, ethmoid, sphenoid, and maxillary) communicate with the nasal fossae and are lined with mucous membranes similar to those that line the nose. Even though it is unlikely that nasal medications penetrate the sinuses, positioning may aid in decreasing inflammation and congestion in the mucous membranes adjacent to the sinuses, thereby indirectly decreasing pressure in the sinuses. To medicate

continues

the mucous membranes adjacent to the frontal sinuses, the client will assume a supine position with the head turned to the affected side to be treated. To medicate the mucous membranes adjacent to the ethmoid sinuses, the client will lie supine with his or her head leaning back over the side of the bed with the client's head supported by the nurse's hand to avoid muscle strain on the client's neck. Although the nose is not considered a clean or sterile cavity, because of its connection with the sinuses, employ medical asepsis when performing nasal instillation.

ASSESSMENT

1. Assess the five rights: right client, right medication, right route, right dose, and right time. **Prevents errors in medication administration.**
2. Assess the client's nasal congestion and nasal obstruction **to determine if the medicine can be inhaled to reach the nasal mucosa and to determine the effectiveness of the medication.**
3. Assess the color, quantity, and odor of the client's discharge and the color and moistness of the nasal mucosa **to check for signs and symptoms of infection, to discern tissue damage, and to establish a baseline for future assessments.**
4. Assess the client's pain and/or discomfort level in the areas of sinuses **because this is another symptom of infection. May determine if the client can use the inhaler or drops.**
5. Assess the client for systemic conditions that may be adversely affected by nasal medications (see manufacturer's information). **Clients with cardiovascular conditions and hypertension may need to use caution with medications containing sympathomimetic ingredients.**

POSSIBLE NURSING DIAGNOSES

Impaired **O**ral Mucous Membrane
Impaired **T**issue Integrity

PLANNING

Expected Outcomes

1. The client will be free of nasal congestion.
2. The client will be free of nasal discharge and odor.
3. The client will breathe freely through the nasal passages.
4. The client will be free of sinus pain and nasal pain.
5. The client's nasal passages will be moist and pink.

Equipment Needed

- Medication in spray, drops, or aerosolized form
- Latex-free gloves
- Tissue as needed
- Dropper as needed

DELEGATION TIPS

The procedure of medication administration is not delegated to ancillary personnel in acute care settings. This may vary in state or federal institutions. Ancillary personnel are generally informed about the medications the client is receiving if adverse effects are anticipated or are being monitored.

IMPLEMENTATION—ACTION/RATIONALE

ACTION

RATIONALE

❋ Check client's identification band ❋ Explain procedure before beginning ❋

ACTION	RATIONALE
1. Cleanse hands. Wear a mask if the client is coughing or sneezing. Don latex-free gloves.	1. Reduces transmission of microorganisms. Respiratory-related microorganisms are easily transferred by the hands and air droplets. Gloves prevent absorption of medication through the skin of health care worker.
2. Explain the position desired for the client.	2. Ensures nose drops will reach the area of treatment by gravity with the client assuming a dependent position.
3. Explain to the client the sensation of the local effects of the medications, such as burning, tingling, and effect on taste buds. If drops are used, explain to the client that a sensation of medications may be felt in the posterior oral pharynx.	3. Some nasal medications cause undesirable tastes. If this occurs, the health care provider may order other medications or encourage mouthwashes after treatment. Prepares the client for sensation that may be felt.

continues

Figure 27-16-1   Positioning a Client for Nose Drop Instillation

4. Have the client clear the nostrils by blowing the nose.

4. Removes discharge that would prevent medication from contacting the mucous membrane.

Nose Drops

5. Ask client to lie supine and hyperextend the neck (Figure 27-16-1). Turn head to the appropriate position described in the Overview.
6. Squeeze some medication into dropper.
7. Have client exhale and occlude one nostril with a finger.
8. Insert dropper about ⅜ inch into the nostril, keeping it away from the sides of the nostril. Ask client to inhale as prescribed dosage of medication is administered.
9. Discard any unused medication remaining in the dropper.
10. Client may blot excess drainage but may not blow the nose, and should remain in position for 5 minutes.
11. Repeat on other nostril if ordered.

5. Allows the nose drops to reach the appropriate area.

6. Makes medication ready to administer.
7. Readies client to inhale as medication is administered.
8. Prevents getting microorganisms back into medication bottle. Medication is distributed better during inhalation.

9. Prevents contamination of medication.

10. Removes discomfort of drainage on face. Allows time for medication to be absorbed.
11. Generally both nostrils are treated.

Nasal Inhalers

12. Repeat Actions 1–4.
13. Explain the manufacturer's directions and how inhalers work.

14. Have the client assume an upright position. Squeeze nose drops into dropper.
15. Have the client exhale and occlude one nostril with a finger.
16. Ask the client to inhale while the spray is administered.

17. Repeat the procedure on the other nostril.
18. Remove all soiled supplies and dispose of them according to Standard Precautions. Remove gloves. Cleanse hands carefully.
19. Evaluate the effect of the medication in 15 to 20 minutes.

12. See Rationales 1–4.
13. Clients will be more compliant if they understand the use of the inhalers and that a fine cold mist will be released into the nasal passage via a pressurized container.
14. The client should be as comfortable as possible. Makes medication ready to administer.
15. Readies the client to inhale as medication is administered.
16. Nasal medications are more effective if instilled during inhalation.
17. Most often both nostrils are treated.
18. Decreases the chance of transmission of microorganisms. Respiratory diseases are especially easily transmitted.
19. Identifies if the medication is effective without adverse side effects.

continues

EVALUATION

- The client is free of nasal congestion.
- The client is free of nasal discharge and odor.
- The client breathes freely through the nasal passages.
- The client is free of sinus pain and nasal pain.
- The client's nasal passages are moist and pink.
- The client is free of adverse side effects secondary to the nasal medication.

DOCUMENTATION

Medication Administration Record

- Time and date medication was given, amount (number of drops may be necessary), and nostril medicated.

Nurses' Notes

- Results of the treatment
- Adverse or unpleasant side effects

PROCEDURE 27-17   Administering Rectal Medications

OVERVIEW

The administration of rectal medications is an important responsibility for nurses in numerous health care settings. Rectal suppositories include medications that produce both local and systemic effects. Suppositories that produce a local effect include laxatives, which promote defecation. Medications to help relieve nausea, fever, or bladder spasms can also be administered via rectal suppository but produce a systemic effect.

ASSESSMENT

1. Assess the five rights: right client, right medication, right route, right dose, and right time. **Prevents errors in medication administration.**
2. Review the health care provider's order and identify the medication to be delivered, verifying dosage, route, time, and correct client. **This ensures safe and correct administration of medications.**
3. Assess the client's need and appropriateness for rectal medication administration and review the client's history for contraindications. **A history of rectal surgery or bleeding may contraindicate use of a suppository.**
4. Consider any adjustments that may need to be taken in delivery of medications resulting from the age of the client. **This allows the nurse to deliver the medication in a correct manner if the client is an infant, child, or adult.**
5. Observe the client for the desired therapeutic effects or any adverse reactions, and document this response appropriately **to determine the effectiveness of the treatment.**
6. Assess the client's knowledge and understanding of the procedure. **Explaining the procedure not only will allay fear and anxiety but also will promote understanding and cooperation. If physically able, the client may wish to self-administer the medication.**
7. Assess the client's rectal area to determine condition of skin, mucosa, and presence of hemorrhoids or other rectal conditions. **Preventive action can be taken to protect injured skin and ensure client comfort.**

POSSIBLE NURSING DIAGNOSES

Constipation
Nausea
Chronic **P**ain

PLANNING

Expected Outcomes

1. The medication will be delivered appropriately and safely following the five rights of medication administration.
2. The desired outcome will be verbalized by the client and documented appropriately by the nurse.
3. The treatment will be completed as quickly and efficiently as possible to decrease discomfort and anxiety.
4. Client will state relief of complaint after medication administration.

Equipment Needed

- Medication (suppository or medicated enema)
- Water-soluble lubricant
- Latex-free gloves
- Tissue or washcloth
- Bedpan if client physically immobile
- Medication administration record
- Towels or pads (such as disposable "Blue pads")

continues

DELEGATION TIPS

The procedure of medication administration is not delegated to ancillary personnel in acute care settings. This may vary in state or federal institutions. Ancillary personnel are generally informed about the medications the client is receiving if adverse effects are anticipated or are being monitored.

IMPLEMENTATION—ACTION/RATIONALE

ACTION	RATIONALE

* Check client's identification band * Explain procedure before beginning *

1. Gather the equipment needed for the procedure before entering the client's room.	1. Prevents numerous trips to gather supplies and helps the procedure flow smoothly.
2. Provide privacy for client.	2. Maintains dignity and self-image.
3. Cleanse hands.	3. Reduces transmission of microorganisms.
4. Apply disposable gloves.	4. Prevents contact with fecal material.
5. Assist client into Sims' (left) position with upper leg drawn up toward chest. Provide protection under client such as towel or pad.	5. The descending colon is on the left side; this is a more anatomically correct position. Exposes the anus to identify placement. Provides comfort to client who may fear soiling linen.
6. Visually assess the client's external anus.	6. Determines presence of any active bleeding.
7. Remove suppository from wrapper and lubricate rounded end along with insertion finger. If a medicated enema is used, lubricate the enema tip if it is not prelubricated.	7. Lubrication decreases friction and decreases discomfort.
8. Tell client a cool sensation and pressure will be experienced during administration. Encourage slow, deep breaths through mouth.	8. Prepares the client for administration. Relaxes the rectal sphincter.
9. Retract buttocks with nondominant hand, visualizing the anus. Using the dominant index finger, slowly and gently insert the suppository through the anus, past the internal sphincter, and against the rectal wall (Figure 27-17-1). Depth of insertion will differ if client is a child or infant. If instilling a medicated enema, gently insert the enema tip past the internal sphincter and instill the contents by slowly squeezing.	9. Slow insertion minimizes pain. Correct placement ensures adequate absorption and less chance for expulsion of medication.

Figure 27-17-1 Inserting a Rectal Suppository

10. Remove finger or enema tip and wipe client's anal area with a washcloth or tissue.	10. Removes lubricant externally. Promotes cleanliness and comfort.

continues

11. Remove and discard gloves.	11. Reduces transfer of microorganisms.
12. Cleanse hands.	12. Reduces transfer of microorganisms.
13. Have client remain in position for 15 minutes.	13. Keeps suppository or medicated fluid in place for better absorption.
14. Place call light in client's reach.	14. Gives client control over situation.

EVALUATION

- The medication was delivered appropriately and safely following the five rights of medication administration.
- The desired outcome was verbalized by the client and documented appropriately by the nurse.
- The treatment was completed as quickly and efficiently as possible to decrease discomfort and anxiety.
- Client stated relief of complaint after medication administration.

DOCUMENTATION

Medication Administration Record

- Name of medication
- Dosage
- Route of administration
- Time administered
- Initials and signature of nurse administering medication

Nurses' Notes

- Time and type of client complaint
- Medication administered
- Outcome of treatment (client response)
- Health care provider notified, if needed
- Nurse's signature

PROCEDURE 27-18   Administering Vaginal Medications

OVERVIEW

Vaginal medications come in the form of creams, suppositories, foams, jellies, or irrigations (commonly known as douches). Vaginal medications are generally used to treat infections, irritations, or pruritis requiring topical treatment. These medications may be prescribed by a physician or nurse practitioner, or many vaginal medications can be purchased over-the-counter (OTC). Irrigations or douches can be used to soothe, cleanse, change vaginal acidity/alkalinity, or disinfect the vagina; however, if used excessively, they can cause vaginal irritation. Most often, creams, foams, or jellies are administered with an applicator or inserter. Suppositories are individually foil-wrapped, oval-shaped solids that require refrigeration. Once the suppository is inserted by an applicator or directly with a finger (gloved hand), body temperature causes the suppository to melt and the medication to be distributed. Clients often prefer to administer their own vaginal medications. Once a vaginal medication is administered, a perineal pad may be placed to collect any drainage and discharge. Pericare and personal hygiene are essential because many vaginal infections cause foul-smelling discharge and irritation. Assess the client's level of pain, pruritis, burning, or general discomfort to establish a baseline for future assessment.

ASSESSMENT

1. Assess the client's comfort level. Evaluate the level of burning, irritation, pruritis, pain, and odor **to establish a baseline for assessment of treatment.**
2. Assess the client's knowledge of the purpose of the medication and treatment. **Enables client to understand and monitor effects of medication.**

3. If the client prefers to self-administer the medication, assess the client's ability to do so, such as ability to manipulate the applicator or insert a suppository the appropriate distance. **Clients may prefer to self-administer vaginal medications for privacy, but if medication is not properly inserted it will not be effective.**

continues

POSSIBLE NURSING DIAGNOSES

*Impaired **T**issue Integrity*
*Ineffective **S**exuality Patterns*

PLANNING

Expected Outcomes

1. Client will experience an absence of vaginal infection, pruritus, burning, or irritation.
2. Client will experience an absence of foul-smelling, curdlike, or blood-tinged discharge.
3. Client will understand the importance of continued treatment until infection is absent.
4. Client will understand the importance of personal hygiene in combination with medication.
5. Client will understand the need to properly clean and store equipment.

Equipment Needed

- Vaginal medication: cream, foam, jelly, or suppository
- Applicator (if needed)
- Water-soluble lubricating jelly (for suppository)
- Nonsterile latex-free gloves
- Perineal pad
- Paper towel, toilet tissue, or tissue paper
- Washcloth and warm water (optional)

DELEGATION TIPS

The procedure of medication administration is not delegated to ancillary personnel in acute care settings. This may vary in state or federal institutions. Ancillary personnel are generally informed about the medications the client is receiving if adverse effects are anticipated or are being monitored.

IMPLEMENTATION—ACTION/RATIONALE

ACTION

❋ Check client's identification band ❋ Explain procedure before beginning ❋

1. Cleanse hands.
2. Ask the client to void.
3. Arrange equipment at client's bedside.
4. Provide privacy by closing door and curtains.
5. Assist the client into a dorsal-recumbent or Sims' position.
6. Drape the client as appropriate, such as over the client's abdomen and lower extremities. Provide towel or protective pad on bed.
7. Position lighting to illuminate vaginal orifice.
8. Don latex-free gloves and assess the perineal area for redness, inflammation, discharge, or foul odor.
9. If using an applicator, fill with medication. If inserting a suppository, remove the suppository from the foil and position in the applicator (applicator is optional). An applicator may be used for suppositories, or a gloved finger may be used. The foil is discarded. Apply water-soluble lubricant to suppository or applicator (optional for applicator).
10. For suppository, with nondominant hand, retract the labia.

RATIONALE

1. Reduces transmission of microorganisms.
2. Provides for client comfort during the procedure.
3. Promotes organization.
4. Protects the client's privacy.
5. Allows for administration and for medication to remain in vagina.
6. Provides privacy. Prevents linen from becoming soiled.

7. Assists in visualization of vagina and proper administration of medication.
8. Decreases transmission of microorganisms and risk of reaction to latex. Provides baseline data.
9. Prepares medication for insertion. Lubricant provides comfort and ease of insertion.

10. Allows visualization of the vaginal orifice and eases insertion of medication.

continues

Figure 27-18-1   Slide the applicator 2 to 3 inches into the vagina.

Figure 27-18-2   Inserting a Vaginal Suppository Along the Posterior Wall of the Vagina

11. With dominant hand, insert the applicator 2 to 3 inches into the vagina, sliding the applicator posteriorly (Figure 27-18-1). Push the plunger to administer the medication. With a suppository, insert the tapered end first with the index finger or applicator along the posterior wall of the vagina (approximately 3 inches) (Figure 27-18-2).

12. Withdraw the applicator and place on a towel.

13. If administering a douche or irrigation:
    • Warm solution to slightly above body temperature (105° to 110°F). Check using the back of the hand or the wrist.
    • Position the client in a semi-recumbent position on a bedpan, on a toilet seat, or in a tub.
    • Apply lubricant to the irrigation nozzle and insert approximately 3 inches into the vagina.
    • Hang the irrigant container approximately 2 feet above the client's vaginal area.

    • Open the clamp and allow a small amount of solution to flow into the vagina.
    • Move the nozzle and rotate around the entire vaginal area. If the labia are inflamed, allow the solution to flow over the labia as well. If the client is on the toilet seat, alternate between closing off the labia and allowing solution to be expelled.

14. Wipe and clean the client's perineal area, including the labia, from the front to the back with toilet tissue. Some clients may prefer that the perineal area is also cleaned with a washcloth and warm water.

15. Apply a perineal pad.

16. Wash the applicator (if reusable) with soap and cool water and store in appropriate container in client's room.

17. Remove gloves and cleanse hands.

11. Medication must be inserted completely to provide coverage of the entire vagina. When medication is deposited at the posterior end of the vagina, gravity will allow medication to move toward the orifice.

12. Reduces transmission of microorganisms.

13.
    • Avoids burning the client. The mucous membranes of the vagina are sensitive.

    • Provides comfort during procedure and allows for appropriate drainage of irrigation solution.
    • Provides comfort.

    • Height is necessary for drainage by gravity. If the container is too high, the flow will be too forceful and uncomfortable.
    • Allows the client to evaluate the temperature.

    • Rotation allows for irrigation throughout vagina. Closing off labia allows medication to stay in and flush total vagina.

14. Provides comfort for client and avoids spread of infective agents to perineal area.

15. Protects client from discomfort of drainage and spread of infection or irritation to perineal area.

16. Applicator can only be used for individual clients; however, some applicators and inducers are reusable and must be appropriately cleaned and stored to prevent reinsertion of infective agents.

17. Reduces transmission of microorganisms.

continues

18. Instruct the client to remain flat for at least 30 minutes.
19. Raise side rails and place the call light in reach.

18. Allows maximum contact between the medication and the vaginal mucous membranes.
19. Provides for client comfort and safety.

EVALUATION

- Client experiences an absence of vaginal infection, pruritus, burning, or irritation.
- Client experiences an absence of foul-smelling, curd-like, or blood-tinged discharge.
- Client understands the importance of continued treatment until infection is absent.
- Client understands the importance of personal hygiene in combination with medication.
- Client understands the need to properly clean and store equipment.

DOCUMENTATION

Nurses' Notes

- Procedure performed and the results
- Unusual findings or client complaints
- Client's response to treatment
- Client's signs and symptoms associated with vaginal condition

Medication Administration Record

- Date and time the medication/treatment was administered

PROCEDURE 27-19 Administering Nebulized Medications

OVERVIEW

A nebulizer is a device that is used to aerosolize medications into a mist for delivery directly into the lungs. Medication that is inhaled in the form of small droplets is absorbed immediately into the mucosa and bloodstream and is available to the body within minutes. This method of medication delivery is one of the fastest noninvasive methods of medication delivery. Many medications can be delivered by inhalation, but currently this delivery method is used primarily for medications designed to ease respiratory distress symptoms such as those seen with asthma.

There are two types of nebulizers: the single-dose nebulizer, which is driven by an air compressor, wall air, or wall oxygen; and the portable metered-dose inhaler. The single-dose, compressor-driven nebulizer delivers smaller droplets, allowing faster, more complete assimilation of the medication. It can be filled with any type of medication that is ordered and can be used by clients who cannot coordinate use of the metered-dose inhaler. The primary drawback of the single-dose nebulizer is its lack of portability. The nebulizer must also be loaded with medication for each use, thus delaying the client's relief.

The metered-dose inhaler has the benefit of being small and portable. It can be carried in the client's pocket. Because the meter dispenses measured doses of the preloaded medication, no special training is needed to prime the inhaler. The primary drawback of a metered-dose inhaler is the need to coordinate dispensing the dose and inhalation.

ASSESSMENT

1. Assess the five rights: right client, right medication, right route, right dose, and right time. **Prevents errors in medication administration.**
2. Assess the client's respiratory status. Note if the client is using accessory muscles for respiration or if there is flaring of the nares. Auscultate the client's chest for wheezes and crackles. **Respiratory distress is the primary reason to administer nebulized medications.**
3. Evaluate the history of this episode of the client's distress. Take a complete history from the client or a reliable informant about the symptoms and length of time the client has had them. Respiratory distress can have many causes. Asthma, bronchitis, a foreign object in the airways, and chronic obstructive pulmonary disease can all cause respiratory distress. **Assessing the client's current symptoms provides more accurate diagnosis and care. The client's history of asthma does not mean that this episode of distress is asthma.**
4. Assess the client's ability to use the nebulizer or metered-dose inhaler. Determine the client's ability to understand and follow the directions, to hold and manipulate the

continues

equipment, and to coordinate the release of the medication with inhalation. **Determines the type of equipment used for the client. Very young children may need a mask instead of a mouthpiece on the nebulizer. The elderly may need specialized dispensers for their metered-dose inhalers.**

5. Assess the medication(s) currently ordered by the health care provider: action, purpose, common side effects, time of onset, and peak of action. **Permits the nurse to anticipate what to observe from the client.**

6. Assess the medications the client is currently taking, including over-the-counter drugs. **Some medications can interact. Beta-blockers (propranolol, atenolol, and betalol) can antagonize the beta agonists and cause or increase asthma symptoms.**

7. Assess the client's knowledge regarding the medications and use of the nebulizer or metered-dose inhaler. **Allows the nurse to determine the need for client education to promote compliance.**

POSSIBLE NURSING DIAGNOSES

Impaired **G***as Exchange*
Ineffective **B***reathing Pattern*
Risk for **S***uffocation*
Deficient **K***nowledge (proper use of the nebulizer or metered-dose inhaler)*
A*nxiety*
F*ear*

PLANNING

Expected Outcomes

1. The client will experience improved gas exchange.
2. The client's breathing pattern will become effective.
3. The client will demonstrate understanding of the need for the medication and use of the nebulizer or metered-dose inhaler.
4. The client will not experience any adverse effects secondary to medication interactions.
5. The client's anxiety level will decrease following treatment.

Equipment Needed

Handheld Nebulizer
• Medication administration record
• Nebulizer set (cup, tubing, cap, T-shaped tube, mouthpiece, or mask) or prepackaged nebulizer and applicator
• Medication(s)
• Saline
• Air compressor, wall air, or wall oxygen
Metered-Dose Inhaler
• Metered-dose inhaler
• Aerochamber, if appropriate

DELEGATION TIPS

The procedure of medication administration is not delegated to ancillary personnel in acute care settings. This may vary in state or federal institutions. Ancillary personnel are generally informed about the medications the client is receiving if adverse effects are anticipated or are being monitored.

IMPLEMENTATION—ACTION/RATIONALE

ACTION   RATIONALE

* Check client's identification band * Explain procedure before beginning *

Single-dose Nebulizer

1. Cleanse hands.
2. Carefully pour the entire amount of the drug(s) into the nebulizer cup.
   • Avoid touching the drug while pouring into the nebulizer cup.
3. Cover the cup with the cap and fasten.
4. Fasten the T-piece to the top of the cap.
5. Fasten a short length of tubing to one end of the T-piece.

1. Reduces transmission of microorganisms.
2. Determines the correct amount of medicine and ensures accurate dosage.
   • Reduces the transmission of microorganisms.

3. Prevents spillage of the medication.
4. Provides a connector for the mouthpiece.
5. Provides dead space to prevent room air from entering the system and medicated aerosol from escaping.

continues

6. Fasten the mouthpiece or mask to the other end of the T-piece.
   • Avoid touching the nebulizer mouthpiece or the interior part of the mask.
7. Identify the medication(s) to the client and clearly explain the therapeutic purpose(s) of the medication.
8. Advise the client to sit in an upright position.
9. Attach tubing to the bottom of the nebulizer cup and attach the other end to the air compressor or wall air.
   • Before turning it on, adjust the wall oxygen valve to 6 liters/min (or less per health care provider's orders).
   • Leave the air on for about 6 to 7 minutes until the medications are used up.
10. Instruct the client to breathe in and out slowly and deeply through the mouthpiece/mask.
    • The client's lips should be sealed tightly around the mouthpiece.
11. Remain with the client long enough to observe the proper inhalation-exhalation technique.
12. Cleanse your hands.
13. When the nebulizer cup is empty, turn off the compressor or wall air.
    • Detach the tubing from the compressor and the nebulizer cup.
    • If the nebulizer is disposable, dispose of the nebulizer in the appropriate container.
    • If the nebulizer is to be reused for this client, carefully wash, rinse, and dry the nebulizer components.
14. Assess the client immediately following the treatment for results or adverse effects from the treatment.
15. Reassess the client 5 to 10 minutes following the treatment.
16. Cleanse hands.

Metered-dose Nebulizer

17. Assess the client for ability to use the metered-dose nebulizer.
18. Cleanse hands.
19. Shake the prepackaged nebulizer.
20. Have the client exhale and place the mouthpiece in his mouth (Figure 27-19-1).

6. Provides a portal for the client to inhale the aerosolized medication.
   • Reduces transmission of microorganisms.

7. Promotes client's cooperation and awareness of the medication's effects.
8. Promotes better expansion of the lungs.
9. Provides a conduit for the compressed air.

   • Drives the medication into a mist or wet aerosol form.

   • Allows the client to receive the entire dose of medication.
10. Promotes better deposition and efficacy of the medication in the airways.

11. Ensures the correct use of the nebulizer to get the full effects from the medications administered.
12. Reduces transmission of microorganisms.
13. Stops the aerosolization.

   • Prepares components for cleaning or disposal.

   • Prevents transmission of microorganisms.

   • Prevents transmission of microorganisms.

14. Determines the effectiveness of the treatment.

15. Some effects may be delayed.

16. Reduces transmission of microorganisms.

17. Ensures client compliance.

18. Decreases transmission of microorganisms.
19. Thoroughly mixes the medication.
20. Prepares for delivery of the medication to the lungs.

Figure 27-19-1   Self-administration with a Metered-Dose Inhaler

continues

21. Have the client press down on the prepackaged dispenser and simultaneously inhale slowly until lungs feel full. Hold breath for 10 seconds and exhale slowly.

22. Observe the client for several minutes to assess for possible adverse effects from the medication.

23. Cleanse hands.

21. Draws medication into the lungs. Allows medication to reach alveoli.

22. Reactions can occur right away.

23. Prevents transmission of microorganisms.

EVALUATION

- The client experienced improved gas exchange.
- The client's breathing pattern became effective.
- The client demonstrates understanding of the need for the medication and the use of the nebulizer or metered-dose inhaler.
- The client did not experience any adverse effects secondary to medication interactions.
- The client's anxiety level decreased following treatment.

DOCUMENTATION

Medication Administration Record

- Name of medication(s)
- Dosage

- Route
- Site
- Time of administration
- Initials of the nurse who administered the medication(s)
- Signature of the nurse identifying the initials

Nurses' Notes

- Client's assessment parameters
- Name of medication, dosage, route, and time of administration
- Amount of oxygen delivered per minute from wall oxygen or air compressor machine
- Signature and initials of the nurse
- Client's response

PROCEDURE 27-20   Applying a Dry Dressing

OVERVIEW

A closed surgical wound can be described as a wound that was caused, revised, or debrided by a surgical intervention. Closed wounds are generally categorized as clean. They may be closed with sutures, staples, or tapes. The general purpose of the closed wound dressing is to cover and protect as well as absorb the minimal drainage that may occur with this type of wound. Dressing care may vary according to the surgeon's preference and institutional policy. General guidelines for the closed surgical wound dressing is covered in this procedure.

There are different approaches to wound care. Cleaning solutions can dry the wound and interfere with wound healing at the cellular level. Furthermore, clients may be allergic or sensitive to these solutions. Although they reduce the risk of infection, frequent application may not be necessary. In many cases, sterile normal saline, sterile water, or pH-neutral solutions will be adequate to cleanse the wound. It is standard for the surgeon to do the first postoperative dressing change. The initial dressing is maintained for 24 to 48 hours postoperatively, unless conditions of the dressing call for contacting the health care provider for a dressing change order. Until the removal of the initial dressing, reinforce the dressing as needed.

The frequency of the dressing change depends on the needs of the wound and the preference of the health care provider. This will usually be specified in the orders. It is important to follow agency guidelines and observe the preferences of the health care provider.

continues

ASSESSMENT

1. Assess the client's comfort level postoperatively upon arrival from the operating room, before wound care, and as needed throughout the postoperative course. **Surgical wounds are painful. If clients are made comfortable with appropriate pain medications and positioning, there will be better tissue gas exchange from deep breathing, coughing, and early ambulation, thereby promoting healing of tissues. Clients will be more cooperative and less anxious during dressing changes if they are comfortable.**

2. Assess the external appearance of the initial postoperative dressing and subsequent dressings. **The initial dressing may need to be reinforced. Excess saturation with drainage, blood, or other bodily fluids, dislodgement, or anything unusual about the dressing should be brought to the attention of the health care provider. The appearance of the external portion of the dressing provides information about needed supplies.**

3. Assess the appearance of the wound and drains once the dressing is removed. **Inspection of the wound is important for assessment of the skin and tissues and for determining dressing supply needs. Assessment includes noting signs of infection as evident by redness, swelling, foul odor, amount of drainage, color of wound exudate (yellow and viscous would indicate purulent), or unusual pain or tenderness; signs of tissue trauma as evident by swelling or ecchymosis; evidence of bleeding or leakage of tissue fluids from the site; and the position of indwelling catheters, drainage tubes, and the sutures or stabilizing devices closing the wound and supporting the drains.**

4. Assess the client's understanding about the postoperative care of the surgical wound site. **It is important to take into consideration the client's ability to understand verbal and written instructions and the cultural and social variations that may affect the delivery of health care and client/family education.**

5. If solutions are to be used on the wound, assess the client's allergy status and test a drop of solution on the skin. **This prevents an adverse reaction.**

POSSIBLE NURSING DIAGNOSES

*Impaired **S**kin Integrity*
*Impaired **T**issue Integrity*
*Risk for **I**nfection*

PLANNING

Expected Outcomes

1. The site will be inspected.
2. The initial postoperative dressing will be reinforced until changed by the health care provider.
3. The site will have the appropriate dressing applied.
4. The client/family will verbalize and/or demonstrate understanding and the ability, if indicated, to perform the dressing change and associated wound care of the surgical wound site.

Equipment Needed

- Clean exam gloves
- Container for proper disposal of soiled dressing
- Sterile 4 × 4 gauze pads
- Washcloth (optional)
- ABD pads (optional)
- 2-inch tape (foam or paper)

DELEGATION TIPS

The application of bandages is not delegated to ancillary personnel. Family members may be taught this before the client's discharge. Occasionally, ancillary personnel will be delegated the task of applying a clean dry gauze as skin protection, but the nurse is responsible for assessing the integrity of the client's skin.

IMPLEMENTATION—ACTION/RATIONALE

ACTION	RATIONALE
* Check client's identification band * Explain procedure before beginning *	
1. Gather supplies.	1. Promotes a smooth work flow.
2. Provide privacy; draw curtains; close door.	2. Maintains client comfort and privacy while body is exposed during procedure.
3. Cleanse hands.	3. Reduces transmission of microorganisms.
4. Apply clean gloves.	4. Promotes infection control and protection from body fluids.

continues

5. Remove dressing and place in appropriate receptacle. Remove soiled gloves with contaminated surfaces inward and discard in appropriate receptacle; apply clean gloves.
6. Assess the undressed wound for signs of redness, foul odor, swelling, irritation, drainage, dehiscence, bleeding, or skin breakdown.
7. Cleanse the skin around the incision if necessary with a clean, warm, wet washcloth.
   • If the suture line requires cleansing, it should be done gently. Use normal saline, half-strength hydrogen peroxide, or betadine swab (consult orders of health care provider and/or institution policy regarding antiseptic agents) and cotton-tip applicators using a rolling motion.
   • Used applicators should not be reintroduced into the sterile solution.
8. Remove gloves and cleanse hands.
9. Apply clean gloves.
10. Grasping just the edges, apply a new dressing using 4 × 4 gauze pads folded in half to the 2 × 4 size. Place the folded gauze pad lengthwise on wound and tape lightly or apply tubular mesh for those with sensitive skin. Initial the dressing, citing date and time it was changed.
    Optional: An ABD pad may be applied on top of the dressing for added protection over sutures or for client comfort.
11. Remove gloves and cleanse hands.
12. Conduct client/family education about the dressing, which may include teaching the dressing technique to the client/family.

5. Dressings and gloves soiled with body fluids are considered contaminated and subject to biohazard disposal in the correct manner per institution protocol.
6. These may be signs of infection or inadequate wound healing.
7. Dried blood or drainage on the surrounding skin can be an irritant and a medium for microbes.
   • The suture line itself should not be disturbed unnecessarily.
   • Avoid betadine if client has iodine allergy.

   • Reintroduction of the soiled applicator into sterile solution will contaminate the solution.
8. Reduces transmission of microorganisms.
9. Promotes infection control.
10. A light dressing of 4 × 4 pads may be the only dressing that is needed to protect the incision from clothing or to collect a small amount of tissue drainage. This maintains a record of the dressing change for the next nurse.

11. Reduces transmission of microorganisms.
12. Educates the client/family and prepares for discharge.

EVALUATION

• Assess client comfort level during dressing change procedure.
• Determine whether the client's privacy was protected during the dressing change.
• Assess whether the correct supplies were brought in for the dressing change and whether any modifications need to be made to the dressing change.
• Determine the effectiveness of client/family education by having the client/family return-demonstrate the dressing or verbally review the steps of the dressing.

DOCUMENTATION

Nurses' Notes

• Date and time dressing done
• Brief description of the wound site
• Brief description of the site care done and dressing applied
• Client comfort before and after dressing change
• Client/family education done and evaluation of the teaching

PROCEDURE 27-21   Applying a Wet to Damp Dressing

OVERVIEW

The purpose of a wet to damp dressing (also known as wet to moist dressing) is to cover and protect the wound, collect exudate, promote healing, and promote light surface debridement. The decision to apply a wet to damp dressing depends on the wound bed, type of tissue and presence of eschar, amount of exudate, stage of wound healing, state of surrounding tissue, and the presence of infection.

   Wound healing is promoted by a warm, moist environment; however, it is imperative to avoid moisture on the surface of the dressing. A wet external dressing can act as a wick with the external environment and draw contamination into the wound. Gentle debridement of a red wound is accomplished with a wet to damp dressing. One must be careful not to apply a dressing so wet that it ends up macerating the surrounding good tissue. Wet dressings are contraindicated in black eschar wounds, where the eschar represents full-thickness tissue destruction, because bacteria will multiply under such a dressing.

   The wet to damp dressing consists of gauze, applied wet and allowed to become "near dry" before the next dressing change. Specifics of the wet to damp dressings vary according to the preferences of the surgeon and wound specialist, institutional policy, and outcome measurement standards used to evaluate the effectiveness of the dressing. General guidelines for a simple wet to damp dressing are covered.

ASSESSMENT

1. Assess the client's comfort level **to assess the need for medication before the dressing change.** Clients will be more cooperative and less anxious during dressing changes if they are comfortable.
2. Assess the external appearance of the dressing **to evaluate dressing adequacy as well as needed supplies.**
3. Assess the appearance of the wound and drains once the dressing is removed, noting redness, swelling, purulent drainage, or ecchymosis **to determine the condition of the wound and the effectiveness of the wet to damp dressing.**
4. Assess the client's understanding regarding the dressing changes and wound care **to determine any client teaching needed.**
5. Assess the client's healing response to previous treatments. The effectiveness of the wet to moist application should be routinely reassessed and the treatment modified if healing is not occurring.

POSSIBLE NURSING DIAGNOSES

*Impaired **S**kin Integrity*
*Impaired **T**issue Integrity*
*Risk for **I**nfection*

PLANNING

Expected Outcomes

1. The site will be inspected.
2. The site will have the appropriate dressing applied.
3. The client/family will verbalize and/or demonstrate understanding and the ability, if indicated, to perform the dressing change and associated wound care of the surgical wound site.

Equipment Needed

- Clean exam gloves
- Container for proper disposal of soiled dressing
- Sterile gloves
- Moisture-proof gown (optional)
- Sterile towel
- Normal saline or ordered solution
- Sterile bowl
- Sterile 4 × 4 gauze pads, multiple
- Cover sponges or fluffs (optional)
- ABD dressing pads
- 2-inch tape (foam or paper)
- Tubular mesh (optional)
- Montgomery straps (optional)

DELEGATION TIPS

Applying a wet to damp dressing requires sterile technique and professional assessment skills and cannot be delegated to ancillary personnel.

continues

IMPLEMENTATION—ACTION/RATIONALE

ACTION	RATIONALE

＊ Check client's identification band ＊ Explain procedure before beginning ＊

ACTION	RATIONALE
1. Review order of health care provider for wound care and gather supplies.	1. Promotes a smooth work flow.
2. Provide privacy; draw curtains; close door.	2. Maintains client comfort and privacy while body is exposed during procedure.
3. Assess need for pain medication. Pain is rated on a scale from 0 (lowest) to 10 (greatest). Assess need based on quality, pain pattern, location, and last pain medication received.	3. Removal of a wet to damp or moist dressing may be painful to the client, so careful assessment of pain medication needs before the dressing change is important.
4. Cleanse hands.	4. Reduces transmission of microorganisms.
5. Apply clean gloves. If there is copious drainage or the wound is infected, wear a gown, a mask, and eye protection.	5. Provides infection control and protection from body fluids.
6. Remove dressing, noting number of gauze pads used and place them in appropriate receptacle. If it is found that the dressing is extremely dry and removal will result in injury, a small amount of saline to loosen that portion of the dressing is indicated (Figure 27-21-1).	6. To counteract the problem of an extremely dry dressing, increase the wetness of the dressing or increase the frequency of dressing changes. Provides number of gauze pads needed to replace the dressing.
7. Observe the undressed wound for healing (granulation and approximation of edges), signs of infection (inflammation, edema, warmth, pain), and drainage.	7. Allows for evaluation of effectiveness of treatment.
8. Cleanse the skin around the incision if necessary with a clean, warm, wet washcloth.	8. Dried blood or drainage on the surrounding skin can be an irritant and a medium for microbes.
9. Remove gloves and cleanse hands.	9. Reduces transmission of microorganisms.
10. Set up supplies in a sterile field, including pouring ordered solutions into appropriate containers if indicated for the dressing.	10. Maintains sterility.
11. Apply sterile gloves.	11. This is a sterile dressing change.
12. Place gauze or packing material in the bowl with the normal saline or specified solution.	12. Wets gauze or packing material for dressing.
• Wring excess solution from gauze or packing. Avoid overwringing the dressing to prevent excessive drying.	• If too wet, wound bed can get soupy, increasing chance of bacterial growth.
• Gently place wet gauze over the area (Figure 27-21-2).	• Dresses the wound.

Figure 27-21-1 If the dressing is too dry and removing it will cause injury, use a small amount of saline to loosen the portion of the dressing that adheres too tightly to the wound.

Figure 27-21-2 Place the gauze on the wound.

continues

Figure 27-21-3 Wrap the wet gauze with an external dressing of dry gauze bandages.

Figure 27-21-4 Montgomery Straps

13. Apply external dressing of dry 4 × 4 gauze pads, cover sponges, fluffs, or ABD pads (Figure 27-21-3).
    • Secure dressing in place with tape, Montgomery straps, or tubular mesh (Figure 27-21-4).

14. Remove gloves and cleanse hands.
15. Mark the dressing with the date and time it was changed. Initial the dressing.
16. Conduct client/family education about the dressing, which may include teaching the dressing technique to the client/family.

13. Prevents excess drying and protects wound.

    • Tape for short-term dressings in clients who are not sensitive to adhesives. For long-term dressings or for those who are sensitive to tape, use Montgomery straps or tubular mesh to prevent skin irritation.

14. Reduces transmission of microorganisms.
15. Maintains a record of the dressing change and provides for continuity of care.
16. Educates the client/family and prepares for discharge.

EVALUATION

• The site was inspected.
• The site had the appropriate dressing applied.
• The client/family verbalized or demonstrated understanding and the ability, if necessary, to perform the dressing change and associated wound care of the surgical wound site.

DOCUMENTATION

Nurses' Notes

• Administration of pain medication before dressing change
• Date and time dressing done
• Brief description of the wound site
• Brief description of the site care done and dressing applied
• Client comfort before and after dressing change
• Client/family education done and evaluation of the teaching

PROCEDURE 27-22   Culturing a Wound

OVERVIEW

Bacterial wound contamination is one of the most common causes of altered wound healing. A surgical wound can become infected preoperatively, intraoperatively, or postoperatively. Nicks or abrasions created during preoperative shaving may be a source of pathogens. The risk for intraoperative exposure to pathogens increases when the respiratory, gastrointestinal, genitourinary, and oropharyngeal tracts are opened. Nonsurgical wounds from trauma, pressure ulcers, or disease can become infected as well.

If the amount of bacteria in the wound is sufficient or the client's immune defenses are compromised, clinical infection may become apparent 2 to 11 days postoperatively. Infection slows healing by prolonging the inflammatory phase of healing, competing for nutrients, and producing chemicals and enzymes that are damaging to the tissues. Identifying the infectious agent in a wound is an important step in wound healing.

ASSESSMENT

1. Assess the wound and the surrounding tissues for signs of infection. Check for heat, redness, inflammation, and drainage. Check the color and consistency of the drainage. Check the smell and color of the wound. **Allows for intervention to detect and treat infection.**
2. Assess the client's overall status, including vital signs, for signs of infection such as fever, chills, or elevated white blood cell count (WBC). **Allows for intervention to detect and treat infection.**

POSSIBLE NURSING DIAGNOSES

Risk for Infection
Impaired Skin Integrity
Disturbed Body Image

PLANNING

Expected Outcomes

1. The wound culture will be collected with a minimum of pain and trauma to the client.
2. The wound culture will be representative of the flora present in the wound, without contamination by flora outside the wound.

Equipment Needed

- Disposable gloves
- Sterile gloves and dressing supplies
- Normal saline and irrigation tray
- Culture tube and swab
- Moisture-proof container or bag

DELEGATION TIPS

Obtaining a wound culture requires nursing assessment and aseptic technique, and is potentially an invasive procedure; therefore, delegation to ancillary personnel is not appropriate.

IMPLEMENTATION—ACTION/RATIONALE

ACTION

RATIONALE

* Check client's identification band * Explain procedure before beginning *

ACTION	RATIONALE
1. Cleanse hands, apply disposable gloves, and remove old dressing. Place old dressing in moisture-proof container and remove and discard gloves. Cleanse hands again.	1. Reduces transmission of microorganisms. Makes the wound accessible for obtaining the culture.
2. Open the dressing supplies using sterile technique and apply sterile gloves.	2. Maintains sterile environment.

continues

Figure 27-22-1   Roll the swab over the area to be cultured.

Figure 27-22-2   Crush the ampule to release the medium inside the culture tube.

3. Assess the wound's appearance; note quality, quantity, color, and odor of discharge.

4. Irrigate the wound with normal saline before culturing the wound; do not irrigate with antiseptic.

5. Using a sterile gauze pad, absorb the excess saline, then discard the pad.
6. Remove the culture tube from the packaging. Remove the culture swab from the culture tube and gently roll the swab over the granulation tissue. Avoid eschar and wound edges (Figure 27-22-1).

7. Replace the swab into the culture tube, being careful not to touch the swab to the outside of the tube. Recap the tube. Crush the ampule of medium located in the bottom or cap of the tube (Figure 27-22-2).
8. Remove gloves, cleanse hands, and apply sterile gloves. Dress the wound with sterile dressing.
9. Label the specimen, place in biohazard transport bag, and arrange to transport the specimen to the laboratory according to institutional policy.
10. Remove gloves and cleanse hands.

3. Provides assessment of the amount and character of the wound's drainage before irrigation. Reddened areas and heavy drainage suggest infection.
4. Decreases the risk of culturing normal flora and other exudates such as protein; an antiseptic may destroy the bacteria.
5. Prevents maceration of tissue caused by excess moisture.

6. Decreases the chance of collecting superficial skin microorganisms.

7. Avoids contamination with microorganisms. Releases the medium to surround the swab.

8. Reduces transmission of microorganisms. Prevents contamination of the wound.
9. Ensures proper handling of specimen.

10. Reduces transmission of microorganisms.

EVALUATION

- Assess whether the wound culture was collected with a minimum of pain and trauma to the client.
- Determine whether the wound culture is representative of the flora present in the wound, without contamination by other bacteria.

DOCUMENTATION

Nurses' Notes

- Time and method of collection of the culture, and what was done with the specimen
- Fill out the lab requisition form with the client's information as well as time and date specimen was collected, location of the culture, and requested tests. Often there are duplicate numbered or coded labels on the lab slips. One copy is placed in the chart.

PROCEDURE 27-23   Irrigating a Wound

OVERVIEW

Wound irrigation is the process of washing debris, drainage, or exudate out of the wound to promote healing. The fluid used to irrigate a wound varies depending on the health care provider's orders. Fluids commonly used include normal saline, betadine, hydrogen peroxide, acetic acid, and specially prepared antibiotic solutions. If cytotoxic solutions are used, then the area must be flushed/irrigated afterward with normal saline. Wounds that require irrigation also vary. They may be simple open lacerations; tunneled pressure ulcers; or complex, open abdominal wounds extending down to the abdominal fascia. Wound irrigation is a sterile procedure. Take care not to contaminate the wound and not to become contaminated with wound drainage.

ASSESSMENT

1. Assess the current dressing **to determine what equipment will be needed to replace it with a clean dressing and whether the dressing has been adequate to protect the wound and contain any drainage or exudate.**
2. Assess the client to determine if able **to understand the need for the wound irrigation and cooperate with the procedure.**
3. Assess whether the client has concerns about pain or body image regarding this wound and the irrigation **to determine what client teaching and support will be most effective.**
4. Assess the client's environment **to plan if the necessary equipment and supplies are available, including irrigant, hand hygiene facilities, and an adequate work area to lay out supplies and establish a sterile field.**

POSSIBLE NURSING DIAGNOSES

Impaired Skin Integrity
Risk for Infection
Acute Pain

PLANNING

Expected Outcomes

1. The wound will be free of exudate, drainage, and debris.
2. The wound will be free of signs and symptoms of infection.
3. The procedure will be performed with a minimum of trauma and pain to the client.

Equipment Needed

- Sterile gloves
- Clean gloves
- Sterile irrigation kit (basin, piston irrigation syringe, solution container)
- Irrigation solution (per health care provider's order)
- Waterproof pad
- Sterile dressing material to redress the wound
- Moisture-proof container or bag for use after the irrigation procedure

DELEGATION TIPS

Wound irrigation requires nursing assessment, aseptic technique, and monitoring of wound healing. This procedure is not delegated to ancillary personnel.

IMPLEMENTATION—ACTION/RATIONALE

ACTION	RATIONALE
* Check client's identification band * Explain procedure before beginning *	
1. Confirm the health care provider's order for wound irrigation and note the type and strength of the ordered irrigation solution.	1. Wound irrigation is a dependent nursing action that requires a medical order stating the type of solution to be used.

continues

Figure 27-23-1 Gently flush the wound.

Figure 27-23-2 Hold the syringe close to the wound, but be careful not to touch the wound with the syringe.

2. Assess the client's pain level and medicate if needed with analgesic 30 minutes before procedure if the medication is to be given po or IM.

3. Place a waterproof pad on the bed. Assist the client onto the pad. Then assist the client into a position that will allow the irrigant to flow through the wound and into the basin from the cleanest to dirtiest area of the wound.

4. Cleanse hands and apply clean gloves; remove and discard the old dressing.

5. Assess the wound's appearance and note quality, quantity, color, and odor of drainage.

6. Remove gloves and cleanse hands.

7. Prepare the sterile irrigation tray and dressing supplies. Pour the room-temperature irrigation solution into the solution container.

8. Apply sterile gloves (gown and goggles if needed).

9. Position the sterile basin below the wound so the irrigant will flow from the cleanest area to the dirtiest area and into the basin.

10. Fill the piston or bulb syringe with irrigant and gently flush the wound. Hold the syringe approximately 1 inch above the wound bed to irrigate. Refill the syringe and continue to flush the wound until the solution returns clear and no exudate is noted or until the prescribed amount of fluid has been used (Figures 27-23-1 and 27-23-2).

11. Dry the edges of the wound with sterile gauze.

12. Assess the wound's appearance and drainage.

13. Apply a sterile dressing.

14. Remove gloves and cleanse hands.

2. Allows time for medication to be absorbed to increase the analgesic effect.

3. Positioning of the client and placement of a waterproof pad will decrease contamination of bed linen.

4. Reduces transmission of microorganisms.

5. Provides assessment of wound status.

6. Reduces transmission of microorganisms.

7. Prevents introduction of microorganisms into the wound. Reduces client discomfort.

8. Promotes sterile environment. Follows Standard Precautions.

9. Decreases possibility of wound contamination.

10. Decreases trauma to granulation tissue, yet provides the ideal pressure for cleansing and removal of debris.

11. Prevents maceration of tissues caused by excess moisture.

12. Provides indication of change in wound status.

13. Protects the wound from microorganisms.

14. Reduces transmission of microorganisms.

EVALUATION

- Assess whether the wound is free of exudate, drainage, and debris.
- Assess whether the wound is free of signs and symptoms of infection.
- Evaluate whether the procedure was performed with a minimum of trauma and pain to the client.

DOCUMENTATION

Nurses' Notes

- Wound's appearance and quality, quantity, color, and odor of drainage
- Client's tolerance of the procedure and any observations regarding the client's body image

Kardex

- Special equipment or techniques required with the client to provide the information to other staff members

PROCEDURE 27-24   Administering Oxygen

OVERVIEW

Administration of oxygen must be ordered by the physician or qualified practitioner. Some areas will have protocols that govern oxygen therapy and allow the nurse to begin therapy independently. Oxygen is a drug, so medication administration criteria are followed in addition to the steps unique to oxygen therapy. Clients unable to maintain adequate PO_2 and O_2 saturation levels on room air are candidates for oxygen therapy. An adequate airway is essential to effectiveness of the treatment. It is best to treat the hypoxia with the lowest oxygen dose possible. Some clients with a normal oxygen level are also given oxygen if they are at risk for complications related to hypoxia; for example, the myocardial infarction client often receives oxygen therapy to prevent dysrhythmias.

The health care provider orders the oxygen delivery system and flow rate, and the nurse monitors response to the therapy. The dosage of oxygen may be ordered as an FIO_2 (fraction of inspired oxygen), which is expressed as a percentage or as liters per minute (L/min). Respiratory therapists may be available to assist in the administration of oxygen therapy and client assessment.

ASSESSMENT

1. Determine client history and acute and chronic health problems. **Clients with carbon dioxide retaining chronic obstructive pulmonary disease (COPD) will need lower amounts of oxygen so as not to obliterate their hypoxic respiratory drive. They may already be on oxygen and need long-term continuous therapy.**
2. Assess the client's baseline respiratory signs, including airway, respiratory pattern, rate, depth, and rhythm, noting indications of increased work of breathing. **Helps determine the client's need for oxygen as well as response to the therapy.**
3. Check the extremities and mucous membranes closely for color. **Gives some indication of oxygenation, although problems with circulation and tissue perfusion can also alter these factors.**
4. Review arterial blood gas (ABG) and pulse oximetry results. **These are the most important determinants of the effectiveness of the pulmonary system and determine the need for therapy as well as changes in therapy.**
5. Note lung sounds for wheezes/crackles. **Secretions will interfere with airway patency and diffusion of oxygen and carbon dioxide across the alveolar-capillary bed.**
6. Assess the nares, behind the earlobes, cheek, tracheostomy site, or other places where oxygen tubing or equipment is in constant contact with the skin **to look for signs of skin irritation or breakdown.**

POSSIBLE NURSING DIAGNOSES

Impaired **G**as Exchange
Ineffective **B**reathing Pattern
Risk for **I**njury
Ineffective **A**irway Clearance
Risk for Impaired **S**kin Integrity
Activity Intolerance

PLANNING

Expected Outcomes

1. Oxygen level will return to normal in blood and tissues as evident by oxygen saturation ≥92%, skin color normal.
2. Respiratory rate, pattern, and depth will be within the normal range for client.
3. The client will not develop any skin or tissue irritation or breakdown.
4. The client will demonstrate methods to clear secretions and maintain optimal oxygenation.
5. Breathing efficiency and activity tolerance will be increased.
6. The client will understand the rationale for the therapy.

Equipment Needed

- Stethoscope
- Oxygen source—portable or in-line
- Oxygen flow meter
- Oxygen delivery device: nasal cannula, mask, tent, or T-tube with adapter for artificial airway
- Oxygen tubing
- Pulse oximeter
- Humidifier and distilled or sterile water (not needed with low flow rates per nasal cannula)

continues

DELEGATION TIPS

The initiation of oxygen therapy requires assessment by a nurse or respiratory care practitioner. All personnel are responsible to maintain fire/safety precautions when oxygen is in use. Ancillary personnel should be instructed to report dyspnea, tachycardia, any changes in the client's activity tolerance, a respiratory rate less than 12 or greater than 20 breaths per minute in the adult client, or changes in mental status. Ancillary personnel should be instructed how to properly reapply respiratory therapy equipment, how to initiate assistance with activities of daily living for the client requiring oxygen therapy, and to report any abnormal client responses.

IMPLEMENTATION—ACTION/RATIONALE

ACTION

RATIONALE

❋ Check client's identification band ❋ Explain procedure before beginning ❋

Nasal Cannula

ACTION	RATIONALE
1. Cleanse hands.	1. Reduces transmission of microorganisms.
2. Verify the health care provider's order.	2. Ensures correct dosage and route.
3. Remind clients who smoke of the reasons for not smoking while O₂ is in use.	3. Increases compliance with procedures. Oxygen supports combustion.
4. If using humidity, fill humidifier to fill line with distilled water and close container.	4. Prevents drying of the client's airway and thins any secretions.
5. Attach humidifier to oxygen flow meter.	5. Allows the oxygen to pass through the water and become humidified.
6. Insert humidifier and flow meter into oxygen source in wall or portable unit. Many institutions also have compressed air available from outlets very similar in appearance to oxygen outlets. Green always stands for oxygen. Be sure to plug the flow meter into the green outlet.	6. Gives access to oxygen. Reduces possibility of inserting into wrong outlet.
7. Attach the oxygen tubing and nasal cannula to the flow meter and turn it on to the prescribed flow rate (1 to 5 L/min). Use extension tubing for ambulatory clients so they can get up to go to the bathroom.	7. Rates above 6 L/min are not efficacious and can dry the nasal mucosa.
8. Check for bubbling in the humidifier.	8. Ensures proper functioning.
9. Place the nasal prongs in the client's nostrils (Figure 27-24-1). Secure the cannula in place by adjusting the tubing around the client's ears and using the slip ring to stabilize it under the client's chin (Figure 27-24-2).	9. Keeps delivery system in place so client receives the amount of oxygen ordered.

Figure 27-24-1 Insert cannula prong into nostrils (gloves are optional).

Figure 27-24-2 Adjust tubing.

continues

10. Check for proper flow rate every 4 hours and when the client returns from procedures.

10. Ensures that client receives proper dose. The nasal cannula is a low-flow system because it administers oxygen while the client also inspires room air. The actual dose of oxygen received by the client will vary depending on the client's respiratory pattern.

11. Assess client's nostrils every 8 hours. If the client complains of dryness or has signs of irritation, use sterile lubricant to keep mucous membranes moist. Add humidifier if not already in place.

11. Dry membranes are more prone to breakdown by friction or pressure from nasal cannula.

12. Monitor vital signs, oxygen saturation, and client condition every 4 to 8 hours (or as indicated or ordered) for signs and symptoms of hypoxia.

12. Detects any untoward effects from therapy.

13. Wean client from oxygen as soon as possible using standard protocols.

13. Oxygen is not without side effects and should be used only as long as needed. Problems with reimbursement may develop if criteria for therapy are not met.

Mask: Venturi (high-flow device), simple mask (low flow), partial rebreather mask, nonrebreather mask, and face tent

14. Repeat Actions 1–6.
15. Attach appropriately sized mask or face tent to oxygen tubing and turn on flow meter to prescribed flow rate. The Venturi mask will have color-coded inserts that list the flow rate necessary to obtain the desired percentage of oxygen. Allow the reservoir bag of the nonrebreathing or partial rebreathing mask to fill completely.

14. See Rationales 1–6.
15. Ensures proper fit; size needed is based on the client's size. Checks the oxygen source and primes the tubing and mask or tent.

16. Check for bubbling in the humidifier.
17. Place the mask or tent on the client's face, fasten the elastic band around the client's ears, and tighten until the mask fits snugly.

16. Ensures proper functioning.
17. Prevents loss of oxygen from the sides of the mask.

18. Check for proper flow rate every 4 hours.
19. Ensure that the ports of the Venturi mask are not under covers or impeded by any other source.

18. Ensures that client is receiving the proper dose.
19. Air must be entrained to mix room air and oxygen coming from source to ensure proper oxygen percentage (FIO_2).

20. Assess client's face and ears for pressure from the mask and use padding as needed.
21. Wean client to nasal cannula and then wean off oxygen per protocol.

20. Provides client comfort and prevents skin breakdown.
21. Oxygen is not without side effects and should be used only as long as needed. The nasal cannula provides a lower FIO_2 than the mask. Problems with reimbursement may develop if criteria for therapy are not met.

EVALUATION

- Oxygen level returned to normal in blood and tissues as evident by oxygen saturation ≥92%; skin color normal for client.
- Respiratory rate, pattern, and depth are within the normal range.
- The client did not develop any skin or tissue irritation or breakdown.
- Breathing efficiency and activity tolerance are increased.
- The client understands the rationale for the therapy.

DOCUMENTATION

Nurses' Notes

- O_2 saturation and respiratory status
- Method of oxygen delivery and rate
- Client's assessment parameters and response to treatment
- Changes in mental status

PROCEDURE 27-25   Performing Nasopharyngeal and Oropharyngeal Suctioning

OVERVIEW

Suctioning secretions is necessary to maintain a patent airway for a client who is unable to effectively clear secretions by coughing. It is considered a sterile procedure, thereby preventing the introduction of microorganisms into the client's airway and lungs.

Suctioning is performed as often as necessary to remove excess secretions, depending on the amount of secretions the client is generating and the client's ability to clear the airway. The client's airway and oxygenation are evaluated to determine the need for suctioning.

Wall suction should be set at 100 to 120 mm Hg for adults, 50 to 100 mm Hg for children, and 40 to 60 mm Hg for infants. Portable suction should be set at 8 to 15 mm Hg for adults, 5 to 8 mm Hg for children, and 3 to 5 mm Hg for infants.

ASSESSMENT

1. Assess respirations for rate, rhythm, depth, and bubbling or gurgling noises **to evaluate airway.**
2. Auscultate lung fields **to evaluate airway and determine need for suctioning.**
3. Monitor arterial blood gases and/or pulse oximetry values **to determine oxygen level and adequate air exchange.**
4. Assess for anxiety and restlessness, **which may be signs of airway distress and/or hypoxia.**
5. Assess the client's understanding of the suctioning procedure **to decrease the client's anxiety.**

POSSIBLE NURSING DIAGNOSES

Ineffective Airway Clearance
Impaired Gas Exchange
Anxiety

PLANNING

Expected Outcomes

1. The client will have no coarse bubbling or gurgling noises with respirations.
2. The client will report breathing comfortably.
3. The client will have no apparent anxiety or restlessness.
4. The client will have arterial blood gases and pulse oximetry values within normal limits.
5. The client will express understanding of the suctioning process.

Equipment Needed

- Suction source (wall or portable with collection bottle)
- Sterile suction kit
- Sterile gloves (if not in kit)
- Sterile water-soluble lubricant
- Small bottle of sterile water or normal saline (if not in kit)
- Tubing connected to suction source
- Personal protective equipment: gown, mask, and goggles or face shield

DELEGATION TIPS

Nasopharyngeal and oropharyngeal suctioning is generally performed by the nurse. Properly trained ancillary personnel may perform oropharyngeal suctioning in some situations.

continues

IMPLEMENTATION—ACTION/RATIONALE

ACTION

RATIONALE

* Check client's identification band * Explain procedure before beginning *

1. Choose the most appropriate route (nasopharyngeal or oropharyngeal) for your client. If nasopharyngeal approach is considered, inspect the nares with a penlight to determine patency. Alternately, you may assess patency by occluding each nare in turn with finger pressure while asking the client to breathe through the remaining nare.

2. Advise the client that suctioning may cause coughing or gagging but emphasize the importance of clearing the airway.
3. Cleanse hands.
4. Position the client in a high Fowler's or semi-Fowler's position.
5. If the client is unconscious or otherwise unable to protect his or her airway, place in a side-lying position.
6. Connect extension tubing to suction device if not already in place, and adjust suction control to between 100 and 120 mm Hg for adult.
7. Put on gown and mask and goggles or face shield.
8. Using sterile technique, open the suction kit. Consider the inside wrapper of the kit to be sterile, and spread the wrapper out carefully to create a small sterile field.
9. Open a packet of sterile water-soluble lubricant and squeeze out the contents of the packet onto the sterile field.
10. If sterile solution (water or saline) is not included in the kit, pour about 100 mL of solution into the sterile container provided in the kit.
11. If gloves are wrapped, carefully lift the wrapped gloves from the kit without touching the inside of the kit or the gloves themselves. Lay the wrapped gloves next to the suction kit, and open the wrapper. Put on the gloves using sterile gloving technique (Procedure 27-2).
12. If a cup of sterile solution is included in the suction kit, open it.
13. Designate one hand as *sterile* (able to touch only sterile items) and the other as *clean* (able to touch only unsterile items).

14. *Using your sterile hand,* pick up the suction catheter. Grasp the plastic connector end between your thumb and forefinger and coil the tip around your remaining fingers.
15. Pick up the extension tubing *with your clean hand.* Connect the suction catheter to the extension tubing, taking care not to contaminate the catheter (Figure 27-25-1).
16. Position your clean hand with the thumb over the catheter's suction port.

1. The oropharyngeal approach is easier but requires that the client cooperate; it may also produce gagging more readily. The nasopharyngeal route is more effective for reaching the posterior oropharynx but is contraindicated in clients with a deviated nasal septum, nasal polyps, or any tendency toward excessive bleeding (low platelet count, use of anticoagulants, recent history of epistaxis or nasal trauma).
2. Promotes cooperation and reduces anxiety.

3. Reduces transmission of microorganisms.
4. Maximizes lung expansion and effective coughing.

5. Protects the client from aspiration in the event of vomiting.
6. Excessive negative pressure can cause tissue trauma, whereas insufficient pressure will be ineffective.

7. Protects nurse from splattering of body fluids.
8. Produces an area in which to place sterile items without contaminating them.

9. Lubricant will be used to further lubricate the catheter tip if the nasopharyngeal route is used.

10. Will be used to lubricate the catheter and to rinse the inside of the catheter to clear secretions.

11. Keeps gloves sterile for handling the sterile suction catheter to avoid introducing pathogens into the client's airway.

12. Will be used to lubricate the catheter and to rinse the inside of the catheter to clear secretions.
13. Usually, the dominant hand is the sterile hand, while the nondominant hand is clean. This prevents contamination of sterile supplies while allowing unsterile items to be handled.
14. Prevents accidental contamination of the catheter tip.

15. The extension tubing is not sterile.

16. Suction is activated by occluding this port with the thumb. Releasing the port deactivates the suction.

continues

Figure 27-25-1 Attach catheter to tubing.

Figure 27-25-2 Insert catheter into nostril. (This nurse is left handed.)

17. Dip the catheter tip into the sterile solution, and activate the suction. Observe as the solution is drawn into the catheter.

18. For oropharyngeal suctioning, ask the client to open his or her mouth. Without activating the suction, use sterile hand to gently insert the catheter and advance it until you reach the pool of secretions or until the client coughs. Do not poke catheter in oropharynx.

19. For nasopharyngeal suctioning, estimate the distance from the tip of the client's nose to the earlobe and grasp the catheter between your thumb and forefinger at a point equal to this distance from the catheter's tip.

20. Dip the tip of the suction catheter into the water-soluble lubricant to coat catheter tip liberally.

21. Use *sterile* hand to insert the catheter tip into the nostril with the suction control port uncovered. Advance the catheter gently with a slight downward slant. Slight rotation of the catheter may be used to ease insertion (Figure 27-25-2). Advance the catheter to the point marked by your thumb and forefinger.

22. If resistance is met, *do not force the catheter.* Withdraw it and attempt insertion via the opposite nostril.

23. With *clean* hand, apply suction by occluding the suction control port with your thumb; at the same time, slowly rotate the catheter by rolling it between your thumb and fingers while slowly withdrawing it. Apply suction for no longer than 15 seconds at a time.

24. Repeat step 23 until secretions have been cleared, allowing brief rest periods between suctioning episodes.

25. Withdraw the catheter by looping it around your fingers as you pull it out.

26. Dip the catheter tip into the sterile solution and apply suction.

27. Disconnect the catheter from the extension tubing. Holding the coiled catheter in your gloved hand, remove the glove by pulling it over the catheter. Discard catheter and gloves in an appropriate container.

28. Discard remaining supplies in the appropriate container and wash your hands.

29. Provide the client with oral hygiene if indicated or desired.

17. Tests the suction device as well as lubricates the interior of the catheter to enhance clearance of secretions.

18. To minimize trauma, do not apply suction while the catheter is being advanced.

19. Ensures placement of the catheter tip in the oropharynx and not in the trachea.

20. Promotes the client's comfort and minimizes trauma to nasal mucosa.

21. Guides the catheter toward the posterior oropharynx along the floor of the nasal cavity.

22. Forceful insertion may cause tissue damage and bleeding.

23. Prolonged suction applied to a single area of tissue can cause tissue damage.

24. Promotes complete clearance of the airway.

25. Allows you to maintain control over the catheter tip as it is withdrawn.

26. Clears the extension tubing of secretions that would promote bacterial growth and could block tubing.

27. Contains the catheter and secretions in the glove for disposal.

28. Prevents transmission of microorganisms.

29. Suctioning and coughing may produce an unpleasant taste.

continues

EVALUATION

- Check breath sounds for a patent airway.
- Ask client if breathing is easier.
- Assess client for signs of dyspnea.
- Review arterial blood gases and/or pulse oximetry results.
- Assess consistency, color, amount, and odor of secretions.

DOCUMENTATION

Nurses' Notes

- Date and time of suctioning procedure
- Client's tolerance of the procedure
- Amount, consistency, color, and odor or secretions
- Arterial blood gases and/or pulse oximetry results

PROCEDURE 27-26   Performing Tracheostomy Care

OVERVIEW

A tracheotomy is an incision made into the trachea with insertion of a cannula for airway management. Tracheostomy is the creation of an opening into the trachea through the neck. The two terms can be used interchangeably. A tracheostomy is performed for the client with potential or present airway obstruction, for ventilatory assistance, to provide pulmonary hygiene, to decrease the anatomic dead space in the client with chronic obstructive pulmonary disease, to avoid prolonged endotracheal intubation, and to provide an airway for clients with severe obstructive sleep apnea syndrome. The tracheostomy is performed below the level of the vocal cords and allows air to enter and exit the tracheostomy rather than through the upper airway. The tracheostomy tube can have a single or double cannula. The determination of the tube design used is based on the needs of the client. The double cannula tube allows for the tube to be cleaned to prevent obstruction caused by dried secretions. During the acute phase after a tracheostomy has been performed, all care must be performed using sterile technique. Once care of the tracheostomy tube becomes a client procedure, a clean technique is used.

ASSESSMENT

1. Assess respirations for rate, rhythm, and depth **to evaluate the airway.**
2. Assess the client's lung sounds **to determine the need for suctioning.**
3. Assess the client's arterial blood gases and/or pulse oximetry values **to evaluate air exchange and blood oxygen levels.**
4. Assess the movement of air through the tracheostomy tube **to evaluate the air exchange through the tube and determine whether there is any obstruction.**
5. Assess the amount and color of tracheal secretions **to evaluate for bleeding, infection, and the need for suctioning.**
6. Assess for anxiety, restlessness, and fear. **Anxiety and restlessness may be symptoms of airway distress and hypoxia.**
7. Assess the client's understanding of the procedure **to determine client education and support needed.**

POSSIBLE NURSING DIAGNOSES

*Ineffective **A**irway Clearance*
*Risk for **I**nfection*
*Risk for **S**uffocation*
*Impaired **S**kin Integrity*
*Impaired Verbal **C**ommunication*
*Deficient **K**nowledge (tracheostomy care)*
***A**nxiety*
*Impaired **G**as Exchange*

PLANNING

Expected Outcomes

1. The client's airway will be free of obstruction.
2. The procedure will be performed with a minimum of client anxiety.
3. The client's skin will remain intact and free of redness and excoriation.
4. The client will remain free of signs and symptoms of infection.

continues

5. The client will have cannulas free of secretions and clean, secure ties.

Equipment Needed

Cleaning the Inner Cannula
- Sterile gloves
- Disposable inner cannula (if available)

- Tracheostomy care kit: 2 basins, tracheostomy brush, tracheostomy ties
- Hydrogen peroxide
- Sterile water or sterile saline

DELEGATION TIPS

Tracheostomy care cannot be delegated by the nurse. Ancillary personnel may assist the nurse in providing care to clients receiving this treatment and should be instructed to report a client experiencing increased secretions, dyspnea, or the need for suctioning to the nurse.

IMPLEMENTATION—ACTION/RATIONALE

ACTION	RATIONALE

◦ Check client's identification band ◦ Explain procedure before beginning ◦

1. Cleanse hands and apply clean gloves.
2. Remove soiled dressing and discard inside gloves as they are removed.

1. Reduces transmission of microorganisms.
2. Prevents contamination of other areas.

Conventional/Reusable Inner Cannula

3. Open tracheostomy care set.
4. Apply sterile gloves.
5. Place hydrogen peroxide solution in one basin and sterile water or saline in a second basin.
6. Dip the applicator in the basin of hydrogen peroxide.
7. Remove inner cannula.
8. Place inner cannula in basin of hydrogen peroxide.
9. Clean the area under the neck plate of the tracheostomy tube using a cotton applicator moistened with hydrogen peroxide (Figure 27-26-1).
10. Rinse area under neck plate with cotton applicator moistened with sterile water or saline.
11. Dry skin under neck plate with cotton-tip applicator.

3. Provides sterile equipment for use in the procedure.
4. Uses aseptic technique.
5. Prepare solutions prior to applying gloves.

6. Prevents contamination of the applicator.
7. Allows for cleaning.
8. Loosens secretions.
9. Decreases microorganisms and removes crusting.

10. Removes hydrogen peroxide from the skin.

11. Prevents skin excoriation from moisture.

Figure 27-26-1   Clean the area under the neck plate with a cotton applicator moistened with hydrogen peroxide.

continues

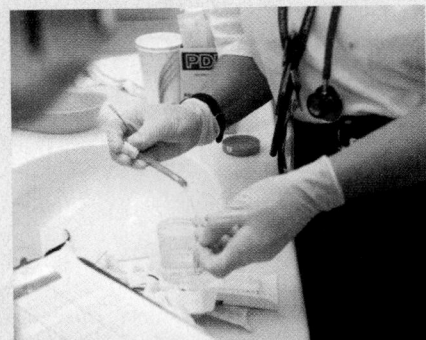

Figure 27-26-2 Use a sterile cotton-tipped applicator to clean the inner cannula area and remove crusted secretions.

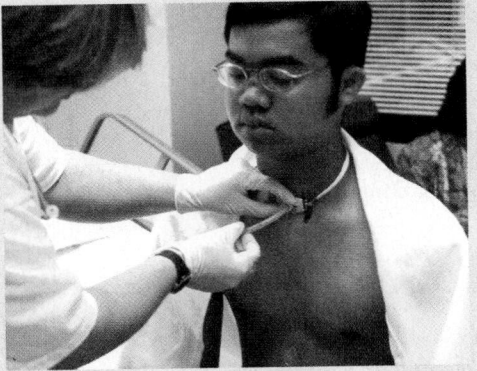

Figure 27-26-3 Carefully reinsert inner cannula and lock into place.

12. Use a tracheostomy brush or sterile cotton-tip applicator to clean inner cannula (Figure 27-26-2).
13. Rinse inner cannula with sterile water or sterile saline.
14. Dry inner cannula.
15. Reinsert inner cannula and lock it into place (Figure 27-26-3).
16. Remove gloves and cleanse hands.

Disposable Inner Cannula

17. Cleanse hands. Open disposable cannula container without touching cannula.
18. Apply sterile gloves.
19. Remove inner cannula and discard.
20. Replace inner cannula with new disposable cannula.
21. Remove gloves and cleanse hands.

Two-Person Technique of Changing Tracheostomy Ties

22. Cut two pieces of twill tape about 12 to 14 inches in length.
23. Make a fold about 1 inch below the end of each piece of twill tape and cut a half-inch slit lengthwise in the center of the fold.
24. Have a second person gently hold the tracheostomy tube in place with fingers on both sides of the neck plate.
25. Untie old tracheostomy ties and discard.
26. Insert the split end of the tracheostomy tape through the opening on one side of the tracheostomy tube neck plate. Pull the distal end of the tracheostomy tie through the cut end and pull tightly.
27. Repeat procedure with second piece of twill tape.
28. Tie tracheostomy tapes with a double knot at the side of the neck.
29. Insert one finger under tracheostomy tapes.
30. Insert tracheostomy gauze under neck plate of tube.

31. Discard all used materials and cleanse hands.

12. Removes crusted secretions.

13. Removes hydrogen peroxide from inner cannula.
14. Prevents introduction of solutions into the trachea.
15. Prevents accidental removal of the inner cannula during coughing.
16. Reduces transmission of microorganisms.

17. Reduces transmission of microorganisms.

18. Uses aseptic technique.
19. Disposable inner cannulas are not to be reused.
20. Provides a clean open cannula.
21. Prevents transmission of microorganisms.

22. Prepares equipment before beginning procedure.

23. Prepares tape for insertion.

24. Prevents accidental movement of the tracheostomy tube resulting in coughing and accidental decannulation.
25. Removes tracheostomy ties.
26. Secures tracheostomy tie within neck plate.

27. Secures tracheostomy tube.
28. Secures tracheostomy tube.

29. Ensures that tube has been tied securely.
30. Prevents irritation of skin from secretions and rubbing of tracheostomy tube.

31. Reduces transmission of microorganisms.

continues

One-Person Technique of Changing Tracheostomy Ties

32. Follow Actions 22–23 and 26–28.
33. Hold the neck plate firmly with one hand; untie and remove old tracheostomy tapes and discard.
34. Place one finger under tracheostomy ties.
35. Discard all used materials and cleanse hands.

32. See Rationales 22–23 and 26–28.
33. Prevents dislodgment while untying and removing old tracheostomy tapes.
34. Checks for tightness and security.
35. Reduces transmission of microorganisms.

EVALUATION

- Airway is free of obstruction.
- Client anxiety was minimal during procedure.
- There is no evidence of infection.
- Airway is patent.
- Cannulas free of secretions, and clean, secured ties.
- Client's skin intact and free of redness and excoriation.

DOCUMENTATION

Nurses' Notes

- Date, time, procedure performed, and client's tolerance of the procedure
- Size and type of tracheostomy tube in place
- Amount and consistency of any secretions
- Condition of the client's skin
- Client teaching and participation

PROCEDURE 27-27   Performing Tracheostomy Suctioning

OVERVIEW

Suctioning secretions is necessary to maintain the airway of a client who is unable to clear his or her own secretions by coughing. Some clients may be able to cough but not effectively enough to expel the secretions. Suctioning the client's airway is considered a sterile procedure. Using sterile technique prevents the introduction of contagion into the client's airway and lungs.

Suctioning is performed as often as necessary to remove excess secretions. The procedure may be performed as often as every 5 minutes or as infrequently as every few hours, depending on the amount of secretions the client is generating and the client's ability to clear his or her own airway. Evaluate the client's airway and oxygenation to determine the need for suctioning. Wall suction should be set at 100 to 120 mm Hg for adults, 50 to 100 mm Hg for children, and 40 to 60 mm Hg for infants. Portable suction set at 8 to 15 mm Hg for adults, 5 to 8 mm Hg for children, and 3 to 5 mm Hg for infants.

ASSESSMENT

1. Assess respirations for rate, rhythm, and depth **to evaluate airway.**
2. Auscultate lung fields **to evaluate airway and determine need for suctioning.**
3. Monitor arterial blood gases and/or pulse oximetry values **to determine oxygen levels and adequate air exchange.**
4. Assess passage of air through the tracheostomy tube **to determine air exchange and obstruction of the tube.**
5. Monitor tracheal secretions for amount, color, consistency, and odor **to assess for evidence of bleeding or signs of infection and need for suctioning.**

6. Assess for anxiety and restlessness, **which may be signs of airway distress and/or hypoxia.**
7. Assess the client's understanding of the suctioning procedure **to decrease the client's anxiety.**

POSSIBLE NURSING DIAGNOSES

Impaired Gas Exchange
Anxiety
Ineffective Airway Clearance
Risk for Infection

continues

PLANNING

Expected Outcomes

1. The client will have no crackles or wheezes in large airways and the absence of cyanosis.
2. The client will report breathing comfortably and will have no apparent anxiety or restlessness.
3. The client will have minimal amount of thin, normal-colored secretions.
4. The client will maintain a patent airway.

Equipment Needed

- Sterile gloves
- Mask, eye protection, and gown if appropriate
- Source of negative pressure (suction machine or wall suction)
- Sterile suction catheter
- Oxygen or Ambu-bag
- Equipment for tracheostomy care or tracheostomy care tray

DELEGATION TIPS

Suctioning a tracheostomy is not delegated by the nurse. Ancillary personnel may assist the nurse in providing care to clients receiving this treatment and should be instructed to report a client experiencing increased secretions, dyspnea, or the need for suctioning to the nurse.

IMPLEMENTATION—ACTION/RATIONALE

ACTION	RATIONALE
* Check client's identification band * Explain procedure before beginning *	
1. Assess depth and rate of respirations; auscultate breath sounds.	1. Determines need for suctioning.
2. Assemble supplies on bedside table.	2. Organizes work.
3. Cleanse hands.	3. Reduces transmission of microorganisms.
4. Position the client in a high Fowler's or semi-Fowler's position.	4. Maximizes lung expansion and effective coughing.
5. Connect extension tubing to suction device, if not already in place, and adjust suction control to between 100 and 120 mm Hg.	5. Excessive negative pressure can cause tissue trauma, hypoxemia, and atelectasis, whereas insufficient pressure will be ineffective.
6. Put on gown and mask and goggles or face shield.	6. Protects from splattering body fluids.
7. Using sterile technique, open tracheostomy care kit. Consider the inside wrapper of the kit to be sterile, and spread the wrapper out carefully to create a small sterile field. Add sterile suction catheter if not in kit.	7. Produces an area in which to place sterile items without contaminating them.
8. If gloves are wrapped, carefully lift the wrapped gloves from the kit without touching the inside of the kit or the gloves themselves. Lay the wrapped gloves down and open the wrapper. Put on the gloves using sterile gloving technique.	8. Reduces introduction of pathogens into the client's airway.
9. Pour hydrogen peroxide in one basin and sterile water or saline in the other.	9. Provides solution to clean inner cannula and to lubricate the catheter and rinse the inside of the catheter to clear secretions.
10. Designate one hand as *sterile* (able to touch only sterile items), usually the dominant hand, and the other as *clean* (able to touch only nonsterile items), the nondominant hand.	10. Prevents contamination of sterile supplies while allowing you to handle unsterile items.
11. *Using your sterile hand,* pick up the suction catheter. Grasp the plastic connector end between your thumb and forefinger and coil the tip around your remaining fingers.	11. Prevents accidental contamination of the catheter tip.
12. Pick up the extension tubing *with your clean hand.* Connect the suction catheter to the extension tubing, taking care not to contaminate the catheter.	12. The extension tubing is not sterile.

continues

13. If client is not receiving oxygen, administer oxygen or use Ambu-bag with *clean* hand before beginning procedure.

13. Hyperoxygenates client and prevents hypoxia during suctioning.

14. Remove inner cannula and place in basin of hydrogen peroxide to loosen secretions, if reusable, or set aside if disposable. Do not dispose of disposable cannula until new inner cannula is securely in place.

14. Allows easier passage of the suction catheter. Retain old cannula until you are sure the new cannula fits correctly.

15. Position your clean hand with the thumb over the catheter's suction port, dip the catheter tip into the sterile solution, and activate the suction. Observe as the solution is drawn into the catheter.

15. Tests the suction device as well as lubricating the interior of the catheter to enhance clearance of secretions.

16. Remove thumb from suction port.

16. Deactivates the suction.

17. Using your *clean* hand, remove the oxygen delivery device from the tracheostomy tube and place it on a clean surface.

17. Permits access to the tracheostomy tube. Placing the oxygen device on a clean surface reduces contamination (the sterile glove wrapper may be used for this purpose).

18. Without occluding the suction control port, insert the catheter tip into the tracheostomy tube and advance it until the client coughs or resistance is met (Figure 27-27-1) and withdraw slightly.

18. Minimizes trauma when suction not applied while the catheter is being advanced.

Figure 27-27-1 Suction Tracheostomy

19. Apply suction by occluding the suction control port with your thumb, while slowly rotating the catheter between your thumb and finger and slowly withdrawing it. Apply suction for no longer than 15 seconds at a time.

19. Prolonged suction can cause tissue damage, atelectasis, and hypoxemia.

20. Repeat step 19 until all secretions have been cleared, allowing brief rest periods between suctioning episodes. Encourage client to breathe deeply between suctioning episodes. Provide oxygen between passes of the suction catheter.

20. Promotes complete clearance of the airway.

21. Withdraw the catheter and dip it into the cup of sterile saline, applying suction.

21. Cleans suction catheter of secretions.

22. Clean inner cannula using tracheostomy brush and rinse well in sterile water or sterile saline. Dry (or open new disposable inner cannula).

22. Removes secretions and maintains patent inner cannula.

23. Reinsert inner cannula and lock into place.

23. Prevents secretions from obstructing outer cannula.

24. Reapply oxygen delivery device.

24. Reoxygenates the client and restores supplemental oxygen and humidification.

25. Dip the catheter tip into the sterile solution and apply suction.

25. Clears the extension tubing of secretions, which would promote bacterial growth.

26. Disconnect the catheter from the extension tubing. Holding the coiled catheter in your gloved hand, remove the glove by pulling it over the catheter. Discard catheter and gloves in an appropriate container.

26. Contains the catheter and secretions in the glove for disposal.

27. Discard remaining supplies in the appropriate container.

27. Follow institutional policy regarding disposal of client care supplies.

continues

28. Cleanse hands.
29. Provide the client with oral hygiene if indicated/desired.

28. Prevents transmission of pathogens.
29. Suctioning and coughing may produce an unpleasant taste.

EVALUATION

- Ask client whether breathing is easier.
- Auscultate breath sounds for a patent airway.
- Review arterial blood gases and/or pulse oximetry values.
- Assess client for signs of dyspnea.
- Evaluate consistency, color, amount, and odor of secretions.

DOCUMENTATION

Nurses' Notes

- Date and time of suctioning procedure.
- Client's tolerance of the suctioning procedure
- Amount, consistency, color, and odor of secretions
- Arterial blood gases and/or pulse oximetry values

PROCEDURE 27-28   Postoperative Exercise Instruction

OVERVIEW

Preoperative teaching of postoperative exercises prepares the client physically and emotionally for the impending surgery. The goal of instruction is to have the client demonstrate the performance of exercises while verbalizing why the exercises are used during the postoperative phase.

Several postoperative exercises help speed recovery from surgery. Turning, deep breathing, and coughing facilitate removal of accumulated pulmonary secretions. Clients may experience their worst postoperative pain while doing these exercises. Inhaled gases and oxygen have a drying effect on the respiratory mucosa, which increases the viscosity of secretions, making them difficult to raise with coughing.

To prevent respiratory complications, teach clients to breathe deeply to achieve sustained maximum inspiration (SMI). SMI promotes the reinflation of the alveoli and the removal of mucus secretions.

Several devices help encourage clients to perform SMI exercises. The breathing devices, called incentive spirometers, measure the client's ventilatory volume and provide the user with a tangible reward for generating an adequate respiratory flow. When the client takes a deep breath, the ball moves upward and the amount of air is measured, thereby making the results visible to the client.

Turning, deep breathing, coughing, and using spirometry prevent respiratory complications by doing the following:

- Promoting pulmonary circulation
- Promoting the exchange of gases by increasing lung compliance
- Facilitating the removal of mucus secretions from the tracheobronchial tree

Postoperatively the client is encouraged to move in bed and perform leg exercises. These exercises assist in preventing circulatory complications that can arise from anesthetic agents that depress the metabolic and heart rates. Early ambulation also increases respiratory function and the return of peristalsis.

ASSESSMENT

1. Assess the client's current understanding of postoperative procedures. **Establishes baseline for teaching.**
2. Assess the client's ability to understand the postoperative exercise instructions. **Establishes baseline for teaching. Affects how the teaching and procedures will be performed.**
3. Assess any preoperative limitations the client may have that would prevent or impair the ability to perform the postoperative exercises accordingly. **Establishes base-** **line for teaching. Affects how the teaching and procedures will be performed. Allows modification of the exercises.**

POSSIBLE NURSING DIAGNOSES

Acute **P***ain*
Impaired Physical **M***obility*
Impaired **G***as Exchange*
Risk for Impaired **S***kin Integrity*

continues

PLANNING

Expected Outcomes

1. The client will be able to successfully demonstrate post-operative exercises, deep breathing, coughing, pillow splinting, turning and proper body alignment, leg and foot exercises, and out-of-bed transfers.
2. The client will be able to successfully demonstrate proper use of the incentive spirometer.

Equipment Needed

- Educational materials
- Pillow
- Tissue
- Nonsterile gloves
- Disposable, volume-oriented incentive spirometer

DELEGATION TIPS

Postoperative instruction requires the assessment and intervention of a nurse. Ancillary staff may reinforce the information and directions taught to the client.

IMPLEMENTATION—ACTION/RATIONALE

ACTION

❖ Check client's identification band ❖ Explain procedure before beginning ❖

1. Cleanse hands and organize equipment.

2. Apply gloves.
3. Place client in a sitting position.
4. Demonstrate deep breathing exercises.
   - Place one hand on abdomen (umbilical area) during inhalation.
   - Expand the abdomen and rib cage on inspiration.
   - Inhale slowly and evenly through your nose until you achieve maximum chest expansion.
   - Hold breath for 2 to 3 seconds.

   - Slowly exhale through your mouth until maximum chest contraction has been achieved.
5. Have the client return-demonstrate deep breathing and repeat 3 to 4 times.
6. Instruct the client on the use of an incentive spirometer (Figure 27-28-1).
   - Hold the volume-oriented spirometer upright.

RATIONALE

1. Reduces the transmission of microorganisms and promotes efficiency.
2. Reduces the transmission of microorganisms.
3. Promotes full chest expansion.
4. Shows the client how to breathe deeply.
   - Exerts counterpressure during inhalation.

   - Promotes maximum chest expansion.
   - Maintains full expansion of the alveoli.

   - Increases the pressure, thereby preventing immediate collapse of the alveoli.
   - Promotes maximum chest contraction.

5. Reinforces learning. Promotes increased air exchange.

6. Reinflates the alveoli and removes mucus secretions.

   - Promotes proper functioning of the device.

Figure 27-28-1 Instruct the client to take a slow, deep breath to elevate the ball in the tube.

continues

- Take a normal breath and exhale, then seal lips tightly around the mouthpiece; take a slow deep breath to elevate the balls in the plastic tube, hold the inspiration for at least 3 seconds.
- The client simultaneously measures the amount of inspired air volume on the calibrated plastic tube.
- Remove the mouthpiece, exhale normally.
- Take several normal breaths.

7. Have the client repeat the procedure 4 to 5 times.

8. Have the client cough after the incentive effort. See the following section.
9. Demonstrate splinting and coughing.

- Have the client slowly raise head and sniff the air.

- Have the client slowly bend forward and exhale slowly through pursed lips.

- Repeat breathing 2 to 3 times.

- When the client is ready to cough, have client place a folded pillow against the abdomen with clasped hands (Figure 27-28-2).

- Have client take a deep breath and begin coughing immediately after inspiration is completed by bending forward slightly and producing a series of soft, staccato coughs.
- Have a tissue ready.

10. Have the client return-demonstrate splinting and coughing.
11. Wash the incentive spirometer mouthpiece under running water and store in a clean container. Disposable mouthpieces should be changed every 24 hours.

- Allows for greater lung expansion; holding the inspiration increases the pressure, preventing the immediate collapse of the alveoli.

- Encourages the client to do respiratory exercises.

- Allows normal expiration.
- Provides the client the opportunity to relax.

7. Encourages sustained maximal inspiration and loosens secretions.
8. Facilitates the removal of secretions.

9. Shows the client how to raise mucus secretions from the tracheobronchial tree.
- Increases the amount of air and helps aerate the base of the lungs.
- Dries the tracheal mucosa as air flows over it. There is a slight increase in carbon dioxide level, which stimulates deeper breathing.
- Loosens mucus plugs and moves secretions to the main bronchus.
- Elevates the diaphragm and expels air in a more forceful cough; supports the abdominal muscles and reduces pain while coughing, if the client has an abdominal incision.
- Removes secretions from the main bronchus.

- Preparation for sputum disposal.
10. Fosters learning.

11. Reduces transmission of microorganisms.

Figure 27-28-2 Use a pillow to support the abdominal muscles when coughing.

continues

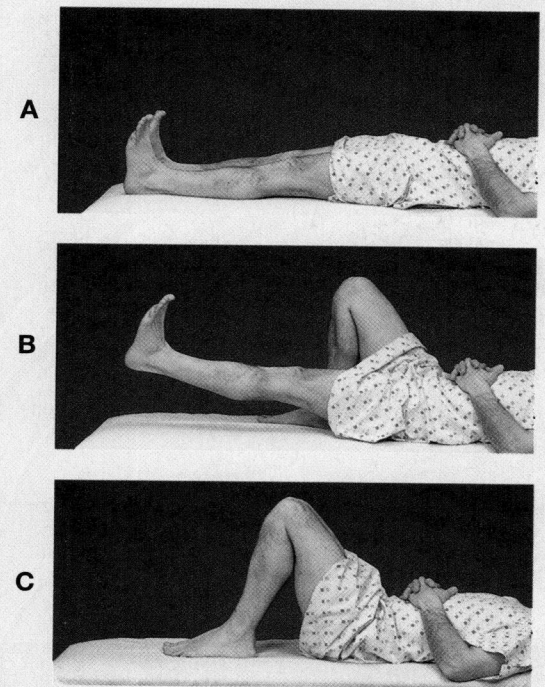

Figure 27-28-3 Leg exercises improve venous blood return.

Figure 27-28-4 Using the hand to splint the incision site when sitting up in bed will reduce pain and pressure at the incision site.

12. Teach the client leg and foot exercises.
- Have the client, with heels on bed, push the toes of both feet toward the foot of the bed until the calf muscles tighten, then relax feet. Pull the toes toward the chin, until calf muscles tighten; then relax feet (Figure 27-28-3A).
- With heels on bed, lift and circle each ankle, first to the right and then to the left; repeat three times, relax (Figure 27-28-3B).
- Flex and extend each knee alternately, sliding foot up along the bed; relax (Figure 27-28-3).

13. Have the client return-demonstrate the leg and foot exercises.

14. Explain how to turn in bed and get out of bed.

15. Instruct the client who has a left-sided abdominal or chest incision to turn to the right side of bed and sit up as follows:
- Flex the knees.
- With the right hand, splint the incision with hand or small pillow.
- Turn toward right side by pushing with the left foot and grasping the shoulder of the nurse or partial side rail of the bed with the left hand.
- Raise up to a sitting position on the side of the bed by using the left arm and hand to push down against the mattress or side rail.

16. Reverse instructions (use left side instead of right) for the client with a right-sided incision according to Action 15 (Figure 27-28-4).

12. To improve venous blood return from the legs.
- Causes contraction and relaxation of the calf muscles.

- Causes contraction and relaxation of the quadriceps muscles.

- Causes contraction and relaxation of the quadriceps muscles.

13. Fosters learning of how to improve venous blood return.

14. Elicits client cooperation.

15. Fosters learning how to turn and get out of bed without putting pressure on the incision line.

16. Same as Rationale 15.

continues

17. Instruct clients with orthopedic surgery (e.g., hip surgery) how to use a trapeze bar.
18. Cleanse hands.

17. Facilitates movement in bed without putting pressure on a leg or hip joint.
18. Reduces transmission of microorganisms.

EVALUATION

- The client is able to successfully demonstrate postoperative exercises, deep breathing, coughing, pillow splinting, turning and proper body alignment, leg and foot exercises, and out-of-bed transfers.
- The client is able to successfully demonstrate proper use of the incentive spirometer.

DOCUMENTATION

Nurses' Notes

- Teaching the client postoperative exercises
- Client's level of understanding and cooperation with the teaching

Preoperative Checklist

- Initial the check-off area for documentation of preoperative teaching.

PROCEDURE 27-29   Performing a Skin Puncture

OVERVIEW

Skin punctures are performed when small quantities of capillary blood are needed for analysis or when the client has poor veins. Capillary puncture is also commonly performed for blood-glucose analysis. The common sites for capillary punctures are:
- Heel—most common site for neonates and infants
- Fingertip—the inner aspect of palmar fingertip used most commonly in children and adults
- Earlob—used when the client is in shock or the extremities are edematous

ASSESSMENT

1. Assess the condition of the client's skin at the potential puncture site **to determine if it is intact, free of bruising, and can be used without causing undue trauma to the site.**
2. Assess the circulation at the potential puncture site **to determine if it is a good site to obtain a sample, and to determine if healing at the site might be compromised.**
3. Assess the client's comfort level regarding the procedure **to determine client education and support needed.**
4. Assess the cleanliness of the client's skin **to determine how much cleansing is needed before the skin puncture.**

POSSIBLE NURSING DIAGNOSES

Risk for Impaired Skin Integrity
Acute Pain
Anxiety

PLANNING

Expected Outcomes

1. An adequate blood specimen will be obtained.
2. The client will suffer minimal trauma during the specimen collection.
3. The specimen will be collected and stored in a manner compatible with the ordered tests.

Equipment Needed

- Antiseptic 70% isopropanol or povidone-iodine
- Microhematocrit tubes or micropipette (collection tubes)
- Sterile 2 × 2 gauze
- Sterile lancet
- Nonsterile gloves
- Hand towel or absorbent pad

continues

DELEGATION TIPS

Properly trained ancillary personnel may perform skin puncture. Agency policy usually dictates certification and recertification requirements for this skill. Proper client and specimen identification are of the utmost importance and must be consistently demonstrated by the ancillary personnel.

IMPLEMENTATION—ACTION/RATIONALE

ACTION

RATIONALE

❖ Check client's identification band ❖ Explain procedure before beginning ❖

1. Cleanse hands.
2. Check the client's identification band if appropriate.
3. Explain the procedure to the client.
4. Prepare supplies:
   • Open sterile packages.
   • Label specimen collection tubes.
   • Place in easy reach.
5. Apply gloves.
6. Select site: lateral aspect of the fingertips in adults/children; heel for neonates and infants.
7. Place the hand or heel in a dependent position; apply warm compresses if fingers or heel are cool to touch.
8. Place hand towel or absorbent pad under the extremity.
9. Cleanse puncture site with an antiseptic, and allow to dry. Use 70% isopropanol if the client is allergic to iodine (Figure 27-29-1).
10. With nondominant hand, apply gentle milking pressure above or around the puncture site. Do not touch the puncture site.
11. Read directions carefully before using the lancet.
    • With the sterile lancet at a 90-degree angle to the skin, use a quick stab to puncture the skin (about 2 mm deep) (Figure 27-29-2).
    • With the automatic unistik, push the lancet into the body of unistik until it clicks. Hold the body of the unistik and twist off the lancet cap. Place the end of the unistik tightly against the client's finger and press the lever. The needle automatically retracts after use.

1. Reduces transmission of microorganisms.
2. Ensures the correct client.
3. Allays anxiety and encourages cooperation.
4. Ensures efficiency.

5. Follows Standard Precautions.
6. Avoids damage to nerve endings and calloused areas of the skin.
7. Increases the blood supply to the puncture site.

8. Prevents soiling the bed linen.
9. Reduces skin surface bacteria; povidone-iodine must dry to be effective.

10. Increases blood to puncture site and maintains asepsis.

11. Provides a blood sample with minimal discomfort to the client.

Figure 27-29-1   Cleanse the puncture site and allow it to dry.

Figure 27-29-2   Use a quick stab to puncture the skin.

continues

Figure 27-29-3   Allow the blood to flow from the puncture site to ensure that an adequate amount can be obtained.

Figure 27-29-4   Collect a small sample of blood.

12. Wipe off the first drop of blood with sterile 2 × 2 gauze; allow the blood to flow freely (Figure 27-29-3).

13. Collect the blood into the tube(s). If blood for a platelet count is to be collected, obtain this specimen first (Figure 27-29-4).

14. Apply pressure to the puncture site with a sterile 2 × 2 gauze.

15. Place contaminated articles into a sharps container.

16. Remove gloves; cleanse hands.

17. Position client for comfort with call light in reach.

18. Cleanse hands.

12. The first drop may contain a large amount of serous fluid, which could affect the results. Pressure at the puncture site can cause hemolysis.

13. Allows blood collection; avoids aggregation of platelets at the puncture site.

14. Controls bleeding.

15. Reduces the risk of needlestick.

16. Reduces transmission of microorganisms.

17. Provides for comfort and communication.

18. Reduces transmission of microorganisms.

EVALUATION

- Specimen is adequate.
- No trauma to client

DOCUMENTATION

Nurses' Notes

- Puncture site and the reason for the puncture
- Test results if the testing is performed at the time of the puncture

---

PROCEDURE 27-30   Assisting with Crutches, Cane, or Walker

OVERVIEW

Mobility is an important part of everyone's life. Being able to move about in the environment can mean the difference between living at home and living in a health care facility. Being able to move independently improves a client's emotional, mental, and physical well-being.

Clients who cannot safely walk unassisted can use devices designed to aid them in walking independently. The three most common devices used are crutches, canes, and walkers.

continues

The appropriate device for each client is determined by the client's health care provider, physical therapist, or nurse. These caregivers often work together to determine which device will be best for the client. This decision is based on the client's ability to bear weight on the legs, upper arm strength, stamina, and the presence or absence of unilateral weakness.

Crutches can be used by clients who cannot bear any weight on one leg, who can only bear partial weight on one leg, and who have full weight-bearing ability on both legs. Several types of crutches are available, depending on the length of time the client will require the assistance and the client's upper-body strength.

A cane is used by clients who can bear weight on both legs but one leg or hip is weaker or impaired. There are several types of canes as well. The standard, straight cane is used most often. There are also canes with three or four legs on the end, called quad canes, to increase a client's stability when walking.

Walkers are used by clients who require more support than a cane provides. Walkers are available with or without wheels. Walkers without wheels provide the most stability, but they must be lifted with each step. Walkers with wheels are somewhat less stable, but a client who does not have the upper-body strength to lift the walker repeatedly can push it along while walking.

ASSESSMENT

1. Assess the reason the client requires an assistive device. Is it a long-term need or a short-term need? **Helps determine which device to use.**
2. Assess the client's physical limitations. How much weight is the client able to bear? Can the client bear weight on both legs or just one? Is the upper body strength good? Does the client tire easily? **Assesses safety and comfort.**
3. Assess the client's physical environment. Is the client at home or in a medical facility? Is the environment suited to assistive needs and the assistive device the client will be using? Are the hallways wide enough? Well lit? Are the doorways wide enough? Are there stairs used frequently, and if so, how many? Do the doors swing open far enough? **Assesses safety and comfort.**
4. Assess the client's ability to understand and follow directions regarding use of an assistive device. Can the client understand the instructions? Can he or she remember them? Has the client used this device in the past? Is there a language barrier that might limit understanding? **Assesses safety, educational, comfort, and effectiveness.**

POSSIBLE NURSING DIAGNOSES

*Impaired Physical **M**obility*
*Risk for **T**rauma*
*Deficient **K**nowledge* (assistive devices for mobility)

PLANNING

Expected Outcomes

1. The client will be able to demonstrate safe and independent ambulation with the assistance of crutches, a cane, or a walker.
2. The client will feel confident and safe while using the assistive device.

Equipment Needed

- Gait belt
- Assistive device: crutches, cane, or walker
- Tape measure
- Nonslip footwear

DELEGATION TIPS

Ambulation of clients with assistive devices is frequently delegated to ancillary personnel. The initial teaching of and ongoing assessment of the proper use of the device is not delegated. The nurse or physical or occupational therapist is responsible to observe the client's technique, reteach if necessary, and document the client's proficiency.

IMPLEMENTATION—ACTION/RATIONALE

ACTION	RATIONALE
* Check client's identification band * Explain procedure before beginning *	
1. Assess client for strength, mobility, range of motion, visual acuity, perceptual difficulties, and balance. *Note:* The nurse and physical therapist often work together on assessment and choosing the correct assistive equipment of ambulation.	1. Helps determine the client's capabilities and amount of assistance required.

continues

Figure 27-30-1   Adjusting the crutches to fit the client will increase comfort and stability.

2. Measure client for size of crutches and adjust crutches to fit. While client is supine, measure client from heel to axilla. When client is standing, the crutch pad should fit 1.5 to 2 inches below axilla (Figure 27-30-1). Adjust hand grip so elbow is at 30-degree flexion.

2. Increases client safety and comfort. Space between crutch pad and axilla prevents pressure on radial nerves. Elbow flexion allows for space between crutch pad and axilla.

3. Provide a robe or other covering as well as nonslip foot coverings or shoes.

3. Provides for privacy and safety.

4. Lower the height of the bed.

4. Allows client to sit with feet on the floor and increases safety.

5. Dangle the client at the side of the bed for several minutes. Assess for vertigo or nausea.

5. Allows for stabilization of blood pressure, thus preventing orthostatic hypotension.

6. Apply gait belt around the client's waist if balance and stability are unknown or unreliable. It is good practice to use a gait belt the first time the client is out of bed.

6. Provides support and promotes safety.

7. Demonstrate to client the method of holding crutches while he or she remains seated. This should be with elbows bent 30 degrees while hands are on the hand grips and pads 1.5 to 2 inches below the axilla. Instruct client to position crutches 4 to 5 inches laterally and 4 to 6 inches in front of feet. With weight on hands, not axilla.

7. Increases comprehension and cooperation, decreases anxiety.

8. Assist the client to a standing position by having client place both crutches in nondominant hand. Then, using the dominant hand, push off from the bed while using the crutches for balance. Once erect, the extra crutch can be moved into the dominant hand.

8. Allows for stability while promoting independence.

9. Instruct the client to remain still for a few seconds while assessing for vertigo or nausea. Stand close to the client to support as needed. While client remains standing, check for correct fit of the crutches.

9. Promotes client comfort, support, and safety. If the client becomes dizzy, sit client back down and wait before trying again.

Two-Point Gait (Figure 27-30-2A)

10. Move the left crutch and right leg forward 4 to 6 inches. Move the right crutch and left leg forward 4 to 6 inches. Repeat the two-point gait.

10. The two-point gait (used for partial weight-bearing) provides a strong base of support. The client must be able to bear weight on both legs. This gait is faster than the four-point gait.

Three-Point Gait (Figure 27-30-2B)

11. Advance both crutches and the weaker leg forward together 4 to 6 inches. Move the stronger leg forward, even with the crutches. Repeat the three-point gait.

11. The three-point gait (used for partial or non-weight-bearing) provides a strong base of support. This gait can be used if the client has a weak or non-weight-bearing leg.

continues

Figure 27-30-2 Various Crutch Gaits: **A,** Two-point gait (partial weight-bearing); **B,** Three-point gait (partial or non–weight-bearing); **C,** Four-point gait (partial or full weight-bearing); **D,** Swing through gait (non–weight-bearing)

Four-Point Gait (Figure 27-30-2C)

12. Position the crutches 4.5 to 6 inches to the side and in front of each foot. Move the right crutch forward 4 to 6 inches and move the left foot forward, even with the left crutch. Move the left crutch forward 4 to 6 inches and move the right foot forward, even with the right crutch. Repeat the four-point gait.

12. The four-point gait (used for partial or full weight-bearing) provides greater stability. Weight bearing is on three points (two crutches and one foot or two feet and one crutch) at all times. The client must be able to bear weight with both legs.

continues

Swing-Through Gait (Figure 27-30-2D)

13. Move both crutches forward 4 to 6 inches. Move both legs forward in a swinging motion past the crutches. Repeat the swing-through gait.

13. The swing-through gait permits a faster pace. This gait requires greater balance, strength, and more practice.

Walking Upstairs

14. Stand beside and slightly behind client. Instruct client to position the crutches as if walking. Place body weight on hands. Place the strong leg on the first step. Pull the weak leg up and move the crutches up to the first step. Repeat for all steps.

14. Prevents weight bearing on the weaker leg. When ascending stairs, crutches should follow the legs, thereby allowing stability if the client's weight shifts down the stairs while moving. This allows the client to catch him or herself instead of falling backward.

Walking Downstairs

15. Position the crutches as if walking. Place weight on the strong leg. Move the crutches down to the next lower step. Place partial weight on hands and crutches. Move the weak leg down to the step with the crutches. Put total weight on arms and crutches. Move strong leg to same step as weak leg and crutches. Repeat for all steps. A second caregiver standing behind the client holding on to the gait belt will further decrease the risk of falling.

15. Prevents weight bearing on the weaker leg. Crutches in front of the legs while descending stairs allow the client more forward stability if his or her weight shifts down the stairs while client is moving. This allows client to catch self before falling forward.

16. Set realistic goals and opportunities for progressive ambulation using crutches.

16. Crutch walking takes up to 10 times the energy required for unassisted ambulation.

17. Consult with a physical therapist for clients learning to walk with crutches.

17. The physical therapist is the expert on the health care team for crutch-walking techniques.

18. Cleanse hands.

18. Reduces transmission of microorganisms.

Sitting with Crutches

19. Instruct client to back up to chair until it is felt with the back of the legs.

19. Allows for less turning, better stability, and increased safety.

20. Place both crutches in the nondominant hand and use the dominant hand to reach back to the chair.

20. Increases safety by giving the client an idea of how far away he or she is from the seat.

21. Instruct client to lower slowly into the chair.

21. Decreases pain and possible injuries.

Walking with a Cane

22. Repeat Actions 1–6.

22. See Rationales 1–6.

23. Have the client push up from the sitting position while pushing down on the bed with arms.

23. Promotes autonomy as well as increases upper body strength.

24. Have the client stand at the bedside for a few moments with cane in hand opposite the affected leg.

24. Allows the client to gain balance. Allows more control of cane.

25. Assess the height of the cane. With the cane placed 6 inches ahead of the client's body, the top of the cane should be at wrist level with the arm bent 25% to 30% at the elbow.

25. A 25% to 30% bend at the elbow provides for better muscle strength and support than if the arm is straight.

26. Walk to the side and slightly behind the client, holding the gait belt if needed for stability.

26. Allows the nurse to provide stability or assistance if the client needs it.

Cane Gait

27. Move the cane and the weaker leg forward at the same time for the same distance (Figure 27-30-3). Place weight on the weaker leg and the cane. Move the strong leg forward. Place weight on the strong leg.

27. The cane helps provide a wide base of support for the body when the weight is on the weaker leg.

Sitting with a Cane

28. Have client turn around and back up to the chair. Have client grasp the arm of the chair with the free hand and lower self into the chair. Be sure to place the cane out of the way but within reach.

28. The cane provides additional support as client lowers self into the chair.

continues

Figure 27-30-3 Move the cane and the weaker leg forward. Cane should be in alignment with client.

Figure 27-30-4 Move the walker and the weaker leg forward.

Figure 27-30-5 Use the arms to support the rest of the weight and move the strong leg forward.

29. Consult with a physical therapist for clients learning to walk with a cane.
30. Cleanse hands.

29. The physical therapist is the expert on the health care team for cane-walking techniques.
30. Reduces transmission of microorganisms.

Walking with a Walker

31. Repeat Actions 1–6.
32. Place the walker in front of the client.

33. Have the client put the nondominant hand on the front bar of the walker or on the hand grip for that hand, whichever is more comfortable. Then, using the dominant hand to push off from the bed and the nondominant hand for stabilization, help the client to an erect position.
34. Have the client transfer hand to the walker handgrips.

35. Be sure the walker is adjusted so the handgrips are just below waist level and the client's arms are slightly bent at the elbow.
36. Walk to the side and slightly behind the client, holding the gait belt if needed for stability.

31. See Rationales 1–6.
32. Positions the walker for use and provides stability when the client is standing.
33. Uses upper body strength and encourages independence.

34. Allows the client to maintain balance while transferring weight.
35. Provides maximum support from the arms while ambulating.

36. Provides stability or assistance if the client needs it.

Walker Gait
37. Move the walker and the weaker leg forward at the same time (Figure 27-30-4). Place as much weight as possible or as allowed on the weaker leg, using the arms for supporting the rest of the weight. Move the strong leg forward and shift the weight to the strong leg (Figure 27-30-5).

37. Provides support for a weak or non–weight-bearing leg by using arm and upper body strength.

Sitting with a Walker
38. Have the client turn around in front of the chair and back up until the back of the legs touch the chair. Have client place hands on the chair armrests, one hand at a time, then lower self into the chair using the armrests for support.
39. Consult with a physical therapist for clients learning to walk with a walker.
40. Cleanse hands.

38. Using the armrests of the chair is a more stable support than using the walker.

39. The physical therapist is the expert on the health care team for walker techniques.
40. Reduces transmission of microorganisms.

continues

EVALUATION

- The client is able to demonstrate safe and independent ambulation with the assistance of crutches, a cane, or a walker.
- The client feels confident and safe while using the assistive device.

DOCUMENTATION

Nurses' Notes

- Type of device the client is using, the level of understanding regarding the use of the device, how far the client is able to walk using the device, and the client's response to the activity

Kardex

- Information that is pertinent to nurses or therapists regarding type of device or a particular client's needs

---

PROCEDURE 27-31   Feeding and Medicating via Enteral Tube

OVERVIEW

Enteral nutrition is a procedure whereby liquid food (formula) is instilled directly into the stomach or small intestines using a tube. Other names for this procedure are tube feedings and gastric gavage. Candidates for tube feedings are clients who have a functional GI tract and will not, should not, or cannot eat. Tube feedings are used for clients who are (or may become) malnourished and in whom oral feedings are insufficient to maintain adequate nutritional status.

Enteral tube feedings maintain the structural and functional integrity of the GI tract, enhance the utilization of nutrients, and provide a safe and economic method of feeding.

Feeding Tubes

Most feeding tubes are made of silicone or polyurethane, which are durable and biocompatible with formulas. They vary in diameter (8–12 French) and length in accord with the route and formula. The health care provider selects the route and type of feeding tube on the basis of the anticipated duration of feeding, the condition of the GI tract, and the potential for aspiration.

A nasogastric, small-bore feeding tube is generally used when the anticipated duration of use is short. See Procedure 28-2.

The gastrostomy tube is placed through an opening in the abdominal wall into the intestines. This is done via an enterostomy, the surgical creation of an artificial fistula into the intestines. Tube enterostomies can be placed at various points along the GI tract and are performed when long-term tube feeding is anticipated or when obstruction makes nasoenteral tube feeding impossible.

Percutaneous endoscopic gastrostomy (PEG) tube placement is performed by the health care provider at the bedside or in the endoscopy room; insertion of a PEG tube does not require general anesthesia surgery. This method of enteral feeding is more common than conventional enterostomies; it is less risky because surgery is not required, and it is more economic.

Administration of Enteral Feedings

Once feeding tube position has been radiographically verified, the formula can be administered as prescribed. There are two typical methods of administering tube feedings. Intermittent feeding is given four to six times a day in the form of a bolus. Intermittent feedings are generally given through a large-bore tube. The bolus (generally 250–400 mL of formula for adult clients) can be given using a large syringe fit into the end of the feeding tube or using a gravity drip over 20 to 30 minutes. The intermittent method is generally practiced in the home care setting because of its ease and need for minimal equipment. Continuous feeding delivers formula with a pump to regulate the rate. Most clients with a small-bore tube receive continuous feeding. One of the advantages of continuous feeding is that it keeps gastric volume small, minimizing residual volume and reducing the risk of aspiration pneumonia; the client is less likely to experience bloating, nausea, abdominal distention, and diarrhea. Continuous feeding is recommended for the seriously ill or comatose client.

continues

Safety Considerations

Clients receiving enteral nutrition through a tube feeding are at risk for aspiration. Auscultate for bowel sounds to determine gastric motility. If the bowel sounds are hypoactive or absent, stop or withhold additional feeding and notify the health care provider.

Always assess placement of the feeding tube before administering any liquids. Clients who are receiving continuous gastric feeding should be assessed every 4 hours for tube placement and residual gastric contents. Aspirate gastric contents with a syringe. Observe and check the pH of the aspirate. If less than 100 mL, replace stomach contents after checking the residual to prevent fluid and electrolyte imbalance.

Client safety and comfort require daily cleansing of the feeding tube exit site. Cleanse the skin with a clean washcloth, soap, and water. Enterostomy tubes require surgical asepsis of the exit site until the incision heals; rotate the tubes within the stoma to promote healing. Report any observations of redness, irritation, or gastric leakage at the site. Between feedings, a prosthetic device may be used to cover the ostomy opening.

The PEG tubes require daily rotation to relieve pressure on the skin. Notify the health care provider if unable to rotate the PEG; it may be an indication of internal embedding of the tube into the gastric wall. When the tube is internally embedded, it can cause gastric acid reflux, which results in skin breakdown, sepsis, and cellulitis. Care must be taken to avoid dislodgment of the tube. Keep it secured to the client's abdomen with tape, being careful not to use excessive tension. The PEG tubes require frequent flushing to prevent clogging. These tubes have small lumens. If a tube becomes clogged, flush it with 60 mL of lukewarm tap water.

ASSESSMENT

1. Assess the client for signs of gastric distress, such as nausea, vomiting, and cramping, **to determine the client's tolerance for the tube feeding.**
2. Assess the feeding tube placement every 4 hours **to confirm tube placement in the intestines.**
3. Assess the client's respiratory status **to evaluate for pulmonary aspiration of gastric contents.**
4. Assess the client's ongoing nutritional status **to evaluate the effectiveness of the tube feeding.**
5. Assess the client's intake and output **to evaluate for fluid deficit or excess.**

POSSIBLE NURSING DIAGNOSES

Risk for Imbalanced Nutrition: Less Than Body Requirements
Risk for Deficient Fluid Volume
Risk for Aspiration

PLANNING

Expected Outcomes

1. The client will receive the correct feeding formula and the correct volume of formula over the correct time period.
2. The client will not experience any undesirable effects: aspiration, nausea, vomiting, abdominal distention, cramping, diarrhea, or constipation.
3. The client's weight and nutritional status will remain stable or improve.
4. The client will not experience any adverse skin or gastrointestinal effects from the gastrostomy or PEG tube.

Equipment Needed

- Asepto syringe or 20- to 50-mL syringe
- Emesis basin
- Clean towel
- Disposable gavage bag and tubing
- Formula
- Infusion pump for feeding tube (if needed)
- Water to follow feeding
- Nonsterile gloves

DELEGATION TIPS

Feedings via gastrostomy tubes may be given by properly trained ancillary personnel if the facility and the state permit. The ancillary personnel must be properly trained in assessing tube placement, proper positioning of the client, and in the administration of the correct type and rate of feeding. All medications must be administered by a nurse.

IMPLEMENTATION—ACTION/RATIONALE

ACTION

RATIONALE

❋ Check client's identification band ❋ Explain procedure before beginning ❋

ACTION	RATIONALE
1. Review medical record for formula, amount, and time.	1. Verifies health care provider's prescription for appropriate formula and amount.

continues

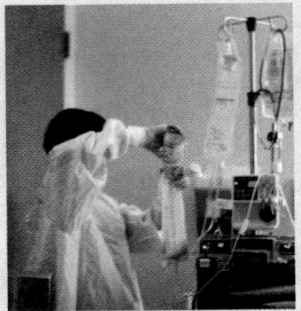

Figure 27-31-1 Fill the bag with the prescribed amount of formula.

Figure 27-31-2 Check that the feeding tube is intact and in place, auscultate for bowel sounds, and look for abdominal distention.

2. Cleanse hands and gather equipment and formula.

3. Assemble equipment. Add color to formula per institutional policy. If using a bag, fill with prescribed amount of formula (Figure 27-31-1).
4. Place client on right side in high Fowler's position.

5. Provide for privacy.
6. Cleanse hands and don nonsterile gloves.
7. Observe for abdominal distention; auscultate for bowel sounds.
8. Check feeding tube (Figure 27-31-2). Insert syringe into adapter port, aspirate stomach contents, and determine amount of gastric residual. If residual is greater than 50 to 100 mL (or in accordance with agency protocol), hold feeding until residual diminishes. Instill aspirated contents back into feeding tube.
9. Administer tube feeding.

Intermittent Bolus

10. Pinch the tubing.
11. Remove plunger from barrel of syringe and attach to adapter.
12. Fill syringe with formula.

13. Allow formula to infuse slowly; continue adding formula to syringe until prescribed amount has been administered.
14. Flush tubing with 30 to 60 mL or prescribed amount of water.

Intermittent Gavage Feeding

15. Hang bag on IV pole so that it is 18 inches above the client's head.
16. Remove air from bag's tubing.

17. Attach distal end of tubing to feeding tube adapter and adjust drip to infuse over prescribed time.
18. When bag empties of formula, add 30 to 60 mL or prescribed amount of water; close clamp.

2. Reduces transmission of microorganisms and promotes efficiency during procedure.
3. Ensures efficiency when initiating feeding. Color will distinguish formula aspirate.

4. Reduces risk of pulmonary aspiration in the event client vomits or regurgitates formula.
5. Places client at ease.
6. Reduces transmission of pathogens.
7. Assesses for delayed gastric emptying; indicates presence of peristalsis and ability of GI tract to digest nutrients.
8. Indicates whether gastric emptying is delayed. Reduces risk of regurgitation and pulmonary aspiration related to gastric distention. Prevents electrolyte imbalance.

9. Provides nutrients as prescribed.

10. Prevents air from entering tubing.
11. Provides system to delivery feeding.

12. Allows gravity to control flow rate, reducing risk of diarrhea from bolus feeding.
13. Prevents air from entering stomach. Decreases risk of diarrhea.

14. Ensures that remaining formula in tubing is administered and maintains patency of tube; prevents air from entering the stomach.

15. Allows gravity to promote infusion of formula.

16. Prevents air from entering stomach. Decreases risk of diarrhea.
17. Allows gravity to control flow rate, reducing risk of diarrhea from bolus feeding.
18. Prevents air from entering stomach and reduces risk for gas accumulation. Maintains patency of feeding tube.

continues

19. Change bags every 24 hours.

19. Decreases risk of microorganism multiplication in bag and tubing.

Continuous Gavage

20. Check tube placement at least every 4 hours.
21. Check residual at least every 8 hours.
22. If residual is above 100 mL, stop feeding.

23. Add prescribed amount of formula to bag for a 4-hour period; dilute with water if prescribed.
24. Hang gavage bag on IV pole. Prime tubing.
25. Thread tubing through feeding pump and attach distal end of tubing to feeding tube adapter; keep tubing straight between bag and pump.
26. Adjust drip rate.
27. Monitor infusion rate and signs of respiratory distress or diarrhea.
28. Flush tube with water every 4 hours as prescribed or following administration of medications.
29. Replace disposable feeding bag at least every 24 hours, in accord with institution protocol.
30. Elevate head of bed at least 30 degrees at all times and turn client every 2 hours.
31. Provide oral hygiene every 2–4 hours.

32. Administer water as prescribed with and between feedings.
33. Remove gloves and cleanse hands.

20. Ensures that feeding tube remains in stomach.
21. Indicates ability of GI tract to digest and absorb nutrients.
22. Reduces risk of regurgitation and pulmonary aspiration related to gastric distention.
23. Provides client with prescribed nutrients and prevents bacterial growth (formula is easily contaminated).
24. Removes air from tubing.
25. Provides for controlled flow rate; prevents loops in tubing.

26. Infuses formula over prescribed time.
27. Prevents complications associated with continuous gavage.
28. Maintains patency of tube.

29. Decreases transmission of microorganisms.

30. Prevents aspiration and promotes digestion and reduces skin breakdown.
31. Provides comfort and maintains the integrity of buccal cavity.
32. Ensures adequate hydration.

33. Reduces transmission of microorganisms.

Instilling Medications into Enteral Tubes

34. Cleanse hands and don nonsterile gloves.
35. Assist the client to high or semi-Fowler's position.
36. Place linen saver over bed linens.
37. Verify NG tube placement (Procedure 28-2).
38. Attach syringe to tube and pour 30 mL of prepared medication into syringe.
39. Open clamp on tube.
40. Hold syringe at a slight angle; add more medication before syringe empties.
41. For two or more medications, give each separately, with 5-mL water rinse between medications.
42. As syringe empties with the last of the medication, slowly add 30 to 50 mL water.
43. Before tube empties of water, clamp the tube, detach and dispose of the syringe.
44. Place clients with an NG tube on the right side with head slightly elevated for 30 minutes.
45. Remove gloves and cleanse hands.

34. Reduces spread of microorganisms.
35. Gravity assists to keep medications down.
36. Prevents soiling during procedure.
37. Ensures tube placement is correct.
38. Readies medication to be given.

39. Allows medication into tube.
40. Allows medication to flow at a slow, steady rate.

41. Ensures each medication is given.

42. Clears medication from the sides and distal end of tube to prevent clogging.
43. Prevents air from getting into the stomach. Disposes of used equipment.
44. Prevents regurgitation.

45. Reduces spread of microorganisms.

EVALUATION

- The client received the correct feeding formula and the correct volume of formula over the correct time period.
- Client did not experience any undesirable effects such as aspiration, nausea, vomiting, abdominal distention, cramping, diarrhea, or constipation.

- Client's weight and nutritional status remained stable or improved.
- Client did not experience any adverse skin or gastrointestinal effects from the gastrostomy or PEG tube.

continues

DOCUMENTATION

Nurses' Notes

- Time, date, formula, and amount of feeding, and client's response
- Amount of residual aspirated before the feeding
- Tube placement checked and method used
- If the dressing at the tube insertion site was changed and the condition of the client's skin
- If the tube was rotated or adjusted
- Any client complaints or adverse effects such as bloating, nausea, vomiting, diarrhea, or constipation

Medication Administration Record

- Date and time the feeding was instilled (per institution specifications)

Intake and Output Record

- Amount of tube feeding instilled and the amount of water used to flush the feeding tube

---

PROCEDURE 27-32   Performing Pulse Oximetry

OVERVIEW

Pulse oximetry is a quick, easy, noninvasive method to assess the arterial blood oxygen saturation of a client by using an external sensor. There are several types of sensors; however, the most common for adult use is a finger sensor. The finger is placed between a clip mechanism. On one side of the clip are light-emitting diodes (a red and an infrared); a photon detector is on the other side. The beam of light goes through the tissue and blood vessels, and the photon detector receives the light and measures the amount of light absorbed by oxygenated and unoxygenated hemoglobin. Unoxygenated hemoglobin absorbs more red light and oxygenated hemoglobin absorbs more infrared light. The amount of each light and, hence, the arterial blood oxygen saturation (SaO_2) is determined by the spectrum of light. Other types of sensors can be used on the toe, nose, ear, forehead, or around the hand or foot and use this same principle of spectrometry. Special sensors are available for the neonatal hand and pediatric toe.

ASSESSMENT

1. Assess the client's hemoglobin level. **Because pulse oximetry measures the percent of SaO_2, the results of the oxygenation status will be affected. The results may appear normal if the hemoglobin level is low because all hemoglobin available to carry O_2 is completely saturated; therefore, it is important to know the hemoglobin level.**
2. Assess the client's color. **If the client has vasoconstriction of the extremities, an inaccurate recording may be obtained.**
3. Assess the client's mental status **because this will assist in general evaluation of oxygen delivery to the brain and indicate a high level of CO_2.**
4. Assess the client's pulse rate. The pulse oximeter measures pulse rate. **Manually assessing pulse can be used as a cross-reference to indicate functioning of the oximeter.**
5. Assess the area where the sensors will be placed **to determine whether it is an area with adequate circulation (no scars or thickened nails).**
6. Remove nail polish and/or acrylic nails, **which interfere with sensor measurements.**

POSSIBLE NURSING DIAGNOSES

*Impaired **G**as Exchange*
*Ineffective **T**issue Perfusion*
*Risk for Impaired **S**kin Integrity*

PLANNING

Expected Outcomes

1. The SaO_2 will be in a normal range for the client (95%–100% in the absence of chronic respiratory disease).
2. The client will be alert and oriented.
3. The client's color will remain normal.
4. The client will tolerate the placement of sensors.
5. There will not be any skin irritation or pressure from sensors.

Equipment Needed

- Pulse oximeter
- Proper sensor
- Alcohol wipe or soap and water
- Nail polish remover if necessary

continues

DELEGATION TIPS

Ancillary personnel routinely perform pulse oximetry. They should be instructed on acceptable parameters and to report any abnormal findings to the nurse.

IMPLEMENTATION—ACTION/RATIONALE

ACTION

RATIONALE

❋ **Check client's identification band** ❋ **Explain procedure before beginning** ❋

1. Cleanse hands.
2. Select an appropriate sensor. Sensors are commonly used for the fingertips.
3. Select an appropriate site for the sensor. Fingers are most commonly used; however, toes (Figure 27-32-1), earlobes, nose, forehead (Figure 27-32-2), hands, and feet can be used. Assess for capillary refill and proximal pulse. If the client has poor circulation, use an earlobe, forehead, or nasal sensor instead. In children, sensors may be used on the hand, foot, or trunk. If elderly clients have thickened nails, pick another site.
4. Clean the site with an alcohol wipe. Remove artificial nails or nail polish if present or select another site. Clean any tape adhesive. Use soap and water if necessary to clean the site.
5. Apply the sensor. Make sure the photon detectors are aligned on opposite sides of the selected site (Figure 27-32-3).
6. Connect the sensor to the oximeter with a sensor cable. Turn on the machine. Initially a tone can be heard, followed by an arterial wave-form fluctuation with each arterial pulse. In most oximeters if the battery is low, a low-battery light illuminates when 15 minutes of battery life are remaining. Oximeters should remain plugged in even when not in use.
7. Adjust the alarm limits for high and low O_2 saturation levels according to the manufacturer's directions. Pulse rate limits most often can also be set. Adjust volume.

1. Reduces transmission of microorganisms.
2. The sensor should be selected based on the size of the person and the site to be used.
3. Decreased circulation alters the O_2 saturation measurement.

4. Polish and artificial fingernails alter the results.

5. Proper application is necessary for accurate results.

6. The tone and wave-form fluctuation indicate that the machine is detecting blood flow with each arterial pulsation.

7. The alarms indicate that the saturation levels or pulse rates are outside the designated levels and alert the nurse of abnormal O_2 saturation levels and pulse rates.

Figure 27-32-1   Pulse Oximeter Sensor Placed on a Toe

Figure 27-32-2   Pulse Oximeter Sensor Placed on the Forehead

continues

Figure 27-32-3 Apply the sensor to the selected site.

Figure 27-32-4 Note the results on the oximeter.

8. If taking a reading, note the results (Figure 27-32-4). If the oximeter is being used for constant monitoring, move the site of spring sensors every 2 hours and adhesive sensors every 4 hours.
9. Cover the sensor with a sheet or towel to protect it from exposure to bright light.

10. Notify the health care provider of abnormal results.

11. Cleanse hands.

8. Prevents skin breakdown from pressure and skin irritation from the adhesive.

9. Ambient light sources such as sunlight or warming lights may interfere with the sensor and alter the SaO_2 results.
10. A low SaO_2 level requires medical attention because permanent tissue damage may result from low oxygen saturation.
11. Reduces transmission of microorganisms

EVALUATION

- The SaO_2 is in the normal range for the client (95%–100% in the absence of chronic respiratory disease).
- The client is alert and oriented.
- The client's color is normal.
- The client tolerates the placement of sensors.
- There is no skin irritation or pressure from sensors.

DOCUMENTATION

Nurses' Notes
- Time pulse oximetry was placed, the location of the sensor, baseline readings, and hemoglobin level

Flow Sheet
- Pulse, oxygen, flow rate, and saturation readings

References/Suggested Readings

Lord, L. (2001). How to insert a large-bore nasogastric tube. *Nursing2001*, 31(9), 46–48.

Metheny, N., & Titler, M. (2001). Assessing placement of feeding tubes, *AJN*, 101(5), 36–45.

Pullen, R. (2003). Caring for a patient on pulse oximetry. *Nursing2003*, 33(9), 30.

ADVANCED PROCEDURES

PROCEDURE 28-1   Initiating Strict Isolation Precautions

OVERVIEW

Occasionally, a client must be placed in isolation to prevent the spread of an infectious process. Barrier protective equipment is put on outside the room before providing any client care. All linens and trash must be double-bagged, according to agency policy, before being removed from an isolation room. Meals are served on disposable dishes.

    Visitors may be limited because everyone entering the room must wear barrier protective equipment. Some clients feel the isolation very profoundly. Paperback books (to be discarded later), TV, and other diversional activities help the client pass the time.

ASSESSMENT

1. Review physician's orders for isolation to ensure proper setup.
2. Assess client's and family's understanding of client's condition and reason for isolation to identify required teaching needed.

POSSIBLE NURSING DIAGNOSES

Social Isolation
Impaired Social Interaction
Deficient Knowledge (disease process, isolation)
Risk for Powerlessness

PLANNING

Expected Outcomes

1. The room will be set up for the appropriate type of isolation.
2. The client and family will understand the client's condition and the reason for isolation.

Equipment Needed

- Isolation sign
- Disposable gowns
- Gloves (nonsterile and sterile)
- Goggles or face shield
- Disposable masks
- Impermeable bags (for linen and trash)
- Tape or bag ties and labels
- Disposable vital signs equipment (single-use thermometers, stethoscope, and sphygmomanometer) if available
- Disposable water pitcher and cups
- Linen
- Room with sink and running water
- Soap and paper towels
- Other supplies relative to client's condition

DELEGATION TIPS

Initiating strict isolation precautions is a nursing responsibility. Properly trained ancillary personnel may provide some client care according to agency policy.

continues

IMPLEMENTATION—ACTION/RATIONALE

ACTION

* Check client's identification band * Explain procedure before beginning *
* NOTE: Barrier protection must be on before checking client's ID *

1. Review physician orders and agency protocols relative to the type of isolation precautions:
   a. Implement protocol related to the type of disinfectants needed to eliminate specific microorganisms.
   b. Alert housekeeping regarding the room number and type of isolation supplies needed in the room.
   c. Make sure the room has proper ventilation (the door will have to remain closed at all times) and that the bed and other electrical equipment are functioning properly.
2. Place appropriate isolation supplies outside the client's room and place isolation sign on the door.

3. Gather appropriate supplies to take in the room:
   a. Soap and paper towels
   b. Linen
   c. Impermeable bags
   d. Disposable vital signs equipment, if available
   e. Wound care supplies, if appropriate
4. Remove jewelry, lab coat, and other items not necessary for providing client care.
5. Cleanse hands and don disposable clothing:

   a. Apply mask by placing the top of the mask over the bridge of your nose (top part of mask has a lightweight metal strip) and pinch the metal strip to fit snugly against your skin.
   b. Apply cap to cover hair and ears completely, if policy requires cap.
   c. Apply gown to cover outer garments completely: Hold gown in front of body and place arms through sleeves (Figure 28-1-1A). Pull sleeves down to wrist. Tie gown securely at neck and waist (Figure 28-1-1B, C).
   d. Don nonsterile gloves and pull gloves to cover gown's cuff.
   e. Don goggles or face shield.
6. Enter client's room with all gathered supplies; if client is to receive medications, bring them at this time.
7. Assess client and family knowledge relative to client's diagnosis and isolation:
   a. Reason isolation initiated
   b. Type of isolation
   c. Duration of isolation
   d. How to apply barrier protection
8. Assess vital signs, administer medications if appropriate, and perform other functions of nursing care to meet client needs. Record assessment data on a piece of paper, avoiding contact with any articles in the client's room.

RATIONALE

1. Ensures compliance without unnecessary stress being placed on the client and family. Allows housekeeping to have the necessary supplies on their cleaning carts. Provides for client comfort and decreases the spread of microorganisms. Limits the number of personnel coming into the client's room and the client's exposure to microorganisms.

2. Ensures staff follows isolation protocol and alerts visitors to check with the nurses' station before entering the room.
3. Provides for organized care, hand hygiene, proper isolation, and client care materials. Decreases the spread of microorganisms and the number of times caregivers have to go into and out of the room.

4. Decreases the spread of resident and transient microorganisms.
5. Disposable garments act as a barrier protecting from contact with pathogens.

   e. Eyeglasses do not offer adequate protection.
6. Prevents trips into and out of client room and keeps supplies clean.
7. Client's and family's understanding of isolation procedures will increase their participation in care.

8. Allows for data collection and the performance of client care measures.

continues

A   B   C

Figure 28-1-1 Donning disposable gowns: **A,** Hold gown in front of the body and place arms through the sleeves. **B,** Fasten neck ties. **C,** Fasten waist ties.

9. Dispose of soiled articles in the impermeable bags, which should be labeled correctly according to contents. If soiled reusable equipment is removed from the room, label bag accordingly.

10. Double-bag soiled linen according to agency policy in an impermeable bag or in plastic linen bag.

11. Replenish supplies before leaving the client's room by having another staff member bring the clean supplies and transfer at the door. Ask client if anything is needed (e.g., juice or personal care items).

12. Before leaving, let the client know when you will return and make sure call light is accessible.

13. Exiting the isolation room:
    a. Untie gown at waist.
    b. Remove one glove by grasping the glove's cuff and pulling down so that the glove turns inside out (glove on glove) and dispose of it. With your ungloved hand, slip your fingers inside the cuff of the other glove, pull it off, inside out, and dispose of it.
    c. Grasp and release the ties of the mask, and dispose of it.
    d. Release neck ties of the gown and allow the gown to fall forward. Place fingers of dominant hand inside cuff of other hand and pull down over other hand (Figure 28-1-2A). With gown-covered hand, pull gown over the dominant hand (Figure 28-1-2B). While gown is still on arm, fold outside of gown together, remove, and dispose of it (Figure 28-1-2C).
    e. Remove cap by slipping your finger under the cap and removing from the front to back and dispose of it.

9. Impermeable bags prevent the leakage of contaminated materials, thereby preventing the spread of infection. Labeling is a warning to other personnel that the contents are infectious.

10. Double-bagging allows the washing of soiled linen without human contact. When linen is double-bagged, the first bag is removed before washing and the second bag goes into the machine with the dirty linen and dissolves.

11. Decreases the number of times staff members have to go in and out of the room.

12. Decreases a feeling of abandonment; provides client with a means of communication.

13. Gloves are removed inside out to avoid contact with skin. The gown is removed and folded with hands touching only the inside of the garment. Only the ties and the inside of the cap are touched with your hands. All articles are disposed of as soon as they are removed.

    c. If a client has an airborne-spread disease, the mask may be removed last.

continues

A   B   C

Figure 28-1-2 Removing disposable gown: **A,** Place fingers of dominant hand inside the cuff of other hand and pull gown down over other hand. **B,** With the gown-covered hand, pull gown down over dominant hand. **C,** As the gown is removed, fold the outside of the gown together and dispose of it.

14. Wash hands for 10 minutes. Don nonsterile gloves and remove bags from the client's room. Exit room and close door. Dispose of bags according to agency protocol. Remove gloves and cleanse hands.

14. Reduces transmission of microorganisms.

EVALUATION

- The appropriate type of isolation was instituted.
- The client and family express understanding of the client's condition and the reason for isolation.

DOCUMENTATION

Nurses' Notes

- Date, time, and type of isolation instituted
- Client response to isolation
- Client and family teaching regarding isolation

PROCEDURE 28-2   Inserting and Maintaining a Nasogastric Tube

OVERVIEW

Nasogastric (NG) tubes are used for several purposes, including feeding for nutrition when the client is comatose, semiconscious, or unable to consume sufficient nutrition orally. Nasogastric suction tubes are used for decompression of gastric content after gastrointestinal surgery, and to obtain gastric specimens for diagnosis of peptic ulcer. Tubes are used for irrigation to clean and flush the stomach after oral ingestion of poisonous substances. Finally, NG tubes are used to document the presence of blood in the stomach, monitor the amount of bleeding from the stomach, and identify the recurrence of bleeding in the stomach.

The two most commonly used NG tubes are the single-lumen Levin's tube and the double-lumen Salem sump tube.

The gastrointestinal tract is considered to be a clean area rather than a sterile one. The procedure to place an NG tube is performed using clean technique unless it is performed in conjunction with gastrointestinal surgery.

continues

ASSESSMENT

1. Assess client's consciousness level **to determine the ability of the client to cooperate during the procedure.**
2. Check the client's chart for any previous medical history of nostril surgery or injury or unusual nostril bleeding. **Reduces risk of injury from the tube.**
3. Use a penlight to assess nostrils for a deviated septum. **Facilitates choice of nostril and size of tube.**
4. Ask the client to breathe through each nostril, occluding the other with a finger. **Facilitates choice of nostril and decreases chance that tube will interfere with respirations.**
5. Assess for latex allergy. **Prevents reaction to latex and determines need to use latex-free tubes and gloves.**

POSSIBLE NURSING DIAGNOSES

Imbalanced **N**utrition: Less Than Body Requirement
Impaired **S**wallowing
Risk for **A**spiration
Risk for **D**iarrhea
Impaired **O**ral Mucous Membrane
Risk for Deficient **F**luid Volume
Acute **P**ain
Impaired **S**kin Integrity

PLANNING

Expected Outcomes

1. Client's nutritional status will improve, as indicated by increased body weight, physical strength, and mental status.
2. Client's nutritional needs will be met with the assistance of tube feeding.

3. Client will maintain a patent airway, as evident by absence of coughing, no shortness of breath, and no aspiration.
4. Client will not have diarrhea caused by nasogastric feeding.
5. Mouth mucous membranes will remain moist and intact.
6. Client will maintain a normal fluid volume, as evident by good skin texture, muscle tone, and blood volume.
7. Client's comfort level will increase.
8. Skin around the tube will remain intact, with no redness or blisters.

Equipment Needed

- Nasogastric tube: adult, 14 to 18 French; child/infant, 5 to 10 French; single-lumen (Levin's tube): feeding; double-lumen (Salem sump tube): feeding, suction, irrigation
- Water-soluble lubricant
- Syringe with catheter tip or adapter, 50 cc
- Glass of tap water with straw, or ice
- Towel or tissue
- Emesis basin with ice chips
- Tongue blade
- pH chemstrip
- Stethoscope
- Disposable, latex-free gloves (nonsterile)
- Hypoallergenic tape, rubber band, and safety pin
- Personal protective equipment: gown, gloves, face shield or goggles, and mask
- Penlight or flashlight
- Disposable irrigation set (if needed)
- Wall mount or portable suction equipment (if needed)
- Administration set with pump or controller for feeding tube

DELEGATION TIPS

Inserting and maintaining a nasogastric tube is the responsibility of a nurse. Oral hygiene for the client may be delegated.

IMPLEMENTATION—ACTION/RATIONALE

ACTION	RATIONALE
⁂ Check client's identification band ⁂ Explain procedure before beginning ⁂	
1. Review client's medical history.	1. To assess for any nostril surgery and abnormal bleeding.
2. Assess client's consciousness and ability to understand. Develop a hand signal.	2. Decreases anxiety and promotes cooperation.
3. Prepare the equipment, putting tissues, a cup of water, and an emesis basin nearby.	3. Facilitates an efficient procedure.

Figure 28-2-1   Measure the distance from nose to ear-lobe to the xiphoid process to determine how much tube will need to be inserted to reach the stomach.

Figure 28-2-2   Gently insert the tube into the naris.

4. Prepare the environment; raise the bed and place it in a high Fowler's position (45 to 60 degrees). Cover the chest with a towel.
5. Cleanse hands and then put on gloves and personal protective equipment.
6. Assess client's nostrils with penlight and have the client blow nose one nostril at a time.
7. Using the NG tube, measure the distance from the tip of the nose to the earlobe and then to the xiphoid process of the sternum and mark this distance on the tube with a piece of tape (Figure 28-2-1).
8. Lubricate first 4 inches of the tube with water-soluble lubricant.
9. Ask the client to slightly flex the neck backward.
10. Gently insert the tube into a naris (Figure 28-2-2).

11. Ask the client to tip the head forward once the tube reaches the nasopharynx—this is usually where the client starts to gag. If the client continues to gag, stop a moment.
12. Advance the tube several inches at a time as the client swallows water or ice chips.

13. Withdraw the tube immediately if there are signs of respiratory distress.
14. Advance the tube until the taped mark is reached.
15. Wipe or wash body oils off tip of nose and allow to dry. Split a 4-inch strip of tape lengthwise 2 inches. Secure the tube with the tape by placing the wide portion of the tape on the bridge of the nose and wrapping the split ends around the tube (Figure 28-2-3). Tape to cheek as well if desired (Figure 28-2-4).
16. Check the placement of the tube:
    • Attach syringe to the end of the tube and rapidly inject 30 cc of air and at the same time auscultate over the epigastric area (upper left quadrant).
    • Aspirate for gastric content, assess the color and quality of the content. If required, measure with pH indicator strip. Follow protocol regarding reinsertion of contents versus discarding.
    • Prepare the client for x-ray checkup, if prescribed.

4. Prevents back strain and facilitates insertion.

5. Reduces transmission of microorganisms. Protects from body fluids.
6. Decreases discomfort and unnecessary trauma by choosing the more patent nostril for insertion.
7. Determines the approximate amount of tube needed to reach the stomach.

8. Facilitates passage into the naris.

9. Makes insertion easier.
10. Promotes passage of tube with minimal trauma to mucosa.
11. Tipping the head forward facilitates passage of the tube into the esophagus instead of the trachea. Tube may stimulate gag reflex. Allows the client to rest, reduces anxiety, and prevents vomiting.
12. Assists in advancing the tube past the oropharynx. The action of swallowing facilitates the insertion process. With each swallow, the tracheal opening is closed to prevent inspiration.
13. Prevents trauma to bronchus or lung.

14. Enables the tube to reach the stomach.
15. Prevents tube displacement.

16. Ensures correct placement. A "whoosh" sound will be heard if the tube is correctly placed. Amount of air varies for pediatric client and if client has had gastric surgery. A pH below 4 indicates the tube is in the stomach; a pH range of 6–7 indicates intestinal sites.

continues

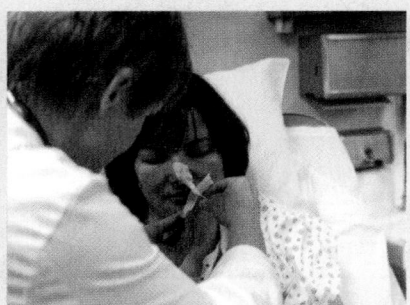

Figure 28-2-3 Secure the tube to the nose.

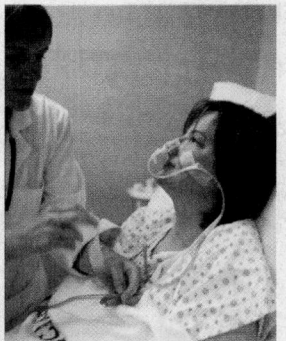

Figure 28-2-4 Tape the tube to the cheek as well, if desired, to provide extra support.

17. Connect the distal end of the tube to suction, draining bag, or adapter according to the purpose of this nursing intervention.
18. Secure the tube with tape, or with rubber band and safety pin, to client's gown.
19. Remove protective equipment, dispose of contaminated materials in proper container, and cleanse hands.
20. Position client comfortably and place the call light in easy reach.

Maintaining a Nasogastric Tube

21. Cleanse hands and apply gloves.
22. Follow the steps in Action 16 to check the proper tubing position before instilling anything per NG tube or at least every 8 hours.
23. Assess for signs that the tube has become blocked, including epigastric pain and vomiting, and/or the inability to pass medications or feedings through the tube.
24. Remember never to irrigate or rotate a tube that has been placed by the health care provider during gastric or esophageal surgery.
25. Provide oral hygiene and assist client to clean nares daily.
26. Remove gloves, dispose of contaminated materials in proper container, and cleanse hands.

EVALUATION

- Client's nutritional status improves, as indicated by increased body weight, physical strength, and mental status.
- Client's nutritional needs are met with the assistance of tube feeding.
- Client maintains a patent airway, as evident by absence of coughing, no shortness of breath, and no aspiration.
- Client does not have diarrhea caused by nasogastric feeding.

17. Establishes an appropriate pathway for intervention.

18. Enhances the level of comfort and secures the tubing system.
19. Implements Standard Precautions.

20. Decreases client's anxiety and provides access to help if needed.

21. Reduces transmission of microorganisms.
22. Prevents complications from dislocation of the tube.
23. Prevents complications from the loss of beneficial effects from the tube.

24. Rotation or irrigation may disturb incisions.

25. Enhances client's comfort and the integrity of skin and nose mucosa.
26. Reduces transmission of microorganisms.

- Mouth mucous membranes remain moist and intact.
- Client maintains a normal fluid volume, as evident by good skin texture, muscle tone, and blood volume.
- Client's stomach decompressed and comfort level increases.
- Skin around the tube remains intact, with no redness or blisters.

continues

DOCUMENTATION

Nurses' Notes

- Type of NG tube inserted, the naris used, how the client tolerated the procedure, and the methods used to verify placement
- Care provided to the client to increase comfort of the NG insertion naris
- Any unusual findings

Intake and Output Record

- Amount of fluid the client drank to aid insertion of the NG tube
- Amount of gastric contents removed for testing
- Amount of gastric suctioning

PROCEDURE 28-3   Performing Venipuncture (Blood Drawing)

OVERVIEW

Obtaining a sample of blood through venipuncture is a commonly used procedure for many diagnostic tests. Blood test results are a source of valuable information to screen for disease, to evaluate the progress of therapy, and to monitor the well-being of the client. The nurse is often required to obtain a variety of specimens. Because some specimens require special handling, it is important to be familiar with the particular test that is ordered.

There are three primary methods of obtaining blood specimens: venipuncture, skin puncture, and arterial stick. Venipuncture is the most common method and involves inserting a large-bore needle into a vein. The nurse attaches either a syringe or a vacutainer tube for the collection of the blood specimen. Skin puncture is the easiest way to obtain a small specimen from the finger, toe, or heel. A lancet is used for the puncture, and a drop of blood is collected through a capillary tube. An arterial stick is the most complicated and requires special assessment skills and techniques.

As with any procedure, it is important to review the employer's policies and procedures as well as the state's nurse practice act.

ASSESSMENT

1. Determine which test(s) is ordered and be familiar with any special conditions associated with the timing of the collection or the handling of the specimen. Many specimens may be collected at very specific times (i.e., before or after administration of a drug, while the client is NPO, or after fasting). Other specimens may require special handling (i.e., ice is used to transport for ammonia level; heparinized collection containers are needed for platelet count; and so on). A blood specimen drawn at the incorrect time or put into an incorrect collection container cannot be used. Test results will be delayed and the client has to be stuck again.

2. Assess the integrity of the veins that may be used in the procedure. Identify any conditions that may contraindicate venipuncture. Avoid veins injured by infiltration or phlebitis or compromised by surgery (i.e., modified radical mastectomy). **Using a damaged vein may cause further injury to the vein. A compromised site may not provide an adequate amount of blood for the specimen and may lead to another venipuncture for the client.** In addition, **drawing samples from sites near IV infusion solutions may alter the composition of the blood sample.**

3. Review the client's medical history to determine if there are any expected complications from the venipuncture. **Clients with a history of abnormal clotting disorders, low platelets, or related disorders (hemophilia) may be at risk for increased bleeding at the site or hematoma formation.**

4. Determine the client's ability to cooperate with the procedure. **Many clients are fearful of needles—especially children—and additional help may be needed. Very young children may need to have the extremity restrained during the procedure.**

5. Review the physician's or qualified practitioner's order. Check for appropriateness of the test as well as the frequency of the test. Critically ill clients may require frequent blood tests and venipuncture. **Combining tests and carefully evaluating frequency may reduce unnecessary blood loss for the client.**

continues

POSSIBLE NURSING DIAGNOSES

*Deficient **K**nowledge* (purpose of blood sample and procedure)
*Risk for **I**nfection*
*Impaired **T**issue Integrity*
***A**nxiety*

PLANNING

Expected Outcomes

1. Venipuncture site will show no evidence of continued bleeding or hematoma.
2. The venipuncture site will show no evidence of signs and symptoms of infection.
3. The blood specimen will be properly acquired and appropriately handled after collection.
4. The client will be able to discuss the purpose of the test and describe the procedure.
5. The client will report minimal anxiety associated with the procedure.

Equipment Needed

- Disposable gloves
- Alcohol swabs
- Rubber tourniquet
- Sterile 2 × 2 gauze pads
- Band-Aid or adhesive tape (precut)
- Appropriate blood collection tubes
- Labels for each collection tube with the appropriate client information included
- Completed laboratory requisition forms
- Needle/equipment disposal container
- Small pillow or folded towel to support the extremity if needed
- Syringe method: sterile needles: 20- to 21-gauge for adults, 23- to 25-gauge butterfly for older adults, 23- to 25-gauge butterfly for children
- Vacutainer method: Vacutainer tube with needle holder; sterile double needles (20- to 21-gauge for adults, 23- to 25-gauge for children)

DELEGATION TIPS

The procedure of performing a venipuncture for the purposes of blood drawing is frequently delegated to properly trained ancillary personnel. Documentation of their competency and skill should be available to the nurse, and periodic reevaluation should occur according to agency and state policy. The ancillary personnel should be reminded to not obtain blood specimens from an extremity above the site of infusing fluids and to report to the nurse any complications or concerns the client might express postprocedure.

IMPLEMENTATION—ACTION/RATIONALE

ACTION

❋ Check client's identification band ❋ Explain procedure before beginning ❋

1. Cleanse hands.
2. Bring equipment to bedside or exam room. Transfer client to the exam room, especially small children.
3. Close curtain or door.
4. Raise or lower bed/table to comfortable working height.
5. Position client's arm; extend arm to form a straight line from shoulder to wrist. Place pillow or towel under upper arm to enhance extension. Client should be in a supine or semi-Fowler's position.
6. Apply disposable gloves.

7. Apply the tourniquet 3 to 4 inches above the venipuncture site. Most often the antecubital fossa site is used. The tourniquet should be able to be removed by pulling the end with a single motion.
8. Check for the distal pulse. If there is no pulse felt, then the tourniquet is applied too tightly and must be reapplied more loosely.

RATIONALE

1. Reduces transmission of microorganisms.
2. Provides an organized approach to the procedure. Keeps their hospital room a "safe haven."
3. Provides privacy.
4. Maintains good body mechanics during the procedure.
5. Helps stabilize the arm. The bed should support the client's body (when possible) in case the client feels faint during the procedure.

6. Reduces the risk of infection to both the client and the nurse (Standard Precautions).
7. Provides improved visibility of the veins as they dilate in response to decreased venous return of blood flow from the extremity to the heart.

8. Impedes arterial flow, preventing venous filling.

continues

9. Have client open and close fist several times, leaving fist clenched before venipuncture.

10. Maintain tourniquet for only 1 to 2 minutes.

11. Identify the best venipuncture site through palpation; the ideal site is a straight prominent vein that feels firm and slightly rebounds when palpated. Palpate potential site.

12. Select the vein for venipuncture. (If the tourniquet has been on too long, release it and let the client rest for 1 to 2 minutes before reapplying the tourniquet.)

13. Prepare to obtain the blood sample. Technique varies depending on equipment used:
    • *Syringe method:* Have syringe with appropriate needle attached.

    • *Vacutainer method:* Attach double-ended needle to vacutainer tube and have the proper blood specimen tube resting inside the vacutainer. Do not puncture the rubber stopper yet.

14. Cleanse the venipuncture site according to agency policy using a circular method at the site and extending 2 inches beyond the site. Allow to dry.

15. Remove the needle cover and warn that client will feel the needlestick.

16. Place the thumb or forefinger of the nondominant hand 1 inch below the site and pull the skin taut.

17. Hold syringe needle or vacutainer at a 15- to 30-degree angle from the skin with the bevel up.

18. Slowly insert needle/vacutainer.

19. Technique varies depending on equipment used:
    • *Syringe method:* Gently pull back on syringe plunger and look for blood return. Obtain desired amount of blood into the syringe.
    • *Vacutainer method:* Hold vacutainer securely and advance specimen tube into needle of holder. Be careful not to advance the needle into the vein. The blood should flow into the collection tube. After the collection tube is full, grasp the vacutainer firmly, remove the tube, and insert additional specimen collection tubes as indicated (Figure 28-3-1).

20. Release tourniquet once blood is flowing into syringe or vacutainer.

9. Increases the venous distension and enhances visibility of the vein.

10. Prolonged time may increase client discomfort and alter some laboratory results (i.e., falsely elevated serum potassium).

11. Straight, intact veins are easier to puncture. A thrombosed vein is rigid, or rolls easily, and is difficult to stick.

12. Increases client comfort and ensures accurate laboratory results.

13.

    • A needle with a very small bore can damage the red cells as the blood is drawn and lead to inaccurate test results.
    • The long end of the needle is used to puncture the vein, and the short end enters the blood tube.

14. Cleans the skin surface of bacteria that may cause infection at the site. Allowing the alcohol to dry reduces stinging. Povidone-iodine must dry to be effective.

15. Clients will be better able to control their reaction if they know what to expect.

16. Helps stabilize the vein during insertion.

17. This angle reduces the chance of penetrating through the vein during insertion. The needle causes less trauma to the skin and vein when the bevel is up during insertion.

18. Prevents puncture through the other side of the vein.

19.

    • If blood does not appear, the needle is not in the vein.

    • Pushing the needle through the stopper breaks the vacuum and causes the flow of blood into the collection tube. Failure of blood to appear in the collection tube indicates the vacuum in the tube has been lost or the needle is not in the vein.

20. Prevents hemolysis.

Figure 28-3-1 Allow the tube to fill with blood. When it is full, remove the tube and insert additional tubes if needed.

continues

21. Apply 2 × 2 gauze over the puncture site without applying pressure and quickly withdraw the needle from the vein.

22. Immediately apply pressure over the venipuncture site with the gauze for 2 to 3 minutes or until the bleeding has stopped. Tape the gauze dressing over the site (or apply the Band-Aid).

23. Syringe method:

   • Using one hand, insert the syringe needle into the appropriate collection tube and allow vacuum to fill. You may also remove the stopper from each vacutainer collection tube, remove the needle from the syringe, fill the tube, and replace the stopper.

24. If any of the blood tubes contain additives, gently rotate back and forth 8 to 10 times.

25. Inspect the client's puncture site for bleeding. Reapply clean gauze and tape if necessary.

26. Assist client into a comfortable position. Return bed to low position with side rails up if appropriate.

27. Check tubes for any external blood and decontaminate with alcohol as appropriate.

28. Check tubes for proper labeling. Place tubes into appropriate bags/containers for transport to the laboratory.

29. Dispose of needles, syringes, and soiled equipment into proper container.

30. Remove and dispose of gloves.

31. Cleanse hands.

32. Send specimens to the laboratory.

21. Helps prevent the skin from pulling with the needle removal.

22. Direct pressure stops the bleeding and minimizes formation of a hematoma. You may avoid using tape or a Band-Aid if after applying pressure no bleeding is present. Many clients are sensitive to tape, and its removal can be painful.

23. Using a one-handed method to fill the syringe helps reduce the chance of needlestick injury.
   • This alternative method allows you to control the speed and amount of fill in the collection tubes.

24. Ensures that the additive is properly mixed throughout the specimen.

25. Keeps site clean and dry.

26. Provides comfort and safety for the client.

27. Prevents contamination to other equipment and personnel.

28. Ensure the specimens are properly identified. Follows Standard Precautions.

29. Prevents spread of disease and needlestick injury.

30. Reduces transmission of microorganisms.

31. Reduces transmission of microorganisms.

32. Facilitates timely handling of specimens and accurate results.

EVALUATION

• Venipuncture site shows no evidence of continued bleeding or hematoma.
• Venipuncture site shows no signs or symptoms of infection.
• The blood specimen is properly acquired and appropriately handled after collection.
• The client is able to discuss the purpose of the test and describe the procedure.
• The client reports minimal anxiety associated with the procedure.

DOCUMENTATION

Nurses' Notes

• Date and time of the venipuncture, the site used for the procedure, any complications, the tests to be run, and the disposition of the specimens
• Client's reaction to the procedure and the condition in which the client was left (i.e., bed lowered with side rails up)

PROCEDURE 28-4

Preparing an IV Solution and Starting an IV

OVERVIEW

An intravenous solution is a method of replacing fluid lost, or correcting an electrolyte imbalance. Clients who are acutely ill, are NPO after surgery, or have severe burns are examples of those who require IV therapy.

The solution in an IV bag is ordered by the health care provider according to the client's needs and is changed at least every 24 hours, or per the institution's policy, to decrease the risk of infection. Tubing is used to connect the solution in the IV bag with the client's IV catheter or needle. Use needleless systems if available. OSHA requires safe devices.

Performing venipuncture in order to establish venous access is a priority for clients with fluid and electrolyte disturbances, clients who are critically ill, clients who are NPO after surgery, or clients who for other reasons are not able to take fluids or food by mouth. Venous access can be used for infusions of IV fluids, emergency medications, parenteral nutrition, blood products, and routine IV medications.

There are a variety of IV needles and catheters. They vary in gauge from small bore to large bore. A 20- to 22-gauge flexible catheter is used for adults, and a 22- to 24-gauge catheter is used for pediatric clients. If large volumes of fluid or blood products are anticipated to be given, a larger bore (18- or 19-gauge) is recommended.

A commonly used angiocatheter has an over-the-needle catheter (ONC) made of plastic, Teflon, or other materials. These flexible catheters have a metal stylet that is used to pierce the skin and vein and a plastic catheter that is threaded into the vein and attached to the IV tubing after the stylet has been removed.

The other type of IV needle is a straight steel needle that is inserted into the vein and secured after being attached to an IV tubing. With an increased emphasis on safety, many health care facilities use a safety-shielded intravenous catheter or retractable needle system when placing a peripheral IV line. This consists of a traditional metal stylet used for the skin puncture covered by the plastic or Teflon angiocatheter. Once the IV line is successfully placed, the person initiating the IV pushes a button and the stylet retracts completely into a protective casing, thereby reducing the risk of needlestick injury.

The Centers for Disease Control and Prevention (CDC) guidelines must be followed to decrease the risk of infection for the client by changing the IV solution every 24 hours, changing the IV site and catheter every 48 to 72 hours, and changing the IV tubing every 48 hours.

ASSESSMENT

1. Check the health care provider's order for the IV solution to be infused and rate of flow **to determine the optimal needle size and type to use and ensure accurate administration.**
2. Review information regarding the solution and insertion of the IV and nursing implications **in order to insert the catheter and administer the solution safely.**
3. Know the agency's policy regarding who may start an IV **because many agencies require that nurses have special training before they can perform this procedure.**
4. Check all additives in the solution and other medications **so that there will be no incompatibilities of additives with the solution.**
5. Assess the client's veins **to optimize planning of the IV site.**
6. Check the client's fluid, electrolyte, and nutritional status **to provide baseline data for comparison with the client's response to IV therapy.**
7. Assess the client's understanding of the purpose of the procedure **so that client teaching can be used to decrease anxiety.**

POSSIBLE NURSING DIAGNOSES

Deficient **K**nowledge (need for IV)
Risk for **I**nfection
Excess **F**luid Volume
Deficient **F**luid Volume
Impaired **S**kin Integrity

PLANNING

Expected Outcomes

1. The appropriate fluids at the ordered dosages will be available for IV infusion.
2. The IV infusion will be sterile, without precipitate or contamination.
3. The IV will be inserted into the vein without complications and will remain patent.
4. Fluid and electrolyte balance will be restored.
5. Nutrition will be restored or maintained.
6. The IV site will remain free of swelling and inflammation.

continues

Equipment Needed

- Appropriate safety needle or catheter for venipuncture
- Tourniquet
- Povidone-iodine swabs (3) or chlorhexidine alcohol (chloroprep)
- Alcohol swab sticks (3) (not needed if using chlorhexidine alcohol)
- Disposable gloves
- Arm board, if needed
- Towel or absorbent drape
- Povidone-iodine ointment (not used in all institutions)
- Gauze dressing
- Tape
- Scissors
- IV solution and tubing
- Medication Administration Record (MAR)
- IV flow sheet

DELEGATION TIPS

Initiating IV therapy via venipuncture involves assessment and the use of medical asepsis. It is an invasive procedure not delegated by the nurse unless other licensed personnel have been trained and certified to perform the procedure. Ancillary personnel who will be caring for the client need to be instructed to handle the extremity with the IV gently and to report any complaints of pain or swelling in the affected extremity to the nurse.

IMPLEMENTATION—ACTION/RATIONALE

ACTION

1. Check health care provider's order for an IV and the solution.
2. Cleanse hands. Apply gloves if required by institutional policy.
3. Prepare solution bag by removing protective cover from bag.
4. Inspect the bag for leaks, tears, or cracks. Inspect the fluid for clarity, particulate matter, and color. Check expiration date.
5. Prepare a label for the IV bag:
   - On the label, note date, time, and your initials.
   - Attach the label to the bag. Keep in mind the bag will be inverted when it is hanging. Make sure the label can be read when the IV is hanging.
6. Remove gloves and cleanse hands.
7. Prepare an IV time tape for the IV bag:
   - On the time tape, note the rate at which the solution is to infuse (Procedure 28-5).
   - Mark the approximate infusion intervals.

   - Attach the time tape to the bag. Keep in mind the bag will be inverted when it is hanging. Make sure the time tape can be read when the IV is hanging.
8. Make sure the clamp on the tubing is closed. Grasp the port of the IV bag with your nondominant hand, remove the plastic tab covering the port (Figure 28-4-1), and insert the full length of the spike into the bag's port (Figure 28-4-2).
9. Compress drip chamber to fill halfway.

10. Loosen protective cap from the end of the IV tubing, open roller clamp, and flush tubing with solution (Figure 28-4-3 A and B).

RATIONALE

1. Ensures accurate administration of the solution.
2. Reduces transmission of microorganisms.
3. Allows for access to the solution container.
4. Prevents infusing contaminated or outdated solution.

5.
   - Communicates when the bag was opened.
   - Labeling the bag upside-down makes identification easier when the bag is hanging.

6. Reduces transmission of microorganisms.
7.
   - Communicates how long before the next IV should be hung.
   - Gives a rough estimate of the accuracy of the infusion rate.
   - Placing the time tape on the bag upside-down makes identification easier when the bag is hanging.
8. Promotes rapid flow of solution through new tubing without air bubbles.

9. Allows the chamber to provide a clear measurement of drip rate when the IV is flowing.
10. Removes air from tubing.

continues

Figure 28-4-1   Open the IV plastic bag and pull down the plastic tab covering the port with one hand while pinching the port with the other hand.

Figure 28-4-2   Remove the cap from the spike and spike the IV port.

A

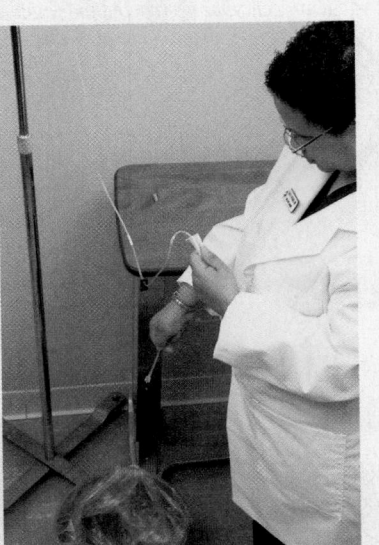

B

Figure 28-4-3 Priming the IV tubing. Open the roller clamp on the tubing to allow the fluid to enter the tube and expel the air.

11. Close roller clamp and replace cap protector.
12. Take prepared fluid and needed equipment to bedside.
13. Check client's identification band and explain procedure.
14. Cleanse hands and put on mask and gown if needed.
15. Inspect potential veins to be used:
    • Place a tourniquet around the upper arm close to the axilla.
    • Examine the veins as they dilate.
    • Palpate the vein to test for firmness (Figure 28-4-4).
    • Release the tourniquet.
16. Select vein for venipuncture:
    • Use most distal part of the vein first.

    • Avoid bony prominences.
    • Avoid client's wrist or hand.
    • Avoid client's dominant hand and arm.
    • Avoid an extremity with decreased sensation.
    • Avoid an area of skin affected by a rash or infection.

11. Prevents fluid from leaking and maintains sterility.
12. Ensures smooth procedure without accidents or contamination.
13. Ensures correct client and decreases anxiety.
14. Reduces transmission of microorganisms.
15. Promotes ease of placement of catheter.
    • Distends vein to allow visual and tactile examination.

    • Evaluates viability of the veins.
    • Determines best site for venipuncture and IV placement.
    • Prevents engorgement of vein.
16.
    • If the vein is later damaged, the proximal part can be used.
    • Increases client comfort.
    • Bending increases risk of infiltration or phlebitis.
    • Allows freedom of movement.
    • Promotes earlier detection of infiltration.
    • Decreases risk of infection.

continues

Figure 28-4-4 Inspect the site for potential veins to use, and palpate to further locate a vein and test for firmness.

Figure 28-4-5 After scrubbing the insertion site with alcohol and povidone-iodine, allow it to dry. *Note:* The tourniquet is released while the site is drying.

17. Select safety shield or angiocatheter that is appropriate for ordered IV fluid. Select the correct size (gauge and length) of catheter.
18. Prepare supplies:
    • Place towel or drape on table for supplies.
    • Place supplies on towel.
    • Open needle adapter end of IV tubing set.
19. Shave hair on skin at site if necessary.

20. Ask client to rest arm in a dependent position, if possible.
21. Put on disposable gloves.
22. Prepare insertion site (Figure 28-4-5):
    • Place absorbent drape under the arm.
    • Scrub the insertion site with 3 alcohol swabs then 3 povidone-iodine swabs.
    • Follow institution protocol. Some facilities use chlorhexidine alcohol instead of iodine.
    • Use separate swab and start in the middle of the site and work outward.
    • Allow the antiseptic solution to air dry.

23. Apply tourniquet 5 to 6 inches above the insertion site.
    • Secure it tightly enough to occlude venous flow, not arterial flow.
    • Check presence of distal pulse.
24. Perform the venipuncture:
    • Anchor the vein by placing thumb over vein and stretching the skin against the direction of insertion 2 to 3 inches distal to the site.
    • Insert the stylet needle at a 20- to 30-degree angle with the bevel up (Figure 28-4-6).
    • Watch for a quick blood return through the flash-back chamber of the ONC.
    • Verify needle placement in a vein, not artery.

    • Advance ONC $^1/_4$ inch into the vein while it is parallel to the skin.
    • Loosen stylet and advance catheter into vein until hub rests at venipuncture site (Figure 28-4-7).

17. Particular intravenous therapies require specific sizes of intravenous access. Age and quality or location of veins can affect choice of size.
18. Provides a clean working surface for an efficiently performed procedure.

19. Ensures adherence of dressing and a less painful removal. Avoid shaving because it causes small abrasions that increase the risk of infection.
20. Allows better venous dilation and visibility.
21. Reduces transmission of microorganisms.
22.
    • Reduces transmission of microorganisms.
    • Alcohol removes fat on the skin and vigorous scrubbing in circular motion with povidone-iodine removes bacteria. Prevents bacteria from being reintroduced to the site.

    • Povidone-iodine or chlorhexidine alcohol must be dry to be effective.
23. Allows the vein to engorge for easier venipuncture.
    • Decreased arterial flow prevents venous filling.

    • Ensures arterial flow is present.
24.
    • Stabilizes the vein for ease of venipuncture.

    • Prevents puncture of posterior wall of vein.

    • Venous pressure from tourniquet causes backflow of blood into catheter or tubing.
    • Some veins are close to an artery. Arterial blood is bright red and pulses.
    • Ensures the catheter is in the vein.

    • Ensures proper placement of the catheter.

continues

Figure 28-4-6 Insert the needle with the beveled side up. Keep the angle low, 20 to 30°.

Figure 28-4-7 Loosen the stylet and advance the catheter into the vein until the hub rests on the skin at the venipuncture site.

- Do not reinsert stylet.

- Hold thumb over vein above catheter tip.

- Release the tourniquet.
25. Attach IV tubing to ONC.
    - Stabilize the catheter with one hand.
    - Remove the stylet from ONC or if using a safety catheter, push the button on the protective casing and stylet will fully retract into the casing.
    - Quickly release pressure over vein and quickly connect needle adapter of IV set to hub of ONC.
    - Begin infusion at slow rate to keep vein open.
26. Secure catheter in place:
    - Place tape over the hub of the catheter.
    - Place transparent dressing over the site and secure.

    - Secure tubing in loop fashion with tape.
27. Regulate flow or, if applicable, attach tubing to infusion device or rate controller if used. Turn on pump and set flow rate (see Procedure 28-5, Setting the IV Flow Rate).
28. Remove gloves and dispose with all used materials.
29. Place label with date and time of insertion and size and gauge of catheter on the dressing. Follow protocol for scheduled dressing change.
30. Cleanse hands.

- Prevents the catheter from being punctured by the stylet.
- Prevents blood from leaking out of vein until IV tubing is connected.
- Reestablishes venous blood flow.
25.
- Maintains catheter placement.
- Provides entry portal for IV fluids. Reduces risk of inadvertent needlestick injury.

- Reduces blood loss.

- Prompt initiation of infusion maintains patency of IV.
26.
- Ensures catheter's safe position.
- Controls bleeding and prevents infection. Allows visualization of site through transparent dressing.
- Prevents dislodgement of IV if tubing is pulled.
27. Sets flow rate at prescribed rate.

28. Reduces transmission of microorganisms.
29. Provides information to schedule next dressing change.

30. Reduces transmission of microorganisms.

EVALUATION

- The appropriate fluids at the ordered dosages were available for IV infusion.
- The IV infusion was sterile, without precipitate or contamination.
- The IV was inserted into the vein without complications and remains patent.
- Fluid and electrolyte balance were restored.
- Nutrition was restored or maintained.
- The IV site remains free of swelling and inflammation.

DOCUMENTATION

Nurses' Notes
- Date and time the IV was inserted
- Type and gauge of catheter
- Date of dressing placement
- Fluid to be infused or if a saline or heparin lock
- Client's reaction to the procedure

PROCEDURE 28-5   Setting the IV Flow Rate

OVERVIEW

Setting the rate of an IV infusion according to the health care provider's order is a nursing responsibility. The flow rate can be controlled by the roller clamp on the IV tubing or by an infusion pump. It is important for the rate to be accurate to prevent complications in fluid balance. A rate that is too fast can result in fluid overload, which is potentially serious in clients with cardiovascular, renal, or neurologic impairment as well as in very young or very old clients. If an infusion is set too slow, the vein may clot or the more serious complication of circulatory collapse in a dehydrated or severely injured client who required large volumes of fluid could develop.

Sudden changes in the rate of infusion may be accidental or positional. A confused client may loosen the roller clamp or get tangled in the IV tubing. A client who gets up to walk may experience an increase in the IV rate. Changes in flow rate can occur with tubing and a roller clamp or infusion devices.

An infusion pump is an electronic device used to deliver a prescribed amount of fluid over a period of time in milliliters per hour. Pumps may have a drop sensor that counts each drop of fluid and sounds an alarm if the flow rate differs from what is programmed. An alarm sounds when the bag is empty or when pressure increases in the system, as in the case of an infiltrated IV.

An IV controller delivers fluid by gravity, so the bag must be at least 36 inches above the IV site. The number of drops per minute as well as the IV tubing size and viscosity of the fluid are necessary to calculate the actual volume delivered per hour. The controller cannot force fluid into the vein like a pump, so infiltrations are detected more quickly; however, the sensitivity of the pump system increases the number of alarms caused by client movement.

A volume-control device is a calibrated chamber placed between the IV bag and the drip chamber so that a small volume of IV fluid (<200 mL) can flow into the chamber and then infuse without danger that the whole bag will be infused into the client.

ASSESSMENT

1. Check the health care provider's order for the IV to be infused and rate of flow **to ensure accurate administration.**
2. Review information regarding the solution and nursing implications **in order to administer the solution safely.**
3. Assess the patency of the IV **to ensure that the solution will enter the vein and not the surrounding tissue.**
4. Assess the skin at the IV site **so that the solution will not be administered into an inflamed or edematous site, which could cause injury to the tissue.**
5. Assess the client's understanding of the purpose of the IV infusion **so that client teaching can be tailored to his needs.**

POSSIBLE NURSING DIAGNOSES

Excess Fluid Volume
Risk for Deficient Fluid Volume
Deficient Knowledge (IV infusion)

PLANNING

Expected Outcomes

1. The fluid will be infused into the vein without complications.
2. The IV catheter will remain patent.
3. The fluid and electrolyte balance will return to normal.
4. The client will be able to discuss the purpose of the IV therapy.

Equipment Needed

- Watch with a second hand
- IV solution in a bag
- IV tubing
- IV infusion pump (optional)
- Volume control device (optional)
- Paper and pencil

DELEGATION TIPS

Setting the rate of the IV after establishing the infusion is the responsibility of the nurse. This procedure is not delegated unless other licensed personnel have been trained and certified to perform the procedure. Ancillary personnel may be instructed to report an infusion that is dripping too fast or an IV bag that is almost empty. It is the nurse's responsibility to monitor the infusion, but ancillary personnel may also be instructed to report observations such as swelling, leaking, or client concerns about pain, numbness, or tingling at the site or in the extremity used for the infusion.

continues

IMPLEMENTATION—ACTION/RATIONALE

ACTION

RATIONALE

* Check client's identification band * Explain procedure before beginning *

1. Check health care provider's order for the IV solution and rate of infusion.
2. Cleanse hands.
3. Prepare to set flow rate:
   • Have paper and pencil ready to calculate flow rate.

   • Review calibration in drops per milliliter (gtt/mL) of each infusion set.

4. Determine hourly rate by dividing total volume by total hours.
   Example 1:
   The order reads 1000 mL D_5W with 20 mEq KCl over 8 hours:
   $$\frac{1000\ mL}{8\ hr} = 125\ mL/hr$$
   Example 2:
   Three liters are ordered for 24 hours:
   $$\frac{3000\ mL}{24\ hr} = 125\ mL/hr$$

5. Mark a length of tape placed on the IV bag with the hourly time periods according to the rate.
6. Calculate the minute rate based on the drop factor of the infusion set:
   $$\frac{mL/hr}{60\ min} = mL/min$$
   $$Drop\ factor \times mL/min = gtt/min$$
   $$\frac{mL\ hr \times drop\ factor}{60\ min} = gtt/min$$
   $$\frac{hourly\ rate \times drop\ factor}{infusion\ time\ in\ minutes} = ggt/min$$

   • Microdrip example:
   $$\frac{125\ mL \times 60\ gtt/mL}{60\ min} = \frac{7500\ gtt}{60\ min} = 125\ gtt/min$$

   • Macrodrip example:
   $$\frac{125\ mL \times 15\ gtt/mL}{60\ min} = 31\ gtt/min$$

7. Set flow rate:
   • *For regular tubing* without a device: Count drops in drip chamber for 1 minute while watching second hand of watch and adjust the roller clamp as necessary (Figure 28-5-1).
   • *For an infusion pump:* Insert the tubing into the flow control chamber, select the desired rate (generally calibrated in cc's per minute), open the roller clamp, and push start button.

1. Ensures accurate administration of the solution.
2. Reduces transmission of microorganisms.
3.
   • A nurse unfamiliar with IV fluid rates should calculate the rate at first.
   • Drops per milliliter vary with manufacturer and tubing type. Macrodrip tubing varies from 10 to 15 gtt/mL. Microdrip tubing generally delivers 60 gtt/mL.
4. Provides a prescribed hourly rate.

5. Provides a visual check of the fluid infused to be sure the rate is correct.
6. Formulas calculate how many drops per minute to be infused.

7.
   • Ensures that infusion is administered as ordered.

   • Pumps the solution through the tubing at the rate set.

continues

Figure 28-5-1 Count the drips in the drip chamber for 1 minute.

Figure 28-5-2 The volume-control device is placed between the IV bag and the client. It is filled with 1 to 2 hours worth of IV fluid.

- *For a controller:* Place IV bag 36 inches above the IV site, select the desired drops per minute, open the roller clamp, and count drops for 1 minute to verify rate.
- *For volume-control device:* Place device between IV bag and insertion spike of IV tubing, fill with 1 to 2 hours amount of IV fluid, and count drops for 1 minute (Figure 28-5-2).

8. Monitor infusion rate and IV site for infiltration.
9. Assess infusion when alarm sounds.

10. Cleanse hands.

- The controller works by gravity.

- The amount of fluid in the volume control chamber depends on the amount of fluid to be infused per hour:
    50 cc/hour = 50 to 100 cc of fluid
    100 cc/hour = 100 to 200 cc of fluid

8. Infusion devices may fail.
9. Sounds when a drip has not been sensed. It can be caused by an empty IV bag, a kink in the tubing, a clotted needle, an infiltrated IV, or another malfunction of the device.
10. Reduces transmission of microorganisms.

EVALUATION

- The fluid is infusing into the vein without complications.
- The IV catheter remains patent.
- The fluid and electrolyte balance returned to normal.
- The client is able to discuss the purpose of IV therapy.

DOCUMENTATION

Flow Sheet

- Date and time IV solution was started
- Rate of infusion in drops per minute and milliliters per hour
- Any changes in the IV rate

Nurses' Notes

- Client's response to the IV therapy
- Changes in condition caused by a complication in the IV infusion

PROCEDURE 28-6 Administering Medications via IV Piggyback

OVERVIEW

A medication is given intravenously when a rapid response to a drug is required or when several medications need to be given IV on a regular schedule. This is best accomplished by using an existing IV to be the basic infusion and adding medications by "piggyback" when they are ordered. It also carries the highest risk of side effects because of the immediate response of the medication and the inability to correct a medication administration error.

The drug is diluted and mixed with a small volume (50 to 100 mL) of compatible solution and then joined to the primary IV line for infusion. The bag is connected to the upper Y-port of the primary infusion line and hung higher than the primary IV bag, thus the name piggyback. The piggyback infusion works because of the backflow valve. When the piggyback infusion starts flowing, the valve stops the flow of the primary infusion. After the piggyback infusion is complete and the solution within the tubing falls below the level of the primary infusion drip chamber, the valve opens and the primary infusion flows.

It is important to note that some medications can be irritating to the lining of blood vessels. Other medications, when injected into a vein that is beginning to infiltrate, will injure the tissue to such an extent that tissue could slough, become abscessed, or become necrotic. No IV medication should be administered through IV sites that are suspected to be inflamed or infiltrated. Use needleless systems if available. Safety needles and syringes are required by OSHA standards.

ASSESSMENT

1. Check the health care provider's order or the medication administration record (MAR) for the medication, dosage, and time and route of administration **to ensure accurate administration.**
2. Review information regarding the drug, including action, purpose, side effects, normal dose, peak onset, and nursing implications, **in order to administer the drug safely.**
3. Determine additives in the solution of an existing IV line **so that the medication will be compatible with the solution.**
4. Assess the placement of the IV catheter in the vein **to ensure that the medication will enter the vein and not the surrounding tissue.**
5. Assess the skin at the IV site **so that the medication will not be administered into an inflamed or edematous site, which could cause injury to the tissue.**
6. Check the client's drug allergy history **because an allergic reaction could occur rapidly and be fatal.**
7. Assess the client's understanding of the purpose of the medication **so that client teaching can be tailored to needs.**
8. Assess the compatibility of the piggyback IV medication with the primary IV solution **to avoid an adverse reaction such as the formation of precipitate in the IV tubing.**

POSSIBLE NURSING DIAGNOSES

*Risk for **I**nfection*
*Risk for **I**njury*
*Impaired **S**kin Integrity*
*Deficient **K**nowledge* (medication)

PLANNING

Expected Outcomes

1. The drug is infused into the vein without complications.
2. The IV site remains free of swelling and inflammation.
3. The client will be able to discuss the purpose of the drug.

Equipment Needed

- Disposable gloves
- Medication prepared in a labeled infusion bag
- Short microdrip or macrodrip tubing set for piggyback (needleless system preferred)
- Safety sterile needles, 21- or 23-gauge, if needleless system not available
- Antiseptic swab
- Adhesive tape
- IV pole
- Medication administration record (MAR)

DELEGATION TIPS

The skill of medication administration is not delegated to ancillary personnel in acute care settings. This may vary in state or federal institutions. Ancillary personnel are generally informed about the medications the client is receiving if adverse effects are anticipated or are being monitored.

continues

IMPLEMENTATION—ACTION/RATIONALE

ACTION

● Check client's identification band ● Explain procedure before beginning ●

1. Check health care provider's order.
2. Cleanse hands. *Gloves are not necessary if you are adding fluids to an existing infusion line.*
3. Prepare medication bag:
   • Close clamp on tubing of infusion set.
   • Spike medication bag with infusion tubing.

   • Open clamp.
   • Allow tubing to be filled with solution to evacuate air from tubing.
4. Hang piggyback medication bag above level of primary IV bag. Use extender found in the piggyback tubing package to lower the primary bag (Figure 28-6-1).
5. Connect piggyback tubing to primary tubing at Y-port:
   • For needleless system, remove cap on port and connect tubing (Figure 28-6-2).
   • If a needle is used, clean port with antiseptic swab and insert small-gauge needle into center of port.
   • Secure tubing with adhesive tape.

RATIONALE

1. Ensures accurate administration of medication.
2. Reduces transmission of microorganisms.

3.
   • Prevents leakage of solution.
   • Provides a method of infusing the medication into the system.
   • Allows the solution to fill the tubing.
   • Prevents air embolus.

4. Relationship between height of the bags affects the flow rate to the client.

5. Ensures medication in piggyback bag is infused.
   • A needleless system is preferred to prevent accidental needlesticks.
   • A small-gauge needle does less damage to the rubber stopper on the port.
   • Prevents accidental removal of tubing.

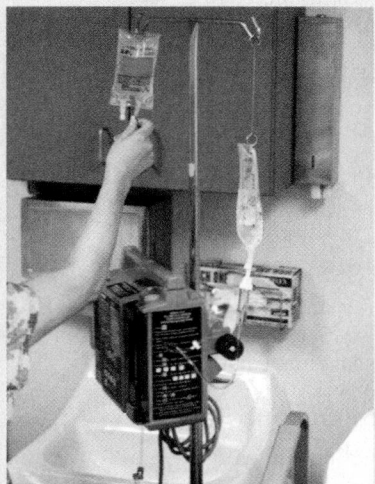

Figure 28-6-1   Hang the piggyback bag higher than the primary IV bag.

Figure 28-6-2   Connect the needleless system tubing.

6. Administer the medication:
   • Check the prescribed length of time for the infusion.

   • Regulate flow rate of piggyback by adjusting regulator clamp (Figure 28-6-3).
   • Observe whether backflow valve on piggyback has stopped flow of primary infusion during drug administration (Figure 28-6-4).

6.
   • Each medication has a recommended rate for IV piggyback administration.
   • Medication infuses through primary line.

   • Prevents backup of medication into primary infusion line.

continues

Figure 28-6-3   Regulate the flow rate of the piggy-back by adjusting the regulator clamp.

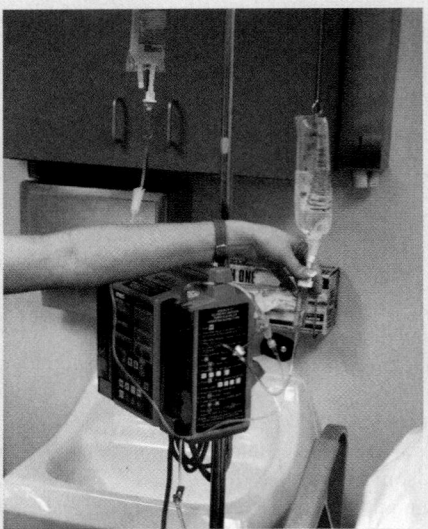

Figure 28-6-4   Double-check that the primary infusion has stopped flowing.

7. Check primary infusion line when medication is finished:
   • Regulate primary infusion rate.
   • Leave secondary bag and tubing in place for next drug administration.
8. Dispose of all used materials and place needles in needle biohazard sharps container.
9. Cleanse hands.

7.

   • Reestablishes primary infusion.
   • Reduces risk for entry of microorganisms by repeated changes of tubing.
8. Reduces transmission of microorganisms.
9. Reduces transmission of microorganisms.

EVALUATION

• The drug was infused into the vein without complications.
• The IV site remained free of swelling and inflammation.
• The client was able to discuss the purpose of the drug.

DOCUMENTATION

Medication Administration Record

• Date, time, dose, and route of medication

Flow Sheet

• Date, time, and volume of fluid infused IV piggyback

Nurses' Notes

• Client's response to the medication
• Any serious side effects and report them to the health care provider immediately

Intake and Output Record

• Amount of fluid infused

PROCEDURE 28-7

Assessing and Maintaining an IV Insertion Site

OVERVIEW

Assessing an established IV site requires knowledge about the length of time since the insertion, the condition of the dressing, and the site itself. The site should be without redness, swelling, pain, or discharge. When palpating the vein, it should have the characteristics of a healthy vein without signs of infection or phlebitis. Knowledge of both the IV solution and medications to be given and their potential side effects on the veins should be included in the assessment. Intravenous solutions with electrolytes and medications can have irritant properties that would require more frequent IV monitoring.

ASSESSMENT

1. Review the order for IV therapy: Identify potential side effects from medication actions, and fluid rate. Consult drug reference books or pharmacists for information. **Decreases the risk of medication errors.**
2. Identify potential risk factors for your client's condition that might indicate fluid and electrolyte imbalances. **Allows targeted assessment and monitoring.**
3. Assess for dehydration: sunken eyes, dry skin, mucous membranes, flattened neck veins, vital sign changes, inelastic skin turgor, decreased urine output, behavior changes, and confusion. **Allows intervention to increase fluids and reduce dehydration.**
4. Assess for fluid overload: periorbital edema, distended neck veins, auscultation of crackles or wheezes in lungs, changes in vital signs, and level of consciousness. **Allows intervention to decrease fluids.**
5. Determine the client's risk for developing complications from IV therapy: very young or very old, heart or renal failure. **Allows the procedure to be modified if needed and promotes targeted assessment to look for signs of risk-related problems.**
6. Observe IV site for complications, that is, signs of infection, phlebitis, or infiltration: redness, swelling, pallor, or warmth at the IV site and surrounding tissue, and bleeding or drainage. **Allows interventions to reduce further damage.**
7. Observe IV site for patency by briefly compressing the IV cannulated vein above the site. Note slowing or momentary cessation of IV rate with a positive blood return. **Provides ongoing assessment of current patency status. Allows early detection of changes.**

8. Assess the client's knowledge regarding the need for the IV therapy. **Allows for teaching, including information and education regarding medications, fluid needs, and signs of IV site irritation or phlebitis.**

POSSIBLE NURSING DIAGNOSES

Impaired **T**issue Integrity
Risk for Impaired **S**kin Integrity
Risk for **I**nfection
Excess **F**luid Volume
Deficient **F**luid Volume

PLANNING

Expected Outcomes

1. The client will have a patent IV, without signs of infection or inflammation.
2. The client's fluid and electrolyte imbalance will return to normal and will be maintained.
3. The client will be able to report signs of inflammation or infiltration.
4. The client's IV rate will be administered and maintained per order.
5. The client's IV dressing will remain intact, clean, and dry.

Equipment Needed

- Clean gloves
- Gauze dressing
- Tape

DELEGATION TIPS

Assessing and maintaining the IV after establishing the infusion is the responsibility of the nurse. This procedure is not delegated unless other licensed personnel have been trained and certified to perform the procedure. Ancillary personnel may be instructed to report an infusion that is dripping too fast or an IV bag that is almost empty. It is the nurse's responsibility to monitor the infusion, but ancillary personnel may also be instructed to report any observations, such as swelling, leaking, client concerns about pain, numbness, or tingling at the site or in the extremity used for the infusion. Ancillary personnel may also be involved in monitoring the client's daily weight, if ordered, along with intake and output. Ancillary personnel should be instructed not to obtain vital signs on an extremity with solutions infusing.

continues

IMPLEMENTATION—ACTION/RATIONALE

ACTION

* Check client's identification band * Explain procedure before beginning *

1. Review health care provider's order for IV therapy.
2. Review client's history for medical conditions or allergies.
3. Review client's IV site record and intake and output record.
4. Cleanse hands.
5. Obtain client's vital signs.
6. Check IV fluid for correct fluid, additives, rate, and volume at the beginning of your shift (Figure 28-7-1).
7. Check IV tubing for tight connections every 4 hours.
8. Check gauze IV dressing hourly to be sure it is dry and intact (Figure 28-7-2).
9. If the gauze is not dry and intact, remove the dressing and observe site for redness, swelling, or drainage.
10. Replace gauze dressing if site is okay.
11. If an occlusive dressing is used, do not remove the dressing when assessing the site.
12. Observe vein track for redness, swelling, warmth, or pain hourly.
13. Cleanse hands.

RATIONALE

1. Ensures accuracy in the administration of IV therapy.
2. Decreases risk of fluid overload and allergic reactions.
3. Assesses for potential problems with fragile IV sites and fluid balance.
4. Decreases transmission of microorganisms.
5. Assesses for changes in cardiovascular system.
6. Ensures client is receiving correct therapy.

7. Ensures that no fluid leaks from tubing and connections.
8. Ensures there is no sign of infiltration or infection at IV insertion site.
9. Ensures there is no sign of inflammation or infection at IV site.
10. Protects IV insertion site.
11. Ensures there is no sign of inflammation or infection at IV site.
12. These are early signs of phlebitis or infiltration.

13. Decreases transmission of microorganisms.

Figure 28-7-1   Check the IV fluid rate, volume, tubing, and additives at the beginning of the shift.

Figure 28-7-2   Check the IV dressing site every hour.

EVALUATION

- IV site observed on an hourly basis to avoid complications of phlebitis and infiltration.
- Client reported no signs or symptoms of redness, swelling, and pain.

DOCUMENTATION

Flow Sheet

- Name of IV solution with additives
- Hourly rate of fluids
- IV site condition
- Time checked
- Initials/signature of nurse

PROCEDURE 28-8   Removing Skin Sutures and Staples

OVERVIEW

Sutures and staples are a surgical means of closing a wound by sewing, wiring, or stapling the edges of the wound together. Most wounds are sutured in layers to maintain alignment of the tissues and reduce scarring. Sutures are generally removed 7 to 10 days after surgery, depending on where the wound is located and how well it is healing. Suture removal requires a health care provider's orders. Timing is important because sutures left in too long can increase the risk of infection and irritation from a foreign substance.

Sutures placed deep within the tissue layers are made of absorbable materials. Surface sutures are made of wire, nylon, or cotton. Continuous sutures are made with one thread, tied at the beginning and end of the suture line. Interrupted sutures are tied individually. Staples are used for large incision areas where the risk of dehiscence is greater, such as in sterneotomies, in clients with increased adipose tissue, abdominal areas, and wounds that fail to heal or adhere.

ASSESSMENT

1. Assess the wound **to determine whether the edges are approximate and healing.** In deep wounds, palpate around the suture site for edema or any evidence of failure of tissue to adhere below the skin's surface.
2. Assess **for any signs of infection,** such as increased warmth, redness, exudate or drainage, and pain.
3. Assess for any conditions **that impede the healing process,** such as age, immunosuppression, diabetes, obesity, smoking, radiation, poor cellular nutrition, infection, and deep wounds.

POSSIBLE NURSING DIAGNOSES

*Impaired **S**kin Integrity*
*Risk for **I**nfection*
*Acute **P**ain*
*Deficient **K**nowledge* (fear of dehiscence)

PLANNING

Expected Outcomes

1. The wound is healing, with the edges of the wound well-approximated.
2. There is no redness or signs of infection.
3. There is an absence of pain.

Equipment Needed

- Suture removal kit or sterile forceps with sterile suture removal scissors
- Gauze size as appropriate for wound area to be covered
- Biohazard bag or appropriate waterproof disposable bag
- Sterile saline, prepackaged antiseptic swabs, or gauze for cleaning if appropriate
- Examination gloves
- Sterile gloves if dressings are to be applied
- Adhesive strips or butterfly adhesive tape as needed
- Sterile gauze to wipe stitches or sutures from forceps and scissors
- Tincture of benzoin as indicated

DELEGATION TIPS

Suture removal is a skill requiring aseptic technique and wound assessment by a nurse and, therefore, is not delegated to ancillary personnel.

IMPLEMENTATION—ACTION/RATIONALE

ACTION	RATIONALE

❋ Check client's identification band ❋ Explain procedure before beginning ❋

ACTION	RATIONALE
1. Cleanse hands.	1. Reduces transmission of microorganisms.

continues

2. Assess the wound to determine whether the edges of the wound are well-approximated and healing has occurred.

3. Close the door and curtains around the client's bed.
4. Raise the bed to a comfortable level.
5. Position the client for comfort with easy access and visibility of the suture line.
6. Drape the client so that only the suture area is exposed.
7. Open the suture removal kit on a clean surface and assemble any supplies needed within easy access.
8. Apply clean gloves to remove the old dressing and place it in a disposable bag.
9. Remove gloves and cleanse hands.
10. If dressings are to be used, assemble equipment and supplies on sterile field.
11. Apply sterile gloves according to institutional policy. Clean the incision with saline-soaked gauze pads, antiseptic swabs, or per institutional policy.

12. When removing an interrupted suture, hold forceps in your nondominant hand and grasp the suture near the knot (Figure 28-8-1).
13. Place the curved edge of the scissors under the suture or near the knot (Figure 28-8-2).
14. Cut the suture close to the skin where the suture emerges from the skin (not in the middle). Pull the long end and remove it in one piece.
15. If the client has a continuous suture, cut both the first and second suture before removing them.
16. Some policies require the removal of every other suture, with the remaining sutures removed at a later time. Assess the suture line to ensure that the edges remain approximated.
17. Discard the sutures onto the gauze squares as they are removed and place the gauze squares in the disposable bag when all the sutures have been removed.
18. Assess the suture line to ensure that the edges remain approximated and that all sutures have been removed.

2. Health care providers often have standing orders for sutures to be removed at a specified date. If the wound is not well-healed, sutures should be left in place longer and the health care provider notified.
3. Provides for privacy.
4. Provides for proper body mechanics.
5. Facilitates removal of the sutures and allows for careful observation of suture line.
6. Provides for privacy.
7. Facilitates removal of sutures.

8. Follows Standard Precautions protocol.

9. Reduces transmission of microorganisms.
10. Protects client from microorganisms.

11. Protects the incision from microorganisms on the nurse's hands. Protects the nurse from possible contact with bodily fluids. Various opinions exist regarding use of cleansing solutions for wound care.
12. Pulls the suture up and away from the client's skin.

13. Facilitates clipping of the suture.

14. Facilitates suture removal. Avoids pulling large amounts of contaminated suture through tissue.

15. Facilitates suture removal without traumatizing the incision line.
16. Any dehiscence should be detected early, and every other suture can be left in place.

17. Decreases transmission of microorganisms and follows Standard Precaution protocol.

18. Detects early signs of dehiscence. Ensures that sutures do not remain in the skin when they are no longer needed.

Figure 28-8-1 Hold forceps in your nondominant hand and grasp the suture near the knot.

Figure 28-8-2 Hold the scissors in your dominant hand. Place the curved edge of the scissors under the suture.

continues

19. Apply adhesive strips or butterfly tape adhesive strips across the suture line to secure the edges. The amount of reinforcement varies depending on the adherence of the suture line and the length of the suture line. Adhesive skin closures may be placed 1 inch apart or closer together.
      Tincture of benzoin may be used.
20. Dispose of the soiled equipment.

21. Remove gloves and cleanse hands.
22. If removing staples:
   • Repeat Actions 2 to 11.
   • Use a staple extractor to remove every other staple. Place the lower tip of staple remover under the staple and squeeze the handles together. The ends of the staple will extract from the skin. Move the staple away from the skin surface and release the staple into a disposal container. Assess the wound for adherence. Move on to the next staple if the skin has adhered well.
   • Repeat Actions 19 to 21.

19. If the suture line pulls apart a little after the sutures are removed, adhesive skin closures can be used to reinforce the suture line.

   Helps adhesive adhere to skin.
20. Reduces odors in the client's room and reduces transmission of microorganisms.
21. Reduces transmission of microorganisms.
22.
   • Prepares for staple removal.
   • When removing staples, it is best to remove every other staple and assess wound adherence before removing all staples. A staple extractor is designed to remove the staple with a minimum of discomfort and trauma to the surrounding skin and tissue.

   • See Rationales 19 to 21.

EVALUATION

•   The wound is intact, edges are adhered, and there are no signs of infection or drainage.
•   Sutures/staples removed with a minimum of pain and trauma to the client.

DOCUMENTATION

Nurses' Notes

•   Procedure and findings at wound site, such as redness, pain, or drainage
•   Time sutures/staples were removed
•   Follow-up instructions and client teaching provided

References/Suggested Readings

Pullen, R. (2003). Removing sutures and staples. *Nursing2003,* 33(10), 18.

SECTION II
ADULT HEALTH NURSING

UNIT
9

Essential Concepts

ANESTHESIA

MAKING THE CONNECTION
Refer to the following chapters to increase your understanding of anesthesia:

Basic Nursing
- **Legal and Ethical Responsibilities**
- **Fluid, Electrolyte, and Acid–Base Balance**
- **Pain Management**

Adult Health Nursing
- **Surgery**

LEARNING OBJECTIVES

Upon completion of this chapter, you should be able to:
- **Define key terms.**
- **Describe the difference between regional and general anesthesia.**
- **Identify the purposes of sedation.**
- **Describe the effects of sedation or general anesthesia on memory and cognitive function.**
- **Discuss the types of monitoring necessary to ensure client safety during sedation.**
- **Describe the signs and symptoms and risks of oversedation.**
- **Discuss the dangers involved in aspiration of gastric contents and how gastric aspiration is prevented during anesthesia.**
- **List the medications that are typically given on the day of surgery.**
- **List and describe the different types of regional anesthesia.**
- **Describe the risks involved with regional and general anesthesia.**
- **Discuss the residual effects of anesthesia on the client.**
- **List three methods of postoperative pain management and explain briefly how each is administered.**

KEY TERMS

amnesia	general anesthesia
analgesia	orthostatic hypotension
anesthesia	regional anesthesia
anesthesiologist	sedation
anesthetist	synergism
capnography	

anesthesia. The delivery of general anesthesia to prevent pain during surgery began in the United States in the 1800s. When surgeons began using anesthesia routinely, they soon realized the need for someone trained in its administration and turned to the nurses with whom they worked daily. Early nurse anesthetists were trained on the job by the surgeons with whom they worked.

Anesthesia is now a specialty of both nursing and medicine. Experienced registered nurses (RNs) with a baccalaureate degree can become certified registered nurse anesthetists (CRNAs) after completing two or more years of graduate education in nurse anesthesia. A new rule, written in November 2001, regarding physician supervision of nurse anesthetists administering anesthesia to Medicare clients allows states to opt out of this requirement (AANA, 2001). According to the AANA (2002), five states have opted out.

Today, there are more than 28,000 CRNAs in the United States (AANA, 2001). Certified registered nurse anesthetists administer 65% of all anesthetics given in the United States every year, often working in groups with anesthesiologists (AANA, 2001). An **anesthesiologist** is a licensed physician educated and skilled in the

INTRODUCTION

Anesthesia refers to the absence of normal sensation. **Analgesia** refers to pain relief without producing

Physical Assessment and Anesthesia
What is the relevance of physical assessment and anesthesia?

Oral Intake Before Surgery

- Clearly explain to clients those things that they will or will not be allowed to eat or drink before surgery.
- Emphasize the need to exactly follow the instructions related to the time at which eating or drinking must cease before surgery.

delivery of anesthesia who also adds to the knowledge of anesthesia through research or other scholarly pursuits. An **anesthetist** is a qualified RN, dentist, or physician who administers anesthetics.

Before administering an anesthetic, the anesthesia provider assesses the client's health status, discusses anesthesia with the client, and plans an anesthetic appropriate for the client and the surgical procedure. Surgical nurses can help prepare clients to talk with their anesthesia providers by encouraging them to ask any questions they have about anesthesia and the care they will receive.

The use of anesthesia is essential to the health and well-being of clients undergoing surgery. While anesthesia prevents any sensation of pain, it also temporarily eliminates or diminishes the client's ability to control many essential physiologic functions such as respiration, heart rate, and temperature regulation. In addition to ensuring adequate levels of anesthesia throughout a surgical procedure, the anesthesia provider monitors and, when necessary, controls physiologic functions such as respiratory rate and blood pressure. Before the end of the surgery, the anesthesia provider administers appropriate medications to ensure that the client is comfortable when emerging from the anesthetic. Pain may be relieved with local anesthetic infiltration, opioid analgesics, or nonopioid analgesics.

PREANESTHETIC PREPARATION

Preparing a client for anesthesia and surgery is a cooperative effort involving the surgeon, the anesthesia provider, and the nursing staff who will care for the client both before and after surgery. The client may be having general (total body) anesthesia, where the control of body functions is temporarily lost; regional anesthesia, where a region of the body is made insensible to

pain; or local anesthesia, where only a small area of the body is made insensible to pain.

Oral Intake

Normally, only air should enter the trachea and lungs. The body prevents foreign material from entering the trachea by coughing forcefully when something other than air enters or by tightly closing the vocal cords to prevent entry of the foreign substance. Anyone who has ever been drinking something and had it go down the wrong "pipe" knows how uncomfortable it is and how hard the body works to cough up the foreign substance.

General anesthesia removes a person's ability to guard the airway by coughing or closing the vocal cords. Passive regurgitation of stomach contents into the back of the throat can occur at any time during the delivery of general anesthesia. Aspiration of gastric contents into the lungs can cause significant illness or death. An important step in preventing aspiration of gastric contents is ensuring that the stomach is as empty as possible. In the past, adults have been instructed not to eat or drink anything for at least 8 hours before surgery, and usually nothing past midnight the night before surgery. More recent information, however, strongly indicates that adults need not go without clear liquids for 8 or more hours before surgery; 2 hours are sufficient (Crenshaw, 1999). In fact, the amount of liquid in a person's stomach at the time of surgery may actually be decreased if water is taken a couple of hours before surgery. Some anesthesia providers still prefer that their clients not have anything to eat or drink for at least 8 hours before surgery; others may allow water up to 2 hours before.

Preoperative Medication

Most scheduled medications that a person receives while in the hospital or takes at home every day will be continued until the time of surgery. Give oral medications with just enough water to swallow them, even

Anesthesia for Pediatric Clients

- Have a parent present when the anesthesiologist examines the child and performs the preoperative assessment.
- Explain the procedure at the child's level of understanding, such as "This mask will help you go to sleep for a while."
- Allow the child to play with a mask.

Fasting: Infants and Small Children
Infants and small children have a high metabolic need and can tolerate only short periods of fasting, 4 hours or less.

PROFESSIONAL TIP

Preanesthetic Care

- Complete the preoperative checklist.
- Make sure all preoperative orders are executed, especially those for blood tests, preoperative medications, and blood from the blood bank.
- Check, verify, and document the presence or absence of drug allergies for each client.
- Administer regular daily oral medications with a small sip of water as ordered.
- Remind the client of the importance of following instructions regarding any eating or drinking restrictions.
- Administer preoperative medications at the ordered time. Timing can be crucial to achieving the desired effect at the correct time.
- If the client responds abnormally to the preoperative medication, notify the anesthesia department immediately.
- Be sure the client's chart is complete when it goes to the operating room with the client. Recent diagnostic test results are especially important to include; otherwise, surgery may be delayed while these results are sought.
- Make sure the client's consents are in order and included in the chart when the client is transported to surgery.

when a client is going to have surgery first thing in the morning. The anesthesia provider usually writes orders specifying how the morning medication should be managed. Cardiovascular medications such as antihypertensives and heart medications are especially important for the client to receive.

Exceptions to the practice of continuing scheduled medications before surgery include administration of drugs such as insulin and oral antihyperglycemics, nonsteroidal anti-inflammatory drugs (NSAIDs) such as aspirin, and anticoagulants such as heparin or coumadin. Because food is being withheld, giving insulin or oral antihyperglycemic drugs is likely to result in a dangerously low blood sugar level. The way insulin and glucose administration is handled will depend on the severity of the client's disease and the preference of the physician and anesthesia provider. Anticoagulants and NSAIDs affect clotting. With some types of surgery, the bleeding caused by aspirin-like drugs or low-dose heparin is more likely. In some cases, no NSAIDs are allowed for 10 days to 2 weeks before surgery. In other circumstances, they may be taken right up until surgery. Low-dose heparin or heparinoids may be given preoperatively to prevent postoperative thromboembolism, but higher doses of heparin and any dose of coumadin will almost certainly be stopped before surgery to allow the return of normal coagulation time.

Additional medications may be ordered to prepare the client for surgery or anesthesia. Surgeons often order prophylactic antibiotics. The anesthesia provider may order a sedative to help the client sleep the night before

surgery or to ease the client's anxiety while waiting for surgery. Opioids like morphine or meperidine (Demerol) may also be used for pain relief or to ease the induction of anesthesia. Some anesthesia providers prefer to give preoperative medications in the operating room to precisely control the medication's effect on the client. This is especially true for very sick clients.

Consent

Consent for anesthesia is usually obtained on the same form as is surgical consent, or a separate anesthesia consent form may be used instead of or in addition to the combined consent. In either case, for informed consent to be obtained, the anesthetic must be discussed with the client by someone with expert knowledge of anesthesia, usually an anesthesia provider or the surgeon.

SEDATION

Sedation refers to a reduction of stress, excitement, or irritability and involves some degree of central nervous system (CNS) depression. Sedation is used to decrease awareness of events, relieve anxiety, control the physiologic changes that often accompany anxiety, and ease the induction of general anesthesia. This is welcome news to many clients who fear local or regional anesthesia because they do not want to be awake and see and hear anything during surgery or a diagnostic procedure.

Different sedatives given in combination have a greater effect on the client than does any one of the sedatives given alone. This phenomenon is called **synergism.** The synergistic effect that occurs when different sedative drugs are administered together makes respiratory depression and unconsciousness more likely. In general, benzodiazepines (diazepam [Valium] and midazolam hydrochloride [Versed]) are better sedatives than are opioids (morphine and fentanyl citrate [Sublimaze]). If a client's anxiety is caused by pain, an opioid is a better choice of sedative because the opioid will relieve the pain that caused the anxiety.

Sedative medications are administered based on the client's physical condition, weight, mental state, and the procedure being performed, with close observation of the effects of the drugs on the client.

The amount of sedation required by a client for comfort is always balanced with the amount of stimulation experienced as a result of pain or anxiety. Sedation and general anesthesia both involve CNS depression; thus sedation and anesthesia exist on a continuum. As sedation becomes deeper and deeper, it eventually becomes general anesthesia. Sometimes, the line between sedation and general anesthesia is very difficult to distinguish. When sedation becomes general anesthesia, all of the risks of general anesthesia are present, including airway obstruction, respiratory arrest, and aspiration of gastric contents. For this reason, all but the lightest sedation should be administered by an anesthetist or another provider skilled and experienced in airway assessment, protection, and management, as well as assessment of oxygenation and ventilation.

Sedation and Monitoring

Sedation is often used to alleviate client anxiety and discomfort during procedures performed under local anesthesia. Properly administered, local anesthetic injection blocks the painful stimulus of small incisions and minor surgical procedures; however, local anesthetic administration can cause significant discomfort because of edema and tissue irritation caused by the acidity of the local anesthetic solution. Most clients are uncomfortable knowing they are undergoing surgery and prefer to be less alert during the procedure. Procedural sedation, formerly called conscious sedation (Carroll, 2002), decreases the client's perception of these physical and mental discomforts.

During local anesthesia and sedation, the client must remain conscious and in control of his own airway and breathing reflexes. Oversedation is likely to result in airway obstruction and places the client at risk for aspiration of gastric contents. Because sedatives are CNS depressants and, thus, respiratory depressants, give supplemental oxygen to clients during sedation. Monitoring during sedation is done through observation by an individual knowledgeable and experienced in the assessment of respiratory volume and airway patency.

The revised Joint Commission on Accreditation of Healthcare Organizations (JCAHO) standards for monitoring clients undergoing procedural sedation require that heart rate and oxygenation be continually monitored by pulse oximetry, and that respiratory rate and pulmonary ventilation adequacy also be continually monitored (JCAHO, 2000). One method of monitoring pulmonary ventilation is **capnography,** which provides breath-to-breath feedback of the client's exhaled CO_2 level with a nasal cannula-like device. It makes a distinct tracing similar to an EKG (Carroll, 2002).

Monitoring should also include an electrocardiogram (EKG) and blood pressure. The individual monitoring the client's breathing and vital signs should be devoted to that task to the exclusion of any other duties.

Residual Effects of Sedation

Sedation usually persists beyond the duration of the surgical procedure. The length of time it takes to recover from sedation depends on the health of the client, the properties of the drugs used, other drugs the client may be taking, and the amount of sedative drugs administered.

Amnesia (inability to remember things) produced by sedatives is commonly found even in clients who appear to be completely recovered. Such clients will probably not remember any instructions given to them during or soon after the procedure. Given that minor procedures and surgery are commonly performed on an outpatient basis, some clients may be discharged before regaining the ability to remember verbal instructions. All instructions should thus be given in writing and explained to the person responsible for taking the client home. Some facilities put the discharge instructions on a CD-ROM or video for the client to take home and review.

If heavy sedation was used or the procedure ends suddenly, the client may remain significantly sedated after the procedure is over because the CNS stimulation ended while the CNS depressant effect of the sedative remains. The client should be closely monitored until the effects of the sedative medications wear off enough for the client to wake and become oriented.

REGIONAL ANESTHESIA

In **regional anesthesia** a region of the body is temporarily rendered insensible to pain by injection of a local anesthetic. Local anesthetics are a class of drugs that temporarily block the transmission of small electrical impulses through nerves. The duration of anesthesia produced by a local anesthetic depends on the drug used, the amount injected, and into which part of the body the drug is injected. The amount of insulation surrounding a nerve fiber, the anatomic location of the fiber, and the diameter of the fiber all influence the ease with which nerve impulses are blocked by local anesthetics.

Types of Regional Anesthesia

There are three types of regional anesthesia: local anesthesia, nerve blocks, and spinal and epidural blocks.

Local Anesthesia

Clinically, the use of local anesthetics to block nerves is identified by different names depending on the amount of local anesthetic used and where it is injected. When a small amount of local anesthetic drug is injected either into the skin and subcutaneous tissues around a cut or at the site of a needle puncture for a central line placement, it is called *local anesthesia.* The anesthetic is not aimed at a specific nerve; rather it anesthetizes all small superficial nerves in the target area. Local anesthesia is most commonly performed using lidocaine (Xylocaine) and lasts approximately 1 hour. Occasionally, for some types of plastic surgery, this type of anesthesia is used over a large area of the body. In this case, longer-acting local anesthetics may be used. Because very small amounts of local anesthetics are generally used, the risk of local anesthetic toxicity is also small.

Topical anesthesia, achieved with direct application of a local anesthetic to tissue, may be desired in some situations (e.g., before insertion of an IV). The anesthetic may take the form of an ointment, lotion, solution, or spray.

 Safety: Preventing Choking and Aspiration
In order to prevent choking and aspiration after the use of an oral anesthetic solution (e.g., viscous lidocaine) or spray, fluids and foods must be withheld until the gag reflex returns.

Nerve Blocks

When a local anesthetic is injected more deeply into the body and/or is directed at a specific nerve or nerves, it is called a *nerve block.* Nerve blocks are often called by the name of the specific nerve or nerves they block. Examples include an ulnar nerve block in the arm or a brachial plexus block of all the nerves in the arm. Nerve blocks are often performed using lidocaine (Xylocaine),

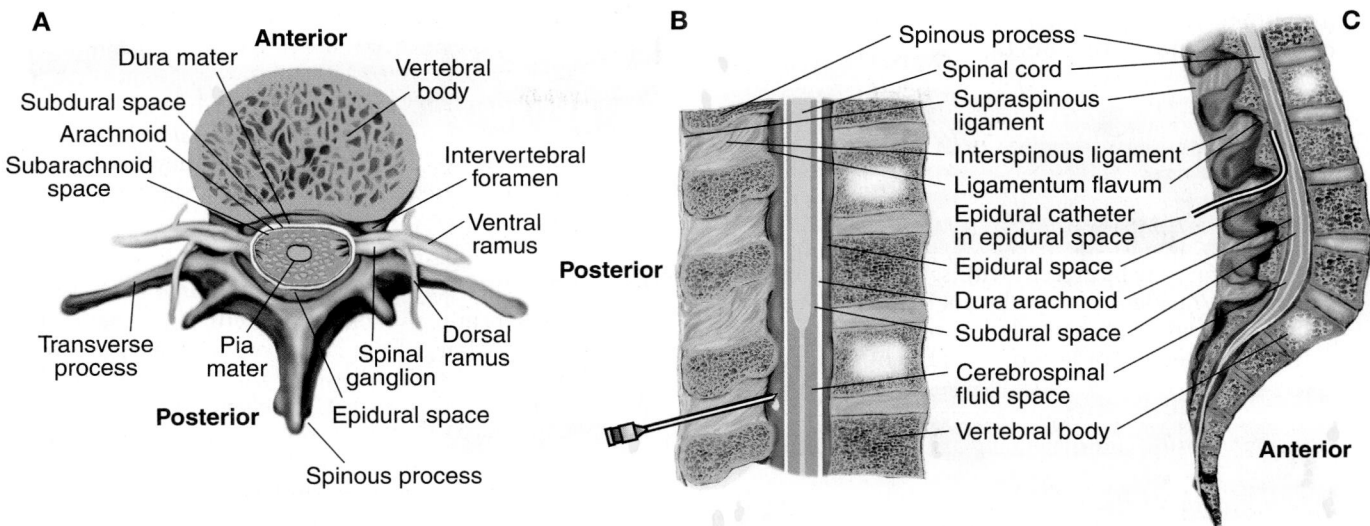

Figure 29-1 *A,* Cross-sectional anatomy of the spine. *B,* Side view of spinal anatomy with the tip of an epidural needle placed in the epidural space. *C,* Side view of spinal anatomy with the tip of an epidural catheter placed in the epidural space.

mepivacaine (Carbocaine), or bupivacaine (Marcaine) and may last from 1 to 12 hours.

Spinal and Epidural Blocks

Blocks may also be identified according to where the local anesthetic is injected. One example is an *epidural block,* for which local anesthetic is injected into the epidural space near the spinal cord to anesthetize several spinal nerves at once. With *spinal blocks* (also called subarachnoid blocks), the local anesthetic is injected into the cerebrospinal fluid, where it can bathe uninsulated spinal nerves as they exit the spinal cord to the periphery of the body (Figure 29-1).

Spinal and epidural blocks are generally used to anesthetize a significant area of the body. They are capable of safely producing anesthesia sufficient for surgery in the abdomen, pelvis, perineum, or lower extremities. When an epidural block is performed, a catheter is usually inserted into the epidural space, making it possible to inject additional doses of drug. The client must either be sitting in a bent-over position or lying on the side with head and knees as close together as possible (Figure 29-2). Either position separates the vertebra, making insertion of the needle or catheter possible. Epidural blocks have an added advantage in that by varying the way the anesthetic is used, the block can produce analgesia (pain relief without producing anesthesia), complete anesthesia, and even profound muscular relaxation (needed for some types of surgery). This allows epidural anesthesia to be used not only for surgical procedures, but also for analgesia during labor and for postoperative pain relief.

Spinal blocks are most often performed using lidocaine (Xylocaine) or bupivacaine (Marcaine) and last from 1 to 3 hours. Epidural blocks are most commonly performed using bupivacaine (Marcaine), and the block can be continued as long as local anesthetic is injected through the catheter into the epidural space.

Figure 29-2 *Correct positions for performing a spinal block or inserting an epidural catheter into the lumbar area. The assistance of trained personnel is crucial to the proper positioning, reassurance, and safety of the client.*

Opioids such as morphine and fentanyl citrate (Sublimaze) may be added to the local anesthetic in either of these blocks to intensify the analgesic or anesthetic effect, or to provide postoperative pain relief after the block has worn off.

One type of complication is peculiar to spinal and epidural regional anesthetics. When cerebrospinal fluid (CSF) leaks out through a hole made in the dural membrane during performance of a subarachnoid block or an accidental dural puncture during the attempted performance of an epidural block, a postdural puncture headache (PDPH) may result. The headache is caused by the loss of CSF from around the brain. The headache is relieved by lying down and returns when the individual sits up or stands. Pain commonly occurs in both the front and the back of the head and is sometimes accompanied by neck and shoulder stiffness. Photophobia or double vision may be present with severe headache. The onset of the headache is usually not immediate and may take 1 to 2 days to become bothersome. Treatment involves adequate hydration to allow the normal production of CSF; analgesics; and bed rest in a supine position. One treatment for significant or persistent PDPH is a procedure called an epidural blood patch, which involves injecting 15 to 20 mL of the client's own blood into the epidural space. Once the blood clots, it plugs the hole in the dural membrane. Another treatment involves connecting an IV infusion to the epidural catheter to replace the lost CSF and treat the headache.

Residual Effects of Regional Anesthesia

All anesthetics wear off as the drug responsible for causing the anesthesia is removed, metabolized, and eliminated. Some anesthetic effects wear off faster than others, and important residual effects may not be detected by casual observation. This is especially true of a regional anesthetic because the client may be wide awake and able to carry on a conversation as if nothing has happened. Three common residual effects are discussed following.

Residual Motor Block

A motor block is a temporary condition caused when local anesthetic blocks nerves that carry instructions to skeletal muscles telling them to contract. Motor block results in the inability to move a body part and is usually the last effect to develop and the first to wear off. It results only when the regional block is very dense and complete.

A complete motor block results in a temporary paralysis, with the client being incapable of moving the blocked part despite tremendous effort. With a complete motor block, there is usually no function in any other type of nerve in the same area. A client with a complete motor block of any part of the body would not likely be released from the recovery area. Clients experiencing residual (incomplete) motor block may be released from recovery. A client who has had any type of block involving the legs should never be allowed to get out of bed without assistance until it can be demonstrated that a complete recovery of motor strength in the legs has been regained. Even a small amount of residual motor block greatly increases the possibility that a client will fall.

As a regional block begins to wear off, motor function begins to return first, sensation begins to return next, and sympathetic nervous function returns last. Motor function and sensation can be detected easily by asking the client to move the blocked part or by touching the skin and asking the client whether it feels normal. The return of sympathetic function is more difficult to detect. Orthostatic hypotension may occur even after motor and sensory function have completely returned and the regional block appears to have worn off. To prevent fainting, clients should not be allowed to get out of bed without the presence of a nurse until after they have been able to do so without any dizziness or significant decrease in blood pressure.

Residual Sensory Block

Normal sensation may not have returned completely upon client discharge from the recovery area. As the regional block wears off, sensation will return gradually. As sensation begins to return, the client may experience a "pins and needles" feeling in an arm or leg that has been blocked and may feel touch or pressure before recovering complete sensation. Until complete recovery of normal sensation, any blocked areas must be frequently checked and carefully protected, as the client may be unaware that a finger or hand, for example, is being pinched or denied blood supply.

Residual Sympathetic Block

The last nerve fibers to recover as a local anesthetic wears off are those responsible for carrying instructions to the muscles that surround blood vessels. When these sympathetic nerves are blocked, veins and arteries dilate, lowering the blood pressure. The venous system has a large capacity, and venous dilation results in the pooling of a large amount of blood. This decreases the amount of blood that returns to the heart, and the blood pressure falls. The amount of blood that pools is greatest in parts of the body that are farthest below the level of the heart. Even in a client who has had a spinal or epidural block and is lying supine, a significant amount of venous pooling occurs, resulting in lower-than-normal blood pressure. If the same client is allowed to sit up, even more venous pooling will occur, less blood will return to the heart, and blood pressure will fall substantially. This phenomenon of having a large drop in blood pressure when sitting up or standing is called **orthostatic hypotension.** *Orthostatic* signifies that it involves body position, and *hypotension* means low blood pressure. Clients who have had a spinal or epidural block are more likely to have orthostatic hypotension the higher in the spinal column the level of their block.

GENERAL ANESTHESIA

General anesthesia involves unconsciousness, complete insensibility to pain, amnesia, motionlessness, and muscle relaxation. With general anesthesia, the body also loses the ability to control many important functions, including the abilities to maintain an airway, control vital functions such as breathing and heart rate, and regulate temperature. These functions are controlled by the anesthesia provider during administration of general anesthesia.

General anesthesia involves four overlapping stages: induction (going to sleep), maintenance, emergence (waking up), and recovery.

Induction and Airway Management

The induction of general anesthesia is a short but critical period during which the client is rendered unconscious, vital functions are controlled, and enough anesthetic drug is introduced into the body to keep the client asleep during surgery. In adults, drugs are usually injected into an IV line to quickly produce unconsciousness, and additional anesthetic is then inhaled.

Immediately after the induction of general anesthesia, the anesthesia provider will usually secure the airway using a cuffed endotracheal tube (ETT) (Figure 29-3). An ETT provides a breathing passage from outside the client to within the client's trachea.

Maintenance

General anesthesia is maintained with some combination of IV and inhaled drugs. Figure 29-4 shows a client connected to an anesthesia machine by a breathing circuit.

Skeletal Muscle Relaxation

Some types of surgery require complete relaxation of skeletal muscles. In these cases, the anesthesia provider administers a skeletal muscle relaxant such as pancuronium bromide (Pavulon) or vecuronium bromide (Norcuron) to completely paralyze the client. These types of drugs prevent clients from breathing on their own, requiring the anesthesia provider to ventilate clients during surgery. Paralysis must be eliminated before emergence from anesthesia in order for the client to be able to breathe independently again.

Inadequate reversal of paralysis may present as anything from total skeletal muscle paralysis to the inability of the client to cough and clear the airway. If the client is having difficulty breathing, basic life support should be provided until the arrival of an anesthesia provider.

Emergence

Emergence from general anesthesia occurs when anesthetic drugs are allowed to wear off. The anesthesia provider carefully controls the timing and amount of anesthetic drug given in order for the client to emerge from general anesthesia at the desired time. The initial phase of emergence is usually quite quick, allowing the client to awaken enough to respond to verbal directions and maintain an airway. After this time, the client's breathing tube can usually be removed, and the client can be taken to the postanesthesia care unit (recovery room). If, for some reason, the client must be left on a ventilator and with a breathing tube in place, the anesthesia provider may take the client to an intensive care unit asleep instead of waking the client up from the anesthetic.

Recovery

Recovery from general anesthesia is not complete simply because the client has regained consciousness. The client may not remember what has happened for minutes or even hours after having received an anesthetic. The ability to think clearly often takes longer to

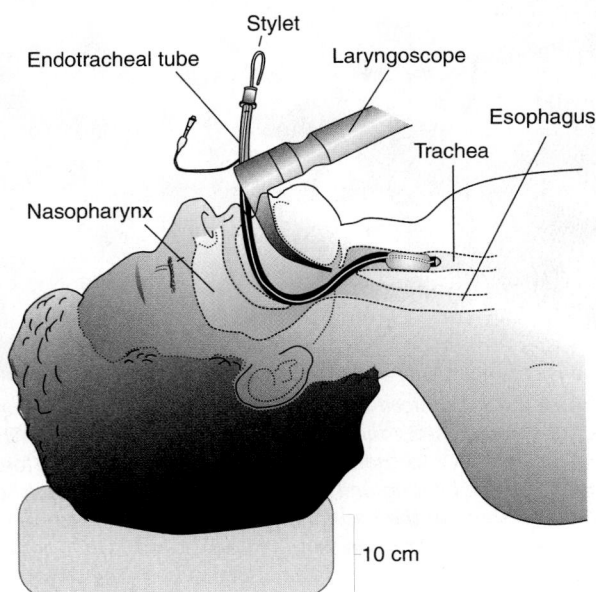

Figure 29-3 *Placing an Endotracheal Tube in the Trachea with Direct Visualization by Laryngoscopy*

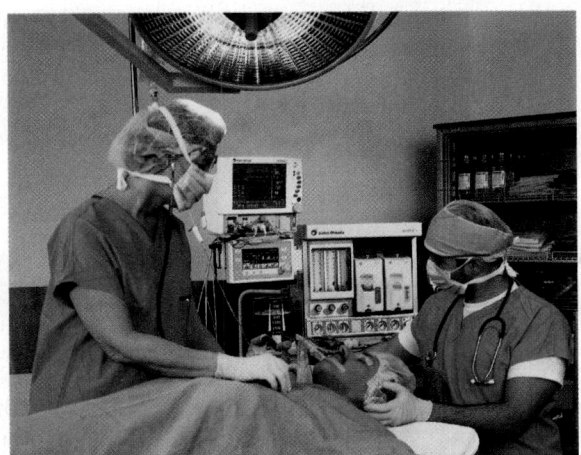

Figure 29-4 *A typical anesthesia machine is a complex equipment set. This machine has anesthetic vaporizers and flowmeters to deliver oxygen, nitrous oxide, and air. It also supports a ventilator and equipment to monitor ventilation, oxygen content of inspired gas, client oxygen saturation, blood pressure, heart rate, and respiration. (Pictured above is the Datex-Ohmeda Aestiva/5 Anesthesia Delivery System equipped with a Cardiocap/5 Monitor. Reprinted with permission of Datex-Ohmeda, Inc.)*

return, with some residual thinking difficulty persisting for several days or even weeks. Inhalation anesthetics are eliminated from the body through the lungs, and very small amounts of anesthetic are still being exhaled for several weeks. Many anesthetic drugs are stored in body fat and released back into the bloodstream very slowly after anesthetic administration has ended. The speed of this release depends on the amount of anesthetic given during the surgery, the length of the surgery, and how deeply the client is breathing.

Oxygenation and Ventilation

Almost all anesthetics are respiratory depressants. Benzodiazepines, opioids, and inhalation anesthetic agents have significant respiratory depressant effects. Any one of these drugs may be used in a dose that causes apnea, or lack of respirations for more than 10 seconds, during a general anesthesia. When used in combination their effect on respiration is at least additive. When the rate or depth of respirations decrease, the elimination of carbon dioxide is retarded, and carbon dioxide builds up in the blood and in the lungs. Oxygen saturation is monitored by pulse oximetry. Even small amounts of supplemental oxygen given to a client whose rate or depth of breathing is decreased adds significantly to the amount of oxygen in the bloodstream. This is the most important reason that oxygen is given to even healthy clients when they are recovering from general anesthesia.

Heart Rate and Blood Pressure

Few direct effects on heart rate (HR) and blood pressure (BP) regulation are seen during recovery from general anesthesia. Some anesthetic techniques that are heavily based on opioids, such as fentanyl citrate (Sublimaze) or sufentanil citrate (Sufenta), can cause a slow HR, but as long as BP is maintained, no specific treatment is necessary. Although most general anesthetics are myocardial depressants, the depressive effects of current agents are mild, especially after anesthetic administration is ended.

Most HR and BP changes seen during recovery result from factors related indirectly to the anesthetic. Both HR and BP increase as a result of sympathetic stimulation. Pain, hypoxia, and fear can all result in sympathetic stimulation with an increase in HR and BP. Discovering and addressing the source of the client's fear often re-

duces the anxiety. When the causes of sympathetic stimulation are addressed, HR and BP should normalize.

Temperature Regulation and Shivering

With general anesthesia, the body loses its natural ability to regulate temperature. General anesthetic agents dilate the blood vessels close to the surface of the body, exposing the client's warm blood to the cool exterior. During anesthetization, the client is mostly uncovered in a cold operating room, and the area of the body to be operated on is cleaned with cold solutions. After this is done, the client's insulating covering (skin and subcutaneous fat) is cut open to expose the warm interior of the body and allow its heat to escape. Room temperature intravenous fluids are infused into the veins, and the client breathes cool gases. Surgical clients lose a great amount of heat at a time when the body is least able to respond to warm the tissues. Hypothermia adds to the CNS depression resulting from any residual anesthetics. Surface warming with a forced-air warming blanket is an effective way to increase the temperature of a client intraoperatively and when recovering from general anesthesia; cloth blankets or heating lamps may also be useful. Figure 29-5 shows use of a forced-air warming blanket.

All potent inhalation agents are associated with shivering during emergence from general anesthesia when the blood level of the anesthetic agent is very low. The

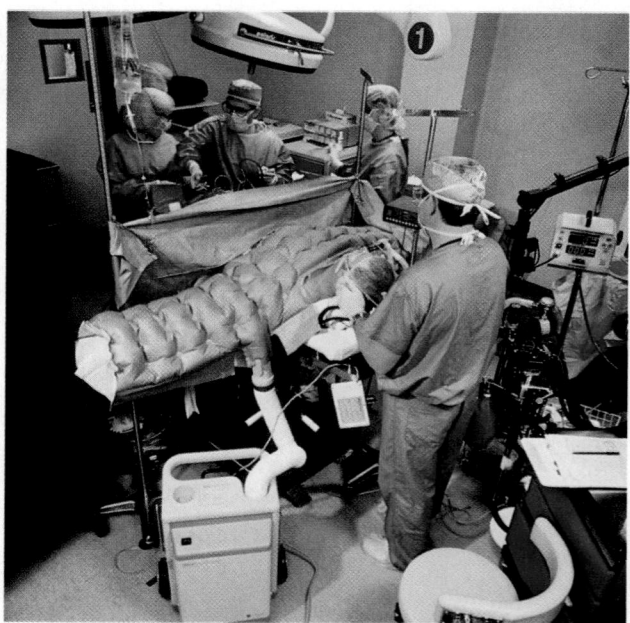

Figure 29-5   *A forced-air warming blanket applied to the upper abdomen, chest, and arms of a client during surgery. The unit on the floor to the left of the anesthesia provider (foreground) is the heating unit, which contains a fan that pushes warm air through the hose and into the blanket, much like a furnace pushes warm air through heating ducts and into a house. Warm air exits hundreds of pinholes on the surface of the blanket and next to the client. (Courtesy of Mallinckrodt Medical, Inc.)*

cause of the shivering is not clear but does not appear to be related to the client's body temperature. (Of course, postoperative clients also shiver when they are cold.) The key to eliminating shivering postoperatively is to ensure client warmth and encourage deep breathing so that the anesthetic is eliminated as quickly as possible.

Fluid Balance

Surgical procedures and the injuries that necessitate them have major effects on the body's distribution of fluid. Appropriate care during anesthesia sometimes necessitates the delivery of a large volume of IV fluid. This IV fluid does not stay in the vascular system long, moving out of the vascular space to replace losses from the interstitial and intracellular spaces.

Trauma, whether caused by an accidental injury or a surgical incision, results in fluid losses or shifts in three general areas as follows: direct blood loss, evaporation through the surgical wound, and fluid shifts. Large volumes of fluid can be lost to the air through the surgical wound, especially during abdominal procedures. A major abdominal procedure, for example, can result in the loss of up to 10 cc/kg/hour of fluid by evaporation.

POSTOPERATIVE PAIN MANAGEMENT

Pain has many causes. Postoperative pain results from tissue injury, release of local and hormonal substances, inflammation, mental outlook, and, perhaps, neural hyperexcitability related to excessive noxious input. As such, baseline postoperative pain, pain from pressure placed on an incision, and pain from client movement may each respond best to different pain-relieving strategies.

The amount of medication needed to relieve pain depends on the intensity and type of pain, the size of the client, and the client's age. The dose requirement for most opioids is dramatically lower for clients who are elderly as compared to younger clients. An 89-year-old needs 50% less opioid analgesic than does a 20-year-old (Scott & Stanski, 1987).

Patient-Controlled Analgesia

Patient-controlled analgesia (PCA) allows clients to self-administer pain medication by pushing a button when they experience pain. After an IV catheter is in place, a client-controlled analgesia pump is connected "piggyback" to the IV line. The pump is programmed to deliver a predetermined dose of morphine, dilaudid, or meperidine (Demerol) when the client pushes a button. It will not, however, deliver unlimited amounts. A set time must pass between each successive dose, and when the total dose of opioid delivered in any hour reaches a preset limit, the pump will not deliver any more medicine until the next hour. This is referred to as lockout.

Properly programmed, PCA allows the client a great deal of control over when pain medicine is received, which is likely to help decrease anxiety. Patient-controlled analgesia also results in a shorter interval between the need for pain medicine and its administration, better pain relief than that obtained with intermittent IM injections, and a reduction in nursing time necessary for the delivery of pain medicine. It does not, however, decrease the need for client assessment while the PCA machine is in use.

Regional Analgesia

Regional analgesia and anesthesia have many applications in the relief of postoperative pain. Regional anesthetics do not cease working when the surgery ends and provide pain relief for a variable period of time afterward. The duration of postoperative pain relief can be extended by continuing the infusion of pain medication into the epidural space or by adding opioids to either epidural or spinal anesthetics.

Local Anesthetics

Local anesthetics, either alone or in combination with opioids, can be administered into the epidural space at low concentrations that do not cause complete anesthesia. This type of pain relief is most commonly used for women in labor who receive epidural analgesia. Local anesthetic in low concentrations is a powerful analgesic. If local anesthetic is administered in a way to relieve pain in the lower extremities, clients are usually confined to bed, because even dilute concentrations of local anesthetic may affect the strength of leg muscles enough to increase the risk of falling. Clients receiving analgesia via an epidural block should be watched carefully to ensure that they do not develop pressure necrosis in the blocked areas.

Opioids

The spinal cord has receptors for opioids, and when opioids are added to a spinal or epidural anesthetic, they provide pain relief even after the anesthetic block has worn off. Morphine added to a spinal or epidural anesthetic can provide hours of postoperative pain relief, often

PROFESSIONAL TIP

Postanesthetic Care

- Immediately report to the anesthesia provider or surgeon any breathing difficulty the client is having.
- Immediately report to the surgeon or the anesthesia department a fall in the client's BP or increase in HR.
- Verify client's ability to stand or walk with normal motor strength and coordination and without any dizziness while in your direct care before allowing the client to get up without assistance.
- Do not allow clients to rub their eyes. Clients who are still drowsy may try to rub out protective eye moisturizer and, in the process, cause painful corneal abrasions.
- Observe clients immediately for bladder distention. Both regional and general anesthesia can sometimes cause temporary urinary retention.
- If clients have an epidural catheter for postoperative pain management, ensure that they change positions from time to time to prevent pressure necrosis. Do not allow the lateral aspect of the leg to rest on the side rails.
- Report to the anesthesia department as soon as possible any headache that gets worse when the client sits up or stands.
- Before giving discharge instructions, verify that the client's ability to remember instructions has returned. Always share discharge instructions with the individual responsible for taking the client home and provide the client with a written copy of the instructions.

---

enough so that no other pain medication is needed; it may even provide better pain relief than do IM injections or intravenous PCA. Opioids may be added to spinal or epidural anesthetics as a single dose or be infused into the epidural space postoperatively. Although spinal and epidural morphine provide excellent pain relief, they may also produce significant respiratory depression. Fortunately, the respiratory depression following spinal or epidural morphine administration is rarely rapid in onset. Respiratory depression is very rare with properly dosed epidural or spinal fentanyl citrate (Sublimaze). With current client selection and dosing protocols, life-threatening respiratory depression is a rare event. When it does occur, it can be detected long before it causes harm, by observing the client frequently, noting respiratory rate and depth, and periodically measuring oxygen saturation by pulse oximetry.

Summary

- In addition to ensuring an adequate level of anesthesia throughout a surgical procedure, the anesthesia provider monitors and controls physiologic functions.
- Some anesthesia providers prefer that clients not have anything to eat or drink for at least 8 hours before

surgery. Others allow water up to 2 hours before surgery.
- Most scheduled medications that a client takes every day will be continued up to and including the morning of surgery.
- Sedation depresses brain activity, decreasing awareness, reducing anxiety, and easing the induction of general anesthesia.
- Oversedation results in respiratory depression, which can cause airway obstruction, and places the client at risk for aspiration of gastric contents.
- Regional anesthesia by the injection of a local anesthetic temporarily renders a "region" of the body insensible to pain.
- General anesthesia produces unconsciousness, complete insensibility to pain, amnesia, motionlessness, and muscle relaxation.
- A person is unlikely to remember what has happened for minutes to hours after sedation or a general anesthetic.
- Intravenous patient-controlled analgesia (PCA) allows clients to self-administer pain medication by pushing a button on the PCA machine. Limits are programmed into the machine to prevent overdose.
- Local anesthetics, alone or in combination with opioids, can be injected into the epidural space at low concentrations to provide postoperative analgesia.
- Spinal and epidural morphine can produce dangerous respiratory depression. This can be detected by frequent observations of the client's respiratory rate and depth and by periodic measurement of oxygen saturation via pulse oximetry.

Review Questions

1. Clients are at risk for aspiration of gastric contents into the lungs when receiving a general anesthetic because:

    a. general anesthesia causes stomach distention.
    b. general anesthesia eliminates protective airway reflexes.
    c. gastric peristalsis is reversed during general anesthesia.
    d. vomiting normally occurs during general anesthesia.

2. The most dangerous result of oversedation is:

    a. lack of response to verbal directions.
    b. longer recovery time and resultant delayed discharge.
    c. prolonged amnesia.
    d. inability to breathe adequately.

3. What is a sign that a client has a postdural puncture headache following a spinal or epidural regional block?

    a. The headache subsides after intake of plenty of liquids.
    b. The headache begins after the surgical procedure.
    c. The headache worsens when the client sits up or stands.
    d. The client is confused in addition to having a headache.

CASE STUDY

Mrs. Pinkerton is in the recovery room following outpatient surgery. She received a general anesthetic and is now awake, breathing deeply, and talking to the staff. She has received meperidine (Demerol) intravenously and is quite comfortable. Before being discharged home from the surgery center, Mrs. Pinkerton rests in an easy chair in the transitional recovery area. The nurse taking care of her notices that she asks questions about things that have already been discussed and has even asked one question three times.

The following questions will guide your development of a nursing care plan for the case study.

1. After making these observations, what nursing diagnoses and goals might the nurse identify for Mrs. Pinkerton?
2. List the nursing interventions to be performed in caring for Mrs. Pinkerton.
3. Identify teaching approaches.

4. After cessation of a general anesthetic, how long might it be before the client can think as clearly as before the client received the anesthetic?

a. before being discharged from the recovery room
b. within 2 hours
c. six hours
d. several days

5. What effect might a spinal or epidural anesthetic block still have after normal sensation and motor function have returned?

a. decrease in pulse rate when the client is lying in bed
b. decrease in blood pressure when the client stands up
c. inhibition of protective airway reflexes
d. sore muscles

References/Suggested Readings

American Association of Nurse Anesthetists (AANA). (2001). *Administration puts politics before patients; Implements cumbersome anesthesia care rule.* [Online]. Available: www.aana.com/capcorner/finalrule_111301.asp

American Association of Nurse Anesthetists (AANA). (2002). *New Hampshire becomes fifth state to opt out of federal anesthesia requirement.* [Online]. Available: www.aana.com/press/2002/061102.asp

American Society of Regional Anesthesia and Pain Medicine (ASRA). (2002). *Regional anesthesia in the anticoagulated patient: Defining the risks.* [Online] Available: www.asra.com/items_of_interest/consensus_statements/page5.iphtml

Berkowitz, C. (1997). Epidural pain control—Your job, too. *RN, 60*(8), 22–27.

Carroll, P. (2002). Procedural sedation: Capnography's heightened role. *RN, 65*(10), 54–62.

Clinical News. (1999). "NPO after midnight" outdated? *AJN, 99*(2), 18.

Connolly, M. (1999). Postdural puncture headache. *AJN, 99*(11), 48–49.

Crenshaw, J. (1999). New guidelines for preoperative fasting. *AJN, 99*(4), 49.

Joint Commission Resources. Joint Commission on Accreditation of Healthcare Organizations. (2000). New definitions, revised standards address the continuum of sedation and anesthesia. *Joint Commission Perspectives, 20*(4), 10.

Kost, M. (1999). Conscious sedation: Guarding your patient against complications. *Nursing99, 29*(4), 34–39.

Kreger, C. (2001). Spinal anesthesia and analgesia. *Nursing2001, 31*(6), 36–41.

Messinger, J. S., Hoffman, L. A., O'Donnell, J. M., & Dunworth, B. A. (1999). Getting conscious sedation right. *AJN, 99*(12), 44–49.

O'Donnell, T., Bragg, K., & Sell, S. (2003). Procedural sedation: Safely navigating the twilight zone. *Nursing2003, 33*(4), 36–41, 44.

Pasero, C., & McCaffery, M. (1999). Providing epidural analgesia. *Nursing99, 29*(8), 34–39.

Scott, J. C., & Stanski, D. R. (1987). Decreased fentanyl and alfentanil dose requirements with age: A simultaneous pharmacokinetic and pharmacodynamic evaluation. *Journal of Pharmacology and Experimental Therapeutics, 240,* 159–166.

Wong, D. (2003). Topical local anesthetics. *AJN, 103*(6), 42–45.

Woomer, J., & Berkheimer, D. (2003). Using capnography to monitor ventilation. *Nursing2003, 33*(4), 42–43.

Resources

American Association of Nurse Anesthetists, 222 South Prospect Avenue, Park Ridge, IL 60068-4001, 847-692-7050, www.aana.com

American Society of Anesthesiologists, 520 N. Northwest Highway, Park Ridge, IL 60068-2573, 847-825-5586, www.asahq.org

American Society of Peri Anesthesia Nurses, 10 Melrose Avenue, Cherry Hill, NJ 08003, 877-787-9696, www.aspan.org

American Society of Regional Anesthesia and Pain Medicine, PO Box 11086, Richmond, VA 23230-1086, 804-282-0010, www.asra.com

Anesthesia Patient Safety Foundation, 4246 Colonial Park Drive, Pittsburgh, PA 15227-2621, 412-882-8040 www.gasnet.org/societies/apsf/

Foundation for Anesthesia Education and Research, Charlton Building 1-128, Mayo Clinic, 200 First Street SW, Rochester, MN 55905, 507-266-6866, www.faer.org

Society for Education in Anesthesia, 520 North Northwest Highway, Park Ridge, IL 60068-2573, 847-825-5586, www.seahq.org

SURGERY

MAKING THE CONNECTION

Refer to the following chapters to increase your understanding of perioperative nursing:

Basic Nursing
- **Legal and Ethical Responsibilities**
- **Communication**
- **Cultural Considerations**
- **Fluid, Electrolyte, and Acid–Base Balance**
- **Assessment**
- **Pain Management**

Adult Health Nursing
- **Anesthesia**
- **Respiratory System**

- **Cardiovascular System**
- **Integumentary System**

Basic Procedures
- **Hand Hygiene**
- **Transferring from Bed to Stretcher**
- **Applying Antiembolic Stockings**

Intermediate Procedures
- **Postoperative Exercise Instruction**

Advanced Procedures
- **Removing Skin Sutures and Staples**

LEARNING OBJECTIVES

Upon completion of this chapter, you should be able to:
- Define key terms.
- List risk factors to be identified in a preoperative nursing assessment.
- List information to include in a general teaching plan for a preoperative client.
- Identify common nursing care for the preoperative, intraoperative, and postoperative phases.
- Describe the principles of asepsis and their application to nursing practice.
- Discuss nursing interventions to prevent or treat postoperative complications.
- Identify information needed by the postoperative client prior to discharge.
- Discuss the physiologic changes of aging that may affect the elderly client's response to surgery.
- Plan care for a postoperative client.

KEY TERMS

Aldrete Score	intraoperative phase
ambulatory surgery	perioperative
asepsis	postoperative phase
aseptic technique	preoperative phase
circulating nurse	scrub nurse
dehiscence	sterile
evisceration	sterile conscience
first assistant	sterile field
informed consent	surgery

INTRODUCTION

Surgery refers to the treatment of injury, disease, or deformity through invasive operative methods. Surgery is a unique experience, with no two clients responding alike to similar operations. Even the same client may respond differently to two separate surgical situations or to the same surgery performed at a later time. Surgery is a major stressor for every client. To a client, there is no such thing as minor surgery; anxiety and fear are normal. Surgery, even when planned well in advance, is a stressor that produces both psychological (anxiety, fear) and physiologic (neuroendocrine) stress reactions. Surgery is a stressful experience because it involves entry into the human body.

Surgeries are classified as minor (presenting little risk to life) or major (possibly involving risk to life) and may

TABLE 30-1   INDICATIONS FOR SURGERY

TYPE OF SURGERY	PURPOSE	EXAMPLE
Diagnostic	Determine cause of symptoms	Biopsy
		Exploratory laparotomy
Curative	Remove a diseased body part or replace a body part to restore function	Cholecystectomy
		Total knee arthroplasty
Palliative	Relieve symptoms without curing disease	Tumor resection associated with cancer
Restorative	Strengthen a weakened area	Herniorrhaphy
Cosmetic	Improve appearance	Face lift
	Change shape	Mammoplasty

be performed for a variety of reasons. Table 30-1 lists indications for surgery.

The term **perioperative** encompasses the preoperative (before surgery), intraoperative (during surgery), and postoperative (after surgery) phases of surgery. Each phase refers to a particular time during the surgical experience, and each requires a wide range of specific nursing behaviors and functions. Perioperative nursing has one continuous goal: to provide a standard of excellence in the care of the client before, during, and after surgery. Nursing activities must be geared to meet the client's psychosocial needs as well as immediate physical needs.

Individuals face surgery with their own values. Each client has specific expectations of the surgical experience and distinct hopes for the outcome of the surgery. The nurse must take an active part in the entire perioperative process to ensure quality and continuity of client care.

PREOPERATIVE PHASE

The **preoperative phase** is that time during the surgical experience that begins with the client's decision to have surgery and ends with the transfer of the client to the operating table.

The outcome of surgical treatment is tremendously enhanced by accurate preoperative nursing assessment and careful preoperative preparation. The client must be assessed by the nurse both physiologically and psychologically. Assessment of the client involves the integration of factors relating to the client's illness, physical condition, related medical conditions, and current surgical diagnosis. Regardless of how minor the surgical procedure, a thorough health history is essential and should be available to the perioperative team throughout the client's surgical experience.

The psychological well-being of the client may have an impact on the surgical outcome. The surgical client is at risk for anxiety related to the surgical experience and the outcome of surgery. Fear and anxiety are normal responses to the stress of surgery and can affect the client's ability to cope with the proposed plan of care. Because individuals differ in their perceptions of the meaning of surgery, the degree of anxiety and fear experienced will vary. If fear and anxiety become excessive, however,

these emotions can interfere with recovery by magnifying the normal physiologic stress response. By assessing and being aware of the fears and anxieties of the surgical client, the nurse can provide support and information so that stress does not become overwhelming. The most common fears related to surgery are:

- Fear of the unknown
- Fear of pain and discomfort
- Fear of mutilation and disfigurement
- Fear of anesthesia
- Fear of disruption of life patterns
  Separation from family/significant others
  Sexuality
  Financial
  Permanent/temporary limitations
- Fear of death/not waking up
- Fear of not being in control

Fear of the unknown is the most prevalent fear before surgery and is the fear the nurse can most easily allay through client education and preoperative teaching.

Preoperative Physiologic Assessment

Physiologic assessment should include a physical examination and a review of the client's laboratory values and diagnostic studies. Laboratory and diagnostic studies may be divided into those that are routine and those that are done specifically to evaluate the client's primary disease process or coexisting condition. The following summarizes common preoperative laboratory tests:

- Hemoglobin and hematocrit (Hgb and Hct)
- White blood cell count (WBC)
- Blood typing and cross matching (screening)
- Serum electrolytes
- Prothrombin time (PT) and partial thromboplastin time (PTT)
- Bilirubin
- Liver enzymes: alanine aminotransferase (ALT) and aspartate aminotransferase (AST)
- Urinalysis
- Blood urea nitrogen (BUN) and creatinine

Although it is common practice to obtain a chest x-ray for many clients admitted to the hospital, this study is increasingly omitted for healthy children and healthy adults younger than age 40 years in whom the physical examination is normal and there is no reason to suspect pulmonary or cardiac disease. Additional radiographic or fluoroscopic examinations, sonograms, radioisotopic scans, magnetic resonance imaging, and computerized tomography scans give useful information about the nature of the disease process and its anatomic location and extent. Any organ that is undergoing major surgery should be adequately evaluated with these techniques before the operation.

Electrocardiograms (EKGs) are routinely performed in middle-age and elderly clients undergoing surgery because of the prevalence of ischemic heart disease in these age groups. It is also of value to have a baseline study for comparison in case subsequent EKGs are needed.

Preoperative testing may be done several days before the date of surgery. The type and amount of screening will depend on the age and condition of the client, the nature of the surgery, and the surgeon's preference. Surgeons (doctors who perform surgery) are coming under increasing economic pressure to minimize routine testing procedures. The current trend is based on cost versus benefits, moving away from extensive testing in the absence of indicative/warranting data from the health history and physical examination.

The nurse's role in preoperative testing is to ensure that the ordered tests are performed, that the results are placed in the client's chart, and that abnormal results are reported to the physician immediately.

The physiologic nursing assessment is completed before surgery. Preoperative assessment can take place in the surgeon's office, in the hospital during hospitalization, or in the hospital or ambulatory surgery unit on the day of surgery. The nurse collects client health data by interviewing the client, the family, significant others, and health care providers. Data collection can also be accomplished through review of the client's records, assessment, and/or consultation. Assessment is essential to establishing nursing diagnoses and predicting outcomes (Association of Perioperative Registered Nurses [AORN], 2002b). When performing the nursing assessment, the nurse screens the client for risks that may contribute to complications in the perioperative period. The nurse's role in the preoperative phase ensures client safety, understanding, and compliance with health care treatment. The variables affecting surgical status are discussed following.

Age

Surgery can be performed on individuals of any age, although persons at both extremes of age (infants and elders) may be at greater risk for complications. Infants can easily become dehydrated or fluid overloaded with resultant electrolyte imbalances. Because their metabolic rate is two to three times that of adults, infants can have formula up to 6 hours before surgery, and breastfed infants may be nursed up to 4 hours before surgery. Infants may then have clear liquids for up to 2 hours before surgery.

Body temperature regulation and the renal, immune, and respiratory systems are different in infants than in

LIFE CYCLE CONSIDERATIONS

Surgery in the Elderly Client

Morbidity and mortality rates for surgical clients older than age 90 years are much higher than for those age 70 to 75 years (Hogstel, 2001). Elderly clients do not tolerate emergency or long, complicated surgery as well as do younger clients because of a lesser ability to adapt to physical and psychological stress.

adults. Renal function in the infant is comparatively less efficient because of a lower glomerular filtration rate and less efficient renal tubular function (Fortunato, 2000). This may lead to retention of anesthesia and medications and to fluid overload. Because of a comparatively larger ratio of body surface area to body mass, infants are also more prone to hypothermia when placed in a cool environment or when large areas of their body surface is exposed. Furthermore, an immature immune system renders the infant more susceptible to infections. Because of a smaller and less developed anatomic structure and enlarged tongue and lymphoid tissue, the infant is also more prone to respiratory obstruction. The nursing process and nursing care must be tailored to meet the unique needs of the infant client.

Elderly clients experience many physiologic changes associated with aging and are more likely to have degenerative disease in many organs. Elders are more likely to become dehydrated and are thus less able to adapt to fluid loss during surgery. The elderly client is also more sensitive to central nervous system depressants used during the perioperative period; however, even elderly clients can favorably tolerate extensive surgery when carefully assessed and managed.

Nutritional Status

Nutritional assessment includes evaluation of individual deficiencies or excesses that can place the client at greater risk for complications during surgery. Surgery increases the body's need for nutrients necessary for tissue healing and resistance to infection.

Nutritional deficiencies place the client at higher risk for fluid and electrolyte imbalance, delayed wound healing, and wound infections. The malnourished individual may have diminished stores of carbohydrates and fats; in such instances, proteins are utilized for energy instead of tissue building and restoration. In addition to carbohydrates and fats, vitamins B complex and C are also significant, because these vitamins are essential to healing. Poor nutritional status can also adversely affect liver and kidney function, leaving the client with a poor tolerance for anesthetic agents and a tendency for bleeding.

Nutritional excesses or obesity increase the risk for respiratory, cardiovascular, and gastrointestinal complications. Obesity makes access to the surgical site more difficult, which prolongs surgical time and increases the amount of anesthetic agents required. Because inhalation anesthetics are absorbed by and stored in adipose tissue and released postoperatively, recovery time from anesthesia is slower in the overweight client. Adipose tissue is less vascular and more difficult to suture, which predisposes the client to wound infection, delayed wound healing, and increased incidence of wound complications, including postoperative incisional hernias. Failure to exercise and ambulate increases the chances of decreased respiratory function accompanied by atelectasis and pneumonia and also may lead to decreased wound healing and an increased risk of thrombus formation. Often, obese clients also have other chronic conditions, such as hypertension or diabetes mellitus, that increase the likelihood of surgical complications. In some surgical situations, such as joint replacement, surgery may be delayed until nutritional status improves and the client loses weight.

Fluid and Electrolyte Status

Dehydration and hypovolemia, with correlating electrolyte disturbances, predispose a client to complications during and after surgery. Both may be caused by diarrhea, excessive nasogastric suctioning, inadequate oral intake, vomiting, and/or bleeding. The complications of fluid and electrolyte imbalance are numerous and varied. Changes in fluid and electrolyte balance affect cellular metabolism, renal function, and oxygen concentration in the circulation. Nursing care focuses on administering parenteral fluids or blood products as prescribed, keeping a detailed intake and output record, and evaluating results of laboratory studies.

Respiratory Status

Respiratory assessment should include detection of acute and chronic problems. Because acute respiratory infections may lead to bronchospasms or laryngospasms, surgery for clients with these conditions may be delayed or contraindicated. Chronic respiratory problems, such as asthma and chronic obstructive pulmonary disease, impair the client's gas exchange and increase the risk associated with inhalation anesthetic agents. Clients with chronic respiratory problems are more likely to develop atelectasis and pneumonia.

Respiratory assessment as performed by the nurse includes assessing breath sounds, color of the skin and mucous membranes, and for shortness of breath (dyspnea) and coughing. All clients, and especially those clients who smoke and have chronic lung disease, should be taught deep breathing, use of incentive spirometry, coughing, and preoperative turning.

Cardiovascular Status

Cardiovascular assessment focuses on such diseases as angina, recent myocardial infarction or cardiac surgery, hemophilia, hypertension, and congestive heart failure. Clients with a history of cardiac disease are prone to developing complications such as dysrhythmias, hypotension, myocardial infarction, congestive heart failure, cardiac arrest, stroke, shock, deep vein thrombosis, thrombophlebitis, or pulmonary embolism.

PROFESSIONAL TIP

Client's Psychological Condition

The client "who fears dying while under anesthesia runs a greater risk of cardiac arrest on the operating table than [do] clients with known cardiac disease" (Fortunato, 2000).

- The psychological condition of the client can have a stronger influence than does the physical condition.
- Encourage clients to express their feelings and fears about receiving anesthetic and having surgery.
- Observe the client for nonverbal clues indicating anxiety.
- To reduce client anxiety, explain what will be happening throughout the surgical experience.

Also assess for anxiety; elevated blood pressure; slow, rapid, or irregular pulse; chest pain; edema; coolness or cyanosis/discoloration of extremities; weakness; and shortness of breath (dyspnea). All clients must be taught postoperative leg exercises to prevent thrombophlebitis. The goal of nursing care is to improve the client's cardiovascular condition to the highest degree possible by promoting rest alternated with activity; encouraging a low-sodium and low-cholesterol diet; administering heart medications; and judiciously administering parenteral fluids and recording intake and output.

Renal and Hepatic Status

Because many medications and anesthetic agents are detoxified by the liver and excreted by the kidneys, renal and hepatic sufficiency constitute a major concern. Renal disease affects fluid and electrolyte balance and protein equilibrium. Liver disease may be accompanied by bleeding tendencies or carbohydrate, fat, and amino acid imbalances that impair wound healing and increase the risk of infection. Assess for symptoms of urinary frequency, dysuria, and anuria, and record the color and amount of the urine. Also assess for a history of bleeding tendencies, easy bruising, nosebleeds, and use of anticoagulants. The most commonly ordered preoperative tests to assess renal function are urinalysis, blood urea nitrogen (BUN), and creatinine. The most common liver tests are prothrombin time (PT), partial thromboplastin time (PTT), bilirubin, and the liver enzymes alanine aminotransferase (ALT) and aspartate aminotransferase (AST). Nursing care focuses on administering fluids and adequate nutrition, monitoring fluid intake and output, and evaluating results of laboratory tests.

Neurological, Musculoskeletal, and Integumentary Status

Assess the client's overall mental status, including level of consciousness; orientation to person, place, and time; and the ability to understand and follow instructions. Note skin condition including turgor and any rashes, bruises, lesions, or previous incisions. Assess

CLIENT TEACHING

Postoperative Leg Exercises

Activity	Instructions
Leg lifts	1. While lying on back or in a semi-sitting position, bend the leg and raise it. 2. Hold for count of five. 3. Lower leg to the bed. 4. Repeat five times then proceed to other leg. Perform every hour.
Dorsiflexion and hyperextension of ankles	1. Flex ankles and raise toes toward head, stretching posterior calf. 2. Hold for count of two. 3. Relax. 4. Repeat five times then proceed to other foot. Perform every hour.
Foot circles	1. Point the toe and raise the leg slightly off the bed. 2. Use the great toe to trace a circle in the air, first to the right and then to the left. 3. Repeat five times then proceed to other foot. Perform every hour.

client mobility and sensation through observation of both range of motion and ability to ambulate and through client statements. Note any abnormalities, injuries, or previous surgery and assess the risk for falls. The presence of internal or external prostheses or implants such as pacemakers, heart valves, or joint prosthesis is also noted, because the presence of these may necessitate preoperative antibiotics.

Thin clients, clients undergoing long surgical procedures or vascular procedures, and elderly clients are the most vulnerable to neurological, musculoskeletal, or integumentary injuries. Some underlying disease processes, such as edema, infection, cancer, osteoporosis, arthritic joints, or neck or back problems, also place a client at higher risk for injury. Clients who are malnourished, anemic, obese, hypovolemic, paralyzed, or diabetic are also prone to skin breakdown. Information gathered about the neurological, musculoskeletal, and integumentary systems is used to prepare the surgical site, for surgical positioning, and as a comparative basis for postoperative assessments and complication screening.

Endocrine and Immunological Status

Clients with diabetes should be scheduled as early in the morning as possible, and a fasting glucose drawn immediately before surgery. Surgery is a stressor, and stress raises the serum glucose level in the client with diabetes. Thus the morning dose of insulin may need to be adjusted.

When anesthetized during surgery, the diabetic client exhibits very few symptoms of glucose imbalance. Serum glucose must therefore be checked frequently during surgery, usually by the anesthesia provider. Stability is attained by the administration of insulin, glucose, or both. Besides hyperglycemia and hypoglycemia, a diabetic client is more prone to fluid and electrolyte imbalances; infection including respiratory and urinary tract infections; neurogenic bladder; impaired wound healing; ketoacidosis; deep vein thrombosis; thrombophlebitis; and pulmonary embolism.

Because the immunological system protects the client from infections, the immunocompromised surgical client is very prone to infection. Clients receiving steroids or chemotherapy, or who have systemic lupus erythematosus, Addison's disease, or acquired immunodeficiency syndrome (AIDS) are considered to be immunocompromised. The immune response in these clients is weakened or deficient, resulting in an increased incidence of infection. Because surgery breaks the integrity of the skin and the normal inflammatory response is suppressed, wound healing may be impaired. Strict adherence to aseptic technique (covered later in this chapter) is thus even more imperative. Prevention of infection is crucial in these clients. The role of the nurse is to communicate the presence of potential immunosuppression to other health care team members involved in the client's care and to help prevent infection by practicing aseptic technique.

Medications

Knowledge of the client's use of drugs for recreational or therapeutic purposes is essential to preoperative assessment. The history of medication usage by the client should include type and frequency of use for over-the-counter, prescription, and street drugs. The use of certain drugs can affect the client's reaction to anesthetic agents and surgery. Some drugs increase surgical risks; these medications usually are temporarily discontinued before surgery. Other medications, such as heart or hypoglycemic medications, may still be given even though the client is to undergo surgery; the surgeon or anesthesia provider will write specific orders in such instances. Dosages of medications may also be adjusted during the perioperative period.

Chronic alcohol use increases surgical risk because it is often accompanied by impaired nutrition and liver disease. Postoperatively, the client may exhibit delirium tremens or acute withdrawal syndrome. Furthermore, pain medication may be less effective.

Psychosocial Health Assessment

The psychosocial health status of the client is also assessed. The nurse elicits the client's perceptions of surgery and the expected outcome. The nurse also ascertains the client's coping mechanisms and the client's knowledge level and ability to understand. The data collected are incorporated into nursing care throughout the perioperative experience.

Cultural beliefs can influence a client's perception of surgery. For example, some cultures believe that surgery is a "final effort" performed only when all other possible treatments have been of no avail. Furthermore, surgeries that cause changes in the appearance of the body can alter body image and self-esteem; the client may worry about being sexually attractive or active after surgery.

Clients should be provided the opportunity to express their spiritual values and beliefs. Many clients wish to see a member of the clergy before having surgery.

Surgical Consent

An **informed consent** is a legal form signed by the client and witnessed by another person that grants permission to the client's physician to perform the procedure described by the physician. An informed consent is needed whenever:

- Anesthesia is used.
- The procedure is considered invasive.
- The procedure is nonsurgical but has more than a slight risk of complications (such as with an arteriogram).
- Radiation or cobalt therapy is used.

Informed consent protects both the client (against unauthorized procedures) and the physician and the health care facility and its employees (against claims that an unauthorized procedure was performed). Although the ultimate responsibility for obtaining the informed consent lies with the physician, the nurse often obtains and witnesses the client's signature and ensures that the client signs the consent form voluntarily and is alert and comprehending of the action.

Most hospitals use a standard preprinted form. The information written by the health care personnel must be specific to the individual client. The client's signature on the consent form indicates the information has been read and is correct. The client has the right to refuse treatment even after the consent has been signed. When this occurs, the nurse must inform the physician immediately of the client's decision.

Preoperative Teaching

The client about to have surgery is at risk for knowledge deficit related to preoperative procedures and protocols and postoperative expectations. The potential benefits of preoperative teaching include reduced anxiety and more rapid recovery with fewer complications and shorter hospitalization. Reduction in anxiety has a secondary benefit: The client usually requires less medication for pain. The purposes of preoperative teaching are to (1) answer questions and concerns about surgery; (2) ascertain the client's knowledge of the intended surgery; (3) ascertain the need or desire for additional information; and (4) provide information in a manner most conducive to learning.

One-on-one sessions constitute the most personal method of instruction, but try to include the family or significant other when possible. The level of learning increases when more than one teaching medium is used. For example, using materials such as videotapes, charts, tours, anatomic models, pictures, and brochures reinforces both visual and auditory learning. Demonstration followed by return demonstration is helpful. Written instructions serve as a reference for later use. Instructions should be simple, using terms the client can understand. Any unfamiliar words or concepts should be thoroughly explained.

Clients are often interested in any information that describes the sights, sounds, tastes, feelings, odors, and temperature of what they are about to experience. For example, the feeling of relaxation from preoperative medications; the sounds of instruments or equipment in the operating room (OR); the pressure from the automatic blood pressure cuff; the warmth or coolness of skin-preparation solutions; or the brightness of the operating room lights are all sensations the client may experience. Analogies or stories of real or fictitious situations of sensory experiences help the client understand. The teaching methods used strongly influence the client's learning and retention of information.

Preoperative teaching should begin as soon as surgery is agreed upon. Instructions given over the phone and/or mailed to the client during the time leading up to surgery are beneficial. Just before surgery, a brief review with additional information tailored to the needs of the client may be given. Give the client an opportunity to ask questions.

Information should always be targeted to the client's needs and according to the client's level of knowledge and anxiety. Mild to moderate anxiety actually heightens a person's alertness and motivates learning. Mildly

CLIENT TEACHING

Preoperative Teaching

- Introduce self
  - Identify role in client's care
- Determine client's knowledge level and need or desire for additional information
- Explain the routine for the day of surgery
  - Restricted food or fluid intake
  - Intravenous fluids
  - Premedication
  - Time of surgery
  - Anticipated length of surgery
  - Transportation to the operating room
  - Special skin preparations
  - Type of surgical incision (Figure 30-1)
- Familiarize the client with the operating room environment
  - Operating room lights and table
  - Accessory equipment
  - Monitoring equipment
  - Anesthesia induction
- Include significant others
  - Time to arrive at the hospital
  - Location of surgical waiting area
  - What to expect when client returns to the unit
- Explain postanesthesia care unit (PACU)
  - Location of recovery room
  - Purpose of recovery room
  - Routine of postanesthesia care
- Identify anticipated dressings, drains, catheters, casts, etc.
- Demonstrate and evaluate client's proficiency with:
  - Coughing and deep breathing exercises
  - Turning
  - Incentive spirometry
  - Extremity exercises
  - Any special transfer procedures or aids required after surgery
- Describe pain management strategies appropriate for the specific surgical procedure

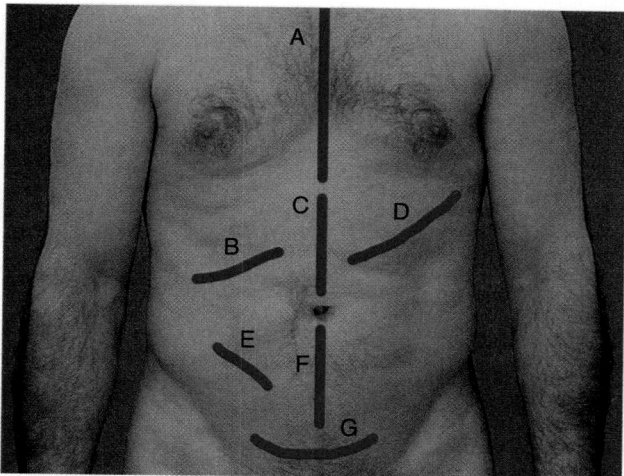

Figure 30-1 *Common Surgical Incisions:* **A**, *Sternal Split;* **B**, *Oblique subcostal;* **C**, *Upper Vertical Midline;* **D**, *Thoracoabdominal;* **E**, *Mcburney;* **F**, *Lower Vertical Midline;* **G**, *Pfannenstiel*

Particular attention should be given to differentiating between right and left operative sites.

Special care is given to the preparation of the operative site to lessen the chance of infection. The operative site is thoroughly cleansed with an antiseptic soap such as povidone-iodine to reduce the number of microorganisms on the skin. Typically, the operative site is not shaved, but if shaving is to be performed, it is done in the operating room immediately before surgery. To reduce the number of bacteria in the gastrointestinal tract for gastrointestinal, peritoneal, perianal, or pelvic surgery, an enema is ordered. Enemas prevent contamination of the peritoneal area by fecal content passed during surgery. The reduction in colon size related to the loss of bulk also helps prevent colon injury and increases visualization of the operative site. Enemas are usually given the night before surgery. If the enema is to be done at home, give the client detailed instructions. Many types of surgery require special preparations. The specific protocol for each surgical procedure is available from the health care facility or the physician.

 Safety: Iodine Allergy, Latex Allergy
- Each client must be asked about allergy to iodine and latex.
- If a client is allergic to either, document the allergy on the client's record and inform the surgeon and OR personnel so that an iodine-free solution and latex-free equipment will be used.

Check the client's vital signs including blood pressure, temperature, pulse, and respirations. Some changes in vital signs are normal as a result of anxiety. If marked differences exist from the baseline data, however, the surgeon must be notified.

Assist the client in putting on a hospital gown, hair cap, and, if ordered, antiembolic hose. The client's legs must be properly measured for the correct size (McConnell, 2002). Institutional policy usually requires that all jewelry be removed. This includes body jewelry

anxious clients should receive the most complete instructions. Moderately anxious clients should receive less information but more attention to specific areas of concern. Severely anxious clients should receive only basic information but should be encouraged to verbalize their concerns. Clients in a state of panic are unable to learn; in such cases no instruction is given, and the surgeon should be notified.

Physical Preparation

Extremely close attention must be given to identifying the proper client both verbally and by reading the identification name band and to verifying the operative procedure. This is completed through client statements, surgeon verification, and the signed surgical consent form.

(AORN, 2001). Hairpins, wigs, and prostheses must also be removed. The nurse is responsible for recording the disposition of any personal items removed for surgery. If policy requires, nail polish (from at least one nail, if dark polish) is removed so that oxygen saturation may be read via pulse oximetry. Makeup is also removed so that skin color can be observed.

Allergies to medication, food, and chemicals (including contrast agents) are verified, as are previous blood reactions. The nurse must differentiate between a medication intolerance and a true allergic reaction. With a medication intolerance, the client may suffer side effects that are unpleasant. For example, many clients experience nausea when given meperidine (Demerol); although unpleasant, this is not a drug allergy. A true allergy produces a skin reaction or anaphylactic reaction, where the client experiences cardiorespiratory reactions that may be life threatening, such as hypotension and pulmonary edema. A client with multiple food allergies is also prone to hypersensitivities to medications. When allergies are identified, the client's chart is marked accordingly, and an allergy wrist band is put on the client. By being aware of and alerting other team members to the client's allergies, client safety and comfort are maintained.

Verify the NPO (nothing by mouth) status of the client for the time specified by the surgeon's order. Restricting oral intake reduces the possibility of aspiration. If surgery takes place in the afternoon, the client may have a clear liquid breakfast if ordered by the surgeon. Careful client instruction is required because surgery may need to be postponed if the client eats or drinks.

In addition to the previously outlined preparations, remove dentures and bridgework to prevent loss, damage, and possible dislodgement and airway obstruction during the surgery. Ensure that the client has an empty bladder by allowing time for the client to void before transfer to surgery.

Identify any sensory deficits of the client and communicate this information to other health care team members. Glasses, contact lenses, and hearing aids are usually removed to prevent loss or damage; if policy allows, however, it is best to leave these items in place so the client is better able to see and hear. Then the nurse is responsible for communicating the presence of these aids to the surgical team members.

The surgeon or anesthesiologist (a doctor trained in providing anesthesia) may order preoperative medica-

LIFE CYCLE CONSIDERATIONS

Preparation for Surgery

For pediatric clients:

- Provide physical and psychological preparation at the child's level of understanding.
- Listen carefully to the child to promote understanding.
- Ask the child to point to the operative site on self or doll.
- Be honest and truthful.

The elder client may have:

- Increased risk of complications including infection
- Increased incidence of coexisting conditions
- Unpredictable response to medications and anesthetics
- Greater need for support from family and significant other
- Increased skin and bone fragility
- Nutritional and financial deficiencies
- Impaired vision and hearing
- Impaired or slowed thought processes and cognitive abilities
- Fear of death, loss of independence, and change in lifestyle

tion. The nurse gives the medication by the prescribed route (intramuscular, intravenous, or oral) at the specified time (typically 1 hour before surgery). Preoperative medications may be ordered "on call," which means that the nurse is notified by a member of the surgical team when the preoperative medication is to be given. Before administering the medication, ask the client to void. After administering the preoperative medication, raise the side rails of the gurney or bed, put the bed in the lowest position, and instruct the client not to get up without assistance.

When the surgical team is ready, the client is transported on a gurney by a member of the OR team, typically an orderly. The client is always transported feet first and with the side rails up to ensure safety and minimize the likelihood of dizziness and nausea. The client may be taken to a preoperative holding area first (Figure 30-2). The nurse instructs the family or significant others where to wait.

The information collected as part of preoperative preparation is documented in the client record, usually on a preoperative checklist. Figure 30-3 illustrates a typical preoperative checklist. This checklist is completed before the client leaves the clinical unit or upon the client's admission to ambulatory surgery. The nurse must also verbally communicate to other health care members any necessary information collected.

INTRAOPERATIVE PHASE

The **intraoperative phase** is the time during the surgical experience that begins when the client is transferred to the operating room table and ends when the client is admitted to the postanesthesia care unit (PACU).

PROFESSIONAL TIP

Implementing NPO Status

- Explain reasons for NPO status to the client.
- Remove any food and water from the client's overbed table and nightstand.
- Mark the client's door and bed with an NPO sign.
- Mark the client's Kardex and other nursing information sources.
- Notify the dietary department.

Figure 30-2 *The holding area is used for clients who are waiting to have surgery.*

Physical Description of the Operating Room Environment

For the purposes of preventing wound infections, the surgical suite is environmentally controlled. Personnel restriction and geographic isolation from other areas of the hospital or clinic are part of this control. Constant filtered airflow and positive air pressure in the operating rooms also aid in environmental control. Clean areas and contaminated areas are separated within the suite. Equipment and supplies needed for each client are in the surgical suite so members of the surgical team do not have to leave the area.

Operating rooms vary in size depending on the amount of equipment needed for each particular type of operation. Supplies and furniture are limited to prevent dust collection and are usually made of stainless steel to withstand corrosive disinfectants. Furniture and equipment are easily movable on wheels. In addition to general illumination from ceiling lights, the operative site is illuminated by overhead operating lights. Figure 30-4 shows a typical operating room. The temperature of the room can be adjusted but usually is maintained at a cool 66°F to 68°F. This provides comfort for the surgical team (the members of which wear gowns, gloves, and masks under hot lights). This temperature also is an unfavorable environment for bacterial incubation and growth.

The client entering the operating room is confronted with an environment that is most likely unfamiliar. The operating room is cold. The surgical team members dress in surgical scrubs and have their hair covered by caps and their faces covered by surgical masks, making them appear impersonal and distant. The sounds of equipment being prepared can be unfamiliar and alarming. The terminology used in conversations among OR personnel may be foreign. These elements combined with the sight of ominous overhead lights and the feel of the hard operating room table may increase the client's fear, anxiety, and feelings of powerlessness.

Members of the Surgical Team

The surgical team is a group of hospital personnel assigned to see a client successfully through an operative procedure. At no other time during hospitalization will the ratio of personnel to client be higher than when the client is undergoing surgery. The surgical team includes **sterile** (without microorganisms) team members: the surgeon, the **first assistant** (a physician or RN who assists the surgeon in performing hemostasis, tissue retraction, and wound closure), and the **scrub nurse** (an LP/VN, RN, or surgical technologist who, under the direction of the circulating nurse, prepares and maintains the integrity, safety, and efficiency of the sterile field throughout the operation). Sterile team members scrub their arms and hands, don sterile gowns and gloves, and then perform their duties in the sterile field. The **sterile field** is that area surrounding the client and the surgical site that is free from all microorganisms. It is created by using sterile drapes to drape the work area and the client. Nonsterile team members include the anesthesia provider (an anesthesiologist or anesthetist) and **circulating nurse** (an RN responsible for management of personnel, equipment, supplies, environment, and communication throughout a surgical procedure). The nonsterile team members perform their duties outside of the sterile field. Each team member has a clearly defined role and duties. Clear communication among team members and coordination of their activities improve the most favorable outcome for the client.

Asepsis

Prevention of infection is the responsibility of the entire surgical team. The environment of the surgical client contains both pathogenic (disease-producing) and nonpathogenic microorganisms. When the skin, a prime barrier to infection, is broken, as during surgery, susceptibility to a bacterial invasion increases. Bacteria carried by dust or nose and throat droplets are easily transported by air currents.

Asepsis is the absence of pathogenic microorganisms. **Aseptic technique** is a collection of principles used to control and/or prevent the transfer of pathogenic microorganisms from sources within (endogenous) and outside (exogenous) the client. For example, scrubbed persons wear sterile gowns and gloves; sterile drapes are used to create a sterile field; items used in a sterile field are sterilized; and those working within a sterile field maintain the integrity of the sterile field. Aseptic technique is applicable to other nursing functions such as changing dressings, inserting a Foley catheter, or preparing for an obstetrical delivery. Thus the practice of aseptic technique is not confined to the OR, but applies to other clinical nursing units and other procedures as well.

The practice of aseptic technique requires the development of **sterile conscience,** an individual's personal sense of honesty and integrity with regard to adherence

CRITICAL THINKING

Sterile Conscience

How can you use a sterile conscience when providing nursing care?

PAGE 1

RUN DATE: 05/15/00 RUN TIME: 0823
Spohn Health Patient Care System "LIVE"
NURSING PROTOCOL DICTIONARY
LAST UPDATE 03/03/99 TIME 1044 USER AGA4642

MNEMONIC SSC-7043
ACTIVE Y
DESCRIPTION PRE-OP CHECKLIST/SURGICAL CHECKLIST

SURGICAL CHECKLIST
(CIRCLE APPROPRIATE CHOICES)

NURSING UNIT
YES | NO | N/A

HISTORY AND PHYSICAL ON CHART; DICTATED; PRE-OP NOTE
IF HAS TAKEN DIET PILLS WITHIN 2 WEEKS; NOTIFY ANESTHESIOLOGIST
ANESTHESIA PRE-OP NOTE
SURGICAL PERMIT: SIGNED AND WITNESSED
ACCEPTANCE/REFUSAL TRANSFUSION INDICATED ON FORM(S)
IF PATIENT IS A DNR THE "DNR STATUS DURING SURGERY" FORM IS COMPLETED & SIGNED
MEDICAL POWER OF ATTORNEY
AUTOLOGOUS BLOOD AVAILABILITY CHECK
ACCEPTANCE/REFUSAL PREGNANCY TEST (FORM SIGNED & ORDER ON CHART IF APPROPRIATE)
LAB ORDERED AND COMPLETE
CBC WITHIN PAST 7 DAYS
PT/PTT
SMA 7
LMB REMOVAL FORM SIGNED #900960
VITAL SIGNS: T____ P____ R____ BP____ FHT____
FINGERSTICK RESULTS: _____ @ TIME ____
ELIMINATION: VOIDED _____ CATHETER ____
MAR ON CHART
02 NEEDED FOR TRANSPORT
TELEMETRY NEEDED FOR TRANSPORT
FISTULA/GRAFT; INFECTION; MASTECTOMY - R OR L
I.D. BAND ON

PATIENT CARE SERVICES
SURGICAL CHECKLIST
DATE: _____
7043 page 1 of 3 pages

PAGE 2

RUN DATE: 05/15/00 RUN TIME: 0823
Spohn Health Patient Care System "LIVE"
NURSING PROTOCOL DICTIONARY
LAST UPDATE 03/03/99 TIME 1044 USER AGA4642

MNEMONIC SSC-7043
ACTIVE Y
DESCRIPTION PRE-OP CHECKLIST/SURGICAL CHECKLIST

SURGICAL CHECKLIST CONTINUED
(CIRCLE APPROPRIATE CHOICES)

NURSING UNIT
YES | NO | N/A

ALLERGY BAND ON: ALLERGIES VERIFIED WITH PATIENT
NPO AFTER: 12M____ BREAKFAST____ OTHER____
PRE-OP: ENEMA____ DOUCHE____ BOWEL PREP____
SHOWER____ SCRUB____ PRE-OP SHAVE____ (LOCATION)
JEWELRY REMOVED/SECURED
DENTURES/PARTIAL PLATE, HEARING AID
GLASSES, CONTACT LENS
OTHER
RAILS UP-BED IN LOW POSITION

PATIENT/FAMILY PATIENT INFORMATION OBTAINED FROM? PT/FAMILY
PRE-OP MEDICATIONS | INT | TIME | ROUTE | SITE

I.V. FLUIDS:
LIDO/WHEAL YES____ NO____ WITH ORDER ONLY: DATE:____
SITE:____ GAUGE:____
SIG/TITLE:____ SIG/TITLE:____
INT: SIGNATURE____ INT: SIGNATURE____ :INT: SIGNATURE____
DATE/TIME____

PATIENT CARE SERVICES
SURGICAL CHECKLIST
DATE: _____
7043 NEW: 04/88 REV: 02/25/99
page 2 of 3 pages

PAGE 3

RUN DATE: 05/15/00 RUN TIME: 0823
Spohn Health Patient Care System "LIVE"
NURSING PROTOCOL DICTIONARY
LAST UPDATE 03/03/99 TIME 1044 USER AGA4642

MNEMONIC SSC-7043
ACTIVE Y
DESCRIPTION PRE-OP CHECKLIST/SURGICAL CHECKLIST

SURGICAL CHECKLIST

GOAL: Patient will verbalize understanding of pre- and post-op routines to reduce anxiety and fear.

IMPLEMENT OR INTERVENTIONS
1. Effective pre-post op teaching, surgery, recovery room, and post op care.

INITIAL/ CIRCLE AREAS OF PRE OP TEACHING INSTRUCTIONS
Length of O.R. and length of recovery room
Type of anesthesia
Instruct family where to wait and return to room
Post Op room location (i.e. return to same room/ new room)
Turn, cough, deep breaths, leg exercises, abdominal pillow
I.V's / antibiotic
PCA and pain control
Foley / continuous bladder irrigation
TED's / pneumatic stockings
Dressings / drains
Open Heart Teaching by:
Other: (Specify)
Phantom Pain
Offer Psychological Counseling
Patient informed of CCTV Pre-Op teaching program

____ Date / time/ instructions given
Initial:____ Patient verbalized understanding of pre- & post-op teaching plan
Initial:____ Initial:____
Signature:____ Signature:____

SURGICAL CHECKLIST
7043
NEW: 04/88 REV: 02/25/99
page 3 of 3 pages

Figure 30-3 Sample Preoperative Checklist (Courtesy CHRISTUS Spohn Health System, Corpus Christi, TX)

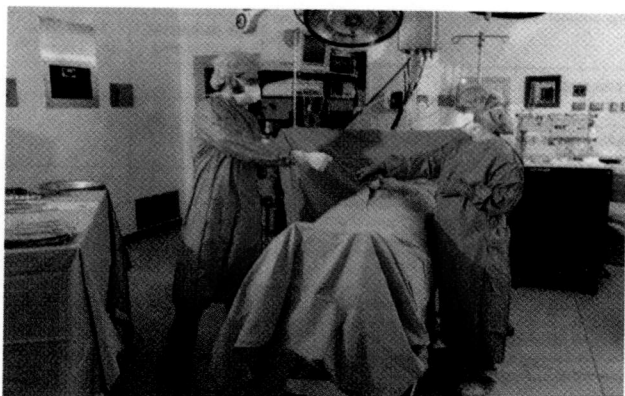

Figure 30-4 *Typical Operating Room and Proper Surgical Attire (Photo courtesy of the U. S. Army)*

Operative site

Figure 30-5 *Skin Preparation at Operative Site*

to the principles of aseptic technique. Aseptic technique must be strictly followed. Doing so requires constant assessment and monitoring of self and others. It is sometimes easier or less expensive to overlook an infraction of aseptic technique rather than to correct that infraction. This must *never* be allowed. Compromising the principles of aseptic technique may increase the likelihood of infection and, thus, harm to the client.

Surgical Hand Scrub

An item is considered sterile when all microorganisms are removed. The skin, however, cannot be sterilized. For this reason, the sterile team members wear gloves as barriers between the sterile field and the skin. Because accidental tearing or puncturing of the surgical glove and resultant introduction of microorganisms into the surgical wound are possible, the sterile team members must take measures to lower the number of microorganisms on their hands and arms. The surgical hand scrub, performed before gowning and gloving, removes soil and transient (not always present and easily removed) microorganisms from the hands and forearms. The antimicrobial soap used lowers the count of resident (almost always present and not easily removed) microorganisms and continues to prevent sudden bacterial rebound or regrowth after the scrub is completed. The surgical scrub thus reduces the possibility of transmission of microorganisms from the surgical team to the client.

Watches, rings, and bracelets are removed before the surgical hand scrub. Fingernails must be short, clean, and healthy. Artificial nails cannot be worn (AORN, 2002a), although unchipped fingernail polish that has been applied within the last 4 days may be allowed (AORN, 2002b). The hands and forearms should be free of breaks in skin integrity.

Surgical Skin Preparation

Like the skin of the surgical team members, the skin surface at the client's incision site also cannot be sterilized. As with the surgical hand scrub, the goal of surgical skin preparation at the client's incision site is to lower the number of microorganisms on and near the incision site.

Typically, the client is asked to shower or to wash the operative site either before arriving at the surgical facility or immediately before surgery. The client is then transferred to the operating room. After general anesthesia induction or regional block completion or before local infiltration of the operative site, the circulating nurse performs the surgical skin preparation. Using aseptic technique, the circulating nurse scrubs the area with an antimicrobial soap. Typically the soap used is povidone-iodine (containing iodine) or chlorhexidine, thus potential allergies to iodine must be verified. The circulating nurse scrubs a generous area surrounding the operative site to allow for extension of the surgical incision if the need arises. The scrub is completed in an ever-widening circular motion from the incision site, which is considered clean, to the periphery, which is considered dirty (Figure 30-5). Once the periphery is reached, the sponge is discarded, never brought back toward the center of the area. The concept of cleansing from the center (incision site) to the periphery also applies to skin preparation for other procedures such as intravenous (IV) insertion, chest tube insertion, thoracentesis, or subclavian catheter placement. Surgical skin preparation lasts 5 to 10 minutes. After the scrub is completed, the area is blotted dry with sterile towels. An antiseptic solution, often also iodine based, is then applied in the same manner.

Intraoperative Nursing Care

The success of nursing care in the operating room is measured by client outcomes. The AORN has established client outcome standards for evaluating perioperative clients upon completion of surgery. These outcomes state that the client is to be free from infection and injury related to positioning, foreign objects, or chemical, physical, and electrical hazards. In addition, skin integrity and fluid and electrolyte balance are to be maintained. Consequently, nursing care in the operating room strives to provide these standards to all clients undergoing surgery.

Although the responsibilities of the circulating nurse and scrub nurse may seem to be a series of tasks or duties, these same tasks and duties provide quality nursing care to the client. The nurse planning for surgery is involved in selection of equipment and supplies, room preparation, and formation of the sterile field before the delivery of actual nursing care.

Safety: Electrical Equipment

- Electrical equipment must be plugged into grounded outlets.
- Electrical equipment must be regularly checked by a bioelectronic technician.
- A grounding pad must be placed under the client and in direct contact with the client's skin.

After completion of surgery, the circulating nurse applies and secures the dressing. When the anesthesia provider is ready, the client is transferred to a stretcher or a gurney. The unconscious or semiconscious client is placed in a side-lying or semiprone position unless contraindicated by the surgical procedure. If the client is supine, the client's head is turned to the side in case the client vomits. The client is then taken to the PACU, accompanied by the anesthesia provider and another surgical team member.

POSTOPERATIVE PHASE

The **postoperative phase** is the time during the surgical experience that begins with the end of the surgical procedure and lasts until the client is discharged not just from the hospital or institution, but from medical care by the surgeon. Upon transfer from the operating room, the client usually goes to the PACU (Figure 30-6). All clients who receive general anesthesia, spinal anesthesia, or regional anesthesia are admitted to the PACU. Occasionally, clients who have undergone surgery with local anesthesia or no anesthesia or who have received only IV sedation are placed in the PACU for a short period to be monitored closely until their conditions stabilize. The PACU is usually located next to the operating room. Typically, it is one large room with individual units for clients along the perimeter of the room. Each of these units has an oxygen delivery system, suction, various other supplies, and cardiac, respiratory, and blood pressure monitoring devices. Curtains can be pulled to provide privacy if

needed, but an open view allows continual assessment of all clients.

Postoperative Nursing Care

The postanesthesia care nurse is an RN specially trained in caring for immediate postoperative clients. The goal of postanesthesia nursing care is to promote recovery from anesthesia and the immediate effects of surgery. The postanesthesia nurse has knowledge and skill in recognizing and treating anesthetic and surgical complications very quickly. The postanesthesia nurse is empathetic and is able to assess and manage pain for the client who may not be able to express himself.

Upon the client's arrival in the PACU, the anesthesia provider verbally reviews the client's anesthesia and operative procedure with the postanesthesia nurse. The postanesthesia nurse begins the following nursing assessment and care in the immediate postoperative period:

- Time of arrival in recovery room
- Patency of airway
- Respirations
- Presence of artificial airway devices
    - Oral airway
    - Nasopharyngeal airway
    - Endotracheal airway
- Oxygen saturation
- Need for supplemental oxygen
    - Mode of administration
    - Flow rate
- Breath sounds
- Color of skin, nail beds, and lips
- Presence of cardiac dysrhythmias
- Other vital signs
    - Blood pressure, pulse
- Skin condition (moist or dry, warm or cool) and skin temperature
- Initiate Aldrete Score
- Intravenous infusion
    - Type of solution
    - Amount in bottle or bag
    - Flow rate
    - Appearance and location of IV site
- Dressings
    - Amount and character of drainage
- Drains and tubes
    - Intactness and function
    - Connection to drainage and/or suction
    - Amount and character of drainage
- Level of consciousness
- Activity level
- Other assessments according to surgical procedure
- Pain

The postanesthesia nurse notes the client's arrival time to the unit and immediately begins to assess the patency of the airway by placing a hand above the client's nose and mouth to feel exhalation. The quality and quantity of respirations are then immediately observed, as is the presence of an artificial airway. The client is attached to a pulse oximeter (Figure 30-7), and breath sounds are auscultated. The color and condition of the skin are noted as part of the respiratory assessment. Peripheral cyanosis may be an indication of hypother-

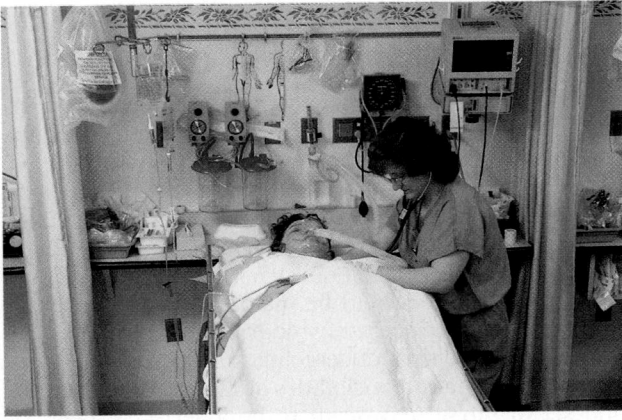

Figure 30-6 *Postanesthesia Care Unit (PACU)*

Figure 30-7 *Client with Pulse Oximeter on Finger*

TABLE 30-2	ALDRETE SCORE/ POSTANESTHETIC RECOVERY SCORE	
Activity	Able to move 4 extremities voluntarily or on command	2
	Able to move 2 extremities voluntarily or on command	1
	Able to move 0 extremities voluntarily or on command	0
Respiration	Able to breathe deeply and cough freely	2
	Dyspnea or limited breathing	1
	Apneic	0
Consciousness	Fully awake	2
	Arousable on calling	1
	Not responding	0
Circulation	B/P ± 20% of preanesthetic level	2
	B/P ± 20% to 50% of preanesthetic level	1
	B/P ± 50% of preanesthetic level	0
Color	Normal	2
	Pale, dusky, blotchy, jaundiced, other	1
	Cyanotic	0

Additional Assessments: Aldrete Score/ Postanesthetic Recovery Score for Clients Having Anesthesia on an Ambulatory Basis

Dressing	Dry and clean	2
	Wet but stationary or marked	1
	Growing area of wetness	0
Pain	Pain free	2
	Mild pain handled by oral medication	1
	Severe pain requiring parenteral medication	0
Ambulation	Able to stand up and walk straight	2
	Vertigo when erect	1
	Dizziness when supine	0
Fasting/ feeding	Able to drink fluids	2
	Nauseated	1
	Nausea and vomiting	0
Urine output	Has voided	2
	Unable to void but comfortable	1
	Unable to void and uncomfortable	0

Courtesy J. Antonio Aldrete, M.D., M.S., Defuniak Springs, FL.

mia rather than respiratory distress. Thus, correlating with the "ABCs" of *a*irway, *b*reathing, and *c*irculation, the respiratory system is assessed first.

Because most clients admitted are unconscious and have received muscle relaxants during surgery, respiratory exchange is often affected. Snoring, stridor, labored chest movement, sternal retractions, cyanosis, and apnea are all signs of respiratory distress. Respiratory distress is the gravest of all complications because respiratory crisis and subsequent death can occur in a matter of minutes if distress is not observed and treated quickly. In the event of any signs of respiratory distress, the postanesthesia nurse must be alert to the possibility of respiratory arrest and be ready to initiate cardiopulmonary resuscitation.

The **Aldrete Score,** also known as the Postanesthetic Recovery Score, is used in PACUs to objectively assess the physical status of clients recovering from anesthesia and serves as a basis for discharge from the PACU (Table 30-2). The Aldrete Score was recently adapted to also assess the readiness of clients for discharge from ambulatory surgery. The first five items are used for discharge from the PACU. Clients are assessed at the time of admission to the PACU and every 15 minutes until discharge. The first five items include assessing activity, respiration, consciousness, circulation, and color (oxygen saturation). Each of the five items is scored from 0 to 2, according to the degree of functional disturbance. The score is expressed as a total score, with 10 being the maximum. Typically, a minimum score of 8 is required for discharge from the PACU.

Fluid intake and output are assessed. The amounts and types of IV solutions hanging are identified, as are any added medications. The IV fluids are infused according to the surgeon's order and are run at a specified rate. The IV site is assessed for patency, redness, and swelling. The client is restrained as necessary to maintain patency of the IV site. All other infusions and irrigations are also assessed.

Dressings and/or peripads are checked for any evidence of bloody drainage and the amount noted so that any subsequent appearance of blood may be accurately evaluated. All drainage tubes are then connected, and the type of drain and the drainage amount are recorded according to physicians' orders. Table 30-3 outlines common types of drains placed in surgery. Urinary output is

TABLE 30-3 DESCRIPTION, USES, AND NURSING CARE OF COMMON DRAINAGE DEVICES PLACED DURING SURGERY

TYPE	EXAMPLE	DESCRIPTION	USES	NURSING CARE
Passive	Penrose	A single-lumen, soft latex tube that works with gravity directly from the surgical incision	To remove drainage when more than a minimal amount of drainage is expected	• Inspect dressing • Check underneath client to ensure drainage has not leaked from the side of the dressing.
	T-tube	A single-lumen tube shaped like a T and made of latex	Used after common bile duct exploration to drain bile from the duct as suture lines heal and swelling decreases	• Always keep a dressing over drain • Check safety pin through end of drain • Attach to a drainage bottle or to a T-tube bag
Active	Hemovac Jackson-Pratt J-Vac Relia Vac Surgivac	Closed wound drainage system with drain and reservoir having self-suction when reservoir is compressed	Used after multiple types of procedures; provides continuous gentle suction of the operative site to increase drainage of serosanguinous fluid and collapse tissue to facilitate healing	• Assess the drainage system as appropriate to client's condition for: 1. Continued drainage 2. Maintained decompression 3. Air-tight tubings 4. Need for emptying • To reactivate suction, wash hands and wear gloves and eye/face protection • Empty reservoirs every 8 hours, when drainage nears the full line, or as ordered by the physician
Passive or active	Davol Sump Axiom Sump	Large, multilumen tube with a larger main port for drainage and/or suction and with smaller side port(s) for irrigation and/or air venting to help prevent tissue from being suctioned against catheter and damaged	To drain intra-abdominal fluids from abscesses, cysts, or hematomas	• Use one of the smaller or sump ports for continuous irrigation • Calculate intake and output carefully with irrigations • Place impervious pads underneath client • Change dressings frequently when saturated • Attach to catheter drainage bag if not attached to suction; do not plug sump ports
	Chest tube ThoraKlex Pleure Vac	Large single-lumen drain attached to closed water-seal drainage system	To drain fluid or air from pleural cavity	• Assess breath sounds and respirations, including depth, rate, symmetry of chest expansion, color of mucous membranes, and presence of crepitus with suction off or tubing clamped • If present, assess amount and type of suction • Ensure that connections are tight and sealed with tape • Keep chest tube drainage reservoir lower than client's chest • Observe for air leaks in air leak indicator or drainage chamber of drainage reservoir • Place petroleum jelly gauze nearby for quick access should the tube become dislodged • Measure drainage at least every 8 hours (more frequently if in a critical care unit or client's condition warrants it) • Clamp or milk the chest tube only if ordered by surgeon • Notify surgeon if drainage is greater than 100 cc/hour • Change drainage system when $2/3$ full

Figure 30-8 *Common Drainage Devices:* **A,** *Penrose Drains;* **B,** *Hemovac;* **C,** *Jackson-Pratt*

also monitored. Scanty urinary drainage (less than 50 cc/hour or as ordered) is reported to the surgeon.

Surgical drains are placed so the wound can drain freely of blood clots, body fluids, pus, and necrotic material that otherwise would collect in the wound and provide a rich medium for bacterial growth. Figure 30-8 illustrates common drainage devices. All drains are inserted at the operative site and exit through the incision or a separate stab wound adjacent to the incision. The type of drain is chosen according to the location of wound, size of wound, and type of drainage anticipated. The use of drains decreases pain and infection and aids wound healing; however, if the wound is draining, the skin is not closed, and a pathway exists for the entrance of microorganisms. Drain sites can thus also be a source of infection. Potential complications of drains include hemorrhage, sepsis, drain loss, and bowel herniation. Nursing care for drains includes assessing the color, character, and odor of drainage; ensuring the patency of the drain (making sure there are no kinks in the tubing); and ensuring that the drain does not accidentally become dislodged. Table 30-4 lists additional nursing care according to surgical procedure.

Part of the neurological assessment involves assessing the activity level or the ability to move extremities voluntarily. The ability to move extremities on command indicates voluntary movement. Hearing is the first sensation to return to the client after having been anesthetized. Clients in the PACU are asked to squeeze the postanesthesia nurse's hands and to plantarflex and dorsiflex the feet.

Continuing Nursing Care in the PACU

After the client has been admitted and assessed in PACU, the postanesthesia nurse checks the surgeon's and the anesthesia provider's orders and initiates any therapy designated for the PACU.

The postanesthesia nurse charts on a separate nursing record for the PACU. Anything unusual must be adequately documented. If vital signs are in the normal range, the postanesthesia nurse checks them every 15 minutes. If vital signs are unstable, they are checked every 5 minutes or as often as necessary until stable. If vital signs fail to stabilize, the surgeon and anesthesia provider are notified. The surgical site is checked at least every 30 minutes. If any initial bleeding has not subsided, the surgeon is notified. Routine checks are continued until the client is discharged from the PACU.

The postanesthesia nurse determines whether the client meets the criteria for discharge from the PACU. Typically, the client's vital signs must be stable and within the client's normal limits. The Aldrete Score must be 8 to 10. If 7 or less, a surgeon's or anesthesia provider's order is required for discharge. Also before client discharge, the dressing must be checked, changed, or reinforced according to orders. All other parameters are reassessed and charted. Institutional protocol dictates minimum stay in the PACU. Adults are typically kept in the PACU for a minimum of 1 hour, except outpatients, who go to the ambulatory surgery unit when they are awake and when postmedication time has been fulfilled. Children are typically kept in the PACU until they are awake, stable, and have an Aldrete Score of 8 to 10. When criteria for discharge are met, the postanesthesia nurse calls the clinical unit or ambulatory surgery unit and reports the client's name, vitals, surgery, and any other pertinent information. The client is then transferred to the appropriate unit.

Later Postoperative Nursing Care

Before the client's arrival in the clinical unit, the nurse has prepared for the client. The linen has been changed, the bed linen folded down, and the room cleared of clutter. Special required equipment, as directed by the postanesthesia nurse, has been gathered. An emesis basin and tissue are available. The nurse is ready to assess the client in an organized manner, focusing on the body system affected by surgery.

Upon the client's arrival in the clinical unit, the nurse assists in transferring the client to the bed. Nursing assessment and care of the client upon admission to the clinical unit includes the following:

- Time of arrival in unit
- Transfer from cart to bed
    - Place bed in lowest, locked position, with side rails up
    - Place client in position of comfort, or as ordered
- Vital signs including airway assessment and breath sounds
- Color of skin, nail beds, and lips
- Skin condition (moist or dry, warm or cool)
- Level of consciousness
- Activity level
- Intravenous infusion
    - Type of solution
    - Amount in bottle or bag
    - Flow rate
    - Appearance and location of IV site
- Dressings
    - Amount and character of drainage
- Drains and tubes
    - Intactness and function
    - Connection to drainage and/or suction
    - Amount and character of drainage

TABLE 30-4 ADDITIONAL NURSING CARE ACCORDING TO CLASSIFICATION OR TYPE OF SURGICAL PROCEDURE

CLASSIFICATION OR TYPE OF SURGICAL PROCEDURE		NURSING CARE
Orthopedic		• Expose wet casts to the air. • Check surgeon's orders for positioning of client; operated extremities typically are elevated. • Check for digital warmth, color, mobility, circulation (pulses), and sensation in affected extremity.
Urologic		• Attach all catheters to drainage. • Closely monitor continuous irrigation to ensure that flow in and flow out are equal; if obstructed, the bladder could rupture. • Increase or decrease irrigation flow rate according to amount of bleeding. • Assess for chills or elevated pulse, possibly indicative of hemolysis or bacterial infection. • Assess abdomen for signs of distension and rigidity and report, especially if client complains.
Oral		• Suction frequently and carefully around sutures. • Observe breathing; ensure that drainage or packing does not obstruct airway. • Apply ice bag, when ordered. • Remove dental packs as ordered and assess every 15 minutes for further bleeding.
Eye, ears, nose, & throat (EENT)	*Eye surgery*	• Assess for facial paralysis • Minimize head movement, coughing, vomiting, and restlessness.
	Ear surgery	• Assess edema and tracheal patency (listening for stridor and observing for restlessness).
	Nose surgery	• Maintain open airway; suction orally; and apply ice.
	Tonsillectomy	• Place on side to facilitate drainage: elevate head of bed; have suction available; and observe closely for bleeding, vomiting, and obstruction.
Neurologic		• Assess level of consciousness; be alert to drowsiness, slurred speech, disorientation, or irritability that differs from that exhibited in the preoperative state. • Observe for pupil changes: inequality, constriction, and nonreactivity to light. • Assess for respiratory changes such as snoring, retraction of cheeks and trachea, shallowness, and slowed rate. • Monitor blood pressure and pulse; an elevated blood pressure coupled with a lowered pulse leads to shock. • Observe extremity movement for weakness, paralysis, and rigidity; observe for unilateral drooping of facial features. • Use caution when medicating.
	Laminectomy or discectomy	• Move only as ordered. • Assess sensation, circulation, and motion of extremities distal to incision.
	Craniotomy	• Position as ordered. • Complete a neurological check. • Use Trendelenburg position only with permission of the surgeon.
Vascular (all grafts, carotid endarterectomy, femoral-popliteal bypass)		• Assess color, sensation, warmth, and mobility of extremity. • Observe presence and strength of pedal and post-tibial pulses. • Complete a neurological check for carotid endarterectomy. • Frequently check all dressings and the area directly beneath the client.
Thoracic		• Closely observe chest tube for patency, amount of bleeding, and air leaks. Tape all connections. Mark drainage container upon client's admission and discharge. Assess fluctuation of drainage in tubing. Attach suction as ordered.

continues

TABLE 30-4 continued

CLASSIFICATION OR TYPE OF SURGICAL PROCEDURE	NURSING CARE
Thoracic— continued	• Observe respirations closely with regard to color change, restlessness, apprehension, dyspnea, or mediastinal shift. • Elevate head of bed 30°, unless contraindicated. • Encourage coughing and deep breathing. • Use caution in administering narcotics, especially morphine sulfate, as client cannot afford respiratory depression.
	Pneumonectomy • Do not turn on nonoperative side. Alternately turn from back to operated side.
	Lobectomy and resection • May turn client to either side.
Gynecologic	• Assess vaginal drainage.

• Urinary output
  Need to void or time of voiding
  Presence of patency and catheter; output/hour
• Pain
  Last dose of analgesia
  Current pain location, intensity, quality
• Compare assessment with PACU report
• Call light within reach
  Reorient client to usage
• Location of family or significant others
• Postoperative orders

A brief assessment including vital signs is completed every 15 minutes for 1 hour; every 30 minutes for 2 hours; and every hour for 4 hours, or as prescribed by the physician. The possibilities of postanesthetic complications continue, but as time passes, different postsurgical complications may develop; the nurse is responsible for managing these.

1. The client is at risk for *Ineffective Airway Clearance* caused by atelectasis and hypostatic pneumonia. Respiratory complications can still occur with any anesthetized client. As in the PACU, the postoperative client is at risk for ineffective airway clearance, ineffective breathing patterns, and aspiration. Now, however, nursing measures are directed toward preventing ineffective airway clearance caused by atelectasis and hypostatic pneumonia, both of which usually occur within the first 48 hours postoperatively. In postoperative atelectasis, the bronchioles of the lungs become plugged with mucus so that air cannot reach the alveoli. The alveoli then collapse. The client develops dyspnea, fever, tachypnea, tachycardia, and cyanosis. In postoperative hypostatic pneumonia, stagnant mucus promotes the growth of bacteria, and atelectasis then develops into a secondary infection. To prevent these complications, actively encourage the client to cough, deep breathe (with and without incentive spirometry), and turn as instructed preoperatively. Encourage the

client to sit up and ambulate as soon and as often as ordered. Ensure adequate pain relief measures so that mobility is well tolerated.

2. The client is at *Risk for Peripheral Neurovascular Dysfunction, Excess/Deficient Fluid Volume,* and *Activity Intolerance.* The client continues to be at risk for decreased cardiac output and fluid volume deficit. Implement measures to prevent deep vein thrombosis, thrombophlebitis, pulmonary embolism, complications of fluid overload, fluid deficit, hypokalemia, and syncope.

    The stress response to surgery, inactivity, pressure related to body position, obesity, and injury to pelvic veins during surgery may contribute to the formation of deep vein thrombosis, thrombophlebitis, or pulmonary embolism. These complications may appear immediately following surgery or 1 to 2 weeks later. Routinely assess for a positive Homan's sign and for warm, tender, reddened, hardened areas in the calves. To assess for Homan's sign, ask the client to forcefully dorsiflex the foot. If pain is felt in the calf of the leg, it is considered a positive Homan's sign; if no pain is felt, it is considered a negative finding. A positive Homan's sign may indicate thrombophlebitis and should be reported to the surgeon. Deep vein thrombosis and thrombophlebitis may lead to a pulmonary embolus, although there may be no warning of pulmonary embolism. When pulmonary embolism occurs, the client may experience dyspnea, chest pain, cyanosis, cough, hemoptysis, tachycardia, and fever coupled with an elevated white blood cell count. If the embolism is large enough, shock may develop rapidly. Pulmonary embolism may be fatal.

    To prevent the formation of deep vein thrombosis, thrombophlebitis, and pulmonary embolism, encourage the client to ambulate to the extent the client is able. When in bed, encourage the client to perform postoperative leg exercises each hour. Anti-embolism stockings may be ordered, or a sequential compression device, which is a boot applied to the legs to simulate walking by alternate inflation. Remove the boots and antiembolism stockings every day so the skin can be cleansed. Antiembolism stockings and the sequential compression device are not substitutes for leg exercises. Leg exercises must still be performed.

When it is ordered, administer low-dose heparin therapy to hemostatically stable clients who are older than 40 years of age and have undergone pelvic, abdominal, or thoracic surgery. Heparin is usually given subcutaneously every 12 hours until discharge. If the drug is administered at low dosage and if preoperative prothrombin time, partial thromboplastin time, and platelet count were within the normal range, no laboratory test is necessary to determine the drug's effect. This regimen is ordered at the surgeon's discretion.

Measure intake and output and monitor laboratory findings (e.g., electrolytes, hematocrit, hemoglobin, and serum osmolality) and signs and symptoms of hemorrhage by assessing vital signs, skin color and condition, dressings, drains, and tubes, as in the PACU.

Clients often experience syncope when changing from a lying position to a sitting or standing position. Assist the client to change positions slowly, proceed in steps, and allow time for the client's internal equilibrium to adjust. Check the radial pulse frequently and ask the client if dizzy or nauseated. If syncope occurs during ambulation, ask for assistance in obtaining a wheelchair for the client, use a nearby chair, or lower the client to the floor until the client recovers. Although frightening for the client, syncope is not physiologically threatening unless the client is injured in a fall.

3. The client may be at risk for *Imbalanced Nutrition: Less than Body Requirements* related to nausea and vomiting, hiccups, abdominal distention, constipation, and NPO status. Gastrointestinal complications become more prevalent after immediate postoperative recovery. The client may also experience pain related to hiccups and slowed gastrointestinal function.

Nausea and vomiting are caused by anesthetic agents, narcotics, hypotension, and the manipulation of the bowel during surgery. Handling of the bowel during pelvic and abdominal surgery causes peristalsis to stop or severely slow. Bowel function normally returns 2 to 5 days following surgery. If bowel inactivity persists, a paralytic ileus may develop. As bowel function resumes, continue to assess the client for bowel sounds and, if a nasogastric tube is present, a reduction in drainage. As peristalsis returns in a discontinuous fashion, the client may experience distention along with flatulence and gas pains. After bowel sounds resume in all quadrants, the client may be removed from NPO status according to the surgeon's orders. Provide good oral hygiene when the client is NPO and administer antiemetics as needed for nausea and vomiting.

Hiccups are caused by irritation of the phrenic nerve. Impulses then cause the diaphragm to contract rhythmically and violently. Abdominal distention, gastric distention, and the presence of a nasogastric tube are common causes, but electrolyte and acid–base disturbances, intestinal obstruction, and intra-abdominal bleeding may also initiate hiccups. Notify the surgeon when hiccups are prolonged.

Gas pains and signs and symptoms of abdominal distention may be minimized by early and frequent ambulation and resumption of oral intake. Gas pains might also be helped by frequently repositioning the client to encourage movement of air through the intestines. As air rises and peristalsis moves from right to left, the client can be moved from lying on the left side (where air will rise on the right), to lying supine, to lying on the right side (where air will rise on the left). If the client can tolerate it and there are no contraindications, lying prone with the head turned to the side places pressure on the abdomen, forcing air to rise and move out through the rectum. Other nursing care measures to relieve abdominal distention might include irrigation of the nasogastric tube, if present. Irrigating the nasogastric tube may also relieve hiccups.

Constipation is a major source of discomfort for the client. Analgesics combined with decreased activity and NPO status are very constipating. Oral fluids and activity should be encouraged. If ordered, the medical regimen of stool softeners and suppositories may be indicated.

4. The client is at risk for developing **Urinary Retention** related to anesthesia, immobility, and pain. The client is also at *Risk for Infection* related to Foley catheter placement. The quantity and quality of urine are more directly related to cardiac output and the perfusion of the kidneys than to anesthesia, immobility, and pain; although a stress response following surgery causes the body to retain fluids for 24 to 48 hours following surgery. Urine output should be at least 30 cc per hour if a catheter is in place. The catheter must be assessed for patency. If not catheterized, the client should void at least 200 cc at the first postoperative voiding. Most clients void within 6 to 8 hours after surgery; however, urinary retention occurs frequently in the postoperative period, especially following abdominal or pelvic surgery. Anesthesia depresses the urge to void. Narcotics, vagolytic agents (anticholinergics), and spinal anesthesia also interfere with the ability to initiate voiding. Facilitate voiding by encouraging fluid intake and assisting the client to void in an anatomically correct position depending on the client's condition. Privacy, running water, indirect bladder pressure (placing a firm hand over the bladder), and warm water over the perineum may also encourage voiding.

If the client has not voided, palpate, inspect, and percuss the bladder. Often, the surgeon orders a Foley catheter to be inserted if the client has not voided after 8 to 10 hours.

5. The client may become at risk for *Disturbed Sensory Perception* related to anesthesia, narcotics, change of environment, fluid and electrolyte imbalances, sleep deprivation, hypoxia, and sensory deprivation or

overload. The client may also experience *Acute **P**ain* related to the surgical incision; ***H**ypothermia* related to anesthesia and surgical environment; and ***H**yperthermia* related to infection. Alterations in neurological function vary and may manifest as pain, fever, or delirium. Assessing the level of consciousness is a priority. A change in level of consciousness may be the first indication of a stroke and/or increased intracranial pressure. Determining the level of consciousness may be difficult, especially in the elderly client or at night, when clients may be groggy from being awakened. Often, thoughts will clear if the client is given the opportunity to thoroughly awaken. Encouraging the presence of loved ones, offering explanations, and listening to the client may decrease sensory perceptual alterations. Encouraging previous sleep patterns, providing uninterrupted sleep, and alternating rest and activity may also be beneficial.

Assess and record subjective data regarding pain location, intensity on a scale of 0 to 10, quality, and duration as well as factors contributing to pain. Objective data such as grimacing and crying are also recorded. Analgesics are usually ordered to be administered via patient-controlled analgesia (PCA) or epidural analgesia or intravenously, intramuscularly, or orally, all on a PRN (as needed) basis. Encourage the client to ask for medication before the pain becomes severe. Offer medication before activity or painful procedures such as wound irrigation. Attend to analgesic requests promptly. Ensuring comfort encourages the client's full participation in coughing, deep breathing, turning, and ambulation.

Hypothermia is common in the first few hours following surgery. Offer blankets as needed. Because of the normal inflammatory response, temperature may later elevate to a low-grade fever. If temperature rises higher than 101°F, notify the surgeon. Atelectasis and dehydration may cause elevated temperature (higher than 101°F) in the first 24 to 48 hours following surgery. After 48 hours, temperature higher than 101°F may indicate a wound, respiratory, or urinary tract infection; thrombophlebitis; or pulmonary embolism.

The nurse's primary role is to prevent infection by using aseptic technique. Once a fever has occurred, follow orders to ascertain the cause of the elevation by taking urine, wound, blood, or sputum cultures. Administer antipyretics as ordered. Providing light covers and clothing, performing frequent linen changes, offering cool washcloths, and ensuring a cool environment are measures that may increase comfort.

6. The surgical client is at *Risk for Impaired **S**kin Integrity* and *Risk for **I**nfection* related to surgical incision. The nurse generally does not remove the primary dressing without an order to do so. Bleeding may be monitored by circling the drainage on the dressing and then reassessing later to ascertain whether the drainage area has increased in size. The dressing may also be reinforced with additional absorbent dressings as needed. In some institutions, the dressing may be changed as necessary after the first dressing change. Dressings may not be necessary if there is no drainage or drains, but this is usually the surgeon's preference.

Drainage on dressings and in drains typically changes from sanguinous to serosanguinous to serous over several hours to several days, depending on the type of surgery. The amount should also decrease over the same time period. Purulent, odorous drainage may be a sign of infection. A sudden increase in drainage may be a sign of impending wound separation. Always notify the surgeon of any excessive or abnormal drainage.

All wounds heal by primary, secondary, or tertiary intention. In primary intention, the wound layers are sutured together and have no gaping edges. The wound generally heals in 8 to 10 days but may take up to 3 months. There is minimal scar formation. Most surgical wounds are of this type.

In secondary intention, the wound heals by filling in with granulation tissue and by contracting where the skin edges are not approximated. This method is used for ulcers when there is not enough tissue to approximate the edges or for infected wounds when drainage is desirable. Wounds healing by secondary intention are assessed according to the presence of granulation tissue having a red, granular appearance. Wound healing is slow, possibly taking many months or years. Thus wound healing by primary intention is preferable.

In tertiary intention, the approximation of tissue edges is delayed. This allows an infection to drain or an area of extensive tissue removal to begin healing. The edges of the wound are closed 4 to 6 days later. Because areas of granulation tissue are brought together at this time, the scar is usually much wider (Figure 30-9).

Wound dehiscence and evisceration are serious complications of wound healing. **Dehiscence** occurs when the wound edges separate. **Evisceration** occurs when the wound separates completely and the viscera protrude from the wound (Figure 30-10). Both are more likely to occur 7 to 10 days following surgery and are preceded by a sudden spillage of serosanguinous drainage. Dehiscence and evisceration are more likely to occur in the very elderly client, the malnourished client, the client with an infection, or the client with abdominal distention who is straining severely. If evisceration occurs, the viscera should be immediately covered with sterile saline dressings and the surgeon notified of the wound disruption.

When dressings are changed, the surgical incision is cleansed to remove debris and bacteria from the incision. The choice of cleansing agent depends on the physician's prescription as well as institutional protocol. It is recommended that isotonic solutions such as normal saline or lactated ringers be used.

The major principles to keep in mind when cleansing a surgical incision are as follows:
- Use Standard Precautions at all times.
- Use a sterile swab or gauze and work from the clean area out toward the dirtier area. Begin over the incision line and swab downward from top to bottom. Change the swab and proceed again on

Figure 30-9 *Wound Healing:* **A,** *Primary Intention;* **B,** *Secondary Intention; and* **C,** *Tertiary Intention*

Figure 30-10 **A,** *Dehiscence;* **B,** *Evisceration*

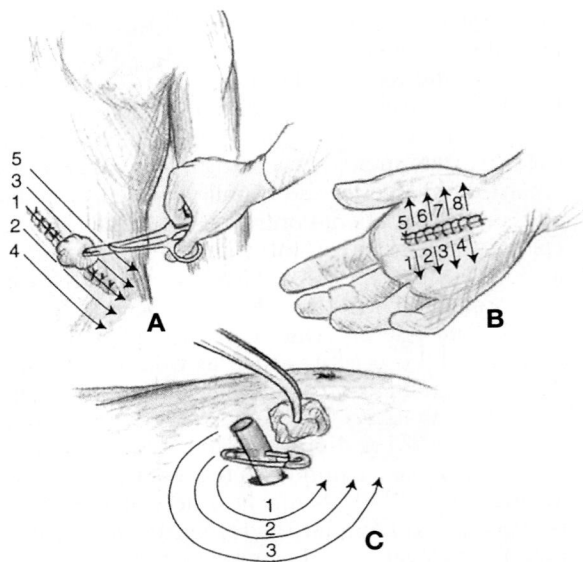

Figure 30-11 *Use a clean, sterile swab for each stroke when cleansing a surgical incision.* **A,** *Gently clean the incision, then each side alternately;* **B,** *Gently wipe swab outward, away from the incision;* **C,** *Clean around a drain site in a circular motion.*

either side of the incision, using a new swab each time (Figure 30-11).

The surface closures, staples, or sutures must be removed as the incision heals. Continuous sutures are made with one thread and tied at the beginning and end of the suture line. Intermittent sutures are each tied individually. In blanket continuous sutures, the single thread is grounded again in the last suture exit (Figure 30-12).

The incisional dressing keeps the incision clean and protects it from physical trauma and bacterial invasion. Generally, the same kind of dressing can be put on as was taken off. As the incision heals and drainage lessens, a small, thinner dressing can usually be applied. Bandages and binders may be applied over the incision dressing to secure, immobilize, or support a body part; to hold the dressing in place; or to prevent or minimize swelling of a body part. Bandages are long rolls of material, such as gauze, webbing, or muslin, designed to be wrapped around body parts. Figure 30-13 illustrates several different methods of bandaging. Binders are bandages made for specific body parts, usually the abdomen, perineal area, or arm (sling) (Figure 30-14). Abdominal binders support the abdomen and are used following abdominal surgery or childbirth. Perineal binders, called T-binders, are used to hold pads or dressings in the perineal area. Because of the urination and defe-

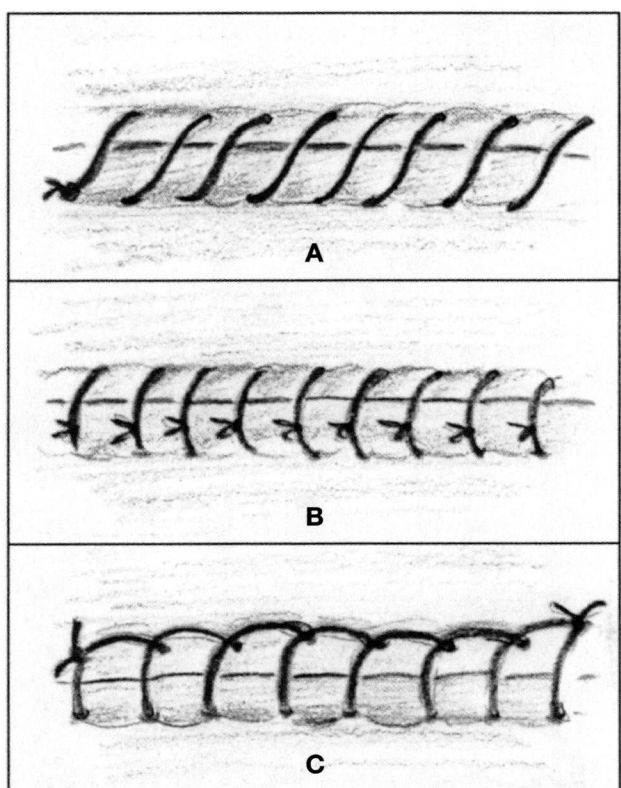

Figure 30-12 *Selected Suturing Methods:* **A,** *Continuous;* **B,** *Intermittent; and* **C,** *Blanket Continuous*

COMMUNITY/HOME HEALTH CARE

Dressing Wounds

- Because of early discharge, clients are often sent home with incisions that need dressing changes.
- Ascertain the client's support system, including caregivers, the home environment, and available resources.
- Teach the client and/or home caregiver the correct method of changing the dressing.
- Have the client and/or home caregiver change the dressing before the client is discharged.
- Provide a list of signs and symptoms of complications of wound healing.
- At times, a referral for home care nursing is necessary.

cation needs of clients, T-binders must be changed regularly. A sling is a cloth support for an injured arm; it wraps around the back of the neck to maintain the arm in a set position.

During dressing changes and after the dressing has been removed, the surgical wound is assessed for skin edge approximation, edema, and bleeding. The skin edges may be slightly reddened and swollen from the normal inflammatory response. Possible signs of a wound infection include increased suture

COMMUNITY/HOME HEALTH CARE

Postoperative Care

For proper home care, the client and family must be given information about the following topics:

- Medication regimen
- Diet
- Activity restrictions
- Follow-up appointments
- Wound care
- Special instructions

The specifics for each topic will vary with each client and will depend on the surgical procedure and the client's age and physical condition.

tension, warmth, erythema, drainage, odor, pain, and induration around the incision site. Wound healing can be enhanced by promoting nutrition, discouraging smoking, and performing proper wound cleansing. The practice of aseptic technique cannot be emphasized enough in preventing nosocomial infections in a surgical incision.

7. Clients are at risk for **A**nxiety or *Ineffective* **C**oping related to disturbance in body image, change in lifestyle, financial strain, or a poor prognosis. Many clients undergo a psychological adjustment to surgery. Taking time to listen to the client as well as offering simple explanations and reassurances may be all the support the client needs to combat anxiety.

As the client recovers and is ready for discharge from the hospital, the client is at risk for *Deficient* **K**nowledge related to home care. Ideally, the client has been instructed routinely about home care since admission. Adequate teaching about home care results in a quicker recovery, fewer complications, and greater independence.

AMBULATORY SURGERY

Ambulatory surgery is defined as surgical care performed under general, regional, or local anesthesia involving less than 24 hours of hospitalization. Other names for ambulatory surgery include same-day, one-day, outpatient, in and out, or short-stay surgery.

The trend in health care is to promote wellness. Clients are encouraged to accept more personal responsibility for their state of health. In the past, the message sent to clients was that the client is sick, and the medical community will provide all care. Today, ambulatory surgery clients are being sent a totally different message: that the postoperative client is not sick and, except for a few minor limitations, can often resume normal daily activities soon after undergoing anesthesia and surgery.

Ambulatory surgery provides the longest period of time for the client to receive skilled postoperative care or monitoring without being formally admitted to the hospital. The practice of ambulatory surgery attempts to

Figure 30-13   *Common Bandaging Methods:* **A,** *Circular turns are wrapped around a body part several times to anchor the bandage or supply support.* **B,** *Spiral turns begin with a circular turn and then proceed up the body part, with each turn covering two-thirds the width of the preceding turn.* **C,** *Spiral reverse turns begin with a circular turn. The bandage is then reversed or twisted, once each turn to accommodate a limb that gets larger as the bandaging progresses.* **D,** *Figure-eight turns crisscross in the shape of a figure eight and are used on a joint that requires movement.* **E,** *Recurrent turns are anchored with circular turns, follow a back-and-forth motion, and are completed with circular turns; they are used to cover a fingertip, head, or amputated stump.*

Figure 30-14 *Common Binders:* **A,** *Abdominal;* **B,** *T-Binders, Female and Male;* and **C,** *Arm Sling*

overcome the risk of premature dismissal while meeting fiscal requirements. The emphasis on cost containment coupled with government reductions in Medicare and Medicaid payments has further promoted the concept of ambulatory surgery.

To further reduce health care costs, few clients are admitted to the hospital before the day of surgery. Most surgical clients are processed through the ambulatory surgery unit. These clients are called "day of surgery" or "A.M. admit" clients. Necessary laboratory work, radiology tests, or other examinations are completed on an outpatient basis before the day of surgery. Even clients undergoing extensive surgeries such as open-heart surgery (a coronary artery bypass), craniotomy, or total joint replacement can be admitted the day of surgery. Then, after discharge from the perioperative suite, the client may either be admitted to the hospital as an inpatient or may be sent home from the ambulatory surgery unit.

In addition to fiscal considerations, the growth of ambulatory surgery can also be traced to technological advances. Clients now require shorter recovery periods as a result of new procedural technology, such as laparoscopic cholecystectomy. The introduction of shorter-acting anesthetic agents also decreases the immediate postoperative recovery time, facilitating the client's ability to function independently upon discharge from the ambulatory surgery setting.

The benefits of ambulatory surgery are many. Ambulatory surgery decreases cost to the client, institution, insurance carriers, and governmental agencies. The risk of acquiring a nosocomial infection is also decreased. The client experiences less disruption to personal life and less psychological distress related to hospitalization. With ambulatory surgery, the client especially benefits from early postoperative ambulation.

Ambulatory surgery is performed in several different settings. Hospital-based integrated facilities are formal ambulatory surgery programs incorporated into existing inpatient surgery programs. Clients are cared for preoperatively and postoperatively in the ambulatory surgery unit but are mixed with inpatients on the operating room schedule. This type of facility also allows preoperative processing of day-of-surgery clients. Hospital-affiliated facilities consist of a separate department with designated preoperative, intraoperative, and postoperative areas. Such a facility may be located within the hospital, adjacent to the hospital, or at a satellite location.

Freestanding facilities are independently owned and operated and are not affiliated with a hospital or medical center. In the past, physicians generally owned such facilities, but today the trend is for health care corporations to own these facilities. Some doctors' offices also have facilities for performing minor ambulatory surgery.

The Aldrete Score has been modified for use with clients having anesthesia on an ambulatory basis. Five assessments were added to the Aldrete Score for this purpose (Table 30-2). Attainment of these criteria indicates that clients should be able to care for themselves at home and accomplish activities of daily living independently and safely. The points are totaled at regular intervals (usually every half hour), and clients may be discharged home when their total score is 18 or higher.

ELDERLY CLIENTS HAVING SURGERY

Elderly clients (older than 65 years of age) are at risk for developing complications from surgery or anesthesia. Unfortunately, because an increased incidence of disease correlates with increasing age, more elderly clients require surgery than does any other age group. As the percentage of elderly persons in the whole population rises, the number of surgeries on elders will also rise. Because of the complex needs of the elderly client undergoing surgery, knowledge in promoting health and rehabilitation in the elderly client is necessary.

Surgery is a stressor. Because of depleted energy sources, the elderly client may not have sufficient resilience to react defensively to this stressor. The risk of complications from surgery further rises in elderly clients who have one or more chronic diseases. In these clients, surgery then can be the source of a downward spiraling effect toward debilitation or possibly death.

Elderly clients vary in their abilities to respond to the stress of surgery. Physiologic changes related to the aging process may inhibit the elderly client from readily coping with surgery. The number of physiologic changes in the very elderly client (older than 80 years of age) is markedly greater than that in those in their sixties and seventies. Breathing capacity, renal blood flow, cardiac output, and conduction velocity of the nervous system all diminish. Table 30-5 lists the physiologic changes in the elderly client along with correlating nursing interventions for postoperative care. Aging affects all body systems, and the nurse must be familiar with these changes and the interventions geared toward each to prevent and detect complications of surgery.

The elderly client has a lifetime of experiences that affects the response to surgery. A lifetime of watching family and friends experience surgery, illness, and death particularly influences personal reactions to impending surgery. Because of the variation in such experiences, each client reacts differently to similar situations. Simply talking with the client to provide information or listening to the client's fears helps prepare the client for upcoming surgery.

Third-party reimbursement policies often require elderly clients to undergo surgical procedures on an outpatient basis. Because many elderly clients have neurological deficits and other chronic disease processes, the elderly outpatient poses a particular challenge. Additional postoperative self-care deficits may result from the surgical procedure and the effects of anesthesia. Elderly clients often live alone and lack the support systems necessary for home care. In order to provide realistic discharge planning, the nurse must assess the ability of the client, family, and friends to provide care at home.

Summary

- Surgery is a major stressor for all clients. Anxiety and fear are normal. Fear of the unknown is both the most prevalent fear before surgery and the fear easiest for the nurse to help the client overcome.
- The outcome of surgical treatment is tremendously enhanced by accurate preoperative nursing assessment and careful preoperative preparation. Information gathered through preoperative assessment and risk screening is later used to prepare the surgical site, for surgical positioning, and as a comparative basis for postoperative assessments and complication screening.
- The teaching methods used by the nurse strongly influence the degree of learning and the retention of information.
- Aseptic technique is a collection of principles used to control and/or prevent the transfer of microorganisms from sources within (endogenous) and outside (exogenous) the client. These principles are practiced in all clinical nursing units. The sterile conscience governs personal behavior with regard to adherence to aseptic technique.
- Nursing care in the operating room focuses on the safety and protection of the client.
- Postoperative nursing assessments are completed in an organized manner, focusing first on the priorities of airway, breathing, and circulation, and then on the body system affected by surgery.
- The nurse can help prevent the formation of deep vein thrombosis, thrombophlebitis, and pulmonary embolism through encouraging early ambulation and postoperative leg exercises and by providing antiembolism stockings and/or sequential stockings, if ordered.
- Ambulatory surgery is defined as surgical care performed under general, regional, or local anesthesia and involving fewer than 24 hours of hospitalization. Cost containment, governmental changes, and technological advances have all promoted the concept of ambulatory surgery.
- Because of the physiologic changes and complex needs of the elderly client undergoing surgery, the nurse must be knowledgeable in promoting health and rehabilitation in the elderly surgical client.

TABLE 30-5 PHYSIOLOGIC CHANGES OF AGING AND RELATED POSTOPERATIVE NURSING INTERVENTIONS

BODY SYSTEM	CHANGES	NURSING INTERVENTIONS
Cardiovascular	• Decreased elasticity of the vascular system • Decreased cardiac output • Decreased peripheral circulation	• Closely monitor vital signs and peripheral pulses • Encourage early ambulation • Use antiembolism stockings • Monitor intake and output, including blood loss • Monitor preoperative response to activity and compare to postoperative response
Respiratory	• Decreased vital capacity • Decreased alveolar volume • Decreased movement of cilia	• Closely monitor respirations • Auscultate breath sounds frequently • Encourage coughing and deep breathing • Turn frequently • Monitor oxygen saturation
Urinary	• Decreased glomerular filtration rate • Decreased bladder muscle tone • Weakened perineal muscles	• Monitor intake and output every 1 to 2 hours • Assist frequently with toileting • Monitor fluid and electrolyte status
Gastrointestinal	• Decreased gastric and intestinal motility • Altered digestion and absorption • Decreased food consumption	• Assess for obesity and malnutrition • Encourage fluids and activity • Encourage high-protein foods and supplements • Assist with meals as needed • Provide companionship during mealtime
Immunological	• Decreased level of gamma globulin • Decreased plasma proteins	• Follow strict aseptic technique • Monitor temperature • Assess incision site
Neurological	• Decreased conduction velocity • Decreased visual acuity • Loss of hearing • Decreased sensation	• Allow use of glasses and hearing aids • Orient to environment • Provide for safe environment • Repeat information as needed • Use medications sparingly • Provide written instructions • Allow for extra education time
Integumentary	• Lack of elasticity • Loss of collagen • Decreased subcutaneous fat	• To prevent shearing forces on skin when positioning client, lift rather than slide client • Pad bony prominences • Use tape that is easy to remove • Use warm prepping solutions, irrigating solutions, and IV solutions intraoperatively • Provide extra blankets • Ensure warm room temperature • Turn frequently • Encourage early ambulation

CASE STUDY

Mr. Glen Stone, a 74-year-old retired schoolteacher who is married and the father of four and the grandfather of six-teen, weighs 275 lbs. He has undergone a right hemicolectomy, wherein the right side of his colon was removed be-cause of cancer. He has a history of smoking but has no other health problems. The surgery was uncomplicated, and he is in the PACU. He has a midline incision with a Penrose drain; a stab wound with a Jackson-Pratt drain is adjacent to the incision. He also has a nasogastric tube attached to low intermittent suction. He is alert and oriented, and he can move all four extremities. His blood pressure is normal for him in comparison to his preoperative levels. He is breathing regularly and easily at a rate of 16 breaths per minute, and his skin color is normal. His oxygen saturation, however, is 86% with additional oxygen being given via mask.

The following questions will guide your development of a nursing care plan for the case study.

1. What risk factors for developing postoperative complications can you identify for Mr. Stone?
2. What is his Aldrete Score at this point?
3. What nursing measures can you institute to promote oxygenation?
4. What type of drainage is expected from the incision and the drains during the first 1 to 2 days?
5. What nursing observations can be made and reported to indicate to the surgen that the nasogastric tube can be removed?
6. What nursing measures can be implemented to prevent deep vein thrombosis, thrombophlebitis, and pulmonary embolism?
7. Write and prioritize three individualized nursing diagnoses and goals for Mr. Stone.
8. What information will Mr. Stone need before discharge?

Review Questions

1. Client education is:
   a. completed when time allows.
   b. started when discharge is scheduled.
   c. always more beneficial when completed in a structured group setting.
   d. directed toward the client's family when the client is unable to learn.

2. The role of the nurse in obtaining consent includes:
   a. judging the quality of the explanation and ascertaining the client's understanding of the consent form.
   b. acting as a witness to the signature of the client.
   c. administering the preoperative medication before the client signs the consent.
   d. ensuring that coercion was used to obtain the client's signature on the consent.

3. Upon the client's admission to the PACU, the nurse knows to first:
   a. take the client's blood pressure.
   b. assess the airway.
   c. assess the client's level of consciousness.
   d. check the incision site.

4. The nurse is making a preoperative assessment on a client. Of the following findings, the most important item to know for a client who is having general anesthesia is:
   a. hearing impaired.
   b. a right-leg amputee.
   c. color blind.
   d. a smoker.

5. The nursing intervention that has the greatest impact on reducing overall surgical risk is:
   a. encouraging activity and early ambulation.
   b. assessing blood pressure.
   c. ensuring adequate nutrition.
   d. monitoring intake and output.

References/Suggested Readings

Aldrete, J. (1995). The post-anesthesia recovery score revisited. *Journal of Clinical Anesthesiology, 7*(1), 89–91.
Association of Perioperative Registered Nurses (AORN). (2001). Patients wearing jewelry. *AORN Online Journal.* [Online]. Available: www.aorn.org/journal/2001/augci.htm
Association of Perioperative Registered Nurses (AORN). (2002a). Artificial nails. *AORN Online Journal.* [Online]. Available: www.aorn.org/journal/2002/juneci.htm

Association of Perioperative Registered Nurses (2002b). *Standards, recommended practices, and guidelines*, Denver, CO: Author.

Brenner, Z. (1999). Preventing postoperative complications. *Nursing99, 29*(10), 34-39.

Bryant, R. A. (Ed.). (2000). *Acute and chronic wounds: Nursing management* (2nd ed.). St. Louis, MO: Mosby.

Burden, N., Defazio-Quinn, D. M., & O'Brien, D. (2000). *Ambulatory surgical nursing.* Philadelphia: W. B. Saunders.

Cizzell, J. (1994). Back to basics: Test your wound assessment skills. *AJN, 94*(6), 34–35.

Crenshaw, J., & Winslow, E. (2002). Preoperative fasting: Old habits die hard. *AJN, 102*(5), 36–44.

Erwin-Toth, P., & Hocevar, B. (1995). Wound care: Selecting the right dressing. *AJN, 95*(2), 46–51.

Fort, C. (2002). Get pumped to prevent DVT. *Nursing2002, 32*(9), 50–52.

Fortunato, N. (2000). *Berry & Kohn's operating room technique* (9th ed.). St. Louis, MO: Mosby.

Gilchrist, B. (1990). Washing and dressings after surgery. *Journal of the Wound Care Society, 86*(50), 71.

Grogan, T. (1999). Bringing bloodless surgery into the mainstream. *Nursing99, 29*(11), 58–61.

Hogstel, M. (2001). *Gerontology: Nursing care of the older adult* Clifton Park, NY: Thomson Delmar Learning.

Ignatavicius, D. D. (2002). *Medical-Surgical Nursing* (4th ed.). Philadelphia: W. B. Saunders.

Lewis, S. M., Collier, I. C., & Heitkemper, M. M. (2002). *Medical–surgical nursing: Assessment and management of clinical problems* (5th ed.). St. Louis, MO: Mosby.

McConnell, E. (2002). Applying antiembolism stockings. *Nursing2002, 32*(4), 17.

Motta, G. (1993). How moisture retentive dressings promote healing. *Nursing 93, 23*(12), 26–33.

Phillips, J. (1998). Wound dehiscence. *Nursing98, 28*(3), 33.

Phipps, W. J., Monahan, F. D., Sands, J. K., Marek, J. F., & Neighbors, M. (2002). *Medical–surgical nursing: Health and Illness Perspectives* (7th ed.). St. Louis, MO: Mosby.

Smeltzer, S. C., & Bare, B. G. (2002). *Brunner and Suddarth's textbook of medical-surgical nursing* (9th ed.). Philadelphia: Lippincott Williams & Wilkins.

Talabiska, D. G. (1995). Malnutrition in the elderly. *Newlines in Multi-Vitamin Infusion, 4*(2), 1, 2, 6.

Vernon, S., & Molnar-Pfeifer, G. (1997). Are you ready for bloodless surgery? *AJN, 97*(9), 40–47.

Winslow, E., & Jacobson, A. (2001). The case against artificial nails. *Nursing2001, 31*(10), 30.

Resources

Association of Perioperative Registered Nurses (AORN), 2170 South Parker Road, Suite 300, Denver, CO 80231-5711, 800-755-2676, www.aorn.org

MAKING THE CONNECTION

Refer to the following chapters to increase your understanding of oncology nursing:

Basic Nursing
- **Legal and Ethical Responsibilities**
- **Loss, Grief, and Death**
- **Pain Management**
- **Diagnostic Tests**

Adult Health Nursing
- **Surgery**
- **Hematologic and Lymphatic Systems**
- **Reproductive System**
- **Integumentary System**
- **Immune System**
- **The Older Adult**

LEARNING OBJECTIVES

Upon completion of this chapter, you should be able to:
- Define key terms.
- Explain how the behavior of cancer cells differs from that of normal cells.
- Describe the role of the nurse in cancer detection.
- Discuss three medical treatments for cancer.
- Describe four complications that can occur in advanced cancer.
- Discuss ways the licensed practical/vocational nurse can aid the client in coping with cancer.

KEY TERMS

alopecia	leukemia
anorexia	lymphoma
antineoplastic	malignant
benign	metastasis
biologic response	neoplasm
modifier	oncology
cachexia	palliative surgery
cancer	radiotherapy
carcinogen	reconstructive surgery
carcinoma	sarcoma
chemotherapy	stomatitis
curative surgery	tumor marker
differentiation	vesicant
extravasation	

INTRODUCTION

Cancer is a disease resulting from the uncontrolled growth of cells, which causes malignant cellular tumors. One in three Americans will develop some type of cancer during their lifetime. Cancer is the second leading cause of death in the United States and can develop in individuals of any race, gender, age, socioeconomic status, or culture. It is not a single disease but, rather, a group of more than 200 different diseases that can attack any tissue or organ of the body.

According to the American Cancer Society (ACS), in the 1930s fewer than one in five cancer clients was alive 5 years after diagnosis. In the 1940s one in four survived 5 years. Today, 62% of people diagnosed with cancer will be alive in 5 years (ACS, 2003). Survival rates are influenced by the type of cancer, the progression of the disease at diagnosis, and the client's response to the treatment.

INCIDENCE

In the United States, men have a 1 in 2 lifetime risk of developing cancer while women have a risk of 1 in 3 (ACS, 2003). Incidence and mortality rates are usually

Estimated New Cases*

MALE	FEMALE
Prostate 220,900 (33%)	Breast 211,300 (32%)
Lung & bronchus 91,800 (14%)	Lung & bronchus 80,100 (12%)
Colon & rectum 72,800 (11%)	Colon & rectum 74,700 (11%)
Urinary bladder 42,200 (6%)	Uterine corpus 40,100 (6%)
Melanoma of the skin 29,900 (4%)	Ovary 25,400 (4%)
Non-Hodgkin lymphoma 28,300 (4%)	Non-Hodgkin lymphoma 25,100 (4%)
Kidney 19,500 (3%)	Melanoma of the skin 24,300 (3%)
Oral cavity 18,200 (3%)	Thyroid 16,300 (3%)
Leukemia 17,900 (3%)	Pancreas 15,800 (2%)
Pancreas 14,900 (2%)	Urinary bladder 15,200 (2%)
All sites 675,300 (100%)	All sites 658,800 (100%)

Estimated Deaths

MALE	FEMALE
Lung & bronchus 88,400 (31%)	Lung & bronchus 68,800 (25%)
Prostate 28,900 (10%)	Breast 39,800 (15%)
Colon & rectum 28,300 (10%)	Colon & rectum 28,800 (11%)
Pancreas 14,700 (5%)	Pancreas 15,300 (6%)
Non-Hodgkin lymphoma 12,200 (4%)	Ovary 14,300 (5%)
Leukemia 12,100 (4%)	Non-Hodgkin lymphoma 11,200 (4%)
Esophagus 9,900 (4%)	Leukemia 9,800 (4%)
Liver 9,200 (3%)	Uterine corpus 6,800 (3%)
Urinary bladder 8,600 (3%)	Brain 5,800 (2%)
Kidney 7,400 (3%)	Multiple myeloma 5,500 (2%)
All sites 285,900 (100%)	All sites 270,600 (100%)

*Excluding basal and squamous cell skin cancer and in situ carcinomas except urinary bladder.

Percentages may not total 100% due to rounding

©2003, American Cancer Society, Inc., Surveillance Research

Figure 31-1 *Leading Sites of New Cancer Cases and Deaths—2003 Estimates (From* American Cancer Society Cancer Facts and Figures, *2003. Reprinted with permission.)*

higher for African Americans than for Anglo Americans. The incidence of cancer is higher in the elderly population than in any other age group. In men, the most common cancers are prostate, lung, colorectal, and urinary bladder; in women, they are breast, lung, colorectal, and uterine cancer (Figure 31-1).

The ACS estimates that 1,334,100 new cancer cases were diagnosed in the United States in 2003. Not included in this estimate are basal- and squamous-cell skin cancers and noninvasive cancers except for urinary bladder cancer. Approximately 1.3 million cases of highly curable basal- and squamous-cell skin cancers were estimated to be diagnosed in 2003 (ACS, 2003).

In 2003, approximately 166,650 cancer deaths were estimated to be caused by tobacco. About one-third of the 556,500 cancer deaths estimated for 2003 are related to nutrition, physical inactivity, obesity, and other lifestyle factors and could be prevented (ACS, 2003).

PATHOPHYSIOLOGY

Cancer is a disease characterized by neoplasia, an uncontrolled growth of abnormal cells. Unlike normal cells, which reproduce in an orderly manner and grow for a purpose, cancer cells develop rapidly, undiscriminatingly, and serve no useful function as they grow at the expense of healthy tissue. **Neoplasms,** any abnormal growth of new tissue, can be found in any body tissue. Neoplasms may be **benign** (not progressive and, thus, favorable for recovery) or **malignant** (becoming progressively worse and often resulting in death).

Benign neoplasms are not cancerous and are usually harmless. They grow slowly, are encapsulated and well-defined, and do not spread to neighboring tissues. Unless their location interferes with vital functions, benign neoplasms are associated with a favorable prognosis.

Malignant neoplasms form irregularly shaped masses with fingerlike projections. They usually multiply quickly and spread to distant body parts through the bloodstream or the lymph system. This process is called **metastasis.** Patterns of metastasis will differ depending on the type of cancer.

Cancers are usually named according to the site of the primary tumor or to the type of tissue involved. There are four main classifications of cancer according to tissue type:

- **Lymphomas** (cancers occurring in infection-fighting organs, such as lymphatic tissue)
- **Leukemias** (cancers occurring in blood-forming organs, such as the spleen, and in bone marrow)
- **Sarcomas** (cancers occurring in connective tissue, such as bone)
- **Carcinomas** (cancers occurring in epithelial tissue, such as the skin)

The exact mechanism that causes cancer is unknown, but most authorities believe that cancer develops from a combination of factors rather than from a single factor. Environmental, genetic, and viral factors have been implicated in the development of cancer. Chemical substances that initiate or promote the development of cancer are known as **carcinogens.** These agents are thought to alter the DNA in the cell nucleus.

RISK FACTORS

Many risk factors, such as environmental, lifestyle, genetic, and viral, may increase an individual's chances of developing cancer.

Environmental Factors

The first environmental carcinogen was discovered in 1760 when Percival Pott noted that chimney sweeps had a very high rate of what is now known to be scrotal cancer because they were exposed to cancer-causing oils in the soot that was rubbed into their clothing. Since that time, hundreds of chemical carcinogens have been identified.

Many individuals come into contact with cancer-causing agents through occupational exposure. Industrial chemicals, such as asbestos or vinyl chlorides, have been found to be carcinogenic. For workers who handle these chemicals, the risk of developing cancers is greatly increased if occupational exposure is combined with cigarette smoking. Tobacco may act synergistically with other substances to promote cancer development. Occupational exposure to coal tar, creosote, arsenic compounds, or radium constitutes a risk factor for development of skin cancer. The effects of carcinogenic agents are usually dose dependent. The larger the dose or the longer the duration of exposure, the greater the risk of cancer development. It is estimated that 80% of all cancers may be associated with environmental exposures and might be prevented if exposure is avoided. For those likely to be exposed to chemical carcinogens at work, safety standards and levels of exposure have been established by the Occupational Safety and Health Administration (OSHA).

In 1993, the U.S. Environmental Protection Agency (EPA) declared secondhand smoke a human carcinogen. Approximately 3,000 nonsmoking adults die each year of lung cancer from breathing secondhand smoke (ACS, 2002).

Lifestyle Factors

Lifestyle factors include the use of tobacco, sun exposure, alcohol consumption, and diet. Tobacco accounts for nearly one in three deaths in the United States (ACS, 2002). Tobacco use includes cigarettes, cigars, pipes, and smokeless forms (snuff and chewing tobacco). The same carcinogens are found in all forms of tobacco, causing cancer of the oral cavity, esophagus, pharynx, and larynx. When tobacco is smoked, it can also cause cancer of the lung, pancreas, uterus, cervix, kidney, and bladder.

Overexposure to the sun's ultraviolet rays over long periods of time is the cause of many skin cancers. The most serious form of skin cancer is melanoma. The ACS (2003) estimates 54,200 newly diagnosed cases of melanoma in 2003. Other factors predisposing a person to skin cancer are family history, multiple nevi, and atypical nevi.

Heavy alcohol consumption has also been implicated in mouth, throat, esophageal, and liver cancers. Alcohol is hypothesized to cause 5% of cancer deaths. Alcohol and tobacco used together greatly increase the risk of oral and esophageal cancers. The combined effect of al-

cohol and tobacco is greater than the sum of their individual effects (ACS, 2003). Despite the epidemiological evidence linking alcohol to cancer, the exact carcinogen in alcohol is yet to be determined. Table 31-1 lists some risk factors for cancer.

TABLE 31-1	RISK FACTORS FOR CANCER
Breast Cancer	• Family history (immediate female relatives) • High-fat diet • Obesity after menopause • Early menarche, late menopause • Alcohol consumption • Postmenopausal estrogen and progestin • First child after age 30
Cervical Cancer	• Multiple sexual partners • Having sex at early age • Exposure to human papillomavirus • Smoking
Colorectal Cancer	• Family history (immediate relatives) • Low-fiber diet • History of rectal polyps
Esophageal Cancer	• Heavy alcohol consumption • Smoking
Lung Cancer	• Cigarette smoking • Asbestos, arsenic, and radon exposure • Secondhand smoke • Tuberculosis
Skin Cancer	• Excessive exposure to ultraviolet radiation (sun) • Fair complexion • Work with coal, tar, pitch, or creosote • Multiple or atypical nevi (males)
Stomach Cancer	• Family history • Diet heavy in smoked, pickled, or salted foods
Testicular Cancer	• Undescended testicles • Consumption of hormones by mother during pregnancy
Prostate Cancer	• Increasing age • Family history • Diet high in animal fat

Dietary Guidelines To Reduce the Risk of Cancer

- Choose most foods from plant sources.
  — Eat five or more servings of fruits and vegetables each day, especially green and dark-yellow vegetables and those in the cabbage family.
  — Consume other foods from plant sources including breads, cereals, pastas, beans (legumes), and soy products.
- Limit intake of high-fat foods, particularly from animal sources.
  — Choose foods low in fat.
  — Limit consumption of meats, especially red meats and high-fat meats.
- Be physically active and achieve and maintain a healthy weight.
  — Physical activity can help by balancing caloric intake with energy expenditures or by other mechanisms.
- Limit or eliminate consumption of alcoholic beverages.

(*ACS, 2002*)

Research suggests that an increase in dietary fiber may help prevent colon cancer. Some studies have suggested that obesity is a significant risk factor for breast, colon, endometrial, and prostate cancers. Studies have also shown that diets high in salt-cured, smoked, and nitrite-cured foods increase an individual's risk for cancer of the stomach and esophagus. Food substances that may reduce cancer risk include cruciferous vegetables (cabbage, broccoli, cauliflower, brussels sprouts, kohlrabi); possibly vitamins A, E, and C; and selenium. Some foods have been found to contain carcinogens in the forms of additives or as by-products of storage. On the basis of current knowledge, the ACS has offered dietary guidelines to reduce cancer risk.

Lifestyle Guidelines to Reduce the Risk of Cancer

- Do not smoke or use tobacco in any form.
- Avoid overexposure to the sun.
- Eat a healthy diet.
- Get plenty of exercise.
- Have a physical examination on a routine basis, including a mammogram, Pap smear, testicular, and colon examinations.
- Get plenty of sleep (6 to 8 hours per night).
- Keep weight within normal limits.
- Practice regular self-examinations and see your physician if any changes are noted.
- Know and follow health and safety rules at the workplace.

Genetic Factors

Some families have a high incidence of certain types of cancer. Breast cancer, for example, occurs more frequently in women whose mothers, grandmothers, or sisters have had the disease. Leukemia and cancers of the colon, stomach, prostate, lung, and ovary may also run in families. Therefore, relatives of persons with these cancers should be carefully monitored.

Viral Factors

Although viruses have been linked to several cancers, their exact role is unclear. It has been theorized that they incorporate themselves into the genetic structure of the cell. Herpes simplex II virus and some of the human papillomaviruses that are transmitted sexually are known to predispose women to cervical cancer. Reducing the number of sexual partners can reduce the risk of contracting these viruses.

DETECTION

When cancer does develop, the earlier it is detected the more likely it is to be controlled. In some cases, diagnosis can be made before symptoms become apparent. Cancer is usually found by the affected individual, who notices a warning sign, or a health care provider during a checkup. A cancer checkup is recommended every 3 years for persons ages 20 to 39 years and annually for those ages 40 years and older. Risk assessment is the first step in cancer prevention. The cancer examination should include both a medical history of exposures to environmental agents and a comprehensive family history.

If cancer is suspected, various diagnostic studies are performed depending on the suspected primary or metastatic site of the cancer. They include laboratory studies or blood tests, radiologic studies, endoscopy, cytology, and biopsy. Nurses must be able to give brief descriptions of such tests as well as assist in client preparation.

Although no one blood test can confirm a cancer diagnosis, some malignancies do alter the chemical composition of the blood. Specialized laboratory tests have been developed to detect **tumor markers,** substances such as specific proteins, antigens, genes, hormones, or enzymes that are found in the serum and indicate the possible presence of malignancy. Tumor markers are not 100% accurate, as benign processes can also cause elevations; they are, however, useful in monitoring response to treatment or detecting a relapse.

Cancer Detection

Which diagnostic tests should a person have as part of a routine physical to detect cancer?

COMMON DIAGNOSTIC TESTS

Commonly used diagnostic tests for clients who present with symptoms of cancer are listed in Table 31-2. See Basic Nursing Diagnostic Tests, for explanation/normal values and nursing responsibilities related to each test.

TABLE 31-2	COMMON DIAGNOSTIC TESTS FOR CANCER DETECTION

Laboratory Tests
- Acid phosphatase (elevated)
- Alkaline phosphatase (elevated)
- Bence Jones protein
- CA-15-3
- CA-19-9
- CA-125
- CEA (carcinoembryonic antigen)
- PSA (prostate-specific antigen)
- Stool for occult blood (Guaiac)
- Serum calcitonin

Radiologic Studies
- X-ray studies
- Computerized axial tomography (CT scan or CAT scan)
- Magnetic resonance imaging (MRI)
- Scans (radioisotope test)
- Ultrasound

Invasive Diagnostic Techniques
- Endoscopy
- Cytology
- Biopsy

STAGING OF TUMORS

Staging determines the extent of the spread of cancer. The TNM classification proposed by the American Joint Commission on Cancer is one of the most frequently used systems. The *T* refers to the anatomical size of the primary tumor; *N*, the extent of lymph node involvement; and *M*, the presence or absence of metastasis (Table 31-3). Use of this internationally recognized staging system for tumors ensures a reliable comparison of clients in many different hospitals. Staging is important because it influences decisions about treatment modalities and helps predict overall prognosis.

GRADING OF TUMORS

Normal body cells have individual characteristics that allow them to perform different body functions. This process is called **differentiation.** Tumor cells that retain many of the identifiable tissue characteristics of the original cell are termed *well differentiated.* Tumor cells having little similarity to the tissue of origin are termed *undifferentiated.* Tumor grading is based primarily on the degree of differentiation of malignant cells. Grading evaluates tumor cells in comparison to normal cells. Pathologists indicate tumor cell grades by using the Roman numerals I through IV; the higher the grade, the higher the number and the worse the prognosis. Thus, a grade I tumor is the most differentiated, and a grade IV tumor is the most undifferentiated (or least differentiated). Tumors containing poorly differentiated cells are more aggressive in growth and may display uncharacteristic behaviors, leading to a poorer prognosis. Grading criteria vary for different neoplasms.

TREATMENT MODALITIES

After cancer is diagnosed, staged, and graded, a medical treatment plan is developed. The most common

TABLE 31-3	STAGING OF TUMORS: EXAMPLES OF TNM CLASSIFICATION		
STAGE	**TUMOR**	**LYMPH NODE**	**METASTASIS**
I	<2 cm diameter Mobile Often superficial Confined to organ of origin	No involvement	No evidence
III b	<2 to >5 cm diameter Mobile or not mobile Localized or extended	>2 to 3 cm diameter Firmer than normal	No evidence
IV c	No evidence to >10 cm diameter	No evidence to >10 cm diameter Fixed and destructive Extension to second or distant stations	Solitary or multiple

treatment methods used today are surgery, radiation therapy, and **chemotherapy** (use of drugs to treat illness); biotherapy and bone marrow transplantation may also be used. These methods may be used alone or in combination.

Surgery

Surgery is the oldest form of cancer treatment and remains the most common method of treatment today. Surgery can be classified as curative, palliative, or reconstructive.

The goal of **curative surgery** is to heal or restore to health; this involves excising all of the tumor, the involved surrounding tissue, and the regional lymph nodes. Surgery most often has curative results when performed in the early stages of cervical, breast, or skin cancer.

Because 70% of clients show evidence of metastasis at diagnosis, cure is not always possible, and **palliative surgery** may be necessary. This surgery is effective in relieving symptoms in more advanced stages of cancer, although it does not alter the course of the disease. It is usually performed in an attempt to relieve complications such as obstructions or to surgically interrupt nerve pathways for intractable pain. It may also be used to insert special access devices or to place tubes for enteral nutrition.

Reconstructive surgery is performed to reestablish function or rebuild for a better cosmetic effect. Reconstructive surgery to areas such as the head, neck, breast, and extremities can minimize deformity. The surgery may be completed all at once or done in stages.

Radiation Therapy — shrink or diminish used in conjunction w/.

Radiation therapy is the second most common method of treating cancer. Radiation therapy, or **radiotherapy,** uses high-energy ionizing radiation to kill cancer. Ionizing radiation has the ability to penetrate tissue cells and deposit energy within them. This intense energy causes breakage in chromosomes within the cell, thus preventing the ability of the cell to replicate. Cell death may occur hours, days, or even years after treatment, depending on the rate of mitosis.

The goal of radiation therapy is to eradicate malignant cells without causing harm to healthy tissues. Some cells are more sensitive to radiation than others. Better vascularized, better oxygenated cells and those that divide rapidly are the most sensitive.

It may be used alone or as an adjunct to other therapies. As a single treatment modality, it is most often used when the disease is localized. Preoperative radiation is frequently used to reduce the tumor mass before surgery. Postoperative radiation therapy is frequently used to decrease the risk of local recurrence following surgery. Some chemotherapeutic drugs increase the sensitivity of cancer cells to radiation and thus are used together with radiation. Radiation therapy can be classified as curative or palliative. It is frequently used to alleviate symptoms of metastasis, such as pain.

There are two types of radiation therapy: external radiation and internal radiation.

CLIENT TEACHING

External Radiation

- Do not wash off the skin markings used to designate reference points for treatment.
- Client is alone in the room during treatment.
- Client must lie absolutely still.
- Treatment typically lasts 1 to 3 minutes.
- Treatment is usually painless.

External Radiation

External radiation, or teletherapy, is performed with special equipment that can deliver high-energy radiation. Treatments are usually administered on an outpatient basis, divided over many days or weeks. Customized shielding blocks may be created to protect healthy tissues, and immobilization devices may be used to maintain the exact position for each treatment. Dyes or tattoos may be used to designate reference points on the skin.

Nursing care should be directed toward client teaching, safety, and carrying out interventions that provide relief from side effects. Undesirable side effects that are most likely to occur include varying degrees of skin reactions and gastrointestinal discomfort such as abdominal cramping, diarrhea, loss of appetite, and fatigue. Treatments have a cumulative effect and may thus produce symptoms after the therapy has been completed.

Internal Radiation

Internal radiation delivers radioactive isotopes directly within the body. Clients treated with internal sources of radiation can be a source of radioactivity. Isotopes may be introduced into the body by sealed or unsealed sources.

With sealed sources, radioactive elements are encapsulated in special containers such as tubes, wires, needles, seeds, or capsules. These containers are implanted close to the cancer cells to deliver a highly concentrated dose of radiation to the cancer cells. Radioactive implants are commonly used in the treatment of cancers of the tongue, lip, breast, vagina, cervix, endometrium, rectum, bladder, and brain.

Because sources are sealed, body fluids are not radioactive. Personnel caring for clients who have sealed sources must still be familiar with the hazards of radiation, however. Generally, the degree of exposure is dependent on three factors:

- The distance between the individual and the source (Figure 31-2)
- The amount of time an individual is exposed
- The type of shielding provided

Safety: Internal Radiation

Client care should be modified based on the three factors related to the degree of exposure to sealed-source radiation by:

- Preparing everything outside of the room so that as little time as possible is spent close to the client

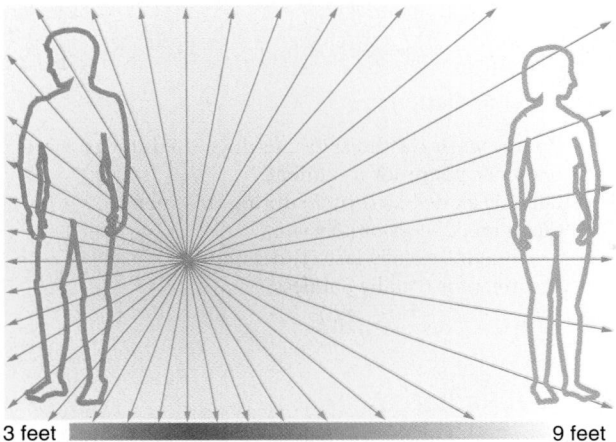

Figure 31-2 *Radiation dose decreases with distance. (Courtesy of the U. S. Nuclear Regulatory Commission)*

3 feet   9 feet

- Having several nurses assigned to care for the client so that the time of exposure for each nurse is lessened
- Wearing a lead apron or other shielding device, as provided

Radioactive isotopes can also be placed in suspensions or solutions as unsealed sources of radiation. They may be given orally or parenterally or be instilled into intrapleural or peritoneal spaces.

Some radioactive elements used in unsealed radiation sources are eliminated in body secretions, including urine and stool; thus health care workers must take special precautions to avoid exposure. Agency policies and procedures as well as Standard Precautions must be followed closely. Unsealed sources are not usually radioactive as long as are sealed sources.

Chemotherapy - *rapid growing cells*

Chemotherapy may be used to cure, prevent, or relieve cancer symptoms. Drugs used in chemotherapy are called **antineoplastics** because they inhibit the growth and reproduction of malignant cells. To understand how anticancer drugs work, one must have a basic understanding of the cell cycle.

Almost all anticancer drugs kill cancer cells by affecting DNA synthesis or function, but they vary in how they exert their activity within the cell cycle. Most chemotherapeutic drugs are classified as cell-cycle specific (CCS) or cell-cycle nonspecific (CCNS).

Cell-cycle specific drugs attack cancer cells when the cells enter a certain phase of reproduction. These agents are most effective against rapidly growing tumors. Many of the drugs are "schedule dependent" because they produce a greater cell kill when given in multiple, repeated doses.

Cell-cycle nonspecific drugs can destroy cancer cells in any phase of the cell cycle and are used for large tumors that have fewer actively dividing cells. These drugs are not schedule dependent but, rather, dose dependent. This means that the number of cells destroyed is determined by the amount of drug given.

Anticancer agents are cytotoxic (toxic to cells) and destroy both normal and abnormal cells. They are most effective against cells that reproduce rapidly, such as those in bone marrow, gastrointestinal lining, hair follicles, and the ova and sperm. Because cells multiply at their most rapid rate at the beginning of the disease, the drugs work best against cancer in its earliest stages.

Many of these drugs are given in combination with or after radiation or surgery to achieve maximum effect. They are usually given intermittently over an extended period. Drug resistance can occur.

The most common routes of administration are oral and intravenous. A few drugs may be given topically, subcutaneously, or intramuscularly. Recently, other methods have been introduced to increase the local concentration of the drug at the tumor site, including intrathecal injection and intracavity instillation. Table 31-4 lists some commonly used drugs.

Careful attention must be given to intravenous administration. Leakage of fluid from the vein into the sur-

COMMUNITY/HOME HEALTH CARE

Home Care Following Chemotherapy

Teach clients receiving chemotherapy to monitor the side effects of therapy at home.

- Inspect the skin daily for any signs of rash or dermatitis, which may signal hypersensitivity to a drug.
- Report taste loss and tingling in the face, fingers, or toes, which may signal peripheral neuropathy.
- Report signs of dizziness, headache, confusion, slurred speech, or convulsions, which may be signs of central nervous system (CNS) toxicity.
- Report signs of unusual bleeding or bruising; fever; sore throat; or mouth sores, which may signal developing myelosuppression.
- Report signs of jaundice; yellowing of the eyes; clay-colored stools; or dark urine, which may signal developing hepatic dysfunction.
- Report a continued cough or shortness of breath, which may signal developing pulmonary fibrosis.

TABLE 31-4   DRUGS COMMONLY USED IN CHEMOTHERAPY

Antimetabolites (CCS)
cytarabine (Cytosar)
fluorouracil (Adrucil)
methotrexate (Mexate)
6-mercaptopurine (Purinethol)

Antibiotics (CCNS)
dactinomycin (Cosmegan)*
daunorubicin (Cerubidine)*
doxorubicin hydrochloride (Adriamycin)*
mitomycin (Mutamycin)*
mithramycin (Mithracin)
bleomycin (Blenoxane)

Antihormonal Agents (CCNS)
flutamide (Eulexin)
goserelin acetate (Zoladex)
tamoxifen (Nolvadex)

Vinca Plant Alkaloids (CCS)
vinblastine sulfate (Velban)*
vincristine sulfate (Oncovin)*

Hormones (CCNS)
diethylstilbestrol (DES)
megestrol acetate (Megace)
medroxyprogesterone acetate (Depo-Provera)
testosterone (Histerone, Testoderm)

Nitrosureas (CCNS)
carmustine (BiCNU)
lomustine (CeeNU)

Alkylating Agents (CCNS)
busulfan (Myleran)
chlorambucil (Leukeran)
cisplatin (Platinol)
cyclophosphamide (Cytoxan)
mechlorethamine hydrochloride
   (Mustargen)*
melphalan (Alkeran)
thiotepa (Thiotepa)

Corticosteroids
dexamethasone (Decadron)
hydrocortisone sodium succinate
   (Solu-Cortef)
prednisone (Deltasone)

Miscellaneous Agents
etoposide (VePesid)
L-asparaginase (Elspar)
procarbazine hydrochloride
   (Matulane)

Frequently Used Combinations

CMF±P	cyclophosphamide, methotrexate, 5-fluorouracil, and prednisone
CAMP	cyclophosphamide, doxorubicin (Adriamycin), methotrexate, and procarbazine
CAE	cyclophosphamide, doxorubicin (Adriamycin), and etoposide
CVP	cyclophosphamide, vincristine, and prednisone
FAC	5-fluorouracil, Adriamycin, and Cytoxan
MOPP	mechlorethamine hydrochloride (Mustargen), vincristine (Oncovin), procarbazine, and prednisone

*= vesicant drug

rounding tissues during infusion is called **extravasation**. Because most chemotherapeutic drugs are irritating to the tissues, extravasation is a potentially serious problem, especially if the drugs being administered are **vesicants**. These agents are so irritating that they can cause blistering and even necrosis. All sites must be monitored carefully. Pain, swelling, redness, and the presence of vesicles are all signs of extravasation. Additional signs include the following:

- Pain or burning at the site or along the vein
- Absent or sluggish blood return
- Redness 6 to 12 hours later
- Swelling
- Diffuse hardening

If extravasation does occur, the drug must be stopped immediately and protocols for treatment initiated.

Safety: Chemotherapy and Contamination
- Any personnel handling blood, vomitus, or excreta from clients who have received

chemotherapy within the previous 48 hours should wear disposable latex gloves and a disposable gown.
- Place contaminated linen in specially marked laundry bags according to agency procedures.

Improved infusion techniques, control of symptoms such as nausea and vomiting, and cost-containment restrictions have reduced the length of hospitalizations for clients undergoing chemotherapy. Teaching clients and family members to monitor side effects in the home setting is thus an essential function of the **oncology** (study of tumors) nurse.

Clients should also be advised that lifestyle may need to be adjusted to accommodate the side effects of chemotherapy. Clients should be instructed to pace themselves according to their energy level and allow time for rest throughout the day. It is also important to inform clients that even between treatments they may not have the same amount of energy as before treatment initiation. Many clients do not experience any adverse effects, but some experience life-threatening toxicity. Nursing care of the client receiving chemotherapy requires not only a thorough understanding of the drugs used to destroy the cancer, but also skills in helping clients and families cope with the side effects of the therapy.

Biotherapy

Biotherapy is performed with **biologic response modifiers** (BRMs), agents that stimulate the body's natural immune system to control and destroy malignant cells. Most BRMs are still being evaluated in trial studies. Biotherapy is used after surgery, radiation, and chemotherapy have removed the bulk of the tumor. Some agents currently being investigated include interferons, monoclonal antibodies, interleukin-2, tumor necrosis factor, *bacillus Calmette-Guérin* (BCG), and colony-stimulating factors. Side effects are usually less severe than those seen in chemotherapy and may include fever, malaise, myalgia, and headache. Because an anaphylactic reaction can occur, the client must be closely monitored.

Bone Marrow Transplantation

Bone marrow transplantation (BMT) is used for cancers that respond to high doses of chemotherapy or radiation therapy. Treatment involves aspirating and storing a fraction of bone marrow, exposing the client to high-dose drug therapy or total-body irradiation, and then reinfusing the bone marrow after the treatment is complete.

The bone marrow used in transplantation can be the client's own marrow (autologous), marrow taken from an identical twin (syngeneic), or marrow taken from a histocompatibly matched donor, preferably a sibling (allogeneic).

According to Otto (2001), the cost of BMT is high. Client expenses may range from $100,000 to $200,000 unless covered or partially covered by insurance. The average length of hospital stay is 35 to 40 days. Complications can be life threatening and include infection, bleeding, gastrointestinal effects, renal insufficiency, veno-occlusive disease (deposits of fibrin obstruct venules of liver), and graft-versus-host disease (new bone marrow cells recognize environment as foreign and try to destroy the host). Clients who undergo autologous BMT do not experience graft-versus-host disease.

SYMPTOM MANAGEMENT

Cancer clients undergoing treatment experience a variety of secondary problems. One of the most important responsibilities of the oncology nurse is to formulate nursing interventions to manage these problems.

Bone Marrow Dysfunction

Cancer treatments kill both malignant cells and normal cells in bone marrow. Blood counts should thus be monitored carefully during and after treatment.

A low white-cell count increases the risk of infection. A decreased neutrophil count (below 500/mm³) is an indicator that special infection prevention measures should be initiated. Scrupulous hand hygiene is the most effective method of controlling bacterial infection. Personnel should maintain strict asepsis when changing dressings or performing invasive procedures. Clients should avoid contact with anyone who is ill. Antimicrobial soaps should be used for bathing clients. The skin and mucous membranes should be inspected daily for signs of infection. Vital signs should be taken every 4 hours and the client observed for fever and chilling.

Clients with a platelet count below 50,000/mm³ should be monitored for bleeding. Their skin should be inspected daily for bruises or petechiae. Shaving should be done with an electric razor to minimize the chance of cutting the skin. Stool and urine should be monitored for occult blood. Observe the client for bleeding from the vagina, rectum, nose, mouth, and venipuncture sites. If bleeding does occur, pressure should be applied to the site for 5 minutes. Any bleeding that does not stop in 5 minutes should be reported. A soft toothbrush may be recommended for oral care. Aspirin or any medication containing acetylsalicylic acid should not be given.

Nutritional Alterations

Cytokines are substances secreted by the tumor in an attempt to cannibalize the body and by the immune system to fight the tumor. Cytokines make the body digest muscle for energy instead of using stored fat for this purpose. This state of malnutrition and protein (muscle) wasting is called **cachexia.** It occurs in conjunction with lung, pancreatic, stomach, bowel, and prostate cancers but rarely with breast cancer.

In some cases, untreated cachexia, rather than the cancer itself, is the cause of death. Untreated cachexia can also decrease the effectiveness of cancer treatments and may increase the side effects of these treatments. Treating cachexia with drugs has met with little success.

A registered dietitian understands cancer cachexia and can identify appetizing foods that are nutrient and calorie dense. Foods that appeal to the client should be eaten anytime. The use of liquid nutritional supplements and a multivitamin is often recommended (Wilkes, 2000).

Hallmarks of malnutrition are a weight loss of 10% or more or a serum albumin level below 3.4 g/dL. Clients unable to maintain sufficient oral intake for long periods may be given enteral or total parenteral nutrition (TPN). Nutritional problems associated with cachexia include

---

CLIENT TEACHING

Increasing Nutritional Intake

- Drink 4 ounces of a nutritional supplement before breakfast.
- Eat breakfast (if desired), and then take a walk. Doing so will help build muscle and increase appetite.
- Drink another 4 ounces of nutritional supplement 1 hour before having a lunch consisting of whatever foods are appealing.
- Have another 4 ounces of nutritional supplement at midafternoon and at bedtime.
- If not hungry for dinner, take another walk.

anorexia, nausea and vomiting, altered taste sensation, mucosal inflammation, and dysphagia.

Anorexia

Anorexia, loss of appetite, is a common complaint among individuals with cancer. It is generally best for these clients to eat small, frequent, high-calorie (carbohydrate and fat-rich) meals. Try to ascertain the client's likes and dislikes. Highly seasoned foods help increase taste. Clients should be encouraged to eat when they are feeling best. Weight should be monitored weekly.

Nausea and Vomiting

Nausea and vomiting usually occur within 3 to 4 hours after chemotherapy is administered and may last up to 72 hours. Antiemetics are given before chemotherapy and continued afterward as needed (Table 31-5). Small, frequent feedings of complex carbohydrates may be beneficial. Liquids should be given 30 to 60 minutes before meals. Although highly seasoned foods may increase taste, they often also increase nausea and vomiting. Cool, bland foods are more easily tolerated. Avoid foods with strong odors. Frequent mouth care can help remove the taste of chemotherapy and increase the likelihood of the client's wanting to eat. The client should be monitored for dehydration and electrolyte imbalances.

Altered Taste Sensation

Taste sensation can be altered because cancer cells release substances that stimulate bitter taste buds, causing a bitter or metallic taste in the mouths of some clients. Some find they no longer enjoy the taste of red meat, and others say they have an aversion to sweets.

Mucosal Inflammation

Stomatitis, or inflammation of the mucous membrane of the oral cavity, occurs in one-half of cancer clients receiving treatment. It usually occurs 7 to 14

days after chemotherapy administration and lasts 2 to 3 weeks. To minimize stomatitis, assess for early signs and symptoms such as edema, ulceration, erythema, excessive saliva, and infection. If the client is receiving a chemotherapy drug that is known to cause stomatitis (e.g., methotrexate) oral care should be administered at least 4 times a day.

Avoid rough, chewy foods and acidic foods. Straws are beneficial because food can be taken in the back of the mouth and swallowed. Popsicles and frozen fruit bars sometimes help numb and lessen pain. Avoid commercial mouthwashes containing alcohol. A saline rinse may be helpful after meals. If the client has dentures, remove them at night. Viscous Xylocaine rinses can be ordered for pain. Lemon and glycerine swabs should not be used because lemon may be irritating to mouth lesions.

Dysphagia

Dysphagia, difficulty in swallowing, often occurs in clients with esophageal cancers, or in those receiving radiotherapy.

Artificial saliva may be ordered for severe dryness. A softer diet along with nutritional supplements may be prescribed. Dry foods such as toast can scratch the delicate tissues of the throat. Food puréed in a blender may be easier to tolerate. Clients should take plenty of time to chew and swallow.

Pain

Approximately 60% to 90% of all individuals with progressive malignancy will experience pain. The pain may be acute, but it is more likely to be chronic (greater

TABLE 31-5	COMMONLY USED ANTIEMETICS

prochlorperazine (Compazine)
metoclopramide (Reglan)
ondansetron hydrochloride (Zofron)
lorazepam (Ativan)
dolasetron (Anzemet)

than 3 months in duration). Pain usually does not occur until the advanced stages of the disease. The most common causes of pain are metastatic bone disease, venous or lymphatic obstruction, or nerve compression.

Pain can cause anxiety, depression, and feelings of helplessness in addition to physical discomfort. It can affect the client's sleeping habits, eating patterns, work, family, and social relationships. Ultimately, pain can affect the client's quality of life.

Noninvasive pain-relief techniques may be useful in pain management. They include cutaneous stimulation (heat, cold, massage), transcutaneous electrical nerve stimulation (TENS), relaxation techniques, imagery, and hypnosis. Most of these techniques are inexpensive and easy to perform. They have few side effects and can usually be done in any environment. They also give the client some control over the treatment of pain. Although not every client will respond successfully to these measures, it is worthwhile to attempt them before using invasive techniques.

The federal government took steps toward ensuring that cancer pain can be treated. The Agency for Health Care Policy and Research (AHCPR, 1994) developed Cancer Pain Guidelines for clients, family members, and health care professionals. Some points emphasized by the guidelines include the following:

- Cancer pain can be managed effectively through relatively simple means in up to 90% of cancer clients in the United States. Skin patches, slow-release tablets, and client-controlled pumps are now available to complement standard drugs.
- The mainstay of pain assessment is the client self-report. Because there is no standard test for pain, the nurse must respect the client's report of pain and regard it as the single most reliable indicator.
- The simplest dosage schedules and least invasive pain management modalities should be used first. Nonopioids are the first step in the analgesic ladder. They should be tried first for mild to moderate pain.
- Morphine is the most commonly used opioid for moderate to severe pain because it is available in a wide variety of dosage forms, it has well-characterized pharmacokinetics and pharmacodynamics, and it is relatively low in cost. Morphine can be given orally, subcutaneously, intramuscularly, intravenously, rectally, and intraspinally. It can also be given in sustained-release preparations.
- Health care providers should work to prevent pain rather than try to treat pain after it has occurred. Analgesics work better when given regularly around the clock before pain becomes severe. A major nursing

responsibility is to teach the client to request pain medication before the pain becomes severe. When medication is ordered around the clock, the nurse should not hesitate to wake the client to administer analgesics.

If pain control cannot be achieved with noninvasive techniques or medications, neurosurgical procedures such as nerve blocks may be performed.

Fatigue

Fatigue occurs as a direct result of cancer treatment or because of anemia, chronic pain, stress, depression, insufficient rest, or inadequate nutritional intake. Although the etiology is not well understood, fatigue is often related to the effects of the tumor itself (Greifzu, 1998). Fatigue may contribute to client noncompliance with the treatment regimen.

Frequent rest periods should be provided for the client. Assess for the presence and pattern of fatigue. Proper planning allows the client to be active when energy level is higher, which may in turn restore a greater sense of control. Evaluate factors that increase or decrease fatigue, such as nutritional intake. Blood count should be monitored for anemia.

Alopecia

Alopecia, the thinning or loss of hair, may be induced by chemotherapy or radiation treatments. The extent of hair loss depends on the dose and duration of the therapy. Scalp hair is most commonly affected, but pubic, axillary, and facial hair, even eyebrows and eyelashes, may also be affected. The treatments cause hair loss by interfering with the growth processes in the hair follicle. This results in weakening of the hair shaft, thereby causing the hair to break off at the surface of the scalp. Hair loss usually begins 2 to 3 weeks after the initial treatment. Drug-induced alopecia is not permanent. Hair usually begins to grow back within 8 weeks after treatment is completed. The color and consistency of the hair may change.

Odors

Unpleasant odors emanating from the cancer client may be a source of embarrassment. These odors are usually associated with drainage, exudates, or incontinence. Fortunately, meticulous nursing care can eliminate most offending odors. Change soiled linens, drainage pads,

CLIENT TEACHING

Alopecia, Threat to Body Image
Encourage client to:

- Buy a wig or hairpiece before treatment actually begins so that it will match the client's normal hair.
- Wear hats, scarves, or bandanas to cope with the change in body image caused by hair loss.
- Focus on other positive aspects rather than on just physical appearance.

and dressings immediately. Wash the client's skin gently with soap and warm water. Protective creams may be used if the areas are not receiving radiation. Room deodorizers can be helpful but should be used cautiously because many clients experience nausea when exposed to the odors from room fresheners. Placing a drop of oil of wintergreen or oil of cloves on a cotton ball near the ventilation system can sometimes lend a light freshness to the environment.

Dyspnea

One-half of all clients with terminal cancer experience dyspnea, or difficulty in breathing. Possible causes include fluid accumulation in the chest, infection such as pneumonia, fibrosis caused by radiation, and anemia. Lungs should be auscultated every 4 hours. Oxygen may be ordered. Fluid may be drained by an invasive procedure called a thoracentesis. High-Fowler positioning helps maximize ventilation. Plan care to keep activity to a minimum to balance oxygen requirements and oxygen supply. Oxygen status can be monitored with a pulse oximeter. Report a sustained reading of less than 90%. Avoid pulling the privacy curtain or shutting the client's door unless absolutely necessary, because either of these actions may reduce air flow and create more anxiety.

Bowel Dysfunctions

Cancer clients frequently exhibit changes in bowel patterns. Constipation, diarrhea and subsequent perineal skin breakdown, and bowel obstructions are common elimination disorders.

Constipation results from decreased motility of the colon. It is frequently caused by chemotherapy, opioid analgesic, or inactivity. Monitor and record the frequency of the client's bowel movements. Constipation can be an early sign of vincristine toxicity. Fluid consumption may be encouraged and a stool softener given daily. Clients at risk for constipation should be started on a high-fiber diet, with increased intake of bran and prune juice.

Common causes of diarrhea include radiation therapy, chemotherapy, antibiotics, tube feedings, hyperosmolar dietary supplements, stress, and fecal impactions. Clients can develop fluid and electrolyte imbalances from constant diarrhea. If the client is receiving a chemotherapy drug known to cause diarrhea (such as fluorouracil [Adrucil] or doxorubicin hydrochloride [Adriamycin]), a low-residue and lactose-free diet should be encouraged. Instruct the client to avoid foods that stimulate the gastrointestinal tract, such as warm liquids and coffee.

Bananas (which are high in potassium) and sports drinks (which contain sodium and potassium) can help replace lost fluids and electrolytes without irritating the gastrointestinal tract.

The perineum should be kept clean and dry after each loose stool. Treat anal irritations cautiously with agents such as heat lamps, ointments, and cornstarch; they may be contraindicated in clients receiving radiation therapy. Note signs of fluid and electrolyte imbalances, such as thirst, dry mucous membranes, and decreased skin turgor. The potassium level should be monitored. Measure and record the amount, frequency, and charac-

teristics of all client bowel movements. Antidiarrheal medications such as Lomotil or Imodium should be given for every loose stool. Sitz baths will help soothe sore or broken-down tissues.

Bowel obstructions occur more commonly in conjunction with advanced abdominal malignancies and should always be suspected if the client has received radiation or has adhesions from prior surgeries. Symptoms include nausea, vomiting, and abdominal pain. Surgery may be required to relieve the obstruction.

Pathological Fractures

Pathological fractures are a major problem in cancers that metastasize to bone. These cancers weaken the bone to the point that normal activities can cause painful breaks. Thus, limbs should be supported and handled gently, and extreme care should be taken when moving clients. Special devices such as splints may be used for extra protection. Weight-bearing restrictions may be ordered.

Ascites

Abdominal cancers may cause ascites, fluid accumulation in the abdomen. Clients may experience abdominal swelling and difficult breathing. Symptoms may be treated temporarily with an invasive procedure called a paracentesis, wherein a small, plastic tube is advanced through the abdominal wall and excess fluid is withdrawn. Chemotherapy drugs sometimes are instilled in an attempt to prevent the fluid from returning. Visually assess the abdomen. A protruding abdomen may indicate ascites as well as intestinal distention and enlarged organs. Measure abdominal girth at the umbilicus daily with a tape measure to monitor changes. Then auscultate the abdomen in all four quadrants. Gurgling bowel sounds heard every 5 to 15 seconds indicate normal peristalsis. Decreased or absent bowel sounds may indicate peritonitis or paralytic ileus. Fluid accumulation can be confirmed by percussing for shifting dullness. When a large amount of fluid is present, fluid waves may be seen. Gentle palpation is used to detect pain and tenderness as well as abdominal masses. The nurse should carefully document any abnormal findings.

Weigh the client daily to monitor weight gain. Fluid consumption may be restricted. Good skin care, especially to the abdomen, is essential. Fowler positioning helps maximize ventilation. Clients should be observed closely for electrolyte imbalance if large amounts of fluids are withdrawn via paracentesis.

Sexual Alterations

Many chemotherapy drugs can interfere with sexual functioning and reproduction. Premenopausal women may become infertile. Those younger than age 35 may regain their fertility after therapy is completed. Men may experience impotence, decreased libido, interrupted sperm production, and ejaculation problems. Women may experience vaginal dryness.

Encourage clients and their partners to express their feelings and concerns to each other and to explore other avenues of sexual expression, such as cuddling, kissing, and stroking. Birth control should be practiced during therapy and for 1 or 2 years after therapy (depending on physician recommendation) to ensure that all chemotherapy drugs have been eliminated and will have no ill effects on a pregnancy. Eggs and sperm may be saved before treatment.

MEDICAL EMERGENCIES

Medical emergencies occur in approximately 20% of clients with advanced-stage cancer. Early recognition and treatment can prevent irreversible complications and improve the quality of life. Four complications with which to be familiar are hypercalcemia, spinal cord compression, superior vena cava syndrome, and cardiac tamponade.

HYPERCALCEMIA

Hypercalcemia occurs commonly and can be a potentially fatal complication if not detected early. It is found most often in clients with malignant tumors that have metastasized to bone, such as breast cancer. The condition occurs when the serum calcium level rises higher than 10.5 mg/dL.

Early symptoms of hypercalcemia, such as nausea, vomiting, constipation, and weakness, may be overlooked because these are common side effects of many cancer therapies. Later symptoms such as dehydration, renal failure, coma, and cardiac arrest may develop swiftly.

Hypercalcemia is treated aggressively with intravenous normal saline and furosemide (Lasix), which increase calcium excretion. Clients may also be given drugs to decrease bone reabsorption. Monitor the serum calcium level when Lasix is being administered. Teach clients early symptoms of hypercalcemia so they can recognize a recurrence. These clients are also at increased risk for pathological fractures because calcium has been released from the bones, leaving them very fragile.

SPINAL CORD COMPRESSION

Spinal cord compression can result in permanent paralysis if not treated promptly. Cancers of the lung, breast, and prostate carry the greatest risk of metastasizing to the spinal cord.

The chief symptom of metastasis to the spinal cord is back pain. The discomfort is aggravated by lying down, coughing, or moving, and may be relieved by sitting upright.

Treatment is aimed at reducing tumor size to decrease pressure on the spinal cord. Radiation, surgery, and steroid therapy may be used. Pain medications should be given frequently, and clients should be supported carefully during transfers.

SUPERIOR VENA CAVA SYNDROME

Superior vena cava syndrome is a collection of symptoms caused by an obstruction of the superior vena cava. It occurs more frequently in conjunction with lung cancer and lymphomas. Typically, clients experience dyspnea and swelling of the face and neck. Edema in the upper extremities, chest pain, and coughing may also occur. Central nervous system symptoms such as headache, visual disturbances, and alteration in consciousness rarely occur.

The goal of treatment is to reduce tumor size. Radiation along with diuretics is usually ordered. Administer oxygen as ordered and provide a calm, restful environment. Encourage the client to limit activities and lie in Fowler's position. Carefully monitor respirations. Lower extremities should not be elevated, as doing so will increase venous return to an already engorged area.

CARDIAC TAMPONADE

Cardiac tamponade is caused by the formation of pericardial fluid, which reduces cardiac output by compressing the heart. Tumor metastasis to the pericardium is associated with lung cancer, breast cancer, Hodgkin's disease, lymphoma, melanoma, gastrointestinal tumors, and sarcoma. Common symptoms of cardiac tamponade include a rapid, weak pulse; distended neck veins during inspiration; ankle or sacral edema; pleural effusion; ascites; enlarged spleen; lethargy; and altered consciousness.

Treatment is aimed at aspirating the fluid constricting the heart (pericardiocentesis). Reassure the client, explain the procedure, and administer medication for pain.

PSYCHOSOCIAL ALTERATIONS

Perhaps of all the problems that clients with cancer experience, none is more challenging than the associated psychosocial alterations. The mere diagnosis of cancer invokes fear and misunderstanding. A myriad of emotions may surface initially. These may range from deep depression to denial and total refusal of treatment. Anxiety, sadness, and withdrawal are common. Some clients may feel that the disease is a punishment for some misguided deed. Each client responds differently to the diagnosis, depending on individual coping mechanisms and support systems.

Research has identified effective and ineffective coping mechanisms. Clients who seek information or share feelings tend to cope more effectively than do those who submit to treatment and procedures without asking questions or who use small talk to avoid discussing threatening issues.

Cancer affects not only the client, but the client's family as well. Responses of family members to the disease will have a significant impact on the client's coping. The

COMMUNITY/HOME HEALTH CARE

Psychosocial Aspects of Cancer

• Clients may see themselves as burdens to their families.
• Family caregivers may be angry that their own needs must go unmet.
• Family caregivers may feel inadequate with regard to caring for the client.
• Medical equipment such as a hospital bed, commode chair, or wheelchair may need to be brought into the home. These may have an impact on family member state of mind and disposition with regard to the family member with cancer.

client and family must face issues such as loss of control, changes in body image, and financial burdens, which can be a huge problem.

The nurse has several roles in this context. The client needs time and space to adjust to the diagnosis. Be available to offer support and reassurance. Answer questions, but do not bombard the client with information. Interpret information given by the physician and help the client formulate questions to ask the physician. Encourage the client to express feelings and fears about the illness.

The initial treatment is very frightening for most cancer clients. Allay anxiety by giving information about the treatment's purpose, adverse reactions, and signs and symptoms to report to the physician. Explaining procedures and answering questions in simple language can help the client and family regain a feeling of some control. Treatment modalities cause many discomforts, but if the client knows what to expect, the distress can generally be handled. Symptom management is critical in preventing lifestyle disruptions.

Families and clients facing the terminal phase of cancer are confronted with a complex set of problems. The client and family must face separation and impending death. Some families will demand that extraordinary measures be taken to keep the client alive. Some will search for meaning in life and will experience a genuine closeness. Give the client and family privacy and time to share feelings. Sometimes, the only psychosocial support the client needs is to have someone sitting by the bedside. Touch, especially at times when words are hard to find, can often be the most comforting intervention.

As the client's condition deteriorates, physical needs become more pronounced. Focus on keeping the client comfortable and free of pain. Hospice care is designed to provide spiritual, emotional, and physical support during the final days of illness. The goal of hospice is to keep the client as comfortable as possible. Pain relief and symptom management are stressed. The focus is shifted from cure to care. Care may be given in an institution, but most hospice care is given in the home. Hospice care is medically managed and nurse coordinated. Members of the hospice team typically include a chaplain, physician, nurse, social worker, physical therapist, and home health aide, as well as various volunteers. The team functions to ensure that the client's plan of care is carried out and that family members receive adequate support. The family is instructed in the area of care to be given. Bereavement counseling is offered to help family members deal with their loss.

NURSING PROCESS

Assessment

Subjective Data

The client interview serves as a forum for ascertaining the client's perception of the illness, treatment, and prognosis; health practices; and health concerns. The client's significant other may also be interviewed to ascertain support systems.

Objective Data

Vital signs are measured, and a head-to-toe assessment is performed. Past hospital records are reviewed along with the current record. Laboratory reports, biopsy results, treatment modalities, and comments from other health care professionals are studied.

CRITICAL THINKING

Nursing Intervention Rationale
What is the rationale for each nursing intervention given for the possible nursing diagnoses given in this chapter?

Nursing diagnoses for a client with cancer may include the following:

Nursing Diagnoses	Planning/Goals	Nursing Interventions
Fear related to cancer diagnosis	The client will express anxieties and fears to family and/or health care providers.	Review the client's previous experience with cancer to ascertain any current misconceptions based on past beliefs.

continues

Nursing Diagnoses	Planning/Goals	Nursing Interventions
		Encourage the client to share feelings regarding the diagnosis to facilitate identification of coping strategies.
		Explain hospital routines and focus on the recommended treatment, including its purpose and potential side effects. Accurate descriptions that convey what the client can expect help ease fears associated with the unknown. A calm, reassuring environment can also enhance coping abilities.
Anticipatory Grieving related to potential loss of body function	The client will express grief to family and/or health care providers.	Open, honest discussions can help the client cope with the situation. Be aware that mood swings, hostility, and other negative behaviors often occur. Discuss the loss of body function with the client. Ask what the loss of body function means to the client.
		Encourage the client to seek help and support from close family members.
Imbalanced Nutrition: Less than body requirements related to side effects of chemotherapy	The client will maintain body weight.	Encourage the client to eat a high-calorie, nutrient-rich diet. Supplements may be useful. Some clients may benefit from frequent, small meals and snacks. Foods high in protein, such as cheese, fish, and poultry, are also recommended.
		Provide oral hygiene before and after meals.
		Administer antiemetics approximately 30 minutes before meals. Mints, hard candies, and saltine crackers may help if the client complains of metallic taste.
		Nondietary interventions may include varying the surroundings, using small plates, eating at a table with friends, and minimizing food odors.
		Monitor intake and output along with daily weight.
Risk for Impaired Skin Integrity related to chemotherapy and radiation	The client will maintain skin integrity.	Assess skin frequently for side effects of cancer therapy. (A reddening or tanning effect may develop with radiation. Skin reactions such as rashes, pruritus, and alopecia develop with chemotherapy.)
		Use lukewarm water and soap to gently wash the client's skin. Skin often becomes sensitive during radiation treatments.
Risk for Infection related to side effects of chemotherapy	The client will remain free of infection.	Monitor vital signs at least every shift. White blood count should be monitored and protective isolation should be instituted if the count falls below 500/mm^3.
		Educate the client, staff, and visitors in all aspects of infection prophylaxis. Thorough hand hygiene is the most important means of preventing and controlling the transmission of organisms. Because fresh flowers and raw fruits and vegetables can transmit microbes, they should be eliminated. The client should not be exposed to anyone who has an infection or who has been recently vaccinated against or exposed to a communicable disease. Visitors should be limited.
Risk for Injury related to altered clotting factors secondary to side effects of chemotherapy	The client will remain free of injury related to bleeding.	Every shift, assess the client for signs of bleeding (petechiae, ecchymoses, hematomas, bleeding gums, epistaxis, tarry stools, hematuria, frank or prolonged bleeding from puncture sites) because transfusions may be indicated.
		Monitor platelet count, which is an indicator of clotting ability. Institute special precautions if the count falls below 50,000/mm^3.

continues

Nursing Diagnoses	Planning/Goals	Nursing Interventions
		Apply pressure to all puncture sites for 3 to 5 minutes. Doing so prevents prolonged bleeding, which can cause damage to underlying tissues such as nerves. Instruct the client to use a soft toothbrush or sponge for oral hygiene to prevent damage to oral mucosa, which is particularly susceptible to bleeding. Instruct the client to use an electric razor when shaving.
Fatigue related to analgesics, anemia, stress, increased metabolism, and chemotherapy	The client will experience less fatigue.	Plan frequent rest periods for the client to restore energy, and schedule activities when the client has the most energy. Monitor nutritional intake, as adequate nutrients are necessary to meet energy needs. Recognize that weakness places the client at increased risk for injury. Because fatigue may make activities of daily living difficult to complete, assistance may need to be provided.

Evaluation Each goal must be evaluated to determine how it has been met by the client.

SAMPLE NURSING CARE PLAN

THE CLIENT WITH LUNG CANCER

Mr. Sanez is a 54-year-old carpenter. He is admitted with pain over his left scapula and radiating to his left arm. He describes having dyspnea and admits that he does have a productive cough. He denies any recent weight loss but does acknowledge experiencing extreme fatigue for the last 2 months. Mr. Sanez has been a chronic smoker for 20 years. A chest x-ray reveals an area of density in the left lung. A needle biopsy confirms small-cell lung cancer. A computerized tomography (CT) scan confirms extrathoracic involvement. His physician referred Mr. Sanez to an oncologist for palliative chemotherapy. Mr. Sanez is to receive his first treatment of cisplatin (Platinol) and etoposide (VePesid). Mr. Sanez states that he is not sure about this treatment given that it will not cure him and he does not know how he will keep breathing. He has never before been hospitalized.

Nursing Diagnosis 1 *Anxiety* related to unfamiliar surroundings and uncertainty regarding change in health status as evidenced by Mr. Sanez's statement that he does not know how he will keep breathing and the fact that he has never before been hospitalized

Nursing Outcomes Classification (NOC)
Anxiety Control
Acceptance: Health Status
Symptom Control

Nursing Interventions Classification (NIC)
Anxiety Reduction
Coping Enhancement
Calming Technique

PLANNING/GOALS	NURSING INTERVENTIONS	RATIONALE
Mr. Sanez will share his feelings regarding his dyspnea.	Ascertain what the physician has told Mr. Sanez and what conclusions Mr. Sanez has reached. Encourage Mr. Sanez to share his feelings concerning cancer.	Helps decrease fear of the unknown. Identifies the source of any misconception that is serving to increase anxiety.

SAMPLE NURSING CARE PLAN

PLANNING/GOALS	NURSING INTERVENTIONS	RATIONALE
Mr. Sanez will express less anxiety about being in the hospital.	Maintain frequent contact with Mr. Sanez. Explain the hospital routine and care Mr. Sanez should anticipate.	Reassures Mr. Sanez that he is not alone. An unfamiliar environment increases anxiety.

EVALUATION Mr. Sanez shares his feelings about his diagnosis and treatment regimen. Mr. Sanez exhibits less anxiety about the change in his health status and being in the hospital.

Nursing Diagnosis 2 *Impaired Gas Exchange* related to decreased lung capacity and increased secretions as evidenced by dyspnea, productive cough, and dense area in left lung

Nursing Outcomes Classification (NOC)	Nursing Interventions Classification (NIC)
Respiratory Status: Gas Exchange	*Airway Management*
Respiratory Status: Ventilation	*Respiratory Monitoring*
Tissue Perfusion: Pulmonary	*Oxygen Therapy*

PLANNING/GOALS	NURSING INTERVENTIONS	RATIONALE
Mr. Sanez will report less dyspnea with oxygen saturation >90%.	Monitor pulmonary status by auscultating breath sounds; checking rate, depth, and pattern of respirations; evaluating skin color for cyanosis; and monitoring pulse oximetry.	Provides information regarding pulmonary status changes indicating either improvement or onset of complications.
	Position Mr. Sanez in Fowler's position.	Promotes expansion of lungs and respiratory muscles.
	Administer oxygen at prescribed level.	Corrects hypoxemia and provides oxygen for metabolic needs.
	Administer opioids with caution.	Opioids can depress the respiratory center.
	Monitor amount, color, and consistency of sputum.	Changes in sputum suggest infection or change in pulmonary status.
	Plan care and treatments within Mr. Sanez's tolerance.	Oxygen demands increase with activity.

EVALUATION Adequate ventilation with oxygen saturation >90% is maintained.

Nursing Diagnosis 3 *Acute Pain* related to tumor growth and tissue destruction as evidenced by verbal report of pain over left scapula radiating to left arm

Nursing Outcomes Classification (NOC)	Nursing Interventions Classification (NIC)
Pain: Disruptive Effects	*Pain Management*
Comfort Level	*Environmental Management: Comfort*

continues

SAMPLE NURSING CARE PLAN

PLANNING/GOALS	NURSING INTERVENTIONS	RATIONALE
Mr. Sanez will report less pain following pain-relief measures.	Provide routine comfort measures such as repositioning and backrub.	Noninvasive pain-relief techniques may be helpful in pain management.
	Teach Mr. Sanez to request pain medication prior to onset of pain.	Keeps pain under control.
	Have Mr. Sanez rate pain on a scale of 0 to 10 (0 = no pain and 10 = worst pain).	Provides a method of evaluating the subjective experience of pain.
	Teach Mr. Sanez relaxation techniques.	May decrease the perception of pain.
	Document Mr. Sanez's response to the pain-control regimen and adjust as needed.	Identifies effectiveness of pain-relief techniques.

EVALUATION   Mr. Sanez reports less pain; <4 on a scale of 0 to 10.

Nursing Diagnosis 4 *Fatigue* related to chronic pain and dyspnea as evidenced by client's description of dyspnea and extreme fatigue for 2 months

Nursing Outcomes Classification (NOC)
Activity Tolerance
Energy Conservation

Nursing Interventions Classification (NIC)
Energy Management
Simple Relaxation Therapy

PLANNING/GOALS	NURSING INTERVENTIONS	RATIONALE
Mr. Sanez will report feeling less fatigued.	Plan care to allow for rest periods.	Helps conserve energy.
	Assess for related factors such as nutritional imbalances, lack of sleep, and causes of stress.	May reduce fatigue.
	Have Mr. Sanez rate fatigue on a scale of 0 to 10 (0 = not tired, 10 = total exhaustion) for a 24-hour period.	Identifies peak energy and exhaustion times.
	Teach energy-conservation strategies such as planning ahead, setting priorities, scheduling rest periods, and resting before a difficult task.	Decreases physical and psychological stress.

EVALUATION   Mr. Sanez exhibits less fatigue in light of having frequent rest periods daily.

Nursing Diagnosis 5 *Anticipatory Grieving* related to loss of body function as evidenced by Mr. Sanez's statement that he does not know how he will keep breathing

Nursing Outcomes Classification (NOC)
Grief Resolution
Coping

Nursing Interventions Classification (NIC)
Grief Work Facilitation
Emotional Support

continues

SAMPLE NURSING CARE PLAN

PLANNING/GOALS	NURSING INTERVENTIONS	RATIONALE
Mr. Sanez will verbalize his loss and develop coping skills as he acknowledges his illness as terminal.	Provide opportunities for Mr. Sanez to express his feelings.	Helps identify Mr. Sanez's coping strategies.
	Answer all of Mr. Sanez's questions honestly.	Helps Mr. Sanez cope.
	Encourage Mr. Sanez's participation in his care.	Gives Mr. Sanez a greater sense of control.
	Encourage family support and visits from friends.	Assures Mr. Sanez that he is not alone and provides time to discuss concerns openly.
	Utilize appropriate referrals to professionals such as clergy, as needed.	Facilitates the grief process and spiritual care.

EVALUATION   Mr. Sanez comes to terms with the reality of his diagnosis and prognosis.

CASE STUDY

Mr. John Dalton is a 70-year-old male with a history of cancer of the prostate, which was treated with palliative hormones and radiation. His admitting diagnosis is adenocarcinoma of the prostate with widespread bone metastasis. Mr. Dalton is married and has one grown daughter, who often helps with his care. His chief complaint is severe back pain. The physician has ordered intrathecal morphine sulfate and aspirin 10 gr for pain relief.

The following questions will guide your development of a nursing care plan for the case study.

1. List symptoms typically seen in clients diagnosed with prostate cancer.
2. Identify the population most at risk for developing prostate cancer.
3. List three possible risk factors for prostate cancer.
4. Discuss why the physician's orders include aspirin along with morphine sulfate.
5. Discuss why benzodiazepines should not be used for pain relief.
6. List the subjective and objective data the nurse would want to obtain.
7. When you walk into Mr. Dalton's room, he greets you with a smile and continues talking and joking with his daughter. While assessing him, you note that his vital signs are normal. You ask him to rate his pain on a scale of 0 to 10. He pauses to think about it, then rates the pain at 8. In the chart, you must record your nursing assessment by circling the appropriate number on the scale. Which number do you think you should circle?
8. Write three individualized nursing diagnoses and goals for Mr. Dalton.
9. Discuss which oncological emergency Mr. Dalton is most likely to develop.

Summary

- Cancer is the second most common cause of death in the United States.
- Most cancers are curable if treated early.
- Benign neoplasms are localized and encapsulated and do not spread.
- Malignant neoplasms spread to neighboring tissues via blood and lymph.
- Biopsy is the most accurate diagnostic test for cancer.
- The most common medical treatments for cancer are surgery, radiation, and chemotherapy. They may be used alone or in combination.
- Surgery is the treatment of choice for early cancers.
- Chemotherapy is the treatment of choice for metastatic cancers. It is also the treatment most responsible for increasing cancer cure rates in recent years.
- Lung cancer is the leading cause of cancer death among men and women. Eighty percent of all cases are related to smoking.
- Quality of life, not quantity of life, is the ultimate goal for clients living with cancer.

Review Questions

1. The nurse carefully monitors the client's intravenous chemotherapy. An early indicator that extravasation may be occurring is when:

   a. the fluid stops infusing.

   b. edema is noted at the site.

   c. blood returns when the bottle is lowered.

   d. burning occurs at the site.

2. A breast cancer client states that the doctor says he is going to prescribe hormone therapy. Which of the following hormones would probably be ordered?

   a. thyroxin

   b. parathormone

   c. progesterone

   d. testosterone

3. A cancer client develops a low white-cell count. She is placed on neutropenic precautions. Which of the following menu selections would be best?

   a. meat loaf, mashed potatoes, green beans, and fruit gelatin

   b. meat loaf, mashed potatoes, marinated carrots, and a garden salad

   c. meat loaf, mashed potatoes, chef salad, and tapioca

   d. meat loaf, mashed potatoes, green beans, fruit salad, and a cookie

4. When stomatitis develops, it is best to encourage the client to:

   a. drink plenty of orange juice.

   b. use lemon and glycerine swabs frequently.

   c. brush teeth before and after eating.

   d. rinse with commercial mouthwash as needed.

5. Clients receiving radiation should be encouraged to:

   a. wash and dry the skin carefully and apply lotion.

   b. not bathe.

   c. not apply deodorants or lotions.

   d. wash the skin with soap and apply baby powder.

References/Suggested Readings

Agency for Health Care Policy and Research. (1994). *Clinical practice guidelines: Management of cancer pain* (AHCPR Publication No. 94-0592). Rockville, MD: U.S. Department of Health & Human Services.

American Cancer Society (ACS). (2000). 2000 Facts and Figures. [Online]. Available www.cancer.org/statistics/cff2000/basicfacts.html

American Cancer Society (ACS). (2002). Cancer news roundup. *Nursing2002, 32*(10), 32hn6–32hn7.

American Cancer Society (ACS). (2003). *Cancer Facts & Figures 2003.* [Online]. Available: www.cancer.org/downloads/STT/CAFF2003pwSecured.pdf

American Pain Society. (1992). *Principles of analgesic use in the treatment of acute and chronic cancer pain* (3d ed.). Skokie, IL: Author.

Baird, S., Donehower, M., Stalsbroten, V., & Ades, T. (Eds.) (1997). *A cancer source book for nurses* (7th ed.). Atlanta, GA: American Cancer Society.

Belcher, A. (1992). *Cancer nursing.* St. Louis, MO: Mosby.

Blackburn, G. (1998). Wasting away: Cancer cachexia. *Health News, 4*(4), 4. Waltham, MA: Massachusetts Medical Society.

Bral, E. (1998). Caring for adults with chronic cancer pain. *AJN, 4*(98), 27–32.

Chapman, D., & Goodman, M. (2000). *Cancer nursing principles* (5th ed.). Boston, MA: Jones & Bartlett.

Chiramannil, A. (1998). Lung cancer. *AJN, 4*(98), 46–47.

Dell, D. (2001). Regaining range of motion after breast surgery. *Nursing2001, 31*(10), 50–52.

Dochterman, J., & Bulechek, G. (2004). *Nursing Interventions Classification (NIC)* (4th ed.). St. Louis, MO: Mosby.

Erickson, J. (1994, November). Update on Hodgkin's Disease. *Nurse Practitioner,* 63–67.

Estes, M. E. Z. (2002). *Health assessment & physical examination* (2nd ed.). Clifton Park, NY: Thomson Delmar Learning.

Fieler, B. K. (1997). Side effects and quality of life in patients receiving high-dose rate brachytherapy. *Oncology Nursing Forum, 24*(3), 545.

Galvan, T. (2001). Dysphagia: Going down and staying down. *AJN, 101*(1), 37–42.

Greifzu, S. (1998). Fighting cancer fatigue. *RN, 61*(8), 41–43.

Harris, L. (2002). Ovarian cancer: Screening for early detection. *AJN, 102*(10), 46–52.

Held-Warmkessel, J. (1998). Chemotherapy complications: Helping your patient cope with adverse reactions. *Nursing98 4*(28), 41–45.

Kediziera, P. (1998). The two faces of pain. *RN, 61*(2), 45–46.

Kohr, J. (1995). Measuring your patient's pain. *RN, 58*(4), 39–40.

Lewis, S., Heitkemper, M., & Dirksen, S. (2000). *Medical–surgical nursing: Assessment and management of clinical problems* (5th ed.). St. Louis, MO: Mosby.

Machia, J. (2001). Breast cancer: Risk, prevention & Tamoxifen. *AJN, 101*(4), 26–35.

McCaffery, M., & Ferrell, B. (1994, July). How to use the new AHCPR cancer pain guidelines. *AJN,* 42–47.

McCarron, E. (1995, June). Supporting the families of cancer patients. *Nursing95,* 48–51.

McConnell, E. (2001). Myth & Facts about dysphagia. *Nursing2001, 31*(7), 29.

Moorhead, S., Johnson, M., & Maas, M. (2004). *Nursing Outcomes Classification (NOC)* (3rd ed.). St. Louis, MO: Mosby.

Myers, J. S. (2000). Chemotherapy-induced hypersensitivity reaction. *AJN, 100*(4), 53–54.

Otto, S. (2001). *Oncology nursing* (4th ed.). St. Louis, MO: Mosby.

Phipps, W. J., Monahan, F. D., Sands, J., Marek, J. F., & Neighbors, M. (2003). *Medical–surgical nursing: Health and illness perspectives* (7th ed.). St. Louis, MO: Mosby.

Porth, C., Kumert, M. A. (2002). *Pathophysiology concepts of altered health states* (6th ed.), Philadelphia: Lippincott Williams & Wilkins.

Researchers say new drug may boost effects of cancer radiation. (1998, May 12). *Corpus Christi Caller Times.*

Resnick, B., & Belcher, A. (2002). Breast reconstruction. *AJN, 102*(4), 26–33.

Sargent, C., & Murphy, D. (2003). What you need to know about colorectal cancer. *Nursing2003, 33*(2), 36–41.

Scherer, J., & Timby, B. (1999). *Introductory medical–surgical nursing* (7th ed.). Philadelphia: Lippincott Williams & Wilkins.

Schweid, L., & Werner-McCullough, M. (1994, September). Will you recognize these oncological crises? *RN,* 23–27.

Smeltzer, S., & Bare, B. (2002). *Brunner and Suddarth's textbook of medical–surgical nursing* (9th ed.). Philadelphia: Lippincott Williams & Wilkins.

Tamoxifen for breast cancer prevention. (1998, December 15). *Healthnews, 4*(15).

Thaler-DeMers, D. (2000). The cancer survival toolbox. *AJN, 100*(4), 52.

U.S. Preventive Services Task Force. (2002). Screening for colorectal cancer: Recommendations and rationale. *AJN, 102*(9), 107–114.

Watson, A., & Coyne, P. (2003). Recognizing the faces of cancer pain. *Nursing2003, 33*(4), 32hn1–32hn8.

Weber, M. (1995). Clinical snapshot: Chemotherapy-induced nausea and vomiting. *AJN, 95*(4).

White, L., & Spitz, M. (1994). Cancer risk and early detection assessment. *Capsules and Comments in Oncology Nursing, 2*(1), 2–3.

Wilkes, G. (2000). Nutrition: The forgotten ingredient in cancer care. *AJN, 100*(4), 46–51.

Woodward, W., & Thobaben, M. (1994). Special home health care nursing challenges: Patients with cancer. *Home Health Care Nurse, 12*(3), 33–37.

Zuckerman, D. (2002). The breast cancer information gap. *RN, 65*(2), 39–41.

Resources

American Cancer Society (ACS), 1599 Clifton Road, NE, Atlanta, GA 30329, 800-ACS-2345, www.cancer.org

National Alliance of Breast Cancer Organizations, 9 East 37th Street, 10th Floor, New York, NY 10016, 212-719-0154, www.nabco.org

National Cancer Institute, Suite 3036A, 6116 Executive Boulevard MSC8322, Bethesda, MD 20892-8322, 800-422-6237, www.cancer.gov

National Coalition for Cancer Survivorship (NCCS), 1010 Wayne Avenue, Suite 770, Silver Spring, MD 20910-5600, 877-622-7937, www.canceradvocacy.org

Y-ME National Breast Cancer Organization, 212 West Van Buren, Suite 500, Chicago, IL 60607, 800-221-2141, www.y-me.org

Nursing Care of the Client: Oxygenation and Perfusion

RESPIRATORY SYSTEM

MAKING THE CONNECTION

Refer to the following chapters to increase your understanding of the respiratory system:

Basic Nursing
- **Assessment**
- **Diagnostic Tests**

Adult Health Nursing
- **Oncology**
- **Cardiovascular System**
- **Hematologic and Lymphatic Systems**

Basic Procedures
- **Performing the Heimlich Maneuver**

Intermediate Procedures
- **Administering Oxygen**
- **Performing Nasopharyngeal and Oropharyngeal Suctioning**
- **Performing Tracheostomy Care**

Delmar's Heart & Lung Sounds CD-ROM: Lung Sounds

Review: Delmar's Anatomy & Physiology CD-ROM: Nose, Thorax & Lungs

LEARNING OBJECTIVES

Upon completion of this chapter, you should be able to:
- **Define key terms.**
- **Describe components of a complete respiratory assessment.**
- **Identify normal parameters for common respiratory diagnostic studies.**
- **Discuss the etiology, medical–surgical management, and nursing care for clients with respiratory disorders.**
- **Prepare a nursing care plan for a client with a respiratory disorder.**

INTRODUCTION

Respiratory disorders account for millions of the dollars spent in the U.S. health care arena. From loss of time on the job because of the common cold to care for those with chronic respiratory disorders, the cost of respiratory disease is staggering. This chapter explores the various respiratory disorders, with a focus on the nursing process.

KEY TERMS

adventitious breath sound
asthma
atelectasis
audible wheeze
bronchial sound
bronchiectasis
bronchitis
bronchovesicular sound
caseation
cavitation
chemoreceptor
coarse crackle
diffusion
emphysema
epistaxis
external respiration
fine crackle
hemopneumothorax

hemothorax
internal respiration
liquefaction necrosis
lung stretch receptor
perfusion
pleural effusion
pleural friction rub
pleurisy
pneumonia
pneumothorax
primary tubercle
respiration
sibilant wheeze
sonorous wheeze
status asthmaticus
stridor
surfactant
ventilation
vesicular sound

ANATOMY AND PHYSIOLOGY REVIEW

The primary function of the respiratory system is delivery of oxygen to the lungs and removal of carbon dioxide from the lungs.

Thoracic Cavity

The chest cage is a closed compartment bounded on the top by the neck muscles and at the bottom by the diaphragm. The walls of the chest cage are formed by the ribs and intercostal muscles laterally, the thoracic vertebrae posteriorly, and the sternum anteriorly. The inside of the chest cage is called the *thoracic cavity.* Contained within the thoracic cavity are the lungs. The lungs are cone-shaped, porous organs separated from the other chest organs by the mediastinum. The lungs lie free, except for their attachment to the heart and trachea, and are encased in the pleura, a thin, transparent double-layered serous membrane lining the thoracic cavity. The layers of the pleura are the parietal pleura, which lies adjacent to the chest wall and produces pleural fluid, and the visceral pleura, which adheres to the surface of the lungs and absorbs pleural fluid. The area between the two pleura is known as the *pleural space.*

The pleural space normally contains 5 to 20 mL of fluid, which allows the layers of the pleura to slide on each other yet hold together. The pressure within the pleural space is less than that of outside air. This difference in pressure creates a suction that prevents the lungs from collapsing on exhalation.

The right lung is larger than the left and is divided into three sections, or lobes: upper, middle, and lower. The left lung is divided into two lobes: upper and lower (Figure 32-1). The upper portion of the lung is referred to as the *apex* (plural, apices). The lower portion is called the *base.* The lungs possess a dual blood supply: bronchial circulation and pulmonary circulation. Bronchial circulation begins with the bronchial artery, which provides the passageways of the lungs with blood to meet nutritional needs and ends when the venous blood enters the pulmonary veins. Pulmonary circulation is the route by which blood is delivered to the alveoli for gas exchange.

Conducting Airways

The conducting airways are tubelike structures that provide a passageway for air as it travels to the lungs. These are the nasal passages, mouth, pharynx, larynx, trachea, bronchi, and bronchioles (Figure 32-1). The conducting airways are lined with epithelial tissue containing serous glands, mucus-secreting Goblet cells, and hairlike projections called *cilia.* The mucus of the Goblet cells together with the cilia form a mucociliary blanket

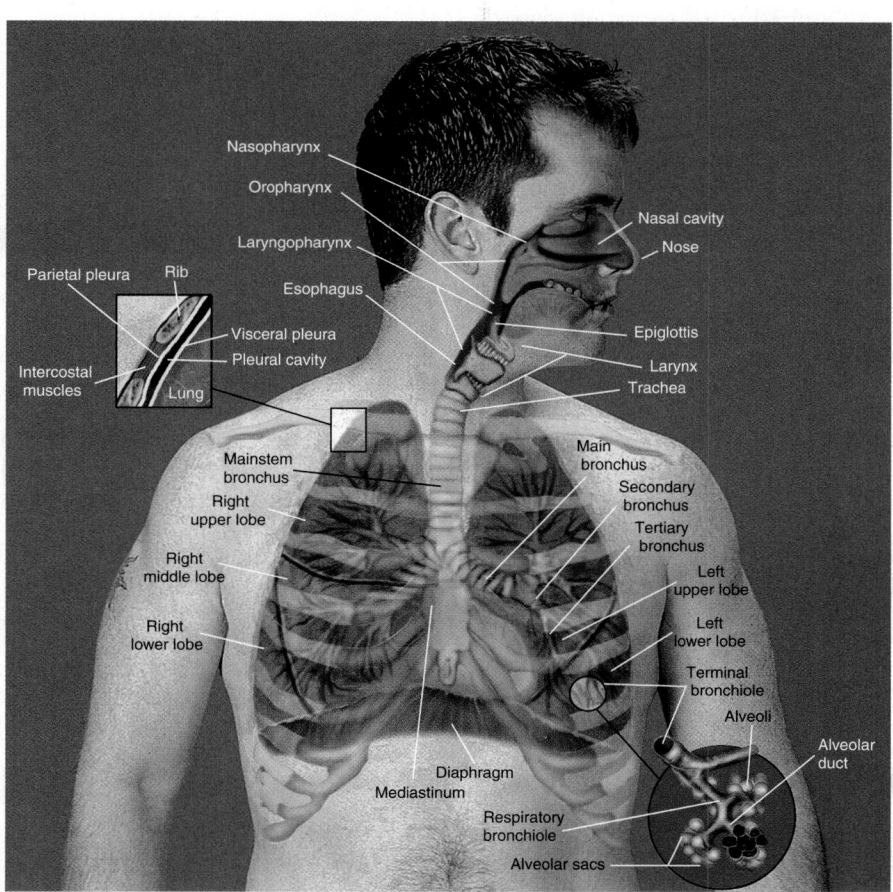

Figure 32-1 *Structures of the Respiratory Tract*

that protects the respiratory system from foreign particles. The constant upward motion of the cilia propels the mucociliary blanket toward the pharynx, where foreign matter may be expectorated.

The nasal passages are the preferred route for air to enter the respiratory tract. In addition to the function of filtering inspired air, the nasal passages are richly supplied with blood vessels that warm and moisten the air. Because the mouth lacks cilia and abundant blood supply, breathing through the mouth reduces the ability to filter, warm, and moisten inspired air.

Connecting the nasal passages and mouth to the lower parts of the respiratory tract is the pharynx. Located behind the oral cavity, the pharynx serves as a passageway for both inspired air into the larynx and ingested food passing into the digestive system. At the distal portion of the pharynx is the larynx, also known as the voice box.

The larynx contains the vocal cords and is the passageway for air entering and leaving the trachea. The larynx is composed of four structures: the uppermost thyroid cartilage (Adam's apple), the cricoid cartilage (which lies at the lower edge of the larynx), the epiglottis (a leaf-shaped structure that covers the larynx during swallowing), and the glottis (the triangular space between relaxed vocal cords).

The trachea, commonly known as the windpipe, is a tube composed of connective tissue mucosa and smooth muscle supported by C-shaped rings of cartilage that extends into the bronchi. The trachea is 2.0 to 2.5 cm wide (approximately 1 inch) and 10 to 12 cm long (approximately 4 to 6 inches). The trachea terminates by branching into two tubes: the right and left primary bronchi. The bronchi are somewhat smaller in diameter than the trachea, and each passes into its respective lung.

The right bronchus is wider and more vertically positioned than the left. This difference in positioning allows foreign matter to enter the right bronchus more easily than the left. Within the lungs, the bronchi branch off into increasingly smaller diameter tubes until they become the terminal bronchioles. These branch further, forming alveolar ducts that end in numerous saclike, thin-walled structures called the *alveoli*. Collectively, the alveoli and the alveolar ducts resemble a cluster of grapes. The branching makes this portion of the respiratory tract resemble an inverted tree, giving rise to the term *bronchial tree* (Figure 32-1).

Respiratory Tissues

The respiratory tissues perform the function of gas exchange. The alveoli constitute the primary site of gas exchange. The alveolar ducts are smooth, muscular tubes containing abundant alveolar macrophages that remove foreign particles (e.g., bacteria). The alveoli, into which the alveolar ducts terminate, consist of interconnected spaces with thin walls, or septa, occupied by a network of capillaries called the *alveolar capillary membrane.*

The alveoli contain two specialized types of cells. Type I alveolar cells are flat, squamous, epithelial cells across which gas exchange occurs. Type II alveolar cells produce a phospholipid substance called **surfactant.** Surfactant coats the inner surfaces of the alveoli, re-

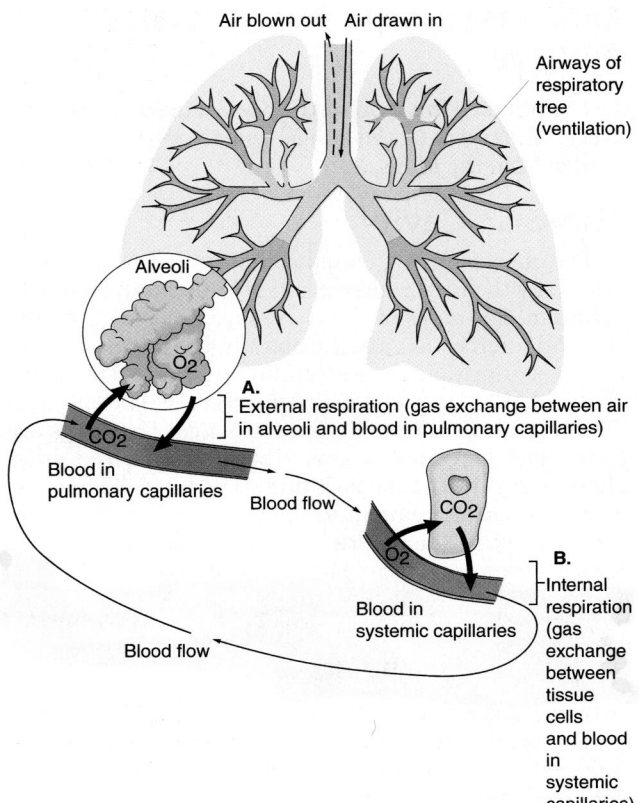

Figure 32-2 *A, External Respiration; B, Internal Respiration*

duces the surface tension of pulmonary fluids, allows gas exchange, and prevents the collapse of the airways. Each lung contains approximately 300 million alveoli.

Respiration

Respiration is a process of gas exchange. This process is necessary to supply cells with oxygen for metabolism and to remove the waste by-product carbon dioxide. There are two types of respiration: external respiration and internal respiration. **External respiration** is the exchange of gases between the inhaled air, now in the alveoli, and the blood in the pulmonary capillaries. **Internal respiration** is the exchange of gases at the cellular level between tissue cells and blood in systemic capillaries (Figure 32-2). These functions depend on the adequacy of ventilation, perfusion, and diffusion. **Ventilation** is the movement of gases into and out of the lung. **Perfusion** is the flow of blood through the vessels of a specific organ or body part. Pertaining to the respiratory system, **diffusion** is the movement of gases across the alveolar capillary membrane from areas of high concentration to areas of lower concentration. Factors that affect ventilation, perfusion, and diffusion affect respiration (Table 32-1).

Neuromuscular Control of Respiration

Unlike the heart muscle, the respiratory muscles must receive continuous neural stimuli to function. Regulation of respiration is integrated by neurons lo-

TABLE 32-1	FACTORS AFFECTING VENTILATION, PERFUSION, AND DIFFUSION
Ventilation	Position: Dependent areas receive majority of air.
	Lung volume: Low volume results in shunting air to lung apices.
	Disease: Bronchial constriction and airway collapse decrease ventilation.
Perfusion	Position: Dependent areas receive majority of blood.
	Hypoxia: Results in vasoconstriction and decreased perfusion.
	Blockage: Results in decreased or absent perfusion to distal areas.
Diffusion	Alveolar capillary membrane: Alterations may occur in thickness and permeability of membrane.

Figure 32-3 *Alveolar Gas Exchange*

cated in the pons and medulla of the brain. The control of respiration is influenced by involuntary (automatic) and voluntary components. Involuntary components include chemoreceptors, lung stretch receptors, and impulses from other sources. **Chemoreceptors** monitor the levels of carbon dioxide and oxygen and the acidity/alkalinity (pH) of the blood. Normally, chemoreceptors initiate respiration in response to an increase of carbon dioxide in the blood. With certain chronic pulmonary disorders, such as emphysema, chemoreceptors become more responsive to a low level of oxygen. This becomes significant when administering oxygen to persons whose drive to breathe depends on a low level of oxygen in the blood. **Lung stretch receptors** monitor the pattern of breathing and prevent overexpansion of the tissues. Many other sources involuntarily send impulses to the respiratory center. For example, if a person becomes frightened or angry, the respiratory rate increases in response to stimuli from the autonomic nervous system. Voluntary components of respiratory control integrate breathing with acts such as talking and speaking.

The diaphragm acts as the primary muscle of respiration. During inspiration, the diaphragm contracts and flattens out in response to stimuli from the respiratory center, increasing the length of the thoracic cavity. At the same time, the intercostal muscles contract, elevating the ribs and increasing the diameter of the thoracic cavity. The total thoracic space increases, reducing the pressure within the thoracic cavity. The pressure within the thoracic cavity then becomes negative in relation to that of atmospheric pressure, and air moves into the thoracic cavity. Upon expiration, the respiratory center signals the diaphragm and intercostal muscles to relax. The thoracic cavity returns to its original size. Aided by the elastic recoil of the lungs, the decrease in size of the thoracic cavity increases pressure, and air moves out of the lungs.

Gas Exchange

Gas exchange occurs at the alveolar capillary membrane. Venous blood from the right ventricle is pumped into the pulmonary arteries and travels to the alveolar capillary network, where it is exposed to the inhaled air. Because of the higher concentration of oxygen in the alveoli, oxygen diffuses into the blood within the alveolar capillary network. The majority of oxygen binds to the iron atoms of the hemoglobin molecule in the red blood cells. Approximately 1% to 3% of oxygen dissolves into the blood plasma.

The exchange of carbon dioxide also occurs within the alveoli. Within the alveolar capillary network, the carbon dioxide detaches from hemoglobin and diffuses into the alveolar space. Carbon dioxide is removed from the alveolar space when exhalation occurs. The blood within the pulmonary capillary network is now oxygenated and travels to the heart via the pulmonary veins. Oxygenated blood is sent to the body via the aorta and the arterial network (Figure 32-3).

ASSESSMENT

To understand the assessment of the respiratory system, the student must be familiar with related terminology (Table 32-2).

Health History

Nursing assessment begins with a complete history. The client should be questioned regarding allergies, occupation, lifestyle, and health habits such as smoking or alcohol use. Ask about other health problems that affect the respiratory system, such as pneumonia or cardiac problems. Symptoms such as dyspnea, decreased exercise tolerance, and cough must be explored in depth. Following a complete history, the nurse completes a physical assessment of the client.

TABLE 32-2	RESPIRATORY TERMS
TERM	**DEFINITION**
Eupnea	Normal breathing
Apnea	Cessation of breathing, possibly temporary in nature
Dyspnea	Labored or difficult breathing, possibly normal if associated with exercise
Bradypnea	Abnormally slow breathing
Tachypnea	Abnormally rapid breathing
Orthopnea	Discomfort or difficulty with breathing in any but an upright sitting or standing position
Kussmaul's respirations	Abnormal respiratory pattern characterized by irregular periods of increased rate and depth of respiration; most often seen with diabetic ketoacidosis
Biot's respirations	Abnormal respiratory pattern characterized by irregular periods of apnea alternating with short periods of respiration of equal depth; most commonly seen with increased intracranial pressure
Cheyne-Stokes respirations	Abnormal respiratory pattern characterized by initially slow, shallow respirations that increase in rapidity and depth and then gradually decrease until respiration stops for 10 to 60 seconds; pattern then repeats itself in the same manner
Anoxia	Without oxygen
Hypoxia	Lack of adequate oxygen in inspired air such as occurs at high altitude
Hypoxemia	Insufficient amount of oxygen in the blood possibly due to respiratory, cardiovascular, or anemia-related disorders
Cyanosis	Bluish, grayish, or purplish discoloration of the skin caused by abnormal amounts of reduced (oxygen-poor) hemoglobin in the blood; not always a reliable indicator of hypoxia
Acrocyanosis	Cyanosis of the fingertips and toes; often caused by vasomotor disturbances associated with vasoconstriction
Circumoral cyanosis	Bluish discoloration encircling the mouth
Oxygen saturation	Amount of oxygen combined with hemoglobin

Inspection

Physical assessment of the respiratory system starts with inspection. Note the client's color, level of consciousness, and emotional state. Respirations are observed for their rate, depth, quality, rhythm, and breathing pattern. Symmetry of chest wall movement is also noted. The nurse observes for use of accessory muscles to aid breathing. The position the client assumes provides information on respiratory status because individuals having trouble breathing often lean forward.

Palpation and Percussion

The next steps in the respiratory assessment are palpation and percussion. These are normally done by the registered nurse or physician. Through the use of palpation and percussion, areas of varying densities in the lung can be detected. The density of lung tissues changes with disease states such as pneumonia, pneumothorax, and pleural effusion.

Auscultation

The client should breathe slowly through the mouth while the listener assesses breath sounds at each location for the length of a complete inspiration and expiration. Breath sounds are assessed for duration, pitch, and intensity.

Normal Breath Sounds

Under normal circumstances, **bronchial sounds** are heard over the sternum. These loud, high-pitched tubular, hollow-like sounds last longer during expiration than during inspiration. When heard in areas other than the sternum, bronchial sounds indicate fluid, exudate, or lung tissue compression. **Bronchovesicular sounds** are heard over the anterior one-third of the chest near the sternum and also around the scapula posteriorly. Bronchovesicular sounds have a medium pitch and intensity with inspiration and expiration being equal in duration. They may be heard in the periphery of the lung when consolidation and fluid are present.

Vesicular sounds are heard over the majority of the lungs. These soft, low-pitched sounds are best heard during inspiration and may be inaudible during expiration.

Adventitious Breath Sounds

Abnormal breath sounds are called **adventitious breath sounds** and include **fine crackles, coarse crackles, sonorous wheezes, sibilant wheezes, pleural friction rub,** and **stridor.** Table 32-3 describes the general characteristics of these adventitious breath sounds.

COMMON DIAGNOSTIC TESTS

Commonly used diagnostic tests for clients with respiratory disorders are listed in Table 32-4. Table 32-5 lists normal values for arterial blood gases.

TABLE 32-3 CHARACTERISTICS OF ADVENTITIOUS BREATH SOUNDS

BREATH SOUND	RESPIRATORY PHASE	TIMING	DESCRIPTION	CLEAR WITH COUGH	ETIOLOGY	CONDITIONS
Fine crackle	Predominantly inspiration	Discontinuous	Dry, high-pitched crackling and popping of short duration: sounds like hair rolled between fingers when held near ears	Possibly	Air passing through moisture in small airways that suddenly reinflate	Chronic obstructive pulmonary disease (COPD), congestive heart failure (CHF), pneumonia, pulmonary fibrosis, atelectasis
Coarse crackle	Predominantly inspiration	Discontinuous	Moist, low-pitched crackling and gurgling of long duration	Possibly	Air passing through moisture in large airways that suddenly reinflate	Pneumonia, pulmonary edema, bronchitis, atelectasis
Sonorous wheeze	Predominantly expiration	Continuous	Low-pitched snoring	Possibly	Narrowing of large airways or obstruction of bronchus	Asthma, bronchitis, airway edema, tumor, bronchiolar spasm, foreign body obstruction
Sibilant wheeze	Predominantly expiration	Continuous	High-pitched and musical	Possibly	Narrowing of large airways or obstruction of bronchus	Asthma, chronic bronchitis, emphysema, tumor, foreign body obstruction
Pleural friction rub	Inspiration and expiration	Continuous	Creaking, grating	Never	Inflamed parietal and visceral pleura; can occasionally be felt on thoracic wall as two pieces of dry leather rubbing against each other	Pleurisy, tuberculosis, pulmonary infarction, pneumonia, lung abscess
Stridor	Predominantly inspiration	Continuous	Crowing	Never	Partial obstruction of the larynx, trachea	Croup, foreign body obstruction, large airway tumor

INFECTIOUS/INFLAMMATORY DISORDERS

Infectious/inflammatory disorders of the upper respiratory tract, pneumonia, tuberculosis, and pleurisy/pleural effusion are discussed in the following sections.

INFECTIOUS/INFLAMMATORY DISORDERS OF THE UPPER RESPIRATORY TRACT

Infectious and inflammatory disorders of the upper respiratory tract are common and usually self-limiting. Among the causal factors of infectious and inflammatory disorders are various viruses (rhino viruses,

TABLE 32-4   COMMON DIAGNOSTIC TESTS FOR RESPIRATORY DISORDERS

Laboratory Tests
- Hemoglobin
- Arterial blood gases (ABGs)
- Pulmonary function tests (PFTs)
- Sputum analysis

Radiologic Studies
- Chest x-ray
- Ventilation-perfusion scan
- Computerized axial tomography (CAT scan)
- Pulmonary angiography

Other
- Pulse oximetry
- Bronchoscopy
- Thoracentesis
- Magnetic resonance imaging (MRI)

TABLE 32-5   ARTERIAL BLOOD GASES: NORMAL VALUES

MEASUREMENT IN BLOOD	NORMAL VALUE
Acidity or alkalinity (pH)	7.3 to 7.45
Partial pressure of oxygen (PaO_2)	80 to 100 mm Hg
Partial pressure of carbon dioxide ($PaCO_2$)	35 to 45 mm Hg
Bicarbonate ion (HCO_3^-)	22 to 26 mm Hg
Arterial oxygen saturation (SaO_2)	95% (at sea level)

influenza viruses) and bacteria (streptococci and pneumococci). Group A *beta-hemolytic streptococci* infections of the upper respiratory system are associated with serious sequelae such as rheumatic fever. Allergic reactions frequently play a role in the development of sinusitis and pharyngitis. Laryngitis is associated with factors such as pollution, smoking, and excessive use of the voice. Breathing cold air decreases local immune responses of the respiratory tract. This fact coupled with closer and prolonged contact with others indoors during the colder months leads to an increased incidence of acute upper respiratory tract inflammatory disorders.

The signs and symptoms that occur with acute upper respiratory tract infection or inflammation are a result of the inflammatory process. Early signs and symptoms include general malaise, low-grade fever, localized redness, and edema of affected tissues. Joint pain is common with viral disorders. The client may complain of nasal or sinus congestion and headache. Drying of the mucous membranes coupled with edema cause local discomfort such as sore throat. Cough and nasal or sinus discharge may occur. Nasal secretions that are thick and purulent indicate bacterial infection.

Medical–Surgical Management

Medical

Most clients with acute upper respiratory tract infections or inflammatory disorders are treated in a clinic or office setting. Unless the disorder becomes chronic or bacterial infection occurs, treatment is symptomatic. When infection is suspected, specimens for culture and sensitivity are obtained, and appropriate antibiotic therapy is initiated.

Surgical

Disorders that develop into chronic conditions (e.g., tonsillitis and sinusitis) may require surgical intervention to remove or drain affected tissues.

Pharmacological

Nonprescription antipyretic, analgesic, anti-inflammatory medications may be used to reduce discomfort, fever, and inflammation. Antitussives may be used to suppress cough and allow for rest. To aid in removal of secretions, expectorants are used. Bacterial infections are treated with various antibiotics according to culture and sensitivity studies. Comfort measures such as saline gargles may be useful.

Diet

Clear fluids are advocated to liquefy secretions and hydrate dry mucous membranes. Nausea may occur if secretions are swallowed as opposed to expectorated. The client should be encouraged to cough up all secretions and dispose of them in a tissue. With severe coughing, emesis may occur. The client should be encouraged to rest before meals and may require an antitussive to reduce coughing.

Activity

Normally, activity does not need to be restricted, but energy level may decrease. The client who is infectious should be encouraged to avoid contact with others. Strenuous activity should be avoided to reduce oxygen requirements and coughing.

Nursing Management

Client teaching about signs and symptoms of a respiratory infection, avoiding items causing an allergic response, and taking all prescribed antibiotics is the main nursing responsibility.

NURSING PROCESS

Assessment

Subjective Data

Subjective data include information about present signs and symptoms, onset of symptoms, exposure to allergens or infected individuals, and frequency of the disorder. Common symptoms include sore throat, dyspnea, and headache.

Objective Data

Objective data include fever and inflammation, redness, edema, and drying of the mucous membranes of the oropharynx. Secretions are evaluated for their color, viscosity, amount, and odor, which will help in identifying the specific illness. The client may have hoarseness and a cough. Culture and sensitivity studies may reveal a causative organism and, thus, guide antibiotic therapy. If infection with group A *beta-hemolytic streptococci* is suspected, an antistreptolysin O (ASO) titer may be done to reveal the presence of antibodies formed in reaction to this bacteria. Nonspecific diagnostic studies include elevated white blood cell count and erythrocyte sedimentation rate.

Nursing diagnoses for a client with an upper respiratory infection or inflammatory disorder may include the following:

Nursing Diagnoses	Planning/Goals	Nursing Interventions
Deficient Knowledge related to signs and symptoms of respiratory bacterial infection, potential allergens, and antibiotic therapy	The client will be able to state the signs and symptoms of bacterial infection.	Educate the client regarding signs and symptoms indicating a respiratory bacterial infection, such as purulent or green secretions, fever.
	The client will be able to identify individual potential allergens.	Assist the physician in allergy testing. Teach the client to avoid those things that precipitate an allergic response.
	The client will complete entire course of antibiotic therapy.	Instruct client to complete the entire course of antibiotics.
Ineffective Airway Clearance related to nasal secretions.	The client will verbalize a decrease or absence of nasal congestion.	Encourage client to blow the nose and not "snuffle" secretions back up into nose.

Evaluation Each goal must be evaluated to determine how it has been met by the client.

PNEUMONIA

Pneumonia is inflammation of the bronchioles and alveoli accompanied by consolidation, or solidification of exudate, in the lungs. It can result from bacteria, viruses, mycoplasms, fungi, chemical exposures, or parasite invasions. Pneumonia can also be caused by aspiration, oversedation, or inadequate ventilation. Pneumonia remains a common cause of hospitalization and is often a cause of death, particularly among the elderly. Under normal circumstances, the alveolar macrophages are able to remove foreign matter. When confronted with overwhelming numbers of virulent microorganisms, however, this protective mechanism fails. The invading organism irritates the walls of the alveoli. In response to this irritation, the alveolar walls secrete exudate (an accumulation of fluid in the pulmonary passageways). Eventually, the alveoli fill with the exudate, resulting in consolidation. The exudate within the alveoli interferes with gas exchange.

Risk factors for the development of pneumonia include immobility, depressed cough reflex (caused by anesthesia or cerebrovascular accident [CVA]), alterations in respiratory function (e.g., chronic obstructive pulmonary disease [COPD]), advanced age, and numerous other chronic debilitating conditions (e.g., congestive heart failure [CHF], diabetes mellitus). Common bacterial causes of pneumonia are *Streptococcus pneumoniae*, *Pneumococcus*, *Staphylococcus aureus*, *Klebsiella pneumoniae*, and *Pseudomonas aeruginosa*. A common, serious viral source of pneumonia is the *Cytomegalovirus*, which affects clients with compromised immune status, such as those taking immunosuppressant medications or those infected with human immunodeficiency virus (HIV). *Pneumocystis carinii* pneumonia can also occur in the immunosuppressed client. The invading organism associated with *Pneumocystis carinii* pneumonia is thought to be a protozoan. The infecting microorganisms that cause

CLIENT TEACHING

Pneumonia

- Discuss pertinent information about medications being taken.
- Instruct in measures to prevent spread of infection (covering the mouth and nose with a tissue when coughing or sneezing).
- Encourage disposal of tissues in a closed paper sack.
- Outline individual's specific risk factors (age, chronic respiratory condition, cardiac condition).
- Instruct in methods to prevent future infection (avoiding crowds and obtaining vaccine).

pneumonia are spread by airborne droplets or direct contact with infected individuals or carriers.

Chemical pneumonia is caused by entry of irritating substances into the pulmonary passageways. A common source of chemical pneumonia is the aspiration of gastric contents. Inhalation of irritating substances can also result in a chemical pneumonia. Pneumonia is now classified according to the causative factor rather than the area of the lung affected. The right middle and lower lobes are affected by pneumonia more frequently than the right upper and left lobes because of the anatomy of the right bronchus and the effects of gravity.

A high fever of sudden onset is often the presenting complaint of the client. The elderly client, however, may be seriously ill and have only a low-grade fever. A productive cough yielding abnormally thick and discolored sputum may be present. Associated respiratory symptoms include dyspnea, coarse crackles, and diminished breath sounds. Most clients complain of pleuritic chest pain, which is stabbing in nature and increases on inspiration. Pain occurs as a result of irritation of the pleura lying adjacent to the affected alveoli.

In the case of bacterial pneumonia, white blood cell count increases and may go as high as 40,000/mm³. Pneumonia caused by viruses or mycoplasms may produce a normal or a lowered white blood cell count. Chest x-ray will reveal consolidation in the affected areas. Bacterial pneumonia is likely to produce isolated areas of consolidation on a chest x-ray, whereas viral and chemical pneumonia appear as more diffuse areas of consolidation. Arterial blood gases (ABGs) may reveal a decrease in PaO_2 or oxygen saturation caused by interference with gas exchange. Pulmonary function tests (PFTs) are usually within normal limits unless the client has an underlying pulmonary disorder such as emphysema.

Medical–Surgical Management

Medical

Clearing the airways of exudate and maintaining adequate oxygenation are the goals of treatment for clients with pneumonia. Postural drainage and percussion may be ordered to aid the client in mobilizing secretions.

COLLABORATIVE CARE

Postural Drainage, Medications

Respiratory therapists work together with nurses in providing postural drainage for clients with pneumonia or other respiratory problems when exudate drainage from the lungs is desired. They also collaborate on administering aerosol or nebulized medications.

Aerosol or nebulization treatments may also be utilized, often with added medications. The client is encouraged to cough and deep breathe, particularly following respiratory treatments. Incentive spirometry, which measures the amount of air inspired in one inhalation, may be ordered to aid the client when coughing and deep breathing are inadequate (Figure 32-4). If the client is unable to mobilize secretions, suctioning of the respiratory tract is indicated. When secretions are overwhelming, the physician may perform a bronchoscopy in order to remove them. Intravenous fluids may be utilized to maintain adequate hydration, especially in the presence of fever. Adequate hydration promotes liquefaction of respiratory secretions and thus aids in their removal. Pulse oximetry or ABGs are done to assess the level of oxygenation. Supplemental oxygen is used when oxygenation is inadequate.

Pharmacological

The treatment of choice for bacterial pneumonia is specific based on a sputum specimen for culture and sensitivity. It should be obtained before initiating an-

LIFE CYCLE CONSIDERATIONS

Respiratory Status in the Elderly Client

- Respiratory effort increases because muscles atrophy, the diaphragm flattens out, costochondral cartilage calcifies, ligaments and joints stiffen, and intervertebral discs degenerate.
- Alveolar gas exchange diminishes because of a decrease in the lung's elastic recoil, which causes air to be trapped, especially in the lower lobes, for a portion of the respiratory cycle.
- The medulla becomes less sensitive to changes in carbon dioxide and oxygen levels, thereby rendering the respiration triggering mechanism less active.
- Ciliary activity diminishes, thereby increasing susceptibility to infection.
- Cough reflex decreases.
- Aspiration risk increases because of the decrease in the cough reflex.

Figure 32-4 *An Incentive Spirometer*

tibiotic therapy. After a specimen has been obtained, the physician may start therapy with a broad-spectrum antibiotic. If laboratory data indicate resistant microorganisms, a specific antibiotic will be started. Antiviral agents, such as acyclovir sodium (Zovirax), are utilized for clients with chronic respiratory problems related to viral pneumonia. Prophylactic antibiotic therapy is often utilized for viral pneumonia to prevent a secondary bacterial infection. To promote opening and clearing of the airways, bronchodilators, and mucolytic agents are administered via aerosol or nebulization by the respiratory therapist or nurse. Expectorants may be given orally. Cough suppressants and pain relievers, especially those containing narcotics such as codeine sulfate, are administered only with discretion, because they may further inhibit the client's ability to clear the airways.

Diet

The client with pneumonia is encouraged to drink fluids to aid in the liquefaction of respiratory secretions. Small, frequent, nutritionally balanced meals are preferred. Respiratory treatments that promote coughing should be avoided immediately before and after meals to prevent nausea and vomiting associated with vigorous coughing.

Activity

Bed rest or limited activity promotes optimal tissue oxygenation; however, range-of-motion exercises and progressive ambulation prevent immobility complications.

Health Promotion

Pneumococcal vaccine (Pneumovax 23), a vaccine that prevents infection caused by *Streptococcus pneumonia*, should be given to clients at risk of developing pneumonia, such as those with chronic respiratory or cardiac conditions, and the elderly. Medicare pays for this vaccine (ALA, 2002).

Nursing Management

Auscultation of lungs for breath sounds, assessment of vital signs, and monitoring pulse oximetry and/or ABGs are nursing responsibilities. Encourage deep breathing, use of incentive spirometer, and the intake of fluids. Reposition clients who are on bed rest at least every 2 hours. Assist with range-of-motion exercises and ambulation when able.

NURSING PROCESS

Assessment

Subjective Data

Data gathered in the history include the onset, duration, and severity of cough; the color, amount, and odor of sputum if present; the onset and duration of elevated temperature; and the presence or absence of night sweats.

Objective Data

The client's level of consciousness should be noted. Evidence of dyspnea, orthopnea, tachypnea, and cyanosis may be present. On auscultation of the lung fields, moist crackles or diminished breath sounds are heard. In the event of obstruction of the airways, sibilant wheezes occur. All vital signs are taken before and after drug therapy to provide information regarding the severity of the illness and the efficacy of treatment. The color, amount, viscosity, and odor of sputum are noted.

Nursing diagnoses for a client with pneumonia may include the following:

Nursing Diagnoses	Planning/Goals	Nursing Interventions
Ineffective Airway Clearance related to inability to remove airway secretions.	The client will have clear breath sounds upon auscultation.	Encourage the client to breathe deeply and cough a minimum of every 2 hours.
		Teach use of the incentive spirometer to encourage lung expansion.
		Administer aerosol and nebulizer treatments as ordered.
		Assess breath sounds and respiratory rate prior to and following respiratory procedures to evaluate their effectiveness.
		Encourage fluids to liquefy thickened secretions.
		For clients who are able, assist in sitting up or ambulating three to four times daily; those on bed rest, turn every 2 hours.
		Administer medications as ordered.
		Provide oral care several times a day.
Impaired Gas Exchange related to inflammatory changes in alveolar capillary membrane	The client will have an oxygen saturation of 92% or greater.	Monitor pulse oximetry and/or ABGs.
		Administer supplemental oxygen as ordered.
Activity Intolerance related to hypoxia secondary to pneumonia	The client will be able to complete activities of daily living (ADL) and activity as ordered and without complaints of fatigue.	Encourage the client to complete ADL according to ability and the physician's orders.
		To prevent client fatigue, alternate periods of activity and care with periods of rest.

Evaluation Each goal must be evaluated to determine how it has been met by the client.

TUBERCULOSIS

Pulmonary tuberculosis (TB) is an infection of the lung tissue by *Mycobacterium tuberculosis*. Infection by tubercle bacilli can occur in other parts of the body, but with less frequency. In pulmonary tuberculosis, the tubercle bacilli are inhaled into the lungs. Whether infection occurs depends on the host's susceptibility, the virulence of the tubercle bacilli, and the number of bacilli inhaled. Tuberculosis is not as highly contagious as once thought. Prolonged exposure to the bacilli is required to produce infection. In addition, persons with uncompromised immune systems are able to combat the bacilli and do not develop the disease. Those at risk for tuberculosis include persons suffering from malnutrition, those living in crowded conditions, persons with compromised immune status, and health care workers providing care to high-risk individuals.

Once inhaled in sufficient numbers, the tubercle bacilli cause an inflammatory response within the alveoli of the lung. A small nodule called a **primary tubercle,** containing tubercle bacilli, forms in the lung tissue. In an attempt to isolate the primary tubercles, the body forms a fibrous outer coating around each tubercle. This fibrous surface interferes with the blood and nutritional supplies to the tubercle. In time, the interior of the tubercle becomes soft and cheese-like as a result of decreased perfu-

sion, a process known as **caseation.** Then the tubercle may become calcified and is called a Ghon's tubercle. **Liquefaction necrosis,** where the tissue dies and changes to a liquid or semi-liquid state, may occur; this fluid may then be coughed up. A cavity is formed at the site where the primary tubercle liquefied and ruptured. This is called **cavitation.**

Following the advent of antitubercular medications in the 1950s, the incidence of TB decreased dramatically until 1985. From 1985 to 1992, TB cases increased 20%, but from 1992 have decreased 39% (ALA, 2001). New forms of TB, resistant to conventional drug therapy, have surfaced. Some of the factors that may be responsible for the increase in TB cases are increased numbers of persons with compromised immune systems (e.g., many AIDS clients also have TB); increased mobility of the world's population (persons from areas of high TB incidence moving to areas of low incidence); widespread IV drug abuse; increased numbers of those with poor access to health care; and increased numbers of those living in impoverished conditions. Direct health care costs for TB are $703.1 million each year (ALA, 2001).

Symptoms of TB develop gradually following infection and include the following: low-grade fever that recurs in a specific pattern, persistent cough, hemoptysis, hoarseness, dyspnea on exertion, night sweats, fatigue, weight loss, and enlarged lymph nodes.

TABLE 32-6	CLASSIFICATION OF THE TUBERCULIN REACTION

CLASSIFIED AS POSITIVE	POPULATION
Induration of 5 mm or more	• HIV-positive persons • Recent contacts of TB case • Persons with chest x-rays consistent with old, healed TB • Clients with organ transplants or other immunosuppressed persons
Induration of 10 mm or more	• Injection drug users • Recent arrivals (<5 years) from high-prevalence countries • Residents and employees of high-risk congregate settings (prisons, nursing homes, mental institutions, residential facilities for AIDS patients, and homeless shelters) • Persons with medical conditions that have been shown to increase the risk of TB, such as silicosis; persons who are 10% or more below ideal body weight; and persons with some hematologic disorders (leukemias and lymphomas) and other malignancies • Mycobacteriology laboratory personnel • Children <4 years of age, or children and adolescents exposed to adults in high-risk categories
Induration of 15 mm or more	*Persons with no risk factors for TB*

TABLE 32-7	TUBERCULOSIS MEDICATIONS

DRUG	MEDICATION PRECAUTIONS AND INFORMATION
First-line Drugs ethambutol hydrochloride (Myambutol)	Monthly vision checks are important for acuity and distinction of red and green colors. Take medication with food.
isoniazid (INH) (Laniazid)	Alcohol ingestion interferes with metabolism and may cause hepatitis. Check baseline and monthly hepatic enzymes. Report signs of neuropathy and hepatitis. Have client take pyridoxine (vitamin B_6) to decrease side effects.
pyrazinamide (PMS Pyrazinamide)	Take medication with food and drink 2 liters of liquids daily. Check baseline and monthly uric acid and liver enzymes.
Rifamate	A combination of isoniazid and rifampin.
rifampin (Rifadin)	Body secretions (urine, sweat, tears) turn orange while taking the medication.
rifapentine (Priftin)	As effective as rifampin but taken less frequently. Body secretions (urine, sweat, tears) turn orange. Drug must be given with at least one other tuberculosis drug.
Rifater	A combination of isoniazid, rifampin, and pyrazinamide.
streptomycin sulfate	Have monthly audiograms to check auditory function. Check baseline and monthly renal function.
Second-line Drugs cycloserine (Seromycin)	Observe for mental alertness. While taking the medication, monitor renal and liver function, drink 2 to 3 liters of fluid daily, and avoid alcohol.
ethionamide (Trecator-SC)	Given with other antitubercular drugs to prevent resistant organisms from developing.
kanamycin sulfate (Kantrex)	Drug may cause steatorrhea and electrolyte imbalance.
para-amino-salicylate (Sodium P.A.S.)	Must be taken with other antitubercular drugs; taken with meals.

The Mantoux skin test is the preferred screening method for TB. Purified protein derivative (PPD) of killed tubercle bacilli 0.1 cc is injected intradermally in the inner forearm. The test is evaluated by measuring the area of induration (palpable swelling) that occurs 48 and 72 hours following injection. A reddened area with no induration is not considered positive. A positive skin test, however, indicates only that the client has been infected with and developed antibodies against the tubercle bacillus (Table 32-6). It is important for clients to know that the test will thereafter always be positive throughout the individual's lifetime.

The bacteria can remain alive but inactive in the body, often for a lifetime, so a client is given prophylactic treatment, usually isoniazid (INH), for 6 to 12 months. Other medications used against tuberculosis are outlined in Table 32-7. If INH has not been given and the person later in life is under physical or emotional stress, which weakens the immune system, the bacteria may become active and cause TB disease. Nine of ten persons who have been infected never develop TB disease (ALA, 2002b).

A negative reaction does not rule out the possibility of TB exposure. Individuals at high risk, such as those who are infected with HIV or who have compromised immune status, may have a negative reaction because they are unable to develop antibodies. Immediately following exposure to TB, a skin test may reveal a false-negative result because it can take up to 10 weeks for an infected individual to develop the antibodies. An additional skin test may be done in 10 to 12 weeks. If the second TB test is positive, the client's history is reviewed for the presence of symptoms suggesting TB, and further evaluation is indicated.

Chest x-ray and sputum specimens are utilized to confirm a diagnosis of TB. Sputum is tested for the presence of acid-fast bacilli (AFB). The sputum specimen is collected when the client arises in the morning to prevent specimen contamination with ingested food and liquids. In most instances, three specimens collected on consecutive days and testing positive for AFB indicate a positive diagnosis of TB. The TB diagnosis is confirmed if the TB bacilli grow in a culture. Individuals who are unable to produce sputum, including children and elderly persons, may have stomach contents aspirated for AFB testing. Chest x-ray may reveal the presence of primary tubercles, calcified lesions, and cavitation in the lung.

Medical–Surgical Management

Medical

Most clients are treated briefly in the hospital, with long-term treatment continuing at home. In the hospital, follow Airborne Precautions in addition to Standard Precautions. The precautions include placing the client in an isolation room with negative air pressure (air inflow is controlled through one vent and air outflow is exhausted through another vent directly to the outside and is not recirculated to other rooms.). The doors and windows of the client's room must be kept closed to maintain control of air flow. Caregivers should wear N95 particulate respirator masks because standard isolation masks do not prevent *Mycobacterium tuberculosis* from passing through (Figure 32-5). The Centers for Disease Control and Prevention recommend periodic TB skin testing for health care personnel.

Figure 32-5 *A particulate respirator must be fitted tightly around the nose and face. (Photo courtesy of Donna Hannum, RN, BSN)*

 Infection Control: Use of a Particulate Respirator
- Follow facility's procedure for fit-testing.
- Use the correct size mask.
- Put on respirator before entering client's room and remove after leaving client's room.
- Ensure that the respirator is free of holes.
- Check that the seal between face and respirator is intact.
- Discard soiled or damaged respirators.
- Have client wear N95 respirator when leaving the room.

 Infection Control: Tuberculosis
- Instruct client to cover mouth and nose when coughing or sneezing.
- Double-bag secretions and dispose of them as infectious waste.
- Use disposable items for care when possible.
- Thoroughly clean and disinfect nondisposable items.

 Safety: Caregivers in Health Care Institutions
- Be aware of risks when caring for a client with TB.
- Follow Standard Precautions and Airborne Precautions.
- Use face and/or eye shield in addition to particulate mask when performing sputum-induction procedure.
- Plan care to limit prolonged exposure to client.

Surgical

In the past, surgical intervention involving the removal of affected lung tissues was common. With the advent of effective chemotherapy (treatment with drugs), however, surgical intervention is now rarely utilized.

 Pharmacological

Multidrug-resistant TB (MDR TB) can develop when a client does not complete the full therapy or is inadequately treated. Active TB is treated with a combination of medications. Three medications—isoniazid (Laniazid, which is most effective), rifampin (Rifadin), and pyrazinamide (Pyrazinamide)—are given for several months. This is followed by a regimen of rifampin and isoniazid for an additional time. The combination

CLIENT TEACHING

Rifampin Side Effects

- Urine, saliva, or tears may turn orange.
- May permanently discolor contact lenses.
- Birth control pills and implants become less effective. Use alternative methods of birth control.

COMMUNITY/HOME HEALTH CARE

The Client with Tuberculosis

Advise the client of the following:

- Keep all clinic appointments.
- Take all medications exactly as directed for duration of treatment.
- Until tested and noninfectious:
  — Put used tissues in a closed paper sack and throw away.
  — Avoid close contact with anyone; wear mask.
  — Sleep alone in bedroom.
  — Air out bedroom often, using a fan in the window to blow air outside.
  — Thoroughly clean articles such as eating utensils.

of three drugs is given initially to rapidly decrease the number of active bacilli in the body and to prevent the development of MDR TB. Long-term therapy is required because TB bacilli have long periods of metabolic inactivity. Those clients with bone and joint infections, meningitis, or resistant forms of TB are treated for longer periods. Clients who are HIV positive require a longer regimen of isoniazid and pyrazinamide; prophylactic treatment with isoniazid is indicated from then on. Ethambutol hydrochloride (Myambutol) and streptomycin sulfate are added to the treatment regimen if the infecting organism is resistant to one of the three normally used medications. Infection with MDR TB requires the use of kanamycin sulfate (Kantrex), capreomycin sulfate (Capastat Sulfate), and cycloserine (Seromycin). The client is considered noninfectious following three negative AFB sputum specimens. At that point, the client may return to work and other normal activities. Prophylactic treatment of high-risk individuals is recommended to reduce their chances of developing the disease following their exposure.

Taking multiple drugs can be confusing and lead to noncompliance. The development of two new drugs has been valuable. These drugs are Rifater, a combination of isoniazid, rifampin, and pyrazinamide, and Rifamate, a combination of isoniazid and rifampin.

Diet

The client with TB often has nutritional deficits. Correcting these deficits assists the client in overcoming the disease process. Dietary management is based on the type of deficiency present. A well-balanced diet is en-

CRITICAL THINKING

TB Prevalence

Why is TB becoming more prevalent?

couraged for all clients with TB. Fluids are encouraged to aid in the liquefaction of respiratory secretions.

Activity

Activity is restricted based on the client's tolerance. The client who is severely compromised from a respiratory standpoint may be placed on bed rest. If the client's condition allows, activity should be encouraged because it promotes lung expansion and aids in the removal of static secretions. The client in isolation whose condition permits it may ambulate in the hallways, as long as a particulate respirator mask is worn by the client while outside of the room.

Health Promotion

Prevention of TB is preferred to treatment. In areas where the disease remains endemic (seldom in the United States), a vaccine containing attenuated tubercle bacilli, *bacillus Calmette-Guérin* (BCG), may be given, but its effectiveness has not been proven. Individuals receiving it will test positive to the tuberculin skin test.

Any person who has had close contact with a client with TB without practicing appropriate protective measures should be tested. Other measures that decrease the likelihood of TB include adequate nutrition, housing, and health care access, and treatment of individuals who have or are at risk for developing TB.

Nursing Management

Assess client for low-grade fever, night sweats, and persistent cough. Teach client and family about the disease process and stress the importance of absolute compliance with the treatment plan.

NURSING PROCESS

Assessment

Subjective Data

The history includes questions about the presence of signs and symptoms of TB, such as night sweats, dyspnea on exertion or at rest in late disease, anorexia, loss of muscle strength, and fatigue. Pleuritic pain occurs when the pleura is involved.

Objective Data

Objective data include weight loss; persistent, low-grade fever; and persistent cough. The cough may be nonproductive early in the disease. Later, the cough is productive and yields thick, purulent sputum. Eventually, hemoptysis (blood spitting) occurs. Auscultation of breath sounds reveals coarse crackles. In the presence of cavitary disease, breath sounds are diminished or absent in the affected areas. Sputum is observed as to amount, color, odor, and consistency.

Nursing diagnoses for a client with TB may include the following:

Nursing Diagnoses	Planning/Goals	Nursing Interventions
*Ineffective **B**reathing Pattern* related to pulmonary infectious process	The client will have color and respiratory rate within normal limits and will not complain of dyspnea.	Assess the client's color, respiratory rate, and respiratory effort and auscultate the breath sounds. Plan care activities to allow the client uninterrupted periods of rest. Assist the client in assuming the position that most aids respiratory effort. Administer medications as ordered. Encourage fluids if not otherwise contraindicated.
*Deficient **K**nowledge* related to disease process and its treatment	The client will verbalize an understanding of the disease process and its treatment.	Teach client and family about the basic pathophysiology of TB, how the infection is contracted, who is at risk of developing an infection, the signs and symptoms of TB infection, and complications that may arise. Present information regarding the actions, side effects, and untoward effects of the drugs being administered. Teach the client signs and symptoms of adverse drug reactions to report to the physician. Emphasize the necessity of long-term therapy to cure TB. Inform the client and family that symptoms decrease and are often gone long before the organism is eliminated from the body.
*Ineffective **T**herapeutic Regimen Management* related to client value system	The client will continue medication regimen for the prescribed length of time.	Include the client and family in making decisions about the care, when appropriate. Allow the client to be an active participant in care decisions, to increase personal responsibility and accountability. Visits from public health or home care nurses may be necessary to monitor the client for compliance. Explore the reasons for noncompliance with the client and family, and identify strategies to increase compliance. Refer the client who is unable to afford the cost of medications to agencies such as the local health department for assistance. Begin directly observed therapy if the client continues to be noncompliant. Directly observed therapy involves sending the nurse or another health care worker to the client to administer the medications and verify that they are taken.

Evaluation Each goal must be evaluated to determine how it has been met by the client.

SAMPLE NURSING CARE PLAN

THE CLIENT WITH TUBERCULOSIS

Mr. Stuart is an 87-year-old male admitted to the hospital with a chief complaint of productive cough and fatigue. Four months ago, Mr. Stuart was placed in a long-term care facility because of his inability to care for himself at home following his wife's death 1 year previously. Since admission to the long-term care facility, Mr. Stuart has lost 15 pounds. The nurses at the facility report that Mr. Stuart has experienced progressive fatigue, dyspnea on exertion, cough, night sweats, and anorexia. Initially, his cough was nonproductive, but it is now productive of moderate amounts of thick, purulent sputum that is occasionally streaked with blood. Vital signs are temperature 99.8°F, pulse 108, respirations 26, and blood pressure 138/86. A TB skin test done at the long-term care facility 1 week ago was evaluated as negative at 6 mm. Sputum specimens

continues

SAMPLE NURSING CARE PLAN

for AFB reveal the presence of active tubercle bacilli, and chest x-ray is positive for TB. Auscultation of breath sounds reveals crackles in the right lower half of the lung. Mr. Stuart says, "I don't understand why I can't breathe good and what all this fuss is about."

Nursing Diagnosis 1 *Ineffective **B**reathing Pattern* related to infectious pulmonary process as evidenced by dyspnea on exertion and productive cough

Nursing Outcomes Classification (NOC)
Respiratory Status: Airway Patency
Respiratory Status: Ventilation
Energy Conservation

Nursing Interventions Classification (NIC)
Airway Management
Ventilation Assistance
Energy Management

PLANNING/GOALS	NURSING INTERVENTIONS	RATIONALE
Mr. Stuart will have respiratory rate, oxygen saturation, and color within normal limits and will not complain of dyspnea.	Initially and periodically assess Mr. Stuart's respiratory status, including color, respiratory rate, respiratory effort, oxygen saturation, breath sounds, level of consciousness, cough, and sputum.	Provides a database from which the plan of care can be formulated and against which the effectiveness of treatment is evaluated. Subsequent assessments evaluate the effectiveness of interventions and may modify the care plan.
	Assist Mr. Stuart in assuming a position that most aids respiratory effort.	Allows for greater ease of respiration and lung expansion.
	Alternate care activities with periods of rest.	Allows Mr. Stuart to compensate for the increased oxygen demand required by activity.
	Encourage activity within Mr. Stuart's tolerance.	Promotes expansion of the lungs.
	Encourage fluids.	Promotes liquefaction of respiratory secretions.
	Administer medications for fever as ordered.	Persistent fever leads to dehydration, which hinders the removal of respiratory secretions.
	Administer oxygen as ordered to maintain an SaO_2 of 95% or greater.	Necessary for optimal cellular function.
	Administer antitubercular drugs as ordered.	Decreases the number of viable tubercle bacilli.

EVALUATION Mr. Stuart verbalizes a decrease in dyspnea and cough. Mr. Stuart's color, respiratory rate, and oxygen saturation are within normal limits.

Nursing Diagnosis 2 *Risk for **I**nfection* spread related to viable bacilli in secretions as evidenced by AFB in sputum

Nursing Outcomes Classification (NOC)
Knowledge: Infection Control

Nursing Interventions Classification (NIC)
Health Education

continues

SAMPLE NURSING CARE PLAN

PLANNING/GOALS	NURSING INTERVENTIONS	RATIONALE
Mr. Stuart will verbalize both those situations that allow for the transmission of the tubercle bacilli and the means to prevent their transmission.	Place Mr. Stuart in a negative air pressure, private room; keep door closed at all times. On the door, place Airborne Precaution signs indicating that Mr. Stuart has an infectious process and asking visitors to see nursing personnel before visiting. Instruct visitors to wear N95 respirators when in Mr. Stuart's room, to limit the length of their visits, to avoid intimate contact, and to wash their hands when leaving the room.	Prevents transmission of the tubercle bacilli in air that has been circulated into and out of Mr. Stuart's room. Prevents inadvertent contact and exposure. The nature of the infection is not revealed publicly to maintain client confidentiality. Visitors are informed of precautions to take to prevent exposure.
	Instruct Mr. Stuart to cover his mouth and nose when coughing and sneezing.	Aids in the containment of the tubercle bacilli.
	Instruct Mr. Stuart to cough up secretions in tissues and to place the tissues in a plastic bag. Dispose of contained secretions as infectious waste.	Aids in preventing the spread of the tubercle bacilli.
	Inform the long-term care facility and family/significant others of the positive results of the AFB studies. Instruct those persons who have been exposed to Mr. Stuart to have a TB skin test.	Known exposure to active tubercle bacilli necessitates testing to identify individuals who may have become infected.
	Observe Standard Precautions and Airborne Precautions.	Decreases the likelihood of transmitting the tubercle bacilli (and other infectious diseases) to staff and other clients.
	Wear a fitted N95 respirator when in Mr. Stuart's room.	Prevents the inhalation of tubercle bacilli, which are able to pass through a simple surgical mask.
	Plan care activities to limit the time spent in close contact with Mr. Stuart.	Decreases the likelihood of infection.

EVALUATION   Persons exposed to Mr. Stuart have been tested for TB. Those with TB are being treated.

Nursing Diagnosis 3 *Deficient **K**nowledge* related to disease process and its treatment as evidenced by client statement: "I don't understand why I can't breathe good and what all this fuss is about."

Nursing Outcomes Classification (NOC)	**Nursing Interventions Classification (NIC)**
Knowledge: Disease Process	*Teaching: Disease Process*
Knowledge: Treatment Regimen	*Teaching: Individual*

PLANNING/GOALS	NURSING INTERVENTIONS	RATIONALE
Mr. Stuart will verbalize an understanding of the disease process and the required medication regimen.	Assess Mr. Stuart's present level of knowledge regarding TB and its treatment.	Provides a database regarding Mr. Stuart's present level of knowledge regarding TB and its treatment. Client education can then be individualized to build and expand on that knowledge base. Misinformation can also be corrected.

continues

SAMPLE NURSING CARE PLAN

Provide information in small amounts and use a variety of approaches (e.g., verbal, written, video).	Increases the likelihood of learning and stimulates the various senses.
Encourage and allow time for Mr. Stuart to ask questions.	Provides a means to clarify information and for the nurse to evaluate learning and correct misconceptions.
Have Mr. Stuart verbalize signs and symptoms of adverse medication effects to report to the staff.	Provides a means of evaluating the effectiveness of teaching.

EVALUATION Mr. Stuart verbalizes individual treatment regimen and its purpose. Mr. Stuart reports adverse effects of medication to health care personnel to allow for early intervention.

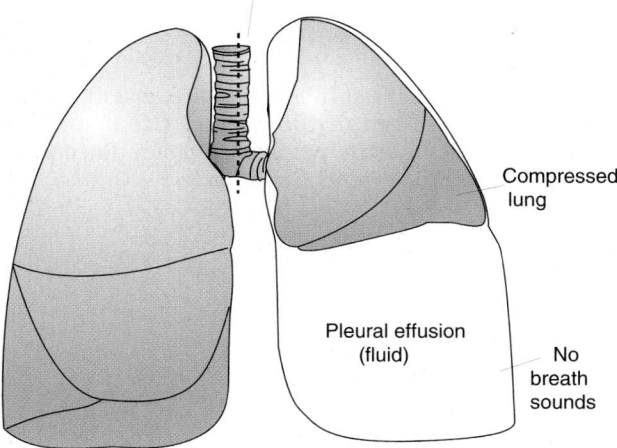

Contralateral mediastinal shift

Compressed lung

Pleural effusion (fluid)

No breath sounds

Figure 32-6 *Pleural Effusion*

PROFESSIONAL TIP

Assessment of Client with a Chest Tube

- Obtain vital signs as ordered.
- Be alert for dyspnea.
- Record and describe amount of drainage.
- Look for loops of tubing containing drainage.
- Monitor water level in the water seal. Fluctuation (called tidaling) should occur with respirations and will stop when lung is reexpanded, tubing is kinked, connections are not tight, or chest tube becomes dislodged.
- Keep chest drainage system below the level of the client's chest.
- Every 2 hours, monitor client's response to coughing and deep breathing.
- If the chest tube is accidentally dislodged, cover opening with petrolatum gauze and apply pressure to prevent air from being sucked back into chest.

PLEURISY/PLEURAL EFFUSION

Pleurisy is a painful condition that arises from inflammation of the pleura, or sac that encases the lung. This pleuritic pain is sharp and stabbing in nature. Pain increases on inspiration as the irritated pleura rub over each other. Inflammation of the pleura occurs with many disorders, such as viral infections, cancer of the lung, trauma, tuberculosis, congestive heart failure, and pulmonary embolism. The inflamed pleura secretes increased amounts of pleural fluid into the pleural cavity, creating a **pleural effusion.** As fluid accumulates within the pleural space, it compresses the lung tissue (Figure 32-6). Collapse, or atelectasis, results if the effusion is left untreated. Those areas of collapsed lung tissue are unable to take part in gas exchange, thereby decreasing oxygenation. Empyema is the term to describe infected pleural exudate.

The primary manifestation of pleurisy is pain on inspiration. Signs and symptoms of pleural effusion depend on the amount of lung tissue compressed and the source of the effusion. With large pleural effusions, the mediastinum (heart, great vessels, and trachea) shifts toward the unaffected side; this can be detected by inspection, and heart sounds will move toward unaffected side. Magnetic resonance imaging (MRI) or computerized tomography (CT) studies are useful in detecting pleural effusions, particularly small ones. A chest x-ray will show pleural effusions of 250 cc of fluid or more. If empyema is suspected, culture and sensitivity studies will identify the presence and type of infection. The client with empyema will also have an elevated temperature and white blood cell count.

Medical–Surgical Management

Medical

Treatment is aimed at eliminating the underlying cause, maintaining adequate oxygenation to the tissues, and preventing complications such as atelectasis and pneumonia. Oxygenation is evaluated by ABGs and/or pulse oximetry. Supplemental oxygen is given to maintain an oxygen saturation of 95% or greater. Respiratory treatments to aid lung expansion such as incentive spirometry are used.

Surgical

Larger pleural effusions require that a thoracentesis be performed by the physician to remove accumulated fluid. After the overlying tissues are anesthetized, a large-bore needle is placed into the pleural space. Fluid is removed (no more than 1500 mL) and may be sent to the laboratory for diagnostic purposes (i.e., culture, cytology). If fluid accumulation continues, a thoracotomy tube is placed into the pleural space to drain fluid continuously. Following administration of local anesthetics, the physician places a large-bore catheter into the pleural space. This catheter is attached to an underwater seal drainage device (Figure 32-7). It prevents the negative pressure within the pleural space from pulling air into the pleural space, and allows for the drainage of accumulated fluid or air. Most devices have a chamber to which suction may be applied to assist in the removal of fluid or air from the pleural space. A chest x-ray is done to evaluate the chest tube's placement and effectiveness.

Pharmacological

If a pleural effusion is small and does not interfere greatly with respiratory function, diuretics are used to promote removal of fluid from the pleural space. Furosemide (Lasix) and bumetanide (Bumex) may be given for this purpose. If empyema is present, specific therapy is used once the causative agent is identified. Pain relief is a high priority. Analgesia that also decreases inflammation is preferred. Ketorolac tromethamine (Toradol) or other NSAIDs are often used. Severe pain may require narcotics. For extensive inflammation, corticosteroids may be utilized.

Activity

The client's activity is limited to prevent fatigue. High Fowler's position assists respirations.

Nursing Management

Assess the client's color, respiratory rate and effort, and level of consciousness. Monitor vital signs and breath sounds. If a chest tube is in place, watch that all tubes are in place and the drainage device is working properly. Empty drainage per agency policy. Encourage the client to use the incentive spirometer.

Figure 32-7 *Underwater Seal Chest Drainage Device*

NURSING PROCESS

Assessment

Subjective Data

A nursing history is obtained from the client regarding onset, duration, and severity of symptoms. The client usually describes both chest pain that increases with each inspiration and difficulty breathing.

Objective Data

The client's color, respiratory rate, and effort are evaluated along with the level of consciousness. Abnormalities in vital signs are noted. Breath sounds over the areas of involvement are diminished or absent. A pleural friction rub may be audible. Dyspnea, cyanosis, and hypoxia occur proportional to the severity of the condition. If a chest tube is in place, the amount and color of drainage are assessed.

Nursing diagnoses for a client with a pleural effusion may include the following:

Nursing Diagnoses	Planning/Goals	Nursing Interventions
Acute Pain related to inflammation of the pleura	Using a scale of 1 to 10, the client will verbalize a decrease in the level of pain.	Administer pain medications as ordered. Assist the client in attaining the position that allows for greatest comfort. Elevate the head of the bed. Provide diversional activities.
Impaired Gas Exchange related to compressed lung	The client will maintain an oxygen saturation of 95% or greater and a respiratory rate of 14 to 22 and will have clear breath sounds.	Monitor vital signs and pulse oximetry. Provide supplemental oxygen as ordered. Encourage the client to breathe deeply or use the incentive spirometer as ordered. Administer diuretics and anti-inflammatory medications as ordered. Assist the physician with the thoracentesis or the placement of a thoracotomy tube. Collect specimen for culture and sensitivity and other studies.
Bathing/Hygiene Self-care Deficit related to mobility restriction	The client will increase self-care activities as mobility increases.	Assist the client with hygiene and self-care needs, but encourage participation in self-care activities within the limits of the physician's orders.
Risk for Activity Intolerance related to hypoxia secondary to pleural effusion	The client will increase activity without complaining of fatigue.	Stagger periods of activity with periods of rest. To prevent fatigue, plan activities around therapies.

Evaluation Each goal must be evaluated to determine how it has been met by the client.

SEVERE ACUTE RESPIRATORY SYNDROME

The first report of severe acute respiratory syndrome (SARS) occurred in February 2003 in Asia. It is caused by the SARS-associated coronavirus (SARS-CoV). Approximately 10% of those affected in this first outbreak died (CDC, 2003a).

It appears that SARS spreads by close personal contact or contact with infectious material (respiratory secretions). This happens when a client with SARS coughs or sneezes droplets onto themselves, others, or nearby surfaces.

The incubation period is generally 2 to 7 days. Then an elevated temperature of more than 100.4°F (>38°C) occurs and may be associated with chills, headache, malaise, body aches, and sometimes respiratory symptoms. After 2 to 7 days, clients may develop a dry, nonproductive cough and dyspnea.

There is no specific treatment for SARS. Support treatment is provided based on the symptoms.

Nursing Management

Follow Standard Precautions (hand hygiene and eye protection), Contact Precautions (gown and gloves), and Airborne Precautions (isolation room with negative pressure and use of N-95 respirators). Monitor client's vital signs. Assess breath sounds. Provide routine care with uninterrupted rest periods.

ACUTE RESPIRATORY TRACT DISORDERS

Acute respiratory tract disorders include atelectasis, pulmonary embolism, pulmonary edema, adult respiratory distress syndrome, and acute respiratory failure.

ATELECTASIS

Atelectasis refers to the collapse of a lung or a portion of a lung. The most common cause of atelectasis is airway obstruction. A bronchiole becomes blocked with secretions, and the alveoli distal to it collapse (Figure 32-8). Airway obstruction of this nature is common after surgery and with immobility problems. Anesthesia, pain, narcotics, and immobility can cause hypoventilation and retention of secretions. Hypoventilation can cause atelectasis, which increases hypoventilation. Atelectasis can occur with compression of lung tissue, as in pleural effusion or pneumothorax. Insufficient surfactant results in increased recoil properties of the lungs, leading to atelectasis.

Signs of respiratory distress are proportional to the amount of lung tissue involved. When large areas of the lung are involved, orthopnea or cyanosis may develop. Breath sounds are diminished or absent over collapsed areas. Chest wall movement may decrease on the affected side. Oxygenation decreases as shown by ABGs or

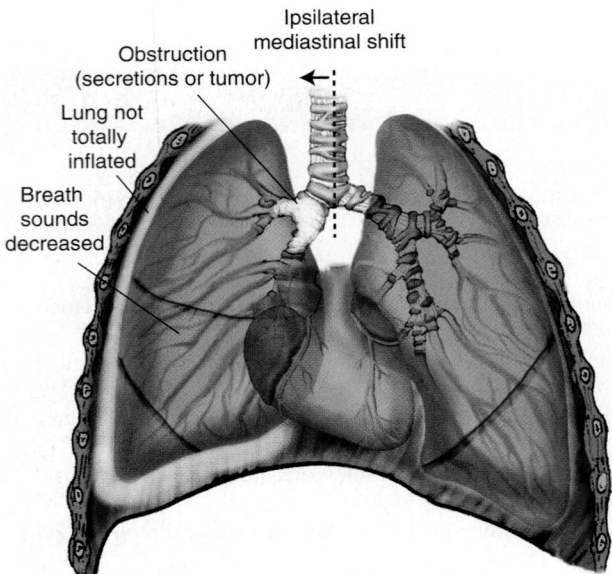

Figure 32-8 *Atelectasis (collapsed lung)*

pulse oximetry. Pulse and respiratory rate increase as the heart and lungs work harder to meet the body's oxygen needs. Trapped secretions are a growth medium for microorganisms. An elevated temperature indicates secondary infection (pneumonia). Chest x-ray shows the areas of collapse. Bronchoscopy (insertion of a bronchoscope into the trachea) is used to directly visualize the area of obstruction and obtain a specimen for diagnostic purposes.

Medical–Surgical Management

Medical

The physician will order incentive spirometry and deep breathing and coughing exercises to promote expansion of the lungs. Postural drainage and percussion aids in the removal of any static secretions. If the client is unable to cough up secretions, suctioning of the respiratory tract is performed. Bronchoscopy may be done to remove secretions and obtain specimens. Arterial blood gases and pulse oximetry are utilized to evaluate the need for supplemental oxygen. Oxygen is administered to maintain an oxygen saturation of 95% or greater.

Surgical

Clients with pneumothorax or pleural effusion as the underlying cause of atelectasis require removal of trapped air or fluid via thoracentesis or placement of a thoracotomy tube (refer to the sections on pleural effusion and pneumothorax). Atelectasis resulting from the growth of a tumor requires removal of the tumor.

🔲 Pharmacological

Adequate pain control aids the client, particularly the surgical client, to breathe deeply and cough. Client-controlled analgesia or a routine schedule of pain medication may be used to provide effective pain management. Bronchodilators may be used to open the airways. Mucolytic agents are used to liquefy secretions. Bronchodilators, such as albuterol sulfate (Ventolin), and mucolytics, such as acetylcysteine (Mucomyst), may also be administered via updraft or nebulizer treatments. The client with an infection requires treatment with an appropriate antibiotic.

Diet

Unless otherwise contraindicated, fluids are encouraged to promote liquefaction of trapped respiratory secretions.

Activity

Activity promotes lung expansion. Immobile clients are turned a minimum of every 2 hours and assisted to do range-of-motion exercises. Surgical clients may do leg exercises as well as deep breathing and coughing. Ambulation is recommended if the client's condition allows. If the client is unable to walk, sitting up in a chair is encouraged. To prevent fatigue, rest periods are planned between activities.

Nursing Management

Monitor for pain, shortness of breath, fatigue, dyspnea, cyanosis, anxiety, and level of consciousness. Assess for Homan's sign. Teach client how to cough, deep breathe, and use the incentive spirometer. Encourage ambulation as client's condition allows. Turn immobile clients at least every 2 hours.

NURSING PROCESS

Assessment

Subjective Data

Clients who smoke, those who are immunocompromised, and those who have known chronic respiratory or cardiovascular diseases are at increased risk of developing atelectasis. The client is asked about the onset, duration, and severity of symptoms such as pain, cough, and dyspnea. The client may complain or show signs of air hunger, shortness of breath, fatigue, and anxiety.

Objective Data

Assess the client for changes in level of consciousness, an early sign of decreased oxygenation. Periodically evaluate for dyspnea, tachypnea, cyanosis, and restlessness. Measure vital signs frequently, with particular attention to respiratory rate and effort. Auscultation reveals diminished or absent breath sounds over the areas of atelectasis. Crackles or sonorous wheezes may be heard if pneumonia develops. Note objective indicators of pain such as facial grimacing, and validate by subjective questioning. Assess the effectiveness of the client's cough. A productive cough is evaluated for amount, color, consistency, and odor of secretions.

Nursing diagnoses for a client with atelectasis may include the following:

Nursing Diagnoses	Planning/Goals	Nursing Interventions
*Deficient **K**nowledge* related to the complications of surgery and/or immobility	The client will verbalize the purpose of deep breathing, coughing, and activity following surgery and will demonstrate deep breathing and coughing.	Teach all preoperative and immobile clients to cough and breathe deeply at least every 2 hours and have the client demonstrate to ensure that learning has occurred. Teach the surgical client to splint the surgical incision to minimize discomfort that might occur with coughing and deep breathing. Instruct clients at risk for developing atelectasis in the use of incentive spirometry. Emphasize the importance of early ambulation and activity to promote lung expansion.
*Impaired **G**as Exchange* related to decreased alveolar–capillary surface	The client will have an oxygen saturation of 95% or greater, a respiratory rate of 14 to 22, and clear breath sounds.	Establish a schedule for coughing and deep breathing. Encourage clients to ambulate and/or sit up in a chair three to four times daily. Turn the immobile client every 2 hours or more frequently. Assess the client's vital signs and breath sounds every 4 hours or more frequently as situation warrants. Encourage fluids if the client's condition allows. Administer respiratory treatments and medications as ordered. Assess secretions (sputum) for color, amount, consistency, and odor.
*Risk for **A**ctivity Intolerance* related to hypoxia secondary to atelectasis	The client will complete activity without complaints of shortness of breath, dyspnea, or fatigue.	Encourage some activity, such as walking, to promote lung expansion, and alternate with periods of rest to avoid client fatigue. Provide assistance with ADL as the client's condition requires. Place the client in a high or semi-Fowler's position to aid lung expansion. Position client on the unaffected side.

Evaluation Each goal must be evaluated to determine how it has been met by the client.

PULMONARY EMBOLISM �

Pulmonary embolism (PE) develops when a blood-borne substance lodges in a branch of a pulmonary artery and obstructs flow. A common source of PE is deep vein thrombus. Other sources are air from intravenous infusions; fat from long-bone fractures; and amniotic fluid. The size and location of the emboli determine the severity and outcome of the condition.

Pulmonary emboli rarely develop before adulthood. As age increases, the risk for pulmonary embolism becomes greater because of the development of arteriosclerosis and other vascular changes associated with aging. Other factors increasing the risk for PE are heredity, smoking, peripheral vascular disease, diabetes mellitus, and oral contraceptive use.

Emboli interfere with gas exchange to the pulmonary circulation distal to the emboli, resulting in hypoxemia. The client describes breathlessness and dyspnea. Pulse oximetry or ABGs will show the degree to which oxygenation has been affected. Obstruction of a main branch of a pulmonary artery can result in lung infarction and necrosis.

All clients at risk for PE should be observed for signs and symptoms of deep vein thrombosis, such as localized calf tenderness or swelling. Measures to prevent thrombus formation should be taken for these individuals. Any signs of thrombophlebitis should be immediately reported to the physician.

Signs and symptoms of PE are abrupt in onset. The client becomes anxious and restless. Sudden, sharp chest pains of a pleuritic nature (worse on inspiration) develop. Dyspnea and cough, along with hemoptysis, occur. Venous return is diminished, resulting in jugular venous distention. The client becomes diaphoretic. A low-grade fever develops in response to inflammation. A high temperature indicates lung infarction. Diagnosis of PE is often done by a ventilation/perfusion lung scan, but the gold standard is pulmonary angiography. Arterial blood gases show hypoxia and respiratory alkalosis. A spiral CT scan of the lungs can be performed in a few seconds and is replacing the ventilation/perfusion scan (Lazzara, 2001).

Medical–Surgical Management

Medical

Preventive measures are instituted for the client at risk of developing deep vein thrombosis. Following surgery, antiembolism stockings and early ambulation are indicated. When hypoxia occurs, supplemental oxygen is given to increase oxygenation. The underlying cause of the PE is treated when identified.

Surgical

In severe cases, the physician may elect to remove the clot via an embolectomy. This procedure is usually done at the time of angiography. Clients who experience successive episodes of PE may require a venacaval plication. This surgical procedure involves placing a sieve-like device in the inferior vena cava to catch emboli before they enter pulmonary circulation (Figure 33-27 in Chapter 33).

Pharmacological

The client at risk of developing deep vein thrombosis and/or PE may be treated with enoxaparin (Lovenox). Lovenox is often used in the postoperative client to prevent clot formation. After PE have developed, anticoagulation is ordered to prevent the formation of further clots. Heparin sodium is initially used to establish anticoagulation and is administered parenterally by either the intravenous or subcutaneous route. After adequate anticoagulation is established, warfarin sodium (Coumadin) therapy is initiated and may be given concurrently with heparin while the client is hospitalized. Coumadin alone is given orally when the client is discharged. If the clot is large or lies in a branch of a main pulmonary artery, fibrinolytic therapy may be used. Fibrinolytics lyse, or dissolve, the clot versus inhibiting the formation of new clots. Examples of fibrinolytic agents are alteplase recombinant (Activase) and streptokinase (Streptase). These agents may be administered intra-arterially at the site of the clot or intravenously to

CLIENT TEACHING

Anticoagulant Therapy (Coumadin)

Stress the importance of:

- Follow-up laboratory testing
- Using a soft toothbrush to prevent trauma to the gums (bleeding)
- Inspecting the skin for bruises or petechiae
- Using an electric razor to avoid scratching skin
- Reporting nosebleeds, tarry stool, hematuria, or hematemesis to the physician
- Eating a consistent amount of green, leafy vegetables daily (differing amounts alter anticoagulant effects)
- Avoiding other medications including aspirin (it has an anticoagulant effect) without approval from physician
- In the female client, monitor menstrual flow for excessive amount

LIFE CYCLE CONSIDERATIONS

Anticoagulant Therapy (Coumadin)

Elderly clients are especially sensitive to Coumadin, therefore, they must be closely monitored.

achieve a systemic effect. Narcotic analgesics such as morphine are used to control pain.

Diet

Fluids are encouraged to prevent hemoconcentration leading to clot formation. Unless contraindicated, fluids should be encouraged for the client at risk of developing PE.

Activity

To prevent the formation of clots, activity is encouraged. After a clot has formed, however, the client's activity is restricted to prevent the clot from moving and becoming an embolus. Activities such as sitting, crossing the knees, or prolonged bending at the hips are to be avoided because they promote venous stasis.

Nursing Management

Assess the abrupt onset of pleuritic chest pain for location, duration, severity, and character. Monitor pulse oximetry, vital signs, jugular veins for distension, peripheral pulses, and capillary refill. Encourage deep breathing and provide supplemental oxygen as ordered. Monitor results of APTT, INR, PT, hemoglobin, and hematocrit.

NURSING PROCESS

Assessment

Subjective Data

The client's history is obtained to identify potential risk factors for the development of PE. Ask the client about the onset, duration, and severity of symptoms. Shortness of breath, dyspnea, and severe pleuritic chest pain are abrupt in onset. Pain is evaluated as to onset, location, duration, severity, and character.

Objective Data

Pulse oximetry measurements are monitored. The client's respirations are rapid and shallow. Pallor progressing to cyanosis develops as oxygenation decreases. The client becomes diaphoretic. Increased anxiety or a change in level of consciousness may be the first indication of PE. The pulse increases in response to anxiety and in an attempt to supply oxygen to the body's cells. Blood pressure may increase or decrease in response to hypoxia, anxiety, and pain. Temperature may elevate in response to inflammation and tissue necrosis. On auscultation, breath sounds may or may not be decreased. The jugular veins are distended.

Nursing diagnoses for a client with pulmonary embolism may include the following:

Nursing Diagnoses	Planning/Goals	Nursing Interventions
Impaired Gas Exchange related to alteration in pulmonary circulation	The client will maintain an oxygen saturation of 95% or greater, have a respiratory rate of 14 to 22, and have color within normal limits.	Assess the client for indications of decreasing oxygenation. Auscultate breath sounds every 4 hours or more often. Assess peripheral pulses and capillary refill. Encourage deep breathing and coughing. Provide supplemental oxygen to maintain oxygen saturation at greater than 95% or as ordered. Administer subcutaneous heparin and coumadin as ordered. Encourage fluids, unless contraindicated, to prevent hemoconcentration.
Acute Pain related to decreased perfusion of lung tissue	Using a scale of 1 to 10, the client will indicate decreased pain.	Administer pain medication as ordered. Assist the client in assuming a position of comfort. If possible, place the client in a high-Fowler's position to aid respiratory effort.
Risk for Injury related to anticoagulation/fibrinolytic therapy	The client will be free of abnormal bleeding and maintain hemoglobin and hematocrit within normal limits.	Assess for evidence of bleeding. Monitor lab reports for activated partial thromboplastin time (APTT), international normalized ratio (INR), prothrombin time (PT), and hemoglobin and hematocrit levels. Evaluate blood pressure and pulse for signs of bleeding (i.e., rapid pulse and low blood pressure). Check stool for occult blood. Assess gums for bleeding.

Evaluation Each goal must be evaluated to determine how it has been met by the client.

PULMONARY EDEMA

Acute pulmonary edema is a life-threatening condition characterized by a rapid shift of fluid from plasma into the pulmonary interstitial tissue and the alveoli (Figure 32-9). As a result, gas exchange is markedly impaired. Pulmonary edema most generally has a cardiac cause such as left ventricular failure or myocardial in-

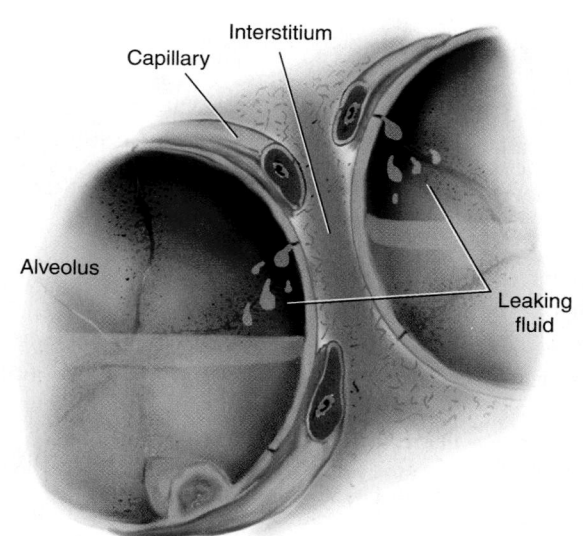

Figure 32-9 *Pulmonary Edema*

farction, or a noncardiac cause such as fluid overload, inhalation of noxious gases, opiate overdose, aspiration, sepsis, or radiation injury (Lazzara, 2001).

The hallmark of acute pulmonary edema is a cough producing a copious amount of frothy, blood-tinged sputum (hemoptysis), often appearing pinkish. The client rapidly becomes dyspneic, orthopneic, and cyanotic. Anxiety ranging from restlessness to panic occurs. Heart and respiratory rate increase. Progressive crackles are heard in the lung fields on auscultation. Initially, fine crackles are present in the posterior bases of the lung. As pulmonary edema progresses, the crackles become increasingly coarser, louder, and more diffuse. Wheezes are heard in the presence of significant airway obstruction by fluid. Left untreated, the client deteriorates rapidly as oxygenation decreases. The client's history is crucial to identify the cause. Noncardiogenic pulmonary edema can quickly become respiratory failure.

Medical–Surgical Management

Medical

The goals of medical management are to remove fluid from the alveoli and pulmonary interstitial space, prevent further influx of fluid, and improve oxygenation. Arterial blood gases and pulse oximetry values are used to assess oxygenation. Oxygen is administered per physician's order when hypoxia is present. Noncardiogenic pulmonary edema often requires ventilation support and treatment of the cause.

Pharmacological

A diuretic such as furosemide (Lasix) is the primary treatment for cardiogenic pulmonary edema. When the pumping force of the left ventricle is impaired, a digitalis preparation is given to improve the contractile force of the myocardium. To prevent further influx of fluid into the lungs, venous pooling is enhanced. This also decreases the workload on the heart by limiting venous return. Morphine is used to promote vasodilation and, thus, venous pooling and to relieve anxiety. Bronchodilators are administered to dilate airways obstructed with fluid.

Diet

A sodium-restricted diet may be ordered to prevent fluid retention. Intake and output as well as daily weight are measured to monitor fluid balance.

Activity

Bed rest reduces the workload on the heart and lungs. High Fowler's position aids respiratory effort and enhances venous pooling. Activities are increased slowly according to the physician's orders and the client's ability to tolerate activity.

Nursing Management

Monitor ABGs and pulse oximetry and administer oxygen as ordered. Assess breath sounds, vital signs, and level of consciousness. Keep client in high Fowler's position. Keep an accurate intake and output record. Monitor client's weight daily.

NURSING PROCESS

Assessment

Subjective Data

The nurse must be aware of the conditions that predispose the client to pulmonary edema. The client may describe feeling anxious, breathless, and fatigued.

Objective Data

Breath sounds are auscultated for the presence of crackles. Report increasingly coarse and diffuse crackles to the physician. Assess the client's level of consciousness, respiratory rate and effort, and color. Dyspnea, tachypnea, cyanosis and/or pallor may be present. Assess oxygenation via pulse oximetry or ABGs. A productive cough may be present, as may symptoms of CHF, such as rapid weight gain and peripheral edema. Pulse may be rapid and weak. Blood pressure may increase in response to anxiety and decreased oxygenation.

Nursing diagnoses for a client with pulmonary edema may include the following:

Nursing Diagnoses	Planning/Goals	Nursing Interventions
*Impaired **G**as Exchange* related to fluid in the lung tissue	The client will maintain an oxygen saturation of 95% or greater and will have respiratory rate and color and blood gases within normal limits and clear breath sounds.	Place the client in high Fowler's or orthopneic position (sitting upright leaning forward).
		Continually assess oxygenation with ABG or pulse oximetry measurements and provide supplemental oxygen to maintain an oxygen saturation of 95% or greater or per physician's order.
		Frequently assess respiratory rate, breath sounds, apical heart rate, and blood pressure. Administer respiratory treatments as ordered.
		Assist the client with activities to reduce the workload on the heart and lungs, and alternate periods of activity with periods of rest to prevent client fatigue. Administer medications as ordered and evaluate the effectiveness of each. Monitor lab reports for electrolyte values.
*Excess **F**luid Volume* related to altered tissue permeability	The client's weight will return to normal.	Weigh client daily. Monitor I&O.
		Frequently assess the client for peripheral edema.
		Provide the client with a low-sodium diet as ordered.
		Administer diuretics per order and evaluate their effectiveness.
		Monitor lab reports for electrolyte values.
		Monitor the rate at which intravenous fluids are given.
		Teach client and family fluid excess symptoms, medication information, and dietary modifications.

Evaluation Each goal must be evaluated to determine how it has been met by the client.

ADULT RESPIRATORY DISTRESS SYNDROME

9-19-07

Adult respiratory distress syndrome (ARDS) is a life-threatening condition characterized by severe dyspnea, hypoxemia, and diffuse pulmonary edema. The condition usually follows a major assault on multiple body systems or severe lung trauma. Underlying causes include trauma, sepsis, coronary artery bypass surgery, major thoracic or vascular surgery, renal failure, severe pulmonary infections, inhalation lung injuries, and acute drug poisoning. Adult respiratory distress syndrome is a noncardiogenic pulmonary edema, caused by damage to the alveolocapillary membranes allowing fluid to leak into the lungs under normal pressure.

Gas exchange is severely impaired by the damage to the pulmonary capillary membrane and the presence of fluid in the alveoli. The surfactant is rendered inactive, resulting in the collapse of the alveoli, further reducing gas exchange. Hypoxemia, resistant to conventional oxygen therapy, develops.

The client with ARDS is critically ill, as reflected by severe dyspnea, tachypnea, and cyanosis. Arterial blood gases will show PaO_2 less than 70 mm Hg, $PaCO_2$ more than 35 mm Hg, bicarbonate ion less than 22 mEq/L, and initially elevated then steadily decreasing pH. The ABGs and pulse oximetry reveal severe hypoxemia and progressive respiratory and metabolic acidosis. On auscultation, the lung fields are filled with diffuse coarse crackles and sonorous wheezes. The client will have a productive cough yielding blood-tinged sputum. Chest x-ray will show widely scattered infiltrates, often referred to as a "white out."

Medical–Surgical Management

Medical

The client with ARDS is cared for in the intensive care unit. The underlying cause of ARDS is ascertained and treated; until that time, supportive care is given. Mechanical ventilatory support is necessary, with multiple other systems often also being supported. A mechanical ventilator allows the oxygen percentage, pulmonary pressure, and lung volume to be controlled. Oxygenation is monitored with ABGs and pulse oximetry. Respiratory secretions are removed by frequent bronchial suctioning. In severe cases, extra corporeal membrane oxygenation (ECMO) may also be used (Dirkes & Winklerprins, 2002).

Pharmacological

Pharmacological therapy includes high doses of corticosteriods such as hydrocortisone sodium succinate (Solu-Cortef) or methylprednisolone sodium succinate (Solu-Medrol). Furosemide (Lasix) and other diuretics are given to remove fluids and increase urinary output. Aminophylline (Aminophyllin) is administered to open the bronchi. While the client is on the mechanical ventilator, pancuronium bromide (Pavulon) is given to suppress the client's own respiratory effort. Blood pressure can fall dangerously low, and vasopressors such as dopamine hydrochloride (Intropin) may be required to maintain the blood pressure within an acceptable range.

Diet

Total parenteral nutrition (TPN) may be given to the client, especially during the acute phase of the illness. When possible, enteral feedings are preferred.

Activity

The client with ARDS will be on bed rest. Special beds that provide movement and pressure adjustment prevent the complications associated with immobility. According to Marion (2001), prone positioning improves oxygenation and may prevent further lung damage.

Nursing Management

Monitor client's level of consciousness, response to stimuli, vital signs, ABGs, pulse oximetry, and breath sounds. Suction excess secretions. Provide frequent oral care. Plan for uninterrupted rest periods. Assess for restlessness and anxiety.

NURSING PROCESS

Assessment

Subjective Data

The client history is typically gathered from family members or significant others because the client is usually too ill to communicate.

Objective Data

The client's level of consciousness and response to stimuli are assessed, and the client is observed for restlessness and anxiety. Vital signs are measured every 15 minutes or more often. Heart rate is increased, and arrhythmias may be present. Blood pressure is usually low. Respiratory rate, rhythm, and effort are assessed for signs of dyspnea, nasal flaring, cyanosis, tachypnea, and other indications of respiratory distress. Arterial blood gases and pulse oximetry values are assessed to evaluate oxygenation and acid–base balance. Diffuse, coarse crackles and wheezes are heard throughout the lung fields.

Nursing diagnoses for a client with ARDS may include the following:

Nursing Diagnoses	Planning/Goals	Nursing Interventions
Impaired Gas Exchange related to pulmonary capillary membrane damage	The client will have an oxygen saturation of 95% or greater, ABGs within normal limits, and respiratory rate and effort within normal limits.	Provide adequate oxygenation and ventilation as ordered. Monitor ABGs and pulse oximetry to evaluate oxygenation and acid–base balance. Assess the client's respiratory rate and effort and auscultate the lungs frequently. Suction the respiratory tract as necessary to remove excess secretions, and provide oral care frequently.
Anxiety related to the condition and mechanical ventilation	The client, if able, will verbalize a decrease in anxiety or will exhibit fewer objective signs of anxiety, such as restlessness and facial grimacing.	Describe care and purposes to the client. Allow rest periods between periods of activity to avoid overwhelming the client with stimuli. Plan care to allow for uninterrupted rest. Allow family and significant others to visit and participate in care, as appropriate. Assess the client for signs of sensory overload/deprivation.

Evaluation Each goal must be evaluated to determine how it has been met by the client.

ACUTE RESPIRATORY FAILURE

Acute respiratory failure is not a disease entity in and of itself; rather, the term is used to refer to conditions wherein there is a failure of the respiratory system as a whole. This condition occurs as a result of the client's literally becoming too tired to continue the "work" of breathing. Mechanical ventilatory support is required during the acute phase. Clients with preexisting pulmonary conditions coupled with acute respiratory tract infections are at risk for developing acute respiratory failure.

CHRONIC RESPIRATORY TRACT DISORDERS

Asthma, chronic obstructive pulmonary disease (COPD), chronic bronchitis, emphysema, and bronchiectasis are discussed following.

✳ ASTHMA

Asthma is a condition characterized by intermittent airway obstruction in response to a variety of stimuli. The epithelial lining of the airways responds by becoming inflamed and edematous. Bronchospasm occurs in the smooth muscles of the bronchi and bronchioles. Secretions increase in viscosity. Elastic recoil decreases. All of these changes result in a reduction of the diameter of the airways, making breathing more difficult. Some clients who develop asthma in childhood experience spontaneous recovery.

LIFE CYCLE CONSIDERATIONS

Asthma and Age

In children:

- Asthma attacks often become less severe and less frequent as the child ages.
- Asthma attacks are usually associated with definite allergens.
- Oral bronchodilators should be taken 30 to 60 minutes before exercise, inhaled bronchodilators 15 to 20 minutes before exercise.

In adults:

- Asthma attacks usually become more severe and more frequent as the individual ages.

- Asthma attacks are usually not associated with definite allergens.

Asthma may be classified as extrinsic or intrinsic. Extrinsic asthma is caused by substances outside the body that precipitate the asthma response, such as pollen, house dust, or food additives. Intrinsic asthma is diagnosed when no extrinsic factor can be identified and the asthma is the result of internal factors such as emotional stress, exercise, or fatigue. An asthma attack that does not respond to treatment and persists is known as **status asthmaticus**.

The hallmark of an asthma attack is sudden onset of wheezing, increasing dyspnea, and chest tightness. Mild asthma can usually be controlled by routine medication. Severe asthma attacks usually occur at night and require extra medication. With severe attacks, wheezing may be audible to the unaided ear. Expiratory wheezes are common as air attempts to escape through the narrowed airways. Both inspiratory and expiratory wheezes may be heard. *Absence of wheezing could indicate complete closure of the airway.* The respiratory rate rises initially, but as the client tires, the rate may decrease. Nasal flaring and costal and sternal retractions may be present, particularly in the young client. The client uses accessory muscles to assist respiratory effort. Cough occurs as the respiratory secretions become thick and block the airways. Cyanosis and a decrease in oxygen saturation occur. Heart rate elevates, as may blood pressure. The client becomes anxious and may complain of a sense of impending doom. These responses are thought to be caused by a release of catecholamines. Values of ABGs indicate hypoxia and respiratory acidosis. Chest x-ray shows hyperinflation of the lungs. Pulmonary function tests reveal an abnormal flow rate and lung volume. With a severe asthma attack, apnea and sudden death can occur in minutes.

Medical–Surgical Management

Medical

The client with allergies should avoid specific antigens that might bring on an attack. Some clients with asthma are aided by controlling psychological stressors. Routine physical exercise is beneficial in treating exercise-induced asthma. The client with asthma should avoid other respiratory irritants such as cigarette smoke and air pollution. Clients who develop asthma later in life show more symptoms as they age.

Pharmacological

The primary treatment for an acute asthma attack is pharmacological. A combination of medications is used to open the narrowed airways. Medications used to dilate the bronchi include bronchodilators such as aminophylline (Aminophyllin) and terbutaline sulfate (Brethine, Bricanyl); beta agonists such as epinephrine (Primatene Mist) and albuterol sulfate (Ventolin); and anticholinergics such as atropine sulfate and ipratropium bromide (Atrovent). Corticosteroids such as prednisone (Delatsone) are utilized to decrease inflammation. Mucolytic agents such as acetylcysteine

(Mucomyst) aid in liquefying secretions. Supplemental oxygen is given when indicated.

Diet

Adequate fluid intake should be maintained to promote liquefaction of secretions.

Activity

Incorporate several rest periods for the client. Use relaxation techniques to manage anxiety. The client should not overexert to the point of dyspnea, wheezing, or fatigue. If overexertion occurs, the client should sit down and sip warm water. This promotes slower, regular breathing; bronchodilation; and loosens secretions.

Nursing Management

Obtain history about previous asthma attacks. Evaluate wheezes for location, duration, and phase of respiration when they occur. Monitor pulse oximetry and ABGs for oxygenation and acid–base balance.

NURSING PROCESS

Assessment

Subjective Data

A detailed history is taken regarding exposure to triggering stimuli before past asthma attacks. Also, the onset, duration, and severity of symptoms such as dyspnea are noted.

Objective Data

Note the effectiveness of ventilation. Wheezes are evaluated as to their duration, location, and the phase of respiration during which they occur (e.g., inspiration). Wheezes heard without the aid of a stethoscope are called **audible wheezes.** Respiratory rate, depth, rhythm and effort; position assumed; and client color are evaluated. Monitor pulse oximetry or lab reports of ABG values to determine oxygenation and acid–base balance. If sputum is produced, note its color, amount, viscosity, and odor.

Nursing diagnoses for a client with asthma may include the following:

Nursing Diagnoses	Planning/Goals	Nursing Interventions
Inefficient **B**reathing Pattern related to narrowed airways	The client will have respiratory rate and color within normal limits, clear breath sounds on auscultation, and ABG or pulse oximetry values within normal limits.	Assist the client in assuming a position that facilitates ventilation. Administer medication as ordered. Assist the client in the use of inhalers and aerosol treatments. Assess oxygenation by ABG or pulse oximetry values and administer supplemental oxygen, as ordered. Frequently assess respiratory rate and effort as well as color as client's condition dictates and auscultate the lung fields for presence of wheezes. If sputum is produced, note its color, amount, viscosity, and odor. Frequently assess vital signs as client's condition dictates. Unless otherwise contraindicated, encourage fluid intake to promote liquefaction of respiratory secretions.
Deficient **K**nowledge related to asthma, asthma treatment, and individual triggers for asthma attacks	The client will verbalize an understanding of both the pathophysiology and treatment of asthma, including the medications taken and their purposes and side effects. The client will also identify individual triggers and means of avoiding these triggers.	Teach client and family about the disease process; the purpose, effect, adverse effects, side effects, and use of all prescribed medications, especially inhalers and respiratory aerosol equipment. Assist client in establishing a medication schedule that will facilitate regular and timely taking of medications. Instruct the client to use the inhaler prior to meals to aid in breathing while eating. If the client is taking steroids, teach to rinse mouth after using the inhaler so as to prevent fungal infection. Encourage exercise because it increases respiratory reserve and improves overall physical condition. Assist client in identifying triggering stimuli and ways to avoid them. Teach client and family signs and symptoms of asthma attacks and respiratory tract infections. Teach client to avoid crowded areas and close contact with persons with infections.
Anxiety related to perceived threat of dying	The client will verbalize a decrease in anxiety.	Provide the client with explanations for all care. Provide care in a calm, unhurried manner. Plan care to allow the client uninterrupted periods of rest. Allow the client to make decisions regarding care, if possible. Provide the client with opportunities to discuss anxiety with staff, family, or significant others.

Evaluation Each goal must be evaluated to determine how it has been met by the client.

CHRONIC OBSTRUCTIVE PULMONARY DISEASE

Chronic obstructive pulmonary disease (COPD), also called chronic obstructive lung disease (COLD), is a term used for two closely related respiratory diseases: chronic bronchitis and emphysema. These two diseases often occur together. Most clients have a long history of heavy cigarette smoking (NHLBI, 2001a). First signs are chronic cough, sputum production, or shortness of breath. It gradually gets worse over time. There is no known cure. In the United States, about 16 million adults have COPD. It is the fourth leading cause of death. In 2000, direct and indirect costs were estimated at $30.4 billion (ALA, 2002d).

CHRONIC BRONCHITIS

Bronchitis is an inflammation of the bronchial tree accompanied by hypersecretion of mucus. The condition becomes chronic if cough and sputum are present on most days for 3 months a year for two consecutive years or for 6 months in one year (NHLBI, 2001b). Constant irritation of the bronchi results in hypertrophy of the mucus-secreting glands. The bronchioles fill with exudate, and subsequent infections are common. There may be narrowing of large and small airways. Environmental factors, especially cigarette smoke, play an important role in the development of chronic bronchitis.

The client usually has a history of recurrent respiratory infections, dyspnea, cyanosis, and chronic or recurrent cough yielding copious amounts of sputum. Often, the sputum is purulent or green in color. Over the course of time, the chest wall configuration becomes slightly distended. Coarse crackles are present throughout the lung fields. Breath sounds may be diminished or absent over the periphery of the lung fields. Elevation of pulmonary artery pressure results in increased workload for the right ventricle and in signs and symptoms of right-sided congestive heart failure (CHF), such as peripheral edema and fatigue. Arterial blood gases reveal increased $PaCO_2$ and decreased PaO_2. The red blood cell count elevates, as do hemoglobin and hematocrit. The increases in the amounts of red blood cells and hemoglobin represent an attempt by the body to compensate for the lower oxygen level. Chest x-ray shows hyperexpansion of the lungs. When CHF occurs, the chest x-ray also shows an enlarged heart.

Medical–Surgical Management

Medical

The goals of medical treatment are to decrease symptoms of airway irritation, decrease airway obstruction related to secretions and inflammation, prevent infection, maintain oxygenation, and increase the client's exercise tolerance. Respiratory therapy includes the use of updraft (nebulizer) and aerosol treatments, along with percussion and postural drainage. Humidification of inspired air helps liquefy secretions. Supplemental oxygen is administered based on ABG or pulse oximetry values. The neurological stimulus to breathe becomes altered in some clients with chronic bronchitis so that breathing is initiated when the blood level of oxygen falls instead of when the level of carbon dioxide rises. Consequently, when the level of oxygen in the blood is relatively high in relation to the level of carbon dioxide, the stimulus to breathe is reduced and further depresses the CNS. When supplemental oxygen is necessary, it is maintained at the lowest possible flow rate to maintain oxygenation and prevent depression of the client's respiratory drive. Evaluate the client with chronic bronchitis and CHF for signs of fluid overload. Daily weight, intake, and output are monitored.

🔲 Pharmacological

Bronchodilators such as theophylline (Theo-Dur), oxtriphylline (Choledyl), terbutaline sulfate (Brethine), and ipratropium bromide (Atrovent) are given to open the airways. Inhalation or aerosol treatments with bronchodilators such as albuterol (Ventolin) or metaproterenol sulfate (Alupent) are often used in conjunction with oral medications. Prednisone (Meticorten), a corti-

costeroid, is given as short-term therapy for acute exacerbations. If steroids are required on a long-term basis, they may be given by inhalation to prevent some adverse systemic effects. Medications that liquefy respiratory secretions are also given. Acetylcysteine (Mucomyst) may be given by inhalation, and guaifenesin (Humibid LA) may be given orally. If infection occurs, broad-spectrum antibiotics are given. Immunization against influenza viruses and *Streptococcus pneumoniae* is recommended.

The client with chronic bronchitis who also has CHF will receive medications to aid the function of the weakened heart. Digoxin (Lanoxin) strengthens the force of the contraction of the heart muscle. Diuretics such as furosemide (Lasix) are given to remove fluid by increasing urinary output. Supplemental potassium chloride (K-Dur, Kay-Ciel elixir) is given if the client's potassium level decreases from effect of the diuretic.

Diet

The client is encouraged to eat a well-balanced diet. If the client also has CHF, sodium intake is restricted. Unless contraindicated, fluids are encouraged.

Activity

Activity is restricted to decrease the workload on the heart and lungs. With acute exacerbations, the client is placed on bed rest. The level of activity is then slowly increased based on the client's tolerance.

Programs of breathing exercises and graded (easy to difficult) exercise regimes assist the client to achieve the maximum level of activity tolerance. Breath-retaining exercises such as coughing techniques, pursed-lip breathing, and diaphragmatic or abdominal breathing are taught. The client is monitored from a respiratory standpoint while exercising. The goal is to increase the client's capacity for all ADLs.

Nursing Management

Obtain history of onset, duration, and severity of symptoms. Note changes in level of consciousness, mental status, respiratory rate and effort, color, and use of accessory muscles. Obtain sputum specimen for culture and sensitivity. Monitor vital signs. Assess for weight gain, peripheral edema, and neck vein distention.

NURSING PROCESS

Assessment

Subjective Data

A thorough past medical history is obtained, including information about the onset, duration, and severity of symptoms. The client may describe fatigue and difficult breathing.

Objective Data

Note changes in level of consciousness or mental status, color, respiratory rate and effort, the position the client assumes to aid respiratory effort, and the use of accessory muscles. Review ABGs or pulse oximetry values. Auscultate lung fields for crackles and diminished breath sounds. Note color, amount, viscosity, and odor of sputum. Obtain specimens for culture and sensitivity, if indicated. Frequently measure vital signs. The pulse may be elevated and irregular. Blood pressure may be elevated or low. An elevated temperature may indicate infection. Assess for peripheral edema, neck vein distention, and rapid weight gain.

Nursing diagnoses for a client with chronic bronchitis may include the following:

Nursing Diagnoses	Planning/Goals	Nursing Interventions
Ineffective Airway Clearance related to thicker and increased amounts of respiratory secretions	The client's color, respiratory rate, and ABG values will be within normal limits.	Frequently assess level of consciousness, mental status, vital signs, respiratory effort, and color and auscultate breath sounds at least every 4 hours.
		Obtain sputum specimens as ordered, and assess sputum for amount, viscosity, color, and odor.
		Assist the client in assuming the position that most aids respiratory effort, usually an upright position.
		Administer oxygen and respiratory treatments as ordered and assess their effectiveness.
		Evaluate the results of diagnostic and laboratory tests (ABGs) and notify the physician of abnormalities.
		Alternate care with periods of uninterrupted rest.
		Administer antibiotics and bronchodilators as ordered.
		Provide the client with a well-balanced diet and unless otherwise contraindicated, encourage fluids.
		Assess the client for signs and symptoms of CHF (i.e., fine crackles heard on auscultation, peripheral edema, weight gain, and fatigue).
		Report any signs and symptoms of CHF to the physician.
Deficient Knowledge related to chronic bronchitis and its treatment and prevention	The client will verbalize signs and symptoms to report to the physician, safety precautions to take with medication and equipment, medication and respiratory treatment regimen, and techniques for facilitating breathing.	Teach the client to avoid respiratory infections, maintain adequate nutrition, increase fluid intake, and obtain adequate rest; the purpose, expected effects, and side effects of medications; and to administer respiratory treatments and medications prior to eating to aid in breathing.
		Instruct client to rinse mouth following use of inhaler.
		Teach the client to self-administer oxygen.
		Provide information regarding both the use of equipment and safety measures for the equipment.
		Refer the client to an established respiratory rehabilitation program. If such a program is not available, instruct the client in breathing techniques.
		Encourage regular exercise within the client's limitations.
		Encourage the client to obtain immunization against influenza viruses and *Streptococcus pneumoniae.*

Evaluation Each goal must be evaluated to determine how it has been met by the client.

EMPHYSEMA

Emphysema is a complex and destructive lung disease wherein air accumulates in the tissues of the lungs. The airways lose their elasticity and the walls thicken, resulting in narrower lumens. Airflow is impeded as it leaves the lungs (i.e., during expiration). The alveoli distal to these airways become overdistended with trapped air (Figure 32-10). Rupture of the alveolar wall may occur. The alveolar capillary membrane is destroyed, resulting in a loss of available area for gas exchange. Cigarette smoking is the most common cause of emphysema. Deficiency in alpha-1-antitrypsin is a familial disorder that leads to the development of emphysema. Alpha-1-antitrypsin is an enzyme that inhibits the activity of the enzyme elactase, which breaks down lung tissue.

Figure 32-10 *Emphysema*

Figure 32-11 *Changes in Chest Configuration and Posture:* ***A,*** *The normal ratio of the anterior posterior diameter to the lateral diameter is 1:2.* ***B,*** *With a barrel chest, the ratio between the diameters is 1:1.*

Emphysema develops slowly over a period of years. The earliest symptom is a daily morning cough with clear sputum. Later, the client notes increasing dyspnea in response to activity. The degree of dyspnea corresponds to the degree of hypoxia, which is usually mild at rest but becomes increasingly severe in response to activity. In advanced stages of the disease, hypoxia is evident even at rest. With infection, a cough yielding purulent sputum occurs. The client's complexion appears ruddy, or reddish in color. The chest becomes barrel shaped (Figure 32-11) as the chest cage enlarges to accommodate distended lung tissues. The respiratory rate elevates. The expiratory phase of respiration becomes increasingly difficult. Accessory muscles are used to aid respiratory effort. Because of destruction of the alveoli, bronchial breath sounds are heard in the periphery of the lungs. As the disease progresses, breath sounds diminish and eventually disappear over the periphery of the lungs. Arterial blood gases reveal the degree of hypoxia depending on the severity of the disease. Hypercapnia, or retention of carbon dioxide, is not as likely as with chronic bronchitis. The extra effort required to breathe increases metabolic need, resulting in weight loss. Chest x-ray reveals hyperinflated lung tissue and a flattened diaphragm, which has been displaced by distended lung tissues. Pulmonary function studies reveal a decrease in expiratory volume. Polycythemia and elevation of hemoglobin and hematocrit occur in response to prolonged hypoxia.

Medical–Surgical Management

Medical

The goals of treatment are to prevent further damage to the lung tissues, maintain adequate oxygenation, prevent infection, and improve the client's activity tolerance. The client who smokes should stop or, at least, decrease the number of cigarettes smoked daily. Supplemental oxygen is given to maintain oxygenation. The client with advanced emphysema and severe, chronic hypoxia may be maintained at PaO_2 of 55 to 59 mm Hg and/or oxygen saturation of 90% or greater. As with chronic bronchitis, the client with emphysema is given supplemental oxygen at the lowest possible flow rate, usually 2 to 3 L/min, to prevent respiratory and CNS depression.

Pharmacological

The client with emphysema receives many of the same medications used to treat chronic bronchitis. To open airways that have become fibrotic, theophylline and similar preparations are used. Steroids may be required for exacerbations. The client with emphysema usually does not need mucolytic agents, unless infection is present. Antibiotics are used to treat and prevent respiratory tract infections. The client should receive immunizations against influenza and *Streptococcus pneumoniae*. The client who smokes may use nicotine gum or transdermal patches to aid in smoking cessation.

Diet

The client with emphysema requires a diet high in carbohydrates to supply the energy necessary for breathing. If a negative nitrogen balance exists because of the client's using muscle tissue to provide energy, a diet high in protein is ordered. Dietary supplements such as Ensure may be needed to supply the necessary calories and nutrients. Unless contraindicated, fluids are encouraged.

CULTURAL CONSIDERATIONS

Skin Color/Cyanosis

- For a client with highly pigmented skin, establish a baseline skin color.
- Observe skin surfaces that have the least amount of pigmentation, such as the palms, the soles of the feet, the abdomen, or the inner aspect of forearms.

Activity

The client is placed on bed rest. Level of activity is increased based on the client's oxygenation. Oxygen saturation is evaluated periodically as the activity level is increased to determine the effect of activity on oxygenation.

Health Promotion

The client with emphysema benefits from a respiratory rehabilitation program. The client is taught breathing exercises similar to those taught to the client with chronic bronchitis. A graded exercise program is also used for the client with emphysema. Group programs that aid in smoking cessation are useful for the client who smokes.

Nursing Management

Review factors that increase client's dyspnea and those that relieve dyspnea. Evaluate client's nutritional status, vital signs, ABGs, pulse oximetry, color, and level of consciousness. Assist with ADLs. Plan for uninterrupted periods of rest.

NURSING PROCESS

Assessment

Subjective Data

Included in the history is information regarding the timing of dyspnea, those factors that exacerbate dyspnea, and those factors that relieve dyspnea.

Objective Data

Assess sputum for color, amount, viscosity, odor, and vital signs. An elevated pulse may indicate hypoxia and/or infection. Auscultation of the lungs will reveal the presence of adventitious, diminished, or absent breath sounds. Note the client's position to aid respiratory effort, color, respiratory rate and effort, and use of accessory muscles to aid breathing. Evaluate the client's nutritional status by weighing the client and measuring nutrient and caloric intake. Review results of laboratory and diagnostic tests.

Nursing diagnoses for a client with emphysema may include the following:

Nursing Diagnoses	Planning/Goals	Nursing Interventions
Impaired Gas Exchange related to destruction of the alveoli	The client's respiratory rate, color, and ABG values will be within normal limits.	Assess the client's level of consciousness and mental status.
		Frequently evaluate the client's respiratory rate, respiratory effort, color and oxygenation with ABG and/or pulse oximetry.
		Assess the effect of activity on oxygenation, particularly when activity is being increased and provide supplemental oxygen as ordered.
		Auscultate the lungs and report abnormalities to the physician.
		Assess the client's vital signs: Heart rate and temperature elevations may indicate infection. An elevated pulse may indicate hypoxia.
		Review the results of diagnostic and laboratory tests and report abnormalities.
		Administer medications and respiratory treatments as ordered.
		Assist the client in assuming the position that offers the most comfort and most aids respiratory effort. Instruct the client in breathing techniques, such as pursed-lip breathing.
Risk for Activity Intolerance related to hypoxia	The client will complete activity without experiencing fatigue or dyspnea.	Assist the client with ADL and hygiene needs.
		Plan care and treatments to allow the client uninterrupted periods of rest. Allow rest before and after meals.
		As activity increases, assess the effects on oxygenation.
Imbalanced Nutrition: Less than body requirements, related to increased energy requirements to maintain respiration	The client will achieve or maintain a weight within normal limits for height.	Assess the client's weight and evaluate in relation to the client's height.
		Evaluate the client's diet for nutritional adequacy and review the client's food likes and dislikes.
		Provide a well-balanced diet based on the client's likes and dislikes. Provide nutritional supplements as ordered.
		Avoid activities or procedures prior to meals that might reduce appetite (e.g., enemas).
		Administer medications and respiratory treatments prior to meals to aid in breathing.

Evaluation Each goal must be evaluated to determine how it has been met by the client.

CHAPTER 32 ■ Respiratory System 881

CRITICAL THINKING ?

COPD Disorders
What are the differences and the similarities of the two disorders classified as COPD?

BRONCHIECTASIS

Bronchiectasis is chronic dilation of the bronchi. The main causes of this disorder are pulmonary TB infection, chronic upper respiratory tract infections, and complications of other respiratory disorders of childhood, particularly cystic fibrosis. The bronchi become distended and eventually lose their elastic recoil property. The mucociliary blanket's function is impaired, and secretions thicken. Secretions accumulate in the bronchi, resulting in a medium for infection. Airflow is hindered, reducing gas exchange.

The client with bronchiectasis describes a frequent or chronic productive cough, dyspnea, weight loss, and fatigue. Sputum is thick and sometimes purulent when infection is present. Crackles, which clear on coughing, are heard scattered throughout the lungs and are more prominent early in the morning. Accessory muscles are used to aid respiration. Over a period of time, right-sided CHF and peripheral edema develop. Arterial blood gases reveal elevated $PaCO_2$, decreased PaO_2, and respiratory acidosis. Polycythemia and elevated hemoglobin and hematocrit levels are present. Chest x-ray shows slight hyperinflation of lung tissue and, in the presence of CHF, cardiomegaly. Respiratory flow rate decreases, and lung volume increases, as demonstrated by pulmonary function studies. Table 32-8 compares asthma, chronic bronchitis, emphysema, and bronchiectasis.

Medical–Surgical Management
Medical

Medical treatment is aimed at removing respiratory secretions, preventing or eliminating infection, and maintaining adequate oxygenation. Percussion and postural drainage are used to aid in the removal of secretions. Aerosol and updraft respiratory treatments may be ordered before percussion and drainage. If the client is unable to expectorate secretions, bronchial suctioning is performed. The physician may perform a bronchoscopy to remove especially tenacious and copious secretions. Arterial blood gases and/or pulse oximetry values are evaluated to assess the need for supplemental oxygen. Daily weight and I&O are performed to detect signs of CHF. Pulmonary function studies evaluate the severity of lung damage.

Pharmacological

Mucolytic agents are given to promote liquefaction of respiratory secretions. Antibiotics are ordered to treat and prevent infection. The client is immunized against influenza and against *Streptococcus pneumoniae* with the pneumococcal vaccine (Pneumovax 23). Bronchodilators are indicated to open the fibrotic airways. Inflammation is treated with oral steroids such as prednisone (Meticorten) and/or by inhalation with beclomethasone dipropionate (Beclovent). The client with cystic fibrosis is required to take pancreatic enzymes, pancrelipase (Pancrease capsules, Cotazym capsules), to replace those that are missing with this disorder. If CHF occurs, the client is treated with digoxin (Lanoxin), furosemide (Lasix), and potassium supplements, as indicated.

Diet

To provide energy for breathing, the diet should be high in carbohydrates and calories. Protein is supplemented if necessary. Dietary supplements such as Ensure may be needed. Fluids are encouraged, unless otherwise contraindicated. Sodium is restricted in the diet of the client with CHF to prevent fluid retention. The diet for the client with cystic fibrosis is restricted in fats because fats are not properly absorbed.

Activity

During acute exacerbations or in the presence of serious infection, activity is limited. The client is placed on bed rest. Activity is progressively increased depending on the client's tolerance. Respiratory rehabilitation and graded exercise programs are useful in the treatment of bronchiectasis. Regular exercise is encouraged, particularly for the pediatric client with cystic fibrosis.

Nursing Management

Review client's history for recent and past respiratory infections, TB, and cystic fibrosis. Monitor vital signs. An increased heart rate may indicate hypoxia and/or infection, and an elevated temperature may indicate infection. Note weight loss and muscle wasting. Monitor breath sounds and suction mucous as necessary.

CHEST TRAUMA

Pneumothorax/hemothorax is discussed following.

PNEUMOTHORAX/HEMOTHORAX

Normally, there is no space between the visceral and parietal pleura. They are held together by surface tension. Thus the pleural space is a closed compartment with a negative pressure compared to the lungs or the atmosphere. When the integrity of the pleura is interrupted, air from the atmosphere or from the lungs moves between the pleura, creating a space. This air in the pleural space is known as a **pneumothorax** (Figure 32-12). The lung tissue underlying the pneumothorax is compressed and unable to fully expand. If the pneumothorax is large enough, the entire lung may collapse from the compression.

A pneumothorax may be referred to as closed, open, spontaneous, or tension. A closed pneumothorax occurs when there is no communication between the pleura

TABLE 32-8   SIGNS AND SYMPTOMS OF ASTHMA, CHRONIC BRONCHITIS, EMPHYSEMA, AND BRONCHIECTASIS

	ASTHMA	CHRONIC BRONCHITIS	EMPHYSEMA	BRONCHIECTASIS
History	Intermittent attacks of dyspnea and wheezing	Recurrent respiratory infections, chronic cough	Insidious onset, dyspnea on exertion to dyspnea at rest	Cystic fibrosis, recurrent respiratory infections, TB
✓**Cough**	Present during attack	Chronic or recurrent productive cough	Present with infections	Frequent or chronic productive cough
✓**Sputum**	Thick	Copious, purulent, green	Scanty mucoid, unless infection present	Thick, tenacious, sometimes purulent secretions
Weight	No weight loss	Slight or no weight loss	Weight loss common	Commonly, weight loss or failure to gain
Appearance	Flushed then cyanotic	Commonly cyanosis ("blue bloater")	Ruddy complexion ("pink puffer")	Clubbing of fingernails
Chest Configuration	Slight overdistention	Slight overdistention	Overdistention prominent ("barrel chest")	Slight overdistention
✓**Breath Sounds**	Audible wheezing Prolonged expiration	Coarse crackles	Bronchial breath sounds in peripheral lung fields Diminished or absent in late disease	Crackles
✓**Edema**	Infrequent	Peripheral edema common, especially in ankles	Infrequent	Peripheral edema in late disease
✓**Right-sided CHF (Cor Pulmonale)**	Infrequent	Frequent	Infrequent	Frequent late in disease
CO Retention (Hypercapnia)	Sometimes	Common	Unlikely	Common in late disease
Hypoxemia	Depends on severity of attack	Possibly severe	Usually mild, especially at rest	Possibly severe in late disease and with infection
Dyspnea	Increases during attack	Progressive	Dyspnea on exertion to dyspnea at rest usually presenting symptom	With respiratory infection and late disease
Accessory Muscles Used for Respiration	Yes	Yes	Yes	Yes
Polycythemia	Uncommon	Late in disease	Yes	In late disease
Respiratory Failure	Possible	Common	Possible	Common

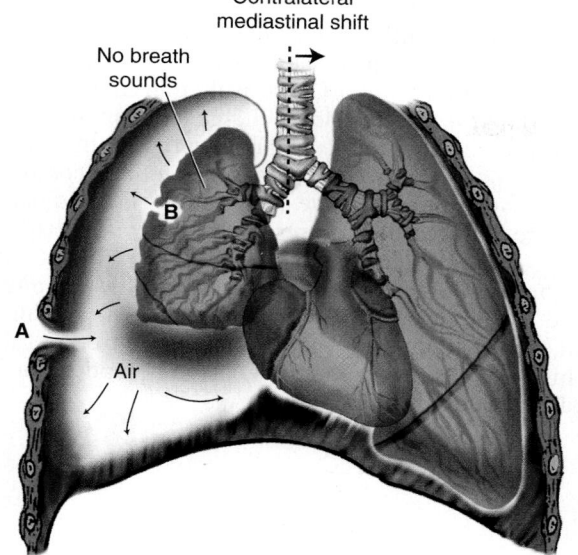

Figure 32-12 *Pneumothorax:* **A,** *Penetrating Wound;* **B,** *Ruptured Bleb on the Lung*

Contralateral mediastinal shift

No breath sounds

B

A

Air

and the external environment. An example of a closed pneumothorax is when blunt trauma to the chest causes a broken rib that pierces the pleura and lung, allowing air to enter between the pleura. An open pneumothorax exists when there is direct communication between the external environment and the pleural space as in a gunshot wound. A spontaneous pneumothorax occurs without an obvious underlying cause. A tension pneumothorax is a life-threatening condition wherein air enters the pleural space on inspiration but is unable to exit on expiration. The air thus continues to accumulate in the pleural space, compressing the underlying structures. If left untreated, a tension pneumothorax will collapse the lung and encroach on the structures on the opposite side. The structures of the mediastinum will shift to the unaffected side as more and more air accumulates in the pleural space. Without intervention, tension pneumothorax will result in cardiopulmonary arrest. Tension pneumothorax is often associated with mechanical ventilation. The pressure exerted by the ventilator on compromised lung tissue interrupts the integrity of the pleura. Air continues to enter the pleural space but is unable to exit as mechanical ventilation continues. In the case of a pneumothorax associated with trauma or surgery, bleeding of adjacent vessels into the pleural cavity often occurs. Blood within the pleural space is referred to as a **hemothorax.** When accompanied by air, the condition is called a **hemopneumothorax.**

The severity of injury and the amount of lung tissue affected determine the signs and symptoms the client exhibits. The client with a small pneumothorax may be asymptomatic or may complain of minor dyspnea, whereas the client with a significant pneumothorax may exhibit signs of severe respiratory distress. Dyspnea, tachypnea, orthopnea, and cyanosis may be present. Oxygenation is impaired. Pleuritic pain is common. Breath sounds are absent in the area of the pneumothorax. The client with an accompanying hemothorax will

exhibit signs and symptoms of shock associated with blood loss.

Medical–Surgical Management
Medical

In order for the affected lung to reexpand, the air and/or blood must be removed from the pleural space. When the blood loss associated with a hemothorax is significant, fluid and blood replacement may be necessary.

Surgical

A thoracotomy tube, or chest tube, is inserted by the physician into the pleural space to drain fluid and air and allow the lung to reexpand. The tube is placed in the midaxillary line at approximately the fifth intercostal space. To drain air alone, the tube is placed in the anterior chest at the midclavicular line and the fourth intercostal space. The thoracotomy tube is connected to an underwater seal drainage device (refer back to Figure 32-7). The underlying cause of the hemopneumothorax then must be treated.

A recurrent spontaneous pneumothorax may require a pleural cortication to prevent further episodes. This involves roughing the adjacent surfaces of the visceral and parietal pleura so the resulting scar tissue will improve adhesion between the two surfaces. Emergency treatment for a tension pneumothorax that is severely compromising the function of the heart and lungs is placing a large-bore needle into the anterior chest at the fourth intercostal space. A thoracotomy tube is then inserted until the lung(s) are fully reexpanded and to prevent a recurrence.

Pharmacological

To control pleuritic pain, narcotic analgesics such as morphine sulfate or meperidine (Demerol) are prescribed. Analgesics may be given orally or parenterally depending on the severity of the pain. Before insertion of a thoracotomy tube, intravenous narcotics may be given prophylactically. Tissues adjacent to the area of the pneumothorax are injected with local anesthetics before insertion of a thoracotomy tube.

Diet

A well-balanced diet with sufficient amounts of protein is encouraged for healing. The client with other injuries and conditions may require TPN or enteral feedings.

Activity

If hypoxia is present, activity restrictions are necessary. The presence of other injuries or conditions may also necessitate activity restrictions. After the client is adequately oxygenated and stable, activity is encouraged to promote expansion of the lungs.

Nursing Management

Gather information about recent chest injuries or falls. Assess level of consciousness, mental status, color, respiratory effort, and chest wall movement. Monitor vital signs. Auscultate for breath sounds. When a chest tube is in place, assess function, patency, and amount and character of drainage.

NURSING PROCESS

Assessment

Subjective Data

Gather information about the source of the pneumothorax. Ask the client about previous pneumothoraces, recent chest injury, falls, and severe coughing. The client often describes being very anxious.

Objective Data

Assess the client's level of consciousness and mental status and the client's color, respiratory effort, and chest wall movement. Chest wall movement is decreased on the affected side. When a large pneumothorax is present, the trachea shifts toward the unaffected side. Dyspnea and cyanosis may occur. The cough is forceful and nonproductive. Respiratory rate and heart rate are elevated. Blood pressure may be elevated because of the presence of pain and anxiety or may be low because of blood loss. Breath sounds are diminished or absent over the affected areas. Note the location, duration, and severity of pain. When a chest tube is inflated, assess for function, patency, and amount and character of drainage.

Nursing diagnoses for a client with a pneumothorax may include the following:

Nursing Diagnoses	Planning/Goals	Nursing Interventions
*Ineffective **B**reathing Pattern* related to decreased lung expansion	The client's respiratory rate and color will be within normal limits, and the client will have clear breath sounds in affected area.	Monitor the amount and character of drainage from the chest tube and note chest tube drainage as output.
		Observe fluctuations (tidaling) in the water seal chamber, which indicates that the tube is in the pleural space.
		Investigate the absence of tidaling because this may indicate that the lung is fully reexpanded or that the tube is occluded or kinked.
		Observe for bubbling in the water seal chamber, which indicates an air leak. Assess the connections and chest tube to determine if leaks are present. If no air leaks are present, notify the physician because the air leak may be within the client's lungs.
		Encourage the client to cough and deep breathe to prevent further respiratory complications.
*Acute **P**ain* related to pleural space irritation	The client will verbalize a decrease in pain on a scale of 1 to 10.	Assist the client in assuming the position that most aids respiration. Most clients find this to be the orthopneic position.
		Assess vital signs and respiratory status.
		Administer pain medications as ordered. Remember that respiratory depression is possible with narcotic medications.
		Provide diversional activities.

Evaluation Each goal must be evaluated to determine how it has been met by the client.

NEOPLASMS OF THE RESPIRATORY TRACT

Neoplasms discussed following include benign neoplasms, lung cancer, and laryngeal cancer.

BENIGN NEOPLASMS

A benign tumor or cyst in the lung has sharply defined edges, as revealed on an x-ray. Peripheral tumors usually have no symptoms. Bronchial tumors may cause obstruction, infection, or atelectasis.

LUNG CANCER

Malignant tumors (carcinomas) of the lung may originate within the lung or may result from metastasis from other tumor sites (e.g., breast, colon, or kidney). Men, especially those older than 40 years of age, are more likely to have lung cancer than are women. The incidence of lung cancer has plateaued among women and is declining among men (American Cancer Society [ACS], 2003). Cigarette smoking is the most important risk factor for lung cancer. Air pollution and exposure to carcinogens such as asbestos are also risk factors, especially among smokers, for developing lung cancer. Prognosis depends on the size of

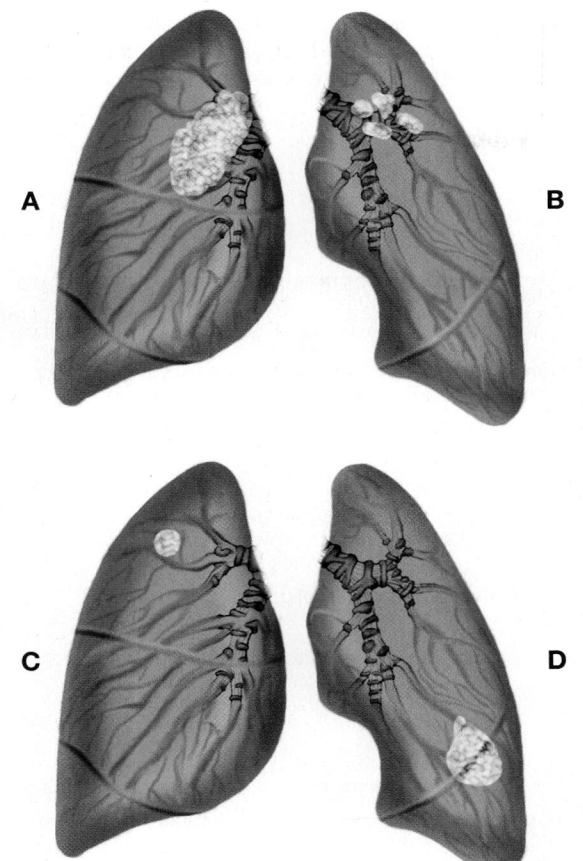

Figure 32-13 *Lung Cancers:* **A,** *Small-cell Carcinoma;* **B,** *Epidermoid (squamous-cell) Carcinoma;* **C,** *Adenocarcinoma;* **D,** *Large Cell (undifferentiated) Carcinoma*

the tumor when diagnosed and the specific cell type (Figure 32-13).

Symptoms develop late in the course of lung cancers. Peripheral lesions generally have few symptoms. Initially, the client may complain of a chronic cough or wheezing. Central lesions cause obstruction and erosion of the bronchi. As the tumor grows and occludes the air passages, the client may experience shortness of breath, dyspnea, and blood-tinged sputum. Pain occurs relatively late in the course of the disease and indicates that the tumor has grown to a significant size to put pressure on adjacent nerves and other structures. Although some tumors can be seen on chest x-ray, many cannot. Low-dose helical CT scans and MRI scans are more reliable studies when assessing soft-tissue structures. To confirm a diagnosis, cytology studies are performed on specimens collected via bronchoscopy, needle biopsy, or mediastinoscopy. Lung scans are occasionally useful for diagnosis. Before initiating treatment, the client is evaluated for metastatic disease using bone and total body scans.

Family members and significant others often need assistance in coping with their feelings.

Medical–Surgical Management

Medical

Treatment of lung cancer depends on the type and stage of the cancer.

Surgical

Surgical intervention involves the removal of the tumor and adjacent lung tissue. Pneumonectomy is the removal of an entire lung. Lobectomy is the removal of a lobe of a lung. Segmental resection is the removal of a segment of a lung. The client will have a thoracotomy tube on the operative side. Radiation and chemotherapy are often used in conjunction with surgery. The incidence of lung tumor recurrence following surgery is high. Surgery is often indicated for early non–small-cell carcinomas.

Pharmacological

The specific type of chemotherapy used depends on the cell type and the extent of tumor growth.

Health Promotion

The foremost method of preventing lung cancer is to avoid smoking or to cease smoking. Avoid the second-hand smoke of others.

Nursing Management

Review client's history for smoking, exposure to carcinogens, and other risk factors. Gather information about onset and severity of symptoms. Assess for pain. Monitor breath sounds, vital signs, and drainage from chest tube. Assist to semi-Fowler's position or lying on the affected side. Monitor ABGs and provide oxygen as indicated. When pain medication is given, monitor for respiratory depression. Aid client to express feelings of grief about diagnosis.

NURSING PROCESS

Assessment

Subjective Data

Review the client's history for smoking, exposure to carcinogens, and other risk factors. Gather information regarding the onset, duration, and severity of symptoms. The client may report hoarseness, chronic cough, pain, and shortness of breath. Assess pain for location, character, duration, and severity.

Objective Data

Note the color, amount, consistency, and odor of sputum. Before surgery, wheezing or decreased breath sounds may be heard on the affected side. Following surgery, breath sounds are diminished or absent on the affected side. Monitor the amount and color of drainage from the thoracotomy tube. Assess the wound for hemorrhage and infection. Respiratory rate and effort may be increased. Pulse rate may be elevated as a result of a variety of factors including decreased oxygenation, hemorrhage, and

infection. Hypotension occurs with significant blood loss. High blood pressure may indicate pain, anxiety, or other underlying pathology such as essential hypertension.

Nursing diagnoses for a client with lung cancer may include the following:

Nursing Diagnoses	Planning/Goals	Nursing Interventions
Ineffective **B**reathing Pattern related to disease process	The client's respiratory rate and color will be within normal limits.	Frequently monitor the client's level of consciousness, vital signs, color, and respiratory effort. Auscultate breath sounds.
		Assess oxygenation and provide supplemental oxygen as indicated.
		Stagger activities with periods of rest to prevent overtaxing the client's reserves.
		Assist the client in assuming the position that maximizes respiratory effort by positioning the client in semi-Fowler's position or lying on the affected side.
		Monitor lab reports for blood gas levels.
Chronic **P**ain related to lung cancer	The client will state pain is decreased on a scale of 1 to 10.	Administer pain medication and monitor for respiratory depression.
		Provide diversional activities.
		Assist the client in assuming a position of comfort.
Anticipatory **G**rieving related to prognosis and perceived separation from significant others	The client will be able to express to significant others and/or staff feelings related to diagnosis and prognosis.	Aid the client in expressing feelings of grief related to the diagnosis.
		Hope should not be eliminated, but false hope should not be encouraged.
		Allow the client and family time to express their feelings.

Evaluation Each goal must be evaluated to determine how it has been met by the client.

LARYNGEAL CANCER

Cancer of the larynx is more common among men than women, an estimated 7,100 and 2,400, respectively (ACS, 2003). Risk factors for cancer of the larynx include smoking, chronic alcohol abuse, chronic laryngitis, and overuse of the voice. Laryngeal cancer is relatively asymptomatic. The client may experience hoarseness or difficulty speaking above a whisper. If either persists for more than 2 weeks, medical care should be sought. Difficulty swallowing is sometimes present. Laryngeal pain radiating to the ear or a lump in the throat are often signs of metastasis.

Medical–Surgical Management

Treatment is determined by the extent of tumor growth.

Surgical

Surgical removal of the larynx, a laryngectomy, is used to treat laryngeal cancer. If the cancer has spread to surrounding tissues, a simple or radical neck dissection

COMMUNITY/HOME HEALTH CARE

Client with Laryngeal Stoma

- Humidify home, especially in winter.
- The client and family must know how to suction the respiratory tract and care for the respiratory equipment.
- Use warm water to clean around the stoma.
- Do not use tissues, linty cotton, or soap for cleansing.
- Wear a bib or dressing over the stoma to filter and warm incoming air.
- Do not swim or splash water in the stoma when showering or bathing.
- Notify the physician if any signs of respiratory infection develop, such as fever, cough, yellow or green mucus, or redness around the stoma.
- Keep follow-up appointments with physician.

may be required. Radiation may be used as an adjunct to surgery or as primary treatment if the tumor is detected in the early stages. Following surgery, a permanent tracheostomy is necessary to allow air to enter the respiratory tract. A small incision is made into the trachea and below the Adam's apple, and a plastic tracheostomy tube is inserted.

Nursing Management

Monitor respiratory status. Suction secretions and provide tracheostomy care. Teach client stoma protection. Keep head of bed elevated and provide extra humidity. Refer client to the American Cancer Society for support.

NURSING PROCESS

Assessment

Subjective Data

Obtain a history of the onset, duration, and severity of symptoms, such as hoarseness or laryngitis and alcohol and tobacco use. The client may describe ear pain and difficulty breathing and swallowing.

Objective Data

Evaluate the client's respiratory status for other respiratory problems that may accompany laryngeal cancer, such as COPD. Examine sputum for the presence of blood.

Nursing diagnoses for a client with laryngeal cancer may include the following:

Nursing Diagnoses	Planning/Goals	Nursing Interventions
Impaired Verbal Communication related to removal of the larynx	The client will be able to communicate needs.	Before surgery, establish a means of communication to be used afterward. If available, a manual or computer word/picture board works well.
		Keep call light by client's bed.
		Avoid mouthing communications, as this is frustrating to the client and is time consuming.
		As possible, ask questions that require only a "yes" or "no" answer.
		Refer the client to the local support group (Lost Chord Club) or the American Cancer Society.
Ineffective Airway Clearance related to tracheostomy tube	The client's respiratory rate and color will be within normal limits, and the client will have clear breath sounds to auscultation.	Suction frequently following surgery to remove static secretions and provide routine tracheostomy care.
		Provide small, frequent feedings of liquid or pureed food to prevent choking.
		Assist client to turn, cough, and deep breathe two to four times an hour.
		Teach client stoma protection.
		Assess respirations two to four times an hour, if secretions are copious. Auscultate lung sounds.
		Keep head of bed elevated. Provide extra humidity.
Deficient Knowledge related to tracheostomy care	The client will verbalize precautions and safety measures for a tracheostomy; how to use equipment; how to suction the respiratory tract; how to change a tracheostomy tube; and actions to take in an emergency.	Teach the client and family how to suction the respiratory tract, care for the tracheostomy, and use respiratory equipment.
		Instruct the client and family in what to do in case of an emergency, such as secretions clogging the tracheostomy tube.
		Advise client not to swim and to avoid aspirating water when showering or bathing.
		Advise client to avoid extremely cold temperatures. Cover tracheostomy site for warming or cosmetic purposes with a porous material without frayed or loose threads.

Evaluation Each goal must be evaluated to determine how it has been met by the client.

DISORDERS OF THE NOSE

The most common disorder of the nose is epistaxis, or nose bleed.

EPISTAXIS

Epistaxis is hemorrhage of the nares or nostrils. It may be either unilateral, which is most common, or bilateral. Epistaxis may be primary in nature, stemming from drying of the nasal mucosa, local irritation, or trauma, or may occur secondary to uncontrolled hypertension or coagulopathies (e.g., thrombocytopenia, anticoagulant therapy). The diffuse vascularity and proximity of blood vessels to the surface of the nasal mucosa make the nares a susceptible avenue for hemorrhage. Blood loss can be minimal to severe. With significant blood loss, hypovolemic shock occurs.

Medical–Surgical Management

Medical

The client with epistaxis usually arrives at an urgent care facility or emergency room after unsuccessful attempts to stop the bleeding. Signs of airway obstruction or aspiration require immediate attention. The goals of treatment are to maintain airway, stop bleeding, identify the cause, and prevent recurrence. Nosebleeds are usually responsive to compression of the nares. Maintain firm pressure for 5 minutes. If bleeding persists, the client should blow the nose and clear the nasal passages. Resume pressure for a full 10 minutes. Epistaxis that continues following these measures requires more aggressive treatment. Bleeding sites that cannot be visualized require a sterile nasal packing inserted after application of a local anesthetic. In severe cases, a nasostat is inserted. This device resembles a Foley catheter and provides direct compression to the site of bleeding via a balloon. Clients with severe nosebleeds may require fluid and blood replacement to prevent hypovolemic shock. Persistent or recurrent epistaxis may require surgical ligation of the artery supplying the area.

Infection Control: Epistaxis

Wear gloves, goggles or a face mask, and a gown when caring for a client with epistaxis. A cough or sneeze can splatter blood.

Pharmacological

Sites of bleeding that can be visualized are cauterized by the physician using silver nitrate sticks. Hemostasis may also be accomplished by packing the affected nostril with epinephrine 1 : 1000 on cotton packing.

Nursing Management

Evaluate overt blood flow and visually examine the posterior oropharynx for hidden bleeding. Monitor vital signs. Have client sit up with head bent slightly forward, breathe through the mouth, and allow blood to run freely from the nose into a container. Then, wearing gloves, compress the nares for 5 minutes. Suction through the mouth to prevent aspiration.

NURSING PROCESS

Assessment

Subjective Data

Ask about the onset, precipitating events, duration, and frequency of epistaxis, as well as associated symptoms such as nausea, vomiting, headache, and lightheadedness. The client with an occult, or hidden, bleed may complain of needing to swallow frequently.

Objective Data

Evaluate blood flow for amount, consistency, color, and rate (or severity). Overt bleeding from the nose may be present. This bleeding can vary in flow, from a continuous drip to a pulsating stream of blood. Visually examine the posterior oropharynx of the client with an occult epistaxis to assess blood flow. Vomiting may be present. Lowered blood pressure and rapid heart rate are signs of hypovolemic shock. Conversely, the client with uncontrolled hypertension has an abnormally high systolic blood pressure. Prothrombin time (PT), APTT, INR, and other clotting studies will be abnormal with underlying coagulopathies. Decreased red blood cell count, hemoglobin, and hematocrit are evidence of significant bleeding.

Nursing diagnoses for a client with epistaxis may include the following:

Nursing Diagnoses	Planning/Goals	Nursing Interventions
Impaired Gas Exchange related to airway obstruction	The client's respiratory rate, color, and blood gases will be within normal limits.	Place the client in a high Fowler's position, with the head bent slightly forward. Instruct the client to breathe through the mouth and allow the blood to escape freely from the nose and into a container. This aids in preventing obstruction of the airway and swallowing of blood.

continues

Nursing Diagnoses	Planning/Goals	Nursing Interventions
		Monitor the client for signs and symptoms of airway obstruction.
		Assess the client's color, respiratory rate and effort, and breath sounds.
		Monitor pulse oximetry and lab reports of ABGs and administer supplemental oxygen as indicated.
Risk for Aspiration related to epistaxis	The client will develop no complications related to aspiration.	Place the client in the position previously described to aid in preventing aspiration of blood. Assess the client for signs of aspiration, such as choking, coarse crackles on auscultation, or elevated temperature.
		Suction the respiratory tract through the mouth to remove secretions and blood.
Deficient Fluid Volume related to blood loss.	The client will maintain adequate fluid volume.	With a gloved hand, compress the nares for 5 minutes. If bleeding persists, have client blow nose to clear passages, then compress nares for 10 minutes.
		If bleeding continues following compression attempts, prepare to assist the physician with procedures such as cautery or insertion of nasal packing.
		Administer medications to control blood pressure, as ordered.
		After hemostasis has been established, the clots formed should not be removed or dislodged, as this will lead to recurrence of bleeding.
		Every 30 minutes, evaluate the blood pressure and pulse of the client who shows signs of volume depletion.
		Assess for orthostatic hypotension as a means of measuring volume depletion. A decrease in systolic blood pressure of greater than 10 mm Hg when the position is changed from lying to sitting or standing indicates hypovolemia.
		Administer intravenous fluids, as ordered.

Evaluation Each goal must be evaluated to determine how it has been met by the client.

CASE STUDY

Mrs. White is a 77-year-old female with a history of smoking two to three packs of cigarettes per day for the past 60 years. Mrs. White has been diagnosed with COPD for the past 4 years. She has required supplemental oxygen at 2 L/min for the last 18 months. Three days ago, Mrs. White was admitted with chief complaints of increasing dyspnea on exertion and a productive cough yielding thick, green-yellow sputum. She states that she does "not know why she is coughing up this awful stuff."

Physical examination of Mrs. White this morning revealed vital signs of T = 101.5°F, P = 124, R = 38, BP = 168/74; and sonorous and sibilant wheezes on expiration and in the posterior lung fields, with superimposed coarse crackles heard in the right posterior lower lung field. She is unable to ambulate to the bathroom or complete other ADL due to the dyspnea. Chest x-ray showed a large area of consolidation in the right lower lobe. Sputum culture is still pending.

The following questions will guide your development of a nursing care plan for the case study.

1. List the clinical manifestations that indicate Mrs. White is experiencing an infection concomitant with her COPD.
2. Explain why COPD predisposes a client to respiratory infection.

continues

CASE STUDY—continued

3. Explain why the physician will increase Mrs. White's oxygen flow to 3 to 4 L/min.
4. List the subjective and objective data the nurse should obtain during the nursing assessment.
5. Identify three nursing diagnoses and client goals that would be pertinent to Mrs. White's care.
6. List the above diagnoses in order of priority, with number one being the highest.
7. Describe client outcomes indicating that Mrs. White's treatment and nursing care regimen have been successful.

Summary

- The primary function of the respiratory system is delivery of oxygen to the lungs and removal of carbon dioxide from the lungs.
- Pneumonia is a lung infection wherein infectious secretions accumulate in the air passages and interfere with gas exchange. Clients with chronic pulmonary disorders or problems of immobility are at increased risk of developing pneumonia.
- Pulmonary TB is an infection of the lung tissue caused by the *Mycobacterium tuberculosis*. Treatment of TB requires the long-term administration of pharmacological agents.
- A common respiratory tract disorder associated with immobility and the administration of anesthetic agents is atelectasis. Clients at risk are encouraged to cough and breathe deeply to aid in preventing atelectasis.
- Obstruction of a pulmonary artery by a bloodborne substance is known as pulmonary embolism. Deep vein thrombosis is a common cause of pulmonary emboli.
- Chronic obstructive pulmonary disease is a collective term used to refer to chronic bronchitis and emphysema, which often occur together.
- Traumatic disorders of the respiratory tract include pneumothorax and hemothorax, wherein the underlying lung tissue is compressed and eventually collapses.
- Cigarette smoking is indicated as a major causative factor in the development of respiratory disorders, such as lung cancer, cancer of the larynx, emphysema, and chronic bronchitis.

Review Questions

1. The physician orders 2 to 3 L/min of oxygen to be delivered to the client with COPD because:
   a. no client ever requires more than 2 to 3 L/min of oxygen.
   b. the client requests it.
   c. a higher flow rate may suppress the client's drive to breathe.
   d. 2 to 3 L/min is the maximum flow that a nasal cannula can effectively deliver.

2. A particulate respirator mask is used by the nurse caring for a client with TB because:
   a. regular masks allow the tubercle bacilli to pass through.
   b. this mask is more comfortable for long-term use.
   c. this type of mask allows the nurse to be in close contact with the client for prolonged periods of time.
   d. there is no need for this type of mask when caring for clients with TB.

3. Incentive spirometry is used to measure the amount of air that:
   a. is exhaled in 1 minute.
   b. is inspired in 1 minute.
   c. is inspired with one inhalation.
   d. is exhaled with one exhalation.

4. Asthma is characterized by:
   a. chronic narrowing of the airways.
   b. intermittent airflow obstruction.
   c. chronic dilation of the airways.
   d. fibrosis of the alveoli.

5. The client with a pneumothorax experiences hypoxia due to:

    a. the entry of air into the thoracic cavity.

    b. compression of the lung tissue underlying the pneumothorax.

    c. impairment of gas exchange.

    d. a lack of surfactant.

References/Suggested Readings

American Cancer Society (ACS). (2003). *Cancer facts and figures 2003*. Atlanta, GA: Author.

American Lung Association (ALA). (2001). *Trends in tuberculosis morbidity and mortality*. [Online]. Available: www.lungusa.org/data/tb/tb1.pdf

American Lung Association (ALA). (2002a). *Fact sheet: Tuberculosis*. [Online]. Available: www.lungusa.org/diseases/tbfac.html

American Lung Association (ALA). (2002b). *Fact sheet: Tuberculosis and HIV*. [Online]. Available: www.lungusa.org/diseases/tbhivfac.html

American Lung Association (ALA). (2002c). *Lung cancer* [Online]. Available: www.lungusa.org/data/lc/CCO2Pt1.pdf

American Lung Association (ALA). (2002d). *Trends in chronic bronchitis and emphysema morbidity and mortality*. [Online]. Available: www.lungusa.org/data/copd/COPD1.pdf

American Lung Association (ALA). (2002e). *Trends in morbidity and mortality: Pneumonia, influenza, and acute respiratory conditions*. [Online]. Available: www.lungusa.org/data/pi/PI_1.pdf

Andrews, C., & Kearney, K. (2002). Preventing air embolism. *AJN, 102*(1), 34–36.

Avalos-Bock, S. (2001). The hard truth about the PPD skin test. *Nursing2001, 31*(6), 56–57.

Carroll, P. (2001). How to intervene before asthma turns deadly. *RN, 64*(5), 52–58.

Centers for Disease Control and Prevention (CDC). (2002). *Core Curriculum on Tuberculosis 2000* (Updated, 2002). Atlanta, GA: Author. [Online]. Available: www.cdc.gov/nchstp/tb/pubs/corecurr/default.htm

Centers for Disease Control and Prevention (CDC). (2003a). *Basic information about SARS*. [Online]. Available: www.cdc.gov/ncidod/sars/factsheet.htm

Centers for Disease Control and Prevention (CDC). (2003b). *Updated interim domestic infection control guidance in the health-care and community setting for patients with suspected SARS*. [Online]. Available: www.cdc.gov/ncidod/sars/infectioncontrol/htm

Chan, S., & Goldrick, B. (2003). Emerging infections. *AJN, 103*(6), 60–62.

Chrisp, D. (2000). Tension pneumothorax. *Nursing2000, 30*(5), 33.

Davies, P. (2002). Guarding your patient against ARDS. *Nursing2002, 32*(3), 36–41.

Diehl-Oplinger, L., & Kaminski, M. F. (2002). Flash pulmonary edema. *Nursing2002, 32*(7), 96.

Dirkes, S., & Winklerprins, A. (2002). Help for ARDS patients. *RN, 65*(8), 52–58.

Dochterman, J., & Bulechek, G. (2004). *Nursing Interventions Classification (NIC)* (4th ed.). St. Louis, MO: Mosby.

Dunn, N. (2001). Keeping COPD patients out of the ED. *RN, 64*(2), 33–37.

Eckler, J. (2002). Keeping pulmonary tuberculosis at bay. *Nursing2002, 32*(12), 70.

Ellmers, K., & Criddle, L. (2002). Cystic fibrosis. *RN, 65*(9), 60–66.

Estes, M. E. Z. (2002). *Health assessment & physical examination* (2nd ed.). Clifton Park, NY: Thomson Delmar Learning.

Finesilver, C. (2001). Perfecting your skills: Respiratory assessment. *Travel Nurse Today* supplement to *RN* (April) 16–26.

Goodfellow, L., & Jones, M. (2002). Bronchial hygiene therapy. *AJN, 102*(1), 37–43.

Hayes, D. (2001). Stemming the tide of pleural effusions. *Nursing2001, 31*(5), 49–52.

Jones, L., & Hannum, D. (1998). Playing it safe with a particulate respirator. *Nursing98, 28*(1), 50–51.

King, M., & Tomasic, D. (1999). Treating TB today. *RN, 62*(6), 26–30.

Lazzara, D. (2001). Respiratory distress. *Nursing2001, 31*(6), 58–63.

Lazzara, D. (2002). Eliminate the air of mystery from chest tubes. *Nursing2002, 32*(6), 36–43.

Lindell, K., & Jacobs, S. (2003). Idiopathic pulmonary fibrosis. *AJN, 103*(4), 32–41.

Little, C. (2002). Chronic bronchitis. *Nursing2001, 32*(9), 52–55.

Marion, B. (2001). A turn for the better: "Prone positioning" of patients with ARDS. *AJN, 101*(5), 26–33.

Marthaler, M., Keresztes, P., & Tazbir, J. (2003). SARS: What have we learned? *RN, 66*(8), 58–66.

McConnell, E. (2002). Providing tracheostomy care. *Nursing2002, 32*(1), 17.

Miracle, V. (2002). Asthma attack. *Nursing2002, 32*(11), 104.

Moorhead, S., Johnson, M., & Maas, M. (2004). *Nursing Outcomes Classification (NOC)* (3rd ed.). St. Louis, MO: Mosby.

National Heart Lung and Blood Institute (NHLBI). (2001a). *Fact sheet on COPD*. [Online]. Available: www.nhlbi.nih.gov/health/public/other/copd_fact.htm

National Heart Lung and Blood Institute (NHLBI). (2001b). *What are chronic bronchitis and emphysema?* [Online]. Available: www.nhlbi.nih.gov/health/public/lung/other/copd/bronemph.htm

O'Hanlon-Nichols, T. (1998). Basic assessment series: The adult pulmonary system. *AJN, 98*(2), 39–45.

Owen, A. (1998). Respiratory assessment revisited. *Nursing98, 28*(4), 48–49.

Perkins, L., & Shortall, S. (2000). Ventilation without intubation. *RN, 63*(1), 34–38.

Phipps, W., Monahan, P., Sands, J., Marek, J., & Neighbors, M. (2003). *Medical–surgical nursing: Health and Illness Perspectives* (7th ed.). St. Louis, MO: Mosby.

Pope, B. (2002). Asthma. *Nursing2002, 32*(5), 44–45.

Pullen, R. (2003). Teaching bedside incentive spirometry. *Nursing2003, 33*(8), 24.

RNWeb. (1999). *Treating TB today*. [Online]. Available: www.RNWeb.com/ce/699/treating.html

RNWeb. (2000). *Trauma! Chest injuries*. [Online]. Available: www.RNWeb.com/ce/199/chestblt.html

Schultz, T. (2002). Community-acquired pneumonia. *Nursing2002, 32*(1), 46–49.

Shortall, S., & Perkins, L. (1999). Interpreting the ins and outs of pulmonary function tests. *Nursing99, 29*(12), 41–47.

Spratto, G., & Woods, A. (2004). *2004 PDR Nurses Drug Handbook*. Clifton Park, NY: Thomson Delmar Learning.

Tasota, F., & Davies, P. (2001). Diagnosing pulmonary embolism with spiral CT. *Nursing2001, 31*(5), 75.

Togger, D., & Brenner, P. (2001). Metered dose inhalers. *AJN, 101*(10), 26–32.

Ulrich, S. A., & Canale, S. W. (2001). *Medical–surgical nursing care planning guides* (5th ed.). Philadelphia: W. B. Saunders Company.

Wallace, C. (1998). Emergency! Acute pulmonary edema. *RN, 61*(1), 37–40.

Wisniewski, A. (2003). Chronic bronchitis and emphysema: Clearing the air. *Nursing2003, 33*(5), 46–49.

Woods, A. (2002). Pneumonia. *Nursing2002, 32*(11), 56–57.

Zorb, S. (2002). Transplantation offers hope. *RN, 65*(9), 66–68.

Resources

American Cancer Society (ACS), 1599 Clifton Road, NE, Atlanta, GA 30329, 800-ACS-2345, www.cancer.org

American Lung Association, 61 Broadway, 6th Floor, New York, NY 10006, 800-586-4872, www.lungusa.org

American Thoracic Society, 61 Broadway, New York, NY 10006-2747, 212-315-8619, www.thoracic.org

Centers for Disease Control and Prevention (CDC), Division of Tuberculosis Elimination, 1600 Clifton Road, Mailstop E-10, Atlanta, GA 30333, 404-639-8120, www.cdc.gov

Cystic Fibrosis Foundation, 6931 Arlington Road, Bethesda, MD 20814, 800-FIGHT-CF (344-4823), www.cff.org

International Association of Laryngectomees, 8900 Thornton Road, Box 99311, Stockton, CA 95209, 866-425-3678, www.larynxlink.com/ (Lost Chord and New Voice clubs are member clubs of this organization.)

CARDIOVASCULAR SYSTEM

LEARNING OBJECTIVES

Upon completion of this chapter, you should be able to:
- **Define key terms.**
- **Describe the anatomy and physiology of the cardiovascular system.**
- **Relate laboratory results to each disorder.**
- **Describe basic heart dysrhythmias.**
- **Explain the pathophysiology of each disorder.**
- **Describe nursing interventions in caring for clients with cardiovascular conditions.**

INTRODUCTION

Since 1900, heart disease has been the leading cause of death in the United States every year except in 1918 (American Heart Association [AHA], 2001b). It is estimated that 61.8 million Americans have one or more types of cardiovascular disease (CVD) (AHA, 2001b).

Even though these facts are astounding, the death rate for cardiovascular disease has been declining in the last 15 years because of public education in modifying and decreasing risk factors such as smoking, high-fat diets, and minimal exercise.

KEY TERMS

aneurysm
angina pectoris
annulus
arteriosclerosis
ascites
atherosclerosis
baseline level
bradycardia
cardiac cycle
cardiac output
cardiac tamponade
depolarization
dyspnea
dysrhythmia
embolus
heart sound
hemolysis
Homans' sign
hypertrophy
implantable cardioverter-defibrillator (ICD)
myocardial infarction
myocarditis

necrosis
orthopnea
palpitation
paroxysmal nocturnal dyspnea
pericardial friction rub
pericardiocentesis
pericarditis
peripheral resistance
phlebitis
phlebothrombosis
primary hypertension
repolarization
sclerotherapy
secondary hypertension
stasis dermatitis
stent
stroke volume
tachycardia
thrombectomy
thrombophlebitis
thrombosis
thrombus

KEY TERMS continued

transesophageal echocardiography (TEE)	vasodilate
	vein ligation
	vein stripping
varicosities	Virchow's triad
vasoconstrict	

This chapter reviews the anatomy and physiology of the cardiovascular system. Pathophysiology, medical management, and nursing interventions related to cardiovascular conditions are discussed with an emphasis on decreasing risk factors and improving lifestyles.

ANATOMY AND PHYSIOLOGY REVIEW

The cardiovascular system consists of the heart and its vasculature and the peripheral vascular system. The heart is located in the lower anterior area of the mediastinum with the apex near the diaphragm. In an average lifetime, the heart will pump 80 million gallons of blood.

The peripheral vascular system consists of arteries, arterioles, capillaries, venules, and veins. The arteries carry oxygenated blood away from the left side of the heart to the body tissues, and the veins carry deoxygenated blood back to the right side of the heart. The capillaries connect the arterioles to the venules. The venules and veins contain 60% to 70% of the body's total blood volume.

The cardiovascular system provides oxygen, nutrients, and hormones to the cells and removes carbon dioxide and waste products of cellular metabolism from body cells. Body temperature is maintained by the distribution of heat throughout the body produced by the metabolic activity of muscles and other body organs.

Structure of the Heart

The heart consists of three layers; endocardium, myocardium, and epicardium. The endocardium is the inner endothelial lining of heart chambers and valves. The myocardium is the thickest part of the heart and consists of cardiac muscle. The epicardium consists of a visceral layer and a parietal layer. The visceral epicardium attaches to the myocardium and is the outer layer of the heart. The parietal epicardium forms the inner layer of a double-walled sac called the pericardium that surrounds the heart.

The heart is a hollow muscular organ containing four chambers that fill and empty of blood with each contraction **(depolarization)** and recovery phase **(repolarization)** of the cardiac muscle. The upper chambers are the atria and the lower chambers are the ventricles (Figure 33-1). When the atria contract, blood is forced into the ventricles. Contraction of the right ventricle pumps blood into the pulmonary arteries and on to the lungs (pulmonary circulatory system). Contraction of the left ventricle pumps blood into the aorta and out to

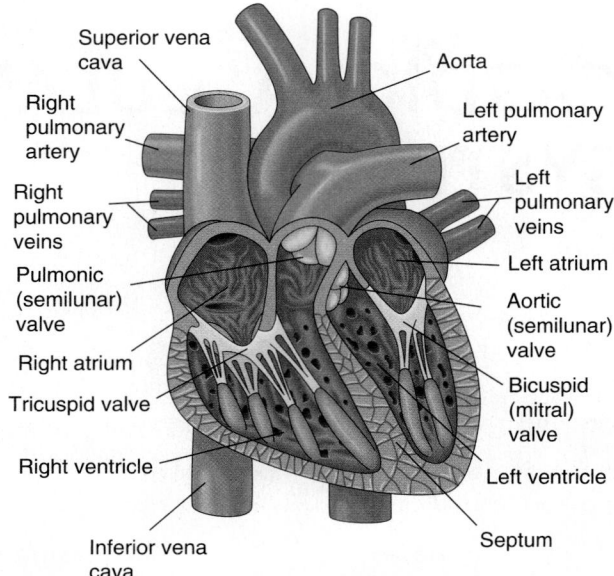

Figure 33-1 *Internal View of the Heart with Aorta, Vena Cava, and Pulmonary Arteries and Veins*

the entire body (systemic circulatory system). The myocardium of the left ventricle is thicker than the right ventricle because more force is needed to pump blood throughout the body.

There are four valves in the heart: tricuspid, bicuspid (mitral), pulmonic, and aortic. One end of fibrous cords called *chordae tendineae* is attached to the cusps of the tricuspid and mitral valves, and the other end is attached to papillary muscles on the walls of the ventricles. The chordae tendineae keep the valves from inverting when the ventricles contract, thus preventing blood from flowing back into the atrium. The pulmonic and aortic valves prevent blood from flowing back into the ventricles from the pulmonary artery and aorta during repolarization.

Circulation of Blood

Blood enters the heart through veins and leaves the heart through arteries. With the contraction of the right ventricle, blood is forced through the pulmonic valve into the pulmonary artery. Blood circulates through the pulmonary circulatory system where carbon dioxide is exchanged for oxygen in the lungs. The blood then returns to the left atrium through the pulmonary veins providing oxygenated blood for systemic circulation. When the left ventricle contracts, blood is forced through the aortic valve into the aorta, beginning systemic circulation. Blood is then distributed throughout the body and returns to the right atrium of the heart through the inferior and superior vena cava.

Each time the heart beats, the ventricle pumps 60 to 80 cc of blood. The volume of blood pumped by the ventricle with each contraction is called **stroke volume.** The volume of blood pumped by the left ventricle per minute is known as **cardiac output** and averages 5 liters for an adult at rest. Stroke volume multiplied by the pulse rate yields the cardiac output. If the heart has a strong ventricular contraction, more blood will be

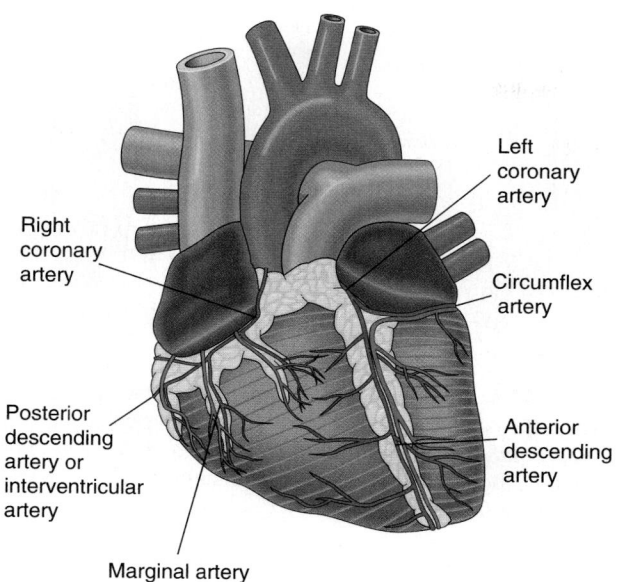

Figure 33-2 *Coronary Arteries that Supply Blood to the Heart Tissue*

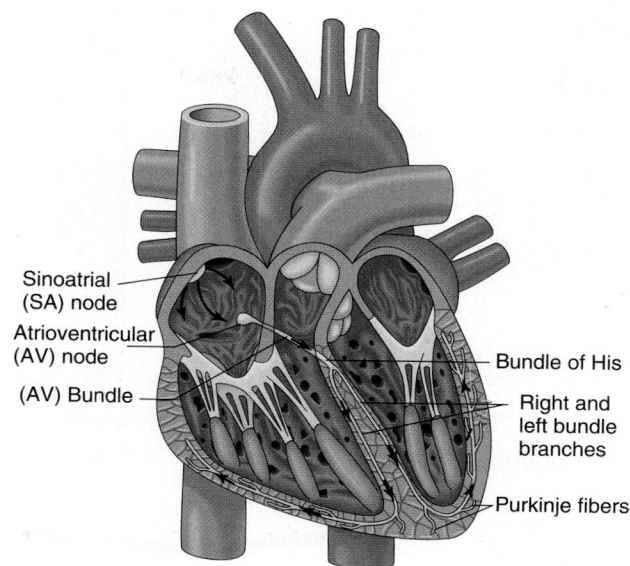

Figure 33-3 *Conduction System of the Heart*

pumped by the heart into the systemic circulatory system. Therefore, cardiac output has a direct effect on the volume of arterial blood being circulated.

Coronary Arteries

Coronary arteries supply nutrients and oxygen to the muscle tissue of the heart. The two coronary arteries, which branch off the aorta, are the right coronary artery and the left coronary artery (Figure 33-2). The right coronary artery divides into the posterior descending artery (interventricular artery) and the marginal artery and supplies blood to the anterior area of the right and left ventricles, the posterior area of the right ventricle, the AV node, and the posterior section of the interventricular septum. The left coronary artery divides into the anterior descending artery and the circumflex artery. The left anterior descending (LAD) artery supplies blood to the anterior section of the interventricular septum, anterior area of the left ventricle, and the lateral aspect of the left ventricle. The circumflex artery nourishes the left atrium and ventricle.

Conduction System

The specialized cardiac muscle cells are capable of conducting electrical impulses from one part of the heart to another. For the heart to beat regularly in a rhythmic sequence, electrical impulses follow a set pattern through the conduction system of the heart. The conduction system, consisting of the sinoatrial node (SA node), atrioventricular node (AV node), bundle of His, bundle branches, and Purkinje fibers, controls the heartbeat (Figure 33-3).

The SA node located in the superior aspect of the right atrium initiates electrical impulses that cause the heart to beat. It is called the pacemaker of the heart. Electrical impulses from the SA node pass through the muscle fibers of the right and left atria, causing the

atria to contract almost simultaneously. Atrial impulses are transmitted to the AV node located in the lower part of the right atrium. There is a short delay in the impulse at the AV node that allows the atria to complete their contraction and empty the blood into the ventricles. The electrical impulse is transmitted from the AV node into a group of specialized conduction fibers called the AV bundle or the bundle of His. Once the impulse leaves the AV node, it travels down the fibers of the bundle of His into the interventricular septum. The fibers separate into right and left bundle branches dividing into smaller and smaller branches, called Purkinje fibers. These terminate in the ventricular muscle, causing the ventricles to contract. When an impulse has completely gone through the conduction system of the heart and the ventricles have contracted, a **cardiac cycle** has been completed.

Heart Sounds

There are two normal **heart sounds** heard on auscultation, called S_1 and S_2. They yield a sound like "lubb-dubb." S_1, or the "lubb," is the sound of the mitral and tricuspid valves closing simultaneously, heard on the left fifth intercostal space. S_2, or the "dubb," is the simultaneous closing of the pulmonic and aortic valves, heard on the right second intercostal space. There is a slight pause after the "lubb-dubb" is heard. Clients with congestive heart failure may have a third sound known as S_3. This low-pitched sound occurs after the S_2 sound, or the "dubb," making the heart sound like the word "Kentucky" ("lubb-dubb-by"). The S_3 sound has also been described as a gallop.

Arterioles and Arteries

The arteries are thick-walled tubes consisting of three layers or tunics (Figure 33-4). The inner layer is called the *tunica intima* and consists of a single layer of smooth

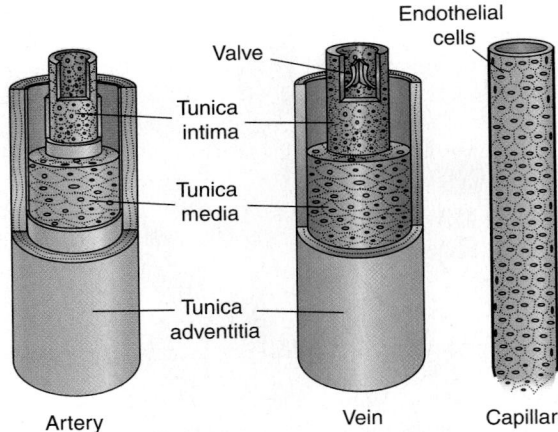

Figure 33-4 *Tunic Layers of Each Type of Vessel*

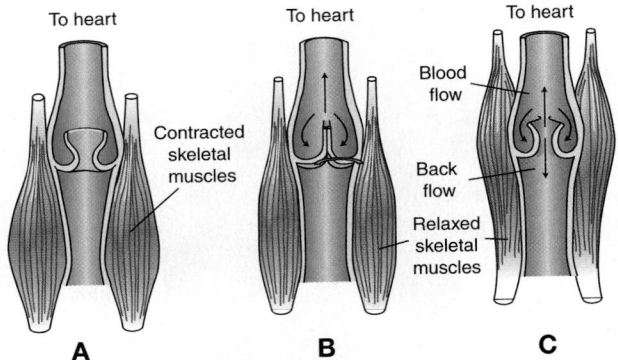

Figure 33-5 *Valves in the veins hold the blood at a certain level in the vein. **A,** Contracted skeletal muscles apply pressure to veins and assist with the circulation of blood. **B,** Valves prevent the backflow of blood. **C,** Incompetent valves allow a backflow of blood.*

endothelial cells. The middle layer is the *tunica media* and is composed of smooth muscle cells. The smooth muscle layer of the artery receives nerve stimulation from the sympathetic nervous system. The suppleness of the smooth muscle allows the vessel to **vasoconstrict** (decrease in diameter) and **vasodilate** (increase in diameter). The outer layer, the *tunica adventitia* or *tunica externa*, consists of a connective tissue sheath with some of its collagen fibers fusing with those of the surrounding tissue to hold the vessels in place. The elastic connective tissue allows the artery to expand and recoil with each contraction of the ventricle as an increased volume of blood is pumped through the vessel. The arteries have thick walls, so they can withstand the increased pressure from the left ventricle pumping blood through the body.

The arteries divide and branch into smaller vessels called *arterioles*. The same three layers are present in the walls, but as the arterioles approach the capillaries their walls become thinner. The outer layer is reduced to a very thin layer of connective tissue.

Capillaries

Capillaries are very tiny thin vessels that connect the smallest arterioles with the smallest venules. They have only one layer of endothelial cells whose cell membranes are the semipermeable membrane that allows oxygen, nutrients, carbon dioxide, and waste products to be exchanged between the tissues of the body and the blood.

Venules and Veins

Venules are small vessels that emerge from the capillaries and gradually increase in size to eventually form veins.

Veins have three layers or tunics like the arteries, but the middle layer of a vein is thinner with less smooth muscle and elastic tissue. This allows the walls of the veins to dilate more easily. Endothelial flaps, called *valves*, are on the inside lining of veins. The valves open and close with each contraction of the surrounding muscles. The valves assist the blood in returning to the heart. Blood is held by the valves at a certain level until skeletal muscle contractions move the blood higher in the vein (Figure 33-5).

HEALTH HISTORY

There are three goals when obtaining a health history from a client: (1) identify present and potential health problems, (2) identify possible familial and lifestyle risk factors, and (3) involve the client in planning long-term health care.

Ascertain the onset of the symptoms, the predisposing factors that cause the symptoms, and the client's treatment of the symptoms. Ask about the client's activity level or limitations in activity. Determine if appetite has increased or decreased. Evaluate the client's ability to sleep, the need for the trunk of the body to be supported with pillows when sleeping, or the need to sleep in a chair.

Major risk factors associated with cardiovascular diseases are age, gender, heredity (including race), smoking, dyslipidemia (presence of increased total serum cholesterol and low-density lipoprotein [LDL]), high blood pressure, physical inactivity, overweight, obesity, and diabetes mellitus. An individual's response to stress may be a contributing factor. Additional contributing factors for women may include menopause, use of birth control pills, and high triglyceride level (AHA, 2001d).

Advancing age, male gender, diabetes, heredity, and family history of chest pain or myocardial infarctions are risk factors that cannot be altered. Alterable risk factors are physical inactivity, smoking, contraceptive method, dyslipidemia, overweight, obesity, and triglyceride level. A change in diet may alter the last four factors.

There are two objectives in assisting the client toward a healthier lifestyle: (1) to educate the client about the risk factors; and (2) to determine what risk factors the client would like to modify. Once this is determined, assist the client to establish goals and determine actions to achieve the goals.

ASSESSMENT

Assessment includes clients' self-report of symptoms as well as physical findings and confirming lab data.

Subjective Data

The typical concerns expressed by a client with a cardiac disorder are chest pain, **dyspnea** (difficulty breathing), edema, fainting, palpitations, diaphoresis, and fatigue. When a client talks about having chest pain, ascertain the time of onset, situation occurring at the onset of pain, location and radiation of pain, severity of chest pain, duration, past episodes of chest pain, and methods used to alleviate pain. Women are more likely to experience atypical discomfort, shortness of breath, or fatigue (Nagle & Nee, 2002).

The client may be experiencing several types of dyspnea. Exertional dyspnea occurs when a person participates in moderate activity and becomes short of breath. This occurs in the early stages of heart failure and indicates that the heart is not able to meet the demands of the body during moderate activity. **Orthopnea** is when a client has difficulty breathing while lying down and must sit upright or stand to relieve the dyspnea. This occurs in a more advanced stage of heart failure. **Paroxysmal nocturnal dyspnea** is when a person suddenly awakens, is sweating, and is having difficulty breathing. This usually occurs 2 to 5 hours after the person has fallen asleep.

A client may have fainting spells for various physical and psychological reasons. Cardiac clients faint because of decreased cardiac output causing decreased blood flow to the brain.

A client may describe a "fluttering" or "pounding" sensation in the chest. This is known as **palpitations.** If these sensations occur during exercise, it is a sign that the heart is having to work harder to meet the demands of the body. Palpitations may also be caused by anxiety, ingestion of a large meal, lack of adequate rest, or a large intake of caffeine.

A cardiac client will usually experience fatigue increasing throughout the day because the heart is not able to keep up with the demands of the body. Frequent rest periods will help alleviate some of the fatigue.

The typical concerns expressed by the client with a peripheral vascular disorder are pain, paresthesia, and/or paralysis in the hands, thigh, calf, ankles, foot, abdomen, or lower back. The quality of the pain (aching, cramping, sharp, or throbbing) and any numbness or tingling should be noted.

Objective Data

In a head-to-toe assessment on a cardiac client, the skin, neck veins, respirations, heart sounds, abdomen, and extremities are carefully assessed. Observe the skin for cyanosis in the earlobes, lips, fingers, and feet. Assessment of skin turgor may indicate fluid volume. If the skin is dry and has poor turgor, the client may be dehydrated from diuretics. If a client has distended neck veins when the head of the bed is at a 45-degree angle or higher, there may be right-sided heart failure. Assess the quality of respirations for rate and ease of breathing, signs of dyspnea, and coughing. Heart sounds are assessed for the normal S$_1$ and S$_2$ sounds. If the typical lubb-dubb is heard, the valves are closing properly.

While listening to the heart, the radial pulse should be palpated to account for every heartbeat. If a heartbeat is heard through the stethoscope but not felt in the radial pulse, the heart has decreased cardiac output to the extremities. If the abdomen is distended, the client may have **ascites,** which is excess fluid in the abdomen. After the heart and lung sounds have been assessed, check the peripheral pulses. Pulses on both sides of the body should be checked at the same time to determine adequate bilateral perfusion. It is important to check pedal pulses in both feet to determine blood flow to each foot. Pulse amplitude can be described as absent, diminished, normal, increased, and bounding (Gehring, 2002).

If the hands and feet are cold or have mottling, this could indicate decreased cardiac output. Capillary refill should be less than 3 seconds in the fingers and toes.

Note if the feet, ankles, or legs are edematous (Figure 33-6). A client may gain 10 pounds before edema can be detected. Weigh cardiac clients with edema daily. The weight must be taken on the same scale, at the same time of day, with the client wearing the same amount of clothing.

Decreased circulation to an area can result in coolness in the ischemic area, pallor, paresthesia, and paralysis. Paresthesia (decreased sensation in an area) and paralysis result from a lack of oxygenated blood and nourishment to the nerves. Symptoms of paresthesia are numbness and tingling.

If an artery in the leg is occluded, the foot and/or leg becomes reddish in color when the leg is in a dependent position, and pale when elevated. As the ischemia progresses,

1+ = disappears rapidly

2+ = lasts 10 to 15 seconds

3+ = lasts more than 1 minute

4+ = lasts 2 to 5 minutes

Figure 33-6 *Edema Rating Scale: Press down for 5 seconds, then time how long indentation remains.*

TABLE 33-1	COMMON DIAGNOSTIC TESTS FOR CARDIOVASCULAR SYSTEM DISORDERS

Laboratory Tests

Arterial blood gasses (ABGs)

Complete blood count (CBC)

Platelet count

Hemoglobin (Hgb)

Hematocrit (Hct)

Electrolytes

Cardiac enzymes

    Serum aspartate aminotransferase (AST)

    Creatine kinase CPK (CK)

    Lactic dehydrogenase (LDH)

Erythrocyte sedimentation rate (ESR)

Glucose

Prothrombin time (PT)

Partial thromboplastin time (PTT)

International Normalized Ratio (INR)

Serum lipids (lipid profile)

    Cholesterol

    High-density lipoprotein (HDL)

    Low-density lipoprotein (LDL)

    Very low-density lipoprotein (VLDL)

    Triglycerides

Radiologic Tests

Chest x-ray

Cardiac positron emission tomography scan

Radionuclide angiography (multiplegated radioisotope scan, multigated aquisition scanning, MUGA)

Technetium pyrophosphate scanning

Thalium scan

Other Diagnostic Tests

Cardiac biopsy

Cardiac catheterization

Echocardiogram

Electrocardiogram (EKG)

Holter monitor

Magnetic resonance imaging (MRI)

Pericardiocentesis

Pulse oximetry

Stress test

Arterial plethysmography (pulse volume recorder)

Venous plethysmography (cuff pressure test)

the leg and/or foot skin becomes mottled, smooth, and shiny. If the veins are occluded, the foot and/or leg becomes cyanotic when in a dependent position, and has a normal coloration when elevated. The anterior area of the lower leg and ankle often have a brown pigmentation with venous involvement.

Clients with decreased circulation to the extremities have hardened and brittle nails. The leg will be cool if there is an arterial circulatory problem but warm if there is a venous circulatory problem. Skin ulcerations may be found around the ankles and toes.

Check the client's ankles for **stasis dermatitis,** an inflammation of the skin caused by decreased circulation. Waste products that normally are carried away by the circulatory system remain in the tissues, causing pruritus and irritation of the skin. At first, the ankle area is reddened and edematous, then vesicles form and start oozing. The skin becomes crusted, thickened, and brown.

A positive **Homans' sign** is present in some cases of deep vein thrombosis (DVT). To test for Homans' sign, dorsiflex the client's foot. If there is pain in the calf of the leg or behind the knee, the Homans' sign is positive and may indicate the presence of a venous clot.

COMMON DIAGNOSTIC TESTS

Commonly used diagnostic tests for clients with symptoms of cardiovascular system disorders are listed in Table 33-1. Beattie (2002) describes new biomarkers that may predict a client's risk of coronary artery disease (CAD). Elevated levels of lipoprotein (a), homocysteine, fibrinogen, and C-reactive protein have been found in clients with CAD.

CARDIAC RHYTHM/DYSRHYTHMIA

As a basis for understanding cardiac dysrhythmias, the normal sinus rhythm must first be understood.

NORMAL SINUS RHYTHM

The electrical conduction of the heart begins with the SA (refer to Figure 33-3) node located in the superior section of the right atrium. From the SA node, the electrical impulse spreads in wave fashion through the atria similar to the ripples from a pebble dropped in water. The firing of the SA node and the electrical impulse spreading across both atria yields a P wave on the EKG. The P wave represents the electrical activity causing the contraction of both atria.

After the atria contract, the electrical impulse reaches the AV node, where it pauses for approximately one-tenth of a second, allowing blood to enter both ventricles. The electrical impulse then starts down the AV bundle, which divides into right and left bundle branches in the interventricular septum. The electrical impulse continues from the right and the left bundle branches to the Purkinje fibers, which transmit the electrical impulse to the myocardial cells, causing contractions of the ventricles. On an EKG the QRS complex represents the electrical impulse as it travels through the AV node, AV bundle, bundle branches, Purkinje fibers, and myocardial cells, ending with the ventricles

Figure 33-7 *An EKG Strip Showing a Normal Sinus Rhythm with the P Wave, QRS Complex, and T Wave Identified*

Figure 33-8 *Sinus Bradycardia*

Figure 33-9 *Sinus Tachycardia*

contracting. The Q wave is not always present on the EKG strip.

The pause after the QRS complex is called the ST segment. This represents the period between the contraction and the beginning of the recovery or repolarization of the ventricular muscles. The T wave represents the repolarization of the ventricles.

After the repolarization of the ventricles, the entire cycle begins all over again at the SA node. In this way the P wave, QRS complex, and T waves are repeated with each heartbeat. Figure 33-7 shows an EKG strip of normal sinus rhythm.

DYSRHYTHMIAS

A **dysrhythmia** is an irregularity in the rate, rhythm, or conduction of the electrical system of the heart. Dysrhythmia can occur in the atria, ventricles, or any part of the conduction system. Specialized cells in the heart muscle have the ability to generate an electrical impulse. Under certain conditions these cells start sending impulses to other cells in the heart, causing irregular beats called *ectopic beats.* The most common causes of dysrhythmias are coronary artery disease (CAD), congestive heart failure (CHF), and myocardial infarction (MI). Other causes of dysrhythmias are electrolyte imbalances and drug toxicity.

Symptoms of a client experiencing a dysrhythmia can vary from asymptomatic to cardiac arrest. The client may experience fainting, seizures, fatigue, decreased energy level, exertional dyspnea, chest pain, and palpitations.

BRADYCARDIA

Sinus **bradycardia** is a heart rate of 60 beats per minute or less (Figure 33-8). Causes of sinus bradycardia are myocardial ischemia, electrolyte imbalances, vagal stimulation, heart block, drug toxicity, intracranial tumors, sleep, and vomiting. The treatment for bradycardia is the administration of atropine. Some clients with bradycardia may require a permanent pacemaker. Asymptomatic bradycardia related to physical fitness is usually not treated.

TACHYCARDIA

Tachycardia is a sinus rhythm with a heart rate ranging from 100 to 150 beats per minute (Figure 33-9).

Causes of tachycardia are exercise, emotional stress, fever, medications, pain, anemia, thyrotoxicosis, pericarditis, heart failure, excessive caffeine intake, and tobacco use. When the heart is beating at this rate, there is limited time for the ventricles to fill with blood, and less blood is pumped to the coronary arteries and throughout the body. The client may experience anginal pain. The treatment for sinus tachycardia depends on the cause.

ATRIAL DYSRHYTHMIAS

Atrial dysrhythmias occur from disturbances in the electrical conduction in the atria, resulting in premature beats or abnormal atrial rhythms. Common causes for atrial dysrhythmias are myocardial infarction, congestive heart failure, electrolyte imbalances, emotional stress, and drugs.

Premature Atrial Contractions

A premature atrial contraction (PAC) is an ectopic impulse not originating in the sinoatrial node, but rather in the atrial tissue. This causes an atrial depolarization to occur earlier in the cycle than expected, thus the term *premature atrial contraction.*

PACs often do not cause physical symptoms depending on how often they occur. Generally they are benign and occur several times a day in healthy individuals. If their occurrence causes an increase or decrease in the pulse rate, they should be evaluated. PACs can be a symptom of myocardial ischemia, developing congestive heart failure, digitalis toxicity, hypokalemia, or an inflammatory condition. Stress, caffeine, and smoking can also cause PACs. PACs can be the first indication that more serious atrial dysrhythmias could occur if not treated properly.

Atrial Tachycardia

Atrial tachycardia is an ectopic impulse that causes the atria to contract at the rate of 140 to 250 beats per minute. This is sometimes referred to as a *supraventricular dysrhythmia*, meaning the impulse causing the dysrhythmia is occurring above the ventricles. This dysrhythmia can occur as a continuous rhythm or as short, sudden eruptions that start and end spontaneously.

Atrial tachycardia occurs with hypokalemia, digitalis toxicity, and ischemia. Potassium supplements are given for hypokalemia. If an increased level of serum digitalis is the cause, digitalis is withheld until the level returns to normal. An artificial pacemaker may be surgically inserted to regulate the atrial tachycardia.

Paroxysmal Supraventricular Tachycardia

Paroxysmal supraventricular tachycardia (PSVT) was previously called paroxysmal atrial tachycardia (PAT). PSVT is a rapid atrial beat accompanied by an abnormal conduction in the AV node. The dysrhythmia occurs suddenly (paroxysmally) and is usually initiated by a premature beat. PSVT can stop as abruptly as it begins. It can be caused by myocarditis, caffeine, alcohol ingestion, smoking, and stress. PSVT may also be present in clients with coronary artery disease, mitral valve prolapse, and acute pericarditis.

Teach the client vagal stimulation procedures such as the Valsalva maneuver and carotid sinus pressure or massage, which usually stops the dysrhythmia.

Atrial Flutter

Atrial flutter, a rapid contraction of the atria, yields a heart rate of 250 to 350 beats per minute (Figure 33-10). The EKG displays a sawtooth wave pattern. The AV node attempts to block some of the atrial impulses, but usually the ventricles are also contracting at a rate of 300 beats per minute. This causes a decreased blood supply to the body because the atria and ventricles are unable to fill with blood when they are contracting at such a fast rate. This requires immediate intervention.

Atrial Fibrillation

Atrial fibrillation is an erratic electrical activity of the atria, resulting in a rate of 350 to 600 beats per minute (Figure 33-11). Atrial depolarization is so uncoordinated during the dysrhythmia that the atria quiver rather than contract. The AV node is bombarded with impulses and randomly transmits the impulses to the ventricles, causing varied irregular contractions of the ventricles with a ventricular rate of 100 to 180 beats per minute. The underlying cause is mitral valve disease or dysfunction, CAD, acute MI, hypertensive heart disease,

Figure 33-10 *Atrial Flutter*

LIFE CYCLE CONSIDERATIONS

Antidysrhythmic Medications

Doses may need to be reduced with the elderly, who may have hepatic or renal impairment.

Figure 33-11 *Atrial Fibrillation*

heart failure, cardiomyopathy, or hyperthyroidism. Because the atria are not contracting properly, blood pools in the atria, predisposing the person to thrombi forming on the walls of the atria. The clots can dislodge and travel to the brain, lungs, and other parts of the body. Most cardiac clients take an aspirin daily to prevent clot formation.

Once the underlying condition is treated, atrial fibrillation may stop. If the dysrhythmia cannot be controlled with medication, cardioversion may be necessary.

VENTRICULAR DYSRHYTHMIAS

Ventricular dysrhythmias originate in the ventricles. They are more life threatening than atrial dysrhythmias because the ventricles supply blood to the lungs and the body. These dysrhythmias must be treated promptly.

Premature Ventricular Contractions

Premature ventricular contractions (PVCs) arise from ectopic beats in the ventricles and are the most common ectopic beats (Figure 33-12). PVCs can easily be identified on the EKG because of the wide, bizarre QRS complexes. No P waves precede the QRS complex.

Coronary artery disease is the most common cause of PVCs. Other causes of PVCs are myocardial ischemia, CHF, electrolyte imbalances, digitalis toxicity, anxiety, exercise, hypoxia, caffeine, and excessive alcohol consumption.

The most common pharmacological treatment for PVCs is lidocaine hydrochloride (Xylocaine HCl). Initially, it is given as an IV bolus and then titrated according to the client's response. Administering oxygen may increase the oxygen perfusion to the myocardial tissue and decrease the frequency of premature beats.

Ventricular Tachycardia

Ventricular tachycardia (VT) is the occurrence of three or more consecutive PVCs. The ventricular rate may go as high as 140 to 240 beats per minute. Underlying condi-

Figure 33-12 *Premature Ventricular Contraction*

tions in which VT occurs are cardiomyopathy, hypoxemia, digitalis toxicity, and electrolyte imbalance.

During VT, the client will have a low blood pressure, weak or absent peripheral pulses, body weakness, and may become unconscious. The ventricle is beating so rapidly that it is unable to fill with blood or eject blood properly. This causes blood to back up in the pulmonary circulation, leading to pulmonary congestion.

It is important that VT be treated promptly because a ventricular tachycardia rhythm may lead into ventricular fibrillation, a life-threatening dysrhythmia. The client is given oxygen, and an intravenous line is inserted if one is not already in place. The drug of choice is procainamide hydrochloride (Procan SR) given intravenously because it slows the electrical conduction in the ventricle. Lidocaine hydrochloride (Xylocaine HCl) is given if PVCs occur with myocardial ischemia or infarct. If the VT is not controlled with medications, the client may be cardioverted if peripheral pulses are present, or defibrillated if peripheral pulses are absent.

Cardioversion

Cardioversion is the delivery of a synchronized electrical shock to change a dysrhythmia to a rhythm that will circulate more blood to the body tissues and improve oxygenation of the tissues. The electrical shock is set to be delivered on the R wave because a shock during ventricular depolarization may cause ventricular fibrillation. Cardioversion is done as an elective or emergency treatment. Electrodes are placed to the right of the sternum below the clavicle and at the apex of the heart. The electrodes are lubricated with a special gel or placed on normal saline pads. The electrical current delivered through the electrodes depolarizes the myocardium and allows the heart's pacemaker to reestablish a sinus rhythm.

The client is NPO for 8 hours before an elective cardioversion. Diuretics and digitalis preparations are withheld 24 to 72 hours before the cardioversion because they make myocardium cells less responsive to conversion to a normal rhythm or may cause a serious dysrhythmia after the cardioversion. Anticoagulants and oral antiarrhythmics are still given before cardioversion. Anticoagulants are given so a thrombus is not released into the system. A sedative such as diazepam (Valium) or midazolam hydrochloride (Versed) is given intravenously before the procedure. Monitor the client's vital signs and EKG strip closely for the first hour afterward and then as ordered by the physician.

Defibrillation

Defibrillation is the delivery of an unsynchronized, high-energy electrical shock during an emergency situation, such as a cardiac arrest or pulseless VT, to convert the life-threatening dysrhythmia or arrhythmia to a sinus rhythm. Defibrillation is done by a physician or a nurse who has had special education to handle emergency situations. Paddles are lubricated with a special gel, or normal saline pads are applied to the skin where the paddles will be placed. The paddles are placed to the right of the sternum below the clavicle and at the apex of the heart. When the electrical shock is delivered to the client, everyone stands clear of the bed to prevent them from also receiving the electrical shock. More than one electrical shock may be delivered in an attempt to convert the rhythm.

If conservative measures do not control the VT and the client has periodic episodes of VT, an **implantable cardioverter-defibrillator (ICD)** is implanted in the client (Figure 33-13). This device senses the dysrhythmia and automatically sends an electrical shock directly to the heart to defibrillate it.

One type of ICD has leads that are attached to the heart muscle. The pulse generator that initiates the shock is placed in a pocket of subcutaneous tissue in the abdominal wall and is powered by lithium batteries. Another type of ICD has an endocardial lead that is guided through a vein into the right side of the heart. The pulse generator may be placed under the skin below the collarbone or in the abdomen.

The ICD detects VT and ventricular fibrillation (VF) through the leads attached to the heart muscle. Once VT or VF is detected, an electrical shock is sent from the pulse generator. The ICD is capable of delivering three more shocks to the heart muscle if the heart does not return to normal sinus rhythm (NSR). Usually, clients are converted to NSR with the first shock. Complications following the insertion of an ICD are atelectasis, pneumonia, pneumothorax, thrombus, and a seroma at the generator site. According to Shaffer (2002), anger and depression are common, expected side effects.

Ventricular Fibrillation

The most common cause for VF is CAD. VF is a disorganized, chaotic quivering of the ventricles. The ventricles are unable to contract, and no blood is ejected into the circulatory system. The EKG reading is a series of jagged, unidentifiable waves (Figure 33-14). The client will not have a pulse, blood pressure, or respirations. This dysrhythmia is serious. Aggressive measures must be taken to initiate CPR and defibrillate the client immediately.

Ventricular Asystole — Flat line

Ventricular asystole is represented only by a P wave or by a straight line on the EKG (Figure 33-15). The ventricles are not contracting, and the client is in cardiac arrest. The client loses consciousness and has no pulse or respirations. Aggressive treatment should be initiated within 1 minute to prevent chemical changes within the body that jeopardize recovery. CPR is started, and the client is defibrillated. Atropine sulfate and epinephrine are given intravenously.

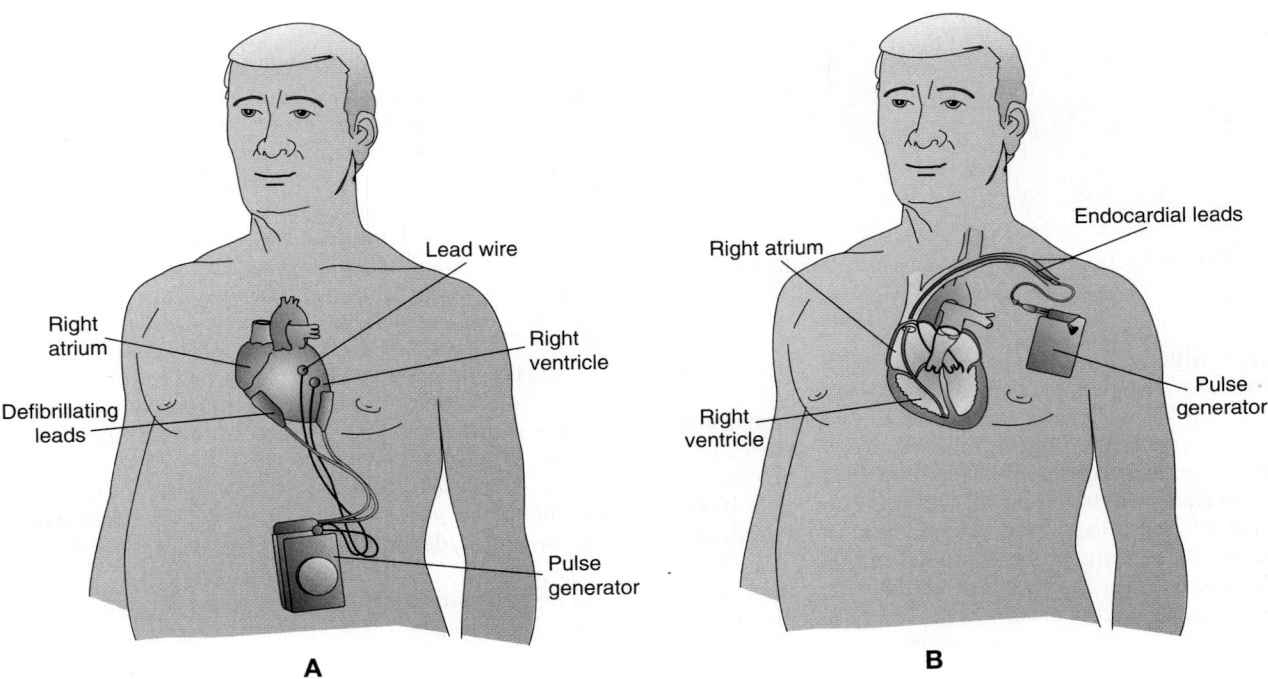

Figure 33-13 *Two Different Types of Implantable Cardioverter-Defibrillators (ICD):* **A,** *Pulse generator implanted in the subcutaneous tissue of the abdomen with lead wires and defibrillating leads going to the heart;* **B,** *Pulse generator implanted below the collarbone with endocardial leads positioned in the heart through a vein.*

Figure 33-14 *Ventricular Fibrillation*

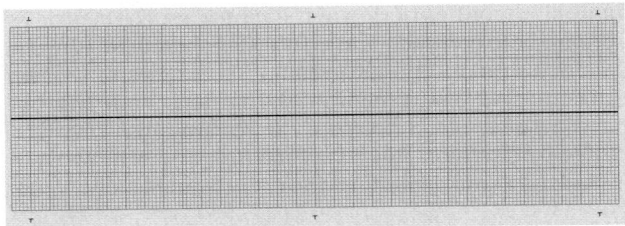

Figure 33-15 *Asystole*

ATRIOVENTRICULAR BLOCKS

In atrioventricular blocks, the electrical conduction is interrupted to some degree between the atria and ventricles at the AV node. The extent of interruption is classified as first degree, second degree, or third degree.

First-Degree AV Block

In first-degree block, the impulse is delayed in traveling through the AV node. The impulse eventually reaches the ventricles but is delayed. There are no physical symptoms or treatment for first-degree block.

Second-Degree AV Block

In second-degree block, some of the impulses pass through the AV node to the ventricles and others are blocked. Symptoms include irregular pulse, vertigo, and weakness. A temporary pacemaker may be inserted until the conduction pattern is stabilized. If the dysrhythmia persists, a permanent pacemaker may be implanted.

When the impulse is blocked, the EKG reveals an extended PR interval that is not followed by a QRS complex.

Third-Degree AV Block

Third-degree heart block is when no impulses are able to pass from the atria through the AV node to the ventricles. The atria and ventricles beat independently of each other. The causes of third-degree block are myocardial ischemia, drug toxicity, and electrolyte imbalances. Atropine sulfate may be given to improve conduction through the AV node. A permanent pacemaker is usually required to control the dysrhythmia.

 Safety: Pacemaker
The client should wear a medical identification tag indicating the presence of a pacemaker.

Pacemaker

- High-tension wires, high-voltage electrical generators, or MRIs may cause pacemaker malfunction.
- Avoid contact sports.
- Pacemakers may activate airport security alarms.

Medical–Surgical Management

Pharmacological

Dysrhythmias originating in the atria are treated with a digitalis preparation while dysrhythmias originating in the ventricles are treated with lidocaine hydrochloride (Xylocaine HCl) or other antiarrhythmic agents.

Diet

The client is usually placed on a low-fat, low-cholesterol diet. Caffeine consumption is restricted.

Nursing Management

Monitor vital signs including apical pulse. Provide rest periods throughout the day. Explain all procedures and treatments. Encourage client to verbalize concerns about condition and potential complications. Teach relaxation methods.

NURSING PROCESS

Assessment

Subjective Data

Inquire if the client has experienced palpitations, lightheadedness, nausea, dyspnea, anxiety, fatigue, or chest discomfort.

Objective Data

If a client is experiencing dysrhythmias, check the heart rate, blood pressure, and respirations. While listening to the apical pulse and respirations, note abnormal heart sounds and monitor breath sounds for crackles. Crackles indicate the lungs are filling with fluid. Observe the skin for pallor and cyanosis. Urine output may decrease.

Nursing diagnoses for a client with dysrhythmias may include the following:

Nursing Diagnoses	Planning/Goals	Nursing Interventions
Decreased Cardiac Output related to inadequate electrical conduction	The client will have increased cardiac output.	Apply electrodes for telemetry monitoring. Balance activity with rest periods, and monitor vital signs during activity and at rest. Listen to the apical pulse, especially noting rate and rhythm. Elevate the extremities so they are not in a dependent position.
Anxiety related to fear of potential diagnosis, treatment regimen, and death	The client will relate fears of potential cardiac problems.	Care for the client in a calm, confident, and efficient manner. Remain with the client and explain procedures and treatments. Encourage client input regarding the care. Encourage the client to verbalize concerns about the dysrhythmia and potential future complications. Teach the client relaxation activities.
Deficient Knowledge related to electrical conduction of the heart and treatment methods	The client will describe electrical disorder and treatment methods.	Explain medication administration times, action, side effects, and symptoms that need reporting. Provide written instructions to the client and family. Explain symptoms of dysrhythmias such as fatigue, edema, palpitations, lightheadedness, nausea, dyspnea, and anxiety. If a pacemaker is needed, explain to client and family the purpose, insertion procedures, and home care.

Evaluation Each goal must be evaluated to determine how it has been met by the client.

INFLAMMATORY DISORDERS

Inflammatory disorders include rheumatic heart disease, infective endocarditis, myocarditis, pericarditis, and valvular heart disease.

RHEUMATIC HEART DISEASE

Rheumatic heart disease is a complication of rheumatic fever and is also linked to group A streptococcus following an upper respiratory infection. Rheumatic fever is a systemic inflammatory disease that occurs 2 to 3 weeks after an inadequately treated pharyngitis caused by the group A *beta-hemolytic streptococcus*. Symptoms of rheumatic fever are a mild fever, polyarthritis, carditis, chorea, and a rash. The endocardium, myocardium, and epicardium can become inflamed, with the most damage occurring to the mitral valve. The mitral valve becomes incompetent because of thickening and stenosis of the valve leaflets. Mitral prolapse (valve leaflets fall into the left atrium during systole) may result.

A person who had rheumatic fever is more likely to have it again. It is treated with intravenous antibiotics, anti-inflammatory agents, corticosteroids, and strict bed rest. The main goal is to treat the inflammation, prevent cardiac complications, and prevent the recurrence of the disease. These clients are placed on prophylactic antibiotic therapy before dental procedures or invasive surgery. Antibiotic therapy has reduced the mortality from 15,000 in 1950 to 3,676 in 1999 (AHA, 2001c).

INFECTIVE ENDOCARDITIS

Infective endocarditis is an inflammation or infection of the inside lining of the heart, particularly the heart valves. The etiology of inflammatory endocarditis is a collagen-vascular disease or rheumatic fever. Infective endocarditis is caused by bacteria, fungi, or virus. As the microorganisms invade the valves, they form fibrinous substances called *vegetations*. Vegetations cause scar tissue on the valves so they become hard and brittle, do not close properly, and blood leaks back to the chamber from which it was pumped. The valve is said to be insufficient. Sometimes the vegetations cause the valve flaps to grow together, resulting in a narrowing of the opening. This is called a *valvular stenosis*. The mitral valve is more frequently affected than any other. When the mitral valve is affected, it is termed *mitral insufficiency* or *mitral stenosis*.

Historically, rheumatic fever was the common cause of endocarditis. More recently, IV drug users, immunosuppressed clients, and clients with valvular heart disease are at risk for endocarditis. Goldrick (2003) reports that endocarditis is now associated with body piercing.

There are two forms of endocarditis: acute and subacute. Symptoms of acute endocarditis are tachycardia, pallor, diaphoresis, and symptoms of a systemic infection, such as temperature of 103°F and shaking chills. Clients with subacute endocarditis have low-grade fever, malaise, weight loss, and anemia. Clients with both types may have murmurs and symptoms of congestive heart failure, such as dyspnea, peripheral edema, and pulmonary congestion.

Endocarditis is diagnosed by the client's history and symptoms. **Transesophageal echocardiography (TEE)** can confirm the diagnosis by ultrasonic imaging of the cardiac structures through the esophagus. The erythrocyte sedimentation rate (ESR) and WBC are elevated. A blood culture and sensitivity is done to determine the causative organism and the most effective antibiotic.

Medical–Surgical Management

Surgical

Surgical repair or replacement of a valve is done in severe cases.

Pharmacological

Clients are treated with antimicrobial drugs (endocarditis) and intravenous antibiotics. The antibiotics are usually continued for 2 to 6 weeks. The most commonly used antibiotics are penicillin V potassium (V-Cillin K), vancomycin hydrochloride (Vancocin), and gentamicin sulfate (Garamycin).

Diet

Provide the client with a well-balanced nutritious diet with between-meal snacks.

Activity

The client is on bed rest to decrease the workload of the heart. Provide a calm, quiet environment.

Health Promotion

Clients who have previously had endocarditis or have a mitral valve prolapse are more prone to develop endocarditis. They should take antibiotics prophylactically before having dental work and genitourinary or gastrointestinal invasive procedures. Amoxicillin trihydrate (Amoxil) 1 hour before the procedure and again after the procedure is the usual order.

Nursing Management

Administer oxygen as needed, and measure blood pressure and pulse before and after activity to monitor toleration. Note apical pulse rate and rhythm and assess breath sounds for adventitious sounds. Balance activity with rest periods. Monitor BUN and creatinine levels if a client is on vancomycin hydrochloride (Vancocin) or gentamicin sulfate (Garamycin) because both of these drugs are nephrotoxic.

MYOCARDITIS

Myocarditis is an inflammation of the myocardium of the heart. Lymphocytes and leukocytes invade the muscle fibers of the heart, causing the chambers to enlarge and the muscle to weaken. This can lead to congestive heart failure. Myocarditis is caused by bacteria, viruses, fungi, or parasites. It can also be an autoimmune reaction such as with rheumatic fever or lupus erythematosus. Usually the cause is a virus. Recently, myocarditis has been more prevalent in clients with AIDS.

Acute myocarditis presents with flulike symptoms of fever, pharyngitis, myalgias, and gastrointestinal complications. The client will also have chest pain and should be monitored for signs of congestive heart failure. A **pericardial friction rub** is often heard if the pericardium becomes involved. The friction rub is a "squeaky" sound heard through the stethoscope when the two inflamed pericardial surfaces rub together with the contraction of the heart.

Myocarditis diagnostic symptoms are nonspecific. They include elevated ESR and elevated LDH, CK, and SGOT levels. The diagnosis of myocarditis can be confirmed with an endomyocardial biopsy.

Medical–Surgical Management
Pharmacological

Digitalis preparations are given to try to prevent congestive heart failure. Broad-spectrum antibiotics are also given to treat the infection. Anti-inflammatory agents may be given to reduce the inflammation. Oxygen is administered as needed.

Activity

The client is placed on bed rest to decrease the workload of the heart.

Nursing Management

Monitor the client for symptoms of congestive heart failure or pericarditis. Place the client in a semi-Fowler's position. Provide a quiet environment and frequent rest periods. Apply a pulse oximeter to monitor oxygen saturation.

PERICARDITIS

When the membranous sac surrounding the heart becomes inflamed, the condition is called **pericarditis.** Causative organisms are viral, bacterial, fungal, or parasitic. Inflammation can also occur from rheumatic or collagen-vascular conditions such as systemic lupus erythematosus. The most common cause of pericarditis is idiopathic, meaning no known cause. Symptoms of pericarditis are severe precordial pain (pain on the anterior surface of the chest over the heart) and a pericardial friction rub. The pain may radiate to the neck, back, or abdomen and become worse when the client coughs or lies on the left side. If the client sits erect and leans forward, the pain is relieved. Pericardial effusion (excess fluid in pericardial space) may develop. **Cardiac tamponade** will result if the fluid rapidly increases and hinders the functioning of the ventricle. The S_1 and S_2 sounds are often muffled and hard to hear because of fluid accumulation.

With inflammation, scar tissue develops in the pericardial sac. Heart movement is limited by the scar tissue and cardiac failure results.

Medical–Surgical Management
Medical

A **pericardiocentesis** is done to aspirate the excess fluid from the pericardial sac. A needle is inserted through the chest wall into the pericardial space.

Surgical

If fibrotic scar tissue in the pericardium hinders heart performance, a pericardiectomy or pericardial window may be done. Pericardiectomy is removal of the pericardium. When a pericardial window is done, a section of the parietal pericardium is cut and tacked back onto itself, allowing fluid to escape from the pericardial sac.

Pharmacological

Clients are given antipyretics, analgesics, and anti-inflammatory agents. The infection is combated with antibiotics. A digitalis preparation and diuretic may also be given to improve the pumping action of the heart and decrease fluid retention.

Nursing Management

Assess the client's apical pulse and blood pressure and monitor the EKG for dysrhythmias. Assess for signs of cardiac tamponade such as decreased pulse and blood pressure, muffled heart sounds, increased respirations, restlessness, and oliguria. Administer oxygen as needed, and assist the client to a position of comfort. Administer analgesics, antibiotics, and anti-inflammatory agents as ordered and monitor the client's responses. Encourage the client to verbalize concerns and fears.

VALVULAR HEART DISEASES

Valvular heart disease occurs when the valves do not open and close properly. When the valve does not close completely, blood leaks back into the chamber from which it was pumped. This is called regurgitation (Figure 33-16). The client with valvular heart disease often has a history of rheumatic fever.

STENOSIS AND INSUFFICIENCY

The definitions, symptoms, diagnostic findings, medical–surgical management, and nursing interventions for mitral and aortic valve conditions are covered in Table 33-2.

MITRAL VALVE PROLAPSE

Mitral insufficiency can lead to mitral valve prolapse in which the valve leaflets, chordae tendineae, and papillary muscle become damaged. The valve leaflets flip back into the left atrium when the left ventricle contracts. This condition affects more women than men. Often the client remains asymptomatic. The symptoms that a client may experience depend on how seriously the mitral valve is affected. Sometimes clients experience palpitations and fatigue caused by decreased cardiac output. They also may experience angina, dizziness, and syncope. Some clients have panic attacks. Often a click or murmur can be heard.

Scar tissue thickens valve, preventing
it from opening the whole way

Scar tissue causes the valve to harden and pull
apart, preventing it from closing completely
and allowing blood to leak backwards

Figure 33-16 A, *Normal Valve;* **B,** *Stenosed Valve;* **C,** *Insufficient Valve*

Figure 33-17 *Types of Artificial Valves:* **A,** *St. Jude Medical Mechanical Heart Valve (St. Jude Medical is a registered trademark of St. Jude Medical, Inc.);* **B,** *Starr-Edwards Silastic Ball Valve, Model 1260 Aortic;* **C,** *Carpentier-Edwards Bioprosthesis Model 2625 Aortic (***A** *courtesy of St. Jude Medical, Inc. All rights reserved;* **B** *and* **C** *courtesy of Edwards Lifesciences.)*

Medical–Surgical Management

Medical

Clients with valvular heart disease are to take antibiotics prophylactically before any dental procedures and genitourinary or gastrointestinal invasive procedures.

Surgical

When the activities of a client with valvular heart disease become curtailed because of decreased cardiac output and the symptoms can no longer be controlled by medical means, surgery may be done. The type of surgery performed will depend on the client's overall condition and on the involved valve.

For the mitral valve, surgery alleviates the symptoms, but it does not cure the condition. Surgeries frequently have to be repeated. A commissurotomy is done for mitral stenosis, which surgically separates the valve leaflets. For mitral regurgitation or insufficiency, a valvuloplasty is becoming the treatment of choice. A percutaneous mitral valvuloplasty is a repair of perforated cusps or torn chordae tendineae. The risk of a thrombus is less with valvuloplasty than with grafts or prosthetic valves. An annuloplasty, a repair of an **annu-**

lus or valvular ring, can also be done. The annulus is tightened with a purse-string suture or an annular ring. The mitral valve is replaced when other repair measures are not feasible.

The aortic valve is not repaired, only replaced, if the symptoms cannot be controlled by medical means.

There are two types of replacement valves: mechanical and biological. The mechanical valves are the caged-ball valve or the tilting-disk valve (Figure 33-17). There is a higher risk of a thromboembolism with a caged-ball valve. Clients remain on anticoagulant therapy with both types of valves. The biological valves come from calves,

TABLE 33-2 MITRAL AND AORTIC VALVE STENOSIS AND INSUFFICIENCY

VALVE CONDITION	DEFINITION	SYMPTOMS	DIAGNOSTIC FINDINGS	MEDICAL–SURGICAL MANAGEMENT	NURSING INTERVENTIONS
Mitral stenosis	The diseased valve becomes narrowed and the leaflets thickened, preventing blood from freely flowing from the left atrium into the left ventricle.	Gradual onset of symptoms: exertional dyspnea, fatigue, orthopnea, paroxysmal nocturnal dyspnea, murmur. **Later symptoms:** peripheral edema, atrial fibrillation, jugular venous distention, hepatomegaly, abdominal distention, hypotension, thrombus from blood pooling in the left atrium.	**Chest x-ray:** hypertrophy and enlargement of left atrium and right ventricle. **EKG:** atrial fibrillation. **Echocardiogram:** fusion of valve leaflets, enlarged left atrium, decreased blood flow through valve.	**Medical management:** diuretics, digitalis, anticoagulants, antidysrhythmics, prophylactic antibiotics for invasive procedures, low-sodium diet, semi-Fowler's position, activity restrictions as needed. **Surgical management:** commissurotomy, percutaneous balloon mitral valvuloplasty, mitral valve replacement	Encourage rest periods, administer oxygen, elevate head of bed, reposition frequently to decrease pressure points, elevate legs, low-sodium diet, monitor for signs of right and left-sided heart failure, teach stress reduction techniques, daily weight.
Mitral insufficiency	The valve leaflets become hard and do not close completely. Blood backs up in both the left atria and ventricle, causing both chambers to hypertrophy.	Gradual onset of symptoms: exertional dyspnea, palpitations, fatigue, atrial fibrillation, loud murmur and gallop.	**Chest x-ray:** hypertrophy and enlargement of left atrium and left ventricle. **EKG:** atrial fibrillation.	**Medical management:** same as mitral stenosis. **Surgical management:** valvuloplasty, mitral valve replacement.	Same as mitral stenosis, teach exercise modification.
Aortic stenosis	The valve cusps become hard and calcify due to rheumatic fever, syphilis, a congenital anomaly, or the aging process.	Syncope, exertional dyspnea, arrhythmias, angina, murmur, and gallop; sudden death may occur. **Later symptoms as the disease progresses:** paroxysmal atrial tachycardia, orthopnea.	**Chest x-ray:** enlargement of left ventricle, calcification of aortic valve. **EKG:** hypertrophy of left ventricle inverted T wave echocardiogram fusion of valve leaflets, regurgitation.	**Medical management:** same as mitral stenosis. **Surgical management:** percutaneous balloon aortic valvuloplasty, aortic valve replacement.	Same as mitral stenosis.
Aortic insufficiency	The valve cusps become so hardened they do not close completely. The blood no longer flows through the aorta but backs up into the left ventricle.	Palpitations, chest pain, exertional dyspnea, nocturnal angina, dizziness, fatigue, decreased activity, intolerance, paroxysmal nocturnal dyspnea, visible pulsation of the neck veins, murmur, lung congestion.	**Chest x-ray:** hypertrophy and enlargement of left ventricle.	**Medical management:** same as mitral stenosis. **Surgical management:** aortic valve replacement.	Same as mitral stenosis, teach exercise modification.

pigs, or humans. The disadvantage of the biological valves is tissue degeneration and calcification of the valve.

Nursing Management

Assess for dyspnea, fatigue, palpitations, lightheadedness, cough, and numbness and tingling in the extremities. Provide rest periods during the day. Encourage smokers to stop. Refer client and family to dietitian for information on low-sodium diets. Encourage client's input regarding care decisions.

NURSING PROCESS

Assessment

Subjective Data

Review past medical history for conditions such as rheumatic fever or streptococcal infections. Document if the client has experienced any dyspnea, palpitations, fatigue, cough, lightheadedness, or numbness and tingling in the extremities.

Objective Data

Take the vital signs and listen to the apical pulse for rate, rhythm, murmurs, and S_3 sound. Auscultate breath sounds for adventitious sounds. Note edema, jugular distention, cyanosis, and equality of peripheral pulses. Test for Homans' sign because dysrhythmias may produce clots.

Nursing diagnoses for a client with cardiac valvular disorders may include the following:

Nursing Diagnoses	Planning/Goals	Nursing Interventions
Decreased **C**ardiac Output related to structural changes in valves	The client will have increased cardiac output.	Administer oxygen as needed.
		Help the client balance activities with rest periods. The pulse should return to the baseline within 10 minutes of activity; if not, activity has been excessive.
		Discourage smoking and refer clients to support groups to assist them to stop smoking.
Excess **F**luid Volume related to decreased cardiac output	The client will have a decrease in edema.	Administer diuretics as needed.
		Support extremities so they are not in a dependent position.
		Encourage the client to maintain a low-sodium diet.
Anxiety related to threat to or change in health status	The client will list ways to cope with stressors.	Calmly explain the procedures before doing them.
		Encourage the client's input to decisions regarding care.
		Assist the client and the client's family in identifying ways to cope with stressors.
		Teach relaxation techniques.
Deficient **K**nowledge related to disease process and treatment	The client will relate the disease process and needed self-care management.	Explain the valvular disease process, medication actions, dosage times, and medication side effects to report.
		Refer the client and family members to the dietitian for low-sodium diet instructions.
		Encourage the client to begin an appropriate exercise program.

Evaluation Each goal must be evaluated to determine how it has been met by the client.

OCCLUSIVE DISORDERS

Occlusive disorders include arteriosclerosis, angina pectoris, and myocardial infarction.

ARTERIOSCLEROSIS

Arteriosclerosis is a narrowing and hardening of arteries. A buildup of lipids, collagen, and smooth muscle cells narrows the lumen of the vessel. Decreased blood flow through the vessel causes decreased perfusion to cells beyond the narrowed or hardened area.

There are three types of arteriosclerosis: atherosclerosis, calcific sclerosis, and arteriolar sclerosis. **Atherosclerosis** is fatty deposits on the inner lining of vessel walls. The fat deposit is called *plaque.* In calcific sclerosis, calcium deposits are on the middle layer of the wall of the arteries. Hypertension causes a thickening of the arterioles and is called *arteriolar sclerosis.* With these conditions, vessels lose their elasticity, resulting in various conditions, such as arteriosclerotic heart disease, angina, myocardial infarction, stroke, and peripheral vascular disease.

ANGINA PECTORIS

When coronary arteries lose elasticity or become narrow as a result of plaque collection, the heart muscle receives less blood and oxygen. Physical exertion, emotional stress, smoking, exposure to extreme cold, heavy meals, or an arterial spasm may cause a temporary inadequate blood and oxygen supply to the heart. Myocardial ischemia and angina pectoris result. Myocardial ischemia is a temporary inadequate blood and oxygen supply to the myocardial tissues. When this temporary condition occurs, the person experiences chest pain or **angina pectoris.**

At first, the person may experience a squeezing pain under the sternum, which radiates to the left shoulder. For some, the pain may radiate to the right shoulder, jaw, or ear. The discomfort may vary from mild discomfort to immobilizing pain. Anginal attacks usually increase in frequency and severity over time. The severity of the condition depends on the amount of collateral circulation that has developed.

Collateral circulation develops as larger vessels gradually narrow or harden. Blood that normally passes through the larger vessels is shunted into surrounding smaller vessels. These vessels enlarge in an attempt to supply blood to the affected area. Collateral circulation increases the blood supply to tissues with an inadequate blood supply. There is a high incidence of angina pectoris in clients with hypertension and diabetes mellitus.

Many people experiencing ischemic attacks do not experience angina. This is called silent myocardial infarct or ischemia. Symptoms are chest pressure or heaviness, restlessness, shortness of breath with increased respiratory rate, a sensation of epigastric fullness with noisy belching, numbness or tingling in both arms or shoulders, physical or mental fatigue, and dizziness. The person may also experience a change in sleep patterns and mental alertness. The person may state that he or she "feels funny."

Two other types of angina are unstable angina and Prinzmetal's angina. Unstable angina occurs at rest or with minimal exertion and is not relieved with nitroglycerin. This client is more susceptible to myocardial infarction and sudden death. Prinzmetal's angina is caused by a coronary artery spasm and occurs at rest.

The diagnosis of angina is made after reviewing the client's history, lifestyle, laboratory tests, and stress test.

Cholesterol, low-density lipoprotein (LDL), and high-density lipoprotein (HDL) levels are evaluated. Angina pectoris can be diagnosed by a stress test, thallium scan, or a coronary arteriogram.

Medical–Surgical Management

Medical

Treatment for angina includes measures to increase the blood supply to the affected area. This can be accomplished by rest and vasodilation medications.

Silent ischemia is treated in the same way symptomatic ischemia is treated. The client needs to be educated about cardiac risk factors, the importance of following the prescribed medical regimen, and maintaining regular physical checkups.

Surgical

A percutaneous transluminal coronary angioplasty (PTCA) may be done if only one coronary artery is involved and if the atherosclerotic material is small and has not hardened. When a PTCA is done, atherosclerotic matter is pressed against the walls of the coronary vessels to improve circulation to myocardial tissue supplied by that coronary artery (Figure 33-18). A guidewire is inserted to the stenosed area, and a special balloon-tipped catheter is placed in the narrowed sclerotic area. When the balloon is inflated, the atherosclerotic material is pressed against the wall of the vessel. The vessel, now open, allows more blood to flow to the myocardial tissue. During this procedure, a piece of the atherosclerotic material may break off and occlude the vessel. If

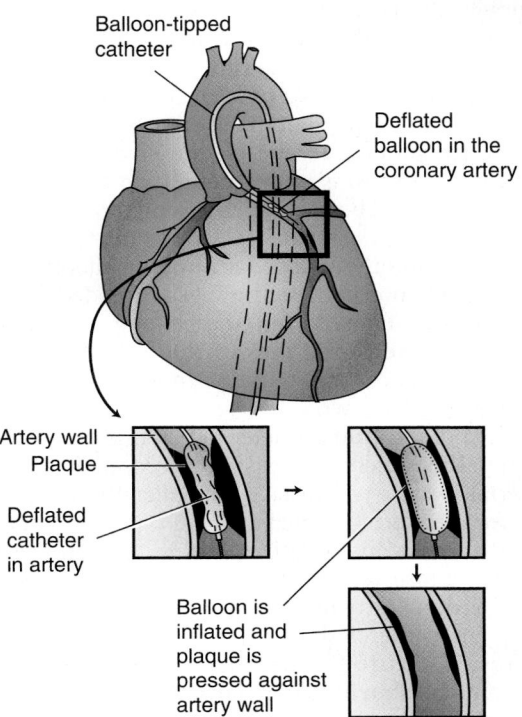

Figure 33-18 *Demonstration of the Function of a Balloon-Tipped Catheter During a PTCA Procedure*

Figure 33-19 *Placement of a Stent in a Coronary Artery:* **A,** *Palmaz-Schatz Stent;* **B,** *Gianturco-Roubin Ex-Stent*

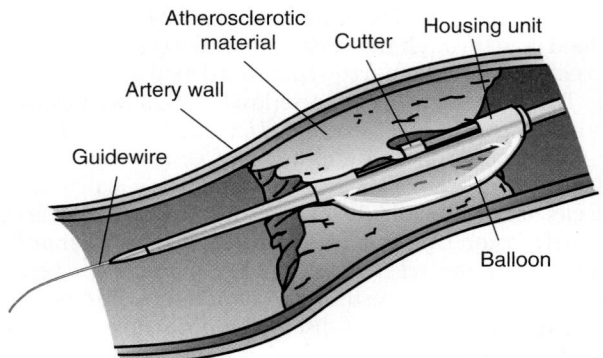

Figure 33-20 *A Simpson Coronary AtheroCath cuts the atherosclerotic material (plaque) away from the artery wall.*

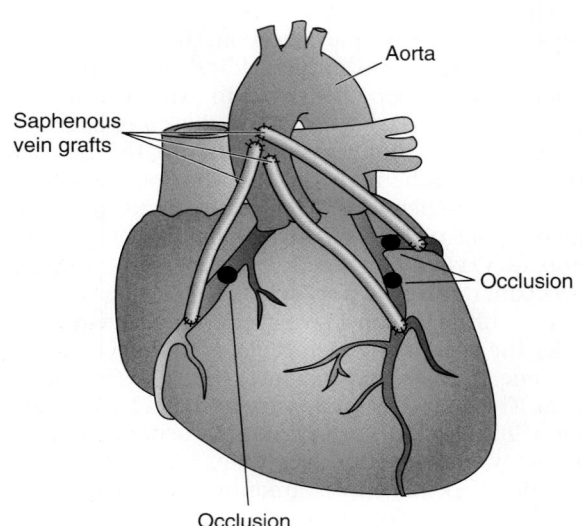

Figure 33-21 *Coronary Artery Bypass Graft (CABG) with the Saphenous Vein*

this occurs, the client would have to undergo immediate coronary artery bypass graft (CABG) surgery. Other complications of the procedure are occlusion of the vessel because of a vascular spasm.

An intracoronary **stent** may be implanted into a stenosed vessel to prevent the vessel from collapsing and to keep the atherosclerotic plaque pressed against the vessel wall. A stent is a tiny metal tube with holes in it (Figure 33-19). The procedure is sometimes done when a vessel collapses after a PTCA or in place of a PTCA. The stent is tightly wrapped around a balloon catheter. When the balloon catheter has been threaded through a vessel to the stenosed area, the balloon is inflated and the stent expands and presses the plaque against the vessel wall. The stent remains in the vessel and the catheter is withdrawn.

Sometimes a transcatheter ablation is done to break up the atherosclerotic areas with a laser. The sclerotic material is broken into pieces smaller than blood cells and excreted through the kidneys.

With a coronary atherectomy, an atherectomy catheter is inserted into the affected coronary vessel to the atheroma (fatty deposit in the vessel wall). The cutter on the catheter shaves the plaque from the wall of the vessel (Figure 33-20). Depending on the type of catheter, the shavings may be saved in the end of the catheter, suctioned out, or shaved so small that they pass through the capillary circulation without damage to the body.

If a CABG is performed, the internal mammary artery, the saphenous vein, or an accordion type of synthetic graft material is used. The vein or synthetic material is grafted to the aorta and passed beyond the obstruction in the coronary vessel (Figure 33-21). The graft provides an increased blood supply to the affected myocardium. The client then has less angina and an increased tolerance for activities.

Pharmacological

Vasodilators, such as nitroglycerin tablets, cause the blood vessels to dilate, providing an increased blood supply to tissues. The client may not need as much analgesic medication if beta-blockers are given. Beta-adrenergic blockers and calcium channel blockers slow the heart rate and decrease the oxygen demand of the heart. Calcium channel blockers also dilate vessels and decrease spasms of the coronary vessels. All of these measures provide an increased blood supply to the myocardium.

Diet

The client is placed on a low-fat, low-cholesterol, sodium-restricted diet. Sodium restriction may vary from no salt to 4 grams daily depending on the ability of the client's kidneys to excrete excess sodium.

Activity

Activity should be slower and for shorter periods of time with more rest periods.

Health Promotion

To prevent coronary artery disease from resulting in angina, it is recommended that a person limit fat intake to 30 grams or less per day and exercise 5 times per week for at least 30 minutes. Simple activities such as parking a car farther from an entrance to increase walking distance and taking stairs instead of an elevator improve circulation and help decrease cholesterol levels. Activities such as gardening or housework are also good.

Nursing Management

Assess pain and medicate client as ordered. Monitor vital signs. Emphasize taking rest periods. Encourage client to always carry nitroglycerin and to get regular exercise as recommended by the physician. Answer questions about the low-fat, low-cholesterol, sodium-restricted diet that is prescribed.

NURSING PROCESS

Assessment

Subjective Data

Ask the client to describe the pain regarding type, radiation, onset, duration, and precipitating factors.

Objective Data

Observe and document the client's actions during the anginal attack. Take vital signs and attach the client to an EKG monitor and observe for any dysrhythmias.

Nursing diagnoses for a client with angina may include the following:

Nursing Diagnoses	Planning/Goals	Nursing Interventions
*Acute **P**ain* related to decreased oxygen supply to the myocardium	The client will experience decreased episodes of angina.	Administer nitroglycerin tablets sublingually. The pain should be relieved within 1 to 2 minutes. If the pain has not stopped after 3 doses 5 minutes apart, notify the emergency personnel. Administer other medication such as beta blockers or calcium channel blockers as ordered and monitor client's response.
Anxiety related to perceived threat of death or change in lifestyle	The client will relate concerns and practice stress reduction techniques.	Assist the client in learning to decrease personal expectations and to live within personal activity limitations. Emphasize the importance of getting adequate rest and stopping before becoming too exhausted.
*Deficient **K**nowledge* related to disease process, medications, and treatment regimen	The client will explain the disease process, medication actions, dosage times and side effects, and self-care practices.	Explain the cause of angina. Teach the client to avoid stressful situations that may produce angina. Other ways to prevent angina are to sleep in a warm room, eat smaller proportions at mealtimes, and not exercise outside in cold weather. Inform the client to always carry nitroglycerin in a tightly closed container. Nitroglycerin may cause orthostatic hypotension, so inform the client to sit after taking it and to change position slowly after taking the medication. Encourage the client to start and maintain a regular exercise program as recommended by the physician.

Evaluation Each goal must be evaluated to determine how it has been met by the client.

MYOCARDIAL INFARCTION

In 2002, an estimated 1.1 million persons in the United States had an acute myocardial infarction (MI), and about 45% died. Half of those who died did so before arriving at a hospital (Nagle & Nee, 2002).

The most common cause for myocardial infarction is atherosclerosis.

A **myocardial infarction** is caused by an obstruction in a coronary artery, resulting in necrosis (death) to the tissues supplied by the artery. The obstruction is usually caused by atherosclerotic plaque, a thrombus, or an embolism. The area most commonly affected is the left ventricle.

Obstruction of a large coronary artery damages the myocardial tissue and affects the pumping efficiency of the heart. A client's prognosis is better if a small coronary artery or arteriole is obstructed and there is good collateral circulation to the heart. If a large vessel is obstructed and the client does not have sufficient collateral circulation, the client may die immediately.

The typical symptoms of an MI in men are feelings of chest heaviness or tightness that progresses to a severe gripping pain in the lower sternal area. The pain is not relieved by rest or nitroglycerin. The client may become short of breath (dyspneic), diaphoretic, and anxious. Women are more likely to have upper abdominal pain, dyspnea, nausea, and fatigue as well as chest pain (Cheek & Cesan, 2003). The client frequently becomes nauseated and vomits. The pulse may be irregular, rapid, and weak, and the blood pressure will be low. The skin will be pale and then turn cyanotic. Even though a person may not experience the typical MI symptoms, the condition can still be serious or fatal. Complications such as heart failure and stroke may also occur.

A myocardial infarction can be diagnosed by client symptoms, EKG tracings, cardiac enzyme values, and a radioactive isotope scan; however, in women the EKG stress test has less diagnostic value than in men. An exercise echocardiography is more reliable for women (Cheek & Cesan, 2003). When an MI is evolving in men, the EKG has an elevated ST segment, which eventually changes into an inverted T wave. The pattern of the rising and falling values of CK, LDH, and AST are significant in diagnosing a myocardial infarction. The CK level rises within 3 to 6 hours of the infarct, peaks within 12 to 18 hours, and returns to normal in 3 days. The higher the CK level rises, the greater the damage to the heart, and the longer the level peaks, the more serious the prognosis. AST value increases in 6 hours, peaks in 12 to 14 hours, and returns to normal in 3 to 4 days. LDH level peaks in 72 hours and slowly returns to normal in 11 to 14 days.

The CK and LDH enzymes can be broken down into isoenzyme (a fragment of an enzyme) fractions of the total values of CK and LDH. A CK-MB fraction, which measures an isoenzyme specific to the cardiac muscle, rises in 3 to 6 hours of the onset of a myocardial infarct, peaks in 18 to 24 hours, and returns to normal in 72 hours. CK studies are done as soon as the client is admitted and then every 8 hours until four samples have been obtained. A CK-MB fraction above 5% indicated myocardial damage. LDH isoenzymes, LDH_1 and LDH_2 are also specific to heart muscle. An LDH_2 is normally higher than an LDH_1 but after an MI, the LDH_1 is higher than the LDH_2 (referred to as "flipped LDH"). An LDH_1 of more than 40% indicates myocardial damage. LDH studies are done upon admission and then every 8 to 12 hours for 24 hours.

Two other important lab values for diagnosing an MI are cardiac troponin I and myoglobin. Cardiac troponin I is a protein found in cardiac cells. When cardiac cells are damaged, this protein is released, resulting in an elevated level (<0.6 mg) for 7 days. Within an hour of an MI, the myoglobin blood level elevates,

peaks in 4 to 12 hours, and returns to normal in 18 hours. If an MI is suspected, this lab value must be obtained quickly.

During the first 3 days after the infarction, the client may have a low-grade fever and an increased white cell count. The infarcted heart tissue is soft and necrotic and incapable of responding to electrical stimuli. Life-threatening dysrhythmias are most likely to occur at this time. Four to seven days after the infarction, the infarcted tissue is the softest and weakest. An aneurysm, or ballooning effect, can occur in the infarcted area with the potential of rupturing. There is a possibility of the ventricle rupturing from the time of the infarct to 2 weeks after the infarct. Collateral circulation begins forming around the edges of the infarct, but it will be 2 to 3 weeks before the collateral circulation functions effectively. Two to three months will pass before the heart muscle regains maximum strength.

Medical–Surgical Management

Medical

Medical–surgical management focuses on reducing oxygen demands, increasing oxygen supply to the myocardium, relieving pain, improving tissue perfusion, and preventing complications and further tissue damage. Immediately after an MI, a client is admitted into a coronary care unit. The client's heart is constantly monitored for dysrhythmias, and vital signs are monitored for any changes.

Three dysrhythmias that may occur following an MI are ventricular fibrillation, bradycardias, and tachycardias. Ventricular fibrillation is treated by defibrillation. Atropine and, if needed, a temporary pacer may be inserted for bradycardias. Two tachycardias that may occur are atrial fibrillation and ventricular tachycardia. Atrial fibrillation is treated with digoxin (Lanoxin) or amiodarone hydrochloride (Cordarone). Ventricular tachycardia is treated with lidocaine or cardioversion. If dysrhythmias continue, magnesium may be given.

Medical complications that can occur following an MI are acute left ventricular failure, cardiogenic shock, pericarditis, embolism and/or thrombosis, and cardiac rupture. The health care team must closely monitor the client for signs of these complications. Women have a worse prognosis and die more often than men after a heart attack or bypass surgery (Cheek & Cesan, 2003).

Surgical

Primary treatment may be PTCA instead of thrombolytic therapy. Along with balloon compression, a stent(s) may be inserted. Clients with multiple vessels occluded, or for whom thrombolytic therapy and PTCA have not been effective, may have the CABG procedure performed.

Pharmacological

Oxygen will be given by a Venturi mask or nasal cannula. Morphine sulfate is given intravenously for pain. Nitrates are also given intravenously or sublingually to relieve pain and dilate coronary arteries. Sedatives may be given to help calm and relax the client. A stool softener is given to prevent rectal straining.

Thrombolytic therapy is sometimes used within 3 to 6 hours of the myocardial infarction to dissolve a clot blocking an artery and reperfuse the area. Medications such as streptokinase (Streptase), anistreplase (Eminase), and alteplase recombinant (Activase) are used. A possible complication from thrombolytic therapy is bleeding. Bleeding problems are rare, but be alert for symptoms of hemorrhaging in the gastrointestinal tract (hematemesis and tarry stools), retroperitoneum (low back pain and numbness in lower extremities), or cerebrum (headache, vomiting, and confusion). Heparin therapy inhibits further clotting. Aspirin and/or clopidogrel (Plavix) is given to prevent vasoconstriction and platelet aggregation.

Diet

Until the client is stabilized, a diet is withheld in case a PTCA or CABG procedure is required. Fluids may be offered during the acute stage. A liquid diet is progressed to a regular low-fat, low-cholesterol, low-sodium diet. The client may tolerate small frequent feedings better than three large meals. Avoid caffeine and extremely hot and cold foods.

Activity

It is vital that the client receive physical, mental, and emotional rest. Less stimuli places less demand on the heart. Explain procedures so the client will understand the care being provided.

The client is usually limited to bed rest during the first 24 hours and progressed to sitting in a chair by the second day. If pain returns or other complications occur, the client is back to bed rest. Early ambulation is encouraged to prevent thrombosis. During and after each activity, the client's tolerance is assessed by monitoring the heart rate for an increase of 20 beats per minute, checking for a decrease in systolic blood pressure, and observing for dyspnea and dysrhythmias. Document verbal and nonverbal statements of fatigue and chest pain.

Before the client is dismissed, low-intensity exercise tests may be done to determine the types of activities in which the client may engage at home. When the client is able to climb two flights of stairs, sexual activity may be resumed.

Health Promotion

A diet of less than 30 grams of fat per day helps reduce the progression of atherosclerosis, but there is no documented evidence that diet will prevent the disease in clients with hereditary hyperlipidemia. Regular exercise, 30 minutes at least 5 days per week, and smoking cessation help prevent an MI.

Participation in a cardiac rehabilitation program provides the client with monitored exercise sessions as well as education and counseling about reducing the risk of future heart problems and coping with a new lifestyle. Because women have a worse prognosis than men, it is critical for women to participate in a cardiac rehabilitation program.

Nursing Management

Assess for pain. Observe for verbal and nonverbal signs of pain. Have client describe symptoms. Monitor vital signs, breath sounds, pedal pulses, and EKG strips. Maintain client on bed rest with call light and other items within reach. Accurately record I&O. Provide a quiet, calm environment. Balance activity with rest periods.

NURSING PROCESS

Assessment

Subjective Data

Note the medications the client has taken, including over-the-counter medications, anticoagulants, and thrombolytic medications. Assess pain regarding onset, duration, intensity, location, radiation, and precipitating factors; ask the client to describe the symptoms. Not all persons having angina or an MI will experience or state having pain. Some may describe feelings of chest heaviness, indigestion, or "something not right." Explore these statements with the client so the client can explain them in more detail. Dizziness, weakness, and shortness of breath may be expressed. Ask how the client tried to relieve pain.

Objective Data

Assess vital signs, skin changes, breath sounds, and EKG rhythm strips. Monitor vital signs for an irregular or increased pulse, hypotension, or slight temperature elevation. The client may have pallor, cyanosis, diaphoresis, vomiting, cool clammy skin, or confusion. Assess breath sounds for lung congestion, and monitor the EKG for dysrhythmias. Note any client clenching of hands or clutching at the chest.

Nursing diagnoses for a client with myocardial infarction may include the following:

Nursing Diagnoses	Planning/Goals	Nursing Interventions
Decreased Cardiac Output related to damaged heart tissue	The client will have increased cardiac output.	Maintain bed rest with head of bed elevated 30° until the condition is stabilized.
		Auscultate breath sounds and palpate pedal pulses every 4 hours.

continues

Nursing Diagnoses	Planning/Goals	Nursing Interventions
		Administer oxygen per mask or nasal cannula at 2 to 4 L/min
		Start an IV so medications such as morphine and antidysrhythmics can be administered.
		If beta-blockers are administered, monitor closely for a drop in heart rate and blood pressure.
		Constantly monitor the client for dysrhythmias. Place a rhythm strip on the chart at least once per shift.
		Monitor I&O.
		Administer medications as prescribed by the physician.
Acute Pain related to decreased oxygenation of myocardial tissue	The client will verbalize decrease in frequency and intensity of chest pain.	Maintain client on bed rest and observe for verbal and nonverbal signs of pain such as grimacing, diaphoresis, or increased heart rate.
		Ask the client to rate the pain on a scale of 0 to 10, 0 being no pain and 10 extreme pain.
		Administer analgesic, usually morphine and oxygen, as ordered.
Risk for Activity Intolerance related to decreased circulation to body tissues	The client will increase activities with decreased symptoms of angina, dyspnea, cyanosis, and dysrhythmia.	Place objects within reach of the client.
		Balance activity with rest periods.
		Assist the client and partner to discuss their fears and feelings candidly about resuming sexual activity.
Death Anxiety related to change in health status and threat of death	The client will verbalize situations that are causing stress.	Encourage the family and client to verbalize their feelings.
		Provide a quiet, calm environment to relax the client and family.
		Administer sedatives to help the client relax and provide periods of uninterrupted rest.
		Since the myocardial client may be in denial, be aware of denial symptoms such as attempting to conduct business over the phone while hospitalized or statements that the pain is really nothing.

Evaluation Each goal must be evaluated to determine how it has been met by the client.

HEART FAILURE

Heart failure (HF) is often the final stage of many other heart conditions. A weakened muscle wall from a myocardial infarction or a heart that has been stressed over a period of time to meet metabolic needs of the body can cause heart failure. Heart failure develops when the heart is no longer capable of meeting the oxygen needs of the body. The muscle of the left ventricle may **hypertrophy** (increases in muscle mass), and often the ventricular chamber enlarges in an attempt to meet the oxygen needs of the body.

Both the right and left ventricles act as pumps for the heart. Each of these pumps can fail separately, resulting in two types of heart failure: right-sided heart failure and left-sided heart failure. Heart failure usually begins on the left side. Some of the causes of right-sided failure are untreated left ventricular failure, right ventricular myocardial infarction, chronic obstructive coronary disease, cor pulmonale, and pulmonic valve stenosis. Left-sided failure is caused by left ventricular myocardial infarction, aortic valve stenosis, prolapsed valve complications, and hyper-

tension. Notice that right- and left-sided failure are caused by a defect of the ventricle or an increased resistance in the path of the blood pumped by the ventricles. This causes an increased workload for the involved ventricle.

When left-sided heart failure occurs, the left ventricle is not able to completely empty of blood or effectively pump blood out through the aorta to the body systems. Usually the right ventricle continues to pump adequate quantities of blood. This causes blood to back up in the left ventricle, left atrium, and pulmonary veins. The lungs become congested with fluid as fluid leaks through the capillaries and fills air spaces in the lungs. The client becomes cyanotic, dyspneic, restless, and coughs up blood-tinged sputum. The breath sounds have moist crackles. Often the client has tachycardia with low blood pressure because the heart is not able to pump sufficient blood to meet the body's demands. The client may have decreased urinary output because enough blood is not being pumped through the kidneys. As the blood oxygen level decreases, the client becomes confused.

As the right side of the heart fails, blood becomes congested in the inferior vena cava, causing edema first in the extremities and then in the trunk of the body. As the condition progresses, the client experiences edema of the ankles, lower legs, thighs, and finally in the abdomen. The excess abdominal fluid causes the client to be anorectic. Hepatomegaly (enlargement of the liver) and splenomegaly (enlargement of the spleen) develop. The jugular veins in the neck become distended when the client is sitting or standing, and pitting edema occurs in the lower extremities. Refer to Figure 33-6. Oliguria occurs as decreased amounts of blood are pumped through the kidneys.

In the early stages of heart failure, the client experiences fatigue, dyspnea with slight exertion, pedal edema, and a slight cough with a small amount of expectoration. The client may also have paroxysmal nocturnal dyspnea.

Medical–Surgical Management

Medical

Goals for treating heart failure are to improve circulation to the coronary arteries and decrease the workload of the left ventricle. To meet these goals, cardiac efficiency is increased with medication; oxygen requirements of the body are decreased through bed rest with head elevated 45 degrees; edema and pulmonary congestion are treated with medications, diet, and restricted fluid intake; and fluid retention is monitored by weighing the client daily. A chest x-ray directly visualizes the ventricles and evidence of lung congestion. An EKG is done and arterial blood gases are evaluated. The client's oxygen saturation level is monitored by pulse oximetry. Depending on the seriousness of the client's condition, a pulmonary artery catheter may be inserted to determine left ventricular function.

In right-sided failure, the symptoms of edema, hepatomegaly, and neck vein distention are significant diagnostic evidence.

Surgical

Two mechanical devices are available: an intra-aortic balloon pump and a ventricular assist device (VAD). An intra-aortic balloon is threaded through the femoral artery to the descending aorta (Figure 33-22). The pump is synchronized with the contractions of the left ventricle so the balloon inflates during diastole and deflates during systole. Inflation of the balloon increases the blood flow to the coronary arteries, thus increasing oxygenation of the myocardium. Deflation of the balloon allows the left ventricle to pump blood to the body tissues with less peripheral resistance.

The left ventricular assist device has a cannula that takes blood from the left atrium to the aorta, bypassing the ineffective left ventricle (Figure 33-23). This gives the left ventricle time to rest and heal. The same process can be done for the right ventricle or both ventricles.

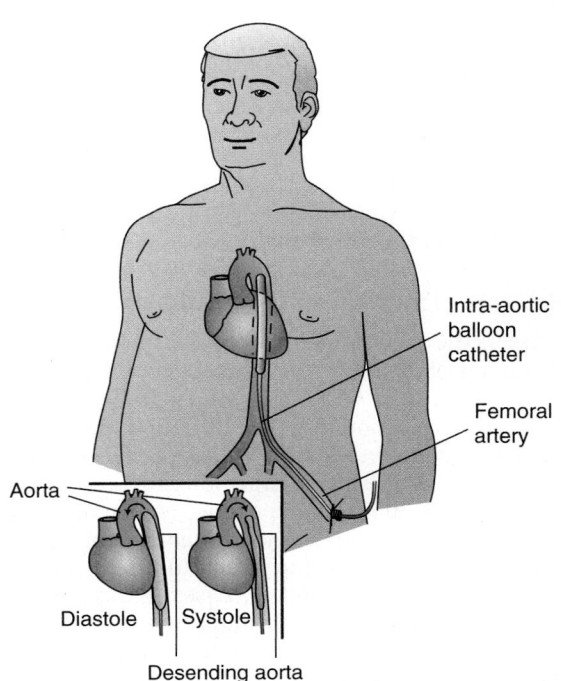

Figure 33-22 *An intra-aortic balloon pump increases circulation to the coronary arteries and decreases the workload of the left ventricle.*

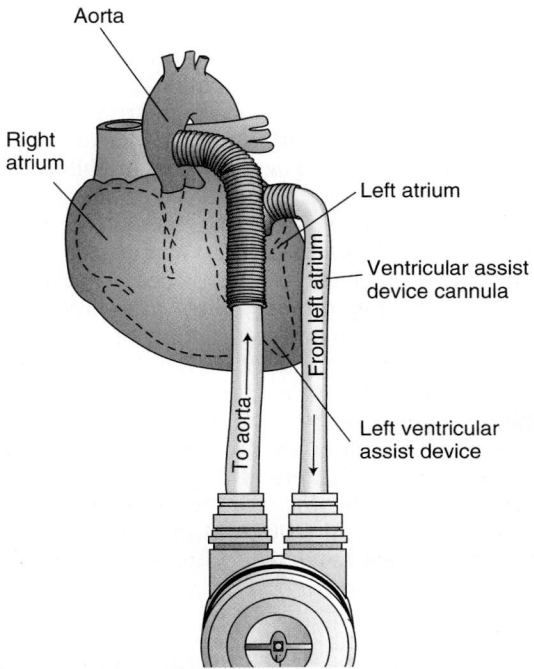

Figure 33-23 *The cannula of the ventricular assist device (VAD) takes blood from the left atrium to the aorta, bypassing the ineffective left ventricle.*

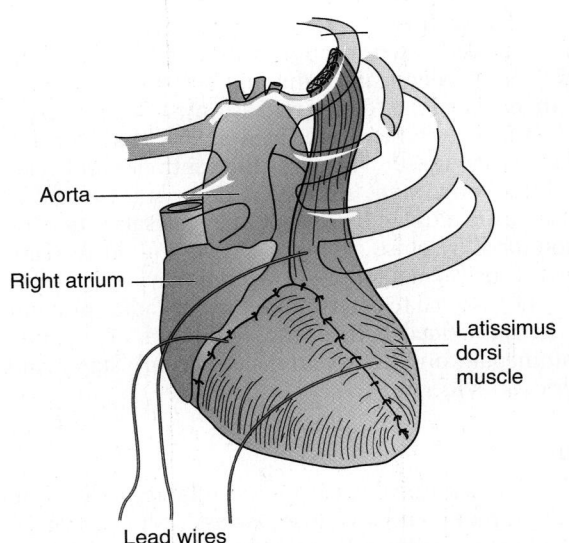

Aorta

Right atrium

Latissimus
dorsi
muscle

Lead wires

Figure 33-24 *Cardiomyoplasty: The latissimus dorsi muscle is wrapped around the heart and stimulated by electrical impulses.*

A cardiomyoplasty may be performed to assist the heart's functioning and improve circulation (Figure 33-24). The latissimus dorsi muscle is wrapped around the heart, and a cardiomyostimulator and leads are implanted to stimulate contractions of the muscle. The stimulator is programmed to begin functioning 2 weeks after the surgery. After 4 months, the muscle stimulation is at either a 1 : 1 or 1 : 2 heartbeat ratio.

Pharmacological

The client with HF will receive diuretics such as chlorothiazide (Diuril) or furosemide (Lasix) to decrease fluid retention. To reduce blood pressure and peripheral arterial resistance and improve cardiac output, angiotensin-converting enzyme (ACE) inhibitors such as captopril (Capoten) or enalopril (Vasotec) are given. Beta-blockers carvedilol (Coreg) and metoprolol succinate (Toprol XL), the only beta-blockers approved for heart failure in the United States, are then added (Ammon, 2001). A digitalis preparation may be required to increase the strength and contractility of the heart muscle. Vasodilators such as nitroglycerin (Cardabid) are given to dilate the veins so the blood will stay in the peripheral vessels and decrease blood return to the right side of the heart, thereby decreasing the workload on the heart. Clients in severe heart failure who are already taking an ACE inhibitor may be given spironolactone (Aldactone) (Ammon, 2001). Morphine sulfate is given in the acute phase to control pain and decrease anxiety.

Diet

A daily weight and strict intake and output are necessary to assess fluid retention. Sometimes fluid intake is limited. The client is generally on a low-sodium diet.

Activity

Activity orders will depend on the client's activity tolerance. The client's activity may vary from strict bed rest to ambulation depending on the severity of the condition. When in bed, the head of the bed should be elevated 45 degrees. Visitation privileges may be monitored to provide rest periods.

Health Promotion

The most common cause of HF is left ventricular failure after a myocardial infarction. To prevent HF following coronary artery disease, a diet low in fat, high in fiber, and balanced in caloric intake to maintain optimum weight is recommended. Stress reduction and a regular exercise program will also decrease the risk of developing HF. Clients with congenital heart defects may not be able to prevent HF, but following the prescribed medical regimen may prevent the early development of HF.

Nursing Management

Monitor client's level of consciousness, skin color and turgor, and jugular veins for distension. Assess breath, heart, and bowel sounds. Check capillary refill and peripheral and abdominal edema. Weigh client daily at same time, on same scale, in same type of clothes. Monitor electrolytes and vital signs. Keep bed in semi-Fowler's position. Maintain accurate intake and output. Provide frequent rest periods and minimal interruptions at night. Teach about disease process, medications, and diet.

NURSING PROCESS

Assessment

Subjective Data

Ask the client about dyspnea, orthopnea, fatigue, anxiety, weight gain, edema, pain, or difficulty in performing activities of daily living.

Objective Data

Assess the client's level of consciousness to determine circulation of blood to the brain. Check skin color for pallor or cyanosis. Assess skin turgor to help determine the level of hydration. Jugular distention indicates right ventricle functioning. Assess breath sounds for adventitious sounds and heart sounds for gallop or murmurs. Bowel sounds may be hypoactive depending on the amount of fluid retention in the abdomen. Check peripheral pulses and capillary refill to assess the level of circulation to the extremities. Assess edema in the extremities and abdomen according to the edema rating scale. Monitor the client's weight daily for possible increase from fluid retention. The physician should be notified if there is a gain of more than 2 pounds in one day. Monitor I & O and assess for oliguria.

Nursing diagnoses for a client with heart failure may include the following:

Nursing Diagnoses	Planning/Goals	Nursing Interventions
Decreased **C**ardiac Output related to mechanical failure of heart muscle	The client's vital signs will remain stable. The client will have decreased adventitious breath sounds.	Take an apical pulse on all cardiac clients, especially checking the rate and rhythm. Monitor the client's heart rate and rhythm by telemetry. Auscultate breath sounds every 4 hours. Administer diuretics, digitalis, and vasodilators as prescribed. Closely monitor the electrolytes, especially the potassium level, as diuretics can deplete the potassium level. Administer potassium supplements as ordered. Take the apical pulse before giving a digitalis preparation. If the heart rate is below 60, withhold the medication and notify the physician. In some institutions the heart rate can drop to 50 before the physician is notified if the client is taking a calcium channel blocker or beta-blocker along with digitalis.
Impaired **G**as Exchange related to decreased cardiac output and pulmonary edema	The client will have increased gas exchange.	Provide oxygen by mask or nasal cannula at 2 to 6 L/min. Apply a pulse oximeter and monitor the oxygenation status. If the pulse oximeter is ≤90%, notify the physician. Elevate the head of the bed to a semi-Fowler's or Fowler's position to relieve pressure on the diaphragm.
Excess **F**luid Volume related to decreased cardiac output and decreased renal output	The client will have less edema of the extremities.	Encourage elevation of the client's legs, not letting them hang in a dependent position. Maintain an accurate intake and output. Weigh daily at the same time each day, on the same scales, and with the client wearing the same type of clothing. If the client is on a fluid-restricted diet, offer hard candies to quench the thirst.
Risk for **A**ctivity Intolerance related to edema, dyspnea, and fatigue	The client will have an increased tolerance for activity.	Schedule nursing care so the client is given frequent rest periods with minimal interruptions at night. Teach the client to take frequent rest periods and to stop activities before becoming tired. Monitor the client's vital signs for an increase or decrease in heart rate or blood pressure, especially after periods of activity. Have an occupational therapist assist the client in energy saving methods. Instruct the client to call the physician if there is more dyspneic, fatigue, less activity tolerance, or weight gain or loss when at home.

Evaluation Each goal must be evaluated to determine how it has been met by the client.

COR PULMONALE

In this condition, the heart is affected because of a lung condition that interferes with the exchange of carbon dioxide and oxygen in the alveoli. The carbon dioxide level increases in the blood. For some unknown reason, the pulmonary arteries vasoconstrict, causing pulmonary hypertension. The right ventricle is forced to pump against increased pulmonary pressure. The right ventricle enlarges and finally weakens in the attempt to pump blood into the lungs. The symptoms the client experiences and medical and nursing care are the same as for right-sided heart failure.

CARDIAC TRANSPLANTATION

Cardiac transplantations are done for cardiomyopathy, end-stage coronary artery disease, and valvular disease. Recipients are evaluated for emotional stability, minimal disease involvement, and a good support system. The heart donor and the recipient's tissues are matched.

The transplant is performed by removing the recipient's heart except for posterior sections of the atria. The posterior sections of the atria are removed from the donor's heart, and then the heart is sutured to the recipient's posterior atria.

The recipient must remain on an immunosuppressant medication for the remainder of life so the donor heart will not be rejected. Some immunosuppressant medications are azathioprine (Imuran), cyclosporine (Sandimmune), antithymocytic globulin, ATG (Atgam), antilymphocytic globulin (ALG), rapamycin, and FK 506 (Prograf).

PERIPHERAL VASCULAR DISORDERS

Disorders in this category include aneurysm, hypertension, venous thrombosis/thrombophlebitis, varicose veins, Buerger's disease, and Raynaud's disease.

ANEURYSM

An **aneurysm** is a localized dilation occurring in a weakened section of an artery's medial layer. The main cause for aneurysms is atherosclerosis (Mayo Clinic, 2002). Some aneurysms occur because of congenital conditions such as Marfan's syndrome or because of trauma to the vessel wall. Two other possible causes of an aneurysm are an increased turbulence in a section of the vessel and a slower production of smooth muscle cells. Clients have a higher tendency to develop an aneurysm if they smoke cigarettes and have hypertension.

Aneurysms can occur in any artery but occur most often in the abdominal aorta. Abdominal aneurysms occur more frequently in men over the age of 55 (Mayo Clinic, 2002). Other involved vessels are the ascending, transverse, and descending aorta, thoracic aorta, popliteal arteries, and femoral arteries.

Deposits of atherosclerotic plaque on the tunica intima cause a hardening of the vessel, and the media layer of the vessel loses elasticity. Atherosclerosis and a lack of elastin in the vessel wall predisposes the vessel to a weakened area, which develops into an aneurysm.

Symptoms of an aneurysm depend on its location. Aneurysms are often asymptomatic until they start leaking or pressing on other structures. A thoracic aneurysm may press on surrounding structures, causing dull upper back pain or deep, scattered chest pain. Pressure on the trachea and bronchus may cause dyspnea, coughing, wheezing, and hoarseness. Pressure on the esophagus causes dysphagia.

The most common location of an abdominal aortic aneurysm is between the renal and iliac arteries. There may be no symptoms, but as it enlarges and presses on other vessels, organs, and nerves, the client may experience abdominal, back, or flank pain. The client may feel a pulse in the abdomen when in a supine position. A tender pulsating mass may be palpated slightly left of the umbilicus. Popliteal and femoral aneurysms may cause decreased pedal pulses. Rupture of an aneurysm is an emergency situation. Signs of rupture may include hypotension, tachycardia, pallor, cool and clammy skin, and intense abdominal, back, or groin pain. An aneurysm is usually diagnosed when a client has an x-ray or ultrasound done for other conditions/symptoms.

Medical–Surgical Management

Medical

If the client has hypertension, control of the hypertension is the focus of care. Aneurysms are monitored for enlargement. Thrombi formation and ischemia may also result.

Surgical

Before elective surgery, the status of the client's carotid arteries and peripheral vessels are checked with a Doppler ultrasound. Cardiac status is usually evaluated by a stress test or cardiac catheterization before surgery is scheduled. The surgeon often orders an angiogram, ultrasound, or CT scan of the affected vessel before surgery to assess the blood supply to the area surrounding the aneurysm. Before surgery, 4 to 8 units of blood are placed on hold because hemorrhage is a possibility. The surgeon clamps the aorta, removes the section of the vessel involving the aneurysm, and replaces it with a section of the client's saphenous vein or a synthetic graft (Figure 33-25). Complications that can occur from clamping the aorta are myocardial infarctions, strokes, and renal damage. Vessels below the repaired aneurysm may become occluded because of decreased blood flow during surgery or from plaque that has broken off from the wall of the vessel. A nasogastric tube may be inserted to decrease pressure on the aneurysm repair site and incision. After surgery, the client may be in the ICU with mechanical ventilator assistance in breathing.

Pharmacological

Clients with aortic aneurysms may be given propranolol hydrochloride (Inderal) to decrease the pressure of the blood coming from the heart. Clients with hypertension are given antihypertensive medications and diuretics. Analgesics are given to control pain.

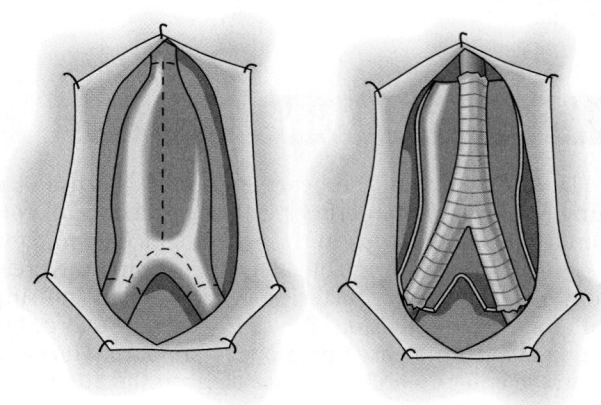

A   **B**

Figure 33-25 A, *Aortoiliac Aneurysm;* **B,** *Bifurcated Synthetic Graft*

Activity

Any activity that increases blood pressure, especially exercise and lifting, can increase pressure in the arteries and should be avoided.

Health Promotion

Clients are encouraged not to smoke. Education for the hypertensive client includes the importance of closely monitoring the blood pressure and taking antihypertensive medication as prescribed.

Nursing Management

Preoperatively, monitor vital signs and peripheral pulses. Assess capillary refill, feet for mottling, and for edema. Postoperatively, add checking operative site frequently. Measure abdomen for increasing size indicating internal hemorrhage. Check function and drainage of NG tube. Measure output hourly for at least 25 to 30 cc of urine.

NURSING PROCESS

Assessment

Subjective Data

Preoperatively, the client may be concerned about an abdominal pulsation when reclining. The client may have chest, back, abdominal, or flank pain depending on the aneurysm location. Postoperatively, listen for statements of pain and assess the level of pain according to a scale of 1 to 10 or the facility-approved scale.

Objective Data

Palpate the abdomen for a pulsating mass, and check vital signs. Immediate intervention is needed if symptoms of bleeding or a rupturing aneurysm occur. Check the peripheral pulses before surgery. Pulses can then be compared preoperatively and postoperatively. Postoperatively, assess the extremities for color, warmth, peripheral pulses, and sensation.

Nursing diagnoses for a client with an aneurysm may include the following:

Nursing Diagnoses	Planning/Goals	Nursing Interventions
Ineffective Tissue Perfusion (Peripheral) related to decreased arterial blood flow	The client will have well-oxygenated tissues as manifested by strong pulses and the skin remaining baseline color and warm.	Monitor for symptoms of an occluded vessel (pain, paleness, cyanosis, and coldness).
		Monitor the temperature, color, and fullness of the peripheral pulses in both extremities and compare them to the preoperative pulses.
		Assess capillary refill and client's feet for mottling and darkened areas on the toes and soles of the feet.
		Notify physician immediately if any of these symptoms occur.
Risk for Deficient Fluid Volume related to hemorrhage	The client will have adequate fluid volume.	Monitor vital signs closely for signs of hemorrhage.
		Check the operative site frequently to make sure the dressing is dry. Turn the client to make sure blood is not pooling under the client's body. Monitor for other signs of hemorrhaging.
		Measure the abdomen for increasing abdominal girth indicating internal bleeding. If the client has low back pain, there may be hemorrhaging in the retroperitoneal space. Other symptoms of hemorrhage are lightheadedness, dizziness, and tachycardia.
		Check for adequate functioning and drainage of the NG tube to decrease pressure on the aneurysm repair site and incision.
Ineffective Tissue Perfusion (Renal) related to interruption of blood flow during surgery	The client will have a urine output above 25 cc/hour.	Measure hourly output to make sure the client has at least 25 to 30 cc of urine per hour. Assess for edema which could indicate fluid overload or a vessel occlusion.
		Provide fluids as ordered.

Evaluation Each goal must be evaluated to determine how it has been met by the client.

HYPERTENSION

Hypertension (HTN), also known as high blood pressure, is defined as an elevated arterial blood pressure. A systolic blood pressure at or above 140 or a diastolic blood pressure at or above 90 indicates hypertension. Fifty million adults in the United States have hypertension (NIH, 2002).

Before age 55, more men than women have hypertension, but after age 55, more women have hypertension (CDC, 2002). Unalterable risk factors include

CULTURAL CONSIDERATIONS

Hypertension

African Americans develop hypertension earlier in life, and it is more severe at any decade of life, than other ethnic groups.

African American, male, aging, postmenopausal women, and family history of hypertension. Modifiable risk factors include smoking, lack of exercise, obesity, stress, low socioeconomic status, diet high in sodium and fat, alcohol intake, and oral contraceptives.

When the cause of hypertension is unknown, it is called **primary hypertension** or "essential hypertension." Ninety-five percent of clients with hypertension have primary hypertension (Woods, 1999). In 5% of the cases, the cause of hypertension is caused by another condition within the body such as renovascular disease, polycystic kidney disease, coarctation of the aorta, Cushing's syndrome, or pheochromocytoma (Woods, 1999); this is known as **secondary hypertension.** Arteriosclerosis, atherosclerosis, hypernatremia (increased sodium in the blood) or prolonged stress may also cause hypertension.

Malignant hypertension is a rapidly progressing, severe elevation of BP (diastolic >120 mm Hg). It damages small arterioles in the major organs. Arteriole inflammation in the eyes is the primary distinguishing finding. It is most common in black males younger than 40 years of age.

Renal diseases may interfere with blood flow to the kidneys, causing them to release an enzyme called *renin.* The released renin interacts with plasma proteins, forming a vasopressor called *angiotensin.* Vasoconstriction caused by angiotensin increases blood pressure when more force is required to push the blood through the vessel. Vasodilation decreases vascular or **peripheral resistance** (pressure within a vessel that resists the flow of blood such as plaque buildup or vasoconstriction). Figure 33-26 depicts how renal disease causes hypertension.

Arteriosclerosis causes the vessel walls to have less elasticity, decreasing their ability to expand and recoil. Because the vessel is not able to expand, more pressure is needed to force the blood through the vessel. The plaque buildup causes resistance to blood flow through the vessel, and more pressure is needed to get the blood through the vessel. Hypernatremia (increased blood sodium) causes vasocongestion, and the heart must pump with more force, increasing the pressure in the arteries, thus causing HTN.

Stress stimulates the sympathetic nervous system, which supplies nerves to the smooth muscles of the arteries, arterioles, veins, and venules. Stimulation of these smooth muscles causes the vessels to constrict, leading to elevated blood pressure.

Some complications of HTN are cerebral vascular accident (stroke), myocardial infarction, heart failure, and renal failure. Table 33-3 lists the recognized classification of blood pressure.

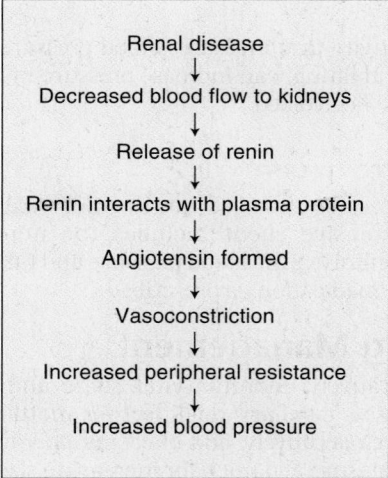

Figure 33-26 *Pathophysiology of Renal Diseases and Hypertension*

TABLE 33-3	CLASSIFICATION OF BLOOD PRESSURE			
CATEGORY	**SYSTOLIC (MM HG)**		**DIASTOLIC (MM HG)**	
Normal	<120	and	<80	
Prehypertension	120–139	or	80–89	
Hypertension				
Stage 1	140–159	or	90–99	
Stage 2	≥160	or	≥100	

From *The Seventh Report of the Joint National Committee on Prevention, Detection, Evaluation, and Treatment of High Blood Pressure,* 2003, Bethesda, MD: National Institutes of Health.)

Medical–Surgical Management

Medical

The main goal for a client with HTN is keeping the blood pressure within normal limits. The regimen is referred to as a stepped-care approach. The first step is to encourage the client to try some diet and lifestyle changes, including losing weight if more than 15% over optimum weight; limiting sodium, saturated fat, cholesterol, and alcohol intake; exercising on a regular basis; stopping the use of nicotine; and maintaining an adequate intake of calcium, magnesium, and potassium. This step is tried for 3 to 6 months, and if the BP then is less than 140/90, these steps would be continued. If the BP still remains high, the second step would be implemented, which would be adding a diuretic or a beta-blocker to the client's care regimen. The client would again be evaluated for a period of time, usually 2 months. If the BP still is not less than 140/90, the third step of in-

COLLABORATIVE CARE

Hypertension

Assisting a client to eliminate hypertension is a multidisciplinary task. Members of the care team most often include physician, nurses, dietitian, fitness center therapist, smoking cessation counselor, and stress management advisor.

CRITICAL THINKING

Lifestyle Changes for Hypertension

How can you best teach the hypertensive client ways to modify the present lifestyle?

creasing the drug dosage, trying another drug, or adding a second antihypertensive drug from another class of drugs would be implemented. If the BP is maintained at less than 140/90, the regimen would be continued. If the BP is still high, the last step would be implemented by adding a second or third antihypertensive drug.

Pharmacological

Diuretics are usually the first pharmacological step in treating HTN. Diuretics increase the renal excretion of sodium and water from the body, decreasing the total fluid volume. When less fluid is in the body, less pressure or force is needed to pump the blood through the body.

Beta-adrenergic blocking agents are given to block the epinephrine and norepinephrine receptor sites. With these receptor sites blocked, the vessels will not constrict and the blood will have less resistance flowing through the vessel. Diuretics and antihypertensive medications may cause impotence.

Diet

A low-fat, low-cholesterol, and low-sodium diet is encouraged. Restricting sodium intake to 2.3 grams of sodium or 6 grams of sodium chloride per day assists in decreasing blood pressure. Avoiding processed foods, carbonated drinks, and most cereals helps decrease sodium intake. The client should have an adequate intake of potassium, magnesium, and calcium. These minerals can be obtained by eating fresh oranges, bananas, broccoli, and collards. Fresh foods are better sources for minerals than frozen foods. Yogurt is a good calcium supplement. The National Committee on Prevention, Detection, Evaluation, and Treatment of High Blood Pressure recommends that clients with hypertension not consume more than 2 ounces of alcohol at a time and no more than twice a week.

Activity

A regular aerobic exercise regimen assists in lowering blood pressure. The client is to gradually increase the exercise period to 30 to 45 minutes three to five times per week with a pulse rate at 75% of the target heart rate (target heart rate = $220 - age \times 0.75$). Walking, swimming, and jogging are excellent aerobic exercises.

Health Promotion

Measures to prevent hypertension are exercising regularly; reducing sodium in the diet; maintaining an optimum weight; reducing and managing stress; maintaining intake of potassium, calcium, and magnesium; decreasing alcohol consumption; and ceasing smoking.

Nursing Management

Monitor BP. Make referrals to assist in lifestyle changes. Explain pathophysiology, risk factors, suggested lifestyle changes, and complications.

NURSING PROCESS

Assessment

Subjective Data

Ask about general lifestyle habits such as smoking, alcohol consumption, exercise routine, dietary intake, and family history of hypertension. Note any dizziness, blurred vision, and headache in the occipital region upon rising in the morning.

Objective Data

The basic assessment is taking the blood pressure. An accurate blood pressure is obtained if the blood pressure cuff bladder surrounds two-thirds of the client's arm, which is supported at heart level. The blood pressure is taken in both arms in supine and sitting positions. Before taking the blood pressure, the client should rest quietly for 5 minutes. If the client has an elevated BP, a repeat blood pressure should be taken 15 minutes later and compared to previous readings. Measure client height and weight, heart sounds, and peripheral pulses.

Nursing diagnoses for a client with hypertension may include the following:

Nursing Diagnoses	Planning/Goals	Nursing Interventions
*Ineffective **H**ealth Maintenance* related to lack of knowledge about lifestyle habits contributing to hypertension	The client will relate needed changes in lifestyle habits to decrease blood pressure.	Make referrals to the appropriate personnel to teach the client lifestyle changes. These may include a dietitian, smoking cessation clinic, fitness center, or stress management seminars. Explain the pathophysiology, risk factors, lifestyle changes, medication actions and side effects, and complications of hypertension.
***N**oncompliance* related to individual's value system (lack of physical symptoms and expense of medication)	The client will keep appointments for regular check-ups and take medications as prescribed.	Regularly inquire about the client's satisfaction in regard to the prescribed regimen of diet, exercise, and prescribed medication(s). If the client cannot afford needed medications, refer the client to financial assistance programs. Encourage the client to become an active participant in the treatment because this will give the client a sense of control over the condition. Encourage the client to record BP readings, weekly weight, exercise activities, and dietary intake as a way of giving a sense of control and encouraging compliance.
*Imbalanced **N**utrition: more than body requirements,* related to excess caloric intake and excess sodium intake	The client will maintain weight at no more than 15 percent over optimum weight and have no more than 2.3 grams of sodium per day.	Give basic dietary instructions as stated under medical management or make a referral to a dietitian. Weigh the client at scheduled appointments.
***S**exual Dysfunction* related to altered body structure or function and side effects of antihypertensive medications	The client will state satisfaction with sexual function while taking antihypertensive medications.	Because diuretics and antihypertensive medications may cause impotence, discuss this effect in an open and candid manner, so the client and spouse will be more open to discuss difficulties in this area.

Evaluation Each goal must be evaluated to determine how it has been met by the client.

SAMPLE NURSING CARE PLAN

THE CLIENT WITH HYPERTENSION

Thomas Liggins, a 28-year-old African American, is in his last year of law school and is clerking for a prestigious law firm. He and his fiancé are planning to be married as soon as he graduates. During the last week he has had four dizzy spells and has had a headache at the base of his skull upon awakening for the last 2 days. His father has a history of hypertension, so Thomas is aware that his symptoms may indicate high blood pressure. Thomas stops by the clinic on his way home from work and asks to have his blood pressure checked. The nursing assessment has the following data.

Subjective data: States he has had four dizzy spells and has awakened with a headache in the occipital lobe the last two mornings. Thomas has been having 1 glass of wine at lunch and 2–3 beers in the evening to relax from the tension of school and work. Most of his meals are at fast-food establishments and have a high fat content. Thomas does not smoke. He used to jog 4 mornings a week but quit when he started clerking. He has had nocturia for the last 3 weeks. He is not taking any medication. Thomas states he is concerned about having hypertension because he does not want to take medication.

Objective data: T 98.6 P 78 R 16 BP 142/92 Wt 190 (optimum weight 160). No edema noted in hands, feet, or legs.

Nursing Diagnosis 1 *Ineffective **H**ealth Maintenance* related to ineffective individual coping as evidenced by high-fat diet, lack of exercise, stressful job, and alcohol intake

continues

SAMPLE NURSING CARE PLAN

Nursing Outcomes Classification (NOC)
Health Promoting Behaviors
Knowledge: Health Promotion

Nursing Interventions Classification (NIC)
Nutrition Management
Support System Enhancement

PLANNING/GOALS	NURSING INTERVENTIONS	RATIONALE
Thomas will change lifestyle habits by engaging in aerobic exercises at least 3 times a week for 30 to 45 minutes, stating three ways to reduce stress, and limiting alcohol consumption to 2 ounces twice a week.	Refer Thomas to a dietitian to learn ways to cut fat and sodium in his diet.	Knowledge encourages compliance.
	Discuss ways Thomas can exercise and still meet responsibilities of work, school, and personal and social life.	Encourages exercise if he sees ways that he can still meet responsibilities of life.
	Explain alcohol content in various beverages.	Encourages compliance.

EVALUATION   Thomas starts exercising with his fiancé 3 times a week. Thomas uses breathing techniques and a hot shower to reduce daily stress. Thomas limits alcohol consumption to 1 beer a day.

Nursing Diagnosis 2 *Imbalanced Nutrition: more than body requirements*, related to excessive caloric intake as evidenced by 30 pounds overweight and high-fat diet

Nursing Outcomes Classification (NOC)
Nutritional Status
Weight Control

Nursing Interventions Classification (NIC)
Weight Management
Weight Reduction Assistance

PLANNING/GOALS	NURSING INTERVENTIONS	RATIONALE
Thomas will lose 30 pounds and maintain a low-fat, low-sodium diet.	Refer Thomas to a weight support group.	It is easier with support of others.
	Encourage Thomas to record a weekly weight and daily intake of fat.	Promotes self-care.

EVALUATION   Thomas and his fiancé are maintaining a diet low in sodium and no more than 30 grams of fat per day. Thomas keeps a weekly record of his weight.

Nursing Diagnosis 3 *Anxiety* related to threat to or change in health status and stress as evidenced by alcohol consumption to relax and statement of not wanting to take medications

Nursing Outcomes Classification (NOC)
Acceptance: Health Status
Coping

Nursing Interventions Classification (NIC)
Teaching: Individual
Coping Enhancement

PLANNING/GOALS	NURSING INTERVENTIONS	RATIONALE
Thomas will state preventive measures to reduce blood pressure.	Have Thomas identify stress factors in life.	Action to cope with stressors can be taken only if stressors are identified.
	Discuss stress reduction techniques with Thomas.	Knowledge promotes compliance.

continues

SAMPLE NURSING CARE PLAN

Discuss risk factors of hypertension and ways to reduce it.	Promotes identification of risk factors in personal life.
Explain to Thomas and his fiancé that hypertension is a chronic condition, possibly without symptoms, but with some potentially serious complications.	Knowledge promotes compliance.

EVALUATION   Thomas states four ways to reduce blood pressure.

VENOUS THROMBOSIS/ THROMBOPHLEBITIS

The terms *phlebitis, thrombosis, phlebothrombosis* and *thrombophlebitis* are often used interchangeably even though each word has a separate meaning and etiology. **Phlebitis** is an inflammation in the wall of a vein without clot formation. The formation of a clot in a vessel is a **thrombosis,** and a formed clot that remains at the site where it formed is a **thrombus.** If the thrombus moves, it becomes an **embolus,** a mass such as a blood clot or an air bubble, that circulates in the bloodstream. **Phlebothrombosis** is the formation of a clot because of blood pooling in the vessel, trauma to the vessel's endothelial lining, or a coagulation problem with little or no inflammation in the vessel. **Thrombophlebitis** is the formation of a clot caused by an inflammation in the wall of the vessel.

In 1846, Virchow listed three factors leading to the formation of a clot: pooling of blood, vessel trauma, and a coagulation problem. These are known as **Virchow's triad.** Risk factors for thrombi formation are prolonged bed rest, leg trauma, oral contraceptives, obesity, varicose veins, hip fractures, and total hip and knee replacement.

There are two types of thrombi: a superficial thrombus and a deep vein thrombus (DVT). A superficial vein thrombus forms in a superficial vein such as the saphenous vein in the leg. A DVT forms in the deep veins of the arms, pelvic area, or legs, but the legs are the most common site. Leg veins in which clots form are the femoral, popliteal, iliac, and deep veins of the calf.

Phlebitis can either form spontaneously or as a result of IV catheters or cannulas, IV medications such as potassium or antibiotics, or direct trauma to a vein. A clot may then form as red blood cells pass over the damaged area, rupture, and start the clotting process.

Phlebitis may manifest as a reddened streak over a vein. If a clot is in a superficial vein, the site becomes reddened, warm, tender, and swollen. A hardening may be palpated in a section of the vein. There may be no symptoms with a deep vein thrombus, or there may be

CLIENT TEACHING

Thrombophlebitis

- Drink 2 to 3 quarts of water per day.
- Do not sit with legs crossed.
- Elevate both legs when sitting.
- Avoid sitting or standing for extended periods.
- Wear support hose.
- When standing, shift weight frequently and occasionally stand on tiptoes to stimulate the calf muscle to pump blood.
- Notify the physician immediately if leg pain, tenderness or swelling, difficulty breathing, or chest pain is experienced.

warmth and tenderness at the site, unilateral edema of the affected extremity, positive Homans' sign, dilation of superficial veins, and cyanosis of the foot. The client may say the leg feels "tight" or "heavy." If the clot is in the calf of the leg, the calf may feel tender. If the swelling restricts the arterial blood flow, the leg may be cool and pale. If there are obvious clinical signs of a thrombosis, Homans' sign should *not* be assessed because the clot may be dislodged and become an embolus.

A complication of a DVT is a pulmonary embolus that may result in death. Symptoms of a pulmonary embolus are sudden and severe chest pain, dyspnea, and tachypnea. Emboli may travel and block other vessels in the heart, brain, or peripheral vessels.

Medical–Surgical Management

Medical

A superficial phlebitis or thrombus may need no treatment, or warm soaks may be applied to the affected area. Acetaminophen or an NSAID is given for pain. Elevating the extremity decreases swelling and improves venous return. Some doctors recommend the application of elastic support hose. If a DVT is diagnosed, the client is placed on bed rest. Once the client improves and becomes ambulatory, below-the-knee compression stockings are recommended.

Surgical

If a clot has formed in a large vein and all conservative methods have failed, the clot may be removed surgically. This procedure is called a **thrombectomy** and is performed only if the tissue in the area becomes ischemic or gangrenous or if the client has a history of thromboemboli.

Another surgical procedure is a vena cava interruption surgery (venacaval plication) in which a Greenfield vena cava filter or umbrella filter is placed in the inferior vena cava to prevent thromboemboli from traveling from the lower extremities to the lungs, heart, or brain. Figure 33-27 shows these filters and their placement in the vena cava. The procedure is done on clients with a history of pulmonary emboli.

Pharmacological

If a client is at risk for a thrombus or phlebitis, anticoagulant therapy can be initiated. A prophylactic heparin dose is given. Enoxaparin injection (Lovenox), a low-molecular-weight heparin, is used prophylactically after hip replacement surgery. It should be used cautiously with clients on oral anticoagulants.

If a clot forms, the client is immediately started on heparin as an IV bolus and then followed with a continuous IV drip of heparin. Before heparin is started, a partial thromboplastin time (PTT) or activated partial thromboplastin time (APTT) and a platelet count are drawn by the laboratory to establish a baseline level. The heparin dose is regulated by the PTT or the APTT. For effective heparin therapy, the client's PTT or APTT level should be 2.5 times the baseline. A **baseline level** is a value at a particular time that serves as a reference point for future value levels.

Clients are usually discharged on Coumadin. Because of rapid hospital discharges, clients are often started on Coumadin the next day after heparin has been initiated. Once the Coumadin dose is regulated, heparin is stopped.

After the initial Coumadin dose, the daily Coumadin dose is regulated by the prothrombin time (PT) or the International Normalized Ratio (INR). The client generally remains on Coumadin for 3 to 6 months.

Thrombolytic drugs, urokinase (Abbokinase), streptokinase (Streptase), and tissue plasminogen activator, t-PA (Alteplase), are used locally and systemically if there is a massive DVT. Streptokinase should only be used on the same client once every 6 months. If the client has had a recent streptococcal infection, streptokinase may not be effective (Spratto & Woods, 2004). The main complication in a client receiving thrombolytic drugs is bleeding. Heparin and Coumadin are given after the thrombolytic drugs to prevent thrombi formation.

Diet

Adequate hydration is important for clients at risk for thrombi. This can be accomplished orally or intravenously.

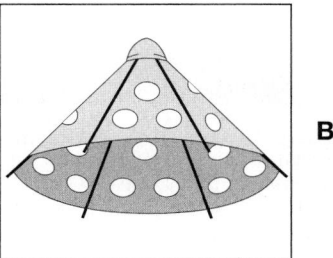

Figure 33-27 *A filter in the vena cava prevents an embolus from traveling to the heart, lungs, or brain: **A,** Greenfield Filter in Place; **B,** Umbrella Filter*

Activity

During the acute stage, the client is placed on bed rest to prevent the clot from dislodging and embolizing. Later, the leg is elevated periodically to improve venous return and decrease swelling. The client's leg should never be massaged because a clot could be dislodged and become an embolus.

Health Promotion

Prevention is the best way to treat a DVT. Early ambulation, adequate hydration, alternating pneumatic compression devices, prophylactic anticoagulants, elevation of legs, leg exercises, and deep breathing exercises all contribute to the prevention of thrombi.

Nursing Management

Monitor vital signs for changes and IV sites for redness and warmth. Check Homans' sign. Measure circumference of affected leg. Assess peripheral pulses and capillary refill. If on anticoagulant drugs, assess for signs of bleeding. When on bed rest, elevate entire affected leg. Remove elastic support or pneumatic compression stockings daily for hygiene.

NURSING PROCESS

Assessment

Subjective Data

Ask the client if there was any recent injury to the extremity, if the affected area is tender to the touch, or if there have been clots previously. Note any chest pain, dyspnea, tachycardia, or hemoptysis.

Objective Data

Check IV sites at least once per shift to see if a phlebitis or reddened area is developing at the insertion site. If a positive Homans' sign is detected during an assessment, notify the physician and do not perform another Homans' sign until a clot has been ruled out. Assess the skin for redness, tenderness, hardness, or warmth, and measure both legs to determine baseline measurements. Measure the circumference of the affected leg every shift to determine an increase or decrease in swelling. Assess peripheral pulses every 4 hours and more frequently if the client experiences increased pain in the leg, cyanosis of the foot or extremity, or increased swelling. These are signs of an occlusion.

Nursing diagnoses for a client with a venous thrombosis may include the following:

Nursing Diagnoses	Planning/Goals	Nursing Interventions
*Ineffective **T**issue Perfusion (Peripheral)* related to decreased venous blood flow and/or clot formation	The client will have adequate tissue perfusion.	Elevate the client's entire affected leg when on bed rest to improve venous return. When elevated, the leg should be slightly flexed at the knee with a pillow under the thigh and calf.
		Apply elastic support or intermittent pneumatic compression stockings on the client.
		If the client has received thrombolytic or anticoagulant drugs, assess for signs of bleeding which include hematuria, bruising, bleeding from the gums, and blood in the stool.
		Monitor pedal pulses and capillary refill and measure thigh or calf circumference daily.
*Acute **P**ain* related to inflammatory process	The client will state absence of pain.	If the client has a phlebitis, apply warm moist soaks to the affected area as ordered.
		Administer acetaminophen or a nonsteroidal anti-inflammatory as ordered for discomfort.
***A**nxiety* related to possibility of the clot becoming an embolus	The client will express anxiety about possible embolus.	Encourage client to discuss the possibility of embolus formation.

Evaluation Each goal must be evaluated to determine how it has been met by the client.

VARICOSE VEINS

Varicose veins, also called **varicosities,** are visibly prominent, dilated, and twisted veins, usually in the lower extremities, but the veins in the esophagus (esophageal varices) and anus (hemorrhoids) can also be affected. Usually, the saphenous vein is affected in the leg. Women are more prone to varicose veins than men. Risk factors for developing varicose veins are a familial tendency, congenital abnormalities, pregnancy, obesity, constrictive clothing, and occupations that require prolonged standing. Pregnancy and obesity cause more pressure in the veins of the legs.

The causes of varicose veins are incompetent valves and veins that have lost their elasticity. The wall of the vessel is weakened from a lack of elastin or collagen and is unable to support the normal pressure of the blood in the vessel. The vein dilates as the blood in it flows backward. As the walls of the vein dilate, the valves become incapable of holding the blood and allow blood to leak backward through the space between the valves. Refer to Figure 33-5C. The client has pain in the feet and ankles, swelling, and ulcers on the skin. Trendelenburg's test is used for diagnosis.

Medical–Surgical Management
Medical

Varicose veins are usually treated conservatively with elastic support hose, elevation of the legs when sitting, not crossing legs, and ankle and leg exercises.

Sclerotherapy involves injecting a chemical into the vein, causing the vein to become sclerosed (hardened) so blood no longer flows through it. A compression bandage or elastic stocking is applied to the extremity for 4 to 5 days. The client wears support hose for 5 more weeks. Complications of the procedure are **necrosis** (tissue death) at the injection site, vasospasm, allergic responses, and **hemolysis** (destruction of red blood cells).

Surgical

In more severe cases, varicose veins can be ligated (tied off) or stripped. **Vein stripping** involves introducing a wire into a vein. The wire has collapsible claws on the end. As the wire is withdrawn, the claws expand and strip the walls of the vein. This measure is used when there is a threat of thrombus or leg ulcers. **Vein ligation** is tying off an involved section of a vein with suture.

Pharmacological

Analgesics are given for leg discomfort. Anticoagulants may be given to prevent clot formation.

Activity

The client is encouraged to exercise regularly. Walking is a very good exercise to improve circulation because the blood circulates faster in response to an increased heartbeat. Muscles in the legs apply pressure to the veins, forcing the blood upward toward the heart. Ankle exercises such as rotating the ankle in circular motions also improves circulation.

Health Promotion

Encourage clients with a familial tendency for varicose veins to elevate their legs 6 to 10 inches on a small stool when sitting in a chair. Frequent position changes and not standing in one spot for extended times also improve circulation.

Nursing Management

Assist the client in elevating the legs above the heart when in bed or elevating the feet 6 to 10 inches on a pillow or stool when sitting in a chair.

After a vein stripping, the client is on bed rest for the first 24 hours. Elastic hose are worn continuously for 5 days to compress the blood into the deeper veins and for 5 weeks after the surgery. Administer pain medication 30 minutes before the client ambulates until walking is tolerated without discomfort. Encourage walking and leg exercises.

After sclerotherapy the affected area may be tender and discolored. Most discoloration will disappear in a few weeks, but a darkened pigmentation may last for 6 to 8 months. Repeated sclerotherapy may be needed. Encourage the client to maintain a walking exercise program to improve circulation to the legs.

BUERGER'S DISEASE (THROMBOANGIITIS OBLITERANS)

Buerger's disease is an inflammatory disease of small and medium arteries and veins that leads to vascular obstruction. Inflammation occurs in the adventitia and media layers of the vessels and may affect only a portion of the vessel or the entire vessel. Hands and feet are mainly involved, but the wrists and lower extremities may also be affected. The distal tips of the hands and feet are pale, but as the disease progresses, the hands and feet become reddened when held in a dependent position. At first, pain in the palm of the hand and arch of the foot is the main symptom. Pain becomes more severe with disease progression, and as ischemia affects the nerves, the client may experience numbness, burning, pain when at rest, and decreased sensation in the hands and lower extremities. The dorsalis pedis, posterior tibia, and ulnar and radial pulses are weak or absent. Skin color changes, cold sensitivity, ulcers, and gangrene may occur in the later stages.

Buerger's disease occurs primarily in men between the ages of 20 and 40 of Israeli, Indian, and Asian descent. There is a correlation between smoking and Buerger's disease. Tests for diagnosis include arteriography and Doppler ultrasound.

Medical–Surgical Management

Medical

The client is encouraged to stop smoking and may be referred to a smoking clinic or seminar. Buerger-Allen exercises are recommended and explained. Buerger-Allen exercises consist of elevating the legs until they blanch and supporting them at that angle for 2 to 3 minutes. The legs are then lowered to a dependent position until they become red and supported at that level for 5 to 10 minutes. The legs are then placed flat on the bed with the client in a supine position for 10 minutes. The exercises are repeated as tolerated by the client.

Surgical

A sympathectomy may be done to relieve pain and prevent vasospasm in the affected area. Digits and toes may have to be amputated if gangrene occurs.

Pharmacological

Analgesics are given to control pain. Vasodilators are given to increase circulation to the affected area.

Nursing Management

Nursing diagnoses and interventions are the same as for other obstructive vascular conditions and are described under Raynaud's disease.

RAYNAUD'S DISEASE/ PHENOMENON

Raynaud's disease or primary Raynaud's is an intermittent spasm of the digital arteries and arterioles resulting in decreased circulation to the fingers and toes. Sometimes the tip of the nose and ears are also affected. The cause of the condition is unknown but seems to be related to vasospastic disorders, a disturbance with the innervation of the sympathetic nervous system, and angiography complications. During a spasm that lasts approximately 15 minutes, the fingers become pale, and then cyanotic. As the circulation returns to the fingers, the fingertips become reddened and the person experiences a tingling or throbbing pain in the fingers. Some people experience only pallor and cyanosis. The episode may last 1 to 2 hours. Symptoms usually occur when the person is exposed to cold or experiences emotional stress. Gangrene is not common but can occur in the fingertips. Ulcerations can also occur and are difficult to heal because of decreased circulation in the fingers.

When associated with a connective tissue or collagen vascular disease, medications, or occupational trauma, the condition is called Raynaud's phenomenon or secondary Raynaud's. Raynaud symptoms may occur 10 years before the related disease is diagnosed. A 2-year history of signs and symptoms with no evidence of underlying disease, especially an autoimmune disease, is necessary for a diagnosis of Raynaud's disease.

Raynaud's is more prevalent in cold climates. Women are nine times more likely to be affected than men (Raynauds Association, 2001). About 75% are diagnosed in women between the ages of 15 and 40 (NIAMS, 2001). Persons who use vibrating hand tools such as air hammers or grinding wheels or who perform repetitive movements such as typing or playing the piano are at risk.

Diagnostic examinations include a complete blood count, digital blood pressure measurement, digital plethysmography waveforms, and a cold-challenge test. A digital blood pressure of 30 mm Hg below the brachial pressure indicates of a digital artery obstruction. A sedimentation rate, antinuclear antibody, and rheumatoid factor are done to determine the presence of autoimmune diseases. During a cold-challenge test, thermistors are placed on the fingers and a baseline temperature is taken. The hands are submerged into ice water for 20 seconds, then removed. The temperature of the hands is then taken every 5 minutes until it returns to the baseline level. Hand x-rays determine the presence of subcutaneous calcium deposits and narrowing of bone in the digits. The diagnostic tests distinguish between Raynaud's phenomenon and Raynaud's disease. If a client has unilateral or single-digit Raynaud's, an obstruction or emboli is suspected.

Medical–Surgical Management
Medical

Raynaud's phenomenon is treated conservatively. The client is assessed regularly for symptoms of autoimmune diseases. If the symptoms of Raynaud's are caused by a vasospastic disease, relief is best achieved with medications. Alternative therapies such as relaxation techniques and biofeedback may be beneficial.

Surgical

A sympathectomy (excision of a nerve, plexus, or ganglion of the sympathetic portion of the autonomic nervous system) is sometimes done to alleviate the client's symptoms; however, it usually provides temporary relief and is not a routine treatment.

Pharmacological

Clients may be given nifedipine (Adalat, Procardia) at night for severe cases of Raynaud's phenomenon. Clients may also take the medication 1 to 2 hours before engaging in an outdoor activity during cold weather. They may not need to take the medication during warmer months. Other medications used to improve symptoms in severe Raynaud's phenomenon are diltiazen hydrochloride (Cardizem), verapamil (Calan), nicardipine hydrochloride (Cardene), and captroprol (Capoten). Pentoxifylline (Trental) is used investigationally to decrease the viscosity of blood and improve the blood flow to peripheral arteries (Spratto & Woods, 2004). Some clients have benefited from topical nitroglycerin and prostaglandin E_2 (NIAMS, 2001). The adrenergic blocker reserpine (Serpasil) may improve circulation.

Beta-blockers, birth control pills, cold medications, and diet pills cause some clients to have Raynaud's phenomenon. Chemotherapy drugs such as bleomycin sulfate (Blenoxane) and cisplatin, CDDP (Platinol), also cause secondary Raynaud's.

Health Promotion

Encourage the client to avoid decongestants, caffeine, exposure to cold, repetitive hand movements, and stressful situations. Also encourage the client to quit smoking and avoid secondary smoke because nicotine is a potent vasoconstrictor. Stress management techniques (e.g., biofeedback) may assist in alleviating some distress from the condition. Wearing mittens in cold weather or when handling cold foods keeps fingers warmer than wearing gloves. Keeping the entire body warm is helpful.

Nursing Management

Assess digits for pallor, blanching, cyanosis, rubor, coldness, and texture. Encourage client to keep indoor temperature at a comfortable level. Teach relaxation exercises to enhance circulation. Encourage use of mitts when handling cold foods, wear mittens and socks to bed, and wear mittens when pushing shopping carts. Apply lotion regularly to prevent dry, chapped skin.

NURSING PROCESS

Assessment

Subjective Data

Ask the client how frequently the vasospastic episodes occur, what symptoms are experienced, what triggers the episodes, which digits are affected during an episode, and how long the incident lasts. Inquire about daily activities the client finds difficult, such as tying shoes, washing dishes, or handling frozen foods. Obtain a history of occupational activities.

Objective Data

Assess the digits for pallor, blanching, cyanosis, rubor, coldness, and texture. If the disease is longstanding, the digits may be tapered and the skin shiny in appearance. There may be ulcerated or gangrenous areas on the fingertips.

Nursing diagnoses for a client with Raynaud's disease may include the following:

Nursing Diagnoses	Planning/Goals	Nursing Interventions
Ineffective **T**issue Perfusion (Peripheral) related to vasospasm of peripheral arteries	The client will have fewer vasospastic episodes and increased circulation in digits.	Encourage the client to use caution when engaging in activities that may cause a cut or scratch because healing may be impaired because of decreased circulation.
		If a client has ulcers, wash the areas with soap and water and administer prescribed medications such as ciprofloxacin (Cipro) and intravenous iloprost.
Acute **P**ain related to decreased circulation in digits	The client will experience decreased pain as vasospasms are controlled.	Teach client to keep the indoor temperature at a comfortable level to avoid ischemic attacks.
		Encourage client to avoid dramatic changes in environmental temperatures (e.g., entering a cold air-conditioned room during hot summer months). Encourage the client to wear woolen or wind-proof gloves or mittens and layered clothes when exposed to colder temperatures. Mittens may be better than gloves so the fingers can obtain warmth from each other. Chemical warming devices may be used inside gloves and shoes.
		Encourage the client to stop smoking and make a referral to a smoking cessation clinic.
		Teach the client relaxation exercises that may decrease the number of ischemic attacks.
Situational Low **S**elf-esteem related to inability of hands to perform activities of daily living	The client will learn ways to handle activities of daily living.	Encourage client to use mitts or potholders when removing items from the freezer or handling cold food to decrease the risk of a Raynaud's episode. Clients can wear mittens or socks to bed. Use of insulated mugs, foam rubber holders, or stemware glasses may reduce ischemic attacks.
		Instruct client to wash vegetables under tepid water instead of cold, to bathe in lukewarm water, and to apply lotion regularly to prevent dry and chapped skin.
		Encourage client to use gloves when pushing shopping carts or operating some vibrating machines because this may decrease the cold sensation and soften the vibration.

Evaluation Each goal must be evaluated to determine how it has been met by the client.

CASE STUDY

Mr. Lance Jeffers, a 55-year-old truck driver, is admitted to the emergency room with a feeling of heavy squeezing pressure in his sternal area. The pain is radiating to his left shoulder. He is diaphoretic, short of breath, and nauseated. He states the sternal pain came on suddenly while watching a football game. He had been mowing his yard and decided to rest. The emergency physician gives Mr. Jeffers a nitroglycerin tablet and connects him to an EKG monitor. Cardiac enzymes with isoenzyme fractions and a chest x-ray are requested STAT. Morphine sulfate 2 mg is given intravenously. Oxygen is given by mask at 4 liters/minute. Mr. Jeffers's apical pulse is 102 and his blood pressure is 130/88. A cardiac catheterization with fluoroscopy is ordered to determine the patency of the coronary blood vessels and functioning of the heart muscle. Three hours after admission, crackles are heard in the lungs.

The following questions will guide your development of a nursing care plan for the case study.

1. List symptoms/clinical manifestations, other than Mr. Jeffers's, a client may experience when having a myocardial infarction.
2. List two reasons morphine sulfate was given to Mr. Jeffers.
3. List two other diagnostic tests that may have been ordered for Mr. Jeffers.
4. List subjective and objective data a nurse would want to obtain about Mr. Jeffers.
5. Write three individualized nursing diagnoses and goals for Mr. Jeffers.
6. Mr. Jeffers is moved from the critical care unit. List pertinent nursing actions a nurse would do in caring for Mr. Jeffers related to:

oxygenation	activity
cardiac output	medications
comfort/rest	teaching

7. List teachings that Mr. Jeffers will need before his discharge.
8. List at least three successful client outcomes for Mr. Jeffers.

Summary

- The function of the heart is to pump blood through the vascular system. Blood is the medium by which oxygen and nutrients are provided to the body cells and carbon dioxide and waste products are removed from the body cells.
- The coronary arteries supply blood to the heart. If the blood flow through these vessels becomes diminished or occluded, ischemia to the heart tissue occurs, resulting in angina or a myocardial infarction.
- Typical symptoms experienced by a person with cardiac problems include chest pain, dyspnea, edema, fainting, palpitations, diaphoresis, and fatigue.
- A lipid profile and cardiac enzymes, including the CK and LDH isoenzymes, provide diagnostic information about the risk of heart disease and the occurrence of a myocardial infarction.
- A dysrhythmia is an irregularity in the rate, rhythm, or conduction of the electrical system of the heart.
- Inflammatory or infectious conditions of the heart include endocarditis, myocarditis, and pericarditis. Endocarditis may cause valvular heart disease with the possibility of the valve needing to be surgically repaired (valvuloplasty) or replaced with a mechanical (caged-ball valve or tilting-disk valve) or biological valve from a calf, pig, or human.
- Atherosclerosis causes a narrowing and occluding of vessels and is a primary cause of angina and myocardial infarction.
- Surgical treatment for angina includes a PTCA, intracoronary stent, transcatheter ablation, or a coronary artery bypass graft.
- Heart failure is often the final stage of many other heart conditions in which the heart is no longer able to fulfill the demands of the body.
- To assess the peripheral vascular system, the nurse assesses pain, pulse, pallor, paresthesia, and paralysis.
- Three factors leading to the formation of a clot—pooling of blood, vessel trauma, and a coagulation problem—are called Virchow's triad.
- A client with a DVT may be asymptomatic or may have warmth and tenderness at the site, edema of the extremity, a positive Homans' sign, cyanosis of the foot, and a sensation of heaviness or tightness in the extremity.
- It is important for the nurse to measure the leg circumference every shift and check peripheral pulses for the client with a thrombus.
- The cause of varicose veins is incompetent valves and veins that have lost their elasticity.

- Primary Raynaud's disease is an intermittent spasm of the digital arteries and arterioles, resulting in decreased circulation to the digits.
- Symptoms of an aneurysm depend on the location of the aneurysm in the body. Aneurysms are often asymptomatic until they start leaking or pressing on other structures.

Review Questions

1. To assess a client with right-sided heart failure, the nurse would:
   a. listen for a pericardial friction rub.
   b. listen for a muffled S_1 and S_2 heart sound.
   c. check for distended neck veins with the bed at a 45-degree angle.
   d. assess for radiation of the squeezing sensation under the sternum.

2. It is important to teach a client with angina to:
   a. take antibiotics before having dental work.
   b. carry nitroglycerin tablets at all times.
   c. perform the Valsalva maneuver daily.
   d. massage the carotid sinuses in the neck.

3. A nursing intervention to improve cardiac output is:
   a. encouraging the client to verbalize fears.
   b. teaching the side effects of new medications.
   c. a referral to a dietitian for low-sodium diet instructions.
   d. administer oxygen per physician orders.

4. Instructions to a client on anticoagulant therapy include:
   a. taking Coumadin twice a day.
   b. watching for symptoms of bleeding.
   c. taking over-the-counter medications as needed.
   d. no dietary or activity limitations.

5. The first step of the stepped-care approach in treating hypertension is:
   a. lifestyle changes.
   b. diuretics.
   c. beta-blockers.
   d. adding a second or third antihypertensive.

References/Suggested Readings

American Heart Association (AHA). (2001a). Cardiovascular disease statistics [Online]. Available: http://216.185.112.5/presenter.jhtml?identifier=4478

American Heart Association (AHA). (2001b). *2002 Heart and Stroke Statistical Update.* [Online]. Available: www.americanheart.org/downloadable/heart/101483280944 61013190090123HS_State_02.pdf

American Heart Association (AHA). (2001c). Rheumatic heart disease statistics [Online]. Available: http://216.185.112.5/presenter.jhtml?identifier=4712

American Heart Association (AHA). (2001d). Women, heart disease and stroke statistics [Online]. Available: http://216.185.112.5/presenter.jhtml?identifier=4787

Ammon, S. (2001). Managing patients with heart failure. *AJN, 101*(12), 34–40.

Baker, S., & Graziano, J. (2003). A new device for heart failure. *RN, 66*(3), 32–35.

Beattie, S. (1999). Cut the risks for cardio cath patients. *RN, 62*(1), 50–54.

Beattie, S. (2002). New biomarkers may predict CAD. *RN, 65*(9), 47–54.

Bither, C., & Apple, S. (2001). Home management of the failing heart. *AJN, 101*(12), 41–45.

Bond, E., Nelson, K., Germany, C., & Smart, A. (2003). The left ventricular assist device. *AJN, 103*(1), 32–39.

Breen, P. (2000). DVT: What every nurse should know. *RN, 63*(4), 58–62.

Bubien, R. (2000). A new beat on an old rhythm. *AJN, 100*(1), 42–50.

Carelock, J., & Clark, A. (2001). Heart failure: Pathophysiologic mechanisms. *AJN, 101*(12), 26–33.

Centers for Disease Control and Prevention (CDC). (2002). *Health, United States 2002,* [Online]. Available: www.cdc.gov/nchs/data/hus/tables/2002/02hus068.pdf

Chase, S. (2000). Hypertensive crisis. *RN, 63*(6), 62–67.

Chavez, J., & Brewer, C. (2002). Stopping the shock slide. *RN, 65*(9), 30–34.

Cheek, D., & Cesan, A. (2003). What's different about heart disease in women? *Nursing2003, 33*(8), 36–42.

Corona, G. (1999). Pacemakers: Keeping the beat today. *RN, 62*(12), 50–55.

Crumlish, C., Bracken, J., Hand, M., Keenan, K., Ruggiero, H., & Simmons, D. (2000). When time is muscle. *AJN, 100*(1), 26–35.

Daniels, R. (2002). *Delmar's guide to laboratory and diagnostic tests.* Clifton Park, NY: Thomson Delmar Learning.

Darty, S., Thomas, M., Neagle, C., Link, H., Wesley-Farrington, D., and Hundley, G. (2002). Cardiovascular magnetic resonance imaging. *AJN, 102*(12), 34–37.

Davis, S. (2002). How the heart failure picture has changed. *Nursing2002, 32*(11), 36–44.

Day, M. (2003). Recognizing and managing DVT. *Nursing2003, 33*(5), 36–41.

Dochterman, J., & Bulecheck, G. (2004). *Nursing Interventions Classification (NIC)* (4th ed.). St. Louis, MO: Mosby.

Fort, C. (2002). Get pumped to prevent DVT. *Nursing2002, 32*(9), 50–52.

Freeman, J., & Hedges, C. (2003). Cardiac arrest: The effect on the brain. *AJN, 103*(6), 50–54.

Gehring, P. (April 2002). Perfecting your skills: Vascular assessment. *Travel Nursing Today* (supplement to *RN*) 16–24.

George, E., & Tasota, F. (2003). Predicting heart disease with C-reactive protein. *Nursing2003, 33*(5), 70–71.

Goldrick, B. (2003). Endocarditis associated with body piercing. *AJN, 103*(1), 26–27.

Goodreau, L. (2003). Coronary stenting—with a twist. *RN, 66*(1), 32–36.

Granger, B., & Miller, C. (2001). Acute coronary syndrome. *Nursing2001, 31*(11), 36–43.

Halm, M., & Penque, S. (1999). Heart disease in women. *AJN, 99*(4), 26–31.

Hays, D. (2003). Picturing reciprocal changes in an MI. *Nursing2003, 33*(5), 53.

Hiller, G. (1999). Atrial fibrillation. *Nursing99, 29*(2), 27–31.

Hurley, M. (2003). The latest hypertension guidelines. *RN, 66*(8), 43–45.

Joint National Committee on Prevention, Detection, Evaluation, and Treatment of High Blood Pressure. (2003). *The Seventh Report of the Joint National Committee on Prevention, Detection, Evaluation, and Treatment of High Blood Pressure* [Online]. Available: www.nhlbi.nih.gov/guidelines/hypertension/index.htm

Kowalczyk, T. (2002). A low-tech approach to venous congestion. *RN, 65*(10), 26–30.

Lazzara, D. (1999). Shocking facts about semiautomatic defibrillation. *Nursing99, 29*(4), 55–57.

Lewis, A. M. (1999). Cardiovascular emergency. *Nursing99, 29*(6), 49–51.

Lewis, S., Heitkemper, M., & Dirksen, S. (2004). *Medical–surgical nursing: Assessment and management of clinical problems* (6th ed.). St. Louis, MO: Mosby.

Linton, A., Matteson, M. A., & Maebius, N. K. (2000). *Introductory nursing care of adults* (2nd ed.). Philadelphia: W. B. Saunders.

Macklin, D. (2003). Phlebitis. *AJN, 103*(2), 55–60.

Malacaria, B., & Feloney, C. (2003). Going with the flow of anticoagulant therapy. *Nursing2003, 33*(3), 36–42.

Mancini, M. E., & Kaye, W. (1999). AEDs: Changing the way you respond to cardiac arrest. *AJN, 99*(5), 26–30.

Marcolongo, E. (2003). Isolated systolic hypertension—not your usual silent killer. *Nursing2003, 33*(1), 32hn1–32hn3.

Martin, T. (2002). How heart failure complicates care. *Nursing2002, 32*(7), 32hn1–32hn5.

Mayo Clinic (2002). *Aneurysms.* [Online]. Available: www.mayoclinic.com/findinformation./invoke.cfm?objectid=FE3FE459-7DIE-405F-95E9339CD2E974B

McAvoy, J. (2000). Cardiac pain: Discovering the unexpected. *Nursing2000, 30*(3), 34–39.

McConnell, E. (2002a). Applying antiembolism stockings. *Nursing2002, 32*(4), 17.

McConnell, E. (2002b). Using an automated external defibrillator. *Nursing2002, 32*(10), 18.

McCormick, J., & Deeg, M. (2000). Pharmacologic treatment of dyslipidemia. *AJN, 100*(2), 55–60.

McGrath, A. (1997). Clinical snapshot: Raynaud's syndrome. *AJN, 97*(1), 34–35.

McKinney, B. (1999). Solving the puzzle of heart failure. *Nursing99, 29*(5), 33–39.

Metules, T. (1999). Cardiac tamponade. *RN, 62*(12), 26–31.

Metules, T. (2003). IABP therapy: Getting patients treatment fast. *RN, 66*(5), 56–62.

Miracle, V. (2001a). Act fast during a hypertensive crisis. *Nursing2001, 31*(9), 50–51.

Miracle, V. (2001b). Putting the brakes on pericarditis. *Nursing2001, 31*(4), 44–45.

Moorhead, S., Johnson, M., & Maas, M., (2004). *Nursing Outcomes Classification (NOC)* (3rd ed.). St. Louis, MO: Mosby.

Mosley, M., Oenning, V., & Melinik, G. (1999). Methemoglobinemia. *AJN, 99*(5), 47.

Nagle, B., & Nee, C. (2002). Acute myocardial infarction. *Nursing2002, 32*(10), 50–54.

National Institute of Arthritis and Musculoskeletal and Skin Diseases (NIAMS). (2002). *Questions and answers about Raynaud's phenomenon.* [Online]. Available: www.niams.nih.gov/hi/topics/raynaud/ar125fs.htm

National Institutes of Health (NIH). (2002). *New Recommendations to Prevent High Blood Pressure Issues* [Online]. Available: www.nhlbi.nih.gov/news/press/02-10-15.htm

Oliver-McNeil, S. (2001). Treating hypertrophic cardiomyopathy without surgery. *Nursing2001, 31*(2), 32cc1–32cc4.

Palatnik, A. (2001). How cardiac drugs do what they do. *Nursing2001, 31*(5), 54–60.

Pope, B. (2002). Heart failure. *Nursing2002, 32*(8), 50–51.

Pope, W. (2002). Angioplasty & stenting in the carotid? *RN, 65*(6), 54–59.

Raynaud's Association. (2001). *About Raynaud's Phenomenon* [Online]. Available: www.raynauds.org/pages/raynaud.htm

Reger, T., & Vargas, G. (1999). The return of the radial artery in CABG. *AJN, 99*(9), 26–30.

Ross, G. K., & DeJong, M. J. (1999). Pericardial tamponade. *AJN, 99*(2), 35.

Ryan, D. (2000). Is it an MI? A lab primer. *RN, 63*(1), 26–30.

Shaffer, R. (2002). ICD therapy: The patient's perspective. *AJN, 102*(2), 46–49.

Sims, J., & Miracle, V. (2001). Getting the lowdown on hypotension. *Nursing2001, 31*(10), 56–57.

Siomko, A. (2000). Demystifying cardiac markers. *AJN, 100*(1), 36–40.

Spratto, G., & Woods, A. (2004). *2004 PDR Nurse's Drug Handbook.* Clifton Park, NY: Thomson Delmar Learning.

Willis, K. (2001). Gaining perspective on peripheral vascular disease. *Nursing2001, 31*(2), 32hn1–32hn4.

Woods, A. D. (1999). Managing hypertension. *Nursing99, 29*(3), 41–46.

Woods, A. (2001). Improving the odds against hypertension. *Nursing2001, 31*(8), 36–41.

Woods, A. (2002). High blood pressure (hypertension). *Nursing2002, 32*(4), 54–55.

Zangerm, D., Solomon, A., & Gersh, B. (2000). Contemporary management of angina: Part II. Medical management of chronic stable angina. *American Family Physician, 61*(1), 129–138.

Resources

American Heart Association, National Center, 7272 Greenville Avenue, Dallas, TX 75231-4596, 800-242-8721, www.americanheart.org

National Cholesterol Education Program Information Center, P.O. Box 30105, Bethesda, MD 20824-0105, 301-251-1222, 301-951-3260, www.nhlbi.nih.gov

National Heart, Lung, and Blood Institute Information Center, Public Health Service, P.O. Box 30105, Bethesda, MD 20824, 301-592-8573, www.nhlbi.nih.gov

President's Council on Physical Fitness and Sports, Department W, 200 Independence Avenue S.W., Room 738-H, Washington, DC 20201, 202-690-5251, www.surgeongeneral.gov/ophs

Raynaud's Association, Inc., 94 Mercer Avenue, Hartsdale, NY 10530, 914-682-8341, www.raynauds.org

The Coronary Club, Inc., 9500 Euclid Avenue, Suite EE37, Cleveland, OH 44195, 216-444-3690

The Mended Hearts, Inc., 7272 Greenville Avenue, Dallas, TX 75231, 214-706-1442, www.mendedhearts.org

HEMATOLOGIC AND LYMPHATIC SYSTEMS

MAKING THE CONNECTION

Refer to the following chapters to increase your understanding of the hematologic and lymphatic systems:

Basic Nursing
- **Fluid, Electrolyte, and Acid–Base Balance**
- **Assessment**
- **Pain Management**

Adult Health Nursing
- **Oncology**
- **Respiratory System**
- **Cardiovascular System**
- **Immune System**
- **Endocrine System**

Basic Procedures
- **Hand Hygiene**

Intermediate Procedure
- **Administering an Intramuscular Injection (Z-track technique)**

Advanced Procedures
- **Initiating Strict Isolation Precautions**

Review: Delmar's Anatomy & Physiology CD-ROM: Lymphatic System

LEARNING OBJECTIVES

Upon completion of this chapter, you should be able to:
- **Define key terms.**
- **Relate anatomy and physiology of the blood and lymph systems to disease processes.**
- **Relate diagnostic test results to the blood and lymph disorders.**
- **Describe nursing interventions in caring for clients with blood and lymph disorders.**
- **Assist in developing a nursing care plan for clients with blood and lymph disorders.**

KEY TERMS

agranulocytosis	hyperuricemia
apheresis	idiopathic
autologous	leukocytosis
bands	leukopenia
blastic phase	lymphoma
erythrocytapheresis	phlebotomy
fibrinolysis	purpura
hemarthrosis	reticulocyte
hematocrit	sickle
hematopoiesis	thrombocytopenia
hemolysis	

INTRODUCTION

The hematologic system of the body consists of blood and blood-forming organs. Blood consists of formed elements (red blood cells, white blood cells, and platelets) and plasma. As blood is pumped through the body, it carries essential substances to the tissues and removes waste products from the tissues. Disorders of the hematologic system usually result from abnormal production or functioning of the cells. Some of these disorders are the result of genetics, environment, or pathogenic organisms.

The lymph system consists of lymph vessels, nodes, and organs. Lymph vessels collect and return lymph fluid to the blood vessels through the right and left lymphatic ducts at the right and left subclavian veins. The functions of the lymph system are to assist with immunity, control edema, and absorb digested fats.

Medical management and nursing diagnoses, goals, and interventions are given for each blood and lymph disorder. It is important to have a complete understanding of the blood and lymph disorders when providing nursing care to clients.

ANATOMY AND PHYSIOLOGY REVIEW

The blood and lymphatic systems are discussed following.

Blood

The heart pumps 5 to 6 liters of blood per minute through the circulatory system of an adult. Blood is an aqueous mixture consisting of plasma and cells (Figure 34-1).

Plasma

Plasma is a straw-colored liquid consisting of approximately 90% water and 10% proteins. The water component assists in transporting body nutrients, hormones, antibodies, electrolytes, and waste; regulating blood volume; and controlling body temperature. The proteins are albumin, globulins, and fibrinogen. Albumin controls the volume of the blood and blood pressure by osmotic pressure that pulls tissue fluid into the capillary system. There are three types of globulins: alpha, beta, and gamma. Alpha and beta globulins are secreted by the liver and are carrier molecules for substances. Gamma globulins are antibodies important in the immune response of the body. Fibrinogen changes into fibrin, a solid, that controls bleeding in the blood-clotting mechanism of the body. The formed elements in plasma are red blood cells (RBCs), white blood cells (WBCs), and platelets.

Red blood cells   Platelets

Granular leukocytes (granulocytes)

Eosinophils   Basophils   Neutrophils

Nongranular leukocytes (agranulocytes)

Lymphocytes   Monocytes

Granular and nongranular white blood cells

Figure 34-1 *The Cells in Blood:* **A,** *Red Blood Cells (erythrocytes);* **B,** *Platelets (thrombocytes);* **C,** *White Blood Cells (leukocytes)*

Red Blood Cells

Red blood cells, also called erythrocytes, are the most numerous blood cells in the body, generally 4.5 to 6.1 million/mm³ in an adult. RBCs are biconcave disks that do not have a nucleus. They are about the size of the smallest capillary but are flexible and capable of changing shape so they can squeeze through the capillaries.

RBCs, in conjunction with the respiratory and circulatory systems, oxygenate body tissues. In the capillary bed of the alveoli, blood receives oxygen (O_2), and carbon dioxide (CO_2) is eliminated. The O_2-enriched RBCs (oxyhemoglobin) carry O_2 to systemic capillaries, where O_2 is exchanged for CO_2. The carbon dioxide–laden blood then returns the CO_2 to the alveoli in the lungs, where it is again exchanged for oxygen. The CO_2 is exhaled from the body with each breath. Hemoglobin is a protein in the RBC that carries O_2 and is responsible for the exchange of O_2 and CO_2.

The average life span for an RBC is 120 days. Blood cells originate from a single stem cell that proliferates and differentiates into lymphoid stem cells or blood stem cells (Figure 34-2). The lymphoid stem cells further divide and differentiate into T cells and B cells. The blood stem cells divide and differentiate into RBCs, WBCs, and platelets. The process of blood cell production and development is called **hematopoiesis.** RBCs are produced daily by the bone marrow according to the demand of the body. When the partial pressure of O_2 drops, a renal hormone, erythropoietin, stimulates the bone marrow to produce more immature RBCs **(reticulocytes),** which are released into the bloodstream. These reticulocytes develop into mature red blood cells. The number of circulating reticulocytes can be used as a diagnostic tool for RBC disorders.

As RBCs age, their outer membrane deteriorates and they are destroyed by large macrophages in the liver and are filtered out of the body by the spleen. The iron from heme in the old RBCs is used in the production of new RBCs.

Hematocrit is the percentage of blood cells in a volume of blood. A normal hematocrit for a female is 38% to 47% and for a male, 40% to 54% (Daniels, 2002).

White Blood Cells

White blood cells, also called leukocytes, fight infection and assist with immunity. The life span of a WBC

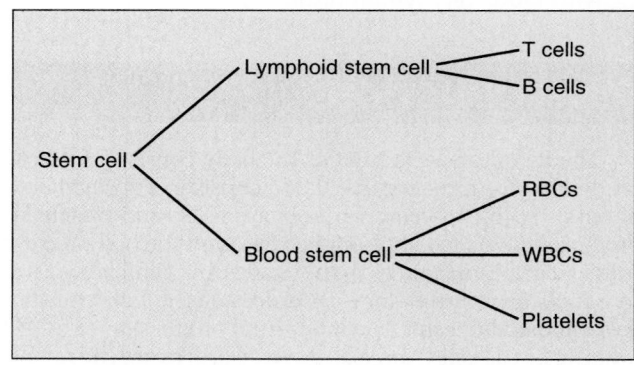

Figure 34-2 *Origin of T cells, B cells, RBCs, WBCs, and Platelets*

varies, depending on the type of WBC. Neutrophils, basophils, and eosinophils live from a few hours to days, whereas lymphocytes and monocytes live from days to years. The normal WBC count is 4,100 to 10,800/mm³ of blood (Daniels, 2002). An increased number of WBCs **(leukocytosis)** may signify the presence of an infection, inflammation, tissue necrosis, or leukemia. A decreased number of WBCs **(leukopenia)** may indicate bone marrow failure, a massive infection, dietary deficiencies, a drug toxicity, or an autoimmune disease.

WBCs are classified as granulocytes or polymorphonuclear leukocytes (PMNs, or polys), and agranulocytes. The granulocytes have granules (grainy substances) in their cytoplasm, and the agranulocytes do not have granules. Granulocytes are divided into three types: the neutrophils, eosinophils, and basophils. Agranulocytes are classified into two groups: monocytes and lymphocytes. Neutrophils are the most numerous WBCs, making up approximately 60% of the total number of WBCs. The main function of neutrophils is to digest and kill microorganisms. If a client has an acute infection, the bone marrow is stimulated to produce more neutrophils, resulting in an increased circulation of immature neutrophils called **bands.** An increased production of neutrophils indicates the presence of an acute infection. An increased number of basophils and especially of eosinophils indicates an allergic response.

Monocytes become macrophages, cells that destroy dead and injured cells and bacteria. There are two types of lymphocytes, T cells and B cells, which are involved in the body's immune response.

Platelets

Platelets (thrombocytes) are not typical cells but nonnucleated, granular ovoid, or spindle-shaped cell fragments. The normal life span of a platelet is approximately 10 days. Platelets are active in the clotting mechanism of the body. When platelets flow over a rough or damaged area in a vessel, they adhere to the area and release thromboplastin and clotting factors that start the blood-clotting process. They also secrete prostaglandins and serotonin, which cause the vessel to constrict, thereby decreasing the blood flow through the area. Prothrombin, thromboplastin, and calcium ions form thrombin, which joins with fibrinogen to form fibrin. The fibrin strands seal the opening or area, and a clot is formed (Figure 34-3).

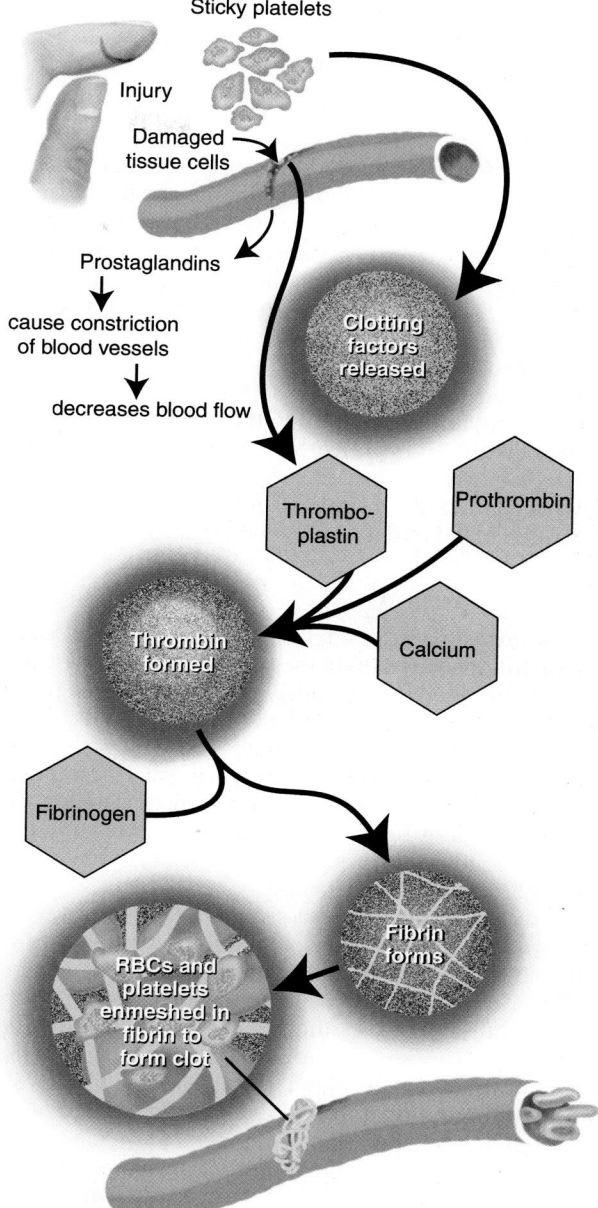

Figure 34-3 *The Process of Clot Formation*

Blood Types

Genetically determined antigens called agglutinogens are located on the surface of RBC membranes. The A and B antigens constitute the ABO blood group. If the A antigen is on the RBC membrane, the client has type A blood. If the B antigen is on the RBC membrane, the client has type B blood. If both an A and a B antigen are present, the client has type AB blood, and if no antigen is present, the client has type O blood.

Type A blood has anti-B antibodies in the serum, and type B blood has anti-A antibodies. If a person with type A blood receives type B blood during a transfusion, the anti-B antibodies will attack the infused RBCs and hemolyze (destroy) them. The hemoglobin released when these cells are hemolyzed can lead to kidney damage.

A person with AB blood has neither anti-A nor anti-B antibodies in the serum. People with AB blood are theoretically universal recipients because they can receive blood from all blood types. Type O blood has no antigens that the antibodies can attack. Persons with type O blood can theoretically give blood to persons having any type of blood. Persons with type O blood are called universal donors. The terms *universal recipient* and *universal donor* are only theoretical because during blood transfusions, blood incompatibilities can occur because of other types of antigens.

There are 14 different blood groups and more than 100 different antigens. The different blood groups vary in number with different ethnic groups.

Rh Factor

Another factor to consider during blood transfusions is the Rh factor. Persons who have Rh antigens (the D antigen) are Rh positive. Those who do not have Rh antigens on their RBC membranes are Rh negative. Approximately 85% of Caucasian people have Rh-positive blood and 15% have Rh-negative blood. The African-American population has 93% and 7%, respectively (Daniels, 2002).

If a person with Rh-negative blood is exposed to Rh-positive blood during a blood transfusion or during childbirth, anti-Rh antibodies form in the blood serum. When a person with Rh-negative blood is exposed a second time to Rh-positive blood, the anti-Rh antibodies will react with the Rh-positive blood and cause hemolysis of the infused blood and a severe blood reaction.

Blood Transfusions

Blood transfusions are given to replace needed blood components because of hemorrhage, anemia, clotting disorders, or blood deficiencies. Transfusable blood products are whole blood, packed red cells, platelets, fresh frozen plasma, and cryoprecipitate. Whole blood is given to increase blood volume and the various blood components. Packed red cells are given for anemia. Platelets assist in controlling bleeding. Fresh frozen plasma is administered for clotting disorders. Cryoprecipitate corrects fibrinogen deficiencies.

Before blood products are given, the lab does a type and crossmatch to check compatibility between the donor's blood type and Rh factor and the client's blood type and Rh factor. The lab also checks all blood products for HIV and hepatitis B and C viruses. Blood must be handled gently so as not to damage the cells. Administration of the blood should begin within 30 minutes of obtaining it from the laboratory refrigerator.

Take baseline vital signs—temperature, pulse, and blood pressure—before administering the blood product. Once the transfusion is started, temperature and pulse are measured after 15 minutes, 30 minutes, and then hourly; blood pressure is measured hourly during the transfusion. Blood is generally administered through a peripheral vein using an 18- or 19-gauge cannula. A large cannula is used so the blood cells do not break when passing through the cannula.

Before the transfusion, two nurses check the compatibility of the blood product with the client's blood. The first 50 cc is given within 5 to 10 minutes. The client is observed closely for a hemolytic blood reaction during this time. If a client experiences any symptoms of a reaction, the infusion must be stopped immediately and the physician notified. Follow institutional protocol.

A blood transfusion should be completed within 4 hours of the start of administration. No medications should be given at the blood administration site during infusion. The only solution given during a blood transfusion is 0.9% sodium chloride to prevent clotting.

Autologous Transfusion If time and the client's condition permit, **autologous** ("from self") blood as opposed to homologous ("from a donor") blood is collected and saved for the client. This may be used for elective surgeries. An alternate procedure is to recover the blood lost during surgery and transfuse it back into the client. The use of autologous blood eliminates the possibility of a transfusion reaction and prevents the transmission of disease.

Lymphatic System

The lymphatic, or lymph, system is a separate vessel system. The two main functions of the lymph system are to transport excess fluid from the interstitial spaces to the circulatory system and to protect the body against infectious organisms.

Lymph Fluid and Vessels

Lymph fluid is pale yellow. Fluid and substances move from the plasma through the capillary walls and become interstitial fluid (Figure 34-4). As fluid accumulates in the interstitial space, pressure within the interstitial

Figure 34-4 *Flow of Fluid from the Blood into the Lymphatic System*

CULTURAL CONSIDERATIONS

Jehovah's Witnesses and Blood

- Many Jehovah's Witnesses will agree to autologous blood transfusions.
- Some Jehovah's Witnesses will allow the use of certain blood volume expanders and will carry a card identifying the expanders to be used.

space increases. The interstitial fluid then diffuses through the lymphatic vessel wall into the lymph vessel.

Semilunar valves in the lymphatic vessels assist the lymph system in returning the interstitial fluid, which is now called lymph, to the venous system. When the valves do not work properly or the vessels become obstructed, edema occurs. The pumping action or contractions of the skeletal muscles and the rhythmic action of the respiratory muscles assist in the movement of the lymph toward the subclavian veins. The right lymphatic duct drains lymph from the right side of the head, neck, thorax, and arm into the right subclavian vein. The lymph from the rest of the body drains into the left subclavian vein through the thoracic duct.

Lymph Nodes

Lymph nodes are scattered throughout the body along the lymph vessels (Figure 34-5) and contain dense patches of lymphocytes and macrophages. Lymphocytes act against such foreign particles as viruses and bacteria. Macrophages ingest and destroy foreign substances, damaged cells, and cellular debris. The superficial lymph nodes in the neck, axilla, and groin can be palpated, especially when infected and swollen. The tonsils in the pharynx and Peyer's patch in the mucosal lining of the ileum are located deeper within the body and cannot be palpated.

As lymph is collected from body tissues, cancer cells may enter the lymphatic system and escape into the cir-

culation or to other body tissues, such as the lungs. Wherever the cancer cells collect, more cancer cells may be produced. In this way, cancer can spread to other body parts. Lymph nodes are biopsied to check for the spread of cancer.

Lymph Organs

The spleen and thymus are lymph organs. The spleen removes old RBCs, platelets, and microorganisms from the blood. Approximately 350 mL of blood are stored in the spleen and approximately 200 mL can be pumped out within a minute into the body as needed (Thibodeau & Patton, 1999). During an infection, the spleen enlarges to produce and release monocytes and lymphocytes. Lymphocytes in the lymph tissue differentiate into T lymphocytes (T cells) and B lymphocytes (B cells).

In infancy and childhood, the thymus gland is large but decreases in size with age. In advanced age, it is replaced with fat and connective tissue. The thymus performs an important role in the special processing and proper functioning of the thymus-derived T lymphocytes (T cells). The T cells are actively involved in immunity.

ASSESSMENT

Information is based on client report, physical examination, and diagnostic tests.

Subjective Data

Biological and demographic data, including age, sex, ethnic background, and race, are important for many hematologic problems. Inquire about the client's occupation and hobbies because there may be exposure to radiation or chemicals. Past military experience is also important because some military personnel have been exposed to toxic chemicals. Obtain a medication history, including prescription and over-the-counter medications. Note recent or recurring infections, night sweats, palpitations, bleeding problems, previous blood transfusions, and any complications.

Assess neurological functioning by asking if the client has experienced any cognitive or mental difficulties or numbness and tingling of the extremities. A headache may indicate a low erythrocyte count or intracranial bleeding. Note hearing or vision difficulties.

Ask about past surgeries and any complications from surgeries; if the client has had a duodenal, gastric, or ileal resection, the absorption of iron and vitamin B_{12} may be affected. Alcohol use may affect vitamin intake and is caustic to the GI tract. Ask about the presence of blood in the stool or urine and any anorexia, nausea, vomiting, oral discomfort, or problems with taste perception. A diet history is helpful when reviewing the erythrocyte level. Inquire if the client has difficulty accomplishing ADLs because of decreased energy.

Objective Data

Begin by obtaining the client's height, weight, and vital signs. An elevated temperature may indicate an infection. Note recent weight gains or losses.

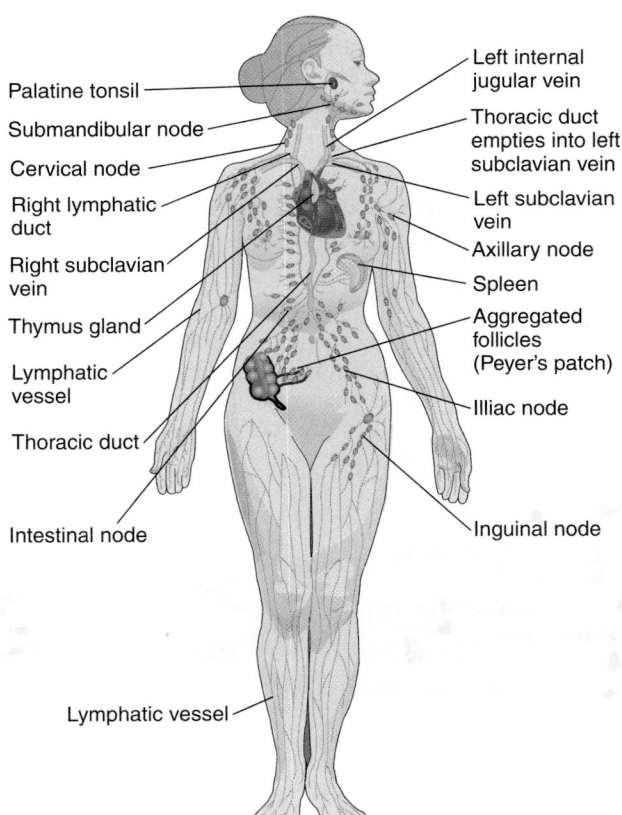

Palatine tonsil
Submandibular node
Cervical node
Right lymphatic duct
Right subclavian vein
Thymus gland
Lymphatic vessel
Thoracic duct
Intestinal node
Lymphatic vessel

Left internal jugular vein
Thoracic duct empties into left subclavian vein
Left subclavian vein
Axillary node
Spleen
Aggregated follicles (Peyer's patch)
Illiac node
Inguinal node

Figure 34-5 *The Lymphatic System*

Laboratory tests are very important when assessing the hematologic and lymphatic systems. It is important to compare past and present laboratory results.

Palpate the lymph nodes in the neck, axillae, and groin; normal findings include small (0.5–1.0 cm) nodes that are freely movable, firm, and nontender. Tender nodes indicate inflammation. Hard, fixed nodes may be malignant.

Next, inspect the skin and extremities for petechiae, bruises, lesions, and brittle nails. Check urine and stool for blood. Note dyspnea, an enlarged abdomen, or swollen joints.

COMMON DIAGNOSTIC TESTS

Commonly used diagnostic tests for clients with symptoms of blood and lymph system disorders are listed in Table 34-1.

TABLE 34-1   **COMMON DIAGNOSTIC TESTS FOR BLOOD AND LYMPHATIC SYSTEM DISORDERS**

Partial thromboplastin time (PTT)
Activated partial thromboplastin time (APTT)
Bleeding time
Blood culture and sensitivity
Coombs' test (direct antiglobulin test)
D dimer test
(Fragment D-dimer, Fibrin degradation fragment)
Erythrocyte sedimentation rate (sed rate, ESR)
Folic acid (Folate level)
Hematocrit (Hct)
Hemoglobin (Hgb)
Hemoglobin electrophoresis
Platelet count
Prothrombin time (PT, Protime)
Red blood cells (RBCs)
Schilling test
Sickledex (Sickle cell test)
Total iron binding capacity (TIBC)
White blood cells (WBCs)
 Differential count
 Granulocytes
  Basophils
  Eosinophils
  Neutrophils
  Bands
 Agranulocytes
  Lymphocytes
  Monocytes
Bone marrow aspiration
Gastric analysis, tube and tubeless test
Radiologic lymphangiogram

RED BLOOD CELL DISORDERS

Red blood cell disorders discussed in this section are anemias and polycythemia vera. The nursing process for anemias is presented after the discussion of sickle-cell anemia because the nursing diagnoses, goals, and interventions are similar for all anemias.

Anemia is a common hematopoietic disorder in which the client has a decreased number of RBCs and a low hemoglobin level. The causes for anemia are a decreased production of RBCs, an increased destruction of RBCs, or a loss of blood. The types of anemia discussed in this section are iron-deficiency anemia, hypoplastic (aplastic) anemia, pernicious anemia, acquired hemolytic anemia, and sickle-cell anemia.

IRON-DEFICIENCY ANEMIA

Iron-deficiency anemia is the most common type of anemia and occurs when the body does not have enough iron to synthesize functional Hgb. The decrease in iron may be caused by dietary deficiency, but the most common cause is a slow, chronic blood loss such as GI bleeding, which generally has no symptoms (Holcomb, 2001). Decreased iron absorption, menstruating women, or an increased need for iron such as during growth periods or pregnancy are also causes. Iron-deficiency anemia is more frequently found in premature or low-birthweight infants, adolescent girls, alcoholics, and the elderly. The symptoms are fatigue, palpitations, tachycardia, exertional dyspnea, and pallor. Clients with chronic anemia may have pica, stomatitis, glossitis, and brittle hair. Diagnostic tests would reveal decreased RBCs, a low Hgb level, a low Hct, a low serum iron, and a high total iron-binding capacity (TIBC).

Medical–Surgical Management

Pharmacological

An oral iron preparation, usually ferrous sulfate (Feosol) is ordered. These preparations are not given with food or milk because they interfere with iron absorption. The administration of iron with orange juice or vitamin C–rich drinks increases iron absorption. Iron dextran (Infed), an intramuscular iron preparation, is given by Z-track technique.

Diet

A diet high in iron is encouraged. Foods rich in iron are red meats, fish, raisins, apricots, dried fruits, dark green vegetables, dried beans, eggs, and iron-enriched whole-grain breads. An increase of vitamin C in the diet assists in the absorption of iron. If the client has a loss of appetite, small frequent snacks may be tolerated better than three large meals.

Activity

Daily activities should be spaced to provide rest periods between times of exercise.

CRITICAL THINKING

Iron-Deficiency Anemia

How are the symptoms of iron-deficiency anemia related to a decreased red blood cell count and decreased hemoglobin?

APLASTIC ANEMIA — *chemical*

When the bone marrow stops making enough blood cells, the client has aplastic anemia. Reduced production of RBCs results in anemia, of WBCs results in infections, and of platelets results in bleeding. In most cases the cause is unknown, but genetic factors are suspected. Other suspected causes include exposure to viruses, chemicals (benzene or airplane glue), radiation, or medications. Some medications that cause aplastic anemia are chloramphenicol (Chloromycetin), mephenytoin (Mesantoin), trimethadione (Tridione), mechlorethamine or nitrogen mustard (Mustargen), methotrexate (Folex PFS), 6-mercaptopurine or 6-MP (Purinethol), and phenylbutazone (Butazolidin). Symptoms include fatigue, weakness, palpitations, headaches, fever, mouth ulcers, petechiae, gingival bleeding, and epistaxis. These clients are extremely ill. Diagnosis is confirmed by a bone marrow aspiration.

Medical–Surgical Management

Medical

The cause of aplastic anemia is removed if possible. Immunosuppressive therapy with antithymocyte globulin or ATG (Atgam) and cyclosporine is given to suppress the reaction causing the aplastic anemia and to allow the client's bone marrow to recover. A client who has a good response will improve in 3 to 6 months. The response rate is 70% to 80% (Aplastic Anemia & MDS International Foundation, 2002). Transfusions of packed red cells and platelets may be given.

Surgical

A bone marrow transplant is done if the client's bone marrow fails to respond to treatment. Cyclosporine (Sandimmune), an immunosuppressant, is given for a bone marrow transplant to decrease the graft rejection. The best response occurs in a young client who has not previously had a transfusion because transfusions increase bone marrow graft rejection. Bone marrow transplants from a human leukocyte antigen- (HLA-) matched sibling donor is the treatment of choice for clients younger than 30 years of age. The treatment of choice for an older adult or a client who does not have an HLA-matched sibling donor is immunosuppression with ATG and cyclosporine. (Bone marrow transplants are discussed in the section on acute myelocytic leukemia.)

Pharmacological

Infections are treated with antibiotics. Steroids and androgens are also sometimes used to stimulate the bone marrow.

PERNICIOUS ANEMIA *lack of intrinsic factor*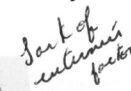

The parietal cells of the gastric mucosa secrete a protein intrinsic factor that is essential for the proper absorption of vitamin B_{12}. The lack of intrinsic factor may be an autoimmune malfunction (Holcomb, 2001). Without the secretion of the intrinsic factor, vitamin B_{12} cannot be absorbed in the distal portion of the ileum.

The onset of the disease occurs around the age of 60. Pernicious anemia occurs most frequently in women of Northern European descent and some African Americans. Pernicious anemia can occur in clients who have had a gastrectomy with the section of the stomach removed that secretes the intrinsic factor. A gastric analysis and Schilling test are confirming diagnostic tests.

Pernicious anemia has an insidious onset because the body can store 3 to 5 years' worth of vitamin B_{12} in the liver. Neurologic changes, paresthesia, and numbness may occur before lab tests identify vitamin B_{12} deficiency (Holcomb, 2001). Symptoms include extreme weakness, a sore tongue, edema of the legs, ataxia, dizziness, dyspnea, headache, fever, blurred vision, tinnitus, jaundice with pallor, poor memory, irritability, and loss of bladder and bowel control. The client may have decreased sensitivity to heat and pain because of neurological involvement. Clients with pernicious anemia are highly susceptible to gastric carcinoma and should be monitored closely for symptoms.

Medical–Surgical Management

Pharmacological

Topical anesthetics are given to relieve oral discomfort during the acute phase of the disease. Vitamin B_{12}, cyanocobalamin crystalline (Rubesol-1000) is given IM until the Hct returns to normal. Then it is given monthly for the rest of the client's life. The frequency of administration will depend on the client's symptoms and response to the medication. Oral administration of vitamin B_{12} is not effective because vitamin B_{12} cannot be absorbed without the intrinsic factor. Folic acid or folate (Folvite) may be prescribed. Encourage the client to increase folic acid in the diet by eating green leafy vegetables, meat, fish, legumes, and whole grains. Iron is usually not prescribed because once the condition is corrected with regular administration of cyanocobalamin, erythrocytes are produced and the Hgb and Hct return to normal.

ACQUIRED HEMOLYTIC ANEMIA

In hemolytic anemias, **hemolysis,** or destruction of RBCs, occurs, and iron and hemoglobin are released.

PROFESSIONAL TIP

Vitamin B_{12} Deficiency

Strict vegetarians are at risk for vitamin B_{12} deficiency. A dietary supplement of Vitamin B_{12} is the treatment.

Several causes for acquired hemolytic anemia are an autoimmune reaction, radiation, blood transfusion, chemicals, arsenic, lead, or medications. Sulfisoxazole (Gantrisin), penicillin, and methyldopa (Aldomet) are medications that can cause hemolysis. A substance produced by the bacterium *Clostridium perfringens* can also cause hemolysis. Symptoms may go unnoticed, or there may be a severe reaction. Symptoms are mild fatigue and pallor. More severe symptoms include jaundice, palpitations, hypotension, dyspnea, and back and joint pain. Diagnostic tests reveal a low Hgb and Hct and an elevated LDH. LDH is an enzyme in the heart, liver, kidneys, skeletal muscle, brain, red blood cells, and lungs. As these tissues are damaged, LDH is released into the bloodstream, causing an elevated LDH.

Medical–Surgical Management

Medical

Treatment is aimed at removing the cause, if possible. The client may be given blood transfusions or **erythrocytapheresis** (a procedure that removes abnormal RBCs and replaces them with healthy RBCs).

Surgical

The function of the spleen is to destroy RBCs. In severe cases of hemolytic anemia, a splenectomy may be done in an attempt to stop the destruction of RBCs.

Pharmacological

Corticosteroids are administered to decrease the autoimmune response. Folic acid may also be given to increase the production of RBCs.

SICKLE-CELL ANEMIA (INHERITED HEMOLYTIC ANEMIA)

Sickle-cell anemia is also known as inherited hemolytic anemia or sickle-cell disease. This genetic disorder has abnormal hemoglobin S rather than hemoglobin A in the RBCs. Sickle-cell anemia is caused by a recessive gene or genes that are passed through the generations (Figure 34-6). The client with one s gene has sickle-cell trait (Hb sA) and is asymptomatic but is a carrier of the disease. The client with sickle-cell anemia has two s genes (Hb ss) and manifests symptoms.

The condition occurs most frequently in African Americans, with an estimated 1,000 babies born with sickle-cell disease each year in the United States (SCDAA, 2002). It also occurs in persons from Asia Minor, India, and the Mediterranean and Caribbean areas.

Sickle-cell tests are done on infants to diagnose sickle-cell trait or disease. A screening test to detect the presence of Hb S is Sickledex or sickle-cell test. If Hb S is present, a hemoglobin electrophoresis is done to distinguish between sickle-cell trait and sickle-cell disease. If the hemoglobin electrophoresis test is negative, the client has the sickle-cell trait and not sickle-cell disease.

Situations that precipitate sickle-cell crisis are dehydration, deoxygenation, acidosis, and temperature

Figure 34-6 *Inheritance of the Sickle-Cell Trait and Sickle-Cell Anemia*

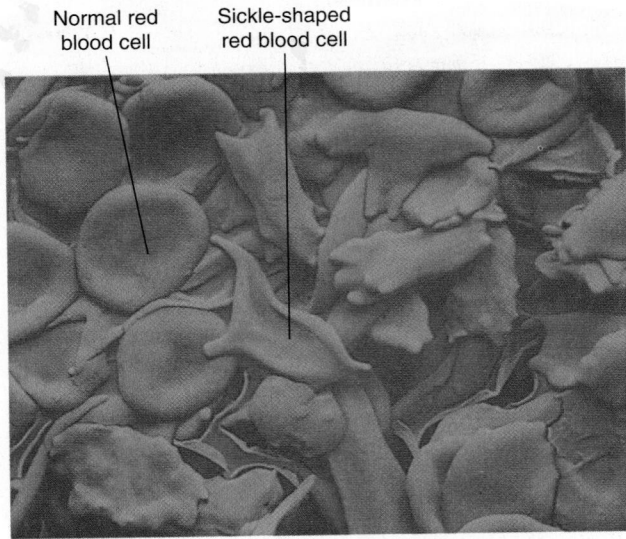

Figure 34-7 *Blood cells magnified through a scanning electron microscope show normal and sickle-shaped red blood cells. (Courtesy of Phillips Electronic Instruments Company.)*

changes (Platt, Beasley, Miller, & Eckman, 2002). In these situations crystallization of hemoglobin is promoted, which forces the RBCs to **sickle** become crescent-shaped and elongated and obstruct vessels, especially capillaries (Figure 34-7) (Platt et al., 2002). The area normally supplied by these obstructed blood vessels becomes infarcted and ischemic. The destruction of sickled RBCs in 12 to 15 days causes chronic anemia; the heart enlarges in an attempt to circulate more blood for adequate oxygenation of body tissues. Other symptoms include fatigue, jaundice, chronic leg ulcers, tachypnea, dyspnea, and arrhythmias. When the client experiences a sickle-cell crisis, there is fever, severe pain, and loss of

CLIENT TEACHING

Sickle-Cell Anemia

- Encourage client to avoid high altitudes and nonpressurized airplanes.
- Encourage adequate fluid intake because dehydration causes a sickle-cell crisis.
- Treat all infections promptly.
- Client should avoid tight-fitting, restrictive clothing, and strenuous exercise, smoking, and cold temperatures.
- Encourage client to receive yearly flu vaccine and pneumococcal vaccine.

CRITICAL THINKING

Anemias

Compare the etiologies and symptoms of iron-deficiency anemia, aplastic anemia, pernicious anemia, acquired hemolytic anemia, and sickle-cell anemia.

blood supply to various organs because of obstructed vessels. Areas most frequently affected are the joints, bone, brain, lungs, liver, kidneys, and penis. Joints become painful, swollen, and immobile. The client may experience cerebrovascular accidents, renal failure, pulmonary infarction, shock, and priapism (a continuous, painful erection).

It is important to assess extremity circulation frequently by doing capillary refill, peripheral pulses, and temperature. Application of warm compresses to painful areas relieves pain. Encourage the client to avoid restrictive clothing and anything that may restrict circulation. It is important for clients to avoid high altitudes and have adequate fluid intake.

Medical–Surgical Management

Medical

Infections are treated promptly with antibiotics. Large amounts of oral and intravenous fluids (3–5 L/day) are given to remove the by-products of broken RBCs. Oxygen is administered based on ABGs to combat deoxygenation. Skin grafting may be necessary for chronic leg ulcers.

Genetic counseling is recommended for clients with sickle-cell trait and sickle-cell anemia. There may be more openness to counseling if the counselor is from the same community as the client.

Pharmacological

Hydroxyurea (Droxia) reduces the frequency of painful crisis and the need for blood transfusions in adults (Spratto & Woods, 2004). Folic acid or folate (Folvite) is administered daily to assist in the production

of RBCs. Pentoxifylline (Trental) reduces blood viscosity and increases RBC flexibility. Blood transfusions may be given during a crisis.

Patient-controlled analgesia (PCA) with morphine is effective during a crisis. The client is progressed from narcotics to nonnarcotic analgesics as indicated.

Nursing Management

Assess weight, vital signs, apical and peripheral pulses, breath sounds, color, abdominal tenderness, and signs of bruising or jaundice. Review client's history for possible familial illnesses. Encourage client to follow treatment regimen. Monitor laboratory test results. Administer blood products as ordered and monitor for a possible reaction.

NURSING PROCESS

Assessment

Subjective Data

Obtain a history of the client's medical problems, including a history of familial hematopoietic illnesses. Some anemias may be caused by drugs and environmental conditions, so information about medications taken and about environmental situations at work and in recreational settings is important. The client should be asked about fatigue, dyspnea with exertion, palpitations, dizziness, pain, petechiae, tingling and numbness in the extremities, blurred vision, and oral discomfort.

Objective Data

The client's weight and vital signs; apical pulse and peripheral pulses; breath sounds; sensation and movement in the extremities; abdominal tenderness; and edema, pallor, and signs of bruising or jaundice must all be assessed. A thorough assessment of the cardiac system is completed because severe anemia can cause cardiac enlargement and arrhythmias.

Nursing diagnoses for a client with decreased erythrocytes and hemoglobin may include the following:

Nursing Diagnoses	Planning/Goals	Nursing Interventions
Deficient Knowledge related to prescribed treatment regimen	The client will relate the prescribed treatment regimen.	Teach the cause of the particular type of anemia and, if possible, ways to avoid the occurrence of that anemia in the future.

continues

Nursing Diagnoses	Planning/Goals	Nursing Interventions
		For iron-deficiency anemia, teach the importance of taking iron and increasing iron in the diet.
		Instruct clients with pernicious anemia to obtain a vitamin B_{12} injection at regularly scheduled times.
		Teach clients with hemolytic anemias the significance of following the prescribed regimens.
*A*ctivity intolerance related to imbalance between oxygen supply and demand.	The client will increasingly tolerate activity.	Assist the client as needed with activities of daily living.
		Teach the client the importance of alternating periods of rest with activity.
Ineffective *T*issue Perfusion (Peripheral) related to a decreased hemoglobin concentration in the blood.	The client will have increased tissue perfusion.	Administer oxygen as needed to relieve symptoms of dyspnea.
		Monitor Hgb, Hct, RBCs, ABGs, electrolytes, vital signs, and mental alertness.
		Monitor for symptoms of obstructed vessels such as pain, leg ulcerations, abdominal tenderness, dyspnea, confusion, and blurred vision.
		Administer blood products as ordered and monitor the client closely after blood transfusions for possible reactions such as chills, fever, dyspnea, pruritus, wheezing, and pain in the lumbar region.

Evaluation Each goal must be evaluated to determine how it has been met by the client.

SAMPLE NURSING CARE PLAN

THE CLIENT WITH SICKLE-CELL ANEMIA

Reggie Thompson, a 19-year-old African American, was diagnosed with sickle-cell anemia 5 years ago. Reggie works for a computer company and has been working 12-hour days to get a system installed. He has felt fatigued lately and decided to relax by playing golf on a warm Saturday morning. After the seventh hole, Reggie experienced dyspnea and tingling and numbness in his legs. After the next hole, he experienced severe pain in his ankles and knees. He was taken to the local medical center, where he was admitted. The physician ordered oxygen by nasal cannula, IV fluids, and a PCA pump with morphine sulfate.

Nursing Diagnosis 1 *Acute* **P***ain* related to occlusion of small vessels by sickled cells as evidenced by severe pain in the knees and ankles

Nursing Outcomes Classification (NOC)
Pain Control
Symptom Control

Nursing Interventions Classification (NIC)
Oxygen Therapy
Heat/Cold Application

PLANNING/GOALS	NURSING INTERVENTIONS	RATIONALE
Reggie will state pain has been relieved.	Assess pain type, location, and intensity.	Identifies where vessels may be occluded.
	Monitor analgesic administration by PCA pump.	Assesses relief from pain.
	Support joints and lower extremities with pillows.	Relieves joint pain.
	Keep bed linens off knees and ankles with a bed cradle.	Keeps linen from putting pressure on painful areas.

continues

SAMPLE NURSING CARE PLAN

EVALUATION   The morphine in the PCA pump relieved Reggie's pain, and oral analgesics were ordered.

Nursing Diagnosis 2   *Ineffective Tissue Perfusion (Cardiopulmonary and Peripheral)* related to a decreased number of RBCs and decreased oxygenation as evidenced by dyspnea and tingling and numbness in his ankles and knees

Nursing Outcomes Classification (NOC)
Tissue Perfusion: Peripheral
Circulation Status

Nursing Interventions Classification (NIC)
Oxygen Therapy
Intravenous Therapy

PLANNING/GOALS	NURSING INTERVENTIONS	RATIONALE
Reggie will experience improved circulation in his extremities.	Elevate the head of the bed. Administer oxygen as needed.	Allows lungs to expand more fully. Oxygen increases blood oxygen level.
	Administer IV fluids as ordered.	Decreases the possibility of RBCs' sickling.
	Encourage Reggie to drink 8 to 10 glasses of water daily.	Prevents RBCs from sickling.
	Monitor for symptoms of obstructed vessels such as pain, leg ulcerations, abdominal tenderness, dyspnea, confusion, and blurred vision.	Vessels supplying blood to other vital organs can become obstructed.
	Administer blood products as ordered.	Improves the blood oxygen concentration.
	Closely monitor for possible blood transfusion reactions such as chills, fever, dyspnea, pruritus, wheezing, and pain in the lumbar region.	Administration of blood products may cause adverse reactions.

EVALUATION   Circulation in lower extremities has improved as manifested by prompt capillary refill and strong pedal and popliteal pulses. Extremities are warm to touch.

Nursing Diagnosis 3   *Activity intolerance* related to imbalance between oxygen supply and demand, as evidenced by weakness, fatigue, dyspnea, tingling, and numbness

Nursing Outcomes Classification (NOC)
Energy Conservation
Symptom Control

Nursing Interventions Classification (NIC)
Energy Management
Oxygen Therapy

PLANNING/GOALS	NURSING INTERVENTIONS	RATIONALE
Reggie will tolerate some activity.	Assist Reggie as needed with activities of daily living.	Conserves energy resources.
	Teach Reggie the importance of alternating periods of rest with activity.	Conserves energy.

EVALUATION   Reggie rests after each period of activity. He states that he had been working too hard and not getting enough rest before hospitalization.

continues

SAMPLE NURSING CARE PLAN

Nursing Diagnosis 4 *Deficient **K**nowledge* related to prescribed treatment regimen as evidenced by a lack of rest and working long hours

Nursing Outcomes Classification (NOC)
Knowledge: Energy Conservation
Knowledge: Treatment Regimen

Nursing Interventions Classification (NIC)
Self-Modification Assistance
Teaching: Individual

PLANNING/GOALS	NURSING INTERVENTIONS	RATIONALE
Reggie will relate the prescribed treatment regimen before discharge.	Teach Reggie the pathophysiology related to sickle-cell disease.	Improves compliance with the medical regimen.
	Encourage Reggie to take medications as ordered.	Improves circulation and postpones sickle-cell crisis situations.
	Explain the importance of avoiding stressful situations and the symptoms of infection.	These situations increase oxygen demands.
	Explain the importance of adequate rest on a routine basis.	Allows adequate oxygenation and reduces stress.

EVALUATION Reggie states his RBCs have Hgb S rather than Hgb A, and a lack of oxygen causes his RBCs to sickle. Sickling is caused by fatigue, lack of oral fluids, emotional and physical stress, infection, exposure to cold and anesthesia. He knows the purpose and side effects of each medication and the times he is to take them. Reggie states he is to avoid high altitudes. Reggie states that he will try to routinely have enough rest.

POLYCYTHEMIA

Polycythemia is a disease in which there is an increased production of red blood cells. Usually the numbers of white blood cells and platelets are also increased. The increase in RBCs increases the blood volume and viscosity and decreases the ability of the blood to circulate freely. There are two types of polycythemia: polycythemia vera (PV) (primary polycythemia) and secondary polycythemia. Polycythemia vera occurs principally in adults older than 50 and in Jewish men of European ancestry (Leukemia & Lymphoma Society, 2000). The "cause" is an acquired mutation, a DNA abnormality occurring in an early marrow cell, which produces all of the blood cells in the individual. The DNA damage is not linked to any specific environmental cause (Leukemia & Lymphoma Society, 2000). Secondary polycythemia is a compensatory mechanism as the body makes more red blood cells in response to low oxygenation caused by long-term hypoxia, as in chronic obstructive pulmonary disease, chronic heart failure, smoking, or living in a high altitude.

Symptoms of the two types are the same. As the blood viscosity and volume increase, the client experiences headaches, dizziness, tinnitus, blurred vision, fatigue, weakness, pruritus, exertional dyspnea, angina, and increased blood pressure and pulse. The client's complexion becomes ruddy (reddish), and the palms, earlobes, and cheeks are flushed. The client is susceptible to thrombi formation because of the increased viscosity of the blood and increase in platelets. The increased destruction of RBCs causes **hyperuricemia** (increased uric acid blood level). The Hgb and Hct increase in the same proportion as the RBCs (Leukemia & Lymphoma Society, 2000).

Medical–Surgical Management
Medical

The treatment for polycythemia is **phlebotomy,** the removal of blood from a vein. Generally 350 mL to 500 mL of blood is withdrawn at regular intervals to decrease RBCs. Radioactive phosphorus (^{32}P) may be used to decrease the production of blood cells in the bone marrow.

Complications include cerebral vascular accident, thrombosis, myocardial infarction, and hemorrhage.

Pharmacological

Antineoplastic drugs such as busulfan (Myleran), chlorambucil (Leukeran), cyclophosphamide (Cytoxan), and mechlorethamine or nitrogen mustard (Mustargen) are also used to decrease bone marrow production.

CLIENT TEACHING

Polycythemia

- Drink at least 3 L of water daily.
- Elevate feet when resting.
- Avoid tight or restrictive clothing.
- Wear support hose.
- Take medications as ordered.
- Report chest pain, joint pain, fever, or activity intolerance to physician.
- Keep appointments for laboratory testing and physician checks.

Aspirin may be given to prevent clot formation, and hydroxyurea (Droxia) helps reduce RBC and platelet counts (Leukemia & Lymphoma Society, 2000). Allopurinol (Zyloprim) is given to decrease the production of uric acid. Pruritus can be relieved with the administration of antihistamines.

Diet

The client is placed on a diet that has increased calories and protein. A diet low in sodium decreases fluid volume. Iron-containing foods should be avoided.

Activity

Activities of daily living may need to be adjusted so the client can have regular periods of rest to relieve fatigue.

Nursing Management

Monitor vital signs, nutritional status, and oxygenation. Keep accurate I&O. Initiate passive or active leg exercises or encourage ambulation. Encourage compliance with regimen.

NURSING PROCESS

Assessment

Subjective Data

Ask about a history of difficulty breathing, chest pain, dizziness, headache, pruritus, tinnitus, blurred vision, and sensitivity to hot and cold. Assess client's nutritional status for an inadequate dietary intake because of GI symptoms of fullness and dyspepsia.

Objective Data

Observe the skin for bruises and changes in skin color. Assess the cardiovascular system by checking for neck vein distention, edema, auscultating the apical pulse, palpating radial and pedal pulses, and checking for Homans' sign. Assess the respiratory system by observing for epistaxis and dyspnea and listening to the breath sounds. Check the central nervous system through pupil response and presence of numbness or tingling.

Nursing diagnoses for a client with polycythemia may include the following:

Nursing Diagnoses	Planning/Goals	Nursing Interventions
Deficient Knowledge related to disease process and treatment	The client will relate disease process and treatment.	Explain the cause of the disease, possible symptoms, side effects of medications, and possible future complications to report. Teach client to report headache, chest pain, dyspnea, or redness, swelling, or tenderness in the arms or legs to the physician or nurse practitioner immediately.
Ineffective Tissue Perfusion (Peripheral) related to decreased blood circulation	The client will have increased circulation.	Administer oxygen as needed for dyspnea. Check vital signs frequently and assess Homans' sign and signs of thrombi formation. Explain phlebotomy process.
Risk for Injury related to dizziness	The client will relate measures to avoid injury.	Encourage the client to change positions slowly to prevent dizziness. Encourage activities of daily living when the client is feeling well. Teach client to avoid activities in which bruising or trauma may occur.

Evaluation Each goal must be evaluated to determine how it has been met by the client.

WHITE BLOOD CELL DISORDERS

White blood cell disorders include leukemia and agranulocytosis.

LEUKEMIA

Leukemia is a malignancy of blood-forming tissues in which the bone marrow produces increased numbers of immature white blood cells that are incapable of protecting the body from infections. The increased number of WBCs crowds out the other cells in the bone marrow, causing a decreased production of RBCs and platelets. Anemia and bleeding result from the decreased number of RBCs and platelets.

Leukemia is divided into 4 categories: acute myelogenous leukemia (AML), acute lymphocytic leukemia (ALL), chronic myelogenous leukemia (CML), and chronic lymphocytic leukemia (CLL). An estimated 30,800 new cases of leukemia were diagnosed in 2002 (ACS, 2003).

Because of the increased production of immature WBCs, clients with acute leukemia generally are fighting persistent infections and have fever and chills. The decreased number of RBCs causes symptoms of anemia such as fatigue, pallor, malaise, tachycardia, and tachypnea. The decreased platelet production causes bleeding tendencies, and the client will experience petechiae, bruising, epistaxis, melena, gingival bleeding, and increased menstrual bleeding. The client may also experience weight loss, night sweats, and swollen lymph nodes. As the malignant cells invade the central nervous system, the client experiences headaches and visual disturbances. Some clients experience bone pain because the rapid production of WBCs crowds the cells in the bone marrow.

ACUTE LEUKEMIA

Acute leukemias have a rapid onset and must be treated quickly for a good prognosis. ALL usually occurs in children younger than age of 15 and has a more rapid onset than AML. The 5-year survival rate overall is 63% and for children 85% (ACS, 2002).

AML occurs most frequently after 55 years of age (Leukemia & Lymphoma Society, 2002). Overall survival rate is 19% and 46% for children (ACS, 2002).

Medical–Surgical Management

Medical

Diagnosis of acute leukemia is confirmed with a CBC and a bone marrow biopsy. A lumbar puncture determines the presence of malignant cells in the central nervous system. An x-ray, MRI, or CT scan of the chest and skeleton determine the presence of infection and bone marrow tissue involvement.

Bone marrow transplantation is used with relapsed ALL clients and AML clients. High doses of chemotherapy and radiation therapy are given to the client to destroy the bone marrow. Leukemic white blood cells and healthy bone marrow cells are both destroyed, placing the client at a high risk for infection and death. Identical human leukocyte antigen (HLA) bone marrow from a sibling, the client, or an antigen-matched donor is given intravenously in a manner similar to a blood transfusion. The transfused bone marrow finds its way to the client's bone marrow and starts producing WBCs, RBCs, and platelets. The bone marrow is matched in a process very similar to the process of crossmatching blood. If the client's own bone marrow is used, it is removed from the client, treated with chemotherapy, and then reinfused into the client.

Maningo (2002) describes a fast-emerging alternative to bone marrow transplantation, peripheral blood stem cell transplantation. The stem cell donor (client or HLA-matched donor) is given growth factors such as granulocyte colony-stimulating factor (filgrastim [Neupogen]) and granulocyte macrophage–colony-stimulating factor (sargramostim [Leukine]) to increase the number of circulating blood stem cells. The peripheral stem cells, collected with a large-bore central vascular access device, are separated out of the whole blood. The RBCs, platelets, WBCs, and plasma are returned to the donor. The stem cells are then infused by gravity. Engraftment occurs in 2 to 4 weeks.

Pharmacological

Initial doses of chemotherapy are called **induction doses.** Small doses of chemotherapy given every 3 to 4 weeks to maintain remission are called **maintenance therapy.**

Leukemic cells can lie dormant in the brain and spinal area because the chemotherapeutic drugs are unable to pass through the blood–brain barrier. Intrathecal (within the spinal canal) administration of methotrexate has decreased recurrences of ALL. Methotrexate is given by a lumbar puncture into the cerebrospinal fluid or through a subcutaneous cerebrospinal reservoir. Sometimes radiation therapy is also used on the brain and spinal area.

AML is treated with chemotherapeutic agents, blood products, and antibiotics. Chemotherapeutic agents used in treating acute leukemia are listed in Table 34-2.

Diet

Avoid extremely hot or cold foods and drinks as well as alcohol. A bland, high-protein, high-carbohydrate diet is usually ordered. MECHANICAL SOFT. — Cocadium in IJR

Activity

Clients should alternate periods of rest with activity and keep frequently used items nearby to conserve energy.

CHRONIC LEUKEMIA

Chronic leukemia generally occurs in adults with a gradual increase in the white cell count over months or years. The prognosis depends on the severity of the disease at the time of diagnosis. Clients with CLL have a relative survival rate of 73% (Leukemia & Lymphoma Society, 2002).

TABLE 34-2 CHEMOTHERAPEUTIC AGENTS TO TREAT LEUKEMIA

LEUKEMIA	CHEMOTHERAPEUTIC AGENTS
Acute lymphocytic leukemia (ALL)	vincristine (Oncovin) prednisone (Deltasone) 6-mercaptopurine or 6-MP (Purinethol) methotrexate (Methotrexate)
Acute myelogenous leukemia (AML)	daunorubicin HCl (Cerubidine) cytarabine or ara-C (Cytosar-U) 6-thioguanine (Thioguanine) doxorubicin HCl (Adriamycin)
Chronic myelogenous leukemia (CLL)	chlorambucil (Leukeran) COP (Cytoxan, Oncovin, and prednisone)
Chronic lymphocytic leukemia (CML)	busulfan (Myleran) hydroxyurea (Hydrea) DAT (daunorubicin, ara-C, thioguanine)

CLL clients have increased abnormal B lymphocytes, with a WBC count between 20,000 and 100,000. CLL develops with advanced age and has a higher incident rate in men than in women (Leukemia & Lymphoma Society, 2002).

CML is characterized by the Philadelphia chromosome, indicating a possible genetic link. Clients with CML have a poor prognosis with a relative survival rate of 34.5% (Leukemia & Lymphoma Society, 2002). The WBC count ranges from 15,000 to 500,000. Most clients feel good and maintain a relatively normal life until later in the disease process, when the chronic recessed phase changes into an intensified stage that resembles an acute phase of leukemia. This acute phase is called a **blastic phase,** in which there is an increased production of WBCs. When this occurs, the general condition spirals downhill and the client soon dies. The most common cause of death in the leukemic client is viral and fungal pneumonia.

Medical–Surgical Management
Medical

Diagnosis of chronic leukemia is confirmed with a CBC and a bone marrow biopsy.

In the CML chronic phase, the HLA-identical allogenic bone marrow is given, and the client's own treated bone marrow is given in the blastic phase. Autologous or allogenic peripheral blood stem cell transplantation may be used.

Pharmacological

Refer to Table 34-2 for chemotherapeutic agents used in treating CLL and CML. Chemotherapy does not extend the length of life but seems to give a better quality of life by prolonging the chronic phase.

Diet

The client is on a diet high in protein, carbohydrates, and vitamins. A bland, nonirritating diet prevents oral mucosal irritation. Alcohol should be avoided.

Activity

It is important for the client to learn methods to conserve energy, such as placing frequently used items nearby.

Nursing Management

Assess for pain. Monitor for symptoms of infection and bleeding. Check platelet count results. Follow proper hand hygiene procedure and teach it to all visitors. Provide frequent oral care with soft toothbrush or cotton swabs. Assist with or provide daily personal hygiene with antimicrobial soap. Monitor vital signs and report any temperature over 100°F. Encourage client to use an electric razor. Administer antiemetics, stool softener, and vitamins as ordered. Encourage client to talk about concerns and fears.

NURSING PROCESS

Assessment

Subjective Data

Ask the client or family about chromosomal abnormalities, exposure to chemicals, viral infections, and previous chemotherapy or radiation therapy. Ask the client to describe the location, type, and duration of pain, especially in bones or joints. Note symptoms of infection such as the presence of a cough or pain or burning on urination. Document a history of bleeding such as epistaxis, gingival bleeding, melena, or hematuria. Fatigue, malaise, and irritability are often described.

Objective Data

Note signs of infection, bleeding, and chemotherapy complications. Common sites for infection include the mouth, pharynx, lungs, skin, bladder, and perianal area. During chemotherapy, the reduced white cell count may stop the formation of pus, so infection may manifest as redness, swelling, and pain.

Assess for bleeding by monitoring the platelet count because bleeding occurs easily if the platelet count falls below 50,000. Clients can bleed from any orifice, so inspect all body discharge. Occult blood may be present in the urine and stool.

Chemotherapy complications are nausea, vomiting, and stomatitis. Alopecia occurs 1 to 2 weeks after treatments are initiated.

Nursing diagnoses for a client with leukemia may include the following:

Nursing Diagnoses	Planning/Goals	Nursing Interventions
Deficient Knowledge related to disease process and treatment	The client will relate treatment methods and possible complications of chemotherapy.	Teach the client to observe for signs of infection and bleeding. Review side effects of chemotherapy and radiation with the client, family members, and significant others.
Risk for Infection related to increased production of immature white blood cells	The client will describe ways to prevent infection.	Follow good hand hygiene techniques. Teach proper hand hygiene to the family and friends who come into contact with the leukemic client. Use antimicrobial soaps for the client's daily bath. Provide frequent oral care with a soft toothbrush and nonirritating mouthwash to prevent open sores and stomatitis. Wash the perianal area after each bowel movement to decrease bacterial contamination and prevent rectal fissures. Avoid taking a rectal temperature and giving suppositories. Monitor the temperature every 4 hours for signs of infection. Report any temperature over 100°F to the physician. Administer antibiotics and antifungals as ordered. Closely monitor respiratory rate and breath sounds.
Risk for Injury related to decreased production of platelets	The client will identify ways to avoid injury and prevent bleeding.	Frequently observe the client for signs of bleeding such as epistaxis, gingival bleeding, petechiae, ecchymoses, hematemesis, enlarged abdomen, hematuria, melena, and confusion, which can occur from intracranial hemorrhage. Administer stool softeners frequently to prevent anal irritation from hard stools. Use cotton swabs instead of a toothbrush for oral care. Encourage the client to use an electric razor. Avoid giving injections as much as possible. If a catheter is needed, lubricate it well to avoid trauma to the mucosal lining of the urethra.
Imbalanced Nutrition: Less than body requirements related to effects of disease process and chemotherapy on gastrointestinal tract	The client will choose nonirritating, high-protein, high-carbohydrate meals and snacks.	Administer antiemetics as ordered to relieve nausea and vomiting. Suggest that the client may tolerate small frequent feedings better than three large meals. Provide the client with a high-protein, high-carbohydrate diet to prevent infection and provide needed energy. Administer vitamin supplements as ordered. Teach the client to avoid raw fruits and vegetables as these foods may contain more bacteria than cooked foods.
Ineffective Coping related to uncertainty about treatment of disease and prognosis	The client will identify ways to cope with concerns about disease process.	Inform the client of the possibility of alopecia from therapy treatments. Encourage the client to voice concerns and fears. Teach the client, family members, and significant others to monitor and report signs of infection and bleeding. Refer to support groups, social workers, and clergy as needed.

Evaluation Each goal must be evaluated to determine how it has been met by the client.

AGRANULOCYTOSIS

A severely reduced number of granulocytes (basophils, eosinophils, and neutrophils) is called **agranulocytosis.** The primary cause is an adverse reaction to medication or medication toxicity, especially with administration of phenylbutazone (Butazolidin), chloramphenical (Chloromycetin), penicillin derivatives, cephalosporins, phenytoin (Dilantin), antihistamines, vincristine (Oncovin), propythiouracil, diuretics, chlorpromazine hydrochloride (Thorazine), fluphenazene (Prolixin), promazene hydrochloride (Sparine), and sulfonamides and its derivatives. Other causes of agranulocytosis are neoplastic disease, chemotherapy, radiation therapy, and bacterial and viral infection. The causative agent suppresses the bone marrow, reducing the production of leukocytes.

The client exhibits the symptoms of infection: headache, fever, chills, and fatigue as well as mucous membrane ulcerations of the nose, mouth, pharynx, vagina, and rectum. The white blood count and neutrophils will be low.

Medical–Surgical Management

Medical

The main goals of treatment are to remove the cause of the bone marrow suppression and either prevent or treat any infection. When the client's temperature is elevated, blood cultures may be performed. Mucosal ulcerations may be cultured. Blood transfusions are given to provide mature leukocytes. Filgrastim (Neupogen), a human granulocyte colony-stimulating factor, may be given. Protective isolation may be instituted.

Pharmacological

Antibiotics specific for cultured microorganisms are given.

Diet

A soft, bland diet high in calories, protein, and vitamins is ordered.

Activity — stay away from crowds

Periods of activity must be balanced with periods of rest to prevent weakness and fatigue.

 Infection Control: The Client with Agranulocytosis
- Perform hand hygiene frequently and follow aseptic technique when caring for the client.
- Keep client's environment very clean.
- The client should avoid crowds.
- Screen visitors so no one with a cold or any type of infection is allowed to see the client.
- Teach client to avoid hot or cold environments.
- Ensure that the client reports any signs or symptoms of infection.

Nursing Management

Assess vital signs and monitor for temperature over 100.6°F. Auscultate lungs for crackles and wheezes. Balance periods of activity with periods of rest. Use strict asepsis for all procedures. Perform thorough hand hygiene before caring for client. Screen everyone coming into contact with the client for signs of infection. Encourage intake of adequate fluids. Monitor WBC count.

NURSING PROCESS

Assessment

Subjective Data

The client may describe having extreme fatigue, weakness, headache, chills, and fever. Inquire about all medications taken, including over-the-counter and prescription drugs.

Objective Data

Assess vital signs especially for a temperature over 100.6°F. Mucosal ulcerations may be reddened. Auscultate the lungs for crackles and wheezes.

Nursing diagnoses for a client with agranulocytosis may include the following:

Nursing Diagnoses	Planning/Goals	Nursing Interventions
*Risk for **Infection*** related to decreased leukocyte production	The client will not have signs and symptoms of infection.	Thoroughly cleanse hands before caring for the client.
		Screen all persons for signs of infection before allowing them near the client.
		Monitor vital signs for signs of infection.
		Use strict asepsis for all procedures.
		Encourage the client to drink an adequate amount of fluids.
		Monitor WBC count.
		Provide personal hygiene to prevent infection.
		Provide client with periods of rest between activities.

Evaluation Each goal must be evaluated to determine how it has been met by the client.

COAGULATION DISORDERS

Coagulation disorders include disseminated intravascular coagulation, hemophilia, and thrombocytopenia.

DISSEMINATED INTRAVASCULAR COAGULATION

Disseminated intravascular coagulation (DIC) is not a disease in itself but a syndrome that occurs because of a primary disease process or condition. A few of the conditions in which DIC may occur are burns, acute leukemia, metastatic cancer, polycythemia vera, pheochromocytoma, shock, acute infections, septic abortion, abruptio placenta, blood transfusion reactions, and trauma.

DIC is a condition of alternating clotting and hemorrhaging. The primary disease stimulates the clotting mechanism, causing many microthrombi (very small clots) to form and block the circulation in the arterioles and capillaries. With the formation of the numerous small clots, the body's fibrinolytic process responds in an attempt to stop the clot formation, thus causing hemorrhaging (Figure 34-8). This can be a very serious and potentially fatal condition.

The occlusion of blood vessels with the clots causes infarcts and necrosis of organs and tissues. The kidneys are the most commonly affected organ.

If a client with a predisposing condition develops **purpura** (reddish purple patches on the skin indicative of hemorrhage), bleeding tendencies, or renal impairment, the nurse should assess for DIC. Symptoms of DIC may present as oozing from a venipuncture, mucus membrane, or surgical wound. The oozing may progress rapidly into a hemorrhage within a few hours to a day. The client may have decreased urine output from decreased blood flow or renal infarction.

Medical–Surgical Management

Medical

DIC is diagnosed by the client's symptoms and laboratory tests. With DIC there is an increased prothrombin time, partial thromboplastin time, thrombin time, and a decreased fibrinogen and platelet count. A laboratory test that confirms the diagnosis is the D dimer, which measures a fibrin split product that is released when a clot breaks.

The primary disease or condition must be treated. For example, if the primary disease is an infection, an antibiotic is given. If cancer is the primary disease, chemotherapy is given.

DIC is treated by administering whole blood or blood products to normalize the clotting factor level. Platelets and packed red cells are given to replace those lost during hemorrhage. Cryoprecipitate or fresh-frozen plasma is given to normalize clotting factor levels.

Figure 34-8 *Pathophysiology of DIC*

Pharmacological

Heparin has no effect on the thrombi that are already formed but may be given to prevent the formation of more microthrombi. The administration of heparin is controversial because of the risk of hemorrhage. After thrombi formation has been controlled with heparin, aminocaproic acid (Amicar) can be given to stop the bleeding because it stops the fibrinolytic process. **Fibrinolysis** is the process of breaking fibrin apart.

Nursing Management

Be aware of precipitating conditions. Monitor I&O closely. Watch for purpura on the chest and abdomen, a common first sign. Monitor vital signs, peripheral pulses, and neurological checks. Avoid giving injections and venipunctures when possible.

NURSING PROCESS

Assessment

Subjective Data

Ask the client about previous conditions such as infectious processes, trauma, or cancer. Client statements of joint pain may indicate bleeding into the joint. Document recent visual changes.

Objective Data

Observe and record the amount of bleeding from any wound or body orifice. Monitor I&O closely. Purpura on the chest and abdomen is a common first sign. Abdominal tenderness is often present. Note presence of pulmonary edema, hypotension, tachycardia, absence of peripheral pulses, confusion, restlessness, convulsions, and coma.

Nursing diagnosis for a client with DIC may include the following:

Nursing Diagnoses	Planning/Goals	Nursing Interventions
Risk for Injury related to altered clotting factors	The client will experience a minimal amount of injury.	Monitor vital signs, peripheral pulses, neurological checks, and urine output.
		Check urine and stool for the presence of blood. Assess for abdominal bleeding by checking for abdominal firmness or rigidity.
		If abdominal bleeding is suspected, measure the abdominal girth every 4 hours.
		Assess surgical wounds and all body orifices for bleeding and apply pressure to any oozing site.
		Assess color, warmth, sensation, and movement of extremities.
		Observe for changes in mental status.
		Avoid giving injections and venipunctures as much as possible.
		Observe for signs of orthostatic hypotension.

Evaluation Each goal must be evaluated to determine how it has been met by the client.

HEMOPHILIA

Hemophilia is an inherited bleeding disorder in which there is a lack of clotting factors. Approximately 17,000 persons in the United States have hemophilia (NHF, 2002). There are two types of hemophilia: hemophilia A is lacking clotting factor VIII, and hemophilia B (Christmas disease) is lacking clotting factor IX, along with an absence of a plasma protein, which results in nonformation of thromboplastin. The hemophilia trait is carried on the recessive X chromosome, so a mother is asymptomatic but can pass the trait to the son, who then manifests the symptoms of hemophilia (Figure 34-9). In the male population, hemophilia A occurs at the rate of 1 : 10,000 and hemophilia B occurs at the rate of 1 : 34,000 (NHF, 2002a & 2002b). Genetic counseling is often advantageous for clients who are carriers or who have hemophilia. There is no family history of hemophilia B in 20% of those with the disorder. These cases result from a new or spontaneous gene mutation (NHF, 2002b). It is rare for a female to have hemophilia, but it can happen if the father has the disease and the mother is a carrier (NHF, 2002a).

There are three classifications of hemophilia: severe (factor level less than 1% of normal), moderate (factor level 1% to 5% normal), and mild (factor level 40% of normal). The main symptom of hemophilia is bleeding. The client with severe hemophilia bleeds with minor trauma to an area but can also bleed spontaneously. **Hemarthrosis** (bleeding into the joints) occurs most frequently, causing pain, swelling, redness, and fever. Spontaneous ecchymoses and bleeding from the mouth and gastrointestinal and urinary tracts may occur. The most common cause of death is intracranial hemorrhage. Clients with mild hemophilia will not have spontaneous muscle and joint bleeding but will bleed after minor or major surgery.

Figure 34-9 *Hemophilia Inheritance Pattern between a Female Hemophilia Carrier and a Male without Hemophilia*

This condition could prove fatal if the diagnosis is not determined promptly.

Medical–Surgical Management

Medical

Hemophilia is diagnosed by a deficient or absent blood level of factors VIII or IX. The prothrombin time (PT), thrombin time, platelet count, and bleeding time are normal, but the partial thromboplastin time (PTT) is usually prolonged.

The National Hemophilia Foundation's Medical and Scientific Advisory Council (MASAC) recommend that hemophilia A be treated with Recombinant (genetically engineered) factor VIII for clients who are HIV seronegative and Immunoaffinity purified factor VIII concentrates for HIV-seropositive clients. Cryoprecipitate is not recommended because of the risk of hepatitis and HIV infections (NHF, 2002a). For hemophilia B, the MASAC

COMMUNITY/HOME HEALTH CARE

Hemophilia

It is important for the client and family to understand the disease process, learn how to recognize signs and symptoms of bleeding, and be able to administer treatments at home. The client should:

- Obtain medical care for trauma, cuts, edema, or pain in muscles and joints.
- Wear a Medic-Alert tag.
- Not take aspirin.
- Use a soft-bristled toothbrush and carefully perform oral hygiene.
- Prevent injuries by wearing gloves and long-sleeved clothing when doing household chores and participating in noncontact sports and activities.

recommends Recombinant factor IX for HIV-seronegative clients and Immunoaffinity purified and recombinant factor IX. About 60% of hemophilia clients treated with plasma concentrates in the early 1980s were infected with HIV (NHF, 2002b).

 Pharmacological

Desmopressin acetate (DDAVP-stimate) can be given to clients with mild hemophilia.

Nursing Management

Assess for signs of bleeding: petechiae, ecchymoses, hematemesis, melena, epistaxis, hematuria, hemarthrosis, and abdominal rigidity. Note edematous or immobile joints. Encourage client to wear Medic-Alert bracelet and avoid activities that may cause trauma. Advise not to take aspirin, and to use an electric razor and a soft toothbrush.

NURSING PROCESS

Assessment

Subjective Data

Assess the client for pain and ask what measures were used in the past to relieve pain and bleeding.

Objective Data

Assess the client for bleeding by checking for petechiae, ecchymoses, hematuria, hematemesis, melena, epistaxis, hemarthrosis, abdominal firmness and rigidity, and frank bleeding. Note edematous or immobile joints.

Nursing diagnoses for a client with hemophilia may include the following:

Nursing Diagnoses	Planning/Goals	Nursing Interventions
Deficient Knowledge related to disease process	The client will relate symptoms to report and treatment methods if bleeding occurs.	Discuss ways to improve the safety of the client's home environment. Advise client not to take aspirin and encourage the client to use an electric razor and soft-bristled toothbrush. Teach family members or significant others administration of clotting factors for prophylactic purposes and if injury occurs. Encourage client to wear Medic-Alert bracelet. Refer for genetic counseling.
Acute Pain related to bleeding into tissues and joints	The client will have minimal pain.	Assess the client for bruising, swelling, and joint discomfort. Apply ice and pressure to bleeding sites. When a joint is hurting, immobilize it in a flexed position with a supportive device. Give analgesics as needed but not aspirin.
Risk for Injury related to altered clotting factors	The client will take precautions to avoid injury.	Transfuse clotting factors as ordered. Encourage the client to avoid activities that may cause trauma. Post emergency medical numbers in convenient places in case of future need.

Evaluation Each goal must be evaluated to determine how it has been met by the client.

THROMBOCYTOPENIA

Thrombocytopenia is a decrease in the number of platelets in the blood. The decrease may be related to:

- Decreased platelet production as in aplastic anemia, tumors, leukemia, and chemotherapy
- Decreased platelet survival as in infection or viral illnesses
- Increased platelet destruction as in DIC or thrombocytopenic purpura that is either drug induced or **idiopathic** (occurring without a known cause)

Withdrawal of the causative drug usually allows the platelet count to return to normal in 1 to 2 weeks. The acute form of idiopathic thrombocytopenic purpura (ITP) is an autoimmune process caused by an autoantibody-destroying platelet antigen.

Petechiae, ecchymoses, and bleeding from mucous membranes are observed. Bleeding may occur in internal organs. The platelet count is very low; the bleeding time is prolonged; Hgb and Hct may be low; and bone marrow aspiration shows mostly immature platelets.

Medical–Surgical Management

Medical

Transfusions of platelet concentrates may be given, or **apheresis** (removal of unwanted components) may be performed on the client's blood to remove the autoantibodies.

Surgical

A splenectomy may be performed because the spleen is the primary site of platelet destruction. This treatment is usually reserved until all other treatments have been unsuccessful.

Pharmacological

Corticosteroids are given to prolong platelet life and strengthen the capillaries. Immunosuppressive drugs, gamma globulin, and vitamin K may be given.

Diet

A high-fiber diet is used to prevent constipation and the need to strain when having a bowel movement.

Activity

Activity should be undertaken thoughtfully and carefully to prevent any trauma.

Nursing Management

Monitor for signs of bleeding (ecchymoses, petechiae, and rigid abdomen). Check laboratory reports for low platelet count, Hgb, and Hct, and prolonged bleeding time. Encourage a high-fiber diet to prevent constipation. Assess pain and administer analgesics as ordered. Monitor vital signs and mental status.

NURSING PROCESS

Assessment

Subjective Data

Ask the client about medications being taken and any recent infection.

Objective Data

Observe for petechiae, ecchymoses, and any signs of blood or internal bleeding.

Nursing diagnoses for a client with thrombocytopenia may include the following:

Nursing Diagnoses	Planning/Goals	Nursing Interventions
*Acute **Pain*** related to hemorrhage	The client will verbalize having less pain.	Assess client's pain on 0 (least) to 10 (most) pain scale and client's ability to cope with pain. Administer analgesic as ordered, and note client's response.
*Risk for **Injury*** related to thrombocytopenia	The client will have minimal injury.	Monitor client's vital signs and neurological and mental status. Assess client's skin and excretions for signs of bleeding. Handle client very carefully when turning, assisting out of bed, and in all other care situations.

Evaluation Each goal must be evaluated to determine how it has been met by the client.

LYMPH DISORDERS

A **lymphoma** is a tumor of the lymphatic system. Two malignant lymphomas discussed in this chapter are Hodgkin's lymphoma and non-Hodgkin's lymphoma (NHL). The overview and medical management of each disease are presented separately. The nursing process for both diseases is presented together because the nursing diagnoses, goals, and interventions are the same.

HODGKIN'S LYMPHOMA

Hodgkin's lymphoma is a rare lymphoma that usually arises as a painless swelling in a lymph node. The diagnosis is confirmed when Reed-Sternberg cells are biopsied from the swollen lymph node. The incidence is highest in ages 20 to 34 and 75 to 84 (Leukemia & Lymphoma Society, 2002). The 5-year survival rate has doubled from 40% in 1960 to 83% in 2001 (Leukemia & Lymphoma Society, 2002). In children, the 5-year survival rate is 93% (Leukemia & Lymphoma Society, 2002).

Risk factors are mostly unknown, but reduced immune function and certain infectious agents are involved. In Africa, Burkitt's lymphoma is partly caused by the Epstein-Barr virus (Leukemia & Lymphoma Society, 2002).

Clients with Hodgkin's lymphoma most commonly have painless enlarged lymph nodes in the neck, in the area above the clavicles, and in the groin. Lymph nodes in the mediastinum may also be enlarged but are not usually diagnosed until the nodes enlarge and press on the mediastinal structures, causing dyspnea and a cough. A chest x-ray or a computed tomography (CT) scan confirms the involvement of the mediastinal lymph nodes. Other symptoms are weight loss, fatigue, pruritus, recurrent high fever, night sweats, anemia, thrombocytopenia, and lowered resistance to infections.

If a client has painless, enlarged lymph nodes and the symptoms of an elevated temperature, night sweats, pruritus, and weight loss of more than 10% of the body weight in a 6-month period, the prognosis is worse than if only enlarged lymph nodes are present. Hodgkin's lymphoma spreads throughout the body in a predictable pattern. From the site of the original swollen gland, the disease spreads to nearby lymph nodes and then to other lymphatic tissue in the body such as the liver, spleen, and bone marrow. The invasion of other nodes and lymphatic tissue determines the prognosis of the disease.

Medical–Surgical Management

Medical

Diagnostic tests include CBC, platelet count, bone marrow aspiration, chest x-ray, abdominal CT scan, lymphangiogram, and lymph node biopsy.

Localized Hodgkin's lymphoma stages I and II are treated with radiation therapy. Clients with massive mediastinal involvement and those who have relapsed after radiation therapy alone are treated with radiation therapy and chemotherapy.

During radiation therapy, the client may experience weight loss, nausea and vomiting, skin reactions, esophagitis, fatigue, and bone marrow suppression. The client's blood count is monitored closely during therapy to check for infection and bleeding tendencies. If the WBC level drops too low, the client will be more susceptible to infections. A decrease in RBCs and platelets causes a bleeding tendency. Long-term complications from radiation therapy include hypothyroidism, radiation pneumonitis, immune system impairment, herpes zoster, and the development of a second cancer.

Generalized Hodgkin's lymphoma, stages III and IV are treated with combination chemotherapy, which is administering a series of combined drugs over a set period. Serious late complications of chemotherapy are infertility and a secondary malignancy or cancer.

Surgical

Sometimes a laparotomy is done to see if the liver and spleen are involved. The rationale of performing the procedure is being questioned since the overall treatment plan is not altered.

Pharmacological

During radiation therapy, antiemetics, such as ondansetron HCl (Zofran), are given for nausea and vomiting. Analgesics can be given for esophagitis discomfort.

Chemotherapy drugs, such as MOPP and ABVD, are often given in combinations. MOPP combines mechlorethamine or nitrogen mustard (Mustargen), vincristine sulfate (Oncovin), procarbazine HCl (Matulane), and prednisone (Deltasone). ABVD combines doxorubicin HCl (Adriamycin PFS), bleomycin sulfate (Blenoxane), vinblastine sulfate (Velban), and dacarbazine (DTIC-Dome). These drugs are usually administered through an implanted venous port. Allopurinol (Zyloprim) is given to prevent uric acid renal stones caused by the rapid destruction of cells during therapy.

Diet

During therapy, the client is on a high-calorie, high-protein diet. Encourage an intake of 2,500 mL of fluid per day to prevent the formation of renal stones.

Activity

Extra rest periods may be necessary to cope with fatigue that occurs with Hodgkin's lymphoma.

NON-HODGKIN'S LYMPHOMA

Non-Hodgkin's lymphoma (NHL) is more common than Hodgkin's lymphoma and is the sixth most common cancer in the United States. Approximately 53,400 new cases are estimated for 2003 (ACS, 2003). The 5-year survival rate has increased from 47% in 1974 to 55% in 2001; in children, the 5-year survival rate was 78% in 2001 (Leukemia & Lymphoma Society, 2002).

NHL originates from the B lymphocytes and the T lymphocytes. NHL arising from the B lymphocyte occurs in the older adult population; NHL arising from the T lymphocytes manifests in malignant skin diseases such as mycosis fungoides or Sezary syndrome. More men are affected than women. NHL does not have the Reed-Sternberg cell present. The incidence for non-Hodgkin's lymphoma increased 80% from 1973 to 1997 (Leukemia & Lymphoma Society, 2002).

Symptoms of NHL are enlarged painless lymph nodes in the neck, axillary, abdominal, and inguinal areas. Other symptoms include fever, night sweats, excessive tiredness, indigestion, abdominal pain, loss of appetite, and bone pain.

Medical–Surgical Management

Medical

The diagnosis of NHL is confirmed by a lymph node biopsy. Physicians use the same staging system as for Hodgkin's lymphoma.

Pharmacological

There are three different chemotherapy regimens, CHOP, CVP, and COPP: CHOP combines cyclophosphamide (Cytoxan), doxorubicin HCl (Adriamycin), vincristine sulfate (Oncovin), and prednisone (Deltasone); CVP combines cyclophosphamide (Cytoxan), vincristine sulfate (Oncovin), and prednisone (Deltasone); COPP combines cyclophosphamide (Cytoxan), vincristine sulfate (Oncovin), procarbazine HCl (Matulane), and prednisone (Deltasone).

Nursing Management

Assess for enlarged, painless lymph nodes. Monitor vital signs, weight, and voice changes. Review blood test results. Encourage deep breathing and adequate fluid intake. Provide a high-calorie, high-protein diet in small, frequent meals.

NURSING PROCESS

Assessment

Subjective Data

Ask if the client is experiencing pruritus, night sweats, weight loss, decreased appetite, fever, fatigue, weakness, or chest pain.

Objective Data

Assess weight, vital signs, and for skin infections; dyspnea; cough; voice changes; enlarged lymph nodes in the neck, axilla, and groin; and edema in the extremities. Bone scan shows fractures and tumor infiltration. Review blood tests for hypercalcemia if bone lesions are present, and a CBC often indicates anemia. When the client is having radiation or chemotherapy treatments, the assessment includes observing for dysphagia, nausea and vomiting, skin rashes, and alopecia.

Nursing diagnoses for a client with Hodgkin's disease or non-Hodgkin's disease may include the following:

Nursing Diagnoses	Planning/Goals	Nursing Interventions
Ineffective **B**reathing Pattern related to tracheobronchial obstruction from enlarged mediastinal nodes	The client will complete activities of daily living without dyspnea.	Elevate the head of the bed to assist the client's breathing. Encourage the client to take frequent deep breaths to expand the lungs and prevent infection; assess the client's breathing pattern every shift and as needed for dyspnea.
Risk for **I**nfection related to radiation/chemotherapy treatments, decreased WBCs and pruritus	The client will remain free of infection.	Monitor the lab results for lowered WBCs. Teach the client the importance of avoiding situations where there is exposure to infections. Provide cool sponge baths or oral medication to relieve pruritus. Assess the radiated skin areas for redness or breaks in the skin. Encourage the client to report symptoms of dyspnea, sore throat, and burning or frequency of urination.
Imbalanced **N**utrition: Less than body requirements related to decreased appetite	The client will consume an adequate amount of a nutritional diet.	Serve attractive high-calorie, high-protein meals in a pleasant environment. Offer six to eight smaller meals throughout the day to decrease a feeling of fullness. A soft, bland diet may be more palatable during radiation or chemotherapy treatments. Avoid hot, spicy foods that may be caustic to mucous membranes and lead to infection. Encourage an adequate intake of fluids to prevent constipation and renal stones. Weigh the client biweekly or more frequently if needed.

continues

Nursing Diagnoses	Planning/Goals	Nursing Interventions
Anxiety related to disease and therapy treatments	The client will cope effectively with disease process and therapy treatments.	Listen to the concerns of the client regarding the effect of the disease on lifestyle, family, and finances. Encourage the family to express their concerns and discuss effective ways to deal with the diagnosis and treatment. Refer the client and family to clergy and social agencies when appropriate.

Evaluation Each goal must be evaluated to determine how it has been met by the client.

PLASMA CELL DISORDER

The main plasma cell disorder is myeloma.

MYELOMA

There were an estimated 14,600 new cases of myeloma diagnosed in 2002, and an estimated 10,800 persons died from it (Leukemia & Lymphoma Society, 2002). More cases occur in men older than age 60.

The plasma cells, mainly in bone marrow, become malignant, crowd out normal cell production, destroy normal bone tissue, and thereby cause pain. The normal production of antibodies is changed, making the client susceptible to infections. The first sign of myeloma is often bone pain, especially in the ribs, spine, and pelvis. The long bones ache; joints are swollen and tender; and a low-grade fever and general malaise are present. The client tires easily and has weakness from anemia. The weakened bones fracture easily. The cause of myeloma is not known.

Diagnosis is made with bone marrow biopsy showing large numbers of immature plasma cells and x-rays showing demineralization and osteoporosis. Bence Jones protein is found in the urine of many clients with myeloma. The client will also have hypercalcemia, hyperuricemia, anemia, and hypercalciuria.

Medical–Surgical Management
Medical

Myeloma is not curable, so treatment is symptomatic. Intensive chemotherapy followed by autologous peripheral blood stem cell transplantation may restore normal blood cell production.

Surgical

A laminectomy may be required if any vertebrae collapse. If the client gets kidney stones from the large amount of calcium in the blood and urine, surgery may be required.

Pharmacological

Steroids such as prednisone (Metcorten) along with antineoplastic drugs such as cyclophosphamide (Cytoxan), chlorambucil (Leukeran), or melphalan (Alkeran) are given. An analgesic is given for pain relief.

CLIENT TEACHING

Myeloma

- Drink 3 to 4 L of fluids per day.
- Exercise to decrease bone demineralization.
- Monitor for symptoms of hypercalcemia and notify physician if symptoms occur.

If the serum calcium level rises above 10 mg/dL, the physician may order an IV of normal saline infused at a high rate followed by diuretics.

Diet

Six small meals per day are often tolerated better than the usual three meals per day; nutritious meals based on the client's food preferences are recommended. A fluid intake of 3 to 4 L per day is essential to minimize the complications of excessive calcium in the blood and urine.

Activity

It is important to keep the client mobile as much as possible. Walking stimulates calcium resorption and decreases demineralization. When the client is in bed, it is important to reposition the client frequently using a lift sheet to decrease the risk of pathological fractures.

Nursing Management

Assess for bone pain. Monitor laboratory test results for hypercalcemia. Provide six small meals each day of client's preferred foods. Encourage fluid intake to 3 to 4 L per day. Encourage ambulation. Monitor vital signs.

NURSING PROCESS

Assessment

Subjective Data

The client describes constant pain that increases with movement. The pain is usually in the back, ribs, or pelvis. Achiness in the long bones and joints and general malaise may also be described.

Objective Data

Assess pain using a 0 (none) to 10 (most) pain scale. Temperature may be elevated. The client's ability to perform activities of daily living may be decreased. Monitor the level of blood calcium.

Nursing diagnoses for a client with myeloma may include the following:

Nursing Diagnoses	Planning/Goals	Nursing Interventions
Chronic Pain related to disease process	The client will express a decrease in pain level.	Assess the client's pain level with pain scale. Administer analgesic as ordered and monitor the client's response.
Risk for Injury related to bone demineralization	The client will have minimal injuries.	Handle client gently and reposition the client using a lift sheet. Keep the client's personal items within easy reach.
Risk for Infection related to disease process and pharmaceutical agents	The client will have few infections.	Thoroughly cleanse hands before caring for the client. Teach the client and family proper hand hygiene. Assist the client with personal hygiene as needed. Screen visitors for signs of infections before allowing them to visit the client.

Evaluation Each goal must be evaluated to determine how it has been met by the client.

CASE STUDY

James Johns, 46, owns a hobby shop. He has had a cold for 3 weeks that has recently settled in his chest. He has been tired lately and takes naps each evening before the evening meal. His wife noticed several bruises on his arms and legs, but James could not recall any particular injury. James has gradually lost 10 pounds over the last 3 months but has not been concerned about it. When James went to the clinic for some antibiotics for his cold, the nurse practitioner completed a physical assessment and ordered a chest x-ray and CBC. The nurse practitioner noticed the WBCs were 250,000/mm³; RBCs, 4.2 million/mm³; and platelets, 100,000/mm³. After several other tests were performed over the next few days, a diagnosis of chronic myelogenous leukemia (CML) was confirmed.

The following questions will guide your development of a nursing care plan for the case study.

1. List the symptoms occurring in James Johns that are typical of CML.
2. List five other typical symptoms of CML that were not stated in the case study.
3. List other diagnostic tests that could be done to confirm the diagnosis of CML.
4. List subjective and objective data the nurse would obtain about James Johns.
5. Write three individualized nursing diagnoses and goals for James Johns.
6. List nursing interventions for James Johns.
7. List community resources specific to locale that could assist James and his family during his illness with CML.
8. List discharge teaching the nurse would give to James and his family.
9. List successful client outcomes for James Johns.
10. List chemotherapeutic agents and side effects of the agents that may be prescribed for James.
11. List other medical treatments that may be ordered for James.
12. What measures could the nurse take to meet the emotional needs of James and his family?

Summary

- The main formed components of the blood are red blood cells, white blood cells, and platelets.
- The lymphatic system is composed of lymph vessels that drain lymph into the venous system, lymph nodes that filter microorganisms in the body, spleen, and thymus.
- Sickledex and hemoglobin electrophoresis are diagnostic tests for sickle-cell anemia.
- Some of the symptoms of anemia are fatigue, pallor, exertional dyspnea, and tachycardia.
- Symptoms of polycythemia vera are headache, epistaxis, dizziness, tinnitus, blurred vision, fatigue, weakness, pruritus, exertional dyspnea, angina, and increased blood pressure and pulse.
- Polycythemia vera is treated with chemotherapeutic agents.
- DIC is not a disease but a complication of a disease or condition that causes the client to alternate between forming many small clots and hemorrhaging.
- Hemophilia is a recessive X chromosome inherited bleeding disorder in which the client is lacking clotting factors. The main symptom is spontaneous bleeding or bleeding caused by trauma.
- The two types of malignant lymphomas are Hodgkin's lymphoma and non-Hodgkin's lymphoma. Clients with both types of lymphoma have enlarged lymph nodes.
- Hodgkin's lymphoma is diagnosed by the presence of the Reed-Sternberg cell in the swollen lymph nodes. Non-Hodgkin's lymphoma arises from the B lymphocytes and T lymphocytes and does not have the Reed-Sternberg cell in the lymph system.

Review Questions

1. For improved iron absorption, a client with iron-deficiency anemia takes Feosol with:

    a. milk.

    b. an orange.

    c. water.

    d. processed cheese.

2. A thorough assessment of the cardiac system on a client with sickle-cell anemia is important because:

    a. the heart enlarges in an attempt to provide the oxygen needs to the body tissues.

    b. cells sickle more easily in the heart chambers.

    c. more cardiac force is needed to pump RBCs with Hbg S.

    d. people with sickle-cell anemia are prone to bradycardia.

3. Clients with leukemia are prone to infections because:

    a. there are too many WBCs.

    b. the bone marrow is not producing WBCs.

    c. the bone marrow is producing too many cells.

    d. the WBCs are incapable of fighting infections.

4. Symptoms that alert a nurse that a client may have DIC are:

    a. tinnitus and numbness and tingling in the extremities.

    b. jaundice, palpitations, and dyspnea.

    c. purpura, bruising, and decreased urine output.

    d. ruddy complexion, epistaxis, and tinnitus.

5. Encourage a client with non-Hodgkin's lymphoma to:

    a. use an electric razor.

    b. take folic acid as prescribed.

    c. apply ice and pressure to bleeding sites.

    d. avoid exposure to infections.

References/Suggested Readings

American Cancer Society (ACS). (2003). *Cancer Facts & Figures 2003.* [Online]. Available: www.cancer.org/downloads/STT/CAFF2003PWSecured/pdf

Aplastic Anemia & MDS International Foundation. (2002). *Aplastic Anemia* [Online]. Available: www.aplastic.org/diseases.shtml

Atassi, K., & Harris, M. (2001). Disseminated intravascular coagulation. *Nursing2001, 31*(3), 64.

Daniels, R. (2002). *Delmar's Guide to Laboratory and Diagnostic Tests.* Clifton Park, NY: Thomson Delmar Learning.

Day, M. (2001). Sickle-cell crisis. *Nursing2001, 31*(5), 88.

Dochterman, J., & Bulechek, G. (2004). *Nursing Interventions Classification (NIC)* (4th ed.). St. Louis, MO: Mosby.

Gioia, K., Kleinert, D., & Hannon, M. (1999). What's wrong with this patient? *RN, 62*(2), 43–45.

Gorman, K. (1999). Sickle cell disease. *AJN, 99*(3), 38–43.

Holcomb, S. S. (2001). Anemia: Pointing the way to a deeper problem. *Nursing2001, 31*(7), 36–42.

Leukemia & Lymphoma Society. (2000). *Polycythemia Vera.* [Online]. Available: www.leukemia-lymphoma.org/all_mat_toc.adp?item_id=9955&Cat_id=1214

Leukemia & Lymphoma Society. (2002). *Leukemia, Lymphoma, Myeloma Facts 2002.* [Online]. Available: www.leukemia-lymphoma.org/attachments/National/br_1033500385.pdf

Maningo, J. (2002). Peripheral blood stem cell transplant. *Nursing2002, 32*(12), 52–55.

McBrien, N. (1997). Clinical snapshot: Thrombocytopenic purpura. *AJN, 97*(2), 28–29.

Mitchell, R. (1999). Sickle cell anemia. *AJN, 99*(5), 36–37.

Moorhead, S., Johnson, M., & Maas, M., (2004). *Nursing Outcomes Classification (NOC)* (3rd ed.). St. Louis, MO: Mosby.

National Cancer Institute (2002). *Lymphoma staging scheme.* [Online]. Available: http://training.seer.cancer.gov/modul_staging_cancer/unit03_sec04_part07_lymphoma.html

National Hemophilia Foundation (NHF). (2002a). *Bleeding disorders information center/hemophilia A.* [Online]. Available: www.hemophilia.org/bdi/bdi_types1.htm

National Hemophilia Foundation (NHF). (2002b). *Bleeding disorders information center/hemophilia B.* [Online]. Available: www.hemophilia.org/bdi/bdi_types2.htm

North American Nursing Diagnosis Association (NANDA). (2003). *Nursing Diagnoses: Definitions & Classification 2003–2004.* Philadelphia: Author.

Platt, A., Beasley, J., Miller, G., & Eckman, J. (2002). Managing sickle-cell pain . . . and all that goes with it. *Nursing2002, 32*(12), 32hn1–32hn7.

Sickle Cell Disease Association of America (SCDAA). (2002). *Who is affected?* [Online]. Available: www.sicklecelldisease.org/affected1.htm

Spratto, G., & Woods, A. (2004). *2004 PDR Nurse's drug handbook,* Clifton Park, NY: Thomson Delmar Learning.

Thibodeau, G. A., & Patton, K. T. (2003). *Anatomy and physiology* (5th ed.) St. Louis, MO: Mosby.

Resources

American Cancer Society (ACS), 1599 Clifton Road, N.E., Atlanta, GA 30329, 800-ACS-2345, www.cancer.org

Aplastic Anemia & MDS International Foundation, Inc., P.O. Box 613, Annapolis, MD 21404, 800-747-2820, www.aplastic.org

BMT (Bone Marrow Transplant) Newsletter, 2900 Skokie Valley Road, Suite B, Highland Park, IL 60035, 888-597-7674, www.bmtinfonet.org

Cancer Information Service (CIS), 800-4-CANCER

Center for Sickle Cell Disease, 202-806-7930

Cooley's Anemia Foundation, 129-09 26th Avenue, #203, Flushing, NY 11354, 800-522-7222

Cure for Lymphoma Foundation, 215 Lexington Ave., New York, NY 10016, 800-CFL-6848, www.cfl.org

The Leukemia & Lymphoma Society, 1311 Mamaroneck Avenue, White Plains, NY 10605, 800-955-4572, www.leukemia_lymphoma.org

National Association for Sickle Cell Disease Inc., 3345 Wilshire Boulevard, Los Angeles, CA 90010, 800-421-8453

National Heart, Lung, and Blood Institute, 9000 Rockville Pike, Bethesda, MD 20892, 301-496-4236

National Hemophilia Foundation, 116 West 32nd Street, 11th Floor, New York, NY 10001, 800-424-2634, www.hemophilia.org

National Marrow Donor Program, 3001 Broadway St. N.E., Minneapolis, MN 55413, 800-627-7692, www.marrow.org

UNIT
11

Nursing Care
of the Client: Digestion
and Elimination

Chapter 35
Gastrointestinal System

Chapter 36
Urinary System

GASTROINTESTINAL SYSTEM

MAKING THE CONNECTION

Refer to the following chapters to increase your understanding of the gastrointestinal system:3

Basic Nursing
- Loss, Grief, and Death
- Wellness Concepts
- Fluid, Electrolyte, and Acid–Base Balance
- Assessment
- Pain Management
- Diagnostic Tests

Adult Health Nursing
- Oncology
- Endocrine System
- Immune System
- Mental Illness

- The Older Adult

Basic Procedures
- Collecting a Stool Specimen
- Applying Abdominal, T-, and Breast Binders

Intermediate Procedures
- Pouching a Stoma
- Irrigating a Wound

Advanced Procedures
- Inserting and Maintaining a Nasogastric Tube

Review: Delmar's Anatomy & Physiology
   CD-ROM: Abdominal and Digestive System

LEARNING OBJECTIVES

Upon completion of this chapter, you should be able to:
- Define key terms.
- Discuss diagnostic tests associated with the digestive system.
- Discuss components necessary for a complete assessment of the digestive system.
- List medical and surgical management for clients with digestive disorders.
- Describe nursing interventions for clients with digestive disorders.
- Assist with the formulation of nursing care plans for clients with digestive disorders.

INTRODUCTION

Disorders and diseases of the gastrointestinal system and accessory organs can affect not only the digestive process and nutrient absorption, but the lifestyle of the individual as well.

KEY TERMS

adhesion
appendicitis
ascites
calculi (calculus, sing.)
cholecystitis
cholelithiasis
cirrhosis
colostomy
constipation
diverticula
diverticulitis
diverticulosis
effluent
gastric ulcer
gastritis
glycogenesis
glycogenolysis
hematemesis
hemorrhoid
hepatitis
ileostomy
intussusception
jaundice
ligation
melena
occult blood test (guaiac)
pancreatitis
peptic ulcer
peritonitis
polyp
postprandial
steatorrhea
stoma
stomatitis
volvulus

ANATOMY AND PHYSIOLOGY REVIEW

The digestive system, also known as the *gastrointestinal (GI) tract* or the *alimentary system,* is responsible for breaking down complex food into simple nutrients the body can absorb and convert into energy (Figure 35-1). This process is known as **digestion.**

Mouth/Esophagus

Digestion begins in the mouth, where the teeth mechanically break food down into smaller pieces by chewing and mixing it with saliva. The chemical breakdown of cooked starches is begun in the mouth by the enzyme ptyalin, a salivary amylase. The food is then swallowed as a small ball or bolus and transported down the esophagus, a hollow, muscular tube approximately 10 inches long. **Peristalsis,** coordinated rhythmic contractions of the muscles, pushes the bolus through the esophagus. The cardiac sphincter, also called the *lower esophageal sphincter (LES),* located at the distal end of the esophagus, relaxes and allows the food to pass into the stomach.

Stomach

Further mechanical and chemical breakdown of the food occurs in the stomach, a J-shaped muscular organ located beneath the diaphragm. The stomach secretes gastric juices that contain hydrochloric acid (HCl) and pepsinogen, a nonactive form of the enzyme pepsin. HCl and pepsin are responsible for beginning the breakdown of protein and continuing the breakdown of starches. Starch digestion in the stomach gradually stops because of the acidic environment. Mucus is secreted to protect the lining of the stomach. The stomach also secretes an intrinsic factor necessary for vitamin B_{12} absorption and gastrin to stimulate HCl release.

The peristaltic movement of the stomach mixes the partially digested food and digestive enzymes into a semi-liquid mass called **chyme.** The chyme will not pass into the small intestine until it is the proper consistency and particles are 1 millimeter or less. On average, the stomach empties in 3 to 4 hours. Carbohydrates are digested most readily, followed by proteins, with fats taking the longest to pass from the stomach. When the chyme has reached the proper consistency, the pyloric sphincter relaxes, releasing a portion at a time of the chyme into the small intestine.

Small Intestine

The small intestine is approximately 20 to 25 feet long and is responsible for absorbing nutrients from the chyme. The small intestine also secretes digestive enzymes, mucus to protect the mucosa, and hormones to aid in the absorption of nutrients.

The chyme enters the duodenum, the first 10 to 12 inches of the small intestine. The duodenum is responsible for absorbing calcium and iron as well as neutralizing the acids in the chyme. Enzymes from the pancreas and bile from the liver enter the duodenum from the common bile duct by way of the ampulla of vater; it is here that fats are digested.

The jejunum, the middle 8 to 10 feet of the small intestine, is responsible for absorption of fats, proteins, and carbohydrates. Vitamin B_{12} and bile salts are absorbed in the ileum, the distal 12 feet of the small bowel.

Large Intestine

The chyme enters the large intestine, also known as the *colon,* through the ileocecal valve into the cecum, a

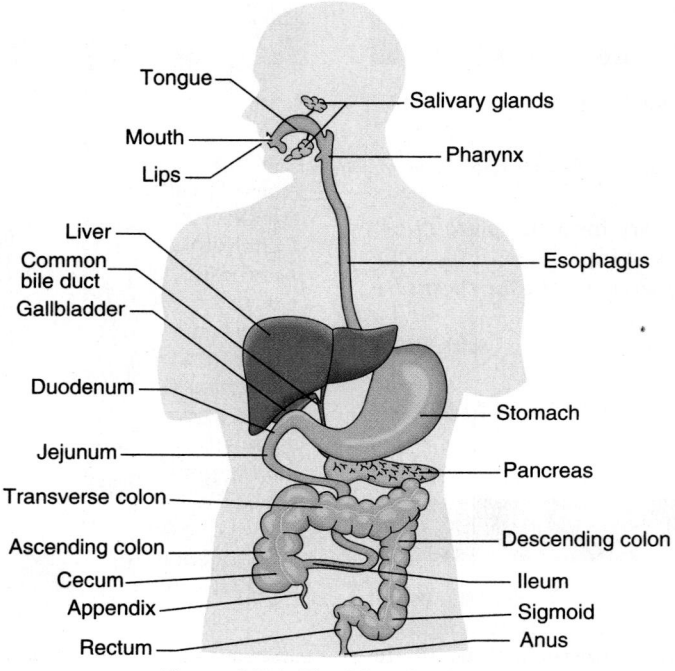

Tongue
Mouth
Lips
Liver
Common bile duct
Gallbladder
Duodenum
Jejunum
Transverse colon
Ascending colon
Cecum
Appendix
Rectum

Salivary glands
Pharynx
Esophagus
Stomach
Pancreas
Descending colon
Ileum
Sigmoid
Anus

Figure 35-1 *The Digestive System*

small pouch to which the appendix is attached. The colon is approximately 4 to 5 feet long and consists of the ascending or right colon, the transverse colon, the descending or left colon, and the sigmoid colon, an S-shaped segment before the rectum. The colon absorbs water, electrolytes, and bile salts.

The last 5 inches of the large intestine comprise the rectum. The distal end of the rectum forms the anal canal composed of muscles that control defecation. The opening to the anal canal is called the *anus.*

Accessory Organs

The digestive system also has accessory organs that aid in the digestion of food. The accessory organs include the pancreas, liver, and gallbladder (Figure 35-2).

Pancreas

The pancreas is a fish-shaped glandular organ 6 to 8 inches long extending from the duodenum across the abdomen behind the stomach. The pancreas has both endocrine and exocrine functions. The endocrine functions, which include the production of glucagon and insulin to regulate the blood sugar level, are presented in the endocrine system chapter.

The pancreas produces three main groups of enzymes in pancreatic juice for its exocrine function. The enzymes are:

amylase—converts carbohydrates into glucose

lipase—aids in fat digestion

protease—breaks down protein

Liver

The liver is the largest glandular organ of the body. It is located in the right upper quadrant of the abdomen. The liver is one of the most vascular organs, filtering

1,500 cc of blood per minute. Some of the many functions of the liver are to:

- Produce and secrete bile, which emulsifies fats
- Convert glucose into glycogen for storage **(glycogenesis)**
- Convert glycogen to glucose when blood sugar level drops **(glycogenolysis)**
- Metabolize hormones
- Break down nitrogenous wastes to urea
- Incorporate amino acids into proteins
- Filter blood and destroy bacteria
- Produce prothrombin and fibrinogen, which are necessary for blood clotting
- Manufacture cholesterol
- Produce heparin
- Store vitamin B_{12} and fat soluble vitamins A, D, E, and K
- Detoxify poisonous substances

Gallbladder

The gallbladder is a pear-shaped sac attached to the undersurface of the liver. The liver produces bile and transports the bile to the gallbladder through the hepatic and cystic ducts. The gallbladder stores and concentrates the bile until it is needed in the small intestine. When fats enter the small intestine, the gallbladder releases the bile through the cystic duct into the common bile duct and finally into the small intestine. The cystic duct, hepatic duct, and pancreatic duct combine to form the common bile duct.

Effects of Aging

As the body ages, several changes may occur in the digestive system (Table 35-1). It is important to educate clients about these changes and ways they can adapt their lifestyles.

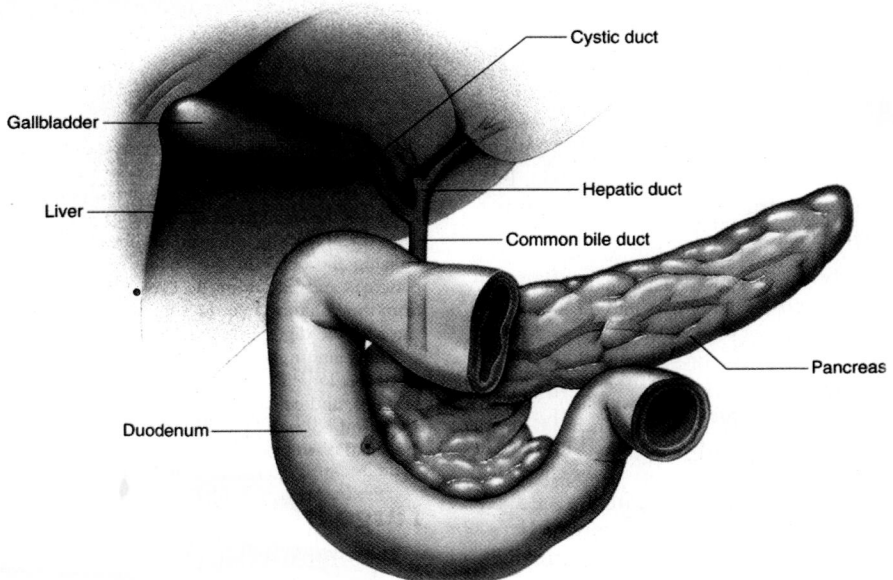

Figure 35-2 *Accessory Organs. Bile travels from the liver to the gallbladder via the hepatic and cystic ducts. The bile is released into the duodenum via the common bile duct. The pancreas releases its digestive juice into the duodenum.*

TABLE 35-1 CHANGES IN THE DIGESTIVE SYSTEM WITH AGING

COMMON CHANGES	RESULT	IMPLICATIONS FOR NURSES
Decrease in peristalsis	Food moves more slowly through digestive system. Bowel movements are more infrequent. Increase in constipation. Feeling full and bloated and may eat less.	Increase fiber and fluid intake. Encourage smaller, frequent meals. Offer fiber supplements.
Oral changes	Dentures are common. Chewing is more difficult. Eating and drinking time may be prolonged. Number of taste buds decreases.	Make sure dentures fit. Cut food into small bites. Teach that softer foods may be better tolerated. Some clients may start using more salt and seasonings to compensate for less flavor; monitor salt usage.
Decrease in enzyme secretion	Food is harder to digest. Increase in indigestion. Intolerance to some food and seasonings.	Encourage water between meals. Avoid foods that are not tolerated while ensuring adequate nutrient intake.
Decrease in saliva	Food is more difficult to chew. Swallowing becomes difficult.	Encourage fluid intake with meals. Have clients chew food well and do two swallows with each bite of food. Have clients sit up to eat.

LIFE CYCLE CONSIDERATIONS

The Aging GI Tract

- Loss of elasticity and slowed motility of the GI tract, accompanied by lack of exercise, make the elderly prone to constipation.
- As the intestinal wall weakens, diverticuli, or scars on the intestinal wall, can develop.
- Decreased liver mass and blood flow alter the pharmacokinetics of various drugs.

ASSESSMENT

A thorough assessment is necessary to collect data on which to make an accurate nursing diagnosis. For clients describing GI symptoms, the assessment should include:

1. History of the present complaint, including length and frequency of symptoms, when symptoms occur, as well as aggravating factors
2. Medication history, including prescribed and over-the-counter (OTC) medications, and their effectiveness. Clients with GI symptoms frequently self-medicate with antacids, laxatives, suppositories, and enemas.
3. A complete nutritional history; a note should be made of any foods that increase or decrease symptoms. Also, assess if meals aggravate symptoms or if symptoms occur within a specific time period after a meal. Note the fiber and fat content of the diet as well as the amount of fluids typically consumed.

4. Psychosocial factors, including compliance and noncompliance with health status. Meal patterns should be evaluated: note if the client eats alone, eats large meals at regular intervals, or snacks all day.
5. Physical examination, including inspection, auscultation, percussion, and palpation of the abdomen. An evaluation of the client's ability to chew and swallow is also important.
6. Bowel elimination patterns, including frequency, consistency, and amounts of bowel movements
7. Evaluation of diagnostic data, including laboratory analysis and radiologic and endoscopic examinations

COMMON DIAGNOSTIC TESTS

Commonly used diagnostic tests for clients with digestive disorders are listed in Table 35-2.

DISORDERS OF THE GASTROINTESTINAL TRACT

Disorders of the gastrointestinal tract include stomatitis, esophageal varices, gastroesophageal reflux disease, gastritis, ulcers, appendicitis, diverticulosis and diverticulitis, inflammatory bowel disease, irritable bowel syndrome, intestinal obstruction, hernias, peritonitis, hemorrhoids, and constipation.

STOMATITIS

Stomatitis is a painful condition characterized by inflammation and ulcerations in the mouth. Stomatitis can be caused by infections, damage to the mucous membranes by irritants, or chemotherapy.

TABLE 35-2 COMMON DIAGNOSTIC TESTS FOR GASTROINTESTINAL DISORDERS

Laboratory Tests
- Complete blood count (CBC) ✓
- Prothrombin time (PT)
- Partial thromboplastin time (PTT)
- Bilirubin ✓
- Albumin
- Globulin
- Total protein
- Alkaline phosphatase
- Lactate hydrogenase (LDH-5)
- Gamma-glutamyl transpeptidase (GGT or GGTP)
- Aspartate aminotransferase (AST/SGOT)
- Alanine aminotransferase (ALT/SGPT)
- Cholesterol
- Triglycerides
- Amylase
- Carcinoembryonic antigen (CEA)
- HAA, now called hepatitis B surface antigen (HBsAG)
- Stool O & P
- Stool occult blood (guaiac) ✓
  Fecal occult blood test (FOBT)
  Hemocult

Radiologic Studies
- Barium swallow
- Upper gastrointestinal tract (UGI) with small bowel follow-through
- Abdominal x-rays ✓
- CT scans ✓
- Ultrasound
- Barium enema
- Gallbladder series

Other
- Flexible sigmoidoscopy
- Esophagogastro-duodenoscopy (EGD)
- Endoscopic retrograde cholangiopancreatogram (ERCP)
- Colonoscopy
- Esophageal motility studies (manometry)
- Gastric secretion analysis
- Liver biopsy
- Peritoneal aspiration

Medical–Surgical Management

Medical

Cultures may be done to determine if an infectious process is present.

Pharmacological

Because the client's mouth can be sore, topical anesthetics such as xylocaine may be used. Analgesics may also be ordered. If an infection is present, the appropriate medication will be ordered.

Diet

Dietary restrictions are based on what the client is able to tolerate. Bland, soft foods or liquids are usually tolerated best. As the sores heal, the diet may be advanced as tolerated. It is important to monitor dietary intake because caloric and fluid intake may be poor as a result of discomfort.

Nursing Management

Monitor caloric and fluid intake for adequacy. Encourage the client to eat soft, bland foods and liquids. Assess for mouth discomfort and check mouth for inflammation and ulcerations. Provide oral care and administer medications as ordered.

NURSING PROCESS

Assessment

Subjective Data

Clients usually describe pain in the mouth and difficulty swallowing.

Objective Data

Observations include inflamed mucosa of the mouth with ulcerations frequently present.

Nursing diagnoses for a client with stomatitis may include the following:

Nursing Diagnoses	Planning/Goals	Nursing Interventions
Acute Pain related to stomatitis	The client will verbalize increase in comfort within 1 hour of initiation of treatment.	Assess the client frequently for discomfort. Administer medications such as topical xylocaine and analgesics as ordered. Allow for rest periods as indicated.

continues

Nursing Diagnoses	Planning/Goals	Nursing Interventions
Imbalanced **N***utrition: Less than body requirements* related to inadequate caloric and fluid intake	The client will maintain caloric intake of 1,500 calories per day within 48 hours of treatment initiation. The client will maintain 2,000 cc per day fluid intake within 48 hours of treatment initiation.	Monitor daily caloric intake and consult with the dietitian to assist with food selection. Administer IV fluids as ordered and monitor I & O.
Impaired **O***ral Mucous Membranes* related to stomatitis	The client will have less inflammation and a decrease in the size of the ulcers by 36 hours after treatment initiation.	Monitor the stomatitis every shift to assess status of condition. Provide oral care every 4 hours. Administer medications as ordered to combat the infection.

Evaluation Each goal must be evaluated to determine how it has been met by the client.

ESOPHAGEAL VARICES

A varix is an enlarged, tortuous vein or, occasionally, an artery. Although varices can occur in any part of the digestive system, they occur most frequently in the distal veins of the esophagus. The varices are often associated with cirrhosis of the liver or any other condition that causes chronic obstruction of drainage from the esophageal veins into the portal veins. Swelling of the veins causes the walls to weaken, making them prone to ulceration and bleeding. Anything that causes increased abdominal venous pressure, such as sneezing, coughing, vomiting, the Valsalva maneuver, swallowing large, poorly chewed pieces of food, and the erosion of vessel walls by gastric acid, can cause the varices to rupture.

Varices have no symptoms, so clients may not be aware of them until they start bleeding. Death may ensue rapidly if the hemorrhaging varix is not treated immediately.

Medical–Surgical Management

Medical

The varices may be treated with sclerotherapy, ligation, or balloon tamponade. Sclerotherapy is a procedure in which a caustic substance is injected into the varix. An esophagogastroduodenoscopy (EGD) is performed and a sclerosing agent is injected through a special needle. Several treatments are necessary to cause formation of scar tissue and to stop the bleeding. After the bleeding has stopped and the client has stabilized, the remaining treatments may be done on an outpatient basis.

Complications to sclerotherapy include mediastinal inflammation secondary to extra esophageal injection, perforation, ulceration, stricture secondary to scar formation, and rebleeding.

Esophageal **ligation,** also called *banding,* involves placing a rubber band, tie, or O-ring on the varix (Figure 35-3). An EGD is performed to guide the placement of the bands. The complications include rebleeding and stricture formation.

In a case where varices are actively bleeding, a three- or four-lumen balloon tamponade, known as a Minnesota or Sengstaken-Blakemore tube, is passed into the esophagus. The balloon is then inflated in the esophagus to put direct pressure onto the bleeding varices. The balloon is periodically deflated to prevent necrosis of the esophageal tissue. Iced isotonic saline lavages may also be administered through the tube. During the procedure, the client must be kept NPO with the head of the bed elevated 30 to 45 degrees. Complications include perforation of the esophagus from pressure from the balloon and necrosis of the surrounding tissue.

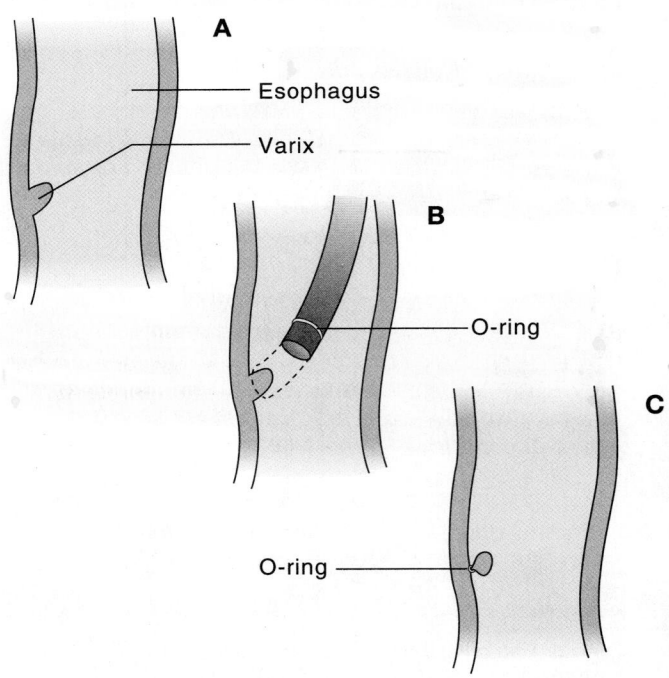

Figure 35-3 *Banding of an Esophageal Varix: **A**, Varix; **B**, Insertion of tube with O-ring; **C**, O-ring is placed around the varix.*

Surgical

A portosystemic shunt may be performed to relieve the pressure on the esophageal veins by redirecting blood from the portal vein to the inferior mesenteric vein. Some of the blood bypasses the liver and reenters the circulatory system (Figure 35-4).

A nonsurgical but invasive procedure, transjugular intrahepatic portosystemic shunt (TIPS), may also be performed. With this procedure, the right internal jugular vein is used to place a cannula into the hepatic and portal veins. A connection is made through the liver tissue between the hepatic and portal veins. A stent is placed in the connection. This allows some of the blood to bypass the liver and relieve pressure in the portal vein. This procedure is done in x-ray and is used with clients who are too unstable for surgery (also refer to Figure 35-9.)

Pharmacological

Octreotide (Sandostatin) may be given by IV to help control the bleeding by decreasing blood flow to the gut, thus lowering pressure in the portal system. Analgesics may be necessary following sclerotherapy if clients have chest discomfort. Clients should avoid NSAIDs, aspirin, and all anticoagulants. Sucralfate (Carafate) liquid may be given to coat the esophagus, protecting it from erosion by gastric acid. IV rehydration as well as blood transfusions may be necessary for clients with active bleeding.

Activity

If varices are bleeding or have recently bled, the client should remain on bed rest. If no active bleeding is present, the client may be ambulatory but should avoid strenuous exercise.

Nursing Management

Monitor vital signs. Explain tests and procedures. Allow time for client to express fears and concerns about the varices. Check laboratory test results for changes. Explain reasons to avoid strenuous activity. Assess for nausea and dizziness.

NURSING PROCESS

Assessment

Subjective Data

Assessment includes history of liver disease or alcohol abuse and nausea. With esophageal varices there is no abdominal pain. The symptom of abdominal pain helps distinguish esophageal varices from bleeding ulcers, which generally do cause pain (Giacchino & Houdek, 1998).

Objective Data

Assessment includes testing stools for **occult blood (guaiac)** and **melena** (black, sticky, tar-like stools containing partially broken-down blood), and assessing for **hematemesis,** or vomiting blood. Review hemoglobin and hematocrit (H & H) to evaluate anemia and liver profile for elevated bilirubin and globulin levels and a decrease in albumin.

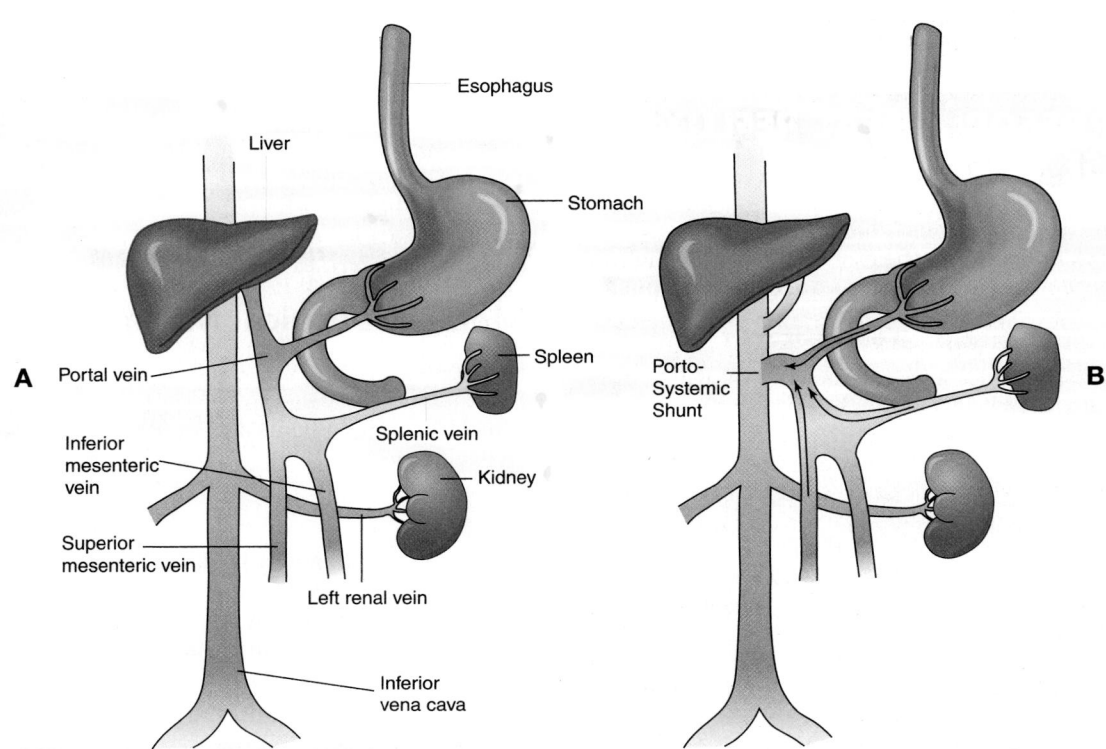

Figure 35-4 A, Normal Circulation of Abdominal Organs; **B,** An Example of a Portosystemic Shunt (may be performed in clients with elevated portal vein pressure that is resistant to medical management).

If cirrhosis of the liver is present, **jaundice,** a yellowing of the skin, mucous membranes, and sclerae of the eyes, is present. Jaundice results when the liver is unable to fully remove bilirubin from the blood. Nutritional status may be poor if the client abuses alcohol.

Nursing diagnoses for a client with esophageal varices may include the following:

Nursing Diagnoses	Planning/Goals	Nursing Interventions
Risk for Deficient **F***luid Volume* related to bleeding esophageal varices (if the varices are not actively bleeding)	The client will maintain adequate fluid volume.	Monitor vital signs every 4 hours including orthostatic blood pressures. Orthostatic blood pressure is obtained by taking the blood pressure when the client is lying down and then when standing. A 20 mm Hg difference in blood pressures from lying to standing would indicate a change in fluid volume, possibly indicating varix bleeding. Monitor for nausea and dizziness. Monitor H & H every 4 to 8 hours as ordered. A decrease in H & H values would indicate bleeding.
Deficient **F***luid Volume* related to bleeding esophageal varices and gastric loss from vomiting	The client will maintain an H & H within normal limits. The client's blood pressure will be within 20 mm Hg of baseline with no orthostatic changes.	Monitor H & H. Frequently monitor vital signs. Administer IV fluids, electrolyte replacement, and blood transfusions as ordered.
A*nxiety* related to change in health status, threat of death	The client will discuss concerns about health status.	Explain all tests and procedures to decrease anxiety. Allow client to express fears and concerns regarding condition.

Evaluation Each goal must be evaluated to determine how it has been met by the client.

GASTROESOPHAGEAL REFLUX DISEASE

In gastroesophageal reflux disease (GERD), gastric secretions flow upward into the esophagus, damaging the tissues. An inability of the lower esophageal sphincter (LES) to fully close contributes to this condition. Environmental and physical factors may contribute to decreased pressure in the LES. Fatty foods, caffeine, nicotine, calcium channel blockers, and NSAIDs decrease the tightness of the sphincter. Symptoms include belching, dysphagia, esophagitis, epigastric pain, heartburn, flatulence, melena, and bleeding. Diagnosis is made by symptoms, a 24-hour pH monitoring, and an esophageal motility test. An endoscopy determines the extent of esophagitis and rules out a malignancy.

Medical–Surgical Management
Medical

GERD is generally treated conservatively with diet and medications. Clients are encouraged to lose weight if they are overweight.

Surgical

A fundoplication may be done to alleviate symptoms. A fundoplication is a laparoscopic procedure in which the LES is tightened by wrapping and suturing the fundus of the stomach around the esophagus.

Pharmacological

GERD is treated conservatively with antacids, H₂ receptor antagonists, proton pump inhibitors, cytoprotective agents, and gastrointestinal motility agents.

CLIENT TEACHING

GERD

- Lose weight as needed.
- Avoid fatty foods, alcohol, nicotine, caffeine, and spicy foods.
- Take medications as instructed.
- Elevate head of the bed 2 to 4 inches on blocks.
- Avoid wearing constrictive clothing.

Diet

A low-fat, high-protein diet is recommended. The client is encouraged to avoid caffeine, milk products, alcohol, peppermint, licorice, and spicy foods.

Nursing Management

Encourage client to avoid foods that increase the symptoms (e.g., caffeine, milk products, alcohol, and fatty foods). Obtain diet history from client. Observe for melena and signs of discomfort or pain.

GASTRITIS

Gastritis is an inflammation of the stomach mucosa occurring when the stomach has been exposed to irritating substances such as medications, smoke, food allergens, or toxic chemicals. Another contributing factor to gastritis may be impaired mucosal defenses, which occur when the epithelial cells of the stomach are not able to secrete an adequate quantity or quality of mucus to protect the stomach. The presence of the bacteria *Helicobactor pylori (H. pylori)* has also been associated with gastritis.

Medical–Surgical Management
Medical

Diagnosis of gastritis is based on history and symptoms. An UGI or EGD may be done to help diagnose the condition. If *H. pylori* is suspected, a biopsy is obtained during an EGD and a culture is performed.

Pharmacological

Treatment for gastritis is primarily pharmacological involving antacids and histamine (H_2) receptor antagonists (also call H_2 blockers). A proton pump inhibitor such as omeprazole (Prilosec) or prostaglandins may be used. If *H. pylori* is present, bismuth preparations may be used to inhibit *H. pylori* growth and antibiotics to eliminate the bacteria (Table 35-3).

NSAIDs such as ibuprofen (Motrin) and indomethacin (Indocin) have been shown to compromise mucosal defenses and increase acid secretion. Clients who are on NSAIDs chronically, such as clients with arthritis, may need to be evaluated to determine if other analgesics would be effective or if a prostaglandin should be taken with the NSAIDs.

Diet

Although studies have shown that dietary modifications have little impact on the rate of gastritis healing, some modifications are indicated. Any foods that aggravate symptoms should be eliminated. Also, foods that increase acid secretions, such as milk, coffee, decaffeinated coffee, tea, colas, and chocolate, should be consumed only in small amounts or eliminated if possible. Bedtime eating should be avoided because it increases nocturnal acid secretions.

TABLE 35-3 MEDICATIONS USED FOR ULCERS AND GASTRITIS

MEDICATION	PURPOSE	NURSING IMPLICATIONS
Antacids • aluminum hydroxide (Amphogel) • aluminum hydroxide and magnesium hydroxide (Maalox) • dihydroxyaluminum sodium carbonate (Rolaids)	Seal impaired mucosa. Neutralize acids.	Antacids containing aluminum hydroxide may cause constipation. Antacids containing magnesium hydroxide may cause diarrhea; monitor serum electrolytes; do not give with other meds.
H_2 Receptor Antagonists • ranitadine HCl (Zantac) • cimetidine (Tagamet)	Decrease gastric acid secretion.	Do not give within 1 hour of antacids.
Proton Pump Inhibitor • omeprazole (Prilosec)	Stop gastric acid secretion.	Give with food. Suspend granules in an acid liquid. Takes 4 days to achieve blood level.
Prostaglandins • misoprostol (Cytotec)	Decrease gastric acid secretion. Enhance mucosal defenses.	Give when NSAIDs need to be continued.
Bismuth Compounds • bismuth subsalicylate (Pepto-Bismol)	Enhance mucosal barriers. Inhibit *H. pylori* growth.	Do not give within 1 hour of H_2 blockers.
Antibiotics • ampicillin (Omnipen) • metronidazole (Flagyl)	Eliminate *H. pylori*.	Some antibiotics will cause N/V if taken with alcohol. Do not give with antacids or meals with the exception of Flagyl, which must be taken with food. Clients usually placed on two different antibiotics simultaneously.

Health Promotion

Smoking and alcohol aggravate the mucosal lining of the stomach and significantly impair gastritis healing. Smoking and alcohol consumption should be minimized or eliminated if possible.

Nursing Management

Encourage client to minimize or eliminate smoking and alcohol consumption (if applicable) and any foods that aggravate symptoms. Teach client about medications.

NURSING PROCESS

Assessment

Subjective Data

Clients with gastritis may have no symptoms or may describe epigastric pain or burning, or nausea. They may also state that certain foods aggravate symptoms.

Objective Data

Stools may test positive for blood.

Nursing diagnoses for a client with gastritis may include the following:

Nursing Diagnoses	Planning/Goals	Nursing Interventions
*Acute **Pain*** related to gastric acid on inflammation	The client will experience less pain within 24 hours of onset of treatment as identified by pain scale.	Administer medications and provide diet as ordered. Assess client for improvement of symptoms. Implement education about lifestyle changes.
*Deficient **Knowledge*** related to condition, therapy, and symptoms of potential complications	The client will verbalize understanding of condition and symptoms of complications and will comply with treatment regimen.	Educate regarding medication regimen and lifestyle changes. If the client smokes or drinks alcohol, provide information on smoking and drinking cessation. Discuss dietary modifications.

Evaluation Each goal must be evaluated to determine how it has been met by the client.

ULCERS

Peptic ulcers are erosions that form in the esophagus, stomach, or duodenum resulting from an acid/pepsin imbalance. **Gastric ulcers** refer to erosions in the stomach and are correlated to exposure to irritants such as NSAIDs, smoking, alcohol, food allergens, toxic chemicals, *H. pylori* infections, and impaired mucosal defenses. Impaired mucosal defenses occur when the epithelial cells of the stomach are not able to secrete an adequate quantity or quality of mucus to protect the stomach.

Clients with gastric ulcers frequently complain of pain 1 to 2 hours after eating. Eating may not relieve pain or may even increase pain. Weight loss is common. Risk factors include alcohol use, stress, and NSAID use.

Stress ulcers are a type of gastric ulcer that form when gastritis becomes erosive and starts bleeding. As the name implies, stress ulcers occur in clients whose bodies are experiencing stress, such as clients who have experienced major surgery, trauma, burns, chemotherapy, or radiation therapy. Clients with chronic respiratory disorders may also experience stress ulcers because hypoxia can lead to impaired mucosa. Bleeding may be massive resulting in significant blood loss or can be slow and insidious. Because of the multiple sites of bleeding, stress ulcers may be difficult to manage.

Duodenal ulcers refer to ulcers in the duodenum. Incidents of duodenal ulcers have been correlated to a high secretion of HCl. Clients with duodenal ulcers frequently complain of pain 2 to 4 hours after eating. Nocturnal pain may be present, occurring between midnight and 3 A.M. Eating frequently relieves symptoms. Weight gain is common. Risk factors include a history of pulmonary disease, cirrhosis, chronic pancreatitis, and/or chronic renal failure.

If an ulcer erodes through a blood vessel, the client may experience a life-threatening hemorrhage. A perforation occurs if the ulcer erodes through the wall of the stomach or small intestine resulting in gastric or intestinal contents entering the abdominal cavity and causing peritonitis.

Diagnosis of ulcers is based on symptoms, history, and an UGI or EGD performed to visualize the ulcer. If an *H. pylori* infection is suspected, a biopsy is obtained during an EGD and a culture is performed.

Medical–Surgical Management

Medical

If an ulcer bleeds, an EGD may be performed, and the ulcer is either injected with epinephrine to cause vasoconstriction or a special electrical probe is used to cauterize or burn the tissue that is bleeding. A nasogastric

(NG) tube may be inserted to remove gastric contents and blood, and iced isotonic saline may be instilled to help cause vasoconstriction and stop the bleeding.

Surgical — Vagotomy

The most commonly performed surgery for peptic ulcers is a vagotomy in which a section of the vagus nerve is cut removing vagal innervation to the fundus of the stomach. This eliminates the production of hydrochloric acid, decreases function of the gastrin hormone, and slows motility of the stomach. A vagotomy eliminates the complications of the more aggressive surgeries, such as gastrectomies.

If the ulcer continues to bleed or if the ulcer has perforated, the client is taken to surgery and a gastrectomy is performed. The portion of the stomach or duodenum that is perforated is removed and the bowel is reconnected with an anastomosis.

Complications from gastrectomies include gastric dumping in which the stomach experiences **postprandial** (after eating) rapid gastric emptying. Clients experience abdominal pain, nausea, vomiting, explosive diarrhea, weakness, and dizziness. Clients with gastric dumping have malabsorption of nutrients because the food passes too quickly to permit absorption, thus leading to malnutrition. In addition, many clients with significant symptoms may limit dietary intake to avoid symptoms, compounding the malnutrition and weight loss issues.

Management of gastric dumping includes small, frequent meals of high fiber and high protein and avoidance of simple carbohydrates.

Pharmacological

Treatment of ulcers is primarily pharmacological involving antacids, histamine (H₂) receptor antagonists (also called H₂ blockers), proton pump inhibitors, or prostaglandins. If *H. pylori* is present, bismuth preparations are generally used to inhibit its growth and antibiotics to eliminate the bacteria (refer to Table 35-3).

NSAIDs such as ibuprofen (Motrin) and indomethacin (Indocin) have been shown to compromise mucosal defenses and increase acid secretion. Clients who are on NSAIDs chronically, such as clients with arthritis, may need to evaluate if other analgesics would be effective or if a prostaglandin should be taken with the NSAIDs.

Diet

Although studies have shown that dietary modifications have little impact on the rate of ulcer healing, some modifications are indicated. Foods that aggravate symptoms should be eliminated. Also, foods that increase acid secretions, such as milk, coffee, decaffeinated coffee, tea, colas, and chocolate, should be consumed only in small amounts or eliminated if possible. Bedtime eating should also be avoided because it increases nocturnal acid secretions.

Health Promotion

Smoking and alcohol aggravate the mucosal lining of the stomach and duodenum and significantly impair ulcer healing. Smokers also experience a higher ulcer recurrence rate. Stress has been shown to increase the rate of peptic ulcers. Although the type or severity of stress may not be significant, the client's interpretation of the events as stressful is. Clients need to develop mechanisms for reducing stress such as exercise, biofeedback, and relaxation.

Nursing Management

Encourage lifestyle changes when necessary regarding smoking, alcohol, and stress. Teach relaxation techniques. Monitor weight and laboratory test results. Discourage having a bedtime snack to prevent acid secretions at night. Assess pain including relationship to eating a meal.

NURSING PROCESS

Assessment

Subjective Data

Clients with gastric ulcers are often asymptomatic or may describe epigastric pain or burning 1 to 2 hours after eating, and nausea or bloating. Clients may experience an increase of symptoms when they eat and therefore may decrease dietary intake. When questioned about lifestyle, NSAID usage, stress, smoking, and alcohol use may be discovered.

Clients with duodenal ulcers may exhibit no symptoms or may complain of pain 2 to 4 hours after eating. Eating will frequently decrease symptoms, so clients will often eat more frequently. When questioned about lifestyle, stress, smoking, and alcohol consumption may be discovered. The client may also have a history of pulmonary disease, cirrhosis, chronic pancreatitis, and/or chronic renal failure.

A client who is actively bleeding from an ulcer will experience an acute onset of epigastric pain, shortness of breath, and nausea.

Objective Data

Clients with gastric ulcers may show a weight loss and stools may test positive for blood. An H & H may show anemia.

Clients with duodenal ulcers may show a weight gain and stools may test positive for blood. An H & H may show anemia.

The client who is actively bleeding from an ulcer will show signs of shock: pale clammy skin, an elevated pulse rate, and a drop in blood pressure. The client may also have hematemesis. Laboratory tests may show a low H & H. Stools may test positive for blood.

Nursing diagnoses for a client with ulcers may include the following:

Nursing Diagnoses	Planning/Goals	Nursing Interventions
Acute Pain related to gastric acid on ulcerated mucosa	The client will experience less pain within 24 hours of onset of treatment as identified on pain scale.	Assess clients for decrease of pain. Administer medications as ordered. Assess for elevated BP.
Deficient Knowledge related to condition, therapy, and symptoms of complications	The client will verbalize understanding of factors related to condition and symptoms of complications. Client will comply with treatment regimen.	Identify client's learning style and provide information in a manner compatible with the learning style. Educate regarding medication regimen, lifestyle changes, and signs and symptoms of possible complications. If indicated, provide client with smoking cessation information and stress reduction techniques such as exercise and biofeedback.
Deficient Fluid Volume related to bleeding ulcer	The client will exhibit normal fluid volume as evidenced by stable H & H and blood pressure within 20 mm Hg of baseline.	Check vital signs every 4 hours and PRN including orthostatic blood pressure. Monitor for dizziness and nausea. Check stool for blood. Administer IV fluids, electrolyte replacement, and blood transfusions as ordered.

Evaluation Each goal must be evaluated to determine how it has been met by the client.

APPENDICITIS

Appendicitis is the inflammation of the vermiform appendix, a 10-cm small, slender tube attached to the cecum. The appendix may be inflamed, gangrenous, or ruptured. If the opening to the appendix becomes blocked with feces, the *E. coli* multiply in the appendix and infection develops with pus formation. If it ruptures, fecal content spills into the abdominal cavity causing peritonitis, which may be fatal. It is most common in young adults, but can occur at any age (Atassi, 2002a).

A barium enema or an ultrasound may be ordered to confirm inflammation in the appendiceal area.

Medical–Surgical Management

Early diagnosis and treatment are necessary for the best client outcome. A white blood count and differential will usually show a WBC above 10,000/mm³ and neutrophils over 75%. An elevated temperature indicates infection. Rebound tenderness in the right lower quadrant (RLQ) of the abdomen (at McBurney's point) is a positive diagnostic finding. An appendectomy may be performed along with other abdominal surgeries as a preventive measure.

Surgical

A surgical procedure called an *appendectomy* is necessary before the appendix ruptures. Appendectomies are the most common emergency surgery and require a hospital stay of 2 to 7 days. If no rupture has occurred, a laparoscopic appendectomy, in which the appendix is removed through a scope, may be done. This requires only a small incision and allows the client to be discharged 24 hours after the surgery.

Pharmacological

Preoperatively, no analgesics are given so that symptoms will not be masked by the medication. Fluids and electrolytes may need to be replaced before surgery. Antibiotics are usually given preoperatively. Postoperatively, analgesics are administered for relief of incisional discomfort. Antibiotics are usually given postoperatively, especially if a perforation is present.

Diet

Preoperatively and initially postoperatively, the client is NPO. If a perforation with peritonitis occurred, the client is kept NPO longer, and an NG tube may be inserted until bowel sounds return. Clear liquids and then full liquids and finally a regular diet is given as normal bowel function returns.

Activity

Initially postoperatively, the client is encouraged to turn, cough, and deep breathe every 2 hours. Next, the client is encouraged to increase ambulation gradually. Activity restrictions depend on the severity of the appendicitis. Driving, exercise, and lifting will be limited for a few weeks to allow for incisional healing.

Nursing Management

Assess pain. Keep client NPO. Monitor vital signs, especially temperature. Assess bowel sounds. Monitor results of CBC especially WBC and neutrophils. Postoperatively, encourage client to turn, cough, and deep breathe every 2 hours. Encourage ambulation. Advance diet from liquid to regular as bowel function returns.

NURSING PROCESS

Assessment

Subjective Data

Clients with appendicitis describe abdominal pain, typically located in the RLQ around McBurney's point (halfway between the umbilicus and the right iliac crest).

Clients also complain of anorexia (a loss of appetite) and nausea.

Objective Data

Clients may have vomiting and fever. Bowel sounds may be diminished or absent. Rebound tenderness, pain that occurs when fingers are pressed into the RLQ and then released suddenly, may be present. A CBC will show WBCs elevated above 10,000/mm³ with neutrophils over 75%.

Nursing diagnoses for the client with appendicitis may include the following:

Nursing Diagnoses	Planning/Goals	Nursing Interventions
Acute Pain related to appendicitis/appendectomy	The client will experience a decrease in pain as evidenced by improved mobility and as identified on pain scale.	Preoperatively, monitor client's pain and check abdomen for rigidity. Provide an ice pack to help relieve pain as ordered; never use heat. Postoperatively, give analgesics as ordered and medicate prior to activities such as ambulation. Teach client to use a pillow to splint the incision when coughing. If client is having difficulty passing flatus, administer enemas or a rectal tube as ordered, and encourage ambulation.
Impaired Skin Integrity related to the abdominal incision	The client will verbalize signs and symptoms of infection and factors that enhance wound healing, by discharge.	Administer antibiotics as ordered. Educate the client that incision may be left open to the air after 24 hours; that showers may be taken, per physician instruction; and signs and symptoms of infection and activity restrictions. If adhesive strips are present, leave in place until they no longer cover the incision (approximately 10 days to 2 weeks).

Evaluation Each goal must be evaluated to determine how it has been met by the client.

DIVERTICULOSIS AND DIVERTICULITIS

Diverticula are saclike protrusions of the intestinal wall. **Diverticulosis** refers to a condition of the colon in which multiple diverticula are present (Figure 35-5). The exact cause of diverticulosis is not known; however, a diet low in fiber is believed to contribute to the formation of the pouches. Diverticulosis affects 30% to 40% of the elderly population (Cameron, 1998). It is asymptomatic unless perforation or hemorrhage occur. **Diverticulitis** refers to the inflammation of one or more diverticula generally in the sigmoid colon. It is a complication of diverticulosis and is thought to be caused by stool impacted in the diverticula.

Medical–Surgical Management

Medical

Diverticulosis is typically asymptomatic and needs no intervention. Most cases of diverticulitis are treated with analgesics, antibiotics, bed rest, NPO to rest the bowel, and IV fluid hydration.

A barium enema or abdominal ultrasound is usually ordered when diverticulitis is suspected. A flexible sigmoidoscopy may also be performed.

Surgical

If bleeding or perforation of the diverticula occurs, or if an abscess forms, surgery is required to remove the affected portion of the bowel. A colon resection is

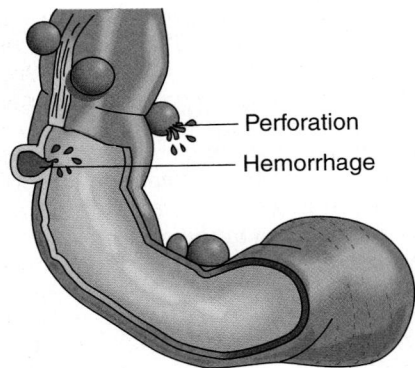

Figure 35-5 *Diverticula in the Sigmoid Colon. Diverticulosis is almost always located in the descending or sigmoid colon.*

Ascending colostomy

Transverse colostomy

Descending colostomy

Sigmoid colostomy

Figure 35-6 *Colostomy Sites (Blue area is colon removed.)*

performed. A colostomy may be required. A **colostomy** is a surgically created opening from the colon through the abdominal wall to relieve either a disease or functional problem in the large intestine.

Stool consistency depends on the placement of the **stoma** (surgical opening between a cavity and the surface of the body) in the colon. A colostomy is named for the part of the colon where it is located. An ascending colostomy takes its name from the ascending colon and would be on the right side of the abdomen. It has a liquid output. A transverse colostomy would be more toward the midline of the abdomen and has a pasty liquid output. A descending colostomy or sigmoid colostomy has a more solid output. Figure 35-6 shows the different colostomy sites.

If a large amount of inflammation is present, a temporary colostomy may be performed to allow the colon to heal. The colon is reconnected at a later time. Sometimes a permanent colostomy needs to be performed.

Pharmacological

Clients who have been identified as having diverticulosis are usually placed on fiber supplements or stool softeners. Clients with diverticulitis are treated with sulfa antibiotics and other antimicrobial agents. Analgesics may also be ordered for discomfort.

Diet

A high-fiber diet is believed to help reduce the occurrence of diverticulosis and diverticulitis. Clients experiencing diverticulitis will be NPO to rest the bowel. Once the diverticulitis begins healing, the client is placed on clear liquids and then advanced to a bland, low-residue diet while the diverticulitis heals.

If surgery is performed, the client is NPO until bowel sounds return. The client is then started on clear liquids, advanced to full liquids as more bowel function returns, and then finally advanced to a regular diet. A high-fiber diet is encouraged for clients once the diverticulitis episode has resolved.

Activity

For clients experiencing diverticulitis, bed rest and decreased mobility are encouraged to allow the bowel to rest. In clients who have had a bowel resection, activity will gradually be progressed postoperatively.

Stoma/Ostomy Management

Assessment

Provide the client with an opportunity to ask questions and begin coping with a possible altered body image. Before ostomy surgery, the surgeon and the enterostomal (ET) nurse talk with the client and explain the reason for the surgery and the possibilities of ostomy surgery. Choosing the site or placement of the stoma depends on the type of ostomy being created, the lifestyle of the client, and the contours of the client's abdomen.

On return from surgery, the new stoma will be edematous and range from deep red to dusky in color. The color of the stoma is checked with a penlight and documented at least once per shift. Color is important because it reveals the status of the blood supply to the stoma. If blood supply to the stoma is inadequate, the stoma will turn black. Notify the physician if the stoma becomes black.

Immediately after surgery there may be a small amount of serosanguineous drainage in the appliance. When the appliance is changed and the stoma is cleaned or touched when swollen, a small amount of bleeding may occur. Reassure the client that a small amount of bleeding is normal.

Bowel function is checked every shift to monitor for any obstruction or ileus. Bowel sounds, distention, and abdominal tenderness are checked every 4 hours.

Complications

Hemorrhage Bleeding or hemorrhage may occur at the incision site or stoma site. It is important to check the incision and stoma site for bleeding and to check the blood pressure and pulse frequently after surgery.

Infection The risk of infection around the stoma is great because of the presence of stool around the new suture line.

Hernia A hernia is the most frequent complication of an ostomy and is caused when a loop of bowel pushes up through the muscle next to the stoma and under the skin.

Obstruction Obstruction of the bowel ostomy may occur as a complication after surgery. Ileostomy clients are instructed to chew their food well before swallowing because large pieces of food such as an olive or large piece of meat may get caught at the opening of the ostomy.

Prolapse The bowel may sometimes telescope out, resembling an elephant's trunk. If the bowel continues to work, this is not an emergency. The physician or ET nurse may be able to replace the bowel back into the abdomen; if not, the mucosa of the bowel may become injured, so the prolapse is corrected surgically. Prolapse can be frightening for the client, and its possibility is discussed in postoperative teaching.

Electrolyte Imbalance An ileostomy with a high output of effluent can cause electrolyte imbalances by loss of large amounts of potassium and protein. The client may have difficulty learning to cope with an appliance that is always filling and the need to take in enough fluid, protein, and potassium to replace the lost nutrients.

Skin Excoriation The skin around a high-output ostomy may become excoriated if an appliance that protects the skin cannot be found. Ileostomy effluent contains digestive juices that, if left on the skin, will start to digest the skin, resulting in red, open areas. To prevent this problem, correct appliance fitting that will stay in place is important for these clients.

Discharge Teaching for the Ostomy Client

Assessment

As the client prepares to go home, it is important to assess the client's or the family's ability to handle ostomy care at home. The client may still be dealing with an altered body image and not want to look at or touch the stoma. The family may have to help with care and be supportive until the client can assume the care.

Appliances

If the client has only one bowel movement per day, a closed appliance that is taken off and emptied once a day will be all that is needed. If the client has several stools per day, an open-ended drainable appliance may be best.

For ileostomies, the one- or two-piece open-end appliance offers ease in emptying. Effluent usually varies from liquid to pasty, so an appliance that can be drained several times per day without taking it off is important. A skin barrier is also necessary for the ileostomy or any ostomy with liquid output.

Irrigation

Irrigation is a means of regulating some colostomies. Descending or sigmoid colostomies may be irrigated daily or every other day for control of evacuation. After irrigation, the client may wear a small security appliance or a gauze pad over the stoma the rest of the day. The disadvantage of irrigation is that it takes about an hour or more to perform. The decision to irrigate is made by the client, with the consent of the surgeon, after healing has taken place. To irrigate a colostomy, a cone tip is needed on the end of the irrigation catheter. Using the cone on the tip of the tubing prevents the end of the tube from poking into the side of the bowel and injuring the bowel and helps hold the fluid in the bowel. The cone will need to be lubricated liberally with lubricating jelly.

Support Person

Upon discharge, the client and family receive the telephone number of the hospital and unit where treatment was received so they may call if questions arise. Seeing the ET nurse again in 4 to 6 weeks is sometimes recommended to check how the client is doing with ostomy care. If there is a local stoma support group, a person from the group may call or visit the client at home and invite the client and family to come to the group sessions.

Having ostomy surgery is no reason to stop any life activity. People with ostomies live full, active, productive lives.

Nursing Management

Assess bowel sounds frequently. Monitor severity of symptoms such as pain, diarrhea, constipation, abdominal distention, anorexia, nausea, vomiting, and fever. Check CBC reports for elevated WBC and low H & H. Explain all tests and treatments and answer questions.

NURSING PROCESS

Assessment

Diverticulosis often has no symptoms, and therefore, clients may not be aware they have it.

Subjective Data

Clients with diverticulitis frequently describe left lower abdominal pain, constipation or diarrhea, bloating, anorexia, and nausea.

Objective Data

Assessment shows abdominal distention with tenderness on palpation, decreased bowel sounds, fever, vomiting, and stools that test positive for blood. A CBC will show an elevated ■ WBC and, if bleeding is present, a low H & H.

Nursing diagnoses for a client with diverticulosis or diverticulitis may include the following:

Nursing Diagnoses	Planning/Goals	Nursing Interventions
Acute **P***ain* related to diverticulitis	The client will verbalize a decrease in pain within 24 hours after intervention as measured by the pain scale.	Encourage bed rest to allow healing. Maintain client as NPO. Administer analgesics and antibiotics as ordered.
Risk for **I***nfection* related to abscess formation or perforation	The client will verbalize understanding of signs and symptoms of possible complications.	Monitor vital signs and pain level every 4 hours and assess abdomen every 4 hours for increased tenderness and distention. Educate the client to notify staff of chills, shortness of breath, or increasing pain.
A*nxiety* related to possible surgery	The client will verbalize fears related to surgery and exhibit decreased anxiety regarding the procedure and follow-up treatment.	Explain all tests and treatments to decrease the client's anxiety level. Answer all concerns and questions. Allow the client to verbalize fears and concerns. If a colostomy is planned, arrange a consult with an enterostomal therapist to help answer concerns.

Evaluation Each goal must be evaluated to determine how it has been met by the client.

SAMPLE NURSING CARE PLAN

THE CLIENT WITH DIVERTICULITIS

Mr. W. is a 67-year-old male admitted to the hospital with abdominal pain that started 2 days ago. The pain has been increasing in intensity and is now accompanied by nausea and anorexia. Physical assessment reveals temperature 101.7, pulse 96, respirations 24, and blood pressure of 162/90. Mr. W.'s abdomen is tender on palpation. He is in obvious discomfort and is unable to lie on his back. Mr. W. states he has not been eating any food or drinking adequate fluids for 24 hours. Skin turgor is poor. An abdominal ultrasound is ordered and identifies diverticulitis. An IV of D5 1/2 NS with 20 mEq KCl, droperidol (Inapsine) IV for nausea, meperidine (Demerol) IM for pain, and IV antibiotics are ordered. Mr. W. is placed on I & O, bed rest with bathroom privileges, and is made NPO. Mr. W. states that he does not understand why all this is being done. His first two voidings are 50 cc each and very concentrated (dark gold colored).

Nursing Diagnosis 1 *Deficient* **K***nowledge* related to diagnosis and treatment regimen as evidenced by statement that he does not understand why all this is being done

Nursing Outcomes Classification (NOC)	Nursing Interventions Classification (NIC)
Knowledge: Disease Process	*Teaching: Disease Process*
Knowledge: Treatment Regimen	*Teaching: Individual*

PLANNING/GOALS	NURSING INTERVENTIONS	RATIONALE
Mr. W. will verbalize understanding of treatment plan.	Assess Mr. W.'s knowledge level of diverticulosis/diverticulitis.	Helps client relate new information and integrate it into his behavior.
	Assess Mr. W.'s learning style and present information in a compatible manner.	Increases understanding and retention.
	Monitor for signs of pain and fatigue.	They impair learning.
	Answer questions and reinforce information.	Reinforces the new information learned.

continues

SAMPLE NURSING CARE PLAN

EVALUATION   Mr. W. verbalizes understanding of the disease process and treatment regimen.

Nursing Diagnosis 2 *Acute Pain* related to diverticulitis as evidenced by tender abdomen

Nursing Outcomes Classification (NOC)
Symptom Control
Pain Level

Nursing Interventions Classification (NIC)
Pain Management
Medication Management

PLANNING/GOALS	NURSING INTERVENTIONS	RATIONALE
Mr. W. will verbalize a decrease in pain within 24 hours of pain intervention.	Assess pain utilizing a scale of 1 (no pain) to 10 (extreme pain).	Provides objective measure of the client's perceived discomfort and effectiveness of analgesics.
	Medicate with analgesics as ordered.	Provides pain relief.
	Encourage Mr. W. to request analgesics before pain gets intense.	Provides better control of pain.
	Monitor effectiveness of pain medication by reassessing the pain 45 minutes after analgesic given.	Provides a measure of analgesic effectiveness.

EVALUATION   Mr. W. demonstrates adequate pain relief as demonstrated by a decrease in pain scale.

Nursing Diagnosis 3 *Deficient Fluid Volume* related to not eating any food or drinking adequate fluids for 24 hours as evidenced by low urine output and poor skin turgor

Nursing Outcomes Classification (NOC)
Hydration

Nursing Interventions Classification (NIC)
Fluid Management
Fluid Monitoring

PLANNING/GOALS	NURSING INTERVENTIONS	RATIONALE
Mr. W. will demonstrate adequate hydration by I & O being nearly equal, normal skin turgor, and electrolytes within normal limits by 24 hours after intervention.	Monitor I & O every shift.	Provides information on Mr. W.'s hydration.
	Administer IV fluids as ordered.	Provides needed hydration.
	Assess skin turgor every shift.	Provides hydration information.
	Monitor electrolytes on laboratory reports.	Provides information on electrolyte balance.

EVALUATION   Mr. W. demonstrates adequate hydration by nearly equal I&O, normal skin turgor, and electrolytes within normal limits.

INFLAMMATORY BOWEL DISEASE

Inflammatory bowel disease (IBD) is the term used to describe Crohn's disease and ulcerative colitis (UC), which are diseases characterized by inflammation and ulcerations of the bowel (Table 35-4). The symptoms of IBD are not confined to the bowel but can affect many of the body's systems. Potential extraintestinal manifestations may be found in other internal organs, eyes, blood, skin, and musculoskeletal system. Thirty percent of IBD clients have at least one extraintestinal manifestation (Rayhorn & Rayhorn, 2002).

Crohn's disease is characterized by lesions that affect the entire thickness of the bowel and can occur anywhere throughout the colon and small intestine. Symptoms include abdominal pain, diarrhea that usually does not contain blood, fever, anorexia, weight loss, and steatorrhea (fatty stools). Electrolyte imbalance, iron-deficiency anemia, and amino acid malabsorption may occur when the disease involves the jejunum and the ileum. Long-term complications of Crohn's disease include bowel obstructions, fistulas, abscesses, and perforation. The risk for colorectal cancer, while not as high as in UC, is still elevated. There is malabsorption of fat and fat-soluble vitamins.

UC is characterized by mucosal lesions occurring typically in the rectal area and sigmoid colon and progressing throughout the colon. Symptoms include fever, anorexia, weight loss, cramping, spasms, abdominal pain, and bloody diarrhea. Long-term complications include fissures, abscesses, and an increased risk for colorectal cancer. (Bloody diarrhea 20/day)

The gold standard for diagnosing IBD is an endoscopic examination with a biopsy.

Medical–Surgical Management

Medical

Treatment for Crohn's disease and UC is similar. Crohn's disease, however, is more debilitating because it involves more of the GI tract. UC is more limited but can still produce significant symptoms.

An endoscopy done on a UC client will reveal continuous mucosal inflammation and ulceration, loss of mucosal vascularity, diffuse erythema, and often purulent exudate. Any granuloma found in the biopsy confirms Crohn's disease (Rayhorn & Rayhorn, 2002).

The goals of treatment are to control inflammation, relieve symptoms, maintain fluid and electrolyte balance, provide adequate nutrition, and prevent complications.

Surgical

In severe cases of UC resistant to medical management, the colon is removed and an ileostomy is performed, curing the disease. An **ileostomy** is an opening created in the small intestine (ileum). The output from an ileostomy is a thin liquid, usually of a yellowish-green color. This thin output is called **effluent.** It generally has no odor, and it may get thicker in time as the body adapts to the need to retain moisture. Many ileostomies have almost constant effluent output. The Kock continent ileostomy has a pouch made inside the abdomen to hold the effluent until the client is ready to empty the pouch. Figure 35-7 illustrates a Kock continent ileostomy.

Most clients with Crohn's disease need surgery at some point to repair the structural damage caused by scarring. Intestinal obstructions and perforations may also occur in Crohn's disease, necessitating further surgery. Surgical intervention, however, does not cure the disease.

TABLE 35-4	COMPARISON OF CROHN'S DISEASE AND ULCERATIVE COLITIS	
PARAMETER	**CROHN'S DISEASE**	**ULCERATIVE COLITIS (UC)**
Involvement	Patchy areas. Can involve small and large intestine.	Starts in lower colon and spreads progressively throughout colon. Affects only the colon.
Tissue affected	Affects entire thickness of bowel.	Affects mucosal lining of bowel.
Long-term complications	Intestinal obstruction, fistulas, abscesses, perforations; cancer risk increases with age.	Fissures, abscesses, increased risk for colorectal cancer.
Surgical intervention	Usually needed at some point to repair structural damage. Does not cure or limit the progress of the disease.	Ileostomy performed in approximately 20% of cases to remove the colon. Cures the disease.
Cause	Unknown: possibly altered immune state.	Unknown: possibly enteric bacterium E. coli.
Stools	3 to 4 semisoft/day; rarely bloody; steatorrhea and mucus present.	15 to 20 liquid/day; blood present; no steatorrhea.

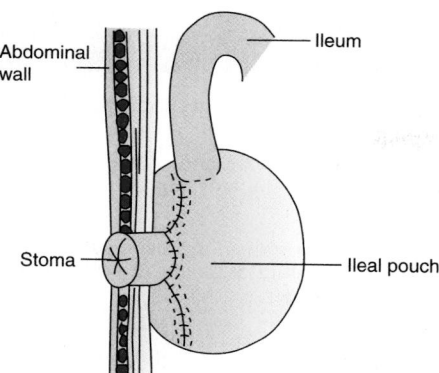

Figure 35-7 *Kock Continent Ileostomy*

Pharmacological

Treatment for both UC and Crohn's disease includes 5-ASA compounds such as sulfasalazine (Azulfidine) or salicylates such as mesalamine (Rowasa) or olsalazine sodium (Dipentum). If inflammation is severe, corticosteroids may also be administered. In cases resistant to the 5-ASA compounds and corticosteroids, immunosuppressors may be used. If an infection is present, antibiotics are administered. According to Rayhorn and Rayhorn (2002), clients are seldom given antidiarrheal medications because they may predispose the client to toxic megacolon.

Clients may need IV fluid and electrolyte replacement during severe flare-ups. In the most severe cases, clients may be placed on total parenteral nutrition (TPN) to allow for complete bowel rest and to improve nutritional status.

Diet

Protein and calorie malnutrition is a concern in clients with IBD. Because of the severe cramping, pain, and diarrhea brought on by foods, these clients typically put themselves on a very restrictive diet that is not nutritionally balanced. Clients with Crohn's disease may also have malabsorption of iron and vitamin B_{12}.

Nutritional support includes modifying the diet to eliminate foods that exacerbate symptoms while maintaining a balanced diet. A high-calorie, low-residue, high-protein, low-fat diet is recommended (Rayhorn & Rayhorn, 2002).

Health Promotion

Although stress has not been shown to exacerbate the symptoms of Crohn's disease or UC, the impact on the client's lifestyle can be significant, especially with Crohn's disease. Support groups can be beneficial. Encourage clients to develop mechanisms to help them cope with the disease process. Exercise, meditation, and biofeedback may be helpful.

Nursing Management

Assess the abdomen for tenderness, distention, and bowel sounds. Monitor weight, vital signs, and stools. Maintain an accurate I&O and calorie count. Provide high-calorie, high-protein small, frequent meals and snacks. Encourage verbalization of feelings.

NURSING PROCESS

Assessment

Subjective Data

Clients may describe mild abdominal spasms and cramping, which may increase to severe abdominal pain, nausea, and anorexia. Clients with UC may have an urge to defecate with the cramping.

Objective Data

Clients have abdominal tenderness on palpation, guarding, distention, weight loss, diarrhea, an elevated WBC count, and fever. In clients with Crohn's disease, steatorrhea and iron-deficiency anemia may be present. In clients with UC, stools may be positive for blood and the H & H may be low. The serum potassium, magnesium, and albumin levels are usually low. Because Crohn's disease is so debilitating, clients may become depressed.

Nursing diagnoses for clients with Crohn's disease or UC may include the following:

Nursing Diagnoses	Planning/Goals	Nursing Interventions
Imbalanced **N**utrition: Less than body requirements related to postprandial pain, bowel hypermobility, and decreased absorption	The client will demonstrate adequate nutritional status as exhibited by maintaining weight within range for height and body type.	Monitor I&O every shift; caloric count and weight daily. Administer IV fluid and electrolyte replacement as ordered.

continues

Nursing Diagnoses	Planning/Goals	Nursing Interventions
		Provide high-calorie, high-protein supplements as ordered along with small, frequent meals.
		Administer TPN, a high-calorie and nutrient-dense IV solution, as ordered. Closely monitor lab reports for electrolytes and glucose level.
Risk for Deficient Fluid Volume related to diarrhea and altered intake	The client will exhibit adequate hydration as evidenced by electrolytes within normal range, moist mucous membranes, and I & O nearly equal within 48 hours of start of intervention. The frequency and amount of diarrhea will decrease within 48 hours of start of intervention.	Administer 5-ASA compounds, corticosteroids, and immunosuppressors as ordered.
		Monitor I&O every shift.
		Administer IV fluid and electrolyte rehydration as ordered.
Powerlessness related to impairment in lifestyle secondary to disease process	The client will verbalize a plan to seek support, by discharge.	Provide client with information on national organizations and local support groups. Arrange social work consult if needed.
		Allow client to verbalize feelings.

Evaluation Each goal must be evaluated to determine how it has been met by the client.

IRRITABLE BOWEL SYNDROME

Irritable bowel syndrome (IBS) refers to a group of symptoms—cramping, abdominal pain, bloating, constipation, or diarrhea. Some clients have both constipation and diarrhea which alternate in appearance. There is no organic cause, but the movement of feces and gas through the colon and the absorption of fluids are affected. When feces stay in the colon too long and too much water is absorbed, constipation results. When feces is pushed through the colon too fast by spasms, little water is absorbed and diarrhea results. Spasms may also temporarily trap gas or feces, preventing them from moving forward, and therefore causing pain.

The colon seems to be more sensitive and reactive especially to certain foods and stress. Since the colon is partly controlled by the autonomic nervous system, it responds to stress. It may contract too much or too little, and too much water or too little water may be absorbed.

In the U.S., one in five persons has IBS, making it one of the most common gastrointestinal disorders. Only a small proportion of people seek medical treatment, while most will treat the symptoms themselves. IBS occurs more frequently in women than in men, and usually begins around age 20 (NIDDK, 2004).

There is no diagnostic test for IBS, but clients presenting with the above symptoms will often undergo testing to rule out other disorders. Criteria for a diagnosis of IBS include:

1. Abdominal pain or discomfort for at least 12 weeks (not necessarily consecutive) out of the previous 12 months.

2. At least two of the following three features must be present:
   - Abdominal pain or discomfort is relieved by having a bowel movement.
   - When abdominal pain or discomfort begins, there is a change in how often the client has a bowel movement.
   - When abdominal pain or discomfort begins, there is a change in the form of the stool or the way it looks.

Medical-Surgical Management

Medical

The goal of treatment is to relieve the symptoms. Foods that make the symptoms worse should be eliminated from the diet. Increasing dietary fiber is often helpful. Anxiety-reducing measures often relieve symptoms. If the client has severe anxiety or depression, counseling may be required.

Pharmacological

Anticholinergic medications may be given before meals. Clients with constipation may be given tegaserod maleate (Zelnorm), usually for 4 weeks. Bulk-forming psyllium hydrophilic muciloid (Metamucil) may also be used.

Clients who primarily have diarrhea and have not responded to other therapies may be given alosetron hydrochloride (Lotronex). It should be used with caution because it can have serious side effects, such as severe constipation or decreased blood flow to the colon.

Diet

The client should be instructed to eliminate from the diet those foods that aggravate the symptoms and discomfort. Foods often associated with making IBS symptoms worse include wheat, rye, barley, chocolate, milk products, alcohol, and caffeinated drinks. Foods high in fiber such as bran, cereal, beans, fruits, and vegetables may reduce symptoms. Large meals may cause cramping and diarrhea.

Activity

Regular exercise may help relieve symptoms. Seldom is weight loss a problem.

Nursing Management

Encourage the client to write down what is eaten, what symptoms are present and when they occur, and which foods always make the client feel bad. Then eliminate those foods causing symptoms or making the client feel bad. Suggest that the client eat five or six small meals instead of three large meals each day. Encourage the client to exercise regularly and practice stress-relieving measures such as progressive relaxation or guided imagery.

NURSING PROCESS

Assessment

Subjective Data

Some clients describe cramping, abdominal pain, and diarrhea during or soon after a meal, others complain of constipation, and still others report alternating diarrhea and constipation. Abdominal fullness, gas, and bloating also often occur.

Objective Data

The client's stools will be either very loose (diarrhea) or very hard and difficult to pass (constipation). Mucus may be passed with the bowel movement. *There is **no** weight loss, bleeding, or fever associated with IBS.*

Nursing diagnoses for a client with irritable bowel syndrome may include the following:

Nursing Diagnoses	Planning/Goals	Nursing Interventions
Diarrhea related to rapid movement of feces through the colon with too little fluid being absorbed.	The client will have normally formed stools.	Encourage frequent, meals. Add high-fiber foods gradually to meals. Teach client to eliminate gas-forming foods and other foods causing symptoms from the diet. Teach stress-reducing measures.
Constipation related to delayed movement of feces through the colon with too much fluid being absorbed.	The client will have regularly passed, soft, formed stools.	Encourage increased fluid intake unless contraindicated, and increase consumption of high-fiber foods. Encourage regular exercise such as walking. Administer medications as prescribed. Teach stress-reducing measures.

Evaluation Each goal must be evaluated to determine how it has been met by the client.

INTESTINAL OBSTRUCTION

An intestinal obstruction occurs when the contents cannot pass through the intestine. Obstructions may occur in the large or the small intestine, with most occurring in the ileum. Obstructions may be mechanical, neurogenic, or vascular in origin.

A mechanical obstruction may be a partial or complete obstruction caused by a tumor; fecal impaction; hernia; **volvulus,** a twisting of the bowel on itself; **intussusception,** a telescoping of the bowel where the bowel slides inside itself (Figure 35-8); or **adhesions,** scar tissue in the abdomen from previous surgeries or disease process such as Crohn's disease.

A neurogenic obstruction, known as a *paralytic ileus,* occurs when nerve transmission to the bowel is interrupted by trauma, infection, or medications, resulting in a portion of the bowel being paralyzed.

A vascular obstruction occurs when blood flow to a portion of the bowel is interrupted, as in atherosclerosis, and that portion of the bowel becomes necrotic.

When the small intestine becomes obstructed, large amounts of fluid, bacteria, and swallowed air build up in the bowel proximal to the obstruction. The normal

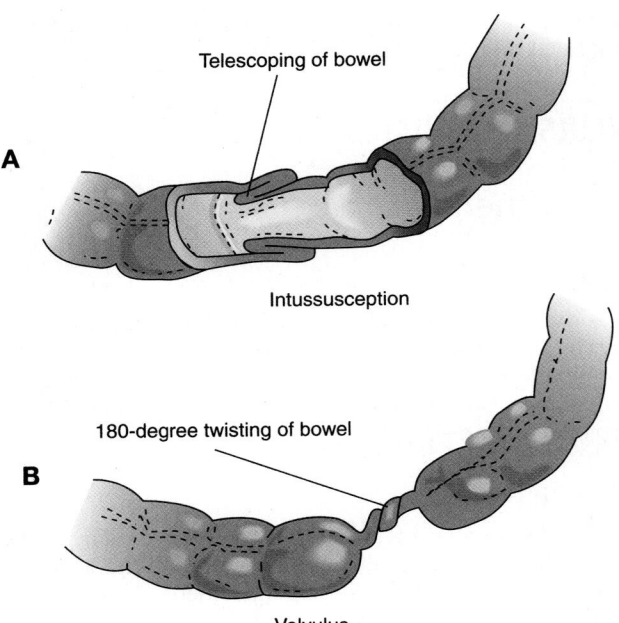

Figure 35-8 *Bowel obstructions can be caused by **A**, an intussusception; **B**, a volvulus.*

process of secretion and absorption of the electrolyte-rich fluid is interrupted. Distention and poor absorption occur when water and salts move from the circulatory system to the lumen of the intestine.

An abdominal x-ray and a barium enema or UGI with small bowel follow-through may be ordered when a bowel obstruction is suspected.

Medical–Surgical Management

Medical

Treatment of the obstruction depends on the cause and location. Some can be treated medically by inserting an NG tube for decompression, providing IV fluids for rehydration, and treating the cause, such as the use of enemas for fecal impaction.

Surgical

Most bowel obstructions require surgery. A bowel resection is performed to remove the portion of the bowel affected by the obstruction.

Pharmacological

Nonnarcotic analgesics are used to avoid the intestinal motility decrease caused by opioids. Antibiotics may also be ordered.

Diet

Clients will be kept NPO until the obstruction is cleared and then slowly progressed from a clear liquid diet to a regular diet as more bowel function returns.

Activity

In cases of paralytic ileus, ambulation should be encouraged to help bowel function return. Encourage clients who have had a bowel resection to turn, cough, and deep breathe every 2 hours initially postoperatively. Activity is progressed the next day.

Nursing Management

Assess abdomen for tenderness, distention, and bowel sounds. Monitor vomiting for fecal material. Assess weight daily. Accurately record I&O. Limit ice chips when NPO. Check laboratory reports for low sodium and potassium and elevated BUN, amylase, and H & H.

NURSING PROCESS

Assessment

Subjective Data

Clients may state symptoms of colicky abdominal pain, nausea, constipation, and bloating.

Objective Data

Objective assessment includes abdominal distention and tenderness on palpation. Vomiting temporarily relieves the abdominal pain. Vomitus may include fecal material, which is a poor prognostic sign (McConnell, 2001b).

Laboratory analysis demonstrates decreased levels of sodium and potassium, elevated BUN, elevated amylase, and elevated H & H caused by hemoconcentration.

Nursing diagnoses for a client with intestinal obstruction may include the following:

Nursing Diagnoses	Planning/Goals	Nursing Interventions
Deficient Fluid Volume related to vomiting, shift in fluids, and NPO status	The client will exhibit adequate hydration within 48 hours of initiation of treatment as evidenced by moist mucous membranes, electrolytes within normal limits, and I&O approximately equal.	Monitor I&O every shift. Administer IV fluid and electrolyte replacements as ordered. Allow limited ice chips to prevent further electrolyte imbalance in clients with NG tubes. Assess weight daily.

continues

Nursing Diagnoses	Planning/Goals	Nursing Interventions
Acute Pain related to distention, edema, or ischemia	The client will verbalize increased comfort within 1 hour of analgesic administration as measured on pain scale.	Administer nonnarcotic analgesics as ordered. In clients with a paralytic ileus, encourage ambulation to encourage return of bowel function. Maintain and monitor NG tube as ordered for abdominal decompression. Check bowel sounds every 4 hours or PRN.
Deficient Knowledge related to disease process, treatment regimen, and possible surgery	The client will verbalize treatment course, possible complications, and possible need for surgery.	Identify client's learning style and present information in a manner compatible with learning style. Include intestinal decompression, need for ambulation, need for good oral care due to fecal drainage, and surgery.

Evaluation Each goal must be evaluated to determine how it has been met by the client.

HERNIAS

A hernia occurs when the wall of a muscle weakens and the intestine protrudes through the muscle wall. Hernias that do not return to the abdominal cavity with rest or manipulation and cause complete bowel obstruction are said to be *incarcerated*. If the blood supply to the hernia is cut off, the hernia is said to be *strangulated*. Immediate surgery is required to restore blood flow. If not done, gangrene develops, which may be fatal.

Several types of hernias exist. In an umbilical hernia, a portion of the bowel protrudes through the umbilicus. In children, these generally resolve on their own once the child begins to walk. Umbilical hernias most commonly occur in a multiparous female or in adults with cirrhosis and **ascites** (abnormal accumulation of fluid in the peritoneal cavity). Because of a high risk for strangulation in adults with umbilical hernias, surgery is usually performed.

Abdominal hernias occur in the midline of the abdomen between the umbilicus and the xyphoid process. Most are asymptomatic, with a few causing pain on exertion that resolves with reclining and rest.

Inguinal hernias, the most common hernia, occur in the groin area. Inguinal hernias frequently occur after activities, such as lifting, that increase intraabdominal pressure; they subside with relaxation. Pain is located lower than in the abdominal hernia.

Femoral hernias occur when the intestine pushes into the passageway carrying blood vessels and nerves to the legs and are more common in women than in men.

A hiatal hernia occurs when a portion of the stomach protrudes into the mediastinal cavity through the diaphragm. Symptoms of hiatal hernias include indigestion and heartburn, especially after eating a large meal.

Upon evaluation and recommendation of a physician, some hernias can be reduced or pushed back into place. This can be accomplished by having the client recline, applying direct pressure to the hernia, and, in some cases, having the client exhale to decrease intraabdominal pressure. The nurse should never try to reduce a hernia.

Medical–Surgical Management
Medical

Some hernias have no symptoms or minimal symptoms, so clients may not be aware they have one or may learn to live with it by reducing it when needed. Clients who are a poor surgical risk may use a truss, a device that applies pressure to the hernia, thus keeping the intestine in the abdominal cavity.

Surgical

Hernias are repaired with surgery called herniorrhaphy. The surgery is typically performed on an outpatient basis, with clients going home the same day. If the surgery is more complicated because the hernia is incarcerated, the client may stay overnight.

If the hernia is strangulated, a bowel resection may be required.

Surgical repair of a hiatal hernia involves reinforcing the esophagus with a portion of the stomach. The surgery is performed laparoscopically, with the client remaining in the hospital 3 to 5 days postoperatively. Initially, the client will have an NG tube. The NG tube is removed 24 to 48 hours later and the diet gradually progressed to a soft diet.

Diet

Clients with hiatal hernias may need to modify their dietary patterns to include small frequent meals, and to avoid eating after supper, lying down for 2 hours after eating, and aggravating foods.

Nursing Management

Assess abdomen for bowel sounds and bulge in abdominal wall. Encourage client with hernia to eat small, frequent meals and avoid lying down for 2 hours after eating.

NURSING PROCESS

Assessment

Subjective Data

Clients may describe pain at the site of the hernia.

Objective Data

Assessment may show a bulge through the abdominal wall. If the hernia is strangulated, the client will have the symptoms of a bowel obstruction.

Nursing diagnoses for a client with a hernia may include the following:

Nursing Diagnoses	Planning/Goals	Nursing Interventions
Acute Pain related to tissue edema	The client will experience less pain within 1 hour of intervention as measured on the pain scale.	Administer analgesics as ordered. Evaluate aggravating activities (e.g., straining to have a bowel movement) and provide information on modification if indicated. Educate regarding signs of complications and when to notify staff of symptoms.
Ineffective Tissue Perfusion (Gastrointestinal) related to strangulation	The client will have minimal tissue necrosis.	Assess abdomen for bowel sounds every 4 hours. Insert NG tube to decrease abdominal distention as ordered. Administer IV hydration as ordered. Prepare client for surgery as ordered. Keep client NPO.

Evaluation Each goal must be evaluated to determine how it has been met by the client.

PERITONITIS

Peritonitis is the inflammation of the peritoneum, the membranous covering of the abdomen. Peritonitis is caused by irritating substances such as feces, gastric acids, bacteria, or blood in the abdominal cavity. A ruptured portion of the digestive system (such as the appendix), a ruptured tubal pregnancy, or invasion of tumors through the gastric wall can lead to peritonitis. Peritonitis can be a serious, life-threatening condition. Complications following peritonitis include adhesions (scar tissue), paralytic ileus, and pneumonia.

Medical–Surgical Management

Surgical

Treatment is primarily surgical with repair of the cause and irrigation of the abdominal cavity with saline and antibiotic solutions. Drains may be left in the abdomen for several days postoperatively to allow any remaining fluid to drain. Because bowel function usually stops as a result of the irritating substances, an NG tube is placed to decompress the abdomen and relieve nausea.

Pharmacological

Analgesics will be ordered postoperatively for discomfort. If an ileus develops, nonnarcotic analgesics will be ordered. Antibiotics will be ordered preoperatively and postoperatively.

Diet

Clients will be NPO preoperatively and postoperatively until bowel sounds return. Clients will then be placed on a clear liquid diet and slowly progressed to a regular diet as more bowel function returns.

Activity

Preoperatively, clients will be placed on bed rest and encouraged to turn, cough, and deep breathe. Because clients tend to breathe shallowly with peritoneal inflammation, pulmonary hygiene is important. Activity should be progressed postoperatively, as soon as tolerated, to increase lung expansion and to encourage bowel function return. Exercise, lifting, and driving are restricted until the incision heals.

Nursing Management

Assess vital signs and administer antipyretics as ordered. Monitor I&O, signs of dehydration, and fluid and electrolyte replacement. Provide comfort measures (cool cloth, oral hygiene, back rub). Maintain patency of NG tube. Encourage coughing and deep breathing and teach incision splinting. Keep client in semi-Fowler's position to help localize purulent exudate. Follow surgical asepsis for wound care. Empty drainage devices as required. If drainage is not into a device, change dressings frequently to keep drainage off skin. If the wound is still draining when the client is discharged, teach client/family aseptic technique for changing dressings.

NURSING PROCESS

Assessment

Subjective Data

Clients may describe abdominal pain, nausea, and constipation.

Objective Data

Assessment may reveal vomiting, absent bowel sounds, a tense or distended abdomen with tenderness on palpation, shallow and rapid respirations, weak and rapid pulse, dry mucous membranes, low urine output, fever, and limited mobility because of pain.

Laboratory analysis will show an elevated WBC. If bleeding is occurring, the H & H will be low. Sodium, potassium, and chloride may be low.

Nursing diagnoses for a client with peritonitis may include the following:

Nursing Diagnoses	Planning/Goals	Nursing Interventions
Deficient Fluid Volume related to gastric losses and restricted intake	The client will maintain hydration as indicated by an I&O that is nearly equal and electrolytes within normal limits.	Monitor I&O every shift. Monitor for signs of dehydration: dry mucous membranes, poor skin turgor, and low urine output. Monitor electrolytes as ordered. Administer IV rehydration and electrolyte replacement as ordered.
Hyperthermia related to inflammatory process and dehydration	The client will maintain temperature within normal limits.	Assess VS including temperature every 4 hours. Administer antipyretics as ordered; probably rectal suppositories due to NPO status. Monitor for dehydration: decrease in urine output, dry mucous membranes, and poor skin turgor. Provide comfort measures: cool cloth to the head or neck, assistance to turn, and a back rub with cooling lotion.
Acute Pain related to abdominal distention	The client will have less pain and improved mobility within 1 hour of receiving analgesics as measured on the pain scale.	Administer analgesics as ordered. Encourage activity such as coughing and deep breathing after analgesics. Teach splinting of incision for cough and deep breathing. Monitor NG tube to decompress abdomen. Maintain patency of NG tube.

Evaluation Each goal must be evaluated to determine how it has been met by the client.

HEMORRHOIDS

Hemorrhoids are swollen vascular tissues in the rectal area. They may be internal or external. Hemorrhoids may be caused by straining with constipation or sitting on the toilet (reading) for an extended time. Hemorrhoids frequently occur with pregnancy. Hemorrhoids can cause burning, pruritis, and pain with defecation. At times, they can bleed, leading to anemia.

Medical–Surgical Management

Medical

Sitz baths or warm compresses on the rectal area for 20 minutes, 4 times a day, often helps decrease swelling.

Surgical

If bleeding continues despite medical intervention, or if discomfort is significant, hemorrhoids can be surgically removed by a hemorrhoidectomy. For external hemorrhoids, surgery is performed on an outpatient basis by placing a band around the hemorrhoid as for esophageal varices, allowing it to necrose and fall off. For internal hemorrhoids, sclerotherapy, cryotherapy, or laser can be done. This usually requires an overnight stay in the hospital. Hemorrhoids can recur after surgical removal if the cause is not eliminated.

Pharmacological

Treatment includes creams and suppositories to decrease inflammation, some with cortisone to decrease swelling. Fiber supplements and stool softeners may be ordered to keep bowel movements soft.

Diet

Bowel movements can be kept soft with a high-fiber diet of 20 to 30 grams of fiber per day and at least 2,500 cc of fluid intake daily.

Nursing Management

Teach client to modify bowel habits (sit on toilet only for short periods), increase fiber in diet to 20 or 30 grams per day, and increase fluid intake to 2,500 cc per day. Provide sitz baths several times a day or teach client how to do it.

NURSING PROCESS

Assessment

Subjective Data

Clients may describe rectal burning, pain, and pruritis with bowel movements; constipation; and, occasionally, bright red bleeding. A dietary history should be obtained to determine fiber and fluid intake.

Objective Data

If hemorrhoids are external, they can be visualized during a physical examination. If chronic bleeding is present, laboratory analysis may show a low H & H.

Nursing diagnoses for a client with hemorrhoids may include the following:

Nursing Diagnoses	Planning/Goals	Nursing Interventions
Acute Pain related to edema and inflammation of swollen vascular tissues	The client will verbalize a decrease in discomfort within 48 hours of initiation of treatment.	Provide sitz baths or warm compresses for 20 minutes, 4 times a day. Administer creams and suppositories as ordered.
		Increase fiber and fluids in diet to keep stools soft to avoid straining.
Deficient Knowledge related to diet, causes of condition, treatment, and potential complications	The client will be able to verbalize treatment regimen and long-term management of hemorrhoids.	Determine client's learning style and present information in a manner compatible with learning style.
		Educate client about increasing fiber in diet to 20 to 30 grams per day, increasing fluid intake to 2,500 cc per day, causes of hemorrhoids, possible complications such as anemia, and modification of bowel habits (such as not sitting on the toilet for long periods).

Evaluation Each goal must be evaluated to determine how it has been met by the client.

CONSTIPATION

Constipation is characterized by hard, infrequent stools that are difficult and/or painful to pass. Constipation can be caused by tumors, low-fiber diet, inactivity, some diseases that interfere with the mechanical functioning of the bowel (such as multiple sclerosis), or some medications (such as narcotics, antidepressants, or anti-Parkinson drugs).

Medical–Surgical Management

Pharmacological

Fiber supplements and stool softeners may be ordered. Laxatives and enemas may be ordered, but long-term use should be avoided because they interrupt normal bowel function. If constipation is caused by medications the client is taking, the client should discuss other options with the physician, such as modifying the dosage or changing medications.

Diet

Fiber should be increased to 20 to 30 grams per day. Fluid intake should be increased to 2,500 cc per day.

Activity

Increase activity level if possible because exercise, such as walking, increases motility in the colon.

Nursing Management

Assess dietary intake of fiber and fluids and activity/exercise level. Review medications client is taking for any causing constipation. Encourage regular schedule for bowel evacuation.

LIFE CYCLE CONSIDERATIONS

Constipation in the Older Client

The slowing of peristalsis, which is part of the aging process, may lead to constipation in the older client. An increase in dietary fiber and fluid intake (water) will help prevent constipation. A regular schedule for bowel evacuation also helps.

NURSING PROCESS

Assessment

Subjective Data

Clients describe infrequent, difficult to pass stools. Dietary assessment of fiber and fluids usually reveals inadequate intake. Assessed activity/exercise level.

Objective Data

Bowel movements will be hard-formed.

Nursing diagnoses for a client with constipation may include the following:

Nursing Diagnoses	Planning/Goals	Nursing Interventions
Constipation related to inadequate intake of fiber and fluids	The client will have soft stools every other day by one week from start of intervention.	Encourage client to increase fiber in the diet to 20 to 30 grams a day and fluid intake to 2,500 cc a day. Administer fiber supplements and stool softeners as ordered. Determine fluid preferences of client and always have fluids at client's bedside within reach. Help the client establish a regular schedule for bowel movements, usually 30 minutes after a meal.
*Deficient **K**nowledge* related to dietary sources of fiber and the importance of adequate fluid intake and exercise	The client will be able to select a menu high in fiber and fluids utilizing nutrients from the food pyramid within 48 hours and verbalize the need for adequate exercise.	Assess client's learning style and present information in a manner compatible with learning style. Teach client about foods that are high in fiber (fruits, vegetables, whole grains) as well as importance of fluid intake. Discuss with client importance of exercise in maintaining bowel function.

Evaluation Each goal must be evaluated to determine how it has been met by the client.

DISORDERS OF THE ACCESSORY ORGANS

Disorders of the accessory organs include cirrhosis, hepatitis, pancreatitis, and cholecystitis/cholelithiasis.

— YES.

CIRRHOSIS

Cirrhosis refers to the chronic, degenerative changes in the liver cells and thickening of surrounding tissue that result from the liver repairing itself after chronic inflammation. Causes of cirrhosis include chronic hepatitis, repeated exposure to toxic substances, disease processes (such as sclerosing cholangitis and hemochromatosis), cancer, and chronic alcohol abuse. Alcohol abuse accounts for most cases of cirrhosis.

Because the liver is responsible for so many functions, complications can be significant and include malnutrition, hypoglycemia, clotting disorders, jaundice, portal hypertension, ascites, hepatic encephalopathy, and hepatorenal syndrome.

Liver dysfunction causes several organ-related complications. Malnutrition results from the liver's inability to absorb fat and fat-soluble vitamins and leads to muscle wasting, weight loss, and fatigue. Hypoglycemia occurs when the liver is unable to perform glycogenolysis efficiently. Clotting disorders result when the liver is not able to produce sufficient amounts of prothrombin and fibrinogen.

Portal hypertension results when blood flow through the cirrhotic liver is inhibited, resulting in blood backflowing in the portal vein. Portal hypertension leads to distention of the esophageal veins, resulting in esophageal varices; distention of rectal veins, resulting in hemorrhoids; and distention of the splenic vein, resulting in splenomegaly.

Because the liver is responsible for metabolizing medications, clients frequently become intolerant to some medications. Jaundice, a yellow discoloration of the skin, is usually present. Jaundice occurs when the liver is unable to convert bilirubin, an end product of red blood cell breakdown, into a water-soluble form that can be excreted in the bile. The extra bilirubin collects in areas that contain elastin, such as the sclera of the eyes, the skin, and the nail beds.

Fluid may accumulate in the pleural cavity in the form of pleural effusions. Fluid may also accumulate in the peritoneal cavity. This condition is called ascites. The cause of ascites is the congestion of blood in the portal system.

Hepatic encephalopathy is a condition in which ammonia accumulates in the brain. Fluid is pulled into the extracellular compartment, accelerating brain stem herniation. Confusion, lethargy, and/or coma may occur. Symptoms of impending hepatic encephalopathy are disorientation and *asterixis* (liver flap), a flapping tremor of the hands. When the client extends the arms and hands in front of the body, the hands rapidly flex and extend.

Hepatorenal syndrome is a complication of cirrhosis in which the client goes into renal failure. Symptoms include oliguria (diminished production of urine), azotemia (excess nitrogen in the blood), anorexia, fatigue, and weakness.

Cirrhosis is a form of end-stage liver disease for which there is no cure. The process of cirrhosis can be slowed by removing the cause (i.e., abstaining from alcohol), but the damage cannot be reversed. Clients in end-stage liver disease may be evaluated to determine if they qualify for a liver transplant.

Medical–Surgical Management
Medical

The physician may perform a paracentesis to remove the fluid from the abdomen and relieve pressure on the diaphragm and lungs. A small incision is made and a trochar inserted into the abdomen to drain the fluid. Albumin may be infused at the same time to pull excess fluid back into the vascular system.

Surgical

If the client continues to develop ascites after medical treatment, a LeVeen or Denver peritoneal venous shunt may be used. The pressure-regulated shunt is implanted in the peritoneal cavity and threaded through the subcutaneous tissue into the superior vena cava, returning the fluid back to the vascular system. As fluid pressure builds in the peritoneal cavity, a valve opens and drains the fluid into the superior vena cava.

If esophageal varices are present, an EGD with sclerotherapy or banding is done to prevent hemorrhage (refer to Figure 35-3).

If portal hypertension cannot be controlled with medications, a portosystemic shunt or a transjugular intrahepatic portosystemic shunt (TIPS) may be performed. The shunt redirects the blood flow, thereby relieving the portal hypertension, and decreases the risk of rupturing distended veins in the esophagus (Figure 35-9).

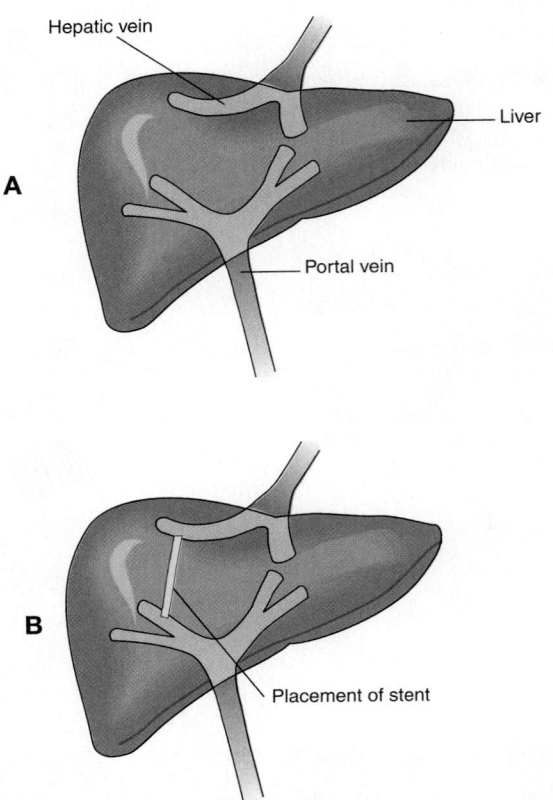

Figure 35-9 A, *Blood Flow Before TIPS;* **B,** *TIPS is performed in radiology on clients deemed too unstable for the surgery necessary for a portosystemic shunt. A stent is placed to redirect the blood flow.*

Pharmacological

A potassium-sparing diuretic, such as spironolactone (Aldactone), is used to decrease ascites and pleural effusion. Lactulose (Cholac) is used to move ammonia from the blood into the bowel. The lactulose acts as a laxative and causes the body to excrete the stool containing ammonia. Tap water enemas may also be ordered to help the body eliminate the ammonia.

Propranolol hydrochloride (Inderal), an antihypertensive medication, may be ordered to lower portal hypertension. All unnecessary medications should be avoided because the liver cannot metabolize them.

Diet

Clients with cirrhosis are placed on a low-protein diet, usually 40 grams per day. If ascites is present, sodium will also be restricted to 2 grams or less per day to decrease the amount of fluid retained by the body. Fluids may also be restricted to 1,000 cc to 2,000 cc per day depending on the severity of fluid accumulation.

Activity

Safety: Cirrhosis

If hepatic encephalopathy is present, precautions should be taken to ensure the client's safety, such as elevating bedrails and allowing the client to ambulate only with assistance, especially if the client's gait is unsteady.

Because fatigue is such a common symptom of cirrhosis, the client's tolerance for activity will be diminished. Plan rest periods during the day, and schedule activities between rests.

Nursing Management

Monitor vital signs and mental status. Restrict fluid intake as ordered. Accurately record I&O. Weigh client daily and measure abdominal girth. Provide low-sodium, low-protein diet. Turn client every 2 hours and monitor for redness and skin breakdown. Assist with or provide frequent oral hygiene.

NURSING PROCESS

Assessment

Subjective Data

Clients describe fatigue, nausea, anorexia, weakness, and indigestion.

Objective Data

Assessment shows ascites, jaundice, enlarged liver and spleen, petechiae (small bruises on the skin), vomiting, weight loss, fever, epistaxis, and decreased breath sounds. Lethargy, confusion, or coma may be present if encephalopathy has occurred.

Laboratory analysis includes a CBC, which will demonstrate low WBCs, RBCs, Hgb, and platelets. A liver panel will show an elevated bilirubin, alkaline phosphatase, GGT, ALT, and AST. Albumin will be low. PT, PTT, and clotting times will be delayed.

Nursing diagnoses for a client with cirrhosis may include the following:

Nursing Diagnoses	Planning/Goals	Nursing Interventions
Disturbed Thought Processes related to elevated serum ammonia level and hepatic coma	The client will experience an improved level of orientation within 48 hours of initiation of treatment.	Administer tap water enemas and lactulose as ordered to eliminate ammonia-rich stools. An NG tube may be placed to give lactulose if client is comatose. Monitor ammonia level. Elevate bedrails to prevent injury. As coma lessens, reorient client frequently.
Excess Fluid Volume related to ascites	The client will have less ascites by discharge.	Weigh daily. Educate client to notify physician of weight gain of $1\frac{1}{2}$ lbs or more in 1 week. Measure abdominal girth daily. Restrict fluid to 1,000 to 2,000 cc per day depending on the severity of the ascites. Provide low-sodium diet of 500 to 2,000 mg a day depending on severity of the ascites. Teach client how to measure fluids and calculate sodium in diet. If a paracentesis is done, check vital signs every 15 minutes during the procedure and after the procedure until the vitals are stable. The amount of fluid removed from the abdomen should be measured and sent to the laboratory.

continues

Nursing Diagnoses	Planning/Goals	Nursing Interventions
*Risk for Impaired **S**kin Integrity* related to accumulation of bile salts in skin, poor skin turgor, ascites, and edema	The client will not experience skin breakdown while hospitalized.	Provide egg crate mattress. Turn client every 2 hours. Monitor skin closely for redness and skin breakdown. Apply lotion to skin frequently, especially to pressure areas. Assist with ADLs to promote good hygiene and conserve client's energy.
*Imbalanced **N**utrition: Less than body requirements* related to inadequate diet, anorexia, or vomiting	The client will eat a balanced diet of 1,500 calories a day.	Offer small, high-calorie meals frequently. Offer high-nutrient supplements if client is unable to maintain adequate caloric intake. Assist and encourage client to eat. Provide frequent oral hygiene. Observe for changes in mental status that would interfere with caloric intake (e.g., increased lethargy).

Evaluation Each goal must be evaluated to determine how it has been met by the client.

HEPATITIS — Hot yet

Hepatitis is a chronic or acute inflammation of the liver caused by a virus, bacteria, drugs, alcohol abuse, or other toxic substances. There is a diffuse inflammatory reaction with liver cells degenerating and dying. The functions of the liver slow down. Because viral infections are the most common cause of hepatitis, emphasis will be placed on viral hepatitis.

Researchers are still learning about the viruses that cause hepatitis. Seven viruses are known to cause hepatitis: A, B, C, D, E, F, and G.

Parini (2001) describes hepatitis F as similar to hepatitis A and E and hepatitis G usually as a coinfection with hepatitis C. Hepatitis F has no serologic test and is diagnosed by seeing the virus with an electron microscope. Hepatitis G is transmitted by blood. Most clients have no symptoms, and 90% to 100% develop chronic infection. The viruses are similar and have almost identical signs and symptoms. Incubation period, mode of transmission, treatment and prognosis vary. See Table 35-5 for a summary of hepatitis viruses A–E.

Medical–Surgical Management

Treatment is focused on resting the liver and early detection of complications. The liver is rested by modifying the diet so that less bile is needed to digest the food. Treatment is related to the signs and symptoms present and the prevention of transmission.

Pharmacological

Antiemetics such as hydroxyzine hydrochloride (Atarax, also Vistaril) or trimethobenzamide hydrochloride (Tigan) may be given before meals for nausea. IV hydration with vitamin C for healing may be ordered. Vitamin B complex may also be ordered to help clients absorb fat-soluble vitamins. Vitamin K may be ordered if clotting time is prolonged. All unnecessary medications, especially sedatives, should be avoided.

Those exposed to hepatitis B by needle puncture or sexual contact should have hepatitis B immunoglobin (HBIG). Vaccines for hepatitis A (HAV) and hepatitis B (HBV) are available. HAV vaccine is recommended for persons 2 years of age and older at risk for exposure to hepatitis A such as homosexuals, IV drug users, travelers to countries with poor sanitation conditions, and laboratory workers who handle live hepatitis A virus (CDC, 2002a). HBV vaccine is recommended as a routine vaccination for all 0 to 18 years olds and for those in high-risk groups (CDC, 2002b). The FDA approved a combined hepatitis A and B vaccine in September 2001. It is recommended for persons younger than age 18 years and those in a high-risk group.

Diet

Diet modifications may include decreasing fat intake to decrease the amount of bile needed in the digestive tract. A low-protein diet may be needed if the liver is no longer able to metabolize the protein. Anorexia is a common symptom that can be treated with small, frequent, high-calorie meals. Fluids may be restricted if the client retains fluids. No alcoholic beverages are recommended for at least 1 year or longer.

Activity

Bed rest is usually recommended for the first several weeks, generally at home unless the serum bilirubin is greater than 10 mg/dL or the PT is prolonged. If either occurs, hospitalization is usually recommended.

Once bed rest is no longer necessary, activity should be increased gradually because fatigue will be present for up to several months. Rest periods should be included throughout the day.

Nursing Management

Follow Standard Precautions with all clients and Enteric Precautions for hepatitis A and E. Teach clients to always follow proper hand hygiene. For hepatitis A and E, be careful about consuming contaminated food and/or water. Hepatitis B spreads through blood and body fluids. Health care workers are at risk for hepatitis B and C. Most clients with hepatitis have flu-like symptoms, weight loss, hepatomegaly, jaundice, dark yellow urine, and light stools. Monitor laboratory test results for elevated bilirubin, GGT, AST, ALT, LDH, and alkaline phosphatase. Clotting time and PT are prolonged. Encourage low-fat, low-protein, high-calorie frequent small meals and fluid intake of 2,500 to 3,000 cc daily. Bed rest is important for the first several weeks and then a gradual increase in activity with rest periods several times a day.

TABLE 35-5 COMPARISON OF DIFFERENT TYPES OF VIRAL HEPATITIS

	A	B	C	D	E
Etiologic Agent	hepatitis A virus (HAV)	hepatitis B virus (HBV)	hepatitis C virus (HCV)	hepatitis D virus (HDV)	hepatitis E virus (HEV)
Transmission	Fecal-oral; contaminated water or food; person to person	Blood or body fluids from infected person	Blood	Only persons with hepatitis B can get hepatitis D; blood and blood products; needlesticks; seldom sexual; rarely perinatal	Oral-fecal route; contaminated water; person to person uncommon
Risk Groups	Household/sexual contact with infected person; international travelers	Infection drug users; sexual/household contact with infected person; infants born to infected mothers; health care workers; multiple sex partners	Blood transfusions or organ transplants prior to 1992; sharing needles; exposure to blood and blood products	Needle sharing; needlesticks	Mainly travel to countries where endemic
Incubation Period	15–50 days	45–160 days	14–180 days	15–60 days	15–60 days
Infectious Period	Usually less than 2 months	Before symptoms appear; lifetime if chronic	Before symptoms appear; lifetime if chronic	Not determined	Not determined
Diagnostic Tests	IgM anti-HAV	HBsAg	EIA-3; RIBA serum ALT increased 10x; HCVRNA-PCR	IgG anti-HDV and/or Igm anti-HDV	None available
Symptoms	Flu-like; jaundice; dark yellow urine; light colored stools	Flu-like; may have jaundice; dark yellow urine; light colored stools	80% have no symptoms; flu-like	Flu-like; may have jaundice; dark yellow urine; light colored stools	Abdominal pain, anorexia; dark yellow urine; jaundice, fever
Prevention	Standard Precautions; enteric precautions; Hepatitis A vaccine (entire series); Immune globulin (for short term)	Standard Precautions; reduce risk behaviors; Hepatitis B vaccine (entire series); Immune globulin (for short term)	Standard Precautions; reduce risk behaviors; no vaccine	Standard Precautions; reduce risk behaviors; hepatitis B vaccine; if client already has hepatitis B no prevention for hepatitis D	Standard Precautions; be sure water safe when traveling; no vaccine
Treatment	Immune globulin within 2 weeks of exposure	Immune globulin (HBIg); Alpha interferon; lamivudine (Epivir-HBV) adefovirdipivoxil (Hepsera)	peginterferon alfa-2a (Pegasys); ribavirin (Virazole)	Alpha interferon	None given

continues

TABLE 35-5 continued

	A	B	C	D	E
Prognosis	Rarely fatal; no chronicity resolves on its own in several weeks	No cure; may become chronic	75% to 85% have chronic infection; 70% develop chronic liver disease	Low risk of chronicity	No evidence of chronicity

Data from Centers for Disease Control and Prevention (CDC) (2002a). *Viral Hepatitis A.* [Online]. Available: www.cdc.gov/ncidod/diseases/hepatitis/a/fact.htm; CDC (2002b). *Viral Hepatitis B.* [Online]. Available: www.cdc.gov/ncidod/diseases/hepatitis/b/fact.htm; CDC (2002c). *Viral Hepatitis C.* [Online]. Available: www.cdc.gov/ncidod/diseases/hepatitis/c/fact.htm; CDC (2002d). *Viral Hepatitis D.* [on-line] Available: www.cdc.gov/ncidod/diseases/hepatitis/slideset/hep-d.htm; CDC (2002). *Viral Hepatitis E.* [Online]. Available: www.cdc.gov/ncidod/diseases/hepatitis/slideset/hep-e.htm; Fried, M.W., Shiffman, M.L. et al. (2002e). Peginterferon alfa-2a plus ribavirin for chronic hepatitis C virus infection. *New England Journal of Medicine,* 347(13), 975; Lau, D. T., Kleiner, D. E., Park, Y., DiBisceglie, A. M. & Hoofnagle, J. H. (1999). Resolution of chronic delta hepatitis after 12 years of interferon alpha therapy. *Gastroenterology, 117*(5), 1229-33; National Institute of Diabetes and Digestive and Kidney Diseases (NIDDK) (2001). What I need to know about hepatitis A [Online]. Available: www.niddk.nih.gov/health/digest/pubs/hep/hepa/ hepa.htm; NIDDK (2001). What I need to know about hepatitis A. [Online]. Available: www.niddk.nih.gov/health/digest/pubs/hep/hepa/hepa.htm; NIDDK (2001b) *What I need to know about hepatitis B.* [Online]. Available: www.niddk.nih.gov/health/digest/ pubs/hep/hepb/hepb.htm; NIDDK (2002a). *What I need to know about hepatitis C.* [Online]. Available: www.niddk.nih.gov/health/digest/pubs/hep/hepc/hepc.htm; NIDDK (2000). *Viral hepatitis A to E and Beyond.* [Online]. Available: www.niddk.nih.gov/health/digest/pubs/hep/hepa-e/hepa-e.htm; Parini S. (2001). Speaking out about the silent epidemic. Nursing 2001, 31(3), 36–42; U.S. Food and Drug Administration. (2002). *FDA approves new treatment for chronic hepatitis B.* [Online]. Available: www.fda.gov/bbs/topics/ANSWERS/2002/ANS01163.html

NURSING PROCESS

Assessment

Subjective Data

Symptoms may include fatigue, anorexia, photophobia, nausea, headaches, abdominal pain, generalized muscle aches, chills, pruritis, and bloating.

Objective Data

The client may have weight loss, hepatomegaly, fever, jaundice, dark amber urine, and clay-colored stools.

CRITICAL THINKING

Hepatitis and Lifestyle

What lifestyle changes are necessary with a diagnosis of hepatitis A, B, C, or D?

Laboratory analysis will show an elevated bilirubin, GGT, AST, ALT, LDH, and alkaline phosphatase. Clotting time and PT will be prolonged. Specific hepatitis test will be elevated (refer to Table 35-5).

Nursing diagnoses for the client with hepatitis may include the following:

Nursing Diagnoses	Planning/Goals	Nursing Interventions
Deficient Knowledge related to disease process, treatment regimen, and mode of transmission	The client will be able to explain disease process, incubation period, and mode of transmission, by discharge. The client will practice precautions to prevent spread of disease. The client will be able to select a menu using foods from the food guide pyramid and maintain a low-fat, low-protein diet.	Assess client's learning style and present information in a manner compatible with learning style. Educate about disease process and incubation period. Teach proper hand hygiene technique and emphasize importance of washing hands after using the bathroom. Emphasize that client cannot donate blood. Emphasize importance of follow-up laboratory analysis. Instruct in selection of low-fat, low-protein diet. For clients with hepatitis A, teach client to disinfect articles contaminated with feces (such as the toilet), not to prepare food for others, and not to share articles such as eating utensils or toothbrushes.

continues

Nursing Diagnoses	Planning/Goals	Nursing Interventions
		For clients with hepatitis B, teach to avoid sexual contact until they test negative for HBsAg or their partners are immunized with the HBV vaccine.
		For clients with hepatitis C, teach that it is unknown whether it can be transmitted through sexual contact, so precautions are recommended until more is known.
Imbalanced Nutrition: *Less than body requirements* related to inadequate caloric intake, fat intolerance, nausea, and vomiting	The client will maintain a caloric intake of 2,000 calories/day.	Monitor I&O every shift. Weigh daily.
		Offer small, frequent, high-calorie, low-fat meals. Encourage low-protein diet of 40 gm of protein. Monitor daily calorie count.
		Offer largest meal in morning, as food tends to be tolerated better in the morning. Encourage fluid intake of 2,500 to 3,000 cc daily.
		Note color and consistency of stools and color of urine.
		Administer antiemetic 30 minutes before meals as ordered.
Fatigue related to decreased energy production and altered body chemistry	The client will verbalize plan to modify activity, by discharge.	Educate client regarding reasons for fatigue and that fatigue may be present for several months.
		Encourage client to maintain bed rest for several weeks. Advise client that when resuming normal activity, rest periods should be included until stamina returns.

Evaluation Each goal must be evaluated to determine how it has been met by the client.

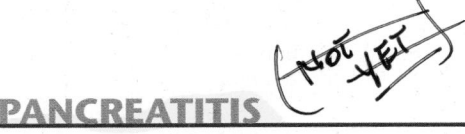

PANCREATITIS

Pancreatitis is an acute or chronic inflammation of the pancreas caused when pancreatic enzymes digest the lining of the pancreas. Pancreatitis occurs when obstruction of the pancreatic duct occurs as a result of gallstones, tumors, exposure to chemicals or alcohol, or injury to the pancreas. In severe cases, the pancreas can hemorrhage, resulting in a life-threatening condition.

Medical–Surgical Management

Medical

Treatment depends on the cause of the pancreatitis. If the pancreatitis results from exposure to chemical or alcohol abuse, treatment is primarily medical. An NG tube is inserted to rest the bowel and relieve abdominal distention.

Surgical

If the pancreatitis is caused by structural changes such as gallstones, an ERCP with stone removal may be performed. Surgery to relieve the pancreatic duct obstruction may be necessary in cases where tumors or injury are the causes of the pancreatitis.

Pharmacological

Insulin may be given if the pancreas is unable to secrete enough to maintain normal blood sugar level. If nausea and vomiting are present, antiemetics may be ordered. Meperidine (Demerol) is ordered for analgesia because morphine sulfate may cause spasms of the sphincter of Oddi. Atropine sulfate or propantheline bromide (Pro-Banthine) may be ordered to decrease pancreatic activity. Antacids or an H₂ receptor antagonist may be ordered to prevent stress ulcers.

Diet

Clients are kept NPO while the serum amylase level is elevated to decrease the demand for digestive enzymes in the bowel. An NG tube may be inserted to decrease pancreatic activity and to prevent nausea, vomiting, and abdominal distention. As the serum amylase level begins to decrease, clients will be started on clear liquids and slowly advanced to a bland, low-fat, high-protein, high-carbohydrate diet. No coffee or alcohol is allowed.

IV rehydration is necessary while the client is NPO. If the pancreatitis is severe and the client must be NPO for a prolonged period, TPN, a high-calorie, high-nutrient IV solution, may be administered.

Activity

Clients are generally placed on bed rest to decrease metabolic rate. Activity can be increased as the serum amylase decreases.

Nursing Management

Monitor and maintain NG tube. Weigh client daily and maintain client on bed rest. Assess pain and administer an analgesic. Monitor vital signs. Provide personal hygiene.

Assess and maintain IV hydration and TPN if ordered. Accurately record I&O. Monitor laboratory results, especially serum amylase, bilirubin, electrolytes, and H & H.

NURSING PROCESS

Assessment

Subjective Data

Clients describe excruciating epigastric pain that radiates to the back. Pain may decrease by leaning forward or lying in a fetal position. Nausea and anorexia are also present.

Objective Data

Assessment includes steatorrhea, vomiting, low-grade fever, tachycardia, and jaundice. Laboratory analysis shows an elevated serum amylase followed by an elevated urine amylase and serum lipase, leukocytosis, and an elevated Hct. Glucose, alkaline phosphatase, and bilirubin may also be elevated.

Nursing diagnoses for a client with pancreatitis may include the following:

Nursing Diagnoses	Planning/Goals	Nursing Interventions
Acute Pain related to inflammation and edema of the pancreas	The client will verbalize a decrease in pain as evidenced by pain scale by 1 hour after initiation of interventions.	Monitor NG tube to decompress the abdomen. Position client in most comfortable position. Assess pain for increasing severity that would indicate worsening pancreatitis. Administer analgesics as ordered and monitor for relief. Monitor serum amylase, WBCs, and H & H for signs of increasing severity of pancreatitis or hemorrhage.
Imbalanced Nutrition: Less than body requirements related to NPO status, nausea, vomiting, and altered ability to digest nutrients	The client will experience no further weight loss during hospitalization.	Monitor I&O every shift. Administer IV rehydration or TPN as ordered. Weigh client daily. Maintain bed rest to decrease the metabolic rate. Insert NG tube to decompress the abdomen as ordered.
Risk for Deficient Fluid Volume related to vomiting, NG tube, or hemorrhage	The client will maintain adequate hydration as evidenced by I&O that is nearly equal, electrolytes within normal limits, and moist mucous membranes.	Monitor I&O every shift. Administer IV hydration or TPN as ordered. Monitor electrolyte levels and H & H as ordered.

Evaluation Each goal must be evaluated to determine how it has been met by the client.

CHOLECYSTITIS AND CHOLELITHIASIS

Cholecystitis is an inflammation of the gallbladder. In more than 90% of the cases, gallstones are present. **Cholelithiasis** is the presence of gallstones or **calculi** (concentration of mineral salts) in the gallbladder. Not all gallstones cause cholecystitis. Some gallstones may pass out of the gallbladder and into the duodenum with the client unaware of the stones. Sometimes gallstones migrate into the cystic or common bile duct causing an obstruction that, in turn, leads to cholecystitis. The exact cause of the formation of these stones is not known.

These two diseases are more common in multiparous women, age 45 and older; obese people; those who use birth control pills or control cholesterol with gemfibrozil (Lopid); and people with a history of a disease of the small intestine such as Crohn's disease. Also, clients on sudden weight reduction diets that are low in fat will cause the bile to pool in the gallbladder, increasing the risk for gallstone formation.

Ultrasound of the gallbladder is ordered if gallstones are suspected.

Medical–Surgical Management

In asymptomatic clients, no intervention is necessary.

Medical

If stones are lodged in the common bile duct, an endoscopic retrograde cholangiopancreatogram (ERCP) may be performed.

Surgical

A sphincterotomy, an incision in the ampulla of vater, may be performed to enlarge the opening of the common bile duct. Stones may then be removed or crushed. If the stones are too large or for clients with repeated episodes of cholelithiasis, a cholecystectomy, the surgical removal of the gallbladder, may be performed. The cholecystectomy may be performed laparoscopically or by making a large abdominal incision.

Laparoscopic cholecystectomies have become the surgery of choice for cholelithiasis and cholecystitis. The gallbladder is removed by making four small incisions and extracting the gallbladder through an endoscope. If the cholecystectomy is performed laparoscopically, it is more difficult to perform an exploration of the common bile duct, especially in clients with cholecystitis. An ERCP may need to be performed if stones remain in the common bile duct (CBD). Clients are ready for discharge 24 hours after the surgery.

The cholecystectomy can also be performed by making a large abdominal incision. A cholangiogram can be performed easily, and therefore this type of procedure is more common in clients with much inflammation of the gallbladder. If damage has occurred to the CBD from severe inflammation or a stone, a T-tube will be left in place to allow the bile to drain into a collection bag. This allows the CBD to heal. Clients are typically ready for discharge 3 to 7 days after surgery.

Pharmacological

In acute cholecystitis, analgesics are ordered to relieve discomfort. Meperidine (Demerol) is preferred because morphine sulfate is believed to increase sphincter spasms. IV hydration may also be ordered if the client is unable to maintain hydration. Antiemetics are ordered for nausea and vomiting.

In clients who have surgery, analgesics will be ordered after surgery to control discomfort.

Diet

In clients with mild or moderate symptoms, a clear liquid diet to rest the bowel, followed by small frequent meals low in fat, may resolve the symptoms.

If clients are to have surgery, they will be NPO before surgery and initially after surgery until bowel sounds return. They will then be started on clear liquids first and then advanced, as tolerated, to a regular diet.

NO Fatty Foods

Activity

In acute cases of cholecystitis, bed rest is recommended to decrease metabolic rate. If surgery is performed, the client will be encouraged to turn, cough, and deep breathe every 2 hours initially after surgery. On the day following surgery, the client should be helped out of bed and encouraged to gradually increase activity. Clients who have had a laparoscopic cholecystectomy may be ambulated the evening of surgery. Clients can typically return to previous activity level 2 weeks after surgery. Clients who have an incision must restrict lifting, driving, and exercise until incisional healing is complete, usually 4 to 6 weeks.

Nursing Management

Monitor vital signs and bowel sounds. Assess pain, nausea, and vomiting and administer analgesic and/or antiemetic. Prepare for surgery by teaching deep breathing, coughing, splinting incision, incentive spirometry use, and leg exercises. Monitor and maintain NG tube if used. Accurately record I&O.

NURSING PROCESS

Assessment

Subjective Data

Clients describe pain in the right upper quadrant radiating to the right scapular area that occurs 2 to 4 hours after a meal containing significant amounts of fat; nausea; flatulence; and indigestion.

Objective Data

Assessment may show vomiting, occasionally a fever, jaundice, steatorrhea, clay-colored stools, and dark amber urine. Laboratory analysis may show elevated alkaline phosphatase, GGT, WBCs, and bilirubin.

Nursing diagnoses for a client with cholecystitis and cholelithiasis may include the following:

Nursing Diagnoses	Planning/Goals	Nursing Interventions
Acute Pain related to inflammation or blocked bile duct	The client will experience less pain as evidenced by pain scale within 1 hour of initiation of treatment.	Keep client NPO or on a clear liquid diet as ordered. Administer analgesics as ordered. Monitor NG tube to decompress the abdomen as ordered. Observe for jaundice and bile flow obstruction.

continues

Nursing Diagnoses	Planning/Goals	Nursing Interventions
*Ineffective **B**reathing Pattern* related to decreased lung expansion because of pain	The client will demonstrate appropriate breathing pattern and will not have respiratory complications while hospitalized.	Assist client to cough and breathe deeply every 2 hours. Teach use of incentive spirometer. Teach splinting techniques for comfort and to facilitate breathing. Turn client every 2 hours and ambulate as soon as indicated.
*Risk for Deficient **F**luid Volume* related to nausea, NG tube, NPO, or bile drainage	The client will maintain adequate hydration as evidenced by I&O that is nearly equal and moist mucous membranes.	Monitor I&O every shift including NG drainage and T-tube drainage if present. Administer IV hydration as ordered. Maintain patency of NG tube.

Evaluation Each goal must be evaluated to determine how it has been met by the client.

NEOPLASMS OF THE GASTROINTESTINAL SYSTEM

Neoplasms of the gastrointestinal system may occur anyplace in the GI system. Signs, symptoms, and treatment vary according to where the cancer occurs. Oral cancer, colorectal cancer, and liver cancer are discussed following.

ORAL CANCER

Oral cancer refers to cancers of the lips, tongue, oral cavity, and pharynx. According to the ACS (2003), 27,700 new cases are expected that year. Risk factors are tobacco use and excessive consumption of alcohol. Symptoms include a mouth sore that bleeds easily and does not heal, a lump, or difficulty chewing, swallowing, or moving tongue or jaw. On the lips, the cancer may be a growth.

Medical–Surgical Management

Surgical

Treatment is primarily surgical and involves removal of the cancer with excision of tissue and lymph nodes surrounding the cancer. In cases of cancer involving the pharynx, a radical neck dissection is performed, which requires reconstruction of the pharynx. Clients undergoing radical neck dissection frequently have a tracheostomy.

Pharmacological

Chemotherapy is not effective against most oral cancers and is, therefore, used only in the most severe cases with metastases. Medications ordered are based on the client's symptoms. If the client is experiencing side effects from the radiation such as nausea, antiemetics will be ordered.

If a client has surgery, analgesics are ordered postoperatively. Analgesics are also ordered if the cancer has progressed and is causing discomfort.

Diet

Because the surgery is in the oral area, it may be difficult to maintain adequate nutrition. Depending on the extent of the surgery, clients may require a soft diet or, in some cases, nutritional supplements to allow the surgical area to heal. Tube feedings, either by a feeding tube or by a gastrostomy tube (a special tube inserted through the abdomen into the stomach), are frequently needed in clients who have undergone a radical neck dissection.

Activity

If the surgery is minor, no activity restrictions will be necessary. If surgery is extensive, postoperatively, the client will need to turn, cough, and deep breathe. Activity will be progressed postoperatively. Clients receiving radiation treatments frequently experience fatigue and need scheduled rest periods.

Other Therapies

In cases where the lesion cannot be surgically removed, radiation or radium implants may be used. High-energy radiation is used to destroy cancer cells. Clients may experience irritated skin, swallowing difficulties, dry mouth, nausea, diarrhea, hair loss, or fatigue. Radiation is usually administered daily for a specified period. If radium implants are used, a radioactive capsule is implanted into the area.

Nursing Management

Encourage all clients to refrain from tobacco use and excessive alcohol consumption. Maintain feeding tube and administer tube feedings as ordered. Preoperatively, teach client to turn, cough, and deep breathe, and encourage client to practice postoperatively. Weigh client daily and accurately record I&O.

NURSING PROCESS

Assessment

Subjective Data

Clients may describe a sore throat, difficulty swallowing, or a painful area in the mouth.

Objective Data

Assessment may find a sore or lesion of the lips or in the oral cavity, and hoarseness.

Nursing diagnoses for a client with oral cancer may include the following:

Nursing Diagnoses	Planning/Goals	Nursing Interventions
Fear related to diagnosis and long-term prognosis	The client will verbalize fear and express plan to cope with diagnosis.	Allow client time alone and with significant others and client and family to express fears and concerns. Answer questions. Encourage contact with support system (e.g., clergy). Discuss past experiences with stress and individual responses to those situations.
Imbalanced Nutrition: Less than body requirements related to oral surgery or radical neck dissection	The client will maintain weight while hospitalized.	Monitor I&O every shift. Weigh client daily. Administer tube feedings and IV rehydration as ordered and introduce fluids, when indicated. Monitor for aspiration.
Disturbed Body Image related to disfiguring surgery	The client will verbalize feelings regarding surgery and altered body image.	Allow client time to verbalize feelings. Answer questions. Discuss options (e.g., plastic surgery or makeup). Provide information on support groups.

Evaluation Each goal must be evaluated to determine how it has been met by the client.

COLORECTAL CANCER

Colorectal cancer is the third most common site of new cancers and deaths in the United States (ACS, 2003). Almost all colorectal cancers arise from **polyps,** an abnormal growth of tissue that protrudes into the colon. Risk factors for colorectal cancer include age 50 or older, history of polyps, family history of polyps and/or colorectal cancer, a history of ulcerative colitis, and a diet high in fat and low in fiber.

Prognosis is very good if caught in the early stages. Recommended routine screenings for early detection include fecal occult blood testing and colonoscopy depending on personal and family history.

A colonoscopy or barium enema may demonstrate the disease. A CBC may show anemia if the cancer is bleeding. A CEA may be effective in detecting recurrent cancer but is not a valid screening test. Signs and symptoms include a change in bowel habits, guaiac-positive stools, and abdominal pain.

Medical–Surgical Management

Surgical

Treatment is surgical to remove the cancer. In class A tumors, a colonoscopy is performed with a polypectomy, the removal of the polyp. In class B or C tumors, a colon resection is done (Figure 35-10). In some cases, a colostomy, either temporary or permanent, is performed. In class D tumors, surgery is done only to relieve symptoms (e.g., bowel obstruction).

Follow-up colonoscopies must be done throughout the client's life to monitor for recurrence of the disease.

Pharmacological

In cases of class B, C, and D tumors, chemotherapy is given following the surgery. Side effects of chemotherapy include nausea, vomiting, weight loss, hair loss, fatigue, and dry skin. Medications to combat some side effects of the chemotherapy are ordered.

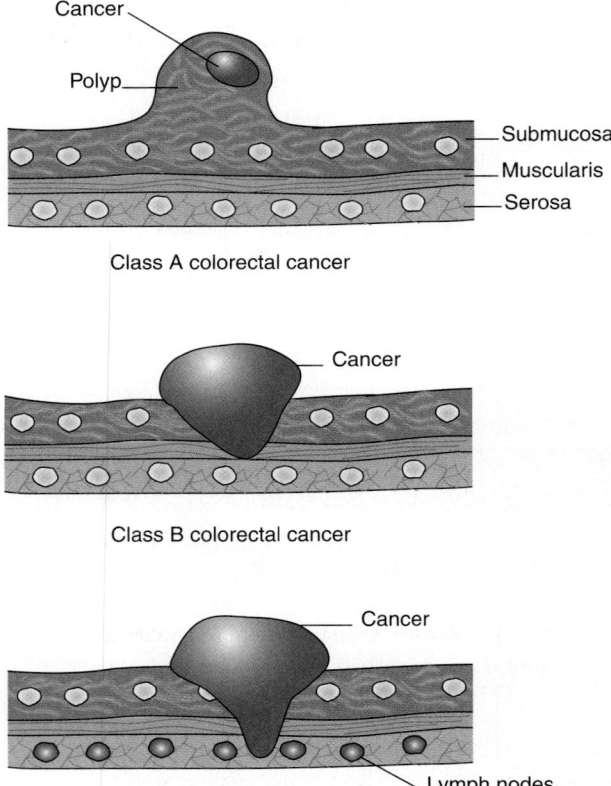

Class A colorectal cancer

Class B colorectal cancer

Class C colorectal cancer

Figure 35-10 *Classes of Colorectal Cancer*

Immunotherapy as an adjunct therapy for class C and D tumors may be ordered to boost the immune system.

Diet

Preoperatively, the client will be NPO. Postoperatively, the client will be NPO and an NG tube will be in place until bowel sounds return. The client is then started on a clear liquid diet and progressed to a high-fiber, low-fat diet.

Activity

Postoperatively, the client is encouraged to turn, cough, and deep breathe every 2 hours. The client is ambulated the next day and activity is progressed.

Other Therapies

No significant benefits have been found with the use of radiation on colorectal cancer; however, radiation may be used on metastatic sites in class D tumors.

Nursing Management

Encourage all clients to have recommended routine screenings, fecal occult blood test, and colonoscopy, based on their personal and family history. Prepare client for side effects (hair loss, fatigue, nausea, and dry skin) when chemotherapy is used. Postoperatively, maintain the NG tube. Assess bowel sounds. Encourage turning, coughing, deep breathing, use of incentive spirometer, leg exercises, and ambulation.

NURSING PROCESS

Assessment

Subjective Data

Clients may describe a change in bowel habits and possibly abdominal pain.

Objective Data

Stools may be guaiac positive for blood. An H & H may show anemia.

Nursing diagnoses for a client with colorectal cancer may include the following:

Nursing Diagnoses	Planning/Goals	Nursing Interventions
Fear related to diagnosis and long-term prognosis	The client will verbalize fear and express plan to cope with diagnosis.	Allow client time alone and with significant others and allow client and family to express fears and concerns. Answer questions and encourage contact with support system (e.g., clergy). Discuss past experiences with stress and identify individual responses to those situations.
Deficient Knowledge related to disease process, treatment options, and follow-up	The client will be able to explain disease process, treatment, and follow-up care.	Determine client's learning style and present information in a manner compatible with the learning style. Educate client regarding disease process and discuss treatment options. Recognize that information may need to be presented more than once.

Evaluation Each goal must be evaluated to determine how it has been met by the client.

LIVER CANCER —No

Primary liver cancer is rare. Most liver tumors are metastatic from other sites in the body. Most cases of primary liver cancer are asymptomatic until later stages. Risk factors for primary liver cancer include a history of cirrhosis, hepatitis B, and exposure to toxic chemicals.

A primary liver tumor can be removed surgically if the disease is not extensive. Metastases cannot be surgically removed and are usually treated with chemotherapy and radiation.

Summary

- The gastrointestinal system is a complex system composed of the digestive tract as well as accessory organs.
- Disorders of the GI tract affect the breakdown and absorption of nutrients, breakdown of wastes and byproducts, and the lifestyle of the individual.
- Because the liver is responsible for so many functions in the body, disorders of the liver can affect other systems significantly.
- Peptic ulcers may be either gastric or duodenal. *H. pylori* is a common cause of ulcers and can be treated with antibiotics.
- Diverticulosis is a commonly occurring disorder in the United States and is believed to be caused by a low-fiber diet.
- Inflammatory bowel disease includes both Crohn's disease and ulcerative colitis. IBD can lead to nutritional imbalances, bowel obstructions, alterations in the structure of the intestine, and affected lifestyle.
- Bowel obstructions have multiple causes and can lead to electrolyte imbalances, dehydration, and possibly sepsis.
- Viral hepatitis is a concern for health care professionals at risk for exposure. Standard precautions must be used to prevent the transmission of the virus.
- Colorectal cancer is one of the most preventable forms of cancer if routine screenings are performed.

Review Questions

1. A client with a bleeding esophageal varix:
   a. should be encouraged to vomit the blood to decrease abdominal distention and pressure.
   b. should have an NG tube placed to suction blood from the stomach.
   c. should have the Minnesota tube deflated every 4 hours.
   d. will not need follow-up once the bleeding has stopped.

2. A client with a perforated duodenal ulcer:
   a. requires an EGD to repair the perforation.
   b. may need diet modification after surgery.
   c. will have a vagotomy performed.
   d. may experience an increased risk for cholecystitis.

CASE STUDY

Ms. R. is a 52-year-old female admitted to the hospital with acute abdominal pain. Ms. R. complains of right upper quadrant pain radiating to the back. She has had prior episodes, usually occurring about 2 hours after eating. This episode, however, is not resolving. Ms. R. also complains of nausea. Her vital signs are BP 152/88, pulse 92, and respirations 24 and shallow. Ms. R. is a slightly obese female who states she has recently been dieting to lose weight. Laboratory analysis includes a CBC with slightly elevated WBCs; elevated bilirubin; and elevated alkaline phosphatase. An IV is started and Ms. R. is given meperidine (Demerol) IM for pain. Ms. R. has been made NPO. An ultrasound of the gallbladder is ordered.

The following questions will guide your development of a nursing care plan for this case study.

1. List subjective and objective data a nurse would want to obtain about Ms. R.
2. List risk factors other than those Ms. R. has that would put a client at risk for developing cholecystitis.
3. List two nursing diagnoses and goals for Ms. R.
4. The ERCP is successful in removing the CBD stone. The decision is made to perform a laparoscopic cholecystectomy. What teaching will Ms. R. need?
5. Why is meperidine (Demerol) the medication of choice for pain control?
6. List at least three successful outcomes for Ms. R.

3. Clients with hepatitis C:

    a. should be instructed that all the mechanisms of transmission are not known.

    b. will have a negative HCV if they are a carrier.

    c. should be instructed that recombinant interferon alpha-2b will cure the hepatitis C.

    d. are not contagious until symptoms develop.

4. Crohn's disease:

    a. can be cured by removing the colon.

    b. usually causes clients to gain weight from the slower metabolism of nutrients.

    c. can be a debilitating disease leading to depression.

    d. is cured as long as the clients remain on 5-ASA compounds.

5. Hernias are a protrusion through the muscle wall and:

    a. can be easily reduced by the nurse applying gentle pressure.

    b. are benign occurrences that do not need any intervention.

    c. can lead to bowel obstructions.

    d. are caused by a lack of exercise.

References/Suggested Readings

American Cancer Society (ACS). (2003). *Cancer Facts & Figures 2003*. Atlanta, GA: Author. [Online]. Available: www.cancer.org/downloads/STT/CAFF2003PWSecured.pdf

Atassi, K. (2002a). Appendicitis. *Nursing2002, 32*(8), 96.

Atassi, K. (2002b). Bleeding esophageal varices. *Nursing2002, 32*(4), 96.

Boekhold, K. (2000). Who's afraid of hepatitis C? *AJN, 100*(5), 26–31.

Brietfeller, J. (1999). Peritonitis. *AJN, 99*(4), 33.

Bunting, T. (2001). Putting the lid on gastroesophageal reflux. *Nursing2001, 31*(6), 46–49.

Cameron, J. L. (1998). *Current surgical therapy* (6th ed.). St. Louis, MO: Mosby.

Carroll, P. (1999). Monitoring the gut to prevent MODS. *RN, 62*(10), 34–37.

Centers for Disease Control and Prevention (CDC). (2001). FDA approval for a combined hepatitis A and B vaccine. *MMWR, 50*(37), 806–807. [Online]. Available: www.cdc.gov/mmwr/preview/mmwrhtml/mm5037a4.htm

Centers for Disease Control and Prevention (CDC) (2002a). *Viral hepatitis A*. [Online]. Available: www.cdc.gov/ncidod/diseases/hepatitis/a/fact.htm

Centers for Disease Control and Prevention (CDC) (2002b). *Viral hepatitis B*. [Online]. Available: www.cdc.gov/ncidod/diseases/hepatitis/b/fact.htm

Centers for Disease Control and Prevention (CDC) (2002c). *Viral hepatitis C*. [Online]. Available: www.cdc.gov/ncidod/diseases/hepatitis/c/fact.htm

Centers for Disease Control and Prevention (CDC) (2002d). *Viral hepatitis D*. [Online]. Available: www.cdc.gov/ncidod/diseases/hepatitis/slideset/hep-d.htm

Centers for Disease Control and Prevention (CDC) (2002e). *Viral hepatitis E*. [Online]. Available: www.cdc.gov/ncidod/diseases/hepatitis/slideset/hep-e/htm

Chene, B., & Decker, A. (2001). Battling hepatitis C. *RN, 64*(4), 54–58.

Clinical Rounds. (2003). Acetaminophen linked to most liver failure cases. *Nursing2003, 33*(3), 34.

Cole, L. (2001). Unraveling the mystery of acute pancreatitis. *Nursing2001, 31*(12), 58–63.

Daniels, R. (2002). *Delmar's Guide to Laboratory and Diagnostic Tests*. Clifton Park, NY: Thomson Delmar Learning.

Dochterman, J., & Bulechek, G. (2004). *Nursing Interventions Classification (NIC)* (4th ed.). St. Louis, MO: Mosby.

Erwin-Toth, P. (2001). Caring for a stoma. *Nursing2001, 31*(5), 36–40.

Estes, M. E. Z. (2002). *Health Assessment & Physical Examination* (2nd ed.). Clifton Park, NY: Thomson Delmar Learning.

Farrar, J. (2001). Acute cholycystitis. *AJN, 101*(1), 35–36.

Fried, M. W., Shiffman, M. L. et al. (2002). Peginterferon alfa-2a plus ribavirin for chronic hepatitis C virus infection. *New England Journal of Medicine, 347*(13), 975.

Galvan, T. (2001). Dysphagia: Going down and staying down. *AJN, 101*(1), 37–42.

Giacchino, S., & Houdek, D. (1998). Ruptured varices! Act fast. *RN, 61*(5), 33–36.

Heitkemper, M., & Jarrett, M. (2001). It's not all in your head: Irritable bowel syndrome. *AJN, 101*(1), 26–33.

Klonowski, E., & Masoodi, J. (1999). The patient with Crohn's disease. *RN, 62*(3), 32–37.

Krumberger, J. (2002). When the liver fails. *RN, 65*(2), 26–29.

Krupp, K., & Heximer, B. (1998). Going with the flow: How to prevent feeding tubes from clogging. *Nursing98, 28*(4), 54–55.

Lau, D. T., Kleiner, D. E., Park, Y., DiBisceglie, A. M., & Hoofnagle, J. H. (1999). Resolution of chronic delta hepatitis after 12 years of interferon alpha therapy. *Gastroenterology, 117*(5), 1229–33.

Lord, L. (2001). How to insert a large-bore nasogastric tube. *Nursing2001, 31*(9), 46–48.

McConnell, E. (1998). Giving medications through an enteral feeding tube. *Nursing98, 28*(3), 66.

McConnell, E. (2001a). Administering total parenteral nutrition. *Nursing2001, 31*(11), 17.

McConnell, E. (2001b). Myths & facts . . . about dysphagia. *Nursing 2001, 31*(7), 29.

McConnell, E. (2001c). What's behind intestinal obstruction? *Nursing2001, 31*(10), 58–63.

Mehta, M. (2003). Assessing the abdomen. *Nursing2003, 33*(5), 54–55.

Metheny, N., & Titler, M. (2001). Assessing placement of feeding tubes. *AJN, 101*(5), 36–45.

Metheny, N., Wehrle, M. A., Wiersema, L., & Clark, J. (1998). pH, color, and feeding tubes. *RN, 61*(1), 25–27.

Metheny, N., Wehrle, M. A., Wiersema, L., & Clark, J. (1998). Testing feeding tube placement: Ascultation vs. pH method. *AJN, 98*(5), 37–42.

Moorhead, S., Johnson, M., & Maas, M., (2004). *Nursing Outcomes Classification (NOC)* (3rd ed.). St. Louis, MO: Mosby.

National Institute of Diabetes and Digestive and Kidney Diseases (2000). *Viral hepatitis A to E and Beyond* [Online]. Available: www.niddk.nih.gov/health/digest/pubs/hep/hepa-e/hepa-e.htm

National Institute of Diabetes and Digestive and Kidney Diseases (2001a). *What I need to know about hepatitis A* [Online]. Available: www.niddk.nih.gov/health/digest/pubs/hep/hepa/hepa.htm

National Institute of Diabetes and Digestive and Kidney Diseases (2001b). *What I need to know about hepatitis B*. [Online]. Available: www.niddk.nih.gov/health/digest/pubs/hep/hepb/hepb.htm

National Institute of Diabetes and Digestive and Kidney Diseases (2002a). *Chronic hepatitis C: Current disease management.* [Online]. Available: www.niddk.nih.gov/health/digest/pubs/chrnhepc/chrnhepc.htm

National Institute of Diabetes and Digestive and Kidney Diseases (2002b). *What I need to know about hepatitis C.* [Online]. Available: www.niddk.nih.gov/health/digest/pubs/hep/hepc/hepc.htm

North American Nursing Diagnosis Association. (2003). *Nursing Diagnoses: Definitions & Classification 2003–2004.* Philadelphia: Author.

O'Brien, B., Davis, S., & Erwin-Toth, P. (1999). G-tube site care: A practical guide. *RN, 62*(2), 52–56.

O'Hanlon-Nichols, T. (1998). Basic assessment series: Gastrointestinal system. *AJN, 98*(4), 48–53.

Parini, S. (2001). Hepatitis C: Speaking out about the silent epidemic. *Nursing2001, 31*(3), 36–42.

Parini, S. (2003). Hepatitis C: Update your knowledge of this silent stalker. *Nursing2003, 33*(4), 57–63.

Perry, J., Jagger, J., & Parker, G. (2003). Statistically, your risk of HCV infection has dropped. *Nursing2003, 33*(6), 82.

Rayhorn, N. (1999). Understanding inflammatory bowel disease. *Nursing99, 29*(12), 57–61.

Rayhorn, N., & Rayhorn, D. (2002). An in-depth look at inflammatory bowel disease. *Nursing2002, 32*(7), 36–42.

RNWeb. (2000). *Oncology today: Colorectal colon* [Online] Available: www.RNWeb.com/ce/199/chestblt.html

RNWeb. (2000). *The patient with Crohn's disease* [Online] Available: www.RNWeb.com/ce/199/chestblt.html

Sargent, C., & Murphy, D. (2003). What you need to know about colorectal cancer. *Nursing2003, 33*(2), 36–41.

Schlapman, N. (2001). Spotting acute pancreatitis. *RN, 64*(11), 54–58.

Spratto, G., & Woods, A. (2004). *2004 PDR Nurse's Drug Handbook.* Clifton Park, NY: Thomson Delmar Learning.

SpringNet (2000). *Caring for a patient with colon cancer* [Online]. Available: www.springnet.com/ce/j801a.htm

SpringNet (2000). *Irritable bowel syndrome* [Online]. Available: www.springnet.com/ce/j801a.htm

SpringNet (2000). *Pancreatitis: Managing a flare-up* [Online]. Available: www.springnet.com/ce/j801a.htm

U.S. Food and Drug Administration. (2002). *FDA approves new treatment for chronic hepatitis B.* [Online]. Available: www.fda.gov/bbs/topics/ANSWERS/2002/ANS01163.html

U.S. Preventive Services Task Force. (2002). Screening for colorectal cancer: Recommendations and rationale. *AJN, 102*(9), 107–114.

Veronesi, J. (2003). Inflammatory bowel disease. *RN, 66*(5), 38–45.

Zimmermann, P. (2002). Triaging lower abdominal pain. *RN, 65*(12), 52–57.

Resources

American Liver Foundation, 75 Maiden Lane, Suite 603, New York, NY 10038, 800-GO-LIVER (465-4837), http://liverFoundation.org

Crohn and Colitis Foundation of America, Inc., 386 Park Avenue South, 17th Floor, New York, NY 10016-8804, 800-932-2423, www.ccfa.org

Hepatitis Foundation International (HFI), 504 Blick Drive, Silver Spring, MD 20904-2901, 800-891-0707, www.hepfi.org

National Digestive Diseases Clearinghouse, 2 Information Way, Bethesda, MD 20892, 301-654-3810, www.niddk.nih.gov

United Ostomy Association, 19772 McArthur Boulevard, Suite 200, Irvine, CA 92612-2405, 800-826-0826, www.uoa.org

URINARY SYSTEM

MAKING THE CONNECTION

Refer to the following chapters to increase your understanding of the urinary system:

Basic Nursing
- Arenas of Care
- Wellness Concepts
- Assessment
- Diagnostic Tests

Adult Health Nursing
- Cardiovascular System
- Reproductive System
- The Older Adult

Basic Procedures
- Hand Hygiene
- Use of Protective Equipment
- Perineal Care

- Routine Catheter Care
- Measuring Intake and Output
- Urine Collection: Closed Drainage System
- Urine Collection: Clean Catch, Female/Male

Intermediate Procedures
- Performing Urinary Catheterization: Female/Male
- Irrigating a Urinary Catheter
- Irrigating the Bladder Using a Closed-System Catheter

Review: Delmar's Anatomy & Physiology CD-ROM: Renal System and Genitourinary System

LEARNING OBJECTIVES

Upon completion of this chapter, you should be able to:
- Define key terms.
- Describe the anatomy and physiology of the urinary system.
- Relate diagnostic test results to urinary disorders.
- Discuss the pros and cons of peritoneal dialysis/ hemodialysis and kidney transplantation, including lifestyle changes for the client receiving dialysis.
- List four drug classifications and two examples of each used in the treatment of urinary disorders.
- State two changes in the urinary system related to the normal aging process.
- Compare and contrast acute and chronic renal failure, including nursing care.
- Assist in formulating a nursing care plan for clients with urinary disorders.

KEY TERMS

anasarca	micturition
azotemia	nephrotoxic
cachectic	nocturnal enuresis
calculus(i)	overflow incontinence
cystitis	pyelonephritis
dialysate	pyuria
dialysis	renal colic
dysuria	residual urine
erythropoiesis	retroperitoneal
fulguration	stress incontinence
ileal conduit	urge incontinence
intravesical	urinary incontinence
litholapaxy	urinary retention
lithotripsy	urolithiasis

INTRODUCTION

Urology is the study of disorders of the urinary system. The National Kidney Foundation estimates that more than 20 million Americans have chronic kidney disease and more than 20 million more are at increased risk (National Kidney Foundation [NKF], 2003). Disorders of the urinary system may seriously affect an individual's health and, thereby, affect the lives of family members. Clients are treated by a urologist, specialist in urinary tract disorders, or a nephrologist, specialist in structure, function, and diseases of the kidney.

According to the National Kidney Foundation (2001a), the warning signs of kidney disease are:

- Burning or difficulty during urination
- Increase in the frequency of urination, especially at night
- Passage of bloody appearing urine
- Puffiness around the eyes, or swelling of the hands and feet, especially in children
- Pain in the small of the back just below the ribs (not aggravated by movement)
- High blood pressure

ANATOMY AND PHYSIOLOGY REVIEW

The urinary system consists of two kidneys, two ureters (upper urinary tract), a urinary bladder, and a urethra (lower urinary tract) (Figure 36-1). The kidneys manufacture urine. Urine normally consists of 95% water; the nitrogenous waste products of protein, which are urea, uric acid, and creatinine; the excessive electrolytes sodium, calcium, potassium, and phosphates; bile pigments; hormones; and metabolized drugs and toxins. Urine moves steadily by peristalsis through the ureters into the urinary bladder. The urine remains in the urinary bladder until capacity has been reached (about 500 mL) or until a desire to empty the urinary bladder (about 250 mL) is felt. The urine is then expelled from the bladder through the urethra, which is shorter in females than in males. **Micturition,** the process of expelling urine from the urinary bladder, is also called urination or voiding.

The kidneys are located beneath the false ribs, in the **retroperitoneal** space (behind the peritoneum outside the peritoneal cavity) of the abdominal cavity. The kidneys also assist in acid–base balance, raise blood pressure by secreting the enzyme renin, and produce the hormone erythropoietin, which is responsible for **erythropoiesis** (the production of red blood cells and their release by the red bone marrow).

Within the kidneys are microscopic units called nephrons, which are responsible for urine formation. The nephron winds into the cortex and medulla of the kidney. Each nephron includes a renal corpuscle, which consists of a glomerulus, a ball-like network of capillaries formed from an arteriole and held within a cuplike Bowman's capsule. The Bowman's capsule is attached to a long, intricate, ultrathin looped and coiled tubular structure called the renal tubule. Continuing on from the glomerulus is an arteriole that forms a capillary network around the tubule. Blood flowing through this system is collected by venioles. The inset in Figure 36-1 illustrates a nephron.

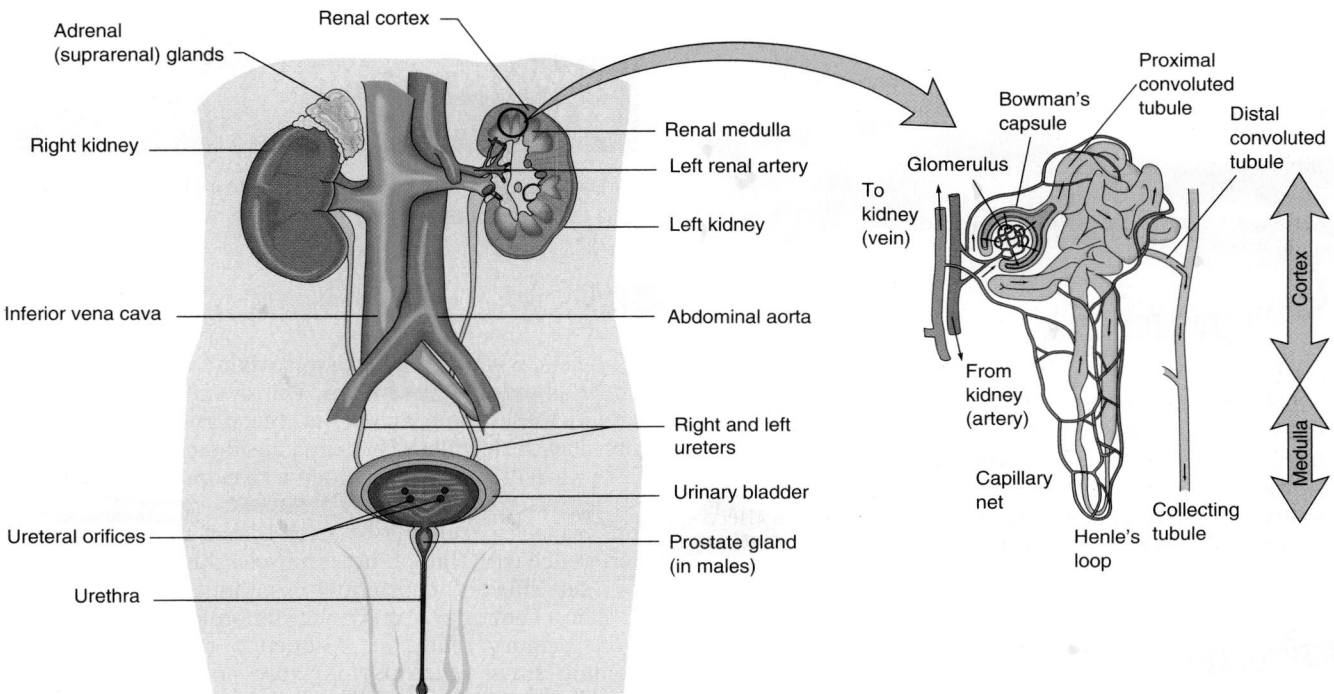

Figure 36-1 *The Urinary System with Inset of a Nephron*

Most of the contents of the blood, except for large molecules and blood cells, are forced out of the blood from the capillaries of the glomerulus and into the Bowman's capsule (glomerulofiltration). This occurs because of the high capillary blood pressure within the glomerulus. The glomerular basement membrane assists with the process of filtration. The material filtered from the blood is called glomerular filtrate, which contains water, electrolytes, glucose, various toxic substances, waste products (urea and creatinine), and just about everything else in the blood except large protein molecules and blood cells. As the filtrate passes through the first parts of the tubular structure, various substances such as necessary amounts of electrolytes, glucose, and water are reabsorbed (tubular reabsorption) back into the circulatory system through the capillaries or into the interstitial fluid. Tubular secretion then removes certain ions, nitrogen waste products, and drugs from the blood in the capillaries and adds it to the filtrate. The remaining filtrate—water, urea, excess electrolytes, toxic substances, and wastes, all of which constitute urine—continues through the tubules into the collecting duct, which collects urine from many nephrons. The urine passes from the collecting duct into the pelvis of the kidney, then through the ureter into the bladder and out of the body through the urethra. The kidneys process about 400 quarts of blood a day to eliminate 2 quarts of waste products and extra water as urine (NIDDK, 2002a).

ASSESSMENT

Assessment of the urinary system is included in the baseline data for all clients. The client may be reluctant to discuss urinary problems. Assist the individual to relax by asking open-ended questions, using familiar terms, and making sure the client understands the medical terms.

A more in-depth assessment is performed when clients are at high risk for renal disease because of exposure to nephrotoxins; an altered health state such as diabetes mellitus, pregnancy, or hypertension; trauma, dehydration, or fluid retention, which can compromise renal function; and those with suspected or active renal disease.

Subjective Data

Ask the client to describe how the symptoms developed and progressed. Is there pain? Is it sharp or a dull ache? Constant or intermittent? Does it radiate to the groin, genital area, or leg? Is the pain associated with urination? Have headaches been experienced?

Next, the client can describe the urine and urination pattern. Is there difficulty starting the stream? Is there urgency, frequency, incontinence, or hematuria? Does the bladder feel empty after voiding? Does the client have pruritis or dry skin?

Objective Data

If edema is present, ask the client if it is always present or if it disappears during the night. Refer to Figure 33-6, Grading Edema. Monitor I&O and vital signs, and palpate the bladder for retention. Weigh the client. Assess mucous membranes for moisture and the skin for dryness and uremic frost. Evaluate urine for color, clarity, and odor. Review diagnostic tests.

Changes with Aging

The following changes are found in the urinary system as a result of aging:

1. Nephrons decrease, resulting in decreased filtration and gradual decrease in excretory and reabsorptive functions of renal tubules.
2. Glomerular filtration rate decreases, resulting in decreased renal clearance of drugs.
3. Blood urea nitrogen (BUN) increases 20% by age 70. The creatinine clearance test is a better index than the BUN of renal function in the elderly.
4. Sodium-conserving ability is diminished.
5. Bladder capacity decreases, causing increased frequency of urination and nocturia.
6. Renal function increases when the client is lying down, sometimes causing a need to void shortly after going to bed.
7. Bladder and perineal muscles weaken, resulting in inability to empty the bladder. This results in residual urine and predisposes the elderly to cystitis.
8. Incidence of stress incontinence increases in females.
9. The prostate may enlarge, causing frequency or dribbling in males.

COMMON DIAGNOSTIC TESTS

Commonly used diagnostic tests for clients with symptoms of urinary system disorders are listed in Table 36-1.

IMPAIRED URINARY ELIMINATION

Disorders in this category include urinary retention and urinary incontinence.

URINARY RETENTION

A person who is unable to void when there is an urge to void has **urinary retention.** This creates urinary stasis and increases the possibility of infection. The urine may overflow the bladder's capacity, causing incontinence.

A variety of causes include a response to stress; obstruction of the urethra by **calculi** (concentration of mineral salts, known as stones), tumor, or infection; interference with the sphincter muscles during surgery; or as a side effect of medications or perineal trauma.

The client may experience discomfort and anxiety from urinary retention. Frequency of urination and voiding small amounts may also occur. A distended bladder can be palpated above the symphysis.

Treatment may include urinary analgesics and antispasmodics to help the client relax. A urinary catheter

TABLE 36-1	COMMON DIAGNOSTIC TESTS FOR URINARY SYSTEM DISORDERS

Urine Tests

Urinalysis

Color	Bilirubin
Odor	Glucose
Albumin (protein)	Specific gravity
Acetone (ketone)	Bacteria
RBCs	Casts
WBCs	pH

Culture and sensitivity (C & S)

Creatinine clearance

Blood Tests

Blood urea nitrogen (BUN)

Serum creatinine

Antistreptolysin O titer (ASO titer)

Serum electrolytes

Sodium	Calcium
Potassium	Phosphorus
Chloride	

Radiographic Tests

Voiding cystourethrography

Kidney-ureter-bladder (KUB) x-ray

Computed tomography (CT)

Magnetic resonance imaging (MRI)

Intravenous pyelogram (IVP)

Renal angiography

Renal scan

Ultrasound

Urodynamic Tests

Uroflowmetry

Cystometrogram (CMG)

Urethra pressure profile (UPP)

Endoscopic Exam

Cystoscopy

may be used to empty the bladder, or surgery may be performed to remove any obstruction.

When the client is able to void, check for residual urine. Immediately after the client voids, insert a catheter. The urine left in the bladder, **residual urine**, should be less than 50 mL.

URINARY INCONTINENCE

Urinary incontinence is the involuntary loss of urine from the bladder. The incontinence may be a com-

plication of urinary tract problems or neurologic disorders and may be permanent or temporary. Medications such as sedatives, hypnotics, diuretics, anticholinergics, antipsychotics, and alpha antagonists may be associated with incontinence.

More than 13 million men and women in the United States experience incontinence, with women twice as often as men (National Institute of Diabetes and Digestive and Kidney Diseases [NIDDK], 2002c). This is not just a physiological problem but also affects the client's emotional, psychological, and social well-being. Incontinence can occur in clients of any age but is more common in older adults. All types of incontinence can be treated at any age. Keeping the perineal area dry and intact is a goal for all clients. Incontinence is classified as stress, urge, overflow, total, or nocturnal enuresis.

Stress Incontinence

Stress incontinence is the most common type of incontinence. It is not a disease or a natural, inevitable effect of aging. Anyone can be affected; however, women are more likely to have this condition than men. In **stress incontinence** there is leakage of urine when a person does anything that strains the abdomen such as coughing, laughing, jogging, dancing, sneezing, lifting, making a quick movement, or even walking.

Medical management depends on the underlying cause. Stress incontinence is treatable and often curable at all ages (NIDDK, 2002c). Treatment may include bladder retraining, medicines such as conjugated estrogens (Premarin Vaginal Cream), or surgery. Surgery may be necessary to restore the support of the pelvic floor muscles or to reconstruct the sphincter but is used after other treatments are unsuccessful. Another possible treatment is having collagen injected into the tissues surrounding the urethra. This closes the urethra enough to prevent urine from leaking out. The procedure is done in a nonsurgical outpatient setting. Several support prostheses and external barriers are available.

The client can be taught pelvic floor exercises (Kegel) to strengthen the muscles, thereby preventing or minimizing stress incontinence. Kegel exercises involve having the client tighten the pelvic floor muscles to stop the flow of urine when urinating, and then releasing the muscles to start the flow of urine again. Once the client can do this, the exercise may be done anytime, anyplace. Practicing the exercise 10 times, 7 or 8 times a day strengthens the muscles.

Bladder retraining begins with assessing the client's voiding pattern and encouraging the client to void 30 minutes before the projected time of incontinence. The schedule is extended until the client can stay dry for 2 hours, gradually increasing the time between voidings until a 3- to 4-hour schedule is achieved.

Urge Incontinence

Urge incontinence occurs when a person is unable to suppress the sudden urge or need to urinate. Sometimes urine may leak without any warning. An irritated bladder is often the cause. Infection or very concentrated urine may irritate the bladder.

LIFE CYCLE CONSIDERATIONS

Elderly Clients and UTIs

- Ten percent to 20% of people older than age 65 have bacteriuria (Marchiondo, 1998).
- Elderly clients are more prone to UTIs because of incomplete emptying of the bladder, fecal incontinence with perineal soiling, and a decrease in urine acidity.
- Incomplete emptying of the bladder in women is caused by bladder or uterine prolapse or loss of pelvic muscle tone; in men it is caused by an enlarged prostate gland.

Treatment includes clearing up an infection, if present, and encouraging the client to have a fluid intake of 3,000 mL per day. This prevents the urine from becoming concentrated. Less fluid does not prevent incontinence but may promote infection.

Overflow Incontinence

When the bladder becomes so full and distended that urine leaks out, it is called **overflow incontinence.** This occurs when a blocked urethra or bladder weakness prevents normal emptying. The blockage may be an enlarged prostate. The distended bladder cannot contract with enough force to expel a stream of urine. Bladder weakness occurs most often in persons who have diabetes, drink a large quantity of alcohol, and have decreased nerve function. Bladder retraining may alleviate the situation.

Total Incontinence

When no urine can be retained in the bladder, it is termed total incontinence. The client may be able to manage with an indwelling catheter. A neurologic problem is usually the cause. Surgery to make a temporary or permanent urinary diversion may be required. Kniest & McGovern (2002) describe the Mitrofanoff procedure, which creates a catheterizable channel between an abdominal stoma and the bladder. Clients can then empty their bladder with a catheter.

Nocturnal Enuresis

Incontinence that occurs during sleep is called **nocturnal enuresis.** Limiting fluid intake after 6 P.M. helps the client remain continent during the night. The total fluid intake for 24 hours, however, should remain the same. The bladder should be emptied immediately before going to bed.

Nursing Management

Identify impaired urinary elimination based on subjective and objective data. Assess vital signs. Encourage adequate fluid intake. Teach Kegel exercises. Initiate bladder retraining.

INFECTIOUS DISORDERS

Infectious disorders of the urinary system are called urinary tract infections (UTIs). There are two types: lower UTIs affect the bladder (cystitis) and urethra, and upper UTIs affect the kidneys (pyelonephritis, and acute and chronic glomerulonephritis) and ureters.

CYSTITIS

Cystitis is an inflammation of the urinary bladder. It is more common in females because their short urethra allows bacteria to ascend through the urethra from the vagina or rectum to the urinary bladder. Also, bacteria from an infected kidney can descend through the ureter into the urinary bladder. Most urinary tract infections are caused by *Escherichia coli*, but some are caused by *Candida albicans*. Other common causes of cystitis are coitus, prostatitis, and diabetes mellitus.

As women age, pelvic floor muscles relax, leading to a decreased ability to empty the bladder completely. This contributes to stasis of urine and promotion of bacterial growth, as in pregnancy or benign prostatic hypertrophy. In men, cystitis usually occurs secondary to another infection such as epididymitis or prostatitis.

Once bacteria enter the bladder, they multiply, causing redness and swelling of the wall of the bladder. These changes result in urinary frequency, dysuria, pyuria, hematuria, and sometimes burning and urgency with urination. These symptoms increase as the bladder distends with even a small volume of urine.

A clean-catch midstream urinalysis showing a bacteria count greater than 100,000 organisms/mL confirms the diagnosis. Microscopic examination of the urine also shows hematuria and pus.

Medical–Surgical Management

Medical

Treatment of cystitis includes medication and fluids. Recurrence of a urinary tract infection usually occurs when it is not effectively treated. Obtaining and sending a urine specimen for C & S before the administration of any urinary antimicrobial is necessary to determine the most effective medication. A repeat urinalysis after 2 or 3 days on medication confirms its effectiveness. Chronic lower urinary tract infections are often a factor in the development of pyelonephritis.

Pharmacological

Cystitis treatment entails the use of antimicrobial medication in conjunction with urinary tract analgesics. Cystitis is generally treated with norfloxacin (Noroxin), nitrofurantoin (Furadantin), ciprofloxacin (Cipro), or sulfonamides such as sulfisoxazole (Gantrisin) or trimethoprim-sulfamethoxazole (Bactrim, Septra). Determine whether the client is allergic to sulfonamides or penicillins before administering the medication. The antimicrobial ordered is determined by the results of the urine culture and sensitivity. The length of treatment is related to the type of cystitis, acute or chronic. Some physicians may order a single dose or short course (3 or 4 days) of antimicrobial therapy rather than the traditional 7- to 10-day course. A single-dose medication, fosfomycin tromethamine (Monurol), is indicated exclusively for UTI treatment (Spratto & Woods, 2003). **Dysuria** (difficult or painful urination) related to a burning sensation when voiding can be alleviated with the use of the urinary tract analgesic phenazopyridine hydrochloride (Pyridium), which causes red-orange urine and stains clothing and toilets.

Diet

Encourage fluid intake. Clients are usually asked to drink between 3 and 4 liters of noncaffeinated fluid per day. The intake of meats and whole grains makes the urine more acidic and may discourage the growth of bacteria in the urinary bladder. Drinking cranberry juice has been advised for years, but how it worked was not understood. Research suggests that condensed tannins in the juice prevent *E. coli* from sticking to the urinary tract. Beneficial results begin within 2 hours and last up to 10 hours (NKF, 2002c).

Activity

Because cystitis causes frequency of urination, call lights must be answered promptly for clients on bed rest or those in need of assistance to the bathroom. Clients on bed rest are generally not able to empty their bladder completely when using a bedpan. Encourage orders for bathroom privileges or using a commode chair. Help allay the client's fears of being incontinent with properly timed bladder management.

Nursing Management

Monitor vital signs. Accurately record intake and output. Encourage fluid intake, especially water and cranberry juice. Encourage the client to void more frequently and women to void after intercourse. Advise clients taking Pyridium that urine will be red-orange and will stain clothing. Encourage cotton-crotch undergarments. Teach those who wear an incontinence control product to change it frequently.

NURSING PROCESS

Assessment

Subjective Data

The client will usually describe having frequency or urgency of urination or nocturia. This is annoying and embarrassing, regardless of age or sex. Burning and pain when voiding are common reasons clients seek medical care. Even clients with an indwelling catheter may complain of dysuria, burning, and frequency. Clients often just do not feel well.

Objective Data

Perineal irritation may be noticed when the client with a catheter pulls on it in hopes of alleviating the bladder pain. The urine will smell foul and appear cloudy. Hematuria may be present. The elderly population in particular may become anorexic and develop a low-grade fever. The urinalysis will indicate the presence of bacteria, and the C & S will identify the specific microorganism causing the urinary tract infection and the medication to which the pathogen is most sensitive.

Nursing diagnoses for a client with cystitis may include the following:

Nursing Diagnoses	Planning/Goals	Nursing Interventions
Impaired **U**rinary Elimination related to urinary tract infection	The client will return to usual pattern of urinary elimination.	Encourage a large amount of fluid intake, at least 3,000 mL each day, especially water and cranberry juice twice a day.
		Administer urinary tract analgesics and antimicrobial medications as ordered.
		Alert the client, if Pyridium is being taken, that the urine will be red-orange and will stain clothing.
Deficient **K**nowledge related to treatment regimen and prevention of recurrence	The client will comply with treatment regimen and practice preventive habits.	Discuss the importance of taking all medication ordered even after the symptoms are relieved.
		Teach or reinforce the following preventive measures.
		Clean the perineum from front to back.
		If nylon undergarments are worn, they should have a cotton crotch.
		Wearing tight-fitting jeans and taking long bike rides may be irritating to the perineum.
		Perfumed perineal products such as menstrual products, douches, powder, or bubble bath may also be contributing factors to bladder infections.

continues

Nursing Diagnoses	Planning/Goals	Nursing Interventions
		Spermicidal contraceptive products can be irritating, thus encouraging a lower UTI.
		Advise the client to void more frequently and not keep urine in the bladder. Advise women to void after sexual intercourse.
		Teach the elderly person who uses incontinence control products, to change the product frequently to prevent cystitis.
		When this client is hospitalized, plan time for frequent ambulation to the bathroom or commode chair.

Evaluation Each goal must be evaluated to determine how it has been met by the client.

PYELONEPHRITIS

Pyelonephritis, also known as pyelitis or nephropyelitis, is a bacterial infection of the renal pelvis, tubules, and interstitial tissue of one or both kidneys. Bacteria generally ascend from the urinary bladder through the ureter and enter the kidney in the renal pelvis. Bacteria can also enter from the blood and lymph. Pyelonephritis can be secondary to ureterovesicular reflux (backflow of urine from the bladder into the ureters) or when urine cannot drain from the pelvis of the kidney because of an obstruction blocking the kidney or ureter. Pyelonephritis may occur during pregnancy, with prostatitis, when bacteria are introduced during a cystoscopy or catheterization, or from trauma to the urinary tract. Pyelonephritis can be an acute illness or a chronic condition leading to the development of high blood pressure and/or chronic renal failure.

Escherichia coli is the microorganism most often cultured. The inflamed kidney becomes edematous and the renal blood vessels become congested. Sometimes abscesses form in the kidney. The urine is usually cloudy, containing mucus, blood, and pus.

Medical–Surgical Management

Medical

Diagnostic tests that may be ordered include an IVP, a urinalysis with a C & S, CBC, BUN, and serum creatinine. Collect urine specimens before the administration of any antimicrobial medication. Medical treatment and care are focused on preventing pyelonephritis from becoming chronic. Follow-up care and treatment may be necessary for up to 6 months.

Pharmacological

Pyelonephritis is generally treated with sulfonamides, such as trimethoprim-sulfamethoxazole (Bactrim) or the antimicrobial ciprofloxacin hydrochloride (Cipro). Cipro may not be indicated if the client has renal damage. Antipyretics are used to reduce fever and analgesics to manage pain.

Diet

As with infections in general, the individual's diet should be light during the febrile stage. Fluids must be increased to 3,000 mL per day by mouth and supplemented intravenously when indicated.

Activity

Because the disease process causes fatigue, bed rest is maintained during the acute phase of pyelonephritis. Diversionary activities are important while on bed rest. When the client is allowed to ambulate, dizziness related to the analgesic medication taken for pain may be a problem.

Nursing Management

Encourage client to verbalize concerns and fears. Answer questions honestly. Monitor I&O and observe output. Encourage fluid intake to 3,000 mL per day and cranberry juice twice a day. Cleanse perineum from front to back. Encourage client to empty bladder frequently. Promote rest periods during the day. Weigh client daily.

NURSING PROCESS

Assessment

Subjective Data

In acute pyelonephritis the client is acutely ill with malaise, urgency in urination, and pain during voiding and in the flank area. **Renal colic,** severe pain in the kidney that radiates to the groin, may occur, impairing urination. The client may describe being hot, with or without chills. In chronic pyelonephritis, only a general symptom of nausea may be present. The client may be very anxious that this kidney infection will cause permanent kidney damage.

Objective Data

Assessment may find the client tender on one or both sides of the lower back. Temperature, pulse, and respiratory rate may all be elevated. The urine is foul smelling and cloudy. The urinalysis results show bacteria and **pyuria** (pus in the urine), and the CBC indicates leukocytosis. The client with chronic disease will have the systemic signs of vomiting, diarrhea, and elevated blood pressure. Some clients with pyelonephritis may be asymptomatic.

Nursing diagnoses for a client with pyelonephritis may include the following:

Nursing Diagnoses	Planning/Goals	Nursing Interventions
Anxiety related to unknown prognosis	The client will verbalize fears and concerns to family and health care team.	Encourage the client to verbalize fears and concerns. Use active listening and observe for behavioral signs of anxiety. Answer questions honestly.
Impaired **U**rinary Elimination related to urinary tract infection	The client will regain normal urinary pattern.	Encourage drinking cranberry juice in the morning and evening. Encourage fluid intake to 3,000 mL per day, especially water. Monitor intake and output. Evaluate kidney function by measuring and observing urine output and monitoring the results of blood and urine tests.
Deficient **K**nowledge related to disease process, treatment regimen, and prevention	The client will verbalize understanding of disease process, treatment regimen, and preventive measures.	Teach or reinforce the hygiene measure of cleansing the perineum from front to back and practice this when doing perineal care on any client. Instruct the client on the importance of taking all the antimicrobial medication as prescribed in order to eliminate the bacteria. Teach the client to refrain from using perfumed perineal products such as menstrual pads, tampons, or douches, and avoid bubble baths and hot tubs because they can be irritating to the tissues of the genital area. Encourage the client to empty the bladder frequently to avoid distention. Promote rest periods, which aid the healing process. Inform the client to call the physician immediately if there is a decrease in urine output or signs of infection (elevated temperature, chills, flank pain, urgency, fatigue, nausea, and vomiting). Teach client to weigh daily and report sudden weight gain (2 pounds/week) to the physician. Emphasize the importance of keeping all appointments with the physician for follow-up care and when signs of infection appear. Teach the client the importance of long-term treatment and monitoring for chronic pyelonephritis.

Evaluation Each goal must be evaluated to determine how it has been met by the client.

ACUTE GLOMERULONEPHRITIS

Glomerulonephritis is a condition that can affect one or both kidneys. In both acute and chronic disease, the glomerulus within the nephron unit becomes inflamed. It is predominantly a disease of children and young adults when the cause is bacterial. The viral form can affect all ages. The prognosis for most clients is a full recovery; however, some may develop chronic glomerulonephritis. Approximately 1% to 2% of people with end-stage renal disease result from acute glomerulonephritis (NIDDK, 2001). Acute glomerulonephritis during childhood is known as Bright's disease.

Clients may develop symptoms 1 to 3 weeks after an upper respiratory infection (tonsillitis or pharyngitis with fever) or skin infection caused most commonly by group A β-hemolytic streptococcus. The infection trig-

gers an autoimmune response and the glomeruli are attacked by antibodies at the site of the glomerular basement membrane, resulting in inflammation. Some clients are asymptomatic. A nephrotoxic drug or systemic disease such as diabetes or lupus may also be a cause (NIDDK, 2002a).

Immunologic effects on the body are not completely understood. Direct effects on the glomeruli result in the reduced ability of the glomeruli to function. The glomeruli become more permeable, resulting in the loss of red blood cells and protein from the blood. These substances escape from the body in the urine. The inflammatory process causes thickening of the membrane of the glomeruli and potential scarring.

Diagnostic tests on blood and urine as well as KUB x-rays will be performed. BUN, serum creatinine, potassium, erythrocyte sedimentation rate (ESR), and antistreptolysin O titer (ASO titer) will be elevated. Urinalysis will show protein and red blood cells.

Medical–Surgical Management

Medical

Prevention of renal complications and complications to cardiac and cerebral functioning is the focus of care. Medical treatment must start as soon as the client is diagnosed to restore kidney function. Management includes drug therapy, diet, and rest. Treatment is correlated with the blood pressure and the results of urine testing for red blood cells and protein. The client is not considered to be free from the disease until the urine tests negative for protein and red blood cells for 6 months.

Plasmapheresis may be indicated if there is no response from other treatments. Between 150 and 400 mL of blood is removed from the client and put in a cell separator. Here the blood is divided into plasma and formed elements which are mixed with a plasma replacement and returned to the client through a vein. Another technique filters the client's own plasma to remove a specific disease mediator (antibody) and then returns the plasma to the client.

Pharmacological

Prophylactic antimicrobial therapy may be administered. The drug of choice is penicillin. Diuretic and antihypertensive medication furosemide (Lasix) may be ordered. Corticosteroids, chemotherapeutic drugs such as cyclophosphamide (Cytoxan), and/or immunosuppressive agents such as azathioprine (Imuran) may be ordered to control the inflammatory response.

Diet

Fluid retention often requires fluid restriction. The restriction is adjusted according to the client's I&O record and daily weight. Protein in the client's diet will be regulated according to the BUN and the creatinine blood levels. The kidneys need to rest; however, particularly in children, it may not be necessary to restrict protein. Potassium will need to be replaced if the diuretic promotes its excretion. Sodium may be restricted to prevent fluid retention. Strict intake and output are necessary to monitor kidney function.

Activity

Physical and emotional rest are essential. Compliance with bed rest may be difficult, especially for a child or the client who feels well. Bed rest is indicated until the inflammation subsides, urinary flow increases, and as long as the client has hematuria or proteinuria. During this time a strict turning schedule needs to be followed because skin breakdown is more likely in the presence of edema. When ambulation is allowed, the client may feel weak from the effects of anemia and inactivity.

Nursing Management

Monitor vital signs and I&O. Assess for headache, flank pain, and edema. Weigh client daily. Assess heart and lung sounds. Monitor results of diagnostic tests. If fluids are restricted, work with client on fluid intake schedule. Encourage client to follow schedule. Assist with or provide oral hygiene several times a day. Refer for dietary consultation if protein and sodium are restricted.

NURSING PROCESS

Assessment

Subjective Data

The health history will likely reveal a recent sore throat, skin infection, flulike symptoms, and a headache. The client describes flank pain as the kidneys become congested. Other symptoms the client may describe are headache, malaise, anorexia, cola-colored "smokey" urine (hematuria), and a marked decrease in the amount of urine (oliguria). Facial edema may be the first sign noticed, may impair vision, and may cause the client to have negative feelings about body image.

Objective Data

Vital signs will generally show an increase in body temperature and blood pressure. Facial (periorbital) edema is present. The edema will progress to dependent areas such as the sacral area and the legs. Monitor daily the location and degree of edema. Ascites may also develop. Assess the general condition of the skin and skin integrity. Weigh the client to establish a baseline weight. Assess heart and lung sounds for signs of heart failure and pulmonary edema (unusual heart sounds and crackles in the lungs). Neck veins may be distended. Dyspnea on exertion or when recumbent, and shortness of breath, may both be noted. Urine output is decreased and hematuria is present (cola-colored to red).

Monitor results of diagnostic tests: urine for red blood cells and protein (albumin) and blood for BUN, serum creatinine, potassium, ESR, ASO titer, and specific gravity, all of which will be elevated.

Nursing diagnoses for a client with acute glomerulonephritis may include the following:

Nursing Diagnoses	Planning/Goals	Nursing Interventions
Fear related to potential permanent damage to the kidneys	The client will communicate fears of kidney damage to the family and the health care personnel.	Provide client and family with ongoing support and understanding. Encourage the client to discuss fears.
		Explain the importance of protecting the client from other infections. Allow no one with an upper respiratory infection to visit the client.
		Discuss the importance of compliance with medications, bed rest, and diet to prevent permanent damage to kidneys.
		Emphasize the importance of keeping the follow-up visits to the laboratory for tests and to the physician's office.
		Arrange consultation with social services to assist the client in arranging time off from work and to help the client and family with their financial needs.
Excess Fluid Volume related to compromised regulatory mechanism secondary to renal dysfunction	The client will have decreased edema and adequate urinary output.	Fluids will be restricted with specific amounts designated throughout the day. For example, 900 mL of fluids for a day might be divided in the following manner: 7 A.M. to 3 P.M. 600 mL; 3 P.M. to 11 P.M. 200 mL; 11 P.M. to 7 A.M. 100 mL.
		Encourage compliance to the fluid amounts. Maintain accurate intake and output records hourly.
		Provide oral hygiene several times a day. Advise that thirst may be relieved by sucking on hard candy or, if allowed, a few ice chips.
		Provide eye care with normal saline to promote comfort from the periorbital edema.
Impaired Social Interaction related to changes in body image	The client will resume social interaction.	Encourage client to keep in contact with friends and relatives by telephone.
		Encourage keeping appointments with the physician and laboratory.
Imbalanced Nutrition: More than body requirements related to the disease process	The client will comply with nutritional restrictions.	Once the client's condition warrants solid foods, arrange a dietary consultation to incorporate food preferences and religious and/or cultural needs. Finances may be an issue if the family has to incorporate foods that are not usually part of its budget.
		Teach client to plan menus and to read food labels in order to comply with the dietary restrictions.
		Before discharge, teach client and family about diet, fluids, and activity restrictions and measuring fluid intake and urine output.
		Provide client with guidelines listing reasons to call the physician.

Evaluation Each goal must be evaluated to determine how it has been met by the client.

CHRONIC GLOMERULONEPHRITIS

The prognosis for acute glomerulonephritis is often good when treatment is begun early; however, chronic glomerulonephritis generally leads to permanent kidney damage. Those who develop chronic glomerulonephritis may have neither symptoms nor a recent history of an infection. Chronic diseases, such as diabetes mellitus or systemic lupus erythematosus, often mask renal symptoms and the client does not seek medical care until kidney function is impaired. It may take up to 30 years for the signs of renal insufficiency to develop.

Chronic glomerulonephritis is a slowly progressive, destructive process affecting the glomeruli, causing loss of kidney function. The kidney decreases in size as glomeruli are destroyed. If end-stage renal disease (ESRD) develops, the client may die quickly.

Nephrons lose their ability to filter nitrogenous wastes from the blood. Protein (albumin) and red blood cells escape into the urine and are present on a urinalysis. Nitrogenous waste remains in the blood, and the blood urea nitrogen (BUN) level increases. As glomeruli are destroyed, the serum level of creatinine also increases. BUN and serum creatinine are checked on a regular basis to monitor renal function. Serum electrolyte levels are also monitored. Anemia is evaluated with a CBC.

Medical–Surgical Management

Medical

Prevention of further renal damage as well as heart or cerebral complications is the focus of care. Management includes drug therapy, diet, and bed rest. Exposure of the client to infection of any kind must be avoided. Blood transfusion may be required for severe anemia. The client may be transferred to a facility where dialysis and/or kidney transplantation can be performed.

Pharmacological

Diuretic and antihypertensive medications are ordered. Antimicrobial therapy is generally given prophylactically. Monitor for side effects from all medications and report to the physician immediately.

Diet

Fluid intake is adjusted according to urinary output. Protein allowed in the diet will be regulated according to the BUN and the creatinine blood levels. As these levels increase, protein will be restricted to decrease the nitrogenous wastes. Sodium and potassium restrictions will be determined by the serum electrolyte levels. Carbohydrates are usually increased in the diet to provide adequate energy.

Activity

Bed rest is indicated when the client has hematuria or albuminuria.

Nursing Management

Assist client with ADLs and encourage bed rest with diversional activities. Monitor vital signs and I&O.

Measure urine hourly or as ordered. Assess color and consistency of urine. Assess lung sounds, edema, speech, and mental functioning. Assist client to reposition frequently and assess skin. Weigh client daily. Monitor laboratory reports.

NURSING PROCESS

Assessment

Subjective Data

Clients may describe a morning headache, pruritis, a decreased ability to concentrate, fatigue, and dyspnea making it difficult to perform ADLs. Facial edema and/or blurring of vision caused by retinal edema may also be reported by clients.

Objective Data

As chronic glomerulonephritis develops, fluid retention becomes evident, leading to shortness of breath, especially at night. Monitor vital signs; hypertension is usually present. Assess lung sounds every shift for crackles, a sign of fluid retention. Monitor weight daily, and note the degree of edema, its location, and if it is pitting or nonpitting. **Anasarca** is generalized edema that appears as the client's condition deteriorates. Assess skin for color, presence of ecchymosis or rash, dryness, and evidence of scratching. Note mental functioning, irritability, tremors, ataxia, or slurred speech.

As nephrons lose their ability to concentrate urine, the urine becomes pale and dilute. Closely monitor I&O because initially, polyuria develops, giving the client a false sense that recovery will be soon. Monitor results of blood and urine tests.

Nursing diagnoses for a client with chronic glomerulonephritis may include the following:

Nursing Diagnoses	Planning/Goals	Nursing Interventions
*Impaired **U**rinary Elimination* related to the failing kidney function	The client will have adequate urine output.	Measure urine output hourly, or every 4 or 8 hours as ordered. Parameters will be set by the physician for immediate notification. Assess and document the color and consistency of the urine.
		Measure intake to determine compliance with the amount of fluids permitted.
		Weigh client daily at the same time each day, on the same scale and with the same clothes.
*Excess **F**luid Volume* related to compromised regulatory mechanism	The client will have decreased edema.	Assess and describe the location of the edema.
		Administer medications as ordered for treatment of the edema.
		Monitor electrolyte values.
		Maintain fluid intake at restricted amount. Document I&O.

continues

Nursing Diagnoses	Planning/Goals	Nursing Interventions
Anxiety related to threat to or change in health status (potential treatment with dialysis)	The client will communicate less anxiety about possible treatment with dialysis.	Assist client to express concerns about possible treatment with dialysis. Arrange for a dialysis nurse to visit client.
Risk for Impaired Skin Integrity related to immobility and edema	The client will maintain skin integrity.	Assess skin every time the client is repositioned. Cleanse the skin frequently, especially when crystals of urea form on the skin, causing itching and dryness.

Evaluation Each goal must be evaluated to determine how it has been met by the client.

OBSTRUCTIVE DISORDERS

Disorders of this type include urolithiasis, urinary bladder tumors, renal tumors, and polycystic kidney.

UROLITHIASIS —STONE

More than 1 million persons in the United States each year have kidney stones (NKF, 2001a). **Urolithiasis** is a calculus, or stone, formed in the urinary tract. A calculus (plural—calculi) is a solid mass of mineral salts occurring within a hollow organ such as the renal pelvis, ureters, bladder, or urethra (Figure 36-2). A urinary calculus can range in size from microscopic to 10 to 20 mm in diameter.

Calculi are formed when minerals precipitate out of solution and collect within hollow areas. The reason stones form has not yet been identified, but individuals who are immobile, hyperparathyroid, or have recurrent UTIs are predisposed. When a person is immobile for long periods, calcium is pulled from the bones into the blood. The nephrons filter the excess calcium out of the blood into the urine. Calculi can also lodge in and obstruct an indwelling catheter. The size and location of the stone within the urinary system greatly affects the degree of pain and other symptoms present. When the stone is in the kidney, the pain is dull and constant mainly in the back just below the ribs near the spine. Stones in the ureter often cause ureteral colic, an excruciating, intermittent pain that begins in the flank and radiates into the groin, inner thigh, or genitalia. It is caused by spasm of the ureter as the calculus moves down the ureter. The client often has nausea and vomiting.

If a calculus becomes lodged anyplace along the ureter and urine cannot pass, a condition called hydronephrosis and/or hydroureter occurs. The kidney and/or ureter become enlarged with the accumulated urine (Figure 36-3).

Tests to confirm the diagnosis and determine the size and location of the stone include KUB, IVP, cystoscopy, and ultrasound. A BUN and serum creatinine indicate whether the calculus has damaged kidney function. A urinalysis with a culture and a CBC may be ordered to determine whether an infection is present. A 24-hour

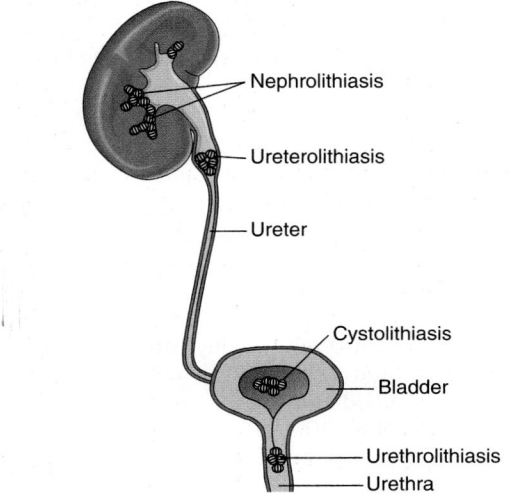

Figure 36-2 *Common Locations of Urinary Calculi Formation*

Labels: Nephrolithiasis; Ureterolithiasis; Ureter; Cystolithiasis; Bladder; Urethrolithiasis; Urethra

urine may be sent to the laboratory to determine whether there is abnormal excretion of calcium oxalate, phosphorus, and uric acid.

Medical–Surgical Management
Medical

All urine is strained whether voided or from an indwelling catheter drainage bag. Urine from a catheter drainage bag is drained and strained every 2 to 4 hours. All strained particles are saved for the physician or sent to the laboratory.

A very small calculus may be flushed out by peristalsis and fluids. The client is encouraged to drink at least 4,000 mL of fluid per day, unless contraindicated by other health problems. The urologist may insert a small, pliable catheter into the ureter or urethra to allow temporary drainage of urine around the calculus.

Extracorporeal shock wave **lithotripsy** (ESWL) is a method of crushing a calculus in the urinary system with ultrasonic waves. The client is placed in a warm-water bath, and ultrasonic waves aimed at the stone break the stone into small pieces. An alternate method is to appropriately place a fluid-filled bag on the client's

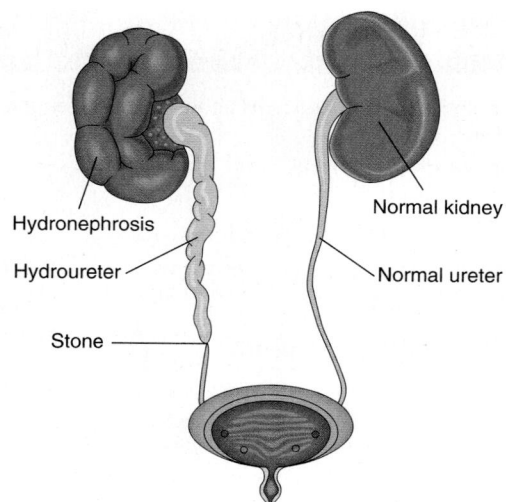

Figure 36-3 *Hydronephrosis and Hydroureter Resulting from a Stone in the Ureter*

Figure 36-4 *Methods of Removing Urinary Stones:* ***A,*** *Nephroscopic removal (percutaneous nephrolithotomy);* ***B,*** *Pyelolithotomy, removal through the renal pelvis;* ***C,*** *Nephrolithotomy, removal through incision into the kidney*

body and aim the ultrasonic waves at the stone through the bag. There is some discomfort and the client may be bruised where the ultrasonic waves hit the body. The urine will be slightly bloody for 24 to 48 hours and must be strained. The client should drink large amounts of fluids (3,000 mL to 4,000 mL per day) unless contraindicated. Clients should avoid taking aspirin and other drugs that affect blood clotting for several weeks before the procedure (NIDDK, 2000).

Ureteroscopy is used for mid- and lower-ureter stones. The small fiber-optic ureteroscope is passed through the urethra and bladder into the ureter. The stone is either removed in a cage-like device or shattered with a shock wave and the pieces removed (NIDDK, 2000).

Surgical

The surgeon may choose from several surgical procedures, depending on the location and size of the calculus. These include nephroscopic removal, pyelolithotomy, or nephrolithotomy (Figure 36-4).

Percutaneous nephrolithotomy is an endoscopic procedure in which a small incision is made in the fleshy area on the client's side between the ribs and the hip. A catheter is inserted and an ultrasonic probe is inserted through the catheter. Ultrasound waves directed at the stone break it into small pieces that can be withdrawn through the catheter. The catheter is left in place until the edema subsides, usually 1 or 2 days.

A bladder calculus may be crushed with special surgical instruments and the fragments washed out through a catheter. This is called a **litholapaxy.**

Pharmacological

Narcotic analgesics are generally prescribed for the severe pain often called renal colic. Antispasmodics such as propantheline bromide (Pro-Banthine) or belladonna preparations may be ordered to relieve ureteral spasms. Antibiotics may be ordered prophylactically.

Drug therapy is specific to stone composition. Allopurinol (Zyloprim) reduces the serum urate level, preventing calcium oxalate stones. Sodium cellulose phosphate (Calcibind) binds with calcium in the bowel and facilitates excretion of calcium. Aluminum hydroxide gel (Amphojel) binds with excess phosphates in the gastrointestinal tract. The phosphates are then excreted.

Diet

Eating foods high in calcium helps prevent calcium stones, but taking calcium in pill form may increase the risk of stones (NIDDK, 2000). When the stones contain uric acid, purine-rich foods (meat, fish, and poultry) are restricted, and organ meats, anchovies, and sardines avoided. Foods rich in oxalic acid (broccoli, asparagus, chocolate, tea, rhubarb, and spinach) are restricted when oxalate stones form. A deficiency of pyridoxine, thiamin, and magnesium may also contribute to the formation of oxalate stones.

CLIENT TEACHING

Urinary System Calculi

A person with a family history of stones or who has had more than one stone is at risk to develop another stone. Instruct these clients to:

- Drink plenty of fluids—water is best—to prevent stone formation.
- Avoid immobility.
- Take medications and modify diet as prescribed.
- Keep a record of intake and output.
- Learn how to strain urine.

Sometimes an effort is made to change the pH of the urine and thus prevent the formation of calculi. Acid-ash or alkaline-ash diets are used. Acid-ash foods are meats, fish, poultry, eggs, cereals, cranberries, and plums. Alkaline-ash foods are vegetables and all other fruits. These diets are often difficult for the client to maintain.

Drinking large amounts of fluid, at least half of it water, dilutes the urine and helps move any microscopic calculi through the system. Up to 4,000 mL per day of fluid is indicated for a client with renal calculi, unless contraindicated by another health problem such as heart failure.

Activity

Exercising regularly helps reduce the formation of calculi and keeps calculi moving through the urinary tract. Clients on bed rest should perform active range-of-motion (ROM) exercises daily in addition to frequent turning and positioning.

Nursing Management

Strain all urine. Monitor I&O. Encourage 4,000 mL per day of fluid intake unless contraindicated. Refer to dietitian for special acid-ash or alkaline-ash diet. Encourage active ROM exercises for clients on bed rest. Assess for pain and administer analgesic as ordered.

NURSING PROCESS

Assessment

Subjective Data

Many individuals are asymptomatic until the calculus begins to move or becomes too large. When the stone moves, the client usually describes intractable pain (pain not relieved by ordinary measures). The pain is often described as beginning in the flank and radiating down to the groin and inner thigh. Nonverbal client behaviors may indicate pain by tossing and turning when in bed or the inability to sit still when out of bed. If the calculus is not moving, the client may describe symptoms of infection such as lethargy, frequency of urination, dysuria, burning on urination, or feeling very warm. Nausea and vomiting are often reported. The client may express feelings of frustration related to the inability to complete daily tasks.

Objective Data

Assess hematuria, vomiting, intake and output, and vital signs. Elevated pulse and blood pressure may indicate pain. Check urine for stones when it is strained.

Nursing diagnoses for a client with urolithiasis may include the following:

Nursing Diagnoses	Planning/Goals	Nursing Interventions
Acute Pain related to irritation of the urinary tract and the mobility of calculi	The client will verbalize a reduction in pain.	Develop a pain management plan. Inquire about intensity, location, duration, and alleviating factors of pain. Observe for nonverbal signs of pain. Provide comfort measures and diversionary activities and administer analgesics and antispasmodics as ordered.
Impaired Urinary Elimination related to blockage of urine flow by the calculi	The client will return to normal urine elimination.	Encourage fluids to dilute the urine and flush out the calculi. Monitor urine for color and amount. Assist client to ambulate, if able. Accurately monitor intake and output. If a ureteral catheter is in place, measure and record the urine output from it separately from the urine output from the bladder.

Evaluation Each goal must be evaluated to determine how it has been met by the client.

URINARY BLADDER TUMORS

The American Cancer Society estimates approximately 57,400 new cases of urinary bladder cancer in 2003 (ACS, 2003). Men are affected four times more often than women. Bladder cancer occurs most frequently after the age of 50. The only early warning signs are increased urinary frequency and painless, intermittent hematuria. The main risk factor is cigarette smoking.

Those individuals who smoke nicotine products have twice the risk of developing bladder cancer as do nonsmokers. Other risk factors are working with dyes, rubber, or leather products; caffeine intake; and the use of certain artificial sweeteners.

Benign papillomas are the most common urinary bladder tumor. Although papillomas are quite small, they should be treated aggressively because they are considered to be premalignant. Cancer cells develop

mainly in the area where the ureters enter the urinary
bladder. The primary sites for metastasis are the liver,
lungs, or bones. Symptoms resulting from obstruction
of the ureters are often the reason the client seeks medical care. Diagnostic studies usually include a urinalysis,
a cystoscopic visualization and biopsy of the lesions, an
IVP, and CT scan.

Medical–Surgical Management

Surgical

Surgical removal of small tumors is generally done
by **fulguration** (a procedure to destroy tissue with
long, high-frequency electric sparks) to burn the lesions off the internal bladder wall. Other surgical procedures used are laser surgery or snaring of the lesion. These procedures are usually performed with
cystoscopic visualization. Several times a year, the
client who has had bladder lesions should be monitored for recurrence of the lesions. A cytologic examination is done on any lesion(s) noted during a cystoscopic examination.

A cystoscopic examination is performed with either
local anesthesia and sedation or general anesthesia.
After the procedure, the client's legs may be sore from
the lithotomy position used. Analgesics will be prescribed for use as needed. After a cystoscopic procedure,
the client may experience urinary frequency, burning on
urination, and the presence of pink-tinged urine.

When the pathology of tissue specimens indicates a
need for more extensive surgery, either a partial or total
cystectomy may be performed. The surgery may be done
in conjunction with radiation therapy or chemotherapy.

Ureters
Ileal conduit
with implanted
ureters
Stoma
Nipple valves
Ileal pouch
Skin
(abdomen)
Bladder

Figure 36-5 *Urinary Diversion—Kock Pouch*

When the urinary bladder is completely removed, a
urinary diversion is necessary. Consideration is made
for age, extent of the disease, and the prognosis. One option is a bilateral cutaneous ureterostomy, in which the
ureters are implanted directly into the abdominal wall.
Another option is for the ureters to be implanted into a
piece of the ileum, which is then attached to the abdominal wall as a stoma. This is known as an **ileal**
("wet") **conduit**.

Other methods of urinary diversion are the implantation of the ureters into the sigmoid colon (ureterosig-
moidostomy) and the creation of a continent stoma with
a pouch of bowel. This urinary diversion is known either
as a Kock (Figure 36-5) or Mainz pouch or a Gilchrist
ileocecal reservoir, depending on which surgical procedure was used.

Pharmacological

One chemotherapy treatment is the instillation of an
antineoplastic drug within the urinary bladder **(intravesical)**. Systemic chemotherapy may also be used.
Medications to relieve symptoms such as pain and nausea are important for the client's well-being.

Diet

If proctitis (inflammation of the rectum and anus) or
diarrhea occurs, a low-residue diet is ordered to facilitate
normal bowel elimination.

Activity

When the client is on bed rest, turning and positioning are important to maintain skin integrity because the
client may be emaciated as a result of significant weight
loss. Activity should be encouraged as the client's condition warrants. During the intravesical instillation of an
antineoplastic drug, the client will have to change positions every 15 minutes, for a period of several hours, to
evenly distribute the chemotherapeutic drug around the
urinary bladder.

Nursing Management

Encourage clients to reduce or eliminate the use of
nicotine products and report urinary frequency and
painless hematuria to their physician. After a cystoscopic examination, administer analgesic as needed for
sore legs from lithotomy position. Encourage client to
have adequate fluid intake and to express fears and concerns, especially if a urinary diversion is performed.
Refer client to local ostomy support group.

COLLABORATIVE CARE

Urinary Diversions
Nurses work together with the enterostomal therapist to
provide the specialized care and teaching required for a
urinary diversion.

NURSING PROCESS

Assessment

Subjective Data

The client will describe having painless, intermittent hematuria and changes in voiding patterns. Fatigue may also be mentioned.

Objective Data

Weakness will be noted if the client has become anemic from the hematuria. Check urine specimen with a reagent strip for blood, review results of diagnostic tests, and assess the client's understanding of current health situation.

Nursing diagnoses for a client with urinary bladder tumors may include the following:

Nursing Diagnoses	Planning/Goals	Nursing Interventions
Deficient **K**nowledge related to surgery and treatment regimen	The client will describe surgical changes and treatment regimen.	If surgical removal of bladder lesions is done as an outpatient procedure, teach the client to observe for pink-tinged urine and to notify the physician if bright red urine is seen.
		Discuss the use of analgesics as ordered for pain of bladder spasms.
		Encourage adequate fluid intake.
		For urinary diversions: Refer the client with a stoma to the enterostomal therapist for specialized care and teaching. The therapist will assist the client with the appliance and skin care protocol.
		Monitor the color and integrity of the stoma daily to ensure that the tissue is receiving adequate circulation. The stoma is normally red and edematous for a time postoperatively. The stoma will remain red in color but will shrink in size during the healing process.
		If the stoma color changes, notify the physician.
		Refer to a local ostomy group for ongoing support and assistance or to the United Ostomy Association, which provides support and literature.
		Teach the signs and symptoms related to potential problems that should be reported to the physician.
		Encourage the intake of fluids, up to 3,000 mL per day, unless contraindicated.
		Teach about the medications to be taken at home.
		Encourage the client to attend all scheduled follow-up visits.
		Assist the client to plan the gradual return to the routines of driving, lifting, sexual activities, and work.
Impaired **U**rinary *Elimination* related to surgical procedure	The client will maintain adequate urinary elimination.	Accurately monitor urine output because this is the major postoperative concern.
		Assist client to discuss feelings about the altered urinary elimination method.
		Assist the client with a bilateral cutaneous ureterostomy to use leg bags for easier ambulation.
		Change the leg bag tubing back to straight bag drainage to promote uninterrupted sleep.
		Teach the client how to use both a leg bag and a straight bag drainage system.

Evaluation Each goal must be evaluated to determine how it has been met by the client.

RENAL TUMORS

The American Cancer Society estimates there were approximately 31,900 new cases of kidney cancer in 2003 (ACS, 2003). A unilateral renal adenocarcinoma is the most common tumor and is seen more often in men between the ages of 50 and 70. Risk factors include smoking, familial incidence, and preexisting renal disorders.

Intermittent, painless hematuria is often ignored by the client, and medical attention is not sought until the malignancy is quite advanced. By this time, the client usually has experienced weight loss, dull flank pain, gross hematuria, and a mass that may be palpable in the flank area. Lymph nodes in the area of the kidney, the renal vessels, and/or the inferior vena cava may become involved. The primary sites for metastases are the lungs, liver, brain, and bone. A pathological fracture may be the reason for admission of the client, resulting in the diagnosis of kidney cancer.

An IVP will detect a renal mass. Other diagnostic studies used to evaluate the kidney or the status of other body systems possibly involved are renal sonography or arteriogram, MRI, CT scan, or a needle biopsy. The painless hematuria contributes to a decreased hematocrit.

Medical–Surgical Management

Medical

The physician may insert a nephrostomy tube into the renal pelvis of each kidney to evaluate their function. Chemotherapy and/or radiation therapy have proved to be of minimal benefit.

Surgical

Usually a radical nephrectomy is performed if the other kidney is healthy and the disease is localized. The surgeon may enter the thoracic as well as the abdominal cavity during this procedure. If the chest is opened, the client will have a closed-chest drainage system postoperatively. A nasogastric drainage tube may be in place and attached to suction. Hemorrhage and compromised respiratory effort are the postoperative problems for which to observe.

Pharmacological

If the client is receiving radiation therapy treatments, antiemetics or antispasmodics may be ordered. Analgesics are ordered to control pain and facilitate respirations and client activity. An antiemetic will usually be ordered to promote comfort and to encourage eating.

Diet

The client having a nephrectomy will have intravenous fluids until food can be tolerated. A well-balanced diet is then ordered. Fluid intake of at least 2,000 mL per day is needed to maintain adequate hydration. The use of alcohol should be avoided. If the client is **cachectic** (in a state of malnutrition and wasting) because of the cancer's pathology, parenteral nutrition may be indicated.

Activity

Encourage ambulation during the client's recovery. Frequent rest periods are necessary even after discharge.

Nursing Management

Encourage client to express feelings and concerns about diagnosis. Observe for signs of grieving. Answer questions honestly. Assess neurologic status, lung sounds, peripheral pulses, and vital signs. Accurately record I & O. Provide preoperative teaching.

NURSING PROCESS

Assessment

Subjective Data

The client will describe having a dull pain in the flank area and noticing blood in the urine intermittently; however, the client often comments that there is no difficulty in urinating. Fatigue and weight loss are also described.

Objective Data

Compare weight with usual weight. Monitor vital signs and diagnostic test results. Assess the client's lung sounds for possible respiratory distress resulting from metastases. Hematuria may be seen. A mass may be palpated in the client's flank area.

Nursing diagnoses for a client with renal tumors may include the following:

Nursing Diagnoses	Planning/Goals	Nursing Interventions
Fatigue related to disease process and treatment	The client will understand reason for fatigue and not feel guilty for taking rest periods.	Discuss with client that fatigue is a result of blood loss in the urine and growth of the tumor. Because there is increased fatigue following any surgery, plan nursing care so the client will have several periods of uninterrupted rest each day.

continues

Nursing Diagnoses	Planning/Goals	Nursing Interventions
Anticipatory **G**rieving related to diagnosis, treatment, and prognosis	The client will maintain open communications with family and health care members.	Actively listen to what the client says. Encourage the client to express feelings about the diagnosis and treatment. Observe for signs of grieving such as crying, denial, anger, or withdrawal. Answer questions honestly. Assist client in identifying strengths and coping skills. Make referrals to other professionals as needed.
Deficient **K**nowledge related to limited information of disease process and treatment regimen	The client will verbalize understanding of information taught.	Inform the client of the assessments to be done: neurological status, lung sounds, the incision, Homans' sign, peripheral pulses, vital signs, and serum electrolyte values. Teach the importance of accurate intake and output records. Provide routine preoperative teaching. Encourage the client to eat a well-balanced diet to enhance healing. Instruct the client not to wash off the skin markings if radiation therapy is being used. Teach the name, purpose, dosage, schedule, and side effects of all medications and the importance of drinking plenty of fluids and ambulating as tolerated. Inform the client and family of community resources and support groups. Point out the importance of following the instructions for care when discharged and keeping physician appointments.

Evaluation Each goal must be evaluated to determine how it has been met by the client.

POLYCYSTIC KIDNEY

Polycystic kidney disease (PKD) may be inherited or acquired. Acquired cystic kidney disease (ACKD) is associated with dialysis and end-stage renal disease. Approximately 90% of clients on dialysis for 5 years develop ACKD (NIDDK, 2002b). In PKD, multiple grape-like clusters of fluid-filled cysts develop in and greatly enlarge both kidneys. They compress and eventually replace functioning kidney tissue. PKD has an insidious onset that becomes obvious between 30 and 50 years of age.

Early symptoms include hypertension, polyuria, and urinary tract infections. Flank pain and headache are common. Recurrent hematuria and proteinuria develop. Diagnosis is made by x-ray or sonogram showing the cysts. BUN and creatinine are used to monitor kidney function.

The goal of medical management is to preserve kidney function, prevent infections, and relieve pain. Hypertension is carefully managed with antihypertensive medications, diuretics, and fluid and dietary modifications. Eventually, dialysis or renal transplantation may be needed.

RENAL FAILURE

According to the NIDDK (2002a), any acute or chronic loss of kidney function is called renal failure and is the term used when some kidney function remains. Total, or nearly total, and permanent kidney failure is called end-stage renal disease (ESRD). It may take only a few days or weeks to lose renal function or it may deteriorate slowly over decades. Disorders of renal failure are either acute or chronic.

ACUTE RENAL FAILURE

The rapid deterioration of renal function with rising blood levels of urea and other nitrogenous wastes (azotemia) is termed acute renal failure (ARF). The nephrons are unable to regulate the fluid and electrolyte or the acid–base balance of the blood. Predisposing factors include acute glomerular disease; severe, acute kidney infection; decreased cardiac output; trauma; or hemorrhage.

There are three major forms depending on the location of the cause: postrenal ARF (disrupted urine flow), prerenal ARF (disrupted blood flow to the kidney), and intrarenal ARF (renal tissue damage). Both postrenal ARF and prerenal ARF are reversible situations if they are identified early and treatment is begun. Undiagnosed postrenal ARF and prerenal ARF lead to intrarenal ARF.

Postrenal ARF

Postrenal ARF is caused by an obstruction. It should be checked out first when a client has an unexplained decrease in urine output or has anuria. Kidney function can be easily restored by removing the obstruction. Urine volume will vary depending on the location and degree of obstruction. Catheterization, ultrasound, and retrograde pyelogram are used to diagnose an obstruction. An obstruction may be caused by renal calculi, blood clots, edema, tumors, urethral strictures, benign prostatic hypertrophy (BPH), or pregnancy. Postrenal failure can be ruled out if there is no obstruction. If an obstruction is confirmed, relief of the obstruction is imperative to minimize renal damage and resolve azotemia. When postrenal failure is prolonged, both blood creatinine and BUN will rise.

Prerenal ARF

Any abnormal decline in kidney perfusion that reduces glomerular perfusion can cause prerenal failure. Fluid volume status does not indicate perfusion. Effective arterial blood volume (EABV) is the amount of fluid in the vascular space that effectively perfuses the kidneys. Even in fluid volume excess situations, such as low cardiac output caused by heart failure, the EABV falls, causing prerenal failure. The kidney interprets a fall in EABV as fluid volume deficit.

The glomeruli are then unable to filter waste from the blood. The renal tubules are structurally intact, and the kidneys can resume normal functioning if perfusion is restored fairly quickly. Ischemia results from prolonged inadequate perfusion, which can cause acute tubular necrosis (ATN).

The client generally has pale, cool skin; orthostatic hypotension; and oliguria. The BUN-to-creatinine ratio rises from 10:1 to more than 20:1. This rise occurs because of greater reabsorption of urea when fluids flow slowly through the tubules. A urinalysis shows a low sodium level (less than 20 mEq/L), high osmolality (more than 500 mOsm/L), and high specific gravity (more than 1.020). This results because the kidneys are retaining sodium and water in an attempt to correct the perceived fluid volume deficit.

When the client truly has a fluid volume deficit, treatment consists of intravenous fluids and albumin, plasma, or blood to restore the EABV. When the cause is inadequate cardiac output, inotropic agents such as dobutamine hydrochloride (Dobutrex) or amrinone lactate (Inocor) are used.

Intrarenal ARF

Tissue damage of the glomeruli and/or tubules causes a loss of renal function known as intrarenal ARF. Glomerulonephritis and ATN are the main reasons for renal tissue damage. The antigen/antibody complexes formed in glomerulonephritis become trapped in the basement membrane, where they cause inflammation. The glomeruli then become more permeable, so red blood cells and protein are allowed to enter the filtrate and ultimately the urine.

Most intrarenal failure cases are caused by ATN and are the most common cause of nosocomial acute renal failure. ATN is the result of ischemia or toxic insult to the renal tubules. Ischemia may result from untreated prerenal failure or severe hypoxemia. Radiographic contrast dye, pigments (myoglobin and hemoglobin), aminoglycoside and cephalosporin antibiotics, and NSAIDs are all **nephrotoxic** (substances that causes kidney tissue damage) and can cause acute tubular necrosis.

CLIENT TEACHING

Acute Renal Failure
Teach clients at risk for ARF (older clients; diabetic clients; and clients with renal, heart, or liver disease) to:

- Immediately report to health care provider signs of fluid retention, pain on urination, and changes in urine output (amount or appearance).
- Avoid chronic use of and high doses of NSAIDs.
- Follow sodium and fluid restrictions as prescribed.
- Advise all health care providers of condition.

The BUN-to-creatinine ratio in acute tubular necrosis is usually normal between 10:1 and 15:1; however, both the BUN and creatinine are greatly elevated. For example, the BUN may be 70 mg/dL and the creatinine 7 mg/dL. Urine sodium is more than 40 mEq/L, urine osmolality less than 300 mOsm/L, and specific gravity less than 1.010.

There are three phases to the clinical course of ATN: oliguric/nonoliguric, diuretic, and recovery. The first phase is either oliguric or nonoliguric depending on the causative factor.

Oliguric/Nonoliguric Phase

A nonoliguric phase is usually seen when nephrotoxic agents are the causative factor. When adequate urine output is maintained, dialysis is needed less often, and the morbidity and mortality rates are lower.

An oliguric phase, which may last 1 to 2 weeks, is seen more often when ischemia is the causative factor. Oliguria, voiding less than 400 mL/24 hours, can cause fluid volume overload; electrolyte imbalance, specifically high potassium and phosphorus, and low sodium and calcium; metabolic acidosis; and uremia.

Diuretic Phase

The diuretic phase is seldom seen because early dialysis keeps extracellular fluid volume at a fairly normal level. If it were seen, there would be a tremendous increase in urine output.

Recovery Phase

As renal function begins to improve, the client's urine output returns to normal and serum and urine laboratory test values move closer to normal. There is usually a short period of rapid improvement and then a period (may be several months) of slower improvement. Some clients will have residual renal insufficiency and a few will require long-term dialysis.

Medical–Surgical Management
Medical

Acute renal failure is often reversible, and complications can be prevented with early diagnosis and treatment. The goal is to have kidney function stabilized and returned to normal. Problems to be alert for are fluid volume overload, electrolyte imbalances, metabolic acidosis, high rate of catabolism, uremia, hemotologic abnormalities, and infection.

Dialysis is now an early treatment in ATN. Homeostasis is maintained while the cause of ATN is determined and treated. Permanent kidney damage may thus be averted. See the section on dialysis later in this chapter.

Surgical

The obstructions causing postrenal failure are often removed surgically. The exact procedure will depend on what type of obstruction is present and its location.

Pharmacological

Drugs used to treat acute renal failure include antihypertensives, diuretics, cardiotonics (inotropics), phosphate-binding antacids, potassium-lowering agents, and electrolyte replacement. It is important to ensure that drugs used are not nephrotoxic. See Table 36-2 for drugs used in acute renal failure.

Diet

Restrictions generally include sodium, potassium, phosphorus, protein, and fluids. The amounts allowed are based on the laboratory tests results. Carbohydrates and fats are increased to be sure energy needs are met and protein will be spared as a source of energy. Clients with a high rate of catabolism often require total parenteral nutrition (TPN) to provide adequate nutrition.

Activity

Because the client is often weak and may also be confused, activity is restricted during the initial phase of acute renal failure. As recovery becomes evident, ambulation is begun.

Nursing Management

Accurately record I&O (often hourly). Monitor vital signs, BUN, creatinine, and serum electrolytes and protein. Weigh client daily. Assess skin turgor, lung sounds, and jugular vein distention. Provide fluids within prescribed limits. Ask dietitian to discuss dietary restrictions with client. Provide or assist with oral hygiene before meals. Listen to client's concerns.

NURSING PROCESS

Assessment

Subjective Data

The client may describe diarrhea; nausea, possibly with vomiting; swelling; loss of appetite; headache; increasing fatigue; and/or a change in mental alertness.

TABLE 36-2 DRUGS USED IN ACUTE RENAL FAILURE

DRUGS	NURSING RESPONSIBILITIES
Antihypertensives methyldopa (Aldomet) minoxidil (Loniten) clonidine HCl (Catapres) hydralazine HCl (Apresoline)	Monitor BP and pulse, weigh daily, monitor for postural hypotension and K, Na, Cl, and CO_2 levels, I&O.
Diuretics furosemide (Lasix) hydrochlorothiazide (HydroDiuril)	Monitor output, maintain fluid restrictions, weigh daily.
Cardiotonics/inotropics digoxin (Lanoxin) amrinone lactate (Inocor)	Assess apical pulse before giving, report blood level of digoxin, monitor BP and P, monitor blood level of potassium.
Phosphate-binding antacids aluminum hydroxide gel (Amphojel)	Administer wtih meals, assess for constipation.
Potassium exchange sodium polystyrene sulfonate (Kayexalate)	Monitor serum potassium, assess BP and P, and for constipation.
Electrolyte replacement calcitrol (Rocaltrol) calcifediol (Calderol)	Monitor blood calcium and phosphate levels, report metallic taste.

Anxiety and fear related to not knowing what is happening is often expressed.

Objective Data

Physical findings will depend on how far the disease process has progressed. Assess for hypertension, GI bleeding and/or bruising, reduction in urine output, anasarca, poor skin turgor, and dry mucous membranes because vomiting or diarrhea can cause dehydration. In a severe stage, the client may be drowsy and have muscle twitching and convulsions.

The BUN and serum creatinine will be elevated, as are the serum electrolytes potassium and phosphorus. The serum electrolyte calcium will be low. Blood level of red blood cells will decrease as the production of erythropoietin decreases. Leukocyte level will increase in the presence of an infection.

Nursing diagnoses for a client with acute renal failure may include the following:

Nursing Diagnoses	Planning/Goals	Nursing Interventions
Excess Fluid Volume related to sodium and water retention	The client will maintain a stable fluid volume.	Monitor BUN, creatinine, and serum electrolyte and protein levels. Accurately measure urine output, often on an hourly basis. Parameters are often set for notification of the physician. Weigh daily to identify weight gain related to fluid retention. One pound of weight gain is equivalent to 500 mL of retained fluid. Assess skin turgor, edema, BP, lung sounds, jugular vein distention, pulse and respiratory rate and quality. Provide fluids within the prescribed limits. Teach client about importance of fluid restrictions.
Impaired Nutrition: Less than body requirements related to anorexia, dietary restrictions, and increased catabolism	The client will have stabilized weight within normal limits.	Arrange for a dietary consultation to provide food in keeping with the prescribed restrictions and client preferences, including cultural and religious factors. Suggest 6 small meals throughout the day. Offer antinausea medications before meals. Provide or assist with oral hygiene prior to meals. Monitor weight and serum albumin level weekly.
Anxiety related to the disease process	The client will verbalize anxieties with the family and health care workers.	Establish rapport with the client. Listen to the client's concerns. Maintain open communications to foster expression of anxieties.

Evaluation Each goal must be evaluated to determine how it has been met by the client.

SAMPLE NURSING CARE PLAN

THE CLIENT WITH ACUTE RENAL FAILURE

Mr. Long, age 65, has had a history of heart trouble for several years. He is admitted because he has urinated very little for 2 days, he gets dizzy when he gets up from lying down, and he cannot get his shoes on because his feet are "fat." He states that he does not know what is happening to him. Results of laboratory tests are BUN 90 mg/dL, creatinine 4 mg/dL, urine sodium 15 mEq/L, and urine specific gravity 1.030.

Nursing Diagnosis 1 *Excess Fluid Volume* related to sodium and water retention as evidenced by "fat feet," urine sodium 15 mEq/L, and urine specific gravity 1.030

Nursing Outcomes Classification (NOC)
Fluid Balance
Electrolyte & Acid–Base Balance

Nursing Interventions Classification (NIC)
Electrolyte Management
Fluid Management

PLANNING/GOALS	NURSING INTERVENTIONS	RATIONALE
Mr. Long will have reduced fluid volume excess.	Accurately measure and record intake and output.	Provides information about retention of intake.
	Weigh Mr. Long daily—same time, scale, clothes.	Allows weight comparisons.
	Assess skin turgor, edema, BP, lung sounds for crackles.	Provides information about fluid in tissue, lungs, or vascular system.

continues

SAMPLE NURSING CARE PLAN

Monitor BUN, creatinine, and serum electrolyte and protein levels.	Gives insight to kidney functioning.
Administer inotropics or cardiotonic medications as ordered.	Strengthens heartbeat, which will give better perfusion to kidneys.
Provide fluids within prescribed limits.	Prevents fluid excess.

EVALUATION   Mr. Long's feet are no longer "fat." His urine sodium is 18 mEq/L and urine specific gravity is 1.027.

Nursing Diagnosis 2 *Anxiety* related to disease process as evidenced by his statement that he does not know what is happening to him

Nursing Outcomes Classification (NOC)
Acceptance: Health Status

Nursing Interventions Classification (NIC)
Teaching: Individual

PLANNING/GOALS	NURSING INTERVENTIONS	RATIONALE
Mr. Long will have less anxiety by understanding what is happening to him.	Establish rapport with Mr. Long.	Begins a nurse–client relationship.
	Encourage him to express his fears and anxieties.	Some people need encouragement to express feelings.
	Provide Mr. Long with information, at his level of understanding, about what is happening to his body, why I&O and weighing daily are important, and what the medications are supposed to do.	Understanding reduces anxieties.

EVALUATION   Mr. Long says that he feels better knowing what is happening.

Nursing Diagnosis 3 *Impaired Urinary Elimination* related to decreased perfusion as evidenced by his urinating very little for 2 days and BUN–creatinine ratio of 22.5:1

Nursing Outcomes Classification (NOC)
Urinary Elimination
Knowledge: Disease Process

Nursing Interventions Classification (NIC)
Urinary Elimination Management
Teaching: Disease Process

PLANNING/GOALS	NURSING INTERVENTIONS	RATIONALE
Mr. Long will increase amount of urination to 1,200 mL/day.	Administer diuretics as ordered.	Increases water elimination by enhancing sodium excretion by the kidneys.
	Accurately measure and record intake and output.	Provides information about fluid movement through the body.

EVALUATION   Mr. Long is urinating 1,000 mL/day. His BUN is 50 mg/dL and creatinine is 3 mg/dL.

CHRONIC RENAL FAILURE/ END-STAGE RENAL DISEASE

Chronic renal failure is a slow, progressive condition in which the kidney's ability to function ultimately deteriorates. This condition is not reversible. The kidneys have an amazing capability to perform effectively, even though most of the nephrons are destroyed.

Renal erythropoietin decreases, causing anemia. Hypertension, acidosis, and glucose intolerance usually are also present. Urea in the blood is extremely elevated. As the disease progresses, uremia develops.

There are three stages of chronic renal failure: reduced renal reserve, renal insufficiency, and end-stage renal disease (ESRD). Symptoms of reduced renal reserve are not apparent until more than 40% of the nephrons fail. A prolonged urine concentration test or a decline in glomerular filtration rate (GFR) may be the only evidence of reduced renal reserve. When 75% of the nephrons stop functioning, renal insufficiency occurs. BUN and creatinine are above normal, and the client may have nocturia and polyuria. The onset of ESRD occurs when at least 90% of the nephrons fail: BUN and creatinine levels rise, polyuria changes to oliguria, and severe fluid and electrolyte imbalances are evident.

When the kidneys become unable to filter blood, an alternate method for filtration is necessary. Lifetime dialysis becomes inevitable unless kidney transplantation is performed and is successful. Life expectancy varies with the initial cause of chronic renal failure and the person's overall health at the time of diagnosis.

According to the National Kidney Foundation (2001c), 370,000 persons in the United States have ESRD, with the number increasing approximately 8% each year. There are numerous causes of chronic renal failure. The four leading causes are diabetes mellitus 38%, hypertension 24%, glomerulonephritis 12%, and cystic kidney 2% (NKF, 2001c). Nephrotoxic drugs, including some over-the-counter drugs, aggravate the situation.

The diagnosis is confirmed when the BUN is at least 50 mg/dL and the serum creatinine level is greater than 5 mg/dL.

CULTURAL CONSIDERATIONS

End-Stage Renal Disease

- African Americans account for 32% of clients with ESRD but make up only 12% of the U.S. population.
- The leading cause of ESRD in African Americans is diabetes, accounting for approximately 43% of new cases in that population (NKF, 2002d).
- End-stage renal disease is four times greater in African Americans than in whites.
- ESRD is increasing rapidly among Native Americans because of the significant increase in the incidence of diabetes in this population.

Medical–Surgical Management

Medical

Chronic renal failure is a multisystem disease process. See Table 36-3 for the effects of chronic renal failure on various body systems. Medical management focuses on preserving the remaining kidney function as long as possible and preventing complications. This helps preserve the integrity of the person's life. Fluid retention increases the risk of complications such as edema (ascites), hypertension, and heart failure. Electrolytes are monitored and regulated.

 Pharmacological

Antihypertensives such as methyldopa (Aldomet) and propranolol hydrochloride (Inderal) are used to control hypertension. Diuretics such as furosemide (Lasix) are used to treat fluid retention; anticonvulsants, phenytoin (Dilantin) to control seizures; antiemetics, prochlorperazine (Compazine) to control vomiting; and antipruritics, cyproheptadine hydrochloride (Periactin) to control itching. Calcium acetate (Phos-Lo) is used to lower the phosphate level in the blood; however, it can be constipating. A low renal erythropoietin level causing anemia is often treated with epoetin alpha (Epogen). An iron supplement is used to decrease the anemia-related symptoms. Multivitamins with folic acid are used because dialysis promotes the loss of water-soluble vitamins.

Diet

Diet restrictions are similar to those in acute renal failure. Sodium, potassium, phosphorus, and protein are restricted. Fluids are also limited. Modifications are made as kidney function deteriorates. With consistent compliance, symptoms decrease, resulting in fewer complications. Resources are available for clients to obtain assistance with dietary restrictions. Meal ideas are published in newsletters such as *NephroNotes*. Long-term dietary compliance is a challenge, and daily activities as well as special events during the year are a continual reminder of the client's dietary restrictions. As with other chronic diseases, those with renal failure need to have all family members and friends encouraging them to adapt to their restrictions. Dietitians can assist the family to incorporate religious and cultural dietary practices. The person with chronic renal failure may also have to incorporate dietary guidelines for additional diagnoses such as diabetes mellitus and/or coronary artery disease.

With the progression of chronic renal disease, dialysis becomes necessary. Fluid restrictions must be followed, and the amount allowed divided throughout the day. The greatest amount of fluid should be allowed during the day, incorporating enough fluids with oral medications. Some fluids should be planned for the evening meal, with a small amount to be allowed during the night; for example, days—500 cc, evenings—200 cc, and nights—100 cc. Protein restriction is closely monitored and regulated with the blood albumin level. The development of hyperkalemia will lead to a diet restricted in potassium. Foods high in potassium include dried fruits or dried beans and peas, peanuts, bananas, sweet potatoes, spinach, products

TABLE 36-3   EFFECTS OF CHRONIC RENAL FAILURE BY BODY SYSTEM

SYSTEM	EFFECT
Urinary	Oliguria from renal insufficiency
	Azotemia
Blood	Anemia from decreased RBC production
	Decreased platelet activity, causing bleeding tendency
Cardiovascular	Hypervolemia and tachycardia
	Hypertension and dysrhythmias from hyperkalemia
Respiratory	Dyspnea, pulmonary edema
	Hyperventilation from metabolic acidosis
	Eventually Kussmaul respirations
Gastrointestinal	Urea in the blood is converted to ammonia by the mouth, causing uremic halitosis
	Hiccups, anorexia, and nausea from edema within the gastrointestinal tract
Skin	Dry skin with pruritis from uremic frost (excretion of urea through the skin with an odor of urine); pallor with anemia
Nervous	Lethargy, headaches, confusion, impaired concentration with disorientation, depression, decreased level of consciousness, sleep disturbances, and uremic encephalopathy resulting in seizures and coma
Sensory	Peripheral neuropathy with numbness and tingling of extremities with complaints of a prickly, crawling feeling in the feet and legs, especially at night
Reproductive	Decrease in libido
	Decreased sperm count
	Amenorrhea
	Impotence
	Delayed puberty
Musculoskeletal	Joint pain and muscle cramping
	Bone demineralization from hypocalcemia
Immune	Greater chance of infections from immunosuppression
	Decrease in antibody production

with tomatoes, oranges, chocolate, artichokes, avocados, pumpkins, and mushrooms.

Activity

The client is encouraged to participate in activities of daily living. Safety becomes a significant factor during periods when the client has weakness, fatigue, or mental confusion. Confusion is seen in clients who have uremic encephalopathy. When bed rest is required, turning, ROM exercises, and skin care are important. As symptoms continue to become more severe, the client will need total assistance for all ADLs.

Nursing Management

Monitor daily weight, skin turgor, vital signs, and lung sounds. Provide prescribed amount of fluids and accurately record intake and output (sometimes hourly). Assist with or provide oral hygiene before meals and as needed. Administer an antiemetic 30 minutes before meals. Arrange for a dietitian to plan meals with the client. Assist with or provide bathing frequently, followed by applying lotion on the skin. Encourage repositioning at least every 2 hours, ROM exercises, and use of an eggcrate mattress or Clinitron bed. Monitor for mental confusion. Refer client and family to the local office of the National Kidney Foundation.

NURSING PROCESS

Assessment

Subjective Data

Inquire about the client's past medical history including treatments for maintenance of renal disease. Take a complete medication history, including the use of over-the-counter drugs. Description of fatigue, joint pain, severe headaches, nausea, anorexia, some chest pain, intractable singultus (hiccups), decreased libido, menstrual irregularities, and impaired concentration is given by the client. The client may feel uncomfortable talking directly to the nurse if uremic halitosis is a problem.

Objective Data

Note changes in the client's neurological status such as reduced alertness and awareness. Kussmaul respirations appear as coma develops. Halitosis with a urine odor and "uremic frost," a white powder on the skin, result from the accumulation of urates.

CRITICAL THINKING

Acute and Chronic Renal Failure

What are the differences between acute and chronic renal failure?

Nursing diagnoses for a client with ESRD may include the following:

Nursing Diagnoses	Planning/Goals	Nursing Interventions
Excess Fluid Volume related to compromised renal mechanism	The client will understand the importance of prescribed (restricted) fluid amounts.	Monitor daily weight, intake and output (maybe hourly), skin turgor, edema, blood pressure, respirations, and lung sounds. Provide prescribed amounts of fluids. Teach client to plan nutritional and fluid intake within the prescribed amounts. Monitor laboratory reports for serum albumin level and serum electrolyte levels.
Imbalanced Nutrition: Less than body requirements related to dietary restrictions, GI distress, anorexia	The client will stabilize weight within normal limits and participate in dietary plan.	Provide or assist with complete mouth care before meals because uremic halitosis leaves a metallic taste in the client's mouth. Provide a clean, quiet, odor-free environment for meals. Suggest 6 small meals throughout the day. Encourage self-feeding. Arrange a consultation with the dietitian to plan alternate ways to prepare foods allowed on the diet. Ask the family to bring favorite foods, within the dietary restrictions, from home. Administer antiemetics 30 minutes before meals to control nausea. Suggest using herbs for flavoring instead of salt or salt substitutes, which often contain potassium.
Risk for Impaired Skin Integrity related to altered metabolic state leading to pruritis from "uremic frost"	The client will maintain skin integrity.	Bathe skin frequently to remove "uremic frost." Encourage the use of emollients and lotions on the skin. Administer antihistamines, as ordered, for the temporary relief of itching. Assist the client to change position every 2 hours. Provide an egg-crate mattress or Clinitron bed.
Ineffective Individual Coping related to uncertainty of long-term compliance of the treatment regimen	The client will verbalize feelings and intention to comply with treatment.	Encourage the client to discuss feelings about long-term lifestyle changes. Refer client to the local office of the National Kidney Foundation for information about client services and treatments for diseases of the kidney. Include the client and family in rehabilitation and discharge planning to ensure compliance. Topics for these sessions include diet, rest, medications, fluid restrictions, intake and output, activities, dialysis, required lab tests, and frequent visits to the physician. Incorporate into the discharge planning and teaching the client's socioeconomic needs, cultural background, role in the family unit, accessibility to medical care, and anticipated follow-up care. Complete referrals before discharge in order to lessen client anxiety. Consider future needs of a newly diagnosed client with end-stage renal disease and include the availability of dialysis, vocational rehabilitation, home health care, financial assistance with medical needs, and psychological therapy for the client and family.

Evaluation Each goal must be evaluated to determine how it has been met by the client.

DIALYSIS

As the kidneys continue to deteriorate, nitrogenous waste products accumulate in the circulatory system. These waste products need to be removed artificially with **dialysis,** a mechanical means of removing nitrogenous waste from the blood by imitating the function of the nephrons. It involves filtration and diffusion of wastes, drugs, and excess electrolytes and/or osmosis of water across a semipermeable membrane into a dialysate solution. The **dialysate** is a solution designed to approximate the normal electrolyte structure of plasma and extracellular fluid.

There are two types of dialysis: hemodialysis and peritoneal dialysis. These treatments can be obtained throughout the country at dialysis centers or at hospital dialysis units.

Hemodialysis

Hemodialysis is performed by a machine with an artificial semipermeable membrane used to filter the blood. This machine is often referred to as an artificial kidney. A graft or fistula is surgically prepared to access the client's circulatory system. Figure 36-6 illustrates several ways this can be done. With each hemodialysis treatment, a catheter is inserted into the graft or fistula. The client's blood is circulated through the semipermeable membrane. Excess fluids are removed by osmosis, and by-products of protein metabolism, especially urea and uric acid, as well as creatinine, drugs, and excess electrolytes, are removed from the blood by diffusion or filtration. In return, the client receives fluids, electrolytes, and blood products, as necessary. The solution (dialysate) is especially prescribed to meet the client's metabolic needs.

For the entire process, Standard Precautions must be followed and strict asepsis maintained. The client is weighed before and after each dialysis session to determine if fluid is being retained. It is important to keep the client comfortable and provide diversionary activities during the treatment. Hemodialysis is usually performed 3 times a week and takes 3 to 4 hours each time.

The graft or fistula site requires strict aseptic care and must be assessed daily for signs of infection: redness, swelling, or drainage. Assess circulation through the site by palpation or feeling the area and/or listening with a (Doppler) stethoscope. A thrill should be felt and/or a bruit should be heard. Lack of these signs may indicate a blood clot, which requires immediate surgical attention. Patency must be documented. Assess pulses peripheral to the graft site.

Blood pressure and blood draws are never done on the extremity where the graft or fistula is placed. Also, restraints or intravenous solutions are never applied to or inserted into that extremity. All health care personnel should know the location of the hemodialysis access site. These sites should not be used for any other purpose than dialysis.

Because most medications are removed during dialysis, they are generally not administered until after the dialysis session. Vancomycin hydrochloride (Vancocin) is not removed during dialysis and so is often used. If the client is

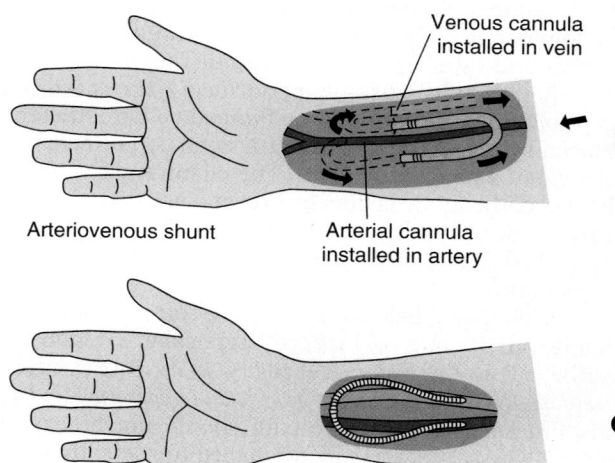

Figure 36-6 *Types of Hemodialysis Access Sites*

hypertensive before dialysis, nifedipine (Procardia) is given because of its fast action.

Possible complications include hemorrhage, infection, and emboli formation. Some factors for the client and family to consider about hemodialysis are the distance they must travel to the dialysis center, the expense, the time involved, and the presence of a permanent arteriovenous (AV) line. Clients can be taught to do their own hemodialysis at a center. Portable units are being developed to make hemodialysis more usable in the client's home. This is a growing trend with home health care.

Continuous renal replacement therapy (CRRT), a slow, gentle form of dialysis, is available (Astle, 2001).

Peritoneal Dialysis

Peritoneal dialysis uses the peritoneal lining of the abdominal cavity as the membrane through which diffusion and osmosis occur instead of the artificial kidney machine. It is usually performed 4 times a day 7 days a week. A Tenckhoff or a flanged-collar catheter is placed by the physician, under aseptic conditions, into the client's peritoneal space. The client must void just before catheter insertion to prevent accidental puncture of the bladder. As with hemodialysis, weigh the client before and after each dialysis session. Also check bowel sounds.

The dialysate, held within a sterile soft container similar to an IV bag, is instilled aseptically through the catheter into the abdominal cavity. *To decrease client discomfort, the dialysate should be at body temperature and not instilled too rapidly.* Severe pain should not be experienced. The container, still connected to the catheter, is then rolled up and the dialysate remains in the abdominal cavity for a specified length of time. The client is free to ambulate during this time. The container is then unrolled and lowered below the abdominal cavity to allow the dialysate to drain, by gravity, back into the container. The dialysate now contains excess fluids, nitrogenous waste, and other impurities. The outflow of dialysate is

inspected for color, sediments, and amount. The fluid should be light yellow and clear enough to read the printing on the bag when placed on a white towel. Usually 2 liters of dialysate are exchanged each time. If the outflow does not at least equal the inflow, the client is asked to turn from side to side to increase the outflow.

Peritoneal dialysis may be performed manually by the nurse, client, or family member as just described; by a cycler machine; or by continuous ambulatory peritoneal dialysis (CAPD). The cycler machine automatically completes dialysis after sterile setup and connection; CAPD is performed by the client. After the dialysate is aseptically installed, the empty bag is rolled up under the clothing, and the client can go about normal activities. Every 6 to 8 hours, the solution is drained into the bag, which is then discarded following standard precaution guidelines. A new bag of dialysate is attached and instilled. This provides continuous dialysis 24 hours per day, 7 days per week. The client's lifestyle is only minimally disrupted. Peritoneal dialysis is less expensive, easier to perform, less stressful for the client, and almost as effective as hemodialysis.

The main complication of peritoneal dialysis is infection. Strict aseptic care of the catheter site is necessary. Standard Precautions are essential in caring for the dialysis client. Figure 36-7 shows a peritoneal dialysis setup.

Fresh dialysate solution

Peritoneal cavity

Tenchkoff peritoneal catheter

Adapter

Used dialysate solution

Figure 36-7 *Peritoneal Dialysis Setup*

KIDNEY TRANSPLANTATION

According to the National Kidney Foundation (2003), 14,000 kidney transplants will be performed in 2003. Transplants are either from a live donor (usually a relative) or a cadaver. There are approximately 50,000 persons on the waiting list for a kidney transplant.

Before being placed on the nationwide donor waiting list, the client with ESRD must be tissue- and blood-typed to determine a compatible donor. Insurance coverage varies for this procedure. Lack of funds does not exclude anyone from needed care. Since 1973, an amendment to the Social Security Act allows Medicare to pay 80% of the cost for treating ESRD clients, regardless of age, including dialysis and kidney transplantation.

When a donor kidney becomes available, the client is transported to the transplant medical center. The donor kidney can be preserved for 36 hours in solution or up to 72 hours if it is attached to an irrigating pump with perfusion maintained while en route to the recipient. Through a lower abdominal incision, the surgeon attaches the donor kidney to the client's blood supply. The donor kidney is usually placed in the iliac fossa anterior to the iliac crest. The donor ureter is anastomosed (surgical connection of tubular structure) to the client's ureter or surgically implanted into the client's urinary bladder. Generally, the client's nonfunctioning kidney is left in place to reduce the postoperative risk of hemorrhage.

After a couple days of bed rest, the client is allowed increasing activities and, if no complications occur, is discharged in 1 to 3 weeks. Routine nursing care includes monitoring urine output, blood tests, vital signs, and level of consciousness. Encourage turning, coughing, and deep breathing. Assess the incision to ensure that wound closure is intact. In addition, assess for rejection.

Organ Rejection

Signs of rejection include generalized edema, tenderness over the graft site, fever, decreased urine output, hematuria, edema (extremities or eyes), weight gain, oliguria or anuria, and/or an increase in feeling tired. The BUN and creatinine will be elevated.

Immunosuppressive drug therapy is begun to decrease the chance of organ rejection. These drugs include azathioprine (Imuran), cyclophosphamide (Cytoxan), cyclosporine (Sandimmune), and corticosteroids such as prednisone (Meticorten). The scheduling and dosage of these drugs vary with acceptance of the donor kidney and the side effects exhibited by the client. People continue to survive many years with a kidney transplant and maintain a quality life.

Complications

The greatest complication in renal transplantation is infection. The immunosuppressive therapy to prevent rejection of the kidney increases the risk and masks the usual signs of infection. The client and family must learn how to recognize these signs of infection. There will be only a slight increase in temperature, development of a cough, low back pain, cloudy urine, or wound drainage. The client must always monitor urine output.

Summary

- The functions of the urinary system are reflected in their relationship with nearly all of the systems in the body.
- Accurate intake and output is imperative for every client with a urinary system disorder.
- Teach proper perineal care, especially to females of all ages, about cleansing from front to back.
- Diet management is important for clients with renal calculi, glomerulonephritis, and renal failure.
- Encourage an adequate intake of fluids for clients unless fluids are restricted.
- Monitor laboratory test results for BUN, creatinine, and electrolytes.
- Level of consciousness, vital signs, lung sounds, and urine characteristics are important to monitor.
- Strict aseptic care is mandatory for dialysis clients.

Review Questions

1. A client has been admitted for chronic pyelonephritis. She is jittery and states she is concerned. Which of the following signs would indicate potential kidney damage?

    a. Urine output is 100 mL on your shift.
    b. Blood pressure is decreased with a rapid pulse.
    c. Blood pressure is elevated with a decreased pulse.
    d. BUN and creatinine clearance are within normal limits.

2. A male client, age 64, has had hematuria for several years. He is admitted to your same-day surgical unit scheduled for cystoscopic fulguration. Postoperatively, which of the following would you anticipate?

    a. Blood in the urine
    b. An elevated temperature
    c. Hypotension
    d. Smoky urine

3. A male client, age 29, had impetigo 2 weeks before his noting a decrease in urine output and urine that "did not look right." His admission diagnosis is acute glomerulonephritis. He is on intake and output with fluid restriction. Which of the following comments indicates knowledge of his nursing care?

    a. "I had my wife empty my urinal."
    b. "My urine still looks pretty bad."
    c. "I put my call light on so you can empty my urinal."
    d. "My wife helped me out of bed, so I urinated in the bathroom."

CASE STUDY

Ruth Andrews, 56, is a client in the extended care facility. She has amyotrophic lateral sclerosis (ALS) with muscle weakness that has progressed and involves her legs and arms. A hydraulic lift is used to transfer her out of bed. A student nurse and a classmate enter with the lift to assist Ms. Andrews OOB, when she asks to use the bedpan. As they help her onto the bedpan, they recall that the staff nurse gave Ms. Andrews the bedpan about a half hour ago. Returning in a few minutes, they help Ms. Andrews off the bedpan and notice the urine is cloudy with a foul odor. Ms. Andrews is not on I&O; however, they notice that there is a very small amount of urine. She tells them that she does not know why she is going to the bathroom so often and why her urine smells bad.

The following questions will guide your development of a nursing care plan for the case study.

1. What subjective data should be gathered? What objective data should be gathered?
2. List diagnostic tests that may be ordered.
3. Write two nursing diagnoses for Ms. Andrews, related to her cystitis/UTI.
4. Write a goal related to each of Ms. Andrews' nursing diagnoses.
5. List pertinent nursing actions for the care of Ms. Andrews for each of the following areas as they relate to the cystitis/UTI:
    elimination—bladder
    diet and fluids
    safety, comfort, and rest
    teaching (client and nursing staff)
6. List two classifications of medications used for the treatment of an UTI.
7. List two successful client outcomes for Ms. Andrews.

4. A female client with chronic glomerulonephritis is discharged home with home health care. As the LP/VN assigned to her case, you are planning her A.M. care. While preparing the bath supplies, she says, "Please do not use any soap. My skin is so dry and flaky." The rationale for this would be:

a. kidney failure leads to uremia.
b. the bladder does not concentrate urine.
c. her blood sugar is elevated.
d. confusion leads to comments of this nature.

5. A male client, in his 50s, is attending classes to be able to do his own peritoneal dialysis. He states he feels well and is eager to continue to learn. He asks if washing his hands before the procedure is important. The best response is:

a. "Yes, only if you have not done so today."
b. "Yes, as you want to keep the procedure as clean as possible."
c. "No, since you just went to the bathroom."
d. "No, because all the equipment is sterile."

References/Suggested Readings

American Cancer Society. (2003). *Cancer Facts & Figures 2003.* [Online]. Available: www.cancer.org/downloads/STT/CAFF2003PWSecured.pdf

American Society of Nephrology (ASN). (1999). *Kidney disease facts & statistics* [Online]. Available: www.asn_online.org/facts/prevalence.html

Arbique, J. (2003). Stop UTIs in their tracts. *Nursing2003, 33*(6), 32hn1–32hn4.

Astle, S. (2001). A new direction for dialysis. *RN, 64*(7), 56–60.

Campbell, D. (2003). How acute renal failure puts the brakes on kidney function. *Nursing2003, 33*(1), 59–63.

Castina, S., Boyington, A., & Dougherty, M. (2002). Urinary incontinence. *AJN, 102*(8), 85–87.

Dochterman, J., & Bulechek, G. (2004). *Nursing Interventions Classification (NIC)* (4th ed.). St. Louis, MO: Mosby.

Gray, M., Ratliff, C., & Donovan, A. (2002). Tender mercies: Providing skin care for an incontinent patient. *Nursing2002, 32*(7), 51–54.

Hayes, D. (2000). Caring for your patient with a permanent hemodialysis access. *Nursing2000, 30*(3), 41–46.

Hayes, D. (2003). Performing peritoneal dialysis. *Nursing2003, 33*(3), 17.

Hess, C. (2001). Calciphylaxis: Taking stock of an unusual wound. *Nursing2001, 31*(5), 66–67.

Innes, C. (2001). An overlooked option for renal patients. *RN, 64*(9), 29–32.

Johnson, S. (2000). From incontinence to confidence. *AJN, 100*(2), 69–76.

Kaplow, R., & Barry, R. (2002). Continuous renal replacement therapies. *AJN, 102*(11), 26–33.

Kearney, K. (2000). Dialysis disequilibrium syndrome. *AJN, 100*(2), 53–54.

Kelly, M. (1997). Acute renal failure. *AJN, 97*(3), 32–33.

King, B. (1997). Preserving renal function. *RN, 60*(8), 34–39.

Kniest, K., & McGovern, P. (2002). Using the umbilicus for catheterization. *RN, 65*(8), 26–30.

Lewis, S., Heitkemper, M., & Dirksen, S. (2000). *Medical–surgical nursing: Assessment and management of clinical problems* (5th ed.). St. Louis, MO: Mosby.

Loughrey, L. (1999). Taking a sensitive approach to urinary incontinence. *Nursing99, 29*(5), 60–61.

Marchiondo, K. (1998). A new look at urinary tract infection. *AJN, 98*(3), 34–38.

Mason, D., Newman, D., & Palmer, M. (2003). Changing UI practice: People have the right to be continent. *AJN, 103*(3), 129.

McConnell, E. (2001a). Applying a condom catheter. *Nursing2001, 31*(1), 70.

McConnell, E. (2001b). Myths & facts . . . about kidney stones. *Nursing2001, 31*(1), 73.

McConnell, E. (2002). Protecting a hemodialysis fistula. *Nursing2002, 32*(11), 18.

Moorhead, S., Johnson, M., & Maas, M., (2004). *Nursing Outcomes Classification (NOC)* (3rd ed.). St. Louis, MO: Mosby.

National Institute of Diabetes and Digestive and Kidney Diseases (NIDDK). (2000). *Kidney stones in adults* [Online]. Available: www.niddk.nih.gov/health/kidney/pubs/stonadul/stonadul.htm

National Institute of Diabetes and Digestive and Kidney Diseases (NIDDK). (2001). *Kidney and Urologic Diseases Statistics for the United States.* [Online]. Available: www.niddk.nih.gov/health/kidney/pubs/kustats/kustats.htm

National Institute of Diabetes and Digestive and Kidney Diseases (NIDDK). (2002a). *Glomerular diseases* [Online]. Available: www.niddk.nih.gov/health/kidney/pubs/glomer/glomer.htm

National Institute of Diabetes and Digestive and Kidney Diseases (NIDDK). (2002b). *Polycystic kidney disease* [Online]. Available: www.niddk.nih.gov/health/kidney/pubs/polycyst/polycyst.htm

National Institute of Diabetes and Digestive and Kidney Diseases (NIDDK). (2002c). *Urinary incontinence in women* [Online]. Available: www.niddk.nih.gov/health/urolog/pubs/uiwomen/uiwomen.htm

National Institute of Diabetes and Digestive and Kidney Diseases (NIDDK). (2002d). *Urinary tract infection in adults* [Online]. Available: www.niddk.nih.gov/health/urolog/pubs/utiadult/utiadult.htm

National Kidney Foundation (NKF). (2001a). *Six warning signs of kidney and urinary tract disease* [Online]. Available: www.kidney.org/general/aboutdisease/warningsigns.cfm

National Kidney Foundation (NKF). (2001b). *Kidney disease: Ten facts.* [Online]. Available: www.kidney.org/general/atoz/content/kidneyfacts.html

National Kidney Foundation (NKF). (2001c). *The problem of kidney and urologic disease* [Online]. Available: www.kidney.org/general/news/problem.cfm

National Kidney Foundation (NKF). (2002). *New studies offer hope to UTI sufferers.* [Online]. Available: www.kidney.org/general/news/newstudy.cfm

National Kidney Foundation (NKF). (2002a). *End-stage renal disease in the United States* [Online]. Available: www.kidney.org/general/news/esrd.cfm

National Kidney Foundation (NKF). (2002b). *National Kidney Foundation releases nutrition guidelines for dialysis patients* [Online]. Available: www.kidney.org/general/news/nutguide.cfm

National Kidney Foundation (NKF). (2002c). *New studies offer hope to UTI sufferers* [Online]. Available: www.kidney.org/general/news/newstudy.cfm

National Kidney Foundation (NKF). (2002d). *Ten facts about African-Americans and kidney disease* [Online]. Available: www.kidney.org/general/news/african-american.cfm

National Kidney Foundation (NKF). (2003). *About kidney disease* [Online]. Available: www.kidney.org/general/aboutdisease/index.cfm

Newman, D. (2003). Stress urinary incontinence in women. *AJN, 103*(8), 46–55.

Newman, D., & Giovannini, D. (2002). The overactive bladder: A nursing perspective. *AJN, 102*(6), 36–45.

North American Nursing Diagnosis Association. (2003). *Nursing Diagnoses: Definitions & Classification 2003–2004.* Philadelphia: Author.

Paton, M. (2003). Continuous renal replacement therapy. *Nursing2003, 33*(6), 48–50.

Rice, J. (2002). *Medications and mathematics for the nurse* (9th ed.). Clifton Park, NY: Thomson Delmar Learning.

Roth, R., & Townsend, C. (2002). *Nutrition and diet therapy* (8th ed.). Clifton Park, NY: Thomson Delmar Learning.

Scherer, J. C., & Timby, B. K. (2002). *Introductory medical–surgical nursing* (8th ed.). Philadelphia: Lippincott Williams & Wilkins.

Schofield, C. (2002). Patient may have a UTI—What next? *Nursing2002, 32*(10), 17.

Schultz, J. (2002). Urinary incontinence: Solving a secret problem. *Nursing2002, 32*(11), 53–55.

Smith, D. (1999). Gauging bladder volume without a catheter. *Nursing99, 29*(12), 52–53.

Stockert, P. (1999). Getting UTI patients back on track. *RN, 62*(3), 49–52.

Williams, L., & Hopper, P. (2003). *Understanding medical surgical nursing.* (2nd ed.). Philadelphia: F. A. Davis.

Zabat, E. (2003). When your patient needs peritoneal dialysis. *Nursing2003, 33*(8), 52–54.

Zellner, K. (1999). Acute tubular necrosis. *RN, 62*(10), 42–46.

Resources

American Association of Kidney Patients, 3506 East Frontage Road, Suite 315, Tampa, FL 33607, 800-749-2257, www.aakp.org

American Foundation for Urologic Disease, 1128 North Charles Street, Baltimore, MD 21201, 410-468-1800, 800-242-2383, www.afud.org

American Society of Nephrology, 1725 I Street N.W. #510, Washington, DC 20006, 202-659-0599, www.asn-online.org

Bard, C.R. Bard, Inc., 730 Central Avenue, Murray Hill, NJ 07974, 800-367-2273, www.crbard.com

Interstitial Cystitis Association, 110 North Washington Street, Suite 840, Rockville, MD 20850, 301-610-5300, 800-HELP-ICA, www.ichelp.org

Medic Alert® Foundation, 2323 Colorado Avenue, Turlock, CA 95382-2018, 888-633-4298, www.medicalert.org

National Association for Continence (NAFC), P.O. Box 8310, Spartanburg, SC 29305-8310, 864-579-7900, 800-BLADDER (800-252-3337), www.nafc.org

National Kidney and Urologic Diseases Information Clearinghouse, 3 Information Way, Bethesda, MD 20892-3580, 800-891-5390, www.niddk.nih.gov/health/kidney/nkudic

National Kidney Foundation, 30 East 33rd Street, Suite 1100, New York, NY 10016, 212-889-2210, 800-622-9010, www.kidney.org

Polycystic Kidney Disease Foundation, 4901 Main Street, Suite 200, Kansas City, MO 64112, 800-753-2873

The Simon Foundation for Continence, P.O. Box 835, Wilmette, IL 60091, 847-864-3913, 800-23-SIMON, www.simonfoundation.org

UNIT
12

Nursing Care of the Client: Mobility, Coordination, and Regulation

MUSCULOSKELETAL SYSTEM

MAKING THE CONNECTION

Refer to the following chapters to increase your understanding of the musculoskeletal system:

Basic Nursing
- **Wellness Concepts**
- **Assessment**
- **Pain Management**
- **Diagnostic Tests**

Adult Health Nursing
- **Oncology**
- **Cardiovascular System**
- **Immune System**
- **The Older Adult**

Basic Procedures
- **Performing Passive Range-of-Motion (ROM) Exercises**

- **Ambulation Safety and Assisting from Bed to Walking**
- **Turning and Positioning a Client**
- **Moving a Client in Bed**
- **Transferring from Bed to Wheelchair, Commode, or Chair**
- **Transferring from Bed to Stretcher**

Intermediate Procedures
- **Assisting with Crutches, Cane, or Walker**

Review: Delmar's Anatomy & Physiology CD-ROM: Bones, Joints, Muscles, Ligaments, & Tendons

LEARNING OBJECTIVES

Upon completion of this chapter, you should be able to:
- Define key terms.
- List the diagnostic tests used in the evaluation of orthopedic disorders and diseases.
- Describe preventive nursing care of the orthopedic client (e.g., positioning, mobility).
- Identify the various types of casts used in the treatment of orthopedic disorders.
- Describe nursing care of clients with orthopedic devices.
- List four types of fractures and their related treatment.
- Discuss the nursing care of the client undergoing a total hip replacement.
- Utilize the nursing process to plan nursing care including physical and emotional needs of the orthopedic client.

KEY TERMS

amphiarthrosis
amputation
arthroplasty
bruxism
closed reduction
contracture
crepitus
diarthrosis
dislocation
fracture
Heberden's nodes
kyphosis
locomotor

lordosis
open reduction
orthopedics
osteoporosis
paresthesia
phantom limb pain
scoliosis
sprain
strain
subluxation
synarthrosis
tophi
windowing

INTRODUCTION

Orthopedics, also spelled orthopaedics, is the branch of medicine that deals with the prevention or correction of the disorders and diseases of the musculoskeletal system. It involves the muscles, skeleton, joints, and supporting structures such as ligaments and tendons.

The prime concern of the nurse caring for a client with **locomotor** (pertaining to movement or the ability to move) disorders is the prevention of **contractures** (permanent shortening of a muscle) or deformities. The objective of all caregivers is to maintain good body alignment, preserve muscle tone, prevent disuse, and continue joint motion for the client with acute or long-term therapeutic or rehabilitative needs. Caring for orthopedic clients also requires an understanding of basic principles that apply to all clients whether they are in traction, casts, or recovering from surgery.

ANATOMY AND PHYSIOLOGY REVIEW

The musculoskeletal system consists of bones, muscles, tendons, ligaments, cartilage, and joints. When it is functioning properly, the musculoskeletal system allows

an individual to stand erect and ambulate. Figure 37-1 identifies the bones of the skeleton.

The skeletal system consists of bones attached to each other by cartilage and strong ligaments. The functions of the skeleton are to:

- Provide the body with structural framework.
- Act as a protective casing for internal organs such as the brain, heart, and lungs.
- Allow movement by muscles attached to the skeleton.
- Store calcium, phosphorus and magnesium and release these minerals when the body requires them.
- Manufacture blood cells in the red bone marrow.

Bones in the skeletal system are classified as long, short, flat, or irregular. Examples include the humerus, a long bone; the phalanges of the finger, short bone; occiput, flat bone; and the vertebrae, irregular bone. Figure 37-2 illustrates these bones.

There are two types of bone. One type of bone is *cancellous*, which resembles a sponge with spaces and is found in the epiphysis or end of the long bones as well as in all other bones. The other type is *cortical* bone, which is compact bone and is found in the diaphysis or shaft of the long bones. Short bones consist of cancellous bone covered by a layer of compact bone. Flat bones are made of cancellous bone layered between compact bone. Generally, the makeup of irregular bones is similar to that of flat bones.

Figure 37-1 *Anterior and Posterior Views of the Adult Human Skeleton*

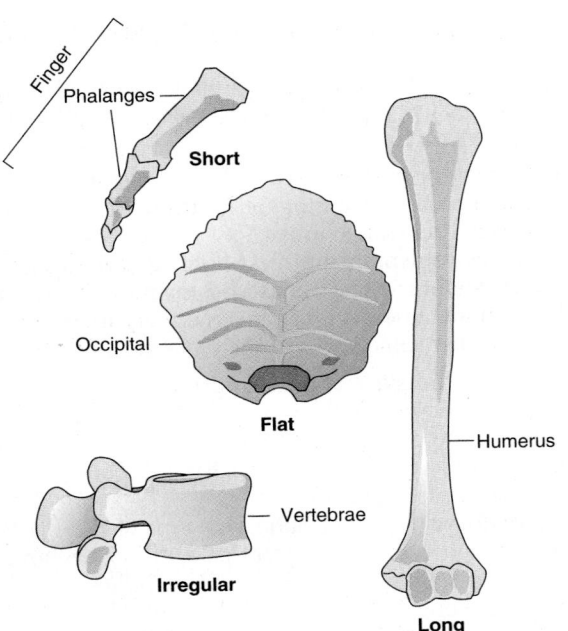

Figure 37-2 *Bone Shape Classification*

cortex. The muscles and the skeleton work together to permit body movement. Muscles are attached to bones by tendons.

The action of muscles is to contract or shorten. Muscles are arranged within the body as opposing pairs to act as antagonists to each other. For example, the biceps flex the forearm and the triceps extend it.

Muscles are surrounded and divided by fibrous envelopes called *fascia*. In the extremities, the muscles surround and give support to main blood vessels and nerves. Muscles also give support to and keep the body erect as well as give shape to the body.

Movement of the muscles may be either voluntary or involuntary. Muscles attached to bone can function at the will of the person (voluntary). Involuntary muscles, found within body organs, regulate the physical activity of the organs so the organs can perform their functions. These actions are not under the person's control. Involuntary muscles are located in the intestinal tract, the pupil of the eye, and in the heart and blood vessels.

A joint is a junction of two or more bones. There are three types of joints: diarthrosis, synarthrosis, and amphiarthrosis. **Diarthrosis** joints are freely movable such as the hinge (elbow, knee), ball and socket (hip and shoulder), pivot (skull and first vertebrae), gliding (wrist), and saddle (thumb). **Synarthrosis** joints are immovable, such as the suture line between the temporal and occipital bones of the skull. **Amphiarthrosis** joints are slightly movable, such as the vertebrae and pelvic bones separated by fibrous cartilage. Figure 37-4 illustrates types of joints.

The muscular system is composed of muscle fibers and tendons innervated by nerves (Figure 37-3). The muscle fibers vary in size and shape and are arranged according to a muscle's function. The muscles act as motors controlled by nerve impulses from the cerebral

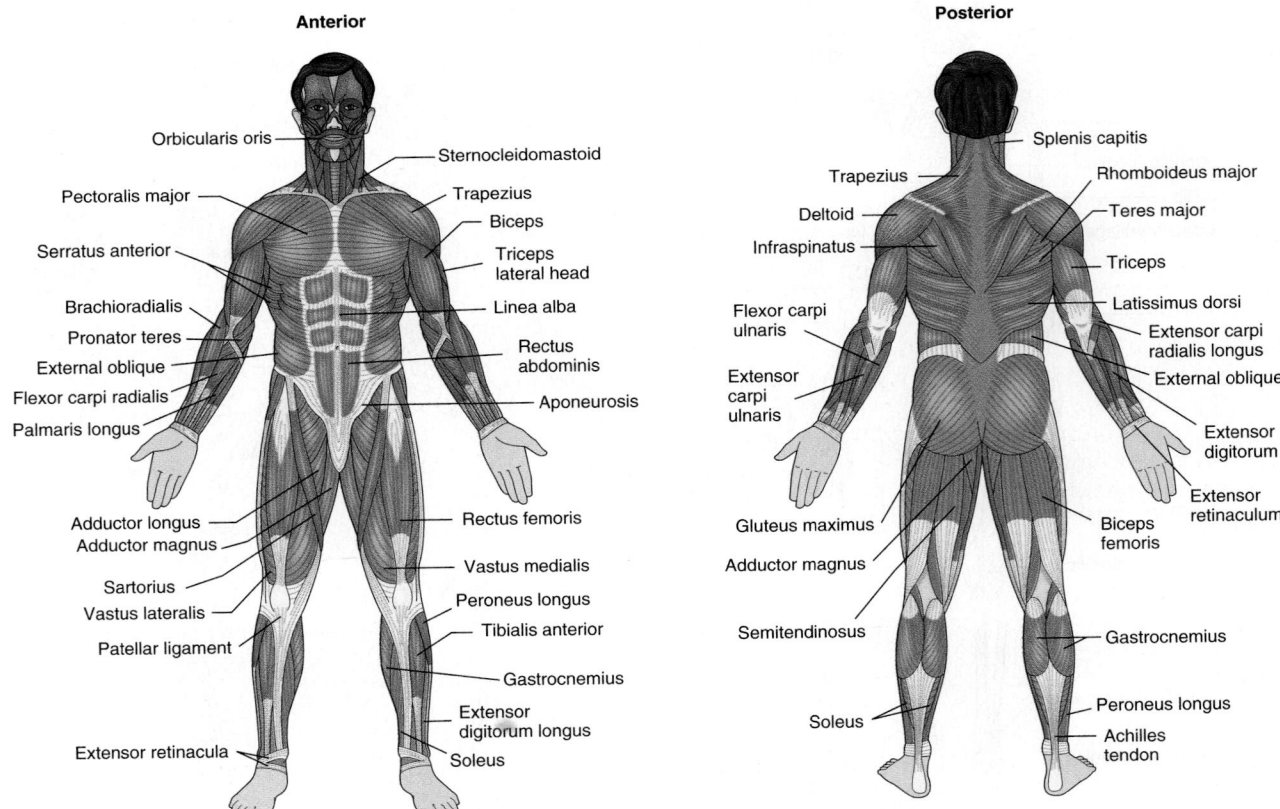

Figure 37-3 *Muscular System: Anterior and Posterior Views*

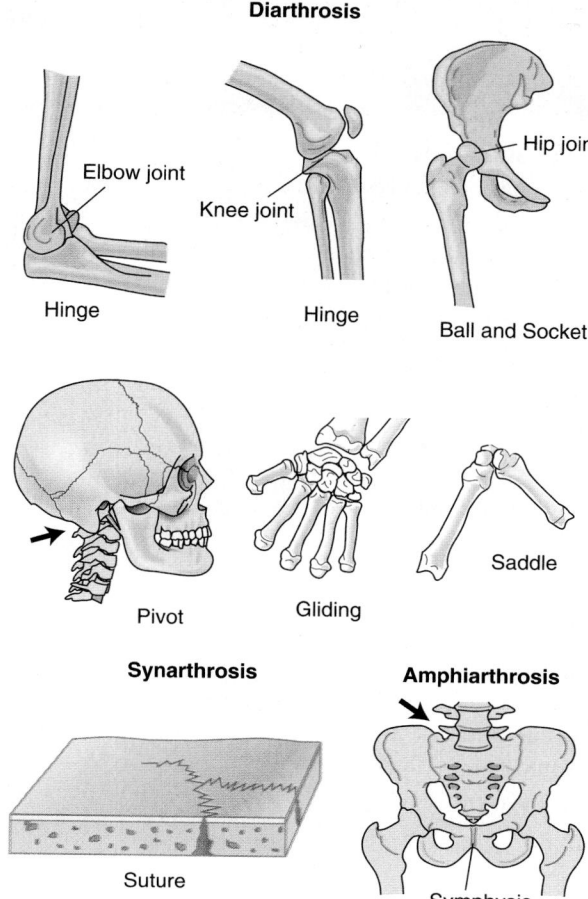

Diarthrosis

Elbow joint

Knee joint

Hip joint

Hinge

Hinge

Ball and Socket

Pivot

Gliding

Saddle

Synarthrosis

Amphiarthrosis

Suture

Symphysis

Figure 37-4 *Joints Classified by the Degree of Movement Permitted*

sess the client's ability to perform basic activities of daily living.

The medical history includes information on any past medical or surgical disorders and any symptoms relative to onset, duration, or location of discomfort or pain. Ask if activity makes symptoms better or worse. A family medical history should also be obtained.

Assessment of the bony skeleton includes notation of deformities, body alignment, abnormal growths, shortened extremities, amputations, abnormal angulation other than at the joints, and **crepitus**, a grating or crackling sensation or sound.

Assessment of the spine necessitates exposure of the client's back, buttocks, and legs for adequate visualization. Note differences in the height of the shoulders or iliac crests. Gluteal folds should appear symmetrical. The vertebral column should be straight and perpendicular to the floor, with the spine convex through the thoracic portion and concave through the cervical/lumbar portion.

Three common spinal curvatures are scoliosis, kyphosis, and lordosis. A lateral curving deviation is known as **scoliosis**. Scoliosis (crooked back) is seen most frequently in school-age children and adolescents. **Kyphosis** (hump back) is seen as an increased roundness of the thoracic spinal curve. This condition is frequently seen in older persons with osteoporosis. **Lordosis** (sway back) is an exaggeration of the lumbar spine curvature as seen in pregnancy as a woman's body adjusts its center of gravity. These three curvatures are illustrated in Figure 37-5.

Assessment of the articular system includes range of motion (limited, active, and passive), stability of joints, deformities and any nodular formation, and pulses in the extremities.

The ends of articulating joints are covered with a smooth articular cartilage. The joint capsule is composed of an outer fibrous layer and an inner synovial layer that secretes synovial fluid. This clear fluid acts as a lubricating fluid for the joints.

Other structures related to the musculoskeletal system include bursa, fascia, tendons, and ligaments. Bursae are sacs filled with fluid that facilitate joint movement by making it possible for muscles and tendons to move or glide over ligaments or bones. Fascia is connective tissue that covers a muscle. Tendons are strong fibrous tissue attaching muscle to bones, providing mobility. Ligaments grow out of the periosteum and lash bones together more firmly.

ASSESSMENT

Assessment of the musculoskeletal system ranges from a basic assessment of functional abilities done by the nurse to a complete physical exam by the physician for diagnosis of specific muscle and joint disorders. The extent of the physical exam depends on the client's symptoms, health history, and any other physical signs.

Inspect and palpate to evaluate bone integrity, posture, joint function, muscle strength, and gait. Also as-

A. Scoliosis

B. Kyphosis

C. Lordosis

Figure 37-5 *Curvatures of the Spine*

Range of motion (ROM) includes assessment of the client's ability to change position, muscle strength and coordination, and the size of individual muscles. When assessing passive range of motion, remember to keep the motion steady and avoid causing any pain.

Joints are examined for excessive fluid. The knee is the most common site for fluid accumulation. Edema and an elevated temperature may be signs of active inflammation in the joint. Normal joint movement is stable and smooth. If there is a snap or crack sound when a joint is passively moved, it may indicate a ligament slipping over a bony prominence.

Deformities may be caused by several factors, including contractures, dislocations, and **subluxation** (a partial separation of an articular [joint] surface). Nodular formations are produced by musculoskeletal diseases such as gout, rheumatoid arthritis, and osteoarthritis.

Pulse points in the extremities are palpated to assess for weak or absent pulses. The strength of the pulse in affected extremities is compared with that of nonaffected extremities. Note skin color and temperature and check capillary refill by pressing down on the client's fingernail or toenail for a few seconds, then release and note the time it takes for the client's nail to return to normal color. The color should return immediately (less than 2 seconds); if a client has an arterial disorder, the color will take longer than 2 seconds to return to normal.

COMMON DIAGNOSTIC TESTS

Commonly used diagnostic tests for clients with symptoms of musculoskeletal system disorders are listed in Table 37-1.

MUSCULOSKELETAL TRAUMA

Trauma to the musculoskeletal system may cause a variety of injuries to clients of all ages. Such injuries include strains, sprains, dislocations, fractures, and compartment syndrome.

STRAIN

A **strain** is an injury to a muscle or tendon caused by overuse or overstretching. A strain may be either acute or chronic. An acute strain may be caused when an individual performs unaccustomed exercises vigorously. A chronic strain may develop after repeated overuse of certain muscles. Individuals with acute strains experience sudden severe pain, whereas the onset is gradual in chronic strains, with the affected part feeling only stiff and sore.

Chronic strains require no specific treatment, but acute strains require rest and possibly immobilization. Immediately following injury, apply cold packs for 20- to 30-minute periods, then remove for 1 hour during a 24-hour period to reduce any edema. Then apply heat for the client's comfort. In the case of a severe strain when

TABLE 37-1   COMMON DIAGNOSTIC TESTS FOR CLIENTS WITH MUSCULOSKELETAL DISORDERS

Laboratory Tests

Antinuclear antibodies (ANA)

Complete blood count (CBC)

- WBC   • Hg

C-reactive protein (CRP)

Erythrocyte sedimentation rate (ESR)

Rheumatoid factor (RF)

Serum calcium

Uric acid
- serum   • urine

Radiologic Studies

Arthrogram/graphy

Computed tomography (CT scan)

Electromyography (EMG)

Magnetic resonance imaging (MRI)

Radiography (x-ray)

Other Tests

Arthrocentesis

Arthroscopy

the muscle may be completely ruptured, surgical repair may be necessary.

SPRAIN

A **sprain** is an injury to ligaments surrounding a joint caused by a sudden twist, wrench, or fall. Symptoms include pain, edema, loss of motion, and ecchymosis. X-ray will reveal soft tissue edema but no evidence of joint or bone injury. Immediate treatment is RICE (rest, ice, compression, and elevation). The client rests and ice is applied to the injured area. The part may then be immobilized with an elastic compression bandage or a brace and elevated. After the edema has decreased significantly, a cast may be applied.

DISLOCATION

Dislocation occurs when articular surfaces of a joint are no longer in contact. The bones are literally "out of joint." The displaced bone may hinder the blood supply, damage nerves, tear ligaments, or rupture muscle attachments. Traumatic dislocations are considered orthopedic emergencies. Congenital dislocations are present at birth, whereas spontaneous or pathologic dislocations are caused by diseases affecting joints.

Symptoms of a dislocation include localized joint pain, loss of function of the joint, and a change in the length of the extremity and contour of the joint. Diagnosis is based on the symptoms, physical exam, and x-rays. X-rays reveal either a complete or partial separation of the articulating surfaces.

FRACTURE

A **fracture** is a break in the continuity of a bone. Fractures occur when the forces from outside the body are greater than the strength of the bone, causing the bone to break. Fractures usually involve soft tissue (edema and bleeding), damaged nerves, and tendons. Most fractures are caused by accidents. These may be the result of direct force, torsion or twisting, or violent contractions of highly developed muscles. Other fractures may be the result of a disease process that weakens the bone. This type of fracture is known as *pathologic* or *spontaneous*. Individuals considered at high risk for fractures include those who have predisposing bone conditions such as metastatic or primary bone tumors or osteoporosis, poor coordination, diminished vision, dizzy spells, or general weakness.

There are more than 90 different classifications of fractures. Some of the more common types include greenstick or incomplete, simple or closed, compound or open, impacted or telescoped, spiral, and comminuted.

In a greenstick fracture, the continuity of the bone is not completely disrupted but has splintering on one side and bending on the other. This fracture is seen most frequently in children. An uncomplicated (clean) fracture in which the skin remains intact is called a closed or simple fracture; the fractured surfaces are not contaminated by outside air. In a compound or open fracture, the bone is broken and the skin is also broken, allowing the bone to protrude and be susceptible to a greater chance for infection. An impacted fracture is also called a telescoped fracture; one portion of a bone fragment is forcibly driven into another. A spiral fracture twists around the shaft of the bone. This type of fracture may occur from a twisting force. In a comminuted fracture, the bone is splintered into many unaligned fragments. Various types of fractures are shown in Figure 37-6.

Healing time for fractures is affected by the age of the client and the type of injury or any underlying disease process, and may take weeks, months, or even years before healing is complete. The sequence of healing takes place beginning with the formation of a hematoma, then granulation tissue formation, callus formation, callus ossification, and ultimately remodeling.

Hematoma formation begins with the formation of a clot that serves as a fibrin network. Bleeding comes from ruptured vessels within the bone as well as from tears in the periosteum and adjacent tissues. The hematoma is not absorbed but develops into granulation tissue. Granulation tissue forms a soft tissue callus that surrounds the fracture site and serves as a temporary splint. Callus ossification is the result of deposits of calcium salts in the callus forming rigid bone in excess as a protective measure. The formation of bone binds the bone ends together. Remodeling is completed by osteoclastic activity, whereby excess bone is gradually reduced and removed by absorption until the original shape and outline of the fractured bone is reestablished. Figure 37-7 outlines the healing sequence.

Complications of a fracture include infection, fat embolism syndrome, and compartment syndrome. Complications may delay healing or be life threatening.

Infections may result from an open fracture in which the bone extends through the skin, allowing contamination from the outside. They may also occur following surgical repair of a fracture using an internal fixation device. Any infection may lead to a delayed union of the bone.

Fat embolism syndrome is usually associated with fractures of the long bones, multiple fractures, or crushing injuries. An embolus usually occurs within 24 to 72 hours following a fracture but may occur up to a week after injury. Much is still unclear about how a fat embolism occurs (Walls, 2002). When a small area of the lungs is involved, the symptoms are pain, tachycardia, and dyspnea. Larger areas of lung involvement produce more pronounced symptoms, including severe pain, dyspnea, cyanosis, restlessness, and shock. Petechiae may appear over the neck, upper arms, chest, or abdomen. Treatment consists of bed rest, respiratory support, oxygen, and IV fluids.

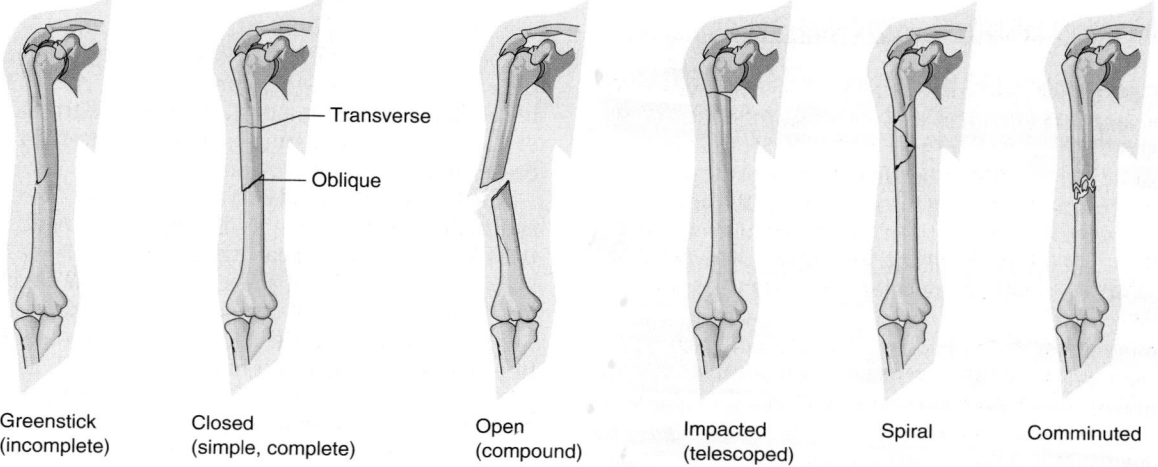

Greenstick (incomplete)   Closed (simple, complete)   Open (compound)   Impacted (telescoped)   Spiral   Comminuted

Transverse

Oblique

Figure 37-6 *Classifications of Common Bone Fractures*

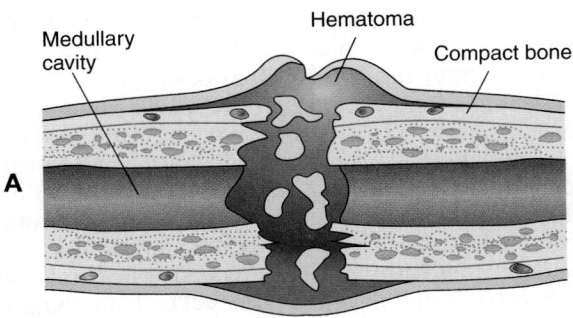

A hematoma forms from blood from ruptured vessels.

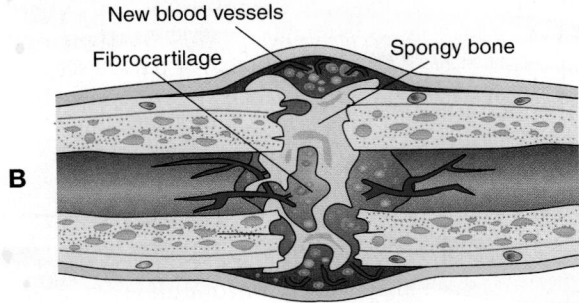

Spongy bone forms close to developing blood vessels; fibrocartilage forms away from new blood vessels.

Bony callus replaces fibrocartilage.

Excess bony tissue is removed by osteoclasts.

Figure 37-7 *Steps of Bone Repair*

RHABDOMYOLYSIS

Crushing injuries most commonly cause rhabdomyolysis. Myoglobin, creatine kinase (CK), and other inflammatory mediators escape from the injured muscle tissue into the circulation. The circulating myoglobin, filtered by the kidneys, can precipitate, causing renal tubular obstruction. About 15% of rhabdomyolysis cases will have acute renal failure (Walls, 2002). Two other major problems are respiratory distress from muscle weakness and fluid and electrolyte imbalance. Standard treatment includes IV fluids to maintain circulating blood volume and renal perfusion so the myoglobin is flushed from the kidneys.

COMPARTMENT SYNDROME

Compartment syndrome is a form of neurovascular impairment that may lead to permanent injury of an affected limb caused by progressive constriction of blood vessels and nerves. It can occur with any orthopedic injury as a result of bleeding into the tissue, tissue edema, or prolonged external pressure (cast or tight dressing). If untreated, in 4 to 6 hours it may lead to irreversible damage to nerves and muscles and within 24 to 48 hours permanent loss of normal limb function. A neurovascular assessment that reveals pain not relieved by narcotic analgesics, greater pain with passive motion than active, diminished capillary refill, weak or unequal pulses, **paresthesia** (numbness or tingling), and paralysis indicates this orthopedic emergency. Treatment consists of relieving pressure by removing the cast or dressing or by performing a fasciotomy. A surgical fasciotomy is an incision into the fascia to relieve pressure on the nerves and blood vessels.

Medical–Surgical Management

Medical

The treatment of a fracture requires immediate attention. The most important objectives are to (1) realign the fracture, (2) maintain the alignment, and (3) regain the function of the injured part. The method of treatment depends on the first aid given; the site, severity, and type of the fracture; and the age and condition of the client.

Closed Reduction Repair of a fracture accomplished without surgical intervention is called **closed reduction.** External manipulation is used to correct bone position. This manipulation requires three maneuvers: traction and countertraction, angulation, and rotation. Following the reduction, x-rays are taken to visualize the fracture alignment. The part is then immobilized by using a cast, bandage, or traction. Local or general anesthesia may be used to make the reduction easier and less painful to the client.

Casts Casts are made either from plaster bandages or synthetic materials such as fiberglass. Synthetic casts are used for non–weight-bearing parts of the body. The cast should include the joint above and below the affected part. The major purposes of casts are immobilization, support and protection of the affected part, prevention of deformities that may be the result of conditions such as arthritis, and the correction of deformities such as scoliosis.

A dry cast should be odorless, shiny in appearance, resonant (produces vibrating sound on percussion) when percussed, and have a temperature similar to the

CLIENT TEACHING

Casts

Because plaster casts dry from the inside out, they should not be covered or dried with a hairdryer or heat lamp. Allow moisture and heat from the drying cast to evaporate naturally. Inform clients that the heat they feel during the application, drying, and setting process is normal and should subside in 10 to 15 minutes. To avoid indentation, a drying cast should be placed on pillows and not on a hard surface. For the same reason, when handling the cast, only the palms of the hands should be used. Synthetic casts dry in minutes.

room air. Moisture occurring from any underlying drainage will give the cast a musty smell, dullness on percussion, a lusterless color, and cool temperature.

Numerous types of casts exist. Long and short arm casts allow the fingers to be visible; long and short leg casts allow the toes to be visible. A spica cast is used for hip, shoulder, and thumb dislocations or injuries. The hip spica has an abduction bar that keeps the cast in the correct position. A walking cast with a cast shoe facilitates client ambulation. Body casts are used to immobilize the spine following surgical spinal fusions, unstable spinal injuries, or for degenerative disorders. Figure 37-8 shows different types of casts.

After the application and drying of a cast, it may be necessary for the doctor to order a cast cut to allow visualization of a body area or to relieve pressure. This procedure is known as **windowing.**

When a cast is removed, the client may become conscious of aches and discomforts caused by the constricted joint structures and immobilized muscles. Minimize the client's discomfort by supporting the joint and maintaining the part in the same position as

it was in the cast. The skin will be cool and pale with mottling and edema present. A yellow exudate, which is part dead skin and part secretions from oil sacs, will be on the skin. This exudate should not be rubbed or forced off.

Traction The principle of traction is to have two forces pulling in opposite directions. Traction consists of weights and counterweights. Countertraction forces can be provided by the weight of the client's body or other weight such as elevating the foot of the bed. Traction may be used to reduce a fracture, immobilize an extremity, lessen muscle spasms, or correct or prevent a deformity.

Types of traction are skeletal, skin, and manual. Skeletal traction requires the surgical insertion of pins (Steinmann) or wires (Kirschner) through the bones. Skeletal traction is continuous and is used most frequently for fractures of the femur, tibia, and cervical spine. Head tongs (e.g., Gardner-Wells tongs) are fixed in the skull to apply traction that immobilizes cervical fractures. Figure 37-9 shows examples of traction devices.

Skin traction is a nonsurgical method of providing necessary pull for shorter periods, such as Buck's traction (Figure 37-10). Materials used include tapes, traction strips, cervical halters, and pelvic belts. Skin traction is frequently used to temporarily immobilize a part or stabilize a fracture. The disadvantage of skin traction for adult use is that it does not adequately control rotation and

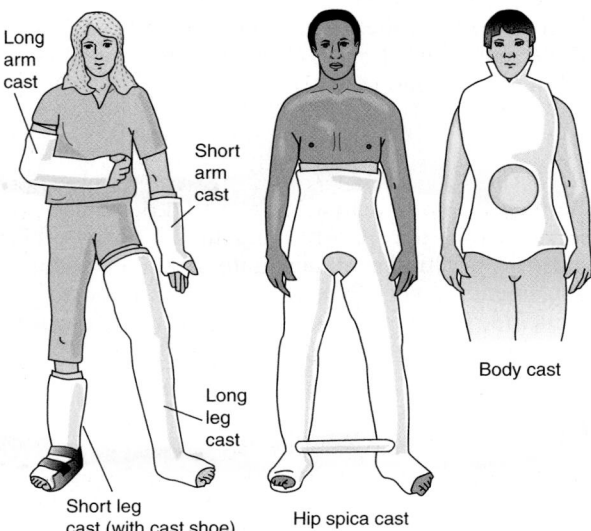

Figure 37-8 *Casts Used to Correct Musculoskeletal Disorders*

Figure 37-9 *Types of Traction Devices: **A,** Skeletal traction; **B,** Head tongs*

Figure 37-10 *Buck's Traction, a Type of Skin Traction*

cannot be maintained for the length of time necessary for adult healing. Tapes and bandages should be applied smoothly to prevent any pressure areas.

A nurse caring for a client in traction should know the purpose of the traction, how it accomplishes its purpose, and any complications associated with the use of the traction. It is also important to know the extent of the injury and the movements and positions allowed. Care of the client should include maintenance of the injured part, general body alignment, the alignment of the traction apparatus, and range of motion in as many joints as possible.

Rehabilitation The physician will determine when the bone has healed sufficiently for rehabilitation. Healing is monitored by periodic x-rays and physical examinations. The major objective of rehabilitation is to assist the client to return to the former level of functioning. Rehabilitation programs vary depending on the injury and the client.

Physical therapy may be started with the use of parallel bars or other exercise equipment before the client is allowed to exercise independently. The nurse has a major role in client education reinforcing the directions of both the physician and the physical therapist. Patience and encouragement are extremely important in assisting the client to feel comfortable in learning self-care techniques. The client should be taught to report any unusual signs or symptoms to the physician.

The client will need to learn proper use of equipment such as crutches, canes, or walkers. Crutches allow ambulation with limited or no weight bearing on the affected extremity. Walkers allow limited weight bearing and provide stability when the client ambulates. Canes allow the client to walk with balance and support.

The tripod position is the basic stance for crutch walking. Tips of the crutches are placed approximately 8 to 10 inches in front of and lateral to the client's feet. The client must place his weight on the handpiece of the crutches and not on the axilla. Crutch gaits depend on the client's disability and are prescribed by the physician.

Canes are held in the hand *opposite* the affected extremity. In normal walking, the opposite arm and leg

COLLABORATIVE CARE

Use of Crutches, Canes, and Walkers
Nurses collaborate with physical therapists to assist clients in the use of crutches, canes, and walkers. Clients generally go to physical therapy to learn how to use the walking aid, and nurses reinforce the teaching when they see clients using their walking aid.

move together. This same action should be done when walking with a cane. Walkers provide more support than canes or crutches. They are especially useful for clients who have poor balance. The client should place the walker 12 to 18 inches in front and walk toward the walker holding onto the hand grips.

Surgical

Open reduction is a surgical procedure that enables the surgeon to reduce (repair) the fracture under direct visualization. When an open reduction/internal fixation (ORIF) is done, orthopedic devices are used to maintain the reduction. Some of the devices used include pins, screws, nails, plates, wires, and rods. These internal fixation devices may be inserted through bone fragments or fixed to the sides of the bones.

The major disadvantage of the open reduction is the possibility of introducing infection into the bone. Possible complications include impaired circulation and accidental injury to major nerves, blood vessels, and bone caused by the fixation devices. X-rays are taken during and after the open reduction to evaluate the alignment of the fracture.

Pharmacological

Analgesics may be given to relieve pain. Muscle relaxants, such as cyclobenzaprine hydrochloride (Flexeril), may also be prescribed for muscle spasms. Severe or continued pain may indicate complications and should be given immediate attention. Stool softeners, such as docusate sodium (Colace), may be given to prevent constipation in the immobilized client.

Diet

The client should be encouraged to eat regular meals. The meals should include foods that provide fiber, protein, calcium, phosphorus, and fluids. For the client whose dietary intake is inadequate, vitamin and mineral supplements, especially calcium and phosphorus, may be included. Consultation with a dietitian regarding client food preferences may be necessary.

Activity

Client activity and exercise are important in maintaining muscle strength and tone and minimizing cardiovascular problems. Joints that are not immobilized should be exercised either actively or passively to maintain function. *Isometric* (maintaining constant resistive force) exercises help maintain muscle strength of immobilized muscles.

Nursing Management

Frequent and accurate assessment of the musculoskeletal trauma area including CMS is very important. Provide comfort measures and administer analgesia as ordered. An important nursing responsibility is the prevention of constipation, skin breakdown, urinary calculi, and respiratory complications from immobility.

NURSING PROCESS

Assessment

Subjective Data

The neurovascular assessment of a client with a fracture may reveal subjective data of pain, especially on movement; muscle spasms; and paresthesia.

Objective Data

Edema, shortening and deformity of the affected limb, and pallor may be found. Check pulses in the affected and unaffected extremity and compare with each other. Take the client's vital signs routinely, and note the client's general physical and mental condition. Check the skin, especially over bony prominences, for color and temperature.

When the client has a cast applied, check all cast edges for smoothness. Also check the cast for spots indicating

---

PROFESSIONAL TIP

Neurovascular Assessment

- Circulation, movement, and sensation (CMS) assessments are performed on clients following musculoskeletal trauma; after surgery, if nerve or blood vessel damage is possible; and following casting, splinting, and bandaging.
- The CMS assessment is performed every 15 to 30 minutes for several hours, and then every 3 to 4 hours.
- All findings must be documented.
- Tingling and numbness may be relieved by flexing fingers or toes or repositioning extremity.
- Remember 6 Ps when performing a CMS assessment:
  1. Paresthesia (unrelieved tingling or numbness)
  2. Pain
  3. Pallor (slow capillary return)
  4. Paralysis
  5. Puffiness (edema)
  6. Pulselessness

---

wound drainage, including the color and amount. Mark the size of the drainage spot on the cast with a ballpoint pen and indicate the date and time. Then an increase in the size of the drainage spot can easily be identified. Assess extremities including fingers, toes, hands, and feet for changes in skin color, pulse, or temperature. Check all traction wires, pulleys, and weights. Weights should hang free.

Nursing diagnoses for a client with musculoskeletal trauma may include the following:

Nursing Diagnoses	Planning/Goals	Nursing Interventions
Acute Pain related to fracture	The client will have relief of pain with medication.	Provide comfort measures. Administer medications for pain as ordered.
Risk for Impaired Skin Integrity related to immobility	The client will experience no skin breakdown.	Change client position, if allowed, maintaining correct body alignment.
		Check bony prominences and keep the client's skin clean and dry.
		For the client in a cast, check the edges of the cast for roughness, keep the exposed skin next to the cast clean and dry.
		Inspect all body pressure points including the head, ears, and heels; turn the client as orders direct; and check for friction rubs.
		Instruct clients not to poke anything under the cast or use objects to scratch, causing skin breakdown or infections.
		Avoid getting the cast wet.
Impaired Physical Mobility related to loss of integrity of bone structures	The client will perform range-of-motion exercises in unaffected joints.	If the client in a cast is allowed to turn, use an overhead trapeze.
		Assist client in performing ROM exercises.
	The client will demonstrate use of adaptive devices to improve mobility.	Assist client in use of adaptive devices.

Evaluation Each goal must be evaluated to determine how it has been met by the client.

INFLAMMATORY DISORDERS

Inflammatory disorders involve inflammation of the joints and include conditions such as rheumatoid arthritis, bursitis, and osteomyelitis.

RHEUMATOID ARTHRITIS

Rheumatoid arthritis is an autoimmune disease of unknown etiology, with recurring inflammation involving the synovium or lining of the joints. It can also affect the lungs, heart, blood vessels, muscles, eyes, and skin. Rheumatoid arthritis is a potentially destructive and disabling disease. The course is variable with either slow or rapid progress and/or periods of remissions. Women are affected more often than men. Rheumatoid arthritis can occur at any age; however, it most commonly affects young adults. In children it occurs in a form known as juvenile rheumatoid arthritis (Still's disease). See the immune system chapter for more information on rheumatoid arthritis.

BURSITIS

Bursitis is inflammation of the bursa, a sac filled with synovial fluid that facilitates joint movement. Major bursae are found in the shoulder, knee, hip, and elbow. The inflammation is usually the result of trauma or repetitive movements. The client experiences painful joint movement. Diagnosis is made from the client's symptoms and x-ray, which shows a calcified bursa. Treatment includes rest of the joint and the administration of anti-inflammatory drugs including salicylates and NSAIDs. For some clients, corticosteroids may be injected into the bursa.

(prednisone)

OSTEOMYELITIS

Osteomyelitis is the inflammation of the bone and bone marrow. The most common cause of osteomyelitis is the introduction of pathogenic bacteria into a penetrating injury such as an open fracture. Bone infections may also result from the spread of infection from another site such as infected teeth, tonsils, or an upper respiratory infection. The most common pathogen causing osteomyelitis is *Staphylococcus aureus*. Other organisms found in osteomyelitis are *Pseudomonas* and *Escherichia coli*. Osteomyelitis may become a chronic disabling prob-

lem affecting the quality of life. The affected bone may have spontaneous fractures.

Local symptoms of an acute infection are sudden pain and tenderness of the affected bone, warmth, redness, edema, and pain on movement. General symptoms with acute severe bone infections may include chills, elevated temperature, rapid pulse, and marked leukocytosis.

Medical–Surgical Management

Medical

The client is placed on bed rest, and the infected bone is kept at rest with the use of sandbags or casts. Antibiotics are given IV as soon as osteomyelitis is suspected. Unless the infective process is controlled early, a bone abscess forms (Figure 37-11). Cultures of the abscess may indicate a need for change in the antibiotic therapy. The abscess may drain naturally; however, it usually requires an incision, allowing it to drain. The abscess cavity of dead bone tissue does not liquefy easily, drain, and heal as in soft tissue abscesses. A bone sheath forms around the sequestrum (dead bone), giving the appearance of healing; however, chronically infected sequestrum has the tendency to produce recurrent abscesses throughout the life of the individual.

Surgical

A sequestrectomy to remove the dead bone tissue may need to be performed. Strict aseptic technique must be maintained when changing any dressings. Because infected bone may be extremely painful, unnecessary movement should be avoided and the affected extremity should be handled very gently.

Pharmacological

Vigorous antibiotic therapy and analgesics are the medications used to treat osteomyelitis. Wound irrigations with antiseptics or antibiotics are often prescribed by the physician. Specific drugs given are determined by the causative organism.

Diet

A high-calorie, high-protein diet is generally ordered for the client with osteomyelitis. Dietary supplements of vitamins and calcium are also given. Fluids should be increased as tolerated.

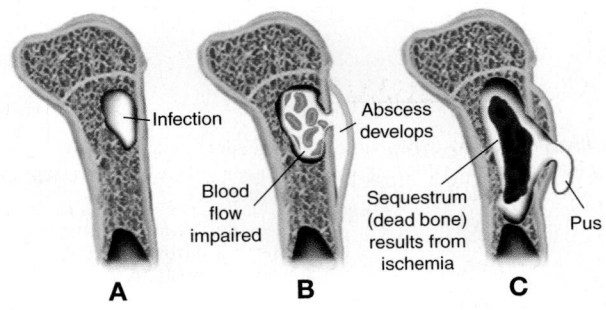

Figure 37-11 A, *Osteomyelitis;* **B,** *Without early treatment, an abscess forms;* **C,** *Bone dies (sequestrum) and pus forms*

Activity

There should be absolute rest of the affected extremity. Avoid excessive handling of the extremity because it is very painful. The extremity should be handled in a smooth, unhurried manner, supporting the joints above and below the affected area.

Nursing Management

Maintain the client on bed rest and the infected bone at absolute rest. Avoid excessive handling of the affected extremity. Administer IV antibiotics, analgesics, and dietary supplements (vitamins and calcium) as ordered. Maintain strict asepsis if wound irrigations are ordered. Encourage the client to drink more fluids and to eat the high-calorie, high-protein diet ordered. Provide for diversional activities.

NURSING PROCESS

Assessment

Subjective Data

Inquire about pain, muscle spasms, and tenderness in the bone. Ask about any traumas, surgeries, and other diseases.

Objective Data

Observe the client for signs of infection, including chills, elevated temperature, pain, redness, and edema of the affected extremity. The client may also experience headaches, restlessness, and irritability.

Nursing diagnoses for a client with osteomyelitis may include the following:

Nursing Diagnoses	Planning/Goals	Nursing Interventions
*Impaired Physical **Mobility*** related to pain	The client will maintain movement of unaffected extremities.	Encourage and assist client to maintain active ROM or perform passive ROM to unaffected extremities.
*Risk for Impaired **Skin** Integrity* related to immobility	The client will maintain skin integrity.	Handle the affected extremity gently, protect it from injury, keep it in good body alignment and level with the body.
		Irrigate wound as ordered. Use aseptic technique when irrigating the affected area and when changing the dressing.
		Assess skin and bony prominences for reddened areas.
		Encourage adequate fluid intake.
*Acute **Pain*** related to inflammation	The client will verbalize reduction of pain.	Protect client from jerky movements and falls.
		Assess wound appearance and new sites of pain.
		Provide diet high in protein and vitamin C.
		Administer pain medications as ordered.

Evaluation Each goal must be evaluated to determine how it has been met by the client.

DEGENERATIVE DISORDERS

Conditions discussed following include osteoporosis, degenerative joint disease, and total joint arthroplasty.

OSTEOPOROSIS

Osteoporosis is an increase in the porosity of bone. It is a common disorder in bone metabolism in which both mineral and protein matrix components are diminished and the bone becomes brittle and fragile. There is an increased susceptibility to fractures of the hip, spine, and wrist.

Ten million individuals in the United States have osteoporosis, and another 34 million have low bone mineral density, which places them at risk for osteoporosis (National Osteoporosis Foundation [NOF], 2002a; National Institute of Arthritis and Musculoskeletal and Skin Diseases [NIAMS], 2000). Of those affected by osteoporosis, 80% are women (NOF, 2002c). More than 1.5 million fractures occur annually related to osteoporosis, including 300,000 hip fractures, 700,000 vertebral fractures, 250,000 wrist fractures, and more than 300,000 fractures of other types (NOF, 2002c).

Osteoporosis has been called the "silent disease" because there are no symptoms of bone loss. As the bone tissue loses density, fractures and kyphosis may occur. Very slight trauma may fracture the brittle bones. With multiple vertebral fractures, the individual may experience a loss of height.

The only way to determine if an individual has osteoporosis is to measure bone mineral density (BMD). There

PROFESSIONAL TIP

Osteoporosis

Risk factors for osteoporosis include being female, having thin or small bones, advanced age, family history of osteoporosis, postmenopause without estrogen replacement therapy, amenorrhea, eating disorders, low calcium intake, inactive lifestyle, smoking, excessive alcohol intake, use of corticosteroids or anticonvulsant medications; and low testosterone level in men.

COMMUNITY/HOME HEALTH CARE

Osteoporosis

- Maintain physical activity—walking, isometric exercises.
- Remove potential hazards—throw rugs.
- Eat a diet high in calcium and vitamin D.
- Be out in the sun 10 to 15 minutes a day.
- Move items down from top shelves of cupboards because it is difficult to see or reach what is up there as a result of curvature changes in the spine.

are several methods of measuring BMD; all are painless, noninvasive, and safe. They include:

- DXA or DEXA (dual-energy x-ray absorptiometry) measures spine, hip, or total body.
- DXA (peripheral dual-energy x-ray absorptiometry) measures wrist, heel, or finger.
- SXA (single-energy x-ray absorptiometry) measures wrist or heel.
- QCT (quantitative computed tomography) measures spine.
- QUS (quantitative ultrasound) measures heel, shin bone, and kneecap (NOF, 2002b).

Medical–Surgical Management

There is no cure for osteoporosis. Prevention through diet, regular exercise, eliminating tobacco and alcohol use, having BMD testing, and taking medication is possible for most people (NOF, 2002e).

Pharmacological

Four medications are approved for postmenopausal women to prevent and/or treat osteoporosis (NOF, 2002c). Estrogen is used both for prevention and treatment. It is the primary choice for prevention in postmenopausal women. Alendronate sodium (Fosamax) is used for prevention and treatment for men and women. Calcitonin (Miacalcin) for treatment of osteoporosis is available as a nasal spray; approved only for women (NOF, 2002d). To obtain its full therapeutic effect, the client should also take calcium and vitamin D supplements. To

prevent osteoporosis, raloxifene (Evista) may be used. It prevents bone loss throughout the body but may cause venous thrombosis.

Testosterone replacement therapy may be used for men with low testosterone levels.

Nonnarcotic analgesics may be prescribed for relief of pain. The client may also be advised to take supplemental calcium.

Diet

Encourage the client to maintain an adequate balanced diet rich in calcium and vitamin D. A reduction in the consumption of caffeine, alcohol, excess protein, and smoking cessation is recommended.

Activity

Encourage the client to practice good body mechanics and posture and to walk, preferably outdoors for the benefits of sunshine (vitamin D). This is effective in preventing further bone loss and stimulating new bone formation.

Nursing Management

Encourage clients to prevent osteoporosis through a diet adequate in calcium and vitamin D, regular exercise, and eliminating tobacco and alcohol use. Teach correct body mechanics and encourage good posture.

NURSING PROCESS

Assessment

Subjective Data

This includes the client's gender, age, and family health history. Note any symptoms the client expresses regarding altered body image or back or neck pain that worsens when coughing, sneezing, straining, or standing. Take a nutritional history. Note lifestyle patterns such as smoking, inactivity, or immobilization. A medical history regarding any medications is also important.

Objective Data

Kyphosis, gait impairment, and poor posture are often noted.

CULTURAL CONSIDERATIONS

Osteoporosis

- Significant risk has been reported in persons of all ethnic backgrounds.
- White women older than age 65 have twice as many fractures as African American women (NOF, 2002c).
- White men are at greater risk for osteoporosis, but osteoporosis is found in men from all ethnic groups (NOF, 2002d).

Nursing diagnoses for a client with osteoporosis may include the following:

Nursing Diagnoses	Planning/Goals	Nursing Interventions
*Chronic **P**ain* related to disease process	The client will express minimal discomfort.	Administer analgesics as ordered; teach the client about the medications. Handle the client carefully; instruct the client to avoid any twisting movements. The bed should have a firm mattress or bed board for support.
*Risk for **I**njury* related to disease process	The client will practice correct body mechanics.	Teach client correct body mechanics.
*Impaired Physical **M**obility* related to disease process	The client will maintain physical activity.	Teach client about types of exercises and physical activities that will help maintain bone mass and isometric exercises to strengthen muscles. Encourage ambulation with the client using a walker or cane if necessary.

Evaluation Each goal must be evaluated to determine how it has been met by the client.

OSTEOARTHRITIS (DEGENERATIVE JOINT DISEASE)

Osteoarthritis (OA) is considered a "wear and tear" disease and is characterized by slow and steady progressive breakdown of cartilage. It is a nonsystemic, noninflammatory disorder causing bones and joints to degenerate. It is the most common type of arthritis. The etiology is unknown, but predisposing factors include increased age, obesity, an injury to a joint, poor posture, or occupations that put strain on joints. Genetics plays a role in OA, especially in the hands (Arthritis Foundation, 2002b). The weight-bearing joints of the lower extremities as well as the hands and cervical and lumbar vertebrae are the joints most frequently affected. The cartilage covering the bone becomes thin and then wears off. The synovial membrane thickens and fibrous tissue around the joint ossifies. The effects of degenerative changes on the knee joint are shown in Figure 37-12.

The onset of osteoarthritis begins during middle age, and by age 65 most people have some degeneration. Symptoms include early morning stiffness and pain after physical activity. There is joint enlargement and characteristic hypertrophic spurs, called **Heberden's nodes**, in the terminal interphalangeal finger joints. More women are affected with OA, especially in the hands. The hips are more affected in men.

Diagnosis is made from the client's symptoms and examination of the joints that are enlarged and tender. X-ray shows a narrowing of joint spaces and gross irregularities of joint structure. A CT scan or MRI may be used to show vertebral joint involvement.

Medical–Surgical Management

Medical

No treatment exists to stop the degenerative process; therefore, treatment focuses on relief of the client's discomfort. Medical management includes lo-

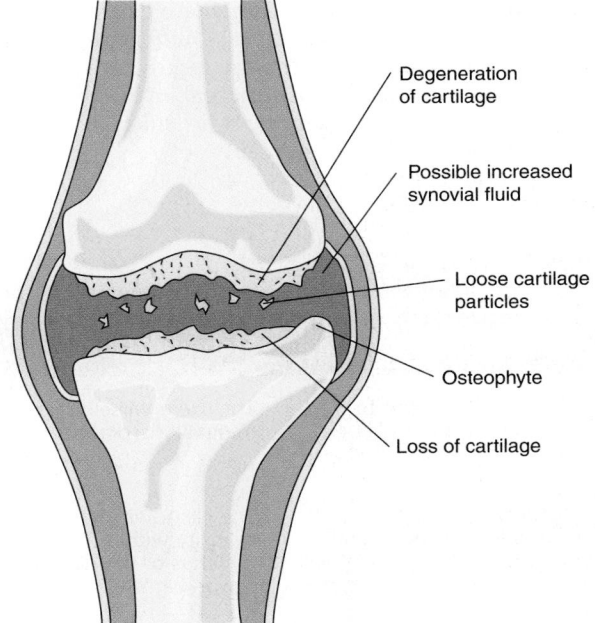

Figure 37-12 *Degenerative Changes in the Cartilage of the Knee due to Osteoarthritis*

cal heat and rest for the affected joint, weight reduction for obese clients to relieve strain on affected joints, and orthotic devices (braces, canes, crutches) to support the joints. Physical therapy can provide exercises to strengthen muscles and keep joints flexible and teach self-management skills.

Surgical

Surgical procedures such as total hip or knee replacement may be recommended for clients with severe osteoarthritis. Osteotomy may help correct malalignment

CLIENT TEACHING

Osteoarthritis

- Set priorities each day, and do the most important activities first.
- Do not plan too many activities for one day.
- Plan rest periods during the day between activities.
- Prevent rushing and stressful situations by planning ahead.
- Lose weight, if necessary.
- When knees or hips are affected, avoid climbing stairs, bending, stooping, or squatting.

situations. Refer to the section on total joint arthroplasty in this chapter.

 Pharmacological

Pharmacological treatment includes the use of aspirin or NSAIDs. Narcotics should be avoided because of the chronic nature of the disease. Steroids may be used and are sometimes injected into a joint to provide immediate relief of pain and to stop the degenerative process temporarily. If the client has vertebral involvement with muscle spasms, cyclobenzaprine hydrochloride (Flexeril) may be given to relax the muscles.

Nursing Management

Encourage clients to maintain a proper weight for height and to practice good posture. Provide rest and heat for the affected joint. Collaborate with physical therapy for muscle-strengthening exercises and self-management skills.

NURSING PROCESS

Assessment

Subjective Data

The client may describe nonspecific symptoms such as general musculoskeletal pain, joint stiffness especially on rising, and joint pain or tenderness. Note weight gain, occupation, and any conditions or situations that may exacerbate the client's joint pain. Some of these situations may include cold weather, overexercising, or extreme fatigue. Assess the client's understanding of the disease and its effect on lifestyle and ability to perform activities of daily and social living.

Objective Data

This includes edema and tenderness around the joints and bony enlargements of distal interphalangeal joints (Heberden's nodes).

Nursing diagnoses for a client with osteoarthritis may include the following:

Nursing Diagnoses	Planning/Goals	Nursing Interventions
*Chronic **P**ain* related to joint tenderness and edema	The client will express minimal discomfort.	Handle the affected extremity gently and apply heat as ordered. Administer prescribed analgesic and evaluate its effectiveness.
*Impaired Physical **M**obility* related to joint deterioration	The client will maintain mobility within the parameters of the disease process.	Coordinate with physical therapy and assist in a planned exercise program as ordered. Advise the client to plan rest periods during the day.

Evaluation Each goal must be evaluated to determine how it has been met by the client.

TOTAL JOINT ARTHROPLASTY

Joint replacement or **arthroplasty** is the replacement of both articular surfaces within a joint capsule. The hip, knee, shoulder, and fingers are the joints most frequently replaced. Replacements consist of metal and polyethylene and may be cemented in the prepared bone with methyl methacrylate, which has properties similar to bone. See Figure 37-13 for knee and hip replacement components.

Newer techniques use porous-coated cementless artificial joint components. These allow bone to grow into the joint component and securely fix the prosthesis. This reduces the incidence of prosthesis failure. Joint replacement is usually an elective procedure, and clients may wish to have autologous blood transfusions whereby they predonate their own blood in case a blood transfusion is needed.

Total Hip Replacement

Total hip replacement is the replacement of a severely damaged hip with an artificial joint. This procedure is usually reserved for clients older than age 60

Figure 37-13 A, *Total hip and knee replacement;* **B,** *Radiograph of a total knee replacement (anterior-posterior view). Because the patella is plastic, it is not visible here.*

with severe pain or irreversibly damaged hip joints; however, with improved prosthetic materials and operative techniques, younger clients with severely damaged hips are being considered for total hip replacement surgery. Potential problems with the hip replacement include dislocation of the prosthesis, excessive wound drainage, and infection.

Following a total hip replacement, the client's hip and leg should be kept in a position of abduction and extension. The knees are kept apart by using foam wedges, several pillows, or an abductor pillow. The client may lie on the unaffected side. When the client turns from the back to a side-lying position, the entire leg should be supported with pillows to keep the hip abducted. The client should be instructed to avoid acute flexion of the hip. The legs should not be crossed nor the hips flexed to pull up a blanket or sheet. A fracture bedpan should be used until the client can ambulate to the bathroom. Use a raised toilet seat in the bathroom. Any specific client turning, movement, and positioning will be ordered by the physician. Vital signs and circulation, movement, and sensation (CMS) checks are done routinely.

Inspect the dressings frequently. If the surgical site is drained with a portable suction device, monitor it for patency and the type and amount of drainage. Initially, drainage might be 200 to 500 cc. Within 48 hours, the drainage should decrease to 30 cc or less and the suction device can be removed.

The goal for clients who have total hip or knee joint replacement is to ambulate independently. Ambulatory activity progresses rapidly for clients with joint replacement. Clients who have total hip replacement are usually out of bed the night of surgery or early the next day. Gait training may begin with the use of a walker and progress to the use of crutches or a cane. The client should avoid hip flexion of more than 90 degrees and stair climbing for at least 3 months.

Total Knee Replacement

Total knee replacement, like the hip replacement, is considered for clients experiencing severe pain and functional disability related to joint destruction. The prosthesis chosen for the replacement provides the client with a painless, stable, and functional joint. Following total knee replacement surgery, clients may use a continuous passive motion (CPM) machine. This machine helps increase circulation to the operative area and promotes flexibility within the knee joint. The surgeon orders the frequency of use and the amount of tension, flexion, and extension produced by the machine.

Following knee arthroplasty, the client's knee may be immobilized with a firm compression dressing and an adjustable soft knee immobilizer. The client may transfer out of bed to a wheelchair with the immobilizer in place. No weight bearing is allowed on the knee until it is prescribed by the surgeon. If ordered, a sequential compression device (SCD) may be used or antiembolism stockings worn to minimize the development of thrombophlebitis.

Rehabilitation generally starts the second day for clients who have total knee arthroplasty. When the client sits in a chair, the knee should be elevated. Ambulation with assistive aids and weight-bearing limits is usually started 1 to 2 days after surgery.

Nursing Management

Perform neurovascular assessment of the affected extremity as well as incision assessment, vital signs, lung sounds, pedal pulses, and I&O. Maintain the client's hip in a position of abduction and extension for 6 to 10 days as ordered. Keep client's skin and bed dry and clean. Encourage the client to cough and deep breathe and to use the trapeze to raise hips off the bed for bedpan use.

NURSING PROCESS

Assessment

Subjective Data

Assess for irritability, restlessness, orientation, and neurovascular assessment of the affected extremity for pain, numbness, tingling, and paresthesia.

Objective Data

Assess the incision for approximation, redness, and drainage and the skin over all bony prominences. Assess for tachypnea, dyspnea, hypoxemia, and crackles and wheezes in the lungs (signs of fat embolism). Vital signs, pedal pulses, and I&O are also assessed.

The client with a total hip replacement should be assessed for position of the affected hip. The hip should be maintained in a position of abduction and extension. The most prominent symptom of a dislocation is a clicking, popping sound. Other symptoms are a sudden sharp pain that is unrelieved by narcotic analgesics, loss of leg motion, and edema of the affected hip. The client should not be moved and the physician should be notified immediately.

Assessment of the client with a total knee replacement includes the neurovascular status of the leg, the dressing and drainage device, keeping the knee elevated, and monitoring the CPM machine. Vital signs, intake and output, and the color and temperature of the extremity are also assessed.

Nursing diagnoses for a client undergoing arthroplasty surgery may include the following:

Nursing Diagnoses	Planning/Goals	Nursing Interventions
Impaired **S**kin Integrity related to immobility and surgical incision	The client's skin will remain free from redness or any other signs of breakdown.	Maintain a clean and dry dressing. If a drainage device is used, assess functioning. Keep client's skin and bed clean and dry. Assess bony prominences for redness. Provide high-protein diet with dairy products and vitamin C.
Impaired Physical **M**obility related to surgery	The client will ambulate following physician's direction.	Keep hip in a position of abduction. Use an abductor pillow or wedge to maintain the position when turning the client. Encourage client to use the trapeze to raise hips off the bed to use the bedpan. Assist the client in accomplishing activities of daily living.
Ineffective **T**issue Perfusion (Peripheral) related to surgery and immobility	The client will have adequate circulation of extremity.	Encourage the client to cough and deep breathe. Monitor vital signs until stable. Assess pedal pulses and capillary refill in both extremities.

Evaluation Each goal must be evaluated to determine how it has been met by the client.

MUSCULOSKELETAL DISORDERS

Musculoskeletal disorders discussed include amputations, temporomandibular joint disease/disorder, and carpal tunnel syndrome.

AMPUTATIONS

An **amputation** is the removal of all or part of an extremity. Amputations are done in response to injuries resulting in extensive laceration of arteries or nerves, or diseases such as malignant tumors, infections, and peripheral vascular disorders. Other disease conditions that may require amputation include extensive osteomyelitis or congenital disorders. In severe trauma situations, an amputation may be done to save the client's life.

Recent advances in microsurgical techniques have allowed replantation (limb reattachment) in some injuries. These procedures involve the use of microscopes and highly specialized instruments to reconnect severed nerves and blood vessels. Amputations involving the hand or wrist are more likely to be considered for replantation rather than an injury involving a large muscle mass because of extensive tissue, bone, and muscle damage. Any amputation creates a major physical and psychological adjustment for the client.

Medical–Surgical Management

Medical

Rehabilitation for the client with an amputation requires the effort of the entire rehabilitation team. The client's physical and psychological responses to the amputation are monitored by all members of the team. If appropriate, counseling and job training will enable many clients to return to their jobs.

Surgical

Before surgery, the surgeon must evaluate the client and make several decisions. These decisions include necessity of an amputation, type of amputation (open or closed), level of amputation, potential for rehabilitation, and type of prosthesis and rehabilitation program.

The surgeon will try to save as much of the limb as possible. A closed amputation is done by using skin flaps to cover the bone end of the extremity. This type of amputation is done when there is no evidence of infection. Sometimes a Guillotine (open) amputation is necessary. This amputation requires a straight cut and allows for free drainage of infectious material. Tissue, bone, and vessels are severed at the same level without skin flaps. The major indication for doing an open amputation is infection.

The level of an amputation is determined by the vascular supply and is never higher than absolutely necessary. If the blood flow at the site of the incision is normal, the amputation is performed at that level. If the bleeding is scant, a higher level of amputation is performed to ensure adequate postoperative healing.

Pharmacological

Narcotic analgesics may be required immediately following surgery. After several days, pain may be controlled with nonnarcotic analgesics. If infection exists, appropriate antibiotic therapy will be ordered.

Diet

A balanced diet with adequate vitamins and protein is essential for adequate wound healing. Many elderly clients are poorly nourished or require special diets. Nutritional care plans should be discussed with the physician and a dietitian.

Activity

Postoperative positioning of the stump will be determined by the surgeon. The stump may be placed in an extended position or elevated on pillows for short periods. Encourage the client to spend some time in the prone position. This position helps stretch the flexor muscles and prevents contractions of the hip. One to two days following surgery, the client may begin bed exercises. These exercises, taught by the physical therapist, are done to pre-

CRITICAL THINKING

Phantom Limb Pain
How would you explain phantom limb pain to a client?

vent contractures and increase muscle strength. Ambulation begins in physical therapy after transfer techniques are learned by the client. Ambulation progresses according to whether the client is to be fitted with a prosthesis immediately or at a later time.

Nursing Management

Perform routine postoperative care by encouraging deep breathing, coughing, and turning; assessing pain on a 1 to 10 scale; and administering analgesics as ordered. Encourage client to eat a balanced diet with extra protein for wound healing. Collaborate with physical therapy regarding bed exercises, transfer techniques, and later ambulation.

NURSING PROCESS

Assessment

Subjective Data

This should include pain, sensations felt on the extremity to be amputated, and the emotional status of the client. If a client has experienced chronic pain before the amputation, pain may seem mild following the surgery. Severe pain may indicate a hematoma or excessive pressure from a cast or elastic bandage on a bony prominence. The client may confuse **phantom limb pain** with the incisional pain. Phantom limb pain is the sensation that there is pain, soreness, tingling, burning, stiffness in the amputated limb. These sensations are thought to be caused by the sensory capacity from the missing limb remaining in the brain. Phantom pain will decrease as inflammation subsides at the incisional site.

Objective Data

This includes the color and temperature of the skin, pulse, and responses to limb movement. The unaffected extremity should also be assessed for function and circulation.

Nursing diagnoses for a client who has an amputation may include the following:

Nursing Diagnoses	Planning/Goals	Nursing Interventions
Impaired **S**kin Integrity related to amputation	The client will remain free from infection.	Inspect the incision for any inflammation, excessive drainage, edema, increased pain, and hypersensitivity to touch. Use aseptic technique for all dressing changes. Monitor vital signs.

continues

Nursing Diagnoses	Planning/Goals	Nursing Interventions
Disturbed Body Image related to loss of limb	The client will participate in the care of the residual limb.	Handle the residual limb gently and treat it as though a prosthesis will be worn. Encourage client to watch dressing change and eventually assist with and do the dressing changes. Encourage the client to express feelings and concerns about the amputation.
Impaired Physical Mobility related to loss of limb	The client will demonstrate improved physical mobility.	Encourage the client to participate in physical therapy and to perform ROM exercises. Assist the client when ambulating with assistive devices.

Evaluation Each goal must be evaluated to determine how it has been met by the client.

SAMPLE NURSING CARE PLAN

THE CLIENT WITH A BELOW-THE-KNEE AMPUTATION

Mrs. Spencer is a 76-year-old resident in a retirement home. She has remained active since her retirement from the secretarial job she held for 20 years. Her health history indicates she has had circulatory problems with inadequate peripheral circulation resulting from atherosclerosis. Her physician has hospitalized her for a planned below-the-knee amputation on the left leg and has ordered an arteriogram to assist in determining the site for the amputation. The arteriogram will help determine the circulatory status of her leg necessary to promote wound healing.

The nurse's assessment of Mrs. Spencer's vital signs indicated B/P 120/68, pulse 72, and respirations 18. Femoral pulses were present in both extremities; however, the pedal pulse in her left foot was barely palpable, and the skin was cool and pale. She stated that lately her left foot is always cold and is a bluish-black color. Mrs. Spencer has expressed concern about her ability to take care of herself after she loses her foot.

Nursing Diagnosis 1 *Disturbed Body Image* related to scheduled amputation as evidenced by statement of concern over losing foot

Nursing Outcomes Classification (NOC)
Acceptance: Health Status
Psychosocial Adjustment: Life Change

Nursing Interventions Classification (NIC)
Body Image Enhancement
Amputation Care

PLANNING/GOALS	NURSING INTERVENTIONS	RATIONALE
Mrs. Spencer will communicate her concerns and feelings about the changes in her body image.	Involve Mrs. Spencer in participating in her daily care.	Gives sense of independence.
	Encourage Mrs. Spencer to voice her concerns.	Helps resolve concerns.
	Provide positive reinforcement when Mrs. Spencer attempts to adapt to body changes.	Encourages her to continue adapting.

EVALUATION   Mrs. Spencer has demonstrated beginning acceptance of body changes by taking an active interest in her appearance.

Nursing Diagnosis 2 *Situational Low Self-Esteem* related to loss of body part as evidenced by expression of concern about ability to care for self

continues

SAMPLE NURSING CARE PLAN

Nursing Outcomes Classification (NOC)
Psychosocial Adjustment: Life Change
Role Performance

Nursing Interventions Classification (NIC)
Self-Esteem Enhancement
Support System Enhancement

PLANNING/GOALS	NURSING INTERVENTIONS	RATIONALE
Mrs. Spencer will identify at least two positive qualities about herself.	Encourage Mrs. Spencer to express her feelings about herself.	Helps Mrs. Spencer identify positive qualities.
	Involve Mrs. Spencer in decision-making regarding her care.	Helps Mrs. Spencer maintain a sense of control over her life.
	Provide Mrs. Spencer with positive feedback.	Gives Mrs. Spencer a feeling of approval.

EVALUATION   Mrs. Spencer has voiced two positive qualities about herself.

Nursing Diagnosis 3 *Anticipatory* **Grieving** related to loss associated with amputation as evidenced by her expression of concern

Nursing Outcomes Classification (NOC)
Psychosocial Adjustment: Life Change
Coping

Nursing Interventions Classification (NIC)
Grief Work Facilitation
Emotional Suppor

PLANNING/GOALS	NURSING INTERVENTIONS	RATIONALE
Mrs. Spencer will express her feelings about the loss of her foot.	Encourage Mrs. Spencer to express her feelings by talking, crying, writing.	Gives several options for expression.
	Spend a specific amount of nonnursing time each shift with Mrs. Spencer to allow for uninterrupted conversation.	Allows expression of feelings and shows concern and understanding.
	Inform Mrs. Spencer and her family about support groups and organizations in the community.	May help Mrs. Spencer find new ways of adapting to loss.

EVALUATION   Mrs. Spencer expresses feelings about her potential loss.

Nursing Diagnosis 4 *Deficient* **Knowledge** related to postoperative care and activity as evidenced by concern about ability to care for self

Nursing Outcomes Classification (NOC)
Knowledge: Treatment Regimen

Nursing Interventions Classification (NIC)
Teaching: Procedure/Treatment

PLANNING/GOALS	NURSING INTERVENTIONS	RATIONALE
Mrs. Spencer will perform stump wrapping correctly.	Encourage Mrs. Spencer to participate in the care of the residual limb.	Helps client adjust to body changes.
	Demonstrate how to wrap her stump, then allow her to do it several times.	Helps client to know how to take care of themselves.

EVALUATION   Mrs. Spencer demonstrated the ability to care for the residual limb by wrapping the stump correctly.

TEMPOROMANDIBULAR JOINT DISEASE/DISORDER

Temporomandibular joint disease/disorder (TMD) is commonly referred to as TMJ. It is a collection of conditions affecting the temporomandibular joint and/or the muscles of mastication. More than 10 million people in the United States have TMD. It affects both males and females, but 90% of those seeking treatment are females between puberty and menopause (The TMJ Association, 2002).

The temporomandibular joint is the articular surface between the mandible and temporal bone of the skull. It is a combined hinge and gliding joint. Normally, the mandible moves smoothly, appears symmetrical, and is without deformity. Causes for TMD include trauma, stress, teeth clenching or grinding **(bruxism),** and joint diseases such as rheumatoid arthritis or osteoarthritis. Common symptoms of TMD include limited jaw movement, clicking or crepitus when the jaw moves, popping when chewing or talking, and radiating pain in the face, neck, or shoulders. The clicking is caused by displaced cartilage. The jaw may lock as a result of muscle spasms.

Diagnosis of TMD may include an x-ray to evaluate the bony structure, a CT scan to evaluate any degenerative changes, an MRI or arthrography, and an evaluation of the teeth and jaw in a bite position. Nursing assessment of the joint includes movement and appearance. If the mandible protrudes, it may indicate a mandibular dislocation.

Medical–Surgical Management

Medical

Medical management consists of moist heat to promote muscle relaxation, cold therapy to reduce muscle spasms, and analgesics or nonsteroidal antiinflammatory drugs. Clients may be fitted with a dental retainer or bite plate to prevent teeth clenching or grinding, or splints to help realign malocclusions.

Surgical

Procedures such as arthroscopy or surgery to reshape the joint may be done in some cases that do not respond to medical treatment.

Diet

A soft diet allows the jaw and muscles to relax. Clients should be advised against chewing gum.

Nursing Management

Encourage clients to practice relaxation techniques. Advise client to see a dentist for an evaluation of the teeth and jaw and to use the dental retainer or bite plate if given one.

CARPAL TUNNEL SYNDROME

Carpal tunnel syndrome occurs when the median nerve in the wrist is compressed by inflamed, edematous

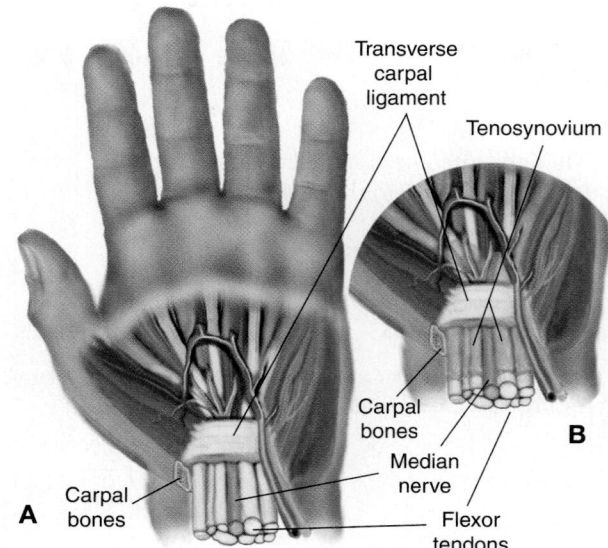

Figure 37-14 *Carpal Tunnel Syndrome:* **A,** *Cross-section of carpal tunnel showing nerves and tendons;* **B,** *Inflamed flexor tendons and tenosynovium put pressure on the median nerve.*

flexor tendons and tenosynovium (Figure 37-14). Symptoms include pain, paresthesia, and weakness of the thumb, index, middle and part of ring fingers but never the little finger. Persons performing assembly line work are especially at risk. Assemblers are three times more likely to have carpal tunnel than data-entry personnel (NINDS, 2002). Arthritis or fractures may also be a cause. Diagnosis is based on a physical examination and the subjective symptoms of the client and may be confirmed by motor nerve velocity studies.

Medical–Surgical Management

Medical

Treatment consists of rest for the hands. Splints to immobilize the hand and wrist may also be used to help relieve some of the discomfort.

Surgical

If conservative treatment does not control the symptoms, surgery may be necessary to relieve the pressure on the median nerve. After surgery, the hand is elevated and may be in a splint for up to 2 weeks. Lifting is restricted for several weeks.

Pharmacological

Anti-inflammatory drugs may decrease inflammation and edema and reduce symptoms. NSAIDs may provide pain relief. If symptoms are not controlled with these measures, cortisone may be injected into the carpal tunnel.

Nursing Management

Encourage clients performing repetitive hand movements to take rest periods from the task.

NURSING PROCESS

Assessment

Subjective Data

This consists of the client's description of tingling in the hands and numbness in the thumb, index, middle and part of the ring fingers. The client may also state that there is a feeling of "puffiness" in the affected hand and that the client is unable to grasp or hold small objects. Waking in the middle of the night with pain and a feeling that the entire hand is asleep is very common.

Objective Data

This may include atrophy of the padded area at the base of the thumb.

Nursing diagnoses for a client with carpal tunnel syndrome may include the following:

Nursing Diagnoses	Planning/Goals	Nursing Interventions
Acute Pain related to inflammation and swelling causing pressure on the median nerve	The client will have less discomfort.	Administer analgesics as ordered and teach client about use, side effects, and dosage. Encourage client to wear wrist brace. Encourage client to refrain from repetitive hand movements.
Risk for Disuse Syndrome related to tingling and numbness of hand and wrist	The client will use fingers and hand.	Teach client to do ROM exercises, and to prevent twisting and turning of wrist.

Evaluation Each goal must be evaluated to determine how it has been met by the client.

SYSTEMIC DISORDERS WITH MUSCULOSKELETAL MANIFESTATIONS

Disorders discussed following include gout and lyme disease.

GOUT

Gout is a metabolic disease of ineffective purine metabolism resulting in deposits of needlelike crystals of uric acid in connective tissue, joint spaces, or both. Middle-aged men are most commonly affected, but it may occur in women after menopause. Gout may be primary (an inherited problem with purine metabolism), secondary (complication from another disease or from use of certain drugs), or idiopathic (unknown cause). Up to 18% of clients with gout have a family history of the disease (NIAMS, 2002b). The excessive use of alcohol interferes with uric acid removal from the body and may contribute to or exacerbate symptoms.

The attack generally begins abruptly with severe constant pain. The joint becomes swollen, red, and tender. The great toe is the joint most frequently involved; however, any joint may be affected. The course of gout is variable, with one to two attacks being severe. If the disease is untreated, the attacks may occur with increasing frequency. Clients with symptoms of gout develop **tophi**, which are subcutaneous nodular deposits of sodium urate crystals appearing in various parts of the body, including the rim of the ears, the knuckles, and great toe. Diagnosis is made from the client's health history and an examination of the affected joint. Aspiration of the joint synovial fluid may show urate crystals. The client should be instructed to avoid foods high in purine, such as liver, sardines, sweetbreads, anchovies, gravies, and asparagus. Oral fluid intake should be increased to 3,000 mL per day to reduce the possibility of urate stone formation in the kidneys.

To reduce inflammation, NSAIDs are given, especially indomethacin (Indocin) and naproxen (Anaprox, Naprosyn). Colchicine may be used if NSAIDs are ineffective. When tophi develop, medicine to reduce hyperuricemia may be used, such as allopurinol (Zyloprim) and probenecid (Benemid).

LYME DISEASE

Lyme disease is caused by a spirochete *Borrelia burgdorferi* carried by deer ticks. In the United States it has been reported in nearly all states, but most cases are in the coastal northeast, mid-Atlantic states, Minnesota, and northern California (National Institute of Allergies and Infectious Diseases [NIAID], 1999).

These ticks should be removed by using a tweezers. Early manifestations occur from spring through late fall. People living in states with a high incidence of Lyme disease should wear protective clothing and check for ticks frequently. Insect repellent containing DEET should be applied to exposed parts of the body and to clothing. Household pets should wear a flea and tick collar or be given monthly preventive medication and also be checked frequently for ticks.

For most individuals, the first symptom is a red rash called erythema migrans. It starts as a red spot at the site of the tick bite and expands, resembling a bull's eye. Other symptoms are headache, neck stiffness, fever, and pain. For those individuals untreated with antibiotics, arthritis (joint swelling and pain), fatigue, and neurological abnormalities such as facial palsy, meningitis, and encephalitis become evident. The antibody test ELISA is used to identify antibodies to *B. burgdorferi* in blood or spinal fluid specimens. Antibiotics such as doxycycline (Vibramycin), cefuroxime exetil (Ceftin), or amoxicillin (Amoxil) speed healing of the rash and may prevent arthritis and neurologic symptoms.

- Compartment syndrome is a serious form of neurovascular impairment. Symptoms include severe pain that is not relieved with narcotic analgesics, sluggish capillary refill, weak pulses, numbness, and paralysis.
- When a client is in traction, it is important to remember to preserve body alignment, maintain continuous pull and countertraction, keep the ropes moving freely through the pulleys, use the prescribed amount of weights, and keep the weights hanging freely.
- Osteoarthritis is characterized by slow progressive degeneration of joint articular cartilage.
- Hips, knees, and fingers are the joints most frequently considered for replacement.
- Following total hip replacement, the hip should be kept in a position of abduction and extension.
- Following total knee replacement surgery, some clients may use a CPM machine that promotes knee joint flexibility and increased circulation to the operative area.
- Individuals at greatest risk for developing osteoporosis are postmenopausal women and older adults who are generally inactive.

Summary

- When assessing the client with a musculoskeletal disorder, the nurse should evaluate any changes in appearance, including alignment, loss of motion, and any signs of circulatory impairment.
- Treatment of a fracture may include any one or more of the following methods: closed reduction, open reduction that may include internal fixation, casts, and traction.

Review Questions

1. The primary goal in the treatment of a fracture is to:
   a. aid in the formation of osteoclasts.
   b. aid in the formation of granulation tissue.
   c. establish a callus between the broken ends of bone.
   d. prevent further injury to the fractured limb.

CASE STUDY

George Ellis, a 40-year-old truck driver, was getting ready to help unload his cargo. He was climbing into the truck when he lost his balance and fell to the ground, twisting his left leg. He stated he was in severe pain and was unable to stand. His coworkers called the emergency ambulance service to transport him to the hospital. Upon arrival in the emergency room, the nurse immediately took Mr. Ellis's vital signs, which were temperature 98.6°F, pulse 92, respirations 24, and blood pressure 158/90. The nurse also noted that Mr. Ellis's face was flushed and his left leg was shorter than his right.

The following questions will guide your development of a nursing care plan for the case study.

1. List five types of fractures.
2. Based on the action of the fall, what type of fracture do you think Mr. Ellis may have received?
3. What diagnostic measures will determine whether or not Mr. Ellis has a fracture of his left leg?
4. What immediate care should have been given to Mr. Ellis?
5. List four nursing interventions for clients in traction.
6. What options may be considered for treatment of Mr. Ellis's injury?
7. List objective and subjective information the nurse would obtain regarding Mr. Ellis's injury.

2. The nurse knows that proper body positioning and alignment of an immobilized client is always maintained to prevent:
   a. scoliosis.
   b. lordosis.
   c. contractures.
   d. atony.

3. One of the first symptoms a client with arthritis may complain of is:
   a. nausea after each meal.
   b. joint stiffness especially on arising.
   c. an increased appetite.
   d. muscle spasms after exercising.

4. Traction is frequently used to treat clients with a musculoskeletal problem. One of the primary reasons for traction is to:
   a. heal a fracture.
   b. maintain a corrected position.
   c. stop muscle spasms.
   d. prevent infection.

5. Osteomyelitis:
   a. affects mainly the hip bone.
   b. is a bacterial infection of the bone.
   c. occurs most often in adults.
   d. causes a great deal of deformity.

References/Suggested Readings

Arthritis Foundation. (2002a). Gout [Online]. Available: www.arthritis.org/conditions/DiseaseCenter/gout.asp

Arthritis Foundation. (2002b). Osteoarthritis. [Online]. Available: www.arthritis.org/conditions/DiseaseCenter/oa.asp

Bailey J. (2003). Getting a fix on orthopedic care. Nursing2003, 33(6), 58–63.

Bryant, G. (2001). Stump care. AJN, 101(2), 67–71.

Burke, S. (2001). Boning up on osteoporosis. Nursing2001, 31(10), 36–42.

Curry, L., & Hogstel, M. (2002). Osteoporosis. AJN, 102(1), 26–32.

D'Arcy, Y. (2002). How to treat arthritis pain. Nursing2002, 32(7), 30–31.

Daniels, R. (2002). Delmar's Guide to Laboratory and Diagnostic Tests. Clifton Park, NY: Thomson Delmar Learning.

Dochterman, J., & Bulechek, G. (2004). Nursing Interventions Classification (NIC) (4th ed.). St. Louis, MO: Mosby.

Estes, M. E. Z. (2002). Health Assessment & Physical Examination (2nd ed.). Clifton Park, NY: Thomson Delmar Learning.

Fort, C. (2002). Getting a fix on long-bone fracture. Nursing2002, 32(6), 32hn1–32hn6.

Fort, C. (2003). How to combat 3 deadly trauma complications. Nursing2003, 33(5), 58–63.

Hayes, D. (2003a). How to wrap an above-the-knee amputation stump. Nursing2003, 33(1), 70.

Hayes, D. (2003b). How to wrap a below-the-knee amputation stump. Nursing2003, 33(2), 28.

Ignatavicius, D. (2002). Catching compartment syndrome early. Nursing2002, 32(11), 10.

Infectious Disease Society of America (IDSA). (2002). Practice guidelines for treatment of Lyme disease. [Online]. Available: www.idsociety.org/newsroom/nr%5Flymepg.htm

Lawrence, B., & Tasota, F. (2003). Detecting neuromuscular problems with electromyography. Nursing2003, 33(4), 82.

Leslie, M. (2000). When the ache is not arthritis. RN, 63(3), 38–40.

Lewis, A. M. (1999). Orthopedic and vascular emergencies. Nursing99, 29(12), 54–56.

Lindgren, V. (2003). When to suspect this bone disorder. RN, 66(6), 32–36.

McClung, B. (2001). Reducing your risk of osteoporosis. A Guide to Women's Health (supplement to Nursing2001), April, 4–8.

McConnell, E. (2001). Myth & facts . . . about gout. Nursing2001, 31(5), 73.

McConnell, E. (2002a). Assessing neurovascular status in a casted limb. Nursing2002, 32(9), 20.

McConnell, E. (2002b). Myths & facts . . . about compartment syndrome. Nursing2002, 32(2), 92.

Moorhead, S., Johnson, M., & Maas, M. (2004). Nursing Outcomes Classification (NOC) (3rd ed.). St. Louis, MO: Mosby.

National Institute of Allergies and Infectious Diseases (NIAID). (1999). Lyme disease [Online]. Available: www.niaid.nih.gov/publications/lyme

National Institute of Arthritis and Musculoskeletal and Skin Diseases (NIAMS). (2000). Osteoporosis: Progress and promise [Online]. Available: www.niams.nih.gov/hi/topics/osteoporosis/opbkgr/htm

National Institute of Arthritis and Musculoskeletal and Skin Diseases (NIAMS). (2002a). Osteoarthritis [Online]. Available: www.niams.nih.gov/hi/topics/arthritis/oahandout.htm

National Institute of Arthritis and Musculoskeletal and Skin Diseases (NIAMS). (2002b). Questions and answers about gout [Online]. Available: www.niams.nih.gov/hi/topics/gout/gout/htm

National Institute of Neurological Disorders and Stroke (NINDS). (2002). Carpal tunnel syndrome fact sheet [Online]. Available: www.ninds.nih.gov/health_and_medical/pubs/carpal_tunnel.htm

National Osteoporosis Foundation (NOF). (2002a). Bone health [Online]. Available: www.nof.org/osteoporosis/bonehealth.htm

National Osteoporosis Foundation (NOF). (2002b). Bone mass measurement [Online]. Available: www.nof.org/osteoporosis/bonemass.htm

National Osteoporosis Foundation (NOF). (2002c). Osteoporosis: Fast facts [Online]. Available: www.nof.org/osteoporosis/stats.htm

National Osteoporosis Foundation (NOF). (2002d). Men and osteoporosis [Online]. Available: www.nof.org/men/index.htm

National Osteoporosis Foundation (NOF). (2002e). Prevention: Four steps to prevention [Online]. Available: www.nof.org/prevention/index.htm

North American Nursing Diagnosis Association. (2003). Nursing Diagnoses: Definitions & Classification 2003–2004. Philadelphia: Author.

O'Hanlon-Nichols, T. (1998). Basic assessment series: Musculoskeletal system. AJN, 98(6), 48–52.

Overdorf, J., Pachuki-Hyde, L., Kressenick, C., McClung, B., & Lucasey, C. (2001). Osteoporosis: There's so much we can do. RN, 64(12), 30–34.

Pauldine, E. (2003). Taking a bite out of Lyme disease. Nursing2003, 33(4), 49–52.

Preboth, M. (2001). Lyme disease: New guidelines. *American Family Physician, 63*(10), 2065–2067.

Rogers, D. (2003). New meaning for safe sex. *RN, 66*(1), 38–41.

Rupert, S. (2002). Pathogenesis and treatment of rhabdomyolysis. *Journal of the American Academy of Nurse Practitioners, 14*(2), 82.

Sauret, J. M., Marinides, G., & Wang, G. K. (2002). Rhabdomyolysis. *American Family Physician, 65*(1), 907.

Spratto, G., & Woods, A. (2004). *2004 PDR Nurses' Drug Handbook.* Clifton Park, NY: Thomson Delmar Learning.

Sullivan, M. P., & Sharts-Hopko, N. C. (2000). Preventing the downward spiral. *AJN, 100*(8), 26–31.

The TMJ Association. (2002). *Changing the face of TMJ* [Online]. Available: www.tmj.org/basics.usp

Wade, C. F. (2000). Keeping lyme disease at bay. *AJN, 100*(7), 26–31.

Walls, M. (2002). Orthopedic trauma. *RN, 65*(7), 52–56.

Yarnold, B. (1999). Hip fracture. *AJN, 99*(2), 36–40.

Resources

American Occupational Therapy Association, Inc., 4720 Montgomery Lane, P.O. Box 31220, Bethesda, MD 20824-1220, 301-652-2682, www.aota.org

American Physical Therapy Association, 1111 North Fairfax Street, Alexandria, VA 22314, 703-684-2782, Fax 703-684-2782, 800-999-2782, www.apta.org

Arthritis Foundation, P. O. Box 7669, Atlanta, GA 30357, 800-283-7800, www.arthritis.org

National Amputation Foundation, 40 Church Street, Malverne, NY 11565, 516-887-3600, www.nationalamputationfoundation.org

National Institute of Arthritis and Musculoskeletal and Skin Diseases (NIAMS), NIAMS/National Institutes of Health, 1 AMS Circle, Bethesda, MD 20892, 301-495-4484, www.niams.nih.gov

National Osteoporosis Foundation, 1232 22nd Street N.W., Washington, DC 20037-1292, 202-223-2226, www.nof.org

Osteoporosis and Related Bone Diseases, National Resource Center, 1232 22nd Street N.W., Washington, DC 20037-1292, 800-624-2663, www.osteo.org

The TMJ Association, Ltd., P.O. Box 26770, Milwaukee, WI 53226-0770, 414-259-3223, www.tmj.org

NEUROLOGICAL SYSTEM

MAKING THE CONNECTION

Refer to the following chapters to increase your understanding of the neurological system:

Basic Nursing
- **Arenas of Care**
- **Assessment**
- **Diagnostic Tests**

Adult Health Nursing
- **Oncology**
- **Cardiovascular System**
- **Musculoskeletal System**
- **Endocrine System**
- **The Older Adult**

Basic Procedures
- **Performing Passive Range-of-Motion (ROM) Exercises**
- **Ambulation Safety and Assisting from Bed to Walking**
- **Turning and Positioning a Client**
- **Transferring from Bed to Wheelchair, Commode, or Chair**

Review: Delmar's Anatomy & Physiology
  CD-ROM: Nervous System

LEARNING OBJECTIVES

Upon completion of this chapter, you should be able to:
- **Define key terms.**
- **Identify basic functional areas of the human neurological system.**
- **Perform a neurological screening and a basic neurological examination.**
- **Prepare a client for common neurological diagnostic examinations.**
- **Derive a Glasgow Coma Scale score for a client.**
- **Recognize common symptoms of neurological disorders.**
- **Plan interventions for a client with a neurological disorder.**

INTRODUCTION

The human neurological system (called nervous system) is highly complex, controlling and integrating all other body systems. This system controls motor, sensory, and autonomic functions of the body. This is accomplished by coordination and initiation of cellular activity through the transmission of electrical impulses and various hormones.

KEY TERMS

affect
agnosia
anosognosia
aphasia
areflexia
ataxia
aura
automatism
autonomic nervous
  system
bradykinesia
central nervous system
cephalalgia
chorea
copralalia
decerebration
dysarthria
dysphagia
emotional lability
encephalitis
fasciculation
Glasgow Coma Scale
graphesthesia
hemiparesis

hemiplegia
homonymous
  hemianopia
Kernig's sign
meningitis
mentation
neuralgia
neurogenic shock
neurotransmitter
nuchal rigidity
nystagmus
orientation
paraplegia
peripheral nervous
  system
postictal
quadriplegia
sclerotic
somatic nervous system
spinal shock
status epilepticus
stereognosis
unilateral neglect
vertigo

ANATOMY AND PHYSIOLOGY REVIEW

The nervous system is divided into the **central nervous system,** consisting of the brain and spinal cord; the **peripheral nervous system,** which consists of the cranial nerves and spinal nerves; and the **autonomic nervous system,** which is part of the peripheral nervous system and consists of the sympathetic and parasympathetic systems.

Central Nervous System

The central nervous system (CNS) comprises the brain and the spinal cord (Figure 38-1).

The Brain

The brain, composed of gray matter and white matter, controls, initiates, and integrates body functions through the use of electrical impulses and complex molecules. The gray matter, on the outer part of the brain, contains billions of neurons. Neurons, the basic cells of the nervous system, have three major components: the cell body, the axon, and the dendrites (Figure 38-2). The axon carries impulses away from the cell body, and the dendrites carry impulses toward the cell body. The cell body controls the function of the neuron. Functions include the conduction of impulses and the release of neurotransmitters. **Neurotransmitters** are chemical substances that excite, inhibit, or modify the response of another neuron (Hickey, 2002).

Figure 38-1 *The central nervous system includes the brain, spinal cord, and meninges.* **A,** *Structures of the brain;* **B,** *Functional areas of the brain.*

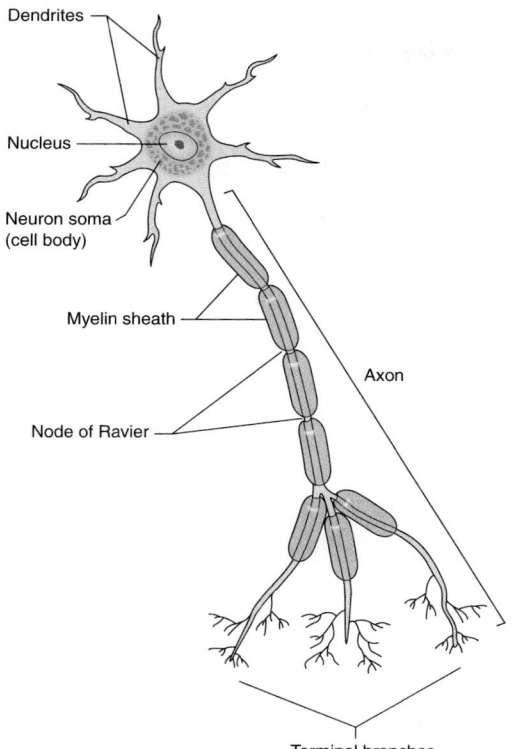

Figure 38-2 *Neuron (Nerve Cell) Structure*

The white matter of the inner structures of the brain contains association and projection pathways that transmit nerve impulses to communicate information to the different areas of the brain. These communication pathways are necessary for integration of brain activity (Hickey, 2002).

The brain is contained within the skull, or cranium, which is a bony, rigid box that protects the brain tissue. There are three coverings of the brain, called meninges. They are the *dura mater, arachnoid mater,* and *pia mater.* These coverings provide protection, support, and small amounts of nourishment. The meninges are separate entities.

The brain is divided into two hemispheres. The right side of the brain receives information from and controls the left side of the body. The left hemisphere receives information from and controls the right side of the body. Both hemispheres of the brain communicate through nerve fibers in the corpus callosum. A predominate hemisphere exists for special tasks so that confusion does not occur. The right side specializes in the perception of physical environment, art, nonverbal communication, music, and spiritual aspects. The left hemisphere generally specializes in analysis, calculation, problem solving, verbal communication, interpretation, language, reading, and writing.

The Spinal Cord

The spinal cord is a continuation of the brainstem. It exits the skull through the *foramen magnum,* an opening in the base of the skull. The spinal cord is approximately 45 centimeters, or 18 inches, in length and is the thickness of one finger. The cord is divided into right and left

halves and has a shallow groove, called the posterior median sulcus, on the dorsal side and a deep groove, called the anterior median fissure, on the ventral side. The cord tapers to a thin tip, called the conus medullaris, at the first lumbar vertebrae, and terminates as a thin cord of connective tissue, called the filum terminale, which continues as far as the second sacral vertebrae (Figure 38-3). The vertebral column provides vertical support for the cord. The meninges cover the spinal cord, providing protection. Reflex activity is initiated within the spinal cord.

There are 31 pairs of spinal nerves originating from the spinal cord. Each pair contains a dorsal, or posterior, nerve root and a ventral, or anterior, nerve root. The dorsal nerve roots carry sensory impulses from the body to the brain; the ventral nerve roots carry motor impulses from the spinal cord to the body. The spinal cord has an H-shaped appearance of gray matter within the white matter. The horns forming the H shape are referred to as the anterior (ventral) horns, the posterior (dorsal) horns, and the lateral horns. These horns contain the cell bodies of neurons that innervate the skeletal muscles.

Cerebrospinal Fluid

Cerebrospinal fluid (CSF) is produced primarily in the choroid plexus. Five hundred milliliters of CSF are produced daily, with excess being reabsorbed by the arachnoid villi in the subarachnoid space. The circulation of CSF is from the lateral ventricles to the third and fourth ventricles. From there, it enters the subarachnoid space to flow around the spinal cord and the brain.

Cerebrospinal fluid absorbs shock and bathes the brain and spinal cord. It contains glucose, protein, urea, and

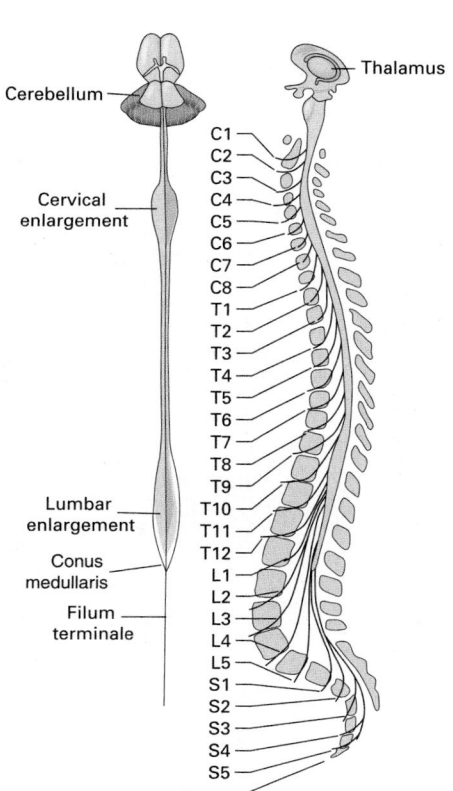

Figure 38-3 *The Spinal Cord*

salts. These nutritive substances are delivered to the CNS cells, and the waste and toxic substances are removed.

Peripheral Nervous System

All of the nerve tissue outside of the CNS is part of the peripheral nervous system (PNS). The PNS consists of the cranial nerves and the spinal nerves and has both sensory and motor components. The PNS can be divided into the **somatic nervous system** and the autonomic nervous system. The somatic portion connects the CNS to the skin and skeletal muscles. It is involved in conscious activities, such as walking. The autonomic portion connects the CNS to visceral organs such as the heart, stomach, intestines, and various glands. It is involved in unconscious activities, such as breathing.

Cranial Nerves

The 12 pairs of cranial nerves have sensory, motor, or mixed functions. Table 38-1 lists functions and describes assessment of cranial nerves. The cranial nerves originate from the brain or brainstem, with most originating from the brainstem. Although always identified by Roman numerals, the cranial nerves also have names.

Spinal Nerves

Thirty-one pairs of spinal nerves exit from the spinal cord through the vertebral column: cervical, 8 pairs; thoracic, 12 pairs; lumbar, 5 pairs; sacral, 5 pairs; and coccyx, 1 pair. The dorsal, or posterior, nerve roots carry sensory impulses to the brain. The ventral, or anterior, nerve roots carry motor impulses from the spinal cord

TABLE 38-1   CRANIAL NERVES

CRANIAL NERVE	FUNCTION	ASSESSMENT	EXPECTED FINDINGS
Olfactory (I)	Sensory: smell	Have client identify smells such as coffee or alcohol, with one nostril occluded; repeat for opposite nostril.	Correct identification of smell or ability to choose smell from a list of choices.
Optic (II)	Sensory: vision	Ask client to read printed material, identify number of fingers held in front of client, or read from Snellen eye chart. Test visual fields by having client identify when the examiner's finger enters visual field.	Vision intact or correctable with lenses. Visual field intact.
Oculomotor (III)	Motor: pupil constriction	Cranial nerves III, IV, and VI are tested together. Inspect for ptosis, or drooping of eyelid. Assess extraocular eye muscles by having client follow the examiner's finger to each quadrant of the visual field. Assess for accommodation by asking the client to look at the examiner's finger held 4 to 6 inches from the client's nose, and then to follow the finger to 18 inches from the client's nose. Ask client about double vision.	Pupils are equal and round and react equally to light. No ptosis or double vision. Eyes move smoothly and consensually inward and downward. As the examiner's finger moves away from the client, the pupil will accommodate by dilating; as the finger moves closer, the pupil will normally constrict.
Trochlear (IV)	Motor: upper eyelid elevation, extraocular eye movement	See oculomotor (III).	Eyes should move smoothly and consensually upward and outward without nystagmus or diplopia.
Trigeminal (V)	Sensory: cornea, nose, and oral mucosa Motor: mastication	Test corneal reflex by lightly touching cornea with a small piece of cotton. Check sensation of face by touching lightly with a cotton ball while the client's eyes are closed and asking the client whether sensation is present. Check motor function by having client clench jaws shut while the examiner palpates the contraction portion of the temporalis and masseter muscles.	Corneal reflex as evidenced by rapid blinking when cotton swept across cornea. Feeling cotton ball on face indicates that facial sensation is intact. Jaw movement symmetrical and able to overcome resistance.
Abducens (VI)	Motor: extraocular eye movement	See oculomotor (III).	Eyes move outward.
Facial (VII)	Motor: facial muscles; Sensory: taste (anterior two-thirds of tongue)	Ask client to smile, show teeth, wrinkle forehead, or whistle. Have client close eyes lightly and keep them closed against the examiner's trying to open them. Have client identify salt and sugar when dabbed on tongue.	Facial movement symmetrical, sense of taste intact.

continues

TABLE 38-1 continued

CRANIAL NERVE	FUNCTION	ASSESSMENT	EXPECTED FINDINGS
Acoustic (VIII)	Sensory: hearing, equilibrium	Assess ability to hear ticking watch or whispered voice. Observe gait for swaying. Perform Romberg test (refer to assessment of motor function).	Sense of hearing intact; no swaying or loss of balance.
Glossopharyngeal (IX)	Sensory: sensation to throat and taste (posterior one-third of tongue) Motor: swallowing	Have client identify taste of salt and sugar on back of tongue. Have client say "ah" and assess for symmetrical position of uvula. Test gag reflex by touching back of pharynx with tongue depressor. Observe swallowing ability and speech patterns.	Taste sensation intact; uvula raises symmetrically; gag reflex intact; swallowing and speech intact.
Vagus (X)	Motor and sensory	Test along with glossopharyngeal nerve.	
Spinal accessory (XI)	Motor: movement of uvula, soft palate, sternocleidomastoid muscle, trapezius muscle	Place examiner's hand on side of client's face and ask client to turn head against resistance; have client shrug shoulders against resistance of the examiner's hand.	Ability to move shoulder and head against resistance.
Hypoglossal (XII)	Motor: tongue movement	Ask client to stick out tongue and observe for symmetry, deviation to side; have client push tongue against tongue depressor and move tongue from side to side.	Tongue should be centrally aligned, able to push against resistance of tongue depressor; no **fasciculations** (involuntary twitching of muscle fibers) should be present.

and brain to the muscles. Motor and sensory impulses are transmitted from the body and internal organs.

Reflex activity is a stereotypical response to a stimulus that is initiated by the nervous system (Hickey, 2002). The three classifications of reflexes are muscle stretch, or deep tendon; superficial, or cutaneous; and pathological (see section on assessment of reflexes). Reflex activity requires the function of five areas in the nervous system: the sensory fibers, the neuron relaying the impulse, the association center in the brain, the neuron relaying the motor impulse from the brain to the body, and the specific organ involved. Disease processes at any of these areas can cause an abnormal reflex response.

Autonomic Nervous System

The main function of the autonomic nervous system (ANS) is to maintain internal homeostasis. There are two subdivisions of the ANS: the sympathetic system and the parasympathetic system. The sympathetic system, activated by stress, prepares the body for the "fight-or-flight" response. The sympathetic system causes increased heart rate, increased blood pressure, vasoconstriction, decreased peristalsis, dilated pupils, increased secretions of epinephrine and sweat, and decreased secretions of digestive juices and saliva (Table 38-2).

The parasympathetic system conserves, restores, and maintains vital body functions, slowing heart rate, in-

creasing gastrointestinal activity, and activating bowel and bladder evacuation.

The sympathetic and parasympathetic systems work antagonistically to regulate the smooth muscles, the heart, and the glands of the body. When one system increases an action, the other system decreases the action. Thus, when one stimulates, the other inhibits; when one dilates, the other one constricts, and so forth. Both systems function simultaneously, but one can dominate the other as needed.

NEUROLOGICAL NURSING ASSESSMENT

A complete health history and a neurological screening assessment allow the nurse to identify areas of dysfunction in order to focus the neurological assessment. Observation (inspection) is necessary for most of the assessment; palpation, auscultation, and percussion are also used.

Health History

A baseline assessment is essential to ascertaining changes in neurological functioning. Any change from the baseline assessment must be identified and early intervention initiated. A thorough health history includes

TABLE 38-2 SYMPATHETIC AND PARASYMPATHETIC RESPONSES

SYSTEM	SYMPATHETIC RESPONSE	PARASYMPATHETIC RESPONSE
Neurological	Pupils dilated Heightened awareness	Pupils normal size
Cardiovascular	Increased heart rate Increased myocardial contractility Increased blood pressure	Decreased heart rate Decreased myocardial contractility Vasodilation
Respiratory	Increased respiratory rate Increased respiratory depth Bronchial constriction	Bronchial relaxation
Gastrointestinal	Decreased gastric motility Decreased gastric secretions Increased glycogenolysis Decreased insulin production Sphincter contraction	Increased gastric motility Increased gastric secretions Sphincter dilatation
Genitourinary	Decreased urine output Decreased renal blood flow	Normal urine output

asking the client about headaches; clumsiness; loss of or change in function of an extremity; seizure activity; numbness or tingling; change in vision; pain; extreme fatigue; personality changes; and mood swings.

Neurological Assessment

The neurological screening involves assessment of level of consciousness and verbal responses to specific questions; selected cranial nerves for eye movement and visual acuity; muscle strength; movement; gait for motor function; and tactile and pain sensation of extremities for sensory screening.

A complete nursing assessment of neurological function includes assessment of the following areas: cerebral function, cranial nerve function, motor function, sensory function, and reflexes. Neurological nursing assessment is discussed in more detail following.

Cerebral Function

Areas of assessment of cerebral function include level of consciousness, mental status, intellectual function, emotional status, pupil reaction, and communication.

Level of Consciousness Level of consciousness is assessed by determining the client's awareness and orientation and is the most important indicator of change in neurological status. **Awareness** is the person's ability to perceive environmental stimuli and body reactions and then respond with thought and action. The client's awareness is assessed through four components: orientation, memory, calculation, and fund of knowledge (Lower, 2002).

LIFE CYCLE CONSIDERATIONS

Neurological Changes with Aging
Remember the following with regard to the elderly client:

- Nerve impulse transmission slows.
- Cardiovascular system changes that lead to a decreased oxygen supply to the brain affect mental acuity, sensory interpretation, and motor ability.
- The amount of neurotransmitters produced diminishes, and the enzyme activity that degrades neurotransmitters increases.
- Changes in neurotransmitters affect sleep, temperature control, and mood.
- The brain tends to atrophy, leaving the cortical bridging veins, which connect the brain to the meninges, vulnerable to trauma and bleeding.

A more objective assessment is made using the **Glasgow Coma Scale,** an objective tool for assessing consciousness in clients, most frequently in clients with head injuries. With the Glasgow Coma Scale, eye opening, verbal response, and motor response are scored using measurable criteria (Table 38-3). The totalled scores indicate coma severity. A score of 15 indicates a fully oriented person. A score of 3 is the lowest possible score, indicating deep coma. A score of 7 or less is considered a state of coma.

TABLE 38-3 GLASGOW COMA SCALE

BEHAVIOR	RESPONSE	SCORE
Eye opening response	Spontaneous	(4)
	To verbal command	3
	To pain	2
	No response	1
Best verbal response	Oriented, conversing	(5)
	Disoriented, conversing	4
	Use of inappropriate words	3
	Incomprehensible sounds	2
	No response	1
Best motor response	Obeys verbal commands	(6)
	Moves to localized pain	5
	Flexion withdrawal to pain	4
	Abnormal posturing— decorticate	3
	Abnormal posturing— decerebrate	2
	No response	1
Total		3 to 15

Test X (handwritten annotations beside Eye opening response, Best verbal response, and Best motor response)

CULTURAL CONSIDERATIONS

Neurological Assessment

- Consider language and cultural norms when performing the mental status assessment.
- An interpreter may be required to ensure that the client understands the questions or directions.

- Adding two numbers, for example, 2 + 6
- Reporting what is on the national news

The nurse determines the client's ability to process thoughts by evaluating the responses to questions such as these. For purposes of comparison, the client's ability to perform these tasks before assessment should be ascertained by asking the family. For example, if the client was math illiterate before the nursing assessment, the client will still not be able to add or subtract.

Emotional Status Emotional status is assessed by observation of the client's **affect** (emotional response or mood). Is affect appropriate for the situation? Is affect labile (prone to rapid change)? Is affect consistent with verbal communication?

Pupil Reaction Size, equality, and roundness of pupils are assessed (Figure 38-4). Size is measured in millimeters. Pupils are evaluated for symmetry of size and for

Changes in the Glasgow Coma Scale indicate changes in client condition. To prevent further damage to the brain in instances of decreasing scores, the nurse must act quickly. The physician must be notified immediately and measures must be taken to decrease intracranial pressure (see section on increased intracranial pressure).

Orientation is the person's awareness of self in relation to person, place, and time. Using open-ended communication techniques, instruct the client to "tell me your first and last name," "tell me the month, day, year and day of the week," "tell me where you are (city, state, hospital)," in order to ascertain the client's level of orientation.

Mental Status Assessment of mental status requires observation of the client's appearance, behavior, posture, mood, gestures, movements, and facial expressions. The nurse compares these behaviors to expected behaviors based on the client's age, health status, educational level, and social position. Mood is assessed by observation and asking the client about moods and feelings.

Intellectual Function Intellectual function is the ability of the brain to perform thought processes. Ability to concentrate, memory function (both long-term and short-term), recall, calculation activities, and fund of knowledge are all aspects of intellectual function.

Nursing assessment of intellectual function involves asking individuals to perform certain tasks, such as the following:

- Repeating a series of numbers, such as 1, 3, 7, 1
- Telling what the individual ate for breakfast

Figure 38-4 A, *Unequal Pupils;* **B,** *Dilated, Fixed Pupils*

reaction to light. The nurse should briefly shine a penlight into the client's eye by passing the light from the outer edge of the eye toward the center of the eye (Figure 38-5). Reaction is assessed as being brisk, sluggish, or nonreactive; consensual reaction (the opposite pupil responding at the same time) is also noted. Accommodation is assessed as described in Table 38-1 under cranial nerve III.

The abbreviation PERRLA is used for documenting pupils that are equal, round, and reactive to light and that demonstrate accommodation. This abbreviation can be used only when pupil reaction is normal. If any part of the assessment is abnormal in one or both eyes, the assessment findings must be written out for clarity.

Communication Both written and oral communication are assessed. Various specialized areas of the nervous system are involved in communication. The inability to communicate verbally, termed **aphasia,** can be caused by the inability to form words or the inability to understand written or spoken words. To assess communication function, various approaches are necessary. Ask the client to follow a simple command such as "Close your eyes." Also use a written card instructing the client to complete a simple task such as "Touch your nose." Note the ability to form words; appropriate use of words; speech patterns, clarity, rate, and flow; and voice modulation. During the health history, ask the client about health care expectations to evaluate the client's ability for verbal expression. Have the client write his name and address on paper to evaluate the ability to write.

Cranial Nerve Function

Cranial nerve function essentially reflects brainstem activity. A complete cranial nerve examination, if required, is usually performed by the physician or advanced-practice nurse.

Motor Function

The neurological screening includes assessment of muscle strength, arm and leg movement, and gait. A complete motor function assessment is performed if a deficit is identified. A complete motor function assessment includes evaluating muscle size, symmetry, tone, and strength; coordination; balance; and posturing.

Muscle Size and Symmetry Muscle size and symmetry are assessed by palpating major muscle groups of the arms and legs and then comparing them to the muscle groups of the opposite side of the body. Unilateral atrophy may indicate a nervous system problem.

Muscle Tone Muscle tone is assessed during palpation of major muscle groups for size and symmetry, while at rest and during passive movement. Muscle tone is described as normal, flaccid, spastic, or rigid. Flaccid muscles are hypotonic, or soft and flabby. Spastic muscles are at first resistant to passive movement, but then release resistance. Rigid muscles may have tremors but are constantly rigid. Rigidity is a more constant state of spasticity, with fewer periods of release of resistance.

Muscle Strength To assess muscle strength, each extremity is placed through passive movement. The client is then asked to move the extremity, first against gravity, by lifting the extremity off the bed, then against resistance, by lifting against slight resistance exerted by the nurse's hand pushing on the extremity. Strength is graded on a scale of 0 to 5 (Table 38-4).

PROFESSIONAL TIP

Assessment of Pupils
To ensure accuracy in assessing direct light reflex and consensual light reflex, the beginning examiner should focus the beam of light a total of four times, twice in each eye.

A

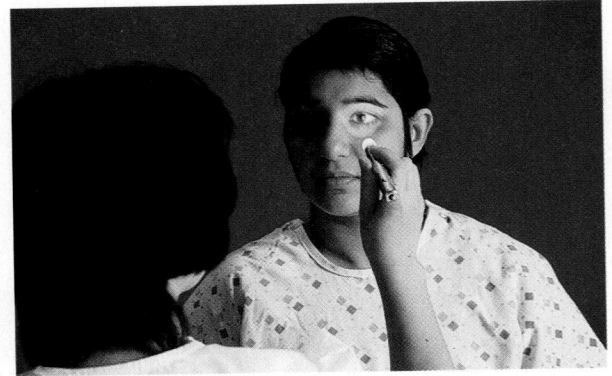

B

Figure 38-5 *Pupil Assessment:* **A,** *Starting position, with penlight to side of pupil;* **B,** *Moving penlight directly in front of pupil*

TABLE 38-4	MUSCLE STRENGTH
SCORE	**DEFINITION**
5/5	Full power of contraction
4/5	Fair or moderate power of contraction
3/5	Just able to overcome force of gravity
2/5	Can move, but cannot overcome power of gravity
1/5	Minimal contractile power
0/5	No movement

Figure 38-6 *Assessment of Coordination: Fingertip-to-Nose Touch*

Figure 38-7 *Assessment of Coordination: Heel Slide*

A

B

Figure 38-8 *Abnormal Posturing:* **A,** *Flexion posturing;* **B,** *Extension posturing (Photo courtesy of John White, Corpus Christi, TX)*

PROFESSIONAL TIP

Assessing Coordination

Ensure that clients who wear eyeglasses have their glasses on before the assessment is performed.

PROFESSIONAL TIP

Assessing Pain and Temperature Sensory Function

- Test upper and lower extremities
- Begin with the upper arms, moving down to the hands; then work from thighs to feet (proximodistal)

Coordination Coordination, a function of the cerebellum, is assessed by asking the client to perform repetitious movement. The client should close her eyes and repeatedly, rapidly touch her own nose with alternate index fingers (Figure 38-6). Lower extremity coordination is assessed by asking the client to run the heel of one foot down the opposite shin, and then repeat with the other heel (Figure 38-7). Inability to perform these movements is termed **ataxia,** incoordination of voluntary muscle action.

Balance Balance is evaluated by using the Romberg test. The client stands with the feet together, arms extended in front, and eyes closed. Balance is observed; a slight swaying is normal.

 Safety: Romberg Test
Always stand in front of the client during the Romberg test, anticipating that the client might fall.

Posturing Abnormal posturing occurs with injury to the motor tract. Two types for which to observe are flexion (formerly decorticate) and extension (formerly decerebrate) posturing (Lower, 2002). Flexion posturing is characterized by flexion of the arms, adduction of the upper extremities, and extension of the lower extremities. Lesions of the cerebral hemispheres or internal structures of the brain cause flexion posturing. Extension posturing is caused by brainstem injury and is characterized by an arcing of the back, backward flexion of the head, adduction and hyperpronation of the arms, and extension of the feet (Figure 38-8).

Abnormal posturing may be present either at all times or in response to stimuli such as loud noises, bright lights, or painful stimuli. The nurse must note whether bilateral or unilateral posturing is present, and, if intermittent, the cause of the posturing. The presence of either type of posturing should be reported at once, because either represents an ominous sign of cerebral dysfunction. Extension posturing represents greater dysfunction than does flexion posturing, and any change from flexion to extension posturing indicates a worsening of condition.

Sensory Function

A subjective examination of sensory function, performed with the client's eyes closed, is generally done only when a dysfunction is suspected. Different pathways are used to transmit different sensory impulses. To evaluate all pathways, the examiner must test tactile sensation, pain and temperature, vibration, proprioception, stereognosis, graphesthesia, and integration of sensations.

Tactile Sensation Tactile sensation is tested by using a cotton ball to lightly touch the client's arms, hands, upper legs, and feet. Comparison is done side to side. The client, with eyes closed, indicates whether the cotton ball is felt.

Pain and Temperature Sensations of pain and temperature are transmitted along the same pathways and are evaluated using a sharp and dull touch. A paper clip or cotton-tipped applicator is used.

Safety: Assessing Pain Sensation
Do not use a safety pin to test pain because skin integrity may be compromised.

Touch the client with the rounded end of a paper clip or cotton-tipped applicator to test for dull sensation, and the pointed end of a paper clip or uncovered end of the applicator to test for sharp sensation. The client's ability to distinguish sharp and dull is noted, again comparing both sides of the body.

Vibration Vibration is tested using a tuning fork. Strike the tuning fork on the palm, holding only the handle, then place the end of the handle first on the client's wrists and then on the ankles and ask whether vibrations are felt (Figure 38-9). The client's eyes should be closed during the test.

Proprioception Proprioception is the sense of joint position in space. With the client's eyes remaining closed, move a joint of the client's finger or extremity up or down in space and ask the client to distinguish the direction of movement of the digit or extremity as being either up or down.

Stereognosis Stereognosis is the ability to recognize an object by feel. Place a familiar object such as a coin or key in the client's hand and ask what the object is. This sensation is a function of the brain, not of the spinal pathways (Figure 38-10).

Graphesthesia Graphesthesia is the ability to identify letters, numbers, or shapes drawn on the skin. Hold the client's hand and, with the stick end of a cotton-tipped applicator or a closed pen, trace an outline on the open palm, ensuring that the letter, number, or shape is right side up for the client (Figure 38-11).

Integration of Sensation Integration of sensation is a higher cortical function. A two-point discrimination test is performed by touching the client simultaneously

Figure 38-11 *Assessment of Graphesthesia*

on opposite sides of the body with a sharp object and asking the client to ascertain the number of objects felt. The normal response is two. If only one is felt, the brain function of integration is abnormal.

Reflexes

Both deep tendon reflexes and superficial reflexes are assessed. Deep tendon reflexes are involuntary contractions of muscles or muscle groups responding to brisk stretching near the insertion site of the muscle (Smeltzer & Bare, 2002). Testing these reflexes is generally the responsibility of the physician or registered nurse, although the LP/VN should be familiar with these assessments, as abnormal reflex responses may be an early indicator of motor or sensory dysfunction.

Superficial, or cutaneous, reflexes are elicited by irritating the skin on the area being assessed. They are diminished or absent with dysfunction of the reflex arc.

The superficial reflex generally assessed is the plantar. To assess the plantar reflex, the handle of the reflex hammer is used to stroke the outer aspect of the sole of the foot from the heel and across the ball of the foot to just below the big toe. Plantar flexion, or curling under of the toes, should occur.

Abnormal Reflexes The absence of deep tendon reflexes in clients is considered an abnormal finding. A fanning of the toes and dorsiflexion of the big toe in response to the assessment of the plantar reflex is called a positive Babinksi's reflex (Figure 38-12). This abnormal response indicates corticospinal disease and is the most important abnormal superficial reflex.

COMMON DIAGNOSTIC TESTS

Commonly used diagnostic tests for clients with symptoms of nervous system disorders are listed in Table 38-5.

HEAD INJURY

Head injuries involve trauma to the scalp, skull, or brain.

Figure 38-9 *Assessment of Vibration*

Figure 38-10 *Assessment of Stereognosis*

Figure 38-12 *Pathologic Reflex: Babinski*

LIFE CYCLE CONSIDERATIONS

Reflexes

The absence of the Achilles reflex in the elderly client is not considered abnormal.

TABLE 38-5	**COMMON DIAGNOSTIC TESTS FOR NERVOUS SYSTEM DISORDERS**

- Lumbar puncture (LP)
- Electroencephalogram (EEG)
- Electromyogram (EMG)
- Imaging procedures: computerized tomography (CT), positron emission tomography (PET), single photon emission computed tomography (SPECT), magnetic resonance imaging (MRI)
- Cerebral angiography
- Brain scan
- Myelogram

SCALP

Scalp injuries bleed profusely because of the abundance of blood vessels in the scalp. As with any break in skin integrity, infection is of major concern. The wound is cleansed and irrigated to remove foreign matter before closing the wound with sutures or butterfly dressings.

SKULL

Skull injuries and fractures of the skull may occur with or without brain injury. A fracture is usually caused by extreme force. Skull fractures are considered closed if the dura mater is intact and open if the dura mater is torn.

The clinical manifestation of skull fracture is localized pain. If the brain is injured, other symptoms may occur.

Types of skull fractures are linear fracture, comminuted fracture, depressed fracture, and basilar fracture. Linear fractures are nondisplaced cracks in the bone. Comminuted fractures occur when the bone is broken into fragments. Depressed fractures have bone fragments pressing into the intracranial cavity. Basilar skull fractures are of the bones in the base of the skull.

Basilar fractures are of particular concern because of the proximity of the fragile sinus bones and the adhesion of the dura mater to this area. The dura mater can easily tear, and CSF can leak from the ears or nose. The internal carotid artery and cranial nerves can also be damaged easily with a basilar skull fracture.

BRAIN

Brain injuries are caused by primary injuries of acceleration–deceleration force, rotational force, or penetrating missile. Acceleration injuries are caused by moving objects striking the head, such as a baseball bat. Deceleration injuries result when the head is moving and strikes a solid object such as a car dashboard. Rotational injuries are hyperextension, hyperflexion, or lateral flexion of the head, which cause twisting of the cerebrum on the brainstem, such as a whiplash injury. Penetrating missile injuries are a direct penetration of an object, such as a bullet, into brain tissue (Thelan, Urden, Lough, & Stacy, 1998).

Open Injury

Skull fractures and penetrating injuries are referred to as open head injuries. Hemorrhaging from the nose, pharynx, or ears; ecchymosis over the mastoid area (Battle's sign); or blood in the conjunctiva may occur in conjunction with open head injuries. Cerebrospinal fluid may leak from the ears or nose. A computed tomography (CT) scan or magnetic resonance imaging (MRI) determines the extent of injury. Neurological deficits depend on the extent and area of injury.

Closed Injury

Closed head injuries are caused by blunt force to the head. Coup injuries are caused by the impact of the head against an object. Contrecoup injuries are caused by the impact of the brain against the opposite side of the skull (Figure 38-13).

Types of closed head injuries are concussion, contusion, and laceration. Concussions are transient neurological deficits caused by shaking the brain. Clinical manifestations may include immediate loss of consciousness lasting from minutes to hours, momentary loss of reflexes, respiratory arrest for several seconds, and amnesia for the period immediately before and after the event. Headaches, drowsiness, confusion, dizziness, irritability, visual disturbances, and unsteady gait may also occur (Hickey, 2002).

Post-concussion syndrome may develop after the injury, as manifested by headache and dizziness. Nervousness, irritability, emotional lability, fatigue, insomnia,

Figure 38-13 *Brain Injuries:* **A,** *Coup/contrecoup;* **B,** *Concussion;* **C,** *Contusion;* **D,** *Epidural hematoma;* **E,** *Subdural hematoma*

loss of **mentation** (ability to concentrate, remember, or think abstractly), and sometimes other neurological deficits occur. This syndrome may last from several weeks up to a year (Hickey, 2002).

Contusions are surface bruises of the brain. Symptoms depend on the area of injury. Frequently, the client is unconscious for a longer period than with a concussion. The client may become conscious only to drift back into unconsciousness. Pulse, blood pressure, and respirations are below normal. Skin is cool and pale.

Cerebral edema may occur with widespread injury (see section on cerebral edema).

Return of consciousness may be followed by cerebral irritability to stimuli. Headache and dizziness may be present for an indefinite period. Permanent damage may cause either changes in mental function or seizure disorders. Prognosis ranges from full recovery to death.

Cerebral laceration is the tearing of cortical tissue. Symptoms of brainstem injury include deep coma from time of impact, extension posturing, autonomic dysfunction, nonreactive pupils, and respiratory difficulty. The ability to relay nerve impulses from high levels in the brain is lost. Diffuse axonal injury (DAI) usually occurs in conjunction with brainstem injuries. This widespread damage to nerve cells in the white matter of the brain causes immediate coma, extension posturing, and increased intracranial pressure.

Hemorrhage

Intracranial hemorrhage is a common complication of any head injury. Bleeding may occur in the epidural space, subdural space, subarachnoid space, or ventricles or intracerebrally. Neurological change is caused by pressure on the brain resulting from the space-occupying hemorrhage. With epidural hematoma (bleeding in the epidural space), momentary unconsciousness is followed by a conscious state of a few hours to a week, depending on the rapidity of the bleeding. As the bleeding continues, neurological status begins to deteriorate, with decreasing level of consciousness; headache; seizures; hemiparesis; **decerebration** (severing spinal cord); and dilated, fixed pupils. Treatment is surgery to evacuate the hematoma, stop the bleeding, and relieve pressure on the brain.

Subdural hematomas (bleeding in the subdural space) cause immediate pressure on the brain. Subdural hematomas are acute (within 48 hours of injury), subacute (from 2 to 14 days following injury), or chronic (from 2 weeks to months following injury). Common symptoms are headache, drowsiness, slow mentation, and confusion. The symptoms slowly progress as the size of the subdural clot increases, causing increased pressure on the brain. Small hematomas are usually reabsorbed. Large hematomas require surgical removal.

Subarachnoid (below the arachnoid) and intraventricular (within the ventricles of the brain) hemorrhages are common in severe head injury. The symptoms include those listed for hematoma, as well as **nuchal rigidity,** stiffness or inability to bend the neck. Blood in the subarachnoid space interferes with the reabsorption of CSF, further increasing intracranial pressure.

Intracranial hematomas from contusions usually occur in the temporal or frontal lobes; from shearing forces, they usually occur deep in the brain. The hematoma usually expands rapidly. The injury may cause immediate unconsciousness. Headache, deteriorating level of consciousness, hemiplegia, and dilated pupils are initial signs of an internal hematoma. As intracranial pressure increases, herniation of the brainstem occurs, causing changes in pupils, respirations, and vital signs. Craniotomy along with evacuation and control of bleeding may be performed depending on the condition of the client, extent of cerebral contusion, and accessibility of the bleeding site.

Signs and symptoms of increased intracranial pressure include a deterioration in level of consciousness; confusion; difficulty in rousing; and, initially, restlessness. Other signs and symptoms are changes in pupil size or reaction to light. The pupil gradually dilates and becomes less responsive to light. Muscle weakness progressing to **hemiplegia,** paralysis of one side of the body, or **paraplegia,** paralysis of lower extremities, and abnormal posturing may occur. Headache and vomiting are experienced by some clients. Vital sign changes generally do not occur until the increased intracranial pressure has progressed to the point of involving the brainstem. An increase in systolic blood pressure and a widening pulse pressure accompanied by a slowing pulse are the effects of pressure on the brainstem.

Cerebral Edema and Increased Intracranial Pressure

The brain is contained in a rigid container, the skull. The only normal opening to the adult skull is the foramen magnum at the base of the skull. Intracranial pressure is a result of the pressure exerted by the contents of the skull, which are the brain, blood, and CSF.

Regulatory mechanisms maintain intracranial pressure between 0 and 15 mm Hg. The Monroe-Kellie hypothesis states that when one component of the cranial contents increases in volume, the volumes of the other components decrease in order to compensate and maintain intracranial pressure between 0 and 15 mm Hg. As long as this ability to compensate remains effective, no neurological changes occur.

In decompensation, the volume increase is so excessive that intracranial pressure cannot be maintained below 15 mm Hg by decreasing the volume of the remaining components. Neurological changes are exhibited because of cellular hypoxia and displacement of the brain, which compresses neurons, especially in the brainstem. These changes include deteriorating level of consciousness; decreased motor response to commands; fixed, dilated pupils; and vital sign changes known as Cushing's triad or reflex. Cushing's triad refers to bradycardia, widening pulse pressure along with increasing systolic pressure, and respiratory irregularities. Respiratory changes include periods of apnea, decreased respiratory rate and depth, and irregular respirations.

Causes of increased intracranial pressure are increased blood volume resulting from vascular vasodilation; increased volume of brain tissue resulting from edema, infection, tumor, or hemorrhage; or increased volume of CSF resulting from overproduction, decreased reabsorption, or interruption of CSF circulation. If intracranial pressure continues to increase, brain herniation will occur at the tentorial notch or through the foramen magnum, resulting in death.

Medical–Surgical Management

Management of head injury is focused on early recognition and treatment of increasing intracranial pressure and maintenance of normal body functions.

Medical

Suctioning may be necessary but is *never* done through the nose on a head injury client because of the possibility of CSF leakage. Oxygen is given to maintain cerebral perfusion. Arterial blood gases (ABGs) are checked.

If the client has an endotracheal tube in place, the $PaCO_2$ level can drop below normal. This causes a slightly alkaline pH, which decreases vasodilation and, thus, intracranial pressure.

Surgical

Decompression is performed surgically by removing a bone flap from the skull to allow room for the expansion of the brain. A space-occupying lesion such as a tumor, hematoma, or abscess may be surgically removed. Excess CSF may be drained from the ventricles.

Pharmacological

Corticosteroids, such as dexamethasone (Decadron), are given to reduce cerebral edema. Antacids, such as Mylanta or Maalox, or histamine receptor antagonists, such as cimetidine (Tagamet), are given to decrease both the side effects of corticosteroids and stress-induced gastric acidity. Osmotic diuretics, such as mannitol (Osmitrol), are administered to rapidly reduce fluid in the brain tissue; muscle relaxants, sedatives, barbiturates, or muscle-paralyzing agents are administered to decrease activity and reduce the oxygen need of the brain.

Antipyretic drugs are used to decrease body temperature and the metabolic needs of the brain, thereby reducing the volume of blood sent to the brain to supply oxygen and glucose. Anticonvulsants are given to prevent or treat seizure activity.

Activity

Activity is limited to keep the metabolic needs of the brain to a minimum. Increased metabolic needs require more oxygen and glucose supplied by increases in blood volume in the cranium, which, in turn, further increases intracranial pressure.

Nursing Management

Frequently monitor level of consciousness, eye movements, pupil changes, vital signs, I&O, and pulse oxime-try. Maintain airway patency and administer oxygen as ordered. Keep head of bed at 30 to 40 degrees and client's head positioned at midline. Watch for signs of arm/leg muscle weakness, muscle twitching, nausea or vomiting, and visual or hearing disturbance. Fluids will often be restricted.

NURSING PROCESS

Assessment

Nursing assessment for any head injury is focused on neurological status.

Subjective Data

Subjective data to be gathered include a history of what happened, including type of trauma (acceleration, deceleration, or missile), site of blow, and any loss of consciousness, including timing, length, and ability to be roused.

Objective Data

A neurological screening is done to obtain a baseline neurological status; then, a more in-depth neurological exam is performed to identify any early signs of increasing intracranial pressure.

Frequent assessment of neurological status, including level of consciousness, motor function, eye movement, pupil size and reaction, protective reflexes, and vital signs, allows for early recognition of and intervention for increasing intracranial pressure. Nursing observation also includes assessing for double vision, headache, nausea, and bleeding from any orifice. Ipsilateral pupil reaction (reaction of the pupil on the same side as the injury or lesion) may occur as a result of pressure on the oculomotor nerve caused by increased intracranial pressure or cerebral edema. Recognition of factors that cause increased intracranial pressure is a necessary aspect of assessment.

For the client undergoing intracranial surgery, an assessment of teaching needs of the client and family must be performed. Emotional and psychosocial needs and support systems are also assessed.

Longer-term care involves assessment of bowel elimination status to prevent the need for straining; skin assessment to prevent skin breakdown, and assessment for complications of immobility.

Nursing diagnoses for a client with a head injury may include the following:

Nursing Diagnoses	Planning/Goals	Nursing Interventions
Ineffective Tissue/Perfusion (Cerebral) related to disruption in cerebral blood flow	The client will demonstrate improvement or maintenance on Glasgow Coma Scale.	Assess neurological status of client every 15 to 60 minutes. Note findings on Glasgow Coma Scale. Compare findings to previous assessments to uncover changes in condition.
		Administer oxygen as ordered to supply a high concentration of oxygen to the brain.

continues

Nursing Diagnoses	Planning/Goals	Nursing Interventions
		Position client with head of the bed at 30 to 40 degrees and client's head at midline to promote venous drainage from the head.
		Minimize physical activity to prevent increasing metabolic demands. Maintain blood $PaCO_2$ between 25 and 30 mm Hg to prevent vasodilation.
*Ineffective **B**reathing Pattern* related to neurological impairment of respiratory status or mechanical ventilation	The client will have an effective breathing pattern.	Assess respiratory status every 15 to 60 minutes. Administer oxygen as ordered to maintain blood oxygen concentration. Provide mechanical ventilation if necessary.
		Continually assess ABG levels or pulse oximeter readings to identify need for assisting respirations to prevent vasodilation in the brain and increasing intracranial pressure.
*Interrupted **F**amily Processes* related to sudden crisis	The client and/or family will demonstrate effective coping mechanisms.	Assess family's coping mechanisms. Involve the family in client care as appropriate.
		Provide information about the client in an ongoing fashion. Provide teaching about the injury and pathophysiology involved.
		Prepare family for possible outcomes of the injury, such as paralysis or death. Collaborate with clergy, social services, mental health counselors, and support groups.
		Teach the family to report increased drowsiness, arm/leg weakness, muscle twitching, nausea or vomiting, visual or hearing disturbances, and so on.
		Inform the family that the client may not be aware of the symptoms and that signs and symptoms of the head injury may not be immediately apparent.

Evaluation Each goal must be evaluated to determine how it has been met by the client.

BRAIN TUMOR

Brain tumors are space-occupying intracranial lesions, either benign or malignant. Classification of brain tumors is by location or tissue type. Intracranial lesions may be primary lesions, which develop initially in brain tissue; extensions of tumors of the meninges, cranial nerves, or pituitary gland; or metastatic lesions from tumors originating in other body systems.

The etiology of primary lesions is unknown. Clinical manifestations differ according to the area of the lesion and the rate of growth. Intracranial pressure increases as compensatory mechanisms are no longer able to balance tumor growth. Clinical manifestations commonly include alteration in consciousness, decreased mental functioning, headaches, seizures, or vomiting (sometimes sudden and projectile). Other signs and symptoms are relative to the functions of areas involved, such as visual problems resulting from occipital lobe tumors.

Diagnostic evaluation is by CT scan, MRI, or electroencephalogram (EEG). Total body scans, chest x-rays, and needle biopsies of the tumor may be performed to identify the type of tumor and, thus, serve as a basis for medical treatment.

Medical–Surgical Management
Medical

Medical management is based on tumor type, growth rate, and assessment of the client. Radiation therapy may be used for specific tumor types or for inoperable tumors. The goal is to destroy the tumor cells, which are more susceptible to radiation than are normal cells. Radiation may be used with surgery and chemotherapy.

Surgical

Surgical intervention removes tumors (benign or malignant) to decrease the space occupied by the lesion or obtains tissue for biopsy. Some CSF may be removed to relieve increased pressure.

Pharmacological

Dexamethasone (Decadron) is given to decrease cerebral edema. Phenytoin (Dilantin) is given to prevent seizure activity. Antacids and H_2 blockers, such as cimetidine (Tagamet), are given to prevent gastric irritation. Analgesics, NSAIDs, or codeine are used for headaches, and stool softeners are administered to prevent straining.

Antineoplastic agents may be administered based on tumor type and whether the client meets the requirements for receiving the drug.

A protective mechanism called the blood–brain barrier prevents many potentially harmful substances from reaching the brain tissue or cerebrospinal fluid. It prevents chemotherapeutic agents from reaching the brain except in very large doses that are not well tolerated by other body systems. Sometimes chemotherapeutic agents are left in the cavity after tumor removal (Williams & Hopper, 2003).

Nursing Management

Prepare client and family for surgery in a caring, compassionate manner. Explain procedures, including shaving the head. The client generally will stay in the ICU for several days.

NURSING PROCESS

Assessment

Subjective Data

Ask the client about fatigue, pain, headache, weakness, and ability to perform daily activities. Note sensory/perceptual alterations such as hearing, visual, tactile, kinesthetic, or olfactory changes. Assess the client's pain and evaluate effectiveness of interventions. A thorough psychosocial assessment, including changes in personality or judgment, serves as the basis for providing emotional support.

Objective Data

Assess functional ability, mobility, and mental status, including motor strength, gait, ability to perform activities of daily living (ADLs), and level of consciousness. Note signs of neurological changes, deficits, or increased intracranial pressure, such as restlessness, changes in logic, changes in vital signs, pupil responses, speech abnormalities, seizure activity, or changes in respiratory patterns.

Nursing diagnoses for a client with a brain tumor may include the following:

Nursing Diagnoses	Planning/Goals	Nursing Interventions
Anxiety related to fear of unknown and treatment plans	The client will demonstrate effective use of coping mechanisms.	Allow client to verbalize feeling of anxiety and discuss coping patterns previously used. Observe for verbal and nonverbal cues of anxiety.
		Provide emotional support by listening and guiding client to explore feelings of helplessness, fear of the unknown, and potential impending death. Maintain a calm demeanor.
		Teach client and family about diagnostic tests, treatments, and expected outcomes.
		Collaborate with pastoral care, physician, social services, and family to provide emotional support.
		Teach relaxation exercises and techniques such as slow, deep breathing and progressive muscle relaxation.
		Administer tranquilizers and sedatives as ordered.
*Disturbed **S**ensory Perception (visual, auditory, kinesthetic, tactile)* related to displacement/compression of brain tissue	The client will recover sensory perceptions.	Maintain communication.
		Provide a safe environment.
		Provide orientation and appropriate stimuli.
		Encourage some social interaction.
*Imbalanced **N**utrition: Less than body requirements* related to side effects of treatment and disease process	The client will maintain weight within 5 pounds of initial weight.	Assess client's weight every other day.
		Provide frequent small feedings of high-calorie and high-protein foods. Offer foods of client's choice. Use nutritional supplements to maintain weight. Offer fluids frequently.

Evaluation Each goal must be evaluated to determine how it has been met by the client.

CEREBROVASCULAR ACCIDENT/ TRANSIENT ISCHEMIC ATTACKS

Cerebrovascular accident (CVA), or stroke is a "brain attack." It happens in the brain rather than the heart and causes a sudden loss of brain function accompanied by neurological deficit. It is a medical emergency and immediate treatment is crucial for the best outcome just as it is for a heart attack (NSA, 2002c). Stroke is the third leading cause of death in the United States, with nearly 160,000 deaths each year (NSA, 2002b). The U.S. stroke mortality rate increased for the first time in four decades in 1993, increased again in 1995, and had a slight decrease in 1997 (NSA, 2002b).

Strokes are caused by ischemia (oxygen deprivation) resulting from a thrombus, embolus, severe vasospasm, or cerebral hemorrhage. Blood supply to the brain is interrupted, causing neurological deficits of sensation, movement, thought, memory, or speech. The loss of function can be temporary or permanent.

Transient ischemic attacks (TIAs) are mini-strokes and frequently precede a stroke. A TIA is a temporary or transient episode of neurological dysfunction caused by temporary impairment of blood flow to the brain. The loss of motor or sensory function may last from a few seconds to minutes to 24 hours. The classic symptoms are sudden blurring of vision or blindness, loss of balance or coordination, difficulty speaking or understanding simple statements, and weakness/numbness/paralysis in the face, arm, or leg (NSA, 2002b).

Clinical manifestations of TIA or CVA vary according to the location of interrupted blood supply in the brain. As with head injury, the specific functions of the involved area of the brain are interrupted, causing the symptoms. Common neurological deficits are motor deficits of hemiplegia (paralysis of one side of the body on the side opposite of the brain lesion), **hemiparesis** (weakness of one side of the body), **dysarthria** (impairment of speech caused by muscle dysfunction), and dysphagia (impairment of swallowing muscles). **Emotional lability** (loss of emotional control), inability to control behavior, and inability to process multiple pieces of information are also common manifestations of a stroke.

Sensory deficits include visual deficits of double vision, decreased visual acuity, and **homonymous hemianopia,** the loss of vision in half of the visual field on the

same side of both eyes. Other possible sensory deficits include decreased sensation to touch, pressure, pain, heat, and cold. The client also may be confused and disoriented.

Intellectual deficits include memory impairment, poor judgment, short attention span, difficulty organizing thoughts, and inability to reason or calculate. Emotional deficits include depression and decreased tolerance to stressors.

Most clients experience initial bowel and bladder dysfunction. With early recognition of the problem and use of bowel and bladder retraining programs, however, most clients regain continence of bowel and bladder.

Differences in the affected side of the brain have been identified. Clients with left-side CVA tend to have communication deficits of aphasia, or inability to communicate. These clients tend to be slow and cautious in behavior and have intellectual impairments such as memory deficits or loss of problem-solving skills. Defects in the right visual field occur, and hemiplegia occurs on the right side.

Clients with right-side CVA have left-sided paralysis and defects in the left visual field. Spatial–perceptual defects, called **agnosia,** cause the inability to recognize familiar objects such as a hairbrush. These clients demonstrate poor judgment and impulsive behavior and are unaware of the deficits. This is called **anosognosia,** which is gross or unconscious denial of the stroke or neurological deficit. Furthermore, these clients are easily distracted and usually show **unilateral neglect,** or the failure to recognize or care for the affected side of the body.

Cerebral edema and increased intracranial pressure may further complicate neurological status. Cerebral edema maximizes in 3 to 5 days following CVA. Neurological deficits begin to resolve within 2 days as cerebral edema decreases. Gradual progression in the re-

Diet

Fluids may be restricted for a few days following a CVA. The client will, however, be given intravenous fluids or tube feedings. The gag reflex must be assessed to identify choking risk and food restrictions implemented accordingly.

Activity

In cases of an embolic or thrombolic stroke, the client's bed is kept flat to increase cerebral perfusion. In the event of a hemorrhagic stroke, the head of the bed is elevated to decrease cerebral perfusion. The type of CVA and the physician's judgment determines the length of time the client stays in bed.

turn of various functions from proximal to distal can occur for 1 to 2 years.

Medical–Surgical Management

Medical

Medical management of the client with CVA is directed toward airway maintenance and supportive therapy during the first 24 to 48 hours. Early diagnosis of the cause and type of stroke is necessary to determine the appropriate treatment. Maintaining adequate cerebral perfusion and preventing cerebral edema reduce neurological deficit. Respiratory failure is treated with mechanical ventilation; temperature is regulated, with the help of a hypothermia blanket if necessary. (See the section on increased intracranial pressure for information on prevention and treatment.)

To prevent further loss of function, a focus on rehabilitation must begin on admission. Self-care and mobility that remain must be maintained.

Surgical

Surgical removal of the thrombus (thrombolectomy) or embolus (embolectomy) may be necessary to relieve pressure on the brain.

Pharmacological

Antihypertensive agents are used to control blood pressure. To prevent further clot formation in cases of stroke caused by thrombi, anticoagulants, aspirin, heparin, or coumadin are used. To dissolve the clot, thrombolytic agents such as alteplase (Activase), anistreplase (Eminase), streptokinase (Streptase), or urokinase (Abbokinase) must be given within 3 hours of the stroke. A stroke caused by bleeding would not be treated with thrombolytic agents. Dexamethasone (Decadron) may be used to reduce intracranial pressure. Anticonvulsants such as phenytoin (Dilantin) may be used if convulsions are present.

Nursing Management

Maintain a patent airway and fluid and electrolyte balance. Administer oxygen and medications as ordered. Monitor vital signs, neurologic status, I&O, pulse oximetry, and ABGs. Ensure adequate nutrition. Provide careful mouth and eye care. Keep client's body in correct alignment, using a footboard to prevent foot drop and contractures. Turn client at least every 2 hours to prevent pneumonia. Perform and assist client to perform ROM exercises using the unaffected side to exercise the affected side. Communicate with the client; even an unresponsive client can hear. Set realistic short-term goals. Involve the client's family in client care when possible.

NURSING PROCESS

Assessment

Subjective Data

Subjective data collected include client statements regarding how the client is feeling, frustration level with limitations, reports of pain, numbness, tingling, and sensory deficits of vision or hearing

Objective Data

Give specific attention to objective findings of assessment of level of consciousness, respiratory status, hemiparesis, hemiplegia, mobility, and cognitive perceptual functioning, including the inability to think clearly and the ability to understand the condition.

Nursing diagnoses for a client with a CVA may include the following:

Nursing Diagnoses	Planning/Goals	Nursing Interventions
Deficient Knowledge related to home care	The client and/or family will verbalize or demonstrate home health care management.	Assess client's and family's needs for discharge teaching, knowledge level about necessary home care. Develop a multidisciplinary plan for client and family teaching. Provide education in verbal, written, and picture forms to accommodate the varying possible impairments from the stroke. Teach small segments of information at a time and reinforce teaching, then, to ascertain effectiveness of teaching, have client and family return demonstrate or verbalize knowledge. Primary areas of teaching are medication administration; dosages, actions, and side effects to report to the physician; mobility needs; self-care needs; safety factors; communication; swallowing; elimination; and skin care.
Impaired Verbal Communication related to neuromuscular impairment	The client will communicate needs to the caregiver.	Assess communication deficits and consult a speech therapist to determine a method of communication, if deficits are apparent. Allow time for the client to attempt to communicate needs; anticipate needs to prevent client frustration in trying to communicate. Use gestures, pictures, and closed questions (those requiring only a "yes" or "no" answer). Provide paper and pencil if dominant side is unaffected.
Unilateral Neglect related to neuromuscular impairment	The client will move paralyzed extremities with assistance from functioning extremities.	Adapt environment to prevent injury of the client with unilateral neglect by positioning water and personal items on the unaffected or unneglected side. Approach the client from the unneglected side. Gradually cue client to remind to tend to the neglected side. Remind client of safety factors such as arm trailing over edge of wheelchair or close proximity of a wall on the neglected side. Teach client and family to place small bites of food on unaffected side and to check for food in the cheek on the affected side after meals. Instruct client to scan environment for safety factors at all times. Teach client how to dress and tend to neglected side. Place arm either in a sling, if client is ambulatory, or on a wheelchair tray, if client is in a wheelchair.

Evaluation Each goal must be evaluated to determine how it has been met by the client.

EPILEPSY/SEIZURE DISORDER

Epilepsy is a disorder of cerebral function in which the client experiences sudden attacks of altered consciousness, motor activity, or sensory phenomenon. Convulsive seizures are the most common type. Most recurrent seizure patterns are caused by epilepsy. Most clinicians and authors use the term "seizure disorder" for epilepsy or seizures (Hickey, 2002).

A seizure is initiated by an electrical disturbance in the neurons, which, in turn, causes an aberrant discharge of electrical activity from any part of the cerebral cortex and possibly from other areas of the brain (Samuels, 1999). This electrical discharge may cause involuntary episodes of loss of consciousness, excessive muscular movement or loss of muscle tone, and changes in behavior, mood, sensation, and/or perception (Smeltzer & Bare, 2002).

The etiology of the electrical disturbance may be birth trauma, hypoxia, infection, tumor, alcohol toxicity, drugs, drug withdrawal, carbon monoxide or lead poisoning, vascular abnormalities such as CVA, hypoglycemia electrolyte imbalance, or fever. Often, the cause is idiopathic, or unknown.

Seizures are classified as generalized or partial. In generalized seizures, the entire brain is affected simultaneously, causing bilateral, symmetrical reactions. Generalized seizures are classified as tonic and/or clonic (grand mal), absence (petit mal), or myoclonic.

Tonic–clonic seizures involve rigid tonic contractions of muscles and loss of postural control followed by a clonic stage of intermittent contraction and relaxation. Incontinence of stool or urine is common. Absence seizures involve loss of conscious activity without the muscular involvement of tonic–clonic seizures. Myoclonic seizures may be very mild, sudden, involuntary contractions of a muscle group or rapid, forceful movements. They usually occur in the trunk or extremities and involve no loss of consciousness.

Partial seizures initiate in a focal point in the brain and involve the function of those specific neurons. Partial seizures are either simple or complex. In simple partial seizures, the area affected may be a hand, a finger, the ability to talk, or a sense such as smell. Consciousness is not lost.

Complex partial seizures generally involve loss of consciousness and may produce cognitive, affective, psychosensory, or psychomotor symptoms. The client may perform inappropriate purposive behaviors, called **automatisms,** or mechanical, repetitive motor behaviors performed unconsciously, such as lip-smacking. **Auras,** peculiar sensations that precede a seizure, may take the form of a taste, smell, sight, or sound; dizziness; or a "funny" feeling. After the seizure, the client typically cannot remember the episode.

Diagnostic testing to determine the type of seizure activity includes the EEG to identify abnormal electrical activity and/or the focal point of the seizure. Sleep and video EEGs are performed to document changes in electrical activity of the brain. Computerized tomography scans are used to identify or rule out lesions, degenerative changes, or vascular abnormalities.

Medical–Surgical Management

Surgical

Surgical intervention may be indicated for a very small percentage of clients. Microsurgery may be utilized to irradiate focal points of abnormal electrical discharge caused by tumor, vascular abnormality, or abscess.

Pharmacological

The primary method of controlling seizure activity is pharmacological. Seizure activity is controlled with an anticonvulsant agent or a combination of anticonvulsants in 75% of clients (Hickey, 2002). Phenytoin (Dilantin), phenobarbital (Phenobarbital), carbamazepine (Tegretol), valproic acid (Depakene), and primidone (Mysoline) are often used. Anticonvulsant agents are started one at a time in gradually increasing doses. The client's blood level is monitored for therapeutic range, and the client is assessed for side effects of the

drug and signs of drug toxicity, such as drowsiness, dizziness, gastric distress, rash, blood dyscrasias, and ataxia.

The goal is to obtain seizure control with minimal side effects. Any anticonvulsant should be gradually discontinued. Abrupt withdrawal can cause **status epilepticus,** an acute prolonged episode of seizure activity lasting at least 30 minutes with or without loss of consciousness (Smeltzer & Bare, 2002). Status epilepticus is a medical emergency that can result in respiratory arrest and irreversible brain damage.

Diet

Nutritionally balanced meals are required. The client should never consume alcohol.

Activity

Adequate rest is required. Driving, operating machinery, and swimming are not allowed until seizures are controlled.

Safety: Precautions During a Seizure
If the client is in bed:
- Be sure the side rails are up.
- Put padding (blankets) on the side rails to prevent injury.

If the client is out of bed:
- Carefully ease the client to the floor.
- Move nearby objects so that the client will not be injured.
- Place a soft item beneath the client's head.

Whether the client is in or out of bed:
- Never leave the client alone.
- Do not restrain the client.
- Do not attempt to put anything in the client's mouth after the seizure has begun.
- Loosen any restrictive clothing around the client's neck.
- Turn the client's head to the side.
- Monitor seizure activity carefully, noting the exact time that the seizure began and ended.

After the seizure:
- Call the client by name and ask to perform a simple command.
- Test the client's memory by asking to remember two words.
- Ask the client whether an aura was experienced before the seizure.
- Check the oral cavity—especially the tongue—for injury.
- Offer comfort and reassurance, as the client may be frightened and embarrassed.
- Document everything observed.

Nursing Management

Monitor for toxic signs of anticonvulsant medications. Stress importance for compliance with prescribed medication schedule. Encourage scrupulous oral hygiene. Warn client not to drink alcoholic beverages.

PROFESSIONAL TIP

Long-Term Use of Dilantin
The client on Dilantin requires good oral hygiene because of hyperplasia of the gums, which become edematous and enlarged.

Encourage client to have anticonvulsant medication blood level checked regularly.

NURSING PROCESS

Assessment

Subjective Data

Include client statements of experiences before the seizure and activity the client was performing when the seizure occurred. Determine whether an aura was experienced and the sensations that were manifested, and ascertain if the client has a prior history of seizure disorder.

Objective Data

Assessment of the nature of the seizure and sequencing of events is important in determining cause and management of seizure activity. During the seizure, assess the client's respiratory status and observe for muscular stiffness or flaccidity, the position of the eyes and head, the size and equality of the pupils, automatism, any cry or sounds made, and incontinence of urine or stool. Note the duration of the phases of the seizure, total duration, and whether unconsciousness occurred. Note if the onset of seizure activity was observed, along with what the client was doing when the seizure began.

After the seizure, observe the client for **postictal** (after a seizure) signs of paralysis of arms or legs, inability to speak, sleep following seizure, difficulty in awakening from sleep, confusion, or general dazed affect (Smeltzer & Bare, 2002; Hickey, 2002). The postictal phase can last from several minutes to hours. Assess the client for signs of injury and vital signs. Clients on anticonvulsant therapy need a thorough nursing assessment because of the wide variety of side effects involving multiple body systems.

Nursing diagnoses for a client with a seizure may include the following:

Nursing Diagnoses	Planning/Goals	Nursing Interventions
*Ineffective **A**irway Clearance* related to mucus accumulation during the seizure and uncontrollable tonic–clonic muscle contractions involving the respiratory muscles	The client will maintain an effective airway during seizure activity.	Following tonic–clonic activity, turn client to the side to allow secretions to drain from the airway. Prepare to suction oropharynx if necessary to clear airway. Assess skin color and respiratory rate and depth during and following seizure. Administer oxygen as needed. Insert oral airway or epistick if client's jaw is not clenched. Never insert an object if the jaw is already clenched. Do not place fingers between client's teeth. Loosen restrictive clothing.
*Risk for **I**njury* related to seizure activity	The client will be free of injury related to seizure activity.	During seizures in bed, use blankets or protective pads to pad side rails. If client is standing or sitting, ease client to the floor when seizure activity begins. Place client in a supine position, but do not physically restrain client. Remove objects from around client so that he or she will not hit them. Following the seizure, turn client to the side to allow secretions to drain from the mouth. Observe client for injuries (e.g., tongue lacerations; broken bones; body lacerations or bruising). Maintain a low-stimulus environment to prevent further seizure activity. Teach client about ways of maintaining a safe environment, including driving restrictions; lying down in a safe area if an aura is experienced; showering instead of tub bathing; either avoiding swimming or swimming with a partner if the physician allows; and wearing a medical identification tag.
*Ineffective **C**oping* related to anxiety secondary to seizure disorder and altered self-concept	The client will verbalize fears and concerns about seizure activity; and will use effective coping methods.	Allow client to verbalize fears and concerns. Explore coping mechanisms with client. Collaborate with mental health counselor or clergy to assist client in development of coping mechanisms.

Evaluation Each goal must be evaluated to determine how it has been met by the client.

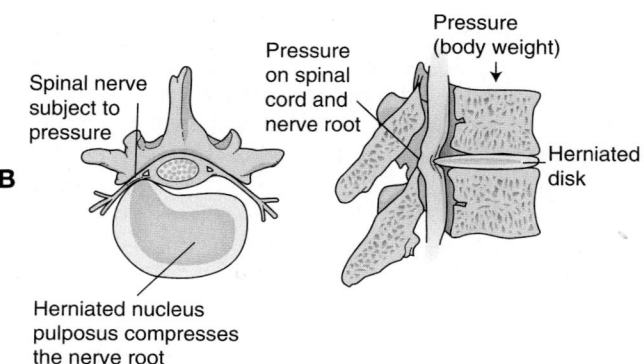

Figure 38-14 *A, Normal Intravertebral Disk; **B,** Herniated Disk*

HERNIATED INTERVERTEBRAL DISK

Herniated intervertebral disks are a major cause of chronic back pain. Most clients with herniated disks are 30 to 50 years of age. Most herniated disks occur in the lumbar or cervical spine because of the flexibility of these regions (Hickey, 2002). This can occur either suddenly from trauma, lifting, or twisting or gradually from aging, osteoporosis, or degenerative changes. Most herniated disks are caused by trauma, such as falls, accidents, or repeated lifting. Degenerative changes related to arthritis, aging, or repeated minor injuries predispose the client to herniated intervertebral disks.

The intervertebral disk is a cartilaginous cushion between vertebral bodies (Figure 38-14). In herniation, or rupture of the disk, the nucleus pulposus protrudes into the fibrous ring, the annulus fibrosus. This protrusion presses on the spinal cord and nerve roots, causing pain, motor changes, sensory changes, and alterations in reflexes.

The nerve root affected and the degree of compression lead to specific symptoms. Ninety percent to 95% of lumbar herniations occur at the L-4 to L-5 and S-1 levels (Hickey, 2002). Low-back pain that radiates across the buttock and down the leg along the path of the sciatic nerve is the most common symptom. The affected leg tingles and is numb. Sneezing, straining, stooping, standing, sitting, blowing the nose, and jarring movements aggravate the pain. Positions of comfort are lying on the back, with knees flexed and a small pillow under the head, or lying on the unaffected side, with the affected knee flexed.

Motor weakness may be experienced. Paresthesia and numbness of the leg and foot occur. Knee and ankle reflexes are diminished or absent. Lasegue's sign, pain experienced upon gentle raising of the fully extended leg of the supine-positioned client to 20 to 60 degrees, stems from stretching of the inflamed sciatic nerve. Inflammation in the nerve roots may also be present as indicated by a positive finding for **Kernig's sign.** To test for Kernig's sign, the client is placed in a dorsal recumbent position and attempts to flex the hip and knee and then extend the knee. Normally, the client should be able to extend the knee to 90 degrees. With a low-back herniated disk, however, the client will be unable to extend the knee because of severe pain radiating down the hip and leg. Symptoms vary with the area and degree of nerve root compression.

Cervical herniation commonly occurs at levels C-5 to C-6 or C-6 to C-7. Symptoms of lateral herniation include pain and paresthesia in the neck, arms, and shoulders. Loss of muscle strength and reflexes may also occur, as may muscle atrophy.

Because of anatomic position, cervical disks may herniate centrally more frequently than do lumbar disks, thereby compressing the spinal cord. Symptoms are weakness of the lower extremities and unsteady gait. Spasticity and hyperactive reflexes may develop in the lower extremities. Difficulty in voiding and sexual dysfunction may occur.

Degenerative spinal cord disease can follow compression from a herniated disk. Spinal cord tumors and herniated lumbar disk are differential diagnoses that are ruled out through the use of MRI or CT scans.

Medical–Surgical Management
Medical

Conservative medical treatment, providing rest, stress reduction and immobility of the spine, and pain relief, is often tried for several weeks.

Surgical

Surgery to remove the herniated disk is done when neurological deficit or pain are not responsive to conservative treatment or when symptoms require immediate surgical intervention.

Pharmacological

Narcotic analgesics, such as hydrocodone bitartrate with acetaminophen (Vicodin), and nonnarcotic analgesics, such as tramadol hydrochloride (Ultram), are ordered for pain control. Antiinflammatory drugs, steroids, or NSAIDs, such as ibuprofen (Motrin) or naproxen (Anaprox), are prescribed to reduce the inflammatory response. Muscle relaxants, such as methocarbamol (Robaxin), are given to reduce spasms of surrounding muscles, which decreases the pain. Antianxiety medications, such as diazepam (Valium), are given to decrease muscle tension and promote rest.

Diet

To decrease the workload on the involved muscles, weight reduction is advocated if the client is overweight. A high-protein diet with calcium, vitamin D, and phosphorus is necessary for bone repair and prevention of osteoporosis. Fiber is necessary for bowel function because constipation is a common side effect of analgesics.

Activity

Bed rest, a support garment (back brace) or cervical collar, a firm mattress, and traction may be used to decrease stress on the affected vertebrae. Postoperatively, log-roll turning is used to prevent injury to the vertebrae and spine.

The client may not lift or carry more than 5 pounds for at least 8 weeks. Twisting movements are to be avoided. The client cannot drive a car until the surgeon permits. Sitting should be limited during the early postoperative period; the client should either stand or lie down. Physical therapy is focused on muscle strengthening and client comfort. Heat therapy, ultrasound, and exercises are often used to promote comfort and healing.

Nursing Management

Preoperatively, monitor neurological status and vital signs. Encourage client to cough, deep breathe, use incentive spirometer, and move legs as allowed. Provide adequate fluids to prevent renal stasis and constipation.

Postoperatively, monitor vital signs, neurovascular status of legs, and check dressing for any bleeding. If drain is in place (e.g., Hemovac), check frequently and empty at end of shift and record on I&O sheet. Use the log-rolling technique for turning the client.

NURSING PROCESS

Assessment

Subjective Data

Assessment includes eliciting client statements about motor and sensory function, pain, and effectiveness of comfort measures.

Objective Data

Assessment entails a neurological evaluation of motor and sensory function of the extremities innervated below the herniated area. Reflex testing may be a part of the nursing assessment in some facilities. Assess range of motion (ROM) of the affected extremity. Assess the client's knowledge about the disease process, the planned treatment including pain management and surgery, and the postsurgical care. Assess bowel and bladder elimination for potential nerve involvement or effects of immobility. Note gait alteration and bending limitations.

Nursing diagnoses for a client with a herniated intervertebral disk may include the following:

Nursing Diagnoses	Planning/Goals	Nursing Interventions
Chronic **Pain** related to nerve compression or surgical intervention	The client will experience increased comfort.	Assess pain intensity and location, as well as activities or position when pain began. Have the client rate pain on a scale of 1 to 10.
		Maintain activity level as ordered by physician. Provide diversional activities.
		Place client in position of comfort, usually on back, with knees slightly flexed and a small pillow beneath head, or on unaffected side, with affected extremity flexed and a pillow between the legs.
		Maintain immobility of vertebrae with corset, brace, or traction.
		Apply moist heat as prescribed and administer medications to relieve pain, relax muscles, and relieve inflammation and anxiety, as ordered. Document effectiveness.
Impaired **Physical Mobility** related to nerve compression or surgical intervention	The client will have no complications of immobility.	Assess for complications of immobility. Turn client every 1 to 2 hours. The client will tend to limit position to one of comfort.
		Assist the client to log roll, that is, move the body as a unit without twisting the back.
		Ambulate as ordered by the physician.

Evaluation Each goal must be evaluated to determine how it has been met by the client.

Figure 38-15 *Spinal Cord—Levels of Injury:* **A,** *Areas of sensory function (dermatomes);* **B,** *Areas of motor function*

SPINAL CORD INJURY

Spinal cord injury (SCI) occurs from trauma to the spinal cord or from compression of the spinal cord caused by injury to the supporting structures. Each year, almost 11,000 new spinal cord injuries occur. Most of the victims are males between the ages of 16 and 30 years. Leading causes of injury are motor vehicle accidents; acts of violence; falls; and sporting accidents (National Spinal Cord Injury Center, 2001).

Numerous classification systems exist for SCIs. Spinal cord injuries may be classified by level of injury, mechanism of injury, or neurological or functional level (Figure 38-15). The injury may be considered complete or incomplete. When injury is complete, no impulses are carried below the level of injury. There is complete disruption of the spinal cord functions, including motor (voluntary) movement, sensation, and reflexes to areas innervated by the spinal nerves at and below the level of the injury. In an incomplete injury, some of the spinal cord tracts are affected while others are able to carry impulses normally.

The mechanism of injury is usually an acceleration–deceleration event that causes hyperflexion, hyperextension, axial loading, or excessive rotation injury (Hickey, 2002). Hyperflexion is the extreme forward movement of the head, which causes compression of the vertebral bodies and damage to the posterior ligaments and intervertebral disks. Hyperextension is the extreme backward movement of the head, causing injury to the posterior vertebral structures and the anterior ligaments. Axial loading or compression occurs when extreme pressure is placed on the spinal column, such as in diving accidents or falls landed on feet or buttocks. Compression of the vertebrae shatters the vertebral body. Compression fractures and posterior ligament injury can also be caused by excessive rotation, or turning the head beyond the normal range.

Classification of injury by cause includes concussion, contusion, laceration, transection, hemorrhage, or damage to blood vessels supplying the spinal cord. Immediately following injury to the spinal cord, an autodestructive process begins, with chemical and vascular changes that lead to ischemia and necrosis of the spinal cord.

Spinal shock (cessation of motor, sensory, autonomic, and reflex impulses) and **areflexia** (the absence of reflexes) occur immediately upon transection of the spinal cord or upon injury to the spinal cord. Flaccid paralysis of all skeletal muscles; loss of spinal reflexes; loss of sensation; and absence of autonomic function below the level of injury also occur. The diaphragm is innervated at levels C3 through C5. Injuries in this area cause partial or complete disruption of respiratory function. The client does not perspire below the level of the injury. Bowel and bladder function may be lost either for a few days to months, or permanently, although this loss generally lasts from 1 to 6 weeks.

As spinal shock resolves, reflex activity returns below the level of injury. The client with a lower motor neuron injury continues to experience flaccid paralysis, areflexia, hypotonic bowel and bladder function, and sexual dysfunction. Lower motor neuron injury causes paraplegia, or paralysis of lower extremities.

Neurogenic shock, a hypotensive situation resulting from the loss of sympathetic control of vital functions from the brain, may occur during spinal shock. This happens in clients with injury above the sixth thoracic vertebra. The client develops orthostatic hypotension, bradycardia, decreased cardiac output, loss of ability to sweat below the level of injury, and subnormal temperature.

Upper motor neuron injury results in spastic paralysis, loss of voluntary skeletal muscle movement, and reflexive bowel, bladder, and sexual responses. Complete upper motor neuron injury results in **quadriplegia,** or dysfunction or paralysis of both arms, both legs, bowel, and bladder. Injuries above C5 affect respiratory function because of innervation of the diaphragm and accessory respiratory muscles. Mechanical ventilation is required to keep the client alive. Fractures below the cervical vertebrae result in diaphragmatic breathing, if the phrenic nerve is functioning.

The client with an injury above the sixth thoracic vertebra is at risk for developing *autonomic dysreflexia* or *autonomic hyperreflexia.* Autonomic dysreflexia is an emergency situation resulting in a hypertensive crisis and possibly stroke or seizure activity. The cause is noxious stimuli such as a full bladder, a fecal impaction, a wrinkle in clothing, menstrual cramps, an erection, an ingrown toenail, a bladder infection, or sitting on catheter tubing. Autonomic reflexes below the level of the injury cause vasoconstriction in this area. The controlling impulses from the higher cortical levels do not transmit past the level of injury but cause bradycardia and vasodilation above the level of injury. Skin above the level of injury is warm and moist, but skin below the level of injury is cold, with goose flesh (Beare & Meyers, 1998; Hickey, 2002).

The noxious stimuli must be removed, if possible, and the client placed in a sitting position immediately. Assess blood pressure immediately and monitor every few minutes until within normal limits (Huston & Boelman, 1995). The drug of choice, nitroprusside sodium (Nipride), may be given if the conservative measure does not work. Prevent autonomic dysreflexia when possible, recognize when it develops, and treat immediately. Once autonomic dysreflexia is relieved, the client may develop hypotension from the decreased sympathetic response and the residual effects of medication and positioning changes. A pattern of individual response to stimuli and of sympathetic response is soon identified for the client; however, the client with an upper motor neuron injury above T-6 is always at risk for developing autonomic dysreflexia. Some clients experience the first episode years after the injury.

The extent of permanent injury cannot be determined immediately because of necrosis, edema, and spinal shock. Functional loss depends on the level, degree, and type of injury.

Medical–Surgical Management

Medical

Medical management of the client with spinal cord injury begins before reaching the hospital. Further damage to the spinal cord is prevented by immobilizing the head, neck, and vertebral column with devices such as rigid cervical collars and splinting backboards. All trauma clients should be treated as potential spinal cord injuries. When the client reaches the emergency room, x-rays of the spine are taken before removing the immobilizing devices.

Respiratory function is continuously assessed, and ventilatory support is provided as necessary. The client may have multiple injuries, necessitating astute diagnostic skills by the emergency room physician. Assessment of the trauma client must involve evaluating for internal hemorrhaging, cardiac contusion, head injury, hemorrhagic shock, and spinal shock resulting from the spinal cord injury. A thorough assessment is done to specifically evaluate the degree of deficit and to establish the level or degree of injury.

Blood pressure monitoring is crucial. A systolic BP below 90 mm Hg should be avoided or corrected as soon as possible because one episode can send the client into shock and cause permanent damage (Baker & Saulino, 2002).

Immobilization of the spinal cord continues to be the focus of care during early medical management of the client. Traction may be used to maintain alignment of the spinal column. Cervical tongs and halo devices are used to apply traction and to immobilize the cervical spine. Under local anesthesia, cervical tongs and halo rings are applied with spring-loaded pins that are embedded into the scalp. Antiseptic solution is used to cleanse the scalp, and a local anesthetic is injected into the insertion sites. Traction weights are applied to the cervical tongs or halo rings after the insertion pins are firmly embedded (Figure 38-16). Body casts, jackets, vests, or braces are used to immobilize thoracic and lumbar fractures.

Surgical

Surgical interventions are performed for decompression, realignment, and stabilization of the vertebral column, depending on the nature of the injury. A laminectomy may be performed to decompress the spinal cord

Figure 38-16 *Halo Vest (Courtesy of DePuy AcroMed)*

COLLABORATIVE CARE

Following a Spinal Cord Injury

The interdisciplinary team works together to optimize the functional capabilities of the client. The physical therapist works on activity level, the occupational therapist on ADLs, the speech therapist on swallowing and communication, and nursing coordinates the team and reinforces what the client has been taught. The focus is to prevent disabilities and maximize and strengthen functional ability.

Activity

Initially, immobilization of the spinal column is necessary. In the acute phase, ROM for all joints is performed to prevent mobility loss and muscle contracture. As the spine is stabilized, the client's activity progresses to sitting up in a chair, performing strengthening exercises, and increasing endurance. The nurse must observe for the complication of orthostatic hypotension.

Orthostatic hypotension is caused by the venous pooling of blood in the lower body and extremities resulting from impairment of the sympathetic nervous system. The client becomes hypotensive and develops bradycardia and syncope. Asystole may even occur. Prevention of orthostatic hypotension also requires the application of full leg support stockings and pneumatic boots and the gradual lowering of the lower extremities. Monitor the client's vital signs throughout the mobilization process to ascertain tolerance to the procedure. After spinal shock has subsided, active rehabilitation begins.

Nursing Management

After stabilization, turn client frequently to prevent embolism, pneumonia, and skin breakdown. Use logrolling technique. Keep call light within client's reach. Provide passive and active ROM exercises as allowed. Maintain adequate nutrition and fluid intake. If client has a halo device, perform pin-site care following facility protocol. For a client with a vest, jacket, or brace, provide skin care under this device. Implement bowel and bladder training regimen. Monitor vital signs.

NURSING PROCESS

Assessment

Subjective Data

Subjective assessment involves eliciting input from the client regarding sensation, pain, and history of the accident. Note how the client is coping with the injury, the resulting disability, and the major lifestyle changes that have occurred. Evaluate how the family or support system is coping with the changes.

with fusion or placement of Harrington rods to stabilize the vertebral column. Realignment is maintained by surgical manipulation of the vertebral column.

If the client has respiratory involvement, an endotracheal tube is put in place to provide mechanical ventilatory support. Following urgent treatment, a tracheostomy will be performed to continue ventilation.

Pharmacological

Steroid therapy with dexamethasone (Decadron) is administered to prevent and reduce edema in the injured spinal cord. To decrease and prevent edema and to improve blood flow, high loading doses of the steroid methylprednisolone sodium succinate (SoluMedrol) are given within 8 hours of the injury, with tapering dosages given over the next 1 to 2 weeks. Mannitol, an osmotic diuretic, may be administered to decrease and prevent cord edema. Hydralazine hydrochloride (Apresoline) or nifedipine (Procardia) is frequently ordered to reduce blood pressure in cases of autonomic dysreflexia. To maintain mean arterial pressure (MAP) between 85 and 90 mm Hg and to improve spinal cord perfusion during the acute phase, vasopressor agents such as dopamine hydrochloride (Intropin) are given.

Objective Data

In the acute phase of care of the client with a spinal cord injury, nursing assessment focuses on the critical factors of airway, breathing, circulation, disability, and exposure.

Assess circulatory status by monitoring vital signs and observing for complications of neurogenic shock; orthostatic hypotension; hypertensive episodes of autonomic dysreflexia; and hemorrhaging.

Assess disability by performing a baseline neurological assessment (as described under the Components of Neurological Assessment section in this chapter).

Exposure refers to removing the client's clothing to perform a thorough assessment of the client's body for skin condition and for entrance and exit wounds. Monitor body temperature because of the neurological deficit in temperature regulation caused by dysfunction of the autonomic nervous system.

Subacute assessment is based on the level of injury and neurological functioning of the client. With upper motor neuron injuries, the client is at higher risk of developing autonomic dysreflexia; thus, assessment includes monitoring for these signs.

Assess all clients with spinal cord injury for skin condition, bowel and bladder function, respiratory status, and signs and symptoms of complications of immobility. Psychosocial assessment is very important to the well-being of the client.

Nursing diagnoses for a client with a spinal cord injury in the subacute phase of care may include the following:

Nursing Diagnoses	Planning/Goals	Nursing Interventions
Risk for Injury related to motor and sensory deficits secondary to spinal fractures	The client will not experience additional injury.	Assess the client's risk factors for additional injury.
		Monitor skin condition for pressure areas or shearing injuries from sliding across sheets or the mats in physical therapy.
		Turn client frequently to prevent pressure areas. Use enough personnel to turn client correctly to maintain alignment of client's spinal column.
		Provide a call light that the client can operate; teach to call nurse for assistance as necessary.
		Reinforce wheelchair safety factors and observe client for use of wheelchair.
		Prevent falls when transferring client to wheelchair. Prevent foot drop.
		Provide passive and active ROM exercises.
		Maintain adequate fluid intake and nutrition.
		Provide routine care for halo device by opening vest on one side to cleanse skin under vest at least daily and to assess for skin breakdown. Repeat procedure on the other side.
		Monitor pin sites of halo device every shift for placement. Perform pin site care using facility protocol.
Powerlessness related to changes in motor and sensory function and in lifestyle	The client will make decisions regarding care, treatment, and future.	Explain all procedures and care options. Allow client to participate in care decisions.
		Establish an open, trusting relationship with client to foster therapeutic communication.
		Allow time for client to express concerns, anger, and fears. Foster a positive environment for client to explore feelings and accept disability.
		Assess for signs and symptoms of depression.
		Collaborate with mental health professional to provide assistance in coping with lifestyle changes.
		Collaborate with family and support people to include them in the plan of care.
Autonomic Dysreflexia related to noxious stimulation secondary to overstimulation of autonomic nervous system	The client will state factors that cause autonomic dysreflexia, describe treatment, and notify the nurse if experiencing symptoms of dysreflexia.	Teach client causes and symptoms of autonomic dysreflexia: increased blood pressure, sudden throbbing headache, chills, pallor, goose flesh, nausea, and/or metallic taste in mouth.
		Prevent bladder distention and fecal impaction by implementing a bowel and bladder training program.

continues

Nursing Diagnoses	Planning/Goals	Nursing Interventions
		Observe for bradycardia, vasodilatation, flushing, and diaphoresis above the level of spinal cord injury. If these symptoms occur, immediately notify the physician and administer medications as ordered to decrease blood pressure. Raise head of bed and lower legs to reduce blood pressure. Then, remove the noxious stimuli, which may include constrictive clothing, shoes, splints, or linens.
		Assess client for a distended bladder and empty the bladder if distended. Observe urine for signs of infection and obtain a urine specimen for culture, if needed to identify the cause of the reaction.
		Check for fecal impaction using xylocaine viscous per physician's order to decrease stimulation.
		Monitor blood pressure every few minutes.

Evaluation Each goal must be evaluated to determine how it has been met by the client.

PARKINSON'S DISEASE

Parkinson's disease is a chronic, progressive, degenerative disease affecting the area of the brain controlling movement. The cause is unknown in most cases, but toxicity, hypoxia, or encephalitis may precede the onset of Parkinson's disease. Vascular and genetic factors have been implicated. Drugs such as cocaine, reserpine (Serpasil), haloperidol (Haldol), and chlorpromazine (Thorazine) may cause a parkinsonian syndrome. The theory is that these drugs interfere with the synthesis or storage of dopamine.

Typical signs and symptoms of Parkinson's disease are muscular rigidity, **bradykinesia** (slowness of voluntary movement and speech), resting tremors, muscular weakness, and loss of postural reflexes. Muscular rigidity along with bradykinesia impairs the person's ability to perform daily activities and speech.

Rigidity is noted along with increased muscle tone when the client is at rest. Stiffness of the trunk, head, and shoulders is present. The rigidity causes loss of arm swing when walking. A cogwheel phenomenon results from the muscle contractions breaking through the muscular rigidity. The alternating rigidity and rhythmic contractions causes a jerking-like movement. Motor impairment progressively affects facial expressions, eye blink, and voice, causing a typical presentation of a mask-like face and a monotone voice.

Resting tremors, usually in the upper extremities, are present when the hand is motionless. The hand moves in a "pill-rolling" motion. When the client is moving or sleeping, the tremors are usually absent. Tremors also occur in other areas, including the feet, lip, tongue, or jaw. The tremors usually begin unilaterally in one area and progress to other areas and then to the opposite side of the body. Anxiety and concentration tend to increase the degree of tremors.

The posture and gait of people with Parkinson's disease is characterized by bowed head, forward-bent trunk, drooped shoulders, and flexed arms. The gait is characterized by shuffling movement and small steps. Balance is affected, resulting in a tendency to fall forward. Figure 38-17 shows the classic posture of a client with Parkinson's disease.

Autonomic dysfunction includes drooling, **dysphagia** (difficulty swallowing), excessive sweating, hyperactivity of oil glands, and constipation. Orthostatic hypotension may occur from loss of the peripheral autonomic response. Urinary incontinence and frequency occur.

Mental changes may also occur. Intelligence is not impaired, but problems with judgment and emotional stability may occur. Dementia, depression, cognitive, perceptual, or memory deficits may occur. The major cause of death is from the complications of immobility or injury. Fatigue increases all signs and symptoms. Because there is no diagnostic test specific for Parkinson's disease, diagnosis is made from clinical signs and symptoms. In cases of early onset, it is important to differentiate from Wilson's disease, an increased absorption of copper, for which testing is available.

Medical–Surgical Management

Medical

The goals of medical management are to control the symptoms, provide supportive therapy and maintenance, maintain function via physiotherapy, and provide psychotherapy as necessary.

Surgical

A surgical procedure to disrupt the transmission of motor impulses is occasionally used to treat the tremors and muscular rigidity. This invasive procedure does not treat the disease but, rather, alleviates the tremors.

Pharmacological

Drug therapy is used to control the symptoms of Parkinson's disease. Levodopa (L-Dopa) is converted into dopamine in the basal ganglia to replace the deficit of dopamine. Dopamine is not given orally because it is metabolized before reaching the brain. L-Dopa, a precursor to dopamine, is given orally and reaches the brain to be converted into dopamine.

Figure 38-17 *Progression of Parkinson's Disease:* **A,** *Flexion of affected arm;* **B,** *Shuffling gait;* **C,** *Need for sources of support to prevent falling;* **D,** *Progression of weakness to point of needing assistance for ambulation;* **E,** *Profound weakness.*

Dopadecarboxylase inhibitors such as carbidopa-levodopa (Sinemet) prevent the conversion of levodopa (L-Dopa) to dopamine in peripheral tissue. Dopamine in the peripheral tissue can cause numerous side effects as well as decrease the amount of L-dopa available to the brain. Dopadecarboxylase inhibitors that do not cross the blood–brain barrier are used to inhibit the enzyme that changes L-dopa to dopamine so that the conversion in the brain is not inhibited.

Anticholinergic drugs, such as trihexyphenidyl hydrochloride (Artane), cycrimine hydrochloride (Pagitane hydrochloride), and benztropine mesylate (Cogentin), are administered to control tremors and rigidity. Anticholinergics are used alone for mild symptoms or if levodopa is contraindicated. In other instances, they may be administered in conjunction with levodopa.

Amantadine hydrochloride (Symmetrel), an antiviral agent, is effective in treating parkinsonian symptoms. The mechanism by which the drug works is not known, but the theory is that it either releases dopamine storage areas or delays the reuptake of dopamine

Ethopropazine hydrochloride (Parsidol), a phenothiazine derivative, is used in combination with other anti-Parkinson drugs to alleviate symptoms. Dopamine agonist-ergot derivatives, such as pergolide mesylate (Permax), directly stimulate the dopamine receptors to improve the use of available dopamine. The monoamine oxidase inhibitor (MAOI) selegiline hydrochloride (Eldepryl) inhibits dopamine breakdown. The tricyclic antidepressants amitriptyline hydrochloride (Elavil) and imipramine hydrochloride (Tofranil) alleviate depression as well as other symptoms.

Diet

Puréed foods or tube feedings may be required because of dysphagia. Maintenance of weight may require high- or low-calorie diets. A diet that discourages formation of free radicals is being researched as a deterrent to progression of the disease. Free-radical formation is thought to be discouraged by diets high in complex carbohydrates (such as those found in whole-grain breads and lentils), low in fat, and high in vitamins A and E. Large doses of supplemental vitamins A and E are also given. A high-fiber diet will help prevent constipation.

 Safety: Mealtime
The client with Parkinson's disease must be monitored for choking while eating because of dysphagia.

Activity

Ambulation with assistance is necessary to maintain joint mobility and prevent injury. The client should not be hurried because the bradykinesia becomes worse when the client attempts to hurry.

Other Therapies

Physical therapy is directed toward maintaining joint mobility, posture, and gait. Occupational therapy focuses on maintaining optimal functioning in achieving ADL. Speech therapy is used to promote communication and maintain swallowing function. Psychotherapy addresses the implications of living with a chronic disease; depression; and the possible psychiatric side effects of the medication regimen.

Nursing Management

Encourage independence. Fatigue may cause more dependence. Assist to establish a regular bowel routine by encouraging the client to drink at least 2,000 mL of liquids daily and eat high-fiber foods. Provide an elevated toilet seat. Assist client and family to express feelings and frustrations.

NURSING PROCESS

Assessment

Subjective Data

Nursing assessment focuses on functional ability and activities. It includes eliciting client statements about symptom control and emotional status. Ascertain bowel and bladder elimination patterns.

Objective Data

Objective assessment involves evaluation of tremors, muscular rigidity, movement, posture, and gait for degree of impairment. Assessment of swallowing ability is necessary to maintain adequate nutrition and prevent aspiration. Evaluate mental/emotional status for signs and symptoms of depression or dementia.

Assess skin for diaphoresis, or excessive oil production; skin integrity; and signs of injury from falls. Obtain supine, sitting, and standing blood pressures to assess for orthostatic hypotension.

Nursing diagnoses for a client with Parkinson's disease may include the following:

Nursing Diagnoses	Planning/Goals	Nursing Interventions
Impaired Physical Mobility related to muscle rigidity, gait disturbance, and bradykinesia	The client will maintain optimal mobility.	Assess degree of muscle involvement by testing ROM, muscular rigidity, tremors, and gait. Perform passive and active ROM exercises to maintain function.
		Administer medications within the time window that provides a constant therapeutic level for symptom control.
		Ambulate, as client is able to tolerate. Frequently turn client when in bed.

continues

Nursing Diagnoses	Planning/Goals	Nursing Interventions
Bathing/Hygiene and Dressing/Grooming Self-care Deficit related to immobility, tremors, and bradykinesia	The client will maintain optimal independence in self-care.	Assess client's ability to perform self-care. Encourage client to perform as much self-care as possible. Consult with occupational therapy for methods to increase the ability to perform self-care. Assist with daily care that the client is unable to perform alone.
Impaired Swallowing related to neuromuscular impairment	The client will swallow with minimal choking and coughing and no aspiration.	Position client sitting upright when eating with client's head slightly forward and never extended to facilitate swallowing. Encourage client to take small bites. Provide small bites of food or pureed foods to prevent client from choking. Have suction equipment available during meals.

Evaluation Each goal must be evaluated to determine how it has been met by the client.

MULTIPLE SCLEROSIS

Multiple sclerosis (MS) is a chronic, progressive, degenerative disease of the central nervous system characterized by a loss of myelin in the brain, spinal cord, or both and by the occurrence of **sclerotic** (hardened) patches (Figure 38-18). The disease interferes with the conduction of impulses. The neurological deficit that occurs depends on which nerve cells are affected. The cause of MS is unclear. Research suggests that it is an abnormal response to the body's immune system. The disease is more prevalent among people of Northern European ancestry (NMSS, 2003). Diagnosis is usually made between the ages of 20 and 50 years. Women are affected two to three times more often than are men (NMSS, 2003).

The white matter of the brain and spinal cord consists of axons covered by a white, lipid substance called myelin. This myelin sheath is an insulator that is involved in the conduction of impulses.

As sclerotic tissue replaces the myelin, neurological function returns. Nerve fibers begin to degenerate as periods of exacerbation become more frequent. Degeneration of the nerve fibers leads to permanent neurological deficits.

Signs and symptoms of MS vary according to the areas of demyelination. The client may have one symptom or a combination of symptoms. Periods of exacerbation and remission also make diagnosis difficult. Symptoms may vary from hour-to-hour or day-to-day. Medical diagnosis is generally based on history and on elimination of other possible diagnoses. Magnetic resonance imaging and CT scan can be used to identify lesions of sclerotic tissue as the disease progresses. Cerebrospinal fluid reveals increased white blood cells, protein, and immunoglobulin (IgG), a diagnostic indicator.

Client symptoms may be sensory, motor, or other disturbances. Sensory symptoms may include visual disturbances, numbness, paresthesia (burning, prickling, tingling), pain, and decreased sense of temperature. Motor symptoms may include decreased muscle strength, spasticity, paralysis, or bowel and bladder incontinence or retention.

Ataxia (loss of balance or coordination), **nystagmus** (constant, involuntary eye movements in any direction), speech disturbances, tremors, and **vertigo** (dizziness) may occur. Other possible symptoms are sexual dysfunction and mood changes ranging from depression to euphoria. Profound fatigue is common.

Exacerbations are frequently precipitated by periods of emotional or physical stress, such as infections, pregnancy,

CLIENT TEACHING

Temperature Sensation

Because the client with MS has a decreased sense of temperature, advise to:

- Be careful when cooking or otherwise around the kitchen stove.
- Use a bath thermometer to test bath or shower water so as to prevent burning
- Use only the low setting on a heating pad.

Figure 38-18 A, *Normal Nerve Fiber and Myelin Sheath;* **B,** *Multiple Sclerosis Destruction of Myelin Sheath* trauma, or fatigue. Hot baths or strenuous exercise may aggravate motor symptoms. Periods of exacerbation may last hours to months. Commonly, the periods of exacerbation become more frequent as the disease progresses. Complications such as urinary tract infection, pneumonia, pressure ulcers, contractures, and depression frequently occur. As the disease progresses and permanent neurological deficits occur, the client may become bedridden, have difficulty speaking and handling oral secretions, and/or develop emotional and intellectual disturbances.

Medical–Surgical Management

There is no cure or specific treatment for MS. Treatment goals are to limit exacerbations, prevent complications, and maintain functional level.

Pharmacological

The treatment of choice for relapsing–remitting MS is interferon beta (Avonex, Betaseron). For 2 or 3 months, clients usually experience flu-like symptoms after each injection. For clients who cannot take either of these two drugs, glatiramer acetate (Copaxone) is an option. The steroids adrenocorticotropic hormone (ACTH) or prednisone (Delasone) are used to decrease periods of exacerbation. Muscle relaxants such as dantrolene sodium (Dantrium) or baclofen (Lioresal) are used for muscle spasticity.

The immunosuppressive agents azathioprine (Imuran), cyclophosphamide (Cytoxan), or cyclosporine (Sandimmune) are administered to decrease immune response. Propantheline bromide (ProBanthine) is often used for urinary frequency and urgency. Bethanechol chloride (Urecholine) may be helpful for the client with a neurogenic bladder. Trimethoprim sulfamethoxazole (Bactrim or Septra) or nitrofurantoin macrocrystals (Macrodantin) is given prophylactically when urinary tract infections are a problem.

Diet

A well-balanced diet complete with roughage is necessary to promote bowel elimination. Plenty of fluids are also necessary. If the client is obese, a dietitian should be consulted for meal planning to help the client lose weight while maintaining adequate nutrition.

Activity

The goal of maintaining the highest possible functional level must be individualized to each client. Daily exercise is necessary for clients with limited motor involvement. Physical therapy may be necessary to prevent contractures, maintain muscle strength, or prevent loss of function from spasticity, or for gait training. Passive/active ROM exercises should be done several times per day. Occupational therapy may be used to maintain or attain self-care. Daily skills of cooking, doing laundry, or maintaining a job may also be encouraged.

Nursing Management

Emphasize avoiding stress, infections, and fatigue. Encourage independence and individualized ways of performing daily activities. Stress the importance of a well-balanced diet, high in fiber to prevent constipation. Encourage adequate fluid intake and regular urination.

NURSING PROCESS

Assessment

Subjective Data

Subjective assessment includes eliciting client statements of symptoms and an historical accounting of exacerbations and remissions. Subjective data should include incidence of visual disturbances, hazy vision, loss of central vision, or diplopia (double vision). Note symptoms of weakness, numbness, fatigue, bowel or bladder problems, sexual dysfunction, emotional instability, vertigo, changes in gait, urinary incontinence or retention, constipation, or difficulty swallowing. Pain is not common.

Objective Data

Objective assessment includes observation of gait for spastic or ataxic gait and a complete neurological examination.

Nursing diagnoses for a client with MS may include the following:

Nursing Diagnoses	Planning/Goals	Nursing Interventions
Impaired Physical Mobility related to muscle weakness, ataxia, spasticity, or perceptual impairment	The client will maintain optimal mobility within physical limitations.	Assess motor status every 4 to 24 hours. Provide active and passive ROM every 8 hours. Ambulate client four times daily with use of assistive devices as necessary. Turn bedridden clients every 2 hours. Use pillows, splints, high-topped (above the ankles) shoes with laces to maintain proper body alignment. Encourage client to perform daily activities as able given the limitations of the disease.
Impaired Urinary Elimination related to changes in innervation of the bladder	The client will have adequate bladder elimination with minimal postvoid residual, urinary tract infections, and episodes of incontinence.	Assess for bladder retention or incontinence. Catheterize as necessary for retention or postvoid residual. Maintain fluid intake of 1,000 cc per day. Develop bladder program to meet individual needs of client. Toilet client at scheduled times even if no urge to go. Assess for signs and symptoms of urinary tract infection, such as elevated temperature and burning on urination.
Situational Low Self-esteem related to neuromuscular and perceptual impairment	The client will verbalize positive statements of self-esteem.	Assess client's concept of self in relation to changes brought about by the disease process. Teach client about the disease process. Allow client to verbalize feelings. Assist client in methods of adapting to change. Collaborate with other health care providers, such as mental health counselors and physicians. Refer client to local support groups (see Resources).
Sexual Dysfunction related to changes in sensation, genitalia, and musculature, and psychological response to diagnosis	The client will seek counseling concerning sexual dysfunction.	Allow client to verbalize concerns. Suggest adaptations (planning time for sexual contact so as to conserve energy, alternatives to sexual intercourse, such as touching or holding). Refer client to appropriate health care providers.

Evaluation Each goal must be evaluated to determine how it has been met by the client.

SAMPLE NURSING CARE PLAN

THE CLIENT WITH MULTIPLE SCLEROSIS

Mrs. Donna Britton, a 37-year-old wife and the mother of two children, ages 3 years and 5 years, was diagnosed with MS 2 days ago. She presents with decreased sensation (paresthesia) in the lower extremities and muscle weakness of the right lower extremity. She has also experienced episodes of loss of central vision. Fatigue has affected her ability to care for her children and perform household tasks. She states, "I do not know what is going to happen to me." She is crying and states, "I do not know about multiple sclerosis or how I am going to take care of my children," and "I cannot get my housework done, and my children need more from me than I can give right now."

Her employer is concerned about her ability to perform her teaching responsibilities, but because he values her excellence as a teacher, he is willing to give her a few weeks off. She has bruises on her thigh, face, and arm from a fall that she experienced several days ago. The client presents in an outpatient clinic for follow-up care.

Nursing Diagnosis 1 *Deficient Knowledge* related to disease process and lifestyle changes as evidenced by client statements, "I do not know what is going to happen to me, I do not know about multiple sclerosis or how I am going to take care of my children"

continues

SAMPLE NURSING CARE PLAN

Nursing Outcomes Classification (NOC)
Knowledge: Disease Process

Nursing Interventions Classification (NIC)
Teaching: Disease Process

PLANNING/GOALS	NURSING INTERVENTIONS	RATIONALE
Mrs. Britton will verbalize knowledge of the disease process, pathophysiology, prognosis, and treatment, including the need to reduce stressors in her life, eat a balanced diet, drink adequate fluids, and get adequate rest.	Assess Mrs. Britton's knowledge of diagnosis, treatment regimen, and lifestyle changes. Ask specific questions.	Provides a frame of reference for Mrs. Britton, helping her to relate new information and integrate it into her behavior.
	Begin teaching information about the pathophysiology and signs and symptoms of MS.	Assists understanding about the disease.
	Discuss needed lifestyle changes, such as planning rest periods, avoiding stressors, eating a balanced diet, and drinking plenty of fluids.	Helps understanding of necessary changes in life.
	Emphasize the importance of keeping a diary of symptoms, activities, and feelings to identify stressors that exacerbate symptoms.	Helps identify activities that exacerbate the symptoms.
	Provide information about the Multiple Sclerosis Society and offer available pamphlets.	Provides resources to strengthen Mrs. Britton's knowledge base.
	Provide the name and telephone number of a contact from the local MS support group or of another client who is willing to share.	Provides a great deal of emotional support as well as practical solutions to problems.

EVALUATION Mrs. Britton verbalizes accurate information regarding the disease process, prognosis, and treatment. She states that by reducing stressors, maintaining a balanced diet, taking in adequate fluids, and obtaining plenty of rest, she can prevent exacerbations of MS.

Nursing Diagnosis 2 *Impaired Home Maintenance* related to fatigue, neuromuscular impairment, and difficulty in performing child care and household tasks as evidenced by client statements, "I cannot keep my housework done, my children need more from me than I can give right now" and by objective data including decreased sensation in lower extremities, muscle weakness, and fatigue

Nursing Outcomes Classification (NOC)
Role Performance
Self-Care: Instrumental Activities of Daily Living (IADL)

Nursing Interventions Classification (NIC)
Support System Enhancement
Energy Management

PLANNING/GOALS	NURSING INTERVENTIONS	RATIONALE
By the next appointment, Mrs. Britton will identify concerns and solutions to accomplishing home maintenance management.	Allow Mrs. Britton to verbalize concerns about home maintenance management.	Plans to organize tasks and responsibilities within her ability to perform home maintenance management can begin.
	Assist Mrs. Britton in identifying areas of concern, items that can be delegated, and possible solutions.	Can then investigate methods of solving her home maintenance problems.
	Assess the extended family's ability to assist with home maintenance management.	May uncover opportunities that she had not considered.

continues

SAMPLE NURSING CARE PLAN

Ask Mrs. Britton to start identifying ways to decrease workload and to set priorities for expending energy.	Helps focus on needed changes.
Collaborate with social services to identify social agencies that can be of assistance.	Gives other possible solutions to achieving home maintenance management.
Plan activities around rest periods.	Conserves strength and prevents fatigue.
Identify peak energy times and plan activities with peak energy in mind.	Allows more to be accomplished.

EVALUATION Mrs. Britton identifies that she is able to care for her children with the assistance of her husband and her mother, but that she does not have the strength to maintain the housekeeping responsibilities. Following further discussion of family commitments and availability of social supports, Mrs. Britton agrees to request weekly assistance from the women's group at her church.

Nursing Diagnosis 3 *Risk for Injury* related to muscle weakness, decreased sensory perception (vision, tactile, kinesthetic), and fatigue as evidenced by recent falls

Nursing Outcomes Classification (NOC)	**Nursing Interventions Classification (NIC)**
Risk Control	*Fall Prevention*

PLANNING/GOALS	NURSING INTERVENTIONS	RATIONALE
Mrs. Britton will remain free of injury.	Teach Mrs. Britton to identify risk factors in the environment.	Avoids injury.
	Teach Mrs. Britton to identify risk factors of the disease process.	Reduces her risk of injury.
	Teach Mrs. Britton to avoid hot baths, hot tubs, saunas, and so on, because muscle weakness and paresthesia can be exacerbated by the heat.	Prevents exacerbation of weakness and decreased sensation, thereby reducing her risk of injury.
	Teach safety factors of wearing well-fitting, oxford-style shoes.	Decreases the risk of falling by providing support for feet.

EVALUATION Injuries have been prevented by increasing Mrs. Britton's awareness of the risks involved with the disease process.

AMYOTROPHIC LATERAL SCLEROSIS (LOU GEHRIG'S DISEASE)

Amyotrophic lateral sclerosis (ALS) is a progressive, fatal disease characterized by the degeneration of motor neurons in the cortex, medulla, and spinal cord. The cause of the disease is not known, but a viral immune response or genetic defect are suggested by current research. Age at onset is 40 to 70 years; men are affected two to three times more often than are women. Average time from onset to death is 3 years, but some clients with ALS have remained active 10 to 20 years after diagnosis.

The upper and lower motor neurons degenerate and deteriorate, causing atrophy of the muscles innervated by those neurons. The involved motor neurons are in the anterior horns of the spinal cord and lower brainstem. The muscles of the hands, forearms, and legs usually atrophy first. As the disease progresses most body muscles are affected. Muscle spasticity and reduced muscle strength result when upper motor neurons are involved. Lower motor neuron involvement causes muscle flaccidity, paralysis, and muscle atrophy. Sensory and intellectual function are not affected. Respiratory function, ability to communicate, and emotional lability are affected as the disease progresses. Drooling, inability to handle oral secretions, and impaired swallowing occur.

Medical–Surgical Management

There is no known cure for ALS. The focus of medical management is to treat the symptoms and to promote independence for as long as possible.

Pharmacological

Muscle relaxants including diazepam (Valium), baclofen (Lioresal), and dantrolene sodium (Dantrium) are used to reduce spasticity. Quinidine is prescribed for muscle cramping. Increased salivation is treated with trihexyphenidyl hydrochloride (Artane), clonidine hydrochloride (Catapres), or amitriptyline hydrochloride (Elavil).

Diet

A regular diet adapted to provide soft, easily chewed food is maintained as long as the client can swallow. Tube feeding may be required to prevent aspiration as chewing and swallowing difficulties arise.

Activity

Ambulation and other activities are encouraged as long as possible.

Other Therapies

Physical and occupational therapy are used to maintain ROM and independence as much as possible. Speech therapy promotes maintenance of communication skills. Mental health counseling assists individual and family coping with the fatal disease.

Nursing Management

Encourage independence as long as possible. Assist with personal hygiene and getting in and out of bed. Provide good skin care, turn client often, keep the bed dry, and use pressure-relieving devices. Position client upright for meals and offer soft, solid foods. When gastrostomy feedings are needed, teach client or family how to administer them.

NURSING PROCESS

Assessment

Subjective Data

Subjective data gathered include the client's and family's emotional status and knowledge status. The client may also indicate chewing or swallowing difficulties as well as dyspnea and fatigue.

Objective Data

Objective assessment includes evaluation of muscle weakness, muscle atrophy, spasticity of upper extremities, flaccid paralysis, difficulty chewing and swallowing, and respiratory status.

Nursing diagnoses for a client with ALS may include the following:

Nursing Diagnoses	Planning/Goals	Nursing Interventions
*Impaired **P**hysical Mobility* related to muscle atrophy, weakness, and spasticity	The client will maintain the highest possible functional ability within limitations of the disease.	Provide active and passive ROM at least twice daily. Use assistive devices to prevent contractures, for ambulation, and for muscle strengthening.
		Assess breath sounds for presence of congestion; skin for pressure areas; and legs for thrombophlebitis.
		Turn every 2 hours.
*Impaired Verbal **C**ommunication* related to weakness of muscles used for speech	The client will communicate verbally or through an alternate communication method as speech muscles deteriorate.	Prolong verbal communication with speech therapy interventions consisting of voice projection and speech devices.
		Develop alternate methods of communicating prior to the loss of verbal skills. Eye-blinking for "yes" and "no"; communication boards, if any arm movement remains; and computer programs can be used.

continues

Nursing Diagnoses	Planning/Goals	Nursing Interventions
*Ineffective **B**reathing Pattern* related to weakness of respiratory muscles and to fatigue	The client will maintain an adequate PaO$_2$ level.	Assess breathing patterns frequently and observe for aspiration and the loss of the swallow reflex. Assess breath sounds every 4 to 8 hours, depending on the progress of the disease. Provide good pulmonary hygiene to prevent aspiration and pneumonia by liquifying secretions and suctioning. Turn from side to side to allow oral secretions to drain from mouth; suction oral pharynx, as necessary. Provide ventilation support, as ordered.
***P**owerlessness* related to loss of control over life; physical dependence; and presence of a fatal disease	The client will inform significant others of wishes while still able to communicate, so as to maintain some control over decisions.	Explore client and family emotional status and coping abilities. Allow client to verbalize feelings while still able to communicate and make decisions in daily care. Promote discussion of client's wishes with family, health care team, and legal representative while client is still able to speak. Provide client education about the disease process, support groups, and counseling to provide support.

Evaluation Each goal must be evaluated to determine how it has been met by the client.

ALZHEIMER'S DISEASE

Alzheimer's disease (AD) is a progressive, degenerative neurological disease wherein brain cells are destroyed. The cerebral cortex atrophies, and neuron loss and changes within the brain cells occur. Identified risk factors are advanced age, female gender, head injury, a history of thyroid disorders, and chromosomal abnormalities.

The cause of AD is unknown. Increasing age is the greatest risk for developing AD (Alzheimer's Association, 2002). The neurons of the frontal and medial temporal lobes are affected, with resultant biochemical and structural changes. Characteristic physiologic changes are neurofibrillary tangles and amyloid plaques (deposits of protein), which interfere with the cells' ability to transmit impulses. These changes are found in the association areas and scattered throughout the cortex. The hippocampus, that part of the limbic system responsible for learning, memory, and emotions, is affected. Those cells most affected are neurons that use acetylcholine as the neurotransmitter. The size of the brain and the amount of acetylcholine both decrease. An increased amount of aluminum is found in the brain tissue on autopsy (Hickey, 2002; Smeltzer & Bare, 2002).

Diagnosis is difficult because of the variety in clinical manifestations and the lack of a test specific to AD. Diagnosis is thus based on the clinical picture and the exclusion of other conditions that can cause similar clinical patterns, such as overmedication, metabolic disorders, depression, thyroid imbalance, or brain tumors. Neuropsychological tests measuring memory, problem solving, attention, counting, and language assist physicians in diagnosing AD (Alzheimer's Disease Education and Referral Center, 2002). Computerized tomography or MRI is used to both measure brain atrophy and rule out other conditions.

The stages of AD are scaled from early to late. Different authors identify from three to six stages of the disease. The time frame for each stage varies from person to person. Table 38-6 lists clinical manifestations of early, middle, and late stages of AD.

In late stages of the disease, an EEG may indicate general slowing of brain waves. Definitive diagnosis is determined on autopsy with a brain biopsy. Although generally a disease of older people, AD does occur in people ages 40 to 50.

The family caring for a member who has Alzheimer's becomes more tied down as the disease progresses. Many clients with advanced Alzheimer's cannot be left alone. Respite care is important for the physical and mental health of the caregiver. With respite care, someone else (e.g., another family member, a friend, or a hired professional licensed practical/vocational nurse or registered nurse) comes in to care for the client with Alzheimer's while the primary caregiver gets away for a time. Respite care should be carried out on a routine basis, such as every 2 or 3 weeks or as often as is feasible.

Medical–Surgical Management

There is no curative treatment for AD. Management of the client is geared toward controlling undesirable symptoms and behaviors.

Pharmacological

Although no drug can stop AD, four are approved for treatment. They are donepezil (Aricept), tacrine (Cognex), revastigmine (Exelon), and gelantamine (Reminyl). About 50% of clients taking one of these drugs show temporary improvement in memory and thinking skills (Alzheimer's Association, 2002). Other medications may be used to treat symptoms such as anxiety, agitation, depression, and insomnia.

Diet

A high-fiber diet is used to prevent constipation. A high-calorie diet is needed for hyperactive clients.

— TEST —

TABLE 38-6   STAGES OF ALZHEIMER'S DISEASE

STAGE	CLINICAL MANIFESTATIONS
Stage 1: Early	Forgetfulness, often subtle and masked by client
	Indecisiveness
	Increasing self-centeredness; decreasing interest in others, environment, social activities
	Difficulty in learning new information
	Slowed reaction time
	Beginnings of compromised performance at home and at work
Stage 2: Middle	Progressing forgetfulness, inability to remember names of family members or close friends
	Tendency to lose things
	Confusion
	Fearfulness
	Easily induced frustration and irritability; sometimes, angry outbursts
	Repetitive storytelling
	Beginnings of communication problems (inability to remember words, apparent aphasia)
	Inability to follow simple directions
	Difficulty in calculating numbers
	Beginnings of getting lost in familiar places
	Evasive or anxious interactions with others
	Physical activity (pacing, wandering)
	Changes in sleep–rest cycle (with frequent activity at night)
	Changes in eating patterns (possible constant hunger or none at all)
	Neglect of ADL and personal hygiene; changes in bowel and bladder continence; and dressing difficulties
	Inability to maintain safety without supervision
	Losses of social behaviors
	Paranoia
Stage 3: Late	Inability to communicate
	Inability to eat
	Incontinence (urine and feces)
	Inability to recognize family or friends
	Confinement to bed
	Total dependence relative to care

COMMUNITY/HOME HEALTH CARE

Safe Environment for the Client with Alzheimer's Disease

- Keep furniture in the same place.
- Orient client to surroundings and reorient as necessary.
- Keep floors free of clutter.
- Provide adequate lighting.
- Monitor temperature of hot water and food.
- Maintain monitoring system to prevent outside wandering.
- Prevent access to sharp items such as knives and razors; hot items such as coffee pot and heaters; poisonous solutions such as cleaning supplies, paints, medications, and insecticides; and hazardous items such as power tools, guns, and electric fans.

CRITICAL THINKING

Parkinson's and Alzheimer's

What are the similarities between Parkinson's disease and Alzheimer's disease?

Frequent feedings of high nutritive value are preferable to three meals a day.

Nursing Management

Maintain a safe, structured environment and a consistent daily schedule for the client. Develop memory aids and cues to help the client remember. Support family in adjusting to the client's altered cognitive ability.

NURSING PROCESS

Assessment

Subjective Data

Data about sleeping and eating habits must be collected. Each client must be assessed for individual signs and symptoms. The client is an expert at hiding these deficits in the early stages of the disease. A family interview may be helpful in ascertaining health and personal history.

Objective Data

An objective neurological examination with particular attention to memory loss and gradual loss of thought processes and impaired judgment is important. Eating patterns, bowel and bladder control, aggressiveness, depression, ambulation, agitation, restlessness, sleep patterns, vision, and hearing should all be assessed. The client's ability to provide self-care, manage finances, drive, prepare meals, use the telephone, perform housekeeping, communicate needs, and perceive the environ-

ment also must be assessed. Attention must be directed to assessing the support system, the family caregiver, support groups, and availability of respite care for the caregiver. The care of the caregiver is often the focus of nursing care of the client with AD.

Nursing diagnoses for the client with Alzheimer's may include the following:

Nursing Diagnoses	Planning/Goals	Nursing Interventions
Risk for Injury related to inability to perceive danger in the environment, confusion, impaired judgment, and weakness	The client will not experience injury.	Assess client's ability to perceive environmental hazards. Teach family to provide a safe home environment.
		Maintain a safe environment: eliminate clutter, position furniture/equipment in same place, monitor temperature of hot water and food, maintain monitoring system to prevent wandering into adverse climate or into traffic, provide adequate lighting, orient client and family to surroundings and reorient as necessary.
		Ensure that the client wears well-fitting tie shoes to reduce risk of falls.
Disturbed Thought Processes related to neuron degeneration, sleep deprivation	The client will maintain optimal cognitive ability.	Assess for cognitive, memory, and communication deficits.
		Develop memory aids and cues to help client remember. Maintain a consistent environment and daily schedule. Approach client in a quiet, nonthreatening manner.
		Do not confront client with reality if it will only upset and agitate him. For example, do not tell a 90-year-old client who wants his mother that she is dead.
		Attend to nonverbal cues for unmet needs (e.g., pacing, grimacing, crying, agitation). The client may be hungry, have a full bladder, or be unable to ask to be repositioned.
		Obtain a photo of client that can be recognized by the client. A current photo of client may appear as a stranger to the client, but a photo of the client at age 20 or 30 may be remembered.
		Give simple, single instructions.
Disturbed Sleep Pattern related to disorientation or irritability	The client will sleep 4 to 5 hours each night.	Advise the client to avoid caffeine.
		Maintain a quiet environment. Provide comfort measures. Provide a night light.
		Increase daytime activities to tolerance and use exercise to tire client.

Evaluation Each goal must be evaluated to determine how it has been met by the client.

GUILLAIN-BARRÉ SYNDROME

Guillain-Barré syndrome (GBS) is an acute inflammatory process involving the motor and sensory neurons of the peripheral nervous system. The cause of Guillain-Barré syndrome is not known, but most cases are preceded by a nonspecific infection. There may be an autoimmune or viral basis for this syndrome. Both spinal and cranial motor nerves can be involved. The demyelination process begins in distal nerves and ascends symmetrically. Remyelination occurs from proximal to distal (Hickey, 2002).

Clinical manifestations occur in differing patterns but include motor weakness and areflexia, or absence of reflexes. Characteristically, motor weakness begins in the legs and progresses up the body. Respiratory failure results from loss of respiratory muscle function. Cranial nerve involvement results in facial muscle deficits, difficulty in swallowing, and autonomic dysfunctions. Autonomic functions possibly affected are cardiac rhythm, blood pressure regulation, gastrointestinal mobility, and urine elimination.

Sensory involvement causes paresthesia and pain in the hands and feet. The pain progresses up the body and may interfere with sleep.

The three stages of Guillain-Barré syndrome are acute onset, lasting 1 to 3 weeks, the plateau period, lasting several days to 2 weeks, and the recovery phase, which involves remyelination and may last up to 2 years.

Diagnosis is based on the clinical picture of a recent viral infection and motor and possibly sensory deficits, along with characteristic diagnostic results. These results include both an elevated protein level in CSF without elevation of red blood cells or white blood cells and electromyelogram (EMG) showing slowed nerve conduction velocity of paralyzed muscles.

Medical–Surgical Management

Medical

The goal of medical management is prevention and treatment of complications such as immobility, infection, and respiratory failure.

Plasma exchanges have been found to decrease the severity and duration of symptoms. Plasmapheresis is performed in severe cases. This complete plasma exchange removes the antibodies affecting the myelin sheath. Three to four exchanges 1 to 2 days apart are initiated within the first 2 weeks of diagnosis of Guillain-Barré. Plasmapheresis may also be used late in the disease process for continued demyelination or lack of progress in remyelination. Mechanical ventilatory support may be required. Blood gas monitoring is used to assess respiratory function.

Surgical

Those who develop respiratory failure may require a tracheostomy along with mechanical ventilation.

Pharmacological

Steroids, such as adrenocorticotropic hormone (ACTH) and prednisone (Detasone), and immunosuppressive agents, such as azathioprine (Imuran) or cyclophosphamide (Cytoxan), may be used to slow the demyelination process. Low doses of anticoagulants, such as heparin, are used to prevent thrombophlebitis.

Diet

A balanced diet is necessary to prevent tissue and muscle breakdown and to promote healing. If severe paralysis is present, a gastrostomy tube may be used to provide adequate nutrition.

Activity

Range of motion and muscle strength are maintained through physical therapy. Occupational therapy activities teach the client to maintain optional self-care within the limitation of the disease process. Pool therapy, or exercising in a swimming pool, is often used to maintain and strengthen muscles.

Nursing Management

Monitor vital signs, LOC, ABGs, and for ascending sensory loss, which precedes motor loss. Turn client frequently and encourage coughing and deep breathing. Provide skin care to prevent skin breakdown and position client to prevent contractures. Perform passive ROM exercises. Apply antiembolism stockings and assess Homan's sign. Provide eye and mouth care every 4 hours if there is facial paralysis. Monitor I&O and encourage adequate fluid intake. Offer prune juice and high-fiber diet to prevent constipation.

NURSING PROCESS

Assessment

Subjective Data

Subjective data collected include client statements about return of sensation; pain; respiratory function; and knowledge.

Objective Data

Assessment includes the status of motor and sensory functions, which are monitored continuously in the acute phase of the illness. Monitor progression of loss of function from distal to proximal with particular emphasis on respiratory status. Decreased depth and quality of respirations and diminished breath sounds may be found. Monitor status of autonomic functions by assessing blood pressure, cardiac rhythm, urinary elimination, and bowel sounds. Assessment for complications of immobility includes breath sounds; signs of thrombophlebitis; loss of ROM; skin condition; and temperature.

Nursing diagnoses for a client with Guillain-Barré syndrome may include the following:

Nursing Diagnoses	Planning/Goals	Nursing Interventions
Ineffective Breathing Pattern related to loss of respiratory muscle function	The client will be adequately ventilated.	Monitor respiratory status of client by assessing breath sounds, respiratory rate, and respiratory quality. Position client to facilitate maximal expansion of the chest wall for optimal breathing.
		Monitor oxygenation by assessing skin color, mental status, pulse oximeter readings, and blood gas values. Administer oxygen as ordered. Report failing respiratory status to the physician. Provide mechanical ventilation for respiratory failure.

continues

Nursing Diagnoses	Planning/Goals	Nursing Interventions
*Impaired **P**hysical Mobility* related to progressive loss of motor function	The client will avoid complications of immobility (pneumonia, thrombophlebitis, pressure areas, and loss of ROM).	Monitor status of motor and sensory functions in an ongoing fashion.
		Have client turn, deep breathe, and cough every 2 hours.
		Suction client as necessary.
		Perform respiratory assessment for diminished breath sounds or congestion.
		Monitor vital signs (blood pressure, pulse, respiration, and temperature) every 4 to 8 hours.
		Assess for calf tenderness, redness, or increased warmth. Monitor for positive Homan's sign, indicative of deep vein thrombosis.
		Perform ROM to lower extremities every 2 to 4 hours.
		Use plexipulse boots, which are intermittent-pumping boots that promote return blood flow from the lower extremities.
		Administer low doses of heparin or other anticoagulants as prescribed.
		Apply antiembolism stockings.
		Assess condition of skin for pressure areas. Massage client's back and pressure points with lotion three times a day.
		Use specialty mattress.
		Assist client to sitting positions in wheelchair two to three times daily. Progress to ambulation as motor function returns. Apply high-topped shoes to keep feet in correct alignment.
*Dressing/Grooming **S**elf-care Deficit* related to decreased motor function	The client will have self-care needs met.	Encourage self-care within the limitations of the neurological deficits. Provide daily care needs that client is unable to perform.
		Maintain muscle strength and ROM with physical therapy. Provide ROM to all extremities three to four times daily.
		Initiate rehabilitation following acute phase of illness with strengthening exercises, occupational therapy, and getting client out of bed several times per day to build strength and endurance.

Evaluation Each goal must be evaluated to determine how it has been met by the client.

HEADACHE

Headache, or **cephalalgia,** the condition of pain in the head, is caused by stimulation of pain-sensitive structures in the cranium, head, or neck. Headaches are symptoms rather than a disease.

The pain-sensitive areas of the intracranial structure include the peripheral nerves, cerebral vasculature, and parts of the dura mater. The external supporting structures of the skin, muscles, and nasal passages are also sensitive to pain. The skull, brain tissue, and most of the meninges are insensitive to pain.

More than 45 million people in the United States each year have chronic, recurring headaches (National Headache Foundation, 2002). Headaches are generally classified as either primary or secondary.

PRIMARY HEADACHES

Primary headaches are not caused by an underlying medical condition. They include tension-type, migraine,

cluster headaches, and rebound headache (American Council for Headache Education, 2001) (Table 38-7).

Tension-Type Headache

The most common type of headache is the tension type, affecting 75% of headache sufferers (ACHE, 2001). The ache is steady rather than throbbing, affects both sides of the head, and occurs frequently, sometimes daily.

Migraine Headaches — Women

Up to 18% of women experience migraine headaches each year, compared to 6% of men (ACHE, 2001). Migraine headaches are vascular and recurrent. The initial vasoconstriction can cause neurological symptoms or an aura before the vasodilation that causes the headache. The aura is a visual disturbance typically consisting of brightly colored or blinking lights or a pattern moving across the field of vision. When only the aura occurs, and there is no pain in the head, the migraine is termed "silent." Migraines generally are a throbbing on

TABLE 38-7   PRIMARY HEADACHE PATTERNS

TYPE	AURA	PAIN	TYPICAL PATTERN	DURATION
Tension ✓	None	Steady ache	Usually begins gradually in frontal or temporal areas; affects both sides of the head; occur frequently, maybe daily	Hours
Classic Migraine ✓	Duration of 15 to 30 minutes; sensory, usually visual (bright spots, zig-zag lines), unilateral or bilateral numbness or tingling in lips, face, or hand; difficulty thinking; confusion or drowsiness; sometimes preceded by premonition 24 hours before	Throbbing, intense; unilateral; tenderness in scalp; muscle contractions in neck and scalp followed by feelings of exhaustion	Periodic, recurrent; usually begins on awakening; begins in childhood or early adolescence; tends to be familial; nausea and vomiting typical; sensitivity to light and sound	Hours to days
Cluster ✓	None	Intense throbbing; unilateral pain in orbitotemporal area	Causes awakening two to three times during the night; accompanied by watering eyes, nasal congestion, runny nose, facial flushing over the throbbing area; after cluster headaches for days, weeks, or months may be free of symptoms for a year or more; same side of head usually involved; usually in men	30 minutes to 2 hours

one side of the head. Other symptoms may include irritability, anorexia, nausea, vomiting, and photophobia. Some migraine headaches may be triggered by certain foods or chemicals.

Cluster Headaches — Men

A cluster headache develops around or behind one eye and is very severe. Generally, it awakens the person from sleep. The affected eye may tear and the nose become congested on the same side. These headaches occur in clusters daily for weeks or months, then disappear for a year or more. Most cluster headaches occur in men. Alcohol often triggers attacks.

Rebound Headache

When pain relievers are overused, headache may "rebound" when the last dose wears off. This leads to taking increasingly more pain relievers. This may occur with tension-type or migraine headaches (ACHE, 2001).

SECONDARY HEADACHES

Secondary headaches are the result of pathological conditions such as aneurysm, brain tumor, or inflamed cranial nerves. The headache is caused by compression, inflammation, or hypoxia of pain-sensitive structures.

Medical–Surgical Management

Medical

Medical management is based on the underlying cause of the headache. A thorough history of headache pattern, dietary pattern, and coping pattern is essential. Underlying pathology of brain tumor, aneurysm, and infection must be ruled out. If pathology is identified, secondary headache is diagnosed and, therefore, treatment is based on findings. If no cause is found, management of primary headache is based on symptoms.

Surgical

Surgical management may include repair of an aneurysm or resection of a brain tumor.

Pharmacological

Management is either abortive, to stop the headache, or prophylactic, to prevent reoccurrence or to decrease frequency of headaches. Abortive therapy for migraine headaches includes naproxen (Aleve), ibuprofen (Advil), sumatriptan (Imitrex), rizatriptan (Maxalt), zolmitriptan (Zomig), naratriptan (Amerge), almotriptan (Axert), and older drugs like cafergot, containing ergotamine and caffeine (McGuire, 2002). Promethazine hydrochloride (Phenergan) is often used to control nausea and vomiting.

Prophylactic treatment includes the beta-blockers propranolol hydrochloride (Inderal) and methysergide maleate (Sansert), which prevent dilation of the blood vessels and interrupt the serotonin mechanism. Clonidine hydrochloride (Catapres) directly affects the ability of the blood vessels to constrict or dilate. Tricyclic antidepressants, such as amitriptyline hydrochloride (Elavil), block the uptake of serotonin.

Diet

A strict food diary should be kept to identify precipitating foods. After all suspect foods have been eliminated from the diet, skin testing for allergies may be performed. Introduction of suspect foods may be done one at a time to identify triggering foods. Alcohol; cured meats containing nitrates; aged cheeses; monosodium glutamate (MSG); citrus fruits; chocolate; and red wines are common precipitating foods.

Activity

Activities that precipitate headaches must be identified and eliminated if possible. Stressful situations are frequently precipitating agents. Biofeedback, relaxation techniques, stress reduction, and development of coping mechanisms are useful in reducing the occurrence of headaches caused by stress and tension.

Nursing Management

Nursing interventions focus on relieving pain and assisting the client in managing the pain. Identifying methods of decreasing pain, such as effective use of medications and managing the environment to minimize stimulation from light, noise, and activity, are also nursing priorities.

Assist the client to develop a plan for accomplishing daily activities when incapacitated by a headache. Teach the client to keep a diary of headache history to determine patterns in headache development. Assist the client in changing lifestyle to decrease the incidence of headaches by minimizing stress, avoiding certain foods, reducing salt intake during premenstrual time frame, and using relaxation techniques.

TRIGEMINAL NEURALGIA (TIC DOULOUREUX)

Trigeminal neuralgia is a condition of cranial nerve V and is characterized by abrupt paroxysms of pain and facial muscle contractions. **Neuralgia** is nerve pain. The pain follows one of the three branches of the trigeminal nerve: the ophthalmic, maxillary, or mandibular. The last two branches are most commonly affected (Figure 38-19).

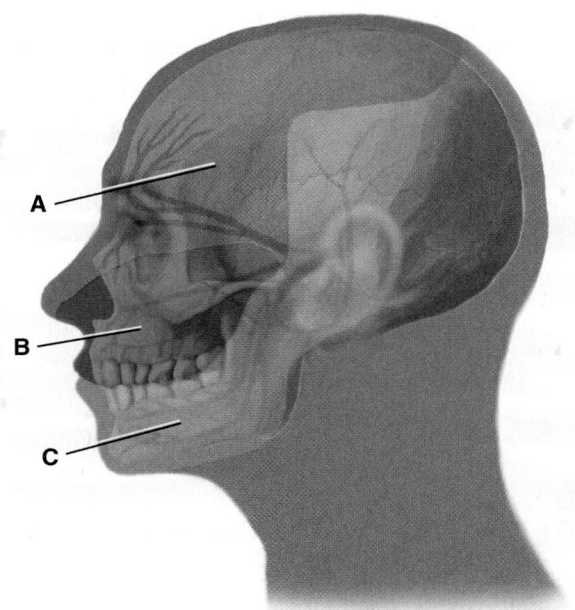

Figure 38-19 *Areas of Face Innervated by the Trigeminal Nerve (CN-I):* **A,** *Ophthalmic;* **B,** *Maxillary;* **C,** *Mandibular*

The etiology of trigeminal neuralgia is not known, but injury, dental caries, dental work, and anatomic position of the nerves have been identified as possible causes. Pain begins when trigger points are stimulated, causing periods of intense pain and facial twitching lasting from seconds to minutes. These periods may last several weeks to months. Periods of remission interspersed with exacerbations occur with increasing frequency with advancing age (Hickey, 2002).

Medical–Surgical Management

Drug therapy, nerve blocks, and surgery are treatment modalities for trigeminal neuralgia.

Surgical

Surgical approaches to relieve pain include percutaneous electrocoagulation with radio frequency. This procedure affects the pain-sensory fibers but causes little

CLIENT TEACHING

Dental Work on the Client with Trigeminal Neuralgia

The client with trigeminal neuralgia should:

- Plan to have dental work done during a period of remission.
- Inform the dentist of the condition.
- Maintain good dental hygiene, especially during remission.

damage to the touch, proprioception, and motor fibers. Longer-term relief or permanent relief may be obtained.

Pharmacological

Phenytoin (Dilantin) and carbamazepine (Tegretol) are used to shorten the length of the paroxysmal pain. Nerve blocks using alcohol and phenol injections into the nerve provide temporary relief for 8 to 16 months.

Nursing Management

Goals of nursing interventions are relief of pain, prevention of injury, prevention of self-care deficits, and promotion of social interaction. The client with trigeminal neuralgia frequently experiences such severe pain that grooming, talking, and eating are avoided. It is especially important to provide good oral hygiene if the client is on phenytoin (Dilantin) because the medication causes hyperplasia of the gums. Teach the client to identify both the trigger points that stimulate the pain and ways to avoid those areas without neglecting daily needs.

The client who has had surgery may have lost the mechanisms that protect the eye from injury, and will need to be taught not to touch his eye and to observe for redness of the eye and conjunctiva. Following surgery, the client may not feel pain caused by dental caries, so routine visits to the dentist for oral examination are needed.

ENCEPHALITIS, MENINGITIS

Encephalitis is inflammation of the brain. **Meningitis** is inflammation of the meninges. The most common cause of encephalitis or meningitis is a virus. Bacteria, fungi, or parasites can also be causative factors. Meningococcal meningitis is highly contagious. Contacts of the client are identified and prophylactic medication is recommended. The virus or other causative agent enters the brain either through the bloodstream as a direct extension of trauma or by nerve pathways.

The inflammatory process causes demyelination of white matter and degeneration of neurons. Cerebral edema, hemorrhage, and necrosis of brain tissue can also occur. Clinical manifestations vary depending on the causative agent, area of involvement, and degree of damage to nerve tissue. Fever, headache, nuchal rigidity, photophobia, irritability, lethargy, nausea, and vomiting are typical signs and symptoms. As the disease progresses, level of consciousness may decrease and other neurological dysfunctions occur, including motor weakness, aphasia, seizures, behavioral changes, or even death. A lumbar puncture is performed to test CSF for the causative agent, presence of white blood cells or red blood cells, and elevated protein level. A complete blood count is done to identify the presence of viral or bacterial infection.

Medical–Surgical Management

Medical

Treatment is supportive and based on presenting symptoms. The aim of treatment is to prevent or decrease increased intracranial pressure and to minimize neurological deficits. Intravenous fluids are given to re-

hydrate the client. Clients are often placed in isolation until the cause of meningitis can be determined.

Pharmacological

Antibiotics or antiinfectives are administered in massive doses as appropriate for the causative agent. They may be given intravenously or intrathecally into the spinal canal. Most viral agents do not respond to antibiotics or antiinfectives. Glucocorticosteroids are administered to prevent cerebral edema. Osmotic diuretics may be used to reduce cerebral edema. To prevent seizures, anticonvulsants are often ordered. Antipyretics are often given to reduce fever.

Diet

Optimal nutritional status must be maintained to promote response to the infection.

Activity

A quiet environment with minimal stimulation from noise, light, or client activity is maintained. Routine turning, ROM exercises, pulmonary hygiene, and skin care are required to prevent the complications of immobility.

Nursing Management

In the acute stage, monitor the client for changes in neurological status, especially for changes in level of consciousness and for signs of increasing intracranial pressure. A quiet environment will decrease external stimulation. Observe the client for seizure activity and protect from injury. Comfort measures such as oral hygiene, tepid baths, and administration of analgesics for relief of headaches should be offered.

HUNTINGTON'S DISEASE

Huntington's disease (HD) is a chronic, progressive hereditary disease of the nervous system. It is characterized by a progressive involuntary choreiform movement and progressive dementia.

The cells of the basal ganglia, which control movement, die prematurely. Cells in the cerebral cortex also die, interfering with thought processes, memory, perception, and judgment. Age of onset is usually 35 to 45 years, with death occurring 10 to 15 years following onset of symptoms (Smeltzer & Bare, 2002). Each child of a person with Huntington's disease has a 50% chance of inheriting the fatal gene. Everyone who has the gene will develop the disease (HDSA, 2002). However, there is no cure for this devastating progressive disease.

Clinical manifestations are **chorea,** abnormal involuntary, purposeless movements of all musculature of the body. Facial tic, grimacing, difficulty in chewing and swallowing, speech impairment, disorganized gait, and bowel and bladder incontinence also occur. Mental or intellectual impairment progresses to dementia. The client may experience paranoia, hallucinations, or delusions. Emotions are labile, from outbursts of anger to profound depression, apathy, or euphoria. A ravenous appetite is usually present, but because of the constant movement, the client is often emaciated and exhausted. Death usually results from heart failure, pneumonia, infection, or choking (HDSA, 2002).

The entire family experiences this disease in an emotional, physical, social, and financial way. Supportive care is required as the family progresses through life with a loved one with Huntington's disease. Because of the hereditary factor, genetic counseling is suggested.

Medical–Surgical Management

Pharmacological

Medications used to decrease choreiform movement are dopamine receptor blockers, chlorpromazine (Thorazine), haloperidol (Haldol), thiothixene (Navane), and reserpine (Serpasil), which depletes presynaptic dopamine. Antidepressants, such as desipramine hydrochloride (Norpramin) and fluoxetine hydrochloride (Prozac), and antipsychotics, such as fluphenazine hydrochloride (Prolixin), are used for emotional disturbances. Many people do better with minimal medication (HDSA, 2001).

Diet

The diet must be high in calories to provide for the high energy needs caused by the continuous movement. Chewing and swallowing difficulties necessitate foods that are easy to chew or foods cut into small pieces to prevent choking.

Activity

Ambulation is maintained as long as possible. A safe environment must be maintained to prevent injury from falls or from sharp objects. Driving is usually restricted when choreiform movement or impaired judgment interferes with the ability to drive safely.

Nursing Management

Nursing interventions include a holistic approach to the client's care. Collaboration with the social worker, the chaplain, the physician, and the mental health worker is necessary.

Teach the client and family about the disease process, the progress of the disease, and the genetic factors involved. Safety factors must be considered. Fall prevention measures, such as removing throw rugs and small objects from the floor, and injury prevention measures, such as removing sharp or dangerous objects such as guns and knives from the home, are implemented. The hazard of choking also must be addressed, by teaching the family to cut the client's food into small pieces and to serve soft foods and by teaching the Heimlich maneuver.

GILLES DE LA TOURETTE'S SYNDROME

Gilles de la Tourette's syndrome is a neurological movement disorder that also has prominent behavioral manifestations. Clinical manifestations include motor tics and involuntary repetitive movements of the mouth, face, head, or neck muscles. The trunk and extremities

may also be involved. Motor tics may take the form of forceful eye blinking or toe touching. Vocal tics or repetitive involuntary vocalizations may take the form of sniffing, grunting, throat clearing, or **coprolalia** (involuntary and inappropriate swearing). Other complex motor and vocal tics that may also be present include copropraxia, involuntary and effectively appropriate use of obscene gestures; echolalia, involuntary repetition of the speech of others; and palilia, involuntary repetition of the person's own speech. The obsessive–compulsive symptoms of repetitive handwashing or checking rituals may also be exhibited. Attention deficit hyperactivity disorder (ADHD) and obsessive–compulsive disorders may also coexist with Tourette's syndrome.

Onset is before age 18 years, with males being more commonly affected than females. Tourette's is an inherited disorder, with the affected individual having a 50% chance of passing the gene on to children.

Medical–Surgical Management

Pharmacological

Tics may be controlled with clonadine (Catapres), haloperidol (Haldol), or primozide (Orap). Coexisting ADHD may be controlled with clonidine (Catapres), methylphenidate (Ritalin), or pemoline (Cylert). Clomypramine (Anafranil) or fluoxetine (Prozac) can be used to keep obsessive–compulsive behaviors under control (Kurlan, 1998). Acetaminophen (Tylenol) may help the discomfort of muscle spasms.

Other Therapies

As they age, clients may learn to suppress tics in social situations. Psychotherapy and family counseling are beneficial in coping with social stigma and adjustment problems.

Nursing Management

The client and the family with Tourette's syndrome need a great deal of emotional support and will benefit from knowing about the availability of support groups for clients with Tourette's syndrome. The nurse should teach about the disease process and expectations for the client. Behavioral modification techniques are generally effective; the nurse must know which modification techniques are being used and must follow through with consistent responses.

Summary

- The nervous system controls all bodily functions, from movement to thinking to processing information to autonomic responses.
- The frontal lobe of the cerebrum specializes in emotional attitudes and responses, formation of thought processes, motor function, judgment, personality, and inhibitions.

CASE STUDY

Mr. Domingo Ochoa, a 76-year-old retired farmer, was admitted to the emergency room with left-sided hemiplegia, difficulty swallowing, and inability to speak. He was awake and watching the staff upon admission. He moved his right arm to indicate that Mrs. Ochoa was his wife, but was unable to speak or form sounds. Mrs. Ochoa stated that her husband was working in the garden, picking tomatoes and cucumbers, when he fell to the ground 30 minutes before admission. The emergency room nurse administered oxygen through nasal cannula at 2 liters per minute and obtained vital signs. His blood pressure was 182/98, pulse was 88, respirations were 20, and temperature was 100.5°F. The emergency room physician ordered an MRI scan of the head, a complete blood count, and prothrombin time (PT). The MRI indicated that Mr. Ochoa experienced a CVA caused by bleeding into the brain.

The following questions will guide your development of a nursing care plan for the case study.

1. List clinical manifestations other than the ones Mr. Ochoa experienced that can occur with a CVA.
2. List subjective and objective data that a nurse would obtain.
3. Identify three individualized nursing diagnoses and goals for Mr. Ochoa.
4. Mr. Ochoa is transferred to a general medical unit for 3 days, then is transferred to a rehabilitation center for intensive therapy. What pertinent nursing actions should a nurse perform in caring for Mr. Ochoa in the acute setting and the rehabilitation setting related to:
    Mobility
    Safety
    Elimination
    Skin integrity
    Comfort and rest
5. What teaching will Mr. Ochoa need before discharge from the rehabilitation facility?
6. List at least three client outcomes for Mr. Ochoa.

- The parietal lobe of the cerebrum is a purely sensory region for interpretation of all senses except smell; the purpose is to analyze sensations, including pain, touch, and temperature, from receptors in the skin.
- The temporal lobe of the cerebrum houses Wernicke's area, the primary auditory association area, where words that are heard are interpreted. Memory is also a function of the temporal lobe, especially memories that are highly detailed or involve multiple sensations.
- A special interpretive area located at the junction of the temporal, parietal, and occipital lobes integrates somatic, auditory, and visual sensory interpretations.
- The occipital lobe of the cerebrum is responsible for visual interpretation and visual association.
- Disorders of the nervous system cause complex dysfunctions; the nurse must use assessment skills and quickly recognize changes in condition.
- Teaching about injury prevention and the effects and prognosis of the disorder are required to meet the physical and psychosocial needs of the client and family.
- Many neurological disorders potentiate injury. Nursing care must include providing the client and family with necessary safety information.
- In order to maintain and restore functional ability, rehabilitation is initiated from the first contact with the client.

Review Questions

1. The most important indicator of change in neurological status is:
    a. level of consciousness.
    b. pupil reaction.
    c. vital signs.
    d. motor function.

2. Assessment of intellectual function requires that the nurse:
    a. have knowledge of the client's prior ability to function.
    b. administer a written test to determine the client's IQ level.
    c. utilize auscultation, percussion, and palpation skills.
    d. observe the client's behavior, posture, and facial expression.

3. Contusion of the brain is a (an):
    a. shaking of the brain.
    b. bleeding into the brain tissue.
    c. open head injury.
    d. bruising of the brain.

4. Benign brain tumors can be:

   a. more anxiety producing than are malignant tumors.

   b. more life threatening than are malignant tumors.

   c. treated with radiation therapy.

   d. the cause of increased intracranial pressure.

5. Miss Webster, a 24-year-old client with Guillain-Barré syndrome, can be told which of the following?

   a. The nerve degeneration continues to slowly progress in this chronic degenerative nerve disease.

   b. The disease is an acute inflammatory process with most clients regaining complete function.

   c. Respiratory failure requiring chronic ventilatory support may occur.

   d. Motor function deficit will occur, but sensation will remain.

References/Suggested Readings

Alzheimer's Association. (2002). *Facts: About Alzheimer's disease.* [Online]. Available: www.alz.org/Resource Center/FactSheets/FSAlzheimerdisease.pdf

Alzheimer's Disease Education and Referral Center. (2002). *Alzheimer's disease fact sheet.* [Online]. Available: www.alzheimers.org/pubs/adfact.html

American Council for Headache Education (ACHE). (2001). *What you should know about headache.* [Online]. Available: www.achenet.org/understanding

Andersen, G. (1998). DX dementia: But what kind? *RN, 61*(6), 26–30.

Barker, E. (1999). Brain attack! A call to action. *RN, 62*(5), 54–57.

Barker, E. (2001). What's your patient's stroke risk? *Nursing2001, 31*(4), 32hn1–32hn5.

Barker, E., & Saulino, M. (2002). First-ever guidelines for spinal cord injuries. *RN, 65*(10), 32–37.

Beare, P. G., & Myers, J. L. (Eds.). (1998). *Principles and practice of adult health nursing* (3rd ed.). St. Louis, MO: Mosby.

Best, J. (2001). Cauda equina syndrome. *Nursing2001, 31*(4), 43.

Bond, C. (2002). Traumatic brain injury: Help for the family. *RN, 65*(11), 60–66.

Costa, M. (1998). Clinical snapshot: Trigeminal neuralgia. *AJN, 98*(6), 42–43.

Crigger, N., & Forbes, W. (1997). Assessing neurologic function in older patients. *AJN, 97*(3), 37–40.

Cross, C. (2002). Spotting concussions in children and in adults. *RN, 65*(7), 72.

Dochterman, J., & Bulechek, G. (2004). *Nursing Interventions Classification (NIC)* (4th ed.). St. Louis, MO: Mosby.

Finesilver, C. (2003). Multiple sclerosis. *RN, 66*(4), 36–43.

Galvan, T. (2001). Dysphagia: Going down and staying down. *AJN, 101*(1), 37–42.

Gendreau-Webb, R. (2001). Acute ischemic stroke. *Nursing2001, 31*(11), 120.

Gray-Vickrey, P. (2002). Advances in Alzheimer's disease. *Nursing2002, 32*(11), 64.

Gumm, S. L. (2000). Straight talk about MS. *Nursing2000, 30*(1), 50–51.

Halper, J., & Holland, N. (1998a). Meeting the challenge of multiple sclerosis (Part I). *AJN, 98*(10), 26–31.

Halper, J., & Holland, N. (1998b). Meeting the challenge of multiple sclerosis (Part II). *AJN, 98*(11), 39–46.

Hickey, J. V. (2002). *The clinical practice of neurological and neurosurgical nursing* (5th ed.). Philadelphia: Lippincott Williams & Wilkins.

Hilgers, J. (2003). Comforting a confused patient. *Nursing2003, 33*(1), 48–50.

Hilton, G. (2001). Acute head injury: Distinguishing subdural from epidural hematoma. *AJN, 101*(9), 51–52.

Huntington's Disease Society of America (HDSA). (2002). *Huntington's Disease.* [Online]. Available: www.hdsa.org/edu/HD_booklet.htm

Huston, C. (1998). Emergency! Cervical spine injury. *AJN, 98*(6), 33.

Huston, C. J., & Boelman, R. (1995). Autonomic dysreflexia. *AJN, 95*(6), 55.

Kurlan, R. (1998). *Current pharmacology of Tourette's Syndrome.* Bayside, NY: Tourette Syndrome Association. [Online]. Available: www.2mgh.harvard.edu/lsa/medsci/medicationsanddosages.html

Lewis, A. M. (1999). Neurologic emergency! *Nursing99, 29*(10), 54–56.

Lower, J. (2002). Facing neuro assessment fearlessly. *Nursing2002, 32*(2), 58–64.

Lower, J. (2003). Using pain to assess neurologic response. *Nursing2003, 33*(6), 56–57.

McCance, K. L., & Huether, S. E. (2001). *Pathophysiology: The biological basis for disease in adults and children* (4th ed.). St. Louis, MO: Mosby.

McGuire, L. (2002). How to treat a migraine. *Nursing2002, 32*(12), 76–77.

Monlus-Swift, C. (2002). Neurological disorders. In P. L. Swearingen (Ed.), *Manual of medical–surgical nursing care: Nursing interventions and collaborative management* (5th ed.). St. Louis, MO: Mosby.

Moorhead, S., Johnson, M., & Maas, M. (2004). *Nursing Outcomes Classification (NOC)* (3rd ed.). St. Louis, MO: Mosby.

Mower-Wade, D., Cavanaugh, M., & Bush, D. (2001). Protecting a patient with ruptured cerebral aneurysm. *Nursing2001, 31*(2), 52–57.

Nadler-Moodie, M., & Wilson, M. (1998). Latest approaches in Alzheimer's care. *RN, 61*(7), 42–46.

National Headache Foundation (NHF) (2002). *Fact sheet.* [Online]. Available: www.headaches.org/consumer/generalinfo/factsheet.html

National Multiple Sclerosis Society (NMSS). (2003). *What is multiple sclerosis?* [Online]. Available: www.nationalmssociety.org/What%20is%20MS.asp

National Spinal Cord Injury Information Network. (2001). *Spinal cord injury: Facts and figures at a glance.* [Online]. Available: www.spinalcord.uab.edu/show.asp? durki=21446

National Stroke Association (NSA). (1999). *Stroke prevention guidelines* [Online]. Available: www.stroke.org/pages/prev_guide.cfm

National Stroke Association (NSA). (2002a). *Stroke in America Campaign* [Online]. Available: www.stroke.org/pages/america_main.cfm

National Stroke Association (NSA). (2002b). *Stroke statistics.* [Online]. Available: www.stroke.org/brain_stat.cfm

National Stroke Association (NSA). (2002c). *Stroke: What it is.* [Online]. Available: www.stroke.org/whats.cfm

North American Nursing Diagnosis Association. (2003). *Nursing Diagnoses: Definitions and Classification 2003-2004.* Philadelphia: Author.

O'Hanlon-Nichols, T. (1999). Neurologic assessment. *AJN, 99*(6), 44–50.

Parini, S. (2001). 8 faces of meningitis. *Nursing2001, 31*(8), 51–53.

Parkinson's Disease Foundation (PDF). (2002). *Parkinson's Disease.* [Online]. Available: www.pdf.org/aboutdisease/overview.html

Pullen, R. (2003). Protecting your patient during a seizure. *Nursing2003, 33*(4), 78.

Rudick, R. (1997). New approaches to multiple sclerosis. *Health News*, 3(17), 1–2. Waltham, MA: Massachusetts Medical Society.

Samuels, M. A. (Ed.). (1999). *Manual of neurological therapeutics* (6th ed.). Philadelphia: Lippincott Williams & Wilkins.

Schweiger, J. L. (1999). Alzheimer's disease. *Nursing99, 29*(6), 34–41.

Smeltzer, S. C., & Bare, B. G. (Eds.). (2002). *Brunner and Suddarth's textbook of medical surgical nursing* (9th ed.). Philadelphia: Lippincott Williams & Wilkins.

Smith, L. (2002). Steady the course of Parkinson's disease. *Nursing2002, 32*(3), 43–45.

Son, G., Therrien, B., & Whall, A. (2002). Implicit memory and familiarity among elders with dementia. *Journal of Nursing Scholarship, 34*(3), 263–267.

Taggart, H. M. (1998, March/April). Multiple sclerosis update. *Orthopaedic Nursing.*

The American Association of Neurological Surgeons & The Congress of Neurological Surgeons. (2002). Guidelines for the management of acute cervical spine and spinal cord injuries. *Neurosurgery, 50*(3), S1.

Thelan, L. A., Urden, L. D., Lough, M., & Stacy, K. (1998). *Critical care nursing: Diagnosis and management* (3rd ed.). St. Louis, MO: Mosby.

Williams, L., & Hopper, P. (2003). *Understanding Medical Surgical Nursing.* Philadelphia: F. A. Davis.

Williams, M., Wood H., & Waxman, J. (2002). How to assess swallowing after a stroke. *Nursing2002, 32*(8), 32hn5–32hn6.

Wilson, R. S., Mendes de Leon, C. F. et al. (2002). Participation in cognitively stimulating activities and risk of incident Alzheimer's disease. *JAMA, 287*(6), 742.

Resources

Alzheimer's Association, 919 North Michigan Avenue, Suite 1100, Chicago, IL 60611, 800-272-3900, www.alz.org

Alzheimer's Disease Education and Referral Center, P.O. Box 8250, Silver Spring, MD 20907-8250, 800-438-4380, www.alzheimers.org

American Academy of Neurology, 1080 Montreal Avenue, St. Paul, MN 55116, 800-879-1960, www.aan.com

American Association of Spinal Cord Injury Nurses (AASCIN), 75-20 Astoria Boulevard, Jackson Heights, NY 11370-1177, 718-803-3782

American Council for Headache Education, 19 Mantua Road, Mt. Royal, NJ 08061, 856-423-0258, www.achenet.org

American Spinal Injury Association, 2020 Peachtree Road, NW, Atlanta, GA 30309-1402, 404-355-9772, www.asia-spinal injury.org

Brain Injury Association, Inc., 105 North Alfred Street, Alexandria, VA 22314, 703-236-6000, www.biausa.org

Coma Recovery Association, Inc., 807 Carmen Avenue, Westbury, NY 11590, 516-997-1826, www.comarecovery.org

Epilepsy Foundation of America, 4351 Garden City Drive, Suite 406, Landover, MD 20785, 301-459-3700, 800-332-1000, www.efa.org

Guillain-Barré Syndrome Foundation, International, P.O. Box 262, Wynnewood, PA 19096, 610-667-0131, www.guillain-barre.com

Huntington's Disease Society of America, 158 West 29 Street, 7th Floor, New York, NY 10001-5300, 800-345-4372, www.gdsa.org

National Headache Foundation, 428 West St. James Place, 2nd Floor, Chicago, IL 60614, 888-643-5552, www.headaches.org

National Institute of Neurological Disorders and Stroke, NIH Neurological Institute, P.O. Box 5801, Bethesda, MD 20824, 301-496-5751, 800-352-9424, www.ninds.nih.gov

National Multiple Sclerosis Society, 733 Third Avenue, New York, NY 10017, 800-344-4867, www.nmss.org

National Parkinson's Foundation, Inc., 1501 N.W. Ninth Avenue, Miami, FL 33136, 305-547-6666, 800-327-4545, www.parkinson.org

National Spinal Cord Injury Association, 6701 Democracy Boulevard, Suite 300-9, Bethesda, MD 20817, 301-588-6959, www.spinalcord.org

National Stroke Association, 9707 East Easter Lane, Englewood, CO 80112, 800-STROKES (787-6537), www.stroke.org

Parkinson's Disease Foundation, William Black Medical Building, Columbia-Presbyterian Medical Center, 710 West 168th Street, New York, NY 10032, 800-457-6676, www.pdf.org

Tourette Syndrome Association, Inc., 42-40 Bell Boulevard, Bayside, NY 11361, 718-244-2999, www.tsa-usa.org

SENSORY SYSTEM

MAKING THE CONNECTION

Refer to the following chapters to increase your understanding of the sensory system:

Basic Nursing
- **Communication**
- **Loss, Grief, and Death**
- **Wellness Concepts**
- **Assessment**
- **Pain Management**
- **Diagnostic Tests**

Adult Health Nursing
- **Surgery**

- **Neurological System**
- **The Older Adult**

Intermediate Procedures
- **Administering Eye and Ear Medications**

Review: Delmar's Anatomy & Physiology CD-ROM: Eyes and Sight: Ears and Hearing

LEARNING OBJECTIVES

Upon completion of this chapter, you should be able to:
- **Define key terms.**
- **Compare and differentiate common disorders of the special senses.**
- **Identify the structure and function of the major parts of the eye and ear.**
- **Explain the purpose of the common diagnostic tests for sensory problems.**
- **List the nursing assessments and common nursing diagnoses related to sensory impairment.**
- **Assist in planning nursing care for clients with sensory disorders.**
- **List some of the common sensory aids for the visual and hearing impaired.**

KEY TERMS

affect	myopia
afferent nerve pathway	nystagmus
arousal	orientation
astigmatism	perception
awareness	presbycusis
cerumen	presbyopia
chalazion	sensation
cognition	sensorineural hearing
conductive hearing loss	loss
conjunctivitis	sensory deficit
consciousness	sensory deprivation
disorientation	sensory overload
efferent nerve pathway	sensory perception
hallucination	strabismus
hyperopia	stye
illusion	tinnitus
judgment	vertigo
keratitis	

INTRODUCTION

From the moment we wake in the morning until we fall asleep at night, we are inundated with information from the outside world through our senses. We depend on visual and auditory alarms to keep us from harm. This chapter reviews the structure and function, identifies appropriate nursing diagnoses, and presents the medical and nursing management for hearing and vision with some discussion of taste, smell, and touch.

SENSATION, PERCEPTION, AND COGNITION

Sensation is the ability to receive and process stimuli through the sensory organs. There are two types of stimuli: external and internal. External stimuli are received and processed through the senses of sight (visual), hearing (auditory), smell (olfactory), taste (gustatory), and touch (tactile). Internal stimuli are received and processed through kinesthetic (an awareness of the position of the body) and visceral (feelings originating from large organs within the body) modes.

Perception is the ability to experience, recognize, organize, and interpret sensory stimuli. **Sensory perception** is the ability to receive sensory impressions and, through cortical association, relate the stimuli to past experiences and form an impression of the nature of the stimulus.

Perception is closely associated with **cognition,** the intellectual ability to think. The processes of organizing and interpreting stimuli depend on a person's level of intellectual functioning. Cognition includes the elements of memory, judgment, and orientation. The well-being of an individual depends on the functions of sensation, perception, and cognition because the person fully experiences and interacts with the environment through these mechanisms.

Sensory, perceptual, and cognitive alterations can be either temporary or progressive in their manifestations and can result from disease or trauma. Whatever the status or cause of the alterations, these conditions usually lead to social isolation and increased dependence on others. In addition, impairment in sensory, perceptual, and cognitive functions can place the individual at risk for injury to self or others.

ANATOMY AND PHYSIOLOGY REVIEW

Sensation, perception, and cognition are neurological functions. The nervous system is composed of two major subsystems: the central nervous system (CNS) and the peripheral nervous system (PNS), which consists of the somatic and autonomic nervous systems. The CNS and PNS act in unison to accomplish three purposes: (1) collection of stimuli from the receptors at the end of the peripheral nerves; (2) transport of the stimuli to the brain for integration and cognition processing; and (3) conduction of responses to the stimuli from the brain to responsive motor centers in the body.

Sensory perception involves the function of both the cranial and peripheral nerves. The cranial nerves arise from the brain and govern the movement and function of various muscles and nerves throughout the body. The peripheral nerves connect the CNS to other parts of the body.

Components of Sensation and Perception

The sensory system is a complex network that consists of **afferent nerve pathways** (ascending pathways that transmit sensory impulses to the brain), **efferent nerve pathways** (descending pathways that send sensory impulses from the brain), the spinal cord, the brainstem, and the cerebrum.

Components of Cognition

Cognition includes the cerebral functions of memory, affect, judgment, perception, and language. In or-

> **PROFESSIONAL TIP**
>
> **CNS Deficits and Illness**
> Specific conditions, such as diabetes mellitus and atherosclerosis, can impair neurosensory pathways and result in deficits in sensation, perception, and cognition. Diseases of the CNS can result in loss of sensory function and paralysis.

> **PROFESSIONAL TIP**
>
> **Effects of Medications on Sensation**
> Certain medications have the potential to alter or depress the neurosensory system. For example, sedatives and narcotics can alter the perception of sensory stimuli. Medications such as analgesics can alter the level of consciousness.

der for these higher functions to occur, consciousness must be present.

Consciousness

Consciousness is a state of awareness of self, others, and the surrounding environment. It affects both cognitive (intellectual) and affective (emotional) functions. An alert individual (one who is aware of self and stimuli) is able to perceive reality accurately and to base behavior on those perceptions. The components of consciousness provide a foundation for behavior and emotional expression, thereby contributing to the uniqueness of each individual's personality. Consciousness may be altered by various metabolic, traumatic, or other factors, such as the pharmacological actions of drugs that affect mental status. The primary components of consciousness are arousal and awareness, both of which must be present before higher cognitive functioning occurs.

Arousal The degree of **arousal** (state of wakefulness and alertness) is indicated by a person's general response and reaction to the environment. People exhibit arousal by behaving in an alert and aware manner and by experiencing periods of wakefulness. The degree of an individual's arousal is indicated by the general response and reaction to the environment. Impaired arousal can exist when a sleep pattern deficit is experienced. There may be an inability to take advantage of opportunities for activity because of inadequate periods of rest.

Awareness **Awareness** is the capacity to perceive sensory impressions and react appropriately through thoughts and actions. An essential element in awareness is **orientation** (perception of self in relation to the surrounding environment). When awareness is impaired, orientation to time is frequently the first area affected. The degree of disorientation is worse when the individual loses awareness of place, self (person), and purpose/situation.

Memory

There are three types of memory: immediate, recent, and remote. Immediate memory is the retention of information for a specified and usually short period of time. The recall of a telephone number long enough to dial it is an example of immediate memory. Recent memory is the ability to recall events that have occurred over the past 24 hours, such as remembering the foods eaten for dinner the previous night. Remote memory is the retention of experiences that occurred during earlier periods of life, such as an adult's memories of childhood or school days. The ability to learn depends on remote memory.

Affect

Affect (expression of mood or feeling) is an important component of cognition in that variations of mood can affect one's thinking ability. For example, a client with a flat affect caused by depression may have difficulty sustaining concentration or attention.

Judgment

Judgment, the ability to compare or evaluate alternatives to arrive at a conclusion based on sound reasoning and supported by evidence, is closely related to reality testing and depends on effective cognitive functioning. Behaviors indicating impaired judgment include impulsiveness, unrealistic decision making, and inadequate problem-solving ability.

Perception

Perceptions are considered in the context of the individual's awareness of reality. Misperceptions of reality can occur in the form of an **illusion** (an inaccurate perception or misinterpretation of sensory stimuli) or a **hallucination** (a sensory perception that occurs in the absence of external stimuli and is not based on reality).

Clients who are anxious and fearful or who are on therapeutic regimens involving the use of certain medications may experience misperceptions of environmental stimuli. For example, a postoperative client, after receiving analgesic medication for pain, may see the belt from his bathrobe lying on the floor and become terrified because he thinks there is a snake in the room. Once the nurse determines that the client is experiencing an illusion, appropriate reassurance and reality orientation can be implemented to reduce the client's anxiety.

Language

Language is one of the most complex of cognitive functions, involving not only the spoken word but also reading, writing, and comprehension. Characteristics of speech are fluency (ability to talk in a steady manner), *prosody* (melody of speech that conveys meaning through changes in the tempo, rhythm, and intonation), and content.

ASSESSMENT

When caring for clients with sensory, perceptual, and cognitive alterations, the nurse must obtain a health history and perform a physical examination to identify existing or potential problems in this area of functioning. The physical examination focuses specifically on the client's ability to hear, see, taste, smell, and touch. For hearing (auditory): Ask about hearing problems, ability to distinguish sounds, buzzing or ringing noises, recent changes in hearing ability, and use of a hearing aid. For seeing (visual): Ask about blurred vision, double vision, blind spots, photosensitivity, rainbows or halos around objects, difficulty seeing far or near, family history of visual problems, use of glasses or contact lenses, and date of last eye examination. For tasting (gustatory): Ask about changes in tasting ability or appetite and ability to differentiate sweet, sour, salty, and bitter tastes. For smelling (olfactory): Ask about changes in the ability to smell and the ability to distinguish common smells. For touch (tactile): Ask about ability to feel temperature changes and pain perception in extremities and the presence of unusual sensations in extremities (tingling or numbness). Refer to the neurologic system chapter for assessment of cranial nerves.

When assessing clients for sensory, perceptual, and cognitive alterations, the level of consciousness (LOC) must also be evaluated. Refer to the neurologic system chapter for the Glasgow Coma Scale, developed to assess LOC objectively.

Safety: Sensory Impairments
Vision—Risk of tripping, falling
Hearing—Lack of awareness of warning sounds such as automobile horns, sirens, smoke alarms
Olfactory—Inability to perceive warning odors such as burning food, escaping gas
Gustatory—Inability to recognize spoiled or contaminated food or beverages
Tactile—Lack of awareness of excessive pressure on a body part; at risk for exposure to extreme temperatures (frostbite, burns)

The Ear

The human ear can be divided into three main anatomical components: the outer ear, middle ear, and inner ear (Figure 39-1). Each part plays a major role in hearing. Similar to other paired organs in the body, dysfunction of part or all of one ear does not affect the function of the other.

Outer Ear

The outer ear is composed of the auricle (pinna), a cartilaginous flap on the temporal sides of the head, and

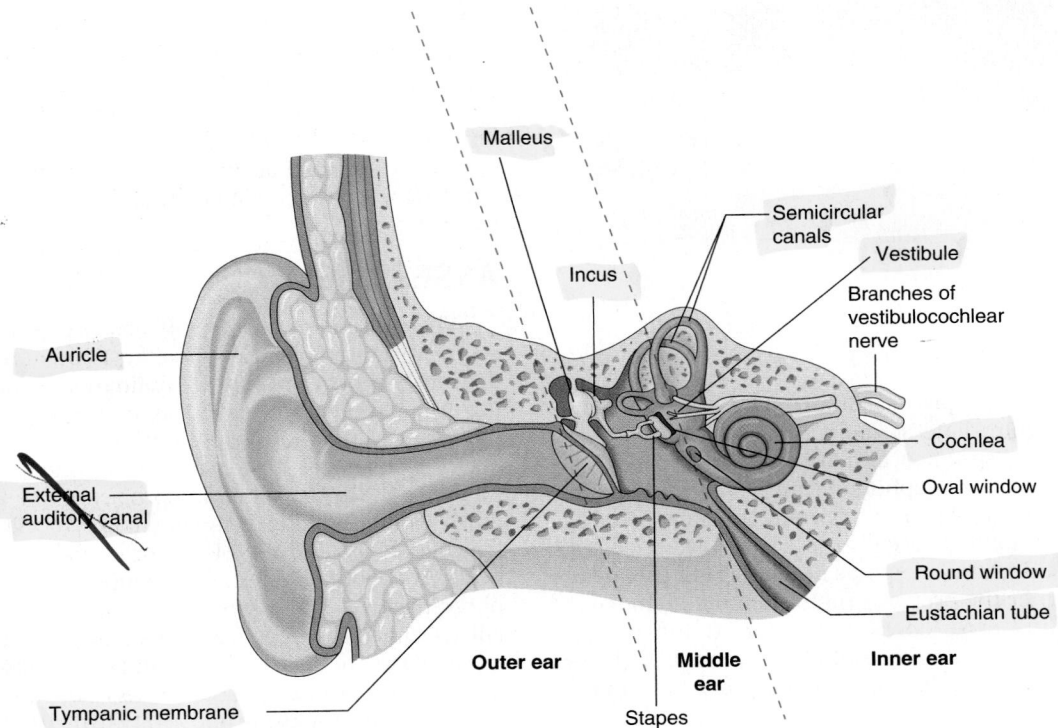

Figure 39-1 *Structures of the Ear*

the external ear canal, or external auditory meatus. The outer ear is responsible for collecting, conducting, and amplifying sound waves. The auricle directs sounds through the external ear canal to the tympanic membrane (eardrum). This canal is lined with ceruminous glands that secrete **cerumen** (ear wax), a yellowish brown protective substance that guards against certain bacteria and small insects, and traps dust and debris that may damage the inner ear. Normally, the cerumen works its way out of the ear as we eat, chew, or speak; however,

cerumen can build up and actually cause significant hearing loss in the affected ear.

The tympanic membrane (TM) serves as a boundary between the outer and middle ear. As sound waves vibrate against the membrane, the motion is transmitted to the bones of the inner ear. In an acute ear infection, fluid fills the middle ear, creating significant pressure on the tympanic membrane.

Middle Ear

The three bones of the middle ear are collectively referred to as the ossicles and include the *malleus* (hammer), *incus* (anvil), and *stapes* (stirrup), so named because they resemble the tools of a blacksmith's trade. The malleus is attached to the upper, inner portion of the tympanic membrane. The head of the malleus connects with the incus, which then joins the stapes. The flat oval bone of the stapes, called the footplate, rests on the oval window (part of the inner ear). The vibration created by sound waves passes through the outer ear canal to the tympanic membrane and then to these three bones.

The eustachian tube opens into the pharynx from the middle ear. It is approximately 3 to 4 cm long, and its primary function is to equalize pressure on both sides of the eardrum by providing a path (via the nasal passages) to relieve the pressure. In addition to pressure equalization, the functions of the middle ear include amplification of the sound waves and stimulation of the oval window to move the fluids of the inner ear.

Tympanic Membrane

The tympanic membrane is normally concave on otoscopic exam, so a convex or bulging tympanic membrane is an important sign of an acute infectious process.

Inner Ear

The inner ear has two main functions: hearing and equilibrium. It consists of a complex series of interconnected, fluid-filled chambers and tubes called the labyrinth. It can be divided into three main parts: the semicircular canals, the vestibule, and the cochlea, all located in the temporal bone. The semicircular canals, which function in providing the sense of balance, open into the vestibule. The vestibule is the central chamber of the inner ear. The cochlea is a snail-shaped structure that contains the auditory organ for the sense of hearing.

Vibration of the stapes creates pressure and causes the nerves to respond to different sounds and initiate neural responses that are sent along the auditory nerve (cranial nerve VIII) to the brain. Thus mechanical information is translated into nerve impulses and sent to the brain, which translates the sound into meaningful impressions and language.

The Eye

The eyes are a pair of spherical organs located in bony orbital cavities in the front of the skull. They are the sensory receptor organs of the visual system that transduce light from the environment into electrical impulses, which the optic nerve (cranial nerve II) then transmits to the brain, where they are interpreted as the sensation of vision. The adult eyeball measures about 1 inch in diameter. Of its total surface area, only the anterior one-sixth is exposed. The remainder is recessed and protected by the bony orbit into which it fits. Anatomically, the eye can be divided into three separate coats, or "tunics": the outer fibrous tunic, the middle vascular tunic, and the inner nervous tunic.

Fibrous Tunic

The fibrous tunic is the outer coat of the eyeball and is composed posteriorly of the sclera and anteriorly of the transparent cornea. The sclera, or "white of the eye," is leathery, white, and relatively thick and is composed of connective tissue. The cornea, or "window of the eye," is a continuation of the sclera and forms a transparent rounded bulge through which light passes.

Vascular Tunic

The vascular tunic is the eye's middle layer and is composed of three portions: the posterior choroid, the anterior ciliary body, and the iris. Collectively, these three structures are called the uveal tract. The choroid carries the blood vessels for the eyeball and contains a large amount of pigment, thus preventing internal reflection of light. Around the edge of the cornea the choroid forms the ciliary body, a thickened structure containing smooth muscle. A thin diaphragm of mostly connective tissue and smooth muscle fibers with an opening in the center is attached around the anterior margin of the ciliary body. The muscles of the ciliary body serve to change the shape of the lens, allowing changes in the focal distance of the eye. The third portion of the vascular tunic is known as the iris and contains the pigment responsible for the color of the eye. The hole in the iris is the pupil, which permits light to enter the eye. Some of the smooth muscle fibers in the iris encircle the pupil and others radiate from it. Contraction of the radial muscle dilates the pupil and contraction of the circular muscle constricts the pupil. By their control of pupil diameter, these muscles regulate the amount of light entering the eye.

Nervous Tunic

The third and innermost tunic of the eye, the retina, translates light waves into neural impulses. An extremely complex structure, the retina contains several layers of nerve cells and their processes, including two types of receptors, the rods for vision in dim light, and the cones for daytime or color vision. Cones are most densely concentrated in the central fovea, a small depression in the center of the macula lutea. The macula lutea, or yellow spot, is in the central part of the retina. The fovea is the area of sharpest vision because the highest concentration of cones are located there. Rods are absent from the fovea and macula, but they increase in density toward the periphery of the retina. The optic disk, where the optic nerve exits the eye, is a weak spot in the fundus (posterior wall) of the eye because it is not reinforced by the sclera. The optic disk is also called the blind spot because it lacks photoreceptors and light focused on it will not be detected.

The interior of the eyeball contains an anterior and posterior chamber separated by the lens. The anterior chamber is filled with a watery fluid called the aqueous humor, which maintains intraocular pressure, provides nourishment, and helps maintain the shape of the eyeball. The posterior chamber is filled with a jelly-like substance called the vitreous humor, which maintains the spherical shape of the eye and supports the inner structures. Both substances are transparent, thus allowing light to pass through the eye to the retina (Figure 39-2).

The lens, located in the anterior chamber of the eye, is a transparent biconvex crystalline body enclosed in an elastic capsule held by suspensory ligaments. The shape of the lens changes to focus the image.

External Structures

The eyeball is protected from the external world by the eyelid, which contains a thin protective layer of epithelium, the conjunctiva (Figure 39-3). The conjunctiva covers the anterior portion of the eyeball and lines the eyelid. Projecting from the border of each eyelid is a row of eyelashes, which protect the eye from foreign particles. The lacrimal gland produces a secretion called tears, which contain a lysozyme, muramidase, to destroy pathogens.

Figure 39-2 *Lateral View of the Interior Eyeball*

Temporal side   Nasal side

Figure 39-3 *External View of the Right Eye*

COMMON DIAGNOSTIC TESTS

Commonly used diagnostic tests for clients with problems in hearing and vision are listed in Table 39-1.

SENSORY, PERCEPTUAL, AND COGNITIVE ALTERATIONS

An individual usually experiences discomfort and/or anxiety when subjected to a change in the type or amount of incoming stimuli. A person can become confused as a result of either overstimulation or understimulation. According to the individual's ability to process the stimuli, confusion (or disorientation) may occur. **Disorientation** is a mentally confused state in which the person's awareness of time, place, self, and/or situation is impaired. When awareness of these four factors is accurate, a person is said to be "oriented × 4."

TABLE 39-1	COMMON DIAGNOSTIC TESTS FOR SENSORY ALTERATIONS

- Weber test (tuning fork)
- Rinne test (tuning fork)
- Audiometric testing (audiogram)
- Speech audiometry (Spondee threshold)
- Caloric test
- Brainstem auditory evoked response (ErA and BAER)
- Tympanometry
- Computed tomography (CT)
- Magnetic resonance imaging (MRI)
- Romberg test
- Otoscopic exam
- Past-point testing
- Color vision tests
- Tonometry
- Slit lamp examination
- Perimetry
- Visual acuity
- Electroretinogram (ERG)
- Ocular ultrasonography
- Ophthalmoscopic examination
- Orbital computerized tomography
- Fluoresce in angiography

A person admitted to a health care agency experiences stimuli that are different from those usually encountered. A change in environment can overwhelm one's ability to perceive and interpret sensory input. As a result, the treatment setting can become a stressor that negatively affects sensory, perceptual, and cognitive functions. If one or more of the factors just discussed causes an alteration in sensation, perception, or cognition, the client may experience problems with perceiving and interpreting stimuli. These problems are manifested by three types of alterations: sensory deficit, sensory deprivation, and sensory overload.

SENSORY DEFICIT

A **sensory deficit** is a change in the perception of sensory stimuli. This deficit can affect all five senses. Examples of sensory deficit are vision and hearing losses such as those caused by cataracts, glaucoma, and presbycusis (steady loss of hearing acuity that occurs with aging).

The client's response to these losses usually depends on the time of onset and the severity of the condition. If the problem occurs suddenly and without warning, the client may have difficulty adjusting to the loss of sensory and perceptual function. If these alterations occur gradually, the client may be able to accommodate the change and actually compensate for it by strengthening one or more of the other senses.

The effects of hospitalization or intensive medical treatments can exacerbate the problems related to sensory deficit. For example, a client with acute hearing loss can feel alone and vulnerable. Clients with sensory deficit are at serious risk of experiencing either sensory deprivation or sensory overload.

SENSORY DEPRIVATION

Sensory deprivation is a state of reduced sensory input from the internal or external environment, manifested by alterations in sensory perception. Individuals can experience sensory deprivation as a result of illness, trauma, or isolation. A person experiencing sensory deprivation misinterprets the limited stimuli with a resultant impairment of thoughts and feelings. Factors that contribute to sensory deprivation include:

- Visual or auditory impairments that limit or prohibit perception of stimuli
- Drugs that produce a sedative effect on the CNS and interfere with the interpretation of stimuli
- Trauma that results in brain damage and decreased cognitive function
- Isolation (either physical or social) that results in a nonstimulating environment

Some contributing factors (such as brain damage or blindness) result in chronic sensory deprivation. Other

factors lead to acute, transient states of deprivation (such as receiving analgesic medications).

Individuals who are sensory-deprived may exhibit any of the following characteristics:

- Inability to concentrate
- Poor memory
- Impaired problem-solving ability
- Confusion
- Irritability
- Emotional lability (mood swings)
- Hallucinations
- Depression
- Boredom and apathy
- Drowsiness

SENSORY OVERLOAD

Sensory overload is a state of excessive and sustained multisensory stimulation manifested by behavior change and perceptual distortion. The individual experiencing this alteration is unable to process the amount or intensity of stimuli being received. Factors contributing to sensory overload are:

- Pain originating from a heightened quality or quantity of internal stimuli
- Invasive procedures that result in an increased amount of external stimuli
- Activity-filled, busy environment that contributes to the amount of stimuli being perceived
- Medications that stimulate the CNS and prohibit the client from ignoring selective stimuli
- Presence of strangers (both health care professionals and others) who contribute to the quantity of stimuli
- Diseases that affect the CNS and maximize the perception of stimuli

DISORDERS OF THE EAR

Disorders of the ear include impaired hearing, Ménière's disease, otosclerosis, acoustic neuroma, otitis media, otitis externa, and mastoiditis.

IMPAIRED HEARING

Hearing loss is the most common chronic disability in the United States, affecting more than 34 million adults (Sommer & Sommer, 2002). It can be seriously debilitating by limiting the ability to socialize and work, or respond to the telephone or alarms, yet relatively few individuals who experience impaired hearing actually seek help. Some may deny the problem and others may feel that a hearing aid is a sign of old age. Family members are often the first to be aware of a hearing deficit.

Types of Hearing Loss

Hearing loss is generally categorized in two ways: conductive and sensorineural. Mixed hearing loss, both conductive and sensorineural, is possible but far less

LIFE CYCLE CONSIDERATIONS

Effects of Aging

Sensory, perceptual, and cognitive function begin to diminish with aging. Decreased visual or auditory senses or impairments in memory are experienced. These changes can have a profound effect on a client's self-esteem and response to life.

likely. Either may occur at birth (congenital), develop later in life, be genetic, or be caused by injury or trauma.

Conductive hearing loss indicates an inability of the sound waves to reach the inner ear. This may be caused by cerumen buildup or blockage, perforated tympanic membrane, or fixation of one or all of the ossicles.

In **sensorineural hearing loss,** the inner ear or cochlear portion of cranial nerve VIII may be abnormal or diseased. A tumor, infection, trauma, or exposure to loud noises may cause destruction of the nerve and result in sensorineural hearing loss.

Sensorineural hearing loss associated with aging is termed **presbycusis.** Higher frequency sounds such as women's voices become especially difficult to hear, and distinguishing words may be a problem. According to Spencer (1998), 95 percent of people with sensorineural hearing loss can be helped by hearing aids.

Behaviors Indicating Hearing Loss

A hearing impairment is a serious disorder that is often debilitating and embarrassing to the client. Hearing is part of the communication process, so the inability to hear may cause the person to do or say the wrong thing in response to a question or command. Persons with hearing impairment may withdraw from conversation or seem indifferent to their surroundings or to those around them.

Alterations in hearing are often manifested by changes in speech habits and patterns. Individuals with hearing impairments may not notice the changes in their own speech pattern until someone constantly asks them to repeat themselves or to speak clearly. Indifference and withdrawal are common behaviors in response to hearing loss. If left undiagnosed and untreated, the person may truly regress, become unhappy, lonely, and possibly even paranoid. Some individuals overcompensate for the hearing loss by becoming very loud and aggressive.

Research on hearing impairment has created many devices to aid speech and sound discrimination. Early diagnosis, treatment, and rehabilitation are essential to help hearing-impaired persons enjoy and appreciate the world they live in.

Hearing Aids/Assistive Devices

Hearing aids today come in a variety of designs and sizes. Some are quite small and tinted to a person's skin

---

PROFESSIONAL TIP

Hearing Specialists

An audiologist evaluates hearing and determines the extent and type of hearing loss, and provides nonmedical treatment such as fitting hearing aids, advice about assistive listening devices, and communication/aural rehabilitative training. An otolaryngologist (ear, nose, and throat physician) provides medical evaluation of hearing disorders and medical and surgical interventions. A hearing aid specialist is licensed to dispense hearing aids but is not a medical doctor.

---

color so as to be virtually unnoticeable. Some are worn in the ear, behind the ear, or are part of eyeglasses frames. Persons with bilateral hearing loss may need *binaural* (worn in both ears) hearing aids.

A hearing aid converts environmental sound and speech into electronic signals that are amplified and converted to acoustic signals. It makes speech and sound louder but not necessarily clearer. Depending on the extent of hearing impairment and preference, the client may need to experiment with several different types of hearing aids. In addition, speech therapy, lip reading, and auditory training may be necessary to help discriminate speech and develop better listening skills.

Many other assistive hearing devices are available for the hearing impaired. Numerous television programs are closed-caption. Advanced technology allows telecommunication through a device called the Telecommunication Device for the Deaf (TDD), also called TTY Typewriter, which sends a printed message onto a small screen. Both sender and receiver must have the typewriter/telephone device. Many hospitals have these to comply with ADA requirements.

Alarm clocks offer strobe lights or vibrators to awaken clients. State-of-the-art receivers give instant access to radio, television, computer, and stereos to enhance receiving and listening systems. For travelers, complete kits are available to provide ready access for smoke alarm, clock, TDD, and door-knock alert in hotels or inns.

Hearing guide dogs are also available. The animals are specially trained to meet the needs of the hearing impaired. At home, the dog responds to alarms, knocking on doors, and babies crying. In public, the dog takes a position between owner and a potential threat. Special identifiers, such as a collar for the dog and ID card for the owner, are available. The dogs are trained to go wherever their master goes, including restaurants, grocery stores, and on public transportation.

Medical–Surgical Management

Medical

The type of hearing loss and underlying etiology determines the best medical or surgical management. The client should undergo a complete physical examination as well as thorough diagnostic hearing tests. Once the etiology is determined, the client and doctor can decide on the best course of therapy.

Surgical

The cochlear implant is a possible treatment for persons with profound deafness. In this procedure, a receiver/stimulator is implanted in the skull and a group of electrodes are planted in front of the round window in the inner ear. The client wears a microphone near the ear that picks up and translates sound into electrical signals. These signals are then transmitted to the brain via the cochlear implant and cranial nerve VIII.

Nursing Management

If the client uses a sign language interpreter, arrange for one to assist with communication. Writing notes, using a TDD, or a computer may be helpful. Approach the client and elicit the client's attention by waving. Make sure all personnel know the client is hearing impaired as well as the client's preferred method of communication. The publication *Pictograms for Hospital Communication* is available from the U.S. Department of Justice.

NURSING PROCESS

Assessment

Subjective Data

Ask the client to describe the initial onset of symptoms and possible familial traits, recent infections of the ears, nose, or upper respiratory system. Determine recent trauma and past surgery as well as medical history such as diabetes, heart disease, or cancer. Ask about allergies to food, drugs, or environmental factors, associated symptoms such as **tinnitus** (ringing sound in the ear), **vertigo** (dizziness), nausea, and vomiting. The client's work history may reveal exposure to loud noises.

Objective Data

Listen closely to the client and note any deterioration of speech, slurring, or dropping of word endings. Document current and recent medications used.

Inspect the outer ear for abnormalities, lesions, or cerumen. Palpate the mastoid process, neck, jaw, and temporal regions of the head for swelling or tenderness to touch. Note the degree of hearing loss as reported by the client and compare it to the diagnostic tests such as the speech audiogram. The client's perception of hearing loss may be significantly different from the diagnostic findings.

A nursing diagnosis for a client with impaired hearing may be:

Nursing Diagnosis	Planning/Goals	Nursing Interventions
Social Isolation related to hearing impairment	The client will participate in conversations and other social situations.	Take time to engage client in conversation. Make sure you have the client's attention and be at eye level. Speak slowly and distinctly. Give the client time to respond. Provide the client and family members written information regarding the availability, variety, and quality of assistive hearing devices. Encourage client to participate in social situations.

Evaluation The goal must be evaluated to determine how it has been met by the client.

MÉNIÈRE'S DISEASE

Ménière's disease, also known as endolymphatic hydrops, is a state of hearing loss characterized by tinnitus and vertigo. Although the exact etiology is unknown, it is thought to be an excessive accumulation of endolymph in the cochlear duct and possible leakage of endolymph into the perilymph caused by increased capillary permeability. Mixing of the two fluids chemically alters the homeostasis of the perilymph and endolymph and could be responsible for the symptoms associated with Ménière's disease.

The major symptoms are the classic triad of vertigo, tinnitus, and unilateral fluctuating hearing loss. The vertigo is often associated with nausea and vomiting. Tinnitus may either be a preceding aura or occur simultaneously with the vertigo. Initially, tinnitus is intermittent, but as the disease progresses, it may be a constant, low-pitched roaring sound. The fluctuating, unilateral hearing loss becomes more profound with each attack.

The symptoms are frequently at their worst during the first attack, which may last from a few minutes to six

PROFESSIONAL TIP

Assisting the Hearing-Impaired Client

- Speak slowly and distinctly after getting the client's attention.
- Face the client and sit or stand to be at eye level with the client.
- Use short, simple sentences and give the client time to respond. Repeat or rephrase if necessary.
- Use written materials when possible to communicate information.
- Keep a notepad and pen or pencil available to write down new or unfamiliar words and concepts.
- If sign language is the client's preferred method of communication, locate a person who understands sign language.
- If the client wears a hearing aid, make sure that the battery is functional, it is turned on, and is adjusted to a comfortable level.

hours. **Nystagmus,** repetitive and involuntary movement of the eyeballs, and diaphoresis may occur during an attack. Subsequent attacks are less severe, but over time may involve both ears and cause permanent bilateral hearing loss. Clients report many different precipitating events, such as stress, weather changes, menstruation, or pregnancy, and various dietary influences, including caffeine, alcohol, and salt. Smoking has also been implicated.

Medical–Surgical Management

Medical

Medical management is the preferred treatment and most helpful to 80% to 85% of persons with this disease. Diagnosis is not difficult and is usually made based on the client's report of symptoms. Diagnosis may also be confirmed with caloric stimulation (although this test is primarily conducted on comatose clients) and an MRI to rule out a tumor. Medical management is symptomatic.

Surgical

Surgical intervention is needed only when the attacks are frequent and debilitating, or when the disease severely affects the quality of life and the ability for self-care. Surgical treatment includes endolymphatic, subarachnoid shunt placement to drain excessive endolymph. With this procedure, hearing is preserved in 60% to 70% of the clients. With a vestibular neurectomy, the vestibular portion of cranial nerve VIII is severed; hearing is preserved in 90% of clients having this procedure. In surgical destruction of the labyrinth, hearing is destroyed but the incapacitating vertigo is completely relieved.

Pharmacological

Several medications are useful to help control the symptoms, such as antihistamines, antiemetics, benzodiazepines, diuretics, tranquilizers, vasoactive agents, and oral niacin. The medications may be prescribed for long-term use or at the onset of symptoms. Because the cause of Ménière's disease is unknown, there is no cure.

Diet

Dietary interventions include strict salt restriction and avoidance of those foods or beverages that precipi-

tate or aggravate an attack. Examples are beer, wine, soda, salty food or snacks, chocolate, and caffeinated coffee and tea.

Activity

Activity is not limited except during or after an attack, when clients may require prolonged bed rest and restriction of activities that may be unsafe, such as driving or operating heavy equipment.

Nursing Management

Advise client against reading and use of glaring lights. Instruct client to avoid sudden position changes and have assistance when getting out of bed or ambulating. Keep side rails up and the call light within the client's reach.

NURSING PROCESS

Assessment

Subjective Data

The history should begin with identifying significant contributory data. Ask the client to describe the initial onset of symptoms including, but not limited to, the classic triad of tinnitus, vertigo, and fluctuating unilateral hearing loss.

Relate questions to recent viral illness; upper respiratory infections; past medical, surgical, and dental history; and any problems related to the neck and face. Document food, drug, or environmental allergies. Record current or recent long-term medications. Identify the client's occupation and hobbies that may contribute to hearing loss.

Objective Data

A thorough physical examination includes looking at the ear for abnormalities, lesions and cerumen blockage, or unusual drainage. Palpate the neck, jaw, and mastoid process for possible lymph node enlargement and tenderness. The nurse may assist with the otologic examination as needed. Audiologic testing determines unilateral or bilateral hearing loss.

Nursing diagnoses for a client with Ménière's disease may include the following:

Nursing Diagnoses	Planning/Goals	Nursing Interventions
Activity Intolerance related to severe vertigo	The client will be able to tolerate activities of daily living.	Provide adequate periods of bed rest. Provide assistance with ambulation and encourage increased activity as tolerated.
		Keep the room dim and quiet when possible. Avoid jarring the bed and caution client to avoid sudden movements.
		Administer antiemetic before symptoms become too severe.

continues

Nursing Diagnoses	Planning/Goals	Nursing Interventions
*Deficient **K**nowledge* related to abrupt onset and unknown progression of the disease	The client will verbalize understanding of the disease process and potential precipitating factors and how to manage or control the symptoms.	Assess the client's current knowledge of the disease process. Review the disease process and underlying etiology of Ménière's disease with the client. Ask the client to identify possible precipitating factors such as stress or dietary habits. Discuss health promotion programs for stress management and healthy cooking classes. Suggest consultations with dietary and social services. Review follow-up appointments, medications, dietary management, activity, and rest parameters. Evaluate client's readiness to discuss progressive hearing loss and current assistive hearing devices available.
*Risk for **I**njury* related to vertigo	The client will not fall or be injured because of vertigo.	Keep side rails up. Teach client to move or turn slowly. Instruct client to sit or lie down when vertigo occurs. Reiterate need to call for assistance when ambulating. Keep call bell within client's reach. Administer medications for vertigo prior to worsening of symptoms. Avoid glaring, bright lights.

Evaluation Each goal must be evaluated to determine how it has been met by the client.

OTOSCLEROSIS

Otosclerosis, the most common conductive hearing loss, is secondary to a pathologic change of the bones in the middle ear. The exact cause is unknown. The ossicles are normally hard, but over time and without warning, the bone becomes softened, spongy, highly vascular, and partially or totally fixed. This fixation reduces or prevents transmission of source waves to inner ear fluids. Although all three bones may be affected, the stapes, which must vibrate on the oval window in order to transmit sound waves, is most commonly afflicted.

Otosclerosis is more common in adults, more often in women, and it is familial in some cases.

The primary clinical manifestations are subtle changes in hearing and low-pitched tinnitus. It becomes more difficult to distinguish a whisper, or to hear in crowded places or understand conversation. Individuals affected by otosclerosis often blame others for speaking too softly or mumbling. Frequently, rather than asking others to speak up or to repeat themselves, the person will be irritable and withdrawn.

Diagnostic testing begins with the Weber and Rinne tuning fork tests. In addition, audiometric testing should be performed. Schwartz's sign, a pink blush, is seen on otoscopic examination. Tympanometry shows stiffness in the sound conduction system.

Medical–Surgical Management

Medical

Treatment for otosclerosis is limited to three options. The individual may choose to do nothing and obtain periodic audiometry to evaluate progression of the disease. The second choice is to use a hearing aid, and the third choice is surgical management with an outpatient procedure known as a stapedectomy.

Surgical

A stapedectomy is the preferred surgical technique for improving hearing loss caused by otosclerosis. A stapedectomy may be done under local or general anesthesia and routinely requires a surgical incision in the posterior ear canal, removal of the stapes, and implantation of a plastic prosthesis. A new technique, laser stapedectomy, may be performed through the ear canal without an incision. The stapes tendon is vaporized, chards are removed with delicate micro instruments, and an opening is made allowing the surgeon to implant a prosthetic piston. This restores normal vibration against the inner ear.

Nursing Management

Postoperatively, instruct the client to turn or move slowly, not to blow the nose for 10 days, to avoid lifting for 1 month, and if sneezing occurs, to keep the mouth open. Administer antibiotics as ordered. Advise the client that hearing may be decreased for 3 to 4 weeks until gel-foam packing dissolves.

NURSING PROCESS

Assessment

Subjective Data

A careful history discovers possible hereditary traits or acquired disease. Ask about recent infections of the ears, nose, or upper respiratory system, and also about past surgery, trauma, or other illnesses such as diabetes, heart disease, or cancer. Identify associated symptoms, such as dizziness, tinnitus, vertigo, and nausea.

Note allergies to foods, drugs, or any environmental factors, such as exposure to loud noises. Record current and recent medications, especially those known to be ototoxic.

Objective Data

Objective data includes a thorough physical examination. Inspect the outer ear for abnormalities, lesions, or impacted ear wax and palpate the mastoid process, neck, jaw, and temporal regions of the head for pain or swelling. Assess the degree of hearing loss. The client may experience vomiting.

Nursing diagnoses for the client with otosclerosis may include the following:

Nursing Diagnoses	Planning/Goals	Nursing Interventions
Anxiety related to decrease or loss in hearing	The client will show evidence of reduced anxiety and verbalize understanding of the disease process and treatment regimen.	Encourage the client to explore feelings of anxiety and to ask questions to clarify concerns. Provide honest and realistic feedback.
		Collaborate with the physician to provide thorough and clear explanations of the disease process, treatment options, and anticipated results.
*Risk for **I**njury* related to vertigo	The client will not fall or be injured because of vertigo.	Keep side rails up. Reiterate need to call for assistance when ambulating and keep call bell within client's reach.
		Instruct the client to move or turn slowly.
		Administer medications for vertigo prior to worsening of symptoms.
		Keep room well lit when client is ambulating.
*Deficient **K**nowledge* related to activities after surgery	The client will demonstrate the ability to change dressing correctly and verbalize knowledge of self-care and follow-up.	Teach client how and when to perform dressing change and have client demonstrate the procedure.
		Instruct client to avoid pressure changes (such as flying in an unpressurized aircraft), avoid heavy lifting (60 lbs) for 1 month, avoid nose blowing for 10 days, and if sneezing occurs, keep mouth open.
		Advise client to keep water out of the ear and keep the ear exposed to air as much as possible for one month. There will be some drainage which is initially red, then pink, and then brownish.
		Tell client to report any greenish, yellowish, or foul-smelling drainage.
		Instruct client to take all antibiotics as prescribed and complete the full course of treatment.
		Advise client there should be very little pain or discomfort but if there is, take prescribed analgesics and notify doctor if pain is prolonged or intense.
		Warn client that hearing may be decreased for 3 to 4 weeks after surgery until gel-foam packing dissolves.
		Inform client that audiometric testing will be conducted 1 month after surgery.
		Instruct client to schedule an appointment with the physician in 1 month but call physician if uncontrolled pain is experienced or a malodorous, greenish discharge comes from the ear.

Evaluation Each goal must be evaluated to determine how it has been met by the client.

ACOUSTIC NEUROMA

Acoustic neuroma is a slow-growing and usually benign tumor of the vestibular portion of the inner ear (cranial nerve VIII). Detection at the onset of symptoms is essential and may be accomplished with an MRI. Presenting symptoms of dizziness, tinnitus, and hearing loss are common to many dysfunctions of the ear, and the possibility of acoustic neuroma must not be overlooked.

Clients who present with dizziness, tinnitus, and hearing loss should have a complete workup for auditory and vestibular (balance) function. Facial weakness may be caused by compression of the tumor on cranial nerve VII. Cranial nerve V may also be affected as the tumor grows, causing paresthesia of the face and loss of the corneal reflex. Large neuromas can cause increased intracranial pressure, papilledema, vomiting, and headache.

Medical–Surgical Management

Treatment is almost always surgical excision of the tumor. Although antihistamines may reduce the dizziness, pharmacologic treatment is only temporary until diagnostic tests are completed and surgery is planned.

Nursing Management

Assist client to express feelings about progressive hearing loss and the changes in activities of daily living, employment, and quality of life issues. Note the family's feelings and ability to cope. Perform postoperative care as ordered.

NURSING PROCESS

Assessment

Subjective Data

Obtain through the client history signs and symptoms, and all contributing data.

Objective Data

Obtain with the physical examination a complete cranial nerve evaluation performed by the physician or audiologist to determine the extent of cranial nerve involvement.

A nursing diagnosis for a client with acoustic neuroma may be:

Nursing Diagnosis	Planning/Goals	Nursing Interventions
Anticipatory **G**rieving related to diminished quality of life, loss of ability for self-care, or possible loss of life	The client will express feelings of grief and demonstrate adaptive coping mechanisms.	Assist the client to express feelings about progressive hearing loss and changes in activities of daily living, employment, and quality of life issues.
		Collaborate with physician and other members of the health care team to provide thorough and clear explanations of the disease process, treatment options, and anticipated results.
		Observe the client's coping styles. Support those that the client finds helpful and explore other coping mechanisms that may prove useful in time (e.g., hobbies and other diversional activities, prayer, reading, and so on).
		Include the family in all interventions that the client desires. Examine the family's feelings and ability to cope.
		Consult social services, pastoral care, or other hospital and community resources when appropriate.

Evaluation The goal must be evaluated to determine how it has been met by the client.

OTITIS MEDIA

Otitis media is an inflammation of the middle ear and a common cause of conductive hearing loss, although usually temporary. Symptoms include ear pain, fever, redness of auricle and ear canal, and sometimes enlarged lymph nodes over the mastoid process, parotids, and upper neck. Otitis media occurs more frequently in children than in adults.

Fluid accumulates behind the eardrum because of blockage of the eustachian tube (Figure 39-4). This may be secondary to an upper respiratory infection, allergies, or acute bacterial infection. On physical examination the tympanic membrane may be retracted, normal, or bulging. A pneumatic otoscope allows the practitioner to blow soft puffs of air against the tym-

CRITICAL THINKING

Hearing Impairment

What modifications would need to be made in the life of a person who could suddenly no longer hear?

panic membrane to assess movement. A stiff, nonmoving, or bulging tympanic membrane may indicate inflammation or fluid accumulation in the middle ear. Visualization of the normal landmarks may be obscured. The Rinne tuning fork test and audiometry confirm a conductive hearing loss.

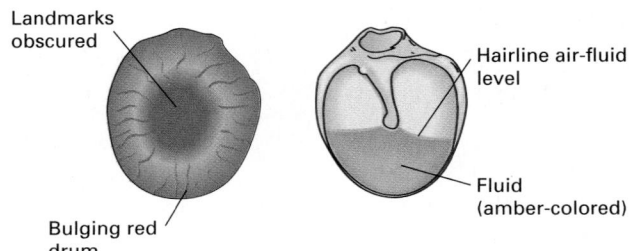

Figure 39-4 *The Tympanic Membrane in the Presence of Otitis Media*

Medical–Surgical Management

Medical

Topical heat and systemic analgesics may be used to control pain. The client should lie on the affected side to facilitate drainage.

Surgical

Surgical management may be necessary for diagnostic or therapeutic reasons. A myringotomy may be performed, in which an incision is made in the eardrum and fluid is aspirated. A polyethylene tube may be placed in the eardrum to equalize pressure and allow drainage of fluid.

A tympanoplasty may be needed if the tympanic membrane is ruptured. If there is a large tympanic membrane perforation, the malleus, which is connected to the tympanic membrane, or other ossicles may be damaged. Ossicular chain reconstruction typically refers to the removal of the actual bones and replacement with a plastic prosthesis. The prosthesis and the tympanic membrane reconstruction often result in a significant improvement in hearing.

Pharmacological

Medications used include decongestants, such as pseudoephedrine hydrochloride (Sudafed); antihistamines, such as diphenhydramine hydrochloride (Benadryl); and systemic antibiotics, such as ampicillin (Omnipen).

Activity

Activity is not restricted unless surgical management is indicated.

Nursing Management

After myringotomy, maintain drainage flow. Sterile cotton may be loosely placed in the external ear to absorb drainage. Change cotton whenever it is damp. Perform hand hygiene before and after ear care. Monitor vital signs. Warn client against blowing nose or getting ear wet when bathing. Encourage client to complete prescribed antibiotics.

NURSING PROCESS

Assessment

Subjective Data

Ask about the onset, duration, and severity of pain and what home remedies have been used. Hearing loss and/or tinnitus and a deep throbbing pain in the ear may be reported.

Objective Data

A watery or yellow discharge may be seen. It may have a foul odor. The client may have a fever.

A nursing diagnosis for a client with otitis media may be:

Nursing Diagnosis	Planning/Goals	Nursing Interventions
Acute Pain related to inflammation in the middle ear	The client will experience pain relief.	Administer antibiotics and analgesics as ordered.
		Teach client and family the importance of administering medications as ordered and to complete full course of prescription.
		Apply heating pad, set on low, for 20 minutes every 2 hours. Do not use on small children.
		Teach client if pain is unrelieved in 48 hours, to contact physician.

Evaluation The goal must be evaluated to determine how it has been met by the client.

OTITIS EXTERNA

Otitis externa, or "swimmer's ear," typically involves a bacterial infection of the external ear canal skin. The canal skin becomes red and edematous. If the swelling is severe enough, it will block the ear passage and cause a mild conductive hearing loss. Also, in most cases there is a discharge. If the discharge is copious and the canal size is constricted, a mild conductive hearing loss may result.

MASTOIDITIS

Mastoiditis (inflammation of the mastoid) is most often the direct result of chronic or recurrent bacterial otitis media. The recurrent infection may find its way into the bone and structures surrounding the middle ear and, if left untreated, can cause severe damage, sensorineural deafness, facial weakness, brain abscess, and meningitis. Symptoms include earache, fever, headache, and malaise. Antibiotics are given for a trial period. If symptoms do not resolve, surgical intervention such as mastoidectomy or meatoplasty may be necessary.

DISORDERS OF THE EYE

Disorders of the eye include cataracts, glaucoma, retinal detachment, infections, refractive errors, injuries, impaired vision, and macular degeneration.

CATARACTS

A cataract is a disorder that causes the lens or its capsule to lose its transparency and/or become opaque (Figure 39-5). The lens is normally clear and transparent and allows light to pass through to the retina. As clouding develops, visual impairment occurs. Cataracts usually affect both eyes; however, the degree of visual impairment is often different in each eye.

Cataracts are typically associated with aging; however, they may be congenital, caused by severe eye injury, or secondary to certain systemic diseases, such as metabolic problems (diabetes mellitus) and chronic eye disease (uveitis). Ophthalmoscopic examination is the primary method of evaluation.

Medical–Surgical Management
Surgical

The only treatment for a cataract is surgical removal of the lens; however, the mere finding of a cataract is not

an indication for surgery. Surgery is indicated when significant vision loss has occurred. The lens may be removed by the intracapsular or extracapsular approach. During the intracapsular cataract extraction, the ophthalmologist removes the lens within its capsule. Extracapsular cataract extraction is the procedure most commonly used (Figure 39-6). The ophthalmologist removes the anterior portion of the capsule and then expresses, or removes, the lens. An intraocular lens (IOL) is generally implanted. Glasses or special contact lenses may also be used.

Most eye surgery is done on an outpatient basis under local anesthesia. General anesthesia can be used at the client's request and for clients who are extremely anxious, deaf, or mentally retarded. A tranquilizer such as diazepam (Valium) is often given to reduce anxiety when receiving injections on the face and around the eye.

Figure 39-5 *A cataract results in the loss of transparency of the lens of the eye. (Courtesy of the National Eye Institute, Bethesda, MD)*

Figure 39-6 *In extracapsular extraction to correct cataracts, the lens is removed, the posterior lens capsule is left intact, and a plastic intraocular lens (IOL) is placed.*

Preoperatively, the client can receive several types of eye medications to prepare the eye for surgery: mydriatic (makes pupil dilate) and cycloplegic (paralyzes ciliary muscle) eyedrops, antibiotic eyedrops as a prophylaxis against infection, and an intravenous infusion of an agent to lower intraocular pressure (mannitol or a carbonic anhydrase inhibitor).

After the anesthesia wears off, the client is discharged. The client is instructed to have a driver available for the trip home. Driving is restricted for a few days.

Postoperatively, the client has a patch over the eye. The patch is removed and reapplied on the first postoperative day, when miotic (makes pupil contract) eye drops are begun. Mild discomfort and scratchiness are expected. Atropine sulfate eyedrops and cold compresses may be ordered to relieve these discomforts.

Nursing Management

Assist with ambulation because depth perception has changed. Maintain eye patch on affected eye. Advise client to sleep with eye patch on as ordered. Teach client or family to administer eyedrops and ointments. Client should avoid heavy lifting, straining during defecation, and vigorous coughing and sneezing.

Dark glasses will relieve glare. Encourage client to keep all follow-up appointments.

NURSING PROCESS

Assessment

Subjective Data

A general medical history as well as a history of symptoms is obtained. Symptoms may include haziness, cloudiness, blurred vision, double vision, altered color perception, and glare when looking at lights, especially with night driving. Fear of losing one's eyesight can be very devastating. There is often a great deal of anxiety when the client seeks an eye examination.

Objective Data

Upon inspection of the eye, the usual black pupil appears clouded, progressing to a milky white appearance, which is a characteristic finding of a mature cataract and indicates significant vision loss.

Nursing diagnoses for a client with cataracts may include the following:

Nursing Diagnoses	Planning/Goals	Nursing Interventions
Disturbed Sensory Perception (Visual) related to ocular lens opacity	The client will demonstrate improved ability to process visual stimuli and communicate visual limitations.	Assess and document baseline visual acuity. Elicit functional description of what the client can and cannot see.
Risk for Injury related to difficulty in processing visual images and altered depth perception	The client will avoid activities associated with increased potential for injury.	Teach the client to change position slowly. Teach the client to avoid reaching for objects to maintain stability when ambulating, as depth perception is altered.
Impaired Home Maintenance related to age, limited vision or activity restrictions imposed by surgery	The client will perform self-care activities in home environment.	Discuss the client's ability to meet self-care needs and activities of daily living. Evaluate how the client's current functional ability will be affected by activity restrictions and postoperative care needs. Help the client decide on a realistic site for postoperative care needs.

Evaluation Each goal must be evaluated to determine how it has been met by the client.

GLAUCOMA

Glaucoma is a disorder characterized by an abnormally high pressure of fluid inside the eyeball (intraocular pressure, IOP). The aqueous humor does not return into the bloodstream through the canal of Schlemm as quickly as it is formed. The fluid accumulates and, by compressing the lens into the vitreous humor, puts pressure on the neurons of the retina. If the pressure continues over a long period, it destroys the neurons and brings about blindness.

There are two primary forms of glaucoma: open-angle glaucoma and closed-angle glaucoma. In open-angle glaucoma (chronic simple glaucoma) there is a gradual rise in IOP, a slowly progressive loss of peripheral vision, and, if not controlled, a late loss of central vision and ultimate blindness. This is the most prevalent form of glaucoma and is usually bilateral. Closed-angle glaucoma (acute glaucoma) is characterized by attacks of suddenly increased IOP, exhibited clinically by a bulging iris, which is an emergency situation. Closed-angle glaucoma is usually unilateral with severe pain and loss of vision caused by acute obstruction of aqueous humor drainage within the eye.

Secondary glaucoma results from ocular or systemic disorders that elevate the IOP. These disorders indirectly disrupt the activity of the structures involved in circulation and/or reabsorption of aqueous humor. This can happen suddenly and without warning.

Medical–Surgical Management

Medical

Medical management for glaucoma is focused on drug therapy, and the main objective is to reduce intraocular pressure. Two mechanisms for reducing this pressure are (1) physically constricting the pupil so that the ciliary muscle is contracted, which allows better circulation of the aqueous humor to the site of absorption, and (2) inhibiting the production of aqueous humor.

Surgical

Surgical intervention to facilitate drainage of the aqueous humor is called an iridectomy. A surgical incision is made through the cornea to remove a portion of the iris to facilitate aqueous drainage.

A laser may also be used to treat various eye disorders. In open-angle glaucoma, a laser is used to create multiple scars around the trabecular meshwork (a supporting or anchoring strand that allows increased outflow of aqueous humor), thereby reducing intraocular pressure. In closed-angle glaucoma, laser energy is used to create a hole in the periphery of the iris, creating an opening between the anterior and posterior chambers for aqueous drainage.

 Pharmacological

Drugs that enhance pupillary constriction are commonly used to treat glaucoma. Miotics and cholinesterase inhibitors such as pilocarpine hydrochloride (Isopto Carpine), carbachol (Carbacel), and demecarium bromide (Humorsol) are frequently used.

Beta-adrenergics such as timolol maleate (Timoptic Solution) are the drugs of choice for decreasing IOP. When used as eyedrops, beta-adrenergics reduce aqueous humor production without pupil constriction.

Carbonic anhydrase inhibitors, such as acetazolamide (Diamox), reduce production of aqueous humor to help maintain a lowered IOP. Side effects reported are numbness, weakness, tingling of extremities, and rashes. Adrenergics such as epinephrine bitartrate (Epitrate) also reduce aqueous humor production. Osmotic agents such as mannitol and glycerin (Osmoglyn) may be administered systemically to the client with closed-angle glaucoma in an emergency as an effort to decrease IOP. The high osmolarity of these agents is used to draw fluid into the intravascular space, which lowers the IOP.

Nursing Management

Administer medications as ordered. Stress client compliance with prescribed medication therapy. Encourage glaucoma screening for all persons older than age 35, especially if there is a family history of glaucoma.

NURSING PROCESS

Assessment

Subjective Data

Obtain a history, noting the presence of risk factors: positive family history (believed to be linked in open-angle glaucoma), eye tumor, intraocular hemorrhage, intraocular inflammation, or contusion of the eye from trauma during cataract surgery.

Symptoms of open-angle glaucoma include gradual loss of peripheral vision, eye pain, difficulty adjusting to darkness, halos around lights, and an inability to detect color. For closed-angle glaucoma, symptoms include sudden onset of severe pain in the eye often accompanied by headache, nausea, vomiting, malaise, rainbow halos around lights, and blurred vision.

Objective Data

Assessment reveals acute increased intraocular pressure (21 to 32 mm Hg) as measured with a tonometer (normal range is 12 to 22 mm Hg).

A nursing diagnosis for a client with glaucoma may be:

Nursing Diagnosis	Planning/Goals	Nursing Interventions
Acute Pain related to closed-angle glaucoma	The client will verbalize relief from discomfort.	Administer prescribed ophthalmic agent for glaucoma.
		Notify physician of the following: hypotension, urinary output less than 240 mL for 8 hours, no relief in eye pain within 30 minutes of drug therapy, and continual diminishing visual acuity.
		Monitor blood pressure, pulse, and respiration every 4 hours if not receiving osmotic agent intravenously and every 2 hours if receiving intravenous osmotic agent.
		Monitor degree of eye pain every 30 minutes.
		Monitor intake and output every 8 hours while receiving intravenous osmotic agent.
		Monitor visual acuity before each instillation of prescribed ophthalmic agent by asking if objects are clear or blurred and if the client can read printed material held at arm's length.
		Remind the client that miotics may cause blurred vision for 1 to 2 hours after use and that adaptation to dark environments is difficult because of the pupillary constriction.

Evaluation The goal must be evaluated to determine how it has been met by the client.

RETINAL DETACHMENT

In retinal detachment, the retina separates from the choroid (Figure 39-7). Partial separation becomes complete, if untreated, with the subsequent total loss of vision. A tear or hole in the retina can extend the separation as vitreous humor seeps through the opening and separates the retina from the choroid. The cause of retinal detachment may be from severe trauma to the eye or from intraocular disorders such as cataract extraction, perforating injuries, or severe **myopia** (nearsightedness). This condition is painless because there are no pain receptors in the retina.

Medical–Surgical Management
Medical

Early corrective intervention to reattach the retina may use one of several techniques. Three procedures can be used to create an inflammatory reaction that,

Torn retina
Sclera
Choroid

Figure 39-7 *Retinal Detachment*

once healing and scarring occur, result in the retina reattaching to the choroid. One such technique is electrodiathermy (heat therapy), which uses an ultrasonic probe to burn (seal) the scleral surface directly over the retinal break. Another technique is cryotherapy, which uses an intensely cold probe applied to the scleral surface directly over the hole in the retina. Laser photocoagulation is also used to seal tears or holes in the retina.

Surgical

A surgical procedure called scleral buckling is sometimes used. This operation reduces the scleral surface and allows contact between the choroid and retina.

Pharmacological

Cycloplegic-mydriatic and antiinfective eyedrops are often ordered following the attachment procedure.

Activity

Bed rest and a patch on one or both eyes restricts activity. If air is injected into the vitreous humor, the client either lies prone or sits forward with the unaffected eye upward.

Nursing Management

Explain surgery routines. *Preoperative:* Level of activity—ocular rest, which includes bilateral eye patching and bed rest to facilitate settling of the retina and prevent detachment from worsening. The client will be NPO after midnight. The affected eye is maximally dilated before surgery to permit adequate visualization of the fundus. *Intraoperative:* Client must lie still during surgery or give surgeon warning if needs to cough or change position. Face covered with drapes. Air and oxygen provided. Monitoring, including frequent blood pressure measurements. *Postoperative:* Positioning (supine with a small pillow under the head), bilateral eye patches, activity restrictions, and need to call for assistance with ambulation until stable and vision is adequate.

NURSING PROCESS

Assessment

Subjective Data

Obtain a medical history for presence of causative factors: trauma, recent cataract surgery, eye tumor, severe myopia, uveitis. The client may describe sudden flashes of light (photopsia), floating spots (caused by bleeding into the vitreous cavity), blurred vision that becomes progressively worse, or complaints of a sensation of a veil in the line of sight.

Objective Data

Ophthalmoscopic examination visualizes the detachment.

Nursing diagnoses for a client with retinal detachment may include the following:

Nursing Diagnoses	Planning/Goals	Nursing Interventions
Anxiety related to sensory visual impairment and lack of understanding about treatment	The client will demonstrate reduction of emotional stress, fear, and depression; and an acceptance of surgery.	Assess degree and duration of visual impairment. Encourage conversation to determine client's concerns, feelings, and level of understanding. Answer questions, offer support, and assist client to devise methods for coping. Orient client to new surroundings. Explain interventions clearly. Announce yourself with each interaction; interpret unfamiliar sounds; use touch to assist with verbal communication. Encourage to carry out ADLs as ability allows. Order finger foods for those who cannot see well enough or do not have the coping skills to use implements. Encourage participation of family or significant others in client care. Encourage participation in social and diversional activities as allowed (visitor, radio, audio tapes, television, crafts, games).
Risk for Injury related to visual impairment or knowledge deficit	The client will not have injury caused by visual impairment.	Assist client when able to ambulate postoperatively until stable and has adequate vision or coping skills (remember that clients with bilateral eye patches are unable to see). Assist client in arranging environment and do not rearrange furnishings without reorienting client. Discuss importance of wearing metal shield or glasses as ordered. Apply no pressure to the affected eye. Use proper procedure to administer eye medications.

Evaluation Each goal must be evaluated to determine how it has been met by the client.

INFECTIONS

Infections of the eye include keratitis, stye, chalazion, and conjunctivitis.

Keratitis

Keratitis is inflammation of the cornea that may be caused by infection, irritation, injury, or allergies. Symptoms associated with keratitis include severe eye pain, red watering eye, photophobia, sometimes reduced vision, and sometimes rash (e.g., herpes simplex, herpes zoster, or rosacea).

Treatment of keratitis includes optical anesthetics to relieve pain and mydriatics to dilate the pupil. Dark glasses should be worn to relieve the photophobia. Antibiotic solutions are prescribed for the specific type of infection.

Stye

A **stye** is also referred to as a hordeolum. It is a pustular inflammation of an eyelash follicle or sebaceous gland on the lid margin commonly caused by staphylococcal organisms. Symptoms include pain, redness, and swelling of a specific area of the eyelid. Treatment consists of warm compresses and topical antibiotic ointments. More severe cases may require incision and drainage. Once the pus drains, the pain is relieved and healing begins.

Chalazion

A **chalazion** is a cyst of the meibomian glands, which are sebaceous glands located at the junction of the conjunctiva and inner eyelid margins. The hard cyst is filled with fatty material from the chronically obstructed meibomian glands. The inherent feature of a chalazion is painless localized swelling that develops over a period of weeks. Treatment usually involves surgical excision if the cyst is large, becomes infected, or interferes with vision or closure of the eyelids. The cyst remains when the inflammation subsides.

Conjunctivitis (Pink Eye)

Conjunctivitis is an inflammation of the conjunctiva (a membrane that lines the inside of the eyelids and covers the cornea) that results from invasion by bacterial, viral, or rickettsial organisms, allergens, or irritants. Symptoms include burning and itching of eyes, discharge, swelling, pain, and redness. Treatment consists of applying warm compresses using saline or boric acid solution and instilling antibiotic or antiviral ointments. When caused by allergens, treatment includes avoiding the allergen, taking antihistamines, or being desensitized.

Conjunctivitis is contagious. Proper hand hygiene must be done by nurse and client. Gloves should be worn when applying compresses or instilling ointment. The client's linen should be disinfected to prevent spread of the infection.

REFRACTIVE ERRORS

Refraction is the deflection or bending of light rays when they pass from a medium of one density to a medium of another density. In the case of the eye, light waves pass through the air (less dense) into the fluids of the eye (more dense) so they can be brought to focus on the retina.

Refractive errors result in changes in visual acuity or vision that is not 20/20. Refractive errors include myopia (nearsightedness), **hyperopia** (farsightedness), **astigmatism** (asymmetric focus of light rays on the retina), **presbyopia** (inability of the lens to change curvature in order to focus on near objects), and **strabismus** (inability of the eyes to focus in the same direction) (Figure 39-8).

With myopia, parallel light rays come to focus in front of the retina because the refractive system is too strong or the eyeball is elongated. Near vision is normal, but distant vision is poor.

With hyperopia, parallel light rays come to focus behind the retina because the refractive system is too weak or the eyeball is flattened. Vision beyond 20 feet is normal, but near vision is poor. Figure 39-9 illustrates where light rays focus for myopia and hyperopia.

Astigmatism is a visual defect caused by unequal curvatures of the refractive surfaces of the eye. Light rays from a point do not come to focus on the retina, resulting in visual distortion.

Figure 39-8 *Strabismus (Courtesy of the Armed Forces Institute of Pathology)*

A

Normal eye
Light rays focus on the retina

B

Myopia (nearsightedness)
Light rays focus in front
of the retina

C

Hyperopia (farsightedness)
Light rays focus beyond
the retina

Figure 39-9 *Refraction: **A**, Normal eye; **B**, Myopia; **C**, Hyperopia*

Presbyopia is the loss of elasticity of the lens of the eye caused by aging that causes the near point of vision to recede. The eye loses the ability to accommodate to near objects but remains accommodated for far objects.

Strabismus occurs when one eye is constantly deviated to the side.

Medical–Surgical Management

Medical

Refractory errors may be corrected by prescription glasses or contact lenses. The corrective lenses bend light rays to compensate for a client's refractive error.

Surgical

Radial keratotomy is a surgical procedure used to correct myopia and astigmatism. Under local anesthesia, incisions that resemble the spokes of a wheel are made in the cornea. After the cuts are made, pressure in the anterior chamber of the eye reshapes the cornea to a normal or near-normal curvature. Both LASIK (laser-assisted in-situ keratomileusis) and PRK (photo-refractive keratectomy) use laser to correct nearsightedness and astigmatism.

Nursing Management

Reassure client that refraction testing is painless and that dilating eyedrops may be instilled. Advise client that it may take a little time to adjust to new glasses and not to wear old glasses after getting new ones.

NURSING PROCESS

Assessment

Subjective Data

Obtain a general medical history as well as a history of symptoms. Symptoms may include blurred vision, headache, or eye fatigue.

Objective Data

The client is asked to view an eye chart while lenses of different strengths are systematically placed in front of the eye. The client is asked if the lenses sharpen or blur vision. The power or strength of the lens necessary to permit focusing of the image on the retina is expressed in measurements called diopters.

A nursing diagnosis for a client with refractive errors may be:

Nursing Diagnosis	Planning/Goals	Nursing Interventions
Anxiety related to impaired vision and having to wear glasses or contact lenses	The client will accept wearing glasses or contact lenses.	Allow client to discuss impact of wearing glasses or contact lenses. Encourage client to wear the glasses or contact lenses as prescribed.

Evaluation The goal must be evaluated to determine how it has been met by the client.

INJURY

Injury to the eye or periorbital area can result from a variety of things, such as chemical sprays, tree branches, slingshots, BB guns, flying debris from lawn mowers, and fireworks. Both children and adults are susceptible to eye injuries, and the importance of protecting the eyes cannot be overemphasized. Injuries to the eyes require immediate attention by an ophthalmologist. Even a few hours' delay in treatment may lead to permanent damage.

Corneal abrasion is the disruption of cells and the loss of the superficial epithelium. The outer surface is easily separated from the underlying layers and can be injured or destroyed by exposure (lack of moisture), chemical irritants that dissolve in the protective tear film, and abrasion from foreign bodies.

 Safety: Avoiding Eye Injury
The eyes can be easily protected from injury by wearing protective goggles when performing tasks that are potentially hazardous to the eyes. Those who wear contact lenses should follow the manufacturer's recommendations for wearing them during certain activities, such as swimming or when sleeping.

Foreign Bodies

Foreign bodies in the conjunctiva or on the cornea may cause excessive tearing and redness. Foreign bodies often become embedded in the conjunctiva under the upper eyelid. The lid must be everted and the client instructed to look up to facilitate inspection and removal. If the particle is not located and removed, sterile fluorescein drops or strips should be instilled to visualize minute foreign bodies that are not readily visible with the naked eye.

Chemical Burns

Emergency treatment of chemical burns to the conjunctiva or cornea includes immediate lavage of the eye with tap water and referral to an emergency room or ophthalmologist. In the emergency room, a specially made lid speculum is placed directly on the eyeball and connected to a minimum of 1 liter of isotonic saline solution for irrigation. A topical anesthetic may be instilled to minimize pain during irrigation. No attempt should be made to neutralize the chemical because the heat generated by the chemical reaction may cause further injury. Both eyes should then be patched to allow more comfort.

IMPAIRED VISION

The term *blindness* evokes an image of total darkness and is used for many legal purposes when central visual acuity is 20/200 or less with corrective lenses, in the better eye. Those who have visual acuity between 20/70 and 20/200 in the better eye, with the use of glasses, are often referred to as partially sighted.

The aids that follow are designed to make the most of the available vision (those in italics can also be used by persons who are blind): magnifying glasses; hand and stand magnifiers; telescopes; large-print books, newspapers, magazines; talking books; *Braille* books; closed-circuit television, which produces highly magnified images; *tactually marked watches and clocks; tactually modified table-top games;* enlarged telephone dials, kitchen implements, tools, medication devices; talking clocks, timers, scales, calculators, computers; *text scanner, which converts text to audio mode or Braille;* speech synthesizer; flashlight eye sonar devices; canes, laser canes, and seeing eye dogs.

MACULAR DEGENERATION

Macular degeneration is atrophy or deterioration of the macula, the point on the retina where light rays meet as they are focused by the cornea and lens of the eye. The person loses central vision but still has peripheral vision.

The most common form of macular degeneration is associated with the aging process and is called age-related macular degeneration. Other forms of this disorder include exudative (wet) macular degeneration (sudden growth of new blood vessels in the area of the macula) and injury, infection, or inflammation that damages the macula.

Medical–Surgical Management

Medical

The treatment of age-related macular degeneration is geared toward assisting the client to maximize the use of

CRITICAL THINKING

Visual Impairment
What modifications have to be made in the life of a person who can no longer see?

the remaining vision. The loss of central vision may interfere with the client's ability to read, write, recognize safety hazards, and drive.

Management of clients with exudative macular degeneration is geared toward halting the initiating process and identifying further changes in visual perception. Fluid and blood may resorb in a small percentage of clients with exudative degeneration. Laser therapy to seal the leaking blood vessels in or near the macula may also limit the extent of the damage.

Nursing Management

Provide a safe environment. Announce your presence when entering the client's room and let the client know when you are leaving. Make sure all personnel know of the client's decreased vision. Respond to the client's call light quickly.

NURSING PROCESS

Assessment

Subjective Data

Obtain a general medical history and a history of symptoms. Symptoms include blurred vision, disturbance in color vision (colors become dim), difficulty in reading or doing close work, distortion of objects (especially those with lines), and an empty area within the central field of vision.

Objective Data

Note coping mechanisms such as turning the head to use peripheral vision.

A nursing diagnosis for the client with macular degeneration may be:

Nursing Diagnosis	Planning/Goals	Nursing Interventions
Disturbed Sensory Perception (Visual) related to macular degeneration	The client will discuss the impact of vision loss on lifestyle and use adaptive measures.	Allow client to express feelings about vision loss such as its impact on lifestyle. Convey a willingness to listen, but do not pressure client to talk.
		Provide a safe environment by removing excess furniture or equipment from client's surroundings.
		Orient client to surroundings and show how to use call light.

continues

Nursing Diagnosis	Planning/Goals	Nursing Interventions
		Provide reality orientation if client is confused or disoriented.
		Always introduce yourself or announce your presence upon entering the client's room; let client know when you are leaving.
		Provide sensory stimulation by using tactile, auditory, and gustatory stimuli to help compensate for vision loss.
		Suggest large-print books, talking books, audiotapes, or radio as preferred by client.
		Give clear, concise explanations of treatments and procedures but avoid information overload.
		Make sure that health care personnel are aware of client's vision loss. Record information on the client's chart or post in room.
		Respond to call light quickly.
		Provide continuity by assigning same staff members to care for client when possible.
		Refer to appropriate community resources.

Evaluation The goal must be evaluated to determine how it has been met by the client.

SAMPLE NURSING CARE PLAN

THE CLIENT WITH MACULAR DEGENERATION

Mr. Datal is a 60-year-old high school Latin teacher. He describes having blurred vision in both eyes with a gradual loss of vision in only the right eye. He has trouble reading and is afraid to drive because he can no longer recognize safety hazards. He denies having pain. He also relates having fallen several times recently at home while going up and down the stairs. The family practitioner referred him to an ophthalmologist, who diagnosed Mr. Datal as having macular degeneration in the right eye.

Nursing Diagnosis 1 *Disturbed* **S**ensory *Perception (Visual)* related to macular degeneration as evidenced by his inability to recognize safety hazards when driving

Nursing Outcomes Classification (NOC)
Vision Compensation Behavior

Nursing Interventions Classification (NIC)
Environmental Management
Communication Enhancement: Visual Deficit

PLANNING/GOALS	NURSING INTERVENTIONS	RATIONALE
Mr. Datal will discuss impact of vision loss on lifestyle.	Encourage Mr. Datal to express feelings about vision loss.	Aids in the acceptance of vision loss.
	Convey a willingness to listen, and discuss Mr. Datal's current ability to meet self-care needs and activities of daily living.	Determines Mr. Datal's awareness of his limitations.
	Educate Mr. Datal in alternative ways of coping with vision loss; care of such adaptive devices as eyeglasses, magnifying glass, and contact lenses.	Client will be better able to cope with vision loss.
	Refer to appropriate community resources.	Helps Mr. Datal and his family cope better with his vision loss.

continues

SAMPLE NURSING CARE PLAN

EVALUATION   Mr. Datal discussed the effects of vision loss on his lifestyle and contacted a local agency that provides assistance to the visually impaired.

Nursing Diagnosis 2   *Risk for Injury* related to difficulty in processing visual images and altered depth perception as evidenced by recent falls

Nursing Outcomes Classification (NOC)	**Nursing Interventions Classification (NIC)**
Risk Control: Visual Impairment	*Teaching: Disease Process*
	Fall Prevention

PLANNING/GOALS	NURSING INTERVENTIONS	RATIONALE
Mr. Datal will not experience injury or visual compromise resulting from a fall.	Advise Mr. Datal that depth perception is changed with macular degeneration.	Information promotes understanding.
	Teach Mr. Datal to avoid reaching for objects for stability when ambulating.	Objects may not be where they are perceived. Excessive reaching alters the center of gravity which can precipitate a fall.
	Advise Mr. Datal to go up and down steps one at a time.	Enhances the sense of balance.

EVALUATION   Mr. Datal has not fallen in 2 weeks.

Nursing Diagnosis 3   *Impaired Home Maintenance* related to limited vision, as evidenced by recent falls at home

Nursing Outcomes Classification (NOC)	**Nursing Interventions Classification (NIC)**
Self-Care: Instrumental Activities of Daily Living (IADL)	*Home Maintenance Assistance*
	Teaching: Individual

PLANNING/GOALS	NURSING INTERVENTIONS	RATIONALE
Mr. Datal will develop a plan for self-care in the desired living environment.	Inform Mr. Datal about required self-care activities: personal care, eyedrop instillation, activities permitted, activity restrictions, medications, and how to monitor for complications.	Knowing what self-care activities are needed will help Mr. Datal plan for his care at home.
	Assist Mr. Datal to determine which activities will require assistance.	Helps Mr. Datal to plan for his care at home.
	Evaluate sources of assistance: friends/family, home health care (skilled nursing care), or home care aids.	Determines availability of assistance.
	Critique the safety of Mr. Datal's home: location of telephone, emergency plan, presence of loose rugs or carpets.	Changes can then be made to make Mr. Datal's home safer.

EVALUATION   Mr. Datal is working on a plan so he can care for himself at home.

OTHER SENSES

Other senses include taste, smell, and touch.

TASTE

The sense of taste (gustation) serves as a protector from rotten or putrid food and provides delightful sensations of creamy chocolate, crunchy carrots, chewy taffy, and fruitful pies. Taste sensors are most efficient at room temperature and respond only to substances in solution. The taste buds are located in four areas of the tongue that sense sweet, salt, bitter, and sour (as shown in Figure 39-10).

Taste sensations can be altered secondary to neurological disorders or trauma. Clients who complain of food not "tasting good" should be evaluated for possible causes, including dietary habits, medication use, smoking and caffeine use, as well as olfactory disturbances. The sense of taste works very closely with the sense of smell for identification of the taste sensations.

SMELL

The sense of smell (olfaction) also serves as a guardian from danger. Our nose warns us of impending danger from gas leaks, smoke, fires, rancid meat or fish, and sour dairy products. Body odors and halitosis are clues for personal hygiene and dental care.

Disorders of the olfactory sense often go unnoticed. New tests such as the University of Pennsylvania Smell Identification Test (UPSIT) allow self-testing of smelling deficiencies. Early identification of the loss of the sense of smell may offer clues to alterations in dietary habits, weight loss or gain, anorexia, malnourishment, and changes in daily habits, such as bathing and brushing teeth. The receptors for the sense of smell are located in the roof of the nasal cavity. If these cells are damaged, the sense of smell is impaired. The body cannot regenerate the olfactory cells.

TOUCH

The sense of touch (tactile) includes sensations pertaining to the skin. The tactile receptors are located throughout the integumentary system. Cutaneous sensations of touch, pressure, vibration, cold, heat, and

LIFE CYCLE CONSIDERATIONS

Aging and Taste Sensation

The ability to taste sweetness remains as one ages, but the ability to taste bitterness declines.

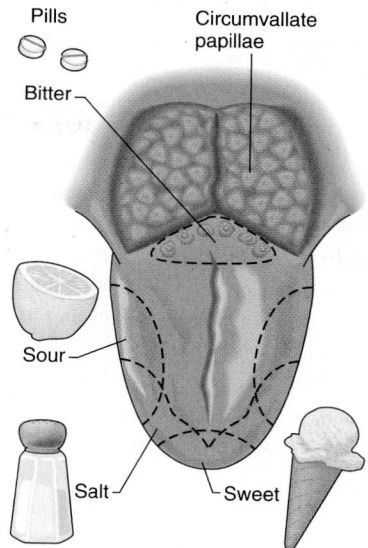

Figure 39-10 *Taste Regions of the Tongue*

pain are examples. Clients who are unable to sense temperature variations should be taught cautionary measures when applying heat or cold therapies, preparing bath water, cooking, or exposing self to hot or cold climates and environmental temperatures.

Clients with reduced or loss of tactile sensation risk injury when their condition confines them to bed. They are unable to sense pressure on bony prominences or the need to change position. The nurse's role in reducing or preventing impairment of skin integrity is crucial. Timely positioning, securing tubes or devices away from the client's body, and using products to minimize skin breakdown are a few of the interventions vital to excellent client care.

Summary

- Hearing loss may be conductive, sensorineural, or a combination of the two. It may also be congenital.
- Ménière's disease is a result of excessive accumulation of endolymph, causing severe vertigo, dizziness, and hearing loss. Treatment is primarily symptomatic.
- Otosclerosis is a conductive hearing loss that may be treated medically with the use of a hearing aid or surgically with a stapedectomy.
- Otitis media is inflammation of the middle ear. Treatment usually includes antibiotics, decongestants, and possibly a myringotomy.
- Cataract surgery is indicated when significant vision loss has occurred.
- Untreated retinal detachment results in total loss of vision.
- Many resources are available for the hearing impaired through community and national agencies.

CASE STUDY

Katie Rollins is a 34-year-old nurse who was diagnosed with a right ear hearing impairment during a routine physical examination. She admitted to her doctor that she noticed she would only use her left ear to talk on the phone and that she had particular difficulty hearing her family or friends in a crowded restaurant or other public settings. She also noted that her husband asked her why she played the television so loud, yet if he turned it down to his normal hearing level, she could not hear it clearly. Her physician ordered an audiogram, which showed a conductive hearing loss of 40% secondary to otosclerosis. Hearing in her left ear was normal.

Katie's doctor gave her three medical treatment options:

1. *Do nothing and monitor her hearing impairment by audiogram every 6 months. If it were to worsen, other options would be considered.*
2. *Be fitted with a hearing aid.*
3. *Have a surgical procedure to correct the hearing loss.*

Katie agreed to have surgery. She thought she would be too self-conscious to wear a hearing aid, after all she was only 34, but she simply could not ignore the problem by doing nothing. Katie was scheduled for same-day surgery.

The following questions will guide your development of a nursing care plan for the case study.

1. How is a conductive hearing loss differentiated from a sensorineural hearing loss?
2. What does an audiogram tell you? What special things should Katie know before she has the audiogram?
3. Describe the surgical procedure that will most likely be used to correct the conductive hearing loss.
4. What will you teach Katie before her surgery about the procedure and expected postoperative course?
5. List four individualized nursing diagnoses and expected outcomes for Katie, and nursing interventions for each diagnosis.
6. Describe the expected discharge instructions that Katie must know related to diet, medications, activity restrictions, and follow-up care.

- The senses of taste, smell, and touch are essential to our enjoyment of life and serve to protect us from danger or harm.

Review Questions

1. In a conductive hearing loss:
   a. the endolymph may cross the capillary membrane and mix with the perilymph, resulting in severe vertigo.
   b. the ossicles of the middle ear fracture, resulting in a tear of the eighth cranial nerve.
   c. sound waves are not transmitted through the ear canal to inner ear fluid.
   d. a tumor in the inner ear blocks the flow of fluid through the bony and membranous labyrinths.

2. A possible nursing diagnosis for a client with Ménière's disease is:
   a. activity intolerance related to impaired hearing.
   b. knowledge deficit related to surgical shunt placement to drain excessive endolymph.
   c. communication, impaired, verbal, related to tinnitus.
   d. risk for injury related to vertigo.

3. Chemical burns of the eye are initially treated with:
   a. local anesthetics and antibacterial drops for 24 to 36 hours.
   b. hot compresses applied at 15-minute intervals.
   c. flushing of the lids, conjunctiva, and cornea with water.
   d. cleansing of the conjunctiva with a small, cotton-tipped applicator.

4. A clinical symptom of a detached retina is:
   a. an increase in tearing.
   b. an area of vague vision.
   c. momentary flashes of light.
   d. pain in the eye.

5. Macular degeneration is characterized by:
   a. purulent periorbital drainage.
   b. pupil dilation.
   c. loss of central vision.
   d. ptosis (droopy lid).

References/Suggested Readings

American Speech-Language-Hearing Association. (2002). *Types of hearing loss.* [Online]. Available: www.asha.org/hearing/disorders/types/cfm

Barnie, D. (2002). Restoring vision in older patients. *RN, 65*(1), 30–35.

Cavendish, R. (1998). Clinical snapshot: Hearing loss. *AJN, 98*(8), 50–51.

Dana, R. (1998, January 27). Dry eye syndrome. *Health News 1,* 3.

Daniels, R. (2002). *Delmar's Guide to Laboratory and Diagnostic Tests.* Clifton Park, NY: Thomson Delmar Learning.

Dochterman, J., & Bulechek, G. (2004). *Nursing Interventions Classification (NIC)* (4th ed.). St. Louis, MO: Mosby.

Estes, M. E. Z. (2002). *Health Assessment & Physical Examination* (2nd ed.). Clifton Park, NY: Thomson Delmar Learning.

Kearney, K. (1997). Retinal detachment. *AJN, 97*(8), 50.

Lucas, L., & Matthews-Flint, L. (2001). Sound advice about hearing aids. *Nursing2001, 31*(2), 59–61.

McConnell, E. (2001a). Instilling ear drops. *Nursing2001, 31*(4), 17.

McConnell, E. (2001b). Myths & Facts . . . about macular degeneration. *Nursing2001, 31*(8), 30.

McConnell, E. (2002). How to converse with a hearing-impaired patient. *Nursing2002, 32*(8), 20.

Moorhead, S., Johnson, M., & Maas, M. (2004). *Nursing Outcomes Classification (NOC)* (3rd ed.). St. Louis, MO: Mosby.

National Institute on Deafness and Other Communication Disorders. (2002). *Cochlear implants.* [Online]. Available: www.nidcd.nih.gov/health/pubs_hb/coch.htm

North American Nursing Diagnosis Association. (2003). *Nursing Diagnoses: Definitions & Classification 2003–2004.* Philadelphia, PA: Author.

Ramponi, D. (2000). Go with the flow during an eye emergency. *Nursing2000, 30*(8), 54–56.

Ramponi, D. (2001). Contact lens removal. *Nursing2001, 31*(8), 56–57.

Shelp, S. (1997). Your patient is deaf, now what? *RN, 60*(2), 37–40.

Smeltzer, S. C., & Bare, B. G. (2002). *Brunner and Suddarth's Textbook of Medical–Surgical Nursing* (9th ed.). Philadelphia: Lippincott Williams & Wilkins.

Sommer, S., & Sommer, N. (2002). When your patient is hearing impaired. *RN, 65*(12), 28–32.

Sparks, S. M., & Taylor, C. M. (1998). *Nursing diagnosis reference manual* (4th ed.). Springhouse, PA: Springhouse Corporation.

Spencer, J. (1998, February 17). Coping with hearing loss. *Health News 2,* 1–2.

Spratto, G., & Woods, A. (2004). *2004 PDR Nurses' Drug Handbook,* Clifton Park, NY: Thomson Delmar Learning.

Tupper, S. (1999). When the inner ear is out of balance. *RN, 62*(11), 36–40.

Walbecker, J. (1997). Knowing the signs. *RN, 60*(2), 40–41.

Resources

Alexander Graham Bell Association for the Deaf, 3417 Volta Place NW, Washington, DC 20007, 202-337-5220, www.agbell.org

American Academy of Ophthalmology, P.O. Box 7424, San Francisco, CA 94120, 415-561-8500, www.aao.org

American Academy of Otolaryngology, Head and Neck Surgery, 1 Prince Street, Alexandria, VA 22314, 703-836-4444, www.entnet.org

American Council of the Blind, 1155 15th Street NW, Suite 1004, Washington, DC 20005, 800-424-8666, http://acb.org

American Foundation for the Blind, Inc., 11 Penn Plaza, Suite 300, New York, NY 10011, 212-502-7600, www.afb.org

American Speech-Language-Hearing Association, 10801 Rockville Pike, Rockville, MD 20852, 800-498-2071, www.asha.org

American Tinnitus Association, P.O. Box 5, Portland, OR 97207, 800-634-8978, www.ata.org

Better Hearing Institute, 515 King St., Suite 420, Alexandria, VA 22314, 703-684-3391

Better Vision Institute, Inc., 1700 Diagonal Road, Suite 500, Alexandria, VA 22314, 703-548-4560, www.visionsite.org

Guide Dogs for the Blind, P.O. Box 15200, San Rafael, CA 94915, 800-295-4050, www.guidedogs.com

Guide Dog Users, Inc., 14311 Astrodome Drive, Silver Spring, MD 20906, 888-858-1008, www.gdui.org

Guiding Eyes for the Blind, 611 Granite Springs Road, Yorktown Heights, NY 10598, 800-942-0149, www.guiding-eyes.org

International Hearing Dog Inc., 5901 East 89th Avenue, Henderson, CO 80640, 303-287-3277, www.ihdi.org

Leader Dogs for the Blind, P.O. Box 5000, Rochester, MI 48308, 888-777-5332, www.leader-dog.org

Lion's International, 300 22nd St., Oak Brook, IL 60523-8842, 630-571-5466, www.lionsclubs.org

National Association for the Deaf, 814 Thayer Avenue, Silver Spring, MD 20910, 301-587-1788 (TTY 301-587-1789), www.nad.org

National Association for Visually Handicapped, 22 West 21st Street, New York, NY 10010, 212-889-3141, www.navh.org

National Society to Prevent Blindness, 500 East Remington Rd., Schaumburg, IL 60173, 800-331-2020, www.preventblindness.org

Recording for the Blind & Dyslexic, 20 Roszel Rd., Princeton, NJ 08540, 866-732-3585, www.rfbd.org

Self Help for Hard of Hearing, 7910 Woodmont Avenue, Suite 1200, Bethesda, MD 20814, 301-657-2248, www.shhh.org

40

ENDOCRINE SYSTEM

MAKING THE CONNECTION

Refer to the following chapters to increase your understanding of the endocrine system:

Basic Nursing
- **Wellness Concepts**
- **Fluid, Electrolyte, and Acid–Base Balance**
- **Assessment**
- **Diagnostic Tests**

Adult Health Nursing
- **Oncology**
- **Cardiovascular System**
- **Hematologic and Lymphatic Systems**
- **Urinary System**
- **Musculoskeletal System**
- **Neurological System**
- **Sensory System**

- **Reproductive System**
- **Integumentary System**
- **Immune System**
- **The Older Adult**

Basic Procedures
- **Measuring Intake and Output**

Intermediate Procedures
- **Withdrawing Medication from a Vial**
- **Administering a Subcutaneous Injection**
- **Performing a Skin Puncture**

Review: Delmar's Anatomy & Physiology CD-ROM: Endocrine System

LEARNING OBJECTIVES

Upon completion of this chapter, you should be able to:
- Define key terms.
- Identify and locate the endocrine glands and list function(s) and hormone(s) secreted by each.
- Differentiate between type 1 and type 2 diabetes in terms of pathophysiology, presenting symptoms and treatment.
- Discuss the roles of diet and exercise in the management of diabetes mellitus.
- Identify signs, causes, and treatment of acute complications of hypoglycemia, diabetic ketoacidosis, and hyperosmolar hyperglycemic nonketotic syndrome.
- Discuss the major long-term complications of diabetes.
- Discuss rationale for the pituitary gland being traditionally called the "master" gland.
- Compare symptoms of the disease process resulting from a hyper- or hyposecretion of an endocrine gland.

KEY TERMS

agranulocytosis	hypoglycemia
autosomal	hypovolemia
Chvostek's sign	iatrogenic
cretinism	insulin
dawn phenomenon	ketonuria
endocrine	lipodystrophy
exophthalmos	myxedema
glucagon	paroxysmal
glycosuria	polydipsia
goiter	polyphagia
gynecomastia	polyuria
hirsutism	Somogyi phenomenon
hormone	tetany
hyperglycemia	Trousseau's sign

- Discuss assessment techniques for a client suspected of having an endocrine disorder.
- Formulate a nursing care plan for the client with an endocrine disorder.

INTRODUCTION

The endocrine system provides the same general functions as the nervous system: communication and control; however, the endocrine system is generally slower and has longer-lasting control over the various body activities and functions. It exerts this control through the secretion of hormones that circulate through the blood. A malfunction of any part of the endocrine system can result in a shift of homeostasis with far-reaching systemic reactions.

Assessment of the endocrine system is difficult. Not only are the components not in direct contact, but only the thyroid gland is close enough to the body surface for direct physical assessment. Still, the nurse needs to be familiar with the normal functioning of the endocrine system. In assessing the client for endocrine dysfunction, the nurse must note negative findings as well as positive ones. Assessment includes results of diagnostic tests as well as any precipitating or aggravating factors.

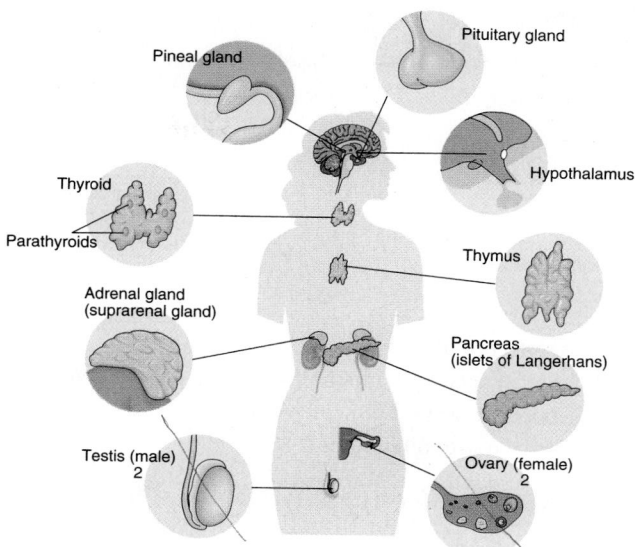

Figure 40-1 *Structures of the Endocrine System*

ANATOMY AND PHYSIOLOGY REVIEW

The endocrine system is unique in that it is composed of a group of various glands scattered throughout the body. The term **endocrine** (*endo*—within, *crin*—secrete) indicates that the secretions formed by these glands directly enter the blood or lymph circulation, rather than being transported via tubes or ducts. These secretions, called **hormones,** are chemical substances that initiate or regulate activity of another organ, system, or gland in another part of the body. The level of hormone in the blood is regulated by the homeostasis mechanism called *negative feedback.* If the blood level for a specific hormone falls below normal, negative feedback causes the specific endocrine gland to produce more of the hormone, which when increased to the normal level causes a decrease in production.

The glands discussed in this chapter that make up the endocrine system are the pancreas, pituitary, hypothalamus, thyroid, parathyroid, and adrenals (Figure 40-1). Several endocrine glands such as the pineal, thymus, ovaries, and testes are of great importance; however, they are discussed in other chapters in connection with the organ system in which they function.

The pancreas lies horizontally behind the stomach at the level of the first and second lumbar vertebrae. The head of the pancreas is attached to the duodenum with the tail reaching to the spleen. It has both exocrine and endocrine functions.

The pituitary gland consists of an anterior and a posterior lobe. It has traditionally been called the "master" gland because so many of its secretions influence other endocrine glands and body systems. It is attached to the hypothalamus by a stalk called the *infundibulum.* The hypothalamus is located in the lower portion of the brain and produces secretions influencing the production and release of the anterior pituitary hormones as well as the posterior pituitary hormones. Both the pituitary and hypothalamus are located in the head. The pituitary, about the size of a pea, is located in the sella turcica, a small depression in the sphenoid bone. Refer to Table 40-1 for specific endocrine hormones and functions.

The thyroid gland is butterfly-shaped and lies in the neck. It consists of two lobes—one on each side of the trachea connected by an isthmus. The gland sits saddle-like starting on the anterior surface of the trachea just below the larynx and surrounds it partway. The thyroid gland stores iodine. The thyroid gland produces thyroid hormones including thyroxine, which is the most abundant, and triiodothyronine. It regulates the metabolic rate for carbohydrates, protein, and fats.

There are usually four parathyroid glands. Two glands are embedded in the posterior portion of each thyroid lobe. They produce parathyroid hormone, parathormone, which regulates the concentration of blood calcium and phosphorus.

The adrenal, or suprarenal, glands are located on top of each kidney. The adrenal cortex secretes mineralocorticoids including aldosterone, glucocorticoids including cortisol, and androgens, which are sex hormones. The adrenal medulla secretes epinephrine or adrenalin and norepinephrine or noradrenalin, which help the body function under stress.

It is important to understand the normal function of the endocrine glands and hormones. Most endocrine disorders are a result of either overactivity or underactivity of these glands.

COMMON DIAGNOSTIC TESTS

Commonly used diagnostic tests for clients with symptoms of endocrine system disorders are listed in Table 40-2.

TABLE 40-1   ENDOCRINE GLANDS AND HORMONES

HORMONE	FUNCTION
Pancreas	
Glucagon	Raises blood glucose
Insulin	Lowers blood glucose
Somatostatin	Inhibits secretion of insulin, glucagon, and growth hormone from the anterior pituitary and gastrin from the stomach
Anterior Pituitary	
Thyroid-stimulating hormone (TSH)	Stimulates thyroid growth and secretion of the thyroid hormone
Adrenocorticotropic hormone (ACTH)	Stimulates adrenal cortex growth and secretion of glucocorticoids
Follicle-stimulating hormone (FSH)	Stimulates ovarian follicle to mature and produce estrogen; in the male, stimulates sperm production
Luteinizing hormone (LH)	Acts with FSH to stimulate estrogen production; causes ovulation; stimulates progesterone production by corpus luteum; in male, stimulates testes to produce testosterone
Melanocyte-stimulating hormone (MSH)	Causes increase in synthesis and spread of melanin (pigment) in skin
Growth hormone (GH)	Stimulates growth
Prolactin or lactogenic hormone	Stimulates breast development during pregnancy and milk secretion after delivery of baby
Posterior Pituitary	
Antidiuretic hormone (ADH)	Stimulates water retention by kidneys to decrease urine secretion
Oxytocin	Stimulates uterine contractions; causes breast to release milk into ducts
Thyroid Gland	
Thyroid hormone (thyroxine T_4 and triiodothyronine T_3)	Increases metabolic rate
Calcitonin	Decreases blood calcium concentration
Parathyroid Gland	
Parathyroid hormone	Increases blood calcium concentration
Adrenal Cortex	
Glucocorticoids (cortisol, hydrocortisone)	Stimulates gluconeogenesis and increases blood glucose; antiinflammatory; antiimmunity; antiallergy
Mineralocorticoids	Regulates electrolyte and fluid homeostasis
Sex hormones (androgen)	Stimulates sexual drive in females; in males, negligible effect
Adrenal Medulla	
Epinephrine (adrenalin)	Prolongs and intensifies sympathetic nervous response to stress
Norepinephrine	Prolongs and intensifies sympathetic nervous response to stress

(handwritten annotations: "Hyperthyroid – loose wt – can't concentrate"; "Hypothyroid – Goiter – thyroid – expanding ENLARGING")

DIABETES MELLITUS

Diabetes mellitus (DM) is a disorder of metabolism. When we eat, most of the food we eat is broken down by digestive juices. Of the food we eat, 100% of carbohydrate and approximately 58% of protein and 10% of fat is broken down to glucose. For the glucose to get into the cells, insulin must be present (Figure 40-2).

Insulin is a hormone produced and secreted by the beta cells of the islets of Langerhans in the pancreas.

Insulin stimulates the active transport of glucose into muscle and adipose tissue cells, making it available for cell use. For glucose to cross the cell membrane, insulin must connect with a receptor on the cell membrane. Some clients with diabetes mellitus have enough insulin but too few functioning receptor sites. Others have inadequate or no insulin production. Blood glucose can always be used by the brain and kidneys. Insulin is not needed for glucose to enter brain cells or cells of the glomeruli.

TABLE 40-2 COMMON DIAGNOSTIC TESTS FOR ENDOCRINE SYSTEM DISORDERS

Pancreas Diagnostic Tests

Blood glucose, Fasting blood sugar (FBS) *YES + Random*

2-hour postprandial glucose (2hPPG) or 2-hour postprandial blood sugar (2hPPBS) *YES ~ +*

Glucose tolerance test (GTT) *— YES*

+ A1C TEST

Pituitary Gland Diagnostic Tests

Adrenocorticotropic hormone (ACTH), Corticotropin

Antidiuretic hormone (ADH), Vasopressin

Follicle-stimulating hormone (FSH)

Growth hormone (GH), Human GH (HGH), Somatotropin hormone (SH)

Growth hormone (GH) stimulation test, GH provocation test, Insulin tolerance test (ITT), Arginine test

Luteinizing hormone (LH) assay

Prolactin level (PRL)

Thyrotropin-releasing hormone (TRH) test, Thyrotropin-releasing factor (TRF) test

Urine specific gravity

Long bone x-rays

Sella turcica x-ray

Computed tomography of head (CT scan of head), Computerized axial transverse tomography (CATT)

Thyroid Gland Diagnostic Tests

Antithyroid microsomal antibody, Antimicrosomal antibody, Microsomal antibody, Thyroid autoantibody, Thyroid antimicrosomal antibody

Calcitonin, HCT, Thyrocalcitonin

Serum-free triiodothyronine (T_3)

Thyroid-stimulating hormone (TSH), Thyrotropin *— YES*
YES

Thyroid-stimulating hormone (TSH) stimulation test *— YES*

Thyroxine index free, FTI, FT_4 Index

Thyroxine, T_4, Thyroxine screen *— YES*

Triiodothyronine, T_3 radioimmunoassay, T_3 by RIA

Radioactive iodine uptake (RAIU), Iodine uptake test, ^{131}I uptake

Thyroid scan, Thyroid scintiscan

Thyroid ultrasound, Thyroid echogram, Thyroid sonogram

Thyroid biopsy

Parathyroid Gland Diagnostic Tests

Parathyroid hormone (PTH), Parathormone

Calcium, total/ionized Ca^{++}

Phosphorus

Adrenal Glands Diagnostic Tests

Adrenocorticotropic hormone (ACTH) stimulation test, Cortisol stimulation test, Cosyntropin test

Cortisol, Hydrocortisone

Dexamethasone suppression test (DST), Prolonged/rapid DST, Cortisol suppression test, ACTH suppression test

Plasma renin assay, Plasma renin activity (PRA)

Progesterone assay

Aldosterone assay

17-Hydroxycorticosteroids (17-OHCS)

17-Ketosteroids (17-KS)

Urine cortisol, Hydrocortisone

Vanillylmandelic acid (VMA) & catecholamines, VMA & epinephrine, Norepinephrine, Metanephrine, Normetanephrine, Dopamine

Adrenal angiography, Adrenal arteriogram

Adrenal venography

Computed tomography of adrenals (CAT scan of adrenals), CT scan of adrenals

---

The amount of glucose in the blood regulates the rate of insulin secretion. When a meal is eaten, the blood glucose elevates and the beta cells of the islets of Langerhans release insulin. As the blood glucose level drops, insulin secretion diminishes. It is important to note that during times of fasting (overnight or between meals), a low level of insulin continues to be secreted along with **glucagon.** Glucagon secreted by the alpha cells of the pancreas stimulates release of glucose by the liver. The balance and interactions of insulin and glucagon maintain a constant serum glucose level.

Other functions of insulin include:

- Promoting conversion of glucose to glycogen for storage in the liver and inhibiting conversion of glycogen to glucose
- Promoting conversion of fatty acids into fat that can be stored as adipose tissue and preventing breakdown of adipose tissue and conversion of fat to ketone bodies
- Stimulating protein synthesis within tissues and inhibiting the breakdown of protein into amino acids

In summary, insulin actively promotes those processes that lower the blood glucose level and inhibits those processes that raise the blood glucose level. A deficiency of insulin results in **hyperglycemia,** or elevated blood glucose. Excess insulin results in **hypoglycemia** (low blood glucose). Diabetes mellitus is actually a group of disorders characterized by chronic hyperglycemia.

DIAGNOSIS AND CLASSIFICATION

The Expert Committee on the Diagnosis and Classification of Diabetes Mellitus (1997) presented to the American Diabetes Association (ADA) new criteria for diagnosis and new classifications for diabetes, which the ADA approved.

Diagnosis

The Committee identified two precursors to diabetes, screening criteria, and diagnostic criteria.

When we eat, food is broken down into chemicals and glucose enters bloodstream.

In response to elevated serum glucose, beta cells of pancreas secrete insulin into bloodstream.

Insulin combines with insulin receptors on cell wall (activating glucose transporters), allowing glucose to enter cell.

● = Glucose
○ = Insulin
∧∧ = Insulin receptors

Figure 40-2 *How Insulin Works*

The two precursors identified are:

1. Impaired glucose tolerance (IGT)—a glucose level of 140 to 199 mg/dL 2 hours after a glucose load
2. Impaired fasting glucose (IFG)—a fasting glucose of 110 to 125 mg/dL

The criteria for who should be screened for diabetes include:

1. Anyone age 45 and older
2. Anyone, regardless of age, with one of the following risk factors:
   - Obesity (body mass index of 27 or greater)
   - Immediate family member with diabetes
   - Member of high-risk ethnic group (African American, Hispanic American, some Native American groups)
   - Having a baby weighing more than 9 pounds
   - History of gestational diabetes mellitus (GDM)
   - Hypertension
   - High-density lipoprotein level of 35 mg/dL or less, or a triglyceride level of 250 mg/dL or more
   - Have either of the two precursors of diabetes

The diagnostic criteria identify when a physician can make a diagnosis of diabetes. The situations are:

- A random blood glucose of 200 mg/dL or greater with the classic symptoms of polyuria, polydipsia, and unexplained weight loss
   or
- A fasting blood sugar of 126 mg/dL or greater
   or

PROFESSIONAL TIP

Diabetes

According to the Centers for Disease Control and Prevention (CDC) (2002a), 11.1 million Americans are diagnosed as having diabetes mellitus. Another 5.9 million are estimated to be undiagnosed. Diabetes was the sixth leading cause of death in the United States and is associated with many serious complications (CDC, 2002a). Diabetes is the leading cause of new blindness among adults, and of new cases of renal failure, and is present in more than 60% of persons experiencing nontraumatic lower extremity amputations (CDC, 2002a).

Diabetes is seen in all age groups and races. About 25% of clients with diabetes are older than age 65. African American, Hispanic, and some Native American populations have a higher incidence of diabetes than the white population (CDC 2002a).

- The 2-hour sample of the oral glucose tolerance test is 200 mg/dL or greater using a load of 75 grams of anhydrous glucose

The committee also recommended not using glycosylated hemoglobin to diagnose diabetes since terminology is confusing, and many methods of measuring glycosylated hemoglobin are used.

Classification

Etiology, not insulin use, is used to classify diabetes into four categories: type 1 diabetes, type 2 diabetes, other specific types, and gestational diabetes mellitus.

Type 1 Diabetes

There are two forms of diabetes resulting from pancreatic beta-cell destruction or a primary defect in beta-cell function, resulting in no release of insulin and ineffective glucose transport. There is usually an absolute insulin deficiency so the clients are insulin-dependent. The two subdivisions of type 1 diabetes are:

- *Immune-mediated*—islet cell or insulin antibodies destroy beta cells. The rate of this destruction is usually higher in children than in adults. Children and adolescents may rapidly develop ketoacidosis. Adults seldom develop ketoacidosis unless they have an infection or other stressor. This is what used to be called insulin-dependent diabetes mellitus (IDDM), or juvenile-onset diabetes.
- *Idiopathic*—no evidence of autoimmunity; the individual just does not produce insulin and is prone to ketoacidosis.

In the absence of insulin, glucose from food eaten cannot be used or stored and remains in the bloodstream, resulting in hyperglycemia. In addition, glucose production from the liver goes unchecked, further elevating the blood glucose level.

As the blood glucose rises, the kidney begins to excrete excess glucose in the urine (**glycosuria**). Glucose

TABLE 40-3 COMPARISON OF THE CLINICAL MANIFESTATIONS OF TYPE 1 DIABETES AND TYPE 2 DIABETES

	TYPE 1 DIABETES	TYPE 2 DIABETES
Etiology	Autoimmune	Genetic susceptibility associated. Usually associated with obesity.
Age of onset	Rare before age 1	Incidence increases with age
Percent of diabetics	5%–10%	90%–95%
Onset	Abrupt, rapid	Gradual, over years
Body weight at onset	Normal or thin	80% are overweight
Insulin production	None	Less than normal, normal, or greater than normal
Insulin injection	Always	Necessary for approximately 30%
Ketosis	Occurs mainly in children and adolescents	Unlikely
Management	Insulin, diet, exercise	Diet and weight loss, exercise, possibly oral hypoglycemics or insulin

eliminated in the urine pulls excessive amounts of water with it (osmotic diuresis), resulting in fluid volume deficit and producing symptoms of excessive thirst (**polydipsia**) and increased urination (**polyuria**).

Insulin deficiency also results in impaired metabolism of fats and proteins. Because of the impaired glucose, fat, and protein metabolism and the inability to store glucose, clients frequently experience protein wasting, weight loss, and increased hunger (**polyphagia**).

Metabolism of fat stores for energy leads to production of acid by-products called ketones, which can be detected in the urine (**ketonuria**). As ketones accumulate, the associated decrease in pH leads to metabolic acidosis, or more specifically a condition known as *diabetic ketoacidosis*, discussed later in this chapter.

Type 2 Diabetes

These clients have insulin resistance with relative insulin deficiency. Most of these clients are obese. When weight is lost, insulin resistance diminishes but reappears if the client regains weight. Age, lack of exercise, history of GDM, hypertension, dyslipidemia, and being of African American, Hispanic American, or Native American origin are all risk factors. A strong family history of diabetes is often evident. Many clients do not require insulin, but eventually one-third will need insulin to maintain a normal glucose level. This is what used to be called noninsulin-dependent diabetes mellitus (NIDDM), or adult-onset diabetes.

Hyperglycemia results when the pancreas cannot match the body's need for insulin and/or when the number of insulin receptor sites are decreased or altered.

Although available insulin may be insufficient to meet the body's metabolic needs and prevent hyperglycemia, there is a sufficient amount of insulin to prevent fat breakdown for energy and the resulting ketoacidosis. Extremely elevated glucose in the type 2 diabetic will result in development of hyperosmolar hyperglycemic nonketotic syndrome (HHNS), discussed later in this chapter. Table 40-3 compares the clinical manifestations of type 1 and type 2 diabetes.

Other Specific Types

This includes conditions such as beta-cell genetic defects, endocrinopathies, and drug- or chemical-induced diabetes. These are in a separate category because there are different disease etiologies.

Gestational Diabetes Mellitus

Occurring during pregnancy, this may be controlled either with or without insulin. Generally, the client's glucose tolerance returns to normal after the infant's birth. The client should be rechecked 6 weeks after the birth to see if the diabetes persists.

Contributing Factors

Persons with a family history of diabetes are at greater risk for developing diabetes. Other factors associated with diabetes include obesity, aging, and ethnic group. The most powerful risk factor for type 2 diabetes is obesity. For persons with a family history of type 2 diabetes, maintenance of an ideal body weight may delay or prevent the onset of diabetes.

Aging can also be considered a contributing factor.

It is known that members of certain racial groups are more likely to develop diabetes. In the United States, there is a greater chance of developing type 2 diabetes for Hispanics, certain Native American populations, and African Americans.

Other groups at risk for development of diabetes include those with a history of gestational diabetes or impaired glucose tolerance (IGT).

Medical–Surgical Management

Medical

There is no known cure for diabetes. The goal of therapeutic management is aimed at the control of blood sugar and the prevention and early detection of the complications associated with diabetes. Diabetes is considered under control if the client maintains ideal body weight and enjoys good health, preprandial glucose levels are less than 140 mg/dL, and postprandial glucose levels do not rise above 180 mg/dL.

Treatment plans vary and are individualized for each client. Control of blood glucose generally involves a balance of a dietary prescription, an exercise plan, and medications. Ultimately, the client is the manager of the treatment plan and, therefore, must be very well informed about diabetes and involved in all aspects of care planning and decision making.

Since the advent of home glucose monitoring devices, urine testing for glucose is rarely used. Testing urine for ketone (product of fatty acid oxidation) production, however, continues to be recommended when the blood glucose level is consistently higher than 240 mg/dL or when any symptoms of ketoacidosis are present.

The client with type 1 diabetes will always require administration of insulin to lower the glucose level and prevent complications of diabetes. Diet and exercise regimens are also important to control the glucose level and maintain health.

Dietary management is the cornerstone of treatment for the person with type 2 diabetes. As the obese person loses weight, the body's insulin requirements decrease, resulting in improved glucose tolerance. Exercise plays an important role in losing weight and lowering the blood glucose level. Type 2 diabetes not controlled by diet and exercise may necessitate administration of medications. Oral hypoglycemic agents or parenteral administration of insulin may be required for optimal control.

Surgical

Pancreas transplantations have been performed and have successfully eliminated the need for exogenous insulin in some clients. At present, pancreas transplants are being performed primarily on clients with type 1 diabetes who also need kidney or other organ transplants because the serious side effects of the antirejection medications do not justify a pancreas transplant alone. Pancreatic islet cell transplants are also being done experimentally with limited success but hold much promise for the future.

💊 Pharmacological

Various pharmacological treatments that are used in the management of type 1 and type 2 diabetes are discussed in the following text.

Insulin Persons with type 1 diabetes always require insulin administration. Persons with type 2 diabetes may not initially require insulin, but it may become necessary as endogenous insulin production decreases or during times of stress or illness.

Historically, insulin has been obtained from beef or pork pancreas. Today, biosynthetic human insulin is used almost exclusively, but some clients still use pork or beef insulin. Human insulin is purer, more effective, and has a much lower incidence of causing insulin allergies and resistance. Insulin is available in very short-, short-, fast-, intermediate-, and long-acting forms that can be injected separately or mixed in the same syringe. Premixed insulins are also available. See Table 40-4 for descriptions of types of insulins and their actions. Insulin is routinely administered subcutaneously. Regular insulin (short-acting) may be administered intravenously when immediate response is desired, as in treatment of greatly elevated glucose levels occurring with diabetic ketoacidosis (DKA) or hyperosmolar hyperglycemic nonketotic syndrome (HHNS). Regular insulin, which is the only clear insulin, is the *only* insulin that can be given intravenously (IV).

The strength of insulin correlates to the number of units of insulin per cubic centimeter. The most common concentrations of insulin used today are U-50 and U-100 insulin (50 and 100 units of insulin per 1 cc respectively). U-500 insulin is available for clients who require very high doses.

Insulin should always be measured in an insulin syringe, which is marked in units. When mixing two types of insulin in the same syringe, it is important that the regular (clear, short-acting) insulin be drawn up first. The policy of many health care institutions requires that two nurses check insulin dosages before administration. Even if the facility does not have such a policy, checking the insulin dosage with another nurse will help protect against an adverse reaction resulting from error.

COMMUNITY/HOME HEALTH CARE

Glucose Monitoring

The availability and use of home glucose monitoring equipment to evaluate serum (blood) glucose has revolutionized self-care for the diabetic client. Also called "fingerstick blood glucose" (FSBG), self-monitoring of blood glucose (SMBG) can be done quickly using capillary blood that provides fairly accurate reading of the current blood glucose. Most often, the glucose level is checked before meals and at bedtime so the client can adjust the treatment plan accordingly. Self-monitoring of blood glucose is recommended for all clients requiring insulin or those with a widely fluctuating glucose level. Symptoms of hypoglycemia at any time warrant immediate evaluation of the blood glucose level.

TABLE 40-4 TYPES OF INSULIN AND THEIR ACTIONS

TYPES OF INSULIN	APPEARANCE	ACTION IN HOURS		
		ONSET	PEAK	DURATION
Very short-acting				
Insulin lispro (Humalog)	clear	$1/4$	$1-1\frac{1}{2}$	5 or less
Short-acting				
Humulin R *Regular*	clear	$1/2-1$	2-4	6-8
Intermediate-acting				
Humulin N *NPH*	cloudy	$1-1\frac{1}{2}$	4-12	up to 24
Humulin L	cloudy	$1-2-\frac{1}{2}$	7-15	22
Long-acting				
Humulin U	cloudy	4-8	10-30	36+
Insulin glargine (Lantus)	clear	1	none	up to 24
Premixed				
Humulin N/Reg				
Humulin 70/30	cloudy	$1/2-1$	4-8	24
Humulin 50/50				

all injectable

Insulin dosages are individually determined, usually requiring two or more injections per day and involving a combination of a short-acting and a longer-acting insulin. Various regimens of insulin administration can be used, each with its own advantages and disadvantages. In general, the more complex the regimen, the more normal the blood glucose level throughout the day. Clients can be taught to use the results of their self-monitoring blood glucose to adjust their insulin doses, allowing more flexibility in their meals and schedules. Recent studies strongly support the theory that intensive insulin regimens that tightly control the blood glucose level delay the onset and progression of complications of diabetic retinopathy, nephropathy, and neuropathy.

Sliding-Scale Insulin During times of surgery, illness, or stress, clients may have their glucose level managed with an insulin sliding scale in lieu of their regular regimen of insulin or oral hypoglycemics. A sliding scale determines insulin dosage based on fingerstick blood glucose level. Regular (short-acting) insulin is used, and a dose is administered every 4 or 6 hours based on the blood glucose level. The sliding scale allows for much flexibility and ensures frequent monitoring of and response to changes in the client's glucose level. An example sliding scale might be:

- 4u Humulin R Insulin for glucose 151–200 mg/dL
- 6u Humulin R Insulin for glucose 201–250 mg/dL
- 8u Humulin R Insulin for glucose 251–300 mg/dL
- 10u Humulin R Insulin for glucose 301–350 mg/dL
- Call physician for glucose >350 mg/dL

Insulin Injections Insulin injections are administered into the subcutaneous tissue. If an inch of skin can be pinched, the needle is injected at a 90-degree angle,

Figure 40-3 *Possible Sites and Rotation for Insulin Administration*

otherwise, at a 45-degree angle. The four main areas for injection are the abdomen, arms, thighs, and hips (Figure 40-3). Factors affecting absorption should be considered when selecting an injection site. Absorption occurs most quickly in the abdomen, followed by the arms, thighs, and hips.

Rotation of sites for injection has traditionally been recommended to prevent **lipodystrophy** (atrophy or hypertrophy in the subcutaneous fat). More recently, some authorities are recommending that the abdomen, which

1. Cleanse the rubber stopper on both vials with an alcohol wipe, then inject the amount of air equal to the dose of the intermediate-acting insulin into the N vial.

2. Inject the amount of air equal to the dose of the rapid-acting insulin into the R vial.

3. Withdraw the correct amount of rapid-acting insulin.

4. Withdraw the correct amount of intermediate-acting insulin by pulling the plunger down to the unit mark that equals the dose of rapid-acting insulin plus the dose of intermediate-acting insulin. The insulins mix immediately in the syringe. If too much intermediate-acting insulin is withdrawn, the entire contents of the syringe must be discarded.

Figure 40-4 *How to Mix Insulin*

provides the most predictable absorption of insulin, be used exclusively for insulin administration.

If sites other than the abdomen are used, site rotation needs to be done systematically to prevent erratic absorption. One system of rotation is to always use the same area of injection the same time each day (e.g., always using the abdomen in the morning and the thigh in the afternoon). Another system of rotation is to use all available injection sites in one area before moving to another.

Areas of lipodystrophy should not be used for injection because absorption may be diminished. Exercise will increase the rate of absorption, so diabetics planning to exercise should not inject insulin into the areas to be exercised.

Vials of insulin not being used should be refrigerated to prevent loss of potency. Vials in use may be kept at room temperature to decrease local irritation at the injection site, which can occur when cold insulin is used. When mixing a short-acting and a longer-acting insulin in the same syringe, the regular (clear) should always be drawn up into the syringe first, followed by the longer-acting (cloudy) insulin. Figure 40-4 illustrates mixing and administering insulin.

It is recommended that insulin syringes be used only once and then discarded.

The visually and/or neurologically impaired diabetic client may benefit from assistive devices available to facilitate drawing up the insulin and administering it.

Clients dependent on others for drawing up their insulin may benefit from prefilled syringes, which are considered stable for up to 3 weeks when stored in the refrigerator.

The nurse should keep in mind that the most important factor in the administration of insulin is consistency in technique. Also, simplification of the procedure may have a major impact on a client's ability to comply and to maintain independence. It is important that the nurse understand the basic principles of insulin administration and thereby remain flexible when teaching new clients or assessing the skills of experienced clients.

Insulin Pumps A portable insulin infusion pump delivers insulin continuously through a subcutaneous needle, usually anchored in the abdomen (Figure 40-5). A continuous, or basal rate, of regular (rapid-acting) insulin is programmed and delivered to closely imitate the body's natural insulin secretion. Additional boluses can be manually administered to coordinate with meal times. The injection site is changed every 24 to 48 hours. The use of the insulin pump prevents multiple injections and allows flexibility in meal size and time. Use of the pump requires a motivated and educated client because intensive self-monitoring of blood glucose is essential.

Complications of Insulin Therapy Complications of insulin therapy include hypoglycemia (discussed later in this chapter), insulin resistance (requiring more than 200 units/day), lipodystrophy, Somogyi phenomenon, and the dawn phenomenon. Lipodystrophy can be minimized by

Figure 40-5 *The Insulin Pump*

using human insulin, using room temperature insulin, and by rotating sites of insulin injection.

The **Somogyi phenomenon** occurs when a rapid decrease in blood glucose (hypoglycemia) causes the release of glucose-elevating hormones (epinephrine, cortisol, glucagon). The hypoglycemia usually occurs during the night but manifests as an elevated glucose in the morning and may be inadvertently treated with an increase in insulin dosage. The Somogyi phenomenon can be diagnosed by checking the blood glucose during the night at about 3 A.M. Adjusting the insulin regimen to avoid the peaking of insulin during the night will correct this effect.

The **dawn phenomenon** is an early morning glucose elevation produced by the release of growth hormone. Administering the evening insulin dose at a later time will coordinate the insulin peak with the hormone release.

Oral Hypoglycemic Agents Oral hypoglycemic agents are used to treat persons with type 2 diabetes who are not controlled with exercise and diet. These agents are meant to supplement diet and exercise, not replace them. Oral hypoglycemics are not insulin and work by other mechanisms.

Sulfonylurea is the original class of oral hypoglycemic medications used for diabetes therapy. The sulfonylureas

---

PROFESSIONAL TIP

Insulin Injection Practices

Fleming (1999) suggests:

- Rolling the insulin vial does not adequately mix lente or NPH insulins; the vial should be shaken carefully.
- Skin preparation with alcohol is unnecessary.
- The angle of injection may vary from 45 to 90 degrees, depending on the client's weight.
- Aspiration before injection, for needle placement, has never been proven in clinical studies.
- Unrefrigerated insulin is effective for 1 month.

---

work primarily by increasing the ability of the islet cells of the pancreas to excrete insulin. To a lesser degree, they increase the cells' sensitivity to insulin and decrease glucose production by the liver.

Metformin (Glucophage), a biguanide, does not increase insulin release but works by making existing insulin more effective at the cellular level. Metformin may be given alone or in combination with other oral hypoglycemics. In some clients, Glucophage works more effectively if given with some dose of Diabeta. Because it does not stimulate increased insulin release, metformin is not associated with episodes of hypoglycemia. The major side effects of metformin are gastrointestinal and include anorexia, nausea, abdominal discomfort, and diarrhea.

Oral hypoglycemics require some production of insulin by the pancreas and, therefore, are not useful in the treatment of type 1 diabetes. See Table 40-5 for a description of oral hypoglycemic agents used today.

Diet

Medical nutrition therapy provides an individualized dietary prescription to meet client and family needs. Consideration is given to usual eating habits and other lifestyle factors, such as dietary likes and dislikes, cultural influences, who prepares the meals, and family finances. It is important that meals remain a social experience, and the person with diabetes not feel isolated or different.

The goals of medical nutrition therapy are (1) maintain as near-normal blood glucose level as possible, (2) achieve optimal serum lipid levels, (3) provide adequate calories to maintain or attain a reasonable weight, (4) prevent complications of diabetes, and (5) improve overall health. Because of the complexity of individualizing medical nutrition therapy, it is recommended that clients be referred early to a registered dietician (RD) for nutritional assessment and education.

Diabetes is a strong risk factor for atherosclerosis and cardiovascular disease. Therefore, reducing serum lipid levels is a goal of medical nutrition therapy. To reduce the risk of cardiovascular disease, the ADA recommendations incorporate a reduction in saturated fat and cholesterol consumption.

It is recommended that individuals taking insulin or oral hypoglycemic agents eat at consistent times synchronized with the actions of the medications used. Distribution of calories over 24 hours, with regular meals and snacks, helps prevent extreme highs and lows in blood glucose.

Consistent-Carbohydrate Meal Plan Current ADA nutrition guidelines suggest using a "consistent-carbohydrate meal plan." The client eats an individually prescribed amount of carbohydrates at each meal or snack. Carbohydrates determine premeal insulin requirements more than the amount of protein or fat in the meal, and they have the greatest effect on the postprandial blood glucose level. Protein and fat intake must be watched to avoid weight gain and increased serum lipid levels.

Protein intake of both animal and vegetable sources should make up 10% to 20% of the daily calorie intake. If nephropathy is present, protein should be 10% of the daily calorie intake.

TABLE 40-5 ORAL HYPOGLYCEMICS			
GENERIC (BRAND)	USUAL DOSE	ONSET TIME (HOURS)	DURATION (HOURS)
First-Generation Sulfonylureas			
Tolbutamide (Orinase), tolazamide, (Tolinase), and chlorpropamide (Diabinese) are seldom used because of their long action, higher incidence of adverse effects, and risk of drug interactions (Cincinnati & Veliko, 2001).			
Second-Generation Sulfonylureas			
glipizide (Glucatrol)	2.5–40 mg single or divided dose	1–1½	10–16
glimepride (Amaryl)	1–4 mg single dose	1	24
glyburide (Diabeta, Micronase)	1.25–20 mg single or divided dose	2–4	24
Biguanides			
metformin HCl (Glucophage)	500–2,500 mg two or three divided doses	24–48	6–12
Alpha-Glucosidase Inhibitors			
acarbose (Precose)	25–100 mg with meals (tid)	1	No data
miglitol (Glyset)	25–100 mg with meals (tid)	2–3	4–6
Thiazolidenediones			
rosiglitazone maleate (Avandia)	4 mg daily	1	
Combinations			
glyburide and metformin HCl (Glucovance)	1.25 mg/250 mg 2.5 mg/500 mg once or twice a day		
rosiglitazone maleate and metformin HCl (Avandamet)	1 mg/500 mg 2 mg/500 mg 4 mg/500 mg		

Total fat intake depends on the goals set by the client and health care provider for desired levels of glucose, lipid, and weight. If lipid level is normal, 30% or less of calories should come from fat with less than 10% from saturated fat. If weight loss is a primary issue, reduction in fat intake is an efficient way to reduce calorie intake. When lipid level is a problem, a decrease of saturated fat intake to less than 7% of the total calories, total fat to less than 30% of total calories, and cholesterol to less than 200 mg per day is recommended.

The remainder of the calorie intake comes from carbohydrates. The amount consumed is more important than the source of the carbohydrate.

Persons with diabetes should follow the same precautions regarding the use of alcohol as applied to the general public. Alcohol may increase the risk for hypoglycemia in people treated with insulin or sulfonylureas, such as acetohexamide (Dymelor), chlorpropamide (Diabinese), or tolazamide (Tolinase).

Activity

The beneficial effects of regular exercise for the diabetic are multiple. Exercise decreases the blood glucose by increasing the uptake of glucose by muscles and improving insulin usage. Exercise also increases circulation, improves cardiovascular status, decreases stress, and assists with weight loss.

Before starting an exercise program, the person with diabetes should have a complete physical and review the exercise plan with the physician or primary health care provider. Regular daily exercise rather than sporadic exercise should be encouraged.

Persons with diabetes need to correlate exercise with their blood glucose, taking care to avoid periods of hypoglycemia or exercising when blood glucose is too high. Exercise potentiates the action of insulin, resulting in lower insulin requirements and an increased risk of hypoglycemia during and after exercise. On the other hand, in the person with diabetes who is insulin-deficient, exercise may cause a further rise in blood glucose and rapid development of ketosis. Diabetics should not exercise at the peak of insulin activity, when their blood glucose is greater than 250 mg/dL, or if they have ketones in their urine.

Health Promotion

The diabetic educator plays a pivotal role in assisting the diabetic client/family to understand diabetes and the necessary lifestyle changes. Some teaching is unique to an individual client and is done one-to-one, whereas some teaching applies to all clients with diabetes and is often done in a class setting. This also allows clients with diabetes to meet each other and share concerns, information, and ideas that have worked for them.

The diabetic educator nurse is part of a team, including the client/family, physician, dietician, and pharmacist, who all work together to help the client understand and comply with the treatment plan.

Sick-Day Management It is important that persons with diabetes have a plan for managing their diabetes in the event of illness. It is important that they continue

Guidelines for Exercising

- Try to exercise at the same time and in the same amount each day.
- Test blood glucose level before, during, and after exercise.
- Do not inject insulin into a limb that you will be exercising.
- Do not exercise at the peak of insulin activity.
- Do not exercise before meals unless trying to lower blood glucose level.
- Do not exercise with a blood glucose level over 250 mg/dL or with ketones in the urine. This indicates severe insulin deficiency and may predispose to hyperglycemia.
- Eat a snack (15 gm carbohydrates) before or during exercise if appropriate, based on blood glucose level.
- Always carry a source of carbohydrates and emergency cash, if away from home, in case hypoglycemia occurs while exercising.
- Always carry personal and medical alert identification.
- Watch for postexercise hypoglycemia. Individuals who have more than usual exercise during the day should increase their carbohydrate intake and test their glucose during the night to detect nocturnal hypoglycemia. (Hypoglycemia can occur 8 to 15 hours following exercise.)

taking their insulin or oral hypoglycemic medication when they are experiencing illness because illness and fever can increase blood glucose and the need for insulin. Some persons with diabetes who do not normally take short-acting insulin may require it during times of fever or illness. Blood glucose should be monitored 4 to 6 times per day and urine should be checked for ketones. Blood glucose greater than 300 mg/dL or ketones in the urine should be reported to the physician.

If the client cannot ingest the planned meal, carbohydrates in the form of soft foods and liquids can be substituted. Extreme nausea and vomiting or diarrhea should be reported to the physician because extreme fluid loss

Fingersticks

- Use shallow skin penetration, just to get enough blood for the meter.
- Rotate sites; use sides of fingertips and thumb.
- Use alcohol sparingly or wash hands with warm soapy water before fingerstick *instead* of using alcohol. The warm water brings more blood into the fingers.
- Apply firm pressure *directly* over the puncture for 10 to 15 seconds; if area is still bleeding, apply pressure until it stops.

can be dangerous. Clients with type 1 diabetes who are unable to retain fluids may need to be hospitalized to avoid ketoacidosis.

Acute Complications of Diabetes

There are three major acute complications of diabetes related to blood glucose imbalance: hypoglycemia, diabetic ketoacidosis (DKA), and hyperosmolar hyperglycemic nonketotic syndrome (HHNS) (Table 40-6).

Hypoglycemia (Insulin Reaction)

Hypoglycemia (low blood glucose) occurs when a client's glucose level drops below 70 mg/dL, with the most severe reactions occurring when it drops below 50 mg/dL. Hypoglycemia can occur any time of the day, but most often will occur before meals or when insulin action is peaking. Factors that can contribute to the development of a hypoglycemic reaction are skipping meals or eating late, unplanned exercise, and administration of excess insulin.

Hypoglycemic symptoms can occur suddenly and unexpectedly and vary from client to client. The cardinal rule is: *Always believe clients who tell you they are having an insulin reaction.* Most persons with diabetes have had hypoglycemic reactions before, so they know the symptoms that precede an insulin reaction. According to Tkacs (2002), some clients with diabetes may have "hypoglycemia unawareness," which refers to the client's inability to recognize the warning symptoms of hypoglycemia. It is usually a complication of type 1 diabetes but can occur in type 2.

When a hypoglycemic reaction is suspected, the nurse must respond immediately according to the institution's protocol. Treatment involves assessing the client, checking blood glucose level, and administering glucose in the most appropriate form. Sammer (2001) suggests using glucose tablets or gel for hypoglycemia. The client taking acarbose (Precose), which slows digestion and absorption of most carbohydrates—including hard candies and many fruit juices—but not glucose, will not have the rapid response to fruit juice or sugar that other clients will have. Hypoglycemic reactions can be fatal, so *leaving the client untreated is more dangerous than causing mild hyperglycemia with overtreatment.* Figure 40-6 provides a sample hypoglycemic protocol.

Persons with diabetes and their families must know the symptoms and treatment for hypoglycemia. Hypoglycemic episodes can be prevented by following a regular pattern of eating, exercise, and insulin administration. Between meals and bedtime snacks can be used to cover times of peak insulin action. Additional food should be eaten when engaging in greater than usual exercise. Blood glucose level should be checked at the first suspicion of hypoglycemia. All clients should wear an identification bracelet or tag indicating that they have diabetes because hypoglycemic reactions can occur unexpectedly.

Diabetic Ketoacidosis

Diabetic ketoacidosis (DKA) is one of the most serious complications of hyperglycemia. Glucose is a hyperos-

TABLE 40-6   SYMPTOMS OF ACUTE COMPLICATIONS OF DIABETES

Symptoms of Hypoglycemia (Insulin Reaction)

Mild hypoglycemia

- Diaphoresis; cold, clammy skin
- Pallor
- Excess hunger

- Palpitations
- Tremors
- Anxious but alert

Moderate hypoglycemia

- Confusion, vertigo
- Slurred speech
- Paresthesia

- Behavior changes
- Irritability

Severe hypoglycemia

- Seizures
- Loss of consciousness
- Shallow respirations
- Nursing Alert: Severe hypoglycemia is a medical emergency. Administer some form of glucose immediately.

Symptoms of Diabetic Ketoacidosis (DKA)

- Same as HHNS plus symptoms of acidosis:
- "Fruity" odor to breath
- Kussmaul's respirations (deep, nonlabored)

Symptoms of Hyperosmolar Hyperglycemic Nonketotic Syndrome (HHNS)

- Polyuria
- Polydipsia
- Skin hot, dry, decreased turgor
- Dehydration—hypotension, increased pulse
- Blurred vision
- Weakness
- Mental status changes, confusion to coma

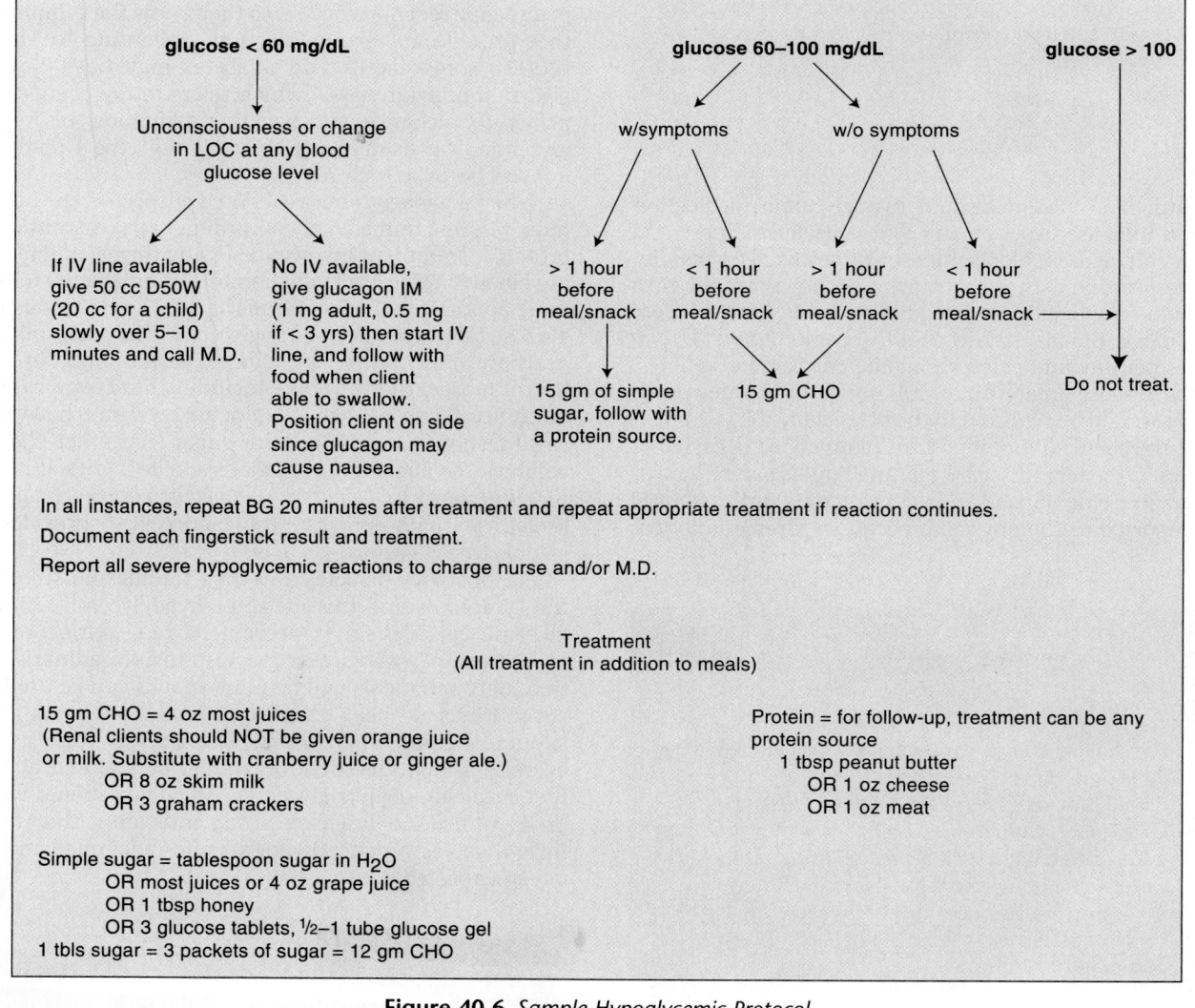

Figure 40-6 *Sample Hypoglycemic Protocol*

molar substance drawing fluid out of the cell and into the circulation, where it is excreted by the kidneys. This oncotic diuresis results in polyuria (increased urine output), dehydration, and electrolyte imbalances. Increased fat metabolism results in accumulation of ketones, resulting in metabolic acidosis. Surgery, stress, or illness may trigger DKA, which usually develops in clients with immune-mediated type 1 diabetes, although it can occur in clients with type 2 diabetes. The client with undiagnosed immune-mediated type 1 diabetes may also present with DKA.

The onset of DKA may be gradual or sudden. Classic symptoms of hyperglycemia (polyuria, polyphagia, polydipsia) usually precede DKA. Other symptoms include nausea and vomiting, abdominal pain from acidosis, headache, weakness, fatigue, and blurred vision. Assessment may reveal hot, flushed skin and signs of hypovolemia or shock. Acidosis will produce signs of hyperpnea (Kussmaul's breathing), fruity odor to breath from respiratory elimination of acetone, and decreased level of consciousness ranging from lethargy to coma.

Laboratory values will reveal blood glucose from 300 to 800 mg/dL and metabolic acidosis. Urine will be positive for glucose and ketones.

Hyperosmolar Hyperglycemic Nonketotic Syndrome

Hyperosmolar hyperglycemic nonketotic syndrome (HHNS) occurs when there is insufficient insulin to prevent hyperglycemia but enough insulin to prevent ketoacidosis. HHNS occurs in persons with type 2 diabetes. Because symptoms of acidosis do not occur, no symptoms may be noticed until the glucose level is dangerously high.

HHNS occurs most often in the elderly client with undiagnosed type 2 diabetes. HHNS can also occur in the poorly controlled client and is usually precipitated by illness or another stressor.

Clinical manifestations of HHNS reflect dehydration and shock. Hyperosmolality eventually results in lethargy, seizures, and coma (Table 40-6). Blood glucose level ranges from 600 to 2,000 mg/dL and serum osmolality greater than 350 mOsm/L.

Medical management of DKA and HHNS involves fluid and electrolyte replacement (particularly potassium), insulin, and treatment of any precipitating factors. DKA and HHNS are associated with significant mortality rates, and the client is usually acutely ill. Treatment will occur in the intensive care setting until the client is stabilized.

Chronic Complications of Diabetes

Long-term complications of diabetes occur 5 to 10 years after diagnosis in both type 1 and type 2 diabetes. The exact pathophysiology is not completely understood but is known to be related to the effects of elevated blood glucose level. Recent studies have shown that intensive insulin therapy and tight glycemic control can reduce or delay the occurrence of many long-term complications associated with diabetes.

Figure 40-7 *Gangrene of the toes and foot as a result of an infection often means eventual amputation.*

Infections

Diabetics, particularly clients who are poorly controlled, appear to be more prone to developing certain infections. Infections of particular concern to diabetics include diabetic foot infections, boils, cellulitis, necrotizing fasciitis, urinary tract infections, and yeast infections. Small cuts on the feet can become gangrenous (Figure 40-7) and require amputation.

Infections increase the need for insulin and can result in ketoacidosis. Infections, once they occur, can often be difficult to treat and heal slowly because of impaired circulation.

CLIENT TEACHING

Guidelines to Healthy Feet

- Wash feet daily and dry them carefully, especially between the toes.
- Inspect feet and between toes for blisters, cuts, and infections. Use a mirror to see the bottoms of the feet. If your vision is impaired, have a family member examine your feet. Remember, because of decreased feeling in your feet, you may have an infection and not know it.
- Avoid activities that restrict blood flow to the feet, especially smoking and sitting with legs crossed.
- Wear shoes that are comfortable, well-fitting, and closed toed. Wear new shoes for short intervals until broken in. Do not walk barefoot.
- Prevent cuts and irritations. Always wear stockings. Look inside shoes for rough edges, nail points, foreign objects.
- Avoid temperature extremes. Test bath water with hands before getting in. Do not use water bottles or heating pads on feet.
- See your physician regularly and make sure that your feet are examined each visit.
- When toenails are trimmed, cut them straight across. When corns or calluses are present, see a physician or podiatrist. *Do not* cut them yourself.

Diabetic Neuropathy

Neuropathy is the most common chronic complication associated with diabetes. The incidence of neuropathy increases with age and duration of disease and is related to elevated blood glucose level. Neuropathy can affect all types of nerves, but the two most common types of diabetic neuropathy are peripheral neuropathy and autonomic neuropathy.

Peripheral neuropathy causes paresthesias and burning sensations, primarily in the lower extremities. Decreased sensations of pain and temperature coupled with decreased peripheral circulation place the client at risk for undetected foot injury.

Autonomic neuropathy can affect almost any organ system, including gastrointestinal (delayed gastric emptying, constipation, diarrhea), urinary (retention, neurogenic bladder), and reproductive (male impotence).

Nephropathy (Chronic Renal Failure)

Diabetic nephropathy develops slowly over many years, progressing eventually to kidney failure. Controlling hypertension and blood glucose level is the key to delaying renal damage. Good hydration before and diuresis following any dye study is valuable in preventing renal damage. Clients with urinary retention should urinate every 3 hours (Plummer, 2001).

Retinopathy

Changes in the small vessels of the retina result in diabetic retinopathy, which is a major cause of blindness among persons with diabetes. Because of the insidious onset of type 2 diabetes, retinopathy is often present at diagnosis. The severity and progression of retinopathy appear to be closely related to glucose and blood pressure control. Persons with diabetes also develop cataracts at an earlier age. Although most clients develop some degree of retinopathy, most do not develop visual impairment. To facilitate early detection,

diabetics should have ophthalmologic evaluations every 6 to 12 months.

Vascular Changes

Diabetes is an independent risk factor for atherosclerotic vessel disease. Atherosclerotic changes that occur in persons with diabetes are similar to those that occur in nondiabetics, but they occur at earlier ages and progress at a more rapid rate.

Cardiovascular Hypertension is twice as common in persons with diabetes and is an important factor in the progression of retinopathy, nephropathy, and vascular (large vessel) disease. The incidence of coronary artery disease, angina, and myocardial infarction is higher when compared to the nondiabetic population. Cerebral vascular disease and cerebral vascular accident are also more common in persons with diabetes.

Therapies aimed at lowering risk factors and effects of atherosclerosis include weight control, low-fat diet, treatment of hypertension and hyperlipidemia, regular exercise, and control of blood glucose level.

Peripheral Vascular Disease Peripheral vascular disease (PVD) occurs most commonly in diabetics with hypertension or hyperlipidemia and in diabetics who smoke. Diabetics have two to three times the incidence of occlusive peripheral arterial disease when compared to the nondiabetic population. Diabetes is present in more than half of persons experiencing nontraumatic lower extremity amputations.

Nursing Management

Monitor vital signs and serum electrolytes. Record I&O, administer fluids as ordered, and encourage oral fluid intake. Teach client about diabetes, use of insulin or oral hypoglycemics, relationship of exercise to diabetes management, and how to perform SMBG. Provide a list of symptoms and treatment for hypoglycemia.

NURSING PROCESS

Assessment

Subjective Data

This includes assessment of the health history, family history, diet, activity regimen, and the understanding of the disease and medical therapies. The client may describe fatigue, weakness, weight changes, mental status changes, polyuria, polyphagia, polydipsia, numbness or tingling of the extremities, blurred vision, and increased appetite.

Objective Data

Objective data should focus on the symptoms of diabetes, the common acute and chronic complications, and the results of diagnostic tests. There may be dependent redness or cyanosis of the lower extremities as well as the absence of hair. A fasting glucose level greater than 126 mg/dL or a nonfasting (random) level greater than 200 mg/dL on two separate occasions is diagnostic of diabetes.

Nursing diagnoses, based on the assessment findings, may be varied and extensive due to the multiple problems and complications caused by diabetes mellitus. Nursing diagnoses may include the following:

Nursing Diagnoses	Planning/Goals	Nursing Interventions
Deficient **K**nowledge diabetes, medical regimen, diet, exercise, self-care management skills (insulin injection, SMBG) related to new diagnosis or changes in treatment	The client will relate basic understanding of pathophysiology of diabetes, and relationship between insulin and hyper-/hypoglycemia.	Teach client about diabetes and the use of insulin to prevent hyper-/hypoglycemia or assist client to enroll in a formal diabetic education program.
	The client will verbalize how/when to take oral hypoglycemics and the side effects to report or will correctly demonstrate how to administer insulin and rotate sites.	Teach client about oral hypoglycemics or insulin, whichever the client will be using.
	The client will relate importance of an exercise program.	Discuss how exercise is related to diabetes management.
	The client will describe the relationship between dietary management and glycemic control; choose foods that comply with diet prescription.	Discuss how dietary management is related to the control of blood glucose and provide an exchange list of foods.
	The client will correctly demonstrate how to use SMBG to determine blood glucose level.	Teach client how to perform SMBG and have client return demonstration.
	The client will verbalize symptoms and treatment of hypoglycemia.	Provide client with a list of symptoms and treatment for hypoglycemia.
Risk for Deficient **F**luid Volume related to hyperglycemia, polyuria, and dehydration	The client will exhibit normal skin turgor, moist mucous membranes, and maintain oral fluid intake of 2,500–3,000 mL/day.	Measure client's intake and output, administer intravenous fluids as ordered, and encourage oral fluids.
	The client will have vital signs within normal limits.	Monitor vital signs and serum electrolytes.
Imbalanced **N**utrition: Less than body requirements related to imbalance between insulin, diet, and activity	The client will have weight within normal range for height and age.	Refer client to dietician to adjust dietary intake in order to maintain weight in normal range.

Evaluation Each goal must be evaluated to determine how it has been met by the client.

PITUITARY DISORDERS

Hyperpituitarism and hypopituitarism are discussed following.

HYPERPITUITARISM

Hyperpituitarism is most commonly diagnosed between the second and fourth decade of life but can appear in infancy and childhood. Although other pituitary hormones may be affected, the most common are the growth hormone and antidiuretic hormone.

Excess secretion of growth hormone (GH) produces different changes depending on the client's age when it occurs. When the excess secretion occurs in childhood before the epiphyses close, gigantism is the result; in adults, acromegaly is the result.

Syndrome of inappropriate antidiuretic hormone and pituitary tumors are also discussed.

GIGANTISM

Gigantism affects infants and children, causing proportional overgrowth of all body tissues. By the time these children reach adulthood, they may be more than 8 feet tall.

Hyperplasia of the anterior pituitary is usually the cause of GH oversecretion. This tissue may develop into a tumor causing other symptoms. Clients with gigantism do not have the strength their size implies.

Medical–Surgical Management

Medical

Irradiation of the anterior pituitary may be the treatment chosen. The child must then be observed for heart failure, hypertension, thickened bones, osteoporosis, and delayed sexual development.

Surgical

If the cause is a tumor, surgery may be performed to remove the tumor (explained under "Acromegaly").

Pharmacological

When the pituitary is either destroyed by irradiation or removed by surgery, pituitary hormone replacement is necessary.

Nursing Management

Monitor children's growth for early identification of a problem. Be understanding and emphasize the positive aspects of being tall.

NURSING PROCESS

Assessment

Subjective Data

Listening to the child's description of the disease process may provide insight into the child's emotional responses.

Objective Data

Frequent measurements of growth indicate a more rapid rate of growth than expected.

ACROMEGALY

Because acromegaly occurs after epiphyseal closure of bones, there is bone thickening with transverse growth and tissue enlargement. This occurs between 30 and 50 years of age. Photographs over years will reveal a progressive enlargement of the face and hands.

Acromegaly involves a gradual onset of clinical manifestations, including visual defects from pressure of the pituitary tumor on the optic nerve, soft tissue swelling, or hypertrophy of the face and extremities. The cartilaginous and connective tissue overgrowths result in a characteristic hulking appearance with thickened ears and nose, and marked projection of the jaw. The jaw can appear enlarged and the tongue may also thicken. The paranasal sinuses can become enlarged. Also laryngeal hypertrophy can occur. The client has thick fingers with tips that appear "tufted" (shaped like arrowheads on x-rays). The client ex-

hibits a characteristic moist, weak, doughy handshake. The heart, liver, and spleen may enlarge. Some other characteristics are diaphoresis (profuse perspiration), oily or leathery skin, fatigue, heat intolerance, weight gain, headache, joint pain, hirsutism (excessive hairiness especially in females), and sleep disturbance. The client may experience decreased libido or impotence, oligomenorrhea (scanty or infrequent menstruation), and infertility.

The client's history and clinical manifestations along with cranial x-rays and a CT scan make a diagnosis of acromegaly. Serum growth hormone level is elevated.

Prognosis depends on the causative factor, hyperplasia or a tumor; however, there is generally a reduced life span. Diabetes mellitus, hypertension, and a higher risk of cardiovascular disease are the most serious health consequences (NIDDK, 2002).

Medical–Surgical Management

Medical

Medical treatment consists of either medication that affects the growth hormone or irradiation of the pituitary gland. Proton beam therapy uses a very low dose of radiation and is much less destructive to nearby tissue than conventional radiation therapy.

Surgical

Surgical treatment for hyperpituitarism is to remove the pituitary gland. Two surgical approaches to remove the pituitary are transfrontal or transsphenoid hypophysectomy. The transfrontal approach is rarely used because it has a high risk of mortality as well as permanent loss of smell and taste and causes severe diabetes insipidus. The transsphenoid approach (Figure 40-8) involves an incision in the superior maxillary gingiva. Surgery may be the treatment of choice or used after attempting medical treatment.

Postoperatively, nasal packing should be checked for clear, colorless drainage. If it occurs, the drainage must be documented and reported to the physician. If this

Figure 40-8 *Transsphenoidal Approach to Hypophysectomy*

drainage is suspected of being cerebrospinal fluid, it should be checked for glucose, which is found in cerebrospinal fluid. The nurse should observe for infection, which includes elevated leukocytes, sudden temperature elevation, or complaint of headache or nuchal rigidity. Analgesics are administered as needed. The client should avoid activities such as coughing, straining, vomiting, or sneezing. The client should be encouraged to use an incentive spirometer instead of coughing. The client should not brush teeth for 2 weeks to avoid problems with the incision. Mouthwash can be used. The client should be instructed to avoid lifting and bending at the waist for 2 to 3 months after surgery.

Pharmacological

Two drugs may be prescribed for acromegaly. Bromocriptine mesylate (Parlodel) is a nonhormonal drug that activates dopamine receptors to inhibit the release of the growth hormone and prolactin. Bromocriptine mesylate (Parlodel) should be given with food to decrease gastric upset. Because this drug can cause drowsiness or dizziness, the client should be instructed to avoid activities that require mental alertness. If the client is on oral contraceptives, alternate contraceptive measures should also be used because bromocriptine can stimulate ovulation.

The other drug, octreotide acetate (Sandostatin), inhibits the growth hormone. Although octreotide is given by injection, it can still cause gastric distress. The injections should be given between meals and at bedtime. Clients with diabetes mellitus should closely monitor their blood sugar level.

Nursing Management

Be supportive. Show respect and acceptance. Assess ability to perform ADLs. Provide soft diet and encourage client to thoroughly chew food and drink fluids often.

NURSING PROCESS

Assessment

Subjective Data

Obtain a thorough nursing history, asking about vision impairment, headache, muscular weakness, and psychological disturbances.

Objective Data

Objective data includes gait changes, vital sign changes (tachycardia or hypotension, which may indicate congestive heart failure), and dyspnea. The jaw is enlarged and projected, so the client may have difficulty in chewing.

Nursing diagnoses for a client with gigantism or acromegaly may include the following:

Nursing Diagnoses	Planning/Goals	Nursing Interventions
Risk for Disproportionate Growth related to increased level of growth hormone	The client will comply with treatment to minimize hyperpituitarism and stop excessive growth with treatment.	Assist client with activities of daily living and range-of-motion exercises. Administer medications as ordered. Remind client to carry medications on person.
Chronic Low Self-Esteem related to irreversible physical changes	The client will acknowledge physical changes, express positive feelings about self, and exhibit ability to cope with altered body.	Encourage client to verbalize feelings. Assist client in setting achievable short-term goals. Offer emotional support and help client to develop coping strategies. Show respect and acceptance of the client as a person. Provide a positive but realistic assessment of the situation. Refer to professional counseling as needed.

Evaluation Each goal must be evaluated to determine how it has been met by the client.

SYNDROME OF INAPPROPRIATE ANTIDIURETIC HORMONE

Syndrome of inappropriate antidiuretic hormone (SIADH) results from an excess of ADH. This causes the kidneys to reabsorb excess water, which decreases urine output and increases fluid volume. The most common cause is "oat cell" lung cancer (NIH, 2002b). Other causes are lymphoid pancreatic, duodenal, thymus, and prostate cancer; central nervous system trauma, infection; chronic obstructive pulmonary disease; acute respiratory failure; mechanical ventilation; and medications such as antineoplastic agents, tricyclic antidepressants, and anesthetics.

The client will have hyponatremia (<130 mEq/L), water retention, weight gain, concentrated urine (urine osmolality >1,200 mOsm/L; specific gravity >1.020), muscle cramps, and weakness. The low osmolality of the blood allows fluid to leak out of vessels and causes brain swelling. If untreated, lethargy, seizures, coma, and death will result.

Medical–Surgical Management

Medical

The underlying disorder must be treated or medications stopped that may be contributing to SIADH. Water restriction will be implemented to prevent further hemodilution. Serious hyponatremia (<120 mEq/L) will usually be treated with intravenous administration of 5% NaCl. The serum sodium level should be increased by 12 mEq/L or less per day.

▣ Pharmacological

Furosemide (Lasix) is given to increase urine output, while demeclocycline hydrochloride (Declomycin) and fludrocortisone (Florinef) are given to enhance sodium retention.

Diet

Fluid restriction will be determined by the serum sodium level.

Nursing Management

Assess client's hydration and neurologic status every 3 to 4 hours. Accurately record I&O. Auscultate lungs every 2 to 4 hours. Explain why fluid intake is restricted. Weigh client daily. Provide frequent mouth care and apply lubricant to lips.

NURSING PROCESS

Assessment

Subjective Data

The client may describe muscle cramps, weakness, anorexia, nausea, and headache.

Objective Data

The client will have weight gain and fluid intake greater than output, may be irritable and disoriented, become progressively lethargic, and have seizures and diminished or absent deep tendon reflexes. Serum sodium and osmolality will be decreased. Urine osmolality and specific gravity will be increased.

Nursing diagnoses for a client with SIADH may include the following:

Nursing Diagnoses	Planning/Goals	Nursing Interventions
Excess **F**luid Volume related to decreased urine output	The client will have increased urine output.	Assess client's weight daily on same scale at same time and vital signs.
		Accurately record I&O. Maintain fluid restrictions.
		Monitor laboratory reports.
		Administer medications as ordered.
Impaired **O**ral Mucous Membrane related to restriction of fluid intake	The client will have moist, intact oral mucous membranes.	Provide frequent oral care, avoiding alcohol-based mouth washes and lemon-glycerine swabs. Allow client to rinse mouth with water, but not swallow any.
		Provide lubricant for client's lips.
		Allow client to choose fluids and times to drink them.

Evaluation Each goal must be evaluated to determine how it has been met by the client.

PITUITARY TUMORS

Pituitary tumors more often affect the anterior pituitary rather than the posterior portion. Adenomas of the pituitary, which are rarely malignant, replace glandular tissue and enlarge the sella turcica. The cause is unknown, but there may be a predisposition toward tumor formation from an inherited **autosomal** dominant trait, meaning it is a dominant characteristic carried on any chromosome other than the one determining sex.

Clinical manifestations frequently start with a headache unrelated to stress or other factors. The next obvious manifestation is visual problems caused by the tumor putting pressure on the optic nerve. Others include personality changes, dementia, amenorrhea, impotence, lethargy, and weakness. The client may complain of cold intolerance, increased fatigue, constipation, and may have seizures. Although the tumor is not malignant, damage is done by tumor invasion of normal tissue.

Treatment is removal of the tumor. Complications of pituitary tumors are endocrine abnormalities if there is no replacement therapy after removal of the tumor. If the hypothalamus is compressed, diabetes insipidus can result. If the tumor has eroded the base of the skull, the client may have rhinorrhea (thin watery nasal discharge). Prognosis depends on the extent of invasion. In most cases, the tumor causes excessive secretion of the anterior pituitary hormones.

Medical–Surgical Management

Medical

Medical treatment of a pituitary tumor would be radiation therapy. This can be used for small tumors or if the client is a poor surgical risk. Radiation can also be used after surgery to shrink tissue remaining after surgical excision. Another alternative to surgery is cryohypophysectomy. This involves freezing the area with a probe inserted via the transsphenoidal approach.

Surgical

Large tumors, especially those impinging on the optic nerve, are generally removed by using the transfrontal approach. Smaller tumors can be resected via the transsphenoidal approach.

Pharmacological

After surgery, the client will need hormone replacement therapy.

Nursing Management

Provide a safe, clutter-free environment. Keep a call light within the client's reach. Provide periods of rest after activity. Adjust room temperature for client's comfort or provide extra blankets. The client will be in ICU for several days if surgery is performed.

NURSING PROCESS

Assessment

Subjective Data

Obtain a thorough client history and assess for manifestations of a tumor, such as visual problems, headache, impotence, lethargy, cold intolerance, fatigue, or constipation. The family may provide insight into any personality changes.

Objective Data

Assess the client for tilting of the head to compensate for visual disturbances, axillary and pubic hair loss, a waxy appearance to the skin, and few wrinkles.

Nursing diagnoses for a client with a pituitary tumor may include the following:

Nursing Diagnoses	Planning/Goals	Nursing Interventions
Fatigue related to decreased ACTH and TSH levels	The client will verbalize an understanding of the relationship between fatigue, the disease, and activity level, and express feeling of increasing energy as treatment progresses.	Explain relationship between pituitary tumor, fatigue, and activity level. Suggest alternating periods of activity with periods of rest. Administer medications as ordered. Encourage completion of all treatments.
Disturbed *Sensory Perception (Visual)* related to altered sensory reception, transmission, and/or integration due to pressure on optic nerve by the pituitary tumor	The client will use adaptive devices and appropriate resources to compensate for visual changes, and regain normal vision with treatment.	Provide information about adaptive devices and resources for visual changes. Provide a safe clutter-free environment. Make certain that the bed is in the low position and the call signal in reach of the client. Use side rails as needed.

Evaluation Each goal must be evaluated to determine how it has been met by the client.

HYPOPITUITARISM

Hypopituitarism is a complex syndrome marked by metabolic dysfunction, sexual immaturity, and growth retardation when it occurs in childhood; Simmonds' disease and diabetes insipidus are examples of hypopituitarism. The most common cause of hypopituitarism is a tumor. Other causes are congenital defects (hypoplasia or aplasia), pituitary infarction (from postpartum hemorrhage), pituitary surgery or irradiation, or chemical agents. Hypopituitarism can be primary (meaning there is no known cause) or secondary. Secondary hypopituitarism can be a result of a deficiency of hypothalamic-releasing hormones. This deficiency can be idiopathic (without a known cause) or a result of infection, trauma, or tumor.

Clinical manifestations develop slowly and generally are not apparent until 75% of the pituitary is destroyed. Specific manifestations will vary with the specific hormone that is deficient.

Deficiency of the growth hormone results in dwarfism, which becomes apparent by 6 months of age as the infant exhibits growth retardation, with chubbiness in the lower trunk and a short stature. As it progresses, secondary tooth eruption is delayed, and later there is a delay in puberty. Growth continues at about half the normal rate until the child reaches about 4 feet in height. Body proportions are normal, as is mental development. Frequently in adulthood, sex organs may not develop normally unless treated with hormones. Clients experience an accelerated pattern of aging, resulting in the life span being shortened by as much as 20 years. If the deficiency occurs in adults, manifestations are not as apparent. There are subtle signs such as wrinkles near the mouth and eyes.

Deficiencies of follicle-stimulating hormone (FSH) and luteinizing hormone (LH) cause differences in clinical manifestations between female and male clients. In the female, symptoms include amenorrhea, dyspareunia, infertility, decreased libido, breast atrophy, sparse or absent axillary and pubic hair, and dry skin. In the male, symptoms include weakness, impotence, decreased libido, decreased muscle strength, testicular softening and shrinkage, and retarded secondary sexual hair growth.

In a child, a deficiency of thyroid-stimulating hormone (TSH) will result in severe growth retardation even with treatment. Other deficiency manifestations include cold intolerance; constipation; increased or decreased menstrual flow; lethargy; dry, pale puffy skin, and bradycardia. Thought processes may also be slowed.

A deficiency of adrenocorticotrophic hormone (ACTH) results in fatigue, nausea, vomiting, anorexia, weight loss, and depigmentation of the skin and nipples. Vital signs taken during periods of stress would show fever and hypotension.

Prolactin deficiency results in absent postpartum lactation, amenorrhea, and sparse or absent axillary and pubic hair. There may also be manifestations of thyroid or adrenal cortex failure.

Findings of hypopituitarism depend on the specific hormone, client's age, and severity of condition when detected. X-rays of the wrist determine bone age, and a skull series will rule out a pituitary tumor. Total failure of the pituitary without treatment is fatal; however, prognosis is good with treatment by the appropriate hormone(s). Treatment is primarily replacement therapy for the deficient hormone(s).

SIMMONDS' DISEASE

Simmonds' disease is defined as a total absence of all pituitary secretions. This is also called *panhypopituitarism.* This disease results from surgery, infection, injury, or tumor. It may also occur after a difficult labor in childbirth because of thrombosis formation during or after delivery.

Clinical manifestations, which vary in intensity, include extreme weight loss, general debility, lethargy, pallor, dry yellowish skin, loss of libido, amenorrhea, and

intolerance to cold. The disease leads to loss of axillary and pubic hair and atrophy of genitalia and breasts. It progresses to bradycardia (slow pulse), hypotension, premature wrinkling of the skin, and atrophy of the thyroid and adrenal glands.

Treatment consists of administration of ACTH, TSH, or thyroid, adrenal, and sex hormones for a lifetime.

DIABETES INSIPIDUS

Diabetes insipidus (DI) is a deficiency of ADH, causing a metabolic disorder characterized by severe polyuria and polydipsia. Diabetes insipidus generally starts in childhood or early adulthood, with a median onset of 21 years. It affects males more often than females. Although a deficiency of ADH is the most common cause (neurogenic), diabetes insipidus can also be caused by failure of the kidneys to respond to ADH (nephrogenic), a defect in or damage to the thirst mechanism (dipsogenic), or during pregnancy (gestational) (NIDDK, 2001).

Neurogenic diabetes insipidus may be caused by injury or ischemia to the hypothalamus or pituitary gland, CNS infections, or sickle cell disease. Nephrogenic diabetes insipidus may be caused by pyelonephritis, chronic renal failure, polycystic disease, or medications such as lithium carbonate (Carbolith), amphotericin B (Fungizone), furosemide (Lasix) or ethycrynic acid (Edecrin). Dipsogenic diabetes insipidus results in an extreme increase in thirst and then fluid intake, which suppresses ADH secretion, increasing urine output. Gestational diabetes insipidus is caused by a placenta enzyme that destroys ADH in the mother (NIDDK, 2001).

Clinical manifestations have an abrupt onset. The client experiences extreme polyuria of 4 to 16 L of dilute urine daily. In some cases, there can be up to 30 L of urine per day. Serum osmolality is >295 mOsm/L and urine osmolality is <150 mOsm/L. Urine specific gravity is <1.005 and serum sodium is >145 mEq/L. The client has extreme thirst, preferring cold beverages. Even though there is an extraordinary volume of fluid intake, weight is lost. Other manifestations include dizziness, weakness, constipation, nocturia, and fatigue that may be a result of inadequate rest because of frequent nighttime voiding and excess thirst.

Complications of untreated diabetes insipidus are **hypovolemia** (abnormally low circulatory blood volume), circulatory collapse, unconsciousness, and central nervous system damage. Prolonged urine flow can cause chronic urinary system conditions such as bladder distension, enlarged calyces, and hydronephrosis.

Prognosis is generally good with fluid replacement in uncomplicated cases. Prognosis also depends on the underlying cause of diabetes insipidus.

Medical–Surgical Management

Pharmacological

In addition to intravenous fluids, several medications can be used to treat diabetes insipidus. For neurogenic and gestational diabetes insipidus, desmopressin acetate (DDAVP), a synthetic antidiuretic hormone that can be given parenterally or nasally, is the drug of choice. Also, vasopressin (Pitressin Synthetic) may be given parenterally or nasally. Make certain that the nasal passage is clear before administering the medication. Monitor intake and output and assess for hypovolemia and electrolyte imbalance. The client should drink fluids or water only when thirsty (NIDDK, 2001).

For nephrogenic diabetes insipidus, a diuretic such as hydrochlorothiazide (Hydrodiuril) may be given alone or with a milorize (Midamor) (NIDDK, 2001).

Nursing Management

Carefully and accurately monitor and record the client's I&O. Assess skin turgor and condition of oral mucous membranes. Weigh client daily. Oral fluids are often restricted. Assess skin on each shift. Apply moisturizing lotion to skin. Provide egg-crate mattress or sheepskin.

NURSING PROCESS

Assessment

Subjective Data

Obtain a thorough client history, including severity of thirst, weakness, fatigue, and lethargy.

Objective Data

Assess for weight loss, constipation, and signs of fluid volume deficit, such as dry skin and mucous membranes, fever, dyspnea, and poor skin turgor. Check urine for color, amount, and specific gravity. Assess weight daily.

Nursing diagnoses for a client with diabetes insipidus may include the following:

Nursing Diagnoses	Planning/Goals	Nursing Interventions
Risk for Imbalanced **Fluid** *Volume* related to polyuria	The client will have sufficient fluid intake to prevent dehydration.	Provide easy access to bedpan/bathroom. Answer call signal promptly. Monitor the client for dizziness and weakness.
		Record client intake and output. Teach client and family how to record intake and output.
		Provide fluids as ordered to cover output.
		Monitor weight daily.
		Provide oral care. Use a soft toothbrush, mild mouthwash, and lubricant for the lips.
		Assess condition of oral mucous membranes.
Risk for Impaired **Skin** *Integrity* related to altered hydration	The client will maintain skin integrity.	Assess skin, especially pressure points, 3 times a day. Apply moisturizing lotion to skin.
		Prevent pressure on skin by turning or ambulating client. Use egg-crate mattress or sheepskin.
		Encourage adequate intake of fluids, protein, vitamin C, and calories.

Evaluation Each goal must be evaluated to determine how it has been met by the client.

THYROID DISORDERS

Worldwide, a deficiency of iodine is the most likely cause of thyroid disorders; however, in countries where iodine in food is plentiful, autoimmune thyroid disease is the most common thyroid disorder (Walpert, 1998). Thyroid disorders are classified as hyperthyroidism, hypothyroidism, tumors, cancer, or goiter.

HYPERTHYROIDISM

Hyperthyroidism is a collective term for a condition marked by increased thyroid activity and overproduction of thyroid hormones thyroxine (T_4) and triiodothyronine (T_3). The thyroid gland may be enlarged. Different forms of hyperthyroidism are Graves' disease, Basedow's disease, Parry's disease, or thyrotoxicosis. Graves' disease is the most common. It generally affects females more often than males; however, it tends to affect males more severely. The highest incidence is in the 20- to 40-year-old group (Walpert, 1998).

In this autoimmune disorder, the immune system triggers the formation of thyroid-stimulating immunoglobulins (TSIs). The TSIs bind with thyroid-stimulating hormone (TSH) receptors and abnormally stimulate thyroid functioning.

Clinical manifestations include two obvious physical changes. The thyroid, palpated for asymmetry and size, may be enlarged 3 to 4 times its normal size. The

Figure 40-9 *Hyperthyroidism with Exophthalmia (From Thyroid and Its Diseases, 6th ed., by DeGroot, 1995, John Wiley & Sons, Inc.)*

LIFE CYCLE CONSIDERATIONS

Hyperthyroid Complications

The older client particularly develops cardiovascular problems such as arrhythmias (atrial fibrillation), cardiac insufficiency leading to cardiac decompensation, and resistance to the usual dose of digoxin.

enlargement of the thyroid gland is called **goiter.** This is generally a result of overactivity of the thyroid gland. The accumulation of orbital fluid behind the eyeball, forcing it to protrude, is called **exophthalmos** (Figure 40-9). This occurs in about half the cases of hyperthyroidism. It produces a characteristic stare.

The increased thyroid hormone production causes an increased metabolic rate. This leads to weight loss despite increased appetite, fatigue, poor tolerance to heat, and profuse perspiration. The client is very nervous, restless, irritable, has difficulty concentrating, is emotionally labile, has mood swings, possible personality changes, and sleep disturbances. The client may have fine tremors of the fingers and tongue, shaky handwriting, clumsiness, trouble climbing stairs, or dyspnea on exertion and possibly at rest. The skin is warm and moist with a velvety texture. The skin may be a characteristic salmon color. The hair is fine and soft with premature graying and increased hair loss. The nails appear fragile with distal nail separation from the nail bed (onycholysis). There may be general or local muscle atrophy and acropachy (soft tissue swelling with underlying bone changes where new bone forms). There is a tachycardia with bounding pulse up to 160 beats per minute and down to 80 beats per minute during sleep. Pulse pressure is widened. There can be muscular weakness and atrophy; osteoporosis; paralysis; vitiligo, milky-white patches on the skin surrounded by areas of normal pigmentation; decreased libido; impaired fertility; and **gynecomastia** (abnormal enlargement of one or both breasts in males).

Diagnostic tests generally include TSH, T_3, T_4, radioactive iodine uptake, and a thyroid scan.

One major complication is thyrotoxic crisis, also called *thyroid storm.* This is a medical emergency that can lead to cardiac, hepatic, or renal failure. Thyroid storm can be precipitated by stressful situations such as surgery, infection, or trauma. Less common causes are cerebrovascular accident (CVA), myocardial infarction, sudden discontinuing of antithyroid medications, subtotal thyroidectomy with excess intake of synthetic thyroid hormone, toxemia, or diabetic ketoacidosis. Any of these events can lead to overproduction of thyroid hormone, causing an increase in systemic adrenergic activity. This causes an overproduction of epinephrine and severe hypermetabolism, leading to rapid cardiac, gastrointestinal, and sympathetic nervous system decompensation. The client will rapidly exhibit severe clinical manifestations of hyperthyroidism.

If the nurse suspects that the client is experiencing thyrotoxic crisis, inform the physician immediately. The client will be transferred to intensive care for closer monitoring of vital signs, EKG pattern, and cardiopulmonary status. Antithyroid therapy will be initiated immediately. The client's temperature is monitored and cooling measures initiated as needed. Acetaminophen may be administered to lower the temperature, but aspirin is not given because it can increase the free T_4 level. Supportive care would be given until the client is out of the thyrotoxic crisis.

Medical–Surgical Management

Medical

The goal of managing hyperthyroidism is to decrease excessive thyroid hormone production. With treatment to decrease the thyroid production of its hormone, the prognosis is good. The client can live a normal life. There can be a combination of treatment methods. The first method is to administer antithyroid medications. This is usually a temporary solution.

Radiation therapy of the thyroid gland could be external radiation to the neck; however, the more accepted method is the oral administration of radioactive iodine, either liquid or capsule, that targets the thyroid tissue. It is most commonly used for women past the reproductive years or clients not planning to have children. The client of reproductive age must sign an informed consent form because small amounts of the radioactive iodine could lodge in the gonads.

Antithyroid medications are stopped 4 to 7 days before treatment. The physician must know if the client is receiving amiodarone hydrochloride (Cordarone), an antiarrhythmic, because it contains large amounts of iodine. The oral ^{131}I should not be given to the client with severe vomiting or diarrhea.

A single dose of oral ^{131} will destroy some iodine concentrating cells that produce the thyroxine. Clinical manifestations decrease in about 3 weeks, with the full effect in about 3 months. Some clients may require a second or third dose.

Safety: Radioactive Iodine

No pregnant nurse should care for the client. The client should expectorate carefully for the first day because the saliva is radioactive. The client should drink plenty of fluids for 2 days to help circulate and eliminate the radioactive iodine. The toilet should be flushed twice after each use for at least 2 days or throughout the hospitalization. Disposable eating utensils should be used by the client. Close contact with children or pregnant females should be avoided for a week after the administration. Females should avoid pregnancy for 6 months after treatment.

The client usually resumes the thyroid hormone antagonist 3 to 5 days after ^{131}I therapy until the physician determines the thyroid to be atrophic (decreased in size). The client may continue to take propranolol hydrochloride (Inderal) for tachycardia, tremor, and diaphoresis. Continued monitoring of thyroid hormone blood levels and physical condition is necessary.

The most common complication is hypothyroidism, which occurs about 2 to 4 months after treatment. The client is then placed on thyroid replacement therapy, generally for life.

Surgical

Generally just a portion of the thyroid gland is removed, but a total thyroidectomy may be performed. This is the most expensive option and has the most risks. A thyroidectomy may also be done for respiratory obstruction by a goiter or thyroid cancer. If a partial thyroidectomy is done, the remaining thyroid tissue should provide adequate amounts of thyroid hormones. If a complete thyroidectomy is done, the client will require thyroid hormone replacement for life.

Clients usually take propylthiouracil PTU for 4 to 6 weeks before surgery and iodine preparations may be prescribed 10 to 14 days before surgery to decrease thyroid vascularity and decrease bleeding. Depending on the symptoms, the client may also be taking propranolol hydrochloride (Inderal). Thyroid function tests and an EKG are performed before surgery to provide baseline information. Informed consent must be obtained.

Preoperatively, the client should be told about activities after surgery. There will be a neck incision, generally with some type of drain. The client may experience a sore throat and hoarseness. The client is kept in high-Fowler's position to promote venous drainage. The client should support the head with a hand when moving the head to prevent strain on the incision. Respiratory problems may occur, such as tracheal collapse, tracheal mucous accumulation, or laryngeal or local tissue edema. *A tracheotomy tray or endotracheal tubes and insertion tray are kept readily available at the client's bedside in case of a respiratory emergency.*

Because the thyroid is so vascular, the dressing must be checked frequently for drainage, especially at the back of the neck. If there is a drain, approximately 50 cc of drainage is expected the first day. If there is no drainage, the drain must be checked for kinks or obstruction. Voice rest is encouraged for 48 hours, with voice checks every 2 to 4 hours as ordered to make certain there is no laryngeal nerve damage.

Because the parathyroid glands could be accidentally removed during the thyroidectomy, the client's blood calcium level is monitored. The client is checked for Chvostek's sign or Trousseau's sign. (These are discussed under hypoparathyroidism.) Analgesics are administered as needed.

Complications of thyroidectomy are respiratory distress and hemorrhage. There can be damage to the laryngeal nerves, affecting the voice. Manipulation of the thyroid gland during surgery can cause a release of large amounts of thyroid hormone causing thyroid storm, which is rare but may occur. Thyroid crisis usually occurs within the first 12 hours postoperative. Hyperthyroid signs and symptoms are exaggerated, plus the client may vomit, have severe hypertension and tachycardia, and sometimes have hyperthermia up to 106°F (41°C). The client may develop congestive heart failure and die. The client must be advised that tetany can occur up to 10 days after surgery. **Tetany** is sharp flexion of the wrist and ankle joints, muscle twitchings, or cramps caused by decreased blood calcium level.

Pharmacological

Antithyroid therapy is used for children, younger adults, pregnant females, the client who refuses surgery, or clients following surgery. Several drugs can be used for antithyroid therapy. Propylthiouracil (PTU) is used frequently, especially in cases of thyroid storm. It reduces the production of the thyroid hormones. It should be given with food. The client must be instructed to avoid foods high in iodine such as shellfish and iodized salt. Over-the-counter preparations must be checked to see if they contain iodine. This drug requires several weeks to exert the full effect, and it may be administered up to 2 years. This drug may cause **agranulocytosis** (a decreased number of granulocytes), so it is important to report signs and symptoms of infection immediately to the physician.

Methimazole (Tapazole) is another antithyroid preparation that interferes with thyroid hormone synthesis. It has a more rapid onset than PTU; however, it does not have as much consistency in effect. It should be administered at evenly spaced intervals with food to prevent gastric upset. This drug can also cause agranulocytosis, particularly in the client older than age 40.

Iodide preparations may be given to the client with hyperthyroidism. Because iodides inhibit the release of thyroid hormones rather than the synthesis, they take effect in 2 days. Two common preparations are saturated solution potassium iodide (SSKI) and a solution of iodine and potassium iodide that is called Lugol's solution. When iodide preparations are administered orally, they should be mixed with milk, juice, or water and

given after meals to decrease gastric upset. Drinking the
preparations through a straw will decrease discoloration of the teeth. These drugs are contraindicated in
the client with acute bronchitis or a known hypersensitivity to iodine.

Clients may be prescribed propranolol hydrochloride
(Inderal) to counteract tachycardia and peripheral effects
of hyperthyroidism. Clients should not smoke while taking this medication. Abrupt withdrawal of the drug can
cause hypertension, myocardial ischemia, or cardiac arrhythmias. Clients should rise slowly from a sitting or lying position in order to prevent orthostatic hypotension.

Topical medications such as isotonic eyedrops may be
ordered to protect the eyes of the client with exophthalmos. Care must be taken that the eyes are not injured or
infected. Some physicians may order high doses of corticosteroids to help reduce exophthalmos.

During a thyrotoxic crisis, antithyroid drugs are given.
Other medications that may be used are propranolol, corticosteroids, and iodine preparations. Individual client
needs could indicate a need for vitamins, nutrients, fluids,
or sedation.

Diet

Because the client has a greatly increased metabolic
rate as well as weight loss, diet is important. The client
may require between 4,000 to 5,000 calories per day.
There is a need for increased protein, vitamins (especially vitamins B and C), and minerals. In addition to 3
meals per day, the client will need additional meals or
snacks. Fluids should be encouraged, but caffeine should
be avoided.

Nursing Management

Provide a high-calorie diet and snacks throughout
the day. Encourage fluids, but avoid caffeine. Keep
client's skin dry and clean and change gown and linens
as needed. Preoperatively, teach the client how to support his head while turning or rising to a sitting or standing position. Inform client that "voice rest" may be enforced for 48 hours and provide paper and pencil for
writing notes.

Postoperatively, keep bed in semi-Fowler's position
with head and shoulders supported by pillows. Keep suction equipment and tracheotomy tray in the client's
room. Monitor vital signs. Inspect dressing, sides and
back of neck, and shoulders frequently for bleeding.
Watch for signs of internal bleeding (apprehension, restlessness, increased pulse, decreased blood pressure, and
fullness feeling in the neck). Watch for signs of tetany
and for signs of edema in the operative area.

NURSING PROCESS

Assessment

Subjective Data

Obtain a thorough client history and ask about the
ability to concentrate, nervousness, insomnia, jitteriness, excitability, emotional lability, or dysphagia.

Objective Data

Assess for rapid pulse, elevated blood pressure, warm
skin, elevated temperature, diaphoresis, or hand
tremors. Female clients may cease to menstruate. Hair is
fine and soft.

Nursing diagnoses for a client with hyperthyroidism may include the following:

Nursing Diagnoses	Planning/Goals	Nursing Interventions
Preoperative		
Imbalanced Nutrition: Less than Body Requirements related to increased metabolism	The client will eat a nu-tritionally balanced diet with enough calories to prevent weight loss.	Arrange a consultation with the dietitian to assist in determining the client's increased nutritional needs.
		Encourage client to eat a well-balanced diet. Provide snacks through-out the day.
Risk for Injury related to exophthalmos	The client's eyes will not be injured from exophthalmos.	Administer isotonic solutions or eye lubricants to keep the eye moist. At night, elevate head of the bed which may assist in keeping the eyelids closed, or cover the eyes with eye guards to prevent drying.
		Suggest to client that dark or tinted wraparound glasses may protect the eyes from wind and airborne particles.

continues

Nursing Diagnoses	Planning/Goals	Nursing Interventions
Postoperative		
Impaired Swallowing related to mechanical obstruction (edema)	The client will have diminished problems with swallowing.	Ensure gag, cough, and swallowing reflexes are present before offering oral fluids. Maintain client in Fowler's position when drinking or eating. Encourage client to drink slowly and chew thoroughly.
Ineffective Airway Clearance related to edema and pain	The client will be able to clear airway.	Keep suctioning equipment ready. Administer analgesic as ordered.

Evaluation Each goal must be evaluated to determine how it has been met by the client.

SAMPLE NURSING CARE PLAN

THE CLIENT WITH HYPERTHYROIDISM

Janey Jackson, 33 years old, has returned to her physician's office to find out results of her tests for hyperthyroidism. She continues to have multiple complaints. "I have lost fifteen pounds in the last month despite eating all the time. I am restless and can't sleep. I feel jittery and irritable. My family says my moods change so rapidly they don't know what to expect from me. I feel so hot most of the time and sweat a lot."

The office nurse notes Mrs. Jackson appears flushed and her eyes protrude slightly. Her vital signs, T.-100.6 orally, P.-120, R.-26, and B/P.-140/88, are slightly elevated from her previous office visit. Her test results confirm that she has hyperthyroidism.

Nursing Diagnosis 1 *Imbalanced Nutrition: Less than body requirements* related to increased metabolism as evidenced by weight loss despite eating

Nursing Outcomes Classification (NOC)
Nutritional Status: Food & Fluid Intake
Nutritional Status: Nutrient Intake

Nursing Interventions Classification (NIC)
Fluid Management
Nutrition Management

PLANNING/GOALS	NURSING INTERVENTIONS	RATIONALE
Mrs. Jackson will eat a nutritionally balanced diet with enough calories to prevent weight loss.	Monitor amount of food ingested and caloric intake.	Provides data to determine if diet is adequate to prevent weight loss.
	Monitor weight daily.	Determines weight gains or losses.
	Provide a diet high in calories, protein, and carbohydrates.	Maintains or increases weight while preventing muscle mass breakdown.
	Advise Mrs. Jackson to avoid highly seasoned or fibrous foods or foods causing flatulence.	Prevents increased peristalsis resulting in diarrhea.
	Provide small frequent meals spread over waking hours.	Provides calories without extremely large meals.
	Obtain nutritional consult as needed.	Ensures nutritional status.

EVALUATION   Mrs. Jackson gained or maintained weight.

continues

SAMPLE NURSING CARE PLAN

Nursing Diagnosis 2 *Hyperthermia* related to increased metabolic rate as evidenced by complaints of feeling hot, flushing, and elevated temperature

Nursing Outcomes Classification (NOC)
Hydration
Thermoregulation

Nursing Interventions Classification (NIC)
Fluid Management

PLANNING/GOALS	NURSING INTERVENTIONS	RATIONALE
Mrs. Jackson's body temperature will be within normal range.	Assess for elevated temperature, heat intolerance, and diaphoresis.	Indicates increased heat production from increased metabolic rate.
	Provide a well-ventilated room with temperature control.	Promotes comfort if heat intolerant.
	Suggest wearing cool, loose-fitting, lightweight clothing.	Provides comfort and prevents overheating.
	Provide frequent bathing and changes in linens or clothing.	Promotes comfort if diaphoretic.
	Provide fluids up to 3 liters per day.	Replaces fluid if diaphoretic.

EVALUATION   Mrs. Jackson maintained her temperature in a normal range.

Nursing Diagnosis 3 *Risk for Impaired Skin Integrity* related to diaphoresis as evidenced by excessive sweating

Nursing Outcomes Classification (NOC)
Nutritional Status
Tissue Integrity: Skin & Mucous Membranes

Nursing Interventions Classification (NIC)
Fluid/Electrolyte Management
Nutrition Management

PLANNING/GOALS	NURSING INTERVENTIONS	RATIONALE
Mrs. Jackson's skin will remain intact and free of injury.	Assess skin for flushing and moisture.	Indicates heat intolerance.
	Assess skin for redness, especially bony prominences.	Indicates potential for breakdown.
	Keep Mrs. Jackson clean and dry.	Prevents skin breakdown.

EVALUATION   Mrs. Jackson maintained an intact skin without impairment.

HYPOTHYROIDISM

Hypothyroidism is a condition in which the metabolic processes are decreased because of a deficiency of thyroid hormones. It is termed primary if the problem arises from a dysfunction solely of the thyroid. It is secondary if the thyroid gland is not stimulated to produce normally or if the target cells fail to respond to normal thyroid functioning. This condition is more common in females than males. There is a significant increase in incidence between the ages of 30 to 60. Hypothyroid conditions include cretinism, myxedema, and Hashimoto's thyroiditis.

CRETINISM

A congenital condition with decreased thyroid hormone production causes defective physical development and mental retardation. This is called **cretinism** and occurs in about 1 of 3,000 live births (NIH, 2002a). The child generally has a large head, short limbs, puffy eyes, thick and protruding tongue, excessively dry skin, and a lack of coordination. If untreated, the child will be permanently dwarfed, mentally retarded, and sterile. This condition is rare in the United States and is diagnosed by the T_4, serum TSH, x-ray of long bones, and thyroid scan.

MYXEDEMA

Myxedema is the term for severe hypothyroidism in adults. A variety of abnormalities lead to decreased thyroid hormone production. The obvious ones are thyroid gland surgery such as thyroidectomy or irradiation of the thyroid gland. Some other causes are chronic autoimmune Hashimoto's thyroiditis, inflammatory conditions (sarcoidosis), pituitary failure to produce TSH, or hypothalamus failure to produce thyrotropin-releasing hormone. There may be an inability to synthesize thyroid hormones related to iodine deficiency (rarely from general diet deficiency) or as a result of taking antithyroid medications.

Clinical manifestations are vague and varied, developing slowly over a period of time, but are primarily related to the reduced metabolic rate. These include an energy loss, fatigue, forgetfulness, sensitivity to cold, unexplained weight gain, hypoventilation, and constipation. As the condition progresses, manifestations include reduced libido, menorrhagia, paresthesias, joint stiffness, and muscle cramping. There is a characteristic alteration in overall appearance and behavior, including decreased mental stability and a thick and dry tongue, causing hoarseness and slow, slurred speech. The skin is flaky and inelastic, and feels cool, dry, rough, and doughy. There is edema of the face, hands, and feet. The hair is dry and sparse, with patchy hair loss including loss of the outer third of the eyebrow. The nails are thick and brittle with visible transverse and longitudinal grooves. The pulse is weak and bradycardic because of the decreased pumping strength of the heart. The thyroid gland may be so small that it may not be palpated unless there is a goiter. The blood pressure is generally lower than normal for the client.

Diagnostic tests generally include TSH, T_3, T_4, radioactive iodine uptake, and a thyroid scan.

Complications affect almost every system. Cardiovascular complications include ischemic heart disease, poor peripheral circulation, enlarged heart, or pleural or pericardial effusion. Gastrointestinal complications include adynamic colon (decreased functioning of the colon), megacolon (massive and abnormal dilation of the colon), or intestinal obstruction. Other complications include conductive or sensorineural deafness, psychiatric disorders, carpal tunnel syndrome, or impotence or infertility. Prognosis depends on the organs involved, duration, and severity of condition.

Myxedema coma or hypothyroid crisis is a rare but serious complication of extreme hypothyroidism. It is life threatening, with symptoms of unresponsiveness, hypothermia, decreased respirations, low blood pressure,

and low blood sugar. It has a gradual onset but is triggered by severe stress such as infection, exposure to cold, or trauma. Abrupt withdrawal of thyroid medication or the use of narcotics, sedatives, or anesthetics can also cause myxedema coma. If myxedema coma occurs, it must be reported to the physician immediately. The client is moved to the ICU, where intubation and mechanical ventilation are instituted. The client is monitored closely for vital signs, EKG changes, and cardiopulmonary status. Wrapping the client in blankets will warm the client, but a warming blanket should not be used because it could cause peripheral vasodilation and shock. Thyroid medications and possibly corticosteroids are administered. Supportive care is given until the client comes out of the myxedema coma. Myxedema coma is often fatal.

Medical–Surgical Management

Pharmacological

Thyroid replacement therapy is lifelong. Thyroid (Armour Thyroid) is a natural form, whereas levothyroxine sodium (Levothroid, Synthroid) is a synthetic. The physician orders thyroid hormone to begin slowly and increases the dosage every 2 to 3 weeks until the desired response is achieved. The medication should be given in the morning to prevent insomnia.

If the client has diabetes mellitus, insulin or oral hypoglycemic dosage might have to be adjusted. The blood sugar level must be monitored closely. If the client is on anticoagulant therapy, thyroid potentiates the anticoagulant action. The client should be taught to watch for excessive bleeding or bruising. Digitalis preparations are also potentiated by thyroid.

Because hypothyroidism impairs the metabolic rate, the client may have difficulty metabolizing medications. The client may have an increased sensitivity to hypnotics, sedatives, or opiates. Dosage may have to be adjusted appropriately. Synthesis of the thyroid hormone can be impaired by drugs such as lithium carbonate (Lithotabs) or aminoglutethimide (Cytadren).

Diet

The client should be instructed to avoid foods high in iodine and foods that interfere with thyroid hormone replacement, such as dried kelp, shellfish, iodized salt, saltwater fish, cabbage, turnips, pears, and peaches. The diet is designed for weight loss and to combat constipation. A high-fiber, high-protein, low-calorie diet is given. Sodium should be decreased to prevent fluid retention. A dietary consultation for meal planning and a list of foods to avoid should be provided to the client.

CLIENT TEACHING

Items Containing Iodine

Check the labels on multivitamins, dentrifices, and non-prescription medications; they may contain iodine.

Nursing Management

Monitor vital signs, heart sounds, lung sounds, I&O, weight, and check for edema. Prevent client fatigue by providing rest periods between activities. Provide a high-fiber diet and encourage intake of oral fluids. Administer stool softener, bulk laxative, or enema as ordered.

NURSING PROCESS

Assessment

Subjective Data

Obtain a thorough client history, asking about lethargy, depression, irritability, impaired memory, and slowing of thought processes. The client may describe speech and hearing problems, anorexia, decreased libido, and constipation.

Objective Data

Assess for hearing and speech deficits, thin hair, dry and thickened skin, enlarged facial features, masklike expression, low and hoarse voice, bradycardia, decreased blood pressure and respirations, and exercise intolerance.

Nursing diagnoses for the client with myxedema may include the following:

Nursing Diagnoses	Planning/Goals	Nursing Interventions
Activity Intolerance related to decreased metabolic and energy level	The client will express understanding to increase activity level gradually. The client will maintain blood pressure, pulse, and respirations within normal limits when active. The client will regain normal activity levels.	Assist the client to gradually increase activity level but encourage rest between activities to avoid fatigue and decrease cardiac oxygen demands. Measure the client's legs correctly so antiembolic hose, which help venous return, will fit properly when worn. Reposition client every 2 hours and encourage client to continue activity when normal activity level is achieved.
Ineffective **T**issue Perfusion (Cardiopulmonary) related to decreased cardiac output	The client will not have chest pain at rest. The client will have a normal heart rate and rhythm. The client will avoid ischemic EKG changes. The client will maintain adequate cardiopulmonary perfusion.	Assess for chest pain and advise client to report any episodes of angina immediately. Monitor the client's vital signs. Monitor cardiac status through EKG and assessment of heart and lung sounds plus checking for edema. Restrict fluid and sodium during the time of cardiac decompensation as ordered. Monitor intake and output and weight.
Constipation related to decreased motility of the gastrointestinal tract	The client will have regular bowel movements.	Provide high-fiber diet. Encourage intake of oral fluids. Assess frequency and character of stool. Administer stool softener, bulk laxative, or enema as ordered.

Evaluation Each goal must be evaluated to determine how it has been met by the client.

HASHIMOTO'S THYROIDITIS

Hashimoto's thyroiditis, the most common cause of hypothyroidism, is an autoimmune disease characterized by the production of antiperoxidase antibodies, which destroy an essential enzyme necessary for production of T_3 and T_4. The disease occurs more often in females than in males, between the ages of 30 and 50, and shows a marked hereditary pattern. There is an increased incidence in clients with Down syndrome and Turner's syndrome.

Clinical manifestations include a thyroid that is enlarged and has a lumpy surface. Generally, the goiter is asymptomatic, but it could cause dysphagia and a feeling of local pressure. The thymus gland is also enlarged. Other clinical manifestations are similar to hypothyroidism.

Treatment of Hashimoto's thyroiditis is similar to that of hypothyroidism. Thyroid hormone replacement is used.

This chronic disorder can be treated but not cured. The client will be on lifetime thyroid hormone replacement.

THYROID TUMORS

There are several neoplasms of the thyroid gland. The benign thyroid cyst and adenoma are firm, encapsulated, noninvasive, slowly growing neoplasms of unknown etiology. Diagnosis of benign neoplasms is done by needle biopsy. These growths tend to be nonfunctioning (not affecting the functioning of the thyroid gland), so there is no treatment other than continued monitoring. If the adenoma is functioning (increasing the functioning of the thyroid gland), then it is treated by radioactive iodine or surgery.

CANCER OF THE THYROID

Cancer of the thyroid is rare and occurs in all age groups. Individuals who have had radiation therapy to the neck are more susceptible. There are four major types of thyroid cancer:

- Papillary carcinoma is the most common type. It can affect any age but is more common in females of childbearing age. It is well-differentiated, grows slowly, is usually contained, and does not spread beyond the adjacent lymph nodes. Cure rate after thyroidectomy is excellent.
- Follicular carcinoma metastasizes to the regional lymph nodes and spreads through the blood vessels to the bone, liver, and lungs. It has a very low cure rate.
- Medullary carcinoma is a solid carcinoma associated with pheochromocytoma. It is curable if detected before signs and symptoms occur. Without treatment, it grows rapidly, metastasizing to the bones, liver, and kidneys.
- Anaplastic or undifferentiated carcinoma resists radiation. It is almost never curable by resection. It metastasizes rapidly, generally causing death by invasion of the trachea and adjacent structures. It generally affects individuals older than age 60.

There are several risk factors, such as radiation exposure, especially in those children and adolescents who received radiation therapy to treat severe cases of acne vulgaris, or to shrink enlarged tonsils, adenoids, and thymus tissue; prolonged secretion of TSH resulting from radiation or heredity; familial disposition; or chronic goiter.

The first clinical manifestation is a painless lump. As it enlarges, it destroys the thyroid, which leads to clinical manifestations of hypothyroidism. Although rare, the tumor could trigger excessive thyroid hormone production, causing the client to display the clinical manifestations of hyperthyroidism. There can be dysphagia, hoarseness, and vocal stridor. There may be a detectable, disfiguring thyroid mass with a firm nodule on palpation.

The thyroid scan shows a "cold" nodule (decreased uptake of ^{131}I) for papillary carcinoma. Follicular carcinoma and benign adenomas show a "hot" nodule. Thyroid function tests are usually normal. A needle biopsy may be done to confirm diagnosis.

Medical–Surgical Management
Surgical

All carcinomas can be treated with surgery (discussed previously). Radioactive iodine or external radiation therapy may also be used. Response of the tumor will depend on early diagnosis and treatment. These methods of treatment may be used individually or in combination. Client care is the same as for hyperthyroidism.

Pharmacological

Exogenous thyroid hormone may suppress thyroid activity. To increase tolerance to surgery or radiation therapy, the physician may prescribe simultaneous exogenous thyroid hormone and adrenergic blocker such as propranolol hydrochloride (Inderal). If there is widespread metastasis, the cancers will be treated with neoplastic chemotherapy.

Nursing Management

The nurse monitors the client's level of anxiety and encourages the client to discuss feelings about the diagnosis and possible surgery. The nurse also assists the client in identifying previously successful coping methods and teaches new coping methods if needed.

GOITER

A goiter is an enlargement of the thyroid unrelated to inflammation or neoplasm. There are three types of goiter. One type is a diffuse toxic goiter found in hyperthyroidism. This type of goiter may be moderate to massively enlarged. The consistency varies from soft to firm and rubbery. It generally feels smooth. It is often associated with exophthalmos.

Another type of goiter is a simple nontoxic goiter. It develops when the thyroid is unable to utilize iodine properly or in response to a low iodine level in the blood. These goiters are more common in females. They develop during times of great metabolic demands such as adolescence or pregnancy. A deficiency of iodine can cause goiter formation. Clinical manifestations depend on the size of the goiter. There is an obvious enlargement of the thyroid gland. A large goiter can compress the esophagus or trachea, causing dysphagia, a choking sensation, or respiratory difficulty. If the goiter impairs venous return from the head and neck, the client may experience dizziness and syncope.

Diagnosis is based on history, clinical manifestations, and results of thyroid function tests. T_3 is generally very low. Treatment concentrates on the underlying cause and may involve thyroid hormone replacement therapy, iodine supplements, or increasing dietary iodine sources. Surgery is done when respiration or swallowing is impaired or for cosmetic effect.

The third type of goiter is the nodular goiter. It is similar to the simple goiter except that palpation reveals multiple nodules causing the enlargement. It is found frequently in females older than 40. It usually is asymptomatic. Treatment varies with the client's age and clinical manifestations.

PARATHYROID DISORDERS

Disorders discussed include hyperparathyroidism and hypoparathyroidism.

HYPERPARATHYROIDISM

Hyperparathyroidism is a condition resulting from overactivity of one or more of the parathyroid glands. It results in increased secretion of parathyroid hormone (PTH), which causes calcium to leave the bones and accumulate in the blood. This cannot be compensated by renal excretion or uptake into the soft tissues. It occurs twice as often in postmenopausal females than males. It occurs frequently between the ages of 35 and 65. Hypercalcemia may also be caused by excessive intake of thiazide diuretics, vitamin D, or calcium supplements.

X-rays will show skeletal decalcification. Blood PTH and alkaline phosphate levels are increased. Serum calcium level is elevated.

It is termed primary if there is an enlargement of one or more of the parathyroid glands, increasing secretion of PTH and thus increasing the blood calcium level. The most common cause is adenoma, but other primary causes include genetics or multiple endocrine neoplasms.

The condition is termed secondary if there is excess compensatory production of PTH stemming from a hypocalcemia-producing abnormality other than the parathyroid gland. Some of these abnormalities are rickets, chronic renal failure, vitamin D deficiency, or osteomalacia caused by laxative abuse or phenytoin (Dilantin).

Many clients are asymptomatic; however, there are several clinical manifestations. The client may have polyuria, chronic low-back pain, bone tenderness, or renal calculi. The client may also experience nausea, vomiting, anorexia, constipation, lethargy, or drowsiness. There can be changes in level of consciousness, disorientation, stupor, coma, or personality changes with a loss of initiative and memory. There may be marked muscle weakness and atrophy especially of the legs, joint hyperextensibility, long bone skeletal deformity, or hyporeflexia.

Without treatment, there can be permanent damage to the skeleton or kidneys. There can be bone and articular problems including pathologic fractures. Renal complications include colic, nephrolithiasis, urinary tract infection, and renal insufficiency leading to chronic renal failure. Other complications may be stone formation in various organs, cardiac or vascular problems, or central nervous system changes.

Medical–Surgical Management

Medical

Medical management is aimed at decreasing overactivity of the parathyroid glands. This may be accomplished by medication or surgery. If there is severe renal involvement, the client may require dialysis.

Surgical

Primary hyperparathyroidism can be treated by surgical removal of three and one-half of the four parathyroid glands. Surgery can relieve bone pain in 3 days but may not reverse renal damage.

Preoperative care includes explanations, encouraging fluids, limiting calcium intake, and administering medications to lower the blood calcium level.

Postoperative care involves administration of magnesium or phosphate. The client may receive calcium supplements for several days. The nursing care is similar to that provided to the client with thyroidectomy (refer to hyperthyroidism). A major complication is airway obstruction.

Pharmacological

Pharmacological treatment is aimed toward correcting secondary hyperparathyroidism, which involves treating the underlying cause. Because hypercalcemia is a major manifestation, medications are geared to decrease the calcium level in the blood. This includes the use of diuretics such as furosemide (Lasix) and ethacrynic acid (Edecrin).

Other drugs that decrease the calcium level in the blood are calcitonin-human (Cibacalcin), plicamycin (Mithracin), and magnesium- or phosphate-based drugs. Phosphate-based drugs lower the calcium level based on the inverse relationship between phosphorus and calcium.

Nursing Management

Preoperatively, encourage oral fluid intake, monitor I&O, strain urine for calculi, and offer cranberry juice to acidify the urine. Postoperatively, carefully monitor I&O, and assess for signs of hypocalcemia (tetany, cardiac dysrhythmias, and carpopedal spasms). Teach client the principles of good body mechanics. Reassure client that bone pain will gradually disappear. Encourage mild exercise as ordered.

NURSING PROCESS

Assessment

Subjective Data

Obtain a thorough client history and ask about muscle weakness, apathy, nausea, mental status, and pain (low back or renal). Ask about increased calcium intake, either dietary or supplements.

Objective Data

Note fatigue, drowsiness, anorexia, constipation, personality changes, renal colic, skeletal deformity, output, hematuria, vomiting, weight loss, hypertension, bradycardia, or dysrhythmias.

Nursing diagnoses for thea client with hyperparathyroidism may include the following:

Nursing Diagnoses	Planning/Goals	Nursing Interventions
*A*ctivity *Intolerance* related to generalized weakness caused by neuromuscular dysfunction	The client will regain and maintain normal muscle mass and strength, maintain maximum joint range of motion, and perform self-care activity as tolerated.	Alternate rest and activity periods. Assist client with pre-scribed, individualized activities. Assist client to identify factors that increase or decrease activity intolerance. Encourage client to perform self-care.
Acute Pain related to musculo-skeletal changes resulting from persistently increased serum calcium level	The client will express relief after analgesics, use comfort measures to decrease pain, and be pain-free when serum calcium level reaches normal.	Administer analgesics as ordered. Provide comfort measures for bone pain, and include turning and repositioning every 2 hours. Assess pain level and compare to serum calcium level. Assess environment for hazards and eliminate them. Assist the client to ambulate. Maintain the bed in a low position with siderails up and call light in reach. Lift and move the client gently to prevent pathologic fractures.

Evaluation Each goal must be evaluated to determine how it has been met by the client.

HYPOPARATHYROIDISM

Hypoparathyroidism is a condition resulting from a deficiency of parathyroid hormone (PTH) secretion by the parathyroids or the decreased action of peripheral PTH. Because the parathyroids normally regulate the serum calcium level, hypoparathyroidism will result in a decreased serum calcium level. PTH normally maintains the serum calcium level by increasing bone resorption and gastric reabsorption. It also maintains the inverse relationship between calcium and phosphorus levels. Hypoparathyroidism can be acute or chronic.

If hypoparathyroidism is idiopathic, it may be the result of an autoimmune disorder or congenital absence of parathyroid glands. Acquired hypoparathyroidism is generally irreversible. The most common cause is accidental removal during thyroid or other neck surgery. It can also result from ischemic infarction during surgery, sarcoidosis, tuberculosis, neoplasms, trauma, or massive thyroid irradiation. Reversible hypoparathyroidism can result from hypomagnesemia-induced impairment of hormone synthesis, suppression of normal gland function because of hypercalcemia, or delayed maturation of the parathyroid glands.

The characteristic sign of hypoparathyroidism is tetany, which is muscle spasms and tremors caused by a lack of calcium. Other clinical manifestations include dry skin, brittle hair, alopecia (loss of hair or baldness), and loss of eyelashes and fingernails. The teeth are stained, cracked, and decayed because of weak enamel. The client may have altered neuromuscular irritability, tingling and twitching of the face and hands, and increased deep tendon reflexes. There may be personality changes or EKG changes.

Two diagnostic assessment tests can be performed. One is the **Chvostek's sign,** which is an abnormal spasm of the facial muscles in response to a light tapping of the facial nerve. The other test is **Trousseau's sign,** which is a carpal spasm caused by inflating a blood pressure cuff above the client's systolic pressure and leaving it in place for 3 minutes (Figure 40-10).

Expected test results include decreased serum calcium, increased urinary calcium, increased serum phosphorus, and decreased urinary phosphorus.

Positive Chvostek's Sign

A

Positive Trousseau's Sign

B

Figure 40-10 *Signs of Hypocalcemia and Hypoparathyroidism: **A,** Chvostek's sign; **B,** Trousseau's sign*

Complications are related to long-standing hypocalcemia, which leads to decreased heart contractility leading to cardiac failure. There can be cataract formation or papillary edema from increased intracranial pressure. There may be bone deformity. In cases of severe tetany, the client can experience laryngospasm, respiratory stridor, anoxia, paralysis of vocal cords, and death.

Medical–Surgical Management

Pharmacological

Calcium gluconate or calcium chloride may be given intravenously. Give very slowly because it is very irritating to the vessel wall. Too-rapid IV calcium infusion can cause cardiac arrest. After the initial IV dose, calcium may be given orally.

Unless the hypoparathyroidism is reversible, the client will require lifelong calcium replacement. Vitamin D may also be given to assist in the absorption of calcium. The calcium supplements should be given 1 to $1^1/_2$ hours after meals to increase absorption. If the client cannot swallow the large tablets, they can be dissolved in hot water and the suspension cooled before administering to the client. The best sources of calcium are from the diet. The client needs to take calcium as ordered and not abruptly stop taking it. The client must be advised that calcium may cause digitalis toxicity. Cimetidine (Tagamet) interferes with normal parathyroid functioning.

Diet

The diet should be high in calcium and low in phosphorus-containing foods. Because many foods that are high in calcium are also high in phosphorus, the client should be given a list of foods that are high in calcium but lower in phosphorus. Foods on this list include vegetables such as asparagus, broccoli, collards, and tomatoes; fruits such as apricots, bananas, cantaloupe, and many berries; and other foods such as kidney beans, lima beans, and brown sugar. Foods that have a high phosphorus content and should be avoided include most legumes, nuts, cheeses, and seafood.

Nursing Management

Monitor vital signs and for signs of hypercalcemia (anorexia, vomiting, disorientation, abdominal pain, and weakness). Assess for respiratory distress. Provide a diet high in calcium-containing foods. Emphasize the importance of having the blood level of calcium and phosphorus checked.

NURSING PROCESS

Assessment

Subjective Data

Obtain a thorough client history, asking the client about recent surgery or irradiation, use of alcohol, numbness or tingling of the skin, anxiety, headache, irritability, depression, or nausea.

Objective Data

Assess for dysphagia, laryngeal spasm, stridor, cyanosis, dysrhythmias, Chvostek's sign, and Trousseau's sign.

Nursing diagnoses for the client with hypoparathyroidism may include the following:

Nursing Diagnoses	Planning/Goals	Nursing Interventions
Risk for Injury related to calcium deficiency	The client will not exhibit signs and symptoms of tetany, and will prevent injury from hypocalcemia.	Monitor Chvostek's and Trousseau's signs, serum calcium and phosphorus levels, as well as EKG changes. Keep tracheotomy tray readily available and maintain seizure precautions. Support the client while walking to prevent injury. Monitor the client taking digoxin for toxicity.
Imbalanced Nutrition: Less than body requirements, related to calcium intake	The client will have adequate calcium intake.	Provide diet with calcium-rich foods. Give calcium replacement as ordered. The client who is taking digoxin must be monitored for toxicity.

Evaluation Each goal must be evaluated to determine how it has been met by the client.

ADRENAL DISORDERS

Disorders in this category include Cushing's disease/syndrome, Addison's disease, and pheochromocytoma.

CUSHING'S DISEASE/SYNDROME (ADRENAL HYPERFUNCTION)

Cushing's *disease*, primary adrenal hyperfunction, is the result of increased pituitary secretion of ACTH, which causes an increased production of cortisol by the adrenal cortex. Cushing's *syndrome* refers to symptoms of cortisol excess caused by other factors. One cause is a corticotropin-producing tumor in another organ, such as oat-cell carcinoma of the lung (secondary adrenal hyperfunction). The most common cause of Cushing's syndrome is prolonged use of glucocorticoid or corticotropin medications for chronic inflammatory disorders such as chronic obstructive pulmonary disease, Crohn's disease, and rheumatoid arthritis. This is **iatrogenic** (caused by treatment or diagnostic procedures) adrenal hyperfunction.

Cushing's syndrome occurs in females more than males, generally between 30 and 50 years of age.

Classic clinical manifestations are adiposity of the face, neck, and trunk, which give rise to the moon-shaped face and buffalo hump. Others include purple striae on the abdomen, hirsutism, and thin extremities caused by muscle wasting. Boys exhibit an early onset of puberty, whereas girls exhibit development of masculine characteristics. The client may complain of fatigue, muscle weakness, sleep disturbances, water retention, amenorrhea, decreased libido, irritability, and emotional lability. There could be petechiae, ecchymoses, decreased wound healing, or swollen ankles.

There are multiple complications of Cushing's syndrome, most of which are produced by the stimulating and catabolic effects of cortisol. There can be increased calcium resorption from the bone, leading to osteoporosis and pathologic fractures. It can cause increased hepatic gluconeogenesis and insulin resistance, causing glucose intolerance and diabetes mellitus. The client may have frequent infections and slowed wound healing. There is a suppressed inflammatory response that can mask severe infections. The client may have decreased ability to handle stress, which can lead to psychological problems from mood swings to psychosis. Other complications include hypertension, ischemic heart disease, congestive heart failure, menstrual disturbances, and sexual dysfunction.

Plasma cortisol level is elevated. Plasma ACTH level may be elevated or low. Adrenalangiography is done for adrenal tumor. Twenty-four-hour urine tests for 17-ketosteroids and 17-hydroxysteroids are elevated.

Prognosis depends on early diagnosis, identifying the underlying cause, and effective treatment. Without treatment, about half of these clients will die within 5 years.

Medical–Surgical Management

Medical

The major goal is to restore hormone balance. Treatment is based on the causative factor. This is accomplished primarily by medications. If there is adrenal cancer, the client may have either radiation therapy to the adrenal gland or surgery on either the pituitary gland or the adrenal glands, or all three treatments.

Surgical

If the underlying cause of Cushing's syndrome is related to the pituitary gland, the client may have a hypophysectomy done. (Refer to hypophysectomy in the section on hyperpituitarism.)

For an adrenal tumor, an adrenalectomy is performed. This could be unilateral or bilateral. During the first 24 to 48 hours after surgery, the client is observed closely for hemorrhage and shock. Vital signs and urine output are monitored. Glucocorticoids are administered with changing dosage until a maintenance dose is established. The client's blood glucose level must be monitored, especially for hypoglycemia.

Pharmacological

Aminoglutethimide (Cytadren) inhibits synthesis of adrenal steroids. It can cause dizziness or drowsiness. The client should be instructed to avoid activities requiring mental alertness or manual dexterity.

Ketoconazole (Nizoral), while classified as an antifungal, inhibits adrenal steroidogenesis and is used in Cushing's syndrome.

Mitotane (Lysodren) directly suppresses the activity of the adrenal cortex. This cytotoxic agent is generally used for inoperable adrenal cortex cancer. It is given for at least 3 months. The client should avoid situations that cause injury or exposure to infections.

If the client had pituitary or adrenal surgery, cortisol therapy may be given before and after surgery to decrease physical stress. Steroid therapy could be a lifetime situation. The client should take the drug with food or antacids to decrease gastric distress. Two-thirds dose of the steroids should be taken in the morning, with the remaining one-third in the early evening to mimic the body's diurnal schedule. Steroids can lead to osteoporosis and the possibility of pathologic fractures. Females should be warned that steroid use can interfere with oral contraceptive effectiveness. There may be an adverse effect on the male's sperm production and count.

COMMUNITY/HOME HEALTH CARE

Cushing's Syndrome

- Carry Medic Alert medal indicating Cushing's syndrome.
- Avoid extreme temperature changes, activities that could result in trauma, and people with infections.
- Wash hands often and protect skin with good care.
- Maintain medication regimen.
- Notify physician if weakness, fainting, fever, nausea, or vomiting occur.

The client with diabetes mellitus may have to adjust insulin dosage because the steroids can affect the glucose level. Steroids can mask severe infections and cause some immunosuppression. Wounds are slower to heal. The client should be instructed to contact a physician before using over-the-counter preparations. The client should not abruptly discontinue the steroid drug; dosage must be tapered before discontinuing.

Diet

The diet should be high in protein and potassium but low in sodium. Foods high in protein include eggs, milk, whole grains, legumes, and meat; however, milk, cheeses, and whole grains are also high in sodium, depending on processing. Many foods high in potassium are also low in sodium. These foods are legumes; fruits such as figs, oranges, bananas, prunes, and raisins; and vegetables such as avocado, potato, and spinach. The client should be advised to read labels for sodium content. Processed foods and many preservatives have high sodium content and should be avoided. Reduced carbohydrates and calories help control hyperglycemia.

Nursing Management

Encourage client to turn frequently and ambulate to prevent pressure on bony prominences. Gently handle client to prevent ecchymosis. Provide elbow and heel protectors and an egg-crate mattress. Provide rest periods during personal hygiene activities.

NURSING PROCESS

Assessment

Subjective Data

Obtain a thorough client history, asking about the use of steroids, stress, methods of coping with stress, irritability, depression, mood swings, loss of libido, and the possibility of suicide.

Objective Data

Assess for thin and fragile skin, petechiae, ecchymoses, delayed wound healing, weight gain, increased abdominal girth, purple striae, hyperglycemia, and hypokalemia. Women may have **hirsutism** (excessive body hair in a masculine distribution), deepening of the voice, and menstrual irregularities.

Nursing diagnoses for the client with Cushing's syndrome may include the following:

Nursing Diagnoses	Planning/Goals	Nursing Interventions
*Disturbed **B**ody Image* related to changes in physical appearance	The client will verbalize feelings about changed appearance.	Encourage the client to verbalize feelings about changed body image. Offer emotional support and a positive realistic assessment of the condition.
*Risk for **I**nfection* related to suppressed inflammatory response from excessive corticosteroid production	The client will take precautions to avoid or decrease exposure to infection.	Advise client to avoid people with infections. Provide a private room with reverse or protective isolation as indicated. Monitor the client's vital signs, intake and output, and weight.

Evaluation Each goal must be evaluated to determine how it has been met by the client.

ADDISON'S DISEASE (ADRENAL HYPOFUNCTION)

Addison's disease, primary hypofunctioning of the adrenals, involves decreased functioning of the adrenal cortex and its secretions—mineralocorticoids, glucocorticoids, and androgens. It can also be called *adrenal hypofunction* or *insufficiency*. It is fairly uncommon, occurring in 1 per 100,000 people in the United States. Although it affects all ages and both sexes, it is less common among the elderly.

Addison's disease occurs when more than 90% of the adrenal gland is destroyed. It is an autoimmune disease in response to conditions such as tuberculosis, histoplas-mosis, HIV, and meningococcal pneumonia. It can be caused by bilateral adrenalectomy, hemorrhage into the adrenal gland related to anticoagulant therapy, or cancer of the adrenal gland. It is termed secondary if it results from decreased pituitary or hypothalamus function or abrupt withdrawal of long-term steroid therapy.

A classical clinical manifestation of Addison's disease is a bronze coloration of the skin resembling a deep suntan, especially in the creases on the hands, elbows, and knees. There may be some areas of vitiligo. The client may complain of fatigue, muscle weakness, lightheadedness upon rising, weight loss, and craving for salty foods. The client may have decreased tolerance even to minor stress. The client is anxious, irritable, and may become confused. The pulse may be weak and irregular. There is hypotension and a variety of GI complaints.

The acute form is called adrenal crisis. It may occur when there is trauma, surgery, other physiologic stress, or abrupt withdrawal of steroids. The clinical manifestations are the same, only more severe with a rapid onset. The crisis requires immediate treatment. The client will be placed on intravenous therapy and IV administration of hydrocortisone (Cortef, Hydrocortone). Measures to maintain a stable blood pressure and normal water and sodium levels are instituted. After the crisis, the client will be placed on a maintenance dose of hydrocortisone.

Expected test results include low serum sodium, high serum potassium, low serum glucose, low cortisol and aldosterone serum levels, and decreased urinary 17-ketosteroid and 17-hydroxysteroid levels.

Medical–Surgical Management

Medical

Treatment is geared toward prompt restoration of fluid and electrolyte balance and replacement of deficient adrenal hormones.

Pharmacological

The client will require lifetime maintenance of steroids. Administration of glucocorticoids such as hydrocortisone (Hydrocortone) and mineralocorticoids such as fludrocortisone acetate (Florinef) are given two-thirds of the daily dose in the morning and one-third in the evening. In times of stress, the dose may need to be doubled or tripled.

Diet

The diet should be high in sodium and low in potassium. It should contain adequate calories and protein. If the client is anorexic, six small meals may increase caloric intake. A late afternoon or evening snack should be available if the client's blood glucose level drops.

Nursing Management

Carefully assess the client's circulatory status. Weigh client daily. Accurately record I&O. Monitor vital signs and skin turgor. Provide a private room and screen visitors for infections. Teach importance of taking medications as prescribed, reporting any illness to the physician, and having regular checkups.

NURSING PROCESS

Assessment

Subjective Data

Obtain a thorough client history, asking about recent synthetic steroid use, adrenal surgery, infection, salt craving, nausea, weakness, vertigo, headache, disorientation, emotional status, anxiety, and apprehension.

Objective Data

Assess for postural hypotension, inability to perform normal activities, syncope, dark pigmented areas on skin and mucous membrane, weight loss, vomiting, diarrhea, and very low or very high temperature.

Nursing diagnoses for the client with Addison's disease may include the following:

Nursing Diagnoses	Planning/Goals	Nursing Interventions
Deficient Fluid Volume related to low sodium level, vomiting, diarrhea, and increased renal losses	The client will regain normal fluid and electrolyte balance.	Monitor the client's vital signs, level of consciousness, intake and output, and weight. Administer IV fluids as ordered and encourage fluid intake.
Risk for Infection related to suppressed inflammatory response	The client will maintain normal temperature and leukocyte count and differential and use precautions to avoid or reduce risks of infection.	Monitor temperature every 4 hours unless elevated, then every 2 hours. Provide a private room with reverse or protective isolation as needed. Screen personnel and visitors for infection. Teach proper hand hygiene. Monitor laboratory test results for WBC and differential.

Evaluation Each goal must be evaluated to determine how it has been met by the client.

PHEOCHROMOCYTOMA

Pheochromocytoma, sometimes known as *chromaffin cell tumor*, is a rare disease characterized by **paroxysmal** (a symptom that begins and ends abruptly) or sustained hypertension caused by excessive secretion of epineph-rine and norepinephrine. Some medical experts estimate that about 0.5% of clients newly diagnosed with hypertension have pheochromocytoma. Although the tumor is generally benign, it can be malignant in 5% to 10% of the cases. It affects all races and both sexes. It is most common in females ages 20 to 50 years.

LIFE CYCLE CONSIDERATIONS

Pheochromocytoma

Pheochromocytoma is frequently diagnosed during pregnancy when the enlarged uterus puts pressure on the tumor, causing more frequent attacks. The attacks could prove fatal to both mother and fetus. Although there is an increased risk of spontaneous abortion, most fetal deaths occur during labor or immediately after delivery.

It is caused by a chromaffin cell tumor of the adrenal medulla, more commonly on the right side. Extraadrenal pheochromocytomas can also occur. Epinephrine overproduction occurs with the adrenal pheochromocytoma; however, norepinephrine overproduction is associated with both adrenal and extraadrenal pheochromocytoma. It is associated with a family history of pheochromocytoma or endocrine gland cancer. It is considered to be inherited on the autosomal-dominant gene in about 5% of the cases.

The classic triad of clinical manifestations is hypertension with diastolic pressure above 115 mm Hg, unrelenting headache, and profuse diaphoresis. Other clinical manifestations include palpitations, visual disturbances, nausea, or vomiting. These attacks may be triggered by activities or conditions that displace the abdominal contents, such as heavy lifting, exercise, bladder distention, or pregnancy. Severe attacks can be precipitated by administration of opiates, histamine, glucagon, and corticotropin. Some attacks may have no precipitating factor. Some other clinical manifestations are mild to moderate weight loss caused by increased metabolism and orthostatic hypotension when arising to an upright position. The client will have tachycardia. The actual tumor is rarely palpable; however, palpation could trigger a hypertensive attack.

The complications are similar to those of severe and persistent hypertension. These complications are stroke, retinopathy, heart disease, or irreversible kidney disease. The client with pheochromocytoma has an increased risk of severe complications or death during invasive diagnostic tests or surgery.

Although pheochromocytoma can be potentially fatal, the prognosis is good with treatment. About 90% of the clients are cured.

Medical–Surgical Management

Surgical

The treatment of choice is surgical removal of the tumor. Sometimes the adrenal gland is also removed. The blood pressure is monitored closely during the immediate postoperative period. The client may have hypotension, but hypertension is more common. About 10% of the clients are not candidates for surgery. They are treated with medications to lower the blood pressure.

Pharmacological

During acute hypertensive attacks, the drugs of choice are phentolamine mesylate (Regitine) or nitro-prusside sodium (Nipride). Phentolamine mesylate (Regitine) and phenoxybenzamine HCl (Dibenzyline) are alpha-adrenergic blocking agents. They are used to control hypertension before surgery or when surgery is contraindicated. The client should be warned about orthostatic hypotension and rise slowly from a supine position to an upright position. The client should not take over-the-counter drugs or alcohol.

Nitroprusside sodium (Nipride, Nitropress) acts on the vascular smooth muscle to cause peripheral vasodilation. The drug is given in an intravenous infusion. An electronic infusion device must be used to monitor the infusion rate. The client's blood pressure is used to titrate the infusion rate per the physician's orders.

Metyrosine (Demser) is used to block catecholamine synthesis. This drug must be continued for life if the tumor is inoperable. Ongoing medications include adrenergic blockers such as propranolol hydrochloride (Inderal), atenolol (Tenormin), prazosin HCl (Minipress), labetalol HCl (Normodyne), or nifedipine (Procardia), a calcium channel blocker. The client's blood pressure must be monitored frequently to determine the effectiveness of the medication.

Propranolol hydrochloride (Inderal) should not be stopped abruptly. The client should not smoke while taking this medication. Atenolol (Tenormin) may enhance the client's sensitivity to cold. Prazosin HCl (Minipress) should be taken on an empty stomach. The initial dose should be given at bedtime. The client should not use cough, cold, or allergy medications without the physician's knowledge. If the client is given parenteral labetalol HCl (Normodyne, Trandate), the client should remain supine for 3 hours to decrease the possibility of orthostatic hypotension. Nifedipine (Adalat, Procardia) should be protected from light and moisture and stored at room temperature. Over-the-counter medications should not be taken.

Diet

The diet should be high in protein with adequate calories. Stimulating foods such as aged cheeses and yogurt; caffeine-containing beverages such as coffee, tea, and soft drinks; and beer and red wine should be avoided (Smeltzer & Bare, 2002).

Nursing Management

The nurse should ask about heat intolerance, severe headaches during hypertensive crisis, anxiety, trouble sleeping, palpitations, nervousness, dizziness, paresthesias, and nausea. The client is assessed for dyspnea, tremors, diaphoresis, glycosuria, hyperglycemia, or dilated pupils. Frequently assess blood pressure, pulse, and respirations for elevations, and observe for signs of anxiety.

Summary

- The endocrine system is composed of glands at various body locations producing secretions (hormones) that directly enter the blood or lymph circulation.

CASE STUDY

Mr. Carnes, a 44-year-old African American male, is admitted to the medical unit from his physician's office. He reports that he has lost 18 pounds over the last month and has been very tired. He also reports symptoms of thirst, frequent urination, and blurred vision. His vital signs are: BP 166/92, P 88, R 16, T 99.2°F. Physical assessment reveals hot, dry, flushed skin. Laboratory exams reveal a blood glucose 490 mg/dL and urine negative for ketones. Mr. Carnes is a truck driver and leads a fairly sedentary lifestyle. History reveals that he is usually 30 to 35 pounds overweight, but has otherwise been in good health. He reports that his mother died from diabetes and renal failure, and an older brother was diagnosed as having type 2 diabetes three years ago.

The following questions will guide your development of a nursing care plan for this case study:

1. List physical symptoms that Mr. Carnes is experiencing that are suggestive of diabetes.
2. Based on history and laboratory values, would you expect Mr. Carnes to be diagnosed with type 1 or type 2 diabetes?
3. Which nursing diagnoses would you identify as priority for Mr. Carnes right now? List two.
4. Mr. Carnes is treated with IV fluids and insulin sliding scale until his blood glucose is stabilized. Describe what an insulin sliding scale is, and when it is used.
5. A 2,000-calorie ADA diet is ordered for Mr. Carnes. Mr. Carnes does not care to eat the apple that came on his breakfast tray and asks if he can exchange it for another serving of scrambled eggs. How would you respond to Mr. Carnes?
6. Mr. Carnes is being discharged and will continue to attend diabetic education classes at a local diabetic treatment center. Assuming Mr. Carnes is to continue on a diabetic diet and will be receiving mixed insulin injections, list the pertinent information Mr. Carnes will need to know about his disease and therapies related to:
   • Diabetes and symptoms of hyperglycemia
   • Role of exercise
   • Effects of diet
   • Self-monitoring blood glucose
   • Insulin injections/technique
   • Symptoms of hypoglycemia
   • Sick-day care
   • Long-term complications

• The endocrine system provides slower and longer-lasting control over various body activities and functions.
• A malfunction of any part of the endocrine system can result in a shift of homeostasis with far-reaching systemic reactions.
• Assessment of the endocrine system can be challenging because the glands are scattered. Negative findings are as important as positive findings.
• Diabetes is a complex chronic disease with multiple acute and chronic complications. It is a systemic disease caused by an imbalance between insulin supply and demand.
• A coordinated program of exercise, diet, and medications is used to achieve diabetic control. Persons with type 1 diabetes always require insulin therapy in addition to dietary control and an exercise program. Persons with type 2 diabetes are managed through diet and exercise and may or may not require oral hypoglycemic agents or insulin.
• The goal of diabetes management is enabling the diabetic to manage the disease by maintaining a blood glucose level within an acceptable range and thereby minimizing the incidence of acute and chronic complications.

• Regardless of disorder, the client should wear a Medic Alert bracelet and be aware that the treatment generally lasts a lifetime.

Review Questions

1. Mrs. Gavin tells the nurse that she is surprised that she developed diabetes at 40 years of age. The nurse knows that the development of diabetes in middle-aged people is most directly the result of:

   a. atherosclerosis.
   b. eating too much sugar.
   c. obesity.
   d. viral infection.

2. When teaching the diabetic client about mixing short- and longer-acting (NPH) insulin in the same syringe, the nurse should teach that:

   a. regular insulin should be drawn up first.
   b. the NPH insulin should be drawn up first.

c.   it does not matter which insulin is drawn up first because they will be mixed anyway.

d.   the two insulins do not mix and should be drawn up
and administered separately.

3.   Which of the following principles is used when planning
for a person with diabetes who is to undergo surgery?

a.   All insulin is withheld until surgery is over and the
client is eating.

b.   Insulin or oral hypoglycemics are given as usual.

c.   Sliding-scale insulin is used to regulate glucose levels during the operative period.

d.   Hyperglycemia poses the most serious danger to the
client during surgery.

4.   Which of the following nursing diagnoses would be most
appropriate for the client with diabetes insipidus?

a.   Alteration in growth and development related to increased growth hormone production

b.   Alteration in thought processes related to decreased
neurologic function

c.   Fluid volume deficit related to polyuria

d.   Hypothermia related to decreased metabolic rate

5.   Meticulous skin care is especially important for the client
with hyperthyroidism because of:

a.   diaphoresis from heat intolerance.

b.   edema from sodium and water retention.

c.   poor nutrition due to nausea and vomiting.

d.   pressure from immobility due to paralysis.

References/Suggested Readings

Anthony, M. (2003). Hypoglycemia. *Nursing2003, 33*(2), 88.

Bacoka, J. (2001). Thyroid storm. *Nursing2001, 31*(12), 88.

Bartol, T. (2002). Putting a patient with diabetes in the driver's
seat. *Nursing2002, 32*(2), 53–55.

Burton, M. (1997). Pheochromocytoma. *AJN, 97*(11), 57.

Caffrey, R. M. (2003). Are all syringes created equal? *AJN,
103*(6), 46–49.

Cameron, B. (2002). Making diabetes management routine.
AJN, 102(2), 26–32.

Centers for Disease Control and Prevention (CDC). (2002a).
National Diabetes fact sheet [Online]. Available:
www.cdc.gov/diabetes/pubs/estimates.htm

Centers for Disease Control and Prevention (CDC). (2002b).
National Diabetes fact sheet 2002 [Online]. Available:
www.cdc.gov/diabetes/pubs/general.htm

Chase, S. (1997). Oral hypoglycemics. *RN, 60*(12), 45–49.

Cincinnati, R., & Veliko, J. (2001). Oral medications. *RN, 64*(8),
30–36.

Clarke, K. (2002). No needles needed. *Nursing2002, 32*(5),
49–51.

Clayton, L., & Dilley, K. (1998). Cushing's syndrome. *AJN,
98*(7), 40–41.

Cypress, M. (2001). Acute complications. *RN, 64*(4), 26–31.

Daniels, R. (2002). *Delmar's Guide to Laboratory and Diagnostic
Tests.* Clifton Park, NY: Thomson Delmar Learning.

Depree, P. (1998). Lispro insulin. *Nursing98, 28*(11), 54–55.

Dochterman, J., & Bulechek, G. (2004). *Nursing Interventions
Classification (NIC)* (4th ed.). St. Louis, MO: Mosby.

Estes, M. E. Z. (2002). *Health Assessment & Physical
Examination* (2nd ed.). Clifton Park, NY: Thomson Delmar
Learning.

Fain, J. (2001). Lowering the boom on hyperglycemia.
Nursing2001, 31(8), 49–50.

Fain, J. (2003). Pump up your knowledge of insulin pumps.
Nursing2003, 33(6), 51–53.

5 tips for finger sticks. (1999). 5 tips for finger sticks.
Nursing99, 29(5), 59.

Fleming, D. (1999). Challenging traditional insulin injection
practices. *AJN, 99*(2), 72–74.

Flood, L., & Constance, A. (2002). Diabetes & exercise safety.
AJN, 102(6), 47–55.

Freeland, B. (1998). Diabetic ketoacidosis. *AJN, 98*(8), 52.

Goldberg, J. (2001). Nutrition and exercise. *RN, 64*(7), 34–39.

Halpin-Landry, J., & Goldsmith, S. (1999). Feet first: Diabetes
care. *AJN, 99*(2), 26–33.

Hardman, L., & Young, F. (2001). Combating hyperosmolar
hyperglycemic nonketotic syndrome. *Nursing2001, 31*(3),
32hn1–32hn4.

Holcomb, S. (2003). Detecting thyroid disease, part 1.
Nursing2003, 33(8), 32cc1–32cc4.

Hutchinson, C., & Peppard, C. (1998). Hypoglycemia.
Nursing98, 28(8), 68–69.

Knight, J. (1998). Inserting an insulin catheter. *Nursing98,
28*(2), 58–60.

LeMone, P., & Burke, K. M. (1999). *Medical–surgical nursing:
Critical thinking in client care* (2nd ed.). New York: Prentice
Hall.

Malchiodi, L. (2002). Thyroid storm. *AJN, 102*(5), 33–35.

McCance, K. L., & Huether, S. E. (2002). *Pathophysiology: The
biologic basis for disease in adults and children* (4th ed.). St.
Louis, MO: Mosby.

McConnell, E. (2002). Myths & Facts . . . about Addison's disease. *Nursing2002, 32*(8), 79.

McConnell, E. (2003). Myths & Facts . . . about diabetes insipidus. *Nursing2003, 33*(6), 84.

Monahan, F. D., & Neighbors, M. (1998). *Medical–surgical nursing: Foundations for clinical practice* (2d ed.). Philadelphia:
W. B. Saunders.

Moorhead, S., Johnson, M., & Maas, M. (2004). *Nursing
Outcomes Classification (NOC)* (3rd ed.). St. Louis, MO:
Mosby.

National Institute of Diabetes and Digestive and Kidney
Diseases (NIDDK). (2001). *Diabetes insipidus.* [Online].
Available: www.niddk.nih.gov/health/kidney/pubs/insipidus/
insipidus.htm

National Institute of Diabetes and Digestive and Kidney
Diseases (NIDDK). (2002). *Acromegaly.* [Online]. Available:
www.niddk.nih.gov/health/endo/pubs/acro/acro.htm

National Institutes of Health (NIH). (2002a). *Congenital hypothyroidism.* [Online]. Available: www.nlm.nih.gov/
medlineplus/ency/article/001193.htm

National Institutes of Health (NIH). (2002b). *Dilutional hyponatremia (SIADH).* [Online]. Available: www.nlm.nih.
gov/medlineplus/ency/article/00394.htm

National Institutes of Health (NIH). (2002c). *Hypothyroidism.*
[Online]. Available: www.nlm.nih.gov/medlineplus/ency/
article/000353.htm

Norris, J. (Senior Ed.). (1998). *Handbook of medical–surgical
nursing* (2d ed.). Springhouse, PA: Springhouse Corp.

North American Nursing Diagnosis Association. (2003).
Nursing Diagnoses: Definitions & Classification 2003–2004.
Philadelphia: Author.

Olohan, K., & Zappitelli, D. (2003). The insulin pump. *AJN,
103*(4), 48–56.

Pickar, G. D. (1999). *Dosage calculations* (6th ed.). Clifton Park, NY: Thomson Delmar Learning.

Plummer, E. S. (2001). Chronic complications. *RN, 64*(5), 34–40.

Robertson, C. (1998). When your patient is on an insulin pump. *RN, 61*(3), 30–33.

Robertson, C. (2001). The untold story of disease progression. *RN, 64*(3), 60–64.

Ruiz, E. (2001). Type 2 disease in children. *RN, 64*(10), 44–48.

Sachse, D. (2001). Acromegaly. *AJN, 101*(1), 69–77.

Sammer, C. (2001). How should you respond to hypoglycemia? *Nursing2001, 31*(7), 48–50.

Schori-Ahmed, D. (2003). Thyroid disease, *RN, 66*(6), 38–43.

Seley, J. (2003). Giving the fingers a rest. *AJN, 103*(3), 73–77.

Shelly, A. (2002). Elderly patients with diabetes. *AJN, 102*(2), 15–16.

Smeltzer, S. C., & Bare, B. G. (2002). *Brunner & Suddarth's textbook of medical–surgical nursing* (9th ed.). Philadelphia: Lippincott Williams & Wilkins.

Spratto, G. R., & Woods, A. L. (2004). *2004 PDR nurses drug handbook.* Clifton Park, NY: Thomson Delmar Learning.

Strowig, S. (2001). Insulin therapy. *RN, 64*(9), 38–44.

Strowig, S. M. (1995, June). Insulin therapy. *RN,* 30–37.

The Expert Committee on the Diagnosis and Classification of Diabetes Mellitus. (1997). Report of the expert committee on the diagnosis and classification of diabetes mellitus. *Diabetes Care, 20*(7), 1183–1197.

Thibodeau, G. A., & Patton, K. T. (2001). *The human body in health & disease* (3rd ed.). St. Louis, MO: Mosby.

Tkacs, N. (2002). Hypoglycemia unawareness. *AJN, 102*(2), 34–39.

U.S. Department of Health and Human Services, National Center for Chronic Disease Control and Prevention, Division of Diabetes Translation (1992). *Diabetes in the United States: A strategy for prevention.* Washington, DC: U.S. Public Health Service.

Valentine, V. (2002). Using a laser to make a point. *Nursing2002, 32*(10), 56–57.

Walpert, N. (1998). The highs and lows of autoimmune thyroid disease. *Nursing98, 28*(12), 58–60.

Watts, S., Anselmo, J., & Smith, M. (2003). Combating hypoglycemia in the hospital and at home. *Nursing2003, 33*(3), 32hn1–32hn5.

Williams, J. (2001). We make foot exams a priority. *RN, 64*(5), 40–41.

Young, J. (1999). Myxedema coma. *Nursing99, 29*(5), 59.

Resources

American Association of Diabetes Educators, 100 West Monroe Street, Suite 400, Chicago, IL 60603, 800-338-3633, www.aadenet.org

American Diabetes Association, Attn: National Call Center, 1701 North Beauregard Street, Alexandria, VA 22311, 800-342-2383, www.diabetes.org

American Dietetic Association, 216 W. Jackson Boulevard, Chicago, IL 60606-6995, 800-877-1600, 312-899-0040, www.eatright.org

Juvenile Diabetes Foundation International, 120 Wall Street, New York, NY 10005-4001, 800-533-2873, www.jdrf.org

National Institutes of Health, 9000 Rockville Pike, Bethesda, MD 20892, 301-496-4000, www.nih.gov/science/campus

National Organization for Rare Disorders, Inc. (NORD), 55 Kenosia Avenue, P. O. Box 1968, Danbury, CT 06813-1968, 800-999-6673, www.rarediseases.org

The Diabetes Insipidus Foundation, Inc., 4533 Ridge Drive, Baltimore, MD 21229, 410-247-3953, http://diabetesinsipidus.maxinter.net

UNIT
13

Nursing Care of the Client: Reproductive and Sexual Health

Chapter 41
Reproductive System

Chapter 42
Sexually Transmitted Diseases

REPRODUCTIVE SYSTEM

MAKING THE CONNECTION

Refer to the following chapters to increase your understanding of the female and male reproductive systems:

Basic Nursing
- **Wellness Concepts**
- **Fluid, Electrolyte, and Acid–Base Balance**
- **Assessment**
- **Diagnostic Tests**

Adult Health Nursing
- **Oncology**
- **Cardiovascular System**
- **Urinary System**

- **Endocrine System**
- **Sexually Transmitted Diseases**
- **The Older Adult**

Basic Procedures
- **Urine Collection—Closed Drainage System**

Intermediate Procedures
- **Irrigating a Urinary Catheter**

Review: Delmar's Anatomy & Physiology
    CD-ROM: Genitourinary System

LEARNING OBJECTIVES

Upon completion of this chapter, you should be able to:
- **Define key terms.**
- **Identify the anatomy of the reproductive systems.**
- **Describe the hormonal mechanisms that regulate the reproductive functions, including the menstrual cycle.**
- **Interpret diagnostic tests for disorders of the reproductive systems.**
- **List the changes in the reproductive systems that occur with aging.**
- **Discuss common problems of the reproductive system.**
- **Differentiate between impotence and infertility.**
- **Discuss contraceptive methods, including actions, side effects, and client teaching.**
- **Utilize the nursing process to develop a care plan for a client with a reproductive system disorder.**

KEY TERMS

abortion	nocturia
amenorrhea	oligomenorrhea
contraception	orchiectomy
cystocele	polymenorrhea
dysmenorrhea	post-void residual
dyspareunia	priapism
endometriosis	prolapsed uterus
hematuria	rectocele
hesitancy	spermatogenesis
impotence	stent
infertility	tenesmus
menopause	urethrocele
menorrhagia	urethrostomy
metrorrhagia	vasectomy

INTRODUCTION

Through modern technology, current medical and nursing knowledge, and health education programs, laypersons have access to much information about their bodies and their reproductive systems. Yet, individuals continue to be seriously affected by health disorders. In some instances they may lack knowledge of how to detect signs and symptoms of these disorders. Often, they simply delay routine medical examinations or avoid seeking medical treatment. In addition, individuals may have difficulty discussing symptoms related to their reproductive system.

Routine health care must be maintained and early diagnosis made in order to reduce the incidence and seriousness of reproductive health disorders. These goals can be facilitated with skilled nursing assessment and client education.

For most people, the reproductive system functions without problems throughout life. For others, minor and major disorders require treatment. Some of the problems are related to alterations in structure; others are related more to altered physiology of the reproductive system. This chapter discusses disorders of the reproductive systems by applying the steps of the nursing process.

ANATOMY AND PHYSIOLOGY REVIEW

The female and male reproductive systems consist of external and internal structures and organs.

External Female Structures

The area known as the vulva includes the external female structures, such as the mons pubis, labia majora, labia minora, and clitoris. The Bartholin glands and Skene's glands, located proximal to the vaginal opening, produce and secrete lubricating fluids. The labia majora and minora serve as protective barriers for the softer internal structures. The clitoris, located proximal to the mons pubis and superior to the urinary meatus, plays a role in sexual arousal in the female and is considered analogous to the male penis. During foreplay, the clitoris engorges and stimulates orgasm or climax in the female. It is covered by a small hood called the prepuce. The perineum is the distal portion of the vulva, located below the vaginal opening and superior to the anus.

The breasts are also a part of the external female reproductive system (Figure 41-1). Their external structures include the nipple, areola, and Montgomery tubercles. The nipples have several openings, or duct, that lead from the lactiferous glands inside the breast. Milk is ejected through the ducts when the infant sucks on the breast. The areola, or the darker area around the nipple, becomes darker in response to the increased hormone levels during pregnancy. Small, mole-like, raised areas around the areola are the Montgomery tubercles. These glands produce a lubricant that keeps the nipple soft and supple.

Internal Female Structures

The vagina is an elastic, tubelike structure leading from the outside of the female body to the cervix. Approximately 2 to 3 inches long, it contains many rugae that allow it to stretch during intercourse and also permit the passage of the baby during delivery. The pH environment of the vagina is normally acidic, providing protection from microorganisms that could cause infections.

The uterus is a 3-inch-long, 2-inch-wide, 1-inch-thick hollow, muscular structure, as seen in Figure 41-2.

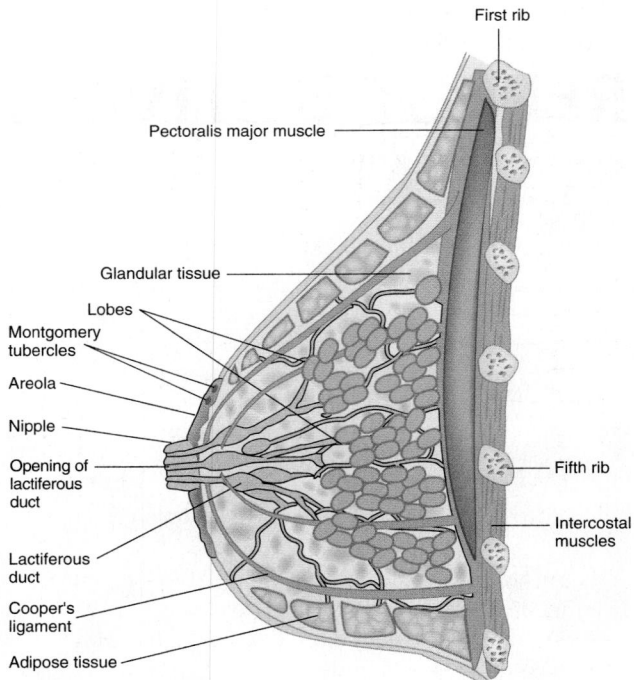

Figure 41-1 *The Female Breast*

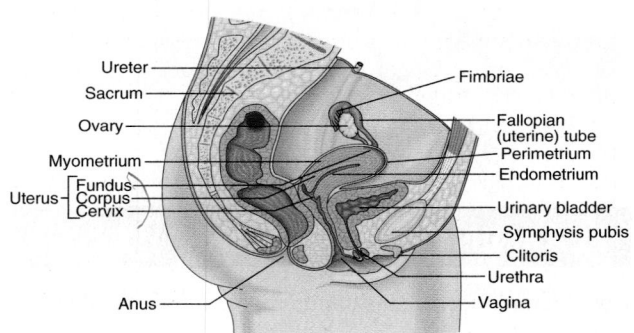

Figure 41-2 *The Female Reproductive System*

The top is the fundus, the middle is the body (corpus), and the lower portion is the cervix. Four sets of ligaments hold the uterus in its normal anteverted (forward) position and permit it the freedom to grow and move during pregnancy. The uterus has three distinct layers. The innermost layer is the endometrium, which sloughs with menstruation each month. The middle layer is the myometrium, which is constructed of many muscle fibers that are interwoven for strength, stretch, and contractility. The outer layer is the perimetrium, which is an external serous membrane covering.

The fallopian tubes are connected to the uterus on either side. They are continuous with the mucous membrane lining of the endometrium on the inside. Billions of cilia line each fallopian tube and make a sweeping motion toward the uterus, especially at the time of ovulation. This sweeping action moves the

Figure 41-3 *Sequence and Approximate Time of Events in the Menstrual Cycle*

Figure 41-4 *The Male Reproductive System*

Male Reproductive Structures

The male reproductive organs and associated structures are illustrated in Figure 41-4. The scrotum is a fleshy structure suspended below the perineum, anterior to the anus. It is divided into two parts, each of which contains a testis, an epididymis, and a portion of the spermatic cord (vas deferens). The left side of the scrotum is usually lower than the right because the left spermatic cord is often longer.

The testes, two smooth, oval endocrine glands, are suspended in the scrotum. This location helps maintain proper temperature and also protects the testes from trauma. Certain cells of the epithelium lining the seminiferous tubules of the testes produce half a billion sperm each day **(spermatogenesis).** They also secrete the androgenic (causing masculinization) hormone testosterone. Spermatogenesis is regulated by follicle-stimulating hormone (FSH), produced by the anterior pituitary gland. The production of testosterone is regulated by luteinizing hormone (LH), also produced by the anterior pituitary gland. After the sperm mature in the epididymis, they travel through the vas (ductus) deferens, a long tube attached to the epididymis. The vas deferens, along with associated nerves and blood vessels, forms the spermatic cord.

The vas deferens travels up and around the bladder and carries sperm from the epididymis to the seminal vesicle, a small pouch that produces secretions that, when mixed with sperm and prostatic fluid, form semen.

The prostate is an encapsulated gland that encircles the proximal portion of the urethra. The prostatic fossa, a depression on the cranial border of the prostate, allows entry of the ejaculatory ducts. Within the prostate is a cluster of 30 to 50 tubuloalveolar glands that secrete prostatic fluid. The prostate gland is of clinical significance because as men age, it is a common site for malignant disease or benign enlargement that can cause urethral obstruction.

The penis is a cylindrical organ through which urine is passed and semen is ejaculated. Half of the penis is located within the body. The external half of the penis is flaccid, unless the male is sexually aroused, at which time it becomes erect because of engorgement with blood. A fold of skin, the prepuce, surrounds the tip of the penis in the uncircumcised male.

ovum along the path toward the uterus. The movement may also impede the progress of the sperm, which must swim upstream against the downward current produced by the cilia.

The cervix is the lower portion of the uterus and extends into the vaginal vault. Like the vagina, the cervix has muscle layers that allow it to stretch to a diameter of at least 10 cm (about 4 inches) during delivery.

An almond-shaped ovary, about 2 inches long and 1 inch wide, is located within the broad ligament on either side of the uterus, just below the fimbriae, the fingerlike projections at the distal end of the fallopian tubes. The ovaries contain all of the ova (eggs) that a woman will have from puberty until menopause. Each month, the ovary responds to hormonal signals from the anterior pituitary gland to ripen one or more ova. Follicle-stimulating hormone (FSH) is released by the anterior pituitary and sends a message to the ovary to release estrogen, which causes the ovum to ripen and enlarge. The entire first part of the cycle is known as the proliferative phase.

Luteinizing hormone (LH) is then released. LH triggers a chain of events that stimulates the ovary to release the ovum. This point in the menstrual cycle is called ovulation. Another hormone, progesterone, causes the glands and blood vessels of the endometrial lining to grow and thicken in preparation for implantation of a fertilized ovum. If fertilization does not occur, the progesterone level decreases, the endometrium sloughs off, and the woman experiences menstruation. If fertilization does occur, the progesterone level remains elevated to ensure the optimal environment for implantation of the zygote about 6 to 8 days after fertilization. Figure 41-3 illustrates the menstrual cycle.

TABLE 41-1   COMMON DIAGNOSTIC TESTS FOR REPRODUCTIVE SYSTEM DISORDERS

Laboratory Tests
- Alpha-fetoprotein (AFP)
- Cultures
- Human chorionic gonadotropin (hCG)
- Pap smear
- Prostate-specific antigen (PSA)
- Prostatic smear
- Serum alkaline phosphatase
- Serum calcium
- Semen analysis
- Segmented bacteriologic localization culture

Radiologic Tests
- Dynamic infusion cavernosometry and cavernosography (DICC)
- Hysterosalpingogram
- Mammography

Surgical Tests
- Breast biopsy
- Dilation & curettage (D&C)
- Endometrial biopsy
- Laparoscopy
- Prostatic biopsy
- Testicular biopsy

Other Tests
- Colposcopy
- Nocturnal tumescence penile monitoring
- Pelvic examination
- Schiller test
- Ultrasound

COMMON DIAGNOSTIC TESTS

Commonly used diagnostic tests for clients with symptoms of reproductive system disorders are listed in Table 41-1.

INFLAMMATORY DISORDERS

Inflammatory disorders discussed include pelvic inflammatory disease, endometriosis, vaginitis, toxic shock syndrome, and epididymitis/orchitis/prostatitis.

PELVIC INFLAMMATORY DISEASE

Pelvic inflammatory disease (PID) is an inflammatory process involving pathogenic invasion of the fallopian tubes (salpingitis) or ovaries (oophoritis), or both, along with vascular and supporting structures within the pelvis, except the uterus. Pathogenic microorganisms such as gonococcus, streptococcus, staphylococcus, and herpes simplex virus II, may cause PID. Infections are usually ascending by nature; that is, the pathogens are introduced into the reproductive system from outside and travel upward from the vagina to the fallopian tubes and then out into the pelvis. Risk factors associated with the incidence of PID include multiple sexual partners, frequent intercourse, IUDs (intrauterine contraceptive devices), and childbirth.

The symptoms of PID include a low-grade fever, pelvic pain, abdominal pain, a "bearing down" backache, a foul-smelling vaginal discharge, nausea and vomiting, **dysmenorrhea** (painful menstruation), **dyspareunia** (painful intercourse), and intense pelvic tenderness upon examination. Peritonitis or pelvic abscesses may develop as complications of PID if the pathogens spread into the pelvic cavity. Future **infertility** (inability or diminished ability to produce offspring) can be related to scarring and strictures of the fallopian tubes, which develop from the chronic inflammatory process within the pelvis. These problems have been associated with ectopic pregnancies because the fertilized ovum becomes trapped inside the fallopian tube before it can complete its trip to the uterus.

PID is often diagnosed during a pelvic examination. Vaginal and cervical cultures are obtained at the time of the exam to determine the causative agent. A pelvic ultrasound may be ordered to rule out other causes of pelvic pain. Instruct the client on the purpose of the procedures and any special preparations that may be required, such as having a full bladder.

Medical–Surgical Management
Medical

The client who is not acutely ill from PID may be treated as an outpatient at home with oral antibiotics and bed rest, unless the infection is herpes simplex virus II. Clients with herpes simplex II infections may require more intensive care in the hospital with IV antibiotic therapy. The physician may also order medicated vaginal suppositories for the vaginal discharge. The acutely ill client may require hospitalization for IV antibiotic therapy.

Surgical

If the inflammation is extensive, or if medical treatment is not successful, the client may require a hysterectomy.

Pharmacological

Antibiotics used may include doxycycline monohydrate (Vibramycin) or metronidazole (Flagyl). IV fluids are frequently administered to promote adequate hydration.

Activity

During hospitalization, the client is placed on bed rest with bathroom privileges. A semi-Fowler's position is preferred because it will facilitate drainage of the pelvis. If vaginal suppositories are used, the client should lie in a supine position for 30 minutes.

Inserting Vaginal Suppositories

- Have the client wash her hands, then cleanse the vulva with a mild soap and warm water to remove any external discharge.
- Client should lie down in a supine position with her knees flexed.
- With one hand, the client can separate the labia and gently insert the suppository high inside the vagina.
- The client should remain supine for a minimum of 30 minutes to ensure adequate absorption of the medication through the vaginal mucosa.

Nursing Management

Support the client with a nonjudgmental attitude. Maintain client in semi-Fowler's position to facilitate drainage. Monitor vital signs and I&O. Teach client proper pericare and hygiene and hand hygiene.

NURSING PROCESS

Assessment

Subjective Data

Obtain information about the client's sexual activity, including the number of partners. Unprotected intercourse is the most frequent method of entry for the microorganisms that cause PID. Also include the client's history of **contraception** (measures taken to prevent pregnancy), previous vaginal infections and treatments, obstetrical history, and normal hygiene practices such as douching and tampon use. Description of nagging pelvic pain and a low-grade fever are often expressed.

Objective Data

Assess for an elevated temperature, flushed, dry skin, the presence of a malodorous vaginal discharge, and positive vaginal or cervical cultures.

Nursing diagnoses for a client with pelvic inflammatory disease may include the following:

Nursing Diagnoses	Planning/Goals	Nursing Interventions
Acute Pain, related to inflammation of the pelvic structures caused by invasion of pathogens	Using a pain rating scale of 0 to 10, the client will report that her pain has decreased.	Assess client's pain level every 4 hours, noting the location, duration, sensation, intensity, and factors that increase or decrease the pain. Administer analgesics as ordered.
Deficient Knowledge, related to the etiology of the pelvic inflammatory process, treatment regimen, self-care, and preventive measures	The client will follow prescribed treatment regimen, self-care, and preventive measures.	If suppositories are ordered, instruct the client in the proper method of insertion. Provide instructions to the client and partner (if available) about the causes of PID and ways to prevent the inflammation.
		Teach proper pericare and hygiene, especially hand hygiene before and after changing sanitary pads. Change sanitary pads every 3 to 4 hours.
		Encourage client to make time for rest periods during the acute phase of the inflammation and to avoid strenuous activities such as straining or heavy lifting.
		Instruct client about pelvic rest, which includes no douching, tampons, or intercourse.
		Advise client to wear underpants with a cotton crotch.
		Teach client to cleanse the perineal area from front to back after each voiding or bowel movement.
		Discuss and encourage the use of safe sexual practices and the use of barrier contraceptives to prevent recurrence of PID symptoms.
		Encourage client to make follow-up appointment.
	The client will contact her health care provider for follow-up and if her symptoms persist, worsen, or return.	Encourage client to notify the NP or physician at the first sign of PID symptoms. Advise client to monitor her own temperature, upon discharge, twice daily for 2 weeks and notify the physician or NP if the temperature increases or remains elevated.
Hyperthermia, related to physiologic responses to the inflammatory or infectious process	The client's temperature will return to normal range after the initiation of therapy.	Monitor client's vital signs every 4 hours.
		Administer antipyretic and antibiotic as ordered by the physician.

Evaluation Each goal must be evaluated to determine how it has been met by the client.

DNC (handwritten)

ENDOMETRIOSIS

Endometriosis is the growth of endometrial tissue, the normal lining of the uterus, outside of the uterus within the pelvic cavity. It occurs most frequently in women 30 years and older and tends to be familial. It predominantly affects Caucasian females who have not given birth and is most common among the higher socioeconomic population. Endometriosis has been called the "career woman's disorder," because it is often diagnosed in the late twenties or thirties when the working woman makes plans for childbearing.

The endometrial tissue implants itself on other pelvic structures (Figure 41-5). Two of the most common areas for endometrial implants are the pouch of Douglas and the ovaries. The tissue implants respond to the monthly hormonal changes in the same way as the endometrial tissue inside the uterus does. Bleeding of the implants during the menses results in the formation of adhesions and scar tissue. The endometriosis appears as brownish or black "powder burns" or larger lesions. If the endometriosis becomes encapsulated in an ovarian cyst it is called a "chocolate cyst."

The disease appears to be progressive and has a tendency to be recurrent. Some women with minimal endometriosis experience severe monthly symptoms, such as lower backache, painful intercourse, a feeling of heaviness on the pelvis, and spotting. Other women have a more extensive disease but have minimal symptoms. Thus the amount of endometriosis present may or may not be correlated with the severity of the client's symptoms.

Endometriosis is one cause of female infertility because of the amount of scar tissue and adhesions around the pelvic organs, ligaments, and fallopian tubes. Pregnancy inhibits the growth and bleeding of the endometrial implants because ovulation and menstruation are suppressed.

Medical–Surgical Management

Medical

Endometriosis may be tentatively diagnosed by palpation of endometrial implants within the pelvis. To confirm the diagnosis, laparoscopy, performed under general anesthesia, is the best method of diagnosis by direct visualization of the pelvic structures. Consideration for treatment depends on the client's age and desire for future childbearing. Sometimes pregnancy relieves the symptoms even after delivery.

Surgical

The older multigravida who is experiencing severe, debilitating symptoms that affect her lifestyle and normal functions, role, or activity may desire a hysterectomy. If the lesions are large or extensive, a laparotomy may be performed for adequate removal; however, if the implants are small and scattered, cauterization or laser vaporization may be most desirable. Lysis of pelvic adhesions would be done at the same time.

Pharmacological

The goals of pharmacological therapy are to suppress ovulation and menstruation, reduce symptoms, and cause the implants to shrink. Medications used in the treatment of endometriosis must effectively suppress the monthly hypothalamic-pituitary-ovarian hormonal stimulation of ovulation. Some medications act on the body as "pseudopregnancy" agents that produce anovulation, breast tenderness, nausea, weight gain, and hirsutism. Other hormonal therapies cause a temporary medically induced menopause state. Oral contraceptives may be administered continuously. Nafarelin acetate (Synarel) is a nasally administered gonadotropin analog that inhibits cyclic hormone release. Danazol (Danocrine) is an androgen hormone that must be taken continuously for at least 6 to 8 months. This medication inhibits the release of gonadotropin. The resulting **amenorrhea** (absence of menstruation) will suppress the growth of the endometrial tissue and is used in moderate to severe cases of endometriosis. Occasionally, Danocrine is given after surgical removal or cauterization of the endometriosis to relieve symptoms from residual disease.

All medications used to treat endometriosis cause mild to moderate side effects that may affect the client's desire to take them or her compliance with continuous usage. Examples of problems that may be experienced include oily skin, fluid retention, weight gain, acne, hot flashes, metrorrhagia, mastalgia, and depression.

NURSING PROCESS

Assessment

Subjective Data

Obtain a description of the pelvic pain, which increases at the time of menstruation. The client may voice concerns about dyspareunia, pelvic discomfort with intercourse. This may result in marital tension if the client avoids sexual intimacy to reduce her pain. Be alert to what the client says as well as what is left unsaid. The client may describe prolonged, excessive menstrual periods that are getting closer and closer together.

Pouch of Douglas
Umbilicus
Sigmoid
Ovary
Utero-ovarian ligament
Rectus muscle
Fallopian tube
Utero-sacral ligament
Round ligament
Uterus
Bladder
Recto-vaginal septum
Labia minora

Figure 41-5 *Common Sites of Endometriosis*

Another sign, although not as significant, is pain with defecation during the menstrual period.

Also note the onset of menses, regularity of cycles, and any changes that client has noted in the frequency, comfort, duration, and amount of menstrual flow. Note the onset of the client's symptoms in relationship to the menstrual cycle, the severity as reported by the client, any alterations in lifestyle related to the pain or other symptoms, and the client's future plans for childbearing.

Objective Data

The nurse's role is usually focused on collecting subjective data from the client interview and assisting the physician during actual procedures.

Nursing Management

Encourage the client to express her concerns and fears. Teach the client about prescribed medications. Emphasize the importance of regular checkups and to report any abnormal vaginal bleeding.

Nursing diagnoses for a client with endometriosis may include the following:

- *Pain* related to bleeding from endometrial implants in the pelvic cavity
- *Anxiety* related to treatment options, possible side effects, and infertility
- *Ineffective Sexuality Patterns,* or *Sexual Dysfunction,* related to altered body function or structure (painful intercourse)
- *Situational Low Self-Esteem,* related to the inability to conceive

VAGINITIS

Several common types of vaginitis are caused by bacteria, protozoa, viruses, and yeasts. The vaginal mucosa is normally protected by an acid mantle. The acidic (pH less than 5.0) environment inhibits the growth of many pathogenic microorganisms. Because the vaginal opening is close to the external environment, microorganisms have an opportunity to invade the reproductive tract. Some organisms that cause vaginitis are transmitted to the female from the male partner during sexual contact. Natural protective barriers may vary with the fluctuating hormonal levels during the woman's monthly cycle because the hormones affect the vaginal pH. At ovulation, the vaginal pH becomes slightly less acidic because of the high level of estrogen. Times when the woman's system has a lower estrogen level, such as immediately after the menses and after menopause, are times when there is a higher risk for infection because the epithelium is less active, no glycogen is present, and the pH may be as high as 7.0.

Diagnosis is made after performing a vaginal examination and obtaining a sample of the vaginal discharge. When the client contacts the physician or nurse practitioner to report symptoms of vaginitis, the nurse should instruct her to avoid douching or using tampons before being examined because douching will wash away the discharge needed to be examined and tampons will absorb it.

Common types of vaginitis include candidiasis caused by *Candida albicans* (a fungus), trichomoniasis caused by *Trichomonas vaginalis* (a protozoan), *Gardnerella vaginalis* (a bacterium), and *Chlamydia trachomatis* (a parasite). Other causes of vaginitis may include streptococcus, staphylococcus, gonococcus, and herpes simplex II. Usually the symptoms depend on the causative agent. The client's description of her symptoms along with the examination of the discharge help confirm the diagnosis. Most infections have a characteristic discharge and irritation with burning or itching that may be internal, external, or both.

Predisposing factors for candidiasis, also called monilia, may include obesity, diabetes, pregnancy, oral contraceptives, antibiotics, bubble baths, and frequent douching. Many of these factors alter the pH of the vagina. Symptoms include a thick, white, cheesy or curdlike discharge with a musty, sweet odor, accompanied by vaginal or vulvar itching and irritation. Upon examination, the vaginal mucosa will have patches of white discharge present. If the patches are scraped off, the tissue underneath will appear reddened and may bleed. Externally, the vulva may be reddened and edematous. The client may have scratches from attempting to ease the itching.

The preferred treatment is vaginal application of antifungal creams or suppositories such as miconazole (Monistat), clotrimazole (Mycelex-G, Gyne-Lotrimin), or nystatin (Mycostatin). Alternative therapies include douching with white vinegar solution (1 tablespoon/1 pint of water) twice a day for a week. This treatment restores the acid balance of the vagina and washes away the *Candida albicans*. Eating cultured yogurt with active acidophilus or applying the yogurt directly to the labia helps restore the normal bacteria and protective mechanisms in the vagina.

Trichomoniasis is frequently passed from partner to partner during intercourse. A copious green-yellow, foul-smelling, frothy vaginal discharge is characteristic. It may produce itching or external burning and irritation. Metronidazole (Flagyl) should be taken orally by both partners.

Flagyl is normally contraindicated in the first trimester of pregnancy, so obtaining a menstrual history or a pregnancy test may be needed before administering this medication. Inform the client and her partner to avoid any alcohol intake during therapy. Flagyl causes a strong antabuse-like effect, which results in severe nausea and vomiting. Clients should read labels on over-the-counter medications being taken concurrently with the Flagyl because many preparations contain alcohol bases.

Instruct the client and her partner to abstain from intercourse during therapy and to finish all of the medication.

Gardnerella vaginalis often produces a gray-white vaginal discharge with a strong fishy odor or is asymptomatic. If itching or burning is present, it may suggest another microorganism. For the treatment of *Gardnerella,* and other bacterial vaginitis, the physician may order Flagyl or an oral antibiotic such as tetracycline hydrochloride (Achromycin) or ampicillin (Omnipen). Sulfa-based creams such as Sultrin, Triple Sulfa, and AVC may be used vaginally in conjunction with the oral

CLIENT TEACHING

Ways to Decrease Risk of Vaginitis

- Wear cotton-crotch underwear.
- Avoid sitting in a wet bathing suit in warm weather for long periods.
- Seek prompt medical attention at the first signs of infection.
- Eat an 8-oz container of yogurt with active cultures daily while taking antibiotics.

medications once or twice a day for 6 to 14 days to completely treat this type of infection.

Chlamydial vaginitis infections are often asymptomatic but have been associated with infertility problems. A culture of vaginal secretions is necessary to specifically identify the organism. The treatment is usually oral antibiotics for at least 7 days. A repeat culture is recommended following treatment to ensure that the parasites have been eradicated.

Postmenopausal vaginitis (atrophic) is caused by a decreased level of estrogen in the vaginal tissue. The client may describe painful intercourse (dyspareunia), itching, burning, or irritation. Estrogen replacement therapy often relieves the symptoms of this type of vaginitis. The medication may be administered orally, vaginally, or by transdermal patch.

NURSING PROCESS

Assessment

Subjective Data

Obtain information from the client regarding the nature of her symptoms, the onset, menstrual history, contraceptive methods, recent or current use of antibiotics or other medications, recent illness, diabetes mellitus, sexual history, pregnancy history, usual hygiene practices such as douching, deodorant sprays, bubble baths, wearing of pantyhose, type of underwear, and use of deodorized tampons or pads.

Objective Data

Observe the vaginal discharge and note any odor. Vaginal or vulvar irritation and possible scratches may be seen.

Nursing Management

Emphasize the significance of hand hygiene before and after applying vaginal medications. Advise client that her sexual partner should also be treated.

Nursing diagnoses for a client with vaginitis, regardless of the etiology, may include the following:

- *Deficient **K**nowledge,* related to the origin of the infection, prevention, and treatment options

- *Impaired **T**issue Integrity,* related to the presence of vaginal discharge, itching, or irritation
- *Sexual **D**ysfunction,* related to discomfort during intercourse or fear of transmitting the infection to the sexual partner
- *Risk for Impaired **S**kin Integrity,* related to internal and external irritation from discharge and itching

TOXIC SHOCK SYNDROME

Toxic shock syndrome (TSS) is a condition most often associated with *Staphylococcus aureus,* which enters the bloodstream. A strong relationship has been found between the use of tampons (especially superabsorbent) during menstruation and the onset of TSS symptoms. It has been hypothesized that the fibers from the tampon lower the level of magnesium in the woman's body and, therefore, produce a favorable environment for the growth of pathogenic microorganisms. The condition was first diagnosed in the mid-1970s, and the incidence increased throughout the 1980s. A high percentage of women who are affected by TSS are younger than age 30. TSS can also occur in nonmenstruating women and men.

The client may present with a temperature of 102°F or greater, vomiting, diarrhea, progressive hypotension, and flulike symptoms of malaise, muscle soreness, sore throat, and headache. There may be a macular erythematous (flat, red) rash followed in 1 to 2 weeks by peeling of the palms and soles. Disorientation may occur from the release of toxins and dehydration.

Medical–Surgical Management

Medical

Blood, urine, genitourinary, and throat cultures may be obtained and are usually negative except for *Staphylococcus aureus.* The goals of treatment are focused on controlling the falling blood pressure, replacing fluid volume, halting the infectious process, and maintaining adequate ventilation efforts. IV fluids are administered per the physician's order. The client may require mechanical ventilation and CPAP (continuous positive airway pressure).

Pharmacological

Broad-spectrum antibiotic therapy is recommended. Culture and sensitivity tests will indicate which type of antibiotic is best. Examples may include dicloxacillin sodium (Dynapen), clexacillin sodium (Tegopen), nafcillin

CLIENT TEACHING

TSS and Tampon Use

Instruct client to avoid tampon use for several cycles. If she chooses to use tampons in the future, they should be changed every 2 to 3 hours. Avoid the superabsorbent types.

sodium (Nafcil), and methicillin sodium (Staphcillin). The medication regimen is continued for at least 2 weeks to ensure control of the pathogens.

Activity

Bed rest is usually prescribed.

Nursing Management

Maintain client on prescribed bed rest. Administer antipyretics and antibiotics as ordered. Monitor vital signs, I&O, and skin turgor. Encourage oral fluid intake.

NURSING PROCESS

Assessment

Subjective Data

Obtain information on recent use of tampons, length of time tampon is left in before changing, sore throat, headache, myalgia, and fatigue.

Objective Data

Assess erythematous rash, edema, peeling of palms and soles, hypotension, level of consciousness, nonpurulent conjunctivitis, and hyperemia of vagina and oropharynx.

Nursing diagnoses for a client with toxic shock syndrome may include the following:

Nursing Diagnoses	Planning/Goals	Nursing Interventions
Hyperthermia, related to inflammatory process	The client will have normal-range temperature within 48 hours.	Administer antipyretics as ordered. Give cooling sponge bath. Encourage oral fluids as tolerated.
Deficient Fluid Volume, related to diarrhea, vomiting, fever, and decreased intake	The client will have normal fluid and electrolyte balance within 24 hours.	Administer intravenous fluids as ordered. Encourage oral fluids if client is not vomiting. Monitor I&O. Administer antiemetic and antidiarrheal medications as ordered. Assess skin turgor and mucous membranes.
Risk for Impaired Skin Integrity, related to dehydration and effects of circulating toxins	The client will maintain skin integrity.	Encourage or assist with position change every 2 hours. Provide or assist with personal hygiene, especially after diarrhea. Assess bony prominences for reddened areas.

Evaluation Each goal must be evaluated to determine how it has been met by the client.

EPIDIDYMITIS/ ORCHITIS/PROSTATITIS

Epididymitis can be a sterile or nonsterile inflammation of the epididymis. A sterile inflammation may be caused by direct injury or reflux of urine down the vas deferens. Urinary reflux that is related to strain exerted by a male while his bladder is full can be caused by lifting heavy objects or doing strenuous exercises. Nonsterile inflammation may occur as a complication of gonorrhea, chlamydia, mumps, tuberculosis, prostatitis, or urethritis. Prolonged use of an indwelling catheter or an invasive procedure can also lead to nonsterile inflammation.

Signs and symptoms of epididymitis include sudden, severe pain in the scrotum, scrotal swelling, fever, dysuria, and pyuria. Treatment includes bed rest, antibiotics, scrotal support (Figure 41-6), and ice compresses to the area. Bilateral epididymitis can cause sterility.

Figure 41-6 *A Bellevue Bridge for Scrotal Support*

Untreated epididymitis leads quickly to testicular tissue necrosis, septicemia, and death.

Orchitis is an inflammation of the testes that most often occurs as a complication of a bloodborne infection originating in the epididymis. Other causes of orchitis include gonorrhea, trauma, surgical manipulation, and tuberculosis and mumps that occur after puberty. In most instances, both testes are involved, and often sterility results. In orchitis, unilateral involvement does not cause sterility. Signs and symptoms of orchitis include sudden scrotal pain with pain radiating to the inguinal canal, scrotal edema, chills, fever, nausea, and vomiting. Treatment includes bed rest, scrotal support, and ice to the area.

Prostatitis, an inflammation of the prostate, is a common complication of urethritis caused by chlamydia or gonorrhea. Infecting organisms may reach the genital tract by direct spread through the urethra or may be borne by blood or lymph. The condition may be acute or chronic, with the chronic form leading to development of fibrotic tissue. This fibrotic tissue causes the prostate to harden, so prostatitis may be difficult to differentiate from prostate cancer. It may take 3 to 6 months for the granulomatous form to resolve. Signs and symptoms of prostatitis include perineal pain, fever, dysuria, and urethral discharge.

Medical–Surgical Management

Medical

When it is suspected that the client currently has urethritis, he should not be catheterized. The infection spreads rapidly to the genital organs because of the trauma of catheterization and the possible spread of bacteria from the nonsterile distal part of the urethra. The physician may order that segmented bacteriologic localization cultures be obtained.

Pharmacological

Treatment of epididymitis and orchitis includes antibiotics and injection of procaine around the spermatic cord. Pharmacological treatment of prostatitis includes antibiotics, analgesics, and stool softeners.

Activity

Treatment of prostatitis includes bed rest. While the client is in bed, his scrotum should be elevated and cold packs applied to the area. Encourage the client to drink a large amount of fluids and use sitz baths for comfort. These interventions are used to reduce inflammation, swelling, and discomfort. Periodic digital massage of the prostate by the physician increases the flow of infected prostatic secretions.

Nursing Management

Monitor vital signs, especially temperature and I&O. Encourage intake of oral fluids. Objectively assess client's pain and administer analgesics as ordered. Maintain client on bed rest. Keep scrotum elevated when the client is in bed and have client use an athletic support when ambulatory. Apply cold pack under scrotum as ordered.

NURSING PROCESS

Assessment

Subjective Data

Ask the client about the presence of urethral discharge or dysuria as well as the nature and location of the pain. A description of pain may include arthralgia, low-back pain, and myalgia. A positive history of recent bacterial or viral infection is of special significance. Ongoing nursing assessment includes monitoring of pain, using a pain scale to objectify data. Ask the client if he is experiencing nausea because this could be a sign that his condition is deteriorating. Assess the client's educational and emotional needs because he may be worrying needlessly about possible sterility or impotence.

Objective Data

Assess vital signs, especially temperature. An increase in temperature may be an indication that the client's condition is worsening. Scrotal edema and purulent urethral discharge may be present. Monitor intake and output. Ask about constipation.

Nursing diagnoses for the male client with an inflammatory disorder may include the following:

Nursing Diagnoses	Planning/Goals	Nursing Interventions
Risk for Injury related to worsening of the inflammatory process	The client will not experience worsening of his condition.	Monitor the client's vital signs, especially his temperature. Report hyperthermia, hypotension, nausea, and tachycardia to the physician immediately.
Deficient Fluid Volume related to nausea and vomiting	The client will maintain fluid balance.	Monitor the client's intake and output. Encourage him to drink plenty of fluids when not nauseated.

continues

Nursing Diagnoses	Planning/Goals	Nursing Interventions
Acute Pain related to inflammation	Using a pain scale of 0 to 10, the client will report pain has decreased to 2 or less within 48 hours after treatment initiation.	Assess client's pain level every 4 hours. Administer analgesics as ordered.
		Encourage the client to maintain bed rest. Provide diversional activities to increase compliance.
		Encourage the client with prostatitis to take a sitz bath, but never the client with epididymitis or orchitis as local heat may increase destruction of sperm cells.
		Fill a plastic glove with crushed ice and place it under the scrotum when heat is contraindicated. Remove the ice for short intervals every hour to prevent ice burns.
Anxiety, related to concerns about possible sterility or impotence	The client will verbalize decreased anxiety.	Reassure the client that with proper treatment, sterility and impotence are not likely complications of prostatitis.

Evaluation Each goal must be evaluated to determine how it has been met by the client.

BENIGN NEOPLASMS

Benign neoplasms include fibrocystic breast disease, fibroid tumors, and benign prostatic hyperplasia.

FIBROCYSTIC BREAST DISEASE

Fibrocystic breast disease (FBD) is also called chronic cystic mastitis or lumpy breast syndrome. It is the most common breast lesion in females and usually occurs between 35 and 50 years of age. Many cases will subside after menopause. The incidence of the potential for developing breast cancer is increased 3 to 4 times with fibrocystic breast disease. There appears to be a familial tendency toward the development of breast cancer.

Lumps may occur as single or multiple cysts that are frequently fluid-filled. It is difficult to differentiate fibrocystic tissue changes from other breast lesions because the dense fibrocystic areas may mask areas of breast cancer. Figure 41-7 shows the differences among cysts, fibroadenomas, and carcinomas of the breast.

The pathophysiology of FBD is found in the formation of fibrous tissue caused by hyperplasia of the epithelial cells in the breast lobules and ducts. The proliferation of the fibrous tissue deviates from the expected normal cyclic response to female hormone shifts during the menstrual cycle.

Routine mammograms provide baseline information and differentiate the palpable breast lumps between benign and malignant types. A computer-directed biopsy may also be performed.

Women should be taught breast self-examination (BSE) as adolescents and encouraged to practice it at the end of each menstrual cycle, when it is easier to palpate the breast tissue. Figure 41-8 provides specific information on how to perform a breast self-examination.

A yellow-greenish, sticky discharge from the nipple is occasionally present with FBD. A Pap smear may be done on the discharge to rule out the presence of malignant

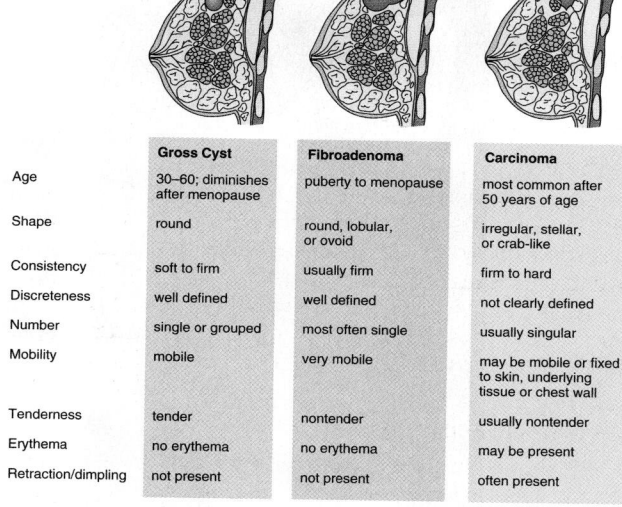

	Gross Cyst	Fibroadenoma	Carcinoma
Age	30–60; diminishes after menopause	puberty to menopause	most common after 50 years of age
Shape	round	round, lobular, or ovoid	irregular, stellar, or crab-like
Consistency	soft to firm	usually firm	firm to hard
Discreteness	well defined	well defined	not clearly defined
Number	single or grouped	most often single	usually singular
Mobility	mobile	very mobile	may be mobile or fixed to skin, underlying tissue or chest wall
Tenderness	tender	nontender	usually nontender
Erythema	no erythema	no erythema	may be present
Retraction/dimpling	not present	not present	often present

Figure 41-7 *Comparison of Breast Neoplasms*

cells. Note the presence of any breast discharge and report it to the health care provider as soon as possible. The physician or nurse practitioner (NP) may perform a biopsy or aspiration of the abnormal areas in the office. If fluid is obtained from the area, it is sent to pathology for examination. If no fluid is obtained, it may be a solid cyst or tumor, and biopsy may be required.

In the office, a breast biopsy may be performed with a local anesthetic. If there is any question of malignancy, or if the physician suspects that the lesion will be malignant on the basis of the mammography report, the biopsy may be performed in the hospital under general anesthetic so that additional tissue may be removed if necessary. A frozen section may be obtained and sent to the laboratory for a preliminary examination to rule out a malignant lesion.

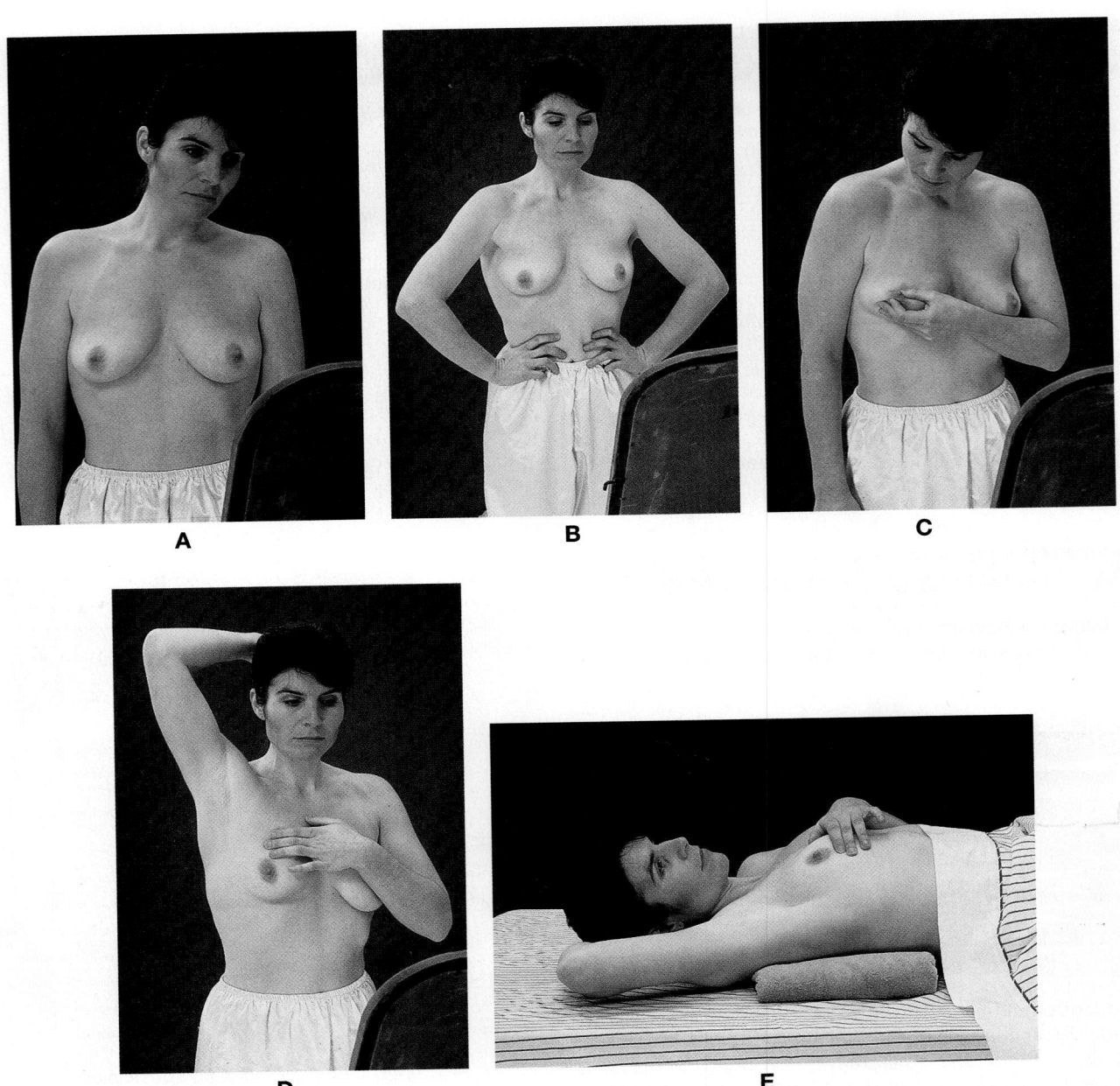

Figure 41-8 *Performing a Breast Self-Examination:* **A,** *Standing in front of mirror, check breasts for puckering, dimpling, scaliness, or discharge from nipples.* **B,** *Clasp hands behind head and press hands forward, watching for changes in the shape or contour of breasts. Press hands on hips and bend toward mirror while pulling shoulders and elbows forward (shown).* **C,** *Gently squeeze each nipple, looking for discharge.* **D,** *Raise one arm and use fingers of other hand to check breast for lumps or masses under skin. Use a pattern of motion (circular, up-and-down, etc.) to cover entire breast.* **E,** *Repeat "D" while lying flat on back with one arm over head and a towel under the shoulder.*

Medical–Surgical Management

Surgical

Aspiration or surgical excision may be indicated for diagnostic or therapeutic reasons. The cystic tissue may be aspirated with a small-gauge needle and syringe. The nurse prepares the client for the procedure and assists the doctor or NP with the procedure. The nurse assists the client into a supine position on the examination table and sets up the equipment and instruments needed. The

---

CRITICAL THINKING ?

Breast Self-Examination

How would you teach a client to do a breast self-examination? Make a teaching plan.

area to be biopsied is cleansed. Upon completion of the aspiration or biopsy, the nurse labels the specimen and sends it to the pathology department.

If the areas of fibrocystic tissue are extensive and have not responded to conservative treatments and methods, or if the risk of cancer is high, the tissue may be excised completely. Removal of fibrocystic tissue does not guarantee that the client will not develop breast cancer in the remaining tissue, and she must continue to perform monthly BSE.

🔀 Pharmacological

Some physicians recommend up to 600 units of vitamin E daily. It is believed that the vitamin supplement helps break down the fibrocystic tissue because it reacts with the polyunsaturated fats in the cell membrane. It may also have some effect on the balance of female hormones.

Diet

Most health care providers recommend limiting or completely eliminating caffeine-containing products from the woman's diet. This would include teas, colas, coffee, and chocolate. These products are all available in caffeine-free forms.

Nursing Management

Emphasize the importance of the client performing BSE one week following menses and having a mammogram as appropriate for age and risk factors. Teach the client how to perform BSE.

NURSING PROCESS

Assessment

Subjective Data

The client may report that the lumps are more tender as she approaches her menstrual period and that there is a greenish, sticky discharge from one or both breasts. Inquire about the client's dietary habits, especially caffeine intake, frequency of BSE, and the date of the most recent mammogram, if applicable.

Objective Data

When examined, single or multiple lumps may be palpated in one or both breasts. The lumps are not always discrete but should be freely movable. Because FBD lumps are more tender near the menses, the client should be seen for an exam the week after her menstrual period. The tissue contains less fluid during that time and palpation is easier and less uncomfortable.

Nursing diagnoses for a client with fibrocystic breast disease may include the following:

Nursing Diagnoses	Planning/Goals	Nursing Interventions
Deficient **K**nowledge, related to the cause of fibrocystic breast disease and method of breast self-examination	The client will verbalize and demonstrate her understanding of the cause of FBD and her role in treatment.	Demonstrate BSE for the client either in person or by video with a follow-up return demonstration by the client.
		Observe the client as she performs the BSE so that immediate feedback can be given. Explain the best timing for the BSE and the rationale for performing the procedure after the menses.
		Assist client with mammogram. Encourage mammography at regular intervals dependent upon the client's age and risk factors.
		Teach the client about dietary modifications, such as limiting caffeine.
Anxiety, related to the underlying potential and risk of breast cancer	The client will display behaviors of decreased anxiety related to the potential for breast cancer.	Explain the differences between malignant breast lesions and FBD to help alleviate the client's anxiety.

Evaluation Each goal must be evaluated to determine how it has been met by the client.

FIBROID TUMORS

Fibroids (leiomyomas) are benign tumors that grow in or on the uterus. A higher incidence is seen with nulliparous women and those who are more than 30 years old. The fibroids may appear below the serosal membrane or the mucosa. An early symptom is often **menorrhagia**, an excessively heavy menstrual flow. Later, the client may experience increasing pelvic pressure as the tumors grow, along with dysmenorrhea, abdominal enlargement, and constipation. Growth of the fibroids is usually slow but can be stimulated by estrogen. During

CULTURAL CONSIDERATIONS

Fibroid Tumors
Fibroid tumors are most prevalent in African Americans and Mediterraneans with dark skin.

pregnancy, when the estrogen and progesterone levels increase dramatically, the tumors grow much faster. Concern arises for the fetus when the fibroids begin to enlarge and crowd the uterus. Overcrowding may compress the fetus or initiate the onset of preterm labor. With either situation, the pregnancy must be monitored carefully.

A medical diagnosis of uterine fibroids may initially be based on the client's symptoms and the findings of the pelvic examination. If on palpation the uterus feels like an irregular mass or several masses, a pelvic ultrasound will be ordered to confirm the diagnosis.

Medical–Surgical Management

Medical
The physician may opt to wait and observe the growth pattern of the fibroids before advising the client to have surgery. This "wait-and-see" attitude may be swayed by the significance of the client's symptoms, size of the fibroids, amount of discomfort the client is experiencing, and amount of menorrhagia and/or **metrorrhagia,** vaginal bleeding between menstrual periods. Reexamination is encouraged at least every 6 months.

Surgical
If the menorrhagia is significant with each menstrual cycle, a dilation and curettage (D&C) may be performed to determine the exact etiology of the bleeding. A my-

omectomy, a surgical procedure to remove the tumor, may be performed if the client desires future pregnancies. In the case of severe menorrhagia, with a dropping hemoglobin level or multiple tumors, the physician may recommend a hysterectomy as the option of choice.

Diet
A diet with many sources of iron helps prevent iron-deficiency anemia, which may result from the extra blood loss.

Nursing Management
Monitor vital signs and hemoglobin level. Assess client's blood loss for amount, color, and clots. Objectively assess pain with a 0 to 10 scale and administer analgesics as ordered. Encourage a diet high in iron-containing foods to prevent iron-deficiency anemia.

NURSING PROCESS

Assessment

Subjective Data
Obtain the client's description of menstrual flow, dysmenorrhea, and/or pelvic pain and pressure. The client may also report difficulty fitting into clothes because of abdominal enlargement, constipation, or urinary frequency or urgency.

Objective Data
Count the number of sanitary pads the client saturates in an hour; observe the presence or absence of clots in the blood, a hemoglobin level of less than 12 mg/dL, and the client's pale skin color. Her blood pressure may be slightly lower than normal and her pulse may be increased as a compensatory mechanism.

Nursing diagnoses for a client with fibroids may include the following:

Nursing Diagnoses	Planning/Goals	Nursing Interventions
Risk for Deficient Fluid Volume, related to excessive blood losses	The client will have a hemoglobin above 12 mg/dL and will maintain fluid balance.	Assess client's blood loss for amount, color, and clots. Provide an accurate count of the saturated sanitary pads, along with the length of time taken to saturate a pad. Monitor vital signs at least every 4 hours, or more frequently if the client is having active blood loss. Monitor laboratory reports for Hgb level.
Acute Pain, related to pressure on pelvic structures caused by growing tumors and cramping during the menses	The client will verbalize less discomfort and pelvic pressure.	Assess pain on 0 (least) to 10 (most) pain scale and note location, onset, and duration. Administer analgesics as ordered.

Evaluation Each goal must be evaluated to determine how it has been met by the client.

BENIGN PROSTATIC HYPERPLASIA

Benign prostatic hyperplasia (BPH) is a progressive adenomatous enlargement of the prostate gland that occurs with aging. More than 50% of men older than age 60 and 90% of men older than age 70 have some symptoms of BPH (NIDDK, 2002). Although this disorder is not harmful, the urinary outlet obstruction that may be associated with the disorder is a problem.

Because the urethra is encircled by the prostate, common early symptoms of BPH are related to partial or complete obstruction of the urethra. Early symptoms include **hesitancy** (difficulty initiating the urinary stream), decreased force of stream, urinary frequency, and **nocturia** (awakening at night to void). However, a temporary reduction of these symptoms may occur as the bladder muscles hypertrophy in response to the increased work they must do to force the urinary stream past the obstruction.

Although this bladder muscle compensatory response may temporarily reduce symptoms, eventually the muscle decompensates, becoming noncompliant and hypotonic. This decompensation leads to atony of the mucous membranes between the muscle bands, which causes stagnant urine to collect in the small compartments (cellules) of the membranes. In addition, the man is unable to completely empty the bladder when voiding **(post-void residual).** Because these changes in urinary function promote urinary alkalosis by increasing the urine pH, a perfect environment for bacterial growth is created. This bacterial growth can cause a urinary tract infection (UTI), which may eventually lead to kidney damage.

Medical–Surgical Management

Medical

The physician performs a digital rectal examination to identify any enlargement of the lateral lobes or nodular lumps on the surface of the prostate gland. Diagnostic tests ordered to learn more about the client's condition may include a prostate-specific anti-

gen (PSA), measurement of residual urine, cystoscopy, intravenous pyelogram, and ultrasonography. The physician will carefully monitor the client's condition to detect any exacerbation of symptoms such as increased hesitancy, urgency, hematuria, or repeated urinary tract infections.

Many alternatives to surgical treatment of BPH have been introduced over the past several years, including balloon dilation of the prostate, a prostate urethral **stent,** as shown in Figure 41-9, and thermotherapy. Balloon dilation of the prostate during an endoscopic examination breaks the prostatic capsule and facilitates decompression of the prostate. A stent is material that is used to hold tissue in place or, in this instance, to provide support to the urethra, which is being compressed by the prostate. Thermotherapy that may be used includes microwave thermotherapy and hyperthermia. Although these minimally invasive treatments are safe, they do not correct the problem of incomplete bladder emptying (NIDDK, 2002).

Surgical

The traditional surgical intervention for 90% of all prostate surgeries for BPH is transurethral resection of the prostate (TURP). This surgery is performed via a resectoscope, an instrument that includes a cutting and cauterization device (Figure 41-10). The client receives either a general or a spinal anesthetic, and the resectoscope is passed through the urethra to remove small pieces of prostate tissue while controlling bleeding. The bladder is continuously irrigated with normal saline or another solution during the procedure. This irrigation is continued during the postoperative period to reduce clot formation that can interfere with urinary drainage.

The traditional surgical alternative to a TURP is open surgery. A suprapubic resection, in which the prostate is removed from around the urethra via the bladder, is per-

Figure 41-9 *Urethral Stent*

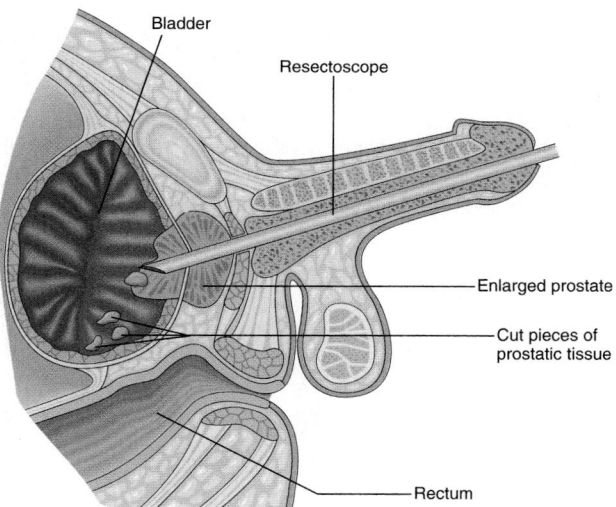

Figure 41-10 *Transurethral Resection of the Prostate Gland via Resectoscope*

formed when the prostate mass is large. In a retropubic prostatectomy, the bladder is not opened but instead is retracted and prostatic tissue is removed through an incision in the anterior prostatic capsule. Both of these alternatives involve an abdominal incision. In a perineal prostatectomy, a perineal incision is made and the prostatic tissue is removed through an incision in the posterior prostatic capsule.

Although these traditional surgeries successfully relieve bladder obstruction, they are costly, and postoperative complications can endanger or seriously affect the quality of a man's life. These complications include hemorrhage, water intoxication, infection, thrombosis, damage to surrounding structures, sexual dysfunction, and urinary incontinence.

Laser prostatectomy, the most recently developed surgical intervention for BPH, is based on thermal action. The transurethral ultrasound-guided laser-induced prostatectomy (TULIP) is performed with a probe that is passed transurethrally into the prostatic urethra. While the adjacent prostate area is visualized by ultrasound, the laser energy is directed at the prostate tissue, resulting in tissue necrosis and sloughing. The client is less likely to experience water intoxication because this surgical method allows blood vessels to seal rapidly, keeping irrigant fluid from being forced into the circulation.

Pharmacological

Finasteride (Proscar) can shrink the prostate in some men. Alpha blockers relax the smooth muscles along the urinary tract without compromising normal urinary control reflexes. Examples are terazosin hydrochloride (Hytrin), doxazosin mesylate, (Cardura) and tamsulosin Hcl (Flomax). They are also used to treat hypertension, so the side effect of orthostatic hypotension is possible. Belladonna and opium (B & O) suppositories are used to reduce postoperative bladder spasms, and narcotic analgesics are used to relieve postoperative pain.

Nursing Management

When inserting a Foley catheter, remove no more than 1,000 mL initially. Provide preoperative care as ordered. Monitor and accurately record I&O to prevent water intoxication; monitor vital signs and color of urine. Provide routine postoperative care. After catheter removal, encourage client to void with the first urge to prevent increased bladder pressure.

NURSING PROCESS

Assessment

Subjective Data

Ask the client about the presence of urinary frequency, hesitancy, dribbling, number of times he gets up at night to void, and the force of the urinary stream. In addition to a careful general medical history, any information pertaining to a history of chronic urinary tract infections needs to be noted.

Postoperative nursing assessment includes assessing for pain (on a 0 to 10 scale) related to bladder spasms. The client's emotional needs should also be assessed, especially for anticipatory grieving, body image disturbance, anxiety, incontinence, or concerns about alteration in sexuality patterns or possible sexual dysfunction. Observe for client behavioral or verbal cues indicating a need for further information or reassurance about his condition and treatment.

Objective Data

Monitor vital signs but *avoid* the use of a rectal thermometer. A bright red urine color persisting for more than a few hours after surgery may be a sign of hemorrhage. Report hemorrhage, hyperthermia, hypotension (low blood pressure), and tachycardia to the physician immediately.

After a TURP, the client will have a three-way Foley catheter and continuous bladder irrigation for at least 24 hours. Accurately record intake and output to ensure that the client has adequate oral intake to promote urinary flow and reduce the infection risk. *In measuring output, the amount of irrigant must be subtracted from the total output in order to determine the actual urinary output.* After the catheter is removed, assess the client for post-void residual and incontinence. Palpate the abdomen for bladder distention, check the bed linens and clothing for signs of incontinence, and ask the client if he is experiencing loss of urinary control.

Assess for water intoxication, which may be the result of absorbing irrigating fluid in addition to the IV fluids. The most common early symptoms of water intoxication are changes in the client's mental status. These may be manifested by agitation, confusion, and, later, convulsions. The client may also have a slow bounding pulse with an increase in systolic and decrease in diastolic blood pressure.

A suprapubic or retropubic prostatectomy does not require a three-way Foley. Instead, the client will have a urethral catheter, a tissue drain from the prostatic fossa, and an abdominal dressing. Assess for incisional pain and do a dressing check. Especially check the linens underneath the client's back for drainage.

Nursing diagnoses for a postoperative client having a TURP for benign prostatic hyperplasia may include the following:

Nursing Diagnoses	Planning/Goals	Nursing Interventions
Acute Pain, related to bladder spasms or incision	The client will state that pain has decreased.	Assess for pain using a pain scale every 2 to 4 hours. Maintain traction on the urethral catheter by anchoring the catheter to the leg with tape, taking care that accidental additional traction will not occur with leg movement. Monitor for signs of bladder spasm pain such as facial grimacing, non-flow of irrigating solution into bladder, and urinating around the catheter. Administer analgesics and antispasmodics as ordered. Teach deep breathing, relaxation techniques.
Risk for Imbalanced Fluid Volume, related to postoperative irrigation	The client will not experience water intoxication.	Accurately record I&O including irrigation fluid. Monitor for changes in the client's behavior, especially confusion and agitation, which may be the first signs of cerebral edema. Monitor for hypertension, bradycardia, weakness, and seizures.
Stress or Urge Urinary Incontinence, related to poor sphincter control after catheter removal after surgery	The client will achieve urinary control after removal of the catheter.	Advise the client that temporary urinary incontinence frequently occurs after surgery, and reassure him that this is normal. Teach the client perineal exercises that will help him regain urinary control. These exercises consist of tightening and relaxing gluteal muscles and are to be used each time the client urinates.
Sexual Dysfunction, related to surgery	The client will regain sexual function postoperatively.	Monitor the client's statements to determine if he has any misunderstanding of the surgery and sexual function. Instruct the client to avoid sexual intercourse until physician approval is given and that it may take time for his previous level of sexual function to return. Encourage the client to use a variety of forms of sexual expression, such as kissing, stroking, and cuddling. Provide the client with opportunities to voice his feelings and ask questions. Advise the client that it is normal and not harmful if his urine has a milky appearance due to retrograde ejaculation.

Evaluation Each goal must be evaluated to determine how it has been met by the client.

MALIGNANT NEOPLASMS

Malignant neoplasms include breast, cervical, endometrial, ovarian, prostate, testicular, and penile cancers.

BREAST CANCER

Breast cancer is the second major cause of cancer death among women. Statistics indicate that 1 woman in 10 will develop breast cancer some time during her life. The American Cancer Society (ACS) estimates that 211,300 new cases were diagnosed in the United States in 2003. The 5-year survival rate is 96% for localized cancer, 78% for cancer that has spread regionally, and 23% for cancers having distant metastases (ACS, 2003). Elderly women (older than 65) have twice the incidence of breast cancer as do younger women. Less than 1% of all breast cancers occur in men; in 2003, approximately 1,300 new cases of breast cancer were diagnosed in men (ACS, 2003).

The key to cure is early detection by physical examination, mammography, and breast self-examination. A painless mass or thickening is the most common presenting symptom.

Because it is so uncommon, breast cancer in men is all the more dangerous. Late diagnosis is quite common; therefore, males need to be educated in the technique of and encouraged to perform breast self-examination (BSE). Signs and symptoms of breast cancer include breast lumps, pain, or discharge from the nipple.

Women at greatest risk for developing breast cancer are those who:

- Had a mother or sibling with breast cancer
- Never had children or had their first child after the age of 30
- Never breast-fed
- Have a history of fibrocystic breast disease

- Started menstruating before age 10
- Are obese
- Consume a high-fat diet and a moderate amount of alcohol
- Smoke
- Experienced a late menopause

A woman generally presents at the health care office after the discovery of a lump in her breast. If she has been performing BE routinely each month, she is likely to be familiar with even minute changes in her breast tissue. Breast cancers often occur in the upper, outer quadrant of the breast and may extend into the tail of the breast and spread upward into the axilla. It is important to teach clients to examine the axillary region as well as the breast during BSE (Figure 41-8).

Women also seek medical advice because they notice a discharge from the breast, dimpling of the skin, retraction of the nipple, pain, a unilateral change in breast size, or an orange-peel appearance (peau d'orange) of the skin. Dimpling and puckering are usually associated with the breast tissue or tumor attaching to the skin or the underlying muscle mass, which does not permit movement. The nurse should not be misled by the client's report of a tender lump or mass and assume it is fibrocystic breast disease (FBD). All new or enlarged lumps or masses in the breast require immediate assessment.

The presence of tiny, palpable clusters of calcium, or "microclusters," may be an early sign of breast cancer. These should be followed closely with mammography every 6 to 12 months to detect subtle changes in shape or size.

The American Cancer Society (2003) recommends that women ages 20 to 39 perform BSE each month and have a clinical breast examination every 3 years. For women age 40 and older, BSE should be performed monthly, a clinical examination every year, and a mammogram every year.

Mammography may be performed by the stereotactic computer-guided technique. This advanced method allows needle biopsies to be taken at the same time if necessary. The physician or nurse practitioner may recommend this method after an initial mammogram has shown suspicious areas. This technique is less costly than excisional biopsy and can be performed with little discomfort to the client. The client is placed in a prone position on the special examination table with the breast hanging down through the opening in the table. The operator moves the position of the table to visualize the entire breast area via computerized guidance.

After the breast has been biopsied and the tissue has been examined by the pathologist, if a malignancy is confirmed, the client may be advised to proceed with surgical removal (lumpectomy or mastectomy) of the affected tissue. Figure 41-11 shows the staging of breast cancer.

Medical–Surgical Management

Medical

Radiation and chemotherapy are used as adjuvant therapy, but surgery is the primary treatment.

Figure 41-11 *Breast Cancer Staging*

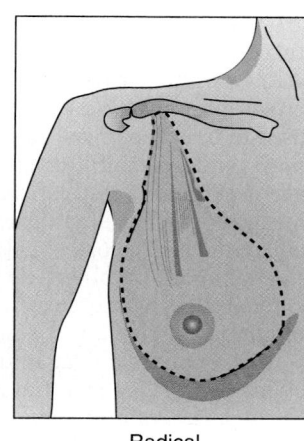

Lumpectomy   Simple mastectomy   Modified mastectomy   Radical mastectomy

Figure 41-12 *Surgical Options for Breast Cancer*

Surgical

There is an abundance of lymphatic vessels proximal to the breast. Malignant cells can thus escape into the general lymphatic system and be spread throughout the body. A lumpectomy is surgical removal of the cancerous mass. A simple mastectomy removes the tumor mass and only a small portion of the adjacent tissue. In the modified mastectomy, the entire breast tissue and nearby lymph nodes are removed; the muscles of the chest wall are left relatively intact. With the radical mastectomy, the entire breast, lymph nodes, and underlying pectoralis muscle are removed. Figure 41-12 shows the various options in the surgical management of breast cancer. The greater the extent of the surgical removal, the longer the client's recovery process and the greater the need for rehabilitation in using the upper extremity on the affected side.

The more lymph nodes that are removed, the greater the chance the client will have lymphedema, an accumulation of lymph in soft tissue. An elastic sleeve may be worn for compression, and ROM exercises may reduce edema. A sodium-restricted diet may be ordered.

Reconstructive surgery after a mastectomy may be determined by the amount of breast tissue and muscle remaining after the initial procedure, the position of the mastectomy scar, and the probability of recurrent breast cancer. Breast reconstruction can help the client deal with the disfigurement that results from the mastectomy.

The client's desire for reconstruction and her psychological status play an important role in determining the personal value of additional surgery. In the United States particularly, the breast is associated with childbearing and female sexuality. It may be difficult for the client to express her concerns to her partner regarding her sexuality and desirability after the mastectomy. She may have difficulty facing the physical alteration immediately after surgery and for some time after. The nurse with good interpersonal communication skills can help the client identify and verbalize her feelings of loss, thus promoting the psychological healing process and acceptance of altered body image.

Breast prostheses constructed to look and feel like real breast tissue are available. The prosthesis fits into a spe-

---

COMMUNITY/HOME HEALTH CARE

After a Mastectomy

- Avoid carrying items in the affected arm or wearing purse straps over the affected shoulder.
- Have vaccinations, blood pressure, and lab tests or blood drawn on the unaffected side only.
- Obtain immediate medical attention for all injuries and infections of the affected side to prevent complications.

---

cial pocket inside the brassiere. Some types are available for swimsuits and strapless tops. The construction of the prosthesis varies from sponge rubber to fluid- or air-filled.

Volunteers from the local cancer society often visit new mastectomy clients to assist them in the physical and psychological transition and adjustment after breast surgery. The American Cancer Society publishes a pamphlet entitled *Help Yourself to Recovery*, which includes simple postmastectomy exercises to perform as a part of the rehabilitation process.

Pharmacological

Some of the agents used to treat breast cancer include antineoplastic drugs such as antiestrogens: megastrol acetate (Megace), medroxyprogesterone acetate (Depo-Provera), tamoxifen (Nolvadex), and aminoglutethamide (Cytadren). Androgens for postmenopausal clients includes testolactone (Teslac); methyltestosterone (Testred), or rotating combinations of chemotherapy agents such as cyclophosphamide (Cytoxan), an alkylating agent, doxorubicin hydrochloride (Adriamycin), an antitumor antibiotic; 5-fluorouracil (Adrucil) and methotrexate sodium (Rheumatrex); antimetabolites; and prednisone (Orasone), a glucocorticoid via intravenous or oral routes. These drugs may be used before or after surgery. These antineoplastic agents act in several ways to either inhibit cellular growth or interfere with DNA replication. A laboratory test called tissue assay determines if estrogen or progesterone stimulates the cancer cells to grow. If the cancerous growth is stimulated by estrogen, antiestrogen drugs are used to treat the breast cancer. When the tumors are not estrogen-dependent, estrogen is used as a chemotherapy agent to treat breast cancers. Examples of two estrogen medications are diethylstilbestrol diphosphate (Stilphostrol) and ethinyl estradiol (Estinyl).

Paclitaxel (Taxol) has demonstrated positive results in clinical trials with breast cancer therapies. It acts by prohibiting cell replication. One of the benefits of this agent is that it causes milder nausea than many of the other chemotherapy agents that are used. It has the potential to cause severe anaphylactic reactions resulting from a histamine release. To avoid this problem, the client should be medicated with the following medications before Taxol infusion therapy: a corticosteroid such as dexamethasone (Decadron), a histamine blocker such as cimetidine (Tagamet), and an antihistamine diphenhydramine hydrochloride (Benadryl).

Tamoxifen (Nolvadex) may be used in certain high-risk women to reduce the incidence of breast cancer (Spratto & Woods, 2004).

Other Therapies

Breast tissue and lymphatic regions may be radiated before or after surgical excision of the tumor. This treatment may be done prophylactically to prevent the metastasis of malignant cells to other areas, or it may be done as a palliative measure to maintain the client's comfort. Figure 41-13 illustrates brachytherapy, the use of radioactive implants at the site of breast cancer.

Nursing Management

Encourage all clients to perform BSE and have a mammogram and clinical evaluation as recommended. Actively listen to client's fears and concerns and reinforce the information from the physician or nurse practitioner. Provide routine preoperative care. Identify the client's support system. Encourage client to contact the local American Cancer Society and Reach to Recovery support groups.

Postoperative care includes monitoring vital signs, drains, and dressing, and for signs of hemorrhage or shock. Encourage client to turn, cough, and deep breathe. If arm is not restricted by the dressing, elevate it with the hand highest to encourage fluid flow through the venous and lymph routes.

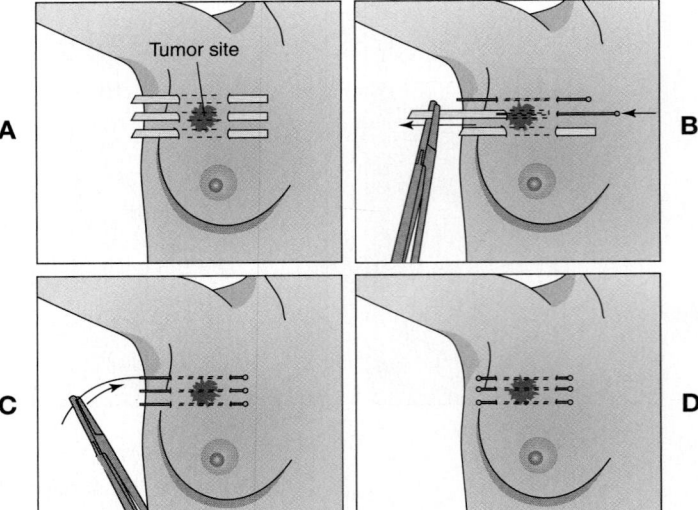

Figure 41-13 *Brachytherapy for Treatment of Breast Cancer:* **A,** *Hollow metal needles are placed at site.* **B,** *Hollow plastic catheters replace metal needles.* **C,** *Radioactive material is placed in catheters, with metal buttons holding the catheters in place.* **D,** *Radioactive implants remain in place for treatment.*

NURSING PROCESS

Assessment

Subjective Data

The client may describe a newly discovered breast lump and other changes in the breast, such as dimpling, puckering, or discharge. Ask how long the lump has been present, whether it is movable, whether it is tender, the frequency that BSE is performed, the date of the most recent mammogram, and current medications being taken. Assess pain using a pain scale to objectify data. Other questions should include the risk factors.

Objective Data

Assess vital signs and weight and review the report of the last mammogram. Examine the breasts for lumps and discharge from the nipples. During the postoperative phase, assess the client's vital signs and incisional site. Monitor client's statements and behaviors to determine emotional status.

Nursing diagnoses for a client with breast cancer may include the following:

Nursing Diagnoses	Planning/Goals	Nursing Interventions
Fear related to breast cancer, possible metastasis, surgery, and disfigurement	The client will express fears. The client will state one positive method of coping.	Encourage client to express specific feelings of fear. Take extra time to clarify or explain procedures and treatments. Provide written information along with verbal information. Encourage support of family members and significant others, and a preoperative visit by a member of the cancer society or Reach to Recovery.

continues

Nursing Diagnoses	Planning/Goals	Nursing Interventions
*Disturbed **B**ody Image,* related to removal of the breast	The client will discuss her feelings related to the loss of her breast and demonstrate acceptance of the change in physical appearance.	Remain attentive to signals from the client indicating readiness to look at the surgical site and encourage doing so when readiness is displayed.
		Be alert for client's comments regarding body changes.
		Encourage client recommended for chemotherapy to obtain a wig before therapy begins. Approximately 80% of clients undergoing chemotherapy will experience hair loss, and, if the client becomes accustomed to wearing a wig before hair begins to fall out, the client may feel more comfortable later.
		Inform client that she may have decreased sensation and lymphatic fluid retention in the arm on the affected side.
		Teach client to keep arm on affected side elevated above the level of the heart to promote lymph drainage, and to wear a properly fitting elastic compression sleeve on the affected arm that will help reduce the lymphedema.
		Anticipate the client's need to grieve the loss of her breast.
		Encourage use of rehabilitation services (Reach to Recovery).
*Ineffective **B**reathing Pattern,* related to the proximity of the surgical incision to respiratory muscles and pain with respiratory effort	The client's breath sounds will remain clear to auscultation. The client will effectively cough and deep breathe every 2 hours.	Preoperatively, teach the client how to turn, cough, and deep breathe.
		Postoperatively, assess the client's breath sounds, rate, and quality of respirations every 4 hours. Monitor O_2 saturation with pulse oximeter. Encourage deep breathing or the use of incentive spirometry every hour. Provide O_2 as needed.
		Medicate the client or encourage use of the PCA pump before performing exercises or deep breathing.
***S**elf-Care Deficist,* related to limited use and range of motion on the affected side and postoperative discomforts	The client will gradually regain ROM and provide self-care.	Begin passive range-of-motion exercises on the first or second postop day as ordered. Demonstrate postoperative exercises for the affected arm or request a consult from the physical therapy department.
		Observe the client as exercises are performed and reinforce correct performance.
		Encourage active ROM as soon as ordered by the physician to strengthen the operative side. This may be difficult at first due to tissue soreness from surgery.
		Encourage client to provide self-care as much as able.

Evaluation Each goal must be evaluated to determine how it has been met by the client.

SAMPLE NURSING CARE PLAN

THE CLIENT WITH BREAST CANCER

Claire Wilder, age 57, is married, with two children ages 24 and 22. During a bath, she noted a small, movable lump in her right breast, grew concerned, and went to see her health care provider. Family history is significant for fibrocystic breast disease and breast cancer on the maternal side (mother, aunt, sister). Personal history: onset of menses at age 10 with regular 28-day cycle, 5-day flow. She is 5 feet 5 inches tall and weighs 175 pounds. Her history is negative for alcohol use, but she smokes one to one-and-a-half packs of cigarettes daily. She did not breastfeed the children. Her last mammogram was 15 years ago. BSE is not practiced routinely. States: "I'm not sure just how to do the exam anyway."

Physical examination reveals a pea-sized lump in the upper right quadrant of the right breast and multiple clusters of lumps throughout each breast. Dimpling is present superior to the nipple. No nipple discharge was noted. The remainder of the exam was unremarkable. Vital signs were within normal limits. A mammogram revealed a suspicious mass, and a biopsy performed using stereotactic visualization was positive for cancer cells. A modified mastectomy was performed the next day with biopsies of adjacent lymph nodes. Six of ten nodes were also positive.

continues

SAMPLE NURSING CARE PLAN

The morning after surgery, Claire displayed behaviors that the nurse interpreted as anxiety. She confided in the nurse that she was afraid she was going to die, as her mother had, from the cancer. Claire had a large chest pressure dressing with two Jackson-Pratt drains in place. She stated that she was glad she had the PCA pump to take care of the pain.

Nursing Diagnosis 1 *Bathing/Hygiene and Dressing/Grooming **S**elf-Care Deficit*, related to temporary altered function of arm as evidenced by large chest pressure dressing and two drains in place

Nursing Outcomes Classification (NOC)
Self-Care: Activities of Daily Living (ADLs)
Comfort Level

Nursing Interventions Classification (NIC)
Self-Care Assistance: Bathing/Hygiene
Self-Care Assistance: Dressing/Grooming
Pain Management

PLANNING/GOALS	NURSING INTERVENTIONS	RATIONALE
Claire will meet her daily hygiene needs before discharge.	Assess Claire's ability to use affected arm to perform ADLs.	Provides baseline information of Claire's abilities and limitations.
	Provide assistance as needed to complete hygiene tasks, such as bathing and grooming.	Assisting with tasks and encouraging Claire to participate will facilitate the return of function and self-esteem.
	Encourage gradual resumption of activities as Claire indicates readiness.	Empowers Claire to help perform her own care, validating her self-image and worth, and she will regain strength and maintain the mobility of the extremity.

EVALUATION   Claire's hygiene needs were met.

Nursing Diagnosis 2 *Fear*, related to removal of the breast as evidenced by her fear of dying as her mother had

Nursing Outcomes Classification (NOC)
Anxiety Control
Coping

Nursing Interventions Classification (NIC)
Anxiety Reduction
Coping Enhancement

PLANNING/GOALS	NURSING INTERVENTIONS	RATIONALE
Claire will have less fear about breast removal.	Encourage Claire and family to verbalize their feelings and concerns related to the diagnosis and treatment.	Relieves fear and perceptions that differ from health care worker's are identified.
	Assess Claire's normal or previously used coping behaviors.	Enables the nurse to help Claire use or change coping behaviors.
	Involve Claire and her family in care planning.	Makes them more likely to feel a part of the team rather than simply accepting a passive "client role."

EVALUATION   Claire verbalized having less fear about the removal of her breast.

continues

SAMPLE NURSING CARE PLAN

Nursing Diagnosis 3 *Acute Pain,* related to surgical manipulation of tissues and excision of tissue as evidenced by client statement that she was glad she had the PCA pump to take care of the pain

Nursing Outcomes Classification (NOC)
Symptom Severity
Pain Level

Nursing Interventions Classification (NIC)
Pain Management
Patient-Controlled Analgesia (PCA) Assistance

PLANNING/GOALS	NURSING INTERVENTIONS	RATIONALE
Claire will verbalize that pain is controlled.	Assess Claire's pain level and response to analgesia every 2 hours.	Alerts the nurse to increasing pain and the client's tolerance of the pain medication.
	Instruct Claire how to use the PCA pump.	Allows Claire control over analgesia and provides consistent pain relief.
	Evaluate the effectiveness of analgesia q 2 hours.	Allows the nurse to identify any untoward effects and effectiveness of the medication.
	Reposition Claire q 2 hours.	Helps improve vascular flow and relieves pressure on bony prominences.
	Elevate the right arm on pillows.	Decreases edema and discomfort due to pressure on nerves in the area.

EVALUATION   Claire reports pain is controlled at less than 2 on a 1–10 scale.

CERVICAL CANCER

An abnormal condition of the cervix known as dysplasia may be an early sign of developing cervical cancer. Dysplasia is a change in the size and shape of the cervical cells, and it is classified as mild, moderate, or severe. An abnormal Papanicolaou (Pap) smear may be the first indication of a problem. Pap smears are classified from 1 through 5. A 1 is considered a normal cervix, and a 5 would indicate a malignant condition.

Cervical cancer is the most preventable gynecological cancer. Sexual habits constitute a major factor in the development of cancer of the cervix. Sexually transmitted disease, particularly the human papillomavirus (HPV), is a particularly significant factor (ACS, 2003). Other factors associated with cervical cancer include a history of multiple sexual partners and maternal use of diethylstilbestrol (DES) during pregnancy. The most common sign of cervical cancer is abnormal bleeding, which progresses from a thin, watery, blood-tinged discharge to frank bleeding. Contact bleeding may also occur after intercourse. Advanced disease is indicated by odor, pain in the lower back and groin, difficulty in voiding, hematuria, and rectal bleeding. The Pap smear is the key to early detection. Promotion of regular pelvic exams and education regarding risk are essential.

Although cervical cancer can occur at any age, it occurs most frequently in women between 35 and 55 years of age. It is insidious because it is asymptomatic. Cervical cancer has a high cure rate in the early stages, and it is easily detected by the routine annual Pap smear. The overall 5-year survival rate is 70% (ACS, 2003).

The nurse should immediately bring any abnormal Pap smear results to the attention of the physician or nurse practitioner so the client can be notified and the appropriate follow-up treatment initiated. A repeat Pap smear may be indicated after treatment with a vaginal antibiotic cream, or a colposcopy may be performed.

Staging of the cancer progresses from I to IV (Figure 41-14). Carcinoma *in situ* (CIS) means that the cancerous cells remain within the cervix and have not yet spread to adjacent areas. The higher the number on the staging table, the more the cancer has metastasized to other structures. Stages II through IV indicate that the cancer cells have invaded the bladder, vagina, or other pelvic organs.

Medical–Surgical Management

Surgical

Treatment modalities may include conization, a surgical excision of a cone-shaped section of the abnormal cervical tissues. This procedure is desirable if

STAGING SYSTEM FOR CANCER OF THE CERVIX	
Stage	Characteristics
I IA IA1 IA2 IB	• Carcinoma is strictly confined to cervix (extension to corpus should be disregarded) • Preclinical carcinoma • Minimal microscopically evident stromal invasion • Microscopic lesions no more than 5 mm depth measured from base of epithelium surface or glandular from which it originates, and horizontal spread not to exceed 7 mm • All other cases of stage I; occult cancer should be marked "occ"
II IIA IIB	• Carcinoma extends beyond cervix but has not extended to pelvic wall; it involves vagina, but not as far as lower third • No obvious parametrical involvement • Obvious parametrical involvement
III IIIA IIIB	• Carcinoma has extended to pelvic wall; on rectal examination, there is no cancer-free space between tumor and pelvic wall; tumor involves lower third of vagina; all cases with hydronephrosis or nonfunctioning kidney should be included, unless they are known to be due to another cause • No extension to pelvic wall, but involvement of lower third of vagina • Extension to pelvic wall, or hydronephrosis or nonfunctioning kidney due to tumor
IV IVA IVB	• Carcinoma has extended beyond true pelvis or has clinically involved mucosa of bladder or rectum • Spread of growth to adjacent pelvic organs • Spread to distant organs

Figure 41-14 *Cervical Cancer Staging*

the client is of childbearing age and wants children in the future.

Laser surgery, cryosurgery (freezing of the cells with liquid nitrogen), or cauterization (burning) may be performed as alternative methods of treatment if the cervical lesions are easily visible for the procedure. A total hysterectomy or radical pelvic surgery may be required to eradicate the cancer. If the spread of the disease has become too extensive, treatment will be directed toward palliative measures.

Other Therapies

The physician may recommend the use of radium implants or radiation therapy before the surgical excision of the cervix. The nurse must be cautious in providing nursing care for the client with radium implants. Pregnant nurses or female nurses of childbearing age should not care for this client or spend extended periods at the bedside. Direct client care should be organized to optimize time spent at the bedside. A sign should be hung on the door to indicate that radiation is being used in the room and provide a warning for visitors to limit their visit time. With the implants in place, the client will remain on complete bed rest.

In addition, chemotherapy may be utilized as an adjunct therapy to help shrink the tumor or slow its growth.

Nursing Management

Provide therapeutic emotional support to the client to help her cope with the diagnosis. After surgery, monitor vital signs and I&O. Encourage client to ambulate as ordered and to turn, cough, deep breathe, and use a spirometer. Assist with active and passive ROM exercises. Provide careful catheter care.

NURSING PROCESS

Assessment

Subjective Data

The client may describe postcoital bleeding (bleeding after intercourse) or spotting between menstrual periods or after menopause and, occasionally, a foul-smelling vaginal discharge. As the disease progresses, she may describe increased or bloody discharge, weight loss, and pain that radiates down the lower back and legs.

Objective Data

Objective data may include the presence and appearance of a vaginal discharge. The cervix may appear eroded or raw and may bleed easily when touched with a cotton-tipped applicator or Pap scraper. Necrotic tissue may be present and cause a foul odor. Pap smear results can indicate dyplasia or Class II through Class IV cell changes. Tissue samples obtained through colposcopic examination may show cellular changes. In advanced

disease, weight loss and anemia may be present. Laparotomy may be performed to stage the disease and along with other laboratory and diagnostic testing to identify metastases, which are most likely to occur in the rectum, vagina, bladder, and pelvis.

Nursing diagnoses for a client with cervical cancer may include the following:

Nursing Diagnoses	Planning/Goals	Nursing Interventions
Anxiety related to unknown outcome and possible treatments	The client will verbalize having less anxiety about treatment and possible outcome.	Be aware of the client's emotional state throughout the course of care and use effective interpersonal communication to facilitate the client's acceptance of her condition and the treatments. Explain diagnostic tests and procedures to client to decrease her anxiety. Provide therapeutic emotional support to client to help her cope with feelings.
Sexual Dysfunction, related to vaginal bleeding, discomfort, and procedures	The client will return to normal sexual function after recovery from treatment for cervical cancer.	Inform client that she may experience dyspareunia related to vaginal dryness after radiation therapy. Instruct client to use a water-soluble lubricant during intercourse or to use lubricated condoms to decrease irritation. Listen to client's concerns.
Impaired **U***rinary Elimination,* related to sensory motor impairment from radiation effects	The client will regain normal urinary elimination.	Assess the function of the Foley catheter to ensure patency and drainage. Provide careful catheter care. Promote urination when catheter is removed. Record I&O, including color of urine. Encourage the client to drink many fluids to flush the kidneys and decrease risk of UTI.

Evaluation Each goal must be evaluated to determine how it has been met by the client.

ENDOMETRIAL CANCER

Postmenopausal women are at the greatest risk for endometrial cancer, especially if they have taken estrogen replacement therapy for several years (usually more than 5 years). Research has shown that unopposed estrogen stimulation of the endometrial lining has a strong relationship with the development of endometrial cancer. During the normal menstrual cycle, estrogen and progesterone rise and fall. These hormonal fluctuations affect the stimulation of the endometrial tissue to grow and be sloughed off. Without the progesterone effects, the endometrial tissue is not sloughed off at regular intervals and may undergo cellular changes, leading to a high risk for endometrial dysplasia or cancer. For this reason, many physicians and nurse practitioners have recommended estrogen-progesterone therapy for clients who experience menopausal symptoms.

In summer 2002, the data and safety monitoring board for the Women's Health Initiative study of estrogen/progestin recommended stopping the trial because of an increased risk of invasive breast cancer (Fletcher & Colditz, 2002). It is recommended that long-term use of this combination be stopped.

Other risk factors associated with endometrial cancer may include never having borne a child, being Caucasian,

being middle class, never having had sexual intercourse, or being of Jewish descent.

Cancer of the endometrium usually does not produce symptoms until it becomes relatively advanced. Routine Pap smear and pelvic examinations are inadequate for early diagnosis. An endometrial biopsy, which examines the tissue from the uterine lining under a microscope, is the best diagnostic tool to identify cellular changes. This may be done on an annual basis when the client has a routine examination. The medical follow-up treatment plan depends on the biopsy results. D&C has a potential for spreading the cancer cells to adjacent tissues because the malignant cells may escape into the bloodstream at the time of the procedure. This is not usually a problem with the biopsy because the amount of tissue removed is so small and blood loss is minimal. A D&C is also more expensive, higher risk, and requires some type of anesthesia. The 5-year survival rate for localized endometrial cancer is 96% (ACS, 2003).

Medical–Surgical Management

Treatments for endometrial cancer may range from radiation, radium implants, chemotherapy, or surgery to a combination of any of the above. The choices of treatment are related to the staging of the cancer.

PROFESSIONAL TIP

Radiation Exposure Risk

Because of the risk of radiation exposure to the caregiver from the radiation implant device, keep procedures that require exposure to the client's perineal area at a minimum.

Medical

Intravenous fluid administration will be implemented to replace fluids lost by the excessive bleeding. A blood transfusion may be ordered for a low hemoglobin. A hemoglobin above 10 gm/dL is preferred before surgical intervention. The physician may order whole blood or packed red blood cells to increase the hemoglobin rapidly.

Surgical

Surgery for endometrial or cervical cancer includes hysterectomy. A total hysterectomy is removal of the cervix and the uterus. In a subtotal hysterectomy, only the uterus is removed and the cervix remains. A radical or pan hysterectomy includes removal of the ovaries, cervix, uterus, fallopian tubes, pelvic lymph nodes, and part of the vagina. Vaginal hysterectomy procedures have been refined with the laparoscopic approach so that many clients are released from the hospital within 24 to 36 hours postoperatively. If the cancer has spread beyond the uterus into the pelvic region, an abdominal hysterectomy may be the best approach for visualization during surgery. The physician may recommend a course of radiation therapy after surgery.

❧ Pharmacological

Hormonal therapy with megestrol acetate (Megace), medroxyprogesterone acetate (Depo-Provera), or hydroxyprogesterone caproate (Prodrox) may be administered to suppress tumor growth when the cancer is considered inoperable or has metastasized, especially if the tumor receptors are estrogen-stimulated.

Other Therapies

There is a tendency for endometrial cancer to confine itself to the uterus, which increases the client's 5-year survival prognosis. Endometrial cancer also usually responds well to the therapies available at this time, including radiation. Radiation may be delivered to the pelvic region via external sources, or it may be delivered via intracavitary devices or implants with radium or cesium. There is a potential danger for injury to adjacent pelvic structures during radiation therapy. The nurse should be alert for signs of complications, such as bleeding from the rectum, moderate to severe abdominal pain, constipation, or diarrhea. New therapies are being developed using protons that are capable of more direct application of radiation, which decreases the chance of injury to other organs or structures.

Nursing Management

One of the earliest symptoms reported by many clients is vaginal bleeding. For the postmenopausal client, it is imperative that all bleeding be investigated immediately unless it is from hormonally induced periods. Late in the progression of the cancer, the client may experience symptoms similar to those discussed with cervical cancer. Pain is often associated with the spread of cancer to adjacent organs and is considered a late sign.

Objective data may be collected from the client's physical exam findings, biopsy reports, and a history of hormone replacement therapy with or without the estrogen-progesterone combination.

OVARIAN CANCER

Ovarian cancer most often originates in the epithelial tissue of the ovary, and, like cervical and endometrial cancer, does not produce symptoms until it is in an advanced, inoperable stage. It is sometimes called "the silent killer." Its symptoms are vague and may be ignored for a long time before the client seeks medical attention.

Ovarian cancer causes more deaths than does any other gynecological cancer, an estimated 25,400 in 2003 (ACS, 2003). The incidence is greatest in women between 45 and 65 years of age. Nulliparity (never having borne a child), smoking, alcohol use, infertility, and a high-fat diet are factors that place the client at higher risk for developing ovarian cancer. Metastasis occurs in more than 75% of cases before diagnosis, and often the cancer has spread beyond the pelvis. The colon is the most frequent site of ovarian cancer metastasis, then the stomach, and diaphragm.

Unfortunately, medical research has not yet developed an early diagnostic or screening tool to detect ovarian cancer. It is believed, however, that there is an increased risk of ovarian cancer for clients with breast cancer and vice versa. A family history of two or more female relatives with breast or ovarian cancer provides a sound rationale for more frequent breast and pelvic examinations. Often, the physician or NP palpates an ovarian mass on a routine bimanual examination. This finding is cause for further investigation by pelvic ultrasound or CT scan to determine the size, character, and consistency (solid or fluid-filled) of the mass and whether other pelvic structures are involved. Some experts believe that there is a link between the occurrence of ovarian cysts and the development of ovarian cancers in certain women.

General diagnostic studies, such as a lower GI series, chest x-ray, intravenous pyelogram (IVP), and laparoscopy may be useful in determining the extent of the primary and secondary lesions. A blood test, CA-125 assay, measures a tumor marker CA-125 that is often higher than normal in women with ovarian cancer (National Cancer Institute, 2002d). If the client develops peritoneal fluid or ascites as the cancer progresses, it may be removed by paracentesis for cytologic examination.

Recurrent disease is common and may occur in 2 years or less. Continued medical surveillance is recommended every 2 months for a period of 2 years for the earliest possible detection of new lesions. The 5-year survival rate is 52% (ACS, 2003).

Medical–Surgical Management

Surgical

Surgical excision of the ovary is rarely successful because of the extensiveness of the disease. A total abdominal hysterectomy with a bilateral salpingo-oophorectomy is performed for most stages of the disease. Most often a combination of radiation, chemotherapy, immunotherapy, and surgery produces the best results, even if they are only palliative for the client. The client must be actively involved and informed of her treatment options as well as her prognosis to enable her to make sound choices in the treatments chosen.

Pharmacological

Chemotherapy drugs that have been used with ovarian cancer treatment include cyclophosphamide (Cytoxan), doxorubicin hydrochloride (Adriamycin), mitomycin (Mutamycin), and paclitaxel (Taxol). These may be administered by regional or intraarterial perfusion techniques. These percutaneous modes direct the drugs to the lesion's vascular supply. If the cancer has not metastasized, a regimen of chemotherapy using a single drug, such as Cytoxan, may be administered over the course of 5 days and repeated again at regular intervals over the course of a year. A combination of the chemotherapy agents, used in a rotating series, is often more effective for reproductive cancers in advanced stages. For example, the client would receive one drug over the course of 5 days, then switch to another drug for 5 days, and then a third drug for 5 days. This series may be repeated over the year in a similar pattern to that used with a single agent.

Sometimes two or three different medications are necessary to achieve pain control. Intravenous medications are often given by a PCA pump with continuous low-dose narcotics. This method seems more effective for the client than IV bolus doses every 4 hours. Medications may also be given slow IV push (an RN procedure), orally in tablets or liquids, intramuscularly, or by transdermal patches (Duragesic). A liquid mixture of syrup, cocaine, morphine, alcohol, flavoring, and water called "Brompton's mixture or elixir" may be ordered. The client may drink up to 20 cc every 3 to 4 hours for pain relief. Most of these methods of narcotic administration are equally effective and may be used in the home care or hospice setting. Other types of medication that may be given include tranquilizers, antiemetics, and laxatives.

Nursing Management

Accurately measure the client's legs to ensure the proper fit of antiembolic stockings. Provide comfort measures of back rub and position change. Teach client about skin care if receiving radiation. Assess bowel sounds and for abdominal distention. Maintain an accurate I&O record.

NURSING PROCESS

Assessment

Subjective Data

The client may describe fatigue, malaise, diarrhea or constipation, pelvic pressure, frequency of urination, loss of appetite, nausea, weight gain or loss, vaginal bleeding or spotting with intercourse, a foul-smelling vaginal discharge, and pain in the lower back. The list of symptoms is very vague and could be related to many reproductive and nonreproductive disorders.

Objective Data

Objective data pertinent to all cancers of the pelvic reproductive organs may include information from the client's previous health history, reproductive history (onset of menses, pregnancies, contraceptive methods, infections, hormonal replacement therapy, and surgeries), the discovery of a palpable mass during a bimanual examination, an abnormal appearance of the cervix or adjacent tissues, abnormal Pap smear results greater than Class II dysplasia, abnormal cervical or endometrial biopsies, increased abdominal girth, or the presence of ascites and pleural effusion.

Diagnostic tests and laboratory studies may include all or some of the following: Pap smear, pelvic ultrasound, chest x-ray, IVP, kidney/ureters/bladder x-ray (KUB), CBC with differential, blood chemistry studies, bleeding and clotting time, endometrial biopsy, cervical biopsy, D&C tissue specimens, Schiller's test and colposcopy, laparoscopy, barium enema, and bone scan.

Nursing diagnoses for a client with endometrial or ovarian cancer may include the following:

Nursing Diagnoses	Planning/Goals	Nursing Interventions
Preoperative *Fear* related to tentative diagnoses, pending surgical procedures, cancer treatment and its side effects, incapacitating or extended illness with resulting dependence, and possible death	The client will verbalize fears and have behaviors consistent with reduced fear before and after surgery.	Facilitate the client's expression of fear by encouraging the client's open discussion of her concerns. Be alert for nonverbal cues as well. Arrange a consultation with a social worker or chaplain, if appropriate.

continues

Nursing Diagnoses	Planning/Goals	Nursing Interventions
*Chronic **P**ain,* related to the spread of cancer throughout the pelvis and adjacent structures	The client will have pain controlled at a level that allows continual functioning in her activities of daily living as long as possible.	Administer analgesics as ordered. Provide comfort measures, such as position changes and back rub.

Nursing Diagnoses	Planning/Goals	Nursing Interventions
Postoperative *Impaired **S**kin Integrity* related to surgical interventions, radiation, and chemotherapy side effects	The client's skin integrity will be maintained.	Provide the client with proper skin care instructions during and after radiation therapy that may include avoiding soaps, creams, powder, deodorants, and other substances around the incision that may irritate the skin; not washing off the radiation markings; and avoiding tight clothing around the area. Teach the client to look for signs of reactions to radiation therapy, such as tenderness, flushed color (like a sunburn), delayed wound healing, and itching. Perform daily cleansing of the incisional area with water only. If the client is on complete bed rest due to radium implant therapy, provide a complete bedbath as well as morning and bedtime skin care. Organize time near the client's bedside to brief periods to avoid overexposure to radiation. Wear rubber gloves when disposing of soiled materials. Put soiled dressings in a biohazard waste container.
*Impaired **U**rinary Elimination, **B**owel Incontinence, or **C**onstipation,* related to the proximity of surgical site to bowel and bladder, spread of cancer to adjacent structures, manipulation of organs during surgery, administration of narcotic analgesics, lack of activity, and changes in dietary intake	The client will have adequate bowel and bladder function during the postoperative period.	Explain dietary modifications designed to reduce residue. The diet should be limited in dairy products, raw fruits, grains, and vegetables. Meats must be well cooked and possibly ground. If the client is not receiving radium implant therapy, weigh her daily on the same scale at the same time of the day. Review the client's normal elimination patterns from the baseline assessment data to help identify early changes in bowel or bladder elimination. Forewarn the client of radiation enteritis and cystitis, and common tissue responses to radiation therapy. Instruct her to report symptoms, such as diarrhea, cramping, frequency, urgency, and dysuria. Assess bowel sounds and abdominal distention at least every 4 to 8 hours. Carefully monitor the client's urinary pattern and maintain an accurate intake and output record. Observe urine and stool for color, consistency, amount, and the presence of blood. Monitor the client for other gastrointestinal problems, such as nausea, vomiting, and **tenesmus** (spasmodic contraction of the anal or bladder sphincter, causing pain and a persistent urge to empty the bowel or bladder).
*Impaired Physical **M**obility,* related to intracavity radiation	The client will not develop deep vein thrombosis.	Accurately measure the client's legs to ensure the proper fit of the hose. Apply thigh-high antiembolic stockings (TEDS) as ordered. Assist client to ambulate when allowed.

Evaluation Each goal must be evaluated to determine how it has been met by the client.

PROSTATE CANCER

Prostate cancer is the second leading cause of cancer deaths in men. According to 2003 estimates by the ACS, 220,900 new cases were diagnosed. Survival rate for all cases is 97%. Incidence increases with age, as 70% of all prostate cancers are diagnosed in men older than age 65. Improved detection methods have greatly increased the number of individuals having positive outcomes. Diagnostic tests that may be performed are measurement of serum prostate-specific antigen (PSA), transrectal ultrasonic examination, and prostatic biopsy. Studies indicate that the PSA alone for routine screening is not especially useful. The American Cancer Society (2003) recommends a yearly PSA level and digital rectal examination to screen for prostate cancer in men age 50 and older with a life expectancy of more than 10 years.

Most prostatic cancers are adenocarcinomas, slow-growing tumors that spread through the lymphatics. Early symptoms include dysuria, a weak urinary stream, and increased urinary frequency. Later symptoms are related to complete urethral obstruction or hematuria. Blood in the urine **(hematuria),** which can lead to anemia, occurs because of the rupture of blood vessels that have been overstretched.

Medical–Surgical Management

Treatment depends on the extent of the disease and the age of the client.

Medical

Radiation is the traditional alternative to surgical removal of the malignant prostate gland; however, radiation may fail to eradicate the tumor or may lead to diarrhea, bowel obstruction, lymphocele formation, edema of the extremities, pulmonary embolism, wound infections, infection, impotence, incontinence, or radiation cystitis. An alternate successful radiation treatment option for early-stage prostate cancer is transrectal assisted radioactive seed implant. With the use of ultrasound, the physician is able to precisely position the rice-sized radioactive seeds inside the malignant prostate gland.

Surgical

Surgical treatment of prostatic cancer involves removal of the entire prostate gland, including the capsule and adjacent tissue. The urethra is then anastomosed to the bladder neck. Sometimes the retropubic approach is used, but the usual approach is perineal with the incision made between the scrotum and the rectum. Because of the proximity of the bladder sphincters to the prostate gland, urinary incontinence may be a complication. Other complications include sexual dysfunction and the universal surgical risks of hemorrhage, infection, thrombosis, and strictures. Removal of the testes **(orchiectomy)** may also be done as a palliative measure to help eliminate the androgenic effect that promotes tumor growth. The client should be 70 years of age or younger, in good health, with a life expectancy of 10 to 12 more years (Held-Warmkessel, 2002).

Cryosurgery (freezing) was used in the 1960s but abandoned because of tissue sloughing and fistula development. With the advent of the transrectal ultrasound and the transurethral warming device, cryosurgery is again a viable alternative. The ultrasound allows the surgeon to selectively freeze prostate gland tissue while the temperature of the prostatic urethra is kept at 44°C by irrigation with heated water. This approach is an option for those who cannot tolerate more extensive surgery, have a localized tumor, or do not have successful radiation treatment. It can be performed more than once, involves a shorter hospital stay, and produces fewer side effects.

Pharmacological

Hormonal agents such as diethylstilbestrol (DES), goserelin acetate (Zoladex), or leuprolide acetate (Lupron) may be used to counteract the production of androgen-dependent hormones. Although systemic chemotherapy has not proved very effective in the treatment of prostate cancer, it may be used for clients who fail to respond to hormone manipulation. Unfortunately, response is limited.

Nursing Management

Encourage all male clients older than age 40 to have an annual rectal examination of the prostate and a PSA serum level. Monitor vital signs (no rectal temperature), urinary output, and fluid intake. Assess urine for signs of bleeding. Objectively assess for pain and administer analgesics as ordered. Keep perineal area clean and dry.

NURSING PROCESS

Assessment

Subjective Data

The client may seek care for BPH, which often accompanies cancer of the prostate. He may describe back pain or sciatica, frequency, dysuria, or nocturia.

Objective Data

Complete a physical assessment including palpation of the abdomen and skin assessment. Palpate the abdomen to determine if there is any bladder distention. Skin assessment is important because the client is at risk for skin breakdown. There may or may not be hematuria present. Vital signs, the incisional site, and intake and output must all be assessed. Report hyperthermia, hypotension, tachycardia, or increased incisional drainage to the physician immediately.

A catheter is used postoperatively to maintain urinary drainage and as a splint for the urethral anastomosis rather than for hemostasis, so there are minimal bladder spasms. Monitor catheter patency by assessing the drainage for color, amount, and presence of clots. If the tubing is not draining freely, reposition or milk it. Call the physician if these measures fail to restore patency. During the first week of the postoperative period, monitor the client for fecal incontinence related to relaxation of the perineal sphincter. This complication occurs when the perineal surgical approach is used because the incision is made between the scrotum and the rectum.

Nursing diagnoses for a client (postoperative) with prostate cancer may include the following:

Nursing Diagnoses	Planning/Goals	Nursing Interventions
Urinary Retention, related to urethral obstruction, secondary to urethral anastomosis.	The client will not experience urinary retention.	Monitor the client's urinary output, noting the amount, color, and presence of clots. The urine should not appear bright red for more than a few hours postoperatively, after which time it should be dark red. Reposition or milk the catheter tubing if not patent. If these interventions fail, notify the physician. Monitor the client's intake, encouraging a fluid intake of 2,500 to 3,000 mL/day.
Bowel Incontinence, related to loss of rectal sphincter control because of perineal incision	The client will achieve rectal sphincter control.	Advise the client that temporary fecal incontinence frequently occurs after a perineal incision. Teach the client perineal exercises that will help him regain bowel control. Avoid the use of rectal thermometers, rectal examinations, and enemas.
Risk for Impaired **S**kin Integrity, related to incontinence	The client will not experience skin breakdown	Keep the client clean and dry, especially if he is experiencing fecal or urinary incontinence and reposition every 2 hours.

Evaluation Each goal must be evaluated to determine how it has been met by the client.

TESTICULAR CANCER

Although testicular cancer accounts for only 1% of all cancer in men, it is the most common cancer in young men between the ages of 15 and 35. According to the ACS (2003), advances in treatment have made the 5-year survival rate 95%. The etiology is unknown, but the incidence is highest in men with undescended testicles and those whose mothers had taken hormones during pregnancy. A small, hard, painless lump is usually the first symptom noted.

Because early diagnosis of testicular cancer is so essential for a positive surgical outcome, men need to be taught how to perform a testicular self-examination (TSE) and be encouraged to routinely perform that examination (Figure 41-15).

TSE is performed as follows:

- Perform TSE after a bath or shower when scrotum is warm and most relaxed.
- Grasp testis with both hands and palpate gently between thumbs and forefingers.
- The testis should feel smooth, egg-shaped, and firm to the touch.
- The epididymis, located behind the testis, should feel like a soft tube.
- Any abnormal lumps or changes in the testes should be reported to a physician.

Medical–Surgical Management

Medical

Testicular ultrasound is used to study the testes for enlargement or lesions. In addition to a testicular ultrasound, the client may have a serum acid or alkaline phosphatase test done. They are both elevated in malignancies.

Surgical

Biopsy of the testis is contraindicated because of the increased potential for metastases. Surgical removal of the testis, spermatic cord, and inguinal canal contents, with examination of the nodes, is indicated for testicular cancers. If unilateral removal of a testis is indicated, the remaining healthy testis will continue to maintain sperm and androgen production.

Figure 41-15 *Performing a Testicular Self-Examination*

Testicular Self-Examination
How would you teach a client to do a testicular self-examination? Make a teaching plan.

Pharmacological

Although chemotherapy and radiation are used as adjuvant treatments, radical inguinal orchiectomy remains the primary intervention. Combination chemotherapy with cisplatin (Platinol), vinblastine sulfate (Velban), and bleomycin sulfate (Blenoxane) is effective.

Nursing Management

Encourage all male clients older than age 15 to perform testicular self-examination monthly. Cancer is suspected in a testicle that is hard. Postoperatively, monitor vital signs and incisional drainage. Maintain strict asepsis when changing dressings. Provide opportunities for the client to voice fears and concerns.

NURSING PROCESS

Assessment

Subjective Data

The client may describe a feeling of heaviness in the scrotum and may mention weight loss. During the postoperative phase, the client needs to be assessed for pain, using a pain scale to objectify data. Assess his emotional and educational needs. Monitor his behaviors and statements for signs of anxiety or depression.

Objective Data

Physical examination should include palpation of the abdomen and assessment of the scrotum. Positive findings in the scrotum include a firm, painless mass in the testis and an enlarged scrotum. Because gynecomastia (breast enlargement) is another symptom of testicular cancer, the client's breast tissue should be assessed for enlargement.

Nursing diagnoses for the client with testicular cancer may include the following:

Nursing Diagnoses	Planning/Goals	Nursing Interventions
Risk for Injury, due to infection and hemorrhage related to surgery	The client will experience minimal bleeding and avoid infection.	Monitor the client's vital signs and incisional drainage. Report hyperthermia, tachycardia, hypotension, increased incisional drainage, and swelling or redness around the incision to the physician immediately.
		Maintain strict asepsis when handling wound dressings.

continues

Nursing Diagnoses	Planning/Goals	Nursing Interventions
*Disturbed **B**ody Image,* related to surgery	The client will maintain or regain a positive body image.	Provide the client with opportunities to voice concerns and ask questions. Monitor the client for statements and behaviors that indicate concern about loss of masculinity.
		Advise the client that unilateral removal of a testis will not cause him to be sterile or demasculinized. Suggest sexual counseling if he does not appear to be resolving these issues. Sperm may be frozen before treatment.
*Deficient **K**nowledge,* related to surgery and post-operative care	The client will demonstrate understanding of postoperative activity restrictions and medical follow-up.	Advise the client that he needs to be on bed rest for 12 to 24 hours postoperatively.
		Instruct the client to wear tight-fitting underwear or an athletic supporter when ambulating and to avoid heavy lifting for 4 to 6 weeks.

Evaluation Each goal must be evaluated to determine how it has been met by the client.

PENILE CANCER

Penile cancer is rare and has a high correlation with poor hygiene and delayed or no circumcision. The bacteria harbored in the foreskin of the uncircumcised male are irritants to the glans penis and the prepuce. The chronic nature of this irritation is thought to be carcinogenic. Males with a history of sexually transmitted diseases (STDs) are also predisposed to developing penile cancer. Symptoms of penile cancer include a painless, nodular growth on the foreskin, fatigue, and weight loss. Metastases are common in the inguinal nodes and adjacent organs.

Medical–Surgical Management

Medical

The primary penile cancer treatment is surgery. Treatment with radiation alone is ineffective, and chemotherapy alone is used only for palliative treatment of penile cancer with deep, distant metastases; however, the client may receive adjuvant therapy with either radiation or chemotherapy.

Surgical

If the tumor is not extensive and no metastases are involved, the remaining penis should be long enough for the client to void standing and avoid soiling himself. If a penectomy is necessary, a suprapubic catheter may be inserted or an ileoconduit may be performed.

Nursing Management

Provide emotional support if penectomy is required. Monitor vital signs and I&O. Elevate the scrotum to prevent edema. Objectively assess pain and administer analgesics as ordered.

NURSING PROCESS

Assessment

Subjective Data

Although the tumor is painless, ask the client if he is experiencing any pain, to rule out other possible diagnoses. Also ask about fatigue or weight loss. Preoperatively, assess the client for emotional and educational needs. Ask questions that can determine his understanding of the surgical procedure and the need for counseling. Postoperative assessment includes monitoring for pain and using a pain scale to objectify data.

Objective Data

The client's physical assessment should include inspection of the penis for the presence of painless, nodular growths. During the postoperative phase, monitor vital signs, incisional site, and intake and output. Hypotension, tachycardia, excessive incisional drainage, redness or swelling around the incision, or bright red or low urinary output could be signs of complications.

Nursing diagnoses for a client with penile cancer may include the following:

Nursing Diagnoses	Planning/Goals	Nursing Interventions
*Risk for **I**njury,* due to infection and hemorrhage related to surgery	The client will experience minimal bleeding and avoid infection.	Monitor the client's vital signs and incisional drainage. Report hyperthermia, tachycardia, hypotension, increased incisional drainage, and swelling or redness around the incision to the physician immediately.
		Maintain strict asepsis when handling wound dressings.

continues

Nursing Diagnoses	Planning/Goals	Nursing Interventions
Anxiety, related to surgery	The client will discuss anxieties.	Provide the client with information about the operative procedure, postoperative and discharge care. When available, a video may be used to present this information, with the nurse being available to answer the client's questions.
Ineffective *Sexuality Patterns,* related to the altered body function or structure	The client will maintain satisfactory sexuality patterns postoperatively.	Advise the client to seek sexual counseling for both himself and his partner if he is unable to maintain normal sexuality patterns.

Evaluation Each goal must be evaluated to determine how it has been met by the client.

MENSTRUAL DISORDERS

Abnormalities of menstruation may be associated with an increase or decrease in secretion from any of the following glands: hypothalamus, pituitary, ovaries, adrenals, and thyroid. The normal menstrual pattern is controlled by a series of hormonal negative feedback mechanisms. The average menstrual cycle occurs every 28 to 30 days when the endometrial lining of the uterus sloughs off in the absence of a fertilized ovum.

DYSMENORRHEA

Painful menstruation, dysmenorrhea, also called "menstrual cramps," is more common in nulliparous women and in women who are not having intercourse. The exact pathophysiology is unknown, but it may be related to endocrine secretions such as prostaglandin F, which causes uterine cramping, irritation, and contractions. Other causes may include uterine anatomical anomalies, chronic illness, or psychological factors.

The primary symptom is pelvic pain before or at the onset of menses that may be caused by spasms of the uterus, narrowing of the cervical canal, emotional factors, endometriosis, pelvic inflammatory disease, or the presence of an intrauterine contraceptive device (IUD). The client may also state that the pain radiates across the lower back and downward into the legs.

The condition is diagnosed on the basis of the client's complaints and description of the timing of the onset of symptoms. Obtain information pertaining to the menstrual history and general health status of the client. A thorough physical exam is performed by the physician, including a bimanual exam to rule out other possible causes. A pelvic ultrasound may be ordered.

One effective preventive intervention may begin before the young woman begins menstruation. A positive parental attitude toward the onset of menstruation can aid the young girl in adjusting to the physiologic and psychological changes that occur with puberty.

Some medications are effective in the treatment of dysmenorrhea. Analgesics such as acetaminophen (Tylenol) and ibuprofen (Motrin) are useful in relieving pain. Oral contraceptives have been used for some clients

to inhibit ovulation, which appears to be an associated cause. Prostaglandin inhibitors such as naproxen sodium (Anaprox) and mefenamic acid (Ponstel) are useful if taken at the earliest sign of discomfort.

AMENORRHEA

Amenorrhea, the absence of menstruation, may be primary or secondary. Primary amenorrhea is defined as the absence of menstruation by the age of 17. Possible causes are related to anatomical or genetic abnormalities (Turner's syndrome). The treatment depends on the cause. Secondary amenorrhea is defined as the absence of menstruation after 6 months of regular periods or after 12 months of irregular periods. Several etiologies are possible for secondary amenorrhea, including anatomic abnormalities, nutritional deficits (anorexia nervosa), excessive exercise with significant decreases in body fat, endocrine dysfunction, emotional disturbances, side effects of medications, pregnancy, and lactation.

Diagnosis is based on the length of menstruation absence. A complete physical examination is performed, including a pelvic examination to rule out many other factors. A progesterone challenge test may be administered in an attempt to force the body to respond hormonally. Medroxyprogesterone acetate (Depo-Provera) is taken orally for 5 to 10 days as ordered by the physician. When the medication is finished, the client should have a menstrual period within 3 or 4 days. A menstrual flow after taking the medication may be an indicator that the client has not been ovulating. If no bleeding occurs, further investigation may be necessary to uncover other causes. Hormonal imbalances, microscopic pituitary tumors, and nutritional deficits are common etiologies of secondary amenorrhea. A microscopic pituitary tumor will cause an elevation in the prolactin level and result in anovulation and amenorrhea. A serum prolactin level should be ordered, especially if the client has noticed any breast discharge. Normal prolactin level should not exceed 15 ng/dL. With pituitary tumors, the prolactin level may exceed 400 ng/dL. In these cases, the drug of choice is bromocriptine mesylate (Parlodel), which had been used in the past to suppress lactation in mothers who did not breastfeed their newborns. A careful examination of the client is needed before administration of Parlodel because of an increased potential for cardiovascular problems associated with this medication. Because of this risk, the medication is no longer used for the postpartum client to suppress milk production. Other medical or surgical interventions depend on the cause of the amenorrhea.

OTHER DISORDERS

Other menstrual disorders include menorrhagia and metrorrhagia. Both types of abnormal bleeding can be problematic for the client and require further investigation. **Polymenorrhea** is a term used to describe short menstrual cycles of less than 21 days in length. The causes are similar to those of the other menstrual disorders. **Oligomenorrhea,** is a diminished menstrual flow, but it is not classified as amenorrhea. It may be associated with low-dose oral contraceptives that inhibit the growth of the endometrium and result in minimal tissue sloughing at the end of the cycle. Other causes may be metabolic or hormonal. Again, treatment is specific to the etiology.

For conditions associated with heavy bleeding or bleeding between periods, a dilation and curettage (D&C) may be performed. In this case, the procedure may be diagnostic and therapeutic. Tissue removed from the uterus is examined microscopically and histologically to evaluate its stage in the menstrual cycle. A hysterectomy may be indicated if abnormalities are discovered or if the bleeding is so excessive that the client is significantly compromised. The client may require a blood transfusion to correct low hemoglobin and hematocrit levels before any other procedures are performed. Supplemental iron generally is prescribed by the physician to also help correct the deficiency.

NURSING PROCESS

Assessment

Subjective Data

Ask the client about the onset of the bleeding and its relationship to the timing of her normal menstruation, the color of the bleeding, amount, number of pads saturated, presence of clots, and presence of pain with the bleeding. A history of current medications, contraception, and the possibility of pregnancy are additional data needed. Explore any preexisting health problems that could affect bleeding and clotting times, as well as life stressors.

Objective Data

Assessment of vital signs may indicate hypertension and tachycardia. Monitor laboratory test results.

Nursing Management

Acknowledge the client's feelings about the problem. Explain diagnostic tests and procedures. Encourage good nutrition, good posture, and exercise. Emphasize the importance of follow-up care.

Possible nursing diagnoses for a client with any of the menstrual disorders discussed in this section may include:

- *Acute **P**ain*, related to uterine cramping or heavy bleeding
- *Decreased **C**ardiac Output*, related to excessive blood loss
- ***F**atigue* related to decreased hemoglobin and hematocrit levels
- *Disturbed **B**ody Image*, related to the absence of menstruation

PREMENSTRUAL SYNDROME

One-third to one-half of women between 20 and 50 years of age experience some of the symptoms known as premenstrual syndrome (PMS). Once, this condition was thought by many physicians to be a psychological problem of women; however, recent research has supported data that many physiologic as well as psychological factors are involved. PMS often occurs during the secretory phase of the menstrual cycle, after ovulation. Risk factors associated with the development of PMS include age (older than 30), multiple life stressors, inappropriate nutritional status, a previous reaction to or side effects from oral contraceptive use, a sedentary lifestyle, marital status, a history of preeclampsia in pregnancy, and multiparity.

More than 150 symptoms have been reported that have been related to PMS. These include weight gain, bloating, irritability, edema, headache, mood swings, inability to concentrate, food cravings, acne, and numerous others. For many women, the PMS symptoms are merely a monthly nuisance, but for others, the symptoms are so incapacitating that they cannot function in their normal roles or responsibilities. The onset of symptoms is usually 7 to 10 days before the menstrual period starts; symptoms end after the menstrual flow begins.

Research has correlated hormonal imbalances of estrogen, progesterone, ACTH, and androgens with the symptoms of PMS. The presence of prostaglandin F in the tissue may also be a cause of some of the symptoms. Prostaglandins are associated with many inflammatory responses in the tissues.

The first step in identifying PMS is a physical examination to rule out other possible disorders of the reproductive system. The client may be asked to keep a monthly calendar of symptoms to see if there are patterns in severity, type, or onset. Blood tests may be ordered to assess estrogen and progesterone levels, as well as checking the glucose level. Low blood glucose level has been associated with irritability that sometimes accompanies PMS symptoms. The client should receive counseling, if needed, to facilitate coping with life stressors that may be complicating the complexity of the PMS symptoms.

Medical–Surgical Management
 Pharmacological

Some physicians and NPs recommend medication such as acetaminophen (Tylenol), naproxen (Naprosyn), mefenamic acid (Ponstel), and ibuprofen (Advil) for the relief of minor discomforts of PMS. Tranquilizers and antidepressants have not proved to be effective for short-term use in PMS; however, in severe cases, they may be a last resort. Several PMS symptoms are thought to be related to a low progesterone level. For some clients, the use of progesterone suppositories or oral progesterone to supplement their own production during the secretory phase of the menstrual cycle has been useful.

Diet

A thorough diet history should be included in the assessment data collected. Certain nutritional deficits or cravings have been linked to the worsening of PMS. Items such as sugar, salt, caffeine, and chocolate are in this category. Many studies have shown that limiting intake of these substances may be helpful. Caffeinated beverages may increase anxiety, irritability, and deplete vitamin B stores in the body. Dairy products interfere with the absorption of magnesium, which helps stabilize the mood. Chocolates have been related to increased sugar cravings, mood swings, fluid retention, and increased vitamin B demands. Oranges and other fruits or vegetables that are highly acidic may worsen PMS. Foods that are recommended are whole grains, nuts, pasta, legumes, root vegetables, fruits such as apples and pears, poultry, and seafood. A good vitamin supplement rich in vitamin B-complex, calcium, magnesium, and zinc should be taken daily, especially during the PMS period. Herbal tea formulas have shown some promise as alternative methods of relieving PMS.

Activity

A regular exercise routine, coupled with the use of stress-management techniques such as deep breathing and relaxation exercises, help the client cope with the increased sense of anxiety or irritability that may accompany PMS. Meditation, positive affirmation, visualization, and imagery may be helpful, as well as acupressure, neurolymphatic or neurovascular massage, and yoga.

Nursing Management

Encourage client to keep a monthly PMS calendar of events. Advise client to limit sodium, sugar, alcohol, caffeine, and nicotine intake to reduce PMS symptoms.

NURSING PROCESS

Assessment

Subjective Data

Ask the client to describe her symptoms and the impact on her lifestyle. Many times, clients will seek medical attention for their PMS symptoms when the emotional impact has caused friction in the home, marriage, work, or family environment. Symptoms described may include weight gain, bloating, irritability, headache, mood swings, inability to concentrate, or food cravings. Ask the client to relate symptoms to time of menstrual cycle.

Objective Data

Assess the client for weight gain and edema. Review laboratory test results.

Nursing diagnoses for a client with premenstrual syndrome may include the following:

Nursing Diagnoses	Planning/Goals	Nursing Interventions
Excess Fluid Volume related to hormonal imbalance and increased sodium or sugar intake	The client's intake and output will be balanced, and edema will be decreased.	Advise client that a certain amount of fluid retention is normal before the onset of the menstrual period and cannot be avoided, but by limiting sodium and sugar intake, she may be able to influence the amount of fluid retained.
Health Seeking Behaviors, related to finding methods to cope with symptoms of PMS	The client will develop effective health-promotion skills to increase coping with PMS symptoms or to decrease symptom severity or frequency.	Teach client how to keep a monthly PMS calendar of events. Discuss prescribed medications with the client, including the dosage, expected effects, and side effects. Discuss relationship of foods to PMS.

Evaluation Each goal must be evaluated to determine how it has been met by the client.

MENOPAUSE

Menopause, or climacteric, is the cessation of menstruation. It may occur as a natural hormonal decline or it may be surgically induced by removal of the uterus and ovaries. Many people think of menopause as the "change of life" and accept it as part of aging. Most women will begin to experience signs and symptoms of approaching menopause around 50 years of age; however, the range of onset is from 45 to 60 years old. Menstrual cycles become further apart and the flow decreases. The onset is usually gradual, and it may take more than a year before the woman has completely ceased menstruation. Reproductive capability is also lost with menopause. For some women this is a sad time perceived as the loss of womanhood; for others it is a welcome relief.

The decreasing level of ovarian hormone production affects women in a variety of ways, more than just the end of menstruation. There may be a relaxation of the pelvic support structures, loss of skin turgor and elasticity, and thinning of the hair on the head, axilla, and pubic regions. Other signs of decreasing hormones (estrogen and progesterone) are vaginal dryness, thinning of the vaginal mucosa, weight gain, dry skin, and stress incontinence. The estrogen level plays an important protective role in maintaining an adequate calcium balance in the bones and preventing coronary artery disease. Without calcium, bones become brittle, and there is an increased risk of fractures and osteoporosis. A baseline bone density study may be recommended before menopause.

Some women experience psychological responses to menopause, such as mild to moderate depression, nervousness, and insomnia. Consultation with a psychologist, minister, or counselor may be useful in facilitating the transition through this period for some women.

Women may also experience mild to moderate periods of profuse perspiration called "hot flashes." These usually move from the waist upward. They are caused by the decreased estrogen level and its effect on the hypothalamus. The sensation may last from a few seconds to 2 to 3 minutes. It appears that many different things can trigger a hot flash—drinking hot beverages, eating spicy foods, smoking, and consuming caffeine and alcohol.

Medical–Surgical Management

Pharmacological

For some women, estrogen replacement therapy is recommended, especially if they are experiencing moderately uncomfortable symptoms. Estrogen replacement therapy (ERT) may help decrease some symptoms, such as insomnia, hot flashes, mood swings, and lack of concentration. Estrogen elevates the high-density lipoproteins (healthy ones) and lowers the low-density lipoproteins (unhealthy) in the circulation. Estrogen may be administered orally, as a transdermal patch, or as a vaginal cream.

Conjugated estrogen (Premarin), estradiol (Estrace), and estropipate (Ogen) are examples of oral estrogens available. Estrogen creams or water-soluble gels such as Lubrifax or K-Y may be used to combat the vaginal dryness and resulting dyspareunia.

Diet

Provide the client with instructions regarding the importance of an adequate daily intake of calcium-rich products, such as dairy products. Many low-fat, high-calcium products are available if the client has a concern about weight gain. Calcium supplements may also be taken in a tablet form. The woman should consult her health care provider before adding a calcium supplement because too much calcium increases the risk for other health problems. Herbal teas, vitamin E, magnesium, and primrose oil have been used as alternative methods to alleviate or decrease hot flashes and promote relaxation for some women.

Activity

One important way that the client can decrease the potential for calcium loss from weight-bearing bones is to exercise. A planned 30-minute program performed at least 3 times per week is adequate to maintain bone density. Exercises such as walking or swimming are excellent. Swimming provides good non–weight-bearing activity and promotes active movement of all extremities. Biking is a good exercise to maintain joint mobility in the lower extremities, but it does not require the use of the same muscle groups as walking.

Nursing Management

Encourage the client to exercise regularly, especially walking. Explain nutritional requirements for vitamins and calcium. Advise the client to try water-soluble gels for vaginal dryness and body lotion to prevent dry skin.

NURSING PROCESS

Assessment

Subjective Data

The client may describe decreasing regularity of menstruation or hot flashes. Obtain information from the client about gynecological and obstetrical history, including menstruation. It is helpful to know when the client began experiencing symptoms in predicting the length of time they may continue.

Objective Data

These include a physical examination and Pap smear. The results of the Pap smear can indicate if there is less estrogen present in the cervical tissue than normal.

Nursing diagnoses for a client experiencing menopausal symptoms may include the following:

Nursing Diagnoses	Planning/Goals	Nursing Interventions
Health-Seeking Behaviors, related to perceived physiological and psychologic impact of decreased estrogen	The client will develop effective health promotion skills to increase coping with menopausal symptoms or to decrease symptom severity or frequency.	Encourage the client to continue to see her health care provider for annual Pap smears and breast examinations. Explain nutritional requirements for vitamins and calcium that increase with menopause. Encourage the client to begin a regular exercise program that includes weight-bearing activities such as walking to prevent loss of calcium from the bones.
Impaired Tissue Integrity, related to vaginal dryness and dry skin	The client will maintain skin integrity, and vagina will not be dry.	Advise the client to try estrogen creams or water-soluble gels such as Lubrifax or K-Y to combat the vaginal dryness and resulting dyspareunia. Encourage the client to use body lotion to prevent dry skin.
Decisional Conflict, related to taking supplemental estrogen therapy	The client will make informed decisions about taking supplemental estrogen.	Discuss the advantages and disadvantages of estrogen replacement therapy with the client. Remind the client that if she has a uterus and takes hormonal replacements, she will continue to have monthly menstrual cycles.

Evaluation Each goal must be evaluated to determine how it has been met by the client.

STRUCTURAL DISORDERS

Structural anomalies are separated into female and male disorders.

CYSTOCELE, URETHROCELE, RECTOCELE, PROLAPSED UTERUS

Cystocele, urethrocele, rectocele, and prolapsed uterus are often associated with relaxation of the pelvic muscles that support the uterus, bladder, and rectum. A **cystocele** is a downward displacement of the bladder into the anterior vaginal wall. A **urethrocele** is a downward displacement of the urethra into the vagina, and a **rectocele** is an anterior displacement of the rectum into the posterior vaginal wall. **Prolapsed uterus** is a downward displacement of the uterus into the vagina (Figure 41-16). Possible causes for the four conditions are multiple pregnancies, third- or fourth-degree perineal lacerations with childbirth, and age-related weakening of the pelvic muscles.

A prolapsed uterus is often accompanied by a cystocele and/or rectocele. With a first-degree prolapse, the cervix is visible at the vaginal introitus, or opening, without straining. With a second-degree prolapse, the cervix extends beyond the vaginal opening to the perineum. With a third-degree prolapse, the uterus protrudes outside of the vagina. This severe condition is called *procidentia uteri*.

Medical–Surgical Management

Medical and surgical interventions for the treatment of each of these conditions are focused on relief of discomfort and restoration of the structure and function of the pelvic organs.

Medical

The pessary is a small molded plastic or rubber apparatus that fits into the vagina behind the pubic bone and in front of the rectum. Its function is to provide an artificial or mechanical support for the uterus. Pessaries are not uncomfortable and should not be felt by the client if properly fitted and in the correct position. The client should be taught how to insert and remove the pessary so it can be cleaned. The pessary may be washed in warm, soapy water once every 1 to 2 weeks. Prolonged use of a mechanical device such as a pessary may result in vaginal necrosis and ulceration. Periodic examination by a health care professional is recommended.

Surgical

Surgery for a prolapsed uterus may require a hysterectomy. If the prolapse is accompanied by a cystocele or rectocele, an A&P repair may also be performed. An A&P repair (anterior/posterior colporrhaphy) may be performed vaginally to replace the bladder, urethra, or rectum in the correct anatomic position. Another procedure, the Marshall-Marchette-Krantz, may be performed to attach the bladder to the inferior surface of the pubic bone. Postoperatively, the client may be sent home with an indwelling Foley catheter because of the potential inability to void. This is a common postoperative situation that usually resolves itself spontaneously within 1 or 2 weeks after discharge.

Figure 41-16 **A,** Cystocele; **B,** Urethrocele; **C,** Rectocele; **D,** Uterine Prolapse

CLIENT TEACHING

Kegel Exercises

- Suggest that the client practice when she has a full bladder. If she can successfully start and stop the flow of urine from the bladder, she is identifying and using the correct muscle groups.
- The muscles should be tightened and held for 5 to 10 seconds and then released slowly.
- Repeat the exercises at least 10 times.
- Kegel exercise can be practiced anytime and anyplace.
- A secondary benefit of increasing the strength and contractility of the pelvic and perineal muscles is seen in an improvement in pelvic sensations for both partners during intercourse.

Activity

The Kegel exercise is performed by tightening and releasing the perineal muscles. An important muscle group, called the "levators," helps lift and support the organs inside the pelvis.

Nursing Management

Teach client Kegel exercise and encourage daily practice. Describe to the client how a high-fiber diet and drinking plenty of fluids will help prevent constipation. Postoperatively, monitor vital signs and I&O. Cleanse perineal area following surgical asepsis. Encourage early ambulation.

NURSING PROCESS

Assessment

Subjective Data

The client often describes stress incontinence, a loss of urine when she coughs, sneezes, laughs, or jumps. She may describe it as "a leaky bladder." She may notice that her panties are damp or that she dribbles urine. Many women complain of frequent urination in small quantities with a feeling of urgency without burning or dysuria. The client may notice constipation or a sense of bearing-down pressure in the pelvis with a rectocele. Many of these symptoms will decrease or subside completely when lying down. Ask about the client's childbearing history, onset of current symptoms, and any other pertinent gynecological data.

Objective Data

These include the visualization of a bulging of the bladder, urethra, or rectum into the vagina. The bulging increases when the client is asked to bear down. Urinalysis results should be evaluated.

Nursing diagnoses for a female client with a structural disorder of the reproductive system may include the following:

Nursing Diagnoses	Planning/Goals	Nursing Interventions
Stress Urinary Incontinence related to relaxation of the pelvic muscles	The client will have less stress incontinence.	Teach the client Kegel exercise and encourage daily practice. Encourage client to empty bladder frequently.

continues

Nursing Diagnoses	Planning/Goals	Nursing Interventions
Constipation, related to relaxation of the anterior rectal wall into the vagina and decreased function	The client will not have constipation.	Encourage client to defecate at same time each day. Encourage client to eat high-fiber foods, drink plenty of fluids, and exercise regularly.
Risk for Infection related to exposure of internal tissues to external environmental factors	The client will be free of signs and symptoms of infection.	Monitor the client's vital signs. Encourage client to practice proper personal hygiene and wear clean undergarments daily.
Sexual Dysfunction, related to discomforts with intercourse	The client will have a fulfilling sexual relationship without discomfort.	Be sensitive to client cues related to her sexual concerns. Help the client set realistic goals during her recovery period to facilitate a new outlook on her relationship. Encourage the client to openly discuss her feelings with her partner.

Evaluation Each goal must be evaluated to determine how it has been met by the client.

HYDROCELE, SPERMATOCELE, VARICOCELE, TORSION OF THE SPERMATIC CORD

A hydrocele is a benign, nontender collection of clear, amber fluid within the space of the testes and the tunica vaginalis or along the spermatic cord. Scrotal swelling may result, which can be painful if it develops suddenly. Inflammation of the epididymis or testis or a lymphatic or venous obstruction may cause this condition. Congenital hydrocele in the newborn occurs when the canal between the peritoneal cavity and the scrotum does not close completely during fetal development. Aspiration of the fluid is only a temporary measure and can lead to secondary infection. Therefore, treatment for the condition is surgery.

A spermatocele is a benign nontender cyst of either the epididymis or the rete testis. It contains milky fluid and sperm. Usually, this condition is painless and does not require medical treatment.

A varicocele is dilation of the veins of the scrotum that occurs when the venous system that drains the testicle lengthens and enlarges. This dilation occurs when incompetent or absent valves in the spermatic venous system permit blood to accumulate, resulting in increased hydrostatic pressure. This condition is most commonly found on the left side because of the increased retrograde pressure of the renal vein, the length, and fewer competent valves. It is theorized that the hyperthermia that occurs with this condition decreases spermatogenesis, resulting in decreased fertility. Symptoms may include a bluish discoloration of the scrotal skin or palpation of a wormlike mass when the male bears down. This condition seldom requires treatment.

Torsion of the spermatic cord occurs when the vascular pedicle of the testis twists, resulting in partial or complete venous occlusion. The three forms of this disorder are (1) rotation of the spermatic cord, (2) torsion of a testicular appendage, or (3) torsion of the spermatic cord and epididymis. Testicular torsion may be related to recent trauma, and the onset of symptoms often occurs suddenly. Symptoms of testicular torsion may include abdominal and scrotal pain, scrotal edema, nausea and vomiting, and, possibly, a slight fever. The pain caused by testicular torsion is not relieved by bed rest or scrotal support.   *INFERTILITY*

Medical–Surgical Management

Medical/surgical management of male structural disorders is specific to the condition. In some newborns, a hydrocele may resolve without medical intervention. Clients of all ages may have aspiration performed to reduce the swelling caused by fluid or a hematoma; however, this solution is usually only temporary, and surgical removal of the sac provides the only permanent solution to the problem. Although a spermatocele usually does not require treatment, sometimes surgical aspiration or excision is necessary.

Because a common complication of a varicocele is male infertility, ligation of the spermatic vein may be performed if infertility is a concern. Sometimes this does not resolve infertility problems because varicoceles may recur after surgery. When fertility is not a concern, the varicocele may be treated simply with scrotal support.

Torsion of the spermatic cord is one disorder that does require immediate surgery to perform surgical detorsion (untwisting) and suturing of the testicle to the scrotum.

Nursing Management

Maintain the client on bed rest with scrotal support and ice to the area. Objectively assess the client's pain and administer analgesics as ordered. Monitor vital signs, incisional drainage, and dressing. Use strict asepsis when changing dressings.

NURSING PROCESS

Assessment

Subjective Data

Ask the client about the type and location of his pain and related symptoms such as alteration in urinary patterns, warmth, fatigue, nausea, or vomiting. Assess the client's knowledge of his condition, treatment, follow-up care, and the implications of sterility and impotence to the client's life.

Objective Data

Inspect and palpate the genitals to detect the presence of scrotal swelling, testicular enlargement, scrotal immobility, redness, and warmth of the scrotum. Large varicoceles may be visible through the scrotal skin as a bluish discoloration.

Nursing diagnoses for a male client with a structural disorder of the reproductive system may include the following:

Nursing Diagnoses	Planning/Goals	Nursing Interventions
Risk for **Injury** related to inflammation and hemorrhage	The client will experience minimal bleeding and avoid infection.	Monitor the client's vital signs and incisional drainage. Maintain strict asepsis when handling wound dressings. Report hyperthermia, tachycardia, hypotension, increased incisional drainage, and swelling or redness around the incision to the physician immediately.
Deficient **Knowledge,** related to the condition and possible complications	The client will demonstrate understanding of the possible complications of his condition.	Monitor statements made by the client to determine if there is any misunderstanding about how the surgery will affect his masculinity and fertility. Provide the client with opportunities to voice his feelings and ask questions.

Evaluation Each goal must be evaluated to determine how it has been met by the client.

FUNCTIONAL DISORDERS AND CONCERNS

Included in this category are impotence, infertility, and contraception.

IMPOTENCE

Impotence is defined as the inability of an adult male to have an erection firm enough or to maintain it long enough to complete sexual intercourse. There are three types of impotence: functional, atonic, and anatomic. Psychological factors that lead to concerns about sexual performance may contribute to functional impotence. These factors include aging and difficulty with communication or relationships.

Atonic impotence may be the result of medications such as antihypertensives, sedatives, antidepressants, or tranquilizers. For example, antihypertensives lower blood pressure in all arteries of the body, and reduction of the blood pressure to penile arteries may lead to failure of the penis to fill sufficiently to achieve erection. The use of alcohol, cocaine, and nicotine can also decrease potency. Disease processes leading to atonic impotence include diabetes and vascular and neurological disorders. Diabetic clients are at increased risk for impotence because of their tendency to develop atherosclerosis and autonomic neuropathy. Vascular and neurological disorders include atherosclerosis, hypertension, spinal cord injuries, and multiple sclerosis. End-stage renal disease and chronic obstructive pulmonary disorders can also decrease potency.

Peyronie's disease is the development of nonelastic, fibrous tissue just beneath the penile skin, leading to anatomic impotence. The resulting loss of elasticity leads to a decreased ability of the penis to fill with and store blood during an erection. Peyronie's disease often causes the penis to bend upward, possibly leading to pain and an inability to penetrate the vagina (Figure 41-17).

Medical–Surgical Management

Medical

The first step in treating impotence is to determine whether the client's lifestyle is a factor. Further assessment may include nocturnal penile tumescence monitoring or dynamic infusion cavernosometry and cavernosography (DICC). Treatment will be based on the

Fibrous plaque

Tunica albuginea

External view   Internal view

Figure 41-17 *Peyronie's Disease:* **A,** *Fibrous plaque causes a curvature of the penis;* **B,** *Cross section of the penis showing plaque.*

Hypotension 7 MEPS
— anidore

assessment findings and test results. Treatment may include changes in lifestyle to reduce the need for medications, manage stress, lose weight, and exercise. These changes often help improve the client's physical health, self-image, and attitude about his ability to function sexually.

External devices can be used to promote an erection. A vacuum constriction device (VCD) may be used to increase the blood supply to the penis, causing engorgement and rigidity. The client inserts his penis into a plastic cylinder and squeezes a pump to withdraw the air from the cylinder, creating a vacuum that draws blood into the penis. Once an erection has been achieved in this manner, a rubber ring is moved from the bottom of the cylinder to the base of the penis. This permits the blood to be safely trapped in the penis for up to one-half hour. Advantages of the VCD over surgical intervention are less expense and fewer complications.

Surgical

Surgical interventions for impotency include revascularization and penile implants. For clients with impotence related to blocked arteries, revascularization is done to bypass blocked arteries and remove veins that are causing excessive drainage. For clients who are not candidates for revascularization, penile prostheses are another option. One type is a semirigid implant, which is a silicone cylinder that may be flexible or inflexible. Another type is a hydraulic implant that has a cylinder that can be inflated by squeezing a pump located in the scrotum or at the end of the penis. Because of its ability to fill and empty, the hydraulic implant, unlike the silicone implant, which is always semirigid, most closely mimics flaccidity and erection. The disadvantages of surgical interventions are expense and postoperative complications, the most serious being postoperative infection.

Pharmacological

Medications that promote erections are available. The one most widely used is sildenafil citrate (Viagra). This drug should not be used by men for whom sexual activ-

ity is not advisable because of underlying cardiovascular problems (Spratto & Woods, 2004). One side effect of drug therapy is prolonged erection that does not occur in response to sexual stimulation **(priapism).** Oral neurotransmitters have been used with variable success, and sublingual apomorphine shows some promise as an erectogenic agent. When administered sublingually rather than subcutaneously, as was done in the past, there are fewer side effects. Self-injections of vasodilators or other drugs may result in serious complications.

NURSING PROCESS

Assessment

Subjective Data

The client may describe a history of illicit and prescribed drug use, and alcohol consumption. Previous diagnoses, lifestyle, sexual functioning, and family disorders must be explored. Assess the client's emotional and educational needs to determine whether anxiety about sexual performance or lack of knowledge are contributing factors to impotence.

Objective Data

If the client has surgery, the nurse needs to monitor vital signs, incisional site, and intake and output.

Nursing Management

Teach client how to take prescribed medications. If an implant has been inserted, teach client the signs of infection such as tenderness, fever, and dysuria.

Nursing diagnoses for a client who is impotent may include the following:

- *Sexual Dysfunction,* related to altered body function or structure
- *Ineffective Sexuality Patterns* related to altered body function or structure
- *Disturbed Body Image,* related to impotence
- *Deficient Knowledge,* related to impotence

INFERTILITY

Approximately one in every six couples experiences infertility, the inability to produce offspring. Infertility may be primary or secondary. In primary infertility, the couple have never achieved a pregnancy or have never carried a pregnancy to viability. Secondary infertility involves problems that arise after the couple has had a successful pregnancy. Many factors may be investigated as causes of infertility in both female and male clients. Forty percent of infertility factors are female-related, 40% are male-related, and 20% are a combination of multiple factors that involve both partners. The more factors that are involved, the more difficult the infertility resolution.

The etiology of infertility may be related to anatomic or endocrine problems. The female anatomic or structural abnormalities may include blocked passages through the cervix or fallopian tubes caused by failed development or by past infections, such as PID, or STDs. Uterine and cervical abnormalities may also occur. The cervix may be too narrow or closed, and sperm are unable to navigate through the passage. The uterus may have a partial or complete septum inside that limits the internal cavity space. Immune problems involve the development of antibodies by the woman's system to the male's sperm. These antibodies may be present in the cervical mucus and kill the sperm on contact. Hyposecretion or hypersecretion of FSH, LH, estrogen, or progesterone have been associated with infertility.

The causes of infertility in males include varicoceles, cryptorchidism, impaired sperm, insufficient number of sperm, and hormonal imbalance. The use of hot tubs or saunas or tight underwear may decrease the sperm count.

The first step in treating an infertile couple is to obtain a history of sexual practices. In addition, detailed health histories need to be obtained and physical examinations performed.

A basic infertility workup may be initiated when the client has been unable to conceive after 6 to 12 months of unprotected intercourse. One simple, noninvasive procedure is the use of a basal body temperature chart. The chart is kept for a minimum of 3 months and then reviewed for normal ovulatory fluctuations in the basal temperature. During the first half of the menstrual cycle, the body temperature may remain below 98°F. At ovulation, there is often a slight decrease in the temperature for a 24-hour period. This is the optimal period of fertility. After ovulation, the woman's basal body temperature should go above 98°F and remain in that range for a period of 14 days. The length of the luteal phase (secretory phase) of the cycle following ovulation is a critical factor in some infertility disorders. Variations in the temperature chart may indicate that the client has had an anovulatory cycle or has a shortened luteal phase. Because the fertilized ovum does not implant in the endometrium until 6 to 8 days after conception, the luteal phase is critical to maintain the blood-rich lining long enough for implantation to occur. A low progesterone level during the luteal phase may result in spontaneous **abortion** (ending a pregnancy before the age of viability) of the fertilized ovum before implantation. Diagnostic tests that may be ordered include the following:

- Endometrial biopsy to detect tissue responses during both phases of the menstrual cycle
- Semen analysis, including sperm count, motility, and morphology
- Testicular biopsy (done when sperm are absent from the semen) to ascertain the presence of sperm
- Endocrine imbalance testing, which measures pituitary, gonadotropin, testosterone, estrogen, and progesterone levels
- Male–female interaction studies (Huhner test) to determine motility and number of sperm 2 to 4 hours after intercourse
- Laparoscopy to discover conditions such as endometriosis, adhesions, or scar tissue that potentially immobilize the fimbriae or polycystic ovarian disease (Stein-Leventhal syndrome)

Medical–Surgical Management

There is no one treatment for infertility problems. The goal of treatment is successful achievement of a pregnancy that is carried to full term and produces a healthy offspring.

Medical

Infertility treatment may include artificial insemination with either the partner's sperm or donor sperm. This method is particularly useful if the male partner has a low sperm count, abnormal sperm, or no sperm production. With the procedure, the semen is placed directly into the cervix or uterus with a small flexible catheter and a syringe.

Surgical

Several methods can be used to accomplish a pregnancy, with each one directed toward a different underlying cause of the infertility. One method is in vitro fertilization. This may be by GIFT (gamete-intra-fallopian transfer) or ZIFT (zygote-intra-fallopian transfer). With the GIFT technique, the female partner receives monthly cyclic hormone injections that cause ova to ripen. The hormones may cause more than one ovum to ripen during each cycle, which enhances the possibility that more than one ovum will be fertilized and implanted in the uterus. A semen specimen is collected from the male partner 1 to 2 hours before the GIFT procedure and the sperm placed into a special catheter. The ripened ovum is obtained from the female via laparoscopy or ultrasound aspiration and is loaded into the catheter in a sequential manner with the sperm and then injected through the fimbrial end of the fallopian tube, also by laparoscopy. This procedure takes approximately 1 hour to complete. Pregnancy is confirmed within 7 to 10 days with a blood hormonal test (Beta hCG) or an ultrasound, or both.

The ZIFT procedure is similar to GIFT; however, several ova are obtained just before ovulation and are placed in a special fluid for several hours while the sperm are prepared. The ova and sperm are then carefully mixed and closely observed for 2 to 3 days. The fertilized ova (now zygotes) are transferred into the fallopian tube or into the uterine cavity. Another name for the ZIFT procedure is IVF-ER (in vitro fertilization and embryo replacement), which more clearly defines what actually occurs.

Both GIFT and ZIFT are relatively expensive procedures (approximately $5,000 or more per cycle) and may or may not be covered by health insurance. For many couples, these are final efforts to conceive.

Pharmacological

Several medications are used in the treatment of infertility disorders, and most are focused on hormone imbalances or deficiencies. Clomiphene citrate (Clomid) stimulates release of follicle-stimulating hormone (FSH) and luteinizing hormone (LH) and is used to induce ovulation. Clomid is administered orally beginning on the fifth day of the menstrual cycle. If ovulation does not occur, the dosage will be increased for 5 days in the next cycle. If ovulation does not occur by the time the dose has been increased 4 or 5 times, it may be considered a Clomid failure. There is some chance of multiple gestation while the client is taking Clomid, and she should be so informed. Most often it is a twin pregnancy, but occasionally triplets may be conceived.

Menotropins (Pergonal) mimics FSH and LH, causing follicular growth and maturation. It is administered by intramuscular injection. Although Pergonal is an expensive drug, it has been shown to increase the possibility for ovulation in clients who have not responded to other medications.

Human chorionic gonadotropin (Pregnyl) may also be administered with the Clomid or Pergonal therapy to help maintain the endometrial lining for implantation. It stimulates the production of progesterone from the ovary until the fertilized ovum implants and the placenta begins to function. Progesterone suppositories may be used vaginally two times per day to help correct a luteal phase defect by lengthening the time from ovulation until the onset of the menses or through implantation and pregnancy. Some clients continue with the progesterone suppositories throughout the first few weeks of the pregnancy to ensure that the endometrium remains intact. If the sperm count or motility is low, testosterone or thyroid extracts may be prescribed.

Health Promotion

Seeking prompt medical treatment for infections that involve the reproductive system is an essential means of preventing infertility problems, especially with STDs and PID. PID causes scarring of the outside of the fallopian tubes, and gonorrhea can result in scarring or strictures of the internal fallopian tube. Either cause can result in an ectopic pregnancy when the fertilized ovum cannot pass through the tube.

Other considerations may include wise choices in contraceptive methods. The use of oral contraceptives has been associated with primary and secondary infertility caused by decreased pituitary function. This condition may resolve spontaneously, or medications may be required to stimulate ovulation in order to conceive.

Multiple sexual partners have also been associated with an increased risk of sexually transmitted disease, infections, and cervical cancer.

CONTRACEPTION

Contraception, or prevention of pregnancy, has been accomplished by many methods over the centuries. In weighing the options, safety, ease of use, effectiveness, and cost should be considered. Both partners' wishes should be considered in this decision-making process.

Contraception may be accomplished by natural means or medical interventions. This section of the chapter discusses a basic overview of the types of contraceptive methods currently available, the advantages

and disadvantages, the effectiveness of each kind, the mechanisms by which they work, and the client education that should accompany the methods (Table 41-2).

NATURAL METHOD

Natural methods of contraception may include what is called the "rhythm method." During the woman's fertile period of the month, usually lasting 7 days (3 days before ovulation to 3 days after), the couple should abstain from intercourse. The determination of the fertile period is based on the time of ovulation. Sperm can live up to 72 hours after ejaculation, and it is possible for sperm to still be in the cervix or uterus if the couple had intercourse 3 days before ovulation. The couple may also decide to maintain a basal body temperature chart to more accurately pinpoint ovulation each month. Another method to determine the approaching ovulation is to monitor the stretchiness of the cervical mucus. This is called "spinnbarkeit." As the woman nears ovulation, estrogen causes the cervical mucus to become clear, thin, and stretchy. This type of mucus provides a favorable environment for the sperm and helps their motility toward the ova. Immediately after ovulation, the cervical mucus becomes hostile to sperm. It becomes thick, cloudy, and more acidic. It also loses its stretchiness. Kits are available for purchase from the local drug store or pharmacy that react to chemicals in the cervical mucus and predict the time of ovulation. The kits are inexpensive and simple to use, much like home pregnancy tests.

HORMONAL METHODS

The many forms of hormonal contraceptives are discussed following.

Oral Contraceptives

The "pill" has been available as a contraceptive method for many years. Since its earliest form, it has been refined and the level of hormones reduced. Oral contraceptives work by suppressing ovulation. In a sense, the body thinks it is pregnant when the pill is used. Some oral contraceptives contain estrogen and progesterone; others contain only progestins.

In response to the pseudopregnancy state, the client may experience mild side effects and discomforts often associated with pregnancy such as nausea, headache, breast tenderness, or weight gain. Major side effects from oral contraceptives may include cardiovascular accidents or thrombophlebitis.

There is approximately a 1 in 200 chance of becoming pregnant while taking the oral contraceptive. If the woman thinks that she might be pregnant, she should stop the pill immediately and contact her physician. When the woman and her partner decide that it is time for a pregnancy, she should discontinue the oral contraceptive for at least 2 to 3 cycles before having unprotected intercourse. This "rest period" will lessen the possibility that pill effects will remain in her system and will allow her body to return to its own natural rhythm.

TABLE 41-2   CONTRACEPTION METHODS: EFFECTIVENESS AND CONCERNS

METHOD	EFFECTIVENESS RATE	RISKS	POSSIBLE SIDE EFFECTS	OTHER ADVANTAGES
Abstinence	100%	None known	Psychological reactions	Prevents infections including HIV
Hormonal				
Oral contraceptives	97%	Cardiovascular complications such as stroke, blood clots, high blood pressure, and heart attacks with the higher-dose combined oral contraceptive	Possible nausea, headaches, dizziness, spotting, weight gain, breast tenderness, chloasma, cramping	Protects against PID, decreases risk of ovarian and endometrial cancer, decreases menstrual blood loss and dysmenorrhea (cramps), decreases benign breast disease, regulates irregular menses, protects bone density, decreases risk of atherosclerosis, lessens the risk of rheumatoid arthritis, decreases uterine fibroids, and decreases ovarian cysts
Depo-Provera	98%	Pulmonary embolism	Headache, depression, hypertension, edema, nausea	Effective to treat obstructive sleep apnea
Lunelle	99%	None known	Breast tenderness, weight gain	None known
Mirena	99.8%	None known	Headache, acne, breast tenderness first few months	Decreases menstrual blood loss, may protect against endometrial cancer
Transdermal patch	99%	None known	Skin reaction at application site	None known
Vaginal ring	97%	None known	Vaginal infections or irritation, headache, weight gain, nausea	None known
Nonhormonal				
IUD	94%	Pelvic inflammatory disease, uterine perforation, anemia	Menstrual cramping, spotting, increased bleeding	None known
Barriers diaphragm cervical cap spermicide	84% 73–92% 79%	Mechanical irritation, vaginal infections, toxic shock syndrome	Pelvic pressure, cervical erosion, vaginal discharges if left in too long	Protects to some degree against sexually transmitted diseases
Condoms	86%	None known	Decreased sensation, allergy to latex, less spontaneity in lovemaking	Protects against sexually transmitted disease, including AIDS; delays premature ejaculation
Sterilization female male	99.6% 99.8%	Infection	Pain at surgical site, psychological reaction with subsequent regret	None known

Some women find that they experience primary or secondary infertility problems after being on the pill for several years because of pituitary suppression. The remedy is often fertility drugs such as clomiphene citrate (Clomid). Women who have never established a regular pattern of menstruation may not be good candidates for oral contraceptives, except as being used to regulate the cycle by artificial means. Other clients who should not take oral contraceptives include women with a history of hypertension, diabetes, cardiovascular disease, or thrombophlebitis. Some physicians may consider oral contraceptives in the newer low-dose combinations for clients who were previously in this high-risk group.

Depo-Provera

The medroxyprogesterone acetate (Depo-Provera) injection is administered intramuscularly (IM) every 12 weeks. It works like oral contraceptives to suppress ovulation. The client may experience breakthrough bleeding after the first injection, but this is not an indication that the hormone is not working. It usually requires about 3 weeks after the first injection before the contraceptive is effective, so the client should be advised to use a barrier contraceptive method during that period. The client must receive the injections at regular intervals to ensure effectiveness. Depo-Provera is a good option for the client who is approaching her forties or who smokes because it contains only progestins, which decreases the risk of cardiovascular problems.

Lunelle

The combination of estradiol cypionate and medroxyprogesterone acetate (Lunelle) is administered by IM injection every 28 to 30 days. It suppresses ovulation, thickens cervical mucus, and thins the endometrial lining. Monthly clinic visits are necessary, or the client must learn self-injection (Akert, 2003).

Mirena

Mirena, a levonorgestrol-releasing intrauterine system device, is placed in the uterus, providing contraception for 5 years. The small, soft T-shaped polyethylene frame has a hormone reservoir on the vertical stem that slowly releases the hormone. Cervical mucus thickens, sperm migration is inhibited, and endometrial growth is reduced. Mirena must be placed and removed by a health care provider (Akert, 2003).

Transdermal Patch

This first contraceptive patch, called OrthoEvra, contains norelgestromin and ethinyl estradiol. A new patch is applied every 7 days for 3 weeks. No patch is worn for the fourth week. Skin reactions are possible at the application site. The patch adheres during exercise, swimming, and hot tub/whirlpool use. It may not be as effective if the client weighs more than 198 pounds (Akert, 2003).

Vaginal Ring

The NuvaRing contains etonogestrel and ethinyl estradiol in a nonbiodegradable, flexible, transparent ring and provides constant delivery of hormones. It is inserted into the vagina and left for 3 weeks and then removed for 1 week. Precise ring position is not critical (Akert, 2003).

NONHORMONAL METHODS

Intrauterine Device

The intrauterine device (IUD) has been used for many years and has undergone several changes. The IUD is a T-shaped device wrapped with copper wire, which acts like a spermicide. The intrauterine device is recommended for women who have had children because the cervix has been dilated. This allows for easier insertion of the device. The IUD is inserted or removed by a clinician while the client is having her period because there is slight dilation of the cervix at that time. A string attached to the distal end of the device hangs out of the cervix into the vagina. The client is instructed to check the string each month after the menstrual period to make sure the device has not been expelled. Some women with an IUD experience more dysmenorrhea and a heavier menstrual flow. The IUD lasts 10 years. Fertility returns immediately upon removal.

Barriers

Methods of barrier contraception include male and female condoms, the diaphragm, and the cervical cap. Barrier devices work by blocking the pathway of the sperm through the cervix into the uterus. This type of contraceptive requires some preplanning on the part of one or both of the partners and may reduce the spontaneity of the sex act.

Spermicides

Spermicides contain a chemical, nonoxynol-9, that kills sperm on contact. If used alone, spermicidal agents have a lower efficacy rate than if used with a condom. The nurse should advise the couple to use a spermicidal gel, foam suppository, or film in addition to another barrier method for the greatest effectiveness. Foam should not be used with the diaphragm because it can result in deterioration of the latex. These agents must be placed in the vagina at least 15 minutes before intercourse to promote the spermicidal reaction. This method is safe and inexpensive but requires a high level of compliance each time or the effectiveness of the method drops significantly.

STERILIZATION METHOD

Sterilization is considered a permanent and very effective method of contraception. In a rare incident, a woman will become pregnant after a tubal ligation or after her partner has had a vasectomy. The female procedure interrupts the pathway through the fallopian tube. Sterilization may be performed on an outpatient basis in a surgical clinic or the outpatient department at the hospital. The tubal ligation is done under a general or epidural anesthetic with laparoscopy. The procedure takes about 30 to 60 minutes. The abdomen is distended with a gas to permit better visualization of the pelvic structures during the procedure.

The male sterilization, **vasectomy** (surgical resection of the vas deferens), is usually performed with local anesthesia on an outpatient basis. Rest, with ice to the scrotum, for 4 hours should follow. The client should not engage in strenuous activity or exercise for 1 week.

It may take up to 6 weeks for the semen to be clear of sperm. The client is instructed to return to the clinic for a sperm count after 20 ejaculations. If he is sexually active, during those ejaculations he should use a condom or some other form of contraception. At 6 months, a sperm count should be repeated and then monitored annually thereafter.

The female sterilization is more expensive and, because it requires more anesthesia, carries a slightly higher risk than the male procedure.

Refined microsurgical techniques have made it possible to reverse sterilization procedures. The reversals are not always successful, and the couple need to consider the odds of success before venturing into the expense of this type of surgery.

Summary

- Potential complications from PID may include sterility or infertility from scarring of fallopian tubes.
- Toxic shock syndrome occurs during the menses, and a strong correlation exists between the onset and use of super-absorbent tampons.
- Common male reproductive system inflammatory disorders include epididymitis, orchitis, and prostatitis. Bilateral epididymitis and orchitis can lead to sterility. Treatment includes antibiotic therapy.
- A BSE is an important method for detecting breast changes and should be practiced each month. Breast cancer is the most common female cancer in the United States.
- Benign prostatic hyperplasia is a common disorder in males older than age 50. Early symptoms include hesitancy, decreased force of stream, urinary frequency, and nocturia.

CASE STUDY

Mr. Able is a 70-year-old Caucasian male with a diagnosis of benign prostatic hyperplasia. Before his hospital admission for a TURP, he had been in good health. He returned from surgery 3 hours ago with a three-way Foley catheter and continuous bladder irrigation. His vital signs 1 hour ago were as follows: temperature 98.9°F, apical pulse 68, blood pressure 130/84, and respirations 18. When the nurse enters his room to take another set of vitals, Mr. Able is restless and moaning and has cool, moist skin; his catheter is not draining properly. His pulse is now 120 and blood pressure is 88/50. The nurse calls the physician to report the change in Mr. Able's condition. The physician orders a STAT hematocrit and a bleeding and clotting time. An increase in the IV fluid drip rate is also ordered. The doctor is planning to arrive at the hospital within the next hour.

The following questions will guide your development of a nursing care plan for the case study.

1. List symptoms and clinical manifestations, other than Mr. Able's, that a client may experience after a TURP.
2. List reasons why the doctor has ordered the STAT blood work and the IV changes.
3. List other diagnostic tests that may have been ordered for Mr. Able.
4. Mentally do a head-to-toe or functional assessment on Mr. Able. List subjective and objective data a nurse would want to obtain.
5. Write three individualized nursing diagnoses and goals for Mr. Able.
6. Upon assessing Mr. Able, the doctor decides to inject additional fluid into the balloon that anchors the indwelling catheter and apply increased traction to the catheter. List pertinent nursing actions a nurse would do following these medical interventions.
   - Medications
   - Comfort/rest
   - Cardiac output
   - Intake and output
   - Activity
   - Teaching
7. List resources within the medical center and the local area that could assist Mr. Able with his postoperative recovery.
8. List teaching that Mr. Able will need before his discharge.
9. List at least three successful outcomes for Mr. Able.

- Cervical cancer is most common in women with multiple sexual partners.
- Endometrial cancer often produces symptoms only after it is widespread. Any unusual vaginal bleeding should be investigated, especially if it occurs after menopause.
- Male cancers related to the reproductive system involve the prostate, testes, breast, and penis. Emphasis should be placed on testicular self-examination and regular physical examinations in order to facilitate early diagnosis and treatment.
- Menstrual disorders are often associated with hormonal imbalances, increased or decreased function of the endocrine glands, or neoplasms.
- Menopause is a normal, gradual decline in the ovarian production of female hormones that occurs around age 50.
- Infertility affects at least 1 in every 4 couples in the United States and is caused by hormonal imbalances and structural or physiologic abnormalities in both male and female clients.
- Women who smoke and are older than age 40 are at greater risk for major complications while using oral contraceptives. Major health risks include cardiovascular accidents and deep vein thrombosis.
- Impotence may be caused by emotional or physical factors. Treatment includes counseling, medications, circulatory aids, and surgery.

Review Questions

1. The female client should perform BSE (breast self-examination)
   a. just before the menstrual period.
   b. just after the menstrual period.
   c. at ovulation.
   d. any time of the month.

2. A dietary element frequently associated with fibrocystic breast disease is:
   a. fats.
   b. protein.
   c. sodium.
   d. caffeine.

3. The characteristic signs of a trichomonas vaginitis are:
   a. thick, white, "cheesy" discharge with itching.
   b. frothy, foul-smelling, yellow discharge with itching and irritation.
   c. creamy, thin, vaginal discharge with a musty or fishy odor.
   d. painful intercourse caused by decreased lubrication.

4. The factor that predisposes males to penile cancer is:
   a. alcohol consumption.
   b. not being circumcised.
   c. advanced age.
   d. circumcision.

5. The nursing intervention that can help alleviate bladder spasms post-TURP is:
   a. increasing fluid intake.
   b. maintaining traction on the urethral catheter.
   c. administering B&O suppositories.
   d. applying ice to and elevating the scrotum.

References/Suggested Readings

Akert, J. (2003). A new generation of contraceptives. RN, 66(2), 54–61.
American Cancer Society (ACS). (2003). Cancer facts & figures—2003 [Online]. Available: www.cancer.org/downloads/STT/CFF2003DUSSecured.pdf
Angelucci, P. (1997). Benign prostatic hyperplasia. Nursing97, 27(11), 54–55.
Baird, S., Donehower, M., Stalsbroten, V., & Ades, T. (Eds.). (1997). A cancer source book for nurses (7th ed.). Atlanta: American Cancer Society.
Choma, K. (2003). ASC-US HPV testing. AJN, 103(2), 42–50.
Conversations with Colleagues. (2003). Endometriosis sufferers risk other diseases. AWHONN Lifelines, 6(6), 502–504.
Crandall, L. (1997). Menopause made easier. RN, 60(7), 46–50.
D'Arcy, Y. (2002). What is postmastectomy pain syndrome? Nursing2002, 32(11), 17.
Daniels, R. (2002). Delmar's Guide to Laboratory and Diagnostic Tests. Clifton Park, NY: Thomson Delmar Learning.
Dell, D. (2001). Regaining range of motion after breast surgery. Nursing2001, 31(10), 50–52.
Dochterman, J., & Bulechek, G. (2004). Nursing Interventions Classification (NIC) (4th ed.). St. Louis, MO: Mosby.
Estes, M. E. Z. (2002). Health assessment & physical examination. (2nd ed.). Clifton Park, NY: Thomson Delmar Learning.
Fink, J. (2003). Beyond the shock of an abnormal Pap. RN, 66(6), 56–61.
Fletcher, S., & Colditz, G. (2003). Editorial: Failure of estrogen plus progestin therapy for prevention. Journal of the American Medical Association, 288(3). [Online]. Available: http://jama.ama-assn.org/issues/v288n3/ffull/jed20042.html
Gordon, S., Brenden, J., Wyble, J., & Ivey, C. (1997). When the Dx is penile cancer. RN, 60(3), 41–44.
Harris, L. (2002). Ovarian cancer: Screening for early detection. AJN, 102(10), 46–52.
Held-Warmkessel, J. (2002). Prostate cancer. Nursing2002, 32(12), 36–42.
Hutti, M. (2003). New & emerging contraceptive methods. AWHONN Lifelines, 7(1), 32–39.
Kessenich, C. (1999). Myths & facts about menopause. Nursing99, 29(4), 67.

Kring, D. (2003). Benign prostatic hyperplasia. *Nursing2003*, *33*(5), 44–45.

Machia, J. (2002). Breast cancer: Risk, prevention, & tamoxifen. *AJN, 101*(4), 26–34.

Marchbanks, P. A., McDonald, J. A. et al. (2002). Oral contraceptives and the risk of breast cancer. *New England Journal of Medicine, 346*(26), 2025.

Marieb, E. N. (2003). *Human anatomy and physiology* (6th ed.). Redwood City, CA: Benjamin/Cummings.

Martini, F. H. (2002). *Fundamentals of anatomy & physiology* (6th ed.). Englewood Cliffs, NJ: Prentice Hall.

Miller, K. (1999). Testicular torsion. *AJN 99*(6), 33.

Moorhead, S., Johnson, M., & Maas, M. (2004). *Nursing Outcomes Classification (NOC)* (3rd ed.). St. Louis, MO: Mosby.

National Cancer Institute (NCI). (2002a). *What you need to know about breast cancer* (NIH Publication No. 00-1556). [Online]. Available: www.nci.nihl.gov/cancerinfo/wyntk/breast

National Cancer Institute (NCI). (2002b). *What you need to know about cancer of the cervix* (NIH Publication No. 95-2047). [Online]. Available: www.nci.nih.gov/cancerinfo/wyntk/cervix

National Cancer Institute (NCI). (2002c). *What you need to know about cancer of the uterus* (NIH Publication No. 01-1562). [Online]. Available: www.nci.nih.gov/cancerinfo/wyntk/uterus

National Cancer Institute (NCI). (2002d). *What you need to know about ovarian cancer* (NIH Publication No. 00-1561). [Online]. Available: www.nci.nih.gov/cancerinfo/wyntk/ovary

National Institute of Diabetes, and Digestive and Kidney Disease (NIDDK). (2002). *Prostate enlargement: Benign prostatic hyperplasia.* [Online]. Available: www.niddk.nih.gov/health/urolog/pubs/prostate/index.htm

North American Nursing Diagnosis Association. (2003). *NANDA nursing diagnoses: Definitions and classification* 2003–2004, Philadelphia: Author.

Otto, S. (2001). *Oncology nursing* (4th ed.). St. Louis, MO: Mosby–Year Book.

Pasacreta, J., Jacobs, L., & Cataldo, J. (2002). Genetic testing for breast and ovarian cancer risk: The psychosocial issues. *AJN, 102*(12), 40–47.

Pickar, G. D. (1999). *Dosage calculations* (6th ed.). Clifton Park, NY: Thomson Delmar Learning.

Resnick, B., & Belcher, A. (2002). Breast reconstruction. *AJN, 102*(4), 26–33.

Sarvis, C. (2003). When lymphedema takes hold. *RN, 66*(9), 32–36.

Spratto, G., & Woods, A. (2004). *2004 PDR Nurse's Drug Handbook.* Clifton Park, NY: Thomson Delmar Learning.

U. S. Food and Drug Administration (FDA). (2002). *Update on advisory for Norplant contraception kits.* [Online]. Available: www.fda.gov/medwatch/safety/2002/norplant.htm

Workman, L. (2002). Breast cancer. *Nursing2002, 32*(10), 58–63.

Wynd, C. (2002). Testicular self-examination in young adult men. *Journal of Nursing Scholarship, 34*(3), 251–255.

Zaccognini, M. (1999). Prostate cancer, *AJN, 99*(4), 34–35.

Zuckerman, D. (2002). The breast cancer information gap. *RN, 65*(2), 39–41.

Resources

American Association of Sex Educators, Counselors, and Therapists, P.O. Box 5488, Richmond, VA 23220-0488, www.aasect.org

American Cancer Society, Inc., 1599 Clifton Road, NE, Atlanta, GA, 30329, 404-320-3333, 800-ACS-2345, www.cancer.org

American College of Obstetricians and Gynecologists (ACOG), 409 12th Street SW, P.O. Box 96920, Washington, DC, 20090-6920, www.acog.org

American Society of Reproductive Medicine, 1209 Montgomery Highway, Birmingham, AL, 35216-2809, 205-978-5000, www.asrm.org

Association of Women's Health, Obstetrical, and Neonatal Nursing (AWHONN), 2000 L. Street NW, Suite 740, Washington, DC, 20036, 800-673-8499, www.awhonn.org

National Breast Cancer Organization, 212 West Van Buren, Suite 800, Chicago, IL, 60601, 800-221-2141, www.y-me.org

National Cancer Institute (NCI), Public Inquiries Office, Suite 3036A, 6116 Executive Boulevard, MCS 8322, Bethesda, MD 20892-8322, 800-422-6237, www.nci.nih.gov

National Ovarian Cancer Coalition, 500 N E Spanish River Boulevard, Suite 14, Boca Raton, FL 33431, 888-682-7426, www.ovarian.org

North American Menopause Society (NAMS), 5900 Landerbrook Dr., Suite 195, Mayfield Heights, OH, 44124, 440-442-7550, www.menopause.org

Older Women's League, 666 11th Street, N.W., Suite 700, Washington, DC, 20001, 800-825-3695, www.owl-national.org

Ovarian Cancer National Alliance, 910 17th Street NW, Suite 413, Washington, DC 20006, 202-331-1332, www.ovariancancer.org

Recovery of Male Potency, Grace Hospital, 18700 Meyers Rd., Detroit, MI, 48235, 800-835-7667

RESOLVE: The National Infertility Association, 1310 Broadway, Sumerville, MA 02144, 888-623-0744, www.resolve.org

SEXUALLY TRANSMITTED DISEASES

MAKING THE CONNECTION

Refer to the following chapters to increase your understanding of sexually transmitted diseases:

Basic Nursing
- Diagnostic Tests

Adult Health Nursing
- Reproductive System
- Immune System

LEARNING OBJECTIVES

Upon completion of this chapter, you should be able to:
- Define key terms.
- List the most prevalent STDs, including causative agents.
- Describe currently used methods of prevention of STDs.
- Describe signs and symptoms, diagnostic aids, and treatment of the common STDs.
- Utilize the nursing process to plan the care of a client with an STD.
- Demonstrate the ability to teach self-care and reinfection prevention measures to the client with an STD.

KEY TERMS

chancre	incidence
exposure	incubation period

INTRODUCTION

Sexually transmitted diseases (STDs) are transmitted or passed from one person to another primarily through sexual contact. The STDs covered in this chapter are chlamydia, gonorrhea, syphilis, genital herpes, cytomegalovirus, genital warts, trichomoniasis, and hepatitis B. Acquired immunodeficiency syndrome (AIDS) is not solely a sexually transmitted disease, although sexual activity is one of the primary modes of transmission. AIDS is discussed in detail in Chapter 44 and will be briefly discussed here.

The **incidence** (frequency of disease occurrence) of STDs has been increasing worldwide, with trichomoniasis, chlamydia, and gonorrhea being the most widespread STDs today. Syphilis has been described as a sexually transmitted disease for centuries. An estimated 15.3 million Americans are diagnosed annually with an STD (National Institute of Allergy and Infectious Diseases [NIAID], 1998). Chlamydia, for example, affects more than 4 million Americans every year, making it 11 times as common as gonorrhea. Syphilis, although less common than either chlamydia or gonorrhea, still affects more than 6,000 people each year in the United States (NIAID 2002a, 2002c, 2002d).

The development of antibiotic treatment for STDs in the 1940s caused a dramatic decrease in the prevalence of STDs, and for awhile it was predicted that STDs would be eradicated completely. But a variety of factors have contributed to the dramatic increase of STDs, such as casual sex, asymptomatic carriers of the disease, the use of nonbarrier methods of birth control, and lack of knowledge of methods of preventing STDs.

Another factor that has contributed to the vast increase in STDs in recent years is the increased consumption of alcohol and the use of illegal drugs. The sharing of needles among intravenous (IV) drug abusers is a factor in the increased incidence of STDs, as is the lessening of inhibitions that occurs with drug and alcohol abuse. The trading of sex for drugs is also a factor in the spread of STDs.

Inadequate reporting of STDs may also cause statistics to be inaccurate. There is no uniformity in reporting requirements for STDs. Regulations differ from state to state and from disease to disease. All states in the United

States require that cases of gonorrhea and syphilis be reported to a health officer in that state. Only 35 states have mandatory HIV reporting (Sharts-Hopko, 1997). The Centers for Disease Control and Prevention (CDC) keeps statistics on reportable diseases.

Public education regarding the causes, methods of transmission, and methods of prevention of STDs is the most important weapon in the battle against STDs. Although many STDs caused by bacterial infection are curable with modern antibiotics, the viruses are not.

Because sexual activity is beginning at earlier ages today, sex education, including information about STDs, is being presented in elementary schools. Many schools have comprehensive education programs already in place to teach about STDs and recommendations to prevent the spread of STDs. Television, especially educational programs, has been helpful in informing the public of the dangers of having sex without protection against STDs.

Many messages have been disseminated to the general public regarding the best methods of prevention of STDs. The only 100% effective method of prevention of STDs is abstinence (refraining from sexual intercourse or mucous membrane–to–mucous membrane contact altogether). Couples who are mutually monogamous are also not at risk, unless one of them was previously infected. The popularity of the birth control pill has decreased consistent condom use. Most current methods of birth control are not effective in preventing the transmission of STDs. Only a barrier method, the latex condom, has been effective in preventing the spread of STDs, although even this method provides only safer sex, not totally safe sex.

Once the diagnosis of an STD is made, identification of all sexual contacts is important. Many people are reluctant to be candid regarding sexual activity and sexual contacts because this is an area of life considered to be extremely private. One of the most difficult aspects in dealing with STDs is that many of the diseases are asymptomatic, especially in women. These asymptomatic partners can both transmit the disease to new partners and/or reinfect a treated partner, if they are not identified and treated.

An overview of the STDs covered in this chapter is presented in Table 42-1.

ANATOMY AND PHYSIOLOGY REVIEW

The major system affected by the sexually transmitted diseases is the reproductive system. Males are generally more symptomatic than females and will seek health care more readily because the signs of disease on the external genitalia are more visible. In females, the sex organs are internal; females, therefore, are more likely to have complications and increased severity of symptoms by the time the disease is identified.

In addition to the reproductive system, any area of sexual contact, such as oral and rectal areas, may also exhibit signs and symptoms of the disease process.

COMMON DIAGNOSTIC TESTS

Commonly used diagnostic tests for clients with symptoms of sexually transmitted diseases are listed in Table 42-2.

TABLE 42-1	SEXUALLY TRANSMITTED DISEASES: AN OVERVIEW	
DISEASE	**CHARACTERISTICS**	**NURSING IMPLICATIONS**
Chlamydia	Asymptomatic or may experience purulent discharge Painful urination Urethral discharge Note: If untreated, pelvic inflammatory disease (PID) can develop.	Instruct client to notify sexual partner(s) of past 2 months of their need for treatment. Instruct client to avoid sexual activity or to use condoms until both client and partner(s) are symptom free. Provide instruction regarding medications prescribed.
Cytomegalovirus (CMV) (Human herpesvirus type 5 [HHV-5])	Often asymptomatic, occasionally fever, fatigue, and weakness Generally acquired during childhood or adolescence 80% to 100% of adults have antibodies to CMV by age 70.	Implicated in some spontaneous abortions or mental retardation Congenital infection produces cytomegalic inclusion disease. May be life threatening in a client with a poorly functioning immune system.
Genital Herpes: Herpes Simplex Virus 2 (HSV-2) (Human herpesvirus type 2 [HHV-2])	Vesicles on penis, vagina, labia, perineum, or anus Can progress to painful ulceration Lesions may last up to 6 weeks Recurrence common Note: May be asymptomatic	Refer sexual partner(s) for examination. Teach that virus can be transmitted even when the person experiences no symptoms. Instruct in use of condoms. Teach females of need for annual Pap smear. Provide instruction regarding medications prescribed.

continues

TABLE 42-1   continued

DISEASE	CHARACTERISTICS	NURSING IMPLICATIONS
Gonorrhea	*Male:* Urethritis (inflammation of the urethra) Purulent discharge Urinary frequency Epididymitis (inflammation of the epididymis) *Female:* Often asymptomatic May lead to PID or salpingitis (inflammation of the fallopian tube) Can occlude the fallopian tubes, resulting in sterility	Instruct client to return if symptoms persist. Sexual partner(s) of past 60 days must be assessed. Instruct client to avoid sexual activity until symptoms subside in both client and partner(s). Provide instruction regarding medications prescribed.
Hepatitis B Virus (HBV)	Varies greatly from asymptomatic state to severe hepatitis to cancer	Partner(s) should receive medical prophylaxis within 14 days after exposure. For client and partner(s), recommend three-dose immunization series when this episode has abated.
Genital Warts (Human Papillomavirus) (HPV)	Fleshy, cauliflowerlike growth on genitalia	Inform and treat sexual partner(s). Provide instruction regarding medications prescribed.
Syphilis	Disease consists of four stages with distinct manifestations as follows: *Primary:* A painless papule on penis, vagina, or cervix (chancre) Usually negative serologic blood test Highly infectious during this stage *Secondary:* Rash, especially prevalent on palms and soles Low-grade fever Sore throat Headache *Early latency:* Possible infectious lesions, otherwise asymptomatic Reactive serologic tests *Late latency:* Possible lesions in central nervous and cardiovascular systems Noninfectious except to fetus of pregnant woman	Interview client to identify sexual contacts. All those exposed to the disease should be given penicillin or other antibiotic if allergic to penicillin. Educate client and sexual contacts about the disease. Provide instruction regarding medications prescribed. Counsel and educate client. Counsel and educate client.
Trichomoniasis	Petechial lesions Profuse urethral or vaginal discharge that is foul smelling, yellow, and foamy	Treat sexual partners simultaneously with metronidazole (Flagyl). Provide instruction regarding medication prescribed.

TABLE 42-2 COMMON DIAGNOSTIC TESTS FOR SEXUALLY TRANSMITTED DISEASES

Blood Tests
- Enzyme-linked immunosorbent assay (ELISA)
- Western blot
- Venereal Disease Research Laboratories (VDRL)
- Rapid plasma reagin (RPR)
- Fluorescent treponemal antibody-absorption test (FTA-ABS)
- Reiter test

Culture
- Tissue: Male urethra, female endocervix
- Discharge
- Tzanck

Urine
- Urine specimen

Other
- Dark field examination of wart scrapings
- Microscopic examination

CHLAMYDIA

Chlamydia is caused by a spherical bacterial organism known as *Chlamydia trachomatis*. Outside the body, the organism has difficulty surviving, but inside the body, chlamydia reproduces rapidly. The mode of transmission in chlamydia must be through intimate body contact because the organism is so fragile that it cannot survive long when outside of the body.

Most chlamydia infections are asymptomatic. Chlamydia is known as the "silent STD" for this reason. If left untreated, chlamydial infections cause tissue inflammation, ulceration, and scar tissue formation in both women and men. Salpingitis (inflammation of the fallopian tubes) or pelvic inflammatory disease (PID) can lead to scarring of the delicate fallopian tubes, ectopic pregnancy, or even infertility.

When symptoms of chlamydia appear in males, they are dysuria and genital discharge. Females may have a grayish white mucopurulent vaginal discharge, itching, and dysuria. *srinky*

Medical–Surgical Management
Pharmacological   *Both partners Tested.*

The treatment of choice is doxycycline (Vibramycin). If compliance with an extended period of drug therapy is thought to be a problem, azithromycin (Zithromax) can be given orally in a single dose. Pregnant women may be treated with erythromycin estolate (Ilosone) or amoxicillin (Amoxil), but they should be cultured again after treatment is completed to confirm the absence of chlamydial infection. Retesting is not required after treatment with doxycycline or azithromycin. It is important that all sexual partners be tested and treated for chlamydia because reinfection is probable if only one partner is treated.

Health Promotion

Persons who have more than one sexual partner, especially women less than 25 years old, should regularly be tested for chlamydial infection even when there are no symptoms. The current use of male latex condoms during sexual intercourse may help reduce transmission (NIAID 2002a).

GONORRHEA

Gonorrheal infections are often seen in combination with chlamydia. Gonorrhea is a serious bacterial infection, caused by the gram-negative bacterial organism *Neisseria gonorrhea*. In 2000, more than 350,000 cases occurred in the United States (NIAID, 2002c). The organism multiplies quickly in warm, moist areas of the body, including the oral cavity, reproductive tract, and rectum. Mouth-to-mouth kissing does not transmit gonorrhea. It is spread during sexual intercourse—vaginal, oral, and anal. The cervix is the usual site of infection in women. The disease progresses in much the same manner as chlamydia and can cause many of the same complications, such as infertility from salpingitis and PID.

Symptoms of infection may occur within 2 to 10 days after **exposure** (contact with an infected person or agent). Again, men are more likely to exhibit symptoms, such as burning on urination and a purulent discharge from the penis. Many women are asymptomatic, but the remainder may have pain or burning on urination and/or a yellow or bloody vaginal discharge.

If a woman is infected with gonorrhea when she gives birth, the infection may be transmitted to the newborn's eyes as the baby travels through the birth canal. In the United States, all infants are treated with an antibiotic ophthalmic ointment within 1 to 2 hours of birth to prevent the gonorrheal-induced eye infection known as ophthalmia neonatorum.

Medical–Surgical Management

Once the presence of gonorrhea has been confirmed, both partners should be treated with a course of antibiotic therapy. Penicillin used to be the drug of choice when treating gonorrhea, but because penicillin has

CLIENT TEACHING

Gonorrhea and HIV
- Infection with gonorrhea increases the risk of HIV infection.
- Prevention and/or early treatment of gonorrhea is critical.

been so widely used against many types of infection, some strains of *Neisseria gonorrhea* have adapted and are no longer affected by penicillin. The current practice is to treat all cases of gonorrhea as though they were resistant to the traditional drug therapies.

Pharmacological

A variety of antibiotics are effective against gonorrhea. One of the most effective therapies includes a single dose of ciprofloxacin (Cipro), followed by a 7-day course of oral doxycycline (Vibramycin). Because almost half of all clients with gonorrhea also have chlamydia, doxycycline (Vibramycin) is an appropriate choice of drug therapy because it combats both infections effectively. For pregnant clients, or those younger than 16 years of age, an injection of ceftriaxone sodium (Rocephlin), followed by oral erythromycin estolate (Ilosone), is recommended. Follow-up cultures to determine the success of the course of treatment are recommended when the treatment has been completed.

SYPHILIS

Syphilis, an STD that was almost eradicated after the discovery of antibiotic therapy in the 1940s, is on the upswing again, with 6,103 cases reported in 2001 (NIAID 2002d). The causative organism of syphilis is a spirochete, a spiral-shaped bacteria known as *Treponema pallidum*, which was first identified in 1905. Transmission of syphilis is either through sexual contact or congenitally (mother to child). Syphilis is often seen with human immunodeficiency virus (HIV) infection, just as chlamydia is often seen with gonorrhea.

Syphilis has four stages. In primary stage syphilis, the **incubation period,** time between exposure to an infectious disease and the first appearance of symptoms, can be 10 to 90 days, with the development of a **chancre** usually occurring within 2 to 6 weeks. A chancre is a clean, painless ulcer, which usually is present at the site of body contact (Figure 42-1). There is usually just one chancre present, but multiple chancres have been known to occur. Chancres may occur on the internal genitalia of women (e.g., the cervix) and thus not be noticed. The chancre will heal within a few weeks, even

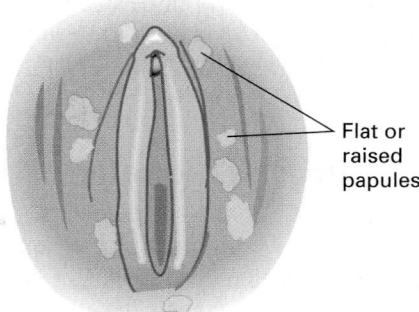

Figure 42-2 *Condyloma latum, a wart-like growth, may be present in the genital area of males and females in secondary syphilis.*

without treatment, and either leave a thin scar or none at all. If not identified and treated, about one-third will progress to secondary syphilis.

In secondary syphilis, the client has a skin rash of penny-sized brown sores that appear approximately 3 to 6 weeks after the chancre. The rash may be on all or any part of the body but almost always involves the palms of the hands and the soles of the feet. Active bacteria are in the sores, so any contact, sexual or nonsexual, with the broken skin of the infected person may spread the infection. The rash heals within several months. Other symptoms, such as low-grade fever, fatigue, headache, sore throat, and generalized lymph node swelling, may occur. Occasionally, a wartlike growth known as condyloma latum may be present in the genital area of both men and women (Figure 42-2). Because this growth is so close in appearance to the condylomata acuminata of human papillomavirus infection, it may be confused with genital warts. Symptoms of secondary syphilis may come and go for 1 or 2 years. Because many of these symptoms are also common to many other diseases, syphilis has often been called "the great imitator."

When not treated, syphilis enters into a latent period when no symptoms are present and the disease is no longer contagious. Only about one-third of those clients with secondary syphilis will develop the symptoms of tertiary syphilis; that is, when the bacteria damages the heart, eyes, brain, nervous system, bones, joints, or any other part of the body. Tertiary syphilis can last for years or decades and may result in heart disease, blindness, neurologic problems, and death.

Figure 42-1 *The chancre usually occurs at the point where the organism contacted the body.*

CLIENT TEACHING

Testing for Syphilis

- Sexually active individuals with a suspicious rash or sore in the genital area should see a health care provider and should avoid sexual contact.
- If treated for another STD, the client should also be tested for syphilis.

Approximately 3% to 7% of untreated persons will develop neurosyphilis (NIAID, 2002d). Symptoms may range from none to headache, fever, seizures, and stroke symptoms. Sometimes it may take 20 years for this progression to occur.

Medical–Surgical Management
Pharmacological

Since the time that syphilis was first treated with antibiotic therapy, penicillin has remained the drug of choice because no cases of penicillin-resistant syphilis have been identified. All types of penicillin are effective, but penicillin G benzathine (Bicillin L-A) is often preferred. Antimicrobial therapy will destroy *Treponema pallidum* at any stage, but any damage done to body organs is irreversible. If the client has a demonstrated allergy to penicillin, alternative medications may be administered, such as doxycycline (Vibramycin), tetracycline HCl (Achromycin V), or erythromycin estolate (Ilosone). For pregnant women who are allergic to penicillin, erythromycin is recommended as the best alternative therapy.

Clients being treated for syphilis must have periodic blood tests to ensure that the infecting agent has been completely destroyed.

GENITAL HERPES

Genital herpes affects an estimated 60 million persons in the United States with an estimated 500,000 new cases each year (NIAID, 1999). It is caused by the human herpesvirus type 2 (HHV-2), commonly called herpes simplex virus (HSV-2). HSV-1 commonly causes sores on the lips (fever blisters, cold sores). HSV-2 causes genital sores. Either can infect the other area following oral-genital sex. Genital herpes is usually acquired through sexual contact with an infected person. That person may or may not be aware of having genital herpes.

When symptoms occur in the first episode, they usually appear in 2 to 10 days after infection and last an average of 2 to 3 weeks. Itching or burning sensations;

Figure 42-3 *Chronic Mucocutaneous Perianal Herpes Infection (Courtesy of Centers for Disease Control and Prevention, Atlanta, GA 30333)*

pain in the genital area, legs, or buttocks; vaginal discharge; or abdominal pressure are the early symptoms. Within a few days, lesions (sores) appear at the infection site (perianal area), in the vagina or on the cervix of females, or in the urethra of females and males.

Small red bumps appear first, change into blisters (Figure 42-3), and then become open sores that crust over in a few days. Other symptoms with the first episode may include fever, muscle aches, headache, dysuria, vaginal discharge, and swollen glands in the groin.

With the first episode, the virus travels through the sensory nerves and remains inactive in nerve cells until the virus travels back to the skin, causing a recurrence. The frequency of recurrences vary greatly (some only 1 or 2 a year), but new sores may or may not be apparent. Symptoms are usually milder than the first episode and last approximately 1 week.

The most accurate method of diagnosis is a viral culture, which takes several days. A blood test detecting HSV antibodies only indicates that the person has been infected at some time.

Medical–Surgical Management
Pharmacological

There is no known cure for the herpes simplex virus at this time. Treatment has been geared toward alleviating symptoms of the disease. Acyclovir (Zovirax) has been utilized in the treatment of herpes. A topical form may be applied to the lesions; the drug may also be taken orally to shorten the duration of the lesions in a primary outbreak. When taken daily, it prevents most recurrences. Famciclovir (Famivir) and valacyclovir (Valtrex) treat later episodes and prevent recurrences.

Cleansing the area of the lesions with mild soap and water, hydrogen peroxide, or Burow's solution often helps reduce the discomfort of the lesions and decrease the chance of secondary infections. The area should be blown dry with a hairdryer, and then the dry skin may be dusted with a cornstarch powder, which aids in decreasing client discomfort.

CYTOMEGALOVIRUS

Another virus in the herpesvirus family is cytomegalovirus (CMV). Figure 42-4 shows an electron micrograph of CMV. Unlike the more commonly recognized herpes viruses, CMV rarely produces noticeable clinical symptoms.

CMV is primarily transmitted from person to person through contact with body fluids such as saliva, urine, and blood. The virus has been identified in semen and cervical mucus, so it can be spread by sexual contact. CMV is incurable; people are infected for life. The inactive virus may reactivate from time to time.

Most people acquire CMV during childhood or adolescence through contact with saliva and respiratory secretions and will not notice any symptoms. Occasionally, a client will present with fever, fatigue, and weakness. These symptoms may persist for several weeks and may lead to a tentative diagnosis of infectious mononucleo-

Figure 42-4   *Electron Micrograph of CMV (Courtesy of Centers for Disease Control and Prevention, Atlanta, GA 30333)*

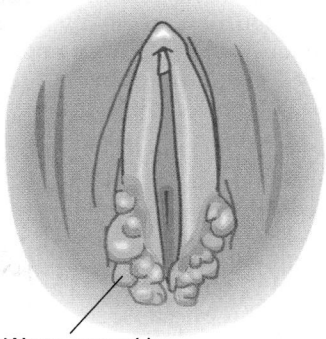

Warts caused by
human papillomavirus (HPV)

Figure 42-5   *Genital Warts (Condyloma acuminatum)*

sis, although the sore throat and swollen lymph nodes of "mono" are not present with CMV.

CMV has been implicated in some complications of pregnancy, such as spontaneous abortion or mental retardation of the neonate. Congenital infection of an infant produces cytomegalic inclusion disease that ranges from an asymptomatic condition to a severely debilitating condition that may even result in death. The central nervous system damage to the infant may be profound, although it occurs rarely. An estimated 6,000 babies each year develop life-threatening complications of congenital CMV at birth or have mental retardation, blindness, deafness, or epilepsy (NIAID, 1998a). CMV can also become a life-threatening illness in a client who has a poorly functioning immune system, such as a client with AIDS.

There is no antiviral agent specifically utilized for this disorder because most of the population will not have any symptoms.

GENITAL WARTS

Another virus that is sexually transmitted is the human papillomavirus (HPV), which causes genital warts, also called condylomata acuminata. These genital warts may occur in the urogenital, perineal, or anal areas and may be either external or internal. The population at risk seems to be teenage girls or young women in their twenties. In the United States, it is estimated that there are approximately 5.5 million new cases of genital warts identified every year, and at least 20 million are already infected with HPV (NIAID, 2001). The incubation period for genital warts appears to be approximately 1 to 2 months, but may be up to 6 months. Unlike genital herpes, genital warts are usually painless, soft fleshy growths appearing most commonly in the genital area. Sometimes many warts may grow together to form a large cauliflower-shaped growth (Figure 42-5).

The greatest health threat that HPV poses to a female client is the possible development of cervical cancer. Although there are more than 100 different types of

HPV, only 30 types are spread through sexual contact, and some of these can cause cervical cancer (NIAID, 2001). Cigarette smoking has been linked to the development of cancerous cervical changes in women with HPV. Women who have HPV should be advised not to smoke. HPV appears to play a role in the development of cervical cancer, along with many other factors. An abnormal Pap test may be the first indication of HPV.

Genital warts are less common in men. If seen, they are usually on the tip of the penis.

Medical–Surgical Management

Because genital warts are caused by a virus, there is no cure for the disease. The focus is on preventing the spread of the disease to sexual partners and reducing the possibility of cancer. Use of a condom during sexual intercourse may provide some protection. Once the genital warts disappear, the disease may lie dormant for many years until there is a recurrence of the outbreak.

Surgical

The warts may be removed under local anesthesia. This is especially recommended if the warts have formed a large, fleshy cauliflower-like growth. Freezing the warts off with cryosurgery, surgical use of extreme cold, is the treatment of choice for small warts. The warts may also be removed with laser surgery or cauterized. Whatever treatment is recommended, it must be remembered that the treatment will not cure HPV, but only provide a palliative effect. The warts may recur after any treatment.

Pharmacological

A topical solution of podophyllum resin (Poddoen) may be applied to the genital warts. It is only recommended for treatment of one or two lesions at a time because it can be toxic if applied to too large an area at one time. Most people report experiencing a good deal of pain from the treatment. After the solution has been in contact with the genital warts for a period of 4 to 6 hours, it is then washed off with soap and water. If not thoroughly washed off, podophyllum may cause chemical burns that heal very slowly and are very painful. This therapy must not be used on a diabetic client, a client with poor circulation, or a pregnant client.

A cream, imiquimod (Aldara), is applied before bedtime and washed off in the morning. It can be used 3 times a week for 16 weeks or less.

AIDS

AIDS, or acquired immunodeficiency syndrome, is not truly a sexually transmitted disease, but it needs to be discussed briefly here because sexual contact is one of the primary modes of its transmission. AIDS is the end stage of the disease process caused by the human immunodeficiency virus (Chapter 44). Similar to the viruses previously discussed in this chapter, AIDS is not curable. Unlike the other viruses, herpes genitalis and genital warts, AIDS is ultimately fatal. AIDS results in a severe disorder of the body's immune system, leading to an inability of the body to fight off disease.

Persons at risk are those who have multiple sexual partners, IV drug users who share needles, and persons with hemophilia. There are three basic modes of transmission: sexual, bloodborne, and from mother to baby either prenatally, during the birth process, or when breastfeeding. When first identified in 1981, HIV infection was primarily found among homosexual men, but by 1990, the disease was moving into heterosexual populations with great rapidity. By the mid-1990s, cases of AIDS were occurring more frequently among women than among men. The greatest growth in AIDS rates among women occurred in African American and Hispanic women. Teenagers also have one of the fastest growing rates of HIV infection.

TRICHOMONIASIS

Trichomoniasis is caused by a parasitic protozoan called *Trichomonas vaginalis*. Trichomoniasis is a very common STD, with an incidence of approximately 3 million new cases every year (NIAID, 1998c). It is seen frequently in combination with gonorrhea. The most common method of transmission is sexual, although the protozoa can survive for a period of time in water, so other modes of transmission are possible.

The incubation period after initial exposure to trichomoniasis ranges from approximately 4 to 20 days. About 25% of women infected with trichomoniasis will have no symptoms, and men almost never have symptoms. In these clients, the *Trichomonas* organisms may remain dormant for years, without becoming an active infection. Precipitating factors that may encourage the growth of *Trichomonas* include pregnancy, sexual intercourse, menstruation, or illness. Vulval and vaginal pruritus are the most common symptoms, with a vaginal discharge of a frothy, copious yellow-green mucus. Only 10% of women will present with the classic symptoms of a *Trichomonas* infection: severe itching of the vulva, redness, swelling of the vulva, pain on intercourse and urination, urinary frequency, and a grayish, malodorous discharge. Males most often have a watery, whitish discharge and difficult or painful urination, but they may also have urethritis and an accompanying inflamma-

tion. In men, *Trichomonas* in the dormant state are usually harbored in the prostate or urethra.

Medical–Surgical Management

Pharmacological

Both partners should be treated with metronidazole (Flagyl) given either orally in a single dose or for a period of approximately 1 week. Metronidazole is effective against both protozoal and bacterial infections. If given vaginally, metronidazole (Flagyl) is not as effective. Pregnant women are usually treated after the first trimester to avoid the possibility of birth defects, because metronidazole is known to cross the placenta.

Adverse effects occur in about 10% of clients taking metronidazole (Flagyl) and usually affect the gastrointestinal system in the form of nausea, vomiting, diarrhea, and abdominal cramping. CNS effects such as headache or dizziness may also be seen.

HEPATITIS B

Hepatitis B, caused by the hepatitis B virus, is now recognized as an STD. Today it is primarily transmitted through sexual contact, as opposed to the oral-fecal or blood contact routes that were far more prevalent 20 years ago (Sharts-Hopko, 1997). An estimated 78,000 cases of hepatitis B occurred in 2001 in the United States (CDC, 2002).

Clients with hepatitis B experience anorexia, vague abdominal discomfort, nausea, vomiting, fatigue, and jaundice. Fever may be mild or absent. Symptoms may progress to chronic liver disease, hepatic cancer, hepatic failure, and death.

Medical–Surgical Management

Medical

There is no specific therapy. Treatment is based on relieving symptoms.

CRITICAL THINKING

Multiple Sexual Partners

What should a client who has multiple sexual partners be taught about sexually transmitted diseases? Make a teaching plan keeping in mind the sensitivity of the information to be shared and the client's receptivity.

Health Promotion

Hepatitis B is the only STD for which a vaccine is available. It is recommended that all newborn infants, 11- to 12-year-old children, and high-risk groups of all ages receive the vaccine (CDC, 2003).

Nursing Management

Follow proper hand hygiene technique. Teach the client hand hygiene to be followed after using the bathroom and every time the penis, vagina, or perineal areas are touched. Provide nonjudgmental support to all clients. Encourage clients to notify past and present sexual partners of the diagnosis and the need to seek medical care. Advise client to wear loose-fitting clothes and cotton underwear for comfort.

NURSING PROCESS

The following is a general nursing process for the client with an STD.

Assessment

Subjective Data

Data to be gathered from a client who presents with a suspected STD are very similar, regardless of the actual STD. A thorough history must be obtained. A relaxed, nonjudgmental attitude will help to elicit accurate information from the client. Confidentiality and privacy are extremely important when dealing with both the history and physical examination for STDs. Gather pertinent information regarding the client's sexual orientation (homosexual, heterosexual, bisexual), any prior treatment for an STD, and the number of sexual partners that the client has had in the last 6 months.

Ask women about symptoms such as vulval or vaginal itching, vaginal discharge, pain or discomfort, skin rashes or pruritus, and any changes in the menstrual periods or other abnormal bleeding. Question men regarding the presence of symptoms such as pain or burning on urination, abnormal penile discharges, skin rashes or itching, or lesions on external genitalia. Ask both men and women about urinary frequency or discomfort and systemic symptoms such as fatigue, malaise, or sore throat. Ask homosexual men about rectal symptoms such as abnormal discharge, itching, lesions, or pain on defecation.

Objective Data

Carefully assess the reproductive, gastrointestinal, and integumentary systems. Determine the presence or absence of skin rashes or lesions and abnormal discharges. Females need a speculum examination of the vagina and cervix to closely observe internal organs for changes consistent with STDs. Examine the rectal area to look for any abnormal discharge, lesions, or tenderness. Palpate inguinal lymph nodes to look for signs of infection.

Nursing diagnoses for the client with an STD may include the following:

Nursing Diagnoses	Planning/Goals	Nursing Interventions
Anxiety related to unknown procedures, embarrassment, or other factors (relates to nearly every client who presents with an STD)	The client will admit lack of knowledge and embarrassment.	Provide a relaxed, nonjudgmental attitude which will aid in reducing client anxiety. Listen actively to both the spoken and unspoken concerns of the client. The nurse must examine own attitudes toward STDs and the clients who suffer from them.
Deficient Knowledge related to mode of transmission of the STD, prevention methods, and risk for spread of the STD	The client will accurately discuss the mode of transmission of an STD and list appropriate measures to avoid reinfection or future infection.	Teach mode of transmission, prevention of further infection, and risk for spread. Take time to make sure the client has a thorough understanding of all necessary aspects of the disease.
Risk for Infection related to incomplete treatment or lack of precautions with untreated, infected partners	The client will state the need for having all sexual partners notified and treated. The client will state understanding of the treatment regimen and of the importance of completing treatment. The client will explain appropriate use of latex condoms, including how and when to apply and remove the device.	Discuss the need for all sexual partners to be notified and treated. Discuss the importance of completing treatment regimen. Teach the importance of abstaining from sexual intercourse until the infection is resolved, or of using appropriate measures, such as latex condoms, to prevent reinfection.

Evaluation Each goal must be evaluated to determine how it has been met by the client.

SAMPLE NURSING CARE PLAN

THE CLIENT WITH GENITAL HERPES

Julie Blackwell is a single woman in her middle twenties who has been coming to the clinic for annual Pap smears and birth control for several years. She is a well-nourished, healthy-appearing young woman of medium height. She rescheduled her annual Pap smear to come into the clinic early because she noticed a cluster of small blisters on the inside of her left thigh that also involves the labia majora. She also reports that she has just gotten the flu as evidenced by headache, fever, and general achiness.

Ms. Blackwell has used birth control pills in the past and reports satisfaction with this method of birth control. She reports that she and her new boyfriend became intimate about 2 weeks ago, so she wants to renew her birth control pill prescription. She also states that intercourse has been uncomfortable since the appearance of the lesions and that she does not feel comfortable with sexual activity while the lesions are present, since they make her feel "ugly."

The assessment determines the presence of a cluster of small blisters as well as swollen, tender inguinal lymph nodes. A Tzanck smear test is obtained.

Nursing Diagnosis 1 *Ineffective Sexuality Pattern related to lesions as evidenced by her comment that intercourse has been uncomfortable since the appearance of the lesions.*

Nursing Outcomes Classification (NOC)
Psychosocial Adjustment: Life Change

Nursing Interventions Classification (NIC)
Sexual Counseling

PLANNING/GOALS	NURSING INTERVENTIONS	RATIONALE
Ms. Blackwell will express her feelings about potential changes in her sexual behavior before leaving the clinic.	Provide a nonjudgmental atmosphere to encourage Ms. Blackwell to express her feelings about this perceived change in her sexual identity.	Demonstrates the caregiver's positive feelings toward Ms. Blackwell and concerns she may have regarding her future sexuality.
	Provide privacy and an uninterrupted amount of time to talk with Ms. Blackwell.	Shows respect and conveys reassurance in discussing sexuality issues and concerns with her.
	Provide accurate information to Ms. Blackwell about genital herpes, and include literature or videos for her to share with her boyfriend.	Helps Ms. Blackwell focus on specific, necessary information and encourages her to ask questions.
	Offer the names of local support groups such as HELP (Herpetics Engaged in Living Productively) or other support persons who can provide information and group support to Ms. Blackwell.	Provides Ms. Blackwell with resources for support once she has returned home and the reality of her diagnosis has set in.

EVALUATION   Ms. Blackwell states that she is still in shock, but thinks that she will be able to deal with her diagnosis. She also states that she will call back to the clinic in a few days with more questions after she has assimilated some of the information.

Nursing Diagnosis 2 *Anxiety related to threatened sexual identity as evidenced by her comment that she is not comfortable with sexual activity while the lesions are present since they make her feel "ugly."*

Nursing Outcomes Classification (NOC)
Acceptance: Health Status

Nursing Interventions Classification (NIC)
Teaching: Individual

continues

SAMPLE NURSING CARE PLAN

PLANNING/GOALS	NURSING INTERVENTIONS	RATIONALE
Ms. Blackwell will be able to express feelings of anxiety and identify support systems to help her cope with these feelings before leaving the clinic.	Explain any procedures clearly and concisely before performing them.	Helps alleviate anxiety.
	Listen attentively to concerns or expressions of anxiety from Ms. Blackwell.	Helps identify anxious behaviors and source of her anxiety.
	Include Ms. Blackwell in as many decisions related to her care and follow-up as is possible.	May reduce her feelings of anxiety and gives her some control.

EVALUATION Ms. Blackwell expresses feelings of anxiety about the diagnosis. States she has a cousin with herpes whom she will use as a resource person. Also states that she has a secure relationship with her boyfriend and will talk to him about herpes. Agrees to call the clinic for any further support or information that she may need.

Nursing Diagnosis 3 *Risk for Infection* related to break in skin integrity as evidenced by the presence of blisters.

Nursing Outcomes Classification (NOC)
Risk Control: Sexually Transmitted Diseases (STD)

Nursing Interventions Classification (NIC)
Teaching: Disease Process
Teaching: Sexuality

PLANNING/GOALS	NURSING INTERVENTIONS	RATIONALE
Ms. Blackwell's herpes blisters will heal without secondary infection within 10 days.	Wear gloves when examining perineal area and when handling exudate from herpes lesions.	Prevents secondary infection in herpes blisters from caregiver's hands and protects caregiver when dealing with wound exudate.
	Teach Ms. Blackwell how to wash hands very thoroughly after using the toilet or handling the area around the herpes lesions.	Prevents spread of herpes infection from genital area to other areas of Ms. Blackwell's body or to another person.
	Instruct Ms. Blackwell in the importance of keeping the herpes lesions clean and dry until they heal.	Helps prevent the occurrence of a secondary infection that may delay healing for up to 6 weeks.
	Instruct Ms. Blackwell to wear cotton underwear and loose-fitting clothing during herpes outbreaks.	Provides air circulation to promote healing and reduce further local irritation.

EVALUATION Ms. Blackwell has been taught to keep blisters clean and dry and states that she will contact the clinic if the lesions develop any signs of a secondary infection. She makes an appointment to return to the clinic in 10 days for a follow-up evaluation.

CASE STUDY

Noelle Landers, a 17-year-old student, has come to your clinic seeking treatment. Noelle is complaining of pain and burning on urination, as well as pain during intercourse. She states that she is infrequently sexually active with her 17-year-old boyfriend and is also seeking a form of birth control. She has not used any form of birth control in the past and neither has her boyfriend. She also complains of a yellowish vaginal discharge and has been wearing a panty liner to deal with this. Upon examination, Noelle complains of some abdominal tenderness, but denies that she has had any tenderness before this time. Noelle is screened for chlamydia and gonorrhea. She denies having had sex with any other partners, but does admit that she and her boyfriend had a fight and broke up temporarily about a month ago. They went back together about a week later. She does not know if he had any other sexual contacts during their period of separation. Noelle is concerned that she has contracted an STD, and states, "I'll die of embarrassment!"

The following questions will guide your development of a nursing care plan for the case study.

1. What other information should be elicited from Noelle?
2. What other sexually transmitted diseases will Noelle most likely be tested for in addition to chlamydia and gonorrhea?
3. Write three nursing diagnoses and goals for Noelle.
4. List the medications that Noelle will be most likely to receive to treat a chlamydial infection.
5. List some complications that Noelle may experience if she does not receive treatment for an active chlamydial or gonorrheal infection.
6. What information will you include when you counsel Noelle regarding sexual activity and forms of birth control? (See the chapter on Reproductive Systems for additional information.)

Summary

- Sexually transmitted diseases are among the most common infections occurring in the United States today.
- Despite massive education efforts, the number of new STD cases identified each year continues to grow.
- Early, intensive education regarding STDs is being utilized to help combat the high incidence of STDs, virtually an epidemic among young, urban-dwelling populations.
- Many STDs, such as gonorrhea, syphilis, and chlamydia, are treatable with antibiotics, but many others are caused by viruses and are not curable.
- Identification of groups at risk for STDs and appropriate prevention teaching are the most effective weapons in the ongoing battle against STDs.

Review Questions

1. The two most effective medications commonly used to treat chlamydia are:
   a. doxycycline and azithromycin.
   b. penicillin and podophyllum.
   c. erythromycin and acyclovir.
   d. doxycycline and penicillin.

2. If a female client with chlamydia fails to complete treatment, complications that may arise in the future include:
   a. fever and headache.
   b. nausea, vomiting, and diarrhea.
   c. infertility and ectopic pregnancy.
   d. urinary retention.

3. When instructing a client with gonorrhea regarding medication, the nurse will be sure to tell the client:
   a. to take the medication until it is gone.
   b. to take the medication until symptoms subside.
   c. to take the medication at bedtime.
   d. to avoid sunlight while taking the medication.

4. When obtaining a health history from a client, the nurse asks the client to report on the presence of which of the following common symptoms of syphilis?

 a. Nausea and vomiting

 b. Fever, cellulitis, and diarrhea

 c. Dysuria and mucopurulent discharge

 d. Painless sore or ulcer in the genital area

References/Suggested Readings

Centers for Disease Control and Prevention (CDC). (2001). *Hepatitis B vaccine—Fact sheet* [Online]. Available: www.cdc.gov/ncidod/diseases/hepatitis/b/vaxfact.pdf

Centers for Disease Control and Prevention (CDC). (2002). *Hepatitis B—Fact sheet* [Online]. Available: www.cdc.gov/ncidod/diseases/hepatitis/b/faab.htm

Centers for Disease Control and Prevention (CDC). (2003). *Recommended Childhood and Adolescent Immunization Schedule, United States, 2003.* [Online]. Available: www.cdc.gov/nip/resc/child-schedule.htm#printable

Choma, K. (2003). ASC-US HPV testing. *AJN, 103*(2), 42–50.

Daniels, R. (2002). *Delmar's Guide to Laboratory and Diagnostic Tests.* Clifton Park, NY: Thomson Delmar Learning.

Dochterman, J., & Bulechek, G. (2004). *Nursing Interventions Classification (NIC)* (4th ed.). St. Louis, MO: Mosby.

Hadley, J. (1999). *Culturally relevant behavioral intervention dramatically reduces STDs* [Online]. Available: www.niaid.nih.gov/newsroom/std.htm

Jagger, J., & Perry, J. (1999). Power in numbers: Reducing your risk of blood borne exposures. *Nursing99, 29*(1), 51–52.

Lammon, C. B., Foote, A. W., Leli, P. G., Ingle, J., & Adams, M. H. (1995). *Clinical nursing skills.* Philadelphia: W. B. Saunders.

Moorhead, S., Johnson, M., & Maas, M. (2004). *Nursing Outcomes Classification (NOC)* (3rd ed.). St. Louis, MO: Mosby.

National Institute of Allergy and Infectious Diseases (NIAID). (1998a). *Other important STDs* [Online]. Available: www.niaid.nih.gov/factsheets/stdother.htm

National Institute of Allergy and Infectious Diseases (NIAID). (1998b). *Sexually transmitted diseases statistics* [Online]. Available: www.niaid.nih.gov/factsheets/stdstats.htm

National Institute of Allergy and Infectious Diseases (NIAID). (1998c). *Vaginitis due to vaginal infections* [Online]. Available: www.niaid.nih.gov/factsheets/stdvag.htm

National Institute of Allergy and Infectious Diseases (NIAID). (1999). *An introduction to sexually transmitted diseases* [Online]. Available: www.niaid.nih.gov/factsheets/std-info.htm

National Institute of Allergy and Infectious Diseases (NIAID). (2001). *Human papillomavirus and genital warts* [Online]. Available: www.niaid.nih.gov/factsheets/stdhpv.htm

National Institute of Allergy and Infectious Diseases (NIAID). (2002a). *Chlamydial infection* [Online]. Available: www.niaid.nih.gov/factsheets/stdclam.htm

National Institute of Allergy and Infectious Diseases (NIAID). (2002b). *Genital herpes* [Online]. Available: www.niaid.nih.gov/factsheets/stdherp.htm

National Institute of Allergy and Infectious Diseases (NIAID). (2002c). *Gonorrhea* [Online]. Available: www.niaid.nih.gov/factsheets/stdgon.htm

National Institute of Allergy and Infectious Diseases (NIAID). (2002d). *Syphilis* [Online]. Available: www.niaid.nih.gov/factsheets/stdsyph.htm

North American Nursing Diagnosis Association (NANDA). (2003). *Nursing diagnoses: Definitions & classification 2003–2004.* Philadelphia, PA: Author.

Novatnack, E., & Schweon, S. (2002). Herpes: A bigger problem than you think. *RN, 65*(6), 31–37.

Sharts-Hopko, N. (1997). STDs in women: What you need to know. *AJN, 97*(4), 46–54.

Spratto, G., & Woods, A. (2004). *2004 PDR Nurses' Drug Handbook.* Clifton Park, NY: Thomson Delmar Learning.

Resources

American College of Obstetricians and Gynecologists (ACOG), 409 Twelfth Street S.W., P.O. Box 96920, Washington, DC 20090-6920, 202-863-2518, www.acog.org

American Public Health Association (APHA), 800 I Street N.W., Washington, DC 20001, 202-777-2742, www.apha.org

American Social Health Association (ASHA), P.O. Box 13827, Research Triangle Park, NC 27709-9940, 877-478-5868, www.ashastd.org

Centers for Disease Control and Prevention (CDC), 1600 Clifton Road N.E., Atlanta, GA 30333, 800-311-3435, www.cdc.gov

National Foundation for Infectious Diseases, 4733 Bethesda Avenue, Suite 750, Bethesda, MD 20814, 301-656-0003, www.nfid.org

National Institute of Allergy and Infectious Diseases, Building 31, Room 7A-50, 31 Center Drive MSC 2520, Bethesda, MD 20892-2520, 301-496-5717, www.niaid.nih.gov

Planned Parenthood Federation of America, Inc., 434 West 33rd Street, New York, NY 10001, 212-541-7800, www.plannedparenthood.org

U.S. Department of Health and Human Services (USDHHS), Public Health Service, 200 Independence Avenue S.W., Washington, DC 20201, 877-696-6775, www.hhs.gov

World Health Organization (WHO), Avenue Appia 20 1211 Geneva 27, Switzerland, www.who.int

Nursing Care of the Client: Body Defenses

Chapter 43
Integumentary System

Chapter 44
Immune System

INTEGUMENTARY SYSTEM

LEARNING OBJECTIVES

Upon completion of this chapter, you should be able to:
- **Define key terms.**
- **Describe common disorders of the integumentary system.**
- **Relate the pathophysiology of each skin disorder.**
- **Discuss the common diagnostic tests used to differentiate skin disorders.**
- **State the usual treatment for each skin disorder.**
- **Assess the nursing care needs of a client with a disorder of the integument.**
- **Plan and implement effective nursing care.**

INTRODUCTION

As an old adage asserts, the health of the skin mirrors the health of the body. Many systemic diseases have skin manifestations. Psychological stress can affect the condition of the skin, and skin rashes can be a complication of drug therapy. As the largest and the most visible system in the body, the integumentary system (skin,

KEY TERMS

alopecia
angiogenesis
angioma
blanching
cyanosis
debride
ecchymosis
erythema
eschar
friction
granulation tissue
hemorrhagic exudate
hemostasis
hyperthermia
hypothermia
inflammation
ischemia
jaundice

keloid
keratin
lipoma
melanin
nevi
pallor
petechiae
purulent exudate
sanguineous
sebaceous cyst
sebum
serosanguineous
  exudate
serous exudate
shearing
telangiectasia
vitiligo
wound

hair, scalp, nails, and mucous membranes) is vulnerable to injury and susceptible to several primary diseases. It is estimated that skin-related problems account for 5% to 10% of all ambulatory client visits in the United States (Deters, 2002). Although the outward appearance of the skin is important for psychological well-being, the healthy, intact status of the skin is also essential for physiologic well-being. Maintaining this status of the integumentary system is, therefore, an important independent nursing function. The focus of this chapter is to describe common skin disorders, identify the usual treatment modalities for these disorders, and discuss measures that nurses can implement to provide effective nursing care for clients with disorders of the integument.

ANATOMY AND PHYSIOLOGY REVIEW

As the external covering of the body, the skin performs the vital function of protecting internal body structures from harmful microorganisms and substances. The skin is continuous with mucous membranes at external body openings of the respiratory tract, the digestive system, and the urogenital tract. As appendages of the skin, the hair and nails also have protective functions. In addition to its vital protective role, the skin also plays other roles in the normal functioning of the human organism. These roles include participating in the regulation of body temperature, functioning as a sensory organ, helping to maintain fluid and electrolyte balance, producing vitamin D, and excreting certain waste products from the body.

Structure of the Skin

The skin is composed of three layers: the epidermis, the dermis, and the subcutaneous fatty tissue (Figure 43-1).

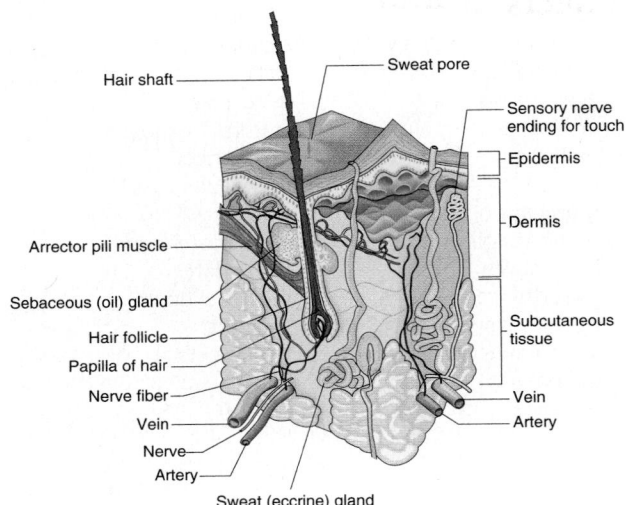

Labels:
Hair shaft
Sweat pore
Sensory nerve ending for touch
Epidermis
Dermis
Arrector pili muscle
Sebaceous (oil) gland
Hair follicle
Papilla of hair
Nerve fiber
Subcutaneous tissue
Vein
Vein
Artery
Nerve
Artery
Sweat (eccrine) gland

Figure 43-1 *Cross Section of the Skin*

Epidermis

The epidermis is a layer of squamous epithelial cells. Most of the cells are keratinocytes that produce a tough, fibrous protein called **keratin.** As new cells are produced in the deep layers of the epidermis, old cells are pushed to the surface of the skin. As these cells move from the deeper epidermal layers to the surface, they undergo a process of keratinization in which they become filled with keratin, thus hardening the outer layer of epidermal cells. The keratin creates a barrier that repels bacteria and foreign matter and is impermeable to most substances. The epidermal cells on the palms of the hands and soles of the feet, areas of the body subjected to increased friction and pressure, contain larger amounts of keratin, resulting in thickened skin and callouses.

The epidermis also contains specialized cells called melanocytes. These cells produce **melanin,** the pigment that gives the skin its color. The more melanin present, the darker the skin color. Moles and birthmarks **(nevi)**, pigmented areas in the skin, are aggregations of melanocytes. In **vitiligo,** melanocytes are destroyed, causing milk-white patches of depigmented skin surrounded by normal skin. Exposure to ultraviolet light (sun) causes an increase in the production of melanin, which darkens (tans) the skin and provides some protection against the harmful effects of suntanning.

Dermis

The dermis is dense, irregular connective tissue composed of collagen and elastic fibers, blood and lymph vessels, nerves, sweat and sebaceous glands, and hair roots. The sebaceous glands secrete an oily substance called **sebum** that lubricates the skin, helping to keep it soft and pliable. Sweat (eccrine) glands are found in the skin over most of the body surface. Another type of sweat gland, apocrine glands, is concentrated in the axillae, anal region, scrotum, and labia majora. These glands secrete an organic substance that is odorless at first but is quickly metabolized by skin bacteria, causing the characteristic odor commonly referred to as body odor (Seeley, Stephens, & Tate, 2002). Intradermal injections, such as the TB skin test, are given in the dermis.

Subcutaneous Tissue

The subcutaneous tissue is primarily connective and adipose (fatty) tissue. Here the skin is anchored to muscles and bones. An individual's nutritional status and genetic makeup dictate the amount of subcutaneous tissue present. Emaciated persons have very little subcutaneous tissue, whereas obese persons may have several inches of subcutaneous tissue. The amount of subcutaneous tissue is an important factor in body temperature regulation.

Functions of the Skin

Understanding the functions of the skin and contiguous mucous membranes guides the nurse in planning and implementing appropriate nursing care. Because intact, healthy skin and mucous membranes serve as the first line of defense against harmful agents, *maintaining skin integrity is one of the most important in-dependent functions of the nurse.* Nursing interventions such as providing daily hygiene care and regularly turn-ing and repositioning dependent clients are aimed at preventing skin breakdown.

Protection

The first and most important function of the skin is protection. As long as the skin is intact and healthy, it is a barrier against microorganisms and numerous sub-stances that could be harmful to the individual. Not only is the skin a barrier to keep harmful substances out, it is also a barrier to keep essential substances such as water and electrolytes inside the body. It also cush-ions internal organs.

Temperature Regulation

The body produces heat as a result of metabolism of food. Exercise, fever, or a hot environment can raise body temperature. Through several mechanisms, the skin can either release or conserve body heat to main-tain normal body temperature. Radiation is the pri-mary means of heat loss. As body heat increases, arte-rioles in the dermis dilate, bringing body heat to the skin surface. By the process of radiation, waves of heat from uncovered body surfaces are released to the envi-ronment. Layering clothes in winter, for example, helps prevent excess loss of body heat by radiation. Heat is also lost by conduction. In conduction, heat is trans-ferred from warmer surfaces to cooler ones. Placing a cool washcloth on a client's forehead is an example of using the principle of conduction. The washcloth be-comes warmer, the forehead cooler. Evaporation is an-other way in which excess body heat is lost. As mois-ture on the skin—either from perspiration or from a tepid sponge bath—dries, the body is cooled. To con-serve (prevent excess loss) body heat, arterioles in the dermis contract to decrease the flow of blood to the skin surface, thus decreasing heat lost by radiation. The phenomenon of "goose flesh" is another method of conserving body heat. Tiny hairs standing on end cre-ate a layer of air insulation decreasing loss of body heat to the environment.

Sensory Perception

The skin contains receptors for pain, touch, pressure, and temperature. The sensory receptors pick up infor-mation to help protect the body from environmental dangers as well as provide sensations of comfort and pleasure. The brain then processes the information and causes the response.

Fluid and Electrolyte Balance

The skin helps maintain the stability of the internal environment by preventing loss of body fluids and elec-trolytes and by preventing subcutaneous tissues from drying out. Skin damage, such as that occurring with se-vere burns, results in rapid loss of large quantities of fluid and electrolytes. This can lead to shock, circulatory collapse, and death.

Structure and Function of Hair

Hair is composed of dead epidermal cells that begin to grow and divide in the base of the hair follicle. As the cells are pushed toward the skin surface, they become keratinized and die. Hair color is genetically determined.

Scalp hair grows for 2 to 5 years, then the follicle be-comes inactive. When the growth cycle begins again, a new hair is produced and the old hair is pushed out. Approximately 50 hairs are lost each day. Sustained hair loss of more than 100 hairs each day usually indicates that something is wrong (Martini, 2000).

There are 5 million hairs covering the entire human body except for the lips, palmar and plantar surfaces, nipples, and the glans penis. The amount and texture of hair vary with age, gender, race, and body part.

Hair on the head protects the scalp from the ultravi-olet rays from the sun and cushions blows to the head. Eyelashes help prevent foreign particles from entering the eyes just as the hairs in the nostrils and external ear canals help keep particles from entering the nose and ears.

Structure and Function of Nails

Nail production occurs in the nail root, an epithelial fold that cannot be seen from the surface (Figure 43-2). The nail plate covers the nail bed. The blood vessels un-der the nail bed give the nails their pink color.

The nails protect the ends of the fingers and toes.

Structure and Function of Mucous Membranes

Mucous membranes have epithelium overlying a layer of loose connective tissue. Specialized cells within the mucous membrane secrete mucus.

The cavities and tubes that open to the outside of the body are lined with mucous membranes. These include the oral and nasal cavities and the tubes of the respira-tory, gastrointestinal, urinary, and reproductive systems. Mucous membranes perform absorptive or secretory functions depending on their placement.

Effects of Aging

With advancing years, the blood flow to the skin is reduced. The skin becomes thinner and is more easily

Figure 43-2 *Structure of the Fingernail*

LIFE CYCLE CONSIDERATIONS

Effects of Aging on the Skin

- Skin vascularity and the number of sweat and sebaceous glands decrease, affecting thermoregulation.
- Inflammatory response and pain perception diminish, increasing the risk of adverse effects from noxious stimuli.
- A thinning epidermis and prolonged wound healing make the elderly more prone to injury and skin infections.
- Skin cancer is more common among the elderly.
- Use of skin lotions containing alcohol can cause drying of the skin, increasing the risk of injury. Moisture-enhancing products should be used instead.

TABLE 43-1	OBTAINING A CLIENT HISTORY OF SKIN PROBLEMS

- When did you first notice this problem?
- Where did the first symptom appear?
- What did the rash/lesion look like when it first appeared?
- Describe what happened in the days/weeks after the first symptom appeared.
- Are the symptoms worse at any particular time? Season?
- Have you experienced any itching or burning sensations?
- Are the lesions painful?
- What do you think might have caused this problem?
- Have you ever had a skin problem like this before?
- Has anyone in your family ever had a problem like this?
- What have you been doing to treat this problem?
- What kind of skin care products do you normally use?
- Have you changed any of your usual products/habits/routines?
- Is there anything else you would like to tell me about this problem?

injured. Older skin breaks down easily from prolonged pressure. The long-accepted rule of thumb is to turn clients every 2 hours, but for the ill older client, every 2 hours may not be often enough. *Significant skin damage can occur in just 1 hour of unrelieved pressure.* Preventing skin breakdown in the elderly client depends on an accurate assessment of both the client's skin condition and mobility status.

Loss of subcutaneous tissue causes skin sagging and wrinkling. The activity of sebaceous and sweat glands diminishes, resulting in dry skin and a decreased ability to adapt to changes in environmental temperature. Extremes in temperature pose hazards for older adults. In very hot weather they are susceptible to **hyperthermia,** a condition in which the core body temperature reaches 106°F. In hyperthermia, the hypothalamus no longer functions appropriately. Sweating stops, the skin becomes dry and flushed, and the person becomes confused and eventually comatose. Each summer many elderly persons die from the effects of hyperthermia. Winter puts older adults at risk for **hypothermia,** a condition in which the core body temperature drops below 95°F. The hypothermic client may become confused and disoriented. As the core body temperature continues to drop, the person becomes comatose. Each winter some older adults die from severe hypothermia (Seeley et al., 2002).

On the hands and face, melanocytes increase in number, causing the age spots commonly seen in older adults. Gray hair occurs from a lack of melanin production. Skin exposed to sunlight ages faster.

ASSESSMENT

Assessing clients with disorders of the integument includes obtaining a health history and performing a physical assessment of the skin, hair, nails, and mucous membranes. The nurse's assessment skills, along with an understanding of the anatomy and physiology of the integumentary system, ensure a complete, factual database from which to plan and implement appropriate

nursing care. Table 43-1 contains a list of questions to use in obtaining a health history.

Assessment of Skin

Seven parameters should be examined when performing a physical assessment of the skin. They are integrity, color, temperature and moisture, texture, turgor and mobility, sensation, and vascularity. Inspection and palpation are the two assessment techniques used when examining the skin. Good lighting is essential for accurate assessment. Table 43-2 outlines these parameters with the normal and abnormal findings.

Any skin lesions should be identified according to type and described regarding color, size, and location. Describe the amount, color, odor, and appearance of any drainage that might be present. Document assessment findings clearly, concisely, and completely. The intent of nursing care is to maintain the integrity of intact skin and to restore damaged skin or mucous membranes to an intact state. Aging changes skin texture, moisture, and mobility, requiring increased nursing vigilance to maintain skin integrity. Daily hygiene products should be selected to meet the client's individual skin care needs.

Assessment of Hair, Nails, and Mucous Membranes

Hair should be smooth, shiny, and resilient. Excess hair loss can result from drugs, radiation, dietary or hormonal factors, stress, and high fever.

Nails should be pink, smooth, and shiny and feel firm yet flexible when palpated. An angle of approximately 160° should be present between the nail body and the eponychium (Figure 43-7).

Mucous membranes normally appear pink and moist.

TABLE 43-2   SKIN ASSESSMENT PARAMETERS

PARAMETER	NORMAL	ABNORMAL
Integrity	Skin intact; no diseased or injured tissue.	Broken skin; open areas such as fissures, ulcers, excoriations. Rash or lesions such as papules, nodules, vesicles, pustules, wheals, scales (Figures 43-3 and 43-4).
Color	Varies with skin type and race: pink, tanned, olive, brown.	**Pallor**—pale skin, especially in face, conjunctiva, nail beds, and oral mucous membranes. **Cyanosis**—bluish discoloration noticed in lips, earlobes, and nail beds. **Jaundice**—a yellowing of the skin, mucous membranes, and sclera. **Erythema**—reddish hue to the skin as in sunburn and inflammation or increased blood flow.
Temperature and moisture	Usually warm and dry, depending on environmental temperature.	Cool, cold, moist, clammy, or warmer than normal.
Texture	Smooth, soft. Thickness varies in different areas.	Loose, wrinkled, rough, thickened, thin, oily, flaking, scaling.
Turgor and mobility	An assessment of skin hydration. Normally skin moves freely. A pinched fold of skin returns immediately to normal position (Figure 43-5).	Taut with edema; slack with dehydration. Rigid in some diseases such as scleroderma.
Sensation	Distinguishes hot and cold, sharp and dull.	Numbness, tingling, insensitive to pressure and sharp objects.
Vascularity	Clear; no discoloration.	**Telangiectasia** (permanent dilation of groups of superficial capillaries and venules); **Petechiae** (pinpoint hemorrhagic spots); **Ecchymosis** (large, irregular, hemorrhagic areas) (Figure 43-6).

COMMON DIAGNOSTIC TESTS

Commonly used diagnostic tests for clients with integumentary disorders are listed in Table 43-3.

PROFESSIONAL TIP

Possible Signs of Physical Abuse

Areas of ecchymosis are one sign of trauma that could be the result of physical abuse. Injuries noted at the base of the skull or on the face, buttocks, breasts, abdomen, or any area such as the top of the back that the client could not reach, are suspicious for abuse. Unusual marks on the skin such as cigarette burns and belt buckle or bite marks may also be signs of abuse. Injuries that are inconsistent with the client's story may also be the result of abuse.

Institutional policies generally relate to reporting and to whom to report when the situation of possible physical abuse is encountered. This is usually based on state laws about reporting physical abuse. Nurses must know the reporting laws of the state in which they are employed.

WOUNDS

A disruption in the integrity of body tissue is called a **wound.**

Physiology of Wound Healing

When an injury is sustained, a complex set of responses is set into motion, and the body begins a three-phase process of wound healing. Understanding these physiological responses will assist the nurse in caring for

TABLE 43-3   COMMON DIAGNOSTIC TESTS FOR INTEGUMENTARY DISORDERS

Biopsy
Patch testing
Tzanck smear
Immunofluorescence (IF testing)
Wood's light examination
Skin scrapings
Culture and sensitivity

NONPALPABLE

(A)

Macule:
Localized changes in skin color of less than 1 cm in diameter
Example:
Freckle

(B)

Patch:
Localized changes in skin color of greater than 1 cm in diameter
Example:
Vitiligo, stage 1 of pressure ulcer

PALPABLE

(C)

Papule:
Solid, elevated lesion less than 0.5 cm in diameter
Example:
Warts, elevated nevi

(D)

Plaque:
Solid, elevated lesion greater than 0.5 cm in diameter
Example:
Psoriasis

(E)

Nodules:
Solid and elevated; however, they extend deeper than papules into the dermis or subcutaneous tissues, 0.5–2 cm
Example:
Lipoma, erythema nodosum, cyst

(F)

Tumor:
The same as a nodule only greater than 2 cm

Example:
Carcinoma (such as advanced breast carcinoma); not basal cell or squamous cell of the skin

(G)

Wheal:
Localized edema in the epidermis causing irregular elevation that may be red or pale
Example:
Insect bite or a hive

FLUID-FILLED CAVITIES WITHIN THE SKIN

(H)

Vesicle:
Accumulation of fluid between the upper layers of the skin; elevated mass containing serous fluid; less than 0.5 cm
Example:
Herpes simplex, herpes zoster, chickenpox

(I)

Bullae:
Same as a vesicle only greater than 0.5 cm
Example:
Contact dermatitis, large second-degree burns, bullous impetigo, pemphigus

(J)

Pustule:
Vesicles or bullae that become filled with pus, usually described as less than 0.5 cm in diameter
Example:
Acne, impetigo, furuncles, carbuncles, folliculitis

(K)

Cyst:
Encapsulated fluid-filled or a semi-solid mass in the subcutaneous tissue or dermis
Example:
Sebaceous cyst, epidermoid cyst

Figure 43-3 *Types of Primary Skin Lesions*

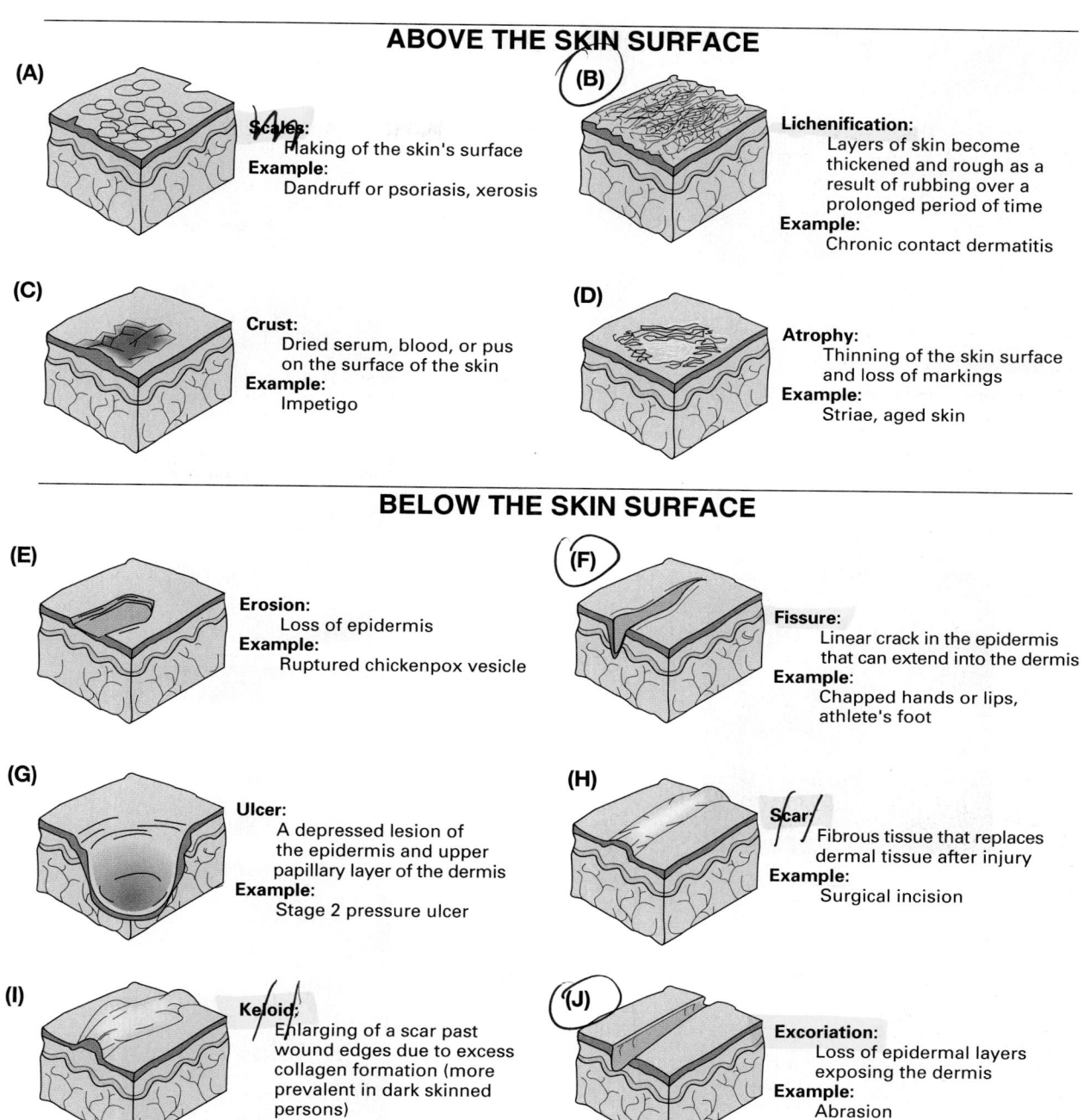

ABOVE THE SKIN SURFACE

(A)
Scales:
  Flaking of the skin's surface
Example:
  Dandruff or psoriasis, xerosis

(B)
Lichenification:
  Layers of skin become
  thickened and rough as a
  result of rubbing over a
  prolonged period of time
Example:
  Chronic contact dermatitis

(C)
Crust:
  Dried serum, blood, or pus
  on the surface of the skin
Example:
  Impetigo

(D)
Atrophy:
  Thinning of the skin surface
  and loss of markings
Example:
  Striae, aged skin

BELOW THE SKIN SURFACE

(E)
Erosion:
  Loss of epidermis
Example:
  Ruptured chickenpox vesicle

(F)
Fissure:
  Linear crack in the epidermis
  that can extend into the dermis
Example:
  Chapped hands or lips,
  athlete's foot

(G)
Ulcer:
  A depressed lesion of
  the epidermis and upper
  papillary layer of the dermis
Example:
  Stage 2 pressure ulcer

(H)
Scar:
  Fibrous tissue that replaces
  dermal tissue after injury
Example:
  Surgical incision

(I)
Keloid:
  Enlarging of a scar past
  wound edges due to excess
  collagen formation (more
  prevalent in dark skinned
  persons)
Example:
  Burn scar

(J)
Excoriation:
  Loss of epidermal layers
  exposing the dermis
Example:
  Abrasion

Figure 43-4 *Types of Secondary Skin Lesions*

clients with impaired skin integrity and promoting optimal wound healing.

Defensive (Inflammatory) Phase

The defensive phase occurs immediately after injury and lasts about 3 to 4 days. The major events that occur in this phase are hemostasis and inflammation. **Hemostasis,** or cessation of bleeding, occurs by vasoconstriction of large blood vessels in the affected area.

Platelets, activated by the injury, aggregate to form a platelet plug and stop the bleeding. Activation of the clotting cascade results in the eventual formation of fibrin and a fibrinous meshwork, which further entraps platelets and other cells. The result is fibrin clot formation, which provides initial wound closure, prevents excessive loss of blood and body fluids, and inhibits contamination of the wound by microorganisms.

Inflammation is a nonspecific cellular response to tissue injury and involves both vascular and cellular

Figure 43-5 *Assessment of Skin Turgor*

Normal nail angle

160°

Figure 43-6 A, *Telangiectasis (Spider Veins);* **B,** *Ecchymosis (bruise)*

Figure 43-7 *Nail Variations (Photos of clubbing and Beau's line courtesy of Robert A. Silverman, MD, Clinical Associate Professor, Department of Pediatrics, Georgetown University)*

responses. During the vascular response, tissue injury and activation of plasma protein systems stimulate the release of various chemical mediators, such as histamine (from mast cells), serotonin (from platelets), complement, and kinins. These vasoactive substances cause blood vessels to dilate and become more permeable, resulting in increased blood flow and leakage of serous fluid into the

surrounding tissues. The increased blood supply carries nutrients and oxygen, which are essential for wound healing, and transports leukocytes to the area to participate in phagocytosis, or the envelopment and disposal of microorganisms. The increased blood supply also removes the "debris of battle," which includes dead cells, bacteria, and exudate, or material and cells discharged from blood vessels. The area is red, edematous, and warm to touch, and it has varying amounts of exudate.

During the cellular response, leukocytes move out of the blood vessel into the interstitial space. Neutrophils are the first cells to arrive at the injured site and begin phagocytosis. They subsequently die and are replaced by macrophages, which arise from blood monocytes. Macrophages perform the same function as neutrophils but remain for a longer time. In addition to being the primary phagocyte of debridement, macrophages are important cells in wound healing because they secrete several factors, including fibroblast activating factor (FAF) and angiogenesis factor (AGF). FAF attracts fibroblasts, which form collagen or collagen precursors. AGF stimulates the formation of new blood vessels. The development of this new microcirculation supports and sustains the wound and the healing process.

Reconstructive (Proliferative) Phase

The reconstructive phase begins on the third or fourth day after injury and lasts for 2 to 3 weeks. This phase contains the process of collagen deposition, angiogenesis, granulation tissue development, and wound contraction.

Fibroblasts, normally found in connective tissue, migrate into the wound because of various cellular mediators. They are the most important cells in this phase because they synthesize and secrete collagen. Collagen is the most abundant protein in the body and is the material of tissue repair. Initially, collagen is gel-like, but within several months it cross-links to form collagen fibrils and adds tensile strength to the wound. As the wound gains strength, the risk of wound separation or rupture is less likely. The wound can resist normal stress such as tension or twisting after 15 to 20 days. During this time, a raised "healing ridge" may be visible under the injury or suture line.

Angiogenesis (formation of new blood vessels) begins within hours after the injury. The endothelial cells in preexisting vessels begin to produce enzymes that break down the basement membrane. The membrane opens, and new endothelial cells build a new vessel. These capillaries grow across the wound, increasing blood flow, which increases the supply of nutrients and oxygen needed for wound healing.

Repair begins as granulation tissue, or new tissue, grows inward from surrounding healthy connective tissue. Granulation tissue is filled with new capillaries that are fragile and bleed easily, thus giving the healing area a red, translucent, granular appearance. As granulation tissue is formed, epithelialization, or growth of epithelial tissue, begins. Epithelial cells migrate into the wound from the wound margins. Eventually, the migrating cells contact similar cells that have migrated from the outer edges. Contact stops migration. The cells then begin to differentiate into the various cells that comprise the different layers of epidermis.

Wound contraction is the final step of the reconstructive phase of wound healing. Contraction is noticeable 6 to 12 days after injury and is necessary for closure of all wounds. The edges of the wound are drawn together by the action of myofibroblasts, specialized cells that contain bundles of parallel fibers in their cytoplasm. These myofibroblasts bridge across a wound and then contract to pull the wound closed.

Maturation Phase

Maturation, the final stage of healing, begins about the 21st day and may continue for up to 2 years or more, depending on the depth and extent of the wound. During this phase, the scar tissue is remodeled (reshaped or reconstructed by collagen deposition and lysis and debridement of wound edges). Although the scar tissue continues to gain strength, it remains weaker than the tissue it replaces. Capillaries eventually disappear, leaving an avascular scar (a scar that is white because it lacks a blood supply).

Types of Healing

Tissue may heal by one of three methods, which are characterized by the degree of tissue loss. *Primary intention* healing occurs in wounds that have minimal tissue loss and edges that are well-approximated (closed). If there are no complications, such as infection, necrosis, or abnormal scar formation, wound healing occurs with minimal granulation tissue and scarring.

Secondary intention healing is seen in wounds with extensive tissue loss and wounds in which the edges cannot be approximated. The wound is left open, and granulation tissue gradually fills in the deficit. Repair time is longer, tissue replacement and scarring are greater, and the susceptibility to infection is increased because of the lack of an epidermal barrier to microorganisms.

Tertiary intention healing, also known as delayed or secondary closure, is indicated when primary closure of a wound is undesirable. Conditions in which healing by tertiary intention may occur include poor circulation or infection. Suturing of the wound is delayed until the problems resolve and more favorable conditions exist for wound healing.

Kinds of Wound Drainage

Chemical mediators released during the inflammatory response cause vascular changes and exudation of fluid and cells from blood vessels into tissues. Exudates may vary in composition, but all have similar functions. These functions include the following:

- Dilution of toxins produced by bacteria and dying cells
- Transport of leukocytes and plasma proteins, including antibodies, to the site
- Transport of bacterial toxins, dead cells, debris, and other products of inflammation away from the site

The nature and amount of exudate vary depending on the tissue involved, the intensity and duration of the inflammation, and the presence of microorganisms.

Serous exudate is composed primarily of serum (the clear portion of blood), is watery in appearance, and has a low protein level. This type of exudate is seen with mild inflammation, resulting in minimal capillary permeability changes and minimal protein molecule escape (e.g., seen in blister formation after a burn).

Purulent exudate is also called pus. It generally occurs with severe inflammation accompanied by infection. Purulent exudate is thicker than serous exudate because of the presence of leukocytes (particularly neutrophils), liquefied dead tissue debris, and dead and living bacteria. The process of pus formation is called suppuration, and bacteria that produce pus are referred to as pyogenic bacteria. Purulent exudates may vary in color (e.g., yellow, green, brown) depending on the causative organism.

Hemorrhagic exudate has a large component of red blood cells (RBCs) because of capillary damage, which allows RBCs to escape. This type of exudate is usually present with severe inflammation. The color of the exudate (bright red versus dark red) reflects whether the bleeding is fresh or old.

Mixed types of exudates may also be seen, depending on the type of wound. For example, a **serosanguineous exudate** is clear with some blood tinge and is seen with surgical incisions.

Factors Affecting Wound Healing

Wound healing depends on multiple influences, both intrinsic and extrinsic. Wounds may fail to heal or may require a longer healing period when unfavorable conditions exist. Factors that may negatively influence healing include age, oxygenation, smoking, drug therapy, and diseases such as diabetes. Such factors reduce local blood supply and impair wound healing. Nutrition and diet can also affect the healing process.

Hemorrhage

Some bleeding from a wound is normal during and immediately after initial trauma and surgery, but hemostasis usually occurs within a few minutes. Hemorrhage is abnormal and may indicate a slipped surgical suture, a dislodged clot, or erosion of a blood vessel. Swelling in the area around the wound or affected body part and the presence of **sanguineous,** bloody, drainage from the surgical drain may indicate internal bleeding. Other evidence of bleeding may include the signs and symptoms seen in hypovolemic shock (decreased blood pressure, rapid thready pulse, increased respiratory rate, diaphoresis, restlessness, and cool clammy skin). A hematoma (localized collection of blood underneath the tissues) may also be seen and appears as a reddish-blue swelling or mass. External hemorrhaging is detected when the surgical dressing becomes saturated with sanguineous drainage. It is also important to assess the linen under the client's wound site because it is possible for the blood to seep out from under the sides of the dressing and pool under the client. The risk for hemorrhage is greatest during the first 24 to 48 hours after surgery.

Infection

Bacterial wound contamination is one of the most common causes of altered wound healing. A wound can become infected with microorganisms preoperatively, intraoperatively, or postoperatively. During the preoperative period, the wound may become exposed to pathogens because of the manner in which the wound was inflicted, such as in traumatic injuries. Nicks or abrasions created during preoperative shaving may also be a source of pathogens. The risk for intraoperative exposure to pathogens increases when the respiratory, gastrointestinal, genitourinary, and oropharyngeal tracts are opened.

If the amount of bacteria in the wound is sufficient or the client's immune defenses are compromised, clinical infection may result and become apparent 2 to 11 days postoperatively. Infection slows healing by prolonging the inflammatory phase of healing, competing for nutrients, and producing chemicals and enzymes that are damaging to the tissues.

Wound Classification

Many different classification systems are used to describe wounds. These systems describe either how the wound was acquired, how clean it is, or which tissue layers are involved. A classification system will assist the nurse in planning wound care management. The following are commonly used classification systems.

Cause of Wound

Intentional wounds occur during treatment or therapy. These wounds are usually made under aseptic conditions. Examples include surgical incisions and venipunctures.

Unintentional wounds are unanticipated and are often the result of trauma or an accident. These wounds are created in an unsterile environment and therefore pose a greater risk of infection.

Cleanliness of Wound

This classification system ranks the wound according to its contamination by bacteria and risk for infection (Schwartz, Shires, Spencer, Daly, Fischer, & Galloway 1999).

- *Clean wounds* are intentional wounds that were created under conditions in which no inflammation was encountered and the respiratory, alimentary, genitourinary, and oropharyngeal tracts were not entered.
- *Clean-contaminated wounds* are intentional wounds that were created by entry into the alimentary, respiratory, genitourinary, or oropharyngeal tract under controlled conditions.
- *Contaminated wounds* are open, traumatic wounds or intentional wounds in which there was a major break in aseptic technique, spillage from the gastrointestinal tract, or incision into infected urinary or biliary tracts. These wounds have acute nonpurulent inflammation present.
- *Dirty and infected wounds* are traumatic wounds with retained dead tissue or foreign material or intentional wounds created in situations where purulent drainage was present.

Depth of Wound

The third classification system is based on the depth of the wound, taking into account the skin layers involved.

- *Superficial wounds* are confined to the epidermis layer, which comprises the four outermost layers of skin.
- *Partial-thickness wounds* involve the epidermis and part of the dermis, which is the layer of skin beneath the epidermis.
- *Full-thickness wounds* involve the entire epidermis and dermis. Deeper structures such as fascia, muscle, and bone may be involved.

Assessment

Nurses are confronted with wounds that are extremely diverse. The wound may have occurred traumatically just before the client presents to the emergency room, or the wound may be a slow-healing chronic ulcer. Approach wound assessment systematically, evaluating the wound's stage in the healing process. Show sensitivity to the client's pain and tolerance levels during assessment and always follow Standard Precautions to prevent transfer of pathogens. Following are some basic criteria for wound assessment.

Location

Assessment begins with a description of the anatomical location of the wound (e.g., "5-inch suture line on the right lower quadrant of the abdomen"). This task often becomes difficult if the client has multiple wounds close to each other, as is common in burn or multiple-trauma victims. Use of a skin documentation form that incorporates drawings of the body allows the nurse to number the location of the various wounds and then describe them.

Size

The length (head to toe), width (side to side), and depth of a wound are measured in centimeters. Single-use measurement guides (tape measures) often come with dressing supplies. To determine the depth of a wound, a sterile cotton swab, moistened with 0.9% saline solution, is inserted into the deepest point of the wound and marked at the skin surface level. Then the swab can be measured and the wound depth in centimeters documented. Tunneling, also called undermining, can be measured by using a cotton swab to gently probe the wound margins. If tunneling is noted, the location and depth are documented. For clarity in describing the location of the tunneling, the hands of the clock can be used as a guide, with 12 o'clock pointing at the client's head. Example: "Tunneling occurs at 1 o'clock and its depth is 2 cm."

For extremely irregularly shaped wounds, the wound edges can be traced on a plastic surface. A plastic bag or piece of plastic sheeting folded in half is placed on the wound, and the wound margins are traced. The side of the plastic placed against the wound is cut off and placed in a biohazard container. The rest of the plastic can be placed in the chart.

General Appearance and Drainage

A general description of the color of the wound and surrounding area helps determine the wound's present phase of healing. Gently palpate the edges of the wound for swelling, and document the amount, color, location, odor, and consistency of any drainage.

Pain

Document and notify the physician of any pain or tenderness at the wound site. Pain may indicate infection or bleeding. It is normal to experience pain in a surgical incision wound for approximately 3 days. Report any sudden increase in pain accompanied by changes in the appearance of the wound to the physician immediately.

Laboratory Data

Cultures of wound drainage are used to determine the presence of infection and the identity of the causative organism. The sensitivity results list the antibiotics that will effectively treat the infection. An elevated WBC count indicates an infectious process. A decreased leukocyte count may indicate that the client is at increased risk for developing an infection related to decreased defense mechanisms. Albumin is a measure of the client's protein reserves; if the albumin is decreased, the client will have decreased resources of protein for wound healing.

Nursing Diagnoses

Nursing diagnoses for clients with wounds focus on prevention of complications and promotion of the healing process through proper wound care and client teaching. Following are NANDA-approved nursing diagnoses with a partial list of related factors:

- *Impaired **T**issue Integrity* related to surgical incision, pressure, shearing forces, decreased blood flow, immobility, mechanical irritants
- *Risk for **I**nfection* related to malnutrition, decreased defense mechanisms
- *Acute **P**ain* related to inflammation, infection
- *Disturbed **B**ody Image* related to changes in body appearance secondary to scars, drains, removal of body parts
- *Deficient **K**nowledge (wound care)* related to lack of exposure to information, misinterpretation, lack of interest in learning

Planning/Outcome Identification

After identifying the nursing diagnoses, establish targeted outcomes for wound healing based on the client's identified needs and individualized to the client's condition. Changes in the health care delivery system have brought about early discharge from the hospital, so clients are often sent home with wounds that need continued care; the goals for clients with wounds generally focus on promoting wound healing, preventing infection, and educating the client.

Implementation

Nursing interventions to promote wound healing and prevent infection include emergency measures to maintain homeostasis (state of internal constancy of the body), and cleansing and dressing of the wound.

Emergency Measures

Assess the type and extent of injury that the client has sustained. If hemorrhage is detected, apply sterile dressings and pressure to stop the bleeding, and notify the physician immediately. Always implement Standard Precautions. Monitor the client's vital signs frequently.

When dehiscence or evisceration occurs, instruct the client to remain quiet and avoid coughing or straining. Position the client to prevent further stress on the wound. Use sterile dressings, such as ABD pads soaked with sterile normal saline, to cover the wound and internal contents. This reduces the risk of bacterial contamination and drying of the viscera. Notify the surgeon immediately and prepare the client for surgical repair of the area.

Cleansing the Wound

The goal of cleansing the wound is to remove debris and bacteria from the wound bed with as little trauma to the healthy granulation tissue as possible. Choice of cleansing agent depends on the physician's prescription as well as agency protocol. It is recommended that isotonic solutions such as normal saline or lactated Ringer's be used to preserve healthy tissue.

Dressing the Wound

Following are the three purposes of a wound dressing:

1. To keep the wound moist and therefore enhance epithelialization
2. To clean the wound or keep it clean
3. To protect the wound from physical trauma or bacterial invasion

Keeping these three purposes in mind, determine an appropriate dressing for the client's wound. There are thousands of different wound care products on the market. The physician may prescribe a specific dressing, or follow agency policy. Remember that dressing plans must be modified as the wound changes.

Monitoring Drainage of Wounds

During the inflammatory response, exudates develop within a wound. When excessive drainage accumulates in the wound bed, tissue healing is delayed. If the outer surface is allowed to heal while the drainage remains entrapped within the wound, infection and abscess may form. To facilitate drainage of any excess fluid, the physician may insert a tube or drain.

Other Therapies

Negative-pressure wound therapy, also called vacuum-assisted closure (VAC), increases healing rates by 40% (Mendez-Eastman, 2002). It supports the wound-healing efforts of the body by increasing cellular proliferation, reducing edema around the wound, and providing a moist, protected wound bed.

Biodebridement or maggot debridement therapy (MDT) is mainly used for chronic wounds. Maggots ingest and digest bacteria and dead tissue and have been used to heal wounds infected with methicillin-resistant *Staphylococcus aureus*. The first intentional use occurred during the Civil War (Martin, 2001). Unintentional use can occur if flies are allowed to land on open wounds.

Electrical stimulation helps speed healing by increasing capillary density and perfusion, improving wound oxygenation, and encouraging fibroblast activity and granulation. Placement of the electrodes varies with the stage of healing. A physical therapist determines electrode placement and polarity (Kloth, 2002).

Evaluation

Evaluate the client's achievement of the goals established during the planning phase to achieve or maintain skin integrity. Goals for clients with wounds generally focus on wound healing, prevention of infection, and client education. If the goals are not achieved, examine the nursing interventions and strategies that were employed and revise the nursing care plan accordingly. Review techniques and procedures, especially those performed by the client or other caregivers in the client's support system.

BURNS

Burns are among the most devastating injuries an individual can suffer. Burns can be painful and disfiguring, requiring long hospitalizations. Many are fatal. Most burns occur in the home and are preventable. Often, the burn injury is the result of the individual's own action. Feelings of anger and guilt can complicate recovery. Often, the individual suffers self-image disturbances, and family relationships can be strained.

Major Causes

There are many different causes for burns to the skin. A major source of burn injury for all ages is overexposure to the sun. Most burn injuries to adults are associated with cigarette smoking and cooking. The elderly are more likely to spill hot liquid on themselves or catch their clothes on fire as they cook or smoke. Young children are especially prone to burn injuries from spilling scalding liquids on themselves and playing with matches or cigarette lighters. Industrial accidents account for a significant number of burn injuries in young adults.

Severity

Burns are classified according to the depth of the burn and the extent of skin surface involved. First- and second-degree burns are partial-thickness (within the epidermis/dermis) burns. First-degree burns involve only the epidermis. The skin is hot, red, and painful. Sunburn is an example of a first-degree burn. First-degree burns heal in about a week without scarring. Second-degree burns damage the dermis and the epidermis. The skin is red, hot, and painful; blisters form and tissue around the burn is edematous. An example of a second-degree burn is spilling boiling water on the skin. Usually, second-degree burns heal in about 2 weeks without scarring; however, if deep layers of the dermis are involved, healing might take months and scarring can occur. Second-degree burns involving deep layers of the dermis may appear white, tan, or red in color.

When the dermis and epidermis are completely destroyed and deeper tissues are involved, burns are classified as full-thickness burns. Third-degree and fourth-degree burns are full-thickness burns. In third-degree burns all dermal structures are destroyed and cannot be regenerated. Subcutaneous tissue is also damaged. Full-thickness burns can be white, tan, brown, black, charred, or bright red in color. Fourth-degree burns, which extend to the underlying muscles and bones, appear white to black or charred with dark networks of thrombosed capillaries visible inside the wound. Fourth-degree burns result from fires, explosions, and nuclear radiation. Figure 43-8 depicts the various layers of skin involved in burn injuries.

Severely burned individuals generally have both partial-thickness and full-thickness burns. Whereas first- and second-degree burns are painful, third- and fourth-degree burns are not painful because sensory nerve endings are destroyed. The client, however, will still be in severe pain. Body movement causes pain in areas of first- and second-degree burns that often surround the full-thickness burns. Skin can regenerate only from the edges of full-thickness burns. Scarring is inevitable. Skin grafting is necessary to promote healing because the section of skin destroyed by the burn cannot regenerate itself.

Prognosis in burn cases depends on the severity of the burn, the surface area of the body burned, and the preinjury health status of the individual. If the client's health status before the burn was good, a burn covering 40% of the body will require a minimum of 40 days to heal (Fritsch & Yurko, 2003). Elderly burn victims whose

A Epidermis

Skin red, dry

First degree, superficial

B Epidermis Dermis

Blistered; skin moist, pink or red

Second degree, partial thickness

C Epidermis Dermis Subcutaneous tissue

Charring; skin black, brown, red

Third degree, full thickness

D Epidermis Dermis Subcutaneous tissue Muscle and bone

Charring; skin white to black with networks of thrombosed capillaries

Fourth degree, full thickness

Figure 43-8 *Skin Layers Involved in Burn Injuries: **A,** First-degree burn; **B,** Second-degree burn; **C,** Third-degree burn; **D,** Fourth-degree burn (Photos courtesy of the Phoenix Society for Burn Survivors, Inc.)*

physiologic reserves are already reduced as an effect of aging will have an extended recovery period and a greater risk of complications.

For years, documenting the extent of burn injuries was done by using the Rule-of-Nines method to estimate the body surface area burned for adults. The body is divided into areas that are about 9% (or multiples of 9%). The head comprises 9% (4.5% anterior and 4.5% posterior). Each arm is 9% (4.5% anterior and 4.5% posterior). The anterior trunk and posterior trunk are each 18%. Each leg is 18% (9% anterior and 9% posterior). The genitalia comprise the remaining 1%.

More recently, Milner (2001), inventor of the "Burn Wheel" (Figure 43-9), incorporated a chart similar to the Rule-of-Nines. His chart has a specific percentage for the upper and lower parts of the arms and legs and for the hands and feet, making a more accurate assessment. One side is for infants and children; the other side is for adults.

Complications

Destruction of the skin renders it unable to fulfill its functions. Vast amounts of internal fluids and electrolytes are lost. The ability to maintain body temperature is altered, and the individual is susceptible to serious infections. Initially, the complications that are the most life threatening are respiratory failure and massive loss of body fluids.

Figure 43-9 *Burn Wheel (Invented by Stephen M. Milner)*

Smoke Inhalation and Carbon Monoxide Poisoning

Heat and smoke can cause serious damage to the respiratory tract. Facial burns, singed nasal hairs, and carbon-tinged sputum are signs that the client may have suffered respiratory tract damage (Hilton, 2001). Inhaling heat and smoke in a closed-space fire causes airway inflammation and edema of the respiratory mucosa. The carbon monoxide that is inhaled along with the heat and smoke attaches to hemoglobin, forming the compound carboxyhemoglobin. A high level of carboxyhemoglobin in the blood means that oxygen is not being delivered to vital body tissues. The client may be stuporous because of cerebral anoxia. Keeping an open airway and administering 100% humidified oxygen are essential for treating these two conditions. Intubation is often necessary.

Shock

Severely burned clients may suffer both hypovolemic shock (a life-threatening condition caused by massive loss of blood and circulating fluids) and neurogenic shock (a form of shock that occurs when peripheral vascular dilation occurs causing hypotension). Fluids and electrolytes must be replaced as fast as they are being lost. Tremendous amounts of fluids are lost through the burn wounds themselves as well as into surrounding tissues in the form of edema. The fluid loss shock that results can lead to circulatory collapse and renal shutdown. The Burn Wheel was developed for use in hospitals and emergency departments (EDs) because the first 24 hours after a burn injury are crucial (Milner, 2001). The Burn Wheel uses the client's weight (in Kg) along with the percentage of area burned to identify the amount of Ringer's lactate solution to be given IV within 2 hours and the amount to be continued for 24 hours. Use of the wheel takes seconds to determine fluid replacement, whereas remembering and figuring formulae may take much longer and mistakes can be easily made. At least two large-bore venous catheters are used to give large volumes of fluid rapidly.

Infection

Once the client has been stabilized, infection poses a serious risk. *Staphylococcus aureus,* an ever-present organism in the environment, is a common cause of infections. Of grave concern is an infection caused by methicillin-resistant *Staphylococcus aureus* (MRSA) because this strain of staphylococcus is resistant to all antibiotics except vancomycin hydrochloride (Vancocin). This antibiotic has serious side effects, especially to the otic nerve and to the liver, and is used only when other antibiotics fail.

All persons coming into contact with the burn client must wear gowns, gloves, masks, and caps to help prevent the introduction of organisms such as *Staphylococcus aureus, Pseudomonas aeruginosa,* or coliform bacilli into burn wounds. Sterile technique is used for wound care and dressing changes. Care in special burn units reduces the chance of infection because of stringent infection control precautions and a carefully controlled environment.

Medical–Surgical Management

Medical

Immediate Care Initially, medical management of the client involves keeping an open airway, maintaining an adequate level of oxygenation, replacing body fluids and electrolytes, monitoring kidney function, controlling pain, and protecting the burns with sterile dressings to minimize the loss of body temperature and the risk of infection. In cases of severe burns, the client usually requires endotracheal intubation and administration of 100% humidified oxygen. A multiport central venous catheter or two large-bore peripheral venous catheters are needed for fluid and electrolyte replacement. A Foley catheter is inserted and urine output measured hourly to help monitor kidney function.

Pain is controlled with small intravenous doses of morphine. Emotional and psychological trauma can intensify pain perception. The client will be anxious about survival, physical appearance, and the effect this injury will have on the family. Prophylactically, the client is given tetanus toxoid.

Stabilized Care Once the client's condition has been stabilized, care focuses on promoting healing, preventing complications, controlling pain, and restoring function. Preventing infection is an important priority. Burn wounds may require daily cleansing and dressing changes. Because of the nature of the injury, burn wounds contain a large amount of dead tissue along with fluids and proteins, making them highly susceptible to infection even with the best of care. Antibiotics and strict aseptic technique are essential. The dead tissue of full-thickness burns forms a dry, dark leathery **eschar** (a scab of denatured protein) within 48 to 72 hours. Infection can often begin under the eschar, causing tissue sloughing. Loose eschar must be **debrided** before skin grafting can occur. Debriding, removing dead and damaged tissue or foreign material within the burn wound, can sometimes be done mechanically by hydrotherapy, either by submersion in a whirlpool bath or by placing the client on a spray table and directly spraying the wound with a hose system that controls both the force and the temperature of the solution (Fritsch & Yurko, 2003). Burn wounds may require surgical debridement. The base of the wound must be free of infection and necrotic tissue before it can be covered with skin grafts.

Infection Control: Debridement
Strict aseptic techniques must be followed during burn debridement procedures.

Use of specialty beds, such as fluidized or alternating air-filled mattresses, minimizes pressure on skin surfaces, thus promoting comfort. Limiting movement and maintaining normal body alignment with the use of splints can also help alleviate client discomfort.

Surgical

Skin grafts cover the burn wound to promote healing. Four types of skin grafts might be used:

1. Autograft—the client's own skin that is removed from an unburned area and applied to the wound

2. Homograft—skin obtained from a cadaver within 6 to 24 hours after death
3. Heterograft—skin obtained from an animal, such as a pig
4. Synthetic skin substitute—a manmade product that has properties similar to skin (Fritsch & Yurko, 2003)

Homografts, heterografts, and synthetic skin substitutes are temporary grafts that facilitate healing. These grafts prevent water, electrolyte, and protein loss. They decrease pain and allow more freedom of movement for the client. When the client's condition is stable and the wound beds have healthy **granulation tissue** (delicate connective tissue consisting of fibroblasts, collagen, and capillaries), permanent closure of the burn wounds is done with autografts. Granulation tissue is red and provides a base for healing (Seeley et al., 2002).

Autografts are taken from areas of healthy skin. They may be either split-thickness grafts or full-thickness grafts. Split-thickness grafts include the epidermis and part of the dermis. They are not so deep as to prevent regeneration of skin at the donor site.

Infection Control: Skin Grafts

Follow strict aseptic care of both the donor sites and the newly grafted burn wounds to prevent infection.

The application of pressure dressings during the rehabilitative phase reduces the development of hypertrophic scarring, a condition in which the scar becomes elevated and has a "Swiss cheese" appearance. Pressure dressings, which may be elastic wraps, stockinettes, or custom-made pressure garments, must be worn constantly and are to be removed only for daily hygiene care. Full maturation of the burn scar may take 1 to 2 years. As the physical wounds heal, so do the emotional and psychological wounds. The client's ability to cope with daily stresses and resume social and work activities typically coincides with the physical healing process.

Pharmacological

Dressing changes, wound debridement, as well as any movement or manipulation, are extremely painful for clients. Many clients become extremely anxious, fearing pain as well as permanent disfiguration and loss of function. Intravenous narcotics, usually morphine, may be administered 10 to 15 minutes before procedures. By decreasing anxiety and fear, daily doses of psychotropic drugs can enhance the effectiveness of pain medications and help the client cope with the prospect of long-term rehabilitation.

Treatment of the burn wound with topical agents can decrease infection and promote healing. Common topical agents used are mafenide acetate (Sulfamylon); silver sulfadiazine (Silvadene); povidone-iodine (Betadine); nitrofurazone (Furacin); and antibiotic agents such as neomycin sulfate (Myciguent), bacitracin (Baciguent), and gentamicin sulfate (Garamycin). Mafenide acetate (Sulfamylon) can penetrate thick eschar and is effective against gram-negative and gram-positive organisms, including *Pseudomonas aeruginosa*. Silver sulfadiazine (Silvadene) is effective against many gram-positive and gram-negative organisms as well as *Candida* organisms. It is painless and somewhat soothing but may cause a skin rash. Povidone-iodine (Betadine) has broad-spectrum microbial action against a wide variety of bacteria, fungi, yeasts, viruses, and protozoa. Application of povidone-iodine to large open areas could lead to elevated serum iodine levels. Nitrofurazone (Furacin) has broad-spectrum activity and is effective against *Staphylococcus aureus*. It is not absorbed systemically and has a low incidence of sensitivity.

Antibiotic ointments are used to decrease infection. Neomycin sulfate (Myciguent) and gentamicin sulfate (Garamycin) can be absorbed systemically and have serious side effects of ototoxicity and nephrotoxicity. Bacitracin (Baciguent) has minimal antimicrobial activity, but it is especially useful to prevent drying of the wound. Topical agents must be applied in a thin layer with a sterile glove. The wound may be left open to air or covered with a gauze dressing, depending on the properties of the medication and the physician's orders. Application of these medications can be painful because of manipulation of the burned tissue. Administration of pain medication may be necessary before providing wound care. The surrounding skin should be assessed for any allergic rashes.

Diet

Following a moderate to severe burn, the need for calories and protein increases. Actual protein loss occurs with the burn injury itself, and some protein is metabolized to meet the increased energy requirements brought on by stress. For tissue repair and healing, daily protein needs may increase by 2 to 4 times the normal daily protein requirement (Fritsch & Yurko, 2003). Twice the normal caloric requirement may be needed to meet the body's energy needs. Supplemental vitamins and minerals are given.

Initially, the client's daily nutritional needs may be met with total parenteral nutrition (TPN) because of a paralytic ileus and gastric dilation. Following a severe burn, decreased enteric circulation leads to slowed or stopped peristalsis. Food and fluids cannot be given orally or by tube feeding until peristalsis is restored. Hearing active bowel sounds is one indication of peristaltic activity in the bowel. Immobility, stress, and the negative nitrogen balance brought on by protein catabolism depress appetite. Curling's ulcer may develop. Meeting the client's nutritional needs can be a challenge. Six to eight small feedings daily and high-protein milkshakes or protein supplements can help meet daily nutri-

---

PROFESSIONAL TIP

Serving Meals

Serve foods attractively and put an occasional small "surprise" on the tray (e.g., a flower, a small, brightly colored seasonal decoration, a funny card) so that the client will look forward to meals.

tional needs. Involving the family in bringing in favorite foods can also stimulate the client's appetite.

Activity

Contractures, among the most serious complications of severe burns, can be prevented with a program of positioning, splinting, exercising, and ambulating. When repositioning, the client's body must be kept in correct alignment. Use pillows to keep limbs in alignment and splints on limbs to prevent contractures or to immobilize joints following skin grafting. Range-of-motion exercises maintain joint mobility. Whenever possible, encourage active rather than passive range-of-motion exercises. Active exercise increases circulation, maintains joint flexibility, and improves muscle tone. As the client recovers, activities of daily living can be increased and ambulation can be initiated.

Nursing Management

Immediate care includes establishing an airway and administering oxygen. (The physician often inserts an endotracheal tube). Initiate IV fluid therapy with Ringer's lactate solution. Insert a Foley catheter and monitor output, which should be 30 to 50 mL per hour. Administer analgesic IV as ordered. Monitor vital signs, noting respiratory pattern, effort, and breath sounds. Assess pulse oximetry, client's color, and level of consciousness. Accurately record I&O. Monitor client's laboratory results, especially electrolytes.

When the client is stabilized, continue monitoring vital signs, I&O, respiratory pattern, daily weight, and for pain. Strictly follow Standard Precautions. Monitor wounds for signs of infection. Assess mental status. If client is on TPN or enteral tube feedings, monitor client's reaction to feedings. Assess abdomen for bowel sounds. Use pillows and splints, if ordered, to keep client's body in good alignment and turn and reposition every 2 hours. Perform passive ROM exercises when able. Explain the healing process to the client and family. Provide opportunities for the client to express feelings. Listen actively. Encourage the client to look at the wounds to see evidence of healing. Maintain an open, honest approach with the client and family. Assist client and family to prepare for discharge.

NURSING PROCESS

Assessment

Subjective Data

Observe for emotional reactions such as anger, self-consciousness, embarrassment, or isolation. Clients with burns are likely to be frightened and anxious. Feelings of guilt, anger, and depression are also common following burns. Ask the client to describe the pain according to location, intensity, and duration, and also to rate the pain on a scale of 0 to 10. Hypoxia or fluid and electrolyte imbalances can cause confusion, disorientation, and decreased level of consciousness. The client may be nauseated.

Objective Data

Assess vital signs, level of consciousness, and breath sounds. If the client has a productive cough, the amount and color of sputum should be noted. Black/gray sputum indicates smoke inhalation. Clients with smoke inhalation may also have crackles, wheezing, or diminished breath sounds. Observe burn wounds for signs of infection such as redness, swelling, purulent drainage, and a foul odor. Measure urine output hourly. Monitor intake and output and daily weight. Routinely check for bowel sounds. As rehabilitation progresses, continue to assess wounds for signs of healing, such as a moist, clean, red wound base and decrease in the size of the wound. Note the client's mobility status and degree of involvement in care. Assess daily dietary intake. Monitor laboratory test results for the following:

- Red blood cell count and hemoglobin level give information about the body's ability to meet oxygen demands of body tissues and organs.
- Creatinine and blood urea nitrogen as well as urine specific gravity give information about kidney function.

- Total protein and albumin levels yield information about the ability to maintain the volume of circulating fluid as well as information about nutritional status.
- White blood cell count indicates the presence of infection and the body's ability to fight it.

- Wound culture and sensitivity data indicate the specific organisms causing infection and the specific antibiotics effective against these organisms.
- Electrolytes yield information about the homeostasis of body fluids. Alterations in pH and electrolyte levels affect cell function in every body tissue, particularly vital body organs such as the heart and cerebrum.

Nursing diagnoses for a client with a burn injury may include the following. Initially, the greatest dangers to the client will be:

Nursing Diagnoses	Planning/Goals	Nursing Interventions
Impaired Gas Exchange related to edema and inflammation of the respiratory tract	The client will achieve a regular respiratory pattern and oxygen saturation level >90%.	Monitor the client's vital signs every 4 hours if stable; otherwise, every 1 to 2 hours. Listen to breath sounds, especially noting respiratory pattern and effort. If the client is on continuous oximetry, note the oxygen saturation reading each time vital signs are assessed. Assess the client's color and level of consciousness. Document assessments and keep the physician informed about the client's condition. Elevate the head of the bed 30 degrees to facilitate full chest expansion with each breath.
Deficient Fluid Volume related to increased capillary permeability with loss of large amounts of fluid through open burn wounds	The client will maintain electrolytes within normal limits and an hourly urine output >30 mL per hour.	Administer intravenous fluids at the ordered rate. Monitor for signs and symptoms of fluid overload such as shortness of breath, crackles auscultated in lung bases, changes in heart rate and/or heart sounds, changes in blood pressure, increased anxiety, or changes in mental status. Measure urine output hourly, report outputs below 30 mL to the physician. Record intake and output. Involve the client and family in keeping a bedside record of fluid intake. Weigh client daily, preferably before breakfast, and in the same type of clothing each day. When the client can tolerate oral fluids, set a fluid intake goal for each shift (e.g., 1,200 mL during the day; 800 mL during the evening; 500 mL during the night). Explain to the client and family the reasons for a high fluid intake. Involve family members in helping the client achieve the fluid maintenance goal. Keep fluids available at the bedside, including within dietary restrictions, the client's favorite fluids. Monitor for signs and symptoms of electrolyte imbalances such as increased muscle weakness, muscle cramps, cardiac arrhythmias, fatigue, nausea, dizziness. Monitor the client's laboratory results.

During the stabilization and recovery period following a burn, the nursing diagnoses may include the following:

Nursing Diagnoses	Planning/Goals	Nursing Interventions
Risk for Infection related to risk factors of tissue destruction and inadequate primary defenses	The client's burn wounds will exhibit signs of healing without serious or life-threatening infections.	Wash hands with an antibacterial skin cleanser before and after gloving. Wear clean gloves when giving client care. Wear an isolation gown over your uniform when giving client care. Whenever the client's wounds are exposed, wear gown, cap, mask, and sterile gloves. Use sterile technique for wound care and dressing changes. Monitor wound daily for signs of infection: redness, swelling, purulent drainage, pain.

continues

Nursing Diagnoses	Planning/Goals	Nursing Interventions
		Assess for signs of systemic infections.
		Observe for increased pulse and respirations, decreased blood pressure, fever, and any changes in mentation such as disorientation and delirium.
		Note urinary output and assess for hypoactive bowel sounds.
		Monitor the client's white blood cell count.
		Assist client with personal hygiene, and keep noninjured areas of the body clean.
Acute Pain related to physical injury	The client will verbalize that pain is controlled at a tolerable level.	Assess for pain every 2 to 4 hours by asking client to rate pain level on a scale of 0 to 10. Observe for nonverbal signs of pain such as grimacing or crying.
		Administer pain medications as ordered, especially prior to wound care or exercise and mobilization activities.
		Monitor and document response to medications.
		Implement comfort and diversional measures: a. Reposition client; use pillows or foam supports to keep all body parts in good alignment. b. Teach client to use progressive relaxation exercises or to use guided imagery. c. Encourage the client to use diversionary activities of his choice such as television or music, or place him so that he can see into the hallway.
Imbalanced Nutrition: Less than body requirements, related to increased caloric requirements and difficulty ingesting sufficient quantities of food	The client will ingest sufficient calories daily to meet increased metabolic needs.	If the client is currently on TPN or enteral tube feedings, administer the ordered nutrients at the correct rate and closely monitor the client's reaction.
		When oral intake is tolerated, encourage the client to eat 90% to 100% of daily diet.
		Provide oral hygiene before meals to stimulate salivation and eliminate any bad taste in the client's mouth.
		Give 6 to 8 small feedings daily of the client's favorite foods within dietary restrictions and encourage family members to bring in home-prepared foods and to eat with the client.
		When permitted, encourage the client to sit up in a chair for each meal.
		Plan care so that painful procedures are not done immediately before meals. A rest period of 20 to 30 minutes before meals helps the client feel more like eating.
		Determine the time of day when the client feels most like eating and does indeed eat most of the meal, and serve the highest calorie/protein nutrients at that time.
Impaired Physical Mobility related to pain and decreased muscle strength	The client will participate in daily activity to maintain joint mobility and prevent contractures.	Perform passive ROM exercises 4 times a day by supporting the limb above and below the joint and performing exercises slowly and smoothly.
		As the client is able, have him perform active ROM exercises every 3 to 4 hours.
		Turn and reposition the client every 2 hours. Use small pillows and foam supports to keep the client's body in good alignment.
		Use splints as ordered by the physician to keep hands, wrists, feet, and ankles in natural alignment and explain the reason for these activities to the client.
		As healing and rehabilitation progress, encourage progressive ambulation and self-care activities.
		Gradually guide and assist the client to resume activities of daily living (ADLs).
		Encourage family members to participate in ADLs and provide positive reinforcement as the client becomes involved in his care.

continues

Nursing Diagnoses	Planning/Goals	Nursing Interventions
Disturbed Body Image related to change in physical appearance with loss of body tissues or body parts	The client will state realistic expectations for recovery and participate in rehabilitation.	Provide time for the client to express feelings (fear, anger, frustration, regret, and depression are commonly expressed by clients with burns) and practice active listening.
		Explain the healing process to the client. Give the client daily updates on the degree of wound healing and on his progress in rehabilitation.
		Encourage the client to look at the wounds, to show evidence of healing. Stress that wound healing following serious burn injuries proceeds slowly and that complete healing with improved skin appearance may take a year or more.
Interrupted Family Processes related to the shift in health status of a family member	The client and family members will verbalize feelings to nurses and each other and will participate in client care.	Involve family members in the client's care and encourage daily visits.
		Encourage family members to express their fears and concerns, especially any feelings of anger, blame, or guilt.
		Guide family members in recognizing and reflecting to the client small, step-by-step progress that is made.
		Maintain an honest, open approach with the client and family but do not give false reassurance.
		Collaborate with counselor, social worker, and chaplain to help the client and family cope with the condition.
		Assist the family to appraise the situation and plan for discharge. What is at stake? What is realistic for the future? What can they expect during the rehabilitation phase? What are their choices? Where can they get help?

Evaluation Each goal must be evaluated to determine how it has been met by the client.

NEOPLASMS: MALIGNANT

Skin cancer is one of the most common malignant neoplasms in the United States and is the most preventable cancer. More than 1 million cases of basal cell carcinoma and squamous cell carcinoma, and 54,200 malignant cases of melanoma make them the three most common skin cancers (ACS, 2003). Skin lymphoma is another type of malignancy. Exposure to the sun is the leading cause of skin cancer. Skin damage from sun exposure is cumulative. The ability of skin to tan is not fully developed until the teenage years, meaning that most of the long-term skin damage from sun exposure occurs during childhood. By age 20, most adults have already experienced significant skin damage; however, it takes 10 to 20 years before unprotected sunbathing results in skin cancer.

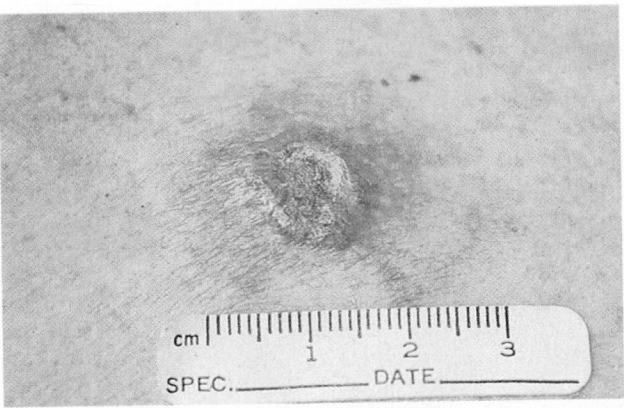

Figure 43-10 *Basal Cell Carcinoma (Courtesy of Robert A. Silverman, MD, Clinical Associate Professor, Department of Pediatrics, Georgetown University)*

BASAL CELL CARCINOMA

Basal cell carcinoma, the most frequent type of skin cancer, arises from the basal cell layer of the epidermis. Prolonged sun exposure, poor tanning ability, and previous therapy with x-rays for facial acne are risk factors for basal cell carcinoma (Figure 43-10). Metastasis are rare.

They are generally found on the face and upper torso, and are scaly in appearance. As the disease develops, it extends into the dermis and may form an open ulcer. Surgical removal cures this type of cancer.

SQUAMOUS CELL CARCINOMA

Squamous cell carcinoma appears as a nodular lesion in the epidermis. It is much less common than basal cell carcinoma. Risk factors include prolonged sun exposure and exposure to gamma radiation and x-rays. The sun-exposed lower lip is a common site for squamous cell carcinoma. Without treatment it can extend into the dermis and ultimately metastasize to other body tissues, causing death (Figure 43-11). The

Figure 43-11 *Squamous Cell Carcinoma (Courtesy of Robert A. Silverman, MD, Clinical Associate Professor, Department of Pediatrics, Georgetown University)*

Figure 43-12 *Lentigo Malignant Melanoma (Courtesy of Robert A. Silverman, MD, Clinical Associate Professor, Department of Pediatrics, Georgetown University)*

lesion may be excised surgically or it may be treated with chemosurgery, which involves application of a dressing with a fixative paste such as zinc chloride. When the dressing is removed, tumor cells trapped in the dressing are also removed. Dressings are reapplied and removed in this fashion until all malignant tissue has been removed (Weaver, 1999).

MALIGNANT MELANOMA

In malignant melanoma, atypical melanocytes are present in both the dermis and epidermis. Malignant melanoma is the most serious of the three types of skin cancers and may begin in a preexisting mole (nevus). These moles have an irregular shape. Contrasted to normal moles, they are larger than 6 mm in diameter and do not have a uniform color. Malignant melanoma can metastasize to every organ in the body through the bloodstream and lymphatic system.

The incidence of malignant melanoma is increasing in the United States as a result of increased sun exposure. At present there is no cure (Deters, 2002). Clearly, the best hope of preventing skin cancer lies in education. Limiting sun exposure and using sunscreen at least SPF 15 on exposed skin markedly reduce damage from ultraviolet rays and ultimately decrease the risk of skin cancer. Figure 43-12 shows lentigo malignant melanoma.

CUTANEOUS T-CELL LYMPHOMA

Cutaneous T-cell lymphoma is also known as mycosis fungoides and skin lymphoma. It is a malignant disease involving T-helper cells that has both skin manifestations and multiple organ system manifestations. In the early stages it resembles psoriasis or seborrheic dermatitis. Later, fissures and skin ulcers develop. Pruritus can be severe. Even if the skin condition can be improved with topical steroids and chemotherapeutic agents, the

disease is ultimately fatal because of the involvement of vital organ systems. Clients with AIDS can develop cutaneous T-cell lymphoma.

Medical–Surgical Management

Surgical

Electrosurgery, cryosurgery, and surgical excision are the primary methods of treatment for malignant neoplasms. Electrosurgery uses electric current to destroy and remove malignant tissue. It is best used for small lesions 1 to 2 cm in diameter. Cryosurgery destroys tumor tissue by freezing it. A special type of needle apparatus directs liquid nitrogen through the tumor until a temperature of $-40°$ to $-60°C$ is reached at the base of the tumor (Deters, 2002). In addition, regional perfusion chemotherapy can be used to treat malignant melanomas of the extremities. The circulation of the involved extremity is isolated, and a high dose of a cytotoxic drug is perfused directly into the tumor area (Deters, 2002). This method of treating just the area of the malignancy minimizes systemic effects of cytotoxic drugs.

Nursing Management

Careful assessment of the client's skin can reveal suspicious skin lesions. Clients with blue eyes, fair complexion, blonde or red hair, and freckles have the greatest risk. Clients who have had one skin cancer are likely to have more. Early referral and prompt care can ensure a good prognosis. Because most skin cancers are treated by excision, client teaching and follow-up care focus on proper wound care to promote healing and prevent infection. Many clients will experience body image disturbance; the nurse can help the client cope with this. All other nursing care should be focused on prevention.

NEOPLASMS: NONMALIGNANT

Benign tumors of the skin include a variety of lesions such as skin tags, lipomas, keloids, sebaceous cysts, nevi (moles), and angiomas. In general, they do not require medical or nursing intervention except for cosmetic reasons or unless they are subject to continual irritation that might predispose to a break in skin integrity and infection. **Lipomas** (benign, fatty tumors) or **sebaceous cysts** (distended sebaceous glands filled with sebum) might cause pressure on surrounding nerves or interfere with normal body function. In these instances they would be surgically removed. A **keloid** is abnormal growth of scar tissue that is elevated, rounded, and firm with irregular, clawlike margins. Surgical removal is not always successful; healing following surgery can again result in a keloid. Steroids or radiation have been helpful in some conditions. **Angiomas,** commonly known as birthmarks, are vascular tumors involving skin and subcutaneous tissue. They can be raised, bright red nodular lesions (strawberry birthmarks) or dark red/purple patches (port-wine angiomas). Cosmetics can be used to camouflage them. Laser treatments are being used on some angiomas with some success.

INFECTIOUS DISORDERS OF THE SKIN

Given an accessible portal of entry and decreased host resistance, virulent organisms can invade the skin, causing inflammation, infection, itching, and pain. Bacteria, viruses, fungi, or parasites can cause infectious disorders of the skin (Figure 43-13). Treating the client's disease is only one aspect of the treatment plan; preventing the spread of infection is the other. Table 43-4 outlines several disease conditions and identifies the organism responsible, clinical manifestations, and the management for each disorder.

Nursing Management

Teach the client and family about preventing the spread of infection. Follow Standard Precautions. Stress the importance of not scratching lesions. Provide emotional support to client and family. Encourage expression of feelings.

NURSING PROCESS

Assessment

Subjective Data

Ask the client how long the problem has existed, if there is any itching or pain, and what treatment has been used. Clients with infectious disorders of the skin may feel shame or embarrassment because of stigmas

A

B

C

D

E

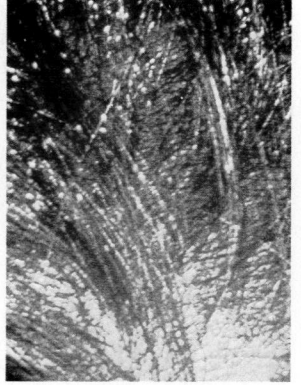
F

Figure 43-13 *Infectious Disorders of the Skin:* **A,** *Impetigo contagiosa;* **B,** *Herpes zoster (shingles);* **C,** *Herpes simplex type 1;* **D,** *Tinea (ringworm);* **E,** *Scabies;* **F,** *Pediculosis (lice) (A, C, and E courtesy of Robert A. Silverman, MD, Clinical Associate Professor, Department of Pediatrics, Georgetown University; B and D courtesy of the Centers for Disease Control and Prevention, Atlanta, GA; F courtesy of Reed and Carnrick Pharmaceuticals)*

TABLE 43-4   INFECTIOUS DISORDERS OF THE SKIN

DISEASE	ORGANISM	CLINICAL MANIFESTATIONS	MANAGEMENT
Bacterial Infections			
Impetigo contagiosa	*Staphylococcus aureus*	Begins as a small vesicle; becomes a weeping lesion; forms a light brown crust. Usually on the face and upper trunk (Figure 43-13A). More common in children. More common in spring and fall. Poor hygiene coupled with warm weather facilitates the spread of the disease.	Cleanse the affected area at least 3 times a day. Apply an antibiotic ointment. Occasionally, systemic antibiotics are needed.
Carbuncle	*Staphylococcus aureus*	Begins as infected hair follicles in the dermis. Symptoms are redness, swelling, pain. Yellow cores of pus develop. Carbuncles usually occur on the nape of the neck and upper back. Obese or malnourished persons with poor hygiene as well as diabetics are most susceptible to carbuncles.	Warm, moist soaks may help "bring the boil to a head." Once the carbuncle ruptures or is incised and drained, pain subsides. Carbuncles tend to recur. The staphylococcus organism may be resistant to topical antibiotics. Systemic antibiotics may be needed.
Viral Infections			
Herpes zoster (shingles)	V-Z (varicella-zoster)	Clusters of small vesicles over the course of a peripheral sensory nerve. Two-thirds of clients have lesions just in the thoracic region. Lesions can occur over the trigeminal nerve, affecting the face, scalp, and eyes (Figure 43-13B). Crusts develop in several days. Symptoms are mild to severe pain, itching, fever, malaise. In older adults, pain can last for months or years. Persons who have not had chickenpox risk contracting the disease if they care for herpes zoster clients with open lesions. Persons who previously had chickenpox, but developed only partial immunity to it, may still be susceptible to herpes zoster.	Acyclovir (Zovirax) is given to clients in severe pain or to immunosuppressed clients. Analgesics help control the pain. Narcotic analgesics are prescribed for severe pain. Antipruritic topical medications decrease the itching.
Herpes simplex, type 1 and 2 (fever blisters, cold sores) Type 2 (genital)	*Herpes simplex virus*	Type 1—a cluster of vesicles on an erythematous base occurring most commonly at the corners of the mouth (Figure 43-13C) or at the edge of the nostrils. Type 2—lesions in the vagina or cervix of a woman or on the penis of a man. The lesions itch, burn, and frequently break open, forming a crust. Healing occurs in about 10 days.	Topical use of antiviral agents such as acyclovir decreases discomfort. Even with treatment, cold sores and fever blisters tend to recur, especially with fever, upper respiratory infections, and stress. Oral administration of acyclovir helps prevent recurrence of genital herpes.
Warts	Human papillomavirus	Seen as small, painless round papules on hands, face, and neck. On the bottom of the feet, warts grow inward from the pressure and are painful (plantar warts). Warts in the anogenital region itch. Genital warts increase the risk of cervical cancer.	No treatment is indicated for painless warts; they tend to disappear eventually. Plantar warts may be removed by cryosurgery or with locally applied chemicals such as nitric acid. Warts are not highly contagious from person to person but may be spread on the person's own body by rubbing or scratching. Genital warts are spread by sexual intercourse.

continues

TABLE 43-4   continued

DISEASE	ORGANISM	CLINICAL MANIFESTATIONS	MANAGEMENT
Fungal Infections			
Tinea (ringworm) Tinea capitis (ringworm of the scalp) Tinea corporis (ringworm of the body) Tinea cruris ("jock itch") Tinea pedis (athlete's foot)	*microscorim audouini*	Tinea is a superficial infection of the skin, called ringworm because of its circumscribed appearance, typically round, and reddened with slight scaling (Figure 43-13D). Lesions of tinea corporis have a pale center. Itching is common with tinea cruris. Itching and burning occur with tinea pedis. Tinea is spread easily. Jock itch and athlete's foot are more common among men than women.	Treat mild infections with a topical antifungal drug such as miconazole nitrate (Micatin) or tolnaftate (Aftate). Severe infections are treated with oral administration of griseofulvin micro-size (Grisactin).
Parasitic Infections			
Scabies	*Sarcoptes scabiei* (female itch mite)	The itch mite burrows under the skin, lays eggs, and deposits fecal material. Short, dark-red wavy lines may be seen on hands, wrists, elbows, axillary folds, nipples, waistline, and gluteal folds (Figure 43-13E). Pruritis is severe and can persist for up to 3 months after treatment. Scratching leads to secondary infection. Scabies is spread by prolonged contact and is frequently seen in several members of a family.	Apply the scabicide, lindane (Kwell), topically to the entire body at bedtime so that the medication remains on the skin 8 to 12 hours. Treat all family members even if they do not have symptoms. Wash all underclothing and bed and bath linens in hot water and dry in dryer. Change linens daily. Items that cannot be washed should be dry-cleaned.
Pediculosis (lice)	*Pediculus capitis* (head lice) *Pediculus corporis* (body lice) *Phthirus Pubis* (pubic lice)	Eggs, or nits, of pediculosis capitis attach themselves firmly to a hair shaft on the head or in a beard (Figure 43-13F). Nits have a gray, pearly appearance. The pubic louse resembles a tiny crab that attaches itself to pubic hair. Body lice live in the seams of clothing. The bite of the louse causes severe pruritis. Scratching leads to secondary infection.	Lindane (Kwell) is applied topically to the hair as a shampoo or to the body as a cream or lotion. Repeat the treatment again in 8 to 10 days. Wash or dry-clean clothing and linens. Disinfect combs and brushes. Vacuum carpets and furniture; then spray with a pediculicide.

attached to some of these conditions, so also note the client's mood.

Objective Data

A complete skin assessment is performed, describing the size, appearance, and distribution of all lesions, as well as any drainage present.

CRITICAL THINKING

Preventing Spread of Skin Infections

How can the spread of skin infections be prevented? Prepare a teaching plan for a client with a skin infection.

CLIENT TEACHING

Herpes Zoster

- Take the full course of prescribed medications.
- Use topical measures along with NSAIDs for pain management.
- Avoid persons who have not had chickenpox, especially pregnant women, so they do not get chickenpox.
- When dark crusts form over pustules, the client is no longer contagious.
- In older adults, pain may last for months or years.

Nursing diagnoses for a client with an infectious disorder of the skin may include the following:

Nursing Diagnoses	Planning/Goals	Nursing Interventions
*Impaired **S**kin Integrity* related to invasion of skin structures by pathogenic organisms	The client will regain skin integrity.	Wear gloves when caring for the client with skin lesions.
		Cleanse the skin thoroughly, but gently. In the case of bacterial infections or lesions with secondary infections, use an antibacterial soap. Gently remove crusts, scales, and traces of old medication before applying fresh creams or lotions. Administer prescribed medications; apply creams and lotions; then monitor their effectiveness.
		Explain what you are doing and why.
*Acute **P**ain,* related to itching, burning, and infection	The client will report less pain.	Instruct the client to keep the environmental temperature cool because warmth increases itching, also cleanse skin lesions with tepid water, not hot.
		Stress the importance of not scratching the lesions.
*Disturbed **B**ody Image* related to unsightly skin lesions and embarrassment	The client will verbalize a positive body image.	Encourage the client to ask questions and to talk about feelings.
		Provide positive reinforcement as the client learns to care for the skin lesions. When possible, suggest ways to camouflage the lesions or minimize their appearance.
		When there is no danger of spreading the infection, encourage the client to participate in social and work activities.

Evaluation Each goal must be evaluated to determine how it has been met by the client.

SAMPLE NURSING CARE PLAN

THE CLIENT WITH SCABIES

Emma Evans, 68, has had a skin rash for the past 2 weeks. The dark red lesions occur mainly on her hands, wrists, and elbows, around her nipples, at her waistline, and in her gluteal folds. The itching has become increasingly intense. She states that she has been scratching the lesions, sometimes until they are open and bleeding. Upon examination, some of the lesions are open with small amounts of serosanguineous drainage. Other lesions are scabbed. She lives with her daughter and two teenaged granddaughters. Because the lesions were getting steadily worse, her daughter finally convinced her to seek medical attention. She was horrified when the doctor told her that she had scabies. She had always associated "the itch" with "dirty people who didn't take care of themselves."

Nursing Diagnosis 1 *Impaired **S**kin Integrity* related to scratching scabies lesions as evidenced by open lesions draining serosanguineous fluid, scabbed lesions, and client statements of scratching the lesions until they bleed

Nursing Outcomes Classification (NOC)
Tissue Integrity: Skin & Mucous Membranes
Self-Care: Hygiene

Nursing Interventions Classification (NIC)
Skin Care: Topical Treatments
Skin Surveillance

continues

SAMPLE NURSING CARE PLAN

PLANNING/GOALS	NURSING INTERVENTIONS	RATIONALE
Mrs. Evans will follow the prescribed treatment protocol to promote healing of skin lesions and regain skin integrity.	Instruct Mrs. Evans to cleanse lesions carefully using an antibacterial soap and tepid water. The lesions can be cleaned 1 to 3 times daily.	Reduces the number of microorganisms present and decreases the risk of infection. Tepid water does not intensify itching as hot water does.
	Teach Mrs. Evans to apply antipruritic lotions as prescribed by the doctor after cleansing the skin.	Lotions applied just after bathing help to retain skin moisture.
	Instruct Mrs. Evans to keep fingernails short with smooth edges.	Less likely to break the skin if the client scratches.
	Teach Mrs. Evans to press itching lesions, and not to scratch them.	Stimulates nerve endings and reduces the sensation of itching. Prevents breaks in the skin, which would be portals of entry for microorganisms.
	Explain that itching can persist up to 3 months following treatment with the scabicide but persistent itching does not mean that treatment was ineffective.	Skin reaction to the toxins and secretions of the itch mite can persist for up to 3 months after the itch mites are killed by the scabicide.
	Keep room temperature between 68° and 72°F and humidity constant at 30% to 35%.	Itching is intensified in hot, humid environments.

EVALUATION   Mrs. Evans's lesions are still red, but none are open and draining. Some lesions are still scabbed. No new open lesions have developed. Mrs. Evans states that the recommended measures "help," but that the itching is still "pretty bad." Goal of promoting healing of skin lesions is being met. Encourage Mrs. Evans to continue outlined protocols. Reassure her that itching will gradually subside as healing progresses.

Nursing Diagnosis 2 *Deficient **K**nowledge (infection control measures),* related to lack of familiarity with treatment and prevention protocols as evidenced by client's inability to recognize the skin lesions as infectious and by statements about scabies happening only to people with poor hygiene

Nursing Outcomes Classification (NOC)	**Nursing Interventions Classification (NIC)**
Knowledge: Infection Control	*Teaching: Disease Process*
	Teaching: Prescribed Medication

PLANNING/GOALS	NURSING INTERVENTIONS	RATIONALE
Mrs. Evans will apply the scabicide correctly and state ways to avoid spreading infection to others.	Assess Mrs. Evans's knowledge of scabies, its treatment regimen and infection control measures. Ask specific questions.	Provides a frame of reference for the client, helping her relate new information and integrate it into her behavior.
	Explain that scabies is transmitted by skin-to-skin contact or by contact with articles freshly contaminated by infected persons and affects persons of all social, economic, and age levels.	Teaching that does not "talk down" to the client communicates respect.

continues

SAMPLE NURSING CARE PLAN

Stress the importance of following treatment protocol exactly. Review salient points such as (1) Shower before applying the scabicide; (2) apply the scabicide to the entire body surface, including skin without scabies lesions; and (3) apply the scabicide at bedtime so that the medication remains on the skin 8 to 12 hours.	Failure to apply the scabicide as directed and/or failure to leave the lotion on the skin for the prescribed length of time will not kill the itch mite.
Give Mrs. Evans step-by-step written instructions.	Enhances compliance with the treatment regimen.
Instruct Mrs. Evans to wash hands under warm running water with plenty of soap (preferably an antibacterial soap) for at least 10 seconds after touching lesions and clean carefully under fingernails while washing hands.	Thorough handwashing is the single most effective means of preventing the spread of infection. Large numbers of bacteria reside under the fingernails.
Advise to not share washcloths, towels, clothing, pillows, or bed linens with other family members.	Disease-causing microorganisms can be spread to well individuals indirectly when their skin comes into contact with contaminated items.
Instruct to wash underclothing and bed and bath linens in detergent and hot water and dry outside in sunlight or in a dryer on the hot setting.	Soap reduces surface tension. When fat or protein substances that shield organisms are broken down, the organisms are exposed to the killing effects of heat. Prolonged exposure to heat or ultraviolet rays from direct sunlight kills microorganisms.
Advise to shower daily, use an antibacterial soap, rinse thoroughly, and dry carefully, especially in skin folds and between toes, using a towel and washcloth only once before laundering it.	Reduces the number of microorganisms on the skin. Moisture encourages the growth of microorganisms. Laundering the towel and washcloth after only one use prevents the indirect transfer of the itch mite.
Assess lesions daily for signs of healing. Report any signs and symptoms of infection in secondary lesions such as redness, swelling, pain, drainage (describe characteristics of the drainage) to the physician or clinic.	Increases the probability of effective treatment with fewer complications.
Teach Mrs. Evans and family members the early signs and symptoms of scabies infection, such as any reddened papules with wavy, threadlike lines visible on the skin around the papules and severe itching, especially at night.	Early recognition and treatment of scabies can minimize the severity of the infection.
Instruct them to assess their skin daily.	A daily examination allows treatment to begin as soon as the problem is identified.

continues

SAMPLE NURSING CARE PLAN

EVALUATION Mrs. Evans and her family did apply the scabicide as prescribed. The client can describe how scabies are transmitted, but continues to express fear that she will give "this awful thing to somebody." Goal of correctly applying scabicide met. Although Mrs. Evans can state how scabies are transmitted, she still has doubts; hence, the goal of stating ways to avoid spreading the infection to others has only been partially met. Reinforce that even though red skin lesions are still visible, the itch mites were killed by treatment and cannot be transmitted to others even if the client does shake hands, hug, or touch someone else.

Nursing Diagnosis 3 *Disturbed **B**ody Image* related to unsightly lesions and embarrassment as evidenced by distribution of lesions on exposed skin areas and client statements of being horrified about the diagnosis and associating scabies with "dirty people"

Nursing Outcomes Classification (NOC)
Body Image

Nursing Interventions Classification (NIC)
Anxiety Reduction
Mutual Goal Setting

PLANNING/GOALS	NURSING INTERVENTIONS	RATIONALE
1. Mrs. Evans will assume self-care of lesions.	Explain that by using the scabicide, lindane (Kwell), as directed and by following measures to prevent secondary infection of the scabies lesions, she can expect complete healing of the lesions without any visible scars within a few weeks.	Reassurance that scabies can be cured enhances the client's self-image.
2. Mrs. Evans will maintain relationships with family and friends.	Encourage Mrs. Evans to express her feelings about herself and her opinions about scabies.	Brings feelings and opinions out into the open where they can be dealt with appropriately.
	Provide information to correct any misconceptions she might have.	Accurate information dispels misconceptions.
	Encourage Mrs. Evans to verbalize the perceptions she has about her family's and friends' feelings about persons with scabies.	A person perceiving derogatory opinions of her is likely to socially isolate herself from them.
	Be alert to verbal and nonverbal messages.	Nonverbal messages give insight into the client's real feelings. Identifying and discussing feelings can lead to behavioral changes.
	Reassure her that she will not infect friends and family members by sitting beside them or being in the same room with them for prolonged periods.	The client will be unlikely to avoid friends or make disparaging remarks about herself when she realizes that she is not a danger to them.
	Share with Mrs. Evans that wearing long-sleeved cotton blouses or dresses will hide most of the visible lesions.	Makes the client less self-conscious and embarrassed. Cotton fabric allows good air circulation. Cool skin itches less.

EVALUATION The client has assumed self-care responsibilities. She does interact with her family but emphasizes that she "doesn't want to get too close to them until these things are completely gone." She has refused to go to church, social gatherings, or activities outside of the house.

Goal has been partially met in that the client does follow proper procedures when caring for her skin lesions, but goal has not been met in so far as maintaining relationships is concerned. Encourage the client to talk about her feelings, particularly feelings of embarrassment. Point out to her the evidence that her lesions are healing. Emphasize that symptoms of intense itching, worsening of present skin lesions, and signs of more skin lesions would be present if the itch mites were alive and still spreading. Encourage her to go on at least 1 outing with her family during the coming week. Reevaluate in 1 week.

INFLAMMATORY DISORDERS OF THE SKIN

Included in this category are dermatitis and psoriasis.

DERMATITIS

By definition, dermatitis is an inflammatory condition of the skin. In current usage, eczema has almost become synonymous with dermatitis, although eczema tends to be used most often to refer to chronic forms of dermatitis. Most clients with dermatitis are treated as outpatients. Patch testing may identify a specific allergen that is causing the dermatitis. Avoiding the allergenic substance may prevent future dermatitis. In some cases, application of a topical corticosteroid is all that is needed. Other types of this inflammatory disorder include contact dermatitis and exfoliative dermatitis.

ECZEMA

Eczema is an atopic dermatitis often associated with allergic rhinitis and asthma. It is a chronic superficial inflammation that evolves into pruritic, red, weeping, crusted lesions (Estes, 2002). See Figure 43-14. Mostly infants get eczema, but older children and adults may have it. The common allergens are chocolate, orange juice, wheat, and eggs. Heredity is a major factor. Elimination of dietary substances is used to identify the client's allergen(s). Tiny cracks in the skin allow body fluid to escape, so skin hydration is the major treatment.

Nursing Management

Nursing management is directed toward promoting healing, providing comfort, preventing infection, and

Figure 43-14 *Eczema (Courtesy of the Centers for Disease Control and Prevention, Atlanta, GA)*

fostering a positive attitude to help the client cope with an altered body image. Nursing diagnoses may include *Impaired Skin Integrity; Risk for Infection; Acute Pain;* and *Disturbed Body Image.*

Affected areas are soaked in warm water for 15 to 20 minutes and then an occlusive ointment is applied, as directed, to retain the water. Following a bath or shower, pat the skin dry and immediately apply the occlusive ointment. Wet dressings may be ordered to maximize skin hydration. Moisturizing lotions such as Curel or Lubriderm may be used as the lesions heal. Client teaching is focused on identifying and avoiding substances that cause dermatitis, care for the lesions, how to prevent infection, and how to cope with the conditions.

CONTACT DERMATITIS

In contact dermatitis the skin reacts to external irritants such as (1) allergens like cosmetics, (2) harsh chemical substances like detergents or insecticides, (3) metals such as nickel, (4) mechanical irritation from wool or glass fibers, and (5) body substances like urine or feces. Symptoms include pruritus, burning, and erythema. Often, a maculopapular rash or a combination of papules and vesicles develops. Scratching the lesions may spread the dermatitis as well as lead to secondary infections of the skin (Figure 43-15).

Treatment of symptoms may include a corticosteroid ointment and an oral antihistamine such as diphenhydramine hydrochloride (Benadryl).

Nursing Management

Assist the client in identifying the causative allergen. Use aseptic technique when caring for open lesions.

Figure 43-15 *Allergic Contact Dermatitis from Poison Oak: Note Linear Pattern to Lesions (Courtesy of the Centers for Disease Control and Prevention, Atlanta, GA)*

Apply dressings wet with Burow's solution as ordered (Weaver, 1999). Advise the client that a cool, moist environment reduces pruritis.

DERMATITIS VENENATA AND MEDICAMENTOSA

Dermatitis venenata is a specific type of contact dermatitis when the allergen is from a plant (e.g., poison ivy, poison oak). The first exposure sensitizes the client's body to form antigens against the allergen. Later exposures lead to inflammation, edema, and vesicle formation.

Dermatitis medicamentosa is a skin reaction to a medication (e.g., penicillin, codeine). Symptoms range from mild to severe erythema and vesicle formation. Respiratory distress may occur.

Nursing Management

For dermatitis venenata, wash the affected area immediately. Calamine lotion relieves the pruritis.

For dermatitis medicamentosa, notify the physician immediately so the medication can be discontinued. Advise the client to wear a Medic Alert bracelet or necklace and to notify all health care members of the allergy.

EXFOLIATIVE DERMATITIS

In exfoliative dermatitis, inflammation of the skin gradually worsens. Localized symptoms include erythema, severe pruritus, extensive scaling, and skin sloughing. Exfoliative dermatitis affects the entire body, not just the skin. Systemic symptoms include chills, fever, and malaise. With the loss of large areas of skin surface, the individual has difficulty maintaining body temperature, loses body fluids and electrolytes, and is susceptible to infection.

In most cases, the cause of exfoliative dermatitis is unknown. Severe reactions to drugs such as penicillin may sometimes cause exfoliative dermatitis. It may also be associated with other types of dermatitis or lymphoma. Exfoliative dermatitis can be fatal, primarily because of overwhelming systemic infections and/or massive loss of body fluids and electrolytes.

Nursing Management

When clients are hospitalized with exfoliative dermatitis, management is directed toward maintaining fluid balance, preventing infection, decreasing inflammation, and

promoting comfort. The client requires intravenous fluids to maintain the volume of circulating fluid, corticosteroids to decrease inflammation, and antibiotics to treat infection. Medicated baths, topical steroids, and mild analgesics may be prescribed to ease the pruritus.

PSORIASIS

Psoriasis, a chronic, inflammatory, noninfectious disease of the skin, affects about 5.5 million people in the United States, especially young adults. The parts of the body most commonly affected are the scalp, elbows, palms, knees, lower back, and soles of the feet (NIAMS, 2002) (Figure 43-16). The exact cause of psoriasis is unknown, although a genetic component may be involved. Emotional stress, infections, trauma, and seasonal and hormonal changes trigger exacerbations of psoriasis. It may improve for a while only to recur. This process of subsiding and recurring continues throughout the client's life. Psoriasis is not curable. In psoriasis the process of keratinization has gone awry. Instead of producing cells that provide a natural barrier against harmful substances and microorganisms, abnormal keratinization causes large, red patches covered with thick silvery scales in the outermost layer of the epidermis (Seeley et al., 2002). If these scales are scraped away, bleeding occurs. When fingernails are affected, pitting and yellow discoloration is seen.

Medical–Surgical Management

Medical

Treatment is directed toward slowing down the rate of cell formation in the epidermis or toward altering the ab-

Figure 43-16 *Psoriasis (Courtesy of Robert A. Silverman, MD, Clinical Associate Professor, Department of Pediatrics, Georgetown University)*

LIFE CYCLE CONSIDERATIONS

Exfoliative Dermatitis
Older adults have a greater risk of fatal complications from exfoliative dermatitis. As body systems age, they are less able to respond quickly and effectively to the stress of illness.

normal process of keratinization. Treatment regimens can be effective in reducing the scaling and itching. The client must recognize that psoriasis can only be controlled, not cured. Furthermore, the client must be committed to lifetime therapy.

Pharmacological

Keratolytic agents such as salicylic acid preparations and coal tar preparations are applied topically to the lesions. Corticosteroids may also be used to reduce inflammation. Ultraviolet light and methotrexate (Mexate) inhibit DNA synthesis in the epidermal cells, thus slowing the rate of cell division and the process of abnormal keratinization. Because of its toxicity to the liver, methotrexate is used only in severe cases of psoriasis that do not respond to any other form of treatment. The Goeckerman regimen, which combines the use of coal tar and ultraviolet light, is one of the oldest treatments available but is effective and is still widely used (Weaver, 1999).

Photochemotherapy is used for severe psoriasis. Photochemotherapy (psorafen ultraviolet A-range, or PUVA) combines the use of methoxsalen (Oxsoralen) with ultraviolet A light waves. The dose of Oxsoralen is based on body weight and must be taken 2 hours before exposure to ultraviolet A light waves. Oxsoralen is a photosensitizing agent that reacts with ultraviolet A light waves to markedly reduce DNA synthesis, thereby slowing cell division in psoriasis lesions and relieving symptoms. Although the treatment is generally effective, the results are not seen immediately (Hill, 1998).

Etretinate (Tegison), a compound related to retinoic acid vitamin A, is used in severe psoriasis not amenable to other therapies. It may be used alone or in combination with ultraviolet A light waves. Etretinate has numerous adverse effects, including liver damage and severe birth defects. The client must be monitored closely. Women of childbearing age must use effective contraception during treatment and for at least 1 month after treatment.

Nursing Management

Assist the client to understand and comply with the treatment. Teach the client proper hand hygiene. Listen to the client's feelings and frustrations.

NURSING PROCESS

Assessment

Subjective Data

Psoriasis lesions are generally very visible and likely to make the client feel self-conscious and uncomfortable. Many clients tend to suffer self-esteem and body image disturbances, and sometimes depression, because psoriasis requires lifelong treatment. The treatment can be time-consuming, bothersome, and, from the client's point of view, not completely effective. Encourage the client to verbalize feelings. Ask about itching, burning, and discomfort, as well as the client's mood.

Objective Data

Check the skin carefully, noting the distribution, size, and appearance of lesions. Note signs of infection such as redness, swelling, pain, or drainage.

Nursing diagnoses for a client with psoriasis may include the following:

Nursing Diagnoses	Planning/Goals	Nursing Interventions
Deficient Knowledge related to psoriasis and its treatment	The client will discuss condition and adhere to treatment.	Help the client gain an understanding of psoriasis and comply with the treatment regimen. Support and encourage the client. Explain the purpose of each medication.
Risk for Infection related to open lesions	The client will not get an infection.	Teach the client how to prevent infections by proper hand hygiene and not scratching the lesions.
Disturbed Body Image related to scaly lesions	The client will identify positive attributes about self.	Listen actively and encourage the client to express feelings and frustrations. Reinforce positive behavior.
Situational Low Self-Esteem related to appearance	The client will demonstrate behaviors that promote self-esteem.	Guide the client in identifying effective coping techniques. Help the client focus on personal attributes that contribute to effective functioning and a positive self-image. Encourage work and social interactions.

Evaluation Each goal must be evaluated to determine how it has been met by the client.

ULCERS

The two most common types of ulcers of the skin are venous ulcers and pressure ulcers.

VENOUS ULCERS

Poor venous circulation, especially in lower extremities, can lead to a condition known as stasis dermatitis (Figure 43-17). The skin changes in texture, turgor, and color. The skin develops a brownish discoloration and a brawny induration—that is, skin in the affected area becomes dry and looks rough; subcutaneous tissue atrophies; and it loses its usual resiliency and feels hard to the touch. Body hair is lost in this area. Pruritus is common. Scratching or small injuries can lead to ulcer formation because of the poor circulation.

Venous ulcers begin as small, tender, inflamed areas above the ankle. Any slight trauma to the area causes an open area that develops into an ulcer. Some edema surrounds the ulcer, which can easily become infected, most often with staphylococcus or streptococcus. Healing is very slow. In an effort to decrease venous congestion and improve circulation, varicose veins, if present, may be removed. Ulcers that do not heal may require surgery. If diagnostic testing reveals adequate circulation, skin grafting will result in the healing of large venous ulcers. In cases that do not respond to treatment, the affected leg has to be amputated.

Figure 43-17 *Venous Stasis Ulcer (Courtesy of Carrington Laboratories, Inc., Irving, TX)*

Medical–Surgical Management

Medical

Vacuum-assisted closure (VAC) therapy may be used for chronic open wounds such as venous ulcers. Applying negative pressure to the wound is painless for the client. The negative pressure stretches or distorts the cells, causing the epithelial cells to multiply rapidly and form granulation tissue. As the vacuum pulls fluid from the surrounding tissues, reducing edema that compressed blood vessels, blood flow to the wound is improved.

Elevation and compression are the keys to reducing edema of the leg and improving blood return to the heart. This reduces venous hypertension and helps the venous ulcer heal. The legs should be elevated 7 inches above the heart at night and for several hours during the day. Many types of compression therapy products are available, including Unna's boot, elastic wraps, compression stockings, compression pumps, and sustained graduated compression using an elastic, multilayered bandage system (Hess, 2001b).

Pharmacological

For healing to occur, the ulcer must have adequate circulation and be free of infection and necrotic tissue. Usually, antibiotics are prescribed. Enzyme preparations such as fibrinolysin and dexsoxyribonucleas (ELASE) or wet-to-dry dressings may be used to debride the ulcer. Normal saline is the solution most often used in wet-to-dry dressings because it is not irritating to healthy tissue.

Diet

A diet high in protein and vitamin C is needed for tissue regeneration. If the client is anemic, lean meats, whole grains, and green, leafy vegetables should be encouraged.

Nursing Management

Maintain peripheral tissue perfusion by encouraging the client to elevate legs when sitting, wear support hose, and not cross legs. Promote comfort by encouraging the client to keep legs elevated, cleansing the venous ulcer as prescribed, and keeping the area covered as ordered. Promote wound healing by reviewing the client's diet and encouraging foods high in iron, protein, and vitamin C.

NURSING PROCESS

Assessment

Subjective Data

Ask the client to describe any pain and rate its severity on a scale of 1 to 10. Note whether the pain is worse with the leg in a dependent position or when the client is standing. Document measures used to relieve the pain. Note if the skin around the ulcer itches, the length of time the client had the ulcer before seeking care, and any palliative measures tried.

Objective Data

Describe the size and location of the ulcer, as well as the appearance of the ulcer and surrounding skin. Observe for necrotic tissue inside the ulcer. It may be yellow and look like thin strands of fibers. The base of the ulcer may have a dark red, "beefy" appearance. Document the color and appearance of the extremity in both a de-pendent and an elevated position as well as any drainage, including its odor and characteristics. Edema may be present, and the lower extremity may appear swollen. Hardened and indurated tissue may surround the ulcer. Tissue farther away from the ulcer may "pit" with firm pressure. Assess peripheral pulses.

Nursing diagnoses for a client with a venous ulcer may include the following:

Nursing Diagnoses	Planning/Goals	Nursing Interventions
Ineffective Tissue Perfusion (Peripheral) related to edema and pooling of venous blood	Client will follow prescribed measures to improve peripheral circulation.	Encourage the client to elevate legs while sitting or when in bed and to avoid standing for more than a few minutes at a time. Advise client to wear elastic stockings when walking and that new stockings should be purchased every few months because continual wear and laundering tend to decrease the elasticity of the stockings. Instruct not to wear garters, tight girdles, or sit with legs crossed. Note the client's hemoglobin level since anemic clients will have difficulty meeting tissue demands for oxygen.
Chronic Pain related to exposed sensory nerve endings and edema	Client will report decreased pain after implementing recommended measures.	Encourage client to elevate legs. Cleanse ulcer with prescribed solutions. Keep ulcer covered with prescribed medications and dressings.
Risk for Infection related to poorly nourished tissue in and around the ulcer and to nonintact skin	Client will describe and implement measures to minimize the risk of infection.	Assess the ulcer daily for signs of healing. Assess the client's ability to care for the ulcer physically and financially. Review diet with the client and instruct in food choices as needed. Encourage foods high in iron such as fortified cereal, lean meats, whole grains, and leafy green vegetables.

Evaluation Each goal must be evaluated to determine how it has been met by the client.

PRESSURE ULCERS

Pressure ulcers, also known as bedsores or decubitus ulcers, are localized areas of tissue necrosis that tend to develop when soft tissue is compressed between a bony prominence and an external surface such as a mattress or chair seat for a prolonged period. Pressure ulcers are caused by **ischemia,** a local and temporary decrease in blood supply, and commonly occur in areas subject to high pressure from body weight on bony prominences.

Physiology of Pressure Ulcers

A pressure ulcer occurs when pressure on the skin is sufficient to cause collapse of blood vessels in the area. Ischemia and redness can occur at the site within 1 hour; when pressure continues for more than 2 hours, necrosis (tissue death) may occur in the involved area. Bony prominences such as the occipital skull, pinna of ears, sacrum, ischial tuberosities, trochanter area of hips, ankles, and heels are the areas most likely to develop a pressure ulcer.

Other forces acting in conjunction with pressure contribute to pressure ulcer formation. **Shearing** is the force exerted against the skin by movement or repositioning. The skin and subcutaneous tissue tend to adhere to the bed surface and remain stationary while deeper underlying tissues pull away and slide in the direction of movement. This action results in stretching and tearing of blood vessels, reduced blood flow, and necrosis.

Friction is the force of two surfaces moving across one another. When a client moves or is pulled up in bed, rubbing of the skin against the sheets creates friction. Friction can remove the superficial layers of the skin, making it more prone to breakdown.

The reduction of blood flow causes **blanching** (white color) of the skin when pressure is applied. When pressure is relieved, the skin takes on a brighter color (reactive hyperemia) because of vasodilation, the body's normal compensatory response to the absence of blood flow. If this area blanches with fingertip pressure or if the redness disappears within an hour, no tissue

Stage 1   Stage 2

Stage 3   Stage 4

Figure 43-18 *Pressure Ulcers (Courtesy of Emory University Hospital, Atlanta, GA)*

damage is anticipated. If, however, the redness persists and no blanching occurs, then tissue damage is present.

Pressure ulcers are staged to classify the degree of tissue damage (Figure 43-18). The National Pressure Ulcer Advisory Panel (NPUAP) (U.S. Department of Health and Human Services [USDHHS], 1992) recommends the following staging system:

- *Stage I:* Nonblanchable erythema of intact skin; the heralding lesion of skin ulceration.
- *Stage II:* Partial-thickness skin loss involving epidermis, dermis, or both. The ulcer is superficial and presents clinically as an abrasion, blister, or shallow crater.
- *Stage III:* Full-thickness skin loss involving damage or necrosis of subcutaneous tissue that may extend down to, but not through, underlying fascia. The ulcer presents clinically as a deep crater with or without undermining of adjacent tissue.
- *Stage IV:* Full-thickness skin loss with extensive destruction, tissue necrosis, or damage to muscle, bone, or supporting structures. Undermining and sinus tracts may also be associated with stage IV pressure ulcers.

The NPUAP (1999) has developed an assessment tool, Pressure Ulcer Scale for Healing (PUSH Tool). It uses three parameters: the surface area of the wound, amount of exudate, and type of tissue present in the wound. The scores for each parameter are added together and plotted to show wound healing or worsening. This PUSH Tool is available on the Internet.

The Braden Scale for Predicting Pressure Sore Risk is a research-based tool that estimates risk level for pressure ulcers and predicts those clients who are most likely to develop pressure ulcers. It can be found on the Internet.

Risk Factors for Pressure Ulcers

Pressure ulcers can be prevented if at-risk individuals are identified and the specific factors placing them at risk are reduced or eliminated. More than 1 million clients

each year have pressure ulcers, and most of these clients are in their 70s and 80s (National Decubitus Foundation, 2002). Both intrinsic and extrinsic factors may influence tissue response to pressure. Intrinsic factors include impaired immobility, incontinence, nutritional status, and altered level of consciousness. Extrinsic factors include pressure, shearing, friction, and moisture. Any condition that decreases tissue perfusion, such as edema, anemia, or atherosclerosis, also increases the risk. Other factors are decreased mental status, diminished sensation, and age-related changes.

Individuals should be assessed for pressure ulcer risk on admission to acute care hospitals and at least every 48 hours, long-term care facilities at least weekly, and home health care at every RN visit (Ayello & Braden, 2001).

Medical–Surgical Management

Medical

Follow sterile technique in the care of all pressure ulcers to prevent secondary infection. Cleanse the wound with normal saline or a noncytotoxic wound cleaner at each dressing change. Such agents as povodine-iodine, iodophor, sodium hypochlorite, hydrogen peroxide, or acetic acid should not be used because they can damage the cells. A 35-mL syringe with a 19-gauge needle or angiocatheter provides enough pressure to cleanse the wound and enhance wound healing without causing trauma to the tissue.

Debridement must be done as needed. Topical enzyme agents may be applied or a mechanical method of wet-to-dry dressings, or hydrotherapy, may be used. Refer to the discussion of VAC therapy in the section on venous ulcers; this therapy can also be used for pressure ulcers.

There are many commercial products available for treatment and dressing of pressure ulcers. Whichever products the physician prescribes, everyone should be taught how to use them and have a commitment to use them properly.

Support Surfaces and Beds A variety of support surfaces and beds are available to support the entire body and evenly distribute pressure. These devices help reduce pressure, but they are no substitute for frequent positioning. There is no evidence that any one support surface works consistently better than any other (USD-HHS, 1992).

In addition to pressure reduction or relief, many support surfaces reduce shear and friction and control moisture. Pressure-reducing support surfaces include overlays filled with foam, gel, or water.

- *Egg-crate mattress:* The egg-crate mattress is composed of thick foam with a unique, egg-crate design. The purposes of the egg-crate mattress include minimizing pressure and shearing force. The open design of the mattress surface allows air to circulate to dissipate heat and moisture. Egg-crate foam is also used as wheelchair cushions, heel-ankle protectors, wrist restraint cushioning pads, and ulnar protectors.
- *Air-filled mattresses:* The air-filled mattress is placed over the mattress of the hospital bed for weight redistribution. Varieties of air-filled mattresses include some with a pump and alternating bands of inflation

Figure 43-20 *Kin Air Bed*

Figure 43-19 *Clinitron® Air-Fluidized Therapy Unit Model C11 (Courtesy of Hill-Rom, Batesville, IN)*

Figure 43-21 *Avoiding Pressure Points with the 30-Degree Lateral Position*

and deflation and some that are inflated continuously with air. Mattresses are covered with a sheet for client comfort. These types of mattresses are frequently used in long-term care situations.

- *Clinitron® bed:* A Clinitron® bed (Figure 43-19) is a specialized bed that has a mattress filled with small glass sand particles. Moisture from urine, stool, or drainage flows through the mattress, preventing moisture exposure to the skin. Because warm air is circulating through the mattress, the accumulation of moisture next to the skin is inhibited. The mattress aids in positioning the client because it is constructed to mold against the client's body.
- *Kin Air bed:* A Kin Air bed, another type of specialized bed, has a mattress of air-inflated pillows divided in sections for the head, back, seat, legs, and feet. The pressure can be adjusted in each of the sections for the client's specific needs. Air flows from the mattress to eliminate moisture. The bed frame can be adjusted for various positions such as Fowler's, Trendelenburg, prone, or supine. A trapeze can be connected to the bed frame (Figure 43-20).
- *Roto Kinetic bed:* A Roto Kinetic bed is a specialized bed that rocks slowly from side to side, thus relieving pressure areas and countering the effects of immobility. The client is placed on the mattress, with dividers between the legs and dividers between the trunk and arms. Clients can be maintained in traction while on this bed.

Regardless of the type of surface or bed on which the client is lying, the 30-degree side-lying position prevents pressure on the sacrum and trochanters. This position is illustrated in Figure 43-21.

PROFESSIONAL TIP

Preventing Pressure Ulcers
- Establish written repositioning/turning schedule for clients, including those on pressure-reducing support surfaces.
- Use 30-degree position when side-lying position is used.
- Prevent direct contact between bony prominences by using pillows and foam wedges.
- Use a lifting sheet.
- Encourage clients in wheelchairs to shift their weight every 15 minutes.
- Raise heels off the bed with pillow lengthwise to support legs.
- Use knee gatch when head of bed is elevated.
- Keep head of bed elevated to less than 30 degrees except at mealtimes.
- Limit sitting time to 1 hour at a time whether in bed, chair, or wheelchair.
- Use proper positioning, transferring, and turning techniques.
- Inspect skin at least once a day.
- Use mild cleansing agent, but avoid hot water for bathing.
- Avoid massage over bony prominences.
- Use moisturizer on skin.
- Use protective barrier on skin if client is incontinent.
- Cleanse skin at time of soiling and at routine intervals.

Surgical

Occasionally, surgical debridement may be necessary.

Pharmacological

Vitamin and mineral supplements may be ordered. Antibiotics may also be ordered.

Diet

Eating a well-balanced diet should be encouraged, including 2 half-cup servings of orange juice or other juice high in vitamin C and 6 ounces of a high-protein drink.

Activity

Active ROM exercises should be performed, if possible. If not, passive ROM exercises should be performed with the client several times a day.

Nursing Management

Assess skin several times a day. Keep linens clean, dry, and free from wrinkles. Provide daily bath and skin care when the client is incontinent of bowel or bladder. Encourage adequate fluid intake, a well-balanced diet, and active or passive ROM exercises. Turn client at least every 2 hours. Position client on unaffected areas and protect skin as ordered. Monitor vital signs, especially temperature.

NURSING PROCESS

Assessment

Subjective Data

Statements such as, "I'm tired of lying on my side"; "I wish I could move more"; or "my hips (back, heels, and so on) are sore" may be expressed.

Objective Data

Symptoms may include any of the risk factors already mentioned; shiny, erythematous area; small blisters or erosions or ulcerations. Check for reddened areas and blanching of those areas.

Nursing diagnoses for a client at risk for pressure ulcers or who has a pressure ulcer may include the following:

Nursing Diagnoses	Planning/Goals	Nursing Interventions
Risk for Impaired Skin Integrity related to immobility	The client will maintain skin integrity.	Assess skin 3 times a day for pressure areas.
		Provide daily bath and skin care as needed for incontinence of urine or stool. Use mild cleansing agents with warm water, moisturizing lotion and minimize exposure to cold and low humidity.
		Avoid massage over bony prominences.
		Keep bed linen clean, dry, and free from wrinkles.
		Encourage adequate fluid intake and a well-balanced diet, including 2 half-cup servings of orange juice or other juice high in vitamin C and 6 ounces of a high-protein drink.
		Encourage active ROM exercises or provide passive ROM exercises.
		Turn and reposition client at least every 2 hours. If reddened area does not blanch when you press it, turn the client more often.
		Use the 30-degree lateral position to avoid pressure on the sacrum and trochanters.
		Use pressure-reducing surfaces. Do not use donut-shaped cushions; they put pressure around the pressure ulcer.
Impaired Skin Integrity related to pressure ulcer formation	The client will show healing of pressure ulcer.	Assess skin daily, identifying the stage of pressure ulcer development (size, color, odor, and exudate).
		Continue all preventive nursing interventions.
		Position client on unaffected areas. Protect skin surface and affected area as per facility protocol or as ordered.
		Monitor temperature. Administer antibiotics as ordered.

continues

Nursing Diagnoses	Planning/Goals	Nursing Interventions
Disturbed Body Image related to trauma or injury (pressure ulcer)	The client will make a positive statement about body image.	Encourage client to discuss meaning of pressure ulcer to the client. Provide information as requested by client.
Anxiety related to threat to or change in health status (pressure ulcer)	The client will discuss concerns about pressure ulcer with caregivers.	Schedule time to be with client, other than care times. Encourage client to discuss fears and concerns. Provide information as requested by client.

Evaluation Each goal must be evaluated to determine how it has been met by the client.

ALOPECIA

Alopecia, which is partial or complete baldness or loss of hair, can be caused by illness, malnutrition, effects of certain drugs such as those used in cancer therapy, hormonal imbalances, or diseases that affect the scalp.

There are many types of alopecia, ranging from head or beard hair loss to loss of all hair over the entire body. Treatment depends on the cause. Hair transplants may be performed on the head, but this is very expensive. In some clients, minoxidil (Rogaine) can promote hair growth, but hair growth stops when the drug is stopped. This is also very expensive.

CASE STUDY

Maude Murphy, age 68, noticed that the skin on the outside of her left lower leg just above the ankle was changing in color and texture. The skin felt rigid and did not move as easily as skin on the upper part of her leg did. Itching was becoming a problem. Inadvertently, she would scratch the area, sometimes causing small excoriations. One day she bumped her leg against the rough edge of the outside steps as she was going into the house. The cut was only an inch long and was not very deep. Over the next few weeks, she noticed that instead of healing, it was getting bigger and was becoming quite painful. The skin around the wound was red and swollen. The yellow drainage coming from the wound had a bad smell. She had never had this kind of problem before. She did have varicose veins in that leg, and while she knew that she was uncomfortable if she was standing for long periods, she did not think the problem was serious. When she went to the doctor, he diagnosed a venous stasis ulcer and cultured the drainage. He ordered the following treatment:

1. Cefaclor (Ceclor) 500 mg p.o. every 8 hours for 2 weeks (culture of the wound identified *Staphylococcus aureus*)
2. Wet-to-dry dressings with normal saline solution. Change every 8 hours.
3. Bed rest with left leg elevated. May have bathroom privileges and be up for meals.

The doctor explained that he would be ordering an Unna's boot after the wound was debrided and the infection controlled so that she could be ambulatory, but that even after the Unna's boot was applied, he would want her to have rest periods during the day with her leg elevated. Mrs. Murphy thought she could learn to change the dressings, but she expressed doubt that she could stay in bed most of the time. She was used to being up and active and getting her work done each day.

The following questions will guide your development of a nursing care plan for the case study.

1. List the clinical manifestations of a venous stasis ulcer.
2. What is the usual medical treatment?
3. List the subjective and objective assessment data that the nurse should obtain from Maude Murphy.
4. Write two to four individualized nursing diagnoses to address these problems.
5. What will be the goals (expected outcomes) of nursing treatment?
6. List appropriate nursing actions for each diagnosis. Include basic nursing care measures. Be specific about client education needs. Address nutrition and pharmacologic implications. Give a rationale for each action.
7. Describe how to evaluate goal achievement for Maude Murphy.

Summary

- Maintaining intact skin and mucous membranes to protect internal body structures from harmful substances and from invasion by microorganisms is an important independent nursing responsibility.
- Burns are devastating, traumatic injuries that can often be prevented.
- In general, skin cancers can be prevented by avoiding excessive sun exposure.
- Treatment of benign skin tumors such as nevi, lipomas, keloids, sebaceous cysts, and angiomas depends on the kind of tumor and its location.
- Psoriasis is a chronic skin condition that can be treated but not cured.
- Skin infections caused by bacteria, viruses, fungi, or parasites can be effectively treated with medications and supportive nursing care.
- Dermatitis, an inflammation of the skin, can have many causes.
- Eczema is a term that is often used for chronic forms of dermatitis.
- Venous ulcers are more common in older persons, heal slowly, and often recur following a slight injury.
- Alopecia, or baldness, can be caused by illness, drugs, hormonal imbalances, or heredity.

Review Questions

1. The skin has a vital role in the normal functioning of the human organism. That role is:

    a. production of antibodies.

    b. protection from invasion by microorganisms.

    c. support for internal organs.

    d. regulation of cellular oxygenation.

2. The nurse charted that the client's skin was loose, wrinkled, and thin with mild scaling. The nurse was describing:

    a. integrity.

    b. texture.

    c. turgor and mobility.

    d. vascularity.

3. An effective nursing intervention related to the care of open burn wounds that require daily dressing changes would be:

    a. keep the head of the bed elevated 30 degrees with all four side rails up.

    b. set a fluid intake goal of 2,500 mL/24 hours (1,200 mL during the day; 950 mL during the evening; 350 mL during the night).

    c. wear a cap, gown, mask, and sterile gloves when providing wound care.

    d. weigh daily, preferably before breakfast, and in the same type of clothing each day.

4. The client has lesions on his scalp and on his arms near his elbows. The lesions appear as red patches covered with thick silvery scales. The most likely cause of these lesions is:

    a. herpes zoster (shingles).

    b. pemphigus vulgaris.

    c. psoriasis.

    d. tinea (ringworm).

5. A nursing care plan for a client with an infectious disorder of the skin would include interventions to teach the client:

    a. how to avoid spreading the infection to others.

    b. how to do range-of-motion exercises to maintain joint flexibility.

    c. ways to conserve energy.

    d. which foods are most likely to cause allergic reactions.

References/Suggested Readings

American Cancer Society (ACS). (2003). *Cancer Facts & Figures 2003.* [Online]. Available: www.cancer.org/downloads/STT/CAFF2003PWSecured.pdf

Ayello, E., & Braden, B. (2001). Why is pressure ulcer risk assessment so important? *Nursing2001, 31*(11), 74–79.

Badger, J. (2001). Burns: The psychological aspects. *AJN, 101*(11), 38–42.

Beare, P., & Myers, J. L. (1998) *Principles and practice of adult health nursing* (3rd ed.). St. Louis, MO: Mosby.

Bjorgen, S. (1998). Herpes zoster. *AJN, 98*(2), 46–47.

Bozinko, G., Lowe, K., & Reigart, C. (1998). A new option for burn victims. *RN, 61*(11), 37–39.

Bryant, R. A. (2000). *Acute and chronic wounds: Nursing management* (2nd ed.). St. Louis, MO: Mosby.

Daniels, R. (2002). *Delmar's Guide to Laboratory and Diagnostic Tests,* Clifton Park, NY: Thomson Delmar Learning.

Davidson, M. (2002). Sharpen your wound assessment skills. *Nursing2002, 32*(10), 32hn1–32hn4.

Deters, G. E. (2002). Management of patients with dermatologic problems. In S. C. Smeltzer & B. G. Bare (Eds.), *Brunner and Suddarth's textbook of medical–surgical nursing* (9th ed.). Philadelphia: Lippincott Williams & Wilkins.

Dochterman, J., & Bulechek, G. (2004). *Nursing Interventions Classification (NIC)* (4th ed.). St. Louis, MO: Mosby.

Drisdelle, R. (2003). Maggot debridement therapy: A living cure. *Nursing2003, 33*(6), 17.

Estes, M. E. Z. (2002). *Health assessment & physical examination* (2nd ed.). Clifton Park, NY: Thomson Delmar Learning.

Fritsch, D. E., & Yurko, L. C. (2003). Management of persons with burns. In W. J. Phipps, F. D. Monahan, J. K. Sands, J. Marek & M. Neighbors (Eds.), *Medical–surgical nursing: Health and Illness Perspective* (7th ed.). St. Louis, MO: Mosby.

Goldsmith, J. (2003). Nit-Picking. *AJN, 103*(9), 22–23.

Hayes, J. (2003). Are you assessing for melanoma? *RN, 66*(2), 36–40.

Hess, C. T. (2001a). Managing a venous ulcer. *Nursing2001, 31*(3), 22.

Hess, C. T. (2001b). Putting the squeeze on venous ulcers. *Nursing2001, 31*(9), 58–63.

Hess, C. T. (2003a). Managing a patient with a venous ulcer. *Nursing2003, 33*(4), 73–74.

Hess, C. T. (2003b). Treating a fungal rash. *Nursing2003*, *33*(9), 20–22.

Hill, M. (1998). Nursing management of adults with skin disorders. In P. G. Beare & J. L. Myers (Eds.), *Principles and practice of adult health nursing* (3rd ed.); 2089–2115. St. Louis, MO: Mosby.

Hilton, G. (2001). Thermal burns. *AJN*, *101*(11), 32–34.

Kloth, L. (2002). How to use electrical stimulation for wound healing. *Nursing2002*, *32*(12), 17.

Leukemia-Lymphoma Society. (2000). *Skin lymphoma.* [Online]. Available: www.leukemia-lymphoma.org/all_mat_toc.adp?item_id=9846

Martin, S. (2001). There's what in the wound? *RN*, *64*(2), 44–47.

Martini, F., & Bartholomew, E. (2000). *Essentials of anatomy and physiology* (2nd ed.). Englewood Cliffs, NJ: Prentice-Hall.

McCain, D., & Sutherland, S. (1998). Skin grafts for patients with burns. *AJN*, *98*(7), 34–39.

Mendez-Eastman, S. (1998). When wounds won't heal. *RN*, *61*(1), 20–23.

Mendez-Eastman, S. (2002). New treatment for an old problem: Negative-pressure wound therapy. *Nursing2002*, *32*(5), 58–63.

Milner, S., Mottar, R., & Smith, C. (2001). The burn wheel. *AJN*, *101*(11), 35–37.

Moorhead, S., Johnson, M., & Maas, M. (2004). *Nursing Outcomes Classification (NOC)* (3rd ed.). St. Louis, MO: Mosby.

Moses, M. (2003). A simple matter of grooming. *AJN*, *103*(9), 11.

National Decubitus Foundation. (2002). Cost savings through bedsore avoidance [Online]. Available: www.decubitus.org/cost/cost.html

National Institute of Arthritis, Musculoskeletal and Skin Diseases (NIAMS). (2002). *Psoriasis.* [Online]. Available: www.niams.nih.gov/hi/topics/psoriasis/psoriafs.htm

National Institutes of Health (NIH). (2002). *Pressure ulcer.* [Online]. Available: www.nlm.nih.gov/medlineplus/ency/article/007071.htm

National Pressure Ulcer Advisory Panel (NPUAP). (1999). PUSH Tool [Online]. Available: www.npuap.org/pushins.htm

Nicol, N. H. (1997). Nursing care of clients with integumentary disorders. In J. M. Black & E. Matassarin-Jacobs (Eds.), *Luckmann and Sorensen's medical–surgical nursing: A psychophysiologic approach* (5th ed.); 1955–1982. Philadelphia: W. B. Saunders.

North American Nursing Diagnosis Association. (2003). *Nursing Diagnoses: Definitions & Classification 2003–2004.* Philadelphia: Author.

Ogden, B. L. (1998). Nursing management of adults with burns. In P.G. Beare & J. L. Myers (Eds.), *Principles and practice of adult health nursing* (3rd ed.); 2117–2142. St. Louis, MO: Mosby.

Regojo, P. (2003). Burn care basics. *Nursing2003*, *33*(3), 50–53.

Roy, D., & Stotts, N. (2002). Targeting cellulitis. *Nursing2002*, *32*(12), 46–47.

Schwartz, S., Shires, G., Spencer, F., Daly, J., Fischer, J., & Galloway, A. (1999). *Principles of surgery* (7th ed.). New York: McGraw-Hill.

Schweon, S., & Novatnack, E. (2002). What's causing that itch? *RN*, *65*(8), 43–46.

Seeley, R. R., Stephens, T. D., & Tate, P. (2002) *Anatomy and physiology* (6th ed.). New York: McGraw-Hill.

Spratto, G., & Woods, A. (2004). *2004 PDR Nurses' Drug Handbook.* Clifton Park, NY: Thomson Delmar Learning.

Thompson, J. (2003). Maximizing your pressure ulcer care. *Travel Nursing Today* (A Supplement to *RN*, April 2003) 16–24.

United States Department of Health and Human Services (USDHHS). (1992). *Pressure ulcers in adults: Prediction and prevention* (Publication Nos. 92-0047 and 92-0050). Rockville, MD: Public Health Service, Agency for Health Care Policy and Research.

Vermette, E. (1998). Emergency! Malignant hyperthermia. *AJN*, *98*(4), 45.

Weaver, V. (1999). Management of persons with problems of the skin. In W. J. Phipps, J. K. Sands, & J. Marek (Eds.), *Medical–surgical nursing: Concepts and clinical practice* (6th ed.). St. Louis, MO: Mosby.

Wiebelhaus, P., & Hansen, S. (1999). Burns: Handle with care. *RN*, *62*(11), 52–57.

Wiebelhaus, P., & Hansen, S. (2001a). Another choice for burn victims. *RN*, *64*(9), 34–37.

Wiebelhaus, P., & Hansen, S. (2001b). What you should know about burn emergencies. *Nursing2001*, *31*(1), 36–41.

Resources

American Burn Association, 625 North Michigan Avenue, Suite 1530, Chicago, IL 60611, 800-548-2876, http://ameriburn.org/home.htm

American Hair Loss Council, 125 Seventh Street, Suite 625, Pittsburgh, PA 15222, 412-765-3666, 888-873-9714, www.ahlc.org

Dermatology Foundation, 1560 Sherman Avenue, Suite 870, Evanston, IL 60201-4802, 847-328-2256, www.dermfnd.org

National Burn Victim Foundation, 246A Madisonville Road, P.O. Box 409, Basking Ridge, NJ 07920, 908-953-9091, www.nbvf.org

National Decubitus Foundation, 4255 South Buckley Road, Suite 228, Aurora, CO 80013, www.decubitus.org

National Pressure Ulcer Advisory Panel (NPUAP), 11250 Roger Bacon Drive, Suite 8, Reston, VA 20190-5202, 703-464-4849, www.npuap.org

National Psoriasis Foundation, 6600 SW 92nd, Suite 300, Portland, OR 97223, 800-723-9166, www.psoriasis.org

Skin Cancer Foundation, 245 Fifth Avenue, Suite 1403, New York, NY 10016, 800-SKIN-490, www.skincancer.org

The Wound Healing Society, 13355 Tenth Avenue North, Suite 108, Minneapolis, MN 55441-5554, 888-434-4234, www.woundheal.org

Wound, Ostomy and Continence Nurses Society, 4700 West Lake Avenue, Glenview, IL 60025, 888-224-9626, www.wocn.org

IMMUNE SYSTEM

MAKING THE CONNECTION

Refer to the following to increase your understanding of immune system disorders:

Basic Nursing
- **Legal and Ethical Responsibilities**
- **Communication**
- **Wellness Concepts**
- **Infection Control/Asepsis**
- **Standard Precautions and Isolation**
- **Fluid, Electrolyte, and Acid-Base Balance**
- **Assessment**
- **Diagnostic Tests**
- **Pain Management**

Adult Health Nursing
- **Oncology**
- **Respiratory System**

- **Cardiovascular System**
- **Hematologic and Lymphatic Systems**
- **Gastrointestinal System**
- **Musculoskeletal System**
- **Neurologic System**
- **Sexually Transmitted Diseases**
- **Integumentary System**
- **Substance Abuse**

Basic Procedures
- **Hand Hygiene**
- **Use of Protective Equipment**

Advanced Procedures
- **Initiating Strict Isolation Precautions**

LEARNING OBJECTIVES

Upon completion of this chapter, you should be able to:
- **Define key terms.**
- **Identify three allergic reactions with a systemic response.**
- **Describe symptoms of anaphylaxis and appropriate first aid.**
- **Recall common diagnostic tests used to evaluate immunological functioning.**
- **Discuss the medical–surgical management of clients with immunological disorders.**
- **Relate signs and symptoms of complications clients with immunological disorders could experience.**
- **Explain the modes of transmission of HIV.**
- **Identify methods of risk reduction of HIV for health care workers.**
- **Use the nursing process to plan the care of clients with immune system disorders.**

KEY TERMS

acquired immuno-
    deficiency syndrome
allergen
allogeneic
anaphylaxis
angioedema
antibody
antigen
autoimmune disorder
autologous
cellular immunity
diplopia
enzyme-linked
    immunosorbent assay
exacerbation
histamine

human immuno-
    deficiency virus
human leukocyte
    antigen
humoral immunity
hypersensitivity
immune response
immunity
immunotherapy
opportunistic infection
ptosis
remission
seroconversion
urticaria
viral load test
Western blot test

INTRODUCTION

Immunity is the body's ability to protect itself from foreign agents or organisms. This occurs through the complex interaction of the tissues within the immune system. Constant surveillance of cells within the body occurs to differentiate self from nonself. Those identified as nonself are then neutralized or destroyed. Dead or damaged cells are eliminated and homeostasis is maintained. When alterations in the system develop, immunological conditions develop. They may be hypersensitivity responses, such as allergies; immunological deficiencies, such as those associated with corticosteroid medications; or **autoimmune disorders,** where the body identifies its own cells as foreign and activates mechanisms to destroy them. Rheumatoid arthritis, systemic lupus erythematosus, and myasthenia gravis are examples of autoimmune disorders. Immunosuppressive disorders suppress the body's natural immune response to an antigen. Kaposi's sarcoma and non-Hodgkin's lymphoma are examples of immunosuppressive disorders.

ANATOMY AND PHYSIOLOGY REVIEW

The human body has a variety of natural physical and chemical mechanisms that enhance immunological functioning. The skin, eyelashes, cilia in the nose and respiratory system, gastric acidity, intestinal mucosa, and pH of vaginal mucosa all act to protect against invading organisms. In addition, all body tissues are linked together via lymphatic ducts and blood vessels to the organs and cells of the immune system.

Organs of the Immune System

The organs of the immune system are classified as primary or peripheral lymphoid organs. Primary lymphoid organs are bone marrow and the thymus gland. Within bone marrow, stem cells, the parent cells for all blood cells, are produced. Peripheral lymphoid organs are lymph nodes, spleen, tonsils, appendix, Peyer's patches of the small intestines, and the liver. Lymph nodes, located throughout the body, connected by an elaborate ductal system, filter lymphatic fluid, removing destroyed matter. Enlargement of lymphoid organs indicates an infectious or malignant process is occurring. The spleen serves as a reservoir for macrophages, lymphocytes, and plasma cells. The tonsils, appendix, and Peyer's patches also contain plasma cells and lymphocytes. The Kupffer cells of the liver house monocytes that ingest and destroy foreign organisms in hepatic circulation.

Cells of the Immune System

Leukocytes, white blood cells (WBCs), are vital components of the immune system. They are formed mostly in the bone marrow and partially in the lymph tissue. After formation, they are transported to different parts of the body, where they fight infectious organisms. There are six types of WBCs normally found in the blood: neu-

TABLE 44-1	PERCENTAGES OF DIFFERENT WBC TYPES
Neutrophils	55%–70%
Eosinophils	1%–4%
Basophils	0.5%–1.0%
Monocytes	2%–8%
Lymphocytes	20%–40%

trophils, eosinophils, basophils, monocytes, lymphocytes, and plasma cells (Guyton & Hall, 2000). Adults have about 7,000 WBCs/mm³ of blood. Each type is a percentage of the total number of WBCs (Table 44-1).

Those cells with granules in the cytoplasm are called *granulocytes,* while those lacking them are called *agranulocytes* (Figure 44-1). Eosinophils, neutrophils, and basophils are granular leukocytes. Monocytes and lymphocytes are agranular leukocytes. Each has its own unique function. Eosinophils come into play during allergic reactions or parasitic invasions. Neutrophils are useful in ingesting bacteria. Basophils secrete **histamine,** a substance released during allergic reactions, and heparin. Monocytes travel to the sites of invading organisms and transform into macrophages, capable of ingesting large quantities of microorganisms and damaged cells, a process known as *phagocytosis.* They also secrete Interleuken-1, which stimulates the activation of specific

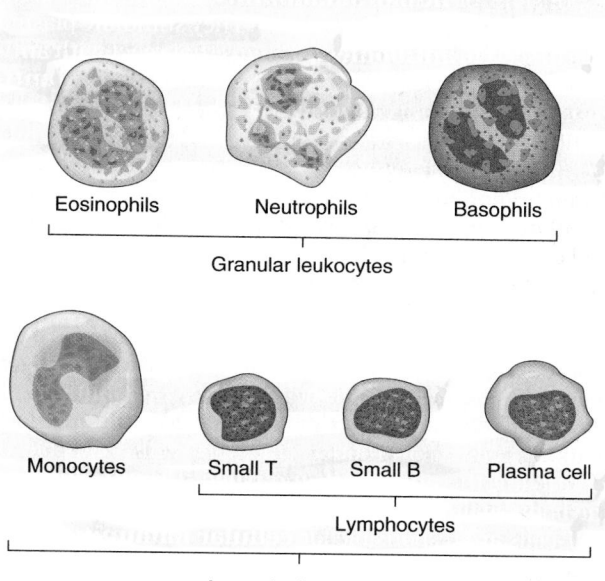

Eosinophils   Neutrophils   Basophils

Granular leukocytes

Monocytes   Small T   Small B   Plasma cell

Lymphocytes

Agranular leukocytes

Wandering macrophage

Figure 44-1 *Cells of the Immune System*

TABLE 44-2	HUMORAL AND CELLULAR RESPONSES
HUMORAL RESPONSE (B-CELL RESPONSE)	**CELLULAR RESPONSE (T-CELL RESPONSE)**
• B-lymphocytes stimulate plasma cells, which manufacture antibodies in response to an antigen and release them into the bloodstream. • Predominant role in response to: Bacteria and some viral infections Allergic reactions Autoimmune diseases	• Plasma cells are transformed into special T-lymphocyte cells, which detect, attack, and destroy invading antigens. • Predominant role in response to: Viral and some bacteria infections Delayed hypersensitivity (TB testing) Transplant rejection Graft-versus-host disease Fungal and parasitic infections Detection and destruction of tumor cells

lymphocytes. Granulocytes, also called *polymorphonuclear leukocytes,* make up the greatest number of WBCs.

B-lymphocytes (or B-cells) and T-lymphocytes (or T-cells) play a vital role in the immune response. B-cells are responsible for **humoral immunity,** or immunity dominated by antibodies (Table 44-2). They stimulate plasma cells to secrete **antibodies** (proteins that react with antigens to neutralize or destroy them) in response to **antigens** (any substance identified by the body as nonself). Antibodies are also called *immunoglobulins.* IgA, IgD, IgE, IgG, and IgM are common antibodies found in plasma. When an antibody-antigen reaction occurs, the complement system, a complex sequential immunological process, is activated. This system is composed of plasma proteins made in the liver. They alter cell membranes in the antibody-antigen reaction, facilitating the cellular breakdown of the invading antigen, and attract macrophages and granulocytes to the antibody-antigen reaction site. When a B-cell identifies an antigen, it places the characteristics of that antigen in a memory bank. B-cells also produce "memory cells" capable of identifying the antigen, if and when it is introduced to the body again.

T-cells are responsible for **cellular immunity,** a type of acquired immunity involving T-cell lymphocytes (Table 44-2). With T-cell mediated immunity, large numbers of activated lymphocytes are formed specifically to destroy the foreign agent. T-cells include helper cells (CD4), suppressor cells (CD8), and killer (cytotoxic) cells. CD4 and CD8 are molecules on the T-helper and T-suppressor cells and are important in understanding how HIV attacks the immune system.

Human immunodeficiency virus (HIV) infection affects the immune system and the brain. In the immune system, the main characteristic of HIV infection is progressive depletion of the CD4-T helper cells. The normal ratio of T-helper cells to T-suppressor cells (CD4:CD8 ratio) is 2:1. As immunodeficiency worsens, it is not uncommon for the CD4:CD8 ratio to fall to as low as 0:1. The altered T-helper cells cause malfunction of the B-cells and macrophages, which leads to collapse of the immune system. HIV also affects the CD4 molecule present on microglial cells in the brain, causing memory loss and other brain dysfunctions.

HIV is a retrovirus. Retroviruses use RNA to make DNA copies that then become part of the genetic material of the human cell. These viruses are called retroviruses because this is a reversal of the usual DNA-to-RNA transcription of genetic information.

Types of Immunity

There are two types of immunity: natural (innate) and acquired (adaptive) (Table 44-3). One is born with natural immunity; it is species specific. For example, humans have an innate resistance to distemper, whereas dogs never develop measles or syphilis. Acquired immunity develops after birth and may be active or passive. Active acquired immunity is the result of exposure to the disease or its vaccine. As a result, the body develops antibodies and memory cells for the causative microorganism. A repeated exposure results in rapid activation of these components of the immune system and annihilation of the invading agent. Passive acquired immunity utilizes antibodies produced by another human being or an animal. Injection of these immunoglobulins temporarily prevents development of the disease after exposure. Transmission of antibodies through fetal circulation is an example of passive acquired immunity.

Factors Influencing Immunity

Although the exact physiological mechanisms involved are unknown, it has been well documented that

TABLE 44-3	COMPARISON OF NATURAL AND ACQUIRED IMMUNITY	
	ACQUIRED IMMUNITY	
NATURAL IMMUNITY	**ACTIVE ACQUIRED IMMUNITY**	**PASSIVE ACQUIRED IMMUNITY**
• Innate immunity • Present at birth • Includes physical and chemical barriers to invading antigens	• Long-term immunity • Antibodies develop as a result of exposure to a disease or vaccine • Antibodies neutralize future invasions of the same antigen	• Temporary immunity • Antibodies obtained from an animal or another human who has been exposed to an antigen • Examples are gamma-globulin or antiserum

several factors influence the **immune response** (body's reaction to substances identified as nonself, neutralization of antigen). These include age, sex, nutritional status, stress, and treatment modalities. As one ages, the immune system becomes less effective. Sex hormones affect immunity; estrogen enhances immunological functioning, while androgen suppresses it. Therefore, women are especially prone to autoimmune diseases, whereas men are more prone to immunosuppressive disorders. Poor nutritional status and emotional stress lead to increased susceptibility to infections. Radiation therapy and a variety of medications, such as corticosteroids and chemotherapeutic agents, suppress the immune system.

ASSESSMENT

Physical assessment of the immune system involves the entire body. The skin and mucous membranes are evaluated for urticaria, inflammation, or bleeding. Superficial head, neck, supraclavicular, axilla, and inguinal lymph nodes are inspected and palpated for redness, tenderness, or swelling. Elevated temperature may indicate infection. Joints must be evaluated for possible tenderness, swelling, or limited range of motion. Changes in the rate and rhythm of respirations, presence of a cough, or abnormal lung sounds may indicate immunological conditions. Cardiovascular status, including rate, rhythm, arrhythmias, and peripheral vascular circulation, must be assessed. Enlarged liver or spleen and gastrointestinal conditions, such as nausea, vomiting, or diarrhea, may have an immunological basis. Alterations in vision, hearing, urinary habits, and neurological function may occur.

COMMON DIAGNOSTIC TESTS

Commonly used diagnostic tests for clients with symptoms of immune system disorders are listed in Table 44-4.

HYPERSENSITIVE IMMUNE RESPONSE

Hypersensitive immune responses include allergies, anaphylaxis, transfusion reactions, transplant rejection, and latex allergy.

ALLERGIES

Allergic disorders are the result of a **hypersensitivity** (excessive reaction to a stimulus) of the immune system to **allergens** (a type of antigen commonly found in the environment). Allergens may be inhaled, injected, ingested, or contacted. There are four types of hypersensitivity reactions based on how tissue is injured.

Type I reactions occur immediately upon exposure to a specific antigen. Upon first exposure to an allergen, IgE antibodies are produced. They adhere to mast cells.

TABLE 44-4	COMMON DIAGNOSTIC TESTS FOR IMMUNE SYSTEM DISORDERS

- Antinuclear antibodies (ANA)
- Complement assay (Total complement, C3 and C4)
- C-reactive protein test (CRP)
- CD4 T-cells
- Enzyme-linked immunosorbent assay (ELISA)
- Erythrocyte sedimentation rate (ESR or Sed Rate Test)
- Human leukocyte antigen DW4 (HLA-DW4)
- Lupus erythematosus test (LE Prep)
- Polymerase chain reaction (PCR)
- Red blood cell count (RBC count)
- Rheumatoid factor (RF)
- Total white blood cell count
  Differential count
  Neutrophils
  —Segs (mature neutrophils)
  —Bands (immature neutrophils)
  Eosinophils
  Basophils
  Lymphocytes
  Monocytes
- Western blot

When a subsequent exposure occurs, these cells attach to the antigen and activate the release of chemical mediators, such as histamine, bradykinin, and serotonin. These chemicals cause vasodilation, enhanced capillary permeability, and bronchoconstriction (Figure 44-2). The most common Type I reactions include allergic rhinitis, urticaria, and angioedema. Anaphylaxis is the most severe and is covered separately.

Allergic rhinitis, also known as *hay fever* or *pollinosis,* is a common allergy in our society caused by airborne allergens such as pollen, mold, animal dander, dust, and ragweed. Symptoms include nasal congestion; thin, clear, watery discharge; sneezing; itching; swelling; and redness of the eyes. Headaches and ear infections may also develop. Approximately 16.7 million office visits to health care providers each year are for allergic rhinitis (National Institute of Allergy and Infectious Diseases [NIAID], 2002a).

Urticaria (hives) are raised pruritic, red, nontender wheals on the skin. They are usually on the trunk and on the areas of the extremities closest to the trunk.

Angioedema, edema of subcutaneous layers and mucous membranes, is painless and only slightly pruritic. Acute urticaria affects approximately 10% to 20% of the U.S. population sometime in their life (NIAID, 2002a).

Drug and food allergies are also Type I hypersensitivity.

Any drug potentially may cause a drug reaction, but common ones include penicillin, cephalosporins, insulin, vaccines, and local anesthetics. Reactions vary from mild to severe. Usually, symptoms do not occur until the client

Allergic response

First exposure

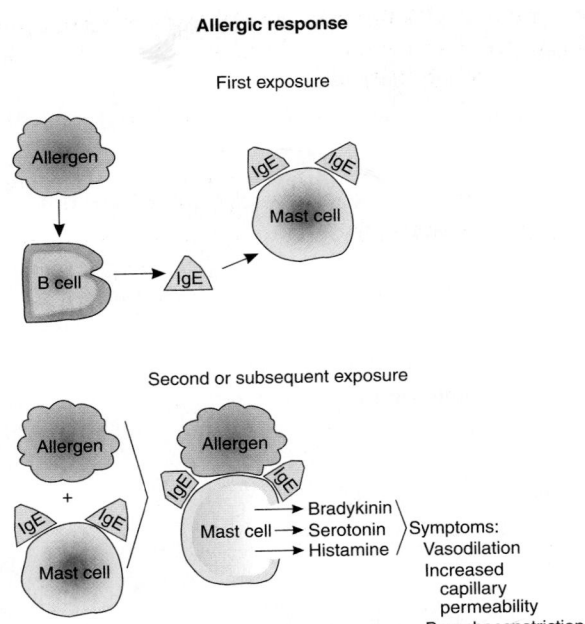

Second or subsequent exposure

Figure 44-2 *Allergic Response*

has taken several doses of the medication, although they can occur at first exposure. The most common reaction is the sudden development of a bright red, itchy rash, often appearing initially on the trunk or arms. Occasionally, a client may develop an anaphylactic reaction. Allergic drug reactions account for 5% to 10% of all adverse drug reactions (NIAID, 2002a).

Although individuals may be allergic to any edible substance, certain foods, such as milk, fish, chocolate, and nuts, are common allergens. Peanut or tree nut allergies affect approximately 3 million persons in the United States and cause the most severe food-induced allergic reactions (NIAID, 2002a). Diarrhea is a result of immunological reaction in the intestinal mucosa. Headache, nausea, vomiting, rash, itching, and wheezing may also develop.

Type II reactions are the destruction of cells or substances with antigens attached that either immunoglobulin G (IgG) or immunoglobulin M (IgM) senses as being foreign. Antibodies cause either lysis of the cells or accelerated phagocytosis. Hemolytic transfusion reactions are this type of reaction. Transfusion reactions are discussed in detail later.

Type III reaction involves IgG immune antigen-antibody complexes. It is a local reaction evident after several hours that may change from red skin to hemorrhage and tissue necrosis. Occasionally, this is noted after penicillin or sulfonamide use.

Type IV is a delayed reaction involving sensitized T-lymphocytes coming in contact with the allergen. Contact dermatitis and transplant rejection are examples of this type of reaction. Poison ivy and poison oak are the most common causes of contact dermatitis. Latex rubber is a more recently discovered cause of contact dermatitis or occasionally a Type I (anaphylactic) re-

action. Transplant rejection and latex allergy are covered separately.

Medical–Surgical Management
Medical

Medical management of clients experiencing an allergic response (reaction to allergen) includes drug therapy to treat symptoms and identification of precipitating agents. Allergen **immunotherapy** (treatment to suppress or enhance immunological functioning) involves repeated injections of the diluted allergen. Decreased levels of histamine are released upon subsequent exposure to the allergen. Venom can be used to treat allergies to bees, wasps, yellowjackets, and hornets.

Pharmacological

Several medications are employed to treat the symptoms of an allergic response. Antihistamines counteract the effects of histamine. They may be taken orally, topically, or intravenously, depending on the type of allergic response and urgency for treatment. Nasal decongestants help relieve respiratory symptoms. Topical corticosteroids effectively relieve inflammation associated with contact dermatitis and dermatitis medicamentosa. Oral or injectable forms of corticosteroids may be used either alone or in combination with antihistamines and nasal decongestants.

Skin testing by a physician can determine the specific causative allergen.

Diet

Individuals who are allergic to certain foods should be taught to check food labels carefully, be aware of how food is prepared, and not eat any product that could lead to a reaction. This includes restaurant foods and foods prepared in another person's home.

Activity

Avoidance of the causative allergen prevents allergic reactions. Activities should be centered around this, if at all possible. For instance, individuals who are allergic to pollen may need to stay in air-conditioned environments on those days when the pollen count is extremely high.

Nursing Management

Advise the client with allergic rhinitis to stay indoors when airborne allergens are present in great numbers. Ask about pets in the house. Encourage the client to read

LIFE CYCLE CONSIDERATIONS

Allergy to Foods

- 8% of children younger than 6 years of age have food allergy.
- 1% to 2% of adults have food allergy (NIAID, 2002).

labels if there are food allergies and to inform all health care personnel if there are drug allergies. Assist the client to plan lifestyle changes to avoid exposure to allergens. Emphasize the importance of following the medication regimen prescribed.

NURSING PROCESS

Assessment

Subjective Data

Take detailed, comprehensive client history, including information about previous allergic reactions, foods eaten or medications taken recently, and contact with environmental pollutants or anything not normally encountered. The client may describe having nausea, pruritis, and being uneasy.

Objective Data

Assess gastrointestinal and respiratory functioning, cardiovascular and neurological status, and the presence of urticaria, angioedema, sneezing, excessive nasal secretions, diarrhea, wheezes, cough, or hypotension.

Nursing diagnoses for clients with allergies may include the following:

Nursing Diagnoses	Planning/Goals	Nursing Interventions
Risk for Injury, related to an allergic reaction	The client will identify factors that increase the potential of a reaction.	Assist client in identifying those factors that increase the potential for a reaction.
Health-Seeking Behaviors related to causative allergen, therapeutic modalities, and/or preventive measures	The client will relate methods to avoid exposure to allergens.	Assist client in planning lifestyle changes that will help in avoiding exposure to allergens.
Deficient Knowledge related to lack of information about allergens, treatment, or preventive measures	The client will demonstrate an understanding of and compliance with therapeutic modalities if a reaction occurs. The client will demonstrate an understanding of and compliance with preventive measures to avoid subsequent allergic reactions.	Teach client about allergy treatments and what to do if a reaction occurs.

Evaluation Each goal must be evaluated to determine how it has been met by the client.

ANAPHYLACTIC REACTION

Anaphylaxis is a type I systemic reaction to allergens and is the most serious type of allergic reaction. It occurs in individuals who are extremely sensitive to an allergen. Symptoms develop suddenly and can progress to severe levels within minutes. Usually, the faster the reaction, the worse it is. Foods, drugs, hormones, insect bites, blood, and vaccines all are associated with anaphylactic reactions. Shellfish, eggs, nuts, berries, and chocolates are the most common foods involved. Any medication has the potential of causing a reaction, but antibiotics (especially penicillin), insulin, muscle relaxants, and x-ray dyes are the most frequent precipitating agents. Bee, wasp, hornet, and snake bites may also cause anaphylactic reactions. At least 40 deaths in the United States each year are the result of insect sting anaphylaxis (NIAID, 2002a).

CLIENT TEACHING

Severe Allergies

- Advise clients with severe allergies to wear a Medic Alert tag.
- Encourage clients who are allergic to insect stings to carry an emergency anaphylactic kit containing epinephrine at all times.

Anaphylactic reactions may be life-threatening. Symptoms involve the skin, GI tract, and cardiovascular and respiratory systems. Clients experience peripheral tingling, flushing, fullness in the mouth, throat/nasal congestion, tearing and swelling around the eyes, itching, cough, laryngeal edema, bronchospasms, severe dyspnea, vasodilation, and cyanosis. If untreated, these catastrophic effects lead to respiratory failure, severe hypotension, anaphylactic shock, and death. Therefore, it is crucial that symptoms be identified early and treatment initiated immediately because death can occur in minutes. Up to 40% have a recurrence of anaphylaxis within 24 hours (Carroll, 2001).

Medical–Surgical Management

Medical

Medical management centers around establishing an intravenous line, administering fluids and emergency drugs, and maintaining an airway. Provide oxygen via a nonrebreather oxygen mask. In severe cases, endotracheal intubation or a tracheotomy may be required.

Pharmacological

Epinephrine is administered subcutaneously as soon as symptoms develop to dilate bronchioles, increase heart contractions, and constrict blood vessels. Antihistamines, such as diphenhydramine hydrochloride (Benadryl), block the effects of histamine in bronchioles, blood vessels, and the GI tract. Corticosteroids are given for their anti-inflammatory effect. Vasopressors, such as norepinephrine bitartrate (Levophed) or dopamine hydrochloride (Intropin), may be needed to increase blood pressure. If bronchoconstriction and spasms are severe, albuterol (Proventil), metaproterenol sulfate (Alupent), and/or aminophylline (Aminophyllin) may be administered.

Diet

Clients will be NPO until normal respiratory and circulatory function have been restored.

Activity

Clients will remain on bed rest until vital signs are stable and normal breathing patterns have been restored. Those experiencing severe anaphylactic responses are generally transferred to intensive care units for continued treatment and observation.

Nursing Management

Monitor vital signs frequently as well as I&O. Administer IV fluids and medications as ordered. Teach client and family the importance of providing the name of the causative agent and a description of the reaction when asked about allergies.

NURSING PROCESS

Assessment

Subjective Data

Client history may reveal a previous anaphylaxis reaction. The client may describe feelings of uneasiness, anxiety, weakness, itching, dizziness, nausea, peripheral tingling, and a generalized warm sensation throughout the body.

Objective Data

Because anaphylaxis is a sudden, unexpected event, be aware that variations in a client's cardiovascular and respiratory status may be signs of an impending anaphylactic reaction. The first symptoms are sweating, sneezing, tachycardia, hypotension, dysrhythmias, cyanosis, edema of tongue and larynx, wheezing, bronchospasms, vascular collapse, and cardiac arrest. Regularly assessing client's vital signs and cardiovascular, respiratory, and neurological status will detect changes before the severe signs of respiratory distress and impending shock develop.

Nursing diagnoses for clients with anaphylaxis may include the following:

Nursing Diagnoses	Planning/Goals	Nursing Interventions
*Ineffective **T**issue Perfusion*, related to increased capillary permeability and vasodilation	The client will have adequate tissue perfusion.	Monitor vital signs frequently. Place client in Trendelenburg position for hypotension. Monitor I&O. Administer IV fluids and medications as ordered.
*Ineffective **B**reathing Pattern* related to bronchoconstriction, laryngeal edema, and increased secretions	The client will have effective breathing patterns.	Monitor vital signs. Maintain patent airway. Suction secretions as needed. Administer oxygen and medications as ordered.
*Deficient **K**nowledge* related to causative allergen, therapeutic modalities, and/or preventive measures	The client will relate causative allergen, therapeutic modalities, and preventive measures.	Teach client and family importance of avoiding allergen and symptoms of anaphylactic reactions. Advise client to provide the name of the causative agent and a description of reaction experienced when asked about allergies. Document allergy on all medical records.

Evaluation Each goal must be evaluated to determine how it has been met by the client.

TRANSFUSION REACTIONS

Blood components, such as whole blood, packed or frozen RBCs, leukocytes, platelets, and plasma, may be administered to clients when their own bodies are incapable of manufacturing them at a rate required to maintain vascular homeostasis. Any client receiving blood products that are **allogeneic,** or from a donor of the same species, may develop a transfusion reaction. For this reason, some clients are arranging to have their own blood collected, saved, and available for infusion, if needed, during or following elective surgeries. This is known as an **autologus** blood transfusion. Immunological reactions do not develop with this type of blood transfusion.

There are five types of transfusion reactions: febrile nonhemolytic, allergic urticarial, delayed hemolytic, acute hemolytic, and anaphylactic. Febrile nonhemolytic reactions are the most common and occur in clients who have had previous blood transfusions as a result of an antibody-antigen reaction to WBCs. Symptoms may develop soon after the infusion has started or up to 5 to 6 hours after completion. Fever is the classic symptom and may be accompanied by chills, nausea, headache, hypotension, and respiratory problems. Clients who have allergic urticarial reactions develop a skin rash during or within 1 hour following the transfusion. A delayed hemolytic reaction may occur days to weeks following the transfusion. The client's hemoglobin level falls because of incompatibility of RBC antigens. This type of reaction is often misdiagnosed and thought to be related to the condition that created the need for blood replacement rather than a transfusion reaction. An acute hemolytic reaction is potentially a life-threatening situation. Symptoms, resulting from the incompatibility of ABO groups, usually occur during the first 15 minutes of administration, but can develop anytime during the transfusion. Clients complain of chills, nausea, and back pain. Fever, drop in blood pressure (hypotension), vomiting, hematuria, or oliguria may be observed. As the condition progresses, chest pain, dyspnea, anuria, and shock develop. Anaphylactic reactions, although rare, are also life-threatening. Symptoms of acute gastrointestinal malfunctioning and cardiovascular and respiratory collapse develop moments after the transfusion has started.

Medical–Surgical Management

Medical

Medical management of clients experiencing a blood transfusion reaction depends on the type of reaction. Treatment of a febrile nonhemolytic reaction includes stopping the blood, infusing normal saline, and treating the symptoms. For clients experiencing an allergic urticarial reaction, the transfusion should be slowed and an antihistamine administered. Delayed hemolytic reactions often go undetected and untreated. Both acute hemolytic reactions and anaphylactic reactions are med-

---

CRITICAL THINKING

Donor Blood Transfusion

What are the pros and cons of receiving a blood transfusion from a donor?

---

ical emergencies. The transfusion must be stopped immediately. Normal saline and emergency drugs are given intravenously.

Pharmacological

If a febrile nonhemolytic or allergic urticarial reaction occurs, diphenhydramine hydrochloride (Benadryl) and a corticosteroid (hydrocortisone or prednisone) are administered to counteract the immunological response. Antipyretics are ordered to control fever. For life-threatening conditions, emergency medications are employed. (Refer back to Anaphylactic Reaction.)

Diet

Clients should not be fed if a reaction is occurring, especially if respiratory symptoms have developed, because aspiration could occur.

Activity

Clients should remain in bed until symptoms of the reaction have subsided.

Nursing Management

Follow agency protocol for use and administration of blood products. Assess vital signs before administration of blood products and at 15-minute intervals four times. Stay with the client for at least the first 15 minutes of administration. When reaction occurs, stop transfusion, but keep saline going for IV access if needed. Notify physician immediately.

NURSING PROCESS

Assessment

Subjective Data

Occasionally, clients verbalize the feeling of something "not being right" or "something strange is going on in my body" before actual symptoms become apparent. They may have itching, headache, or low-back pain.

Objective Data

Assess for any signs of a transfusion reaction, such as fever, chills, or respiratory problems.

A nursing diagnosis for clients with transfusion reactions may be:

Nursing Diagnoses	Planning/Goals	Nursing Interventions
*Risk for **Injury*** related to infusion of allogeneic blood components	The client will not have injury from infusion of allogeneic blood products.	Follow protocol for blood products and administration.
		Check client's identification and blood product with another nurse.
		If a reaction occurs, stop transfusion immediately, then call the physician.
		Administer medications as ordered.
		Send blood tubing and a urine specimen to the lab for analysis.
		Monitor and document client's condition.
		Teach client who has a blood transfusion reaction to inform health care providers whenever questioned about allergies.

Evaluation Each goal must be evaluated to determine how it has been met by the client.

TRANSPLANT REJECTION

In 2002, more than 24,000 organ transplants were performed in the United States (UNOS, 2003). The success of these procedures is directly related to matching antibodies and antigens of the donor and recipient and to the effectiveness of immunosuppressive medications in preventing rejection. Immunosuppressive medications make the client prone to the development of infections and cancers. Clients must have a regular medical checkup, including cancer screening tests.

Medical–Surgical Management

Medical

Although blood components are the most common type of tissue transplants, today it is possible to transplant bone marrow, corneal tissue, skin, kidneys, pancreas, hearts, livers, and lungs. Bone marrow and blood components often employ autologous donations. Allogeneic donations may be from living related donors or living nonrelated donors. Cadaveric donations are harvested from individuals after they are pronounced clinically dead. It is important to match ABO blood groups and **human leukocyte antigen** (antigens present in human blood) to prevent rejection when allogeneic and cadaveric donors are used.

Pharmacological

A combination of immunosuppressive medications is used to hinder rejection. Steroids such as prednisone (Deltasone) and methylprednisolone sodium succinate (Solu-Medrol) decrease the inflammatory response. Cyclosporine (Sandimmune), antithymocyte globulin (equine), ATG (Atgam), and tacrolimus (Prograf) inhibit T-cells. Azathioprine (Imuran) inhibits purine synthesis. Muromonab-CD3 (Orthoclone, OKT 3) prevents acute rejection in kidney transplant clients. Clients taking immunosuppressive medications are especially prone to developing infections. Antibiotics may be prescribed prophylactically.

Steroids cause fluid and sodium retention, low potassium level, elevated blood pressure, moon face, muscle wasting, elevated glucose level, impaired wound healing, mood swings, and masculinization in women. Cyclosporine may be toxic to the kidneys and liver. Imuran may cause hair loss and lower platelet level. OKT 3 also causes fluid retention.

Activity

Activity depends on the type of transplant. Clients who receive a major organ, such as a heart, lung, pancreas, or liver, are placed in reverse isolation in the hospital setting for at least 2 weeks. They are carefully observed for signs of rejection. Exposure to others is limited. Before discharge, they are taught to avoid contact with anyone who may have an infection and to wear a mask whenever out in public.

Nursing Management

Monitor vital signs, fluid balance, nutritional status, mental status, and cardiovascular and respiratory functioning. Prevent contact with anyone who may have an infection. Teach client and family proper hand hygiene. Emphasize the importance of taking all medications as prescribed.

NURSING PROCESS

Assessment

Subjective Data

Client history may reveal fear of possible transplant rejection. The client generally describes tenderness at the transplant site.

Objective Data

Following transplantation, carefully monitor clients' vital signs, nutritional status, fluid balance, urinary output, mental status, and respiratory and cardiovascular functioning. Weigh client daily. Check wound sites frequently. Signs of rejection include fever, weight gain, and swelling or tenderness at the transplant site.

Nursing diagnoses for clients with organ transplants may include the following:

Nursing Diagnoses	Planning/Goals	Nursing Interventions
Fear related to possible transplant rejection.	The client will relate less fear regarding rejection.	Allow client to verbalize concerns and develop realistic expectations. Set aside time to sit down and talk to client.
Deficient Knowledge related to home care following transplantation	The client will discuss signs and symptoms of rejection. The client will demonstrate an understanding of the side effects of immunosuppressive drugs and lifestyle changes to adapt to their effects.	Teach client and family about signs of rejection and infection. Teach client and family ramifications of taking immunosuppressive medications. Teach client to watch for side effects and report them to physician.
Risk for Infection related to immunosuppressive medications	The client will demonstrate appropriate wound care. The client will be free of infection.	Teach client and family appropriate wound care and proper hand hygiene. Teach client importance of taking antibiotics as ordered, wearing a mask whenever out in public, and regular checkups, including cancer screening tests.

Evaluation Each goal must be evaluated to determine how it has been met by the client.

LATEX ALLERGY

Since 1987, when universal precautions (now called Standard Precautions) were mandated, exposure to latex by health care workers has dramatically increased. Today, as many as 17% of health care workers and 6% of the general population have a systemic latex allergy (Lenehan, 2002).

The latex proteins can enter the body through the skin and mucous membranes, intravascularly, and by inhalation. The cornstarch powder on gloves absorbs the latex proteins and becomes airborne when the gloves are put on or taken off. From the air, the latex proteins may be inhaled or may be in contact with the skin and mucous membranes. Anyone, client or health care worker, who after exposure to latex develops red, watery, itchy eyes; sinus or nasal irritation; hives; shortness of breath; dry cough; wheezing; chest tightness; or flushing, tachycardia, and hypotension should be suspected of latex allergy. More than 20,000 medical products contain latex (Burt, 1998). Synthetic versions of products are often available. An individual product may be "latex free," but an environment is "latex safe" only when all items of latex that might come in contact with the allergic individual are removed.

 Safety: Latex Allergy
A Medic Alert tag stating "latex allergy" should be worn by any individual with a latex allergy.

AUTOIMMUNE DISEASES

Disorders in this category include rheumatoid arthritis, systemic lupus erythematosus, and myasthenia gravis.

RHEUMATOID ARTHRITIS

Rheumatoid arthritis (RA) is a chronic, systemic autoimmune disease characterized by joint stiffness. It affects 2.1 million people in the United States, including 1.5 million women and 600,000 men (Arthritis Foundation, 2002). It affects people of all races, usually beginning in middle age but often occurs in the 20s and 30s (Arthritis Foundation, 2002).

The cause of RA is unknown, but there seems to be a genetic predisposition (susceptibility) in many, but not all, persons affected. It is believed that something must trigger the disease process such as a virus, bacterium, hormonal factors, or stress. The person's immune system attacks the cells inside the joint(s), producing substances that act as antigens. Immune complexes are formed within the joint, causing inflammation, swelling, and increased synovial fluid. As this chronic, systemic condition progresses, surrounding cartilage, tendons, and ligaments become involved. Thickening of synovial tissue eventually leads to calcification of the joint, joint pain, limited mobility, and deformity.

It is believed that the damage to the bones begins within the first two years of the onset of RA. Early diagnosis and aggressive treatment are important to control the disease. Usually, the joints of the hand and wrist are affected initially. As the disease progresses, shoulder, elbow, hip, knee, ankle, and cervical spine joints become affected. The pattern of joint involvement is symmetrical (i.e., if a joint is affected on the right side of the body, the same joint will also be affected on the left side) (Arthritis Foundation, 2002). Other areas of the body where connective tissue is present may also be involved, such as blood vessels, lining of the lungs, and pericordial sac.

Clients experience periods of **remission,** a decrease or absence of symptoms, and **exacerbations,** an increase in symptoms. Both physical and emotional stressors lead to increased symptomatology. This means that simple tasks such as answering the telephone or buttoning clothes may become very challenging.

Medical–Surgical Management

Medical

Medical management centers around reducing inflammation, relieving pain, slowing down or a stopping joint damage, and promoting general health. Therapeutic regimen includes medications, exercise, rest, hot and cold applications, and stress management.

Surgical

Hip, knee, and finger joints may be surgically replaced. Refer to the Musculoskeletal System chapter for a discussion of joint replacement.

Pharmacological

Nonsteroidal anti-inflammatory drugs (NSAIDs) and salicylates have the potential to relieve symptoms such as joint pain, stiffness, and swelling but do not control the disease. Disease-modifying antirheumatic drugs (DMARDs) have the potential to modify the disease and should be given early in the disease to control progression. The commonly used DMARDs include prednisone (Deltasone), gold salts, and sulfasalazine (Azulfidine EN-Tabs) (Table 44-5). Because of the large doses required to control inflammation and the long-term use because of the chronicity of this condition, side effects often

---

TABLE 44-5   MEDICATIONS USED TO TREAT RHEUMATOID ARTHRITIS

DRUG	USE/ACTIONS	SIDE EFFECTS	NURSING CONSIDERATIONS
Salicylates • aspirin	Inhibit prostaglandin synthesis resulting in decreased pain. (Analgesia) antipyretic and anti-inflammatory effects.	GI upset, tinnitus, easy bruising, nausea, prolonged bleeding time.	Instruct client to take with food or take enteric coated aspirin and to report ringing in ears. Do not give to clients on oral anticoagulants. Assess for bleeding/bruising.
Nonsteroidal Anti-inflammatory Drugs (NSAIDs) • ibuprofen (Motrin, Rufen) • naproxen (Naprosyn) • phenylbutazone (Butazolidin) • nabumetone (Relafen)	Inhibit prostaglandin synthesis. Reduce joint swelling stiffness. Analgesic and antipyretic properties.	GI irritation, nausea, vomiting, heartburn. GI bleeding and ulceration, dizziness, headache, liver toxicity.	Administer with food. May prolong bleeding time, may require frequent blood count.
Indole Analogues • indomethacin (Indocin) • sulindac (Clinoril)	Analgesic anti-inflammatory effect.	Gastric bleeding, headaches, dizziness, psychiatric disturbances.	Administer with food. Instruct client to report any bleeding (tarry stools, hematemesis). Avoid giving aspirin.
Corticosteroids • prednisone (Deltasone)	Decreases inflammation.	GI irritation, muscle weakness, fluid retention, moon face, muscle wasting, impaired wound healing.	Administer with food. Weigh daily. Monitor BP, sleep pattern, and serum potassium.
Antimalarials • hydroxychloroquine sulfate (Plaquenil Sulfate)	Not a drug of choice.	Visual disturbances, nightmares, skin lesions, nausea, diarrhea, low blood count.	Monitor CBC and liver function tests. Discontinue after 6 months if no beneficial effects noted.

continues

TABLE 44-5 continued

DRUG	USE/ACTIONS	SIDE EFFECTS	NURSING CONSIDERATIONS
Gold Salts • auranofin (Ridaura)	Anti-inflammatory effect.	Diarrhea, nausea, vomiting, jaundice.	Remind client to keep all physician appointments. Beneficial effects may take 3 months to appear.
Chelating Agent • penicillamine (Depen)	Palliative when other medications have failed.	Bone marrow depression, fever, rashes, blood dyscrasias, liver toxicity.	Give on empty stomach. Have epinephrine 1:1,000 handy for anaphylaxis. Fluids to 3,000 mL/day to prevent renal failure.
Sulfonamide • sulfasalazine (Azulfidine EN-TABS)	For clients who do not respond well to NSAIDs.	Anorexia, headache, nausea, vomiting, gastric distress, reversible oligospermia.	Give with food. May discolor urine or skin yellow-orange. Take at least 2–3 L/day of water. May increase sensitivity to sun.

develop. In severe cases, azathioprine (Imuran), hydroxychloroquine sulfate (Plaquenil Sulfate), D-penicillamine (Depen), or methotrexate sodium (Rheumatrex) may be used. These medications also have serious side effects.

Diet

Clients should eat a nutritious, well-balanced diet. Poorly nourished individuals are prone to infections. For clients with RA, an infection results in exacerbation of symptoms. Foods high in iron are encouraged when RBCs are low.

Activity

Because joint mobility is a major problem, occupational and physical therapists are part of the therapeutic team. Range-of-motion exercises, resting splints, and assistive devices such as canes and hand rails are often employed to promote mobility.

Nursing Management

Encourage the client to practice relaxation techniques and take a warm shower to relieve joint stiffness and pain. Emphasize the importance of doing ROM exercises several times a day and to have planned rest periods. Teach the client to use assistive devices such as handrails, tools to pick up objects, raised toilet seat, walker, or cane.

NURSING PROCESS

Assessment

Subjective Data

Client history frequently reveals a gradual development of symptoms, beginning initially with early-morning stiffness and pain in finger joints. Eventually, other joints become involved. Fatigue, weight loss, temperature elevation, and anemia develop, along with malaise, loss of appetite, fatigue, and muscle weakness. Obtain information about periods of remissions and exacerbations as well as the client's understanding of and compliance with the treatment regimen.

Objective Data

Assessment of the hands may reveal the classic deformities associated with RA: boutonniere deformity (fixed flexion of the proximal interphalangeal joint and hyperextension of the distal interphalangeal joint), ulnar drift (deviation of the fingers to the ulnar side of the hand), and swan-neck deformity (fixed flexion of the distal interphalangeal joint and hyperextension of the proximal interphalangeal joint). Figure 44-3 illustrates these changes in the hands.

Skin may show the presence of ulcers, caused by vasculitis, and moveable, subcutaneous skin nodes, known as *rheumatoid nodules.* Eye tissue may be inflamed. Reduction in tear and saliva production can occur, causing dryness of the eyes, mouth, and mucous membranes. This is known as Sjögren's syndrome. The client may have weight loss and an elevated temperature.

Figure 44-3 *Arthritic Hands (Courtesy of the Arthritis Foundation)*

X-rays demonstrate the amount and degree of deformity. No specific laboratory test confirms a diagnosis of RA, although alterations in the following may occur: RBCs decrease (anemia) as the disease progresses, eleva- tion of WBCs, erythrocyte sedimentation rate (ESR), antinuclear antibodies (ANAs), C-reactive proteins, and platelet count. The rheumatoid factor (RF) is present in about 75% of adult clients with RA (Daniels, 2002).

Nursing diagnoses for clients with rheumatoid arthritis may include the following:

Nursing Diagnoses	Planning/Goals	Nursing Interventions
Chronic **Pain** related to swollen, inflamed joints	The client will relate appropriate use of anti-inflammatory medications. The client will relate methods to decrease pain.	Teach client about prescribed analgesics and anti-inflammatory medications Encourage client to practice relaxation techniques and take warm shower to relieve early morning joint stiffness and pain. Use hot and cold packs to decrease muscle spasms. Teach client proper body alignment and to avoid using pillows under the knees, which leads to pooling of blood in the feet.
Impaired Physical **Mobility** related to edema, and joint immobility	The client will demonstrate measures to maintain joint mobility. The client will demonstrate use of adaptive devices.	Teach hospitalized clients to use the overhead trapeze when moving in bed and to change position frequently. Assist with ROM exercises and maintain planned rest periods. Teach client use of assistive devices, such as handrests, tools to pick up objects, or three-legged canes, as needed. Check with occupational and physical therapists for available equipment. Assist client to use handrails in tub, shower, and toilet; raised toilet seat; and rubber-tipped walker or cane.
Bathing/Dressing/Grooming **S**elf-care Deficit related to joint inflammation or deformity	The client will bathe, dress, and groom to abilities.	Encourage client to stop and rest when tired. Teach self-care using assistive devices, as required. Recommend shoes with Velcro® closures. Assist with routine plan for ADLs.
Fatigue related to chronic inflammatory process	The client will state less fatigue. The client will establish priorities for daily activities. The client will balance daily activities with periods of rest.	Explain that fatigue is a common symptom of autoimmune disorders. Plan rest periods between activities. Allow the client to express feelings about altered lifestyle. Inform client of community services such as Meals on Wheels. Help identify activities client should perform and what can be delegated. Instruct client to record level of fatigue and activities performed on an hourly basis for 24 hours. One method uses 0 to 10 scale (0 = not tired, peppy; 10 = totally exhausted). Help plan important tasks during high-energy periods and distribute difficult ones throughout the week.

Evaluation Each goal must be evaluated to determine how it has been met by the client.

SYSTEMIC LUPUS ERYTHEMATOSUS

Systemic lupus erythematous (SLE) is a chronic, progressive, incurable autoimmune disease affecting multiple body organs. It is characterized by periods of exacerbation (flares) and remission. SLE occurs most commonly in women during their childbearing years and is 2 to 3 times more common in African Americans, Hispanics, Asians, and Native Americans (Lupus Foundation of America [LFA] 2001). In clients with SLE, abnormal B-lymphocyte cells produce autoantibodies that destroy body cells. Immune complexes are formed and circulate in serum, causing inflammation and tissue damage in the skin, brain, kidney, lung, heart, or joints. Production of these autoantibodies is influenced by genetic predisposition, medications, infections, stress, and sunlight (ultraviolet light rays).

No single test is conclusive for a diagnosis. The American College of Rheumatology has established criteria for SLE. These criteria include a malar rash (over cheeks); discoid rash; photosensitivity; oral ulcers; arthritis; serositis (pleuritis or pericarditis); excessive protein or cellular casts in the urine; seizures or psychosis; hemolytic anemia, or leukopenia, or lymphopenia, or thrombocytopenia; and positive for LE cells, or anti-DNA antibody, or anti-Sm, or a false-positive syphilis test. If four or more of these criteria are present, a client is diagnosed with SLE.

Medical–Surgical Management

Medical

Medical treatment is aimed at decreasing tissue inflammation and destruction. A knowledgeable client can assist in controlling the disease process through stress management, rest, exercise, taking medications as prescribed, and immediately reporting symptoms to the health care provider. During acute exacerbations, plasmapheresis may be used. This treatment modality involves removal of the client's plasma, processing it through a special machine to eliminate various cellular elements, and reinfusing the cleansed plasma. In SLE, autoantibodies are removed.

Because clients with SLE are prone to a variety of complications, they are carefully monitored for renal, cardiac, pulmonary, hematological, and neurological damage. A large percentage of SLE clients eventually develop renal failure, requiring dialysis to maintain life.

Pharmacological

NSAIDs are used for muscle and joint pain. The lowest possible dose of corticosteroid is used to suppress immune system activity. During periods of exacerbations, higher doses may be required. Prolonged use of these medications leads to multiple side effects. Hydroxychloroquine sulfate (Plaquenil sulfate), an antimalarial agent, is used. Although the exact mechanism involved is unknown, it does work effectively in decreasing joint and skin problems. It can lead to the development of retinal toxicity; therefore, clients should have yearly eye exams. Cyclophosphamide (Cytoxan) or azathioprine (Imuran) may be used for severe SLE (Litton, 2003).

Diet

Clients on corticosteroids are prone to developing hypernatremia, hyperglycemia, hypokalemia, and fluid retention. Diet should be low in sodium and glucose and high in potassium. Excessive fluid intake should be discouraged.

Activity

Clients should be encouraged to sleep at least 8 hours a night and rest periodically during the day. Regular exercise helps prevent muscle weakness and fatigue.

Nursing Management

Teach the client the importance of avoiding direct sunlight and the use of protective clothing and sunscreen (SPF 15 or higher). Encourage the client to balance rest and activity and to eat a balanced diet with reduced sodium. Emphasize the signs of exacerbation (rash, fever, cough, or increased joint and muscle pain) and early signs of infection. Provide emotional, psychosocial, and spiritual support.

NURSING PROCESS

Assessment

Subjective Data

Ask when the disease began, what symptoms have developed, and how they have been treated. Note information about medications the client is taking and side effects, activity level, and degree of fatigue. Determine client's understanding of the disease process, how lifestyle has changed, and how effectively client is coping. The client may describe having malaise, photosensitivity, pain in joints, irregular menses, irritability, confusion, or hallucinations.

Objective Data

Most common findings include joint swelling and pain, fever, swollen glands, nausea, vomiting, anorexia, hypertension, respiratory and cardiac infections, renal involvement, enlarged liver and spleen, and skin lesions, especially the classic "butterfly" rash. Figure 44-4 shows an individual with a "butterfly" rash. If exposed to the cold, Raynaud's phenomenon (intermittent attacks of diminished blood supply to fingers, toes, ears, and nose) may develop.

Laboratory tests frequently reveal serum antinuclear antibodies (ANA) and anti-DNA antibodies. Lupus erythematosus cells (LE cells) are present in most clients. Anemia, leukopenia, and thrombocytopenia are evident.

Figure 44-4 *Butterfly Rash (Courtesy of the American Academy of Dermatology)*

Nursing diagnoses for a client with SLE may include the following:

Nursing Diagnoses	Planning/Goals	Nursing Interventions
Impaired Skin Integrity related to presence of butterfly rash, skin lesions, Raynaud's phenomenon, and/or oral ulcers	The client will participate in a plan to promote wound healing.	Teach client to clean and dry area prior to application of topical corticosteroids.
		Warn client that sunlight and ultraviolet rays increase symptoms and tanning sessions are contraindicated.
		Encourage client to wear protective clothing, sunscreen of at least SPF 15, and sunglasses. In cold weather, client should wear a hat and gloves.
		Encourage client in regular oral care to promote healing of mouth sores.
Deficient Knowledge related to adapting lifestyle with treatment and prevention of complications	The client will describe disease process, factors contributing to symptoms, and regimen for control.	Teach client effects of disease and methods to control complications.
		Teach stress management techniques. Allow client to vent feelings.
		Help client plan methods to adapt lifestyle.
		Encourage client to visit the physician on a regular basis to monitor for early symptoms of major organ involvement.
		Advise client to have regular eye exam if taking Plaquenil Sulfate.
		Inform client of community support groups available through the Lupus Foundation of America, Inc. (see Resources).

Evaluation Each goal must be evaluated to determine how it has been met by the client.

MYASTHENIA GRAVIS

Myasthenia gravis (MG) is an autoimmune disease characterized by extreme muscle weakness and fatigue caused by the body's inability to transmit nerve impulses to voluntary muscles. It is thought that clients with MG develop antibodies that act to decrease the number and effectiveness of acetylcholine receptor sites at neuromuscular junctions. Voluntary muscles are most commonly involved, especially those innervated by cranial nerves. Muscle weakness increases during periods of activity and improves after a period of rest.

Severity of symptoms varies. In mild conditions known as Group I ocular myasthenia, only the eye muscles are involved. As severity increases, symptoms of Group II generalized myasthenia develop: Facial, neck, skeletal, and respiratory muscles become affected. The thymus gland is enlarged in most clients. Anti-ACh receptor antibodies are produced in this organ. MG affects men more frequently than women, with the onset of symptoms after age 50. Periods of remission and exacerbation occur, usually during the first few years.

There are three possible complications: respiratory distress, myasthenic crisis, and cholinergic crisis. Clients need to be carefully monitored for early signs of respiratory distress, such as dyspnea, tachypnea, tachycardia, and diaphoresis.

Myasthenia crisis is an acute emergency characterized by increased muscle weakness; difficulty swallowing, chewing, or talking; and respiratory distress. It occurs in newly diagnosed clients who are not responding to anticholinesterase medications following infections, surgery, or delivery of a child.

Cholinergic crisis is the result of an overdose of anticholinesterase medications. Physical symptoms of both myasthenia crisis and cholinergic crisis are the same. An edrophonium chloride (Tensilon) test is used to differentiate between the two. Tensilon is administered intravenously; symptoms of clients experiencing a myasthenia crisis will be relieved within seconds, whereas clients in cholinergic crisis will show no response. Atropine is administered to counteract the effects of excessive amounts of anticholinesterase drugs. The treatment goal for both is restoration of normal respiratory functioning and alleviation of symptoms.

Medical–Surgical Management

Medical

Medical management involves the use of anticholinesterase medications and plasmapheresis, which removes anti-ACh receptor antibodies. Because it affords only temporary relief of symptoms, it is used primarily for clients in acute crisis who are not responding to drug therapy or before a thymectomy. A client's relief of symptoms is a good indicator of how successful surgery might be.

Surgical

Surgical removal of the thymus gland has shown the best results in young people early in the course of the disease. In some people, the weakness may completely disappear, but it varies with each client.

Pharmacological

Anticholinesterase medications, such as pyridostigmine bromide (Mestinon), neostigmine bromide (Prostigmin), and ambenonium chloride (Mytelase), are prescribed early in the course of the disease and act to increase acetylcholine at the neuromuscular junction. Dosages need to be individually determined. Early side effects of overdosage include nausea, abdominal cramping, vomiting, diarrhea, increased saliva, diaphoresis, and low pulse rate. Variation may occur in muscle group responses for the same client. Steroids may slow down the immunological response.

Diet

Clients need to be encouraged to eat a snack before taking anticholinesterase medications to avoid GI irritation. If the client's ability to chew and swallow is affected,

---

PROFESSIONAL TIP

Myasthenia Gravis

Clients with myasthenia gravis experience problems similar to those with RA and SLE (e.g., fatigue and impaired physical mobility). Although the cause, in this case, is weakness of voluntary muscles, client goals and nursing interventions are the same.

food should be chopped, mashed, or pureed. A commercial thickener can be added to liquids to reduce the risk of aspiration. Sit upright when eating and do not talk.

Activity

Symptoms of MG increase with exercise. Clients should avoid excessive muscular activity and should rest periodically throughout the day. ROM exercises, braces, splints, and walkers assist in keeping the client independent.

Nursing Management

Teach the client airway protective techniques (e.g., double swallowing, chin tuck). Encourage the client to change daily activity pattern for minimal energy expenditure, and to do ROM exercises to help maintain muscle function. Emphasize the need to see the physician at the first sign of an upper respiratory infection. Advise client to avoid crowds during cold and flu season and anyone known to have either.

NURSING PROCESS

Assessment

Subjective Data

Client describes muscle weakness, fatigue, and possibly difficulty chewing or swallowing.

Objective Data

Assess muscle groups affecting the eyes, face, neck, and chest, looking for **diplopia** (double vision), **ptosis** (drooping upper eyelids), and facial symmetry. Note chewing or swallowing problems and weakness in arm and legs muscles as well as muscles used for breathing. Assess vocal tones and breath sounds.

ACh receptor antibody and LE cell tests are often positive. X-rays and CT scans of the thymus gland are used to detect enlargement. Electromyogram (EMG) determines the extent of muscle damage.

Nursing diagnoses for a client with MG may include the following:

Nursing Diagnoses	Planning/Goals	Nursing Interventions
*Ineffective **B**reathing Pattern* related to muscle weakness	The client will have normal respiratory rate and rhythm and normal breath sounds bilaterally.	Monitor client's respiratory rate and rhythm and breath sounds frequently. Administer oxygen as ordered. Notify physician immediately if respiratory problem develops. Elevate head of client's bed.
*Risk for **A**spiration* related to impaired swallowing	The client will not experience aspiration.	Have client eat in a sitting position or with head of the bed elevated. Teach client to chew food well and swallow only small bites. Request a special diet of thickened, soft foods. Suction oral secretions as required. Teach client to suction secretions as needed.
*Deficient **K**nowledge* related to disease process and understanding of methods to control disease and prevent complications	The client will describe disease process, factors contributing to symptoms, and regimen for control. The client will practice health behaviors needed to manage the effects of MG and methods to prevent complications.	Teach client stress management techniques and methods to avoid infections. Teach clients to take medications at regularly scheduled times to maintain appropriate level. Encourage client to wear a Medic Alert bracelet indicating the name and dosage of medications being taken. Refer to the Myasthenia Gravis Foundation for information and support groups (see Resources).

Evaluation Each goal must be evaluated to determine how it has been met by the client.

SAMPLE NURSING CARE PLAN

THE CLIENT WITH MYASTHENIA GRAVIS

Mrs. Henry, a 29-year-old mother of two preschool children, was diagnosed with myasthenia gravis 2 years ago. Initially, she had double vision and drooping eyelids, but after beginning a course of pyridostigmine bromide (Mestinon), she went into remission. Recently, she has been experiencing facial, neck, and chest muscle weakness and is now admitted to the hospital for evaluation. Occasionally, she has difficulty swallowing and breathing. Her thymus gland is enlarged. She has asked the nurse to teach her some strategies for managing this chronic illness.

Nursing Diagnosis 1 *Ineffective **B**reathing Pattern* related to respiratory muscle fatigue as evidenced by facial, neck, and chest weakness

Nursing Outcomes Classification (NOC)
Respiratory Status: Ventilation
Neurological Status

Nursing Interventions Classification (NIC)
Airway Management
Energy Management
Neurologic Monitoring

PLANNING/GOALS	NURSING INTERVENTIONS	RATIONALE
Mrs. Henry's respiratory rate and rhythm and breath sounds will remain within normal limits.	Assess Mrs. Henry's breathing patterns q2h.	Detects early signs of respiratory distress.
	Ask Mrs. Henry to notify the nurse immediately if she has any breathing difficulties.	May be reluctant to call the nurse and needs to be encouraged to do so.
	Notify physician immediately if respiratory problems develop.	Physician must determine the cause and if a tracheostomy is needed.

continues

SAMPLE NURSING CARE PLAN

EVALUATION Mrs. Henry's respiratory rate and rhythm have remained within normal limits.

Nursing Diagnosis 2 *Risk for Aspiration* related to impaired swallowing as evidenced by difficulty swallowing

Nursing Outcomes Classification (NOC)
Neurological Status
Respiratory Status: Ventilation

Nursing Interventions Classification (NIC)
Aspiration Precautions
Neurologic Monitoring

PLANNING/GOALS	NURSING INTERVENTIONS	RATIONALE
Mrs. Henry will not experience aspiration.	Position Mrs. Henry to eat in a sitting position.	Promotes passage of food into the stomach.
	Teach Mrs. Henry the importance of thoroughly chewing food, and swallowing only small bites.	Can cause aspiration.
	Have oral suctioning equipment at the bedside.	Readily available if required.

EVALUATION Mrs. Henry has not aspirated. She makes a point of always sitting up when eating.

Nursing Diagnosis 3 *Deficient Knowledge*, related to disease process and understanding of methods to control effects of myasthenia gravis and prevent complications as evidenced by verbalization of need for future teaching

Nursing Outcomes Classification (NOC)
Knowledge: Disease Process
Knowledge: Energy Conservation

Nursing Interventions Classification (NIC)
Teaching: Disease Process
Teaching: Individual

PLANNING/GOALS	NURSING INTERVENTIONS	RATIONALE
Mrs. Henry will practice health behaviors needed to manage the effects of MG and prevent complications.	Assess Mrs. Henry's prior knowledge of MG and methods of controlling the effects of prescribed medications and preventing complications.	Provides a basis for planning teaching.
	Include Mrs. Henry's family members in teaching sessions.	Fosters implementation of regimen at home.
	Teach Mrs. Henry and family members basic information about MG, the actions of anticholinesterase medication, the need to take it on a regular basis with a snack, side effects of overdose, and the importance of notifying the physician of any signs of respiratory problems or infection.	Information about one's disease, medications, and when to notify the physician is essential knowledge the client and family members need in order to effectively manage this chronic illness.
	Encourage Mrs. Henry to wear a Medic Alert bracelet, which lists here name, diagnoses, and dosage of prescribed medications.	Provides accurate information to medical personnel in case of an emergency.
	Provide Mrs. Henry with the address and telephone number of the Myasthenia Gravis Foundation and encourage her to contact them for additional information and support.	Facilitates future attainment of knowledge and possible involvement with a support group.

EVALUATION Mrs. Henry and her husband related information about MG, action and side effects of Mestinon, signs and symptoms to watch for, and when to notify the physician. She has obtained a Medic Alert bracelet and has contacted the MG Foundation. She plans to attend the next local chapter meeting.

INADEQUATE IMMUNOLOGICAL RESPONSE

This category includes HIV/AIDS; pulmonary, gastrointestinal, oral, gynecological, and central nervous system opportunistic infections; and opportunistic malignancies.

HIV/AIDS

Although allergies are hypersensitive immune responses, and autoimmune diseases literally have the body attacking itself, acquired immunodeficiency syndrome (AIDS) is a disease that causes an inadequate immunological response by the body. The human immunodeficiency virus (HIV) may be acquired anytime after conception.

The **human immunodeficiency virus** (HIV), a retrovirus that causes **acquired immunodeficiency syndrome** (AIDS), was first reported in the United States in 1981. AIDS is a progressively fatal disease that destroys the immune system and the body's ability to fight infection. By the end of 2002, it was estimated that 42 million people in the world were living with HIV/AIDS (National Institute of Allergy and Infectious Diseases [NIAID], 2002b). In the United States, 816,149 cases of AIDS had been reported by the end of 2001, and as many as 950,000 may be infected with HIV (NIAID, 2002b).

Following exposure to HIV and an incubation period of 2 to 4 weeks, some individuals, but not all, will experience flulike symptoms such as fever, sweats, headache, myalgia, neuralgia, sore throat, GI distress, and photophobia (Figure 44-5). Many persons, if tested at this time, will test negative because antibodies may not yet be present in the blood. In 2 or 3 weeks, these symptoms disappear. Infected individuals are very infectious during this period, with large quantities of HIV present in genital secretions.

Most individuals will remain symptom free for years (10 or more), but some may begin to have symptoms in a few months. During this "asymptomatic" period, HIV is multiplying, infecting, and killing the CD4 T-cells of the immune system.

A variety of symptoms become evident as the CD4 T-cells disappear. Lymph nodes enlarged for more than 3 months are one of the first symptoms. Others may include weight loss, lack of energy, fevers and sweats, persistent skin rashes or flaky skin, persistent or frequent oral or vaginal yeast infections, PID that does not respond to treatment, and short-term memory loss. Oral, genital, or anal herpes infection or shingles may also develop.

When the CD4 T-cell count is less than 200 cells/mm^3 (healthy persons have 1,000 or more CD4 cells/mm^3) and the individual has 1 or more of the 26 clinical conditions that affect persons with advanced HIV disease, the individual is considered to have AIDS. Most of the AIDS-defining conditions are **opportunistic infections** (infections in persons with a defective immune system that rarely cause harm in healthy individuals). *Pneumocystis carinii* pneumonia is the most frequent AIDS-defining diagnosis in the United States and Europe (Lisanti & Zwolski, 1997).

The **enzyme-linked immunosorbent assay** (ELISA) is the basic screening test to detect antibodies to HIV. A positive test result is always retested to rule out false-positive results and/or technician error. A confirmatory test, the **Western blot** test, is always employed when the ELISA test is positive. Results of both the ELISA and Western blot taken together have an extremely high accuracy rate.

Obtaining a signed informed consent for testing is often a nursing responsibility. Most states mandate a consent form solely for HIV testing. Some states allow verbal consent and a statement of the client's consent signed by the health care provider.

The FDA has approved the OraQuick Rapid HIV-1 Antibody Test, which provides results with 99.6% accuracy in 20 minutes (FDA, 2002).

Demographics of AIDS in the United States

Demographics are viewed in terms of clients' age, gender, and race.

Age

AIDS mainly affects people during the most productive years of their life. As of December 2001, AIDS is the fifth leading cause of death among persons ages 25 to 44 (NIAID, 2002b). The estimated number of new cases of AIDS among individuals younger than 13 in the United States fell from 954 in 1992 to 101 in 2001 (NIAID, 2002b).

Gender

Trends in HIV-related mortality reflect changes in the demographic patterns of the HIV epidemic. Although more men than women are infected with HIV, the num-

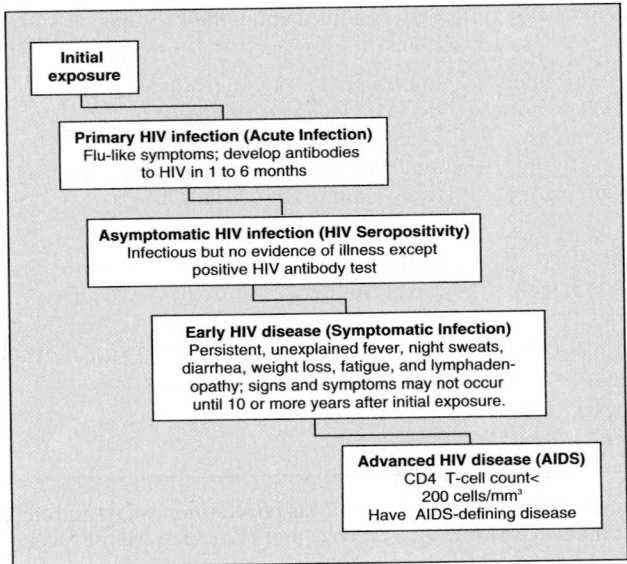

Figure 44-5 *Continuum of HIV Disease*

ber of AIDS cases in women in the United States has increased from 7% in 1985 to 25% in 2001.

Race

Of the new AIDS cases reported in the United States in 2001:

- African Americans accounted for 76.3/100,000 population.
- Hispanic Americans accounted for 28.0/100,000 population.
- Whites accounted for 7.9/100,000 population.
- American Indian/Alaska Natives accounted for 11.7/100,000 population.
- Asian American/Pacific Islanders accounted for 4.8/100,000 population (NIAID, 2002b)

The HIV/AIDS epidemic is growing most rapidly among some minority populations and is a leading cause of death of African American males ages 25 to 44 (NIAD, 2002b).

Modes of Transmission

There are many way to become infected with HIV. The virus may be found in blood, semen, vaginal secretions,

---

PROFESSIONAL TIP

HIV Testing

Although physicians are responsible for client counseling, the nurse must know the information to be able to answer questions and clarify the client's knowledge. Pretest counseling should include the following:

- Ask why the client believes the test should be done.
- Explain the meaning of a positive or negative test result and the possibility of a false-negative result.
- Discuss risk reduction and ways to modify behavior.
- Share state reporting requirements.
- Ensure confidentiality of test results.
- Explain that there is often stress related to test results and possible reactions to learning the results, such as depression or anxiety.
- Discuss the potential negative social consequences of positive results.
- Assist the client in making a decision about testing.
- Arrange a return appointment for the client to receive test results.

Post-test counseling should include the following:

- Review the test results with the client.
- Assess the client's understanding of the test results.
- Allow the client to express feelings about the test results.
- Review routes of HIV transmission.
- Assess the client's psychological condition including the risk for suicide.
- Assess the client's risk behavior and strategies for reducing risk.
- Provide information about support groups and national/local resources.

---

and breast milk of infected individuals. There is no evidence that HIV is spread through sweat, tears, urine, or feces. The saliva of infected individuals has the virus, but there is no evidence that it is spread to others through kissing. The risk of infection from "deep kissing" and oral sex is unknown. Tissue transplantation (including artificial insemination), blood transfusion, and needlesticks are high-risk situations but are relatively rare methods of transmission in the United States today. Having another sexually transmitted disease such as chlamydia, genital herpes, syphilis, or gonorrhea seems to make an individual more susceptible to becoming infected with HIV during sexual intercourse with an infected partner. Theoretically, HIV is present in sufficient quantities in amniotic fluid, cerebrospinal fluid, pleural fluid, peritoneal fluid, and pericardial fluid whereby infection could occur with exchange of these body fluids, particularly in health care settings where contact with these fluids may occur. Behaviors associated with increased risk of sexual transmission of HIV by infected persons include unprotected sexual intercourse, multiple sex partners, failure to disclose HIV status, and trading sex for money or drugs. Transmission of HIV can also take place by having contact with infected blood or sharing needles or syringes; it may also transmit from mother to fetus during pregnancy or birth.

Sexual intercourse (anal, oral, vaginal) without using a condom is the most frequently reported risk behavior for infection with HIV. Injection-drug use is the second most frequently reported risk behavior for infection with HIV. When HIV seropositive women take zidovudine (AZT) during pregnancy and labor and zidovudine is given to the newborn, perinatal transmission is significantly reduced.

Medical–Surgical Management

Medical

The goal of care is to keep the disease from progressing for as long as possible. The client's chance of disease progression can now be monitored by a **viral load test** that measures copies of HIV RNA. The approved viral load test is the Amplicor HIV-1 Monitor test, better known as the *polymerase chain reaction (PCR) test* (AIDS Treatment Data Network, May 1999). It can be used to see if individuals with HIV are at risk for getting sick, for checking the effects of drugs taken by individuals with HIV to see if they are working against the virus, and to distinguish the difference between actual HIV infection in a newborn and maternally acquired antibodies. The "ultra-sensitive" PCR test can measure as few as 50 copies/mL of HIV RNA. There is no "safe" level of viral load. The risk is less, but HIV can be passed to another person if the viral load is undetectable. Only about 2% of HIV is in the blood; the rest is in body tissues and cannot be measured (New Mexico AIDS Info Net, 2002).

Pharmacological

The goal of anti-HIV treatment is to keep the viral load as low as possible for as long as possible, ideally below what the viral load test can detect. Currently available antiretroviral drugs do not cure HIV/AIDS. Treatment is usually begun at the time of **seroconversion** (evidence of antibody formation in response to disease or vaccine). In high-risk occupational exposures, treatment may be started immediately.

One group of drugs, called *nucleoside analog reverse transcriptase inhibitors (NRTIs)*, interrupt HIV's life cycle at an early stage. The spread of HIV in the body may be slowed and the onset of opportunistic infections may be delayed by NRTIs, but these drugs *do not* prevent HIV transmission to other individuals. This group includes zidovudine (Retrovir), formerly known as AZT, zalcitabine (Hivid), didanosine (Videx), stavudine (Zerit), lamivudine (Epivir), and abacavir (Ziagen). A combination of zidovudine and lamivudine (Combivir) is available. Zidovudine (Retrovir) may cause depletion of red or white blood cells. If this depletion is severe, the drug must be discontinued. Painful nerve damage and pancreatitis may be caused by didanosine (Videx).

Non-nucleoside reverse transcriptase inhibitors (NNRTIs) are available to be used only in combination with other antiretroviral drugs. These include delavirdine (Rescriptor), nevirapine (Viramune), and efavirenz (Sustiva).

The protease inhibitors interrupt HIV's life cycle at a later step. These include ritonavir (Norvir), saquinavir mesylate (Fortovase, Invirase), indinavir sulfate (Crixivan), and nelfinavir mesylate (Viracept). Nausea, diarrhea, and other GI symptoms are common side effects of protease inhibitors.

HIV can become resistant to any of three drugs, so combination treatments are necessary to effectively suppress the virus. When NRTIs and protease inhibitors are combined, it is referred to as highly active antiretroviral therapy or HAART. Researchers credit HAART with significantly reducing the number of AIDS deaths in the United States (NIAID, 2002c). Current guidelines recommend drug therapy for any client with symptomatic HIV disease (evidence of opportunistic infections or tumors). For asymptomatic HIV-positive clients, drug therapy is recommended if:

- Viral load test results are greater than 500 copies/mL, *or*
- The client's CD4 T-cell count is under 500 cells/mm³ (Kirsten & Whipple, 1998).

Health Promotion

The CDC and the Occupational Safety and Health Administration (OSHA) have developed Standard Precautions to reduce the risk of health care personnel exposure to blood and body fluids. Personal protective equipment should be worn while caring for all clients when there is a reasonable likelihood of contact with any blood or body fluids.

CRITICAL THINKING

HIV and Lifestyle

How might a person's lifestyle change after receiving a diagnosis of being HIV positive?

PULMONARY OPPORTUNISTIC INFECTIONS

Conditions discussed following include *pneumocystis carinii* pneumonia, histoplasmosis, and tuberculosis.

PNEUMOCYSTIS CARINII PNEUMONIA

Pneumocystis carinii pneumonia (PCP) accounts for 70% of opportunistic infections associated with advanced HIV disease (Coyne, Lyne, & Watson, 2002). A marked decrease in the number of AIDS clients diagnosed with PCP is a result of initiation of prophylactic treatment when the CD4 T-cell count is 200 or less/mm³. Although *Pneumocystis carinii* is found primarily in the lungs, it has also been reported in the adrenal glands, bone marrow, skin, thyroid, kidneys, and spleen of persons with AIDS.

Clinical signs and symptoms include fever, dyspnea, nonproductive cough, and crackles. Initial diagnosis is made by chest x-ray, which shows diffuse infiltrates. Fiberoptic bronchoscopy is the procedure of choice to obtain a definitive diagnosis. During the bronchoscopy, sputum is obtained to demonstrate the presence of the organism.

Current standard treatment for PCP includes either intravenous pentamidine isethionate (Pneumopent, Pentam 300) or sulfamethoxazole-trimethoprim (Bactrim, Septra), given orally or intravenously. Oral sulfamethoxazole-trimethoprim is the treatment of choice; however, approximately one-third of people with AIDS eventually develop hypersensitivity reactions and must switch to pentamidine for primary therapy. Prophylaxis against PCP is a therapeutic necessity for all persons infected with HIV when the CD4 T-cell count is 200 or less. Primary prophylaxis refers to therapy for those considered at risk for PCP based on the CD4 count to prevent infection with PCP. Secondary prophylaxis refers to therapy to prevent recurrences in clients who have already had PCP. Current guidelines recommend either oral sulfamethoxazole-trimethoprim or aerosolized pentamidine for prophylaxis. For those allergic to sulfamethoxazole-trimethoprim, pentamidine diluted in sterile water administered by a Respigard II nebulizer can be used.

HISTOPLASMOSIS

Histoplasmosis is an infection caused by the fungus *Histoplasma capsulatum*. The fungus has been isolated in bird droppings, dirt from chicken coops, and caves. The spores from the fungus are introduced into the body by inhalation. Histoplasmosis is not specific to the lung. In most clients with HIV disease, histoplasmosis is disseminated (spread out). Histoplasmosis should be suspected if the person presents with fever of uncertain origin, cough, and malaise.

The diagnosis is confirmed by culture or biopsy of the bone marrow, blood, lymph nodes, lungs, or skin. Initial treatment of histoplasmosis is usually IV amphotericin B. Oral ketoconazole (Nizoral) can be used for maintenance therapy. Prophylaxis against recurrence of histoplasmosis is provided by itraconazole (Sporanox).

TUBERCULOSIS ← *Road*

Mycobacterium tuberculosis, an acid-fast aerobic bacterium, is the cause of tuberculosis (TB). It is spread through airborne particles and enters the body by inhalation. The particles usually lodge in the apex of the lungs; however, one-half to two-thirds of cases of HIV-associated or AIDS-associated TB involve organs outside the lungs as well.

Clinical manifestations include fever, night sweats, cough, and weight loss. People with AIDS will commonly present with a productive cough and pleuritic pain. Diagnosis is made by a combination of tests: skin testing with purified protein derivative (PPD); examination and culture of sputum, urine, and other fluids; x-rays; and other tests such as IVP.

The most common test for exposure to TB is the Mantoux skin test, which consists of injecting 0.1 mL of (PPD) intradermally. A negative reaction does not rule out infection. HIV-positive clients with a CD4 count lower than $200/mm^3$ may no longer have an immune response to the PPD. The chest x-ray may reveal middle and lower lobe infiltrates. A sputum specimen is smeared and stained with an acid-fast stain, then examined under the microscope for acid-fast bacillus (AFB). Other body fluids such as urine, blood, and stool may also be tested for AFB.

The risk of transmission of TB to health care workers is highest during and immediately after procedures that induce coughing. In the home and health care setting, cough-inducing procedures should be performed only in well-ventilated areas.

Infection Control: TB

A densely woven, snug-fitting mask (particulate respirator) should be worn by all persons in contact with the person who has TB until the person has received treatment for 2 to 3 weeks. Persons with TB should also be taught to cover their mouths while coughing and should wear a particulate respirator when they are out of their room for tests.

Because of the upsurge of multidrug-resistant TB (MDR-TB), the CDC recommends treating with multiple medications. Treatment is provided in two phases. In the initial treatment phase, the client receives isoniazid (Laniazid), rifampin (Rifadin), pyrazinamide, and ethambutol Hcl (Myambutol) or streptomycin sulfate for 2 to 6 months, depending on whether *Mycobacterium tuberculosis* is identified outside the lungs. In the continuation phase, treatment with two to four of the medications used in the initial phase is indicated for 4 to 6 months longer.

Px - TB.

Nursing Management

Monitor vital signs and laboratory test results. Encourage fluid intake of 2.5 to 3 mL per day. Administer oxygen and medications as ordered. Encourage the use of an incentive spirometer, unless contraindicated. Reposition client at least every 2 hours. Plan for client rest periods during the day.

NURSING PROCESS

Assessment

Subjective Data

Assess the client's ability to dress, bathe, ambulate, and so on. Note the client's perception of breathlessness.

Objective Data

Assess the client's respiratory rate, depth, and breath sounds. Note cough (productive or nonproductive), cyanosis, dyspnea, use of accessory muscles, and fever. Monitor arterial blood gas (ABG) results for decreased PaO_2, increased $PaCO_2$, and decreased pH.

Nursing diagnoses for the HIV-positive client with pulmonary disorders may include the following:

Nursing Diagnoses	Planning/Goals	Nursing Interventions
Ineffective **A**irway Clearance, related to chronic, unrelieved cough, pain, or viscous secretions	The client will mobilize secretions effectively.	Administer 2.5–3 L of fluid per day (oral or IV) to decrease thick secretions and medications as ordered to suppress cough and decrease pain. Reposition client every 2 hours and PRN.
Impaired **G**as Exchange related to inadequate ventilation/oxygenation	The client will maintain an $SaO_2 > 90\%$	Administer oxygen as ordered. Encourage use of incentive spirometer, if not contraindicated.
Ineffective **B**reathing Pattern, related to fatigue	The client will pace activities to minimize fatigue.	Plan care to allow rest periods.

Evaluation Each goal must be evaluated to determine how it has been met by the client.

GASTROINTESTINAL OPPORTUNISTIC INFECTIONS

Disorders discussed following include *Mycobacterium avium* complex, cytomegalovirus, cryptosporidiosis, hepatitis, and HIV-wasting syndrome.

MYCOBACTERIUM AVIUM COMPLEX

Mycobacterium avium and *Mycobacterium intracellulare* are two closely related mycobacteria that are grouped together and called *Mycobacterium avium* complex (MAC). The source of exposure to MAC for humans is contaminated water, although it has been isolated from soil, dust, sediments, and aerosols. In persons with AIDS, MAC involvement of the bowel is usually extensive, suggesting that the gastrointestinal tract may be the site of initial infection, with spread to other organs after that. The microorganism can fill the bone marrow and lymph nodes.

The most common symptoms of MAC include chronic fever, malaise, anemia, weight loss, diarrhea, and abdominal pain. Often the client will appear cachectic because of malabsorption. Because the symptoms are nonspecific, MAC is often difficult to distinguish from other AIDS-related infections. MAC is usually disseminated at the time of diagnosis. Diagnosis is made by tissue biopsy and cultures of the lung, bone marrow, lymph nodes, liver, or blood.

Treatment for MAC infection may include one or more of the following medications: clarithromycin (Biaxin Filmtabs) to treat disseminated MAC; and a combination of amikacin sulfate (Amikin), azithromycin (Zithromax), ciprofloxacin hydrochloride (Cipro), cycloserine (Seromycin), and ethionamide (Trecator-SC). For persons with AIDS who have a CD4 count of less than 75/mm^3, rifabutin (Mycobutin) is recommended for prevention of disseminated MAC.

CYTOMEGALOVIRUS

Cytomegalovirus (CMV) belongs to the herpes virus group. Thus it shares the same phenomena of latency and reactivation. The virus lies dormant in tissues waiting to be reactivated in the immunocompromised client. The potential for infection with CMV is increased during two periods: the perinatal period through the preschool years, and later during the sexually active years.

CMV causes disease by destroying the brain, lung, retina, and liver. CMV infection has been identified in all parts of the gastrointestinal tract from the oral cavity to the perianal area. CMV can be life-threatening for persons with suppressed immune systems. Persons with HIV infection or AIDS may develop severe infections, including CMV retinitis that can lead to blindness.

Signs and symptoms of CMV include weight loss, fever, diarrhea, and malaise. The diagnosis of CMV is based on microscopic identification of CMV from specific organs such as the brain, lung, liver, or adrenal gland. Ganciclovir sodium (Cytovene) is the drug of choice for treating individuals infected with CMV. Maintenance therapy is required to prevent relapse. Intravenous foscarnet sodium (Foscavir) has been approved as an alternative therapy.

CRYPTOSPORIDIOSIS

Cryptosporidium, a protozoan causing cryptosporidiosis, usually infects the epithelial cells that line the digestive tract. Transmission is often by the fecal-oral route, but can be spread from animal to person as well as person to person. *Cryptosporidium* can also be spread by ingesting contaminated food and water.

Clinical signs and symptoms include profuse watery diarrhea. Abdominal pain, serious weight loss, abdominal cramping, anorexia, low-grade fever, dehydration, electrolyte imbalance, and malaise may also be present. Diagnosis is made by identifying the organism in fresh stool specimens.

There is no effective treatment for cryptosporidiosis. Antidiarrheals such as diphenoxylate hydrochloride with atropine sulfate (Lomotil), loperamide hydrochloride (Imodium), and opium tincture (Paregoric) should be given on a programmed schedule rather than PRN. Treatment is palliative and focused toward the symptoms. This includes fluid and electrolyte replacement (orally if possible), analgesics, and occasionally the use of total parenteral nutrition (TPN). Anticryptosporidial agents are under investigation. Protecting the integrity of the client's perianal skin is extremely important. A low-residue, high-protein, high-calorie diet helps maintain nutritional status.

HEPATITIS

Only hepatitis B virus (HBV), hepatitis C virus (HCV), and hepatitis D virus (HDV) are commonly seen with HIV infection. All three viruses have been associated with chronic infection and have similar transmission and risk factors. Risk factors include exposure to blood or blood products, exposure to contaminated needles and syringes, and multiple sexual contacts.

Signs and symptoms include malaise, weakness, anorexia, nausea, vomiting, and right upper quadrant pain. Abnormalities in bilirubin and hepatic enzymes may also occur. Diagnosis is made by serologic assays identifying antigens and antibodies.

Interferon has been approved for treatment of chronic HBV and HCV and is being investigated for the treatment of HDV. Response to therapy varies but is decreased with HIV infection. Clients with a CD4 count greater than 400 mm^3 respond best to this therapy (Parr, 1994).

HIV-WASTING SYNDROME

HIV-wasting syndrome is defined as unexplained weight loss of more than 10% of body weight accompanied by weakness, chronic diarrhea, and fever in those infected with HIV. Weight loss and malnutrition are related to reduced food intake, malabsorption of nutrients, and altered metabolism of nutrients. Some of the factors related to reduced intake include anorexia, oral or esophageal lesions, nausea, neurologic or psychiatric conditions, fatigue, inadequate finances, and side effects of medications. Nutritional malabsorption is related to injury of the small intestine caused by opportunistic infections or by HIV infection of the cells in the gastrointestinal tract. Opportunistic infections produce fever that depletes the body's energy stores and causes weight loss.

Signs and symptoms of HIV-wasting syndrome are anorexia, diarrhea, nausea, vomiting, changes in taste and smell, aphthous ulcers of mouth and esophagus, and abdominal pain.

Symptom control is the major focus for HIV-wasting syndrome. Medications to control nausea and vomiting should be given routinely, not PRN. Treatment of anorexia includes megestrol acetate (Megace) or dronabinol (Marinol). Antimotility drugs such as loperamide hydrochloride (Imodium), luminal acting agents such as kaolin and pectin mixture (Kaopectate) and hormonal agents such as octreotide acetate (Sandostatin) are used to treat diarrhea. This makes eating much easier. Oral nutritional supplements are most frequently used for weight loss. TPN is usually considered a final option except in cases of severe malnutrition, because of the risk and expense involved.

Nursing Management

Monitor stools for blood, fat, and undigested food. Keep perirectal area clean and protect with ointment as ordered. Have a schedule for turning the client. Encourage the client to drink fluids between meals and to use hard candy or chewing gum to stimulate saliva production. Monitor laboratory test results. Provide a prescribed diet in small frequent meals at room temperature. Assist with oral hygiene before and after meals. Weigh client daily. Administer antiemetics and antidiarrheals as ordered.

NURSING PROCESS

Assessment

Subjective Data

Ask the client about bowel habits and what causes and relieves diarrhea. Inquire about alcohol consumption because excessive alcohol intake depletes B vitamins and provides no nutrition. Note activities that cause fatigue. Discuss food likes/dislikes, food intolerances, and food intake for the previous 3 days.

Objective Data

Assess the client's skin integrity, including temperature, moisture, color, vascularity, texture, lesions, areas of excoriation, and wound healing. Note fever, weight, and daily nutritional intake. Monitor laboratory values of nutritional status, including serum albumin, total protein, hemoglobin, and hematocrit, as well as stool specimens for ova and parasites.

Nursing diagnoses for the HIV-positive client with gastrointestinal disorders may include the following:

Nursing Diagnoses	Planning/Goals	Nursing Interventions
Deficient Fluid Volume related to nausea, vomiting, diarrhea, or inadequate oral intake	The client will have normal skin turgor and decreased frequency and amount of stools.	Suggest client use hard candy or chewing gum to stimulate saliva production if mouth is dry. Encourage client to drink liquids between (not with) meals.
		Monitor and record intake and output. Monitor client for evidence of electrolyte imbalance (hypokalemia, hypochloremia, confusion, muscle weakness).
Imbalanced Nutrition Less than Body Requirements related to anorexia, dysphagia, malabsorption, or side effects of medications	The client will eat 75% of prescribed diet and maintain current weight.	Provide the prescribed diet (usually low-residue, high-calorie, high-protein) in small frequent meals at room temperature. Provide oral hygiene before and after meals to enhance taste sensation.
		Offer commercially prepared nutritional supplements between meals. Weigh client daily.
		Administer supplemental vitamins and minerals as prescribed.
		Administer antiemetics and antidiarrheals as ordered.
		Advise client to keep a food diary and a log of exacerbation and remission of signs and symptoms.
Risk for Impaired Skin Integrity, related to diarrhea, malnutrition, decreased mobility	The client will maintain skin integrity.	Monitor stool for presence of blood, fat, undigested food and stool cultures for evidence of new infections.
		Protect the perirectal area by keeping it clean and using compounds such as Aloe Vesta cream.
		Avoid prolonged pressure on bony prominences by a scheduled turning plan. If nonambulatory, provide client with a pressure relief mattress. Use soft sheets on the bed and avoid wrinkles.
		Teach client to use nondrying soaps and to pat skin dry.

Evaluation Each goal must be evaluated to determine how it has been met by the client.

ORAL OPPORTUNISTIC INFECTIONS

Candidiasis and leukoplakia are discussed following.

ORAL AND ESOPHAGEAL CANDIDIASIS

Oral candidiasis (thrush) is a fungal infection caused by *Candidia albicans* (Figure 44-6), which occurs in more than 90% of AIDS clients (Lisanti & Zwolski, 1997). Many clients complain of an unpleasant taste or mouth dryness. Other clinical signs and symptoms include creamy, white oral plaques and mucosal tenderness. When the white oral plaques are wiped off, they leave an erythematous or even bleeding mucosal lesions. Esophageal candidiasis, an AIDS-defining disease, causes dysphagia and painful swallowing.

These symptoms may interfere with the client's eating, nutrition, and weight. Diagnosis is established by the presence of the characteristic lesions in the oral cavity. Microscopic examination of oral or esophageal lesions reveals budding yeast cells.

Treatment for esophageal candidiasis is oral fluconazole (Diflucan). Oral candidiasis is treated with nystatin suspension (Mycostatin) and clotrimazole (Mycelex Troches). Another medication used to treat candidiasis is ketoconazole (Nizoral). Amphotericin B (Amphotericin B) is used to treat disseminated candida infection. The antiulcer drug sucralfate (Carafate) may be used as a slurry to relieve mouth pain before eating. Tx - Yogurt
TX = NYSTATIN   Tx = D.fluCAN

ORAL HAIRY LEUKOPLAKIA
- immune compromised   Looks like Mold

Oral hairy leukoplakia (OHL) usually appears as a white patch on the lateral borders of the tongue as shown in Figure 44-7. It is caused by the Epstein-Barr virus. The lesions are rarely in other areas of the mouth and are different in appearance from candidiasis. The irregular surface of the lesion appears as projections that resemble hairs and cannot be scraped off. Diagnosis is made by visual inspection of the lesion. OHL is not usually bothersome to the client and may regress spontaneously. No treatment is necessary for most cases of OHL; however, oral acyclovir (Zovirax) may be given to selected clients.
Avoid Mouthwash w/ (Alcohol)

Nursing Management

Assess oral cavity frequently. Assist with oral hygiene before and after meals. Administer prescribed medications. Teach client to avoid mouthwashes containing alcohol or glycerine because they are very drying.

Figure 44-6 *Oral Candidiasis (Thrush)*

Figure 44-7 *Oral Hairy Leukoplakia (Courtesy of Dr. Joseph Konzelman, School of Dentistry, Medical College of Georgia)*

NURSING PROCESS

Assessment

Subjective Data

Assess the client's symptoms and oral hygiene habits. Ask about recent nutritional intake, use of alcohol and tobacco, and current medications.

Objective Data

Assess the client's lips, tongue, and buccal mucosal surfaces for lesions, white cheesy patches, and bleeding. Note any difficulty swallowing.

A nursing diagnosis for an HIV-positive client with oral manifestations may be:

Nursing Diagnoses	Planning/Goals	Nursing Interventions
Impaired Oral Mucous Membrane, related to oral lesions	The client will be free from oral lesions.	Administer prescribed medications. Frequently assess the oral cavity. Provide oral hygiene with a small soft toothbrush before and after meals. Instruct client to avoid commercial mouthwashes containing alcohol or glycerine.

Evaluation Each goal must be evaluated to determine how it has been met by the client.

GYNECOLOGICAL OPPORTUNISTIC INFECTIONS

Gynecological infections discussed include vaginal candidiasis and cervical intraepithelial neoplasia.

VAGINAL CANDIDIASIS — Plain Yogurt

Vaginal candidiasis is a fungal infection caused by *Candida albicans*. It is the most common initial infection occurring in HIV-infected women. Clinical manifestations include a white, clumped-appearing vaginal discharge, vaginal wall inflammation, and vaginal itching. Diagnosis is made by microscopic identification of yeast.

Most cases of vaginal candidiasis are treated with topical antifungal agents such as clotrimazole (Gyne-Lotrimin). For clients who do not respond to treatment with clotrimazole, ketoconazole (Nizoral) or fluconazole (Diflucan) is recommended.

CERVICAL INTRAEPITHELIAL NEOPLASIA

Women infected with HIV have a much higher incidence of cervical intraepithelial neoplasia (CIN) than women who are not infected. CIN and cancer of the cervix are considered to be on a continuum of abnormal cervical cells, ranging from mild abnormality (Grade I) to severe abnormality and cancer (Grade III). CIN in HIV-infected women progresses more rapidly and is less responsive to standard treatments than in noninfected women. Factors related to increased risk of CIN in HIV-positive women include a decreased number of CD4 T-cells and infection with human papilloma virus (HPV). It is thought that HIV activates HPV, causing cellular abnormalities.

The early stages of CIN have no symptoms. Clinical manifestations of cervical cancer include painless post-coital bleeding and blood-tinged vaginal discharge. As CIN progresses, back pain, abdominal or pelvic pain, weight loss, anorexia, and leg edema caused by obstruction of lymph nodes may occur. Initial diagnosis is made by Pap smear to determine the presence of abnormal cells. Clients with abnormal Pap smears are referred for cervical biopsy and colposcopy.

Treatment for CIN includes laser therapy, conization, and hysterectomy. Treatment for invasive cervical cancer depends on the stage of the disease and may include chemotherapy, surgery, and radiation.

Nursing Management

Encourage the client to have a Pap test every 6 months, to keep vaginal area clean and dry, and to wear loose-fitting cotton underwear. Inquire about bleeding following sexual intercourse, pelvic and abdominal pain, and vaginal itching or discharge.

NURSING PROCESS

Assessment

Subjective Data

Assess the client's history of symptoms, and ask the client about bleeding after intercourse, abdominal and pelvic pain, and vaginal itching or discharge.

Objective Data

Assess vaginal discharge for white or blood-tinged secretions. Note weight loss and edema.

Nursing diagnoses for a female HIV-positive client with gynecological manifestations may include the following:

Nursing Diagnoses	Planning/Goals	Nursing Interventions
Impaired Tissue Integrity related to vaginal mucosal lesions	The client will be free of vaginal infections.	Teach the client to have Pap smears every 6 months. Assess the frequency and consistency of vaginal discharge. Teach client to keep the vaginal area clean and dry and to wear loose-fitting cotton underwear to prevent irritation.
Disturbed Body Image related to chronic vaginal infections or surgery, radiation, or removal of cervix	The client will verbalize feelings and concerns about body image.	Encourage client to verbalize feelings and concerns about body image. Refer client to a support group for women with HIV.

Evaluation Each goal must be evaluated to determine how it has been met by the client.

CENTRAL NERVOUS SYSTEM OPPORTUNISTIC INFECTIONS

Disorders covered include AIDS dementia complex, toxoplasmosis, and cryptococcosis.

AIDS DEMENTIA COMPLEX

The most common central nervous system complication in persons with AIDS is AIDS dementia complex (ADC). This disorder is chronic and progressive, with cognitive, motor, and behavioral dysfunction. ADC is caused by infection of glial cells in the brain with HIV. Signs and symptoms are sometimes vague during the initial stages of ADC. Early signs include poor concentration, forgetfulness, loss of balance, leg weakness, apathy, and social withdrawal. Clients with advanced ADC may exhibit psychotic behaviors and delirium and progress to a catatonic-like state with minimal responsiveness to the environment.

Diagnosis is made by neurological testing of cognitive, motor, and behavioral functioning. Other diagnostic tests include brain imaging to look for cerebral atrophy. Cerebrospinal fluid analysis can show elevated proteins and will exclude other pathogens. Clients treated with zidovudine (Retrovir) have shown improvement in cognitive and motor skills, but the effect lasts only about 12 months (Lisanti & Zwolski, 1997).

TOXOPLASMOSIS

Toxoplasmosis is caused by the protozoan *Toxoplasma gondii*. Cats and other animals serve as a reservoir for this organism. It is spread to humans by ingestion of oocytes found in contaminated water, soil, or food, especially raw or undercooked meat. After entering the body, *Toxoplasma gondii* reproduces and spreads via the blood or lymph system. A person with an intact immune system may have no symptoms or mild symptoms, and the organism may remain dormant for years. In the immunocompromised person, the infection may be reacti-

vated (secondary) or occur with the ingestion of oocytes from contaminated sources. Clinical signs and symptoms may be vague and nonspecific, or range from a mild headache, fever, and lethargy to poor coordination, seizures, and coma. Diagnosis is made by identification of a lesion through brain imaging (computerized tomography or magnetic resonance imaging), presence of serum antibodies to *Toxoplasma gondii*, and recent onset of a neurologic abnormality.

The treatment of choice is oral pyrimethamine (Daraprim) and sulfadiazine (Microsulfon). Lifelong suppressive therapy of pyrimethamine plus sulfadiazine and leukovorin calcium (Wellcovorin) is needed.

CRYPTOCOCCOSIS

Cryptococcosis is a fungal infection caused by *Cryptococcus neoformans*. Cryptococcosis is the most life-threatening fungal infection associated with AIDS (Lisanti & Zwolski, 1997). The organism is acquired in the environment, usually from bird droppings. In the noncompromised host, the fungus is inhaled and contained in the lungs. In the immunocompromised host with AIDS, *Cryptococcus neoformans* can be disseminated, remain in the lungs, or infect the brain and meninges. Clinical manifestations include fever, headache, nausea and vomiting, dizziness, photophobia, mental status changes, seizures, and a stiff neck. Detection of cryptococcal antigen in cerebrospinal fluid, urine, or blood can be used for diagnosis. If untreated, this condition is fatal.

Treatment for acute cryptococcal infections includes intravenous amphotericin B (Fungizone Intravenous) to be given for at least 2 weeks, followed by fluconazole (Diflucan) for 10 to 12 weeks. Once treatment for acute infection is complete, lifelong suppressive therapy with oral fluconazole daily is recommended (Lisanti & Zwolski, 1997).

Nursing Management

Monitor client for forgetfulness, poor concentration, loss of balance, leg weakness, social withdrawal, apathy, stiff neck, seizures, nausea, and headache. Assess vital signs. Provide cues for orientation (e.g., calendar, clock) and a structured environment and activities for social interaction.

NURSING PROCESS

Assessment

Subjective Data

Ask the client about forgetfulness, missing appointments, ability to complete activities of daily living, and if there have been any recent falls or accidents. Ask the client's family and significant others about behavior changes such as social withdrawal or unusual behavior.

Objective Data

Assess the client for subtle mental status changes such as poor concentration and inability to remember instructions or previous conversations. Assess the client for motor impairment such as dropping things, poor coordination, or changes in writing ability. Assess the client's ability to remember usual medication schedule. Observe the environment for safety.

Nursing diagnoses for an HIV-positive client with central nervous system manifestations include the following:

Nursing Diagnoses	Planning/Goals	Nursing Interventions
Disturbed Thought Processes, related to mental status changes	The client will maintain cognitive functioning.	Assess client's mental and neurologic status and emotional, cognitive, and motor skills. Provide cues for orientation (clock, calendar). Monitor client for adherence to medical regimen.
Social Isolation related to alteration in mental status	The client will have contact and interact with significant others.	Encourage family and significant others to visit client. Provide structured activities and environment for social interaction. Encourage client to verbalize feelings and concerns.

Evaluation Each goal must be evaluated to determine how it has been met by the client.

OPPORTUNISTIC MALIGNANCIES

Kaposi's sarcoma and non-Hodgkin's lymphoma are discussed.

KAPOSI'S SARCOMA

Kaposi's sarcoma (KS) is a vascular malignancy that can occur any place in the body, including internal organs. The first lesions often appear subtly on the face or in the oral cavity. The more immunosuppressed the person is, the more aggressive the spread of KS. Clinical manifestations of KS are red to purple lesions, which are painless, nonblanching, and palpable (Figure 44-8). These lesions are sometimes mistaken for bruises. Edema in the face, penis, scrotum, and legs can occur as a result of blockages in the lymphatic system. KS can also be found in the GI tract and lungs. Diagnosis is made by tissue biopsy.

Treatment involves a variety of options depending on whether the lesions are local or systemic. Radiation therapy, intralesional therapy with interferon alpha 2a or 2b (Roferon A, Intron A) or vinblastine sulfate (Velban), laser therapy, and cryotherapy are used on single or iso-

Figure 44-8 *Kaposi's Sarcoma (Courtesy of Daniel J. Barbaro, MD, Fort Worth, Texas)*

lated KS lesions. For clients with advanced widespread symptomatic disease, single or combination chemotherapeutic regimens include vinblastine sulfate (Velban), vincristine sulfate (Oncovin), etoposide (VePesid), bleomycin sulfate (Blenoxane), doxorubicin Hcl (Rubex), and mitoxantrone Hcl (Novantrone).

NON-HODGKIN'S LYMPHOMA

Lymphomas are malignant tumors of the immune system. B-cells are the origin of malignancy for most clients with AIDS-related non-Hodgkin's lymphoma (NHL). Clinical manifestations are nonspecific and may include fever, night sweats, and weight loss. Confusion, lethargy, and memory loss may be present in persons with CNS involvement.

Diagnosis of NHL is complicated because of the nonspecific symptoms. Examination of tissue is the recommended diagnostic procedure. There is no standard treatment of NHL. Individualized treatment may include a combination of chemotherapy, antiretroviral agents, prophylaxis against opportunistic infections, and colony-stimulating factors to enhance bone marrow production of blood cells; however, in many clients with advanced HIV disease, treatment of NHL is withheld because it is not tolerated well and may even lead to earlier death.

Nursing Management

Assess client for fever, night sweats, weight loss, confusion, lethargy, memory loss, and ability to perform ADLs. Emphasize no scratching of skin lesions, not using drying soaps, and making sure clothing and linens are thoroughly rinsed of detergent. Encourage significant others to participate in the client's care. Provide access to clergy, social worker, or HIV counselor.

NURSING PROCESS

Assessment

Subjective Data

Ask the client about frequency, onset, and persistence of current symptoms. Note the effect of current symptoms on ability to perform activities of daily living and relationships with others, as well as the effect of treatment plan on quality of life.

Objective Data

Assess skin lesions. Document increased frequency, intensity, or recurrence of nonspecific symptoms, including fever, night sweats, and weight loss.

Nursing diagnoses for an HIV-positive client with a malignancy may include the following:

Nursing Diagnoses	Planning/Goals	Nursing Interventions
Risk for Impaired Skin Integrity, related to lesions or treatment	The client will maintain skin integrity.	Teach client to avoid scratching skin lesions, to avoid drying soaps, and to make sure clothing and linen have been thoroughly rinsed of detergent.
Social Isolation related to change in appearance	The client will maintain usual social interactions and identify factors that enhance quality of life.	Facilitate the client's interaction with others.
		Keep client and significant others aware of treatment plan. Encourage significant others to participate in the care of the client.
		Encourage physical closeness between the client and significant others.
		Provide client with access to clergy, social worker, or HIV counselor. Encourage the client to join a support group or obtain peer support.
		Assist client in identifying positive coping strategies.

Evaluation Each goal must be evaluated to determine how it has been met by the client.

CASE STUDY

Jim Hayes, a 37-year-old male, suspects that he is HIV positive. He enters the medical unit with chronic symptoms such as fever, night sweats, diarrhea, weight loss, shortness of breath, and a nonproductive cough. On the initial assessment, he is alert and oriented, color is pale, temperature 100.6°F, pulse 92, respirations 36, and blood pressure 140/70. He has generalized lymphadenopathy. His height is 5'11", and his weight is 125 pounds. Jim states that he is not currently taking any medications, although he is "familiar" with the drug zidovudine (Retrovir).

The following questions will guide your development of a nursing care plan for the case study.

1. List symptoms/clinical manifestations, other than Mr. Hayes's, that a client may experience when HIV positive.
2. List two reasons zidovudine (Retrovir) may be initiated for Mr. Hayes.
3. List two diagnostic tests that will confirm the diagnosis of HIV.
4. List subjective and objective data the nurse would want to obtain about Mr. Hayes.
5. Write three individual nursing diagnoses and goals for Mr. Hayes.
6. List pertinent nursing actions the nurse would perform in caring for Mr. Hayes related to:
   hydration
   fatigue
   nutrition
   oxygenation
   medications
7. List resources that could assist Mr. Hayes with his diagnosis.
8. List teaching Mr. Hayes will need before leaving the medical unit.

Summary

- The immune system identifies substances as self or nonself and protects the body by neutralizing or destroying foreign organisms.
- Immunity to a disease is either natural or acquired.
- Age, sex, nutritional status, medications, and stress influence the immune response.
- Clients receiving blood transfusions must be carefully monitored, especially during the first half-hour, for signs of a reaction.
- Anaphylactic reactions, which may occur as a result of exposure to foods, medications, blood, or insect bites, can potentially be life-threatening.
- Organ transplant clients must understand the implications of taking immunosuppressive medications.
- Clients with rheumatoid arthritis must be taught methods of adapting to the effects of synovial joint inflammation, immobility, and deformity.
- Systemic lupus erythematosus affects multiple body systems.
- Clients with myasthenia gravis experience extreme muscle weakness and fatigue and must be carefully monitored for signs of respiratory distress, and myasthenic or cholinergic crisis.
- Diagnosis of HIV/AIDS is made by the ELISA and Western blot test. These tests determine the presence of antibodies to HIV, not the virus itself.

- *Pneumocystis carinii* pneumonia is the most common opportunistic infection associated with HIV.
- Oral candidiasis can be painful and interfere with the client's nutritional status.
- AIDS dementia complex is a progressive disorder with cognitive, motor, and behavioral dysfunction.

Review Questions

1. Ms. Caldwell has just been diagnosed with syphilis and has an order for 1,000,000 units of penicillin IM. She has no history of allergies to medications. She has never had penicillin. When giving her the injection in the right upper outer quadrant of her buttocks, you note a tattoo. Several minutes after receiving the injection, she tells you she feels anxious and weak. You note she is diaphoretic, scratching her forearm, and is breathing faster than normal. Based upon this assessment data, you would conclude:

   a. she is embarrassed because you saw her tattoo.
   b. she is probably anxious since you know she has a sexually transmitted disease.
   c. her syphilis is getting worse.
   d. these are early signs of an anaphylactic reaction.

2. Which of the following statements shows that the client understands a diagnosis of HIV positive?

   a. "Being HIV positive means that I have AIDs."

b. "Since I am only HIV positive, I cannot infect others."

c. "Because I am HIV positive, I have the virus that causes AIDS."

d. "I became infected by donating blood."

3. The nurse is caring for a client who is experiencing diarrhea and weight loss. Which of the following nursing interventions is appropriate for him?

a. Encourage fluids with meals.

b. Substitute a milk shake for lunch.

c. Offer small, frequent meals.

d. Suggest he eat more sweets.

4. The nurse is caring for a client who asks when zidovudine (Retrovir) is normally started. Which of the following would be the nurse's correct response?

a. When the client becomes symptomatic

b. When CD4 level reaches $500/mm^3$

c. After the client's first opportunistic infection

d. As soon as the client is diagnosed as HIV positive

5. The nurse is discussing transmission of HIV with a client. Which of the following statements indicates that the client needs more education?

a. "I should not share needles with anyone."

b. "I can spread the virus through sexual contact."

c. "I can no longer donate blood."

d. "I should not hug or kiss anyone."

References/Suggested Readings

Aids Treatment Data Network. (1999, May). *Viral load tests* [Online]. Available: www.aidsinfonyc.org/network/simple/viral.html

Arnold, L. (2001). Living with AIDS. *Nursing2001, 31*(10), 53.

Arthritis Foundation. (2002). *Rheumatoid arthritis* [Online]. Available: www.arthritis.org/conditions/DiseaseCenter/ra.asp

Arthritis Foundation. (2003). *Systemic lupus erythematosus (SLE)*. [Online]. Available: www.arthritis.org/conditions/DiseaseCenter/lupus.asp

Barbarito, C. (1999). Anaphylaxis. *AJN 99*(1), 33.

Barroso, J. (2002). HIV-related fatigue. *AJN, 102*(5), 83–86.

Bradley-Springer, L. (2001). HIV Prevention: What works? *AJN, 101*(6), 45–50.

Bursaw, M., Keenan, K., & Ehrhart, M. (2001). HIV update. *Nursing2001, 31*(2), 62–63.

Burt, S. (1998). What you need to know about latex allergy, *Nursing98, 28*(10), 33–39.

Carroll, P. (2001). Anaphylaxis. *RN, 64*(12), 45–49.

Cohen, S. (2001). Myths & Facts . . . about latex allergy. *Nursing2001, 31*(2), 76.

Coyne, P., Lyne, M., & Watson, A. (2002). Symptom management in people with AIDS. *AJN, 102*(9), 48–55.

D'Arcy, Y. (2002). How to treat arthritis pain. *Nursing2002, 32*(7), 30–31.

Daniels, R. (2002). *Delmar's Guide to Laboratory and Diagnostic Tests*. Clifton Park, NY: Thomson Delmar Learning.

Daughtry, L., Bankston, J., & Deshotels, J. (2002). HIV meds: Keeping trouble at bay. *RN, 65*(2), 31–35.

Dochterman, J., & Bulechek, G. (2004). *Nursing Interventions Classification (NIC)* (4th ed.). St. Louis, MO: Mosby.

Estes, M. E. Z. (2002). *Health Assessment & Physical Examination* (2nd ed.). Clifton Park, NY: Thomson Delmar Learning.

Food & Drug Administration (FDA). (2002). *FDA approves new rapid HIV test kit*. [Online]. Available: www.fda.gov/bbs/topics/NEWS/22002/NEW00852.html

Guyton, A. C., & Hall, J. E. (2000). *Textbooks of medical physiology* (10th ed.). Philadelphia: W. B. Saunders.

Halzemer, W. (2002). HIV and AIDS: The symptom experience. *AJN, 102*(4), 48–52.

Ignatavicius, D. D., & Workman, M. L. (2002). *Medical–Surgical Nursing: Critical Thinking for Collaborative Care* (4th ed.). Philadelphia: W. B. Saunders.

Jones, S. (2001). Taking HAART: How to support patients with HIV/AIDS. *Nursing2001, 31*(2), 36–41.

Jurewicz, M. (2000). Anaphylaxis: When the body overreacts. *Nursing2000, 30*(7), 58.

Kirsten, V., & Whipple, B. (1998). Treating HIV disease: Hope on the horizon. *Nursing98, 28*(11), 34-39.

Lenehan, G. (2002). Latex allergy: Separating fact from fiction. *Nursing2002, 32*(3), 58–63.

Lenehan, G. (2003). Latex allergy. *Nursing2003, 33*(6), 54–55.

Lisanti, P., & Zwolski, K. (1997). Understanding the devastation of AIDS. *AJN, 97*(7), 27–34.

Litton, K. (2003). Defenses gone awry: Lupus. *RN, 66*(3), 53–59.

Lupus Foundation of America (LFA). (2001). *Lupus Fact Sheet* [Online]. Available: www.lupus.org/education/factsheet.html

Mahot, G. (1998). Rheumatoid arthritis. *AJN, 98*(12), 42–43.

Moorhead, S., Johnson, M., & Maas, M. (2004). *Nursing Outcomes Classification (NOC)* (3rd ed.). St. Louis, MO: Mosby.

Mumu, R. D., Lyons, D. A., Borucki, M. J., & Pollard, R. B. (1994). *HIV manual for health care professionals*. Norwalk, CT: Appleton & Lange.

Myasthenia Gravis Foundation of America, Inc. (2001a). *Facts about autoimmune myasthenia gravis for patients & families*. [Online]. Available: www.myasthenis.org/information/facts.pdf

Myasthenia Gravis Foundation of America, Inc. (2001b). *Nutrition and myasthenia gravis*. [Online]. Available: www.myasthenia.org/information/Nutrition/pdf

National Heart, Lung, and Blood Institute (NHLBI). (1999, July) *Use of autologous blood* [Online]. Available: www.nhlbi.nih.gov/nhlbi/blood/transf/prof/transhc.htm

National Institute of Allergy and Infectious Diseases (NIAID). (2002a). *Asthma and Allergy Statistics* [Online]. Available: www.niaid.gov/factsheets/allergystat/htm

National Institute of Allergy and Infectious Diseases (NIAID). (2002b). *HIV/AIDS statistics* [Online]. Available: www.niaid.nih.gov/factsheets/aidsstat.htm

National Institute of Allergy and Infectious Diseases (NIAID). (2002c). *HIV infection and AIDS* [Online]. Available: www.niaid.nih.gov/factsheets/hivinf.htm

National Institute of Neurological Disorders and Stroke (NINDS). (2001a). *Myasthenia gravis*. [Online]. Available: www.ninds.nih.gov/health_and_medical/disorders/myasthenia_gravis.htm

National Institute of Neurological Disorders and Stroke (NINDS). (2001b). *Neurological sequelae of lupus* [Online]. Available: www.ninds.nih.gov/health_and_medical/disorders/lupus_doc.htm

New Mexico Aids Info Net. (2002). *Viral local tests*. [Online]. Available: www.aidsinfonet.org/articles.php?articleID=125

North American Nursing Diagnosis Association. (2003). *Nursing Diagnoses: Definitions & Classification 2003–2004*. Philadelphia: Author.

Paar, D. P. (1994). Hepatitis. In R.D. Mumu, M. J. Borucki, D. A. Lyons, & R. B. Pollard (Eds.). *HIV manual for health care professionals* (pp. 77–86). Norwalk, CT: Appleton & Lange.

Putman, J., & May, K. (2001). Relief for patients with severe allergies. *RN, 64*(6), 26–30.

Spratto, G., & Woods, A. (2004). *2004 PDR Nurses' Drug Handbook.* Clifton Park, NY: Thomson Delmar Learning.

Trzcianowska, H., & Mortensen, E. (2001). HIV and AIDS: Separating fact from fiction. *AJN, 101*(6), 53–59.

Ungvarski, P. J., & Flaskerud, J. H. (1999). *HIV/AIDS: A guide to primary care management* (4th ed.). Philadelphia: W.B. Saunders.

United Network for Organ Sharing (UNOS). (2003). *Home page: Statistics.* [Online]. Available: www.unos.org

Veronesi, J. (2003). Rheumatoid arthritis. *RN, 66*(8), 46–52.

Yee, C. (2002). Getting a grip on myasthenia gravis. *Nursing2002, 32*(1), 32hn1–32hn4.

Resources

AIDS Treatment Data Network, 611 Broadway, Suite 613, New York, NY 10012, 212-260-8868, www.atdn.org

The American Academy of Allergy, Asthma, and Immunology, 611 E. Wells Street, Milwaukee, WI 53202, 414-272-6071, www.aaaai.org/

American Association of Blood Banks, 8101 Glenbrook Road, Bethesda, MD 20814-2749, 301-907-6977, www.aabb.org

American College of Rheumatology/Association of Rheumatology Health Professionals, 1800 Century Place, Suite 250, Atlanta, GA 30345-4300, 404-633-3777, www.rheumatology.org

American Latex Allergy Association, P. O. Box 13930, Milwaukee, WI 53213-0930, 888-972-5378, www.latexallergyresources.org

Arthritis Foundation, P.O. Box 7669, Atlanta, GA 30357, 800-283-7800, www.arthritis.org

Association of Nurses in AIDS Care, 11250 Roger Bacon Drive, Suite #8, Reston, VA, 20190-5202, 800-260-6780, www.anacnet.org

Asthma and Allergy Foundation of America, 1233 Twentieth Street, N.W., Suite 402, Washington, DC 20036, 800-7ASTHMA, www.aafa.org

CDC National STD & AIDS Hotlines, 800-342-2437; Spanish, 800-344-7432; Deaf, 900-243-7889

Lupus Foundation of America, Inc., 1300 Piccard Drive, Suite 200, Rockville, MD 20850-4303, 800-558-0121, 301-670-9292, www.lupus.org

Myasthenia Gravis Foundation of America, 5841 Cedar Lake Road, Suite 209, Minneapolis, MN 55416, 800-541-5454, www.myasthenia.org

National Institute of Arthritis and Musculoskeletal and Skin Diseases (NIAMS), 1 AMS Circle, Bethesda, MD 20892-3675, 877-226-4267, www.niams.nih.gov

United Network for Organ Sharing, P. O. Box 2484, Richmond, VA 23218, 888-894-6361, www.unos.org

UNIT
15

Nursing Care of the Client: Physical and Mental Integrity

Chapter 45
Mental Illness

Chapter 46
Substance Abuse

MENTAL ILLNESS

LEARNING OBJECTIVES

Upon completion of this chapter, you should be able to:
- Define key terms.
- Identify and describe the components of a therapeutic nurse–client relationship.
- Cite nursing interventions for working with clients who are angry, aggressive, homicidal, and/or suicidal.
- Detail nursing interventions for working with clients who are experiencing anxiety.
- Identify and explain the potential side effects associated with antianxiety medications.
- Recount nursing interventions for working with clients who are depressed.
- Identify and explain the potential side effects associated with antidepressant medications.
- Detail nursing interventions for working with clients who have schizophrenia.
- Identify and explain the potential side effects associated with antipsychotic medications.
- Detail nursing interventions for working with clients who have bipolar disorder.
- Identify and explain the potential side effects associated with mood stabilizers.
- Cite nursing interventions for working with clients who have attention-deficit/hyperactivity disorder.
- Recount nursing interventions for working with clients who have been neglected or abused or who have been exposed to domestic violence.
- Discuss nursing interventions for working with clients who have an eating disorder.

KEY TERMS

abuse
actively suicidal
affect
anger-control assistance
anxiety
anxiolytic
auditory hallucination
brief dynamic therapy
cognitive-behavior therapy
command hallucination
crisis
cycling
delusion
depression
domestic violence
electroconvulsive therapy
empathy
euphoric
flashback
genuineness
hallucination
hypervigilant

hypomania
mania
mental disorder
mental illness
mood
neglect
paradoxical reaction
physically aggressive
pressured speech
psychoanalysis
psychosis
psychotherapy
rapport
respect
seclusion
serum lithium level
startle response
suicidal ideation
tolerance
trust
verbally aggressive
visual hallucination
word salad

INTRODUCTION

Because they will encounter clients who are emotionally disturbed and/or mentally ill, it is imperative that nurses understand and feel comfortable working with such individuals—not just on psychiatric units, but in all types of circumstances and settings. This chapter is designed to give LP/VNs a beginning knowledge base regarding mental health and illness and to better prepare them for working with individuals who are in a state of crisis or who have emotional needs and/or psychiatric problems.

As the nurse becomes more knowledgeable about mental illness, opportunities arise to increase self-awareness and to examine any personal experiences, preconceived ideas, or prejudices that might negatively affect the nurse's ability to work effectively with clients. For example, the nurse who has some unresolved issues regarding sexuality or becomes embarrassed when discussing sexuality will probably be uncomfortable talking about the potential problems in sexual functioning secondary to antidepressant therapy. Examining personal ideas and prejudices before working with clients will facilitate a positive nurse–client relationship.

MENTAL HEALTH AND ILLNESS

In general, a person is considered mentally healthy when he possesses knowledge of himself; meets his basic needs; assumes responsibility for his behavior; has learned to integrate thoughts, feelings, and actions; can successfully resolve conflicts; maintains relationships; communicates directly with others; respects others; and adapts to change. **Mental illness** occurs when an individual is not able to view self clearly or has a distorted view of self; is unable to maintain satisfying personal relationships; and is unable to adapt to the environment (Frisch & Frisch, 2002). The American Psychiatric Association defines **mental disorder** as "clinically significant behavior or psychological syndrome or pattern that occurs in an individual and is associated with present distress (i.e., negative response to stimuli that are perceived as threatening) or disability (i.e., impairment in one or more important areas of functioning) or with a significantly increased risk of suffering, death, pain, disability, or an important loss of freedom."

One of the ways to conceptualize psychiatric disorders is to think of a continuum, with mental health being situated at one end and mental illness at the other (Figure 45-1). Between these two extremes lie a variety of psychiatric disorders ranging in nature from mild to severe. The fourth edition of the *Diagnostic and Statistical Manual of Mental Disorders* (better known as the *DSM-IV*) (American Psychiatric Association [APA], 2000) is the reference tool used to identify and establish psychiatric diagnoses. The psychiatrist is the individual most often involved in this process, although other mental health care practitioners may give input and make recommendations for diagnoses.

One of the primary roles of the nurse in working with clients who have mental illness is that of teaching. The

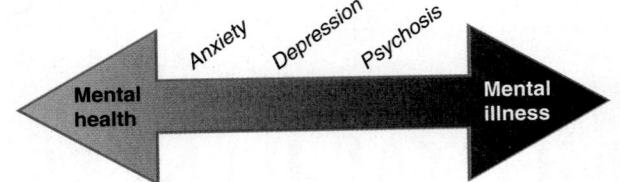

Figure 45-1 *Mental Health Continuum*

nurse is responsible not only for teaching clients about their illnesses, including the probable courses of their given disorders, but also for adequately preparing and educating the client's family. The nurse is usually the first individual to have contact with the family and is most often the one with whom family members maintain consistent contact. Because of the highly personal and sensitive nature of mental disorders, the concept of confidentiality, the nondisclosure of the identity of or personal information about an individual, is vitally important in psychiatric nursing.

RELATIONSHIP DEVELOPMENT

Psychiatric nursing differs from some of the other fields of nursing in that the primary skill the nurse employs is what is referred to as "the therapeutic use of self." Many theorists such as Rogers and Peplau have been instrumental in identifying and exploring the factors that significantly influence the development of therapeutic relationships. Townsend (2000) identifies five components necessary to the development of a therapeutic working relationship and of particular importance in the therapeutic nurse–client relationship. These five components are trust, rapport, respect, genuineness, and empathy.

Trust

Trust is the ability to rely on an individual's character and ability. Trust must be present for help to be given and received. A therapeutic relationship is firmly rooted in trust. Three major activities facilitate the development of trust: consistency, respect, and honesty. Consistency includes following through on plans, adhering to the schedule, being straightforward with no hidden motives, and seeking extra time for client interaction. Respect includes addressing clients the way they wish to be addressed (e.g., Mr., Mrs., Ms., first name), listening to the clients, and providing clear explanations. Honesty includes keeping promises and maintaining confidentiality. Being consistently trustworthy is an expression of the nurse's personal integrity and builds the foundation for nursing effectiveness (Figure 45-2).

Many clients with emotional and/or psychiatric problems have great difficulty trusting and having confidence that others will be good to their word. They may have been lied to or hurt in the past, and this makes it difficult for them to trust again, even with health care professionals who are trying to help them. It is very important, therefore, that the nurse fulfill any promise made to the client.

Figure 45-2 *Spending time with the client one-to-one helps promote a trusting relationship.*

Figure 45-3 *Through empathic listening, the nurse can reach an understanding of the client's experience and help the client see the positive aspects of the experience.*

Rapport

Rapport is a bond or connection between two people that is based on mutual trust. Such a bond does not just happen spontaneously; it is planned by the nurse, who purposefully implements behaviors that promote trust. The nurse sets the tone of the relationship by creating an atmosphere wherein the client feels free to express feelings. When seeking to develop trust, the nurse acts in a manner that indicates recognition of the client as a unique individual and reinforces that individuality. Such actions, which serve to humanize the client, are therapeutic. To establish rapport, the nurse must show that the client is important. Actions are implemented to boost the level of the client's self-esteem. Nonverbal interventions are of utmost importance in helping establish rapport. Interacting with family and significant others is also helpful in establishing rapport with the client. Recognizing the importance of the family and its influence on the healing process allows the nurse to bond with those who will encourage and support the client during recovery.

Respect

Respect is the acceptance of an individual as is, in a nonjudgmental manner. The concept of respect is an integral component of the nurse–client relationship. Respect means caring for clients whose value system may differ greatly from that of the nurse. To show respect, the nurse must not react with shock, surprise, or disapproval toward a client's lifestyle, dress, or behaviors. The nurse respects the client's choices and actions yet sets limits on unhealthy or undesirable behavior.

Genuineness

Genuineness (sincerity) is an attribute easily perceived by the client and can be the most significant aspect of the nurse–client relationship. Nurses are often concerned about whether they will say the right thing to a client; though saying the right thing is important,

more important is that the nurse be honest and genuine in communications with the client.

Empathy

Empathy (the ability to perceive and relate to another's personal experience) is an important quality necessary to successful nurse–client interactions. The empathic nurse understands that the client's perception of the situation is real to him. By perceiving the client's understanding of his own needs, the nurse is better able to assist the client in determining what will work best. Empathy enables the nurse to assist the client to become a fully participating partner in treatment, rather than a passive recipient of care. Through empathy, the nurse validates the experiences of the client (Figure 45-3).

THE CLIENT EXPERIENCING A CRISIS

In psychological terms, a **crisis** is a stressor that forces an individual to respond and/or adapt in some way. Emotions may intensify during a crisis situation or serious illness, and any situation or illness can potentially become a crisis if the stressors are severe enough. The understanding of crisis is particularly important in psychiatric and mental health nursing. A crisis taxes the individual's coping resources, and each person responds differently to seemingly identical situations. Crisis requires that an individual call on all of her personal skills as well as on the outside social and familial supports that she has built through her life (Frisch & Frisch, 2002). Each individual has personality strengths, interpersonal networks, and socioeconomic resources that offer some protection against the threat of crisis. When any (or all) of these protections are weak, however, a person's response to crisis may be dysfunctional, and the result may be one or more symptoms of mental illness. Although theories differ in their definitions of crisis and stress, it is generally accepted that most psychiatric problems result from or are strongly influenced by the interaction of stress and overwhelmed coping mechanisms (Frisch & Frisch, 2002). The client experiencing crisis may be anxious, angry, aggressive, homicidal, suicidal, psychotic, or any combination of these.

ANXIETY

Anxiety is a state wherein a person feels a strong sense of dread frequently accompanied by physical symptoms of increased heart and respiratory rates and elevated blood pressure in the absence of a specific source or reason for these emotions or responses. Nurses frequently encounter clients and family members who are anxious because of alterations in or threats to health and physical well-being. Peplau (1963) identifies four escalating stages of anxiety beginning with mild anxiety, moving to moderate anxiety, followed by severe anxiety, and, finally, to the stage of panic, if not effectively treated. Intervention can occur at any point along the continuum, preferably before the stages of severe anxiety or panic are reached.

MILD ANXIETY

The mildly anxious client is beginning to experience some of the signs and symptoms of anxiety, such as irritability and restlessness; however, the person is still able to concentrate and focus on the task at hand. In fact, *mild* anxiety can actually benefit an individual as far as enhancing performance ability (Townsend, 2000).

MODERATE ANXIETY

The individual with moderate anxiety experiences additional physiologic and cognitive symptoms. Blood pressure, pulse, and respirations increase, and the client becomes diaphoretic. The moderately anxious individual begins to have difficulty concentrating or learning new material. This is important to recognize before teaching a client about a medication or test, or performing a procedure. Before teaching can be effective, the client must be assisted in lowering the level of anxiety (Townsend, 2000).

SEVERE ANXIETY

Severely anxious clients are significantly impaired in several areas. Their ability to cognitively process material may drastically diminish, they may experience tunnel vision, their focus may become very limited, and the physiologic symptoms of anxiety become much more pronounced. Clients at this high level of anxiety are often very fearful and may be irrational in their thought processes (Townsend, 2000).

PANIC

The individual experiencing panic may begin to manifest symptoms of **psychosis** (losing touch with reality), such as **delusions** (false beliefs that misrepresent reality) and/or **hallucinations** (perceptions that something is present when it is not, e.g., hearing voices that are not really there). The individual with this level of anxiety requires constant reassurance, monitoring, and supervision to maintain safety (Townsend, 2000).

ANXIETY DISORDERS

Some of the most common psychiatric diagnoses related to anxiety are Generalized Anxiety Disorder, Panic Disorder, Obsessive-Compulsive Disorder, and Post-Traumatic Stress Disorder. It is estimated that 19 million adult Americans have an anxiety disorder (Anxiety Disorders Association of America, 2002a).

GENERALIZED ANXIETY DISORDER

The client with generalized anxiety disorder (GAD) exhibits symptoms of excessive anxiety or dread. Clients usually realize that their symptoms are out of proportion to any real threat. The symptoms include three or more of the following: restlessness, easy fatigue, difficulty concentrating, irritability, muscle tension, and sleep disturbance. For anxiety to be termed excessive, clients must experience symptoms frequently over a period of 6 months or more.

PANIC DISORDER

Panic disorder is diagnosed when the client experiences at least two panic attacks followed by at least 1 month's concern about having another panic attack (ADAA, 2002c). These attacks begin abruptly and peak within 10 minutes and are characterized by a set of any four of the following symptoms: palpitations or rapid heart rate, sweating, trembling, shortness of breath, sensation of choking, chest pain, nausea, dizziness, fear of losing control, fear of dying, numbness or tingling, chills or hot flushes, and some sense of altered reality. The client has a strong desire to run away or escape from the situation that triggered the attack. In some individuals, the attack is brought about by specific stimuli or a particular setting, for example the dentist's office. In others, the attacks come on "out of the blue."

OBSESSIVE-COMPULSIVE DISORDER

In obsessive-compulsive disorder (OCD), the individual has persistent, recurring thoughts or impulses (obsessions) that are intrusive or inappropriate, causing anxiety or fears leading the individual to perform repetitive behaviors or rituals (compulsions) to neutralize the anxiety caused by the obsession. The obsessions and/or compulsions must take up at least 1 hour a day and interfere with the individual's normal routine, occupation, social activities, or relationships (ADAA, 2002b).

POST-TRAUMATIC STRESS DISORDER

Clients suffering from post-traumatic stress disorder (PTSD) have experienced a serious trauma. Being severely beaten or emotionally, physically, or sexually abused or living through or witnessing a catastrophic event or natural disaster such as a flood, earthquake, hurricane, or plane crash might lead to PTSD. The response to the trauma must have been one of fear or helplessness, and the event is persistently reexperienced through recurrent recollections, dreams, or hallucinatory-like flashbacks. Individuals with this disorder have symptoms for more than 1 month and exhibit impairment of social functioning, anxiety symptoms, avoidance of stimuli associated with the trauma, and a general numbness. More than 5 million Americans are diagnosed with PTSD (ADAA, 2002d).

Medical–Surgical Management

Medical

Psychotherapy (the treatment of mental and emotional disorders through psychological rather than physical methods) continues to be widely used in the treatment of anxiety disorders. Psychotherapy can be viewed as falling into two general categories: those therapies based on helping individuals achieve insight into *why* they feel anxiety and those that emphasize behavioral means of controlling the anxiety.

Psychotherapy based on insight into symptoms may sometimes be valuable, especially for highly motivated individuals whose symptoms are not disabling. **Psychoanalysis** (therapy focused on uncovering unconscious memories and processes) is among the best known of the insight therapies and has been widely employed to assist persons with anxiety.

In contrast, there is strong empirical evidence that behaviorally based treatments are effective in treating at least some anxiety disorders. Cognitive-behavior therapy often results in significant benefit for persons suffering from panic attacks. **Cognitive-behavior therapy** assumes that clients can learn to identify the common stimuli that create their anxiety, develop plans to respond to those stimuli with nonanxious responses, and problem solve when unanticipated anxiety-provoking situations arise. Although insight is very much involved in this process, it is not insight into deep psychological causes, as in psychoanalysis, but rather, practical, commonsense problem solving. Treatment appears both to be effective during the relatively brief course of therapy and to remain effective for some months after therapy finishes. Sometimes medical and psychological follow-up are important to ensure satisfactory improvement.

CLIENT TEACHING

Antianxiety Medications

Be sure to instruct each client taking an antianxiety medication in the following:

- Do not increase the dose or frequency of the medication without consulting your physician.
- Tolerance develops quickly with the medication, and unsupervised use can lead to addiction.
- Do not drink alcohol while on the medication.
- Do not take any other medications unless prescribed by your physician.
- Do not stop taking the medication abruptly.
- Do not drive or operate heavy machinery while on the medication.

Pharmacological

The drugs of choice for treating clients with anxiety are usually the **anxiolytics,** or antianxiety agents (Table 45-1). Some of the antianxiety medications such as alprazolam (Xanax) and lorazepam (Ativan) may also be helpful in alleviating the symptoms of anxiety, nervousness, and sleeplessness frequently associated with panic disorder and PTSD.

Most of these medications can be used on either a routine or as-needed (PRN) basis and belong to the family of benzodiazepines. Onset of action for the benzodiazepines usually occurs within 30 minutes after oral administration, and most individuals respond favorably to these medications; that is, a reduction or cessation of the symptoms of anxiety is experienced.

Clients should be warned about the potential risk of addiction associated with antianxiety medications. These particular medications should be used with extreme caution because long-term use can lead to an increased **tolerance,** acquired resistance to the effects of the drug. Tolerance results in the need to increase the frequency and amount of medication in order to achieve the same benefit. Over time, this may cause a dependency on the medication, actually creating another serious problem for the client. Therefore, the antianxiety agents are usually indicated for short-term management of anxiety rather than for long-term use. The benefits of a particular medication for the client must always be weighed against the possible risk of addiction, particularly if long-term use is or may be indicated. The *one exception* is buspirone hydrochloride (BuSpar), a nonbenzodiazepine antianxiety medication, which does not appear to have any addictive potential; however, the therapeutic effectiveness of BuSpar is not reached for approximately 7 to 10 days; thus, although it can be given as a regularly scheduled antianxiety agent, BuSpar has absolutely no value as a PRN medication. When initiating therapy with BuSpar, another antianxiety medication such as alprazolam (Xanax) or lorazepam (Ativan) may be given concurrently until the therapeutic level is reached; then the other medication can be gradually decreased.

TABLE 45-1	ANTIANXIETY MEDICATIONS		
GENERIC NAME	**TRADE NAME**	**TYPE**	**POTENTIAL SIDE EFFECTS**
alprazolam	Xanax	Benzodiazepine	Dizziness, drowsiness, lethargy, physical and psychological dependence, tolerance
buspirone hydrochloride	BuSpar	Nonbenzodiazepine	Blurred vision, chest pain, clamminess, dizziness, drowsiness, excitement, fatigue, headache, insomnia, nasal congestion, numbness, myalgia, nausea, nervousness, palpitations, paresthesia, skin rashes, sore throat, syncope, tachycardia, tinnitus, incoordination, weakness
cloneazepam	Klonopin	Benzodiazepine	Ataxia, behavioral changes, drowsiness, physical and psychological dependence, tolerance
diazepam	Valium	Benzodiazepine	Dizziness, drowsiness, fatigue, hypotension, hypertension, CV collapse, dependence, tolerance
lorazepam	Ativan	Benzodiazepine	Agranulocytosis, CV collapse, dizziness, drowsiness, lethargy

Data from *2004 PDR Nurses' Drug Handbook*, by G. Spratto and A. Woods, 2004, Clifton Park, NY: Thomson Delmar Learning.

Activity

The anxious client's activity level may be negatively affected by both the anxiety disorder and the side effects of the prescribed medication. The side effects of sedation and drowsiness can pose safety hazards for certain activities and must be emphasized to the client.

Nursing Management

Remain with the client while fear level and/or anxiety level is high and speak in a calm, soothing voice. Reassure the client that she is in a safe place. Explore with the client what things are relaxing and calming. Teach the client relaxation exercises. Encourage participation in recreation or sports activities.

Do not touch the client with PTSD without permission. If the client is confused or disoriented, orient the client to reality.

NURSING PROCESS

Assessment

Subjective Data

Clients experiencing anxiety report problems concentrating, and fear that something dreadful is about to happen. They may verbalize an overwhelming feeling of impending doom. They may also report that the anxiety is very frightening to them and that they are afraid of losing control. Table 45-2 lists questions that may help in identifying a client's anxiety.

Clients with PTSD may describe unwanted memories of an event, express suicidal ideation, or express fantasies of retaliation toward the identified source of trauma. The client with PTSD may describe feeling extremely fearful and "on guard" at all times and may report having **flashbacks** (reliving of the original trauma as if currently experiencing it) along with recurrent dreams and/or nightmares.

Objective Data

Changes in vital signs, such as an increase in blood pressure, pulse, and respirations, as well as restlessness, irritability, pacing, and agitation may become more pronounced as anxiety level increases.

PROFESSIONAL TIP

Achieving a State of Relaxation

Clients who are anxious and feeling overwhelmed will often require assistance in achieving a state of relaxation. Help the client identify activities that are relaxing, such as listening to favorite music, watching television, reading a book, playing a game, drawing a picture, working a puzzle, or whatever is calming to the client. Teach the client a variety of stress-management techniques such as deep-breathing exercises, progressive deep-muscle relaxation, and guided imagery. All of these can assist the client in reaching a greater state of relaxation. Explore with the client the possibility of enrolling in a course such as Tai Chi. In addition to providing physical activity, it assists the client in achieving a state of balance and an increasing ability to focus.

TABLE 45-2 ASKING CLIENTS ABOUT SYMPTOMS OF ANXIETY DISORDERS

Following are questions that have proven useful in eliciting information from clients about symptoms of anxiety disorders. You may find that you prefer to word these questions somewhat differently, but the important thing is to ask them. Many clients experience anxiety symptoms for years before a doctor, nurse, or psychologist takes the time to ask about these symptoms.

Generalized anxiety disorder	Do you find yourself worrying frequently about a number of different things, such as the way things are going for you at home, work, or school?
	Do you find yourself feeling anxious or tense much of the time without any obvious reason?
Panic disorder	Have you ever experienced sudden, intense fear for no reason?
	Have you found yourself experiencing intense physical symptoms of chest pain, shortness of breath, dizziness, or sweating, along with a sense that something terrible or life threatening was happening to you?
Post-traumatic stress disorder	Have you ever had a particularly traumatic experience such as witnessing or experiencing violence or a catastrophic event (such as a flood or fire)?
	Have you ever found yourself reexperiencing a violent or catastrophic event through dreams or waking "flashbacks"?

From *Psychiatric Mental Health Nursing,* by N. Frisch and L. Frisch (2nd ed.). 2002, Clifton Park, NY: Thomson Delmar Learning. Copyright 2002 by Thomson Delmar Learning.

PROFESSIONAL TIP

Flashbacks

The client experiencing a flashback is usually not aware of current surroundings and often does not recognize familiar individuals. For the duration of the flashback, the client is actually reexperiencing and reliving the original trauma once again. For this reason, it is extremely important to never touch a client during a flashback, as the client may perceive you as dangerous and react to you as if you are trying to inflict harm. Talk to the client in a soft, calm voice and gently let the client know who you are, where the client is, and what is happening.

Clients with PTSD may exhibit an exaggerated **startle response** (overreaction to minor sounds or noises), or they may be **hypervigilant** (constantly scanning the environment for potentially dangerous situations). Clients with PTSD may react with survival responses appropriate for the trauma they survived. For example, abused children may seek to placate adults and female incest victims may become flirtatious or seductive with men.

Nursing diagnoses for the client with anxiety may include the following:

Nursing Diagnoses	Planning/Goals	Nursing Interventions
Anxiety related to a subjective sense of uneasiness and tension	The client will learn how to demonstrate and utilize new and more effective methods of managing anxiety.	Teach the client relaxation exercises. Explore with the client those things that are calming and relaxing.
		Encourage physical movement or participation in some type of recreational or sporting activity to release excess energy.
Fear related to a specific object (e.g., hospitals)	The client will report feeling less fearful.	Remain with the client while level of fear is high. Talk to the client in a calm, soothing voice. Reassure the client that he is in a safe place.

continues

Nursing Diagnoses	Planning/Goals	Nursing Interventions
Post-Trauma Syndrome related to anxiety felt following a significant life-threatening event	The client will experience a decrease in frequency and intensity of symptoms.	Orient the client to reality, if the client is confused, disoriented, or experiencing flashbacks.
		Do not touch the client without permission.
		Teach the client, family, and significant others about the symptoms of PTSD, including flashbacks, amnesia, memory loss, and nightmares.

Evaluation Each goal must be evaluated to determine how it has been met by the client.

DEPRESSION

Depression is the state wherein an individual experiences feelings of extreme sadness, hopelessness, and helplessness. Several symptoms may be seen with depression, which can range anywhere from mild to severe and be manifested in many different ways.

It involves an imbalance of neurotransmitters and is treatable. The direct cause of depression is unclear; however, changes in body chemistry caused by experiencing a traumatic event, hormonal changes, altered health habits, presence of another illness, or substance abuse can bring on depression (Depression and Bipolar Support Alliance [DBSA], 2003b).

Symptoms of depression include prolonged sadness; significant changes in appetite and sleep patterns; irritability, agitation, anxiety, worry; pessimism; loss of energy; feelings of guilt, worthlessness; inability to concentrate; inability to take pleasure in former interests; unexplained aches and pains; and recurring thoughts of death or suicide. Approximately 20 million adult Americans of all ages, races, ethnic groups, and social class experience depression every day (DBSA, 2003b). Clients can experience mild, moderate, or severe depression with varying degrees of symptomatology.

MILD DEPRESSION

Individuals with mild depression may notice a difference in the way they are feeling and their ability to function in certain situations, but they may not be able to identify the problem at this point in time. Although they are still able to function and carry on their daily routines, doing so may put quite a strain on them both physically and mentally.

MODERATE DEPRESSION

Moderate depression interferes with the individual's life in a variety of ways. A decrease in the ability to perform on the job may be noticed. Relationships are affected as the individual becomes increasingly withdrawn and isolated and disinterested in things that previously were pleasurable, such as hobbies and leisure-time activities. Interventions performed at this stage are most effective in arresting the depression before the individual's mental health deteriorates any further.

SEVERE DEPRESSION

When depression progresses to a severe state, the individual becomes seriously impaired. The individual with severe depression may experience psychosis, or a loss of contact with reality, in addition to the symptoms of depression.

DEPRESSION DISORDERS

Some of the psychiatric diagnoses associated with depression include Major Depressive Disorder and Dysthymic Disorder.

MAJOR DEPRESSIVE DISORDER

To qualify for the diagnosis of Major Depressive Disorder, *DSM-IV* requires the presence of at least one major depressive episode that (1) lasts at least 2 weeks, (2) represents a change from previous functioning, and (3) causes some impairment in a person's social or occupational functioning. Five or more symptoms of depression must also be present. One of these symptoms *must* be either depressed mood or loss of interest in previously enjoyable activities. The other four symptoms may include changes in appetite or weight; sleep disturbance (usually trouble staying asleep); fatigue or loss of energy; feelings of worthlessness or guilt; difficulty concentrating, thinking, or making decisions; or recurrent thoughts of death or suicide.

Some individuals, particularly adolescents, exhibit irritability or crankiness rather than sadness. Family members or close friends will notice a change in the individual, most commonly a social withdrawal and a neglect of activities that previously brought the person pleasure.

Major depressive episodes frequently develop over a few days or weeks, and without treatment commonly last longer than 6 months (Frisch & Frisch, 2002).

DYSTHYMIC DISORDER

Whereas the essence of Major Depressive Disorder is discrete episodes of depression, persons with Dysthymic Disorder feel depressed nearly all of the time. The *DSM-*

IV criteria for Dysthymic Disorder include "depressed mood for most of the day, for more days than not . . . for at least 2 years." A person with Dysthymic Disorder must also have at least two of the following symptoms: appetite disturbance, sleep disturbance, fatigue, low self-esteem, poor concentration or difficulty making decisions, and feelings of hopelessness. As with Major Depressive Disorder, the symptoms must cause clinically significant distress or impairment in social or occupational functioning. Dysthymic Disorder is somewhat rarer than Major Depressive Disorder, occurring during a lifetime in approximately 6% of persons (Frisch & Frisch, 2002).

Medical–Surgical Management

Medical

Psychotherapy refers to any of more than 250 types of largely verbal techniques designed to help individuals surmount psychological stresses including depression. Psychotherapy based on psychoanalytic interventions emphasizes helping clients gain insight into the causes of their depression. This approach is long term and requires much motivation on the part of the client to invest considerable time, effort, and money (Frisch & Frisch, 2002).

Brief dynamic therapy focuses on core conflicts from personality and living situations. The goal is to resolve depressive symptoms by improving these conflicts and resolving stresses. The therapist in this approach takes an active role to direct sessions toward resolution of conflicts. Techniques of confrontation and interpretation of behaviors and events are frequently used. Conflicts, their meanings, and individuals' choices are emphasized. This type of therapy can be done either with individuals or in a group format.

Cognitive therapy focuses on removing symptoms by identifying and correcting perceptual biases in clients' thinking and correcting unrecognized assumptions. The therapy concentrates on changing negative thoughts and behaviors into alternatives that do not sustain depression.

Electroconvulsive therapy (ECT) is used for clients with severe depression who have not responded to medications. The client under anesthesia is treated with pulses of electrical energy sufficient to cause a brief convulsion or seizure. Muscle-depolarizing agents are also given so that no actual convulsive movements occur; the primary effect of ECT is on the brain. Studies show that clients do not find the actual ECT treatment frightening, painful, or unpleasant. Although deaths have occurred from ECT, particularly in elderly clients or those with heart disease, the risk is quite low. Side effects depend on the specific technique used but are mostly limited to memory deficits (Frisch & Frisch, 2002).

Pharmacological

The main classification of medications usually prescribed for treatment of depression is the antidepressants. Within this classification are several groups, including the tetracyclic and atypical antidepressants (Table 45-3), the selective serotonin reuptake inhibitors (SSRIs) (Table 45-4), the tricyclic antidepressants (Table 45-5), and the monoamine oxidase inhibitors (MAOIs) (Table 45-6). These antidepressant families have unique properties, as do the individual medications within each. Many of these medications must be taken at bedtime. It is a nursing responsibility to adequately educate the client and family about the prescribed medications.

Diet

The client experiencing depression often has a disturbance in eating patterns. Some individuals will not be hungry and will eat very little or sometimes not at all,

TABLE 45-3 TETRACYCLIC AND ATYPICAL ANTIDEPRESSANTS

GENERIC NAME	TRADE NAME	TYPE	POTENTIAL SIDE EFFECTS
mirtazapine	Remeron	Tetracyclic	Agranulocytosis, drowsiness, dry mouth, nausea, suicidal ideation
nefazodone hydrochloride	Serzone	Antidepressant	Constipation, dizziness, dry mouth, insomnia, nausea, weight loss
venlafaxine hydrochloride	Effexor	Antidepressant	Abnormal dreams, altered taste, anorexia, constipation, diarrhea, dizziness, dry mouth, dyspepsia, headache, nausea, nervousness, paresthesia, rectal hemorrhage, rhinitis, seizures, sexual dysfunction, visual disturbances, vaginal/uterine hemorrhage, weakness, weight loss

Data from *2004 PDR Nurses' Handbook*, by G. Spratto and A. Woods, 2004, Clifton Park, NY: Thomson Delmar Learning.

TABLE 45-4   SELECTIVE SEROTONIN REUPTAKE INHIBITORS (SSRIs)

GENERIC NAME	TRADE NAME	POTENTIAL SIDE EFFECTS
fluoxetine hydrochloride	Prozac	Headache, abnormal dreams, anxiety, diarrhea, drowsiness, excessive sweating, insomnia, nervousness, palpitations, pruritus, seizures, tremors, visual disturbances, weight loss
fluvoxamine maleate	Luvox	Constipation, convulsions, impotence, dry mouth, drowsiness, dyspepsia, headache, heart failure, insomnia, MI, nausea, nervousness, weakness
paroxetine hydrochloride	Paxil	Anxiety, constipation, diarrhea, dizziness, drowsiness, dry mouth, ejaculatory disturbance, headache, insomnia, nausea, seizures, sweating, weakness, tremors
sertraline hydrochloride	Zoloft	Diarrhea, dizziness, drowsiness, dry mouth, fatigue, headache, increased sweating, insomnia, nausea, palpitations, sexual dysfunction, tremors, vomiting when given with pimozide (Orap) raises pimozide concentration by about 40% (FDA, 2002).

Data from *2004 PDR Nurses' Handbook,* by G. Spratto and A. Woods, 2004, Clifton Park, NY: Thomson Delmar Learning.

TABLE 45-5   TRICYCLIC ANTIDEPRESSANTS

GENERIC NAME	TRADE NAME	POTENTIAL SIDE EFFECTS
amitriptyline hydrochloride	Elavil	Arrhythmia, blurred vision, constipation, dry eyes, dry mouth, heart block, hypotension, lethargy, MI, sedation, stroke
imipramine hydrochloride	Tofranil	Arrhythmia, blurred vision, constipation, drowsiness, dry eyes, dry mouth, fatigue, hypotension, seizures, urinary retention

Data from *2004 PDR Nurses' Handbook,* by G. Spratto and A. Woods, 2004, Clifton Park, NY: Thomson Delmar Learning.

TABLE 45-6   MONOAMINE OXIDASE INHIBITORS (MAOIs)

GENERIC NAME	TRADE NAME	POTENTIAL SIDE EFFECTS
isocarboxazid	Marplan	Arrhythmia, blurred vision, diarrhea, dizziness, headache, orthostatic hypotension, insomnia, restlessness, seizures, weakness; these medications usually have the side-effect of lowering blood pressure. A potentially fatal hypertensive crisis can result when MAOIs are taken in combination with certain foods and drugs such as broad beans, certain cheeses (e.g., brie, cheddar), liver, caffeine, figs, dry sausage (pepperoni), tea, yogurt, amphetamine, cocaine, dopa, and many OTC cold products, hay fever medications, and nasal decongestants.
phenelzine sulfate	Nardil	
tranylcypromine sulfate	Parnate	

Data from *2004 PDR Nurses' Handbook,* by Springhouse Corporation, 2003, Springhouse, PA: Springhouse.

whereas others will overeat. A nutritional assessment should be done as part of the health history obtained by the nurse, and if any significant problem areas are identified, a dietary consult may be indicated.

When a client is started on antidepressant therapy, the client and family must be educated regarding any special dietary needs, depending on the type of medication prescribed. The client receiving SSRI therapy may experience an initial loss of appetite during the first part of therapy, because of the gastrointestinal (GI) side effects frequently associated with these medications (Table 45-4). Anorectic clients or those at risk for weight loss must be closely monitored. The client receiving MAOI therapy must be especially alert to the dietary restrictions associated with this particular type of medication (Table 45-6).

PROFESSIONAL TIP

Antidepressant Therapy

Before initiating antidepressant therapy, a baseline electrocardiogram (EKG) is needed to determine whether any preexisting underlying cardiac problems are present. If the client develops cardiac difficulties during antidepressant therapy, another EKG is obtained and compared to the original to assist in ascertaining whether the antidepressant exacerbated the cardiac condition.

CLIENT TEACHING

Tricyclic Antidepressants

Be sure to instruct each client taking a tricyclic antidepressant medication in the following:

- Do not drink alcohol while on the medication.
- Do not take any other medications unless prescribed by your physician.
- Drowsiness and sedation may impair the ability to drive and operate heavy machinery.
- Some of the side effects may diminish in intensity once your body adjusts to the medication.
- Do not stop taking the medications without physician approval.
- Increase fluid intake to assist in combating dry mouth and constipation.
- Sugarless candy and gum can help decrease the side effect of dry mouth.
- Increase dietary fiber to decrease the side effect of constipation.
- Rise slowly from a lying position to prevent dizziness and a sudden drop in blood pressure.

Activity

Clients suffering from depression often experience a significant decrease in level of activity and report feeling tired and lethargic. Clients experiencing depression will often require encouragement to engage in any type of physical activity.

Nursing Management

Spend time with the client one-on-one to build rapport and develop a therapeutic relationship. Encourage the client to initiate conversation and interact with others. Guide the client to bathe, groom, and wear clean clothes. Praise the client verbally for conversing and interacting with others and for taking care of hygiene and grooming.

CLIENT TEACHING

Potential Adverse Drug–Drug Reactions with MAOIs

A serious drug–drug reaction can occur when an MAOI is taken concurrently with certain other medications. The combination of an MAOI and some common prescription or OTC medications can result in a hypertensive crisis that is often fatal. Some of the most dangerous reactive medications include meperidine (Demerol), stimulants, decongestants, and weight-reduction aids.

CLIENT TEACHING

Tetracyclic and SSRI Antidepressants

Be sure to instruct each client taking a tetracyclic, atypical, or SSRI antidepressant medication in the following:

- Take the medication *only* as directed by your physician.
- Do not take the medication unless prescribed by your physician.
- Do not take fluoxetine (Prozac), paroxetine (Paxil), or sertraline (Zoloft) on an empty stomach.
- Mirtazapine (Remeron) does not need to be taken with food.
- Ability to drive and/or operate heavy machinery may be impaired while taking the medication.
- Do not drink alcohol while taking the medication.
- If female, advise your physician if you are breastfeeding, suspect you are pregnant, or are planning a pregnancy while taking the medication.
- Wear sunscreen and protective clothing while outdoors, as fluoxetine (Prozac), paroxetine (Paxil), and sertraline (Zoloft) increase susceptibility to sunburn.
- The medications may cause drowsiness.
- If taking fluoxetine (Prozac), mirtazapine (Remeron), or nefazodone (Serzone), rise slowly from a lying position to prevent dizziness and a sudden drop in blood pressure.
- Utilize good oral hygiene in conjunction with sugarless candy or gum to minimize the discomforting side effect of dry mouth associated with fluoxetine (Prozac), mirtazapine (Remeron), nefazodone (Serzone), paroxetine (Paxil), and sertraline (Zoloft).
- Monitor weight, as mirtazapine (Remeron) may cause an increase in appetite.
- Do not take any over-the-counter (OTC) cold medications with mirtazapine (Remeron).
- If taking mirtazapine (Remeron), inform your physician of the medication regimen prior to surgery.
- If taking venlafaxine (Effexor), fluvoxamine (Luvox), or nefazodone (Serzone), inform your physician if signs of allergic reaction occur.

CLIENT TEACHING

MAOIs

Be sure to instruct each client taking an MAOI antidepressant medication in the following:

- *Do not take any other medications, including OTC medications,* unless prescribed by your physician.
- Take the medication exactly as prescribed.
- Do not drink alcohol while on the medication.
- Rise slowly from a lying position to prevent dizziness and a sudden drop in blood pressure.
- *Avoid all foods containing tyramine,* including alcoholic beverages, especially beer and wine; aged cheeses; avocados; bananas; caffeine; chocolate; and smoked or pickled meats (such as salami, pepperoni, smoked fish, and summer sausage).

CRITICAL THINKING

Coworker Depression

What actions would you take if you felt a coworker was suffering from depression?

NURSING PROCESS

Assessment

Subjective Data

The client may verbalize overwhelming feelings of sadness, thoughts of suicide, a loss of interest and pleasure in activities that were previously enjoyable, and problems with memory, recall, and concentration. In addition, a decreased libido, extreme lethargy, and having insufficient energy to complete activities of daily living (ADLs) and needed tasks may be reported. The depressed client who has become increasingly withdrawn and socially isolated may experience problems in intimate, personal, and social relationships.

Objective Data

The client may manifest a noticeable decline in personal hygiene and grooming, possibly because of a lack of energy and an inability to perform even the simplest of tasks. Weight loss resulting from the client's failure to eat may also be noted.

Nursing diagnoses for the client with depression may include the following:

Nursing Diagnoses	Planning/Goals	Nursing Interventions
Social Isolation related to inability to engage in satisfying personal relationships	The client will increase the number of interactions with other individuals.	Build rapport and develop therapeutic relationship with client. Spend time with client individually. Encourage client to initiate conversation and interact with others. Verbally praise client for increasing interactions and initiating conversation.
Bathing/Hygiene, Dressing/Grooming, and Feeding Self-care Deficit related to lack of concern or regard toward self	The client will attend to own basic health care needs.	Encourage client to bathe and wear clean clothes. Teach client the importance of balanced nutrition. Praise client for each activity done on own.

Evaluation Each goal must be evaluated to determine how it has been met by the client.

THE CLIENT WHO IS POTENTIALLY VIOLENT

In today's society, violence has become increasingly common and widespread. The media routinely and graphically reports the numerous violent crimes and acts that occur on a daily basis. Nurses may come face to face with angry clients and their families and significant others and, perhaps, even angry colleagues. When con-

fronted by someone who is angry, the natural reaction is to respond in a like manner or, perhaps, to feel intimidated. In such difficult situations, it is important to maintain objectivity and not get "hooked" into the client's anger and respond in an inappropriate manner.

Nurses may encounter clients who are **verbally aggressive** (prone to saying things in a loud and/or intimidating manner), **physically aggressive** (prone to threatening or actually harming someone), or a combination of the two. Mind-altering substances such as alcohol and phencyclidine (PCP) often increase the risk of aggression. **Anger-control assistance** is defined as a nursing intervention aimed at facilitation of the expression of anger in an adaptive and nonviolent manner (McCloskey & Bulechek, 1996). Anger control includes establishing a basic level of trust and rapport with the client and using a calm and reassuring manner. The nurse should use every means possible to learn from the client (or his family/friends) those situations that are likely to bring on anger, and should encourage the client to inform the nursing staff when he is feeling tension. Although the nurse has a responsibility to help the client learn to deal with his anger, she also has a clear duty to assess for inappropriate aggression and to intervene before such aggression is expressed.

Some of the techniques used in anger control include limiting access to frustrating situations, providing physical outlets for expression of anger or tension (such as punching bags, large motor activities [sports], and anger journals), and ensuring that a client for whom anger is a problem is given enough personal space that he does not have to feel encroached upon by others when he is unable to tolerate environmental stimuli.

HOMICIDAL INTENT

The client who is homicidal is planning or threatening to harm or kill another individual or individuals. It is the responsibility of health care personnel to attempt to ascertain the seriousness of the intent; that is, whether the individual is actually threatening someone else or just "blowing off steam." Once aware of an individual's threat or intent to harm someone else, the nurse must inform the individual(s) at risk of the potential for harm and/or notify the proper authorities and enlist their help. The first step in such a situation is to contact the supervisor and offer an accurate appraisal of the situation.

SUICIDAL INTENT

Purposefully taking one's own life, or suicide, is the ultimate form of self-destruction. Clients who are suicidal often feel overwhelmed by life events and decide that the only relief will come from ending their own lives. Intense feelings of fear, loss, anger, or despair can drive individuals to commit suicide, and the effects of an attempted or completed suicide can be devastating and long lasting. Nurses must learn to recognize the danger signs of clients at risk for suicide and know the appropriate interventions to help clients preserve their health and dignity.

"Suicide is the eleventh leading cause of death in the United States, claiming almost 30,000 lives each year" (CDC, 2003). The populations at greatest risk are individuals with diagnosed mood disorders such as Major Depressive Disorder, elders, and those with serious or life-threatening medical illnesses such as cancer or human immunodeficiency virus.

SUICIDAL IDEATIONS

The client experiencing **suicidal ideations** has thoughts of hurting or killing himself but may or may not be planning to act on these thoughts. It is important to understand the difference between thoughts and actions; that is, having a thought does not necessarily mean that the behavior will follow. When confronted with a client's verbalization of possible suicide, however, it is always wise to take the client's expression of intent seriously. Because suicide is a leading cause of death in the United States, nurses must know how to evaluate a client for the likelihood of a completed suicide. It is critical to thoroughly assess the client and attempt to accurately ascertain the degree of danger the client is experiencing. Once this is done, take the precautions necessary to maintain the client's safety (Table 45-7).

ACTIVELY SUICIDAL

The **actively suicidal** client is intent on hurting or killing himself and is in imminent danger of doing so. This situation requires immediate and appropriate action to protect the client from potentially fatal self-destructive behavior. If the client is in a supervised setting, it is the nurse's responsibility to maintain the safety of the client and to inform other staff members of the client's suicidal intentions. The client at risk for self-inflicted injury must be monitored closely (per institutional policy and the frequency as ordered by the physician).

The frequency of client observation is determined by the degree of suicide risk and is written as a specific order from the physician. Observations of the client are documented. Some clients must be checked a minimum of once every 15 minutes. Other clients may require more frequent observation and monitoring. If the client is *actively* suicidal and/or homicidal and is indicating an imminent intent to harm self or others, a specific staff member will be assigned to that client at all times on a one-to-one basis.

All pertinent observations such as verbalizations and behaviors that indicate self-harm potential should be documented in the client's record. Any changes in the client's condition should be reported immediately to the

---

PROFESSIONAL TIP

Assessing for Risk of Violence

- Be aware of those clients with past history of violence and poor impulse control.
- Observe the client's body language: Notice changes in behavior, words, or dress.
- Assess for aggressive behaviors, increasing tension, clenched fists, loud or angry tone of voice, narrowed eyes, and pacing.
- Remember that hostility tends to be contagious. Do not reciprocate with anger and hostility!

TABLE 45-7 ASSESSMENT OF RISK FOR SUICIDE

The following areas are to be assessed in all potentially suicidal clients:

1. Does the client have a *plan* to commit suicide?

Example: Client plans to "end it all" after wife leaves for work on a Monday.

Rationale: Some clients may be experiencing thoughts of wishing they were dead or killing themselves, but may not have a plan for doing so. *The client who has a plan for committing suicide is at increased risk.*

2. How *specific* is the plan to commit suicide?

Example: Client states he plans to overdose on sleeping pills.

Rationale: *A specific plan increases the risk of completing a suicide.*

3. Does the client have access to the *means* to commit suicide?

Example: Client states he will use his spouse's sleeping pills to overdose.

Rationale: *Easy availability of the means to kill oneself increases the risk of suicide.*

4. How *lethal* is the intended means to commit suicide?

Example: Client states he will "blow his brains out" with a gun.

Rationale: Some means of suicide are more likely to result in a completed suicide. *Gunshots are the most common cause of completed suicide.* The lethality of guns makes the potential for a successful intervention very slim. Intervention in light of means that are less lethal may yield a more favorable outcome (e.g., overdose, cutting of wrists).

PROFESSIONAL TIP

Providing a Safe Environment

When a client verbalizes an intention to inflict self-harm, measures must be taken to ensure the client's safety. One way is to provide and maintain a safe, secure environment for the client. This may require a change in items allowed in the client's surroundings and living space. For example, a pencil or pen could be used as a dangerous weapon; an empty soda can could be used to deeply cut the wrists or to seriously injure someone else; and the broken glass from a bottle of make-up could cause great harm. These and all other potentially dangerous items must be removed from the client's immediate area.

out the reason restraints or seclusion was indicated for use with the client.

Physical Restraints Physical restraints, usually leather straps, are used to immobilize a person who is clearly dangerous to self or others and who poses sufficient risk of harm. Physical restraints may be applied only under the direction and supervision of a registered nurse (RN) and must comply with state laws regarding their use. In almost all cases, there must be a physician's order to apply the restraints, and there must be clearly documented evidence that the restraints were needed. Some of the observable behaviors indicating that restraints are necessary include increased motor activity, verbal and/or physical threats, overresponsiveness to stimuli, and actual physical assault (Frisch & Frisch, 2002).

Seclusion Seclusion is the process of confining a client to a single room. The room may be locked or unlocked, and it may or may not have furnishings. The purpose of seclusion is to provide security, to remove the client from a situation of escalating anger and violence, or to remove the client who is hypersensitive to environmental stimuli from the stimulation of a hospital unit. Seclusion, like the use of physical restraints, can be used only when all other avenues for control have been exhausted. The client must be told what is happening and why. He must not be left alone; a staff member should be assigned to observe the client, usually from the doorway. Seclusion is an enforced "time-out," where the client is removed from the situation only long enough to allow him to calm down, regain a sense of control, and then reenter the unit.

Therapy Psychotherapy is often indicated and initially may focus on personal and social conditions that bring about and/or perpetuate suicidal thoughts. Cognitive-behavioral therapy may be particularly useful, as may techniques to deal with frustration and anger. Substance use and abuse are often involved and may require separate outpatient or inpatient interventions.

Pharmacological

The severely agitated, aggressive, suicidal, and/or homicidal client who is violent or threatening violence

physician. The conversation with the doctor, as well as any new orders or changes in orders, must also be documented in the client's record (Eskreis, 1998).

Medical–Surgical Management

Medical

The client who is severely agitated, aggressive, actively suicidal, and/or homicidal and who is exhibiting or threatening violent acts may need to be restrained or placed in seclusion in order to be safely contained. The physical holding of someone or use of mechanical restraints severely restricts movement and can constitute a violation of the client's rights unless sufficient clinical justification exists. Thus, all of the client's comments and behaviors plus any nursing interventions must be documented in the client record per agency policy. This documentation provides the necessary justification for the use of restraints or seclusion. In addition, the physician must write a specific, time-limited order that spells

PROFESSIONAL TIP

No-Suicide Contract

Obtaining a "No-Suicide Contract" from the client is one way to help reduce the risk of suicide attempts. There are several guidelines to follow in working through this process:

- Ask the client whether he is able to make a promise *to himself* that he will not do anything to harm himself. ***Rationale:*** It is important for the client to make the contract with himself, because if the contract is made with someone else, such as a nurse, and the client later becomes angry or upset with that person, he may then harm himself in order to "get back" at that person.
- If the client is unable to commit to the No-Suicide Contract for the rest of his life, work with him on establishing a time frame to which he can commit, for example, 1 week, 24 hours, 8 hours, or some other time frame. Always meet with the client at the end of the allotted time frame and review/renew the contract at that time. ***Rationale:*** The suicidal individual may feel overwhelmed at the thought of promising *never* to harm himself, but may be able to sincerely commit for a shorter length of time.
- Ask the client whether he is able to maintain the No-Suicide Contract *no matter what happens.* ***Rationale:*** Some clients will leave a way out of the contract. For example, the suicidal client may outwardly make a promise to not commit suicide but inwardly think "unless something really bad happens, like if my wife leaves me." If the wife then files for a divorce, the client may feel that he has "permission" to kill himself. Adding the *no matter what happens* clause blocks off this avenue of escape from the contract.
- Ask the client whether he can make a promise to himself that if thoughts of suicide return, he will talk to someone before taking any action. ***Rationale:*** If the client talks to someone regarding his thoughts of suicide *before* he attempts suicide, a successful intervention and suicide prevention are more likely.
- Assist the client in developing a detailed plan of action regarding those persons he will contact in the event that he again experiences suicidal thoughts. Include names and phone numbers of all significant and supportive individuals. ***Rationale:*** During a crisis, the suicidal individual is not able to think rationally and will behave and act in an impulsive manner. Having a well-developed plan of action increases the likelihood that the suicidal individual can follow these guidelines.
- At the bottom of the list, put the name and phone number of the local suicide crisis hotline and/or local emergency number (911). ***Rationale:*** Including these numbers ensures that there will always be someone available for the suicidal client to talk to 24 hours a day, 7 days a week, 365 days a year.
- Assist the client in putting the No-Suicide Contract in writing and in his own words. Give the client the original and put a copy in the client's chart. ***Rationale:*** When the contract is in writing and the client has a copy, he will be more likely to follow through with his promise to not commit suicide.

may require a medication with strong anxiolytic (antianxiety) and/or sedative properties, such as one of the antianxiety agents or a sedative-hypnotic (Table 45-1). Additionally, the suicidal client who is depressed may be evaluated for treatment with one of the many available antidepressants such as fluoxetine hydrochloride (Prozac), sertraline hydrochloride (Zoloft), paroxetine hydrochloride (Paxil), fluvoxamine maleate (Luvox), mirtazapine (Remeron), or one of the many others (Tables 45-3, 45-4, 45-5, and 45-6).

Diet

Foods are not restricted because a client is severely agitated, aggressive, actively suicidal, and/or homicidal, but may be restricted depending on the medications being taken. The food tray should be inspected for any potentially dangerous objects such as glassware or silverware. Even plasticware can be broken in such a way as to yield a very dangerous weapon for hurting self or others.

Activity

The activity level of the client who is severely agitated, aggressive, actively suicidal, and/or homicidal

may need to be restricted for a period of time in order to maintain the client's safety and the safety of others.

Nursing Management

Assess the client for suicidal thoughts. If the client has a specific plan, evaluate the degree of risk for the client and contact the physician. Assess the environment for potentially dangerous items. Increase the level of client observation.

NURSING PROCESS

Assessment

Subjective Data

The client may argue, yell, curse, and make numerous verbal threats in a loud voice. The suicidal client may indicate intentions verbally, nonverbally, or a combination of the two. The client contemplating suicide may verbalize his thoughts either directly or indirectly. A direct statement may be something as straightforward as

"I am planning to kill myself." An indirect statement might be "I'm not going to be around here anymore" or "Everyone will be better off without me."

Objective Data

The client may exhibit restlessness, pacing, and "poor impulse control"; may be physically intimidating; and may use or try to use items in the environment, such as books, furniture, or a coffee pot, as weapons. A nonverbal signal of possible intentions of suicide may be seen in the client who begins making arrangements for people and pets to be taken care of, putting personal affairs in order, and giving away personal possessions, especially treasured items.

Nursing diagnoses for the client who is severely agitated, aggressive, actively suicidal, and/or homicidal may include the following:

Nursing Diagnoses	Planning/Goals	Nursing Interventions
Risk for Self-Directed Violence related to risk factors such as mental health, emotional status, or suicidal plan.	The client will not harm self.	Assess for the presence of suicidal thoughts and whether a specific plan is present.
		Evaluate the degree of risk associated with the client's verbalization of suicide intent.
		Contact the attending physician or psychiatrist and inform of the client's intentions and current condition.
		Assess and evaluate the client's surroundings and environment for any potentially dangerous items or objects that could be used for self-harm. Remove or secure any potentially harmful items.
		Increase the level of observation so that the client is frequently monitored.
		Assist the client in developing a No-suicide Contract.
Risk for Other-Directed Violence related to risk factors such as history of violence against others, suicidal behavior, impulsivity.	The client will not harm anyone.	Assess for the presence of homicidal ideations.
		If the client is verbalizing a plan to harm someone, immediately notify the proper authorities so they can alert this individual.

Evaluation Each goal must be evaluated to determine how it has been met by the client.

SAMPLE NURSING CARE PLAN

THE SUICIDAL CLIENT WITH MAJOR DEPRESSION

Alice is a 27-year-old female who was brought to the emergency department of a county hospital by ambulance following a serious suicide attempt via ingesting a bottle of insecticide. After being treated in the emergency room, she spent 2 days in the intensive care unit (ICU) and then was transferred to a locked adult inpatient psychiatric unit for evaluation and treatment. Alice reports she became suicidal following the recent ending of a 4-year relationship with her boyfriend and decided to take her life because she felt "completely hopeless," that "there was nothing left to live for," that "no one would miss her" if she were dead, that she "would never be loved," and that she "could never be happy again." Before the suicide attempt, Alice reports that she had not been eating, had only been sleeping 1 to 2 hours per night, and had been crying almost continuously throughout the day. Since admission to the psychiatric unit, Alice has been started on sertraline (Zoloft).

Nursing Diagnosis 1 *Risk for Self-Directed Violence* related to recent loss, feelings of abandonment, and impulsive behavior as evidenced by suicide attempt of drinking bottle of insecticide, verbalizations that "there was nothing left to live for" and that "no one would miss her" if she were dead

continues

SAMPLE NURSING CARE PLAN

Nursing Outcomes Classification (NOC)
Depression Level
Suicide Self-Restraint

Nursing Interventions Classification (NIC)
Self-Esteem Enhancement
Coping Enhancement

PLANNING/GOALS	NURSING INTERVENTIONS	RATIONALE
Alice will verbalize that she is no longer at risk of harming herself.	Assist Alice in developing a No-Suicide Contract. Obtain in writing if possible, make a copy for her chart, and give her the original.	May help deter self-destructive behavior in the future.
	Explore with Alice factors that contributed to her becoming suicidal.	Can be the first step in preventing another.
	Encourage Alice to verbalize her feelings related to the recent break-up and to explore any unresolved past issues that this loss might have triggered.	Current feelings of loss and abandonment are often magnified and intensified by unresolved past situations and circumstances that were never effectively handled.
	Explore with Alice her usual methods of coping with stressful situations and whether these have been effective for her.	Can lead to a better understanding of those behaviors that must be changed.
	Assist Alice in identifying and then developing stress-management methods as alternatives to attempting suicide.	Assists the client in recognizing alternate methods of managing stressful situations.
	Assist Alice in developing a suicide-prevention plan and in identifying supportive individuals and resources that she can turn to in the event that she begins to again have suicidal thoughts.	Plans to prevent suicide must be developed ahead of time, because individuals contemplating suicide are impulsive and unable to problem solve or think clearly. They may, however, be able to follow through with a previously defined plan of action.
	Teach Alice about possible side effects associated with sertraline (Zoloft), such as nausea and GI upset, and encourage her to have something to eat prior to taking this medication.	Medication education is an integral part of treatment.
	Emphasize the importance of taking this medication as prescribed and not stopping the medication on her own, even if she starts to feel better and thinks that she no longer needs it.	If medications are discontinued prematurely, symptoms usually reappear and are often much more serious.
	Encourage Alice to keep a journal to reflect on her thoughts and feelings.	Writing in a journal can be a safe and effective method of identifying, expressing, and releasing feelings and emotions.
	Encourage Alice to keep follow-up appointments for medication to monitor progress.	Recommended to evaluate effectiveness and to monitor for any side effects.
	Assist Alice in setting up an appointment for outpatient counseling/therapy upon discharge per recommendation from the treatment team. Encourage Alice to keep counseling appointments.	Recommended after a suicide attempt in order to address the underlying issues and to prevent future attempts.

continues

SAMPLE NURSING CARE PLAN

EVALUATION   At the time of discharge from the adult inpatient psychiatric unit, Alice was no longer actively suicidal or intent upon harming herself. She still had occasional suicidal ideations; however, she did not feel compelled to act on them. She had made a promise to herself that she would never try to kill herself again no matter what happened, and that if those thoughts returned, she would find someone to talk to before she did anything. She also had developed a written list of friends and relatives she could call if she again experienced thoughts of suicide.

Nursing Diagnosis 2 *Hopelessness* related to feelings of loss about her life and future as evidenced by verbalizations of feeling: "completely hopeless," that she "would never be loved," and that she "could never be happy again"

Nursing Outcomes Classification (NOC)
Depression Control
Mood Equilibrium

Nursing Interventions Classification (NIC)
Suicide Prevention
Patient Contracting

PLANNING/GOALS	NURSING INTERVENTIONS	RATIONALE
Alice will be less hopeless as indicated by verbalizations of plans for her future.	Develop a therapeutic nurse–client relationship with Alice utilizing the components of trust, rapport, respect, genuineness, and empathy.	Fosters the development of a therapeutic nurse–client relationship.
	Encourage Alice to become involved in activities on the unit, for example, interacting with staff and other clients and attending and participating in therapy groups and recreational activities.	Helps distract the mind from a preoccupation with losses, overwhelming feelings of depression, and suicidal ideations.
	Provide things for Alice to do when she is feeling down, for example, go for a walk with the staff, read a newspaper or book, or play a game.	Provides time to allow for something to shift for her, to see the situation as not so utterly and permanently hopeless or for her to begin to feel better and think differently once she has started responding to medication.
	Assist Alice in identifying the irrational beliefs or thoughts that she is having, for example, when she says no one will *ever* love or want her again.	Changing the way a person thinks by replacing irrational thoughts with rational or healthier ones, will change the way the person feels.

EVALUATION   Alice continued to have fleeting thoughts of hopelessness as far as ever having another significant relationship or being in love again; however, she now was beginning to catch herself and could identify these thoughts as being irrational and negative in nature and not helpful to her in any way.

THE CLIENT WHO IS PSYCHOTIC

Psychosis is a state wherein an individual loses the ability to recognize reality. A psychotic person may experience hallucinations, wherein he hears voices or sees images of persons or things that others cannot see or hear. A psychotic person is frequently unable to care for basic needs of safety, security, nutrition, and so on. Such an individual is hospitalized for his own safety and to initiate treatment (usually involving some form of medica-

tion) to bring the symptoms under control. A psychotic person may slip into and out of reality.

Psychosis can be a component of several illnesses, including Schizophrenia and Bipolar Disorder.

SCHIZOPHRENIA

The client with schizophrenia can be very difficult to understand and treat because the symptoms of schizophrenia can be confusing and frightening to caregivers. Clients with schizophrenia frequently have belief systems that have become distorted, so that they hold firmly to false ideas or delusions, even when presented with evidence to the contrary. When confronted with an opposing belief system, they may become even more entrenched in their mistaken views and begin to believe others are "against them," when, in fact, they are not. This makes them even more paranoid and suspicious, adding to their already distorted views of reality. As a result, these individuals are often struggling to determine the difference between that which is real and that which is unreal or delusional.

Hallucinations can occur in relation to any of the five senses (hearing, sight, touch, taste, and smell), but the most common types of hallucinations are auditory and visual. Individuals experiencing **auditory hallucinations** hear someone talking to them, when, in reality, no one is. The voice may be that of someone the individual recognizes, or the voice may be unknown to the person. If the voice or voices are comforting, the individual will be very resistant to "giving them up." Most of the time, however, the voices are derogatory in nature, telling the person that there is something wrong with him.

The individual experiencing a **visual hallucination** perceives or sees someone or something that is not actually there. Depending on the nature of the hallucination and whether the individual perceives it as threatening, the situation can be very frightening.

The most serious type of hallucination is referred to as the **command hallucination**, which occurs when the voice or voices tell the individual to harm himself or someone else. For example, the voices may tell the individual to jump off a bridge or building, step in front of a moving motor vehicle, or take an overdose of medication. These hallucinations are extremely dangerous because the demands are so strong that the individual is very likely to act on them.

Medical–Surgical Management

Medical

At this time, there is no cure for schizophrenia; however, it is possible for some clients with schizophrenia to lead functional lives with minimally debilitating symptoms through psychosocial treatments.

The goals of psychosocial treatment can be divided into three categories: clinical and family support services, rehabilitative services, and humanitarian aid/public safety. Clinical support involves outpatient management and family/community services. Rehabilitation involves increasing clients' capacities, both for social interactions and for productive activity (including gainful employment, when feasible). Humanitarian interventions are those efforts that maximize an individual's independence and quality of life within the bounds of the mental disability. Public safety involves balancing personal liberty with the recognition that some social control may be needed to prevent harm, both to the individual and to society.

Pharmacological

The most commonly prescribed classification of medications for the client experiencing schizophrenia is the

antipsychotics (Tables 45-8 and 45-9). This group of medications is given to reduce the signs and symptoms of psychosis, with a long-term goal of the client eventually being symptom free. If this is not possible, the goal is to reduce symptoms to a manageable level.

TABLE 45-8 ATYPICAL ANTIPSYCHOTICS

GENERIC NAME	TRADE NAME	POTENTIAL SIDE EFFECTS
clozapine	Clozaril	Agranulocytosis, angina, constipation, dizziness, orthostatic hypotension, increased salivation, leukopenia, NMS, drowsiness, seizures, tachycardia, weight gain
olanzapine	Zyprexa	Agitation, acute renal failure, amblyopia, constipation, CVA, dizziness, dry mouth, headache, NMS, orthostatic hypotension, restlessness, rhinitis, sedation, seizures, tachycardia, TD, tremors, weakness, weight gain
quetiapine fumarate	Seroquel	Dizziness, headache, NMS, seizures, TD, weight gain
risperidone	Risperdal	Acute renal failure, constipation, cough, decreased libido, diarrhea, dizziness, dry mouth, dysmenorrhea/menorrhagia, headache, increased dreams, increased sleep duration, insomnia, itching/skin rash, MI, nausea, NMS, pharyngitis, rhinitis, sedation, visual disturbances.

Data from *2004 PDR Nurses' Handbook,* by G. Spratto and A. Woods, 2004, Clifton Park, NY: Thomson Delmar Learning.

TABLE 45-9		PHENOTHIAZINES (ANTIPSYCHOTICS)
GENERIC NAME	TRADE NAME	POTENTIAL SIDE EFFECTS
chlorpromazine, hydrochloride	Thorazine	Agranulocytosis, blurred vision, constipation, dry eyes, dry mouth, hypotension, laryngeal edema, NMS, photosensitivity, sedation, TD
fluphenazine hydrochloride	Prolixin	Agranulocytosis, EPS, photosensitivity, TD
thioridazine hydrochloride	Mellaril	Agranulocytosis, blurred vision, constipation, dry eyes, dry mouth, hypotension, NMS, photosensitivity, sedation, TD

Data from *2004 PDR Nurses' Handbook,* by G. Spratto and A. Woods, 2004, Clifton Park, NY: Thomson Delmar Learning.

CLIENT TEACHING

Adverse Reactions to Antipsychotic Medications

- *Extrapyramidal side effects:* a common adverse reaction of some antipsychotic medications (especially the older ones) involving muscle rigidity and involuntary muscle movements; reversible if the dose is lowered or an antiparkinson agent is administered
- *Tardive dyskinesia:* irreversible reaction to antipsychotics (usually associated with high doses over a long period) consisting of involuntary muscle and body movements
- *Neuroleptic malignant syndrome:* a rare and potentially fatal reaction to antipsychotic medications characterized by a very high fever, severe muscle stiffness, and changes in sensorium progressing to coma

Because several side effects are associated with the antipsychotics, client teaching is an important part of the nurse's role. In addition to common side effects, some antipsychotic medications also have the potential for causing adverse reactions such as extrapyramidal symptoms (EPS), tardive dyskinesia (TD), and neuroleptic malignant syndrome (NMS).

One of the most important factors in symptom management for schizophrenia is medication compliance. In most cases, individuals who are schizophrenic must take some type of antipsychotic medication for the remainder of their lives. Clients suffering from

CLIENT TEACHING

Phenothiazines

Be sure to instruct each client taking a phenothiazine medication in the following:

- Do not drink alcohol while on the medication.
- Do not take any other medications unless prescribed by your physician.
- Do not stop taking the medication abruptly.
- The ability to drive and/or operate heavy machinery may be impaired while taking the medication.
- Be aware of possible side effects of the medication.
- Increase fluid intake to minimize the side effects of dry mouth and constipation.
- Increase dietary fiber to minimize the side effect of constipation.
- Rise slowly from a lying position to prevent dizziness and a sudden drop in blood pressure.
- These medications are contraindicated during pregnancy and lactation. Female clients should advise their physicians immediately if they are either pregnant or planning to become pregnant.
- Wear sunscreen and protective clothing while outdoors, as the medication increases susceptibility to sunburn.
- Some of the side effects may diminish in intensity after an initial period of adjustment.
- The medication may increase your risk of developing EPS, TD, and NMS.

schizophrenia are often extremely resistant to taking their medications as prescribed and usually require multiple repeat hospitalizations for stabilization. Multiple reasons exist for noncompliance, one being the client's denial of the diagnosis or the illness or of the seriousness of the illness. As a result of denial, the individual with schizophrenia resists taking medication, because to the client, taking medication equates to acceptance of having a serious mental disorder. Clients may also become noncompliant after a period of time on medication; once they start to feel better, they think the medication is no longer needed and stop taking it. After a short time of being off the prescribed medication, however, most individuals with schizophrenia will experience a return or significant worsening of their previous symptoms.

Probably the most common reason for medication noncompliance, however, is the number of troublesome side effects and potentially dangerous adverse reactions historically associated with antipsychotic medications. Fortunately, newer antipsychotic medications are now available that have fewer side effects and are much better tolerated. Even with the advent of these newer and more effective medications, however, many individuals are unable to benefit from them because of the high cost and the difficulties sometimes associated with accessing these medications.

Atypical Antipsychotics

Be sure to instruct each client taking an atypical antipsychotic medication in the following:

- Do not drink alcohol while taking the medication.
- Do not take any other medications, prescription or OTC, unless prescribed by your physician.
- Do not stop taking the medication without authorization from your physician.
- Do not stop taking the medication abruptly.
- The ability to drive and/or operate heavy machinery may be impaired while taking the medication.
- Rise slowly from a lying position to prevent dizziness and a sudden drop in blood pressure.
- The medication is contraindicated during pregnancy and lactation. Reliable contraception should be utilized while taking the medication. Female clients should advise their physicians immediately if they suspect they are either pregnant or planning to become pregnant.
- Be aware of the potential side effects of the medications.
- Notify your physician immediately of unexplained fever, sore throat, bleeding, bruising, or petechiae.
- Wear sunscreen and protective clothing while outdoors, as olanzapine (Zyprexa) and risperidone (Risperdal) increase susceptibility to sunburn.
- Avoid temperature extremes if taking olanzapine (Zyprexa), quetiapine fumerate (Seroquel), or risperidone (Risperdal), as the body's ability to regulate internal temperature is affected by these medications.
- Utilize good oral hygiene in conjunction with sugarless candy or gum to minimize the discomforting side effect of dry mouth associated most frequently with clozapine (Clozaril) and olanzapine (Zyprexa).
- Beware of associated risks including EPS, NMS, and a high risk of agranulocytosis and seizures with clozapine (Clozaril); EPS, TD, and NMS with olanzapine (Zyprexa), quetiapine (Seroquel), and risperidone (Risperdal); and seizures with olanzapine (Zyprexa) and quetiapine fumerate (Seroquel).
- Treatment with clozapine (Clozaril) requires *weekly* white blood cell (WBC) monitoring to assess for onset of agranulocytosis. Medication is dispensed in 7-day increments to maintain policy compliance and prevent this potentially life-threatening occurrence.

Diet

Some of the antipsychotics such as clozapine (Clozaril), olanzapine (Zyprexa), quetiapine fumerate (Seroquel), and risperidone (Risperdal) can cause weight gain over time. For the individual who has schizophrenia and its multiple associated problems, weight gain can constitute yet one more stressor. Teaching for the client who is at risk for gaining weight must therefore emphasize the importance of being cognizant of and conservative with regard to caloric and fat intake, avoiding a sedentary lifestyle, and increasing physical activity.

Refrain from Making Judgments

Changing the words we use may help the client and family feel less defensive and may open the door for more effective communication. One example of an often-used term that carries negative connotations is *noncompliance.* Ward-Collins (1998) encourages nurses to consider using another term such as *nonadherence,* which does not carry the same degree of negative connotations.

Activity

Clients with schizophrenia tend to be tired and lethargic, probably because of multiple factors including the disease process and, possibly, the sedative properties associated with some of the antipsychotics, especially some of the older ones such as chlorpromazine (Thorazine) and thioridazine (Mellaril).

Nursing Management

Carefully observe the client's behavior. Listen to the client but neither agree nor disagree with what the client is saying. Accurately document what is seen and heard. Include the family in client care. Encourage the client to perform ADLs.

NURSING PROCESS

Assessment

Subjective Data

The client may be very frightened, confused, and have disorganized thought processes, using a nonsensical combination of words that is meaningless to others **(word salad),** talk out loud even when no one is present, or respond to internal stimulation or hallucinations.

Objective Data

The client may be isolated, withdrawn, experience great difficulty in any type of social interaction or situation, and stay in bed and sleep. Thus, the client may require a great deal of assistance and encouragement to perform ADLs and complete basic hygiene needs.

Nursing diagnoses for the client with schizophrenia may include the following:

Nursing Diagnoses	Planning/Goals	Nursing Interventions
Disturbed Sensory Perception (Visual, Auditory) related to altered sensory perception	The client will experience a decrease in the intensity and frequency of symptoms.	Assess for the presence of hallucinations. Assist the client in beginning to exert some control over the hallucinations. Educate the client about ways to decrease the intensity and power of the hallucinations.
Deficient Knowledge related to medication therapy	Client will verbalize an understanding of the disorder and the ongoing need for medications.	Educate the client and family about the disorder of schizophrenia, the need for antipsychotic medications, and the importance of continuing the prescribed medication regimen.

Evaluation Each goal must be evaluated to determine how it has been met by the client.

BIPOLAR DISORDER

Bipolar Disorder (previously known as manic–depressive disorder) is characterized by wide fluctuations in **mood** (the way an individual reports feeling, e.g., depressed, elated, happy, sad) and **affect** (the objective or outward manifestation of the way an individual is feeling). More than 2 million Americans have bipolar disorder (DBSA, 2003a). In addition to having a wide range of both affect and mood, the individual with bipolar disorder may experience fluctuations between depression and **mania** (extremely elevated mood with accompanying agitated behavior). The client with bipolar disorder may experience these fluctuations in mood and affect in varying degrees and over varying time frames. For example, an individual may experience changes in mood and affect every few years, at certain times of the year, every few months, every few weeks, or even every few days. The alterations in mood between depression and mania are often referred to as **cycling**. Individuals who suffer what is known as rapid cycling may experience multiple swings between depression and mania in the same day. There are also several degrees of both depression and mania that the individual can experience. As is the case with depression, an individual can experience mild, moderate, or severe mania. The degrees of mania range on a continuum from **hypomania** (a mild form of mania without significant impairment) to severe or delirious mania (DBSA, 2003a).

An individual in the depressed phase of bipolar disorder will manifest the same signs and symptoms as an individual with depression. The client in the manic phase of bipolar disorder may be very irritable and agitated and can be intimidating toward others, both verbally and physically. The client exhibiting manic behavior is often hyperactive, unable to sit down or remain still, and may display a **euphoric** (being elated out of context to the situation) affect and mood. Once in the manic phase of illness, clients will often exhibit behaviors incongruent with their usual personalities. For example, the manic client may dress in a flamboyant and provocative manner; spend money and buy things in a very lavish fashion; and become sexually promiscuous and engage in risky behaviors that would otherwise be out of character. After a while, the client may experience a great deal of conflict in social, familial, and personal relationships. It often becomes the responsibility of a significant other or family member to seek professional assistance for the individual. This already difficult situation is compounded by the fact that the client in the manic phase of bipolar disorder is frequently in denial about the illness, does not perceive the erratic behavior as problematic, and enjoys the "high" created by the disorder. As a result, the individual often refuses any type of help, and the family may be required to seek involuntary hospitalization in order to obtain the much-needed treatment.

Medical–Surgical Management
Medical

The severely agitated client in the manic phase of bipolar disorder may need to be secluded and/or restrained in order to protect against self-inflicted injury and/or the risk of injury to others.

Psychotherapy may be helpful to the client experiencing bipolar disorder, but it is not recommended as the only intervention. These clients typically require some type of medication management for the remainder of their lives in order to function adequately.

Pharmacological

The drug of choice for treatment of bipolar disorder is lithium carbonate (Lithonate) (Table 45-10). Lithium is a naturally occurring salt that has proven highly effective for many individuals in managing the severe mood swings associated with bipolar disorder. Lithium is referred to as a "mood stabilizer," meaning that it helps level or even out the wide mood swings associated with the disorder; however, some individuals either cannot tolerate lithium therapy or become resistant to its therapeutic effectiveness after a period of time. Fortunately, some other medications are often prescribed for clients who cannot take lithium. These include the anticonvulsants valproic acid (Depakene) and carbamazepine

TABLE 45-10 MOOD STABILIZER: ANTIMANIC

GENERIC NAME	TRADE NAME	POTENTIAL SIDE EFFECTS	SIGNS AND SYMPTOMS OF TOXICITY
lithium carbonate	Eskalith, Lithonate	Abdominal pain, acneiform eruption, anorexia, arrhythmia, bloating, diarrhea, dizziness, drowsiness, EKG changes, fatigue, folliculitis, GI upset, headache, hypothyroidism, impaired memory, irritability, leukocytosis, muscle weakness, nausea, polyuria, seizures, tinnitus, tremors	Ataxia, change in level of orientation, confusion, diarrhea, drowsiness, excessive urination, lack of coordination, muscle weakness, tremors, vomiting

Data from *2004 PDR Nurses' Drug Handbook,* by G. Spratto and A. Woods, 2004, Clifton Park, NY: Thomson Delmar Learning.

TABLE 45-11 MOOD STABILIZERS: ANTICONVULSANTS

GENERIC NAME	TRADE NAME	POTENTIAL SIDE EFFECTS
carbamazepine	Tegretol	Agranulocytosis, aplastic anemia, ataxia, drowsiness, drug-induced hepatitis, thrombocytopenia
valproic acid	Depakene	Depression, dizziness, indigestion, hepatotoxicity, leukopenia, nausea, thrombocytopenia, vomiting, weight gain

Data from *2004 PDR Nurses' Drug Handbook,* by G. Spratto and A. Woods, 2004, Clifton Park, NY: Thomson Delmar Learning.

CLIENT TEACHING

Lithium

Be sure to instruct each client taking lithium in the following:

- Do not drink alcohol while taking this medication.
- Do not take any other medications, prescribed or OTC, unless authorized by your physician.
- Do not stop taking this medication without authorization from your physician.
- Female clients should utilize a reliable form of contraception while taking this medication. Immediately inform your physician if pregnancy is suspected.
- Drink 2,000 to 3,000 cc of fluid (10–12 glasses) per day.
- Maintain a consistent level of salt in the diet.
- The ability to drive or operate heavy machinery may be impaired while on this medication.
- Serum lithium level must be checked at scheduled intervals throughout therapy.
- Be aware of signs and symptoms of lithium toxicity.

LIFE CYCLE CONSIDERATIONS

Creatinine Clearance

Because elders have reduced creatinine clearance, they are at a greater risk for developing toxicity while taking lithium (Andresen, 1998).

(Tegretol) (Table 45-11) and the anxiolytic/anticonvulsant clonazepam (Klonopin).

Lithium has a very narrow range of therapeutic effectiveness. The amount of lithium the individual has available and whether this level is appropriate is measured by a blood test called **serum lithium level.** The acceptable therapeutic range for the serum lithium level is 0.4 to 1.0 mEq/L; however, the value may vary slightly depending on the laboratory that is performing the test (Spratto & Woods, 2004). A lithium level that is too low will not produce any benefit, and one that is too high may be toxic, or poisonous. It is therefore critical that the serum lithium level be obtained every 5 days until the client is stabilized on the medication. Blood should then be drawn monthly for as long as the client is taking the medication (Spratto & Woods, 2004). Before initiating lithium therapy, a 24-hour urine creatinine clearance test is done to evaluate the functioning of the kidneys and their ability to adequately excrete the lithium.

Diet

Because lithium is a salt that is chemically similar to sodium chloride (table salt), lithium and sodium compete for absorption at receptor sites. This relationship is inversely proportional; thus, any changes in the body's sodium level will directly affect lithium level. Adequate fluid intake is very important for the client on lithium therapy. It is recommended that the client taking lithium consume a minimum of 2,000 to 3,000 cc of water per day. Because of the stimulating effects of caffeine, clients taking lithium should avoid any beverages containing caffeine.

CLIENT TEACHING

Anticonvulsants

Be sure to instruct each client taking an anticonvulsant medication in the following:

- Do not drink alcohol while taking the medication.
- Do not take any other medications, prescribed or OTC, unless authorized by your physician.
- Take the medication exactly as prescribed.
- Do not stop taking the medication without authorization from your physician.
- Do not stop taking the medication abruptly.
- The medications are contraindicated during pregnancy and lactation. Female clients should advise their physicians immediately if they are either pregnant or planning to become pregnant.
- Carbamazepine (Tegretol) can impair the effectiveness of hormonal forms of contraception. Female clients should practice an alternate form of birth control while on this medication.
- The ability to drive or operate heavy machinery may be impaired while on the medication.
- Laboratory tests monitoring complete blood count (CBC), platelet count, bleeding time, and hepatic functioning must be performed periodically throughout therapy.
- Notify your physician immediately of unexplained fever, sore throat, bleeding, bruising, or petechiae.
- Serum level must be checked at scheduled intervals throughout therapy.

Activity

The balance of sodium chloride to lithium can also be affected by the client's level of activity. An increase in activity, especially in hot and/or humid conditions when excessive perspiration is likely, can deplete the client's sodium level, thereby causing a drastic increase in lithium level and, potentially, lithium toxicity. A sudden increase in a client's activity level requires close monitoring and replacement of both fluid and electrolytes in order to prevent a sudden increase in the lithium level.

Nursing Management

Include the family in client education about the disease process, illness progression, medications, and importance of taking the medications as prescribed (even if the client's condition improves dramatically). Emphasize the need to keep follow-up appointments and to have lab work done for lithium level. Encourage the family to help the client maintain a regular eating and sleeping schedule.

NURSING PROCESS

Assessment

Subjective Data

The client may deny having a problem or may view the problem as residing in other people. The client may also be quite loud, flamboyant, and grandiose in verbalizations and manifest very quick and **pressured speech** (rapid, intense speech).

Objective Data

The client may be sleeping very little or not at all and may not be eating or drinking, if in the manic phase. The client may at times be very irritable, agitated, quick to anger, and, possibly, violent. Clients with bipolar disorder often have extreme difficulty in interpersonal and social relationships because they have no personal boundaries. They may also be invasive and intrusive in their interactions with others, both verbally and physically.

Nursing diagnoses for the client with bipolar disorder may include the following:

Nursing Diagnoses	Planning/Goals	Nursing Interventions
Disturbed Sleep Pattern related to sensory alterations	The client will sleep 6 hours per night.	Provide a quiet, peaceful environment. Decrease external stimulation and environmental distractions.
		Teach client relaxation exercises.
Noncompliance (medication and treatment regimen) related to health beliefs	The client will demonstrate increased compliance with medication and treatment.	Educate the client and family about the disease process and the progression of the illness over time, prescribed medication, indications for use, dosage, times, and any possible side effects or untoward reactions, and the importance of taking the medication as prescribed.
		Teach the client to continue taking medication and to not miss doses *even if the condition improves dramatically.*

Evaluation Each goal must be evaluated to determine how it has been met by the client.

THE CLIENT REQUIRING SPECIAL CONSIDERATION

Several disorders require special attention and consideration on the part of the nurse. These include disorders commonly associated with childhood and adolescence and with individuals who have been violated in some manner, such as via neglect and/or abuse.

ATTENTION-DEFICIT/ HYPERACTIVITY DISORDER

The *DSM-IV* identifies 18 diagnostic criteria for Attention-Deficit/Hyperactivity Disorder (ADHD) that fall under the categories of *inattention, hyperactivity,* and *impulsivity* (APA, 2000). There are three varieties of Attention-Deficit/Hyperactivity Disorder listed in the *DSM-IV:* Attention-Deficit/Hyperactivity Disorder, Predominantly Hyperactive-Impulsive Type; Attention-Deficit/Hyperactivity Disorder, Predominantly Inattentive Type; and Attention-Deficit/Hyperactivity Disorder, Combined Type. The child with ADHD may exhibit one or more of these behaviors in any combination (inattention, hyperactivity, and impulsivity). The problematic behaviors associated with these disorders vary in severity for each individual. Once thought to be a disorder only of childhood, it is now known that ADHD may continue well into adulthood. Individuals with ADHD are extremely sensitive to their environments and surroundings and respond immediately to any type of stimuli or distraction that most individuals would not even notice.

PREDOMINANTLY HYPERACTIVE-IMPULSIVE TYPE

Hyperactivity is the hallmark feature of Predominantly Hyperactive-Impulsive Type ADHD, which is usually diagnosed in childhood when the symptoms first manifest. The pediatric client with ADHD may be referred for evaluation and treatment by parents or teachers because of impulsive and disruptive behavior in the classroom and/or at home. Research indicates that among children with ADHD, the ratio of males to females ranges anywhere from 4 : 1 to 9 : 1 (APA, 2000). In many cases, there seems to be a familial or possible genetic link, as seen in health histories, which often reveal a parent or immediate family member as having had a similar problem as a child.

PREDOMINANTLY INATTENTIVE TYPE

In some children with ADHD predominantly inattentive type, the symptom of hyperactivity is not always present. The children have problems primarily with attention span. The inattentive child cannot maintain attention on one task, does not appear to listen when spoken to, and is easily distracted and forgetful.

COMBINED TYPE

Children with ADHD of the combined type exhibit symptoms of hyperactivity, impulsivity, and inattention. The characteristics must typically be exhibited for a period of at least 6 months in order to qualify for the diagnosis.

Medical–Surgical Management

Medical

Counseling and therapy are often recommended to the client and family to assist in managing the child. The parents will require assistance in developing an effective behavior-modification program, such as a token-economy system that rewards desired behaviors, to help manage some of the child's problematic behaviors.

Pharmacological

The central nervous system (CNS) stimulants, which include methylphenidate hydrochloride (Ritalin), pemoline (Cylert), dextroamphetamine sulfate (Dexedrine), and amphetamine sulfate (Adderall), are usually prescribed to treat ADHD (Table 45-12). When one of the CNS stimulants is given to someone with ADHD, however, it has the opposite effect, or **paradoxical reaction.** Thus, instead of making someone with ADHD more hyperactive, it actually helps calm him. Because most of the symptoms of the child with ADHD, such as hyperactivity and the inability to concentrate and remain on task, are manifested in the classroom, any improvement will likely first be noted in this setting. When a child begins a new medication, it is vitally important that the family communicate openly with the child's teacher to ensure close monitoring of the child's response to medication. The child with ADHD who has been hyperactive, unable to stay on task, or complete assignments before receiving medication may now be less disruptive in the classroom and better able to remain on task and complete assignments. In addition, the medication can be a useful adjunct to facilitate the child's ability to develop and strengthen internal mechanisms for improving behavior.

TABLE 45-12   CENTRAL NERVOUS SYSTEM STIMULANTS

GENERIC NAME	TRADE NAME	POTENTIAL SIDE EFFECTS
dextroamphetamine sulfate	Dexedrine	Anorexia, headache, hyperactivity, hypertension, insomnia, palpitations, physical and psychological dependence, restlessness, tachycardia, tolerance, tremors, urticaria, weight loss
amphetamine sulfate	Adderall	Anorexia, hyperactivity, insomnia, palpitations, physical and psychological dependence, restlessness, tachycardia, tremors
methylphenidate hydrochloride	Ritalin	Anemia, anorexia, hyperactivity, hypertension, insomnia, leukopenia, physical and psychological dependence, restlessness, skin rash, suppression of weight gain, tolerance, tremors
pemoline	Cylert	Insomnia, anorexia, aplastic anemia, decreased growth, drug-induced hepatitis, nausea, physical or psychological dependence, seizures, stomachache, tolerance, weight loss
atomoxetine hydrochloride	Strattera	Fatigue, decreased appetite, aggression, nausea, vomiting, postural hypotension

Data from *2004 PDR Nurses' Drug Handbook*, by G. Spratto and A. Woods, 2004, Clifton Park, NY: Thomson Delmar Learning.

Teaching the client and family about the prescribed medication is very important, as there are some common side effects associated with the CNS stimulants, such as insomnia. To help decrease the risk of insomnia, these medications are usually given in the morning at breakfast, and if more is needed, another dose is given again at lunchtime. In some cases, a late-afternoon dose may be needed after school; however, this decision must be made very cautiously, because the later in the day that the dose is given, the greater the risk of insomnia that night for the child.

The client on CNS stimulants must be monitored for any vocal or motor tics, which might indicate the development of Tourette's syndrome. The CNS stimulant should be discontinued immediately if these symptoms are noted.

Diet

One potential problem associated with the CNS stimulants is that of decreased appetite, which can become serious if the child begins losing weight as a side effect of the medication. If this occurs, the medication may be given immediately after a meal to decrease the chance of appetite suppression. The family can adjust the timing and amount of food intake, such as eating larger meals later in the day, when the effects of the medication have worn off, or having a larger snack in the evening before bedtime.

The role and importance of diet in the management of ADHD continues to be highly controversial; however, some data supports the restriction of certain foods as an effective method of managing this disorder. Foods that contain sugar and caffeine are sometimes recommended to be excluded from the diet of the child with ADHD. The theory behind this recommendation is that sugar and caffeine tend to energize and increase any child's activity level, and in the case of some children with ADHD, this effect seems to be even more accentuated. Another controversial issue surrounding the significance of diet is that of food sensitivities and allergies. Food allergies sometimes manifest in symptoms such as irritability and hyperactivity, which may then be confused or misdiagnosed as ADHD.

Activity

The child with ADHD will usually respond best to a highly structured environment, which includes clear expectations and firm, consistent limits as well as appropriate consequences for unruly and disruptive behaviors. For example, a "time-out" may be used when the child must be temporarily removed from a setting or the environment.

Nursing Management

Monitor growth (height and weight) and development. Explain to the client what are acceptable behaviors. Provide positive reinforcement for appropriate behavior. Teach the client and family about prescribed medications.

NURSING PROCESS

Assessment

Subjective Data

The child or adolescent frequently verbalizes feeling "bad" about being unable to control hyperactive and disruptive behaviors and feeling like a failure, especially in the classroom. After only a single dose of medication, however, the child sometimes states a noticeable difference in the ability to remain centered and focused.

Objective Data

Although usually described as being hyperactive, unable to concentrate, unable to focus, and unable to remain on task, children with ADHD may sometimes be able to concentrate and remain quite attentive and focused. This usually happens in situations that the child enjoys and sometimes in situations that are new to the child. It can be quite frustrating for parents to bring in their child for an evaluation or screening, only to have

the child not exhibit any of the usual problematic behaviors. The knowledgeable practitioner or evaluator will be aware of what is happening and will obtain the necessary information from the parental report of the child's health history.

Nursing diagnoses for the child with ADHD may include the following:

Nursing Diagnoses	Planning/Goals	Nursing Interventions
*Deficient **K**nowledge (medications and disease process)*, related to new diagnosis of disorder and treatment regimen	The child and parents will verbalize an increased understanding of the disorder. The child and parents will verbalize an understanding about the role medications can play in treatment.	Educate the child and family about the disorder, including signs and symptoms, about the medication, including indications for use, dosages, when to take the medication, possible side effects, and the benefits that can be expected with the particular medication. Emphasize the importance of taking the medication as prescribed.
*Impaired **S**ocial Interaction* related to unaccepted social behaviors	The child will demonstrate an increase in appropriate peer interactions.	Explain to the child those behaviors that are acceptable. Observe the child in social situations with peers. Provide positive reinforcement for demonstration of appropriate behaviors. Immediately intervene when unacceptable behaviors are observed.

Evaluation Each goal must be evaluated to determine how it has been met by the client.

NEGLECT AND/OR ABUSE

There are many types of **neglect** (a situation wherein a basic need of the client is not being provided) and **abuse** (an incident involving some type of violation to the client). Neglect can be quite evident, such as a lack of

adequate food, clothing, or shelter, or less tangible, such as emotional neglect or an absence of nurturing. Abuse can be physical, emotional, psychological, financial, or sexual in nature, or any combination of these. Abuse can also take the form of **domestic violence,** which is aggression and violence involving family members. Neglect and abuse often go hand in hand.

A client experiencing neglect or abuse is usually dependent on another individual for the meeting of basic care and needs. In many neglectful or abusive situations, the clients are vulnerable individuals such as children, adolescents, or elders. Others who are neglected or abused include individuals with some type of illness or incapacitation. Neglect and abuse can take many shapes and forms, ranging anywhere from mild cases to situations so severe that death is the end result.

ELDER ABUSE AND NEGLECT

Elder abuse became nationally recognized in 1981 after the House Select Committee on Aging issued its landmark report *Elder Abuse: An Examination of a Hidden Problem*. The committee found that elder abuse was simply "alien to the American ideal." Because it is such a difficult concept to come to grips with, even abused elders are reluctant to admit that their loved ones have abused them.

The committee defined the following types of elder abuse: physical, passive physical, financial, psychological, sexual, and violation of rights. There is no federal legislation to protect elders from abuse, neglect, or exploitation. All 50 states, including the District of Columbia, have some form of elder abuse prevention laws (AoA, 2003). Adult abuse and protection laws are based on the legal premise that society (represented by the state) has the authority to act in a parental capacity for persons who are unable to care for and protect themselves and thus prevent them from suffering from abuse, neglect, or exploitation by those responsible for their care or from self-abuse (Frisch & Frisch, 2002). The purposes of adult protection service laws are to facilitate the identification of functionally impaired elders who are being abused, neglected, or exploited by others; to encourage expeditious reporting; and to extend protective services while protecting the rights of the abused. In most states, the adult protective services (APS) agency is the principal agency designated to receive and investigate allegations of elder abuse and neglect. In most jurisdictions, the county departments of social services maintain the APS unit.

The National Elder Abuse Incidence Study of 1996 found that almost 450,000 persons age 60 and older ex-

perienced abuse and/or neglect in domestic settings. Only 16% were reported to APS; that is, less than 1 out of 5 cases were reported. Persons age 80 and older were abused and neglected two to three times their proportion of the elderly population. When the perpetrators of the neglect and abuse were known, 80% were family members and two-thirds of those were adult children or spouses (AoA, 2002, 2003).

DOMESTIC VIOLENCE

Domestic violence is a pattern of controlling behavior and assaults, including physical, sexual, and psychological attacks and economic control, that adolescents and adults use against their intimate partners. It is common and lethal, affecting people of all ages, cultures, religions, sexual orientations, educational backgrounds, and income levels (Family Violence Prevention Fund [FVPF], 2001b).

Domestic violence occurs in relationships where conflict is the continuous result of power inequality between partners. One of the partners is afraid of and harmed by the other. In all cultures, the perpetrators are most often men and the victims are most often women (National Coalition Against Domestic Violence [NCADV], 2003). In the United States, 31% of women report being sexually or physically abused by a boyfriend or husband at some point during their life (FVPF, 2001a).

In all states, domestic violence is a crime, but the laws in each state are a little different (American Bar Association [ABA], 2001). The nurse is responsible for knowing the laws, especially mandatory reporting, about domestic violence in the state of employment. Each state has a coalition against domestic violence, which are valuable resources. The National Domestic Violence Hotline is 800-799-7233 (SAFE).

LIFE CYCLE CONSIDERATIONS

Abuse of Elders

Because of a loss of independence and a forced reliance on others, elders are vulnerable to being abused in several ways. Morris (1998) defines a vulnerable adult "as a person with a physical or mental condition—such as Alzheimer's disease or an infirmity related to aging—that substantially impairs his ability to care for himself." Laws have been developed to protect elders from abusive situations, and agencies such as APS have been established to facilitate this process.

PROFESSIONAL TIP

Caring for the Abused Client

When questioning clients about the possibility of interpersonal violence or sexual assault, the nurse must quickly develop a rapport and create an environment indicating that personal experiences are acceptable topics to discuss. This allows them the opportunity to express their fears and concerns. This can be done by:

- Treating them with dignity and concern.
- Giving priority to them over nonemergency clients.
- Placing them in quiet and private areas.
- Not leaving them alone.
- Speaking quietly and in a nonjudgmental manner.
- Using active and empathic listening skills.
- Not acting shocked or surprised at the details of their experiences.
- Reassuring them that the abuse was not their fault.
- Explaining any delays in treatment.
- Asking permission to call family members, friends, or in the case of rape, rape crisis advocates.
- Providing information about community resources.

CRITICAL THINKING

Domestic Violence

What are your feelings about domestic violence? How would you react to a client who was a victim of domestic violence? Would you be able to respond appropriately? What if the client refuses your attempt to assist her to leave the abusive situation?

RAPE

Rape is a legal term, not a medical entity. It is a crime of violence. Rapists use sexual violence to dominate and degrade their victims and to express their own anger. It is not an act of lust or an overzealous release of passion done to satisfy a sexual urge (Frisch & Frisch, 2002).

There are three basic types of rape: (1) rape by a person known to the survivor, for example, father, former and current friends (date rape), neighbors, partner or separated partner, dissatisfied clients of prostitutes; (2) gang rape; and (3) stranger-to-stranger rape. The latter, which women fear the most, follows an identifiable pattern. Such rapists look for women who are vulnerable, even though they differ on defining who is vulnerable. They might attempt to rape elders, people who are developmentally, physically, or mentally challenged, or intoxicated people. They might look for environments that are easy to enter and relatively safe (e.g., women's bedrooms) and where they will not be interrupted. They often select their victims long before they approach them

PROFESSIONAL TIP

Interviewing the Survivor of Abuse or Violence

The type of questions will depend on the type of violence and whether survivors have told you they have been abused. If they have told you they have been abused, you must ask specific questions about the abuse. If they have not, you must ask more open-ended questions to allow them to disclose sensitive information. Generally speaking:

- Inform the client that it is necessary to ask some very personal questions.
- Use language appropriate for the age and developmental level of the survivor.
- Use conversational language or street language.
- Keep questions simple, nonthreatening, and direct.
- Pose questions in a manner that permits brief answers.
- Indicate sensitivity to and acceptance of the client's state of confusion.
- Avoid using leading statements that can distort the client's report.
- Do not criticize the client's family.
- Do not promise not to report the abuse; indicate that you are required by law to report the abuse.

and repeat the same pattern of victim selection over and over again. All types of rape can be an emotionally terrorizing experience for the survivors.

Medical–Surgical Management

Medical

Planning care for survivors of neglect and abuse and their families requires input from the clients and a survey of their resources to ensure that care is in line with their expectations and commitments. Nursing interventions directed at primary prevention of interpersonal violence are those that reduce or control the causative factors associated with interpersonal violence and sexual assaults. By identifying families at risk for abuse, nurses can help the family plan efforts to modify those risk factors.

Health Promotion

Primary prevention includes empowering survivors of abuse by helping them learn to care for and protect themselves from the imposition by others. For example, children can be taught in health care settings or schools those things to do if they are being abused. It also includes changing the family's perceptions of violence as an acceptable mode of conflict resolution (Clark, 2000).

Provide anticipatory guidance. For example, by anticipating the challenges of toddlerhood, acknowledge that this can be a difficult period for parents and provide practical advice about constructive discipline. Teach college freshmen about date rape and to avoid vulnerable situations. Encourage families with dependent elderly members to use respite care services and day care programs. Such support and anticipatory guidance can enhance the family's and client's competence and diminish the likelihood of violence or abuse.

Nursing Management

Know the mandatory reporting laws in your state of employment. When assessing clients, ask about bruises, scars, and burns when seen. Provide anticipatory guidance for challenging events in a client's family life that will enhance the family's competence and diminish the probability of abuse or violence.

NURSING PROCESS

Assessment

Subjective Data

There is no comprehensive assessment tool that offers conclusive evidence that neglect, abuse, or violence has occurred. Act like detectives when assessing clients, given that clients or their abusers will rarely admit to abuse or violence. Make direct observations of the client and family members (e.g., Does the child seem afraid of the caregiver? Does the caregiver hit the child?). These observations are clues that more probing is necessary.

In order to properly assess survivors of abuse, the symptoms that are commonly seen in interpersonal violence and sexual assaults and the common characteristics of the abusers must be known. Many of the symptoms are subjective, so the health care team must piece together the evidence to ascertain whether interpersonal violence has occurred or clients are at risk for violence. Psychological abuse is a particularly difficult area to assess because emotional relationships are very culture bound, and words and emotions that may be harmful in one family are not necessarily so in another family.

Objective Data

A more extensive examination is warranted when the history or behavioral symptoms indicate interpersonal abuse. Clients need to have physical examinations to assess the extent of their injuries and to collect forensic evidence to prove who assaulted them. A traumagram, or body map (a drawing of the front and back of a nude human figure), is generally used to mark the location of all visible injuries. Each state has legally mandated procedures for collecting evidentiary material, and it is a nursing responsibility to be sure that the legal "chain of evidence" pertaining to collection of forensic samples is unbroken. The medical record should document the injuries and nursing and medical treatment that may serve as legal evidence of the client's condition.

Nursing diagnoses for the client experiencing neglect or abuse may include the following:

Nursing Diagnoses	Planning/Goals	Nursing Interventions
Interrupted Family Processes related to neglect	The client will not experience any further neglect.	Provide support for the client. Document the evidence of neglect with which the client presents via written observations, laboratory reports, and/or pictures, if indicated. Report the case of neglect to the proper authorities: police, child protective services (CPS), APS, and any others that might be indicated.
Fear related to abuse	The client will verbalize being less fearful.	Reassure the client that the client is in a safe place and that you are there to help in any way that you can. Provide emotional support to the client in a nonjudgmental manner.
Risk for Injury related to abusive home life	The client will not experience any further injury or abuse.	Address the client's safety needs and attempt to assess whether abuse is occurring. If you suspect that abuse is occurring notify your supervisor so the proper authorities can be notified (Ladebauche, 1997).

Evaluation Each goal must be evaluated to determine how it has been met by the client.

EATING DISORDERS

Eating disorders include anorexia nervosa and bulimia nervosa. Anorexia nervosa is characterized by self-imposed starvation by restricting caloric intake and compulsive exercising. Bulimia nervosa is characterized by periods of binge eating of up to 10,000 calories at one time followed by self-induced vomiting and other forms of purging such as laxative and diuretic abuse. In bulimia nervosa, the client's weight is normal or above normal. In anorexia nervosa, body weight is low and keeps getting lower. Most clients with these disorders are female and younger than age 30.

Complications can be serious and include cardiac abnormalities such as bradycardia, hypotension, arrhythmias, CHF, and cardiovascular collapse; oral and esophageal erosions and dental caries from vomiting; renal abnormalities that affect the kidney's ability to filter urine; skin rashes from malnutrition; and bruising from vomiting.

Clients with anorexia nervosa tend to be high achievers, perfectionists, have a distorted body image in that they see themselves as fat, and are rigid and ritualistic.

Bulimia nervosa occurs more frequently than anorexia nervosa, with clients experiencing a fear of not being able to stop eating. Clients often experience guilt and depression after a binge.

Medical–Surgical Management
Diet

During severe cases, clients may be admitted for enforced feeding, including the placement of a feeding tube or TPN, IV fluid rehydration, and electrolyte replacement. Clients need to be monitored for refeeding complications such as pancreatitis and gastric dilation. Small quantities are given at first, and very gradually the amount is increased.

Other Therapies

Treatment is primarily psychiatric, involving the client and family, and is typically done on an outpatient basis.

Nursing Management

Monitor weight, calorie intake, I&O, and exercise program. Assess behavior around mealtime. Administer IV fluid and electrolyte replacement. Check vital signs and laboratory test results.

NURSING PROCESS

Assessment

Subjective Data

Clients with either anorexia nervosa and bulimia nervosa may verbalize feelings of helplessness and being out of control, and may exhibit low self-esteem. They may also have overprotective parents. Clients with anorexia nervosa may also describe bad dreams and cold intolerance.

Objective Data

Clients with anorexia nervosa are underweight, usually lost over a short period of time, reluctant to eat with others, move food around the plate without eating it, hypotensive, have heart irregularities, and altered thinking patterns.

Clients with bulimia nervosa have normal weight, tooth erosions and dental caries, puffy face, callused knuckles, broken blood vessels in the eyes and face, reluctance to eat with others, and going to the bathroom immediately after eating.

Laboratory analysis will include a CBC, which may show low Hgb, Hct, and platelets; electrolytes, which may show low sodium, potassium, and chloride; an SMA-22 that shows low protein, phosphate, and magnesium; and elevated BUN.

Nursing diagnoses for a hospitalized client with anorexia nervosa or bulimia nervosa may include the following:

Nursing Diagnoses	Planning/Goals	Nursing Interventions
Imbalanced Nutrition: Less than body requirements related to psychological restriction of food intake, excessive activity	The client will demonstrate increased consumption of nutrients as evidenced by weight gain daily and improved laboratory values.	Weigh daily. Monitor calorie intake. Monitor I&O every shift. Administer IV rehydration, electrolyte replacement, and TPN or tube feedings as ordered. Monitor behavior at and around meal time, such as going to the bathroom right after eating. Monitor exercise patterns.
Risk for Deficient Fluid Volume related to inadequate intake of liquids, self-induced vomiting, laxative and diuretic use	The client's intake and output will be approximately equal by the fourth hospital day. The client's electrolytes will be within normal limits, by the third hospital day. The client's fluid intake will be at least 2,000 mL per day.	Monitor I&O every shift and bowel movements for diarrhea (a sign of continued laxative abuse). Monitor laboratory reports for electrolyte levels as ordered. Administer IV fluid and electrolyte replacement as ordered.
Ineffective Coping (Individual) related to maturational crisis and attempting to control environment	The client will verbalize feelings regarding disease process and hospitalization, by discharge. The client will identify current coping strategies, by discharge. The client will identify personal strengths, by discharge.	Provide opportunities for the client to express feelings regarding hospitalization. Encourage client to identify coping mechanisms and strengths. Give positive feedback regarding identified personal strengths.

Evaluation Each goal must be evaluated to determine how it has been met by the client.

Summary

- The components of a therapeutic nurse–client relationship include trust, rapport, respect, genuineness, and empathy.
- An individual's anxiety level may range anywhere from mild to panic level.
- The nurse often encounters clients and/or family members who are angry, aggressive, homicidal, and/or suicidal in the midst of a crisis situation.
- The depressed individual must be evaluated for risk of suicide.
- The individual with schizophrenia may be out of touch with reality and influenced by delusions and/or hallucinations.
- Individuals with bipolar disorder may experience wide mood swings ranging from depression to mania.
- Neglect and abuse can occur among any age group.
- Anorexia nervosa and bulimia nervosa are psychological disorders affecting mostly women. Severe nutritional imbalances can occur leading to serious effects on the cardiovascular system.

Review Questions

1. The client who is experiencing severe or panic level anxiety should:
   a. be left alone to calm down.
   b. be taught new information.
   c. never be left alone.
   d. be given an antidepressant immediately.

2. A nurse who is aware of a client's plan to kill someone else should:
   a. do nothing; it is not her responsibility.
   b. contact the physician and alert the proper authorities.
   c. discourage the client from following through with the plan.
   d. continue preparing the client for discharge per orders in the chart.

3. The client who is contemplating suicide may:
   a. give away prized personal possessions.
   b. buy new personal items.
   c. purchase an expensive item.
   d. purchase an inexpensive item.

4. Signs and symptoms of schizophrenia include:
   a. hyperactivity and decreased concentration.
   b. crying spells and decreased appetite.
   c. compulsive rituals.
   d. hallucinations and/or delusions.

5. The client experiencing abuse will:
   a. always tell the truth about what is happening.
   b. often lie about what is happening in order to protect the abuser.
   c. always contact the authorities.
   d. never withhold significant information from health care providers.

References/Suggested Readings

Administration on Aging (AoA). (2002). *National Elder Abuse Incidence Study.* [Online]. Available: www.aoa.gov/abuse/report/H-Conclusions.html

Administration on Aging (AoA). (2003). *Fact sheets: Elder Abuse Prevention.* [Online]. Available: www.aoa.gov/press/fact/alpha/fact_elder_abuse_pf.asp

American Bar Association (ABA). (2001). *Know your rights: Domestic Violence.* [Online]. Available: www.abanet.org/domviol/knowrights.pdf

American Psychiatric Association. (APA). (2000). *Diagnostic and statistical manual of mental disorders* (4th ed.). (DSM-IV-TR [text-revision]) Washington, DC: Author.

Andresen, G. (1998). Assessing the older patient. *RN, 61*(3), 46–55.

Anxiety Disorders Association of America (ADAA). (2002a). *Anxiety Disorders.* [Online]. Available: www.adaa.org/AnxietyDisorderInfor/OverviewAnxDis.cfm

Anxiety Disorders Association of America (ADAA). (2002b). *Obsessive-Compulsive Disorder (OCD).* [Online]. Available: www.adaa.org/AnxietyDisorderInfor/OCD.cfm

Anxiety Disorders Association of America (ADAA). (2002c). *Panic Disorder.* [Online]. Available: www.adaa.org/AnxietyDisorderInfor/PanicDisAgor.cfm

Anxiety Disorders Association of America (ADAA). (2002d). *Post-Traumatic Stress Disorder (PTSD).* [Online]. Available: www.adaa.org/AnxietyDisorderInfor/PTSD.cfm

Berlinger, J. (2002). Domestic violence: How you can make a difference. *Nursing2001, 31*(8), 58–63.

Centers for Disease Control and Prevention (CDC), National Center for Injury Prevention and Control (NCIPC). (2003). *Suicide in the United States.* [Online]. Available: www.cdc.gov/ncipc/factsheets/suifacts.htm

Clark, M. J. (2000). Violence. In *Nursing in the community* (3rd ed.). Stamford, CT: Prentice Hall.

Cole, M. (1999). Bipolar disorder: Illness or eccentricity? *Nursing Spectrum (NY NJ), 11A*(2), 4–5.

Cole, M. (1999). Bridging the great divide: Management of the patient with bipolar disorder. *Nursing Spectrum (NY NJ), 11A*(3), 8–9.

Daniels, R. (2002). *Delmar's Guide to Laboratory and Diagnostic Tests.* Clifton Park, NY: Thomson Delmar Learning.

Depression and Bipolar Support Alliance (DBSA). (2003a). *Bipolar Disorder.* [Online]. Available: www.dbsalliance.org/info/bipolar.html

Depression and Bipolar Support Alliance (DBSA). (2003b). *Depression.* [Online]. Available: www.dbsalliance.org/info/depression.html

DiVitto, S. (1998). Empowerment through self-regulation: Group approach for survivors of incest. *Journal of the American Psychiatric Nurses Association, 4*(3), 77–86.

Dochterman, J. C., & Bulechek, G. M. (2004). *Nursing interventions classification (NIC)* (4th ed.). St. Louis, MO: Mosby.

Eskreis, T. R. (1998). Seven common legal pitfalls in nursing. *AJN, 98*(4), 34–41.

Family Violence Prevention Fund (FVPF). (2001a). *Get the Facts: Domestic Violence and Health Care.* [Online]. Available: www.endabuse.org/programs/display.php3?DocID=25

Family Violence Prevention Fund (FVPF). (2001b). *Get the Facts: Domestic Violence and the Workplace.* [Online]. Available: www.endabuse.org/programs/display.php3?DocID=70

Ferri, R., Sofer, D., & Zolot, J. (2003). Depression in America, *AJN, 103*(9), 17.

Frisch, N. C., & Frisch, L. E. (2002). *Psychiatric mental health nursing.* (2nd ed.). Clifton Park, NY: Thomson Delmar Learning.

Gale, G. (2002). A useful screening tool. *RN, 65*(9), 41–43.

Harrison, B., & Kaarsemaker, B. (2000). Continuous quality improvement to an electroconvulsive therapy delivery system. *Journal of Psychosocial Nursing Mental Health Services, 38*(3), 27–37.

Hinkle, P. (2000). Bipolar illness in primary care: An overview. *Lippincott's Primary Care Practice, 4*(2), 163–173.

Incredibly Easy! (2002). Reviewing anxiety and mood disorders. *Nursing2002, 32*(6), 76–77.

Isaacs, A. (1998). Depression & your patient. *AJN, 98*(7), 26–31.

Koschel, M. (2003). Is it child abuse? *AJN, 103*(4), 45–46.

McGlotten, S. (2003). Attempted suicide. *Nursing2003, 33*(4), 96.

Mohr, W. (1998). Updating what we know about depression in adolescents. *Journal of Psychosocial Nursing and Mental Health Services, 36*(9), 12–19.

Moorhead, S., Johnson, M., & Maas, M. (2004). *Nursing Outcomes Classification (NOC)* (3rd ed.). St. Louis, MO: Mosby.

Morris, R. (1998). Elder abuse: What the law requires. *RN, 61*(8), 52–53.

National Coalition against Domestic Violence (NCADV). (2003). *The Problem.* [Online]. Available: www.ncadv.org/problem/what.htm

North American Nursing Diagnosis Association (2003). *Nursing Diagnoses: Definitions & Classification 2003-2004.* Philadelphia: Author.

Orbanic, S. (2002). Understanding bulimia. *AJN, 101*(3), 35–41.

Peplau, H. E. (1962). Interpersonal techniques: The crux of psychiatric nursing. *AJN, 62*(6), 50–54.

Peplau, H. E. (1963). A working definition of anxiety. In S. Burd & M. Marshall (Eds.), *Some clinical approaches to psychiatric nursing.* New York: Macmillan.

Peplau, H. E. (1991). *Interpersonal relations in nursing.* New York: Springer.

Ponech, S. (2000). Telltale signs. *Nursing Management, 31*(5), 32–38.

Romme, M. (1998). Listening to the voice hearers. *Journal of Psychosocial Nursing and Mental Health Services, 36*(9), 40–44.

Rother, L. (2003). Electroconvulsive therapy sheds its shocking image. *Nursing2003, 33*(3), 48–49.

Ryan, B. (2003). Do you suspect child abuse? *RN, 66*(9), 73–77.

Spratto, G., & Woods, A. (2004). *2004 PDR Nurses' Drug Handbook.* Clifton Park, NY: Thomson Delmar Learning.

Sullivan, G. H. (1998). Getting informed consent. *RN, 61*(4), 59–62.

Sundeen, S., Stuart, G. W., Rankin, E. A. D., & Cohen, S. A. (1998). *Nurse–Client interaction: Implementing the nursing process* (6th ed.). St. Louis, MO: Mosby.

Townsend, M. C. (2000). *Psychiatric mental health nursing: Concepts of care* (3rd ed.). Philadelphia: F. A. Davis.

Townsend, M. C. (2003). *Nursing diagnoses in psychiatric nursing: A pocket guide for care plan construction* (5th ed.). Philadelphia: F. A. Davis.

U. S. Food and Drug Administration. MedWatch. (2002). *Zoloft (sertraline hydrochloride).* [Online]. Available: www.fda.gov/medwatch/SAFETY/2002/safety02.htm#zoloft

U. S. House of Representatives, Select Committee on Aging (1981, April 3). *Elder Abuse (an examination of a hidden problem)* (Comm. Pub. No. 97–277). Washington, DC: U. S. Government Printing Office.

U. S. Preventive Services Task Force (2002). Screening for depression: Recommendations and rationale. *Annals of Internal Medicine, 136*(10), 760.

United States Code Annotated, Title 42, The Public Health and Welfare, Chapter 67, Child Abuse Prevention and Treatment and Adoption Reform; Subchapter 1, Child Abuse Prevention and Treatment; Definitions; Title II, Victims of Child Abuse Act of 1990; Subtitle D, Federal Victims' Protection and Rights; Section 226, Child Abuse Reporting. St. Paul, MN: West.

Vernarec, E. (2002). The hidden threat to our nation's kids. *RN, 65*(9), 36–40.

Ward-Collins, D. (1998). "Noncompliant": Isn't there a better way to say it? *AJN, 98*(5), 27–32.

Woods, A. (2003). Depression. *Nursing2003, 33*(3), 54–55.

Wuerker, A. (2000). The family and schizophrenia. *Issues of Mental Health Nursing, 21*(1), 127–141.

Yamashita, M., & McNally-Forsyth, D. (1998). Family coping with mental illness: An aggregate from two studies, Canada and United States. *Journal of the American Psychiatric Nurses Association, 4*(1), 1–8.

Resources

Administration on Aging (AoA), 200 Independence Avenue SW, Washington, DC 20201, 202-619-0724, www.aoa.gov

American Anorexia/Bulimia Association, 165 W 46th Street, Suite 1108, New York, NY 10036, 212-575-6200, www.4woman.gov

American Psychiatric Association, 1000 Wilson Boulevard, Suite 1825, Arlington, VA 22209-3901, 703-907-7300, www.psych.org

American Psychiatric Nurses Association, 1555 Wilson Boulevard, Suite 515, Arlington, VA 22209, 703-243-2443, www.apna.org

Anxiety Disorders Association of America, 8730 Georgia Avenue, Suite 600, Silver Spring, MD 20910, 240-485-1001, www.adaa.org

Depression and Bipolar Support Alliance, 730 North Franklin Street, Suite 501, Chicago, IL 60610-7204, 800-826-3632, www.dbsalliance.org

Family Violence Prevention Fund (FVPF), 383 Rhode Island Street, Suite #304, San Francisco, CA 94103-5133, 415-252-8900, www.endabuse.org

National Alliance for Research on Schizophrenia and Depression (NARSAD), 60 Cutter Mill Road, Suite 404, Great Neck, NY 11021, 516-829-0091, www.narsad.org

National Alliance for the Mentally Ill (NAMI), Colonial Place Three, 2107 Wilson Boulevard, Suite 300, Arlington, VA 22201, 800-950-6264, www.nami.org

National Association of Anorexia Nervosa and Associated Disorders, P.O. Box 7, Highland Park, IL 60038, 847-831-3438, www.altru.net/site/anadweb

National Center on Elder Abuse, 1201 15th Street, N.W., Suite 350, Washington, DC 20006, 202-898-2586, www.elderabusecenter.org

National Coalition against Domestic Violence (NCADV), P. O. Box 18749, Denver, CO 80218, 303-839-1852, www.ncadv.org

National Domestic Violence Hotline, 800-799-7233 or TTD 800-787-3224

National Eating Disorders Association, 603 Stewart Street, Suite 803, Seattle, WA 98101, 800-931-2237, www.nationaleatingdisorders.org

National Institute of Mental Health, 6001 Executive Boulevard, Room 8184, MSC 9663, Bethesda, MD 20892-9663, 301-443-4513, www.nimh.nih.gov

Parents Anonymous, The National Organization, 675 W. Foothill Blvd., Suite 220, Claremont, CA 91711-3475, 909-621-6184, www.parentsanonymous.org

Recovery, Inc.: The Association of Nervous and Former Mental Patients, 802 N. Dearborn Street, Chicago, IL 60610, 312-337-5661, www.recovery-inc.com

Victims of Incest Can Emerge Survivors (VOICES), P.O. Box 13, Newtonsville, OH 45158 800-786-4238, www.voices-action.org

SUBSTANCE ABUSE

MAKING THE CONNECTION

Refer to the following chapters to increase your understanding of substance abuse:

Basic Nursing
- **Legal and Ethical Responsibilities**
- **Wellness Concepts**
- **Assessment**

Adult Health Nursing
- **Respiratory System**
- **Gastrointestinal System**
- **The Older Adult**

LEARNING OBJECTIVES

Upon completion of this chapter, you should be able to:
- **Define key terms.**
- **Differentiate among dependence, abuse, and intoxication.**
- **Describe issues related to drug testing.**
- **Discuss substances frequently abused.**
- **Use assessment skills to identify possible substance abuse.**
- **Describe nursing interventions in working with substance abusers.**
- **Describe stages of alcoholism and the impact on the individual, family, and society.**
- **Discuss medications frequently used in the treatment of substance abuse.**
- **Describe an impaired nurse.**
- **Identify goals of programs for impaired nurses.**

KEY TERMS

abuse	Johnsonian intervention
addiction	misuse
behavioral tolerance	opisthotonos
codependent	relapse
confabulation	reverse tolerance
cross-tolerance	substance
dependence	synthesiasis
detoxification	teratogenic
hallucination	tolerance
intoxication	withdrawal

INTRODUCTION

Substance use has taken place for many centuries. It is not a new problem for society. A **substance** is a drug, legal or illegal, that may cause physical or mental impairment. With the great increase in world population, there are more people involved in substance abuse. Today's speed of travel and communication has facilitated the broad distribution of substances.

Many street drugs are "cut" (mixed) with substances that should not be consumed, such as talcum powder, rodent exterminating powder, or even strychnine. The purity (strength) of the drug is then not known and overdose easily occurs. Fatalities can occur from the substance with which the drug is cut.

In the United States, substance disorders affect males and females, all ethnic groups, and persons of all levels of education and income. From the newborn to the elderly, all ages can be affected.

Substance disorders may be classified as intoxication, abuse, or dependence (addiction); definitions are based on the criteria presented in the American Psychiatric Association's *Diagnostic and Statistical Manual of Mental Disorders,* fourth edition *(DSM-IV).* The reversible effect on the central nervous system (CNS) soon after the use of a substance is termed **intoxication. Abuse** is the misuse, excessive, or improper use of a substance, the abstinence of which does not cause withdrawal symptoms.

Dependence (addiction) is reliance on a substance to such a degree that abstinence causes functional impairment, physical withdrawal symptoms, and/or a psychological craving for the substance.

According to NIDA (2003l), substances interfere with normal brain function creating powerful feelings of pleasure and having long-term effects on brain metabolism and activity. At some point, changes in the brain turn substance abuse into addiction, a chronic, relapsing illness. Table 46-1 shows diagnostic criteria for abuse and dependence.

HISTORICAL PERSPECTIVES

Nearly 6,500 years ago, ancient Egyptians used opium for pain relief. Later they used it for recreation when they discovered it provided anxiety relief, a pleasurable experience, and an escape from reality. Drug problems began in the United States with the Civil War in 1861. Wounded soldiers were given their own supply of morphine. Its use was uncontrolled. Dependence-producing drugs such as cocaine, heroin, and morphine were given freely to clients by doctors. Patent medicines, many containing alcohol, cocaine, and heroin, were said to cure almost any ailment a person might have.

The Pure Food and Drug Act of 1906, requiring accurate labeling of drugs, was the first measure designed to control drugs in the United States. In 1914, The Harrison Act made the use of certain narcotics illegal. Physicians then became unwilling to give individuals these drugs and drug use actually increased as those persons already using drugs turned to illegal markets for a supply. In 1919, Congress passed the 19th Amendment to the Constitution declaring the making and selling of alcohol illegal. Prohibition lasted until 1933, when the 19th Amendment was finally repealed because it had not controlled drunkenness or alcoholism as it was intended.

TABLE 46-1   DIAGNOSTIC CRITERIA FOR SUBSTANCE DEPENDENCE AND ABUSE

SUBSTANCE DEPENDENCE

A maladaptive pattern of substance use, leading to clinically significant impairment or distress, as manifested by three (or more) of the following, occurring at any time in the same 12-month period:

(1) tolerance, as defined by either of the following:

    (a) a need for markedly increased amounts of the substance to achieve intoxication or desired effect

    (b) markedly diminished effect with continued use of the same amount of the substance

(2) withdrawal, as manifested by either of the following:

    (a) the characteristic withdrawal syndrome for the substance (refer to Criteria A and B of the criteria sets for Withdrawal from the specific substances)

    (b) the same (or a closely related) substance is taken to relieve or avoid withdrawal symptoms

(3) the substance is often taken in larger amounts or over a longer period than was intended

(4) there is a persistent desire or unsuccessful efforts to cut down or control substance use

(5) a great deal of time is spent in activities necessary to obtain the substance (e.g., visiting multiple doctors or driving long distances), use the substance (e.g., chain-smoking), or recover from its effects

(6) important social, occupational, or recreational activities are given up or reduced because of substance use

(7) the substance use is continued despite knowledge of having a persistent or recurrent physical or psychological problem that is likely to have been caused or exacerbated by the substance (e.g., current cocaine use despite recognition of cocaine-induced depression, or continued drinking despite recognition that an ulcer was made worse by alcohol consumption)

SUBSTANCE ABUSE

A. A maladaptive pattern of substance use leading to clinically significant impairment or distress, as manifested by one (or more) of the following, occurring within a 12-month period:

    (1) recurrent substance use resulting in a failure to fulfill major role obligations at work, school, or home (e.g., repeated absences or poor work performance related to substance use; substance-related absences, suspensions, or expulsions from school; neglect of children or household)

    (2) recurrent substance use in situations in which it is physically hazardous (e.g., driving an automobile or operating a machine when impaired by substance use)

    (3) recurrent substance-related legal problems (e.g., arrests for substance-related disorderly conduct)

    (4) continued substance use despite having persistent or recurrent social or interpersonal problems caused, or exacerbated by the effects of the substance (e.g., arguments with spouse about consequences of intoxication, physical fights)

B. The symptoms have never met the criteria for Substance Dependence for this class of substance.

Reprinted with permission from the *Diagnostic and Statistical Manual of Mental Disorders,* Fourth Edition. Copyright 2000 American Psychiatric Association.

Many medical, law enforcement, and legislative efforts in the 1930s slowed narcotic abuse and addiction. Then marijuana flooded the market. The Marijuana Tax Act of 1937 was intended to raise revenue, identify the persons involved in its use, and discourage the recreational use of marijuana. Marijuana was removed in 1941 from the official list of drugs U.S. physicians could prescribe. World War II disrupted supply routes of drugs from Asia and Europe, and large-scale drug use disappeared in the United States.

The 1960s saw drug use move into the mainstream of life in the United States. Drugs were used as a form of relaxation. The Comprehensive Drug Abuse Prevention and Control Act was passed in 1970; it is commonly referred to as the Controlled Substance Act. This act regulates the manufacture, distribution, and dispensing of controlled substances. To enforce the provisions of this act, the Drug Enforcement Administration (DEA) was organized.

There are five classifications or schedules of controlled substances. The categories are based on the drugs' potential to cause psychological and/or physical dependence, and also on their potential for abuse. Table 46-2 identifies and explains the five schedules.

In the 1980s, marijuana and other drug use declined, especially among high school students. Cocaine and its derivative, crack, were the new drugs of choice. The increased supply hooked many people into heavy drug use. The early 1990s saw an increase in the use of all substances. By 2002, illicit drug use had decreased or remained stable in high school students (National Institute on Drug Abuse [NIDA], 2003).

FACTORS RELATED TO SUBSTANCE ABUSE

Many factors interact to influence a person's substance abuse. Many people who have stopped substance abuse **relapse** (return to a previous behavior or condition) because of these same factors. These factors may be categorized as individual, family, lifestyle, environmental, and developmental.

Individual Factors

Genetic factors are being researched as a possible reason for a person's susceptibility to substance abuse. Research suggests that variations in the intensity of the flow of neurotransmitters may cause certain individuals to be more susceptible to addiction. The personality traits of sensation seeking and being impulsive may make it easier for the person to experiment with substances.

Family Patterns — "*Peer Pressure*"

Substance abuse, especially in the adolescent, seems to be related to family relationships. Close family relationships, with the parents involved in their children's activities, appear to discourage substance abuse. Families with positive relationships between parents and children generally have less use of illicit drugs. Parent–child interactions that show a lack of closeness, lack of involvement in the children's activities, lack of or inconsistent discipline, and low aspirations for the children's education contribute to the prediction of substance abuse by the children.

Families of adolescent substance abusers generally have negative communication patterns. That is, there is a lack of praise and a great deal of blaming and criticism. Often there are unreal expectations of the children by the parents, inconsistent or unclear behavioral limits, and a pattern of self-medication by family members.

Lifestyle — $

All dimensions of a person's life that influence how that person lives are termed *lifestyle*. First is the physical dimension, which includes food, clothing, shelter, and health care. The second is the social dimension, which includes friends, organizations, and activities with others. Third is the intellectual/emotional dimension, including education, parental support of education, self-esteem, and how the individual is treated by others. The fourth dimension is spiritual and includes a belief in a "higher being," caring and compassion for others, and being in touch with the inner self. Substance use, abuse, or dependence may be the coping mechanism used by an individual who has problems in any dimension of lifestyle.

Environmental Factors

Many environmental factors may encourage or predispose an individual to substance abuse. The social

TABLE 46-2	SCHEDULES OF CONTROLLED SUBSTANCES
Schedule I (C-I)	High abuse and dependence potential. No accepted medical use in the United States. Includes heroin, mescaline, LSD, marijuana, and other hallucinogens and certain opiates. Can be obtained legally for limited research programs.
Schedule II (C-II)	High abuse and dependence potential. Have currently accepted medical use. Includes narcotics, barbiturates, and amphetamines. Obtained only with physician's prescription, nonrefillable.
Schedule III (C-III)	Less abuse potential, moderate dependence likely. Includes nonbarbiturate sedatives and some narcotics in limited doses. Prescription refills good for 6 months. Fewer controls than for Schedule II.
Schedule IV (C-IV)	Even less abuse potential, limited dependence likely. Includes some sedatives and antianxiety agents and nonnarcotic analgesics.
Schedule V (C-V)	Limited abuse potential. Includes cough medicines containing codeine and antidiarrheals. May be sold over-the-counter in pharmacies to persons over 18 years old. A record is kept of the buyer's name.

environment in which persons find themselves, the groups, clubs, gangs, sororities, fraternities, and other organizations influence the acceptance or rejection of substance abuse. Stresses in a person's life, including accidents, disabilities, illnesses, stressful family relations, frequent job changes, divorce, death, or precarious financial conditions may be too much for that person to handle. The maladaptive coping of substance abuse offers temporary relief. Because the symptoms of the stressors are reduced, substance abuse is reinforced.

Advertising can influence people in subtle ways to become involved in substance use and abuse. Landau (1995) describes how use of Camel cigarettes by the 18- to 24-year-old age group soared when the character Joe Camel was introduced in advertising promotions in 1988. It was "cool" to be associated with Joe Camel. Other advertising connects caffeine, nicotine, or alcohol with success, sexuality, and power.

Social traditions, especially in the use of alcohol, may open the door for abuse in certain individuals. Examples of these social traditions are having wine with meals, making toasts at weddings and other celebrations, serving "holiday cheer," and going to "happy hour." For some individuals, these situations may predispose them to alcohol abuse or dependence.

Peer activities, especially during adolescence, may result in substance abuse. Even adults often feel they must go along with certain activities, such as drinks after work or cocktail hour, to get ahead in their careers.

Some occupations, like health care, seem to be more associated with substance problems than others. Physicians and nurses, particularly, have access to many substances that can be abused.

Developmental Factors

Many individuals have not had good role models in their lives. They have not learned to identify with others and do not understand that their behavior affects others. Not learning the skills and attitudes of problem solving leaves individuals unable to apply personal resources to situations, and escape seems the only answer. Substances provide that escape.

Learning the intrapersonal skills of self-discipline, self-control, and self-assessment helps the individual cope with tension and stress. These skills also work to prevent dishonesty with self, inability to defer gratification, and low self-esteem. A lack of interpersonal skills results in dishonesty with others, resistance to feedback, and inability to share feelings and give or accept help. Not learning to take responsibility or adapt one's behavior to a situation results in irresponsibility, not accepting the consequences of behavior, and seeing oneself as a victim of circumstances. Individuals who do not view themselves as empowered may choose substance use as a means of gratification.

PREVENTION

Prevention of substance abuse must be a proactive process to empower people to constructively confront stressful situations in adaptive ways. There are three levels of prevention. *Primary prevention* focuses on preventing the initial use or preventing further uses that may lead to abuse or dependence. This is usually aimed at school-age children. Children need to hear the message that drugs are not good for them. Education about substances and their effects must also emphasize personal, social, and health risks. Children need role models to teach them how to cope with life without drugs, to resist social and peer pressure, and to make effective decisions.

Secondary prevention focuses on preventing ongoing use from becoming a situation of abuse or dependence. If abuse is already evident, the focus is to return the client to a state of abstinence or at least reduced use.

Tertiary prevention focuses on returning the client to a drug-free state. If this is not possible, the goal is then to prevent physical and psychosocial problems from getting worse.

DIAGNOSTIC TESTING

Clients who have a problem with substance abuse or dependence often have abnormal liver function tests and electrolyte levels. Diagnostic criteria for specific substance-related disorders can be found in *DSM-IV*.

Tests may be done with either a blood or urine specimen. A positive test indicates only that the person has been exposed to the substance. It does not indicate abuse, addiction, or intoxication (except alcohol). Positive screening tests should be confirmed by a more specific test using a different process. Drugs for which tests can be done include alcohol, benzodiazepines, barbiturates, cocaine, crack, amphetamines, opiates, synthetic narcotic analgesics, marijuana, and PCP.

Urine is usually the body fluid tested because it is easily obtained and tested. When obtaining a urine specimen for drug screening, the client should be observed to prevent adulteration of the specimen by the client, such as substituting another person's drug-free urine. A "chain of custody" is maintained by having each person who handles the specimen sign an attached paper until the specimen has been tested.

Detection of a substance depends on the amount used and the time since last used. Most substances are detectable for less than 7 days. Chronic marijuana use, however, may be detected for up to 30 days. Cocaine, barbiturates, amphetamines, and opiates are detectable for less than 2 days and alcohol less than 1 day. A false negative may result if the client's drug level falls below the threshold of sensitivity for the test.

Positive results for reasons other than substance abuse can occur. This is called a false positive. Poppy seeds may give a positive result for opiates for up to 60 hours after ingestion. Using a Vicks® inhaler or over-the-counter diet aids may give a positive result for amphetamines. The client should be asked about the use of these items.

Breath specimens can be used to determine alcohol levels. Law enforcement officials do this with the breathalyzer tests. If hair is not cut, hair analysis can detect substance use for up to a year after the person has used a drug for only 2 or 3 days. Testing meconium (first stools) from a newborn can detect illicit drug use by the mother during pregnancy.

TREATMENT/RECOVERY

Treatment depends on many factors, including the amount and frequency of substance use, age, health, diet, and overall lifestyle of the individual. Infection from the use of unsterile needles and/or tissue or organ damage caused by the substance used, such as lung damage from smoking crack or marijuana or using inhalants, will also require treatment.

Recovery requires abstinence along with intrapersonal and interpersonal changes. Most individuals need professional treatment and participation in a self-help program. There are four areas of recovery: physical recovery, psychological and behavioral recovery, social and family recovery, and spiritual recovery.

Physical recovery means eliminating the substance from the body. This is termed **detoxification.** If the client cannot stop using the substance or if withdrawal symptoms are present, admission to a detoxification unit is usually necessary. After detoxification, treatment must focus on restoring the client's physical health and dealing with the cravings for the substance now removed from the client's body. It helps if environmental cues such as drug paraphernalia and alcohol bottles or cans are removed.

Psychological and behavioral recovery becomes evident when the client no longer denies the problem and accepts the inability to consistently control the substance abuse. The client will have developed a desire for abstinence and accepted the need for long-term recovery and support. Emotional stability will be restored when the client learns to cope with uncomfortable emotional states without the use of the abused substance.

Social and family recovery occurs when the client no longer denies the impact on the family and makes amends to family members and significant others who have been negatively affected by the substance abuse. The client works to improve family relationships and develops a recovery support system. Also, the client learns to resist social pressures to use alcohol or other drugs and participates in healthy leisure-time activities. The client's family should also attend a program for recovery. If a client returns to a dysfunctional family, it may be difficult for the client to maintain recovery.

Spiritual recovery is attained when the client has resolved the feelings of guilt and shame and developed a meaning for life and a relationship with a higher power.

SUBSTANCE USE PATTERNS

Patterns of substance use have changed throughout the years. Coffee (caffeine) and cigarettes (nicotine) are legal in our society and widely used. Although many people still drink coffee, more are using decaffeinated coffee. Cigarette use has decreased in the older population as the addictive nature and negative effects of nicotine have become more evident; however, cigarette use has increased in the adolescent population.

The substance of choice is alcohol, which is legal and easily obtained. Many high school seniors have been drunk and some are already regular drinkers. There are

still more alcoholic men than women, but the number of identified women alcoholics is increasing.

Elderly persons are more commonly addicted to prescription medications, especially minor tranquilizers and sleeping pills. Alcohol may be used by the elderly to soothe feelings of isolation and loneliness. Depression and paranoia may be misidentified as senility rather than a problem with alcohol.

Moderate consumption of alcohol may have been influenced by Mothers Against Drunk Driving (MADD) and Students Against Drunk Driving (SADD). Laws that make bars and individuals liable if they let guests leave and drive while drunk, and famous people like Betty Ford and Liza Minelli sharing with the public their illness and recovery, are other influences.

The National Institute on Drug Abuse (2003l) report on the ongoing study of illicit drug use among 8th-, 10th-, and 12th-grade students, which shows a decline in use. This is the sixth year of stable or decreased use.

CNS DEPRESSANTS

Central nervous system depressants usually decrease the heart and respiratory rates as well as voluntary muscle responses. Substances in this category include alcohol, benzodiazepines, and marijuana.

ALCOHOL

Low doses of alcohol depress areas of the brain that are inhibitory, causing diminished self-control and impaired judgment. Continued alcohol ingestion may cause unconsciousness and even death. According to the National Institute on Alcohol Abuse and Alcoholism (NIAAA) (2003), 31.1% of all traffic crash fatalities were alcohol-related.

The active ingredient in alcoholic beverages is ethanol. Depending on the alcoholic beverage consumed, varying amounts of ethanol are ingested. It is metabolized at an average rate of 10 mL/hr. Table 46-3 shows the alcohol content in some beverages.

One ounce of alcohol provides 200 Kcal but no other nutrients. It is not converted to glycogen. The blood alcohol level depends on the size of the person, the amount ingested, and the time since ingestion. Most states have set the legal limit for blood alcohol while driving a motor vehicle at 0.08%, but driving skills are affected at a much lower level (NIAAA, 1999).

TABLE 46-3	ALCOHOL CONTENT IN SELECTED BEVERAGES	
BEVERAGE	**PERCENT ALCOHOL**	**EQUIVALENT AMOUNTS**
Beer	4	12 ounces
Wine cooler	4	12 ounces
Wine	14	4 ounces
Hard liquor	40	$1^1/_2$ ounces

Incidence

Several national surveys have found that approximately two-thirds of the population have more than an occasional drink. Men are likely to drink more frequently and in greater quantity than women. Most individuals with an alcohol problem are blue- or white-collar men and women. Some alcoholics drink little or nothing in public or with friends. They are "at home" or "hidden" alcoholics and are more likely to be women. It often takes a family quite awhile to realize that one of its members has an alcohol problem.

The individual with an alcohol problem often learns **behavioral tolerance,** a compensatory adjustment made by an individual under the influence of a particular substance. The person under the influence of alcohol learns how to compensate for the deterioration of motor performance and speech.

Signs and Symptoms

The ingestion of alcohol causes a feeling of euphoria, relaxation of skeletal muscles, changes in mental activity such as altered judgment, and reduced self-control. It has a diuretic effect that, in heavy drinkers, may cause increased loss of electrolytes, especially potassium, magnesium, and zinc. An increased level of alcohol depresses the cardiovascular and respiratory systems and produces a toxic effect on the intestinal mucosa, resulting in decreased absorption of thiamine, folic acid, and vitamin B_{12}. Excess long-term consumption of alcohol often results in a severe lack of nutrient intake.

Psychosocial aspects include memory blackouts, secretive drinking, rationalization of drinking behavior, trouble with family and employer, loss of outside interests, neglect of food intake, impaired thinking, and moral deterioration. **Confabulation,** making up information to fill in memory gaps, is used by individuals abusing or depending on alcohol. Alcohol may be detected in the blood for 6 to 10 hours.

Potential for Addiction

The potential for addiction is high. Alcohol is not a scheduled or controlled drug.

Associated Problems/Disorders

Excessive and prolonged alcohol intake can affect numerous body systems.

Liver Deterioration

Chronic alcohol abuse causes three distinct diseases of the liver: *fatty liver,* an accumulation of triglycerides in the liver caused by obesity, excessive alcohol consumption, and certain drugs; *alcoholic hepatitis,* an acute toxic liver injury from excess alcohol consumption; and *cirrhosis,* a chronic degenerative liver disease that can be caused by alcohol consumption. Fatty liver is reversible, but alcoholic hepatitis and cirrhosis are not. Liver cells will not function once the scar tissue of cirrhosis develops. In 1999, 68.7% of deaths from cirrhosis of the liver were related to alcohol consumption (NIAAA, 2000). Esophageal varices are associated with cirrhosis and could cause death if they bleed.

Gastrointestinal Disturbances

Alcohol damages the lining of the stomach and esophagus by irritating the mucosa and causing inflammation or ulcer formation. Aspirin with alcohol can result in greater irritation and bleeding in the gastrointestinal (GI) tract. Gastric pain, vomiting, and diarrhea are common in alcohol abuse and are often what brings the individual to the health care system.

Pancreatitis

An alcoholic has a higher risk of developing pancreatitis than an abstainer. Severe pancreatitis can result in death.

Wernicke's Encephalopathy

This inflammatory hemorrhagic and degenerative condition of the brain is caused by a thiamine deficiency. It is characterized by delirium, memory loss, unsteady gait, a sense of apprehension, and an altered level of consciousness. Thiamine intake improves the situation.

Korsakoff's Psychosis

Disorientation, amnesia, insomnia, hallucinations, and peripheral neuropathologies characterize this psychosis. Both thiamine and B_{12} deficiencies contribute to the degeneration of the brain and peripheral nervous system. Frequently, there is bilateral foot drop and pain over the long nerves. Thiamine and B_{12} intake may improve the situation.

Cardiovascular Disturbances

Moderate amounts of alcohol cause cutaneous vasodilation (flushed skin). This causes rapid heat loss, and the core temperature may drop to a dangerous level. Blood pressure decreases with intoxicating doses of alcohol. There may be irregularities in cardiac rhythm. Hematologic alterations such as bone marrow depression, anemia, leukopenia, or thrombocytopenia may also occur.

Fetal Alcohol Syndrome

Fetal alcohol syndrome is caused by the **teratogenic** (causing abnormal development of the embryo) effects of alcohol related to the amount of alcohol ingested and the stage of pregnancy when the alcohol is ingested. Even a small amount of alcohol can be detrimental and have lifelong consequences for the infant. For a diagnosis of FAS, the infant must meet these criteria:

- Prenatal and/or postnatal growth retardation (weight, length, or head circumference below the 10th percentile)
- CNS involvement (signs of neurologic abnormality, developmental delay, or intellectual impairment)
- Craniofacial anomalies, at least two of the following (microcephaly or head circumference below 3rd percentile, microophthalmia or short palpebral fissure, poorly developed philtrum, thin upper lip, or flattening of maxillary area)

If only some of the FAS criteria are met, it is called fetal alcohol effects (FAE). The only treatment for FAS or FAE is prevention. Women who are pregnant or are trying to get pregnant should abstain from alcohol consumption.

Withdrawal

Withdrawal refers to the symptoms produced when a substance on which an individual has dependence is no longer used by that individual. Alcohol withdrawal syndrome (AWS) appears when the blood alcohol concentration of the alcoholic decreases. The onset of symptoms usually occurs 6 to 12 hours after drinking stops and may last up to 8 days. Chronologically, how long the drinking has occurred and the amount of alcohol consistently consumed are factors in the severity of the withdrawal symptoms. Figure 46-1 shows alcohol withdrawal patterns.

Alcohol withdrawal has three stages:

- *Stage 1* (minor withdrawal) includes restlessness, anxiety, sleeping problems, agitation, and tremors; other signs include low-grade fever, tachycardia, diaphoresis, and hypertension.
- *Stage 2* (major withdrawal) includes stage 1 signs and symptoms plus visual and auditory hallucinations, whole-body tremors, pulse greater than 100, diastolic BP greater than 100, pronounced diaphoresis, and possibly vomiting.

Figure 46-1 *Alcohol Withdrawal Patterns*

- *Stage 3* (delirium tremens) includes a temperature over 37.8°C (100°F); disorientation to time, place, and person; global confusion; and inability to recognize familiar objects or persons. Only about 5% of clients progress to this stage (Compton, 2002). This is a medical emergency with a mortality rate of 2% to 5% (NIDA, 2003d).

If alcohol abuse continues, symptoms of subsequent withdrawals are generally more severe. It is recommended that withdrawal be medically monitored to decrease the chance of fatality.

Treatment/Rehabilitation

Many treatment programs are based in hospital or residential treatment centers. These are generally called inpatient programs and last 30 days. Many insurance companies are encouraging clients to participate in lower-cost outpatient programs. Currently, there is no evidence that inpatient programs are more effective than outpatient programs.

Many outpatient programs have both day and evening sessions so clients can maintain their usual occupations. The programs usually consist of a 4-week intensive session with follow-up sessions for 6 to 24 months. The first part of either type of treatment program is detoxification.

Detoxification

The goal of detoxification (DETOX) is to halt or control the neuronal overactivity that occurs when the alcohol level is reduced or alcohol is no longer present in the client's body. This is done by substituting a pharmacologically similar drug and gradually reducing the dose given. The benzodiazepine drugs, chlordiazepoxide (Librium), diazepam (Valium), lorazepam (Ativan), and clorazepate dipotassium (Tranxene), are the most commonly used.

During DETOX, other problems such as malnutrition, vitamin deficiencies (B vitamins, especially thiamine), dehydration, and potassium and magnesium deficiencies must also be treated. A client with hypoglycemia should be given thiamine before administering dextrose to prevent Wernicke's encephalopathy. Ignoring these problems complicates the management of detoxification.

Psychologic Intervention

The classic psychologic intervention technique was originally described by Johnson in 1973 (1990). Although several modifications have been published and used since then, the technique is still used and is known as **Johnsonian intervention,** which is a confrontational approach to a client with a substance problem that lessens the chance of denial and encourages treatment before the client "hits bottom." The client's significant others (spouse, teenage or older children, one or two close friends, possibly employer) meet with a professional addiction counselor. This group rehearses so that they may present a united front when confronting the client. They present specific examples of painful or embarrassing behaviors by the client while intoxicated that caused problems and concerns. It is difficult for the client to maint denial in this situation. Then the group encourages the client to accept professional help. If the client refuses help, each individual of the group must plan to minimize codependent behavior in the future. This technique can also be used for substances other than alcohol. Examples of confrontations may be found in Johnson's books (1990, 1989). Codependency is discussed later in the chapter.

Education

The abuse of or dependence on alcohol is a maladaptive way to cope with life stressors. Learning basic life skills to improve personal competence and provide adaptive coping mechanisms helps the individual resist the use of alcohol.

One adaptive coping mechanism is exercise. Assist clients to become active in an exercise program and encourage them to participate. Exercise helps relieve feelings of stress and promotes feelings of well-being.

Teach clients about the Food Guide Pyramid for an adequate, balanced diet. Most alcoholics have, in the past, received most of their calories from alcohol. They must now learn how to maintain health by eating nutritious foods.

The interaction of alcohol with other drugs should also be taught. Some effects can be life-threatening. Table 46-4 shows the interaction of alcohol with some classifications of drugs.

TABLE 46-4   ALCOHOL INTERACTION WITH OTHER DRUGS

DRUG CLASSIFICATIONS WITH EXAMPLES	INTERACTION	DRUG CLASSIFICATIONS WITH EXAMPLES	INTERACTION
Narcotic analgesics • meperidine hydrochloride (Demerol) • proproxyphene HCl (Darvon) • hydromorphone HCl (Dilaudid)	• Loss of effective breathing (respiratory arrest) • Can be fatal	Antidepressants • imipramine HCl (Tofranil) • desipramine HCl (Pertofrane) • perphenazine and amitriptyline HCl (Triavil)	• Reduces CNS functioning • Chianti wine may cause hypertensive crisis
Nonnarcotic analgesics • aspirin • acetaminophen (Tylenol)	• Stomach and intestinal bleeding • Liver damage	Antihistamines • Most cold remedies • pseudoephedrine HCl and triprolidine HCl (Actifed) • chlorpheniramine maleate and acetaminophen (Couricidin)	• Increased calming effect • Person becomes very drowsy • Driving is hazardous
Anticoagulants • warfarin sodium (Coumadin, Panwarfin) • dicumarol	• Increases drugs' ability to stop blood clotting • May cause life-threatening or fatal hemorrhage		
Antihypertensives • reserpine (Serpasil) • methyldopa (Aldomet)	• Orthostatic hypotension	Antipsychotics • thioridazine HCl (Mellaril) • chlorpromazine HCl (Thorazine)	• Added CNS depression and impairs voluntary movements • Causes respiratory depression • Can be fatal
Antimicrobials • metronidazole (Flagyl) • cefotetan disodium (Cefotan) • rifampin (Rifadin)	• Possible disulfiram-like reaction, nausea, cramps, vomiting, headache, flushing or hepatotoxicity	Sedative-hypnotics • glutethimine (Doriden) • pentobarbital (Nembutal)	• Reduces CNS functioning • Sometimes causes coma and respiratory arrest • Can be fatal
CNS stimulants • Most diet pills • dextroamphetamine sulfate (Dexedrine) • caffeine (No Doz) • methylphenidate HCl (Ritalin)	• May reverse depressant effect of alcohol and give a false sense of security	Antianxiety agents • diazepam (Valium) • chlordiazepoxide (Librium)	• Reduces CNS functioning • Decreased alertness and judgment • Can lead to household and driving accidents
Diuretics • chlorothiazide (Diuril) • furosemide (Lasix)	• May reduce blood pressure and cause dizziness		

Self-Help Groups

Alcoholics Anonymous (AA), begun in 1935, is the model for other self-help groups such as AL-ANON for adults, AL-ATEEN for teenage children, and AL-ATOT for younger children in the family of an alcoholic. The holistic approach of AA to the individual with alcohol problems is described in the Twelve Steps (Table 46-5).

Disulfiram

Disulfiram (Antabuse) may be given to some alcohol abusers as a deterrent to drinking. It inhibits the enzyme needed to metabolize alcohol. Drinking alcohol with disulfiram in the body causes flushing of the neck and face, blurred vision, nausea, vertigo, anxiety, palpitations, tachycardia, and hypotension. Clients must be instructed not to use cologne, mouthwash, aftershave, over-the-counter cold preparations, cough syrups, vitamin-mineral tonics, as well as candies, sauces, and foods made with alcohol. These items will cause the same reaction as if the person took a drink of alcohol.

Therapy should not be started until at least 12 hours after the last drink of alcohol. The effects of disulfiram with alcohol can occur for 6 to 12 days after taking the disulfiram. As with any drug, there are side effects such as drowsiness, fatigue, and impotence. Garlic-like breath occurs frequently and is sometimes used as an indicator of compliance in taking the disulfiram. Disulfiram is contraindicated in clients with cardiovascular disease, hypothyroidism, suicide ideation, and in clients receiving antihypertensives or monoamine oxidase inhibitors (MAOI).

BENZODIAZEPINES AND OTHER SEDATIVE-HYPNOTICS

With the introduction in 1961 of chlordiazepoxide (Librium), the benzodiazepines have replaced most of the short-acting barbiturates and other nonbarbiturate sedative-hypnotics that were in use before that time. Examples of benzodiazepines include diazepam (Valium), secobarbital (Seconal), paraldehyde (Paral), and flunitrazepam (Rohypnol). Rohypnol when mixed with alcohol can incapacitate and prevent the person from resisting sexual assault or remembering what she experiences under the effects of the drug. It is known as the "date rape drug" (NIDA, 2003b). Street names include roofies, tranks, ludes, and barbs.

Incidence

Benzodiazepines are not commonly used as recreational drugs but are widely prescribed and are thus available for abuse. Statistics are not available because some clinicians still deny that addiction to these drugs occurs. Withdrawal symptoms are subtle and delayed, and the symptoms are not always connected to the benzodiazepines.

Barbiturates and other sedative-hypnotics are more abused but less prescribed. These are available on the illegal market.

Signs and Symptoms

Benzodiazepines in low doses produce drowsiness or sedation. Larger doses produce sleep, but surgical anesthesia cannot be induced. Respirations are not depressed, and there is little effect on the cardiovascular system unless extremely large doses are taken. Then a decrease in systolic blood pressure and an increase in heart rate may result. Side effects may include motor incoordination, ataxia, increased hostility or rage, confusion, metallic-like aftertaste, headache, and blurred vision. **Tolerance** (a decreased sensitivity to subsequent doses of the same substance; an increased dose of a substance is needed to produce the same desired effect) to other benzodiazepines and **cross-tolerance** (a decreased sensitivity to other substances in the same category) to other CNS depressants occur with chronic use. In some clients, particularly pediatric, geriatric, or autistic, a paradoxical reaction can occur. They show agitation, emotional lability, and sometimes rage instead of the expected calming effect (Gutierrez, Roper & Hahn, 2001).

Barbiturates depress all areas of the CNS, some selectively according to the dosage. They do not reduce pain. Respirations are depressed but not significantly when therapeutic doses are taken. When a barbiturate is given to a client in pain, excitement rather than sedation may occur. Side effects may include drowsiness, residual

---

TABLE 46-5 ALCOHOLICS ANONYMOUS

1. We admitted we were powerless over alcohol—that our lives had become unmanageable.
2. Came to believe that a Power greater than ourselves could restore us to sanity.
3. Made a decision to turn our will and our lives over to the care of God *as we understood Him.*
4. Made a searching and fearless moral inventory of ourselves.
5. Admitted to God, to ourselves and to another human being the exact nature of our wrongs.
6. Were entirely ready to have God remove all these defects of character.
7. Humbly asked Him to remove our shortcomings.
8. Made a list of all persons we had harmed, and became willing to make amends to them all.
9. Made direct amends to such people wherever possible, except when to do so would injure them or others.
10. Continued to take personal inventory and when we were wrong promptly admitted it.
11. Sought through prayer and meditation to improve our conscious contact with God, *as we understood Him,* praying only for knowledge of His will for us and the power to carry that out.
12. Having had a spiritual awakening as the result of these steps, we tried to carry this message to alcoholics, and to practice these principles in all our affairs.

The Twelve Steps are reprinted with permission of Alcoholics Anonymous World Services, Inc. Permission to reprint the Twelve Steps does not mean that A. A. has reviewed or approved the contents of this publication, nor that A. A. agrees with the views expressed herein. A. A. is a program of recovery from alcoholism only. Use of the Twelve Steps in connection with programs and activities that are patterned after A. A., but address other problems, or in any other non-A. A. context, does not imply otherwise.

effects on motor skills, and especially in the elderly, excitement, irritability, or delirium. An overdose of barbiturates causes decreased respirations, rapid and weak pulse, cyanosis, coma, and sometimes respiratory paralysis. Tolerance results from chronic use or abuse. Benzodiazepines may be detected for 1 to 6 weeks.

Potential for Addiction

The potential for addiction is high for all of these substances. Benzodiazepines are schedule IV drugs; barbiturates may be either schedule II, III, or IV drugs; and methaqualone is a schedule I drug.

Withdrawal

Symptoms of withdrawal for benzodiazepines, which may not manifest for a week or more, include cramping, sweating, disorientation, confusion, tremors, depression, hallucinations, and paranoia. Barbiturate withdrawal symptoms include anxiety, weakness, anorexia, insomnia, tremors, delirium, and seizures that occur within 72 hours of the last use. Withdrawal reactions related to other sedative-hypnotics include nausea, headache, cramping, toxic psychosis, insomnia, and convulsions.

The withdrawal pattern is the same as for alcohol.

Treatment/Rehabilitation

Ideally, treatment for benzodiazepine abuse is a gradual reduction in the amount taken until the client is no longer taking any. A cross-tolerant drug such as phenobarbital is sometimes given to control symptoms and then its dosage is reduced. Hospital treatment is likely to be needed. Treatment for barbiturate and other sedative-hypnotics overdose or withdrawal is symptomatic.

Rehabilitation that focuses on teaching clients alternative methods of coping with the anxiety and stressors in their lives is necessary. Supportive individual psychotherapy or a self-help recovery group is almost always advisable. The goal is to assist the client to identify the consequences of the behavior and to understand the risks of relapse.

MARIJUANA (CANNABIS)

Marijuana is the most common type of cannabis used. It is composed of dried leaves, stems, and flowers of the plant *Cannabis sativa* and can be smoked or added to food. Hash or hashish is a potent concentrate of the resin from the flowers. Hash oil is extremely concentrated, made by boiling hashish in a solvent and filtering out the solid matter. Street names include grass, pot, reefer, smoke, weed, and Mary Jane. "Blunts" are cigars emptied of tobacco and refilled with marijuana. It is the most commonly used illicit drug in the United States (NIDA, 2003h). Often, it is the "gateway" drug leading to the abuse of other drugs.

Incidence

Use in the United States began in the early 1900s, peaked in the period 1978 to 1980, and has steadily decreased since. According to Johnston, O'Malley, and Buchman (1991 and 1998), the prevalence of marijuana use by high school seniors increased from 20% in the class of 1969 to 60.4% in the class of 1979 and fell to 50.2% in the class of 1987 and fell again to 40.7 percent in the class of 1990. Use increased between 1990 and 1997 but declined in 1998 to 49%. It has remained stable through 2001 (NIDA, 2003h).

Signs and Symptoms

Short-term effects of marijuana use include memory and learning problems; distorted perception; difficulty in thinking and problem solving; loss of coordination; and increased heart rate, anxiety, and panic attacks. Long-term use produces changes in the brain similar to those seen after long-term use of other major drugs of abuse (NIDA, 2003h). A **reverse tolerance** can develop whereby a smaller amount of marijuana will elicit the desired psychic effects. Marijuana may be detected for up to 5 weeks.

Potential for Addiction

The potential for psychologic addiction is moderate. More than 220,000 persons seek treatment each year for their primary marijuana addiction (NIDA, 2003h). Marijuana is a schedule I drug.

Associated Problems/Disorders

Critical skills related to attention, learning, and memory are impaired in heavy marijuana users even 24 hours after the last use. Also, persons below college age who use marijuana tend to be more accepting of deviant behavior, have more aggression and delinquent behavior, act more rebellious, and have poorer relationships with parents (NIDA, 2003h).

Withdrawal

Nausea, myalgia, restlessness, irritability, nervousness, insomnia, and depression may appear after ceasing marijuana use. Symptoms may not appear for up to 1 week after the last use.

Treatment/Rehabilitation

Treatment focuses on relapse prevention and the development of new coping mechanisms, ways of living, and means of having fun without drugs. Weekly group therapy sessions to maintain a commitment to abstinence and enhance interpersonal skills are often used. Participation in a self-help group is encouraged.

CNS STIMULANTS

Drugs that stimulate the CNS include cocaine, amphetamines, caffeine, nicotine, and methylphenidate hydrochloride (Ritalin). They increase cortical alertness and electrical activity in the brain and spinal cord. There is tachycardia and an increase in blood pressure.

COCAINE

Cocaine is extracted from the leaves of the coca plant, *Erythroxylum coca*. It may be heated and the fumes inhaled. This is termed *free-basing*. As a white powder, cocaine is snorted by inhaling it through the nose or heated to a liquid state and injected intravenously. Crack is a crystallized form of cocaine that is melted in a water pipe and smoked. Street names include coke, crack, flake, rocks, snow, "C," and blow.

Incidence

Cocaine abuse and dependence was the major illicit drug problem for the United States in the 1980s. The introduction of crack dramatically increased cocaine abuse among the poor. Crack is low cost and gives an intense "high." It is estimated that 3.6 million persons in the United States are chronic cocaine users (NIDA, 2002a).

Signs and Symptoms

The immediate reaction, less than 10 seconds, is an intense euphoria that lasts 10 to 15 minutes. This short response time leads people to repeatedly use cocaine trying to maintain the euphoria.

The heart rate increases, blood pressure goes up, pupils dilate, peripheral blood vessels constrict, and temperature increases. Normal pleasures are magnified, anxiety decreases, self-confidence increases, social inhibitions are reduced, communication is facilitated, and sexual feelings are enhanced. Other psychological effects are inability to concentrate, insomnia, reduced sense of humor, antisocial behavior, hallucinations, and compulsive behavior.

An overdose may occur with the first use because there is little quality control of drug strength in the street drug culture. A client with an overdose may have arrhythmias, tremors, convulsions, respiratory failure, cardiovascular collapse, and death. Cocaine may be detected for up to 4 days.

Potential for Addiction

The potential for addiction is high. Cocaine is a schedule II drug.

Associated Problems/Disorders

Many types of heart disease are linked to cocaine use, especially ventricular fibrillation, heart attack, and hypertension. When cocaine is snorted regularly, respiratory problems occur, including loss of sense of smell, nosebleeds, hoarseness, and respiratory failure.

When cocaine is taken with alcohol, the two drugs are converted in the body to cocaethylene, which is more toxic than either drug alone (NIDA, 2002a).

Withdrawal

The crash, a period of exhaustion, occurs with symptoms of depression, anxiety, and a great need for sleep. The depression may be to the point of suicidal behavior. The client has no energy, shows little interest in the surroundings, and seems to have little ability to experience pleasure. These symptoms are the most intense during the first 3 days but continue for 1 to 4 months. An intense craving for cocaine is felt, including dreaming about cocaine. Then there is a period of less intense craving for cocaine called extinction, which may last months

or even years. Withdrawal does not result in a medical emergency as seen with alcohol.

Treatment/Rehabilitation

Treatment is aimed at reducing the craving and managing the severe depression. Careful monitoring of the client is necessary to identify and prevent actions aimed at carrying out the idea of suicide. An individual with a history of cocaine usage has an intense craving for cocaine and a strong denial that cocaine is addicting. This creates a problem in engaging an individual in treatment. Inpatient programs are necessary for some clients with cocaine dependence, whereas other clients can be effectively treated in outpatient programs.

Medications

Bromocriptine mesylate (Parlodel) in small doses seems to reduce the withdrawal symptoms. Amantadine hydrochloride (Symmetrel) also has some success in treating cocaine withdrawal. Desipramine hydrochloride (Pertofrane) seems to reduce the craving for cocaine.

Education

Individual or group therapy should focus on helping the client feel pleasure again, improve energy level, and reduce cocaine craving. Peer support groups and self-help groups, such as Cocaine Anonymous, may be very effective. Random and regular urine testing is an external support to promote abstinence.

AMPHETAMINES —Sch. II

Amphetamines (also called uppers, speed, bennies) include dextroamphetamine sulfate (Dexedrine), amphetamine sulfate (Amphetamine), and methamphetamine hydrochloride (Desoxyn). Medically they are used to treat attention deficit hyperactivity disorder (ADHD), narcolepsy, and obesity.

Incidence

Amphetamines have been abused since the early 1930s. World War II greatly increased use and abuse when military personnel used amphetamines to decrease fatigue and increase alertness. Today, abuse ranges from truck drivers and college students who want to ward off sleep and increase alertness to the heavy abuser who injects or smokes homemade methamphetamine, known as meth, chalk, ice, crystal, crank, and glass. An estimated 4.9 million people in the United States have tried methamphetamine at some time (NIDA, 2003i).

Signs and Symptoms

Besides suppressing fatigue and increasing alertness, amphetamines enhance psychomotor performance, induce a temporary state of well-being, and give an instantaneous euphoria. Like cocaine, after several days the person becomes exhausted and lapses into a long period of sleep and depression (crash). The action of amphetamines lasts much longer than that of cocaine, and there is a greater potential for adverse reactions and severe toxicity.

High abuse doses may cause insomnia, tachycardia, headache, arrhythmias, hypertension followed by hypotension, nausea, vomiting, cramping, diarrhea, hyperreflexia, convulsions, and death. The psychologic effect is termed *amphetamine psychosis* and closely resembles paranoid schizophrenia. Symptoms include paranoid ideation, confusion, compulsive behaviors, and visual and auditory hallucinations. Tolerance does develop. Amphetamines may be detected for up to 2 days.

Potential for Addiction

The potential for addiction is high. Amphetamines are schedule II drugs.

Associated Problems/Disorders

Cardiovascular problems occur, including irregular and rapid heartbeat; hypertension; and irreversible, stroke-producing damage to small blood vessels in the brain (NIDA, 2003i). Injecting the drug may damage blood vessels and cause skin abscesses, and if injection equipment is shared, there is an increased risk of HIV/AIDS and hepatitis B and C transmission.

Withdrawal — will lead paranoia

There are no physical manifestations of withdrawal. Psychological changes include apathy, irritability, depression, disorientation, anxiety, paranoia, aggression, and an intense craving for the drug.

Treatment/Rehabilitation

Urinary acidifiers, such as ascorbic acid (vitamin C), increase the excretion of amphetamines. Diazepam (Valium) is given for sedation to ease the withdrawal crash. Bromocriptine mesylate (Parlodel) or levodopa (Dopar) may help decrease the craving. A quiet environment is also helpful.

Behavioral therapy is used to help the client recognize and accept the need to stop using amphetamines. Supportive individual or group therapy, and especially self-help groups, aids the client to stay abstinent and in treatment.

CAFFEINE

Caffeine is found in coffee, tea, cola beverages, cocoa, chocolate, and some nonprescription drugs.

Incidence

Caffeine is probably the best known and most frequently used and abused CNS stimulant.

Signs and Symptoms

Caffeine causes relaxation of smooth muscles in blood vessels and bronchi, diuresis, an increased gastric acid secretion, suppression of appetite, increased feeling of energy, and constriction of cerebral blood vessels. An increased level of caffeine intake causes jitteriness, rest-

lessness, nervousness, excitement, flushed face, palpitations, and nausea.

Potential for Addiction

The potential for addiction is moderate. Caffeine is not a scheduled drug.

Withdrawal

Withdrawal produces headache, irritability, and tremulousness.

Treatment/Rehabilitation

A gradual reduction of caffeine intake can reduce or eliminate the withdrawal symptoms. The client can then drink decaffeinated coffee and tea and caffeine-free soft drinks. The intake of cocoa and chocolate should be greatly reduced or eliminated. Caffeine can be avoided by reading labels and not using nonprescription products that contain caffeine.

NICOTINE

Nicotine is found in tobacco in a 1% to 2% concentration. There is no therapeutic use for nicotine. Smoking and other uses of tobacco have been in and out of favor several times during the past five centuries. This century has seen the greatest degree of abuse. Reasons for this increase are related to the mass production of tobacco products, mass advertising campaigns, and the psychological dependence produced by nicotine. Tobacco, even when used in moderation, will likely produce disease and death. Tobacco kills more than 430,000 U.S. citizens each year. That is more than alcohol, cocaine, heroin, homicide, suicide, car accidents, fire, and AIDS combined (NIDA, 2003a).

Incidence

About 28% of the population age 12 and older uses tobacco (NIDA, 2003a). Among students ages 12 to 17, 18% were current smokers in 1998 (NIDA, 2003a).

Signs and Symptoms

Nicotine causes decreased skeletal muscle tone, decreased sensitivity of some receptor sites (pain, heat, taste buds), reduced appetite, vasoconstriction, decreased body temperature, and increased blood pressure. Tolerance develops so the daily intake must increase to continue the desired effect.

LIFE CYCLE CONSIDERATIONS

Smoking

- Menopause generally occurs earlier in women who smoke.
- The older smoker is often less motivated to quit because of the feeling that "I've survived this long."

Potential for Addiction

The potential for addiction is high. Even first-time users can become dependent within weeks of their initial use. Nicotine is not a scheduled drug.

Associated Problems/Disorders

Other ingredients in the smoke (tar, carbon monoxide, and incompletely burned waste products) are largely responsible for the negative health consequences.

Respiratory

Chronic obstructive pulmonary disease is caused by the many changes tobacco use makes in the respiratory system. Smokers are more prone to developing pneumonia, and asthma is exacerbated by smoking. Chronic exposure to smoke inhalation gives children higher rates of otitis media and respiratory illnesses.

Cardiovascular

Ischemic heart disease is twice as likely to develop in a smoker than in a nonsmoker. Cerebrovascular accidents and peripheral vascular disease are strongly associated with smoking. Cessation of smoking, about 10 years, reduces the risks for these three vascular diseases to the nonsmoker's level.

Cancer

Many cancers—oral, pharyngeal, laryngeal, esophageal, lung, pancreatic, kidney, and bladder—are strongly associated with tobacco. Secondhand smoke causes lung cancer in nonsmoking adults. Cigarette smoking is by far the most important risk factor in lung cancer development (American Cancer Society, 2003).

Withdrawal

Short-term effects of nicotine withdrawal include nausea, diarrhea, headache, drowsiness, insomnia, irritability, and poor concentration. Increased appetite along with an intense craving for tobacco may persist for 6 months or longer.

Treatment/Rehabilitation

Nicotine replacement therapy by patch, nasal spray, inhaler, or gum helps individuals break the habit. It is important that the client not smoke while using the patch. Serious adverse effects may be experienced with a high serum nicotine level. It can be toxic. Later, a gradual withdrawal of the nicotine patch can be accomplished. The first non-nicotine prescription drug to treat nicotine addiction, bupropion (Zyban), was approved by the Food and Drug Administration in 1996.

An exercise program will help with stress management and minimize possible weight gain. Relaxation techniques will also reduce stress. Support by family and significant others for the person quitting tobacco use may help the process. A lack of support may greatly increase the difficulty of quitting for the individual. The rate of relapse is highest in the first few weeks and diminishes considerably after 3 months.

METHYLPHENIDATE HYDROCHLORIDE (RITALIN)

SCH. II

Currently, there is an increase in the use (misuse and overuse) of Ritalin that is becoming a growing problem. Ritalin is an accepted treatment for children with attention deficit hyperactivity disorder (ADHD). Although Ritalin is a CNS stimulant, there is a paradoxical calming effect on children with ADHD. Many children are being given Ritalin without thorough testing to eliminate other causes of attention deficit. These children have the potential for dependence. Ritalin is also used for narcolepsy. It can be detected for 1 to 2 days and is a schedule II drug.

HALLUCINOGENS

Hallucinogens refers to a group of naturally occurring and synthetic agents that produce essentially the same mind-altering effects.

Psilocybin and psilocin are naturally occurring organic compounds found in some mushrooms that grow in the United States and Mexico. These mushrooms have been used for centuries in southern Mexico, primarily in religious ceremonies. Fresh or dried mushrooms, sometimes mixed with food, are ingested orally.

Dimethyltryptamine (DMT) and diethyltryptamine (DET) are found in tropical plant leaves and seeds. For centuries they have been dried and powdered and used as snuff. They are not orally active. Sometimes the powder is added to tobacco or marijuana.

There are several amphetamine-like hallucinogens. Probably the two best known are 2,5 dimethyl-4-ethyl-amphetamine (DOM) and methylene-dioxyamphetamine (MDMA, ecstasy), which are chemically manufactured compounds. These are usually taken orally but may be injected intravenously or inhaled.

LYSERGIC ACID DIETHYLAMIDE

Lysergic acid diethylamide (LSD), a manufactured chemical compound, is perhaps the most widely known and used hallucinogen. In the past, LSD has been used as a legitimate medication and in research. In the 1960s, when its abuse became so widespread, the manufacturer refused to supply it for research. It had already been discontinued as a useful medication. It is generally taken orally but can be injected intravenously.

Incidence

The use of hallucinogens declined throughout the 1980s. In the early 1990s, LSD made a comeback. The 1990 and 1991 annual survey of high school seniors found that for the first time since 1976, more seniors had used LSD than cocaine in the previous 12 months. The 1998 survey showed a slight downward movement in LSD use (NIDA, 2003g). Other names for LSD are acid and microdot.

CULTURAL CONSIDERATIONS

Mescaline

Mescaline is the active ingredient in peyote cactus found growing in the southwestern United States and Mexico. It is the only legally used hallucinogen. Members of the Native American Church of the United States may use it for religious purposes. It is ingested orally. A cross-tolerance to LSD and psilocybin occurs.

Signs and Symptoms

The functioning of both the peripheral nervous system and the central nervous system is altered by LSD. Physical effects include hypertension, increased temperature, sweating, loss of appetite, dilated pupils, and dry mouth. Time and distance are distorted, rational judgment is impaired, and visual **hallucinations** (perceiving things that are not really there) and delusions along with **synthesiasis** (hearing colors and seeing sounds) occur. A state of either euphoria or depression is experienced. The depression with feelings of anxiety, panic, or suicidal tendencies is termed a "bad trip." Flashbacks occur suddenly days or years after LSD use. Their occurrence and frequency are unpredictable but seem to happen in times of high stress. LSD may be detected up to 8 hours after use.

Potential for Addiction

LSD is not considered an addictive drug, but it does produce tolerance. It is a schedule I drug.

Associated Problems/Disorders

Personality changes occur with LSD use and may happen after a single LSD experience. Acceptable social behaviors seem to diminish with use.

Withdrawal

There is no withdrawal seen.

Treatment/Rehabilitation

A person on a "bad trip" should be carefully watched to prevent self-injury. Reassurance, support, and "talking down" should be done in a quiet, pleasant manner. The person should be encouraged to sit up or walk. Closing the eyes intensifies the "bad trip." The person should be reminded that the drug is causing the effects, which will soon go away.

After cessation of chronic LSD use, long-term psychotherapy is usually required to determine what needs were fulfilled by the use of this drug. A 12-step program and family assistance are usually necessary to reinforce the decision to remain abstinent. If the client is upset by flashbacks or the fear of flashbacks, an anxiolytic drug such as diazepam (Valium) may be ordered.

PHENCYCLIDINE   *Sch I & II*

Phencyclidine (PCP) was made for use as an anesthetic agent, but it produced such adverse reactions that it was withdrawn from clinical trials; however, it can easily be manufactured in an unsophisticated laboratory from simple materials. The degree of purity varies widely. It is often found as a contaminant in other street drugs. The anesthetic is used in veterinary medicine.

Incidence

PCP is primarily used by adolescents and young adults, with the first use between the ages of 13 and 15 years. Approximately 12.8% of those between the ages of 12 and 17 years had used PCP in 1979. The use decreased to 2.4% in 1992 and increased to 3.9% in 1997 (NIDA, 2003j). Other names for PCP are angel dust, ozone, wack, and rocket fuel. Marijuana combined with PCP is called killer joints or crystal super grass.

Signs and Symptoms

There are usually four phases, with the symptoms dose related. Acute toxicity is characterized by visual disturbances, auditory hallucinations, combativeness, catatonia, convulsions, and coma, and lasts about 3 days. The toxic psychosis phase has visual and auditory hallucinations, agitation, paranoid delusions, and disturbed judgment, and lasts about 7 days. The third phase has psychotic episodes, including thought disorders, paranoid ideation, and affect disorders much like schizophrenia and lasts a month or more. Depression is the fourth phase that may end in suicide. The use of other street drugs may alleviate the depression. Behavior is highly unpredictable. Death can occur from respiratory depression. For 2 to 8 days, PCP can be detected.

Potential for Addiction

Even chronic use does not produce physical dependence. Psychological dependence does develop as evidenced by a craving for PCP. It is a schedule I and II drug.

Associated Problems/Disorders

Seizures are a common occurrence with PCP. Hypertension and hyperthermia must be treated before they become a crisis situation. **Opisthotonos,** a complete arching of the body with only the head and feet on the bed, usually is relieved as the blood level of PCP decreases. Cardiac arrhythmias may need interventions by a cardiologist. Acute renal failure may result from the use of PCP. Strokes also have been reported. In adolescents, PCP interferes with hormones related to normal growth and development (NIDA, 2003j).

Withdrawal

PCP is fat soluble and its effects are felt weeks after the last use as it is gradually released from the fatty tissue into the circulation.

Treatment/Rehabilitation

Treatment should begin in an inpatient setting because of the high risk of suicide. The goal is to keep the client from resuming drug use. Sedatives may be used, and urinary acidifiers such as ascorbic acid may be given to increase excretion of PCP. Minimal confrontation should be used in a nonthreatening, nonstimulating, supportive environment. No effort should be made to "talk down" or calm the individual. Diazepam (Valium) may be ordered.

Vocational counseling and training may enhance self-esteem. Body awareness, yoga, and progressive relaxation help the client focus and improve attention span and concentration. Participation in a self-help group such as Narcotics Anonymous (NA) should be encouraged, although initial involvement is usually minimal.

OPIOIDS .

Opioids is a term used to refer to naturally occurring opiates, semisynthetic opiates, synthetic opiates, and agonist-antagonists. Table 46-6 provides examples of these opioids. Heroin is the most abused and the most rapid acting of the opioids (NIDA, 2003e).

Incidence

Kleber (1999) described the 1990s as the decade of heroin. Cocaine addicts switched to heroin. Heroin was easily available, the purity was higher than in decades, and it could now be sniffed or smoked instead of injected (NIDA, 2003e). By 1999, the use of heroin by 12- to 17-year-olds was 2.2% (NIDA, 2003e). Other names for heroin are horse, smack, "H," skag, and junk.

TABLE 46-6	OPIOIDS
TYPE	**EXAMPLE**
Natural Opiates	morphine sulfate
	codeine sulfate
Semisynthetic Opiates	heroin
	hydromorphone hydrochloride (Dilaudid)
	oxymorphone hydrochloride (Numorphan)
	oxycodone (in Percodan)
	hydrocodone (in Hycodan)
Synthetic Opiates	meperidine hydrochloride (Demerol)
	methadone hydrochloride (Dolophine)
	propoxyphene (Darvon)
Agonist-Antagonists	pentazocine (Talwin)
	nalbuphine hydrochloride (Nubain)
	butorphanol tartrate (Stadol)

Signs and Symptoms

All of these drugs affect the central nervous system, causing mental changes, euphoria, drowsiness, analgesia, constricted pupils, and depressed respirations. These changes become more pronounced as the dose is increased.

Opioids increase stomach tone, decrease intestinal peristalsis, and increase the tone of the anal sphincter. This all adds up to constipation. Prolonged drug use may result in a fecal impaction.

Peripheral blood vessels are dilated by opioids, and orthostatic hypotension frequently occurs. The work of the heart is not changed by opioids, so they are frequently used to treat the severe pain of a myocardial infarction.

Tolerance may develop to one or more of the effects of opioids but not to others. For example, morphine addicts will always have pinpoint pupils even when the euphoric effects are not experienced. Tolerance to one opioid usually means tolerance to other opioids as well. Withdrawal symptoms from one opioid can be suppressed by using another opioid.

Potential for Addiction – sch. I.

The potential for addiction is high. Heroin is a schedule I drug; methadone, schedule II; morphine, schedule II or III; and codeine and opium are schedule II, III, or IV.

Associated Problems/Disorders

Chronic heroin injection may cause scarred and collapsed veins, bacterial infections of heart valves and blood vessels, abscesses, and liver or kidney disease. Pneumonia may result from the respiratory-depressing effect of heroin. Additives to street heroin may clog blood vessels or cause immune reactions, leading to arthritis or other rheumatologic conditions. Sharing injection equipment can lead to infections of hepatitis B and C, HIV, and other blood-borne viruses, which can be passed on to sexual partners and children.

Withdrawal

Withdrawal symptoms depend on drug purity, dose, and route of administration. Withdrawal is characterized by a rebound excitability of those functions that had been depressed. Symptoms include stomach cramps, nausea, vomiting, diarrhea, diaphoresis, hypertension, aching of bones and muscles, lacrimation, rhinorrhea, cold flashes with goose bumps, yawning, mydriasis, anxiety, irritability, restlessness, and sometimes paranoia, violence, fear, or depersonalization.

Morphine withdrawal symptoms begin within 8 to 12 hours after the last dose, and the acute phase is over in about 10 to 14 days. Figure 46-2 illustrates the signs and symptoms of morphine withdrawal. This is the basic pattern of withdrawal for all opioids.

Codeine withdrawal symptoms may be a little less severe than those of morphine withdrawal. Dilaudid and heroin withdrawal may begin slightly earlier than morphine withdrawal. Meperidine (Demerol) withdrawal begins within 3 hours and peaks in 8 to 12 hours. Propoxyphene (Darvon) withdrawal is considerably milder.

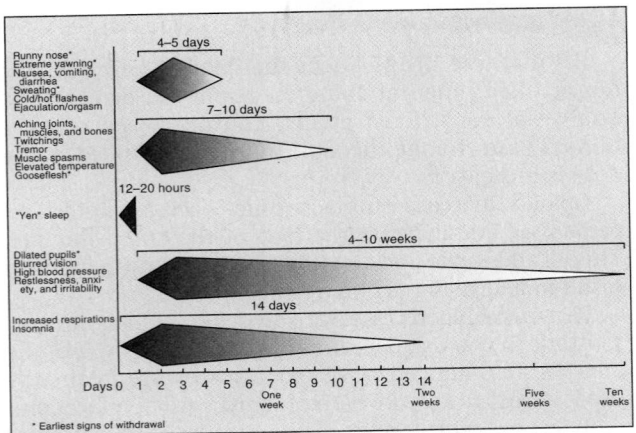

Figure 46-2 *Duration of Morphine Withdrawal Signs and Symptoms (Basic pattern for all opioids)*

Methadone withdrawal is slower to develop and lasts longer. Symptoms may not occur for 1 to 2 days, with acute symptoms lasting 2 to 3 weeks but not disappearing until 6 weeks after abstinence begins. Symptoms of fatigue, sluggishness, and irritability may last up to 6 months.

Withdrawal from the agonist-antagonists begins in 6 to 8 hours and is usually over in 8 days. The symptoms are the same as for morphine only in a milder form.

Treatment/Rehabilitation

Initial treatment is symptomatic and supportive of vital functions until the acute phase is over.

Detoxification

Several methods currently used for opioid detoxification are methadone, LAAM, and naltrexone.

Methadone Methadone is given and the dose adjusted to keep withdrawal symptoms under control. The daily dose is gradually reduced over a period of 3 to 6 months. Routine and random urine testing is usually done to ensure no other drug use.

Levo-alpha-acetyl-methadol Levo-alpha-acetyl-methadol (LAAM) is a synthetic opiate, like methadone, used to treat heroin addiction. It blocks the effects of heroin for up to 72 hours, so it need be taken only 3 times a week.

Naltrexone Naltrexone (ReVia) blocks the effects of morphine, heroin, and other opiates. Its effects last 1 to 3 days depending on the dose. The pleasurable effects of heroin are blocked, making it useful to treat highly motivated individuals. It is also used to prevent relapse in former opiate addicts.

Counseling/Self-Help Groups

Individual and/or group counseling must go hand in hand with the detoxification to help the client learn new methods of coping with life's stresses. Participation in Narcotics Anonymous (NA) helps the client maintain abstinence from drugs.

Behavioral Therapy

Contingency management therapy employs a voucher system. Clients earn "points" for having negative drug tests. These can be exchanged for items encouraging healthy living (NIDA, 2003e).

INHALANTS

Inhalants are inexpensive and easy to obtain. Examples are toluene (glues), gasoline, kerosene, isopropyl alcohol, lacquer thinner, acetone, benzene, naptha, carbon tetrachloride, fluorocarbons (aerosol propellants), correction fluid, and nitrous oxide. They are rapidly absorbed into the brain and stored in body fat.

Incidence

In 1997, 21% of 8th graders, 18.3% of 10th graders, and 16.1% of 12th graders reported using inhalants at least once. By 2002, 15.2% of 8th graders, 13.5% of 10th graders, and 11.7% of 13th graders reported using inhalants at least once (NIDA, 2003f). Inhalants are not scheduled drugs.

Signs and Symptoms

The desired effect of euphoria is followed by nausea, headache, and amnesia. Other effects of using inhalants include dizziness, unsteady gait, slurred speech, auditory and visual hallucinations, drowsiness, hypotension, heightened sexual response caused by profound vasodilation, stupor, unconsciousness, and coma. Heavy use can lead to hypoxia, multiple organ damage, and death. Airway freezing and/or laryngospasm can be caused by nitrous oxide.

Behaviors that may indicate inhalant abuse include decreased school performance; loss of interest in extracurricular, family, and social activities; and the onset of legal problems.

Potential for Addiction

The potential for addiction is high for psychological dependence only.

Associated Problems/Disorders

Chronic pulmonary irritation and/or chemical pneumonitis may be caused by the use of inhalants. Toluene may cause renal tubular acidosis, hearing loss, and brain damage. Fluorocarbons sensitize the myocardium to catacholemines and may cause arrhythmias.

Withdrawal

There are no withdrawal symptoms.

Treatment/Rehabilitation

Initial treatment is to provide oxygen and respiratory support. Participation in a traditional chemical dependency program is often needed. An adolescent 12-step group is very helpful. Individual and family counseling are essential.

ECSTASY

Ecstasy, also called MDMA (3,4-methylene-dioxymethamphetamine), is a complex drug having similarities to methamphetamine, a stimulant, and mescaline, a hallucinogen (NIDA, 2001b). It produces stimulant effects and distorted time and perception rather than true hallucinations. Ecstasy tablets also often contain one or more of the following: caffeine, methamphetamine, dextromethorphan, ephedrine, or cocaine.

Incidence

The 2000 Monitoring the Future survey indicated that MDMA use increased among 8th-, 10th-, and 12th-grade students (NIDA, 2001a).

Signs and Symptoms

Ecstasy provides an enhanced sense of pleasure and self-confidence; feelings of peacefulness, acceptance, and closeness with others; and increased energy. Research has shown that ecstasy can lead to disruptions in body temperature and cardiovascular regulation. It also damages the nerves in the brain's serotonin system and appears to produce long-term deficits in memory and cognition (NIDA, 2001b). It appears that the more ecstasy taken, the greater the deficit (NIDA, 2001a).

Potential for Addiction

There is little data available, but animal studies support the possibility of addiction (NIDA, 2001a).

Associated Problems/Disorders

MDMA interferes with the metabolism of other drugs, including some that may be in the tablet with the ecstasy.

ANABOLIC STEROIDS

Anabolic steroids are synthetic derivatives of testosterone. They cause both androgenic (masculinizing) and anabolic (tissue-building) effects. Most people use anabolic steroids for their anabolic effects. Medically, they are used in the treatment of some anemias and in some cancer therapies. The use of anabolic steroids is banned by the International Olympic Committee and the National Collegiate Athletic Association.

Incidence

Primary users are athletes seeking to improve their performance. Other people use anabolic steroids to improve their physical appearance. In 1997, 1.8% of 8th graders, 2% of 10th graders, and 2.4% of 12th graders had used anabolic steroids. In 2000, 3% of 8th graders, 3.5% of 10th graders, and 2.5% of 12th graders had used anabolic steroids. (NIDA, 2003k).

Signs and Symptoms

The commonly perceived effects of anabolic steroids are an increase in skeletal muscle mass, enhanced physical performance of the skeletal muscles, and improved athletic ability; however, there is no conclusive evidence that these perceived effects are medically accurate.

Potential for Addiction

The potential for addiction is moderate. Anabolic steroids are schedule III drugs.

Associated Problems/Disorders

Other effects found when anabolic steroids are used include hepatocellular damage, cholestasis, hepatoadenoma, hepatocarcinoma, acne, hirsutism, male-pattern baldness, a deepening of the voice, increased cholesterol level, increased blood pressure, decreased glucose tolerance, mood swings, aggressiveness, depression, psychosis, and hepatitis or HIV infection if needles are shared. In males, there is also testicular atrophy, oligospermia, impotence, prostatic hypertrophy, prostatic carcinoma, and gynecomastia. In females, there is also amenorrhea, clitoromegaly, uterine atrophy, breast atrophy, facial hair growth, and teratogenicity.

These effects seem to be reversible when the anabolic steroids are no longer taken, except for the male-pattern baldness, liver tumors, and gynecomastia in males and clitoral enlargement, virilization, and male-pattern baldness in females. The increased aggressiveness and euphoria are probably beneficial during athletic competitions but otherwise may cause severe social problems.

Withdrawal

Symptoms of withdrawal include lethargy, abdominal muscle cramps, constipation, headache, and depression.

Treatment/Rehabilitation

Treatment of withdrawal focuses on providing symptom relief for the client and counseling to build self-esteem and self-confidence in abilities without the use of anabolic steroids.

NURSING PROCESS

Nursing care is an essential component of the multidisciplinary approach to substance abuse treatment.

Assessment

The subjective and objective data given are related to substance abuse and dependence in general.

Subjective Data

The client will often describe being very relaxed; feeling wonderful; or having a headache, fatigue, depression, sleep disturbance, suppression of appetite, dizziness, hallucinations, paranoia, anxiety, emotional lability, memory loss, heightened sexual desire (with early use), or loss of sexual desire (with continued use). Problems in various areas of life are common, such as frequent job changes; marital conflict, separation and/or divorce; work-related accidents, lateness, absenteeism; and legal problems, including arrest for driving while intoxicated. The client may describe having falls or fights and financial problems. Normal diet pattern and the presence of any disease conditions should be noted.

The client should be asked, "How often do you use drugs/alcohol? How much do you usually use? Have you ever used drugs/alcohol more than you use them now? When? Under what circumstances? What substance did you last use?" The information received from the client may not always be accurate. Validation with the family or significant other is helpful.

Objective Data

Neglect of health and personal care is often evident. The client may have dental caries, bad breath, gingivitis, unkempt appearance, and be undernourished or malnourished. If substances have been inhaled, there may be irritation and bleeding of the nasal mucosa, destruction of the nasal mucosa and cartilaginous structures, or depression of respirations. If substances have been injected intravenously, there will be scarring of veins (needle marks, track marks), possibly skin infections, enlarged lymph nodes, and hematomas.

The client may appear older than the stated age and have a chronic cough producing brown to black sputum, dilated or pinpoint pupils, tremors, slurred speech, lack of coordination, frequent episodes of sexually transmitted diseases, jaundice, or vomiting. There may be tachycardia, hypertension, ascites, or petechiae.

Nursing Diagnoses

Nursing diagnoses for a client with substance abuse or dependence may include the following:

- *Imbalanced **N**utrition: Less than Body Requirements*
- ***S**elf-Care Deficits*
- *Risk for **I**njury*
- *Disturbed **S**leep Pattern*
- ***A**ctivity Intolerance*
- *Impaired Physical **M**obility*
- *Disturbed **S**ensory Perception*
- *Impaired Verbal **C**ommunication*
- *Risk for **I**nfection*
- *Excess or Deficient **F**luid Volume*
- *Disturbed **T**hought Processes*
- *Ineffective **C**oping*
- *Situational Low **S**elf-Esteem*
- *Risk for **V**iolence (Other Directed or Self-Directed)*
- ***A**nxiety*
- *Impaired **S**ocial Interaction*
- ***H**opelessness*
- ***P**owerlessness*
- *Compromised Family **C**oping*
- *Defensive **C**oping*

Planning/Outcome Identification

There are several overall goals for the care of a client with a substance abuse problem. The client will do the following:

1. Abstain from using psychoactive substances.
2. Adhere to the treatment plan.
3. Make lifestyle changes to maintain abstinence.
4. Engage in behaviors that foster good health.

Possible outcomes from Nursing Outcomes Classification (NOC) include:
Distorted Thought Control
Risk Control: Alcohol Use
Risk Control: Drug Use

Nursing Interventions

Nursing interventions include active listening, providing care in a nonjudgmental manner, teaching health promotion, and referral to self-help groups or individual counseling. Other nursing interventions must be specific for the goals and nursing diagnoses identified for the individual client. Examples might include the following:

1. Provide a well-balanced diet. Monitor intake and results of lab tests. Assess for GI bleeding.
2. Assist with personal hygiene. Encourage self-care.
3. Administer medications as ordered to decrease or prevent symptoms of withdrawal. Keep call light in client's reach. Keep siderails up.
4. Provide warm milk at bedtime. Plan with client a time for bed. Encourage use of relaxation techniques. Reassure client that insomnia will improve.
5. Encourage client to do active ROM exercises.
6. Assist client to turn in bed. Assist client to ambulate as able. Answer call light promptly.
7. Do not argue with a client having hallucinations. Remind client of day, time, and place.
8. Watch client's nonverbal communication.
9. Encourage good personal hygiene. Inspect skin for integrity.
10. Administer antibiotics as ordered. Monitor vital signs. Monitor I&O. Monitor results of lab test.
11. Administer vitamins as ordered. Provide cues as needed. Encourage adequate diet intake.
12. Assess coping patterns to identify strengths and weaknesses. Actively listen to client. Refer to appropriate community agencies.

LIFE CYCLE CONSIDERATIONS

Substance Misuse or Abuse

In the elderly:

- **Misuse** (using a legal drug for something other than intended or exceeding the recommended dose of a drug) is more common than abuse or dependence.
- Substances that decrease respirations can increase the frequency of mental confusion.
- Decreased coordination from alcohol or other substances is associated with falling more often and fracturing the wrist, back, and hips.
- Chronic medical conditions can be made worse from even minimal use of alcohol or other drugs because these substances can change the effect of prescribed medications.
- Unrealistic expectations of retirement may lead to use of mood-altering substances to relieve depression and boredom.

13. Assist client to identify areas of low self-esteem. Encourage client participation in group therapy. Refer to individual counseling as needed.
14. Monitor client closely. Use restraints as ordered. Keep bed in low position and side rails up.
15. Introduce client to other recovering persons. Encourage client to participate in self-help group.
16. Provide spiritual support if asked.
17. Involve client in decision making when possible. Give positive reinforcement for abstinence.
18. Encourage family to participate in treatment program.

Possible interventions from Nursing Interventions Classification (NIC) include:

  Delusion Management
  Hallucination Management
  Anxiety Reduction
  Delirium Management
  Mood Management

Evaluation

Each goal must be evaluated to determine how it has been met by the client.

CODEPENDENCY

Codependency was first recognized by those working with families of alcoholics. It is a learned pattern of feeling and behaving, a problem with relationships. In healthy relationships, people share love, concern, and respect for each other. There is equal give-and-take. This is termed *interdependence*. In unhealthy relationships, people are often out of touch with their own needs and feelings. They may be unwilling or unable to take care of themselves and have little self-esteem. Only by fulfilling the expectations of others do they feel good about themselves. This is termed *codependence*. **Codependent** persons live based on what others think of them. They always try to meet the needs of others, demand love from others, and manipulate and control the lives of others.

Serious family problems like addictions, abuse, family secrets, or other major stresses cause confusion and put a family at risk. Codependent behavior thrives when fear, guilt, blame, and low self-esteem become evident. When family members do not relate to each other in positive ways or when their interactions do not provide a healthy environment, the family is called *dysfunctional*. Many children grow up in dysfunctional families and learn to be codependent.

Codependency tends to run in families. Parents cannot teach their children how to cope in healthy ways if they do not know how themselves. Without intervention or a conscious change by the individual, a pattern of codependent behavior will continue in other relationships.

Characteristics

Persons who are codependent have specific characteristics or traits. They have low self-esteem, never feel they are good enough, and often feel shame. Emotions are denied. They are out of touch with their own feelings and deny their own needs. Their smile is phony much of the

TABLE 46-7   CHARACTERISTICS OF THE CODEPENDENT PERSON

Caretaking	"I always give to others. No one gives to me."
Obsession	"I can't stop worrying about __ problems."
Denial	"I pretend I don't have problems."
Poor communication	"No one understands me."
Lack of trust	"I don't trust myself."
Anger	"I resent feeling controlled and manipulated."

From *Mental Health Concepts* (5th ed.), by C. Waughfield, 2002, Clifton Park, NY: Thomson Delmar Learning. Copyright 2002 by Thomson Delmar Learning. Adapted with permission.

time. Problems with communication become evident as they have trouble expressing their needs and feelings. Often they say the opposite to hide their true feelings. They expect others to read their minds. Relationship problems occur because they are afraid of being hurt or that others might learn of their secret feelings and reject them. They cannot risk loving and losing. Relationships are desired, but walls are always put up.

Codependent persons live through others. They are people pleasers who would rather give than take. The approval of others means they are okay. They think they can fix others. The feeling of powerlessness occurs because they give power to others by looking to them for approval. They go to extremes. For a while they will try very hard for approval, and then they will not try at all or they will keep negative feelings inside with a smile on their face and then blow up over some little thing. Table 46-7 lists some characteristics of the codependent person.

Treatment

Professional help is usually necessary to change codependent behavior. The goal of treatment is to help the codependent person feel happy and good about himself or herself. Therapy sessions focus on identifying and reconnecting with the true self, dealing with feelings, learning how to communicate feelings, learning to trust, setting boundaries for relationships, and taking charge of their own life.

THE IMPAIRED NURSE

Most states now have peer assistance programs to help nurses who are impaired by either alcohol or other substances. Substance abuse and dependence are greater problems among nurses than among the general public because nurses have access to many controlled substances. The impaired nurse often requests to give medications, makes medication errors, and "wastes" drugs frequently. This nurse may wear long sleeves and spend an extraordinary amount of time in the bathroom.

CRITICAL THINKING

Drug Testing

Should drug testing of all health care workers be required? How would you feel if you were requested to comply?

Substance-Abusing Client

How would you respond to a client who is a substance abuser?

Peer assistance programs first appeared in 1980. They have been formed through the state nursing association or the state board of nursing, or through joint effort of both. The goals of the peer assistance programs are to assist the impaired nurse to receive treatment; protect the public from impaired nurses; help the recovering nurse reenter the nursing workforce in a planned, safe manner; and monitor the nurse's recovery for a time. The state board of nursing may restrict access to controlled substances for the recovering nurse for some period.

Before the peer assistance programs, impaired nurses were generally just dismissed from employment. Then they would find employment at another health care agency where substance abuse or dependence would continue. This pattern often went on for years.

As the name implies, peer assistance programs are staffed with nurses to help nurses. Many of the staff are volunteers who work in psychiatric nursing or substance abuse centers or who are themselves recovering from substance abuse. It is best not to cover up for a colleague with a substance abuse problem; rather, the nurse should report the situation to a supervisor, who can arrange for the nurse to receive help. Some boards of nursing will discipline a nurse for failing to report a fellow nurse who is abusing drugs.

CASE STUDY

Joe, age 19, quit school 3 years ago. He has a part-time job at a fast-food place but has been tardy or absent quite often lately. Sometimes he is easy to get along with, and sometimes he is aggressive and difficult. His mother, with whom he lives, says he is a good boy and does not give her any trouble. Joe was brought to the emergency room by a friend after he passed out. His temperature is 99°F, respirations 10, and pupils are pinpoint. There are track marks on both arms.

The following questions will guide your development of a nursing care plan for the case study.

1. List signs and symptoms, other than Joe's, that a client may experience as a heroin addict.
2. List diagnostic tests that may be ordered.
3. List subjective and objective data the nurse should obtain.
4. Write three individualized nursing diagnoses and goals for Joe.
5. List resources within the medical center and local area that could assist Joe.
6. Describe the use of methadone in heroin addiction.
7. List teaching that Joe will need as a part of his rehabilitation.

Summary

- Substance abuse and dependence have been problems for centuries.
- Factors related to substance abuse include individual, family patterns, lifestyle, environmental, and developmental factors.
- A false-positive result on a drug screening test may be caused by ingestion of poppy seeds, use of a Vicks® inhaler, or use of over-the-counter diet aids.
- Detoxification is the first step in the treatment and rehabilitation of a substance abuser.

- Street drugs vary in strength and purity. Higher-priced drugs are often mixed with drugs that are cheaper or easier to obtain.
- Neglect of health and personal care are often evident in substance abuse and dependence.
- Nurses have a higher incidence of substance abuse and dependence than the general public.
- Most states have peer assistance programs for impaired nurses.

Review Questions

1. Schedule II substances:

   a. can be sold as over-the-counter drugs.
   b. have high abuse and dependence potential.
   c. can have prescription refilled for 6 months.
   d. have no accepted medical use in the United States.

2. Prevention of substance abuse must be focused on:

   a. parents.
   b. children.
   c. teenagers.
   d. young adults.

3. The substance most often chosen for abuse or dependence is:

   a. heroin.
   b. cocaine.
   c. alcohol.
   d. marijuana.

4. Alcoholics Anonymous is:

   a. the newest self-help group.
   b. a short-term temporary help group.
   c. a government agency to help those with an alcohol problem.
   d. a self-help group providing a holistic approach to abstinence.

5. The use of inhalants:

   a. can be fatal.
   b. includes only glue and paints.
   c. has severe withdrawal symptoms.
   d. is a harmless activity of young male teenagers.

References/Suggested Readings

Alcoholics Anonymous. (1939). *Alcoholics Anonymous.* New York: Alcoholics Anonymous World Services.

American Cancer Society (ACS). (2003). *Cancer facts & figures* [Online]. Available: www.cancer.org/downloads/STT/CAFF2003PWSecured.pdf

American Psychiatric Association. (2000). *Diagnostic and statistical manual of mental disorders* (4th ed.). T-R (text revision). Washington, DC: Author.

Biggs-Stewart, K., & Richards, A. (2000). Recognizing and managing your patient's alcohol abuse. *Nursing2000, 30*(2), 56–59.

Compton, P. (2002). Caring for an alcohol-dependent patient. *Nursing2002, 32*(12), 58–63.

Crigger, N. (1998). Defying denial: Clues to detecting alcohol abuse. *AJN, 98*(8), 20–21.

Daniels, R. (2002). *Delmar's guide to laboratory and diagnostic tests.* Clifton Park, NY: Thomson Delmar Learning.

Dochterman, J., & Bulechek, G. (2004). *Nursing Interventions Classification (NIC)* (4th ed.). St. Louis, MO: Mosby.

Doe, J. (2003). My journey through addiction. *Nursing2003, 33*(1), 32hn6–32hn8.

Fletcher, A. (2002). *Sober for good.* New York: Houghton Mifflin.

Gutierrez, M., Roper, J., & Hahn, P. (2001). Paradoxical reactions to benzodiazepines. *AJN, 101*(7), 34–39.

Haack, M. (1998). Treating acute withdrawal from alcohol and other drugs. *Nursing Clinics of North America, 33*(1), 75–92.

Haddad, A. (2000). Ethics in action: Treating pain in substance abusers. *RN, 63*(1), 21–24.

Hess, D., & DeBoer, S. (2002). Ecstasy. *AJN, 102*(4), 45–47.

Johnson, V. (1989). *Intervention: How to help someone who doesn't want help.* New York: New American Library.

Johnson, V. (1990). *I'll quit tomorrow: A practical guide to alcoholism treatment.* San Francisco: Harper San Francisco.

Johnston, L., O'Malley, P., & Bachman, J. (1991). *Drug use among American high school seniors, college students and young adults 1975–1990.* Rockville, MD: National Institute on Drug Abuse, U.S. Department of Health and Human Services, Alcohol Drug Abuse, and Mental Health Administration.

Johnston, L., O'Malley, P., & Bachman, J. (1998). *Drug use by American young people begins to turn downward* [Online]. Available: www.isr.umich.edu/src/mtf

Kleber, H. (1999). Opioids detoxification. In M. Galanter & H. Kleber, *Textbook of substance abuse treatment.* (2nd ed.). Washington, DC: American Psychiatric Press.

Landau, E. (1995). *Hooked: Talking about addictions.* Brookfield, CT: The Millbrook Press.

Mathre, M. L. (2001). Therapeutic cannabis. *AJN, 101*(4), 61–69.

Moorhead, S., Johnson, M., & Maas, M. (2004). *Nursing Outcomes Classification (NOC)* (3rd ed.). St. Louis, MO: Mosby.

Munson, B. (2001). Propellant inhalation. *Nursing2001, 31*(10), 104.

National Institute on Alcohol Abuse and Alcoholism (NIAAA). (1999). *Alcohol: What you don't know can harm you* [Online]. Available: www.niaaa.nih.gov/publications/harm-al.htm

National Institute on Alcohol Abuse and Alcoholism (NIAAA). (2000). *Unadjusted death rates for cirrhosis with and without mention of alcohol, United States, 1970–99* [Online]. Available: www.niaaa.nih.gov/publications/surveillance60/cirr99.htm

National Institute on Alcohol Abuse and Alcoholism (NIAAA). (2003). *Traffic crashes, traffic crash fatalities, and alcohol-related traffic crash fatalities, United States, 1977–2000* [Online]. Available: www.niaaa.nih.gov/databases/crash01.txt

National Institute on Drug Abuse (NIDA). (2001a). *Ecstasy: What we know and don't know about MDMA, a scientific report* [Online]. Available: www.drugabuse.gov/Meetings/MDMA/MDMAExSummary.html

National Institute on Drug Abuse (NIDA). (2001b). MDMA/Ecstasy—A drug with complex consequences. *NIDA Notes, 16*(5) [Online]. Available: www.drugabuse.gov/NIDA_Notes/NNVol16N5/Consequences. html

National Institute on Drug Abuse (NIDA). (2002a). *Cocaine abuse and addiction* [Online]. Available: www.nida.nih.gov/ResearchReports/Cocaine/cocaine.html

National Institute on Drug Abuse (NIDA). (2002b). *Criteria for substance dependence diagnosis* [Online]. Available: www.nida.nih.gov/DSR.html

National Institute on Drug Abuse (NIDA). (2002c). *Heroin: Abuse and addiction* [Online]. Available: www.nida.nih.gov/ResearchReports/Heroin/Heroin.html

National Institute on Drug Abuse (NIDA). (2002e). *Nicotine addiction* [Online]. Available: www.nida.nih.gov/researchreports/nicotine/nicotine.html

National Institute on Drug Abuse (NIDA). (2003a). *Cigarettes and other nicotine products* [Online]. Available: www.nida.nih.gov/Infofax/tobacco.html

National Institute on Drug Abuse (NIDA). (2003b). *Club drugs* [Online]. Available: www.nida.nih.gov/Infofax/Clubdrugs.html

National Institute on Drug Abuse (NIDA). (2003c). *Diagnosis and treatment of drug abuse in family practice* [Online]. Available: www.nida.nih.gov/Diagnosis-Treatment/Diagnosis.html

National Institute on Drug Abuse (NIDA). (2003d). *Ecstasy* [Online]. Available: www.nida.nih.gov/Infofax/ecstasy.html

National Institute on Drug Abuse (NIDA). (2003e). *Heroin* [Online]. Available: www.nida.nih.gov/Infofax/heroin.html

National Institute on Drug Abuse (NIDA). (2003f). *Inhalants* [Online]. Available: www.nida.nih.gov/Infofax/inhalants.html

National Institute on Drug Abuse (NIDA). (2003g). *LSD* [Online]. Available: www.nida.nih.gov/Infofax/lsd.html

National Institute on Drug Abuse (NIDA). (2003h). *Marijuana* [Online]. Available: www.nida.nih.gov/Infofax/marijuana.html

National Institute on Drug Abuse (NIDA). (2003i). *Methamphetamine* [Online]. Available: www.nida.nih.gov/Infofax/methamph.html

National Institute on Drug Abuse (NIDA). (2003j). *PCP (Phencyclidine)* [Online]. Available: www.nida.nih.gov/Infofax/pcp.html

National Institute on Drug Abuse (NIDA). (2003k). *Steroids (Anabolic)* [Online]. Available: www.nida.nih.gov/Infofax/steroids.html

National Institute on Drug Abuse (NIDA). (2003l). *Teen drug abuse—High school and youth trends* [Online]. Available: www.nida.nih.gov/Infofax/HSYouthtrends.html

National Institute on Drug Abuse (NIDA). (2003m). *Understanding drug abuse and addiction* [Online]. Available: www.nida.nih.gov/Infofax/understand.html

Nichols, R. (2003). Pain management in patients with addictive disease. *AJN, 103*(3) 87–90.

North American Nursing Diagnosis Association (NANDA). (2003). *Nursing diagnoses: Definitions & classification 2003–2004.* Philadelphia: Author.

Santomier, J., & Hogan, P. (1992). Health implications of alcohol and other drug use. In M. Naegle (Ed.), *Substance abuse education in nursing* (Vol. 1). New York: National League for Nursing.

Spratto, G., & Woods, A. (2004). *2004 PDR Nurses' drug handbook.* Clifton Park, NY: Thomson Delmar Learning.

Substance Abuse and Mental Health Services Administration, Office of Applied Technologies. (2002). *2001 National household survey on drug abuse* [Online]. Available: www.samhsa.gov/oas/nhsda/2K1nhsda/vol1/toc.htm

Waughfield, C. (2002). *Mental health concepts* (5th ed.). Clifton Park, NY: Thomas Delmar Learning.

Resources

Al-Anon Family Group, 1600 Corporate Landing Parkway, Virginia Beach, VA, 23454-5617, www.al-anon.org

Alcoholics Anonymous (AA), P.O. Box 459, Grand Central Station, New York, NY 10163, 212-870-3400, www.alcoholics-anonymous.org

American Council for Drug Education, www.acde.org

Codependents Anonymous (CODA), P.O. Box 33577, Phoenix, AZ 85607-3577, www.codependents.org

Drug Abuse Resistance Education (DARE), Local Police Department, www.dare-america.com

Drug Enforcement Administration (DEA), Mailstop: AXS 2401 Jefferson Davis Highway, Alexandria, VA 22201, 202-307-7423, www.usdoj.gov/dea

Families Anonymous, (Families of Substance Abusers), Box 3475, Culver City, CA 90231-3475, 800-736-9805, www.familiesanonymous.org

Mothers Against Drunk Driving (MADD), 511 E. John Carpenter Freeway, Suite 700, Irving, TX 75062, 214-744-6233, or 3601 SW 29th, Topeka, KS 66614, 800-438-6233, www.madd.org

Narcotics Anonymous (NA), World Service Office, P.O. Box 9999, Van Nuys, CA 91409, 818-773-9999, www.na.org

National Clearinghouse for Alcohol and Drug Information, Box 2345, Rockville, MD 20857, 301-468-2600, www.health.org

National Council on Alcoholism and Drug Dependence, 20 Exchange Place, Suite 2902, New York, NY 10005, 212-269-7797, www.ncadd.org

Students Against Driving Drunk (SADD) Inc., P.O. Box 800, Marlboro, MA 01752, 877-723-3462, www.saddonline.com

Toughlove, P.O. Box 1069, Doylestown, PA 18901, 215-348-7090, www.toughlove.org

UNIT
16

Applications

47

RESPONDING TO EMERGENCIES

MAKING THE CONNECTION

Refer to the following chapters to increase your understanding of emergency situations:

Basic Nursing
- Holistic Care
- Legal and Ethical Responsibilities

Adult Health Nursing
- Respiratory System
- Cardiovascular System
- Gastrointestinal System
- Urinary System

- Musculoskeletal System
- Neurological System
- Sensory System
- Reproductive Systems
- Integumentary System
- Mental Illness
- Substance Abuse

LEARNING OBJECTIVES

Upon completion of this chapter, you should be able to:
- Define key terms.
- Describe the emergency medical services.
- Explain the role of the nurse in emergency situations.
- List personnel needed to respond to an in-hospital emergency.
- Discuss the steps in assessing an emergency client.
- Cite the different levels of triage.

KEY TERMS

chain of custody
disaster
emergency
emergency medical
  technician (EMT)
emergency nursing

Glasgow Coma Scale
paramedic
shock
trauma
triage

INTRODUCTION

An **emergency** can be defined as a medical or surgical condition requiring immediate or timely intervention to prevent permanent disability or death. Emergency nursing has developed rapidly over the years in response to the changing environment and expectations of the community. Many advancements in emergency care can be attributed to the military. In order to manage vast numbers of injured soldiers, the military had to develop a systematic method of treating and responding to **trauma** (wound or injury). Casualties caused by wartime situations created the need for advancements in the care of large numbers of clients with injuries,

wounds, and illness. Methods of caring for multiple clients were developed and implemented as a result of military influence.

In the United States, trauma is the number-one killer of those younger than age 37 and the fourth leading cause of death overall. Motor vehicle collisions kill more than 43,000 people each year, with more than 4 million car crash victims cared for in emergency departments (EDs).

Emergency nursing is the care of clients who require emergency intervention. The emergency nurse must be capable of rapid assessment and history taking and immediate intervention formulation and implementation utilizing the nursing process. This role carries great responsibility. Throughout the assessment and care of the client, the emergency nurse must plan and teach prevention and health promotion, as well as rapidly develop rapport with the client and family, including assisting with emotional needs. Clinical knowledge, communication, client teaching, and empathy skills are essential to effective emergency care. Although LP/VNs are seldom hired for EDs, they may at times be required to float or help during emergency situations; therefore, a brief overview of emergency nursing is justified.

A **disaster** is a situation or event of greater magnitude than an emergency that has unforeseen, serious, or immediate threats to public health. They may be *natural* events such as large fires, earthquakes, floods, hurricanes, or tornadoes; or *man-made* events such as war, terrorism, or overwhelming contamination of the environment (Gebbie & Qureshi, 2002).

EMERGENCY/DISASTER PREPAREDNESS

In order to be prepared for emergencies or disasters, it is necessary to identify *who* needs to know *how* to do *what*. To this end, Gebbie and Qureshi (2002) have outlined the following core competencies for nurses that were modeled after the CDC's core emergency preparedness competencies for public health workers:

- *Describe* the agency's role in responding to a range of emergencies that might arise.
- *Describe* the chain of command in emergency response.
- *Identify* and locate the agency's emergency response plan (or the pertinent portion of it).
- *Describe* emergency response functions or roles and *demonstrate* them in regularly performed drills.
- *Demonstrate* the use of equipment (including personal protective equipment) and the skills required in emergency response during regular drills.
- *Demonstrate* the correct operation of all equipment used for emergency communication.
- *Describe* communication roles in emergency response within your agency, with news media, with the general public, and with personal contacts.
- *Identify* the limits of your own knowledge, skills, and authority and identify key system resources for referring matters that exceed these limits.
- *Apply* creative problem-solving skills and flexible thinking to the situation, within the confines of your role, and *evaluate* the effectiveness of all actions taken.
- *Recognize* deviations from the norm that might indicate an emergency and *describe* appropriate action.

PROFESSIONAL TIP

Golden Rules of Emergency Care
1. Establish the safety of the scene.
2. Remove the client from danger.
3. Establish airway, breathing, and circulation.
4. Manage shock.
5. Attend to eye injuries.
6. Treat skin injuries.
7. Call for help.

- *Participate* in continuing education to maintain up-to-date knowledge in relevant areas.
- *Participate* in evaluating every drill or response and *identify* necessary changes to the plan.

APPROACHES TO EMERGENCY CARE

There are three general approaches to emergency care: hospital triage, disaster triage, and the emergency medical services. To care for the emergent client, one must first determine the severity of illness.

Hospital Triage

Each hospital with an ED has an established "triage" system in effect. **Triage** refers to classification of clients to determine priority of need and proper place of treatment. Triage is typically utilized in the ED to establish priorities and levels of care needed by the clients. Although clients and their families define emergency according to their perceptions, it is the triage nurse's responsibility to sort and prioritize the clients as they arrive in the ED.

The simplest method of triaging clients is to utilize the American Heart Association's basic life support principles: Airway, Breathing, and Circulation (ABCs). By utilizing this method, those clients with airway problems would be immediately assessed and would become a top priority of care. If any of the ABCs were not functioning, either the Heimlich maneuver or cardiopulmonary resuscitation (CPR) would be initiated.

 Infection Control: Mouth-to-Mouth Resuscitation
When delivering care to any client, the nurse should be careful to practice Standard Precautions. Direct mouth-to-mouth breathing should not be administered; instead, use of a bag-valve-mask for resuscitation is more effective in both protecting the health care worker and the client from possible infection and in administering respirations.

Most hospitals have a triage system established in order to provide expedient care to those requiring it first. Although the term *emergency department* implies emergency care, the client utilizing this department does not always require immediate care. In 2000, there were 108 million visits to hospital EDs (McMahon, 2003). The most commonly used triage classifications are emergent, urgent, and nonurgent and are recognized by the Emergency Nurses Association (McMahon, 2003) (Table 47-1). Emergent clients require immediate care in order to sustain life or limb. Examples of emergent conditions include foreign bodies in the eye, shortness of breath, impending birth, and cardiopulmonary arrest. Urgent clients require care within 1 to 2 hours to prevent worsening of their conditions. Examples of urgent situations include acute abdominal pain and compound fractures. For nonurgent clients, care can be delayed without the risk of permanent consequences. Contusions and sprains are examples of nonurgent complaints.

TABLE 47-1	TRIAGE CATEGORIES	
CATEGORY/ PRIORITY	CLIENT NEEDS	EXAMPLES
Emergent	Immediate intervention is required to sustain life or limb.	Cardiac arrest Multiple trauma
Urgent	Care is required within 1 to 2 hours to prevent deterioration of condition.	Compound fractures Persistent vomiting and diarrhea
Nonurgent	Care may be delayed without risk of permanent sequelae.	Contusions Minor sprains and fractures

Developed from Military Standard Operating Procedure (SOP) for General Hospitals.

TABLE 47-2	DISASTER TRIAGE	
CATEGORY/ PRIORITY	CLIENT NEEDS	EXAMPLES
Immediate	Simple injuries requiring immediate care	Chest wounds Crush injuries Burns
Delayed	Multiple injuries requiring extensive care	Open fractures of the long bones
Minimal	Minor injuries (the walking wounded)	Sprains Contusions Minor cuts
Expectant	Severe injuries likely leading to death	Massive head trauma Spinal cord injuries

Developed from Military Standard Operating Procedure (SOP) for General Hospitals.

Principles of first aid, developed for emergency medicine, are part of the triage process and include what are referred to as the golden rules of emergency care. The first of these rules cautions the health care worker to assess the physical environment for self-protection. That is, safety at the scene must be established before rescue is attempted (Figure 47-1). The next rule is to remove the client from danger, such as that presented by passing vehicles. These first two rules typically apply to emergencies occurring outside of an institutional setting.

Once the safety at the scene and of the client have been established, assessment turns to the ABCs—*a*irway, *b*reathing, and *c*irculation. When these functions have been stabilized, the client should be assessed for shock. Eye and skin injuries should be evaluated next. The last thing to do is to call for help.

Disaster Triage

Disaster triage systems represent a second approach to emergency care. These systems are utilized in the event of a community disaster, either natural or man-made, such as a train accident, tornado, hurricane, or terrorism. Given the possibility of large numbers of casualties as a result of disasters, a different approach to triaging from that of the hospital system is utilized (Table 47-2).

Most communities have disaster/mass casualty committees. These committees include all hospitals, the emergency medical services (EMS) system, and citizens needed to alert the community of an impending or real disaster.

Emergency Medical Services

Before admission to the ED, the client may have been cared for by an **emergency medical technician** (EMT) or **paramedic** in the EMS (Figure 47-2). An EMT is a health care professional trained to provide basic lifesaving measures before arrival at the hospital. A paramedic is a more specialized health care professional trained to provide advanced life support to the client requiring emergency interventions. Both are part of the EMS and are essential to prehospital care of the emergency client.

SHOCK

Shock is a condition of profound hemodynamic and metabolic disturbance characterized by inadequate tissue perfusion (the body's inability to meet tissue demand for oxygen) (Table 47-3). Shock can result from trauma, injury, or insult. Recognizing and immediately treating shock are critical to the client's survival. There are four major types of shock: hypovolemic shock, cardiogenic shock, distributive shock, and obstructive shock (Chavez & Brewer, 2002).

Figure 47-1 *Establishing the safety of the scene is the first priority in emergency care, as in this scene of a motor vehicle accident, where rescue workers may be in danger from oncoming vehicles. (Courtesy of David J. Reimer, Sr.)*

Figure 47-2 *Emergency medical technicians (EMTs) and paramedics are often the first to arrive at an emergency scene.*

Hypovolemic shock is usually easily recognized. It results from severe fluid volume depletion through vomiting, dehydration, diarrhea, or blood loss. Severe external bleeding may be obvious, but internal bleeding, such as that from a gastric ulcer, is not readily observable.

Cardiogenic shock may be caused by several different heart conditions that result in loss of the contractile property of the heart muscle. The most common of these is acute myocardial infarction (heart attack). Severe heart failure and certain arrhythmias may also cause shock.

There are three types of distributive shock: septic, anaphylatic, and neurogenic. In all of these, shock results from vasodilation and an abnormal fluid distribution within the circulatory system.

Septic shock is usually caused by overwhelming infection. Certain organisms may cause severe reactions resulting in collapse of the circulatory system. Toxic shock syndrome, gram-negative shock, and urogenic shock are types of septic shock.

Anaphylactic shock is a severe allergic reaction to a toxin to which a client has been exposed. Causes of anaphylactic reaction include insect bites and certain medications.

Neurogenic shock is the body's response to extreme pain or trauma to the spinal cord. As with the other forms of shock, it results in inadequate supply of oxygen, electrolytes, and other essential chemicals to the tissues.

Obstructive shock is the result of indirect pump failure that leads to decreased cardiac function and reduced circulation. Conditions causing obstructive shock include pulmonary embolism, pulmonary hypertension, arterial stenosis, and cardiac tamponade.

In all types of shock, diminished blood flow causes the signs and symptoms. There is usually no clinical evidence of shock in the *early stage*. There may be an increase in heart rate (above client's baseline), restlessness, and the client may have a sense of impending doom. In the *compensatory stage*, respirations and heart rate increase; pulses may be weak; urinary output decreases; skin is cold and clammy, mottled, and pale; pupils dilate; bowel sounds are hypoactive, and there is hyperglycemia. Interventions at this stage reduce the possibility of permanent damage. If shock advances to the *progressive stage*, the client's condition noticeably deteriorates. The pulse may be too rapid to count, blood pressure falls

TABLE 47-3	**TYPES OF SHOCK**		
TYPE	**CAUSES**	**SIGNS AND SYMPTOMS**	**TREATMENT**
Hypovolemic	Hemorrhage,* burns	Increased heart rate; hypotension, cold, clammy skin; profound thirst	Replace fluids
Cardiogenic	Myocardial infarction*	Increased heart rate; hypotension; cold, clammy skin	Initiate drug therapy for myocardial infarction; replace fluids; consider possible emergency coronary bypass surgery
Septic	Overwhelming infection	Hot, dry, flushed skin; hypotension; increased heart rate	Locate source of infection and treat with broad-spectrum antibiotic; replace fluids
Anaphylactic	Medications,* insect bites or stings, foods	Throat edema in conjunction with increasing difficulty breathing; hypotension; increased heart rate	Manage ABCs; administer epinephrine (Adrenalin); administer diphenhydramine hydrochloride (Benadryl)
Neurogenic	Spinal cord injury, head trauma	Slowed heart rate; hypotension	Replace fluids, administer drugs to increase blood pressure and heart rate
Obstructive	Arterial stenosis, pulmonary embolism, pulmonary hypertension, cardiac tamponade	Increased heart rate, dyspnea	Treat underlying cause

*Most common cause

below 80 mm Hg, peripheral pulses disappear, there is metabolic acidosis, peripheral edema, pulmonary crackles and wheezes are heard, and the client may be unresponsive. In the *refractory stage*, there is too much cell death and tissue damage from inadequate oxygenation. The client does not respond to treatment. Multiple organ failure occurs, which generally results in death.

Medical–Surgical Management

Medical

Management of shock is supportive in nature during initial resuscitation. The immediate priority is maintenance of the ABCs. Active bleeding should then be stopped. Blood may be administered in the event of major blood loss. After the client is stabilized, the underlying cause of shock must be identified and treated.

Pharmacological

Initial treatment involves the administration of oxygen and the insertion of two large-bore intravenous (IV) lines. Intravenous lines must be instituted to establish lifelines through which lifesaving drugs and fluids may be administered. Fluid resuscitation and oxygen delivery are critical to management of the client in shock. Medications, including epinephrine, may be administered to improve circulation.

Nursing Management

The focus is to identify the type of shock and initiate interventions as soon as possible. For hypovolemic shock, the treatment goal is to restore volume. Administer IV solutions such as Ringer's lactate or normal saline, or packed red blood cells, serum albumin, plasma, or dextran as ordered. Excessive fluids dilute clotting factors and worsen bleeding.

For cardiogenic shock, treatment focuses on improving myocardial function. Medications for hypotension are frequently ordered. Provide oxygen. Monitor the client's respiratory and cardiac status.

Septic shock is the most common type of distributive shock. Administer IV antibiotics and fluids as ordered. Monitor vital signs.

Clients in neurogenic shock generally have hypotension, bradycardia, hypothermia, and dry warm skin. Administer medications as ordered for hypotension and bradycardia. Monitor vital signs. Provide warmth.

For clients in anaphylactic shock, talk with family (or client if able) to identify the cause. After assessing ABCs, administer IV fluids, epinephrine, and antihistamines as ordered. Monitor vital signs.

Obstructive shock is managed by identifying the source of the obstruction and treating it. Administer fluids cautiously. Seldom are diuretics used.

NURSING PROCESS

Assessment

Subjective Data

Determine whether the client is responsive and able to respond to questions, or is unconscious. When the client is alert and stabilized, assessment includes obtaining a history of the events leading to the injury or illness, including any food consumed or medication taken and any unusual event (such as a bee sting) that precipitated the shock state. Ask the client to describe any pain with regard to intensity, location, and duration.

Objective Data

Immediate assessment involves evaluating the ABCs. Take vital signs, because many clients in shock will present with hypotension, tachycardia, tachypnea, and pale, diaphoretic, clammy skin.

Nursing diagnoses for a client in shock may include the following:

Nursing Diagnoses	Planning/Goals	Nursing Interventions
Risk for Deficient Fluid Volume related to acute blood loss/vomiting/diarrhea	The client will maintain adequate fluid balance.	Initiate and maintain fluid replacement with two large-bore IV access lines. Administer blood as ordered.
Ineffective Tissue Perfusion related to decreased oxygen-carrying hemoglobin secondary to blood loss and fluid depletion	The client will maintain adequate tissue perfusion as manifested by stable vital signs.	Assess vital signs at least every 30 minutes. Administer oxygen per physician order.
Anticipatory Grieving related to grave nature of illness/injury	The client will cope with illness/injury by cooperating with care provided by health care workers and will discuss outcomes with nurse and family.	Communicate with client and family. Explain all interventions as they occur, to decrease acute anxiety. Allow client and family to express their fears and worries about the situation. Answer questions about care.

Evaluation Each goal must be evaluated to determine how it has been met by the client.

CARDIOPULMONARY EMERGENCIES

Cardiopulmonary emergencies are those emergencies that jeopardize the function of the heart and lungs. These emergencies can result from trauma or illness. Cardiopulmonary emergencies such as drowning, foreign body obstruction of the airway, chest trauma, and chest pain are grouped together, because the effects, medical management, and nursing priorities are similar.

Near-drowning episodes occur most frequently in the summer. Many clients will suffer other related injuries associated with drowning, such as head and spinal cord injuries (Table 47-4).

Foreign body obstruction of the airway most commonly occurs in the larger, right main bronchus. The most common source of airway obstruction is the tongue. Other sources of airway obstruction include hot dogs, candy, steak, and coins (especially in children).

Penetrating or blunt trauma to the chest can cause multiple injuries. Penetrating injuries are insults that puncture the chest, such as gunshot or knife wounds. Blunt trauma is more likely caused by falls or by forceful contact with a blunt object, such as a baseball bat or steering wheel. Injuries associated with pneumothorax include cardiac tamponade, fractured ribs, fractured sternum, and flail chest.

One of the most common complaints evaluated in the ED is chest pain. Those clients presenting with the symptom of chest pain must be clearly and carefully evaluated. Chest pain has a multitude of potential causes and can be frightening to the client until the cause is confirmed.

Medical–Surgical Management

Medical

Management of all cardiopulmonary emergencies is directed at maintaining the ABCs. If indicated, intubation is part of resuscitation in cardiopulmonary emergencies. Establishment of an IV line is essential for medical management, because the line provides access for administration of lifesaving medications.

After resuscitation has been achieved, other treatment modalities must be instituted. Obtain chest x-rays, electrocardiograms (EKGs), and blood tests. Initiate pain control. Morphine sulfate is the drug of choice for clients with these types of emergencies, because morphine decreases both pain and anxiety in the client, which, in turn, leads to improved breathing.

Pharmacological

With the near-drowning client, mannitol (Osmitrol) and furosemide (Lasix) are occasionally indicated in the event of fluid overload. Pain medication is essential for the client with chest injury, because hypoventilation may occur as a result of the pain associated with deep breathing. Pain control is also essential for the client experiencing chest pain. Pain medications can vary from sublingual nitroglycerine to IV morphine sulfate.

Activity

Most clients with cardiopulmonary emergencies are initially confined to bed and must be frequently rolled from side to side. Encourage deep breathing and coughing to prevent stasis of fluid and development of pneumonia.

Nursing Management

Initiate CPR if indicated. Remain with the client to reduce anxiety. Administer pain medication as ordered. Suction as necessary to keep airway patent. Monitor vital signs and lung sounds. Encourage turning and deep breathing.

NURSING PROCESS

Assessment

Subjective Data

Evaluate for restlessness, an early sign of hypoxia. Note pain description. Other areas to include in assessment are fatigue, anxiety, and level of consciousness. Ability to give a brief history of events before the cardiopulmonary emergency should be evaluated.

TABLE 47-4	FRESH-WATER VERSUS SALT-WATER NEAR-DROWNING		
TYPE	**CLIENT SYMPTOMS**	**PATHOPHYSIOLOGY**	**SIGNS**
Fresh-water	Fatigue, anxiety, difficulty breathing, fear	Water in lungs causes changes in surfactant, which in turn causes alveolar collapse.	Hypoxia, collapsed alveoli
Salt-water	Fatigue, anxiety, difficulty breathing, fear, rales, rhonchi	Hypertonic salt water pulls fluid into the alveoli.	Hypoxia, pulmonary edema

Objective Data

Immediately assess airway and breathing. Note any cough, stridor, cyanosis, or inability to talk. Initial vital signs are essential for a baseline.

Nursing diagnoses for a client with a cardiopulmonary emergency may include the following:

Nursing Diagnoses	Planning/Goals	Nursing Interventions
Ineffective Breathing Pattern related to injury to the chest and inability to fully expand the lungs	Client will regain spontaneous respiration within normal rate and pattern.	Initiate CPR, if indicated. Administer pain medications as ordered to ease the work of breathing. Note response to pain medications. Remain with the client during episodes of respiratory distress, because being left alone at these times escalates both the anxiety and breathing problems. Explain all procedures.
Ineffective Airway Clearance related to accumulation of fluid and blood in the airway and to the client's inability to cough	Client's lungs will be clear bilaterally to auscultation.	Maintain airway and breathing with suctioning, if secretions accumulate. Turn client frequently to mobilize secretions. Encourage deep breathing and coughing. Listen to lungs hourly or more frequently to evaluate secretions and suctioning.

Evaluation Each goal must be evaluated to determine how it has been met by the client.

NEUROLOGICAL/ NEUROSURGICAL EMERGENCIES

Head injuries are the most common type of neurological trauma. Spinal cord trauma can also occur as a result of injuries sustained in a head injury. Head trauma most often results from motor vehicle collisions (MVCs) (Figure 47-3). Head injuries vary from very minor contusions to major head trauma.

Clients experiencing a cerebrovascular accident, or stroke, must be immediately admitted to the health care system for prompt evaluation and care. Strokes are now considered "brain attacks" requiring the same initial consideration given to myocardial infarctions, or "heart attacks."

Figure 47-3 *Motor vehicle collisions are the most common cause of head trauma. (Courtesy of David J. Reimer, Sr.)*

Medical–Surgical Management
Medical

As with all trauma, management is aimed at maintaining the ABCs. In addition, if head, neck, or spinal cord trauma is suspected, the client should be placed on a backboard, with the head and neck immobilized. Blood alcohol level should be determined. Intravenous access should be initiated early in the resuscitation phase. Radiological examination is necessary to determine the extent of damage. If the client does not have spontaneous respirations, the injury has probably occurred at C-4 or above, meaning that the client will not be able to independently maintain respirations. The client should be continuously monitored for increased intracranial pressure. Early signs of increased intracranial pressure include a headache; later signs include widened pulse pressure, dilated pupils, and spontaneous emesis without warning. Hiccups are an ominous sign and thus should be reported immediately. Utilization of the **Glasgow Coma Scale,** a neurological screening test that measures a client's best verbal, motor, and eye response to stimuli, is indicated (Figure 47-4).

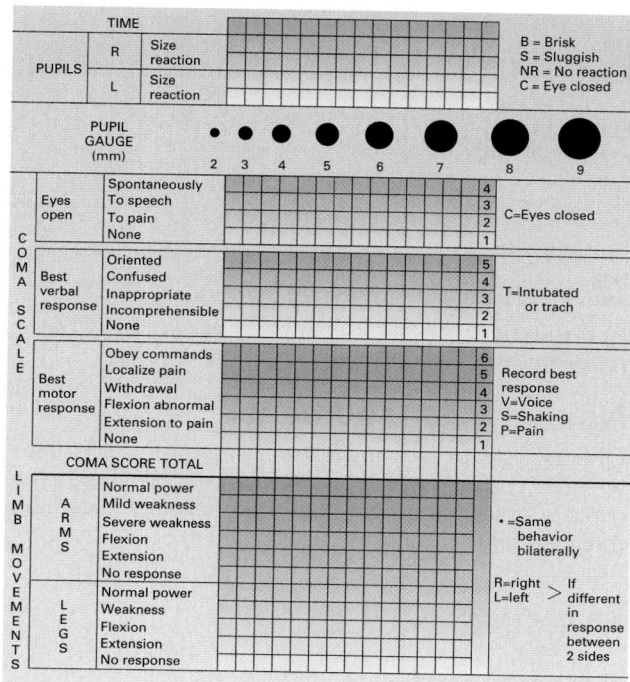

Figure 47-4 *Neurological Flow Sheet, Including Glasgow Coma Scale*

Pharmacological

Increased cranial pressure and buildup of carbon dioxide will complicate the client's condition; oxygen will most often alleviate the resultant complications. Thus, administer oxygen immediately. Pain management is accomplished through IV access.

Activity

Clients with head injuries should be placed in semi-Fowler's position to decrease edema and intracranial pressure.

CRITICAL THINKING

Motor Vehicle Crash

You come upon an MVC involving several vehicles and no emergency response vehicles have yet arrived. What steps can you take to secure the accident site and aid the victims until emergency services arrive?

Nursing Management

Immediately administer oxygen as ordered. Monitor vital signs. Assess Glasgow Coma Scale score. Maintain in semi-Fowler's position or as ordered. Orient to date and time as needed.

NURSING PROCESS

Assessment

Subjective Data

Obtain a history of the accident and the mechanism of injury. Evaluate the client's perception of what happened and the client's emotional response. The client may describe having a headache and difficulty seeing.

Objective Data

Assess the client's vital signs and Glasgow Coma Scale level. Note cerebrospinal fluid leaks, such as clear fluid coming from the nares or ear. Document unequal pupillary response, trouble making self understood, or difficulty swallowing.

Nursing diagnoses for the client with a neurological/neurosurgical emergency may include the following:

Nursing Diagnoses	Planning/Goals	Nursing Interventions
Excess Fluid Volume (Cerebral) related to accumulation of fluid/blood in cranium	The client will remain conscious, maintain a Glasgow Coma Scale score of 15, and experience no further increase in cranial fluid volume.	Monitor intracranial pressure. Maintain the client in semi-Fowler's position. Document vital signs hourly. Assess Glasgow Coma Scale level and record hourly. Administer oxygen.
Impaired Verbal Communication related to injury to speech center	The client will be able to communicate with the nurse and family.	Orient the client frequently to date and time. Explain all nursing interventions. Modify communication methods, such as use of a message board, depending on the client needs. Encourage client to verbalize feelings about condition; offer support.

Evaluation Each goal must be evaluated to determine how it has been met by the client.

ABDOMINAL EMERGENCIES

Abdominal emergencies can be diverse in nature. Trauma to the upper body and torso can result in multiple abdominal injuries, from a simple contusion and bruising to a ruptured spleen. Clients presenting to the ED with complaints of abdominal pain require careful evaluation. Illnesses causing abdominal pain range from gastroenteritis to gastrointestinal bleeding.

Abdominal injuries can result from blunt or penetrating trauma. It is important to determine the mechanism of injury, because certain causes, such as MVCs, often result in multisystem trauma. Blunt trauma, for instance from falling on the abdomen, usually results in injury to internal organs, such as the kidneys or spleen. Penetrating injuries such as gunshot wounds can affect any internal organ. Hemorrhage is a potential complication of both types of trauma.

Medical–Surgical Management

Medical

Initial management of abdominal emergencies is IV access with large-bore catheters. Oxygen should be administered immediately, and standard protocol calls for managing the ABCs. Blood products or plasma expanders may be administered in the event of large-volume blood loss. Insertion of a nasogastric tube decompresses the stomach. A peritoneal lavage may be performed to check for blood in the abdominal cavity of clients with abdominal trauma. Presence of blood indicates a need for immediate surgical intervention. A computed tomography (CT) scan of the abdomen may be indicated as well. Blood work should be drawn, and a urinalysis should be done. Hematuria must be evaluated, and x-rays may be indicated.

> **PROFESSIONAL TIP**
>
> **Open Abdominal Wound**
> If loops of intestines are exposed to outside air, cover with sterile saline-soaked gauze.

Pharmacological

If the client is in severe pain and has been evaluated, narcotics may be indicated.

Nursing Management

Administer oxygen and follow agency protocol for managing ABCs. Initiate IV access. Administer analgesics as ordered. Monitor vital signs, bowel sounds, and abdominal girth. Administer medications and ambulate as allowed.

NURSING PROCESS

Assessment

Subjective Data

Ask about the location, duration, severity, and radiation of pain. Obtain history of nausea, vomiting, and diarrhea. Note the times of the client's last meal, bowel movement, and urination.

Objective Data

Assess vital signs, active bleeding, abdominal girth, and weight. Inspect the abdomen for bruises, edema, and wounds.

Nursing diagnoses for the client with an abdominal emergency may include the following:

Nursing Diagnoses	Planning/Goals	Nursing Interventions
Deficient Fluid Volume related to active bleeding	The client will stabilize, and vital signs and fluid balance will return to normal.	Establish IV access with at least two large-bore catheters. Monitor vital signs frequently, at least hourly. Evaluate abdominal girth and bowel sounds hourly.
Risk for Infection related to penetrating injury	The client will not experience an elevated temperature or show signs and symptoms of infection.	Administer antibiotics as ordered to reduce the risk of infection. Monitor temperature at least every 2 hours. Change saturated dressings as needed. Note amount and quality of any drainage.
Activity Intolerance related to pain and bleeding	The client will ambulate with assistance 1 day after surgical correction.	Turn client hourly from side to side. Assist client to ambulate when able to prevent stasis of fluid and to diminish the risk of infection.

Evaluation Each goal must be evaluated to determine how it has been met by the client.

GENITOURINARY EMERGENCIES

Rape is a legal term and is not considered a medical condition. It is defined as sexual penetration of a forceful and threatening nature with a nonconsenting person. Included under this legal term is penetration of persons who are unable to consent because of intoxication or mental illness. *Alleged sexual assault* is the terminology used by most centers for rape survivors. Because of the many legal implications and the fact that there are not only physical symptoms, but also long-lasting psychological consequences of sexual assault, accurate and methodical care must be given to the survivors of sexual assault. Most communities have hospitals designated to care for rape survivors. These facilities are staffed with registered nurses and doctors familiar with the medical, psychological, and legal issues particular to caring for the client who has experienced a sexual assault.

Straddle injuries are another type of genitourinary emergency. These injuries occur when a client falls while straddling an object, such as a fence or metal bar, thereby injuring the perineum. Though not a very common injury, it is imperative to assess the client and promptly initiate treatment. These injuries can occur with multiple trauma or as a single injury.

Medical–Surgical Management

Medical

As with all emergencies, the ABCs must be managed first. Intravenous access should be established, and blood and urine specimens should be obtained. Rape crisis intervention is essential for the sexual assault victim. Those with straddle injuries must be evaluated for fractures. If blood is seen at the external urethral meatus, a urethral tear should be suspected, and catheterization should be avoided because it will further damage the urethra. Radiological examination should be done to confirm injury.

Surgical

Certain injuries such as urethral or vaginal tears may require surgical repair.

Pharmacological

Douching and bathing for the sexual assault survivor should be delayed until all specimens are collected and all examinations are performed. For the sexual assault client, antibiotics are usually prescribed for possible sexually transmitted disease. Blood tests for baseline human immunodeficiency virus (HIV) and acquired immunodeficiency syndrome (AIDS) and a pregnancy test are usually part of the protocol. In addition, a "morning after" pill such as diethylstilbestrol diphosphate (DES) may be prescribed in the event of a possible pregnancy.

PROFESSIONAL TIP

Chain of Custody

Care should be taken in handling the clothing and belongings of a survivor of sexual assault, as these items may become valuable in legal proceedings. For purposes of potential future litigation, it is thus imperative to maintain a strict chain of custody of evidence. The **chain of custody** is the documentation of the transfer of evidence from one worker to the next in a secure fashion. This means that to follow the rape protocol, each person handling the client's clothing or lab work must sign the document used by the facility to indicate receipt and release of items. The fewer the names on the chain, the more secure the integrity of evidence.

Diet

The client should be designated nothing by mouth (NPO) in case of the need to go to immediate surgery. Fluids can be given intravenously.

Activity

The sexual assault survivor may return to full activity as soon as able, although counseling may be needed before the client regains the desire to resume activities of daily living. Those with straddle injuries need bed rest and careful observation until testing is complete. Clients should be encouraged to resume sexual activities only when they feel physically and emotionally ready.

Nursing Management

Manage the ABCs and establish IV access. Obtain blood and urine specimens. Monitor output and test urine for blood. Make a list of the client's clothing worn during the assault and keep the clothing for evidence in case of legal proceedings. Instruct client to delay bathing or douching until all examinations are completed and all specimens are collected.

NURSING PROCESS

Assessment

Subjective Data

Obtain a description of the rape or assault. A history of menstrual cycles, including date of last menstrual period, is vital in determining the potential for pregnancy.

Objective Data

Assess all bruises, scrapes, or abrasions caused by the assault. Make a list of the client's clothing worn during the assault, and keep the clothing for evidence in case of legal proceedings.

Nursing diagnoses for the client with genitourinary emergencies may include the following:

Nursing Diagnoses	Planning/Goals	Nursing Interventions
Impaired Urinary Elimination related to break in urethra	Client will void clear urine before discharge and will regain normal pre-injury elimination patterns.	Closely monitor output. Test urine for blood using dipstick. Note and report hematuria. Offer bladder retraining and encourage client to resume pre-assault elimination patterns.
Risk for Infection (Sexually Transmitted Disease) related to alleged sexual assault	Client will have negative outcomes on all lab specimens obtained.	Obtain all specimens as ordered. Teach the client how and when to obtain further specimens, as needed. Keep the client informed about all test results.
Rape-Trauma Syndrome related to alleged sexual assault and violence of event	Client will state awareness of help groups for therapy and follow-up care.	Maintain open and nonjudgmental communication with the client. Call rape crisis center for immediate referral and assistance for the client. Refer the client to crisis help per community offerings. Teach the client that the trauma does not resolve overnight and that help is available at all times.

Evaluation Each goal must be evaluated to determine how it has been met by the client.

OCULAR EMERGENCIES

Most eye emergencies are urgent to emergent in nature. Foreign bodies can cause damage to vision very rapidly and thus require immediate attention. Clients with objects impaled in the eye must be immediately evaluated by an ophthalmologist. An eyeball may be avulsed, or forcibly torn out of its socket, either by blunt or penetrating trauma; such an injury requires immediate referral to and treatment by an ophthalmologist. Retinal detachment is a surgical emergency, as it is one of the leading causes of accidental blindness.

Medical–Surgical Management
Medical

The primary goal of care is restoring the health of the eye. The foreign body or impaled object must be removed as soon as the client's condition allows and the effects on the eye of removal of the object have been determined. The client's eye must be protected until definitive treatment is provided. Protective dressings are needed. In the event of ocular avulsion, the eyeball must be protected with a warm saline dressing. Because both eyes move together, patching of the opposite eye will help decrease movement of the affected eye, allowing it to heal more quickly.

Surgical

Immediate surgical intervention is needed for retinal detachment.

Pharmacological

As a prophylactic measure, all eye trauma must be treated with an antibiotic eye medication.

Diet

There should be no modifications to the diet of the client with a foreign body in the eye. Clients with avulsed eyes must be kept NPO in case immediate surgical intervention is needed.

Activity

Because sensory and depth perceptions may be altered when one eye is patched, activity should be limited initially. Clients are maintained in semi-Fowler's position to prevent or alleviate intraocular edema.

Nursing Management

Maintain the client in semi-Fowler's position. Instill eye medications and apply an eye patch (sometimes both eyes are patched to decrease eye movement). Assist the client to ambulate while wearing an eye patch.

NURSING PROCESS

Assessment

Subjective Data

Obtain both the client's perception of what has happened to the eye and a history of the accident, including the time it occurred. Document care given to an avulsed eye, such as placement in a plastic bag with water.

Objective Data

Assessment includes visual acuity testing and observation of tearing and/or redness of the eye.

Nursing diagnoses for the client with an ocular emergency may include the following:

Nursing Diagnoses	Planning/Goals	Nursing Interventions
Disturbed Sensory Perception (Visual) related to impaired vision	The client will regain partial pre-injury vision.	Maintain the client in semi-Fowler's position in cases of ocular avulsion or retinal detachment.
		Assist the client to walk while wearing an eye patch and discuss problems that may be encountered and ways to accommodate decreased vision.
		Ask the client to name one resource person to assist with decreased vision at home.
Risk for Infection related to trauma caused by foreign body	The client will not develop ocular infection.	Instill initial eye medication and apply initial eye patch for the client.
		Teach the client to instill eye medication and apply eye patch.
		Instruct the client to immediately report any visual changes or drainage.
		Be alert and listen to the client's concerns.

Evaluation Each goal must be evaluated to determine how it has been met by the client.

MUSCULOSKELETAL EMERGENCIES

Musculoskeletal emergencies can vary from simple muscle strains to major trauma. A muscle strain is the overstretching of a muscle. A sprain is defined as a twisting of the joint with partial rupture of ligaments, which can cause injury to surrounding tissue. Sprains often occur in the wrist and ankle. A dislocation is the displacement of a bone from its joint. The most common sites of dislocation are the fingers and toes. A fracture is a break in the continuity of a bone. In the event of a long-bone fracture, care must also be given to the cardiopulmonary system: Fat emboli from the fracture site can develop and cause severe respiratory problems if they settle in the pulmonary system.

Medical–Surgical Management

Medical

Initial treatment of simple strains and sprains can be managed utilizing the "RICE" formula, meaning *r*est, *i*ce, *c*ompression, and *e*levation. Fractures must be immediately immobilized, with attention also being given to body areas proximal to the fracture. Radiological examination is indicated to validate the diagnosis. Dislocations must be immediately reduced. Many fractures and dislo-cations can be reduced in the ED using procedural sedation. Tetanus toxoid should be given to any client with an open injury.

Surgical

Some fractures require immediate surgical intervention. Most open, compound fractures fall into this category. Debridement is often indicated, because most fractures are trauma related, and dirt and other matter may imbed in the wound.

Pharmacological

Pain control is a major consideration in relation to musculoskeletal system injuries. Reduction and immobilization often significantly decrease pain. Those clients with minor sprains and strains respond well to anti-inflammatory medications such as ibuprofen (Advil, Motrin) and other nonsteroidal anti-inflammatory drugs (NSAIDs). Those with major or multiple fractures may initially require narcotic relief.

Diet

Clients with sprains, strains, and simple fractures do not need special diets. Those with major fractures and trauma must be kept NPO pending surgical intervention.

Activity

Depending on the site of the fracture, activity may be limited because of casting or immobilization. To help strengthen the muscles and minimize atrophy in cases of immobilization, teach the client to contract and release those muscles immobilized in the casting.

Nursing Management

Immobilize the affected part. Administer analgesic as ordered. Elevate the injured area. Apply ice packs, as ordered. Assess pulse, skin color, capillary refill, ability to move fingers or toes, and sensation in the injured area.

NURSING PROCESS

Assessment

Subjective Data

The client will initially verbalize intense pain, tingling, and loss of use of the injured part.

Objective Data

Obvious deformities, edema, cool skin, and decreased capillary refill will be present on the affected part. Note breaks in the skin and visual bone fragments.

Nursing diagnoses for the client with a musculoskeletal emergency may include the following:

Nursing Diagnoses	Planning/Goals	Nursing Interventions
Acute Pain related to traumatic fracture/ dislocation	The client's pain will decrease with immobilization and pain medications.	Administer pain medications as ordered. Immobilize affected body part. Elevate injured extremity. Apply ice packs, as directed. Listen attentively to the client's concerns and verbalizations of pain.
Ineffective Tissue Perfusion related to edema and fracture/ dislocation	The client's pulses will be equal bilaterally, and capillary refill will be less than 2 seconds at the affected site.	Assess the client's pulse, skin color, capillary refill, and ability to move the fingers and toes every 30 minutes. Ask the client about sensation in the injured body part. Instruct the client to move the toes and fingers. Apply an elastic bandage for compression in cases of a sprain.
Impaired Physical Mobility related to limitations of pain and immobilization of fracture/dislocation	The client will demonstrate the ability to mobilize with cast or other assistive devices.	Teach the client to care for the cast. Teach the client exercises to minimize muscle atrophy and crutch walking, if needed.

Evaluation Each goal must be evaluated to determine how it has been met by the client.

SOFT-TISSUE EMERGENCIES

Most soft-tissue injuries are very common. Minor abrasions, lacerations, puncture wounds, contusions, bites of all varieties (human, insect, animal, and snake), and burn injuries fall into this category. Although most such injuries do not require emergency care, some are more severe than others and some are potentially fatal. Clients will seek medical attention for these injuries because of fear.

Medical–Surgical Management

Medical

Skin emergencies require prompt intervention. All injuries must be cleansed or debrided. Infection is a major consideration, and prophylactic treatment must therefore be initiated immediately. If a laceration is large, suturing may be necessary. Bites, unless extremely large, are usually not sutured because of the increased risk of infection presented by suturing these lacerations, which provide an excellent growth medium for bacteria. Burns can sometimes be treated in an ED, with follow-up care being provided at home. Cool water will decrease the pain associated with minor burns. Careful debridement using running cool water and antiseptic solution should follow. Because burns are painful, debridement should be performed after administration of pain medication. A silver sulfadiazine (Silvadene) dressing is usually applied after debridement.

Major burns may require client resuscitation with rapid EMS transport to a burn center. Initially, the ABCs must be established. "Packaging" the client for transport to a burn unit usually involves insertion of at least two large-bore IV lines, insertion of a nasogastric tube, intubation, Foley catheterization, sterile wrapping, and temperature regulation/monitoring.

Snakebites do not always result in envenomation (poisoning). A rubber band (not a tourniquet) above the site is the best intervention to control rapid spreading of the venom. Most snakebites occur in the foot, so a rubber band is easy to apply. In managing snakebites, it is best to establish the ABCs and, once the type of snake is identified, start antivenom treatment, as necessary.

Pharmacological

All clients with soft-tissue injuries, including those with burns, must be current with regard to immunizations, especially the diphtheria and tetanus (Td) immunizations. Pain medication should be given to alleviate pain related to lacerations, bites, and burns. Topical antibiotic agents must be applied to all injuries. Silver sulfadiazine (Silvadene) is the most widely used topical agent for burn injuries. Systemic antibiotics are often included in the treatment regimen.

Activity

Movement may be somewhat limited depending on the location of injury. Because muscle weakness and atrophy can occur rapidly, physical therapy must be initiated immediately for clients who are immobilized.

Nursing Management

Determine the client's immunization status. Use aseptic technique when cleansing soft-tissue injuries. Administer analgesic, immunization(s), and antibiotic as ordered. Encourage the client to keep the wound and dressing dry and clean, but instruct how to remove and change the dressing when dirty or wet.

NURSING PROCESS

Assessment

Subjective Data

Elicit the client's report of the injury. Evaluate and document the client's level of pain.

Objective Data

Obtain vital signs. Assess the wound or damaged area with regard to depth, location, and size (in centimeters). In the event of a bite, note the location and source of the bite.

Nursing diagnoses for the client with a soft-tissue injury may include the following:

Nursing Diagnoses	Planning/Goals	Nursing Interventions
Impaired Skin Integrity related to break/wound in skin	The client's wound will heal.	Prepare client for cleansing and possible suturing of wound.
		Assist with possible suturing.
Risk for Infection related to imbedded dirt/bacteria in the wound	The client's wound will heal without evidence of infection.	Cleanse wound thoroughly with soap and water.
		Administer tetanus intramuscularly (IM), if ordered.
		Teach the client to keep the wound and sutures dry and clean.
		Apply a topical antibiotic and clean dressing, if indicated.
		Teach the client to remove and change the dressing if it becomes dirty or wet.
		Tell the client to return for additional care if wound becomes red, edematous, or painful or exhibits purulent discharge.

Evaluation Each goal must be evaluated to determine how it has been met by the client.

SAMPLE NURSING CARE PLAN

THE CLIENT WITH A SOFT-TISSUE INJURY

Mr. Perez, a 23-year-old Hispanic rancher, was brought to the ED after an accident at his ranch. He was riding his horse and fixing fences. The horse threw Mr. Perez over its head and stomped Mr. Perez's left upper abdomen with its right forefoot. Mr. Perez, who states that he has never been hurt or in the hospital before, presents with a large, 6-centimeter-by-3-centimeter-by-2-centimeter in depth, jagged laceration imbedded with dirt and other foreign material. There are no other associated injuries. A large pressure bandage that is saturated with bright-red blood is controlling the bleeding.

Nursing Diagnosis 1 *Deficient Fluid Volume* related to active bleeding from traumatic abdominal laceration as evidenced by a large, jagged laceration measuring 6 centimeters by 3 centimeters and a large, bulky, saturated dressing.

Nursing Outcomes Classification (NOC)	**Nursing Interventions Classification (NIC)**
Fluid Balance	*Wound Care*
Hydration	*Fluid Monitoring*

PLANNING/GOALS	NURSING INTERVENTIONS	RATIONALE
Mr. Perez will lose no more blood.	Apply clean pressure dressing.	Controls amount of bleeding.
	Prepare Mr. Perez for suturing of the laceration.	Provides Mr. Perez with knowledge of what is to happen.
	Monitor vital signs.	Identifies the client is going into shock from blood loss. Increased pulse and respiration and hypotension require immediate attention and intervention.

EVALUATION   Mr. Perez's wound was sutured. The dressing applied after suturing is clean and dry and showed no further evidence of bleeding at discharge.

Nursing Diagnosis 2 *Impaired Skin Integrity* related to abdominal injury as evidenced by a jagged laceration measuring 6 centimeters by 3 centimeters and 2 centimeters in depth.

Nursing Outcomes Classification (NOC)	**Nursing Interventions Classification (NIC)**
Tissue Integrity: Skin & Mucous Membranes	*Wound Care*
Wound Healing: Primary Intention	*Infection Protection*

PLANNING/GOALS	NURSING INTERVENTIONS	RATIONALE
Mr. Perez will have regained skin integrity with sutures.	Prepare sterile environment for suturing.	Prevents additional bacteria from contaminating the wound.
	Assist physician with suturing of Mr. Perez's wound.	The nurse is responsible for assisting the physician, who is suturing.

EVALUATION   Mr. Perez had intact skin integrity, with 22 sutures in place.

Nursing Diagnosis 3 *Risk for Infection* related to laceration as evidenced by dirt and other foreign material imbedded in abdominal wound.

continues

SAMPLE NURSING CARE PLAN

Nursing Outcomes Classification (NOC)
Treatment Behavior: Illness or Injury
Immune Status

Nursing Interventions Classification (NIC)
Immunization/Vaccination Management
Infection Protection

PLANNING/GOALS	NURSING INTERVENTIONS	RATIONALE
Mr. Perez's wound will not become infected.	Administer tetanus booster.	All wounds require that the client be current with regard to tetanus booster.
	Cleanse Mr. Perez's wound thoroughly after local anesthesia has been administered.	Wound is cleansed with the least discomfort to Mr. Perez.
	Remove as much dirt and foreign material as possible.	Prevents inflammation and infection at the wound site.
	Cleanse sutured wound and demonstrate care to Mr. Perez.	Removes old blood and other debris from the suturing. Teaches Mr. Perez how to cleanse wound at home.
	Give Mr. Perez explicit directions regarding taking oral antibiotics after discharge.	It is imperative that Mr. Perez takes the full course of the antibiotics to prevent infection.
	Teach Mr. Perez to care for wound.	Provides Mr. Perez with knowledge to remove the dressing when it becomes wet or dirty and apply a new and clean dressing.
	Teach Mr. Perez the signs and symptoms that require a return visit to the doctor (redness, inflammation, increased pain, purulent drainage).	Provides Mr. Perez with knowledge to identify if the wound does become infected.

EVALUATION Mr. Perez was given a tetanus booster because he remembered having received his last at the age of 15. He verbalized the need to take the complete course of antibiotics when he went home.

Nursing Diagnosis 4 *Anxiety* related to reaction to fall and large laceration as evidenced by client's verbalizing that he had never been injured before

Nursing Outcomes Classification (NOC)
Coping
Acceptance: Health Status

Nursing Interventions Classification (NIC)
Coping Enhancement
Teaching: Individual

PLANNING/GOALS	NURSING INTERVENTIONS	RATIONALE
Mr. Perez will demonstrate decreased anxiety.	Allow Mr. Perez to talk about injury.	Gives him the opportunity to verbalize his fears and thoughts about the injury.
	Provide explanations for all procedures.	Assists Mr. Perez in understanding why certain things are being done.
	Give Mr. Perez simple choices to make.	Allows him to participate in his care and gives him some sense of control.

EVALUATION Mr. Perez viewed his injury with the use of a mirror before and after suturing. He was amazed to see that the laceration was completely closed following suturing. He was concerned about the bruising and edema to the area. Mr. Perez was not able to assist with the care of his sutures. His wife was taught how to clean and dress the wound.

POISONING AND OVERDOSES

Poisoning and overdoses can be accidental or intentional. Poison control centers are the best source of antidote information for the client suffering from poisoning or overdose.

There are many types of poisonings and overdoses and several different entry routes. Ingested poisonings are most common. It is important to obtain a clear history of the route of entry: inhalation, ingestion, topical, or injection. In addition, the client must be evaluated for any associated injuries, such as lacerations from a fall.

Medical–Surgical Management

Medical

In treating overdoses, the ABCs must be managed. Oxygen must be immediately initiated, and IV access established. In addition, institute cardiac monitoring. Obtain blood and urine samples for toxicology screening. After the client has been stabilized, try to identify the substance to minimize or reverse the effects.

Pharmacological

If the substance has been ingested, and institutional protocol dictates, administer activated charcoal. Give clients who have ingested caustic products copious amounts of water to dilute the substance.

Diet

The client who has overdosed is typically kept NPO.

Nursing Management

Assess ABCs, initiate IV access, and administer oxygen. Begin cardiac monitoring. Obtain blood and urine samples. Keep client NPO. Obtain a history of the entire incident. Maintain a calm, supportive environment.

NURSING PROCESS

Assessment

Subjective Data

Ask about the timing and the route of overdose. Evaluate mental status to establish whether the exposure was intentional. Document other incidences related to an overdose, such as an altercation with a loved one.

Objective Data

The client's vital signs are critical for baseline data. Try to identify the substance involved, as well as the amount.

Nursing diagnoses for the client with an overdose may include the following:

Nursing Diagnoses	Planning/Goals	Nursing Interventions
Risk for Poisoning related to ingestion of toxin	The client will recover with no residual effects of poisoning.	Manage the ABCs and stabilize the client. Monitor baseline laboratory work and ECG. Administer antidotes to toxins. Document the client's response.
Risk for Self-Directed Violence related to harmful ingestion of toxic substance	The client will not harm self and will participate in help groups to work through issues.	Encourage the client to share reasons for overdose. Maintain a supportive, calm, reassuring environment for the client. If overdose was accidental, discuss exposure to toxin and ways to avoid exposure in the future. Teach varying methods of coping. Refer to help groups.
Interrupted Family Processes related to ingestion of harmful toxin	Client will begin to discuss problems with family.	Encourage client and family to discuss their problems openly and supportively and assist them in identifying different methods of coping. Encourage family counseling.

Evaluation Each goal must be evaluated to determine how it has been met by the client.

ENVIRONMENTAL/ TEMPERATURE EMERGENCIES

Exposure to extremes of heat and cold can be potentially life threatening. Severe cold, or hypothermia, can occur both in very cold weather and from prolonged submersion in cold water. Heart rate and metabolic rate fall, and cardiac arrest may follow. Frostbite is another potentially dangerous result of exposure to cold (Table 47-5). The most common sites of frostbite are the fingers, toes, ears, and nose. Initially, frostbite causes paleness and numbness to the affected areas. If exposure continues, frostbite can progress to blistering and loss of feeling. The

TABLE 47-5   DEGREES OF FROSTBITE SEVERITY

DEGREE	SYMPTOMS	TREATMENT
Mild	Skin is cold to touch, pale, tingling, and numb, with a prickly sensation	Use blankets, warm clothing to warm cold flesh
Moderate	Affects deeper body tissue; skin appears waxy and is puffy to touch and itchy and burning with pain	Use gloves, blankets, warm clothing to warm cold flesh, observe closely for deeper injuries
Severe	Blistering, damage to all layers of soft tissue; flesh appears lifeless and is hard to the touch; no pain sensation in or ability to move frozen area	Initiate emergency rewarming in an ED using warm-water baths at 40.6°C (105°F); observe carefully for increased edema

TABLE 47-6   COMPARISON OF HEAT INJURIES

TYPE	SYMPTOMS	TREATMENT
Heat cramps	Muscle cramps in arms, legs, and abdomen	Move client to cool, shady area. Slowly administer copious amounts of water. Reevaluate.
Heat exhaustion	Diaphoresis, with pale, moist, cool skin, headache, weakness, dizziness; muscle cramps, nausea, chills, tachypnea, confusion, tingling of hands and feet	Move client to cool, shady area. Loosen/remove constrictive clothing. Pour water over client; place client near fan. Encourage client to slowly drink water. Elevate client's legs. Reevaluate.
Heat stroke (a medical emergency)	Red, flushed, hot, dry skin; no diaphoresis	Reduce client's body temperature by removing client's clothing and pouring cool water over client. Start two large-bore IV lines. Use fan to cool client. Place client on cardiac monitor. Elevate client's legs. Assess client's vital signs, especially core (rectal) temperature. Check for neurological signs (confused, combative, disoriented). Check client's core (rectal) temperature frequently.

Developed from U.S. Army Training Support Command Protocols.

client may lose voluntary control over the affected body part. Rewarming in an emergency setting is imperative.

Extreme heat can also cause potentially serious problems, especially in very young or elderly clients. As temperature rises, the body's ability to cool lessens. Table 47-6 compares heat injuries.

Medical–Surgical Management
Medical

For those exposed to extreme cold, rewarming is essential to resuscitation. The body's core (rectal) temperature must be taken. Gradual warming must be initiated using warm blankets, warmed oxygen, warmed IV fluids, warmed nasogastric tubes, and, in extreme instances, warmed enemas. Resuscitation should continue until the body has reached a core temperature of at least 34.4°C (94°F).

For frostbite, rewarming of the exposed body part is indicated. If the frostbite is severe, rapid rewarming is essential. This involves placing the frozen area in warm-water baths not exceeding 40.6°C (105°F). Tetanus should be administered. Acute pain should be treated with analgesics.

For heat injuries, rapidly reducing the body's temperature is vital. Supplemental oxygen may be administered. Pouring cool water over the client, chilling IV fluids, and fanning the client will accelerate the cooling process.

PROFESSIONAL TIP

Frostbite

Do not massage or rub frostbite injuries, as doing so can increase severity of damage to tissue. Caffeine, alcohol, and smoking should be avoided because they decrease circulation to the damaged tissue.

Pharmacological

For heat and cold injuries, establishment of at least two large-bore IV lines is essential. Supplemental oxygen should be administered. Replacement of fluid and electrolytes is essential.

Diet

In the event of heat injuries, fluids, especially water, should be encouraged, if the client is able.

Nursing Management

Initiate CPR if needed. Monitor vital signs. Establish IV access. Provide oxygen and administer fluid and electrolytes as ordered. Warm or cool body as indicated. Monitor cardiac response.

NURSING PROCESS

Assessment

Subjective Data

Ask the client to give a history of the heat/cold injury, if able, and any current medications taken.

Objective Data

Measure and document core (rectal) body temperature and vital signs. Record skin color and temperature. Initiate cardiac monitoring to track any cardiac response to the heat or cold stress to the body. Evaluate pupillary response because neurological problems may result from the heat/cold injury.

Nursing diagnoses for the client with a temperature/environmental injury may include the following:

Nursing Diagnoses	Planning/Goals	Nursing Interventions
Hypothermia related to exposure to cold environment/long submersion in cold water	The client will regain normal core body temperature.	Administer supplemental oxygen. Monitor cardiac response carefully. If CPR is in progress, continue until the client's core temperature reaches 94°F and cardiac status is evaluated. Administer warmed IV fluids. Place warmed blankets on the client.
Hyperthermia related to environmental exposure to heat	The client will regain normal core body temperature.	Remove the client's clothing. Pour cool water over the client. Use large fan to cool the client. Administer chilled IV fluids and supplemental oxygen. Initiate cardiac monitoring. Evaluate client's neurological status with reference to orientation to time, person, and place. Measure core temperature every 30 minutes to assess progress.

Evaluation Each goal must be evaluated to determine how it has been met by the client.

MULTIPLE-SYSTEM TRAUMA

Multiple-system trauma is injury sustained in more than one body system. During the initial care of the emergent client, the mechanism of injury is determined. Blunt injuries and penetrating trauma are most likely to result in multiple-system involvement.

Medical–Surgical Management

Medical

Immediate management of the ABCs is imperative. Bleeding must be stopped using pressure. Two to four large-bore IV lines should be started. Remove all clothing for visualization of bleeding and injuries. Obtain blood and urine specimens. Radiographic studies must be done. Tetanus should also be administered.

Nursing Management

Assess and manage ABCs. Establish IV access. Remove the client's clothing for visualization of injuries. Obtain blood and urine specimens. Assess level of consciousness. Monitor vital signs and neurological status.

NURSING PROCESS

Assessment

Subjective Data

Assess for level of consciousness and orientation to time, person, and place. Evaluate verbalizations of pain. Ask the client for an account of the accident.

CRITICAL THINKING

Multiple-System Trauma

Under what circumstances might a client present with multiple-system trauma? How would you proceed with the assessment of such a client? What immediate actions should be taken to maintain the stability of this client?

Objective Data

Airway, breathing, and circulation should be immediately assessed. Assess vital signs and neurological status utilizing the Glasgow Coma Scale. Assess and control active bleeding.

Nursing diagnoses for the client with multiple-system trauma may include the following:

Nursing Diagnoses	Planning/Goals	Nursing Interventions
Impaired Spontaneous Ventilation related to major trauma and severe hypotension	The client will breathe without assistive devices.	Maintain open airway. Initiate rescue breathing. Ventilate per CPR protocol. Assist with insertion of endotracheal tube. Maintain pulse oximetry reading at 94% to 99%. Start multiple large-bore IV lines.
Powerlessness related to the inability to sustain life without emergency interventions	The client will survive emergency and within several hours will be able to indicate simple choices about care.	Explain all nursing/medical interventions to client. Provide emotional and physiological support to client and family as much as possible throughout resuscitation. Allow the client to make simple choices about care.

Evaluation Each goal must be evaluated to determine how it has been met by the client.

TERRORISM

Terrorist acts can appear in many forms; the events of September 11, 2001, is one example. Nuclear, chemical, and biological terrorism are other forms.

NUCLEAR TERRORISM

According to Kilpatrick (2002), the threat of nuclear terrorism is real. One example is the use of a radiation dispersal device (RDD), a so-called dirty bomb, which has nuclear waste in a conventional bomb. Another example is an attack on a domestic nuclear weapon facility. The effects of either example would be severe and widespread.

The source of radiation on contaminated clients is on the body or clothing, or has been ingested, or absorbed through a skin opening. The amount of radiation absorbed determines the effects on the client. Absorbed radiation, now measured by the gray (Gy), is equal to 100 Rads (old measurement) (Kilpatrick, 2002). When less than 0.75 Gy are absorbed, clients are not likely to have any symptoms, clients with 8 Gy would die, and 30 Gy is always fatal. The Occupational Safety and Health Administration (OSHA) requires that hospitals have an emergency plan for treating clients contaminated with radioactive substances. A decontamination area is set up in or near the ED.

The client who absorbs more than 0.75 Gy can develop acute radiation syndrome (ARS). Symptoms of ARS depend on the dose of radiation and include:

- *Hematopoietic.* Deficiency of WBCs and platelets leading to bleeding, anemia, infections, impaired wound healing, and immunodeficiency
- *Gastrointestinal.* Loss of mucosal barrier and cells lining intestines leading to fluid and electrolyte loss, vomiting, diarrhea, loss of normal flora, and sepsis
- *Cerebrovascular/CNS.* Cerebral edema, hyperpyrexia, hypotension, confusion, and disorientation
- *Skin.* Loss of epidermis and possibly dermis

Signs and symptoms in one or more of these areas appear immediately after exposure. This is the *prodromal phase.* In a day or so, all symptoms generally disappear for a few days to a few weeks. This is the *latent phase.* Next is the *illness phase,* in which the signs and symptoms reappear and intensify. After the peak of the illness phase, the client either begins to recover or dies from infection or other complications.

CHEMICAL TERRORISM

Several types of agents can be used in chemical terrorism, including nerve agents, pulmonary agents, cyanide agents, vesicant agents, and incapacitating agents. All clients exposed to chemical agents must be decontaminated.

Nerve Agents

Nerve agents include taubin (GA), sarin (GB), sonan, cyclosarin (GF), and one called VX (Armstrong, 2003; Yergler, 2002; Reilly & Deason, 2003). These are the most toxic of chemical agents and can cause death within minutes. Clinical effects depend on dose and route of exposure, either inhalation, skin contact, or ingestion. Inhalation is the most dangerous. These agents cause acetylcholine to accumulate either by preventing its breakdown or by desensitizing the receptor sites.

Symptoms range from increased saliva production, chest pressure, rhinorrhea, and vomiting to muscle weakness, incontinence, and convulsions. Symptoms may take up to 18 hours to appear with low exposure.

The antidotes are atropine and pralidoxime (2-PAM). Seizures are treated with diazepam (Valium).

Pulmonary Agents

Pulmonary agents include chlorine (CL), phosgene (CG), diphosgene (DP), and chloropicrin (PS). These agents, when inhaled, destroy the alveoli and capillary bed, resulting in pulmonary edema. There may be a 2- to 24-hour latent period before pulmonary edema occurs. The fluid in the lungs leads to hypovolemia and hypotension (Armstrong, 2002; Reilly & Deason, 2003).

Cyanide Agents

Hydrogen cyanide (AC) and cyanogen chloride (CR), which forms cyanide when metabolized, can be either ingested or inhaled. Cyanide prevents the transfer of oxygen from the blood to tissues. A client in severe respiratory distress but not cyanotic probably was exposed to cyanide. It has a pungent odor like bitter almonds or peaches. Death occurs in 5 to 10 minutes when exposed to a high concentration. Amyl nitrite is the antidote (Reilly & Deason, 2003).

Vesicant Agents

Sulfur mustard (HD), lewisite (L), and phosgene oxime (CX) are in the vesicant group. Phosgene oxime causes skin lesions not vesicles, as do the other two. These agents are more lethal than pulmonary agents and cyanide agents because they can remain in the environment for weeks, providing a continuing source of exposure to populations. Sulfur mustard smells like mustard or garlic, lewisite smells like geraniums, and phosgene oxime has a peppery smell.

All three agents affect the skin, eyes, and airway. Sulfur mustard, in large quantities, damages the bone marrow. Lewisite is immediately irritating, causing vesicles that progress to severe tissue necrosis and sloughing. Symptoms from sulfur mustard exposure appear in 4 to 8 hours, but cellular damage begins in 2 minutes (Reilly & Deason, 2003; Armstrong, 2002). Supportive care is primary treatment.

Incapacitating Agents

BZ, a glycolate anticholinergic compound, and Agent 15, a BZ "copy" made by Iraq, impair rather than kill or seriously injure victims (Armstrong, 2002). The effects are understimulation of organs similar to those of high doses of atropine. Hyperthermia, hallucinations, illusions, and erratic behavior are the greatest risks.

The antidote is physostigmine sulfate (Eserine sulfate) or physostigmine salicylate (Antilirium).

BIOTERRORISM

Bioterrorism is deliberate releasing of pathogenic microorganisms such as viruses, bacteria, fungi, or toxins into a community. Many biologic agents are easily made and disseminated and can potentially injure or kill many people. The CDC has categorized these agents into three categories (Persell et al., 2002).

- *Category A* agents are easily disseminated or transmitted, have a high mortality, cause public panic, and require special public health management.
- *Category B* agents usually spread through water and food, have moderate morbidity and low mortality.
- *Category C* agents have not yet been weaponized (put into a form for mass destruction) but cause high morbidity and mortality.

The category A agents are the ones considered most likely to be used in a bioterrorism attack. Included are anthrax, smallpox, plague, botulism, viral hemorrhagic fevers (VHF), and tularemia. Many of these diseases begin with flulike symptoms and are difficult to identify early. Knowledge about these diseases, careful observation for the sudden appearance of a disease or symptoms occurring at an unusual time, and some critical thinking may help identify a bioterrorist attack. An example is if many people suddenly have flu symptoms in the middle of summer (Steinhauer, 2002).

Anthrax

Anthrax is caused by *Bacillus anthracis*. It may manifest as a cutaneous, inhalation, or gastrointestinal disease. Cutaneous anthrax develops when spores enter a break in the skin. A pruritic macule or papule becomes vesicular and then forms a black, depressed scab. It is completely curable with treatment. Inhalation anthrax has an incubation period up to 60 days. Mild flulike symptoms improve for 1 to 2 days and are followed by acute, severe dyspnea; stridor; and cyanosis. Gastrointestinal anthrax is unlikely because aerosolizing anthrax is easier than sabotaging food supplies.

Use Standard Precautions. No isolation is necessary.

Treatment recommendations include ciprofloxacin (Cipro) or doxycycline calcium (Vibramycin, Monodox) given orally for cutaneous anthrax. These two drugs are initially given IV for inhalation anthrax along with one or two other antimicrobials, such as rifamin (Rifadin), vancomycin HCl (Vancocin), imipenem (Primaxin), penicillin, ampicillin, clindomycin HCl (Clocin), or clarithromycin (Biaxin) (Steinhauer, 2002). Later, clients can be given the medications orally.

Smallpox

Smallpox, caused by variola virus, is easily transmitted from person to person by direct contact or inhalation of respiratory droplets. It has an incubation period of 7 to 19 days and is most contagious during the first week. This disease produces lesions in a body area in the same level of development. They progress from macules to vesicles to pustules and then scabs. Smallpox can be transmitted until all scabs fall off. This is unlike chicken pox, which has some lesions at each level of development in a body area at the same time.

Postexposure vaccination may decrease disease severity if given within 3 to 4 days of exposure.

Standard Precautions, as well as isolation, airborne, and contact precautions, must be observed.

Treatment is supportive with adequate hydration. All laundry and wastes must be autoclaved before washing or incinerating (Persell et al., 2002).

Plague

Plague, also called "black death," is caused by *Yersinia pastis.* When it is transmitted from an infected rodent to humans by an infected flea bite, it is called bubonic plague. Transmission from an infected individual to an uninfected individual by inhalation of respiratory droplets is called pneumonic plague. Terrorists would probably aerosolize the bacteria to cause pneumonic plague. Symptoms would be mainly respiratory.

The incubation period for pneumonic plague is 1 to 6 days. Clients must be treated with antibiotics within 24 hours of the first symptoms. Recommended antibiotics are streptomycin IM or gentamicin sulfate (Garamycin). For postexposure prophylaxis, doxycycline calcium (Vibramycin), ciprofloxacin (Cipro), or tetracycline HCl (Sumycin, Tetracyn) may be used.

Standard Precautions including gown, gloves, mask, and eye protection should be used. Droplet precautions should also be followed for the first 48 hours of antibiotic therapy and until clinical improvement occurs.

Botulism

Botulism is caused by a toxin made by *Clostridium botulinum,* which paralyzes muscles. The toxin, one of the most poisonous substances known, is usually food borne. Terrorists would probably aerosolize the toxin for inhalation. The absorbed toxin irreversibly blocks cholinergic synapses, resulting in bilateral descending paralysis. There is no elevation of temperature, and clients retain complete cognitive functioning, although they may appear comatose.

Standard Precautions are used.

Passive immunization with botulinum antitoxin may be used if botulism is recognized early. Care is supportive and may involve intensive care.

Viral Hemorrhagic Fevers

Viral hemorrhagic fevers (VHF) include Ebola, Lassa, Marburg, Crimean-Congo, Argentine, Yellow fever, and Dengue fever. Fever onset is sudden with signs and symptoms of circulatory compromise. All are infectious by aerosol except for Dengue fever. Ebola, Marburg, Lassa, and Crimean-Congo can be spread from person to person, especially during later stages of the disease.

Isolation in a negative-pressure room is recommended. Caregivers should use a personal respirator, gown, gloves, face shield, and shoe and head covers.

Care is supportive. There is no treatment or proven cure.

Tularemia

Tularemia, caused by *Francisella tularensis,* is not nearly as deadly as anthrax or plague. Inhalation of the bacteria is the likely route used in bioterrorist acts. Terrorists are believed to have developed antibiotic-resistant strains, so the number of fatalities could be high (Persell et al., 2002). There are currently no methods of rapid identification.

Standard Precautions should be followed.

For small outbreaks, parenteral therapy with either streptomycin or gentamicin sulfate (Garamycin) is recommended. When there are large outbreaks or for postexposure prophylaxis, oral doxycycline calcium (Vibranycin) or ciprofloxacin (Cipro) are the drugs of choice.

LEGAL ISSUES

Emergency medicine allows medical personnel to care for clients without obtaining informed consent. In life-threatening and emergency situations, consent is implied. In addition, the Good Samaritan Law, one of the laws and regulations enforced for the benefit of both the caregiver and the client, provides protection against malpractice to persons who stop at the scene of an accident and render care. It should be noted, however, that the Good Samaritan Law offers protection only to those who provide safe and appropriate care; it does not protect those charged with gross negligence or willful misconduct.

There are other legal issues specific to emergency care. Several injuries/illnesses must be reported to proper authorities. For instance, most states require that police be notified of MVCs, assaults, or rape. Likewise, animal control authorities require that animal bite reports be filed to facilitate follow-up on the possibility of rabies.

DEATH IN THE EMERGENCY DEPARTMENT

Death can occur in the ED at any time as a result of trauma, sudden illness, or even extended illness. This creates a delicate situation because the death is usually unexpected. Family members may have a difficult time dealing with sudden death. If their loved one is being resuscitated in the ED, there is little time for health care personnel to comfort the family because the personnel are very busy providing care to the client. In the event of sudden death, the family is usually in a state of shock and will need further assistance to cope with the death of their loved one. Special support groups are available for this assistance and should be contacted for the family.

CASE STUDY

Joe fell from a fishing boat into deep, cold water. He was wearing a life vest and was rescued within 10 minutes, at which time he was immediately dried, placed in a blanket, and brought to the ED. He is alert and oriented to person, time, and place, but is shivering uncontrollably and pale in color. His core temperature is 93°F.

The following questions will guide your development of a nursing care plan for the case study.

1. List the assessments in the order that they should be performed.
2. Identify the priority nursing diagnoses for Joe.
3. List nursing interventions in the order that they should be performed.
4. Identify the goal of treatment for Joe.

Summary

- Clients in shock need immediate assessment and intervention.
- Rapid assessment and observation of ABCs is essential in treating all cardiovascular emergencies.
- Evaluation of abdominal emergencies should include taking a history of the onset of pain because this is critical to outcome and survival.
- Ocular emergencies can be a threat to vision and thus require immediate assessment and treatment.
- Musculoskeletal and soft-tissue injuries can be painful but manageable with rapid assessment and treatment.
- In cases of poisoning or overdoses, the ABCs must first be established, then the agent to which the client was exposed must be immediately identified so that prompt treatment can be initiated.
- Major trauma is a life-threatening and unexpected occurrence for both client and loved ones.
- Nurses must be aware of the legal issues related to emergency care, such as Good Samaritan Laws and mandated reporting.

Review Questions

1. Triage is a system of:
   a. identifying clients by disease.
   b. prioritizing client care.
   c. counting clients waiting for care.
   d. medical diagnosing.

2. A client with a small branch sticking out of the right midchest arrives at the ED during a hurricane. There is bubbling and oozing at the site. Medical personnel should first:
   a. remove the branch and save it.
   b. administer pain medication to the client.
   c. start the ABCs of CPR.
   d. stop the bleeding and take vital signs.

3. An example of a nonurgent client is one with:
   a. CPR in progress.
   b. fractures of both legs.
   c. heat stroke.
   d. a sprained ankle.

4. The ambulance brings a client with a large, bleeding laceration of the upper leg to the ED. Vital signs are as follows: blood pressure, 78/62; pulse, 112; and respirations, 26. A priority nursing diagnosis is:
   a. *Deficient **F**luid Volume.*
   b. *Risk for **A**spiration.*
   c. *Risk for **I**nfection.*
   d. *Disturbed **B**ody Image.*

5. Interventions for a client in shock include:
   a. pain control and assessment of vital signs.
   b. administration of oxygen and IV fluids.
   c. insertion of a nasogastric tube.
   d. calling the physician.

References/Suggested Readings

American Heart Association. (1997). *Advanced cardiac life support.* Dallas, TX: Author.

Arbour, R. (1998). Aggressive management of intracranial dynamics. *Critical Care Nurse, 18,* 30–40.

Armstrong, J. F. (1998). Bombs and other blasts. *RN, 61*(11), 26–29.

Armstrong, J. (2002). Chemical warfare. *RN, 65*(4), 32–39.

Blank-Reid, C. (1999). Strangulation. *RN, 62*(2), 32–35.

Bowen, T., & Bellamy, R. (Eds.). (1998). *Emergency war surgery. United States Department of Defense.* Washington, DC: United States Government Printing Office.

Carroll, P. (1999). Chest injuries. *RN, 62*(1), 36–43.

Chavez, J., & Brewer, C. (2002). Stopping the shock slide. *RN, 65*(9), 30–34.

Coleman, E. (2001). Anthrax. *AJN, 101*(12), 48–52.

Coleman, E. (2002). Tularemia. *AJN, 102*(6), 65–69.

Coleman, E., & Yergler, M. (2002). Botulism. *AJN, 102*(9), 44–47.

Dochterman, J., & Bulechek, G. (2004). *Nursing Interventions Classification (NIC)* (4th ed.). St. Louis, MO: Mosby.

Easter, A. (2002). Ebola. *AJN, 102*(12), 49–52.

Estes, M. E. Z. (2002). *Health assessment & physical examination* (2nd ed.). Clifton Park, NY: Thomson Delmar Learning.

Gebbie, K., & Qureshi, K. (2002). Emergency and disaster preparedness: Core competencies for nurses. *AJN, 102*(1), 46–51.

Harrison, T., Gustafson, E., & Dixon, J. (2003). Radiologic emergency: Protecting schoolchildren & the public. *AJN, 103*(5), 41–48.

Hayes, L. (2000). Poison emergency. *Nursing2000, 30*(9), 34–39.

Huston, C. (2001). Dog bite. *Nursing2001, 31*(7), 88.

Kilpatrick, J. (2002). Nuclear attacks. *RN, 65*(5), 46–51.

Laskowski-Jones, L. (2000a). Responding to summer emergencies. *Nursing2000, 30*(5), 34–39.

Laskowski-Jones, L. (2000b). Responding to winter emergencies. *Nursing2000, 30*(1), 34–39.

Laskowski-Jones, L. (2002). Responding to an out-of-hospital emergency. *Nursing2002, 32*(9), 36–42.

Lewis, A. M. (1999). Neurologic emergency. *Nursing99, 29*(10), 54–56.

McMahon, M. (2003). ED triage. *AJN, 102*(3), 61–63.

Moorhead, S., Johnson, M., & Maas, M. (2004). *Nursing Outcomes Classification (NOC)* (3rd ed.). St. Louis, MO: Mosby.

National Association of Emergency Medical Technicians. (1998). *PHTLS. Basic and advanced pre-hospital trauma life-support* (4th ed.). St. Louis, MO: Mosby.

North American Nursing Diagnosis Association. (2003). *Nursing Diagnoses: Definitions & Classification 2003-2004,* Philadelphia: Author.

Persell, D., Arangie, P., Young, C., Stokes, E., Payne, W., Skorga, P., & Gilbert-Palmer, D. (2002). Preparing for bioterrorism. *Nursing2002, 32*(2), 36–43.

Pettinicchi, T. A. (1998). Lightning strike. *Nursing98, 28*(7), 33.

Quinn, S. (1998). ED triage. *RN, 61*(9), 53–60.

Ramponi, D. (2000). Go with the flow during an eye emergency. *Nursing2000, 30*(8), 54–56.

Rebmann, T., Carrico, R., & English, J. (2002). Are you prepared for a bioterrorist attack? *Nursing2002, 32*(9), 32hn1–32hn6.

Reilly, C. (2002). Plague. *AJN, 102*(11), 47–50.

Reilly, C., & Deason, D. (2002). Smallpox. *AJN, 102*(2), 51–55.

Reilly, C., & Deason, D. (2003). How would you respond to a chemical release? *Nursing2003, 33*(1), 36–42.

Ruffolo, D. (2002). Hypothermia in trauma. *RN, 65*(2), 46–51.

Schulmerich, S. C. (1999). When nature turns up the heat. *RN, 62*(8), 35–38.

Sibley, C. (2002). Smallpox: Vaccination revisited. *AJN, 102*(9), 26–32.

Siwula, C. (2003). Managing pediatric emergencies. *Nursing2003, 33*(2), 48–51.

Sommers, M. (1998). Missed injuries. *RN, 61*(10), 28–31.

Spratto, G., & Woods, A. (2004). *2004 PDR Nurses' Drug Handbook.* Clifton Park, NY: Thomson Delmar Learning.

Stacy, P. (1998). On-scene care. *RN, 61*(9), 50–52.

Steffen, K. (2003). When your trauma patient is over 65. *Nursing2003, 33*(4), 53–56.

Steinhauer, R. (2002). Bioterrorism. *RN, 65*(3), 48–54.

Talbert, S., & Talbert, P. (1998). Flight nursing: Summary of strategies for managing severe traumatic brain injury during early posttraumatic phase. *Journal of Emergency Nursing, 24,* 254–257.

TRAUMA! (1998). *RN, 61*(9), 49.

Veenema, T. (2002). The smallpox vaccine debate. *AJN, 102*(9), 33–38.

Veenema, T. & Daram, P. (2003). Radiation. *AJN 103*(5), 32–40.

Wiebelhaus, P., & Hansen, S. (2001). Burn emergencies. *Nursing2001, 31*(1), 36-41.

Woods, A. (2002). New threat from an ancient microbe: Anthrax. *Nursing2002, 32*(1), 44–45.

Yergler, M. (2002). Nerve gas attack. *AJN, 102*(7), 57–60.

Resources

American Association of Critical Care Nurses (AACN), 101 Columbia, Aliso Viejo, CA 92656, 949-362-2000, www.aacn.org

American Red Cross, 431 18th Street, NW, Washington, DC, 20006, 202-303-4498, www.redcross.org

American Society for Microbiology: Biological Weapons Control and Bioterrorism Preparedness Information and Resources, www.asmusa.org/pcsrc/bioprep.htm

Centers for Disease Control and Prevention, Agency for Toxic Substances and Disease Registry, www.atsdr.cdc.gov

Centers for Disease Control and Prevention, Chemical Agents Listing, www.bt.cdc.gov/Agent/agentlistchem.asp

Centers for Disease Control and Prevention, Public Health Emergency Preparedness Response, 800-311-3434, 770-488-7100 (24-hour emergency hotline), www.bt.cdc.gov

Emergency Nurses Association (ENA), 915 Lee Street, Des Plaines, IL 60016, 800-900-9659, www.ena.org

International Nursing Coalition for Mass Casualty Education, www.mc.vanderbilt.edu/nursing/coalitions/INCMCE

Johns Hopkins University, Center for Civilian Biodefense Strategies, 410-223-1667, www.hopkins-biodefense.org

Oak Ridge Institute for Science and Education, Radiation Emergency Assistance Center/Training Site, P.O. Box 117, MS 39, Oak Ridge, TN 37831-0117, 865-576-3131, www.orau.gov/reacts/default.htm

Salvation Army USA National Headquarters, P.O. Box 269, 615 Slaters Lane, Alexandria, VA 22313, 703-684-5528, www.salvationarmyusa.org

U. S. Food and Drug Administration, 888-463-6332, www.fda.gov/oc/opacom/hottopics/bioterrorism.html

THE OLDER ADULT

MAKING THE CONNECTION
Refer to the following to increase your understanding of the older adult:

Basic Nursing
- **Communication**
- **Fluid, Electrolyte, and Acid–Base Balance**

Adult Health Nursing
- **Surgery**
- **Respiratory System**
- **Cardiovascular System**
- **Gastrointestinal System**
- **Urinary System**

- **Musculoskeletal System**
- **Neurological System**
- **Sensory System**
- **Endocrine System**
- **Reproductive Systems**
- **Integumentary System**
- **Mental Illness**
- **Substance Abuse**

LEARNING OBJECTIVES

Upon completion of this chapter, you should be able to:
- **Define key terms.**
- **Describe stereotypes associated with older adults.**
- **Discuss the biological and psychosocial theories of aging.**
- **Cite the normal physiologic changes that occur with aging.**
- **List the normal functional changes that occur with aging.**
- **Describe key factors of optimal health maintenance in the aging adult.**
- **Identify funding and policy changes that have influenced elder care.**
- **Identify common disorders related to aging.**
- **Detail nursing interventions for each disorder.**
- **Discuss areas wherein the nurse can advocate for older adults on the individual, community, state, and national levels.**

KEY TERMS

activities of daily living
delirium
dementia
gerontological nursing

gerontologist
gerontology
polypharmacy

INTRODUCTION

Gerontology is the study of the effects of normal aging and age-related diseases on human beings. It is a general term used by all health care and social services disciplines. Aging (senescence) is a complex phenomenon that occurs on the continuum of human life, beginning with birth and continuing throughout the life span, and on into the end stages of life and death.

The phrase *older adult* is very subjective and has historically meant persons who are 65 years of age and older. However, there is a great deal of debate among **gerontologists** (gerontological specialists in advanced-practice nursing, geriatric psychiatry, medicine, and social services) as to whether this specific age delineation should continue to be used. The practice of using 65 years of age as a dividing line for social welfare benefits began in the 1880s when Otto von Bismark randomly selected that age for benefits in Germany. It should be noted that there was no standardized clinical basis for establishing this age as the dividing line between young and old. Longer average life-expectancy rates (76.9 years for both genders, 73.6 years for men, and 79.4 years for women) (National Council on Aging [NCOA], 2002) along with a decline in the average number of children per family since the late 1960s have changed U.S. demographics. As a result, there is a great need to support and strengthen independence among older adults, and to value and utilize their life experiences in the areas of career, family, and community.

Retirement age is now less consistently determined by a mandatory age limit. Rather, retirement frequently is offered when the employee meets a formula of combined age and years of service. Since the 1990s, benefit penalties have been imposed on Social Security beneficiaries up to 70 years of age and who continue to earn incomes over a minimum amount. This was changed in April 2000 when the Senior Citizens' Freedom to Work Act of 2000 was signed into law by the president. This eliminates the Social Security retirement earnings test in and after the month in which a person is 65 years of age (the current full retirement age) (Social Security Administration [SSA], 2000).

Currently, the clinical delineation of an older adult is still someone who is 65 years of age or older; older-old adults are defined as those individuals 85 years of age or older. In 1900, there were a total of 3.1 million individuals older than age 65 in the United States; by 1996, there were 33.2 million, 3.8 million of whom were older than age 85 years (AARP, 1998). In 2001, there were 4.2 million people aged 85 and older in the United States (NCOA, 2002). It is projected that by the year 2030, the number of older individuals in the United States will reach 70.3 million (Figure 48-1) including 8 million older than age 85 (National Council on Aging [NCOA], 2002). The most rapid increase is expected to occur in the years 2010–2030, when the "baby-boomers" reach age 65.

The future will also place demands on those who were born from the late 1950s to the late 1960s. Many in this age group chose to focus first on career, delaying marriage and childrearing until in their thirties. They have thus been labeled "the sandwich generation" to denote the challenges they will face in meeting social and financial responsibilities later in life as they work to provide for children entering college and for aging parents and, sometimes, grandparents and, in a few instances, great-grandparents.

This chapter presents an overview of influences on the older adult, including the social impacts of aging. Also examined are theories of aging; myths and realities of aging; health promotion and aging; physiologic and functional changes that normally occur with aging; and some common disorders of aging along with nursing interventions to assist clients to achieve optimal outcomes related to those disorders.

As caregivers for older adults, nurses and other members of the health care team must understand the budgetary and policy decisions that can affect the care they will provide to their clients. Thus, this chapter concludes with a short discussion on health care financing for elder care in the 21st century.

GERONTOLOGICAL NURSING

The acceptance of **gerontological nursing** as a separate nursing specialty that addresses and advocates for the special care needs of older adults has not been realized without a struggle. In 1961, gerontological nursing attained national recognition with the creation of its own division of nursing within the American Nurses Association (ANA). Nurses in the United States who were aware of the trends toward an aging population realized the importance of taking such a step. The charter members of the Division of Gerontological Nursing deserve a great deal of credit for their vision and commitment to developing gerontology education and recognizing the special nursing care needs of older adults. The major topics addressed in the expanding scope of practice for gerontological nursing included:

- The historical evolution of gerontological nursing practice based on population statistics
- The way that ageism in U.S. society has affected the profession of nursing, the health care delivery system, and the care of older adults
- Nursing education and care of older adults with a perspective derived from studies of the attitudes and interests of nursing personnel and nursing students
- The delineation of various aspects of nursing care of older adults, including clinical practice based on the ANA Standards of Nursing Practice; select theories of nursing applied to the care of older adults; and the expanding scope of gerontological nursing, in general, and the roles of clinical nurse specialists and geriatric nurse practitioners, in particular
- Trends in gerontological nursing and long-term care.

The battle continues against stereotyping older adults, both in the health professions and in the community at large. Health professionals, in particular, must be diligent in avoiding age prejudice. Believing stereotypes can influence interactions between older adults and caregivers. The caregiver may treat the older adult as a child in an old body. This approach is demeaning to elders and strips them of their self-esteem and dignity. Clients with cognitive or expressive deficits cannot always process questions

Number of persons 65+: 1900 to 2030

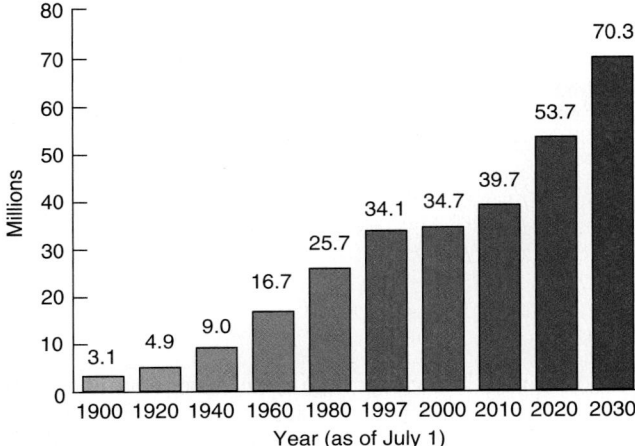

Figure 48-1 *Number of Persons Older Than Age 65: 1900–2030 (Data from AARP, 1998; and The National Council on Aging, 2002.)*

Figure 48-2 *The aging process is a normal and natural part of growth and development.*

or comments quickly or follow through with responses. Nurses and caregivers must never make the mistake of believing that clients do not understand verbal and, especially, nonverbal messages. Elders are a diverse group; they deserve respect and, through their memories and life examples, can teach a great deal to younger persons about life and survival and coping skills. Learning from clients and their families and assisting clients to find activities that enhance the quality of life (regardless of state of health) make caring for older adults a rewarding and satisfying experience.

Aging is universal, progressive, and irreversible and eventually leads to death. The aging process itself, however, is very individualized and is independent of chronological age. The way an individual ages is influenced by genetics; lifestyle; availability and quality of health services; cultural beliefs; and socioeconomic status. Certain physiologic changes are expected with aging (Figure 48-2), although there exists considerable variation in the time of onset, rate, and degree of these changes. In order to render effective and compassionate care to elderly clients, nurses working in gerontology must be familiar with the normal processes as well as the common disorders of aging.

THEORIES OF AGING

At this time, no single theory of aging has been universally accepted by practitioners in gerontology. Aging is a complex issue that takes into account the psychosocial, cultural, and experiential aspects of living. Several biological theories of aging have been proposed to explain the physiologic and functional changes that are observed in older adults. Psychosocial theories of aging strive to explain the behaviors and social interactions of older adults. These theories are summarized in Table 48-1.

TABLE 48-1   THEORIES OF AGING

BIOLOGICAL THEORIES

Title	Major Premise
Somatic mutation theory	Radiation or miscoding of enzymes causes changes in the DNA. Changes associated with aging are the result of decreased function and efficiency of the cells and organs.
Programmed aging theory	The life span is programmed within the cells. This genetic clock determines the speed at which the person ages and eventually dies.
Cross-linkage, or collagen, theory	Collagen is the principal component of connective tissue and is also found in the skin, bones, muscles, lungs, and heart. Chemical reactions between collagen and cross-linking molecules cause loss of flexibility, resulting in diminished functional mobility.
Immunity theory	The thymus becomes smaller with age. The ability to produce T-cell differentiation decreases. This impairs immunologic functions and results in increased incidence of infections, neoplasms, and autoimmune disorders.
Stress theory	Stress throughout the lifetime causes structural and chemical changes in the body. These changes eventually cause irreversible tissue damage.

PSYCHOSOCIAL THEORIES

Title	Major Premise
Activity theory	Roles and responsibilities change throughout the lifetime. Life satisfaction depends on maintaining an involvement with life by developing new interests, hobbies, roles, and relationships.
Disengagement theory	There is decreased interaction between the older person and others in his social system. The disengagement is inevitable, mutual, and acceptable to both the individual and society.
Continuity theory	Successful methods used throughout life for adjusting and adapting to life events are repeated. Characteristic traits, habits, values, associations, and goals remain stable throughout the lifetime, regardless of life changes.

Also, as more knowledge is garnered from scientific studies (e.g., the study of the impact on cells of auto-oxidization by free radicals and the study of dietary chemical exposure) and gene sequencing efforts (e.g., the human genome project), it is likely that the biological theories of aging will change as well.

MYTHS AND REALITIES OF AGING

Myths are fictitious ideas. Myths about elders are abundant and do not reflect the reality of the aging population. Following are some common myths associated with aging, based (in part) on data from the U.S. Bureau of Census and *A Profile of Older Americans* developed by the American Association of Retired Persons (AARP) in 1998.

Myth: Senility is an expected result of aging.

Reality: Senility is an outdated term once used to refer to any form of dementia that occurred in older people. Dementia is a result of disease, can affect adults of all ages, and is not a natural consequence of aging. Although some slight declines are noted in short-term memory from the age of 40 on, most people adjust through the use of memory aids such as lists and calendars. Long-term memory can actually become clearer with age. Even for a client with dementia, long-term memory can remain somewhat intact long into the disease process. Thus, nurses and caregivers find that interventions such as reminiscence, memory photo books, and activities that draw on the client's long-practiced skills provide positive client outcomes.

Myth: Incontinence is an expected result of aging.

Reality: Incontinence is not an expected outcome of aging and, in most cases, can be reversed through assessment and treatment. The challenge is that many people are embarrassed to discuss this problem with family or primary providers. Also, in long-term care settings, both the belief in this myth and the historically low staffing levels have served to dissuade clinical efforts at providing the needed nursing interventions (prompted voiding; consistent, nonhurried, timed voiding) to reverse urinary incontinence. In settings where care is provided to older adults, lack of funding, lack of policy support and education, and inconsistent enforcement of adequate staffing levels have often had a negative impact on client health outcomes. By developing urinary incontinence treatment programs, care facilities could improve clinical outcomes for clients and also reduce health care costs.

Myth: Older adults are no longer interested in sexuality or sexual activity.

Reality: Sexuality is a lifelong need. Elders can be and are sexually active, regardless of age. Although sexual function may be affected by changes in the reproductive systems, persons of both genders are capable of orgasm into old age. Despite interest and desire, physiologic or psychological problems and medication side effects may present barriers to intercourse. In such situations, sexuality without coitus can provide elders with love and intimacy. It is important to remember that human beings are social beings. Just as small babies can fail to thrive without human touch (hugs, nurturing, companionship, valuing of the individual), so can older adults fail to thrive without these same human interactions and support (Figure 48-3).

A national survey by NCOA in 1998 revealed that half of those age 60 and older were sexually active. Approximately 72% of those were as satisfied or more satisfied with their sex lives compared to when they were in their forties (NCOA, 2001).

The medication sildenafil citrate (Viagra) has proven beneficial to many older couples as they work to meet their sexual health needs. The debate over the acceptance and funding of this medication for erectile dysfunction sheds light on just how far U.S. society still has to go in debunking this myth and replacing it with the truth that normal human sexuality needs continue throughout the life span.

Myth: Most people spend the last years of their lives in nursing homes.

Reality: According to NCOA (2002), in 2000 only 4.5% of those older than age 65 lived in nursing homes. The percentage rises steeply with age, however (1.1% of those 65 to 74 years of age, 4.7% of those 75 to 84 years of age, and 18% of those older than 85 years of age). For many, that stay will involve rehabilitation following surgery, a fracture, or stroke before returning home after a short hospital stay. The late 1990s saw a growing interest in the use of alternative care options for elders (retirement communities, assisted living centers, group homes, respite care, and partial hospitalization/adult day programs); however, most older adults continue to live in communities with varying levels of assistive services or support as they age. The projected trends in long-term

CULTURAL CONSIDERATIONS

Aging

It is important to assess the older client's religious beliefs, traditions, and culture and to evaluate the ways that these may influence the client's health beliefs and health practices. Caregivers can make the mistake of not fully assessing the client's beliefs about health in elders, and can also be misled by myths about aging that exist in U.S. society.

Figure 48-3 *Individuals of all ages benefit from intimacy and companionship.*

CRITICAL THINKING

Myths/Stereotypes

What myths or stereotypes have you observed that affect the elderly?

care needs are for continued use of alternate settings that will support interventions to meet residents' physical, psychosocial, cultural, spiritual, cognitive, and mental health needs.

Traditionally, elders in long-term care facilities have been taken from home environments where they have likely experienced the highest level of independence they have had in their lifetimes (to choose when to get up, eat, go to bed, and the like), and have been placed in settings where very few, if any, choices, including care decisions, are made based on their preferences. Gerontological nurses have an ongoing responsibility to help re-create the way care is provided to elderly clients and to advocate for individual choices for older clients in long-term care facilities. Nurse leaders must learn to think in new ways about long-practiced trends in elder care in the United States and to work with older clients and their families to envision and create better trends.

Myth: All elderly persons are financially impoverished.

Reality: Income range varies among those older than 65 years of age, just as it does among those in younger groups; however, the high costs of medications does disproportionately affect those older than age 65, who are more likely to have one or more chronic conditions that require management with medication. In the past, lack of reimbursement for preventive assessment, treatments, and medications led many elders to go without medications or to delay care until they were too ill to wait any longer. This resulted in increased use of acute care services in hospitals.

In 2001, families headed by persons older than 65 years of age had a median income of $33,938 (AoA, 2002). The challenge for most elders below the median (especially older women, who often have lower retirement incomes) is that most of their assets are tied up in the family home or in other nonliquid holdings. Thus, when an acute illness strikes, there is little financial reserve to help cover costs.

HEALTH AND AGING

Like all age groups, elders can do much to adopt a healthy lifestyle that will enhance their remaining years.

Activities of Daily Living

Being well groomed enhances the self-esteem of all older adults. Adaptive devices and techniques are available for those who need assistance with the **activities of daily living** (ADLs), basic care activities that include mobility, bathing, hygiene, grooming, dressing, eating, and toileting.

Mobility

Many assistive devices are available to help the older client maintain mobility and independence. Handrails can decrease the risk of falls while the person is walking; they are also useful in the tub and, when used in conjunction with a plastic riser, can help the older adult get on and off the toilet safely.

Bathing

Skin dryness increases with aging; thus, it may be preferable for older adults to bathe or shower only two to three times per week and to take sponge baths in between. A gentle soap should be used sparingly for the bath, after which a moisturizing lotion should be applied. The individual or caregiver should be instructed to inspect the skin during bathing for any indication of skin breakdown, lumps, or changes in moles.

With aging, oil secretion decreases in the scalp, and hair can thus become dry. Shampooing one or two times per week is usually adequate for most elders, and a simplified hairstyle may be helpful to those with limited mobility in the arms. The use of mild shampoos and conditioners can also enhance hair texture.

Hygiene

Fingernails may become more brittle with aging. Keeping the client's fingernails clean and short can prevent accidental injury or scratches to fragile older skin. Impaired circulation is common among older adults, so special attention should be given to care of the feet and lower extremities. Because toenails frequently become thick and tougher with aging, soaking the feet before trimming the toenails may ease the task. For clients with circulation or skin integrity problems of the feet and toes or for clients with diabetes, a referral to a podiatrist should be made for nail trimming. During bathing, monitor the client's feet for discomfort; inflammation; broken skin; color changes such as redness, pallor, or cyanosis (blue or purple discoloration resulting from lack of circulation); heat or coldness; cracking between toes; and corns or calluses.

The need for adequate oral care does not diminish with aging. Dental problems can result in poor eating habits and inadequate nutrition. Inadequate brushing and dental check-ups can lead to gingivitis (bleeding and edematous gums), which, if left untreated, can progress to periodontal disease that can destroy connective tissue, alveolar bone, and periodontal ligaments. Monitor clients for proper oral care. Yoneyama et al. (2002) reports that nursing home residents who received oral hygiene after each meal and professional cleaning once a week were two times less likely to get pneumonia and two times less likely to die from it. For those clients with dentures, inspect the dentures for cleanliness and proper fit. Clients with dentures must brush the dentures and the gums regularly with a soft brush and a mild cleanser. It is helpful to label dentures with the client's name to facilitate identification of the

Figure 48-4 *Good grooming for the older adult includes choosing personal items such as jewelry and clothing.*

dentures in the event that the client is admitted to a hospital or an assistive care setting.

Grooming

Good grooming is important in promoting the older client's self-esteem and confidence. Keeping the hair neat and tidy, choosing attractive clothing and jewelry, and making decisions about makeup and other personal care practices will all contribute to the older client's sense of well-being and independence (Figure 48-4).

Male clients may feel much better with a clean-shaven face. Infection-control principles demand that each razor (either electric or blade) be used for only one individual and that that razor be marked with the client's name. Women may also require attention to facial hair, as estrogen levels decrease after menopause. It is not uncommon for older women to notice hairs on the chin or upper lip that were not there in younger days. Also, both men and women are likely to notice

Figure 48-5 *Assistive devices such as these for pantyhose and buttons are available to help older adults dress independently. (Courtesy of Maddak, Inc.)*

graying and diminished hair on legs, underarms, and pubic areas as they age.

Dressing

Dressing may be difficult for clients who have restricted joint movement, paralysis, or limited endurance because of health problems. Many choices are available to ease dressing, such as elastic waists, velcro fasteners, and assistive reaching and dressing devices (Figure 48-5).

Eating

Many older adults are able to maintain the ability to self-feed, thereby promoting independence and self-esteem. Neurological and musculoskeletal alterations may, however, affect the ability to self-feed. Dysphagia, or difficulty swallowing, may place the older client at increased risk of choking, and diminished taste sensation may affect the desire to eat.

Toileting

Toileting habits also change with aging. Bowel elimination problems can often be prevented as clients age by:

- Ensuring adequate fiber intake
- Ensuring adequate fluid intake
- Ensuring regular daily exercise
- Developing regular elimination habits

For the client in the hospital or a long-term care facility, it is helpful to:

- Maintain previously effective habits such as drinking warm liquids upon arising
- Assist the client to the toilet approximately 30 minutes after eating, to take advantage of the gastrocolic reflex

As a result of the physical changes that occur with aging, increased frequency of urination may be noted in elders of both genders. It is not uncommon for older adults to self-limit fluid intake because of a fear of incontinence. This habit is unhealthy and should be discouraged. Assess cases of incontinence to determine the cause and type, so that appropriate interventions and treatment can be implemented. Timing the use of prescribed diuretics in the morning rather than the evening

> ### PROFESSIONAL TIP
>
> **Bowel Patterns in Older Adults**
>
> It is extremely important that caregivers of older adults monitor bowel patterns. Long periods of constipation (> 2 to 3 days) should alert caregivers to the need for interventions to minimize the likelihood of bowel impaction, which can ultimately be life threatening if left untreated. Evacuation aids such as laxatives, lubricants, stool softeners, and enemas all have side effects and should thus be avoided if at all possible. Dietary changes or an exercise regimen should be introduced first.

Figure 48-6 *Exercise is important to all clients and should be tailored to interests and ability levels.*

can prevent the increased need for urination at night, which is especially helpful to older clients who are being treated for congestive heart failure (CHF).

Exercise

What was once accepted as the normal deterioration of old age is now considered the result of disuse through sitting and bed rest. Research indicates that high-intensity, progressive resistance training can improve muscle strength and muscle size in frail elderly clients. Walking and all other maneuvers required for ADLs are also beneficial. Individually plan exercise programs taking into consideration the older person's:

- General health status (Figure 48-6)
- Physiologic disorders (if present)
- Preference for solidarity or group activity
- Physical environment
- Financial status

Nutrition

For many older adults, cultural heritage, religious rites, ethnic practices, and family traditions are linked to food. The physiologic, psychological, sociological, and economic changes of aging may compromise nutritional status. Elders must follow a balanced diet, often with lowered intakes of sugar, caffeine, and sodium. There are no universally accepted dietary guidelines specific to older adults. A dietitian can determine the needed food intake for a specific individual by taking into account the individual's height, ideal weight, activity level, and disease processes.

Older adults need 1,000 mg to 1,500 mg of calcium per day for both men and women. Calcium supplements should also contain vitamin D to provide for optimal metabolism by the body. The need for additional supplements depends on the older individual's nutritional status and ability to maintain an adequate diet. Growing discussion supports the needs for adequate protein intake, to maintain both skin integrity and bone density; and moderate carbohydrate intake because carbohydrates metabolize to sugars.

It is important to know about community services designed to help older clients meet their nutritional needs. Such services include grocery transportation and delivery services, homebound meals (e.g., Meals on Wheels), group meals at senior food sites, and the Food Stamp program. Nurses and caregivers should also realize that socialization and companionship are necessary components of adequate dietary intake, and should ensure that these areas are addressed as part of any food-assistance intervention.

Psychosocial Considerations

Older adults, like all individuals, have psychosocial and cognitive needs for lifelong learning. Many colleges have developed education program options for elder students (often at no tuition), and employers are beginning to recruit older workers for part-time positions (recognizing their historically good work ethic and experience). Many elders continue to volunteer countless hours each year, offering to help meet the social service needs of their communities. These efforts can result in feelings of productivity and self-worth for the older adult. Mental activity and emotional involvement are as necessary to the overall well-being as is physical activity. Older clients can benefit from building on their long-practiced skills to develop interesting and stimulating activities or hobbies. Such activities may be of an individual or group nature. Socialization with people of all age groups can help not only the older participants, but also the young and middle-aged participants, by illustrating that aging is not a disease but rather, a rich and natural part of the life process.

Strengths

Older adults generally have suffered many losses over the years. Some losses are slight and require only minor adaptation, whereas others may significantly affect the person. Physiologic changes or disease processes may result in losses, causing impairments in:

- Communication
- Vision and learning
- Mobility
- Cognition
- Psychosocial skills

If the impairment is severe, the individual could lose some degree of independence, and adaptations may be required. Furthermore, losses can cascade for the older client, as one loss contributes to another. For example, if an elderly person with diabetes were to lose her driver's license because of impaired vision related to diabetic retinopathy, socialization might be restricted, which in turn might increase her feelings of loneliness and diminished self-esteem. If, however, her spouse provides caregiving and transportation, these adaptations might allow her to remain active socially while still living in her home. If her spouse later dies, and her health continues to decline, a move to an assisted living facility may become necessary, if other community adaptations are unavailable. She would then be faced with adapting to the loss of both her home and her spouse.

Health care professionals should remember that persons who have lived for many years are survivors and can adapt to life changes better if they are allowed to utilize their existing strengths. They are often much stronger and more ingenious and enterprising than they are given credit for. Identify the strengths of each individual (including past coping skills) and use them when planning care and assisting the older client to find new ways to adapt and maintain optimal independence in a new setting.

Health Promotion and Disease Prevention

Older adults must be alerted to ways of preventing disease and reducing risks. Being knowledgeable about self-care and participating in screening tests are important for health maintenance. For older men, an annual prostate examination and a prostate specific antigen (PSA) level lab test, which can detect prostate cancer in the early stages, are recommended every 1 to 2 years.

For older women, the annual mammogram may be delayed by the physician depending on the client's risk factors. If a client's Pap smears have been negative (normal) for 5 consecutive years, they can be done less often. Men and women older than age 50 should have a yearly stool test for occult blood performed. A colonoscopy may be recommended to monitor for colon cancer. Teach the clients habits for healthy living and inform them of signs and symptoms that require medical investigation. Older clients who have been exposed to environmental chemicals, tobacco, or extensive alcohol use over many years often experience serious health consequences as they reach older age. Older clients of any age can benefit from healthy lifestyles and from disease-prevention interventions, such as being inoculated yearly against influenza and every 6 years against pneumonia; assessment of tuberculosis (TB) status; and adequate safe food and clean water intake.

In many cases, by the time a person reaches 65 to 70 years of age, that person has been prescribed medication to address at least one ongoing (chronic) medical problem (e.g., hypertension, heart disease, diabetes, allergies, gastrointestinal disorders). The challenge many elders face is that side effects from one medication are often treated with another prescription medication. If the client then goes to different doctors, these doctors may prescribe even more medications to address the same or other health concerns. This is called **polypharmacy,** or the problem of clients taking numerous prescription and over-the-counter medications for the same or various

---

PROFESSIONAL TIP

Identifying Strengths of Older Adults as Part of Assessment

Assessment should include the identification of strengths as well as problems. Strengths are utilized to achieve or maintain optimal physical, mental, and emotional function. All of the following can be considered strengths:

- Cognitive health
- Freedom from or successful adaptation to deficits or impairments
- A history of healthy lifestyle with regard to diet, sleep, stress management, exercise, and chemical abuse (none)
- Adequate functional ability to carry out ADLs
- Freedom from incapacitating physical discomfort and pain
- A physically safe living environment
- Feelings of security in present environment
- Realistic knowledge about capabilities
- Pattern of avoiding dangerous situations and unnecessary risks
- Compliance with health care regimen
- Capability with regard to managing own environment
- An intact support system
- Satisfying relationships with others
- Opportunities for sexual expression
- Access to transportation
- Adequate functional mobility
- Successful adaptation to life changes and crises

- History of relinquishing roles as phases of life require and replacing them with satisfying new roles
- A pattern of successful mourning for losses
- Participation in groups: religious, community, hobbies
- Membership in family whose members respect each other and are willing to give and receive help when necessary
- Successful problem-solving skills
- Willingness to seek information to improve situation
- Evidence of initiative and self-confidence in abilities and judgment
- Participation in self-care by making decisions and accepting responsibility for decisions
- A well-defined value system
- Acceptance of that which cannot be changed
- Successful use of assertive skills
- Strong spiritual beliefs and ability to find comfort and strength in spiritual and religious practices
- Enthusiastic appreciation for aging, with demonstrative embrace of the positive aspects and adaptation to the negative aspects
- Participation in healthy reminiscing; evidence of few regrets about life past
- Joyful appreciation for nature, art, music, hobbies, and activities
- A well-developed sense of humor

disease processes, with unknown consequences from the resulting combinations of chemical compounds and cumulative side effects. In many settings, primary care providers, nurses, clinical pharmacists, and social workers collaborate to assist the older client and the family to oversee the client's medication management and other health needs.

Among the biggest challenges facing older clients are shorter hospitalization stays and reduced time with physicians in the physician's offices. There is less time to ensure that the follow-up services the client will need are understood and in place and less time to educate client and family about medication regimens, including timing and possible interactions with other prescription and over-the-counter drugs or herbal remedies that the client may also be taking. The nurse, as part of the interdisciplinary team, plays a vital role as client advocate when ensuring that older clients have the teaching, services, and follow-up care they need.

PHYSIOLOGIC CHANGES ASSOCIATED WITH AGING

Although the aging process brings with it many physiologic changes, it should be remembered that aging and disease are not synonymous. Whereas the physiologic changes of aging described following are normal for most people, the medical disorders described are not considered normal.

Respiratory System

The following respiratory changes result from the aging process:

- The muscles of respiration become less flexible, causing decreased vital capacity of the lungs.
- Decrease in functional capacity results in dyspnea on exertion or stress; usual activity does not affect breathing.
- Effectiveness of the cough mechanism lessens, increasing the risk of lung infection.
- The alveoli thicken and decrease in number and size, causing less effective gas exchange and, in individuals who also have chronic lung disease, intensifying respiratory deficits.
- Structural changes in the skeleton, such as kyphosis (seen in clients with osteoporosis as an often asymetrical convex curve of the spine) can decrease diaphragmatic expansion. Kyphosis in older clients can lead to a need for small, more frequent meals to balance nutritional requirements and respiratory function because of the restriction of adequate space for expansion and contraction of the diaphragm. It can

also create skin integrity risks because the bony prominences of the client's back press against the backs of chairs.

Common respiratory disorders related to aging include the following:

- Respiratory tract infection (RTI)
- Chronic obstructive pulmonary disease (COPD)
- Pulmonary tuberculosis (TB)

Nursing Management: Respiratory Tract Infections

1. Advise discussing the pneumovaccine with the primary care provider.
2. Advise obtaining annual influenza vaccine.
3. Assist the client to assume a position of comfort and assist with medications and respiratory treatments, as ordered.
4. Avoid distention of bowel, bladder, or stomach, any of which can increase breathing discomfort.
5. Allow adequate time for nursing care.
6. Administer humidified oxygen therapy, as prescribed.
7. Administer analgesics and antipyretics, as prescribed.
8. Assess for signs of dehydration and ensure that fluids are accessible to the client, unless contraindicated.
9. Review diagnostic data and monitor lung sounds and intake and output every 8 hours or as needed given changes in the client's condition. Weigh the client daily, assessing for fluid retention.
10. Monitor for any signs of respiratory distress (cyanosis of lips, mucous membranes, or nailbeds) and obtain pulse-oximetry readings, as needed.

Nursing Management: Chronic Obstructive Pulmonary Disease

1. Assist the client to a position of comfort.
2. Teach the client to use pursed-lip breathing to avoid hyperventilation when short of breath.

PROFESSIONAL TIP

TB in the Older Adult
Elders can be vulnerable to TB because of:
- An ineffective cough reflex and the resulting inability to clear the lungs
- An altered immune system and a reduced response to extrinsic antigens. Not only are elders at increased risk of infection via a new contagion, but older clients who contracted TB years ago and have been in remission since can experience reexacerbation. The risk of reexacerbation increases in cases where the initial infection was remote and healed (encapsulated) such that the immune system's memory of the T cells has been lost. Facilities where health care is provided to older clients and to immune-compromised clients thus must regularly assess the TB status of both their clients and their employees.

3. Teach the client diaphragmatic breathing for use when active.
4. Teach proper use of inhalers. Steroid inhalers should be used first, with a full 60-second wait between puffs; after waiting 3 minutes, any bronchodilator inhalers that are prescribed should then be used, also with a 60-second wait between puffs.
5. Teach the client to cough and clear the airway.
6. Adminster chest physiotherapy (e.g., percussion, postural drainage), if prescribed.
7. Establish a schedule for ambulation, gradually increasing the distance ambulated.
8. Assist with active assistive range-of-motion exercises.
9. Monitor for signs and symptoms of infections (e.g., fever, blood-tinged or thick, greenish colored sputum, and diminished lung sounds) and immediately report same to the registered nurse and the primary care provider.
10. Monitor breathing and pulse rate and administer oxygen, if necessary, during periods of increased activity.
11. Suggest smoking cessation programs, if the client is a smoker.

Safety: Oxygen and Smoking
Ensure that no smoking is allowed around clients on oxygen therapy.

Nursing Management: Pulmonary Tuberculosis

1. Monitor clients for TB status and for symptoms including fever, night sweats, weight loss, and cough producing blood-tinged sputum.
2. Inform the client, family, and caregivers of the need for adequate isolation techniques.

Infection Control: TB
Remember that TB is spread through droplets when a client sneezes or coughs (direct and indirect contact). Consult the infection-control nurse on the client's interdisciplinary team and work to protect the client and others from transmission of *Mycobacterium tuberculosis* and other infections.

3. Evaluate the client's risk for infection with the human immunodeficiency virus (HIV) and related pneumocystic pneumonia.

4. Monitor that the client's psychosocial needs are being adequately met while the disease is being pharmacologically addressed with medications like isoniazid (Laniazid). Tell the client and family that the entire course of medication must be completed.
5. Monitor the client's nutrition intake and provide supplements as necessary to maintain adequate body weight.
6. Provide for rest periods throughout the day. Encourage the older client with TB to monitor activity level and length of visits by family so as not to become overtired.

Cardiovascular System

The following cardiovascular changes result from the aging process:

- Cardiac output and recovery time decline. The heart requires more time to return to a normal rate after a rate increase in response to activity.
- The heart rate slows.
- Blood flow to all organs decreases. The brain and coronary arteries continue to receive a larger volume than do other organs.
- Arterial elasticity decreases, causing increased peripheral resistance and, in turn, a rise in systolic blood pressure and a slight rise in diastolic blood pressure.
- Veins dilate, and superficial vessels become more prominent.

Common cardiovascular disorders related to aging include the following:

- Peripheral vascular disease (PVD)
- Hypertension
- Chronic CHF

Nursing Management: Peripheral Vascular Disease

1. Assess the lower extremities, including the peripheral pulses, for signs of arterial or venous insufficiency.
2. Evaluate lifestyle factors that may aggravate or advance atherosclerosis, such as a high-carbohydrate, high-fat diet and little exercise.
3. Teach the client about the disease, including treatment, medication actions and side effects, and signs of thrombosis.
4. Educate the client and caregivers about the care and inspection of the lower extremities.
5. Provide instructions on interventions specific to the client's type of PVD (arterial or venous).

Nursing Management: Hypertension

1. Evaluate food intake patterns, especially of cholesterol, fats, sodium, and carbohydrates. Make recommendations based on findings.
2. Evaluate for fluid retention.
3. Recommend a smoking cessation program, if necessary.
4. Advise the client to avoid alcohol use.

CLIENT TEACHING

Digoxin Toxicity

Possible signs and symptoms of digoxin toxicity include the following:
- Disturbances in cardiac rhythms
- Fatigue
- Listlessness
- Anorexia
- Nausea
- Visual disturbances (halos around lights)
- Shaking
- Unsteady gait
- Confusion

5. Recommend and facilitate a consistent and appropriate exercise program.
6. Discuss the relationship of stress to hypertension and provide resources from which the client can learn relaxation techniques.
7. Provide information on medications and the importance of taking daily blood pressure medications as prescribed, regardless of health status on any given day.
8. Arrange for and encourage regular blood pressure checks and teach the client or significant others proper use of blood pressure equipment, if applicable.

Nursing Management: Chronic Congestive Heart Failure

1. Frequently monitor serum digitalis level and monitor for any signs of digoxin toxicity, for which older clients are at increased risk because of the decreased rate of renal clearance of the drug. Withhold the digoxin and immediately contact the registered nurse and the physician if abnormal serum level or signs and symptoms of toxicity are present.
2. Take the apical pulse for a full 1 minute before administering digoxin. Withhold the medication if the apical pulse is below 60, and consult the registered nurse and the physician if this or any other significant changes in vital signs are noted.
3. Monitor the client's blood pressure and lung sounds.
4. Monitor electrolyte levels, blood urea nitrogen (BUN), and creatinine level to observe system changes including decreased kidney efficiency.
5. Monitor for signs of fluid retention such as intake and output (output too small), weight gain, shortness of breath, or coughing.
6. Encourage alternating periods of activity with periods of rest.
7. Encourage the client to maintain a level of exercise/physical activity appropriate to physical condition.
8. Teach the client and family about the safe use of the prescribed medications.
9. For clients on diuretics, which deplete potassium, monitor fluid intake and level of potassium, ensur-

ing adequacy of each. Encourage administration of diuretics early in the day, unless contraindicated, to prevent increased urination at night.

Gastrointestinal System

The following gastrointestinal changes result from the aging process:

- Tooth enamel thins.
- Periodontal disease rate increases.
- Taste buds decrease in number, and saliva production diminishes.
- Effectiveness of the gag reflex lessens, resulting in an increased risk of choking.
- Esophageal peristalsis slows, and the effectiveness of the esophageal sphincter lessens, causing delayed entry of food into the stomach and increasing the risk of aspiration.
- Hiatal hernia may occur.
- Gastric emptying slows. Food remains in the stomach longer, decreasing the capacity of the stomach.
- Peristalsis and nerve sensation of the large intestine decreases, contributing to constipation.
- The incidence of diverticulosis increases with age.
- Liver size decreases after age 70.
- Liver enzymes decrease, slowing drug metabolism and the detoxification process.
- Emptying of the gallbladder lessens in efficiency, resulting in thickened bile, increased cholesterol content, and increased incidence of gallstones.

Common gastrointestinal disorders related to aging include the following:

- Over-/undernutrition
- Constipation
- Dehydration
- Dental disorders

Nursing Management: Over-/Undernutrition

1. Assess nutritional status.
2. Provide nutritional instruction based on assessment findings.
3. Advise on community nutrition programs (e.g., Meals-on-Wheels, senior center food sites, food pantries, and Food Stamp program).

Nursing Management: Constipation

1. Assess food and fluid intake.
2. Make recommendations based on assessment findings (e.g., increase fiber intake, increase fluid intake).
3. Discuss the relationship of exercise to bowel activity.
4. Discuss the importance of routine for regular bowel elimination.
5. Advise avoiding the overuse of laxatives.
6. Monitor adequate bowel elimination and provide interventions (e.g., prune juice, senna bars, milk of magnesia, as ordered) to assist the client in returning to a normal bowel elimination routine.

Nursing Management: Dehydration

1. Identify the reason for dehydration (i.e., inadequate fluid intake or excessive fluid output).

PROFESSIONAL TIP

Determining Alterations in Nutrition

- Height and weight: Record actual body weight, usual body weight, and ideal body weight. If usual weight has varied significantly from the ideal for several years, the use of height/weight tables may be meaningless. Compare actual body weight to usual body weight to determine present status.
- Review laboratory values: hematocrit, hemoglobin, total iron-binding capacity, total protein, BUN.
- Determine whether client is on a weight-loss diet.
- Determine whether client was edematous when initially weighed and has lost weight with treatment.
- Evaluate cognitive status. Cognitively impaired clients may be unaware of hunger or be unable to attend to the task of eating.
- In clients with central nervous system damage, evaluate the presence of sensory–perceptual deficits that interfere with eating.
- Evaluate ability to pick up utensils and glasses and to get items from table to mouth.
- Evaluate dental/oral status: status of teeth/dentures, gums, presence of oral dryness (xerostomia).
- Determine presence of impaired swallowing.
- Determine whether client has distaste for certain food groups.
- Assess knowledge in regard to nutrition and food purchase and preparation.
- Determine whether client is taking medications that interfere with taste or food absorption.
- Determine whether financial status interferes with food purchasing.
- Evaluate for history of compulsive eating.

COMMUNITY/HOME HEALTH CARE

Nutritional Status

Evaluate the following when assessing a client's nutritional status in the home:
- Ability to shop for and prepare meals
- Mealtime environment, for unpleasant odors, noises, and visual stimuli
- Table setting, for appealing table cover, centerpiece, colorful dishes
- Appropriateness of food storage system (cabinets, refrigerator, freezer)

Urinary System

The following urinary changes result from the aging process:

- Nephrons in the kidneys decrease in number and function, resulting in decreased filtration and gradual decrease in excretory and reabsorbtive functions of the renal tubules.
- Glomerular filtration rate decreases, resulting in decreased renal clearance of drugs.
- Blood urea nitrogen increases. The creatinine clearance test is a better indicator than is BUN of renal function in elders.
- Sodium-conserving ability diminishes.
- Bladder capacity decreases, causing increased frequency of urination, including nocturia.
- Renal function increases when the older client lies down, sometimes causing a need to void shortly after going to bed.
- Bladder and perineal muscles weaken, resulting in the inability to empty the bladder and predisposing the elderly client to cystitis.
- Incidence of stress incontinence increases in older females.
- The prostate may enlarge in older males, causing urinary frequency or dribbling.

Common urinary disorders related to aging include the following:

- Incontinence
- Urinary tract infections (UTIs)

Nursing Management: Incontinence

1. Complete an assessment for bladder management (Figure 48-7).
2. Identify the type of incontinence present (Table 48-2).
3. Implement an appropriate bladder management program (Table 48-3).
4. Frequently monitor for skin impairment.
5. Offer absorbent incontinent pads or briefs that draw the moisture away from the skin.
6. Teach all caregivers, the client, and the family the importance both of adequate cleansing of the genital area (proper retraction and cleansing of the foreskin

2. Identify the reason and corresponding interventions for inadequate fluid intake:
   - Fluids are inaccessible because of the client's physical limitations: offer fluids on a regular basis throughout the day.
   - The client dislikes water or other available fluids: identify fluid choices.
   - The client restricts fluids because of a fear of incontinence: explain the relationship of decreased fluid intake to bladder infections and arrange for assistance, as needed, for toileting.
3. Identify the reasons for any excessive fluid output and treat accordingly.

Nursing Management: Dental Disorders

1. Teach the oral hygiene procedures of brushing and flossing and facilitate and encourage brushing of the teeth and gums and flossing of the teeth, as tolerated.
2. Inspect the mouth regularly for signs of dental disorders.
3. Advise regular dental checkups.

To be completed and reviewed every 90 days or as frequently as needed based on outcome and response.

CLIENT_____ Adm No. _____ Date_____ Diagnoses_____ Birthdate_____

Bladder function: History of infection or other urinary problem._____ Urinalysis: Date_____

Protein____ Glucose__ Ketones__ RBC__ WBC__ Bacteria__ Crystals__ Sp.Gr.__ Culture: Date_____ Result_____

Treatment_____

BUN____ Ser.Creatinine____ Tot.Pro.____ FBS____ To be completed after 2-week assessment period

Frequency of voiding_____ Average amount_____ Is client aware of need to void?_____ Urgency?_____ Dribbling?_____

Incontinence preceded by laughing, sneezing_____

Medications affecting bladder function/continence_____

Mental status: Short-term memory_____ Orientation_____ Able to express self_____

   Able to follow directions_____ Reaction to incontinence_____

Hydration baseline: Daily average fluid intake: Days_____ Eve._____ Night_____

Mobility/self-care skills: Ambulatory/self_____ Cane_____ Walker_____ Requires assist of one or two_____

   Weight-bearing_____ Propels self by w/c_____ Transfers self_____ Requires assistance_____

   Can manage clothing_____ Cleanses self after toileting_____ Washes hands_____

Figure 48-7 *Assessment for Bladder Management*

TABLE 48-2	TYPES OF URINARY INCONTINENCE
TYPE	**CHARACTERISTICS**
Functional	Bladder emptying is unpredictable but complete. Incontinence is related to impairment of cognitive, physical, or psychological functioning or to environmental barriers.
Urge	Incontinence occurs immediately after the sensation to void is perceived.
Reflex	Incontinence is related to neurogenic bladder and central nervous system or spinal cord injury. Bladder fills, and uninhibited bladder contractions cause loss of urine.
Stress	Increased abdominal pressure is higher than urethral resistance. Stress associated with coughing or laughing causes incontinence.
Total	Unpredictable, unvoluntary, continuous loss of urine.

TABLE 48-3	BLADDER MANAGEMENT TECHNIQUES
PROGRAM	**DESCRIPTION**
Kegel exercises	Used for stress incontinence in cognitively alert persons. Exercises strengthen pelvic floor musculature.
Scheduled toileting	Client is on a fixed schedule of toileting—usually every 2 hours. Technique can be used to facilitate voiding and emptying of the bladder.
Habit training	Client is toileted according to individual pattern of voiding. Several days must be spent assessing pattern.
Bladder retraining	Restores normal pattern of voiding/continence. Requires accurate assessment before establishing schedule with progressive shortening or lengthening of toileting intervals. Client must be cognitively alert.
Prompted voiding	Client is prompted to toilet at regular intervals and is given social reinforcement for appropriate toileting behavior.

in the older uncircumcised male and proper cleansing of the skin folds of the older female), legs, and back and of the use of clean linens, to ensure that the client's skin is kept clean and dry. Apply a moisture barrier cream as needed to prevent skin maceration from excessive exposure to moisture.

7. Teach and employ effective infection-control techniques (e.g., wipe and clean [from front to back only] after toileting and when bathing).
8. Encourage referral to discuss medical options (in addition to nursing interventions) for treatment of incontinence.
9. Allow the client to voice concerns over incontinence and assist to overcome any adverse effects on psychosocial functioning.

Nursing Management: Urinary Tract Infections

NOTE: Elderly persons frequently do not present with the usual signs and symptoms of UTIs. Falling or signs of acute confusion (more than usual) may often be the major clinical manifestations.

1. Monitor fluid intake and output. Increase intake unless contraindicated. Offer cranberry juice frequently, per ordered diet.
2. Teach and encourage client to empty the bladder every 3 to 4 hours.
3. Encourage the client to take all medication as prescribed.
4. Use proper infection-control techniques to minimize the risk of infection, including maintaining sterile technique for any urinary catheterization procedure (for urinalysis, assessment for bladder retention, or insertion of indwelling catheter), to prevent unnecessary introduction of bacteria into the bladder.
5. Teach female clients to wipe from front to back only; cleanse thoroughly after bowel movements; avoid bubble baths, colored toilet paper, douches, and vaginal sprays; and wear underwear made from cotton rather than synthetic fibers.
6. Teach the client and caregivers that hematuria (blood in the urine) and fever indicate the need for immediate assessment and intervention, as these signs and symptoms can signify a potentially serious infection or condition. Any signs and symptoms of bladder infection should be immediately reported to the registered nurse and the physician.

Musculoskeletal System

The following musculoskeletal changes result from the aging process:

• Muscle mass and elasticity diminish, resulting in decreased strength, endurance, coordination, and increased reaction time.
• Bone demineralization occurs, causing skeletal instability and shrinkage of intervertebral disks. The flexibility of the spine lessens, and spinal curvature often occurs.
• Joints undergo degenerative changes, resulting in pain, stiffness, and loss of range of motion.

Common musculoskeletal system disorders related to aging include the following:

• Osteoporosis
• Degenerative arthritis
• Fractured hip

Nursing Management: Osteoporosis

1. Make dietary recommendations to ensure adequate intake of calcium, protein, and vitamin D.
2. Recommend a smoking cessation program, if necessary.
3. Advise the client to avoid alcohol.
4. Encourage the client to take a calcium supplement in conjunction with vitamin D, as ordered by the client's primary care provider.
5. Recommend consultation with the primary care provider regarding either estrogen replacement therapy (ERT) options for females or the use of medications like alendronate sodium (Fosamax) to address bone density loss associated with osteoporosis.
6. Teach the client, family, and caregivers about measures to reduce the risk of falling and sustaining fractures.
7. Recommend evaluation (via x-ray) for the presence of stress, or compression, fractures of the spine in cases of severe back pain that occurs with or without a fall. In clients with osteoporosis, these fractures can occur more easily because the vertebrae are compacted by shrinkage of the intervertebral spaces as a consequence of aging.
8. Provide adequate pain control for back pain or other musculoskeletal discomfort.
9. Monitor for adequate dietary intake of calories and fluids and for effective elimination patterns.
10. Teach, encourage, and assist clients to establish exercise programs appropriate to their capabilities. Especially promote exercise programs that include walking or other weight-bearing activities, as tolerated.

Nursing Management: Degenerative Arthritis

1. Suggest a schedule for alternating periods of activity and rest.
2. Advise a weight reduction plan, if necessary, to eliminate extra strain on affected joints.
3. Teach, assist, and encourage the client to establish an exercise program that emphasizes gentle stretching and movement of all joints. For those clients who are more independent, exercise programs in warm water can have positive outcomes.
4. Provide adequate pain control. Teach clients and caregivers to monitor for gastrointestinal distress related to arthritis medications such as nonsteroidal anti-inflammatory drugs (NSAIDs) and to be aware that enteric-coated medications cannot be crushed because they are designed to protect the stomach by dissolving in the duodenum.
5. Encourage the client to seek ongoing evaluation by the physician, as new arthritis medications such as celecoxib (Celebrex) are continually being developed and trialed.

Nursing Management: Fractured Hip

NOTE: Nursing interventions may vary depending on whether the older client has an open reduction/internal fixation fracture (ORIF) or total hip arthroplasty (THA).

1. Maintain postoperative positioning as appropriate to the client's form of treatment.
2. Provide adequate pain control before physical therapy and on an ongoing basis throughout the recovery process.
3. Prevent complications, including skin breakdown, RTIs, infections at the surgical site, and dislocation of the prosthesis or internal fixation device.
4. Facilitate and monitor with the registered nurse the client's consistent use of antiembolism stockings as ordered and the administration of anticoagulant medications and the related monitoring of lab values, to decrease the risk of pulmonary embolism (which can be a significant risk to older clients after hip fracture and/or hip replacement).
5. Teach the client about fall prevention. Evaluate the client's environment (home, room, bathroom) for safety with regard to mobility and make recommendations for rectifying any threats to safety.

Neurological System

The following neurological changes result from the aging process:

- Neurons in the brain decrease in number, resulting in decreased production of neurotransmitters and, thus, reduced synaptic transmission.
- Cerebral blood flow and oxygen utilization decrease.
- Time required to carry out motor and sensory tasks requiring speed, coordination, balance, and fine-motor hand movements increases.
- Short-term memory may somewhat diminish without much change in long-term memory.
- Night sleep disturbances occur because of more frequent and longer wakeful periods.
- Deep-tendon reflexes decrease, although reflexes at the knees remain fairly intact.

Many disorders that affect the neurological system are not unique to elders; however, the risk of acquiring one of these disorders increases with age. One of the most common diagnoses among elders in long-term care facilities is dementia, particularly one form of dementia called Alzheimer's disease (AD). **Dementia** is an organic brain pathology characterized by losses in intellectual functioning. The clinical manifestations associated with dementia are never considered normal aging changes.

PROFESSIONAL TIP

Neurological System in the Older Adult

In the absence of pathology, intellect and capacity for learning remain unchanged with aging.

PROFESSIONAL TIP

Mental Health in the Older Adult

Mood disorders including depression, bipolar disorder, anxiety disorders, late-onset psychosis, sleep disorders, substance abuse, schizophrenia (chronic and late-onset), and other psychiatric diseases certainly occur among older clients and often go unaddressed or are ineffectively treated. Appropriate assessment, treatment, and clinical management of these clients require effective interdisciplinary teams comprising a geriatric psychiatrist; a neurologist; a clinical nurse specialist specializing in gerontology and mental health; a licensed social worker; a clinical pharmacist; other multidisciplinary team members (including direct care nurses and staff and activity therapists); and the client's family and, whenever possible, the client.

It is important for care providers to assess the length of onset of confusion or cognitive changes in the client. Generally, dementia describes declines that have a slow onset of greater than 6 months, whereas **delirium** (or acute confusion) describes cognitive changes that have a shorter onset of 6 months or less. Acute confusion can occur independently or as an exacerbation of a current dementia-related disorder in the client. Acute confusion can result from many stresses such as infections, medication side effects, drug interactions, metabolic imbalances, dehydration, or injuries from falls (e.g., subdural hematomas). Elimination of the causative factor can often turn the acute confusion around in a relatively short period to the preexacerbation level of functioning, unless further pathology to the brain has occurred.

Nursing Management: Alzheimer's Disease

1. Before diagnosis, encourage a medical and psychological diagnostic workup including a mental status examination.
2. Facilitate orientation in the early stages of the disease with calendars, lists, and consistent schedules.
3. Arrange an environment that is therapeutic, consistent, calm, and safe and that alternates rest with activities that require the use of long-practiced skills.
4. Encourage and facilitate access for the client and family to support groups where they can independently share their feelings and concerns and have questions addressed.
5. When assistance is needed with ADLs, implement consistent routines with consistent caregivers but allow for delay of care if needed because of client stress or irritability. Encourage independence of the client while assisting with ADLs (e.g., offer a warm washcloth for client to wash the face and assist with those ADLs that the client cannot complete without assistance).
6. Monitor general health status. Treat any underlying medical problems. Provide adequate pain control, as

needed, and monitor for lack of sleep to minimize the risk of violent behavior. Observe for the client's better times of the day, and plan activities or interventions accordingly.

7. Build a trusting relationship with the client. Use clear, simple directions and treat clients with respect and as individuals, building on their strengths and their unique interests and histories. Doing so demonstrates appreciation for the individual and can help build the client's self-esteem.

8. Be aware that as much is communicated to the AD client through the caregiver's nonverbal behavior and tone and volume of voice as is communicated through actual words. A calm attitude allows the client time to process and retrieve information when spoken to or asked a question.

9. Support the client's mobility within a safe environment, recognizing that as the disease progresses, baseline wandering often increases as a coping skill, whereas verbal communication often decreases. Beanbag chairs, low mattresses, bed and chair alarms, positional (antisliding) wedges for chairs, merry walkers that support independent mobility, and assisted-ambulation programs to build leg strength are all therapeutic interventions for AD clients as the disease progresses and represent preferable alternatives to the use of restraints.

10. Monitor for changes in baseline behaviors and for intensity of wandering (both pacing or lethargy), as either often indicates underlying infections, metabolic imbalances, or stress. Encourage clients to alternate periods of activity and rest.

Nursing Management: Depression

1. Assess for signs of a physical basis for any fatigue (e.g., infection, pain, altered nutritional status, or shortness of breath upon exertion).

2. Administer treatment for underlying physiologic problems, if applicable.

3. If symptoms persist, encourage the client to have a medical diagnostic workup with a geriatric psychiatrist, if such a workup has not yet been done.

4. Monitor for verbal or nonverbal signs of suicidal thoughts/intent. Determine whether the client has a plan.

5. Provide one-on-one supervision of the client as needed and assure the client that the caregiver will keep him safe. If appropriate for the client, seek an agreement that he will not try to harm himself.

6. Administer antidepressant medication as ordered. Provide client and family education regarding medication, including length of time before therapeutic results should occur, and potential side effects. Report immediately to the registered nurse and primary care provider any extrapyramidal side effects (e.g., tremors, drooling, pin rolling of the fingers, shuffling gait) that are observed.

7. If the client is not assessed as being at risk for suicide but is isolating in his room, establish small goals with the client (e.g., coming out of the room and sitting safely in the hallway with the nurse for 5 minutes two times per day and for meals). Advance to

more challenging goals as the client demonstrates increased tolerance for social interaction.

8. Facilitate the client's reintegration into a healthy support system and provide small community group time for the client to share his views.

Nursing Management: Transient Ischemic Attack

1. Assess for risk factors for stroke and for the existence of any previous carotid vascular tests for potential blockage (stenosis).

2. Provide client and family education explaining the relationship between risk factors and TIA and stroke.

3. Provide teaching to assist in reducing risk factors.

4. Monitor orthostatic blood pressure and encourage clients to change positions slowly to decrease the risk of falling.

Sensory Changes

The following sensory changes result from the aging process:

Vision

- With aging, the lens becomes less pliable and less able to increase its curvature in order to focus on near objects, causing presbyopia (trouble seeing objects up close) and decreased accommodation. The lens also yellows, causing distorted color perceptions, with greens and blues washing out and warm colors such as reds and oranges becoming more distinct. The incidence of cataracts also increases.

- Accommodation of pupil size decreases, resulting in both decreased adjustment to changes in lighting and decreased ability to tolerate glare. For instance, high-gloss tile floors in hallways can appear like hills and valleys to older clients, especially those with perceptual deficits; this may increase anxiety and safety risks.

- Vitreous humor changes in consistency, causing blurred vision. Changes in the anterior chamber may increase the pressure of the aqueous humor, resulting in glaucoma.

- Lacrimal glands secrete less fluids, causing dryness and itching. Entropion or ectropion (turning of the eyelids inward or outward) occasionally occurs in older clients. These conditions can not only impact vision, but can also increase the risk of infection caused by dryness and ineffective blinking. In these conditions, obtaining an order for artificial tears, lacrilube, and eye drop treatments for dryness or infection may be necessary.

Infection Control: Eye Care
To decrease infection risks, all caregivers should wash from the nose outward when washing clients' eyes.

Common vision disorders related to aging include the following:

- Presbyopia
- Cataract

- Glaucoma
- Age-related macular degeneration

Nursing Management: Visual Impairment

1. Teach visually impaired clients adaptive techniques for ADL, such as extra lighting.
2. Advise regular examination by an ophthalmologist.
3. Provide preoperative and postoperative care and teaching to clients undergoing cataract surgery, including lifting and bending restrictions as well as measures to prevent infection.
4. Teach proper eye drop administration techniques to all clients who are prescribed eye drops, including holding the drop in the eye with the lid closed for 30 seconds after administration.
5. Ensure that older clients have their glasses on when needed to decrease perceptual and spatial deficits.

Hearing

- As aging occurs, the pinna becomes less flexible, the hair cells in the inner ear stiffen and atrophy, and cerumen (earwax) increases.
- The number of neurons in the cochlea decrease, and the blood supply lessens, causing the cochlea and the ossicles to degenerate.
- Presbycusis, the impairment of hearing in older adults, is often accompanied by a loss of tone discrim-

ination. High-frequency tones are lost first; thus, keeping the voice low and calm and decreasing any background noise can improve the client's comprehension of the caregiver's message.

Nursing Management: Hearing Impairment

1. Assess for ear pain; drainage; inflammation; abnormalities; surgeries; perforations; or impacted cerumen.
2. Evaluate medication regimen and assess for ototoxicity, if medication history reveals such a risk.
3. Advise hearing testing by an audiologist, if the previous assessments are negative.
4. Monitor the care and use of a hearing aid by the older client with unilateral or bilateral aids. Provide teaching and assistance as needed for cleaning the hearing aid(s) and replacing batteries.
5. Instruct caregivers and family about the communication and socialization needs of the client. For some older clients, either the use of a small erasable board to augment verbal questions or communication with written text represents a therapeutic intervention for hearing impairment. If writing dexterity or ability is also impaired, a story board that has pictures indicating the client's needs (e.g., bathroom, food, rest) can assist the client to independently communicate needs to caregivers.

SAMPLE NURSING CARE PLAN

THE CLIENT WITH ALZHEIMER'S DISEASE (AD)

Mrs. Jane Rodriguez, 64 years old, was admitted to the Alzheimer's unit of a long-term care facility. Last month, Mrs. Rodriguez was visiting her daughter in another state and wandered away from the daughter's home. Mrs. Rodriguez was found 60 miles away, unharmed but completely disoriented and agitated. Mrs. Rodriguez had worked as a nursing assistant before she retired. She is a widow and has two children in the same community where the nursing home is located, in addition to the daughter who she was visiting in another state. Unless reminded, Mrs. Rodriguez does not shower or change clothes. She awakens at least once each night and asks for breakfast.

Nursing Diagnosis 1 *Disturbed Thought Processes* related to progressive dementia as evidenced by disorientation to time and place, loss of short-term memory, inability to concentrate, and periods of agitation

Nursing Outcomes Classification (NOC)
Memory
Cognitive Ability
Cognitive Orientation

Nursing Interventions Classification (NIC)
Dementia Management
Environmental Management

continues

SAMPLE NURSING CARE PLAN

PLANNING/GOALS	NURSING INTERVENTIONS	RATIONALE
Mrs. Rodriguez will remain calm and will not experience agitation and anxiety as a result of her disorientation and memory loss.	Provide Mrs. Rodriguez with clues for orientation: "Good morning, Mrs. Rodriguez. My name is Jean, and I will help you today." Avoid putting her on the spot.	Helps Mrs. Rodriquez cope with her environment.
	Place a large sign on Mrs. Rodriguez's door with her name printed in large letters.	Helps her find her room.
	Have family bring in snapshots and photos taken in past years.	Stimulates reminiscing and allows her to recall happy times.
	Avoid changing Mrs. Rodriguez's room. Always put items back in the same place.	Consistency reduces frustration.
	Consult with activities staff in planning self-expressive, non-fail activities that require little concentration (e.g., painting with nontoxic paints, modeling with nontoxic clay).	Prevents boredom, which can lead to irritation.
	If Mrs. Rodriguez is resistant to care, provide clear, simple, nonthreatening instructions and delay care as needed until she is calmer.	Often, delaying care for even 10 to 15 minutes when resistance is encountered improves client outcomes.

EVALUATION   Mrs. Rodriguez remained calm and showed no signs of agitation or anxiety.

Nursing Diagnosis 2 *Risk for Injury* related to risk factors of mode of transportation and cognitive and affective factors as evidenced by wandering behavior, impaired judgment, and disorientation

Nursing Outcomes Classification (NOC)	**Nursing Interventions Classification (NIC)**
Safety Behavior: Personal	*Environmental Management: Safety*
Safety Behavior: Home Physical Environment	*Dementia Management*

PLANNING/GOALS	NURSING INTERVENTIONS	RATIONALE
Mrs. Rodriguez will remain free of injury while retaining as much independence and freedom as possible.	Keep only nonpoisonous plants on the unit. Arrange furniture so that walkways are open. Pad sharp corners of tables and chests. Cover electrical outlets and hot radiators. Place electrical cords and telephone wires out of reach.	Does not recognize unsafe acts or conditions due to loss of impulse control and loss of judgment. Does not comprehend cause and effect.
	Provide assurance during fire drills.	Agitation increases especially when noise level is increased.

EVALUATION   Mrs. Rodriguez has experienced no injury.

Nursing Diagnosis 3 *Bathing/Hygiene and Dressing/Grooming Self-Care Deficit* related to perceptual or cognitive impairment (memory loss and sensory–perceptual deficits) as evidenced by needing a reminder to shower and change clothes

Nursing Outcomes Classification (NOC)	**Nursing Interventions Classification (NIC)**
Self-Care: Bathing	*Self-Care Assistance: Dressing/Grooming*
Self-Care: Hygiene	*Self-Care Assistance: Bathing/Hygiene*
Self-Care: Dressing	
Self-Care: Grooming	

continues

SAMPLE NURSING CARE PLAN

PLANNING/GOALS	NURSING INTERVENTIONS	RATIONALE
Mrs. Rodriguez will complete ADLs with minimal assistance now and with increasing assistance as the disease progresses.	Use verbal cues and hand-over-hand assistance with ADLs. Instruct staff to avoid doing tasks that Mrs. Rodriguez can do by herself. Watch for signs of frustration and irritation and intervene when appropriate.	Minimizes the need for assistance, thereby increasing feelings of self-esteem.
	Ask family to bring in clothing that is easy to manipulate. Set clothing out in the order it is to be put on.	Allow Mrs. Rodriquez to be more independent.
	Consider tub baths rather than showers. Provide privacy, check the temperature of the bathroom, and do not leave the client alone.	Showers may be threatening or confusing to persons with Alzheimer's disease. Tub baths are more relaxing.

EVALUATION   Mrs. Rodriguez participates in ADLs.

Nursing Diagnosis 4 *Disturbed Sleep Pattern* related to disorientation as evidenced by wakefulness at night

Nursing Outcomes Classification (NOC)	Nursing Interventions Classification (NIC)
Information Processing *Mood Equilibrium*	*Sleep Enhancement* *Simple Massage*

PLANNING/GOALS	NURSING INTERVENTIONS	RATIONALE
Mrs. Rodriguez will experience fewer periods of wakefulness during the night. If she awakens, she will remain calm and free of agitation.	Avoid stimulating activities prior to bedtime. Establish a consistent bedtime routine. Take Mrs. Rodriguez to the bathroom and allow sufficient time for complete bladder emptying.	Overstimulation prior to bedtime may increase anxiety, preventing sleep. A consistent bedtime routine is helpful.
	Help Mrs. Rodriguez with a sponge bath and with oral care; give her a back rub using warm lotion and slow, smooth strokes.	Provides relaxation.
	Provide a light snack of a warm, noncaffeinated beverage and a plain, easily digested cracker, cookie, or a piece of toast. Be patient and do not rush her.	Hunger or overeating can interfere with sleep.
	Question family concerning previous bedtime routines and sleeping habits.	Allows same routine to be followed.
	Repeat bedtime routine when Mrs. Rodriguez awakens during night.	Makes Mrs. Rodriguez think it is time to go to bed.
	Encourage a short nap early in the afternoon.	Sleep pattern disturbances may result from overfatigue.
	Avoid the use of sleeping medications.	Prevents confusion, disorientation, and restlessness.

EVALUATION   Mrs. Rodriguez sleeps through the night several times a week.

Endocrine System

The following endocrine changes result from the aging process:

- Alterations occur in both the reception and the production of hormones.
- Release of insulin by the beta cells of the pancreas slows, causing an increase in blood sugar.
- Thyroid changes may lower the basal metabolic rate.

The most common endocrine disorder related to aging is diabetes mellitus type 2.

Nursing Management: Diabetes Mellitus Type 2

1. Arrange for a consultation with a dietitian to assess nutritional status and to provide food-management instruction.
2. Teach the client, family members, or caregivers (as appropriate) the procedure for blood glucose monitoring specific to the equipment the client will be using.
3. Develop a personal exercise program with the client based on the client's physical condition, mental status, resources, and interests.
4. Provide information on prescribed oral hypoglycemic medications.
5. Teach the causes, signs, and treatment of hypoglycemia and hyperglycemia.
6. Advise on self-care and on careful monitoring of the extremities and of sores on the skin, to minimize threats to skin integrity.
7. Encourage the client to wear shoes and to have nails trimmed by a podiatrist, if unable to safely perform self-care.

Reproductive System: Female

The following reproductive changes result from the aging process:

- Estrogen production decreases with the onset of menopause.
- Ovaries, uterus, and cervix decrease in size.
- The vagina shortens, narrows, and becomes less elastic, and the vaginal lining thins. Secretions decrease and become more alkaline, resulting in increased incidence of atrophic vaginitis. These changes may result in discomfort during coitus, which can often be rectified with the use of a water-based lubricant. As at any age, protected intercourse (safe sex) through the use of a latex condom should be advised with new partners.
- Supporting musculature of the reproductive organs weakens, increasing the risk of uterine prolapse.
- Breast tissue diminishes, and nipple erection lessens during sexual arousal.
- Libido and the need for intimacy and companionship in older women remain unchanged (Figure 48-8).

Common female reproductive system disorders related to aging include the following:

- Breast cancer (the risk of which increases with age)
- Altered sexuality patterns related to physiologic changes, medications, changes in body image, or psy-

Figure 48-8 *Sexuality and companionship remain important throughout the life span.*

chosocial changes such as the loss of significant other or a move to a setting that provides some level of assistive care (i.e., group home, assisted living center, or care facility)

Nursing Management: Female Reproductive System Disorders

1. Teach and encourage monthly breast self-exams and yearly mammograms for early detection and treatment of disorders.
2. Establish rapport and encourage the client to verbalize feelings and concerns related to sexuality, body image, and self-esteem.
3. Complete a sexual history and recommend interventions based on findings. Support the client's needs for companionship and intimacy throughout the life span.
4. Recommend that a bone density scan (Dexa-Scan) be discussed with the client's primary care provider to allow for early detection and treatment of osteoporosis.
5. Encourage annual gynecological examinations with the client's primary care provider.

Reproductive System: Male

The following reproductive changes result from the aging process:

- Testosterone production decreases, resulting in decreased size of the testicles.
- Sperm count and viscosity of seminal fluid decrease.
- Although more time is required to obtain erection, the older man often finds that he and his partner can enjoy longer periods of lovemaking (greater control) before ejaculation. As at any age, protected intercourse (safe sex) through the use of a latex condom should be advised with new partners.
- The prostate gland may enlarge.
- Impotency may occur. Medications and other medical interventions have been successful in reversing impo-

tency problems in many older males. A thorough evaluation by the primary care provider and a urologist can provide clients with available options given health status and current medication regimen.

- Libido and the need for intimacy and companionship remain unchanged in older males.

Common male reproductive disorders related to aging include the following:

- Altered sexuality patterns related to physiologic changes, medications, changes in body image, or psychosocial changes such as the loss of significant other or a move to a setting that provides some level of assistive care (i.e., group home, assisted living center, or care facility)
- Benign prostatic hypertrophy (BPH)

Nursing Management: Male Reproductive System Disorders

1. Establish rapport and encourage the client to verbalize feelings and concerns related to sexuality, body image, and self-esteem.
2. Complete a sexual history and recommend interventions based on findings. Support the client's needs for companionship and intimacy throughout the life span.
3. Provide client and family education regarding the signs and symptoms of prostate disorders (e.g., difficulty in starting the urine stream, a smaller urine stream, frequent urination, frequent nighttime awakening for the purpose of urinating, or, in severe cases, the failure or inability to urinate).
4. Teach and encourage monthly testicular self-exam and yearly digital rectal examinations of the prostate gland by a primary care provider. The benefits of a PSA lab test performed every 1 to 2 years to facilitate early detection and treatment of prostate cancer are being researched and debated.

Integumentary System

The following integumentary changes result from the normal aging process:

- Subcutaneous tissue and elastin fibers diminish, causing the skin to become thinner and less elastic.
- Ability of melanocytes to produce even pigmentation diminishes, resulting in hyperpigmentation or liver spots, typically on the hands and wrists (Figure 48-9).
- Eccrine, apocrine, and sebaceous glands decrease in size, number, and function, resulting in diminished secretions and moisturization and, thus, pruritis.
- Body temperature regulation diminishes because of decreased perspiration and, many times, decreased circulation.
- Capillary blood flow decreases, resulting in slower wound healing.
- Blood flow decreases, especially to lower extremities.
- Vascular fragility causes senile purpura.
- Cutaneous sensitivity to pressure and temperature diminishes.
- Melanin production decreases, causing gray-white hair.

Figure 48-9 *Hyperpigmentation is a normal result of the aging process.*

- Scalp, pubic, and axillary hair thin, and women display increased facial hair on the upper lip and chin.
- Nail growth slows, nails become more brittle, and longitudinal nail ridges form.

Common integumentary disorders related to aging include the following:

- Pressure ulcers (alteration in skin integrity)
- Herpes zoster (shingles)
- Skin cancer (included because the risk of skin cancer increases with age)

Nursing Management: Alteration in Skin Integrity

1. Perform a pressure ulcer risk assessment upon the client's admission to the health care setting (Figure 48-10).
2. Implement pressure ulcer prevention protocol for clients at risk for pressure ulcer formation. It is important to consider and document pressure relieving interventions for all surfaces that the client will sit or lay on during the course of the day (Table 48-4).
3. Encourage adequate intake of protein and fluids to help ensure good skin integrity.

 Infection Control: Skin Integrity

It is a nursing responsibility to educate caregivers (including other staff members, as necessary) about the need to thoroughly wash and dry the client's perineal area and to keep linens and clothing clean and dry, especially when incontinence is a problem. Such education may also include instruction on maintaining client privacy; properly retracting, cleansing, and repositioning the foreskin of an uncircumcised older male client; and proper cleansing of the skin folds of an older female client's perineal area. Clients and caregivers should also be instructed to cleanse front to back only and to not rinse and reuse washcloths again or use them on other body areas. These simple hygiene and infection-control guidelines can help maintain the client's skin integrity and can also prevent unnecessary infections.

Date of assessment: _____ Nurse: _____
Pressure ulcer present on admission: No _____ Yes _____ Stage _____

A score of 11 or more places a client at risk for pressure ulcer formation. Preventive protocol should be established.

Activity		Total
Ambulant without assistance	0	
Ambulant with assistance	2	
Chairfast	4	
Bedfast	6	_____
Mobility—Range of Motion		
Full range of motion	0	
Moves with minimal assistance	2	
Moves with moderate assistance	4	
Immobile	6	_____
Skin Condition		
Hydrated and intact	0	
Rashes or abrasions	2	
Decreased turgor, dry	4	
Edema, erythema, pressure ulcers	6	_____
Predisposing Disease Process		
No involvement	0	
Chronic, stable	1	
Acute or chronic, unstable	2	
Terminal	3	_____

Level of Consciousness		Total
Alert	0	
Slow verbal response	1	
Responds to verbal or painful stimuli	2	
Absence of response to stimuli	3	_____
Nutritional Status		
Good (eats 75% or more of required intake)	0	
Fair (eats less than 75% of required intake)	1	
Poor (minimal intake, consistent weight loss)	2	
Unable/refuses to eat/drink, emaciated	3	_____
Incontinence—Bladder		
None	0	
Occasional (fewer than 2/24 hours)	1	
Usually (more than 2/24 hours)	2	
Total (no control)	3	_____
Incontinence—Bowel		
None	0	
Occasional (formed stool)	1	
Usually (semi-formed stool)	2	
Total (no control, loose stool)	3	_____

Figure 48-10 *Pressure Ulcer Risk Assessment*

Nursing Management: Herpes Zoster

1. Treat the pain.
2. Treat the ulcer with medications (e.g., acyclovir [Zovirax] topical cream), as ordered, to reduce the length of time of the outbreak.
3. Develop a plan to ensure continuity in meeting the client's psychosocial needs, and allow the client time to share concerns.

Infection Control: Herpes Zoster
Prevent cross-infection from drainage from the vesicular eruptions by practicing proper hand hygiene and implementing appropriate isolation procedures, especially if the client is in the hospital or another health care facility.

Nursing Management: Skin Cancer

1. Teach clients and caregivers both cancer prevention methods and skin self-examination to detect lesions early. Early detection and treatment of skin cancers are essential to optimal client outcomes.
2. Provide information in both verbal and written form and in collaboration with the client's multidisciplinary team, regarding treatment (surgery, chemotherapy, radiation, and other options).
3. Monitor for signs of infection at the lesion site.
4. Ensure that the client's psychological, psychosocial, spiritual, and dietary needs are also addressed.

FINANCING OLDER ADULT CARE

Since the 1960s, the U.S. Congress has developed and implemented a series of national entitlement programs to help ensure adequate income, housing, and access to medical care for older Americans. As the number of older clients (those older than age 65, particularly those older than age 85) continues to rise, caregivers and advocates for elder care should strive to understand the budgetary policies that have influenced and continue to influence the U.S. health care delivery system.

Medicare

Medicare (Title XVIII) is a nationwide health insurance program for Americans who are 65 years of age or older, for persons who are eligible for Social Security disability payments for longer than 2 years, and for certain workers and dependents who need kidney transplants or dialysis. The Health Care Financing Administration (HCFA) was the federal agency in charge of administering the Medicare program. Since July 2001, the HCFA is now the Centers for Medicare and Medicaid Services (CMS). More than the name has changed. Now there is an increased emphasis on responsiveness to beneficiaries and providers, and quality improvement (CMS, 2001).

The program was enacted as part of the Social Security Act of 1965 and became effective on June 1, 1966. It consists of two separate but coordinated pro-

TABLE 48-4   PROTOCOL FOR CLIENTS AT RISK FOR PRESSURE ULCERS

OBJECTIVE	INTERVENTIONS	OBJECTIVE	INTERVENTIONS
Relieve pressure	• Establish positioning schedule. • Place pressure relieving mattress on bed, cushions on chair. • Teach client wheelchair exercises. • Stand and/or ambulate client in chair frequently. • Use wheelchair for transporting only. • Allow client to sit on bedpan, commode, or toilet for only brief periods. • Check areas of pressure under casts, braces, splints, slings, prostheses.	Prevent spasticity and contractures	• Avoid quick, rough movements. • Do range-of-motion exercises at least twice daily. • Assess for synergy patterns when positioning. • Administer oral antispasmodics if ordered.
Relieve friction and shearing	• Use turning sheet for positioning in bed and chair. • Keep head of bed lower than 30 degrees unless contraindicated. • Use supportive devices to prevent sliding in chairs. • Use appropriate transfer techniques. • Do not use powder on skin. • Place bed cradle under top covers.	Maintain hydration/ nutritional status	• Assess nutritional status. • Investigate causes of anorexia. • Correct underlying nutritional deficits. • Encourage additional fluids, unless contraindicated. • Give high protein supplement, if necessary. • Monitor weight weekly.
Prevent moisture/ maceration	• Implement scheduled toileting or bladder retraining program. • Use absorbent incontinent briefs or pads. • Check incontinent clients frequently. Wash and rinse thoroughly. Apply moisture barrier. • Avoid use of plastic/rubber sheets, protectors.		Continue with routine skin care. Do skin checks with each position change.

grams: hospital insurance (called part A) and medical insurance (called part B), which covers physician's services, outpatient services, some medical supplies, and some skilled nursing and home health services. Medicare provides basic protection for the cost of health care but does not cover all expenses. Among the expenses *not* covered by Medicare for older Americans are those associated with the following:

• Home health care that does not require skilled personnel (e.g., as of February 1998, expenses for a home health visit [skilled] for the purpose of obtaining a blood sample are not covered)
• Nursing home care (except for skilled care for a limited time)
• Some routine medical checkups and related tests
• Prescription drugs
• Eye and hearing tests and eyeglasses and hearing aids
• Routine dental care and checkups

In the late 1990s, many insurance policies were available to supplement at varying levels the benefits paid by Medicare. This led many older clients to "stack" insur-

ance policies or to buy numerous overlapping policies for fear of being underinsured. The insurance industry and Congress worked together to outlaw stacking of Medicare supplement policies.

Although there has been some improvement in insurance coverage for preventive screening tests such as mammograms, the lack of reimbursement for prescription drugs continues to significantly burden older Americans, many of whom must choose between costly medications and food.

In 2001, more than 34 million older adults (age 65 and older) and more than 5 million disabled persons were enrolled in Medicare (CMS, 2002). Medicare Part B payments for 2001 were more than $59 billion (CMS, 2003).

Medicaid

The Medicaid program was also enacted as part of the Social Security Act of 1966 and is often referred to as Title XIX. This program, which is federally aided and state operated and administered, provides medical benefits to certain indigent, or low-income, Americans.

Nursing home bills represent a staggering burden for many older Americans who require nursing care. In 1995, nursing home bills averaged $22,000 per person per year, and projections showed that two-thirds of elders who lived alone would run out of savings after 13 weeks in a nursing home (Gallo, Paveza, Fulmer, 2003). Medicaid takes into account government-determined poverty levels when providing benefits, with coverage being extended to persons who are at certain percentages of the poverty level (e.g., 200% of poverty level, 150% of poverty level, and 100% of poverty level). Long-term care facilities serve both private-pay clients (those whose expenses are paid by themselves, their families, or their long-term care insurance policies) and Title XIX- (Medicaid-) funded clients. Medicaid coverage for long-term care is not available until a person's assets have been depleted to a certain set level. Elder care advocates continue in their efforts to protect the assets of the spouse who is able to stay in the family home after the other spouse must be placed in a nursing home.

To some in the United States, the debate over Social Security, Medicare, and Medicaid financing is viewed as someone else's priority; however, the moral responsibility for providing access to quality services and care for our country's elderly is shared by all Americans. Elder care services should be developed to promote independence yet should provide assistance when needed.

Omnibus Budget Reconciliation Act

The Omnibus Budget Reconciliation Act (OBRA), first enacted in 1987 and reenacted in 1990, sought to ensure quality services for older Americans. The act included guidelines for services that were required to be made available to seniors and promoted the rights of seniors. As was the case with all health care costs, however, elder care costs continued to rise in the United States, and discussions and proposed legislation for financial reforms intensified.

Balanced Budget Act of 1997

Among the most significant influences on the financing of elder care is the Balanced Budget Act (BBA) of 1997. The BBA replaced cost-based reimbursement for care provided in skilled nursing facilities (SNFs) with a prospective payment system (PPS) based on client assessment within a resource utilization group system (RUGS). Reimbursement for home health services also shifted to a PPS.

The BBA also states that discharge from hospitals to SNFs or home care for 10 common but as yet unpublished diagnosis-related groups (DRGs) is to be considered as a transfer for payment purposes. Medicare's goal was to make a single blended payment that combined the traditional hospital DRG payment and the payment for postacute care services to be shared by the providers.

The intended implications for practice included reduced reimbursement to some SNFs, fewer discharges from hospitals to independent facilities for subacute care or home care, and, thus, encouraged the creation of integrated delivery systems and managed care. In reality, however, it has become more difficult to find placement in SNFs for clients with complex needs, because the new

CRITICAL THINKING

Nurse Advocate
How can you, as a nurse, advocate for your older clients?

reimbursement system simply does not fund all of their health care needs.

These reimbursement and regulatory changes surely represent only the beginning of such efforts to balance resources and need as the U.S. population continues to age. Certainly, significant work lies ahead for advocates of quality elder care in the United States and the world. Nurses will play a vital role in the ensuing debates, for they will see firsthand the positive and negative outcomes of their clients.

Summary

- The elderly population is rapidly growing.
- Although many stereotypes and myths are associated with aging, elders are in fact very diverse in their characteristics.
- Health maintenance is as important for older adults as it is for younger persons. A healthy lifestyle can enhance the quality of life.
- Many changes are associated with aging. The disorders commonly seen among elders are often the results of pathology and are thus not considered a normal part of aging; however, the risk of acquiring these disorders increases with age.
- Nurses knowledgeable about aging can plan interventions that will prevent complications for which elders are at risk.
- Nurses have a responsibility to advocate for their older clients. Nurses should be active legislatively and should work collaboratively to develop elder-care services that are affordable, provide equal access for all older Americans, and promote optimal wellness and independence.

Review Questions

1. Which of the following statements is true?
    a. All people eventually become senile if they live long enough.
    b. People lose interest in sex as they age.
    c. Most elders are financially impoverished.
    d. Incontinence is not an expected or normal change of aging.

CASE STUDY

Mr. Jack Baroni, a 72-year-old male, was admitted to the skilled care facility for rehabilitation following an open reduction, internal fixation of the right hip. Mr. Baroni had fallen while going up the stairs of his home, suffering an intertrochanteric, comminuted fracture of the right femur. He has no recollection of what caused him to fall. He is married and, until his surgery, was working part time as a school-crossing guard. While in the hospital, Mr. Baroni exhibited mental status changes including disorientation and confusion. His wife reports that he never had this problem prior to the surgery. He is continent of bowel and bladder. Mr. Baroni was in relatively good health until the fall. He and his wife agree that he should return home after rehabilitation is complete.

The following questions will guide your development of a nursing care plan for the case study.

1. Identify specific admission assessments that would be required for Mr. Baroni because of his age and condition.
2. Identify complications for which Mr. Baroni is at risk.
3. List interventions to prevent each complication.
4. Cite possible reasons for Mr. Baroni's fall.
5. Describe methods for assessing Mr. Baroni's mental status.
6. Describe possible reasons for his altered mental status.
7. Write three individualized nursing diagnoses and goals for Mr. Baroni.
8. List nursing actions related to altered mental status.
9. List four successful outcomes for Mr. Baroni.
10. Develop a teaching plan for Mr. Baroni.
11. List the community resources Mr. Baroni may need after discharge.

2. The programmed aging theory states that:
   a. stress causes structural and chemical changes in the body, which, in turn, cause aging.
   b. a genetic clock determines the speed at which people age.
   c. changes in collagen are the cause of aging.
   d. the decreasing ability to produce T-cell differentiation causes aging.

3. The elderly individual can reduce the potential for acquiring RTIs by:
   a. obtaining an influenza vaccine each year.
   b. staying inside throughout the winter.
   c. avoiding exercise.
   d. limiting fluid intake.

4. Research indicates that:
   a. weight-bearing exercise is not recommended for elders.
   b. high-intensity resistance training can improve muscle strength in elders.
   c. muscle deterioration in elders is to be expected.
   d. walking is the only healthy exercise for elders.

5. Integumentary changes associated with aging include:
   a. increased glandular secretions.
   b. increased capillary blood flow.
   c. increased melanin production.
   d. increased vascular fragility.

References/Suggested Readings

Administration on Aging (AoA). (2001). *The Administration on Aging and the Older American's Act.* [Online] Available: www.aoa.dhhs.gov/aoa/pages/aoafact.html

Administration on Aging (AoA). (2002). *Income and poverty among the elderly.* [Online]. Available: www.aoa.gov

American Association of Retired Persons (AARP). (1998). *A profile of older Americans.* Washington, DC: Department of Health and Human Services.

Andersen, C. (1999). *Antecedents, correlates, and impact of violent behaviors in the elderly VA client.* Unpublished thesis, University of Iowa, Iowa City, IA.

Andersen, C. F. (1998). *Nursing student to nursing leader: The critical path to leadership development.* Clifton Park, NY: Thomson Delmar Learning.

Centers for Medicare & Medicaid Services (CMS). (2001). *Introducing CMS.* [Online]. Available: http://cms.hhs.gov/about/reorg.asp

Centers for Medicare & Medicaid Services (CMS). (2002). *Medicare aged and disabled enrollees by type of coverage.* [Online]. Available: http://cms.hhs.gov/statistics/enrollment/natltrends/hi_smi.asp

Centers for Medicare & Medicaid Services (CMS). (2003). *Medicare Part B physicians supplier data.* [Online]. Available: http://cms.hhs.gov/data/betos/cy2001.asp

Collins, J. (2002). Helping an older patient eat well to stay well. *Nursing2002, 32*(11), 32hn6–32hn8.

Dochterman, J., & Bulechek, G. (2004). *Nursing interventions classifications (NIC)* (4th ed.). St. Louis, MO: Mosby.

Estes, M. E. Z. (2002). *Health assessment & physical examination* (2nd ed.). Clifton Park, NY: Thomson Delmar Learning.

Gallo, J., Paveza, G., Fulmer, T. (2003). *Handbook of geriatric assessment.* Gaithersburg, MD: Jones & Bartlett.

Hamilton, S. (2001). Detecting dehydration & malnutrition in the elderly. *Nursing2001, 31*(12), 56–57.

Hogstel, M. (Ed.). (2001). *Gerontology: Nursing care of the older adult.* Clifton Park, NY: Thomson Delmar Learning.

Kimbell, S. (2001). Before the fall: Keeping your patient on his feet. *Nursing2001, 31*(8), 44–45.

Logue, R. (2002). Self-medication and the elderly: How technology can help. *AJN, 102*(7), 51–55.

Moorhead, S., Johnson, M., & Maas, M. (2004). *Nursing Outcomes Classification (NOC).* (3rd ed.). St. Louis, MO: Mosby.

National Council on Aging (NCOA). (2001). *Sexual Survey.* [Online]. Available: www.ncoa.org/content.cfm?sectionID=109&detail=134

National Council on Aging (NCOA) (2002). Facts about older Americans. [Online]. Available: www.ncoa.org/content.cfm=sectionID.106

Peskin, B. (1999). *Beyond the zone.* Houston, TX: Noble.

Social Security Administration (SSA). (2000). The president signs the "Senior Citizens' Freedom to Work Act of 2000." [Online] Available: www.ssa.gov/legislation/legis_bulletin_040700.html

Steffen, K. (2003). When your trauma patient is over 65. *Nursing2003, 33*(4), 53–56.

Stein, A. (2003). Aging is more than skin deep. *Nursing2003, 33*(2), 32hn7–32hn8.

Victor, K. (2001). Properly assessing pain in the elderly. *RN, 64*(5), 45–49.

Wilkinson, J. (1999). *A family caregiver's guide to planning and decision making for the elderly.* Minneapolis, MN: Fairview Press.

Resources

Administration on Aging (AoA), Washington, DC 20201, 202-619-0724, www.aoa.gov

American Association of Geriatric Psychiatry, 7910 Woodmont Avenue, Suite 1050, Bethesda, MD 20814-3004, 301-654-7850, www.aagpgpa.org

American Association of Retired Persons (AARP), 601 E Street N.W., Washington, DC 20049, 800-424-3410, www.aarp.org

American Geriatrics Society, The Empire State Building, 350 Fifth Avenue, Suite 801, New York, NY 10118, 212-308-1414, www.americangeriatrics.org

American Nurses Association (ANA), Council on Gerontological Nursing Practice, 600 Maryland Avenue S.W., Suite 100W, Washington, DC 20024, 800-274-4262, www.nursingworld.org

National Council on Aging, Inc. (NCOA), 300 D Street, S.W., Suite 801, Washington, DC 20024, 202-479-1200, www.ncoa.org

INTEGRATION

MAKING THE CONNECTION

Through careful study of Basic Nursing and Adult Health Nursing, a knowledge base was developed in preparation for the critical thinking exercises in this chapter. Each critical thinking exercise begins with an index of the body systems relevant to the case study. It may be useful to refer back to these chapters while working through the case study.

LEARNING OBJECTIVES

Upon completion of this chapter, you should be able to:
- **Integrate how a condition affects several body systems and causes multiple clinical problems.**

INTRODUCTION

The format of this chapter is different than that of the other chapters. It provides an opportunity to use critical thinking skills and problem-solving techniques to several case studies in which the condition affects more than one body system. Application of information learned in previous chapters is needed to integrate a holistic view of how multiple body systems are affected. An example is diabetes that affects other body systems such as the integumentary, nervous, musculoskeletal, cardiac, vascular, blood, gastrointestinal, urinary, and reproductive.

Read the case study, then analyze how the condition affects other body systems. It may be helpful to first outline the condition presented in the case study by making a grid of the signs and symptoms, pathophysiology, diagnostic studies, and nursing interventions. Refer to the grid when answering the questions.

The case study questions can be completed alone, in a study group, or in a classroom setting. When completed, share the answers and charts with the entire group to enhance everyone's learning experience. Remember, each student or group of students may arrive at the answers or present the answers in a different manner. The process followed is less important than the opportunity to integrate all aspects of the condition and use critical thinking skills, as long as sound, logical nursing judgment is utilized in obtaining an appropriate answer. This is an opportunity to think creatively and freely.

SYSTEMS REVIEWED IN DIABETES EXERCISE

- Cardiovascular system
- Urinary system
- Neurological system
- Sensory system
- Endocrine system
- Reproductive systems
- Integumentary system

DIABETES EXERCISE

Mr. Brannen, a 46-year-old insurance salesman, is admitted to the hospital with the diagnosis of diabetes type 1.

- List the etiological risk factors for diabetes type 1.
- Brainstorm subjective and objective data that would be included in the assessment of Mr. Brannen.
- Develop a patho-flow diagram identifying the symptoms Mr. Brannen may have been experiencing on admission and relate the pathophysiology of diabetes to the symptoms (see the examples of a patho-flow diagram in Figure 49-1 and an interrelationship chart in Figure 49-2).
- What diagnostic tests could the physician have ordered to confirm the diagnosis of diabetes?
- Relate the possible results of the diagnostic tests to the pathophysiological cause of the results on the patho-flow diagram.
- If Mr. Brannen had been diagnosed with diabetes type 2, how would the pathophysiology and nursing care vary?

A couple of days after Mr. Brannen was diagnosed with diabetes he said to the nurse, "One of my friends at work said there are a lot of future problems with diabetes. I am concerned about this. What are some of the problems? What can I do not to have these problems?"

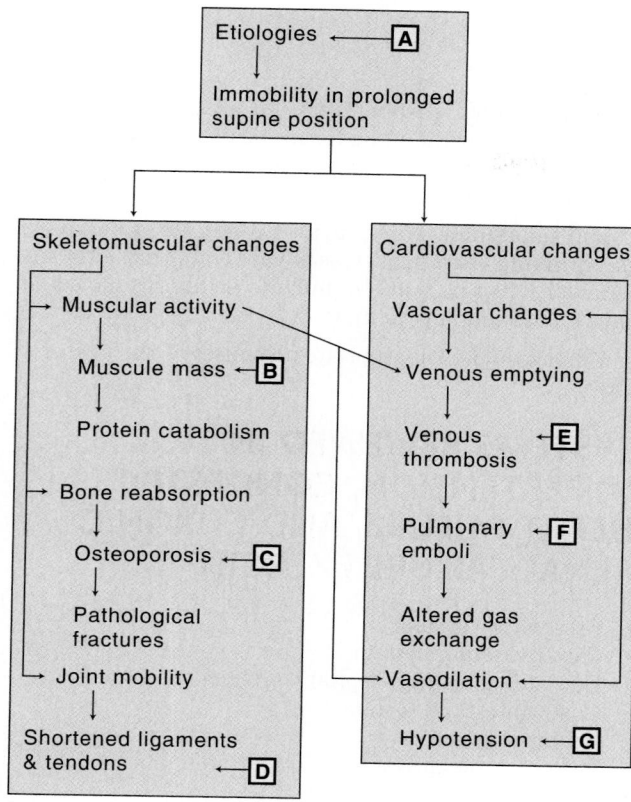

Figure 49-1 *An example of a patho-flow diagram of skeletomuscular and cardiovascular changes caused by immobility. Complete the following instructions corresponding to the letters located at specific points along the pathophysiologic sequence of events.* **A,** *List the risk conditions that may lead to immobility.* **B,** *Name the assessment data at this point.* **C,** *List the interventions that would minimize calcium loss.* **D,** *Name the outcome criteria associated with effective nursing interventions at this point.* **E,** *State the assessment data at this point.* **F,** *List the interventions that may prevent the development of this complication.* **G,** *List the nursing interventions to minimize this consequence. (Courtesy of the* Journal of Nursing Education*)*

- What would be appropriate responses of the nurse?
- List local resources or support groups where Mr. Brannen and his family could be referred.

The discharge teaching included insulin administration, diet, exercise, foot care, and eye exams.

- What is important to include in the discharge teaching regarding:

insulin administration
diet
exercise
foot care
eye exams

- Develop a care plan for Mr. Brannen.

Eight years after Mr. Brannen was diagnosed with diabetes, he had a routine physical examination. At that time his BP was 174/96. The physician monitored the BP

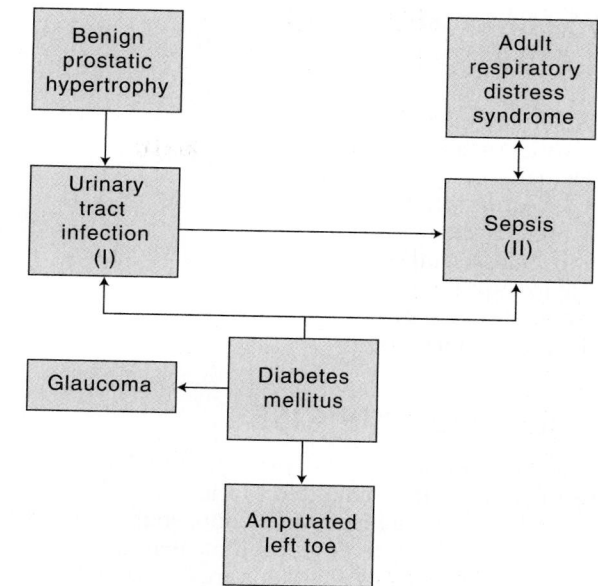

Figure 49-2 *Interrelationships of Conditions and Symptoms. (Courtesy of the* Journal of Nursing Education*)*

for 3 weeks and then placed Mr. Brannen on enalapril maleate (Vasotec). His urine had a trace of albumin.

- Physiologically, what could be occurring to cause Mr. Brannen to have hypertension, which is a common complication of diabetes?
- How does the action of enalapril maleate (Vasotec) lower the BP?
- What is the rationale for placing Mr. Brannen on enalapril maleate (Vasotec) rather than propranolol hydrochloride (Inderal), verapamil (Calan), or clonidine hydrochloride (Catapres)?
- What other complications could have a circulatory etiology?
- What could be the possible long-term renal complication from diabetes mellitus?
- Explain the pathophysiology of renal complications as they relate to diabetes. Relate these to the patho-flow diagram previously developed.

One evening, Mr. Brannen was massaging his foot while watching television. He noticed an ulcerated area between his third and fourth toe.

- State possible reasons Mr. Brannen may not have felt pain from the ulcerated area. Relate these to the patho-flow diagram previously developed.

During a yearly physical, Mr. Brannen relates difficulty obtaining an erection.

- Explain the rationale for this complication.
- What nursing interventions would be appropriate at this time?

In later years, Mr. Brannen may experience some symptoms from autonomic neuropathies.

- List symptoms that may occur and relate the symptoms to the pathophysiological etiology.

SYSTEMS REVIEWED IN CIRRHOSIS EXERCISE

- Respiratory system
- Cardiovascular system
- Hematologic and Lymphatic systems
- Gastrointestinal system
- Urinary system
- Musculoskeletal system
- Neurological system
- Endocrine system
- Integumentary system

CIRRHOSIS EXERCISE

Ben Whitehorse, a 60-year-old male of Native American descent, is admitted to the hospital with hematemesis. He has a history of alcohol abuse. Ben's wife and two daughters accompany him. Ben is 5'10" tall and weighs 140 lbs. His vital signs are T 98.2, AP 98 and slightly irregular, R 24, BP 152/88. He is lethargic, confused, and jaundiced. When the nurse assesses his lung sounds, she hears pulmonary crackles in all lobes. His abdominal girth measures 44 inches. His wife states he has not gone to the bathroom all morning. He has +3 edema in his feet and ankles. Ben's primary diagnosis is hematemesis with a secondary diagnosis of cirrhosis.

- Brainstorm other subjective and objective data that are important to include in the assessment of Ben Whitehorse.
- Relate the pathophysiology of cirrhosis to the assessed symptoms and other symptoms Ben may have experienced. Develop a patho-flow chart relating the symptoms to the pathological cause.
- List diagnostic tests that would be appropriate for the physician to order for Ben. What abnormal laboratory results would be typical of cirrhosis?
- Relate the possible results of the diagnostic tests to the developed patho-flow chart.
- Besides alcohol abuse, what are some other causes of cirrhosis?
- List complications of cirrhosis caused by chronic alcohol abuse.
- Explain the pathophysiology of portal hypertension as it relates to cirrhosis. Relate these to the patho-flow chart previously developed.
- List diuretics that may be ordered for Ben to decrease the ascites.
- How does the action of lactulose (Cephulac) lower the level of ammonia in the blood?
- What other complications result from portal hypertension?
- Explain the rationale for the complication of pleural effusion.
- Identify possible nursing diagnoses for Ben.
- What nursing interventions would be appropriate at this time?
- Develop a care plan for Ben Whitehorse.
- If Ben's condition improved and he was scheduled for discharge, what is important to include in the discharge teaching regarding:

bleeding tendencies

exercise
nutrition
skin care

- Develop diet instructions for Ben Whitehorse. Consider cultural influence in the diet instructions.
- List local resources/support groups where Ben and his family could be referred.

Ben's daughter, Mary, says, "I wish Dad would have quit drinking years ago. I was always embarrassed by his behavior when he had too much to drink. His life could have had so much potential."

- What would be appropriate responses of the nurse?

SYSTEMS REVIEWED IN HYPERTENSION, CONGESTIVE HEART FAILURE, AND CHRONIC RENAL FAILURE EXERCISE

- Respiratory system
- Cardiovascular system
- Hematologic and Lymphatic systems
- Gastrointestinal system
- Urinary system
- Musculoskeletal system
- Neurological system
- Endocrine system
- Reproductive systems
- Integumentary system
- Immune system

HYPERTENSION, CONGESTIVE HEART FAILURE, AND CHRONIC RENAL FAILURE EXERCISE

Mary Butler, a 40-year-old African American female, has a 20-year history of hypertension. She has been noncompliant in taking her antihypertensive medications that were prescribed by her physician. She has recently developed symptoms of congestive heart failure and renal failure.

- Brainstorm some reasons for Mary's noncompliance.
- Name some medications that may have been prescribed to treat Mary's hypertension. List the advantage and disadvantage of each medication.
- Using Table 36-3 (page 1023) Effects of Chronic Renal Failure by Body System, develop a concept map showing the relationship of hypertension to the effects of renal failure on each listed system.
- What is the relationship between hypertension, increased peripheral resistance, cardiac hypertrophy, and congestive heart failure?
- What is the relationship of blood pressure (hypotension and hypertension) and renal failure?
- What is the relationship between the heart's decreasing ability to pump blood through the blood vessels and pulmonary edema?
- Explain the relationship between fluid in the alveoli and dyspnea.

- Physiologically, what is occurring in Mary's body to cause an increased rate of respiration?
- List laboratory results that would indicate that Mary is developing chronic renal failure.
- List symptoms that would indicate Mary is developing chronic renal failure.
- List subjective and objective data for which the nurse would assess for symptoms of chronic renal failure.
- List laboratory results that would indicate that Mary is developing congestive heart failure.
- List symptoms that would indicate Mary is developing congestive heart failure. Give the cause/etiology for each symptom.
- List subjective and objective data for which the nurse would assess for symptoms of congestive heart failure.
- Identify possible nursing diagnoses for Mary.
- List nursing interventions and give rationale for each intervention.

Mary's abdomen is distended and she has lost her appetite for the last 2 days. She has had hiccups constantly for 2 hours. She says, "I am so tired of these hiccups. Why am I having them?"

- Explain to Mary the cause for her hiccups.

SYSTEMS REVIEWED IN PARKINSON DISEASE EXERCISE

- Respiratory system
- Gastrointestinal system
- Urinary system
- Musculoskeletal system
- Neurological system
- Sensory system
- Integumentary system

PARKINSON DISEASE EXERCISE

Mr. Kane is a 76-year-old man who has been exposed to several chemicals during his farming career. For the last 7 years, he has walked with his arms flexed, leaning forward with his head bowed. Recently, he has had some difficulty rising from a chair and balancing himself when he walks. He fell twice when doing odd jobs around the house. He has started making a "to-do list" because he has difficulty remembering. He may go to the store for three items but return with only two. His wife noticed that he has a slight tremor in his hand when he eats and often rolls his forefinger and thumb together in a circular motion.

- Use deductive reasoning and identify Mr. Kane's possible diagnosis.
- With these symptoms, what diagnostic tests may the doctor order?

Mr. Kane shared his symptoms with his family physician. After some tests were completed and results of referrals to specialists were returned, the physician told Mr. Kane he was suspecting Parkinson disease. Mr. Kane said, "Tell me about Parkinson disease."

- Relate what Mr. Kane could be taught about Parkinson disease.
- List objective and subjective data needed to make an appropriate and thorough assessment on Mr. Kane.

- List etiological causes of Parkinson disease. What possible etiological factors does Mr. Kane have?
- Explain the function of dopamine, a neurotransmitter, to the symptoms displayed in a client with Parkinson disease.
- List drugs that interfere in the synthesis and storage of dopamine.
- List the signs and symptoms of Parkinson disease. Think of a client with Parkinson disease, and relate his or her symptoms to the textbook symptoms.
- Develop a patho-flow map relating the pathophysiology of Parkinson disease to the systems that could be affected and the typical symptoms of that system.
- List drugs that Mr. Kane may receive, and relate the drugs to the symptoms that may be controlled. List the symptoms and side effects that need monitoring with each of the drugs listed.

Mr. Kane is becoming more rigid, having difficulty swallowing food, falling frequently, reaching for items to assist in ambulating, experiencing frequent incontinence, complaining of his eyes itching, and having severe memory loss. His voice has become soft, and his speech is slurred.

- List Mr. Kane's autonomic symptoms.
- Develop diet instructions for Mr. Kane and his wife.
- What possible surgical procedures could be done to relieve Mr. Kane's symptoms.
- Develop a nursing care plan for Mr. Kane listing nursing diagnoses, goals, and nursing interventions to address each symptom.
- Using the Internet, research new therapies for Parkinson disease, and share them with other students.

After a year, Mr. Kane is unable to walk and has to be lifted from his bed to his wheelchair. He is unable to verbally communicate. He no longer has bladder control. When he was fed his lunch, he started coughing and perhaps aspirated some food.

- List appropriate subjective and objective data needed in a nursing assessment.
- Reevaluate the previously developed nursing care plan and revise appropriately.

Summary

This may be the first time anatomy and physiology were related to a disease process, or understanding was gained as to why clients have particular symptoms with a specific disease or condition. Ill clients rarely have only one problem but several inter-related problems. These exercises provide an opportunity to think through situations before they are encountered in a clinical situation. The case studies asked pertinent questions, evaluated clinical situations, and allowed the student to make clinical decisions, much the way it is done in the clinical environment. Analyzing and synthesizing skills were utilized to work through these questions. Perhaps a renewed interest and amazement at the complexity of the body was gained while discovering the inter-relatedness of the body systems. Hopefully, these integration exercises and the critical thinking experience are catalysts to becoming a proficient, critical thinking nurse.

SECTION III
MATERNAL &
PEDIATRIC NURSING

Unit 17: Nursing Care of the Client:
Childbearing

Unit 18: Nursing Care of the Client:
Childrearing

UNIT
17

Nursing Care of the Client: Childbearing

PRENATAL CARE

MAKING THE CONNECTION

Refer to the following chapters to increase your understanding of prenatal care:

Basic Nursing
• **Basic Nutrition**

Adult Health Nursing
• **Reproductive Systems**

LEARNING OBJECTIVES

Upon completion of this chapter, you should be able to:
• **Define key terms.**
• **Discuss historical factors affecting pregnancy and childbirth.**
• **Describe fetal development from conception to birth.**
• **Identify the physical and psychological maternal changes during pregnancy.**
• **Describe the assessments to be performed at each prenatal visit.**
• **Discuss the nutritional needs of a woman during pregnancy.**
• **List the discomforts of pregnancy and one way a client might alleviate each.**
• **Use the nursing process to plan care for a pregnant client.**

KEY TERMS

abortion	linea nigra
age of viability	meconium
amenorrhea	morula
amnion	multigravida
anticipatory guidance	multipara
ballottement	nesting
blastocyst	nulligravida
Braxton-Hicks	nullipara
contractions	para
Chadwick's sign	physiologic anemia
chloasma	of pregnancy
chorion	pica
coitus	placenta
colostrum	postterm
copulation	prenatal care
cotyledon	preterm
couvade	primigravida
decidua	primipara
ductus arteriosus	pseudocyesis
ductus venousus	psychoprophylaxis
fertilization	quickening
foramen ovale	striae gravidarum
fundus	supine hypotensive syn-
funic souffle	drome
Goodell's sign	teratogen
GP/TPAL	term
gravida	umbilical cord
Hegar's sign	uterine souffle
implantation	vernix caseosa
lanugo	Wharton's jelly
Leopold's maneuvers	zygote

INTRODUCTION

For centuries, birth was part of family life and took place at home. Women learned about pregnancy and childbirth by asking female family members or friends and by being present when other women gave birth. In the United States in 1900, more than 90% of births were in the home.

In 1908, the American Red Cross and the Maternity Center Association offered the first formal programs for prenatal education. These early classes taught women about pregnancy, nutrition, and health care during pregnancy. By the 1950s, the classes included preparation for birth. In 1960, the American Society for

Psychoprophylaxis in Obstetrics (ASPO/Lamaze) and the International Childbirth Education Association (ICEA) were founded. They both promote the idea that birth is a healthy process and that parents should have choices about the process.

In 1969, the Nurses Association of the American College of Obstetricians and Gynecologists (NAACOG) was formed with a goal of improving the health of women and newborn infants. The organization was renamed the Association of Women's Health, Obstetric and Neonatal Nurses (AWHONN) in 1993. In conjunction with the American Nurses Association, AWHONN offers certification examinations for nurses engaged in obstetrical-gynecological nursing.

Today, many couples postpone pregnancy to obtain advanced education or establish careers; they may expect to participate in every aspect of the pregnancy, including decision making, and are much more informed than in the past of the educational offerings available. Today's nurse must have a firm understanding of the physical and psychological changes brought about by pregnancy, as well as the application of the nursing process in meeting the needs of the childbearing family.

PRECONCEPTION EDUCATION AND CARE

It has long been known that prenatal education and care identifies and reduces some problems in pregnancy and improves many outcomes. Yet, the United States ranks 27th in infant mortality rankings of industrialized nations in the world (CDC, 2001). More perinatal health experts are recognizing that a healthy pregnancy begins before conception.

Preconception education and care are focused on helping a couple prepare to conceive and identifying their reproductive risks before conception. The main goal is to protect the fetus during embryogenesis. Unhealthy habits can harm the fetus before the mother knows she is pregnant. Adopting a healthy lifestyle before pregnancy means eating a low-fat, high-fiber diet rich in vegetables and fruits; exercising at least 3 times a week; and getting to within 15 pounds of one's ideal weight. To prevent neural tube defects, all women who could possibly become pregnant should have an intake of 400 mcg of folic acid from a vitamin supplement and/or fortified foods and eat a healthful diet (Hasenau & Covington, 2002). Another goal is to help the couple identify genetic factors that may affect a pregnancy. Several of the topics covered in preconception visits are discussed following.

Immunizations and Disease Status

Immunization status should be confirmed, and testing for infectious diseases such as syphilis, hepatitis, HIV, chlamydia, gonorrhea, human papilloma virus, and herpes simplex should be performed. These diseases can be treated to minimize adverse effects on the mother and fetus. Some states, such as New York, also test for group B streptococcus. Needed immunizations, especially rubella and hepatitis B, should be completed before a pregnancy is begun. Chronic diseases such as hypertension, cardiac

disease, diabetes, epilepsy, thyroid dysfunction, asthma, renal disease, and phenylketonuria should be under control for the best outcome of pregnancy.

Medications

Known teratogens to be avoided are warfarin (Coumadin), gold salts, isotretinoin (Accutane), valproic acid (Depakene), lithium (Eskalith), diazepam (Valium), phenytoin (Dilantin), tetracycline, diethylstilbestrol, DES (stilphostrol), live-virus vaccines, and folic acid antagonists. Taking any medication, either over-the-counter (OTC) or prescription, should first be discussed with the health care provider. It is best to have the system cleared of medications before conception, if possible.

Smoking, Alcohol, and Illicit Drugs

Smoking, alcohol, and illicit drugs all have negative effects on pregnancy. Smoking is associated with major risk factors for pregnancy and low-birth-weight infants. There is no safe level of alcohol consumption in pregnancy (Allard-Hendren, 2000). Use of illicit drugs can lead to any number of fetal anomalies or disorders. The newborn can experience withdrawal syndrome depending on what substance the mother uses, the amount taken, and when taken relative to the birth of the infant. Clients should be encouraged to discontinue use of these substances before and throughout pregnancy.

Genetic Risk Factors

A review of family history helps identify genetic risk factors. If any are identified, the couple is encouraged to have genetic counseling. Genetic services may be used preconceptually to determine the risk to a fetus of a particular disorder that has appeared in either parent's family, or by individuals believed to be at risk for a genetic dis-

CRITICAL THINKING

Pregnant Drug Addict or Alcoholic

What are your feelings about caring for a pregnant drug addict?

What approach might you use when caring for a pregnant alcoholic?

CULTURAL CONSIDERATIONS

Childbearing

Caring for a pregnant client from another culture can be a very rewarding experience for the nurse who takes time to learn and who shows sensitivity and respect toward cultural differences. Journal articles may be found about the childbirth practices of other cultures, such as those listed in the suggested readings at the end of the chapter.

order but who have no symptoms, and by individuals who have clinical findings indicative of a genetic disorder.

Male Contributions

A lower birth weight, mean deficit of 88 g, has been found in the infants of fathers who smoked and whose mothers did not (Martinez et al., 1994). Also, smoking affects spermatogenesis and sperm mobility. Male exposure to occupational chemicals has been associated with spontaneous abortion, stillbirth, preterm delivery, and small-for-gestational-age babies (Robaire & Hales, 1993). Because spermatogenesis is continuous so that a new supply of sperm are generated every 12 weeks, men can avoid smoking and exposure to occupational chemicals for the period when the couple is planning a pregnancy, and thus eliminate their effects.

PREGNANCY

Pregnancy refers to the condition of carrying an off-spring within the body. It is a form of reproduction that unites the cells of two individuals to form a unique new individual who embodies characteristics of both parents.

Fertilization

Pregnancy typically begins as a result of **coitus** or **copulation,** which is the sexual act that delivers sperm to the cervix by ejaculation of an erect penis. Sperm entering the vagina by other means such as artificial insemination may also result in fertilization. **Fertilization** or conception occurs when a sperm and ovum unite. This union generally occurs in the distal third of the fallopian tube. The fertilized ovum is now called a **zygote.**

The gender of the zygote is determined at the time of fertilization. When the ovum and sperm each contribute an X chromosome, the result is a female. When the ovum contributes an X chromosome and the sperm a Y chromosome, the result is a male.

Cell division occurs as the zygote travels the fallopian tube to the uterus. It takes 3 to 4 days of cell division, or mitosis, for the zygote to become a **morula,** which resembles a mulberry. The morula entering the uterus is now called a **blastocyst.** The cells have differentiated into an inner mass of embryonic cells, which becomes the embryo, and an outer layer called the trophoblast, which is involved in implantation, hormone secretion, and membrane and placental formation (Figure 50-1).

Implantation

About 7 days after ovulation or 5 days after fertilization, the trophoblast burrows into the endometrium, usually in the upper part of the uterus. This process is called **implantation,** or embedding of the fertilized egg into the uterine lining. The endometrium is now called the **decidua.** The trophoblast puts out villi, fingerlike projections, to anchor the blastocyst.

Multiple pregnancy occurs when more than one fetus develops at the same time. When twins result from two ova being fertilized by two sperm, the twins are fraternal or dizygotic. They are nonidentical and may be two males, two females, or one male and one female. There are two amnions, two chorions, and two placentas.

If one ovum is fertilized by one sperm and the inner cell mass of the blastocyst splits in two to form two embryos, the twins are identical or monozygotic. They may be two males or two females. There are two amnions, one chorion, and one placenta. The genetic makeup is identical in each fetus (Figure 50-2).

The outer fetal membrane is the **chorion,** formed from the trophoblast. The chorionic villi degenerate,

Figure 50-2 *Formation of Twins:* **A,** *Fraternal (nonidentical);* **B,** *Identical*

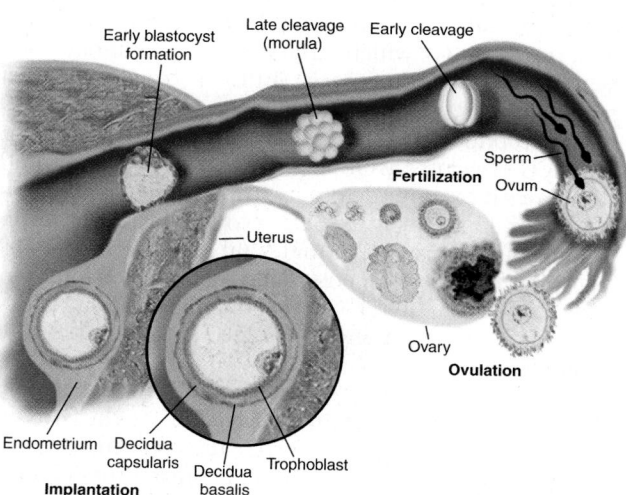

Figure 50-1 *Ovulation, Fertilization, and Implantation*

except for those attached to the uterine wall, which become the maternal side of the placenta. The inner membrane (fetal side), the **amnion,** originates in the blastocyst during the early stages of development. The amnion expands as the fetus grows until it slightly adheres to the chorion. These two fetal membranes form the amniotic sac or bag of water (BOW).

Amniotic Fluid

The amniotic fluid is formed by the secretions from the amniotic cells, lungs and skin of the fetus, and fetal urine. It is 98% water, but also contains glucose, protein, sodium, urea, creatinine, **lanugo** (fine hair covering body of fetus), and **vernix caseosa** (white, creamy covering on the fetus's body). Amniotic fluid is slightly alkaline. Approximately every 3 hours, the fluid is replaced. The amnionic cells and the fetus urinating and swallowing regulate the secretion and reabsorption of the fluid.

The amniotic fluid has several important functions in that it:

- Equalizes the pressure around the fetus.
- Cushions the fetus from external compression.
- Provides a constant temperature and fluid for the fetus to swallow.
- Allows freedom of movement for the fetus.
- Lubricates the membranes and the fetus.

The yolk sac develops as a second cavity in the blastocyst. It forms primitive red blood cells until the liver is able to take over the process in about 6 weeks. Gradually, the yolk sac is incorporated into the umbilical cord.

Placenta and Umbilical Cord

The chorionic villi at the base of the implanted fertilized ovum and the decidua basalis, the endometrium at the site of implantation, form the placenta. The **placenta** is a membranous vascular organ connecting the fetus to the mother, which produces hormones to sustain a pregnancy, supplies the fetus with oxygen and food, and transports waste products out of the fetal system. The development of the placenta, stimulated by progesterone secreted by the corpus luteum, begins about the third week following fertilization. The placenta is fully functional by the 12th week.

There is a maternal side to the placenta and a fetal side. The maternal side is irregular and is divided into subdivisions called **cotyledons.** It resembles liver both in color and texture. The fetal side is covered by the amnion, so it is smooth and shiny.

The chorionic villi contain blood vessels that join to form larger and larger vessels, eventually becoming the umbilical cord. The **umbilical cord,** a structure that connects the fetus to the placenta, has two arteries and one vein. It is surrounded and protected by a thick substance called **Wharton's jelly** and covered by the amnion. The two umbilical arteries carry deoxygenated blood from the fetus to the placenta, where carbon dioxide and other waste products are eliminated. The one umbilical vein carries oxygenated blood to the fetus along with nutrients, hormones, antibodies, and whatever drugs or toxic substances the mother may have in her body. This is one instance in which arteries carry deoxy-

genated blood and a vein transports oxygenated blood. Generally, the cord is attached to the center of the placenta, but it can be attached any place on the placenta.

The circulatory systems of the mother and fetus are separate. Maternal blood enters the intervillous spaces of the placenta. Fetal blood is in the vessels of the chorionic villi. Thus the cells of the fetal blood vessels and the chorion keep maternal blood and fetal blood separate (Figure 50-3).

The placenta has three major functions: transport, endocrine, and metabolic. All are necessary to maintain the pregnancy and promote normal fetal growth and development. The placenta provides the respiratory and excretory functions for the fetus as well as providing nutrition to the fetus.

Transport There are several mechanisms by which the placenta transports substances.

- Substances may move by diffusion from an area of higher concentration to an area of lower concentration. Those substances transported by this mechanism are oxygen, carbon dioxide, carbon monoxide, water, electrolytes, fat-soluble vitamins, anesthetic gases, and drugs.
- Facilitated diffusion uses a carrier system to move molecules more rapidly than simple diffusion. Some glucose and oxygen are transported by this method.
- Active transport allows molecules to move from an area of lower concentration to an area of higher concentration. Substances moved across the placenta by active transport are amino acids, glucose, iron, calcium, iodine, and water-soluble vitamins.
- Pinocytosis transfers larger molecules such as albumin, globulins, antibodies, and viruses through cell membranes.
- Osmotic pressure and hydrostatic pressure move most of the water.

Very large molecules such as insulin, heparin, IgM, and blood cells do not move across the placenta unless there is a tear in the placenta.

Endocrine The placenta secretes five hormones that are essential to pregnancy: human chorionic gonadotropin (hCG), which is the basis for pregnancy tests; human placental lactogen (hPL); estrogen; progesterone; and relaxin.

The trophoblast secretes hCG during early pregnancy. The hCG prevents involution of the corpus luteum and stimulates it to continue producing progesterone and estrogen for 11 to 12 weeks. Eight to ten days after fertilization, hCG is present in maternal blood serum; a few days after the missed menstrual period, hCG is found in maternal urine. After 11 weeks, the placenta is producing enough estrogen and progesterone to maintain the pregnancy.

Human placental lactogen makes a sufficient supply of protein, glucose, and minerals available to the fetus by stimulating changes in maternal metabolism. Human placental lactogen is an insulin antagonist, thus decreasing maternal metabolism of glucose. It also ensures that the mother's body is prepared for lactation.

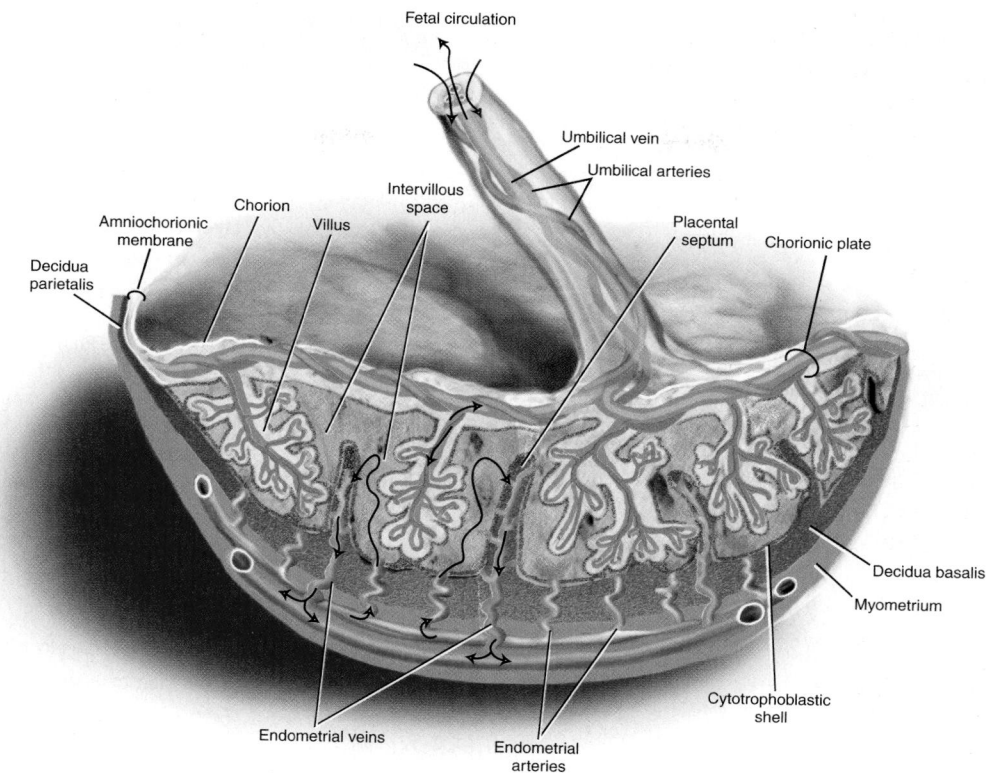

Figure 50-3 *Placental Circulation*

The placenta secretes primarily the estrogen estriol. Essential precursors from the fetal adrenal glands are used by the placenta for conversion to estriol. Estrogen stimulates development of uterine and breast tissues in the mother. It also increases vascularity and vasodilation in the villous capillaries.

After 11 weeks of pregnancy, the placenta takes over the production of progesterone from the corpus luteum. Progesterone, a smooth muscle relaxant, prevents uterine contractions by decreasing its contractility. It also maintains the endometrium.

Relaxin causes changes in collagen. The connective tissue of the symphysis pubis and sacroiliac joints are softened and become slightly flexible.

Metabolic The placenta produces fatty acids, glycogen, and cholesterol for fetal use and hormone production. The enzymes required for fetoplacental transfer are also produced by the placenta. It breaks down epinephrine and histamine and stores glycogen and iron.

FETAL DEVELOPMENT

Fetal development is divided into three stages. The preembryonic or germinal stage is the first 14 days after fertilization. The second stage, the embryonic stage, is from the beginning of the third week (day 15) through week eight. The fetal stage is from week 9 until 38 to 40 weeks or full term.

Development occurs in a systematic manner from head to toe (cephalo-caudal), from proximal to distal (close to body–farthest from body), and from general to specific. This means that the head develops before the arms and the arms develop before the legs; the arms and legs develop before the fingers and toes; and the fetus moves its arms before grasping with the hands.

Fetal development is sometimes described in general terms of trimester. The first trimester is the first 12 weeks, second trimester weeks 13 through 27, and third trimester weeks 28 to 40.

Pregnancy generally lasts 10 lunar (28 days) months, 40 weeks, or 280 days. It is calculated from the first day of the mother's last menstrual period (LMP). Table 50-1 identifies stages of fetal development and gives the weight and length (crown-rump length, or C-R) or crown-heel (C-H) beginning in week 4.

System Development

All systems in the fetus have begun forming by the eighth week. They grow, develop, and mature at different rates, and some do not mature until years after birth.

Cardiovascular System

With the primitive heart beginning to beat on the 21st day following conception, the cardiovascular system is the first to function in the embryo. Most congenital malformations of the heart and great vessels develop during the sixth to eighth weeks.

Fetal Circulation Fetal circulation has several unique features. Oxygenated blood comes from the placenta and enters the fetus, at the umbilicus, through the umbilical vein. It divides at the liver with a small branch

TABLE 50-1   STAGES OF FETAL DEVELOPMENT

STAGE	FETAL DEVELOPMENT	STAGE	FETAL DEVELOPMENT
Preembryonic or Germinal Stage		**Fetal Stage—continued**	
Weeks 1 and 2	Rapid cell division and differentiation.	Week 11	Tooth buds appear.
	Germinal layeers form.		Liver secretes bile.
			Urinary system functions.
Embryonic Stage			Insulin forms in pancreas.
Week 3	Primitive nervous system, eyes, ears, red blood cells present. Heart begins to beat day 21.	Week 12 Wt 45 g (1.5 oz) L 9 cm (3.5 in) (C–R) 11.5 cm (4.5 in) (C–H)	Lungs take shape. Palate fuses. Heart beat heard with Doppler. Ossification established. Swallowing reflex present. External genitalia, male or female distinguished.
Week 4 Wt 0.4 g L 4–6 mm (crown–rump, C–R)	Half the size of a pea. Brain differentiates. GI tract begins to form. Limb buds appear.		
Week 5 L 6–8 mm (C–R)	Cranial nerves present. Muscles have innervation.	**Second Trimester**	
		Week 16 Wt 200 g (7 oz) L 13.5 cm (5.5 in) (C–R) 15 cm (6 in) (C–H)	Meconium forms in bowels. Scalp hair appears. Frequent fetal movement. Skin thin, pink. Sensitive to light. 200 mL amniotic fluid. (Amniocentesis possible.)
Week 6 L 10–14 mm (C–R)	Fetal circulation established. Liver produces red blood cells. Central autonomic nervous system forms. Primitive kidneys form. Lung buds present. Cartilage forms. Primitive skeleton forms. Muscles differentiate.		
		Week 20 Wt 435 g (15 oz) L 19 cm (7.5 in) (C–) 25 cm (10 in) (C–H)	Myelination of spinal cord begins. Peristalsis begins. Lanugo covers body. Vernix caseosa covers body. Brown fat deposits begun. Sucks and swallows amniotic fluid. Heart beat heard with fetoscope. Hands can grasp. Regular schedule of sucking, kicking, and sleeping.
Week 7 L 22–28 mm (C–R)	Eyelids form. Palate and tongue form. Stomach formed. Diaphragm formed. Arms, legs move.		
Week 8 Wt 2 g L 3 cm (1.5 in) (C–R)	Resembles human being. Eyes moved to face front. Heart development complete. Hands and feet well formed. Bone cells begin replacing cartilage. All body organs have begun forming.	Week 24 Wt 780 g (1 lb, 12 oz) L 23 cm (9 in) (C–R) 28 cm (11 in) (C–H)	Alveoli present in lungs, begin producing surfactant. Eyes completely formed. Eyelashes and eyebrows appear. Many reflexes appear. Chance of survival if born.
Fetal Stage		**Third Trimester**	
Week 9	Finger and toe nails form. Eyelids fuse shut.	Week 28 Wt 1200 g (2 lb, 10 oz) L 28 cm (11 in) (C–R) 35 cm (14 in) (C–H)	Subcutaneous fat deposits begun. Lanugo begins to disappear. Nails appear. Eyelids open and close. Testes begin to descend.
Week 10 Wt 14 g (1/2 oz) L 5–6 cm (2 in) crown-heel (C–H)	Head growth slows. Islets of Langerhans differentiated. Bone marrow forms, RBCs produced. Bladder sac forms Kidneys make urine.		

continues

TABLE 50-1   continued

STAGE	FETAL DEVELOPMENT	STAGE	FETAL DEVELOPMENT
Third Trimester—continued		**Third Trimester—continued**	
Week 32 Wt 2,000 g (4 lb, 6.5 oz) L 31 cm (12 in) (C–R) 41 cm (16 in) (C–H)	More reflexes present. CNS directs rhythmic breathing movements. CNS partially controls body temperature. Begins storing iron, calcium, phosphorus. Ratio of the lung surfactants lecithin and sphingomyelin (L/S) is 1.2:2.	Week 38	L/S ratio 2:1
		Week 40 Wt 3,000–3,600 g (6 lb, 10 oz– 7 lb, 15 oz) L 50 cm (20 in) (C–H)	Lanugo only on shoulders and upper back. Creases cover sole. Vernix mainly in folds of skin. Ear cartilage firm. Less active, limited space. Ready to be born.
Week 36 Wt 2,500–2,750 g (5 lb, 8 oz) L 35 cm (14 in) (C–R) 48 cm (19 in) (C–H)	A few creases on soles of feet. Skin less wrinkled. Fingernails reach fingertips. Sleep-wake cycle fairly definite. Transfer of maternal antibodies.		

going to the liver and the other branch, the **ductus venosus,** entering the inferior vena cava. The blood is now partially deoxygenated by the blood coming from the lower part of the fetus's body.

This blood enters the right atrium and moves through the **foramen ovale** (a flap opening in the atrial septum that allows only right-to-left movement of blood) to the left atrium and then to the left ventricle. A small portion of this blood passes into the right ventricle. The left ventricle pumps the blood out through the aorta.

Blood entering the right atrium from the superior vena cava flows to the right ventricle. It is pumped out through the pulmonary arteries. Most of this blood goes into the aorta through the **ductus arteriosus,** a fetal vessel connecting the pulmonary trunk to the aorta. Normally this closes at birth. A small amount of blood goes to the lungs to nourish the lung tissue.

The aorta and its branches supply blood to the rest of the body. The two umbilical arteries branch from the internal iliac arteries and return blood to the placenta to be oxygenated. Figure 50-4 shows fetal circulation.

Hematologic Development The formation of blood goes along with cardiovascular development. About day 14, primitive blood cells are formed in the yolk sac. It is the fifth week of gestation before the fetal liver begins hematopoiesis.

Fetal hemoglobin (Hgb F), found only during gestation and the early neonatal period, has a great attraction for oxygen. This ensures an adequate oxygen supply. Blood type is genetically determined at conception.

Gastrointestinal System

During the fourth week of gestation, the gastrointestinal tract begins forming. The fetus begins swallow-

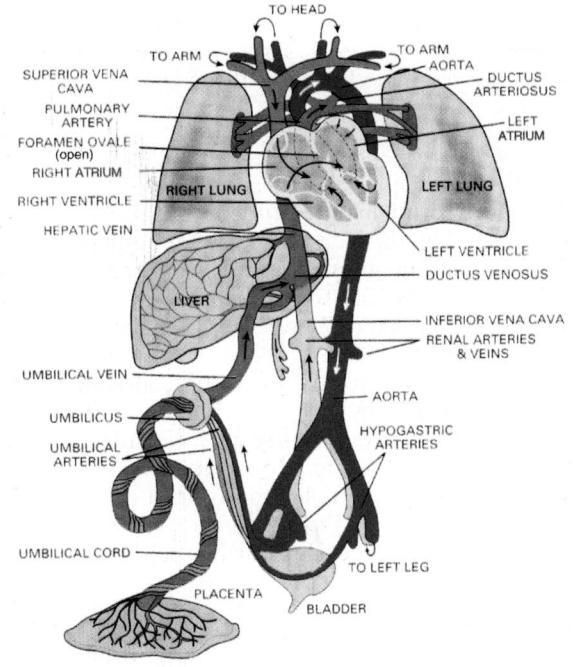

Figure 50-4 *Fetal Circulation. Red is arterial (oxgenated) blood, light purple is venous (unoxygenated) blood, and dark purple is mixed arterial-venous blood.*

ing amniotic fluid by the 20th week, but there is no coordination of the swallow and suck reflexes until about 34 weeks.

Meconium (fecal material stored in the fetal intestines) begins to form about week 16; however, there should not be passage of meconium in utero. If the fetus encounters hypoxic stress, the anal sphincter may relax and meconium may be passed, causing meconium staining of the amniotic fluid.

Musculoskeletal System

Limb buds appear late in the fourth week and development is complete by the eighth week. Growth of the skeleton is determined by genetics and maternal supply of calcium and phosphorus. Cartilage is noted about 5 weeks and ossification begins about 12 weeks but is not completed until after puberty, when growth is complete.

By the end of the 12th week, skeletal muscles begin involuntary movements. Skeletal muscle development depends on an adequate volume of amniotic fluid to allow plenty of fetal movement.

Genitourinary System

Kidneys begin forming at about 3 weeks and pass through several changes. Around 12 weeks, they begin to produce a hypotonic urine. The placenta and the maternal kidneys are still responsible for fetal waste removal. All the nephrons are in the kidneys at birth.

The reproductive system develops at the same time as the urinary system. Testes can be seen in the abdomen by 7 weeks and begin descending to the scrotum about 30 weeks. The ovaries develop in the abdomen and stay in the pelvic cavity. All of the ova a female will ever have are in the ovaries at birth. Visual determination of fetal gender can be made through ultrasound by the end of week 12.

Integumentary System

The skin protects the underlying tissues. Vernix caseosa protects the skin, with the amount present decreasing as the pregnancy progresses. Creases form on the palms, fingers, and soles during week 11, with permanent designs formed by week 17. Skin color is genetically determined.

Lanugo appears during week 20 and slowly disappears; most is gone by birth. Tooth buds for the deciduous (baby) teeth appear during week 6 while tooth buds for permanent teeth do not appear until week 10. Second and third permanent molar tooth buds do not appear until after birth.

Mammary glands develop during the sixth week.

Respiratory System

Lung buds begin forming during week 6, with bronchi forming by week 16. Primitive lungs are formed by 23 weeks, but there are not enough alveoli for sufficient gas exchange. Surfactant production begins between weeks 20 and 24. Surfactant reduces the surface tension of the fluid lining the alveoli in the lungs, thus facilitating breathing. Surfactant production matures between weeks 35 and 37. After 23 weeks' gestation, the lungs are capable of borderline support of extrauterine respiration. Therefore, the **age of viability,** or gestational age at which a fetus could live outside the uterus, is considered to be 24 weeks. Adequate lung functioning also depends on surfactant production and neurologic maturation.

Immunologic System

Between the 12th and 15th weeks, immune capability begins developing. It functions very minimally because the fetus lives in a sterile environment. The fetus produces small amounts of the immunoglobins IgG, IgA, and IgE before 20 weeks. IgG provides the most immunity. Maternal IgG is actively transported across the placenta to provide passive immunity against many infectious diseases. Blood group antibodies are a type of IgG. They can move across the placenta by active transport and cause hemolytic disease of the newborn.

Factors Affecting Fetal Development

Many factors influence fetal development, especially during the first trimester. Even before the mother knows she is pregnant, many factors are affecting embryonic development. One of the very first is the quality of the sperm and the ovum and the genetic code. **Teratogens** (any agent, such as radiation, drugs, viruses, or other microorganisms, capable of causing abnormal fetal development) exert the greatest influence on cells undergoing the most rapid growth. Each organ has a period when teratogenic agents or other insults can cause physical and functional defects.

A well-provided maternal environment is also important. Maternal malnutrition, acute and chronic diseases, drugs, alcohol, and smoking all can exert potentially harmful effects on the fetus before birth.

PHYSIOLOGICAL CHANGES OF PREGNANCY

Many physiological changes take place when a woman is pregnant. Every system of the mother's body undergoes some change during pregnancy.

Reproductive System

The most obvious physiological changes occur in the reproductive system.

Uterus

The most dramatic change occurs in the size of the uterus. Before pregnancy, it is a small, pear-shaped, thick-walled, muscular organ weighing 60 g (2 oz). At the end of pregnancy, it is a large, thin-walled organ weighing 1,000 g (2 lb). Its capacity has increased from 10 mL to 5 L. The uterus enlarges mainly by hypertrophy of the muscle cells stimulated by estrogen and the growing fetus. There are three layers of smooth (involuntary) muscles in the uterus (Figure 50-5). The outer layer is made of longitudinal muscles. The muscle fibers of the middle layer are interlaced in a figure eight pattern. Circular fibers that form sphincters at the openings of the fallopian tubes and at the internal os of the cervix make up the inner layer of uterine muscle. This configu-

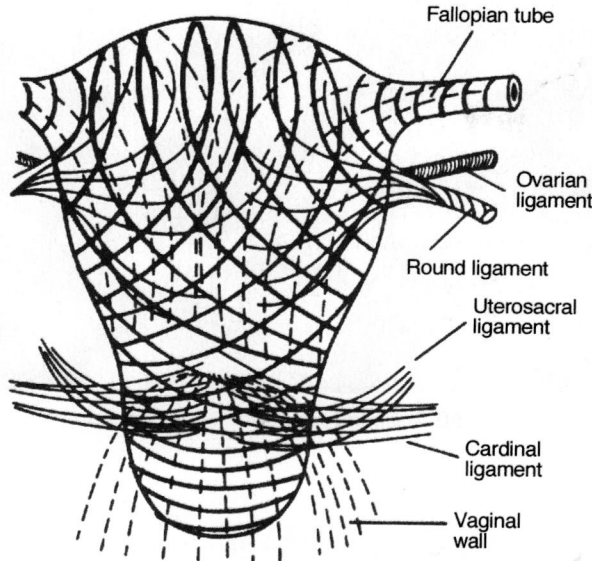

Figure 50-5 *Muscle Layers of the Uterus*

ration of muscle layers allows the uterus to expand evenly in all directions during pregnancy. One-sixth of the mother's blood volume is in the vascular system of the uterus by the end of pregnancy.

Irregular uterine contractions occur throughout pregnancy. About 16 weeks or later, the mother may become aware of these **Braxton-Hicks contractions**. These generally painless contractions assist in uterine and placental circulation. Pain is an individual perceptual experience. A softening of the uterine isthmus about the sixth week of pregnancy, noted during a pelvic exam, is called **Hegar's sign.**

Cervix

The cervix increases in cell number by the influence of estrogen. It secretes a thick, sticky mucus that forms a plug in the cervix. This plug prevents microorganisms from entering through the vagina. During labor, as the cervix dilates, this mucus plug is expelled. **Goodell's sign** (softening of the cervix) and **Chadwick's sign** (a purplish-blue color of the cervix and vagina caused by the increased vascularity) are both noted at about 8 weeks.

Ovaries

Follicles do not mature and ovulation does not occur during pregnancy. The corpus luteum produces progesterone and estrogen for about 12 weeks, at which time the placenta takes over the production.

Vagina

Estrogen causes a loosening of connective tissue and an increase in vaginal secretions. The acidic secretions prevent bacterial infections. The increased level of glycogen in cells may enhance growth of organisms such as *Trichomonas vaginalis* or *Candida albicans*.

Breasts

In addition to breast enlargement from hormonal influence, the nipples become more erect, the areolas darken, and Montgomery's tubercles enlarge. **Colostrum,** an antibody-rich yellow fluid, is secreted by the breasts during the last trimester and first 2–3 days after birth, and gradually changes to milk a few days after delivery.

Cardiovascular System

Blood flow increases to the uterus and kidneys, where the workload is increased. The pulse increases by 10 to 15 beats/minute by the end of pregnancy. Cardiac output increases 30% to 50% early in pregnancy. Blood pressure decreases, is lowest during the second trimester, and increases gradually to near the prepregnant level during the third trimester. This occurs because of the progesterone's relaxing effect on the smooth muscles.

Stasis of blood in the lower extremities, caused by the enlarged uterus interfering with return blood flow, may lead to dependent edema and varicose veins of the legs, vulva, or rectum.

Supine hypotensive syndrome, also known as vena caval syndrome, occurs when the mother lies supine. The enlarged, heavy uterus presses on the inferior vena cava, causing a reduced blood flow back to the right atrium (Figure 50-6). The mother experiences dizziness, clammy-pale skin, and a lowering of her blood pressure. This decreases placental perfusion, which can affect fetal reserve. The situation is relieved when the mother lies on her side.

Maternal blood volume increases 30% to 50%, reaching its peak at about 30 weeks. There is some increase in red blood cells, but most of the increase is plasma. This hemodilution is manifested by a lower hematocrit (34% to 40%) and is termed **physiologic anemia of pregnancy.**

The white blood cell count begins to increase by about 8 weeks and may reach 18,000/mm³ by the time of delivery. Platelets, fibrin, fibrinogen, and coagulation factors VII, IX, and X increase. This increase with possible venous stasis in late pregnancy increases the risk of venous thrombosis.

Figure 50-6 *Supine Hypotensive Syndrome. Enlarged uterus presses on vena cava when mother is supine. Side-lying position relieves pressure.*

Respiratory System

Progesterone decreases airway resistance, allowing an increase in oxygen consumption. The depth of respirations increases, causing a mild respiratory alkalosis, which is compensated by increased renal secretion of bicarbonate (Littleton & Engebretson, 2002). The enlarging uterus presses upward on the diaphragm. The rib cage flares and the chest circumference expands to keep the intrathoracic volume the same as when not pregnant. Estrogen causes edema and vascular congestion of the nasal mucosa.

Musculoskeletal System

The relaxation of the pelvic joints in preparation for delivery is caused by relaxin. As pregnancy progresses, the mother's center of gravity gradually changes because of the increased size and weight of the uterus anteriorly. To compensate, the mother increases the curve of the lumbosacral spine (lordosis), which frequently results in a low backache, and may cause the woman to have a waddling gait. Figure 50-7 illustrates this change throughout pregnancy.

Gastrointestinal System

Nausea and/or vomiting, known as "morning sickness," are common in early pregnancy but usually disappear by 12 weeks. The smooth muscle relaxation effect of progesterone results in delayed gastric emptying and decreased peristalsis. The enlarging uterus displaces the stomach and intestines. All of these changes contribute to constipation. Relaxation of the cardiac sphincter may allow reflux of acidic gastric contents into the esophagus, giving the mother heartburn.

Urinary System

Urinary frequency occurs in the first trimester as the enlarging uterus presses on the bladder and in the third trimester as the fetus settles into the pelvis and presses on the bladder. Progesterone causes the ureters to relax and dilate. Glomerular filtration rate (GFR) begins rising in the second trimester. Tubular reabsorption also increases.

Glycosuria (excretion of glucose in the urine) may develop if the kidneys are unable to reabsorb all of the glucose filtered by the glomeruli. Any amount more than a trace of glucose in the urine should be investigated.

Figure 50-8 *Linea Nigra and Striae Gravidarum*

Integumentary System

Several skin pigment changes generally occur during pregnancy. The nipples, areola, vulva, and perineal area darken. **Linea nigra** is a pigmented line on the abdomen from umbilicus to symphysis pubis. **Chloasma,** also called "mask of pregnancy," is a darkening of the skin of the forehead and around the eyes. It is generally more pronounced in dark-haired women. **Striae gravidarum,** or "stretch marks," are reddish streaks frequently found on the abdomen, thighs, buttocks, and breasts. They are the result of separation of the underlying connective tissue of the skin (Figure 50-8). As the skin stretches, the client may experience itching.

Endocrine System

The anterior pituitary hormone prolactin is responsible for initial milk production. The posterior pituitary hormone oxytocin causes uterine contractions and the ejection of milk from the breasts (let-down reflex) after delivery.

The placental hormones, especially hPL, are insulin antagonists, so a greater insulin production is required. This puts an increased stress on the islets of Langerhans in the pancreas to put out more insulin. A woman with a marginally functioning pancreas may show signs of gestational diabetes.

A slight increase in the size of the thyroid often occurs, as well as an increase in its capacity to bind thyroxine. Maternal thyroxine is important for fetal neural development throughout pregnancy, especially during the first trimester. This results in a higher level of serum protein-bound iodine (PBI).

Metabolism

The metabolic rate of the mother increases during pregnancy as the demands of the growing fetus increase. The mother must meet her own and the fetus's nutritional needs.

SIGNS OF PREGNANCY

The many physiological changes that a woman experiences during pregnancy can be categorized as presumptive, probable, or positive signs of pregnancy.

12 Weeks   20 Weeks   28 Weeks   36 Weeks   40 Weeks

Figure 50-7 *Lordosis increases throughout pregnancy.*

Presumptive Signs

Changes that the woman experiences and reports are termed presumptive or subjective signs. They may be caused by other conditions, so are not diagnostic of pregnancy. Presumptive signs include:

- **Amenorrhea** (absence of menses), usually the first sign that a woman notices causing her to think she is pregnant
- Nausea and vomiting, often referred to as "morning sickness" but can occur any time of the day. This sign usually disappears by 12 weeks of pregnancy.
- Breast changes, tenderness, or tingling
- Urinary frequency, as the growing uterus presses against the bladder, giving the woman the sensation of needing to urinate
- Excessive fatigue, often noted after the first missed menstrual period. It may last for several months.
- Abdominal enlargement usually noticed by the woman, generally after 12 weeks
- **Quickening**, perception of fetal movement by the mother, usually between 16 and 20 weeks. It begins as a fluttering sensation and gradually gets stronger and more frequent.

A positive diagnosis of pregnancy is usually made before these last two signs are noted by the woman; however, there is a condition called **pseudocyesis** or false pregnancy, in which the woman believes so strongly that she is pregnant that she appears to have all the early presumptive signs of pregnancy.

Probable Signs

The examiner can identify these objective changes, but since they can be caused by conditions other than pregnancy, they are not diagnostic of pregnancy.

Pelvic Signs

Goodell's sign (softening of the cervix), Hegar's sign (softening of the uterine isthmus), and Chadwick's sign (purplish discoloration of the vagina, cervix, and vulva) can be identified by the examiner during the first 12 weeks of pregnancy.

Uterine enlargement can be identified after the eighth week of pregnancy. The fundus is palpable just above the symphysis at 12 weeks and at the umbilicus at 20 weeks (Figure 50-9). If these uterine enlargement milestones are reached earlier, multiple pregnancy should be suspected.

Braxton-Hicks Contractions

After the 28th week, these contractions can be felt by the examiner and also by the client.

Increased Pigmentation

The nipples and areola darken. Linea nigra may appear on the abdomen, chloasma may mark the face, and striae gravidarum may be noticed on the breasts and abdomen.

Ballottement

During the fourth or fifth month, if the fetus is pushed upward through the vagina or abdomen, the floating fetus rebounds against the examiner's fingers; this is known as **ballottement** (Figure 50-10). This occurs only while the fetus is small in comparison to the amount of amniotic fluid.

Pregnancy Test

The basis for a pregnancy test is the presence of hCG in either the urine or blood of the woman. A test of the blood is positive 8 days after conception, and a test of the urine is positive 10 to 14 days after conception.

Positive Signs

A positive sign of pregnancy proves conclusively that the woman is pregnant. No other condition can cause these signs to appear. There are only three positive signs of pregnancy: hearing the fetal heartbeat, visualization of the fetus, and the examiner feeling fetal movement.

Figure 50-9 *Fundal Height Milestones*

Figure 50-10 *Ballottement*

Figure 50-11 *Fetoscope in Use*

Hearing the Fetal Heartbeat

The fetal heartbeat can be detected at 10 to 12 weeks using the Doppler ultrasound method. A fetoscope can detect the fetal heartbeat by 18 to 20 weeks (Figure 50-11).

When auscultating the abdomen over the uterus, a soft, blowing sound may be heard. The sound occurring at the same rate as the mother's pulse is called the **uterine souffle,** caused by the blood pulsating through the uterus and placenta. The sound occurring at the same rate as the fetal heart rate is called the **funic souffle,** caused by blood pulsating through the umbilical cord.

Visualization of the Fetus

An abdominal ultrasound examination can detect a pregnancy by the sixth week after the last menstrual period (LMP). An endovaginal ultrasound examination, using a vaginal probe, can detect a gestational sac 10 days after implantation.

Examiner Feeling Fetal Movement

Fetal movement felt by the examiner, not the mother, is a positive sign of pregnancy.

PSYCHOLOGICAL ADAPTATION TO PREGNANCY

Pregnancy is often viewed as a developmental stage having its own developmental tasks. Both the expectant mother and father deal with significant changes and major psychosocial adjustment.

Developmental Tasks

Four major developmental tasks have been identified for pregnancy. They are pregnancy validation, fetal embodiment, fetal distinction, and role transition. These developmental tasks are met in this order. The rate at which they are met will vary. According to Malnory (1996), completion of the developmental tasks is critical to positive parenting.

Pregnancy Validation

During the first trimester, the pregnant woman's task is to validate and accept the pregnancy. Until the woman meets this task, she cannot meet the rest of the developmental tasks. Even when pregnancy is planned, there are normal feelings of ambivalence and disbelief about the pregnancy. Many women become introspective or have mood swings caused by hormone fluctuations.

Fetal Embodiment

Fetal embodiment occurs as the mother incorporates the growing fetus into her body image. The physical changes she is experiencing, especially the growing uterus, help her meet this task. She feels that the fetus is a part of her. Self-involvement, depression, or regressive behavior may be signs of difficulty in meeting this task.

Fetal Distinction

When fetal movement is felt, it becomes easier for the mother to think of the fetus as a separate being. She may daydream about what the baby will be like and think about the kind of mother she wants to be.

Role Transition

The last trimester is a time of preparation. Many expectant parents attend childbirth classes to learn about and prepare for labor, delivery, infant care, and self-care. Preparing a nursery, buying baby clothes, and selecting a day care are all ways of preparing for the infant's arrival. Role transition also includes parents exploring together the meaning of fathering and mothering, learning parenting skills, the amazing skills of a newborn for interactions, and the physical maturing and behavioral changes of the first 12 months of life. Another aspect is learning to enjoy watching the other parent interact with the newborn.

At the end of pregnancy, many mothers experience a surge of energy and see to it that the entire household is organized for the coming of the infant. This is called **nesting.** All of these preparations assist the pregnant woman in the transition to her new role of mother.

Partners' Tasks

Fathers and other partners must meet the same developmental tasks as the expectant mother but in a more ab-

CULTURAL CONSIDERATIONS

Preparation for the Infant

A lack of preparation for the birth of the baby may indicate a problem in meeting the task of role transition; however, some cultures or families do not actually purchase any items for the baby until after birth because this practice is believed to bring bad luck. The nurse must be sensitive to cultural practices different from her own and not assume that the couple who has not established a nursery before the birth is not eagerly awaiting the new baby's arrival.

stract way. Accepting the fact that *they* (as a couple) are pregnant and announcing it to family and friends meets the first task. The partner may also have ambivalent feelings about the pregnancy. By accepting the changes in the pregnant partner, both physical and psychological, the task of fetal embodiment is met. Fetal distinction is generally met when the partner hears the fetal heartbeat and feels the fetus moving. Role transition is met in virtually the same way as is done by the pregnant woman.

Factors Affecting Psychological Response

Factors that contribute to a woman's psychological response to her pregnancy include body image, financial situation, cultural expectations, emotional security, and support from significant others.

Body Image

The mother's body image, or perception of her own body, may change in several areas. The noticeable changes in body shape and the speed with which those changes occur may be very threatening to some women. Some women feel "fat" and "ugly" when they are pregnant, and others feel "so good" and "beautiful" when they are pregnant.

The physical discomforts of pregnancy may cause the mother to feel a lack of control over her own body. For example, urinary frequency or urinary incontinence may increase negative feelings about the pregnancy.

Pregnant women often feel restricted in their physical activities. As long as there is no problem with the pregnancy, they should be encouraged to continue their regular activities, keeping in mind that moderation is the key.

Financial Situation

A poor financial situation may be the cause of anxiety about paying bills, buying needed items for infant care, or having enough and proper foods for good nutrition. Financial consideration may also be a significant concern for the expectant mother's partner.

Cultural Expectations

Cultural expectations of the family may cause conflicts for the pregnant woman and her partner if their ideas are different from their families' expectations. Conflicts may also occur if the cultural expectations of the mother are different from the cultural expectations of the father or partner.

Emotional Security

A pregnant woman's satisfaction with herself and her life situation will also have an impact on how she responds to being pregnant. If the woman is secure in her feelings about herself and her perceived abilities as a mother, the pregnancy is more likely to be enjoyable. A pregnancy that was planned or long anticipated will likely be received with joy and excitement, whereas an unexpected or unwanted pregnancy may be met with fear, dread, or uncertainty.

Support from Significant Others

It is important for the nurse and the expectant mother to also take into consideration the psychological responses of significant others, namely, the father/partner, siblings, and grandparents.

Father/Partner The expectant father or partner must shift thinking from being a person without children to a person with a child. He may feel left out, neglected, or resent the attention focused on the expectant mother.

Couvade is the development of physical symptoms by the expectant father such as fatigue, depression, headache, backache, and nausea. Longobucco and Freston (1989) found that men who show couvade have greater paternal role preparation.

Siblings A new baby may be seen by siblings as a threat to their relationship with the parents. Siblings should be included in the pregnancy and preparations for the new baby on an age-appropriate basis. Feeling the fetus kick or hearing the heartbeat are often helpful activities for siblings. Parents must be sure to maintain some special time just for the siblings. Many areas have classes for siblings to help them understand what is happening in their lives.

Grandparents Grandparents are usually the first ones told about the pregnancy. It is often difficult for grandparents to know how much to become involved in the process. Some grandparents feel they are not ready or are too young to become grandparents.

Practices of childbearing and childrearing often change greatly from one generation to another. Some areas have classes to provide information to grandparents about these changes.

PRENATAL EDUCATION AND CARE

Prenatal care (care of a woman during pregnancy, before labor) is credited with the reduction of perinatal mortality over the last 50 years. The earlier prenatal care is begun, the better. This provides an opportunity for the health care provider to obtain baseline data on physical assessments and laboratory test results. Beckmann, Buford, and Witt (2000) found that cost and length of time at an appointment were the major barriers to prenatal care.

Anticipatory guidance (providing information, teaching, or guidance to a client in anticipation of an expected event) is probably the most important aspect of prenatal care. It is based on the assessment of mother and fetus and knowledge of the normal process of pregnancy and possible complications.

Prenatal Care

The goals of prenatal care are as follows:

- A healthy, prepared mother having minimal discomforts
- Identification of potential problems or complications as early as possible
- Safe delivery of a healthy infant
- A prepared father or partner who participates as much or as little as the couple desires
- Prepared siblings and grandparents

CULTURAL CONSIDERATIONS

Beliefs Influencing Pregnancy

Some cultural practices may not always be observed by a client, but some general practices that have cultural influences include the following:

- Muslim women are to keep hair, body, arms to the wrist, and legs to the ankles covered at all times. Also, a Muslim woman may not be alone in the presence of a man other than her husband or a male relative, including during a physical examination (Hutchinson & Baqi-Aziz, 1994).
- Korean women defer to elders, especially the mother-in-law, for care decisions (Schneiderman, 1996).
- Native American women should not look at a deformed, injured, or blind person, or the baby will have the same defect (Cesario, 2001).
- Koreans do not like having their name written in red ink because red ink is used for the deceased (Howard & Berbiglia, 1997).
- Guatemalan women believe that a pregnant woman and her unborn child are physically and spiritually weak and may be vulnerable to illnesses and evil forces (Callister & Vega, 1998).
- In Malawi, Africa, the father determines family size and the timing of the pregnancies (Gennaro et al., 1998).

TABLE 50-2 TERMS USED IN DESCRIBING A PREGNANT CLIENT

Abortion Loss of pregnancy before the age of viability (usually 20 to 24 weeks' gestation)

GP/TPAL Gravida, para/term, preterm, abortions, living

Examples: Mary Jo is G2 P1/T2 P0 A0 L2; second pregnancy, one delivery/two infants at term (twins), both living.

Susan is G4 P2/T1 P1 A1 L2; fourth pregnancy, two deliveries/one term infant, one preterm infant, one abortion, two living children.

Gravida Pregnancy, regardless of duration, includes present pregnancy

Para Delivery (birth) after 24 weeks' gestation, whether infant born alive or dead or number of infants born

Preterm Delivery after 24 weeks' gestation but before 38 weeks (full term)

Term A pregnancy between 38 and 42 weeks' gestation

Nulligravida Never been pregnant

Primigravida Pregnant for first time

Multigravida Pregnant two or more times

Nullipara Never having delivered an infant after 24 weeks' gestation

Primipara Has delivered once after 24 weeks' gestation

Multipara Has delivered twice or more after 24 weeks' gestation

Postterm Delivery after 42 weeks' gestation

Initial Visit

A comfortable environment, open communication, and the nurse's attitude will help put the woman at ease during the initial prenatal visit. The first visit is often quite lengthy. A complete history is recorded to identify factors that may negatively affect the pregnancy, and a physical examination is performed. If the woman did not seek preconception care, all of the topics covered in that section would then be discussed at the first prenatal visit. Important terms used in describing a pregnant client are provided in Table 50-2.

Initial History The history provides the health care provider with the client's past and present health. Figure 50-12 shows a sample health history summary.

Estimating Duration of Pregnancy Every family wants to know the "due date," the estimated date when the infant is to be born. The estimated date of birth (EDB) or estimated date of delivery (EDD) is 40 weeks from the first day of the woman's LMP. Many women do not keep track of their menstrual periods, or have irregular periods; but an EDB can be identified based on other factors such as uterine size, date of quickening, date when the fetal heartbeat is heard, and ultrasound fetal measurements.

Naegele's Rule Naegele's rule is the most common method of calculating the EDB. The rule is: Take the date of the first day of the last menstrual period, subtract 3 months, and add 7 days. For instance, if the LMP was June 28, the calculation would be as follows:

Month	Day
6 (June)	28
−3 months	+ 7 days
3 (March)	35

Because there are 31 days in March, the EDB moves forward to April 4.

Gestation Calculator A gestation calculator, in the shape of either a chart or a wheel, allows a quick EDB calculation. The wheel generally provides other information also, such as fetal weight and body length for each week (Figure 50-13).

Fundal Height Fundal height generally indicates gestational age through the second trimester (refer back to Figure 50-9). The **fundus** (top of the uterus) is measured in centimeters from the top of the pubic symphysis to the top of the uterine fundus (McDonald's method). This is fairly accurate between 18 and 30 weeks' gestation. The fundal height, for example, is generally 20 cm (at the umbilicus) at 20 weeks' gestation and 25 cm at 25 weeks' gestation in the average-height woman. Evaluating the visit-to-visit fundal height measurements provides a general pattern of fetal growth. A sudden increase may indicate twins or hydramnios (excessive amount of amniotic fluid), whereas a smaller increase may indicate growth retardation (Figure 50-14).

Other Indicators Additional assessments that indicate the gestational week of pregnancy include ultrasound, fetal heartbeat, and quickening.

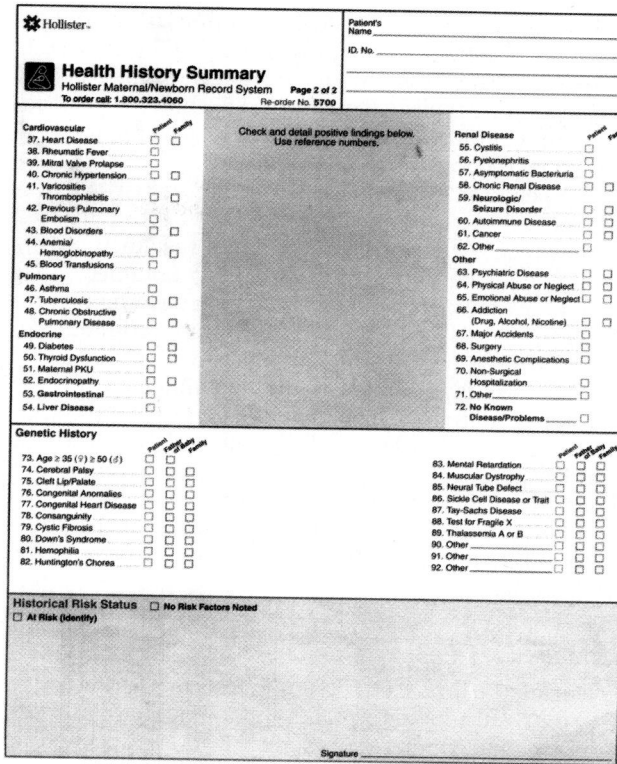

Figure 50-12 *Representative Health History Forms (Permission to use this copyright material has been granted by the owner, Hollister Incorporated.)*

Figure 50-13 *Gestation Calculation Wheel. Place arrow labeled first day of LMP on that date. Read date at arrow labeled expected delivery date.*

Figure 50-14 *Measuring Fundal Height*

- *Ultrasound:* Five to six weeks after the LMP, an ultrasound can detect a gestational sac. It shows fetal heartbeat activity at 9 to 10 weeks' gestation. By 12 to 13 weeks, the biparietal diameter (BPD), or distance between the parietal bones of the fetal skull, can be measured.
- *Fetal Heartbeat:* The fetal heartbeat is generally heard by 10 to 12 weeks with the Doppler device, but may be heard as early as 8 weeks' gestation. It is usually 18 to 20 weeks before the fetal heartbeat can be heard with a fetoscope.
- *Quickening:* Fetal movement is usually felt by the mother at about 20 weeks' gestation. Women may identify these movements as early as 16 weeks or as late as 22 weeks. Typically, the woman will detect this movement earlier with a second pregnancy than with a first.

Physical Examination The physical examination begins with measuring the client's height and weight and vital signs. A head-to-toe examination is performed by the health care provider. Special attention is given to the assessment of the heart, lungs, pelvis, breasts, and nipples. Figure 50-15 shows an initial pregnancy profile form, and Figure 50-16 shows a prenatal flow record.

The pelvic examination is performed last. The external genitalia are examined for scars, lesions, or infection. A Pap smear for cervical cancer and a specimen of cervical mucous for gonorrhea are usually obtained. A bimanual examination is performed to determine uterine changes (Figure 50-17) and pelvic size to estimate adequacy of the pelvic opening for delivery.

Pelvic size is estimated by the examiner during the manual examination. The diagonal conjugate (distance from the lower border of the pubic symphysis to the sacral promontory) is an estimate of the pelvic inlet. It is generally 11.5 cm. The anteroposterior diameter (9.5 to 11.5 cm), measured from the lower border of the pubic symphysis to the tip of the sacrum, is an estimate of the pelvic outlet.

Screening Tests

During the first visit, screening tests are performed to determine the mother's health and to have baseline data with which to compare subsequent test results. The tests may vary for a specific client but generally include those listed in Table 50-3.

Return Visits

Return visits for an uncomplicated pregnancy generally are:

- Every 4 weeks for the first 28 weeks
- Every 2 weeks during weeks 29 to 36
- Every week, after 36 weeks, until birth of infant

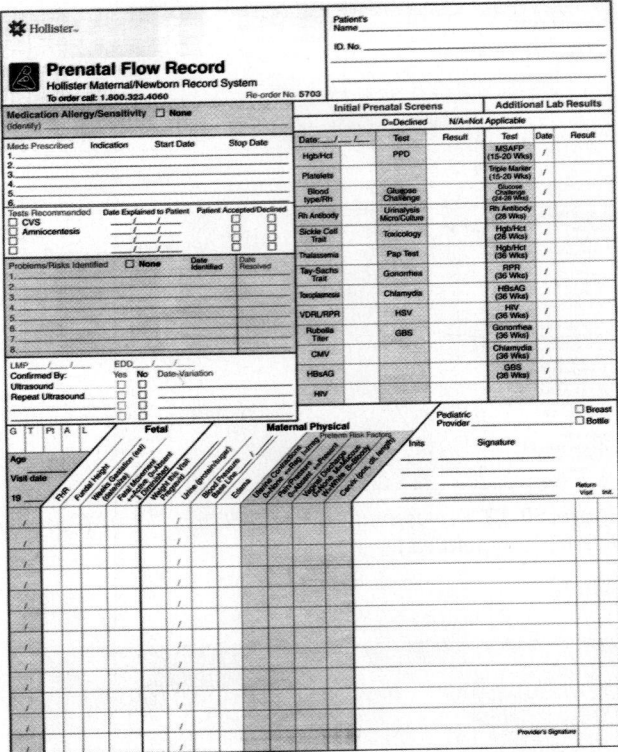

Figure 50-16 *Representative Prenatal Flow Record (Permission to use this copyright material has been granted by the owner, Hollister Incorporated.)*

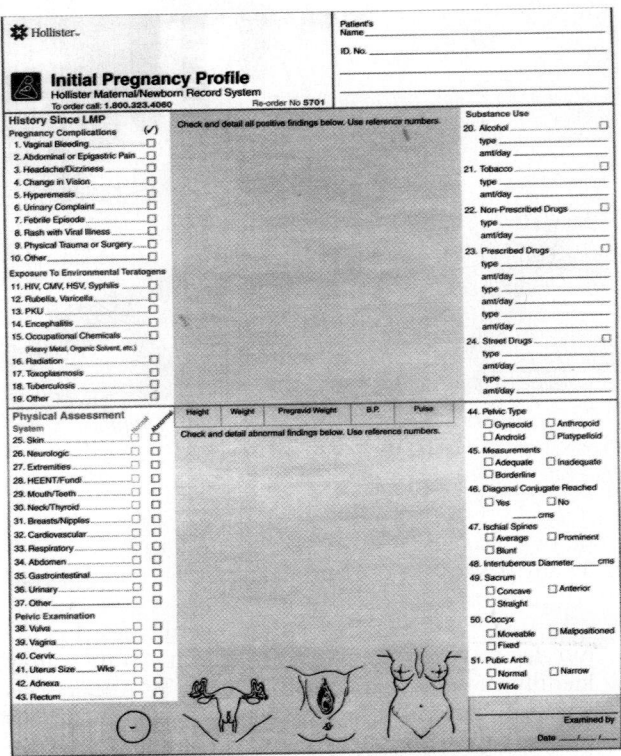

Figure 50-15 *Representative Initial Pregnancy Profile (Permission to use this copyright material has been granted by the owner, Hollister Incorporated.)*

Figure 50-17 *Bimanual Examination to Determine Uterine Changes*

TABLE 50-3	SCREENING TESTS IN PREGNANCY
TEST	**RESULTS**
Complete Blood Count	
RBC	3.75 million/mm^3 due to hemodilution.
WBC	Rises to 18,000/mm^3 by late pregnancy. Mostly an increase in neutrophils.
Hemoglobin (Hgb)	May decrease to 11.5g/dL later in pregnancy due to hemodilution. Repeat at 28 and 36 weeks.
Hematocrit (Hct)	33% lowest acceptable, due to hemodilution.
Blood Type	A, B, AB, or O
Rh factor	Positive or negative. If negative, do indirect Coomb's test. Check father's Rh.
Coomb's Test	Should remain negative. Retest Rh negative women at 28 weeks.
Rubella Titer (HAI)	>1:10 indicates immunity. <1:10, immunize after birth of infant.
Blood Glucose	Should be 60–110 mg/dL. Retest at 24 and 32 weeks.
VDRL or RPR (Syphilis)	Should be negative.

Cervical/Vaginal Culture
   Gonorrhea
   Chlamydia
   Group B *Streptococcus*
	Should be negative.

Hepatitis B Surface Antigen (HB$_s$Ag)	Positive indicates either active hepatitis or carrier state.
Antibody Titer HB$_s$Ag	Positive indicates immunity to hepatitis.
HIV (many states mandate that it be offered)	Should be negative.
Tuberculosis Skin tests: Mantoux or Tine	Should be negative. If positive, do chest x-ray.

Urinalysis
   Color, specific
   Gravity, pH, ketones, albumin, glucose
	Same as nonpregnant. Repeat at 28 weeks. Trace of glycosuria may occur in pregnancy.

Alpha-fetoprotein (AFP)	Check with laboratory for normal range for each week of gestation. If elevated, may have neural tube defects. If decreased, may have Down syndrome.

Subjective Data The following subjective data should be collected at each return visit:

- How the client is feeling
- Any discomforts, concerns, or questions the client may have
- Any body changes noticed by the client
- How developmental tasks are being met

At an early return visit, the mother's expectations for childbirth should be discussed. Closer to the EDB, preparations for the baby should also be covered.

Objective Data On each return visit, the following objective data should be collected and compared to data collected on previous visits and to prepregnant data, if known.

Blood Pressure Any increase of 30 mm Hg systolic or 15 mm Hg diastolic from one visit to the next should be reported to the health care provider. If there is no previous BP to compare to, a blood pressure of 140/90 should be reported.

Weight Total weight gain should be approximately 25 to 35 pounds, distributed as follows:

- Weeks 1 to 12:   2 to 4 pounds
- Weeks 13 to 40:   1 pound/week

Uterine Size The fundal height in centimeters indicates the weeks of gestation between 18 and 30 weeks.

Edema A small amount of dependent edema is often present in the last few weeks of pregnancy. Edema of the hands and face should be reported to the health care provider. Sometimes it is difficult to detect small amounts of edema in the hands, so ask the client if her rings are tighter or if she has had to remove her rings.

Fetal Position Assessment of fetal position is performed using **Leopold's maneuvers,** a series of specific palpations of the pregnant uterus to determine fetal position and presentation. The client is placed in the supine position with knees bent, and the examiner stands at the client's right side facing her head.

- First, the examiner palpates to determine which fetal part is in the fundus. Generally, it is the breech (buttocks).
- Second, the examiner moves hands to the sides of the uterus and determines on which side of the mother the fetal back is located.
- Third, the examiner's right hand is placed above the symphysis pubis to note whether the head or breech is near the pubic symphysis (this should correlate with the first maneuver).
- Fourth, the examiner changes position to face the client's feet, and palpates the sides of the abdomen to determine on which side the cephalic prominence presents (Figure 50-18).

Fetal Heartbeat After Leopold's maneuvers have determined fetal position, the fetal heartbeat should be assessed over the location of the fetal back. The rate should be 110 to 160 beats/minute. The rate is recorded, indicating the abdominal quadrant in which the heartbeat was noted.

Laboratory Tests At each visit, a urine sample is tested with a dipstick for protein, glucose, and ketones. If

First maneuver   Second maneuver

Third maneuver   Fourth maneuver

Figure 50-18 *Leopold's Maneuvers*

the results are positive for any of these three, the health care provider must be notified.

Anticipatory Guidance

Many of the nursing interventions during pregnancy are anticipatory guidance (teaching). The order in which topics are covered and the time frame when topics are covered may vary from client to client, depending on when prenatal care was begun and if there are any complications.

Environmental Hazards

Any chemicals, metals, anesthetic agents, antineoplastic and viral drugs, and x-ray examinations should be avoided. Excessive heat from saunas, hot tubs, or exercise in hot, humid weather should be avoided to prevent maternal hyperthermia (core temperature above 38.9°C/102°F). This has been associated with neural tube defects. Rogers and Davis (1995) report that the time needed to reach this core temperature is 15 minutes in a 39°C (102.2°F) tub and 10 minutes in a 41.1°C (106°F) tub.

Discomforts of Pregnancy

The physiological changes in pregnancy often cause discomforts to the woman. Table 50-4 identifies the common discomforts of pregnancy, possible causes, and interventions the client can try to alleviate or reduce the discomfort.

Test

TABLE 50-4 DISCOMFORTS OF PREGNANCY

DISCOMFORT	CAUSE	CLIENT INTERVENTIONS
Nausea/vomiting	Elevated hCG level Decreased gastric emptying time due to progesterone Ambivalence about pregnancy Fatigue	Limit fluid intake at meals and upon waking. Eat crackers or toast upon waking. Eat small amounts more frequently. Avoid fried, spicy, odorous, or gas-forming foods.
Heartburn	Gastric reflux—cardiac sphincter relaxed due to progesterone	Avoid overeating. Eat small, frequent meals. Avoid greasy foods. Sit up for 1 hour after eating. Take antacid only with health care provider's approval.
Urinary frequency	Pressure of uterus on bladder (early and late in pregnancy) Urinary tract infection	Empty bladder when urge is felt. *Do not* restrict fluid intake. Avoid fluids containing caffeine.
Breast tenderness	Effect of estrogen and progesterone	Wear well-fitting, supportive bra.
Flatulence	Relaxation of GI tract due to progesterone	Eat small meals. Omit gas-forming foods from diet. Have regular elimination.
Constipation	Bowel sluggishness due to progesterone Pressure of uterus on bowel Decreased activity and fluid intake Inadequate fiber in diet Iron supplement	Have regular schedule for bowel movement. Increase activity and fluid intake. Increase fiber in diet (raisins, prunes, fresh fruits and vegetables).
Hemorrhoids	Constipation Straining to have bowel movement Pressure of gravid (pregnant) uterus on veins Prolonged standing	Prevent constipation (see above). Apply ice packs. Use topical anesthetic ointments. Take sitz bath. Gently push hemorrhoids back into rectum.
Ankle edema	Prolonged standing or sitting Sodium and water retention from hormonal influence Increased capillary permeability	Dorsiflex feet when prolonged standing or sitting necessary. Elevate legs when sitting or resting. Increase number of rest periods.
Varicose veins (legs)	Increased blood volume Congenital predisposition to weak vascular walls Relaxation of vessel walls due to progesterone Inactivity Poor muscle tone Prolonged standing Obesity	Rest with feet and legs elevated. Avoid crossing legs, standing still, garters and restrictive clothing. Wear support hose.
Backache	Relaxation of joints due to estrogen and relaxin Exaggerated lordosis from change in center of gravity	Get adequate rest. Use proper posture. Use proper body mechanics.

continues

Test

TABLE 50-4 continued

DISCOMFORT	CAUSE	CLIENT INTERVENTIONS
Backache—continued	Wearing high-heeled shoes Excessive weight Fatigue Poor body mechanics	Wear low-heeled shoes
Dyspnea	Supine hypotensive syndrome Decreased lung capacity from pressure of uterus on diaphragm	Lie on either side. Sleep in semi-Fowler's position. Maintain proper posture.
Leg cramps	Calcium/phosphorus imbalance Pointing toes Fatigue or muscle strain Pressure of gravid uterus impairs circulation to legs	Evaluate diet for adequate calcium and phosphorus intake. Pull toes up toward knees. Rest with legs elevated.
Dizziness and fainting	Supine hypotensive syndrome Sudden change of position Standing for long period in warm area Hyperventilation Hypoglycemia Anemia	Lie on either side, not on back. Arise slowly. Avoid standing in warm area. Practice slow, deep respirations. Drink orange juice for fast-acting sugar.
Bleeding gums, nasal stuffiness, and epistaxis	Increased estrogen level Increased blood volume Lack of vitamin C	Avoid use of decongestants. Use cool vaporizer or humidifier. Use saline nasal spray several times a day. Drink orange juice. Have dental checkup.
Vaginal discharge	Increased estrogen causes more cervical mucous	Bathe or shower daily. Avoid douching. Wear absorbent cotton underwear.
Itchy skin	Tissue stretching Soap use Dehydration	Use lotion on skin. Change soap, rinse well. Drink more fluids.
Mood swings	Hormonal changes Inadequate rest Inadequate diet Ambivalence about pregnancy	Get more rest. Eat balanced diet. Express fears, feelings, and concerns.

Warning Signs

The client should be taught to immediately report to the health care provider the warning signs listed in Table 50-5. They may indicate complications of pregnancy. Generally, the sooner interventions are begun, the better the outcome.

Nutrition

There is very little change needed in the diet of a pregnant woman if she is already following the food guide pyramid. A woman eating a balanced, adequate diet needs to add only 300 kcalories a day to her diet when pregnant and 500 kcalories a day when breastfeeding.

The addition of two milk servings and one meat serving will meet the 300 kcalorie increase as well as the increased need for calcium and protein.

Many health care providers have their pregnant clients take a multivitamin with calcium and iron to ensure an adequate intake of these essential nutrients. Folic acid in the multivitamin prevents neural tube defects, calcium is needed for bone and teeth, and iron is needed to prevent anemia in mother and fetus. Based on a nutritional assessment, suggestions can be made to the client for a more adequate dietary intake, taking into account personal and cultural preferences.

Some pregnant women eat substances that are not considered edible and have no nutritive value. This is called **pica.** Substances generally eaten in the United States are laundry starch, dirt, clay, and freezer frost. Eating laundry starch interferes with absorption of nutrients. Clay, dirt, and laundry starch contribute to constipation and possible fecal impaction.

Factors that place a woman at risk for nutritional inadequacy during pregnancy include:

- Adolescence, due to demands for own growth and pregnancy; possible poor dietary habits; and possibility of trying to hide pregnancy

- Inadequate nutritional intake
- Pica
- Low income
- Smoking, alcohol use, or drug addiction
- Short interval between pregnancies—no time to replenish nutrient stores
- Medical conditions such as diabetes or kidney problems
- Depression

Self-Care

Physical care during pregnancy generally involves minor adjustments in or moderation of normal habits.

Breast Care

Proper support of the breasts is important during pregnancy whether the woman is planning to breast-feed or bottle-feed her baby. A properly fitted maternity or nursing bra promotes comfort, retains breast shape, and prevents back strain if breasts are very large.

Cleanliness of the breasts is very important. Washing with water is sufficient because soap removes the natural lubricant provided by Montgomery's tubercles, causing drying and possible cracking of the nipples. If leakage is experienced, a nursing pad can be worn inside the bra, and the pregnant woman encouraged to rub the fluid into the nipple to lubricate the skin. Air-drying the nipples after leaking will also promote breast health.

Personal Hygiene

Daily bathing is important because the pregnant woman generally has increased perspiration and vaginal mucous. Either a tub bath or shower may be taken, depending on the woman's preference and facilities available. Later in pregnancy, a tub bath may require that the

TABLE 50-5 WARNING SIGNS DURING PREGNANCY	
WARNING SIGN	**POSSIBLE CAUSE**
Vaginal bleeding (any), "bloody show"	Abortion (miscarriage), placenta previa, placenta abruptio, lesions of cervix or vagina
Sudden gush of fluid from vagina	Rupture of membranes
Persistent vomiting	Hyperemesis gravidarum, infection
Severe, continuous headache	Hypertension, preeclampsia
Swelling of face, hands, legs, feet when arising in morning	Preeclampsia
Visual disturbances: blurring, double vision, flashes of light, spots before eyes	Hypertension, preeclampsia
Dizziness	Hypertension, preeclampsia
Fever over 100°F (37.8°C) and chills	Infection
Pain in abdomen or cramping	Ectopic pregnancy, abortion (miscarriage), placenta abruptio, labor
Epigastric pain	Preeclampsia
Irritating vaginal discharge	Vaginal infection
Dysuria	Urinary tract infection
Oliguria	Dehydration, renal impairment
Noticeable reduction or absence of fetal movement	Fetal distress, fetal death

Exercises for Pregnancy

Specific exercises can be taught to clients to help strengthen muscle tone in preparation for birth.

- The pelvic tilt reduces back strain and strengthens the abdominal muscles. Figure 50-19 illustrates how to perform the pelvic tilt in both a standing and kneeling position. Exhale, roll the hips and buttocks forward, hold for a count of five, then inhale and relax.
- Abdominal muscle tightening with every breath increases abdominal muscle tone. This can be done anywhere in any position. While slowly taking in a deep breath, expand the abdomen. Then exhale slowly while pulling the abdomen in until the muscles are completely contracted. Relax a few seconds and repeat the exercise.
- Kegel's exercises strengthen and tighten the perineal muscles. Tighten these muscles and pull them up toward the vagina as if trying to stop urination midstream. This exercise also can be done anytime, anyplace.
- The tailor sit (cross-legged sit) stretches the inner thigh muscles; adding arm reaches stretches the sides and upper body and helps relieve upper backache. Sit cross-legged and stretch one arm high over head, then release and exhale and repeat on the other side. Figure 50-20 illustrates the tailor sit and arm reaches.

Figure 50-19 *Pelvic Tilt*

Figure 50-20 *Tailor Sit and Arm Reaches*

mother have help in getting out of the tub. Douching should not be done because it changes the pH of the vagina and alters the normal flora.

Activity/Rest

The pregnant woman should have some type of regular physical activity. Walking, swimming, and cycling are perhaps the best activities for most women. Women who routinely participate in exercise before pregnancy should continue and nonexercising women should begin exercising. Fatigue should be avoided. Exercise during pregnancy could reduce the risk of cesarean birth (Bungum, Peaslee, Jackson, and Perez, 2000). They should avoid hyperthermia and drink plenty of water before and after exercise to prevent dehydration. Exercise is contraindicated during pregnancy when the following are present: pregnancy-induced hypertension, preterm rupture of membranes, preterm labor during a prior or present pregnancy, incompetent cervix, persistent second or third trimester bleeding, or fetal growth restriction (Bungum et al., 2000).

Adequate rest is important for the pregnant woman. It may be a challenge to find rest time during the day, especially for women who work outside the home or have small children. More sleep is needed, especially during the first and last trimester. Most women experience significant sleep problems throughout pregnancy (Mindell and Jacobson, 2000).

Clothing

Clothing is an important aspect of a woman's self-image, especially during pregnancy when the physical changes may have a negative impact on her self-image. The clothes should be attractive, yet loose and nonconstricting. Maternity clothes are often shared among friends because they are worn for a relatively short time and can be expensive. The pregnant woman should avoid wearing knee-high or thigh-high stockings or garters because they can interfere with circulation in the legs.

Wearing low-heeled shoes is usually recommended. If the woman has no problem with backache *and* can maintain her balance, there is no medical reason for not wearing slightly higher-heeled shoes. Edema in the feet toward the end of pregnancy may require wearing a larger size shoe.

Employment

How long to work when pregnant depends on the type of work done by the woman and how the pregnancy is progressing. The major factors to consider are whether there are teratogenic hazards in the work environment, if the woman will be subject to physical strain or overfatigue, and if there are obstetrical or medical complications of the pregnancy. Rest periods should be available during the workday.

Travel

Unless there are obstetrical or medical complications, travel need not be restricted. When traveling by car, the pregnant client should be encouraged to stop every 2 hours and walk around for 10 minutes or so. It is imperative always to wear the seat belt, both lap and shoulder, and to keep the lap belt snug below the abdomen. Possible bladder trauma, in case of an accident, can be decreased by keeping the bladder empty. Travel by air should be considered for long trips. Clients should be aware that many airlines and cruise ships will not accept passengers past a certain week of pregnancy.

Dental Care

Regular oral hygiene should continue during pregnancy. Dental care can be performed during pregnancy. The woman should inform her dentist that she is pregnant. If possible, x-rays should be delayed until after the infant is born. If x-rays must be done, a lead apron must be used.

Sexual Activity

There is no reason to limit sexual activity in a healthy pregnancy. Only when the woman has a history of preterm labor, there is bleeding, or the membranes have ruptured is sexual intercourse contraindicated. As always, barrier protection should be used to prevent sexually transmitted diseases.

The expectant woman's sexual desire may decrease during the first trimester because of fatigue, nausea/vomiting, and breast tenderness. Often, during the second trimester, when the discomforts have lessened, she has greater sexual satisfaction than when not pregnant. By the third trimester, the discomforts of fatigue, dyspnea, urinary frequency, and painful pelvic ligaments may decrease her sexual desire.

After the fourth month, the woman should not lie flat on her back during intercourse because of supine hypotensive syndrome. A pillow can be placed under her right hip to displace the uterus or an alternate position used. ✳ Vagus nerve pressure

Men may find a change in their desire too. This may be related to their feelings about their partner's changing appearance, concern about hurting her or the fetus, and having sexual intercourse with a pregnant woman.

CHILDBIRTH EDUCATION

Many health care providers recommend that their clients attend a prepared childbirth class. When a woman understands what is happening in her body, she has less fear and is less tense. She will then be more relaxed during labor and will be able to help more effectively during the birth process.

Several persons have gained recognition for developing childbirth education programs. The three most commonly known are Dick-Read, Bradley, and Lamaze. The most popular is the Lamaze method, or more accurately, some adaptation of the Lamaze method.

Dick-Read

In the 1930s, Dr. Grantly Dick-Read proposed the fear-tension-pain syndrome. That is, the woman during childbirth experiences fear because she does not understand what is happening in her body. This causes tension, which causes the woman to perceive pain more intensely. Classes based on this method include the physiology of childbirth, exercises for the abdomen and perineal muscles, and relaxation techniques. Classes also focus on teaching the woman to visualize what is happening inside her body, and to use abdominal breathing, not chest breathing.

Bradley

Dr. Robert Bradley stressed that labor is a normal process and focused on environmental variables. He felt that husband or partner support is most important.

During early labor, diversionary activities are encouraged. When not walking, the tailor sit or Sims position are encouraged. During a contraction, the woman is to close her eyes and relax with slow, deep abdominal breathing. The husband/partner is to be supportive, touch the laboring woman, and put a hand on her abdomen during a contraction.

Lamaze

Dr. Fernand Lamaze introduced the childbirth preparation method called **psychoprophylaxis** (mental and physical preparation for childbirth). It combines controlled muscle relaxation and breathing techniques. The pregnant woman is taught to contract a specific group of muscles and relax the rest of her body. This conditions her to relax when the uterus contracts.

Abdominal effleurage, light stroking of the abdomen, is used to relieve mild pain but not intense pain. Back pain can be relieved by putting pressure on the sacrum.

NURSING PROCESS

The nurse's role centers on helping the client maintain a healthy pregnancy and preparing the client for childbirth and delivery.

Assessment

The information presented in this chapter encompasses the possible subjective data and objective data that may be gathered about a specific client.

Nursing Diagnoses

Nursing diagnoses applicable to a pregnant client may include:

- *Activity Intolerance*
- *Anxiety*
- Disturbed *Body Image*

- *Ineffective **B**reathing Pattern*
- ***C**onstipation*
- *Ineffective **C**oping*
- *Readiness for Enhanced Family **C**oping*
- ***F**atigue*
- ***F**ear*
- *Deficient **F**luid Volume*
- *Excess **F**luid Volume*
- *Ineffective **H**ealth Maintenance*
- ***H**ealth Seeking Behaviors (specify)*
- *Risk for **I**njury*
- *Deficient **K**nowledge (specify)*
- *Impaired Physical **M**obility*
- ***N**oncompliance*
- *Imbalanced **N**utrition: Less Than Body Requirements*
- *Disturbed **S**leep Pattern*
- ***S**exual Dysfunction*

Planning/Outcome Identification

At least one goal must be set with the client to meet the need of the client as identified by the nursing diagnoses.

Nursing Interventions

Nursing interventions must be individualized and specific for the client based on the assessment, nursing diagnoses, and goals. Nursing interventions for prenatal care are focused on teaching the client and providing anticipatory guidance.

Evaluation

Each goal must be evaluated to determine how it has been met by the client.

SAMPLE NURSING CARE PLAN

PRENATAL CARE

Penny, age 23, first pregnancy, states she has been nauseated and has not eaten for about 3 weeks, feels very tired all the time, takes a nap after work, and then has trouble sleeping because she has to go to the bathroom frequently. Her LMP was six weeks ago, menstrual periods have always been regular every 28 days. She smokes 1 pack/day and drinks beer on the weekends. She does not like to cook, so most meals are eaten out. She has lost 3 pounds in the last month. She is unmarried, lives alone, and did not plan to get pregnant.

Nursing Diagnosis 1 *Knowledge Deficit (Self-Care in Pregnancy)* related to inexperience as evidenced by eating, drinking, and smoking habits

Nursing Outcomes Classification (NOC)
Knowledge: Pregnancy

Nursing Interventions Classification (NIC)
Prenatal Care

PLANNING/GOALS	NURSING INTERVENTIONS	RATIONALE
Penny will competently care for herself during pregnancy.	Teach physiology of pregnancy, discomforts of pregnancy, things she can do to relieve the discomforts, self-care aspects, and fetal development.	Provides reasons for Penny to take care of herself.
	Gather more data about her work environment and psychosocial aspects of nutrition, smoking, and drinking.	Provides data for additional teaching.

EVALUATION   Penny states that she now understands the changes pregnancy makes in her body.

Nursing Diagnosis 2 *Imbalanced **N**utrition: less than body requirements* related to inadequate food intake as evidenced by nausea and weight loss

Nursing Outcomes Classification (NOC)
Nutritional Status: Energy
Nutritional Status: Nutrient Intake

Nursing Interventions Classification (NIC)
Nutrition Management
Teaching: Individual

continues

SAMPLE NURSING CARE PLAN

PLANNING/GOALS	NURSING INTERVENTIONS	RATIONALE
Penny will have sufficient nutritional intake during pregnancy	Teach basic nutrition, food guide pyramid, and nutritional needs during pregnancy.	May encourage changes in Penny's eating pattern.

EVALUATION   Penny follows the food guide pyramid most of the time and is drinking 4 glasses of milk a day.

Nursing Diagnosis 3 *Risk for Injury* related to teratogenic substances as evidenced by smoking and alcohol consumption

Nursing Outcomes Classification (NOC)	**Nursing Interventions Classification (NIC)**
Risk Control: Tobacco Use	*Teaching: Individual*
Risk Control: Alcohol	*Risk Identification: Childbearing Family*
Risk Control: Unintended Pregnancy	

PLANNING/GOALS	NURSING INTERVENTIONS	RATIONALE
Penny will stop smoking and drinking alcohol.	Teach effects of smoking and alcohol on fetal development.	May encourage Penny to abstain from both.

EVALUATION   Penny has cut her smoking in half and only drinks one beer on the weekend.

CASE STUDY

Beth, age 30, and John, age 30, have been married 4 years. Beth's LMP was 12 weeks ago, but her menstrual periods have always been very irregular. She is tired all the time and nauseated every day, her clothes are very tight around her waist, and her abdomen is protruding.

The following questions will guide your development of a nursing care plan for the case study.

1. What other data would you collect about Beth?
2. What diagnostic tests would you anticipate the health care provider performing or ordering?
3. What anticipatory guidance would be appropriate for Beth?
4. When should Beth return for a checkup?

Summary

- Ideally, planning for pregnancy should begin before conception.
- Fetal development proceeds in an orderly and predictable manner.
- Prenatal care involves all aspects of the couple's life.
- A complete history for a pregnant client includes her own medical and obstetrical history, family history, and the fetus's father's history.
- Nutrition increase for pregnancy is 300 kcalories/day. Two extra glasses of milk and one extra serving of meat will meet this need and supply the extra calcium and protein needed.
- Anticipatory guidance comprises the majority of nursing interventions when caring for a pregnant client.

Review Questions

1. Using Naegele's rule, when is a client expected to deliver if her LMP began on March 15?

    a. November 15
    b. November 23
    c. December 8
    d. December 22

2. A client pregnant for the first time is termed a:

    a. primipara.
    b. multipara.
    c. primigravida.
    d. multigravida.

3. Which of the following should the nurse recognize as the desired weight gain during pregnancy?

    a. 25 to 35 pounds
    b. 12 to 20 pounds
    c. 15 to 28 pounds
    d. 10 to 15 pounds

4. Which of the following should the nurse recognize as a positive sign of pregnancy?

    a. ballottement
    b. hearing fetal heartbeat
    c. a positive pregnancy test
    d. increase in abdominal size

5. Which of the following lunches would the nurse encourage for a pregnant woman?

    a. bologna sandwich, potato chips, cola
    b. cold chicken, french fries, roll, milk
    c. bowl of bean soup, crackers, glass of ice tea
    d. cottage cheese, tossed salad and cracker, orange, water

References/Suggested Readings

Allard-Hendren, R. (2000). Alcohol use and adolescent pregnancy. *MCN*, 25(3), 159–162.

Beckmann, C. A., Buford, T. A., & Witt, J. B. (2000). Perceived barriers to prenatal care services. *MCN*, 25(1), 43–46.

Brucker, M. C., & Reedy, N. J. (2000). Nurse-midwifery: Yesterday, today, and tomorrow. *MCN*, 25(6), 322–326.

Bryan, A. (2000). Enhancing parent-child interaction with a prenatal couple intervention. *MCN*, 25(3), 139–144.

Bungum, T., Peaslee, D., Jackson, A., & Perez, M. (2000). Exercise during pregnancy and type of delivery in nulliparae. *JOGNN*, 29(1), 258–264.

Callister, L., & Vega, R. (1998). Giving birth: Guatemalan women's voices. *JOGNN*, 27(3), 289–295.

Centers for Disease Control and Prevention (CDC), National Center for Health Statistics (2001). *Health, United States* (Table 26: Infant Mortality Rates). [Online]. Available: www.cdc.gov/nchs

Cesario, S. (2001). Care of the Native American woman: Strategies for practice, education, and research. *JOGNN*, 30(1), 13–19.

Cordero, S. (2003). Assessing fetal heart sounds. *Nursing2003*, 33(10), 54–55.

Dick-Read, G. (1933). *Natural childbirth*. London: Heinemann.

Dick-Read, G. (1944). *Childbirth without fear*. New York: Harper & Row.

Dickason, E., Silverman, B., & Kaplan J. (1998). *Maternal-infant nursing care* (3rd ed.). St. Louis, MO: Mosby-Year Book.

Dochterman, J., & Bulechek, G. (2004). *Nursing Interventions Classification (NIC)* (4th ed.). St. Louis, MO: Mosby.

Freda, M. (1998). Confronting the myths. *MCN*, 23(2), 107.

Gennaro, S., Kamwendo, L., Mbweza, E., & Kershbaumer, R. (1998). Childbearing in Malawi, Africa. *JOGNN*, 27(2), 191–196.

Giarelli, E. (2001). A legal look at genetic testing. *RN*, 64(10), 73–75.

Hall, S. (2002). Amniotomy: Necessary intervention or bad habit. *AWHONN Lifelines*, 5(6), 10–13.

Hasenau, S., & Covington, C. (2002). Neural tube defects: Prevention and folic acid. *MCN*, 27(2), 87–91.

Howard, J., & Berbiglia, V. (1997). Caring for childbearing Korean women. *JOGNN*, 26(6), 665–671.

Hutchinson, M., & Baqi-Aziz, M. (1994). Nursing care of the childbearing Muslim family. *JOGNN*, 23(9), 767–771.

Jones, S. (1996). Genetics: Changing health care in the 21st century. *JOGNN*, 25(9), 777–783.

Ladewig, P., Moberly, S., Olds, S., & London, M. (2001). *Contemporary maternal-newborn nursing care* (5th ed.). Menlo Park, CA: Addison-Wesley Longman.

Lamaze, F. (1965). *Painless childbirth*. New York: Dimon & Schuster.

Littleton, L., & Engebretson, J. (2002). *Maternal, neonatal, and women's health nursing*. Clifton Park, NY: Thomson Delmar Learning.

Longobucco, D., & Freston, M. (1989). Relation of somatic symptoms to degree of paternal-role preparation of first-time expectant fathers. *JOGNN*, 18, 482.

Malnory, M. (1996). Developmental care of the pregnant couple. *JOGNN*, 25(6), 525–532.

Martinez, F., et al. (1994, Sept.). The effect of paternal smoking on the birthweight of newborns whose mothers did not smoke. The Health Medical Associates. *Am. J. Public Health*, 84, 1489–1491.

Matthews, T. J. (1998). Smoking during pregnancy 1990-1996. *National Vital Statistics Reports*, 47(10), 1–12.

Mindell, J., & Jacobson, B. (2000). Sleep disturbances during pregnancy. *JOGNN*, 29(6), 590–597.

Moorhead, S., Johnson, M., & Maas, M. (2004). *Nursing Outcomes Classification (NOC)* (3rd ed.). St. Louis, MO: Mosby.

Nasso, J. (1997). Planning for pregnancy—A preconception health program. *MCN*, 22(3), 142–146.

North American Nursing Diagnosis Association. (2003). *Nursing diagnoses: Definitions & classification 2003–2004* Philadelphia: Author.

Pletsch, P., Morgan, S., & Pieper, A. (2003). Context & beliefs about smoking & smoking cessation. *MCN*, 28(5), 320–325.

Reifsnider, E., & Gill, S. (2000). Nutrition for childbearing years. *JOGNN*, 29(1), 43–55.

Remich, M. (1997). Promoting a healthy pregnancy. In E. Q. Younkin & M. S. Davis (Eds.), *Women's health: A primary care clinical guide* (2d ed.). Norwalk, CT: Appleton & Lange.

Rentschler, D. (2003). Pregnant adolescent's perspectives of pregnancy. *MCN*, 28(6), 377–383.

Rhodes, A. (1995). Liability for failure to offer prenatal AFP testing. *MCN*, 20(3), 169.

Robaire, B., & Hales, B. (1993, August). Paternal exposure to chemicals before conception. *BMI, 307,* 341–342.

Rogers, J., & Davis, B. (1995). How risky are hot tubs and saunas for pregnant women? *MCN, 20*(3), 137–140.

Rossner, S. (1998). Obesity and pregnancy. In G. Bray, C. Bouchard, & W. James (Eds.). *Handbook of obesity* (pp. 575–590). New York: Marcel Dekker.

Schneiderman, J. (1996). Postpartum nursing for Korean mothers. *MCN, 21*(3), 155–158.

Simpson, K., & Creehan, P. (2001). *AWHONN perinatal nursing* (2nd ed.). Philadelphia: Lippincott Williams & Wilkins.

Todd, S. T., LaSala, K. B., & Neil-Urbon, S. (2001). An integrated approach to prenatal smoking cessation interventions. *MCN, 26*(4), 185–190.

Wisborg, K., Kesmodel, U. et al. (2003). Maternal consumption of coffee during pregnancy and stillbirth and infant death in first year of life: Prospective study. *British Medical Journal 326*(7386), 420.

Resources

American Dietetic Association, 216 West Jackson Boulevard, Chicago, IL 60606-6995, 800-366-1655, www.eatright.org

Association of Women's Health, Obstetric, and Neonatal Nurses (AWHONN), 2000 L Street N.W., Suite 740, Washington, DC, 20036, 800-673-8499 (U.S.), 800-245-0231 (Canada), www.awhonn.org

Food and Nutrition Information Center, Agricultural Research Service, USDA, National Agricultural Library, Room 105, 10301 Baltimore Avenue, Beltsville, MD 20705-2351, 301-504-5719, www.nal.usda.gov

March of Dimes, 1275 Mamaroneck Avenue, White Plains, NY, 10605, 888-MODIMES (663-4637), www.modimes.org

COMPLICATIONS OF PREGNANCY

MAKING THE CONNECTION

Refer to the following chapters to increase your understanding of the complications of pregnancy:

Basic Nursing
- Loss, Grief, and Death

Adult Health Nursing
- Cardiovascular System
- Hematologic and Lymphatic Systems
- Endocrine System
- Sexually Transmitted Diseases
- Substance Abuse

Maternal & Pediatric Nursing
- Prenatal Care
- The Birth Process

Basic Procedures
- Hand Hygiene
- Use of Protective Equipment
- Taking Blood Pressure
- Measuring Intake and Output

Intermediate Procedures
- Surgical Asepsis: Preparing and Maintaining a Sterile Field
- Performing Open Gloving
- Performing Urinary Catheterization: Female

LEARNING OBJECTIVES

Upon completion of this chapter, you should be able to:

- Define key terms.
- Discuss therapy for a client with hyperemesis gravidarum.
- Compare and contrast the etiology, medical–surgical management, and nursing care for the bleeding situations in pregnancy.
- Describe the development, medical–surgical management, and nursing care of a client with pregnancy-induced hypertension.
- Describe the nursing care for a client with a chronic medical problem: diabetes, hypertension, heart disease, maternal PKU.
- Discuss the effects of infection on a pregnant woman and her fetus and ways of preventing the infections.
- Compare and contrast the etiology, medical–surgical management, nursing care, and effect on the fetus of Rh incompatibility and ABO incompatibility.
- Describe the effects of multiple pregnancies on the mother, fetuses, and family.
- Describe the effects of addiction on the mother and fetus.
- Summarize the needs of a woman in preterm labor.

KEY TERMS

abortion	incompetent cervix
abruptio placenta	kernicterus
amniocentesis	late deceleration
early deceleration	macrosomia
eclampsia	miscarriage
ectopic pregnancy	oligohydramnios
euglycemia	placenta previa
fetal biophysical profile	preeclampsia
HELLP syndrome	surfactant
hydatidiform mole	tocolysis
hydramnios	variable deceleration
hyperemesis gravidarum	

INTRODUCTION

It is truly impressive that most pregnancies have no complications. For those clients who do have complications, it can be a very frightening and guilt-ridden situation. Regular prenatal care is the best way to identify clients who have high-risk factors. These clients can then be assessed and monitored more closely, and signs

TABLE 51-1	HIGH-RISK FACTORS IN PREGNANCY		
GENERAL	**OBSTETRICAL**	**MEDICAL**	**OTHER**
Age (under 15 or over 35 years)	Previous problems	Chronic diseases	Smoking
Unmarried	Abortion	Diabetes	Drug abuse
Low socioeconomic group, little education	Excessive size of infant	Hypertension	Alcohol abuse
Prenatal care begun 27 weeks or later	Cesarean birth	Sickle-cell anemia	Nutritional deficit
	Preterm/Postterm birth	Thyroid disease	
	Incompetent cervix	Sexually transmitted disease	
	Abnormal fetal presentation	Cervical neoplasia	
	Rh negative and sensitized	Urinary tract infection	
	Preeclampsia	Neurological problem	
	Multiple pregnancy	Psychiatric problem	

and symptoms of complications detected as early as possible. Medical–surgical management and effective nursing care can then be implemented. Many of the high-risk factors in pregnancy are given in Table 51-1.

This chapter covers the common complications of pregnancy including etiology, medical–surgical management, and the nursing process.

ASSESSMENT OF FETAL WELL-BEING

When complications arise in a pregnancy, more intense and specific assessments of the fetus are required.

Ultrasound

Ultrasound allows visualization of the uterine contents. The fetal assessments described in the Prenatal Care chapter are also to be used. High-frequency, inaudible sound waves are directed toward the uterus. The sound waves reflected back are converted into a visual image (Figure 51-1).

Figure 51-1 *Ultrasound provides a visual image of uterine contents.*

Ultrasound provides the following information.

First Trimester

- Early positive diagnosis of pregnancy about 5 or 6 weeks after LMP
- Identification of more than one fetus
- Observation of cardiac activity at 21 days and respiratory movements about 11th week of gestation
- Diagnosis of an ectopic pregnancy

Second and Third Trimester

- Measurement of biparietal diameter, femur length, overall length (crown-heel and crown-rump), gestational age, and intrauterine growth retardation (IUGR)
- Detection of some fetal anomalies, especially anencephaly and hydrocephalus
- Detection of hydramnios (excessive amniotic fluid, or polyhydramnios) or **oligohydramnios** (deficiency of amniotic fluid), either of which is frequently associated with fetal anomalies
- Identification of amniotic fluid pockets; a vertical pocket of 2 cm is associated with normal fetal status
- Location of the placenta, which is necessary before an amniocentesis and to determine placenta previa
- Determination of fetal position and presentation
- Detection of fetal death; fetal heart beating is not visualized, and the bones in the fetal head separate

Transabdominal Ultrasound

The mother is asked to have a full bladder when the ultrasound is performed. This allows the other structures to be assessed in relation to the bladder. The transducer is moved slowly over the abdomen while the client lies on her back. This position may cause shortness of breath. The procedure takes about 20 to 30 minutes.

Endovaginal Ultrasound

A probe is inserted into the vagina, putting it close to the structures being imaged. This produces a clearer image. The client is in the lithotomy position and has an empty bladder.

Nonstress Test

A nonstress test (NST) requires an electronic fetal monitor to record fetal movement and fetal heart rate (FHR) accelerations (short-term increases in fetal heart rate caused by fetal movement). Specific equipment may vary. The mother reclines in a chair or in bed in semi-Fowler's or side-lying position. This noninvasive test is used once or twice a week after 30 weeks' gestation in high-risk clients (Figure 51-2).

The test is reactive if there are two accelerations of 15 beats/minute, lasting 15 seconds in a 20-minute period. This indicates that the fetus has adequate oxygenation and an intact central nervous system.

The test is nonreactive if the criteria for reactive are not met. This may indicate that the fetus is asleep or is having problems.

An unsatisfactory test is identified if there is inadequate fetal activity or the data cannot be interpreted. If decelerations of the FHR are noted, the health care provider should be notified.

Fetal Acoustic Stimulation Test and Vibroacoustic Stimulation Test

The fetal acoustic stimulation test (FAST) and vibroacoustic stimulation test (VST) are used in conjunction with the NST. A small battery-operated device is placed on the mother's abdomen over the fetal head. A low-frequency vibration and a buzzing sound are emitted from the device to stimulate the fetus who had a nonreactive NST. The sounds emitted last no more than 3 seconds and are repeated every minute if no accelerations occur.

Two FHR accelerations of 15 beats/minute, lasting 15 seconds, in a 10-minute period are considered to be a reactive test. Some institutions use the FAST and VST instead of an NST.

Fetal Biophysical Profile

The **fetal biophysical profile** (FBPP) assesses five biophysical variables: fetal breathing movement, fetal movements of body or limbs, fetal tone (extension/flexion of extremities), amniotic fluid volume, and reactive NST (Table 51-2). The first four are assessed by ultrasound. A score of 8 or more shows probable fetal well-being.

Fetal Movements

From the time of quickening (16 to 20 weeks), fetal movement is reassuring to the mother. Counting fetal movement daily provides evidence that the fetus is not having difficulty.

One method is to count fetal movements for 10 minutes three times a day. Another, which is the Cardiff

Figure 51-2 *Nonstress Test (NST) to Assess Fetal Well-being*

TABLE 51-2 BIOPHYSICAL PROFILE		
	SCORE 2	**SCORE 0**
Fetal Breathing	One or more episodes lasting 30 seconds in 30 minutes	Not present or not lasting 30 seconds
Fetal Movement	Three or more body/limb movements in 30 minutes	Two or fewer body/limb movements in 30 minutes
Fetal Tone	One or more episodes of active flexion/extension	Slow extension with return to partial flexion, or movement absent
Fluid Assessment	One or more pockets of amniotic fluid 1 cm in two perpendicular planes	No pocket, or no pocket 1 cm in two perpendicular planes
Fetal Reaction	Reactive NST	Nonreactive NST

method, requires the mother to count fetal movements at the same time each day until 10 movements are felt. The start and stop times are recorded.

The health care provider should be contacted if there are:

- fewer than 10 movements in 12 hours
- no movements for 8 hours
- sudden violent movements followed by reduced movements

Biochemical Assessments

Three tests include maternal serum alpha-fetoprotein, estriol, and human placental lactogen.

Maternal Serum Alpha-Fetoprotein

Maternal serum alpha-fetoprotein (MSAFP) identifies some birth defects and chromosomal anomalies during the antepartum period. AFP is found in maternal serum about 7 weeks' gestation and rises steadily until the last trimester. All women should have the test between 16 and 18 weeks' gestation. Because there is a normal range for each week of pregnancy, a correct gestational age is important to the interpretation of the test.

If the MSAFP level is high, it may indicate a fetal open neural tube defect, multiple gestation, Rh isoimmunization, maternal diabetes mellitus, or fetal distress and death. If the MSAFP level is low, the fetus may have Down syndrome or there may be a maternal hypertensive state.

Estriol

Maternal estriol level indicates fetoplacental function. Essential precursors from the fetal adrenal glands are converted by the placenta to estriol. The level in maternal serum and urine usually increases throughout pregnancy, so there must be a series of tests throughout pregnancy. The gradual increase in the maternal estriol level indicates that the fetal adrenal glands and the placenta are functioning normally.

Human Placental Lactogen

Human placental lactogen (hPL) increases throughout pregnancy correlating with increased fetal weight.

Amniocentesis

Amniocentesis is a procedure in which a needle is inserted through the abdomen into the amniotic sac. Amniotic fluid is withdrawn and sent to the laboratory for testing. At 14 to 16 weeks' gestation, an amniocentesis may be performed for diagnosis of genetic diseases or birth defects if the mother is older than 35 or either parent has a family history of genetic disease (Figure 51-3).

Later in pregnancy, amniocentesis is most often used to determine fetal lung maturity. In a problem pregnancy when preterm delivery of the fetus is a possibility, the physician will often try to maintain the pregnancy until the lungs are mature.

The nurse assists the physician performing the amniocentesis and provides emotional support to the client.

Figure 51-3 *Amniocentesis: A small amount of amniotic fluid is withdrawn for study.*

Safety: Amniocentesis
- Wash hands.
- Wear goggles or face mask, splash apron, and disposable gloves.
- Label specimen clearly so laboratory personnel can use appropriate precautions.
- Wash hands after removal of gloves.

Tests on Amniotic Fluid

Both the fluid and the cells in the amniotic fluid are used for testing. The fluid should be clear, colorless, and may have flecks of vernix caseosa floating in it.

Lecithin/Sphingomyelin Ratio Surfactant is phospholipids in the lungs that lower surface tension and stabilize the alveoli so they do not collapse on exhalation. The ratio of two phospholipids that are components of surfactant, lecithin and sphingomyelin (L/S ratio), determines the maturity of the lungs.

Early in pregnancy, the lecithin level is low and the sphingomyelin level is high. About 32 weeks' gestation, this relationship begins to change. By 35 weeks' gestation, the lecithin level is twice as high as the level of sphingomyelin. An L/S ratio of 2:1 is considered indicative of lung maturity.

Some conditions may accelerate lung maturation, such as severe pregnancy-induced hypertension (PIH), chronic maternal hypertension, or prolonged rupture of membranes. Diabetes and Rh isoimmunization seem to delay fetal lung maturity.

Phosphatidylglycerol Another phospholipid in surfactant, phosphatidylglycerol (PG), appears in the amniotic fluid when the lungs are mature, about 35 weeks' gestation.

Bilirubin In clients with Rh incompatibility, there is bilirubin in the amniotic fluid. The level of bilirubin corresponds to the degree of fetal anemia.

Sex Determination The sex of the fetus can be accurately determined by cell studies. This is important in sex-linked genetic abnormalities.

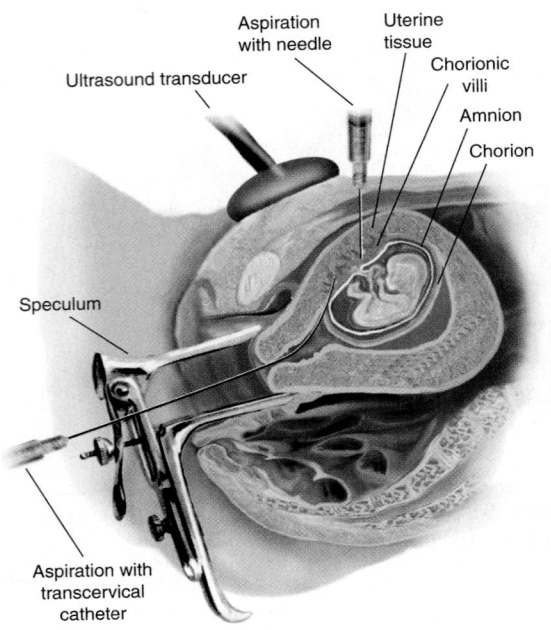

Figure 51-4 *Chorionic Villi Sampling (performed between 8 and 10 weeks' gestation)*

Chorionic Villi Sampling

In chorionic villi sampling (CVS), samples of chorionic villi from the developing placenta are obtained to assess for the same genetic disorders as in amniocentesis. CVS is performed between 8 and 10 weeks' gestation. Either a vaginal or abdominal approach may be used (Figure 51-4).

Contraction Stress Test

A contraction stress test (CST) evaluates the respiratory function of the placenta. During a uterine contraction, blood flow to the intervillous spaces is momentarily reduced, thus decreasing oxygen available to the fetus. A healthy fetus tolerates this well. Fetal hypoxia, myocardial depression, and a decrease in fetal heart rate (FHR) occur if the placenta's reserve is not sufficient.

This test is used with clients who have heart disease, hypertension, pregnancy-induced hypertension (PIH), sickle-cell anemia, previous stillbirths, Rh sensitization, or a nonreactive NST. It is most often performed on the client with diabetes (chronic or gestational).

The vascular changes that take place in diabetes will also affect the placenta. Vascular changes in the placenta cause placental insufficiency, so the fetus will not tolerate a CST well. Contraindications for use of this test are placenta previa, abruptio placenta, premature rupture of membranes, a history of preterm labor, or previous cesarean birth.

The uterine contractions are induced by either intravenous oxytocin or breast self-stimulation. An electronic fetal monitor provides continuous information of the FHR and uterine contractions. A 15-minute baseline recording on the fetal monitor is obtained before contractions are stimulated. Intravenous oxytocin is given

piggyback to another IV so it can be stopped when necessary. When three uterine contractions lasting 40 to 60 seconds occur in 10 minutes, the oxytocin is stopped. If three late decelerations occur, the oxytocin is stopped.

For nipple stimulation, warm washcloths are applied to the breasts and/or one nipple is manually rolled by the client. When three uterine contractions lasting 40 to 60 seconds occur in 10 minutes, the stimulation is discontinued. If a decrease in FHR occurs with a contraction, the nipple stimulation is stopped.

A negative CST with no late decelerations is the desired result. The fetus is able to tolerate the hypoxia of uterine contractions. A positive CST with late decelerations that occur with more than half of the contractions is not the desired result.

Electronic Fetal Monitoring

Electronic fetal monitoring (EFM) provides a visual record of the FHR in relation to the uterine contractions. It allows early detection of fetal distress and abnormal uterine activity. High-risk clients and clients with a problem in their pregnancy are candidates for EFM. Some birthing places routinely have all clients on EFM.

External (Indirect) Monitoring

A tocodynamometer (for uterine activity) is placed on the mother's abdomen near the fundus. A strap around the mother holds it securely in place. A Doppler transducer (ultrasonic device) is placed on the mother's abdomen and moved around until the fetal heart is heard the best. A strap around the mother holds it in place also (Figure 51-5A). Sound waves are bounced off the fetal heart and picked up and displayed by the monitor.

Internal (Direct) Monitoring

This is a more reliable method then external monitoring. An EKG electrode to directly monitor FHR is attached to the fetal presenting part (head) (Figure 51-5B). For this to be initiated, the membranes must be ruptured, the cervix must be dilated at least 2 cm, the presenting part must be down against the cervix, and the presenting part must be known. Only a person specially trained for this procedure should perform it.

Either the external tocodynamometer or an intrauterine catheter may be used to assess uterine contractions. A thin, flexible polyethylene catheter filled with sterile, distilled water is inserted into the amniotic fluid in the uterus. The increased pressure on the fluid during a contraction is translated into an electrical signal. This provides reliable information about the contractions. Sterile technique is used when inserting both the scalp electrode and the catheter.

Interpretations

New definitions have been recommended by the National Institute of Child Health and Human Development Research Planning Workshop. These are being tested and so may be found in practice in specific institutions.

The interpretations currently in use will be presented here.

Figure 51-5 *Fetal Monitoring:* **A,** *External (indirect). The top transducer picks up the uterine contractions and the lower transducer picks up the fetal heart tones and transmits the signal as an electrical impulse to the monitor where they are recorded;* **B,** *Internal (direct). The EKG electrode on the fetus's scalp picks up the fetal heart tones and the intrauterine catheter picks up uterine contractions.*

Baseline Rate Baseline rate is the average FHR during a 10-minute period. The normal rate is 110 to 160 beats/ minute. A rate above 160 beats/minute is tachycardia, and a rate below 110 beats/minute is bradycardia.

Baseline Variability Short-term variability is the beat-to-beat change in FHR. Long-term variability is the waviness (called cycles) that occurs 3 to 5 times per minute.

Accelerations Accelerations are short-term increases in FHR usually caused by fetal movement. This is the basis for the NST.

Early Deceleration **Early decelerations** are reductions in fetal heart rate that begin early with the contraction and typically mirror the contraction. Head compression during contractions causes a decrease in cerebral blood flow, which shows as early deceleration. No intervention is required (Figure 51-6).

Late Deceleration **Late decelerations** are reductions in fetal heart rate that begin at the peak of the contraction and increase to the baseline level after the contraction has ceased, caused by uteroplacental insufficiency. Oxygen administered to the mother may be

started. Late decelerations should be reported to the health care provider (Figure 51-6).

Variable Deceleration **Variable decelerations** are reductions in fetal heart rate that have no relationship to contractions of the uterus. They occur when compression of the umbilical cord reduces blood flow between fetus and placenta. A change in the mother's position may take pressure off the cord. These should also be reported immediately (Figure 51-6).

HYPEREMESIS GRAVIDARUM

Hyperemesis gravidarum is excessive vomiting during pregnancy. The cause is unknown but may be related to an increased estrogen level, gonadotropin production, or trophoblastic activity. Psychological factors

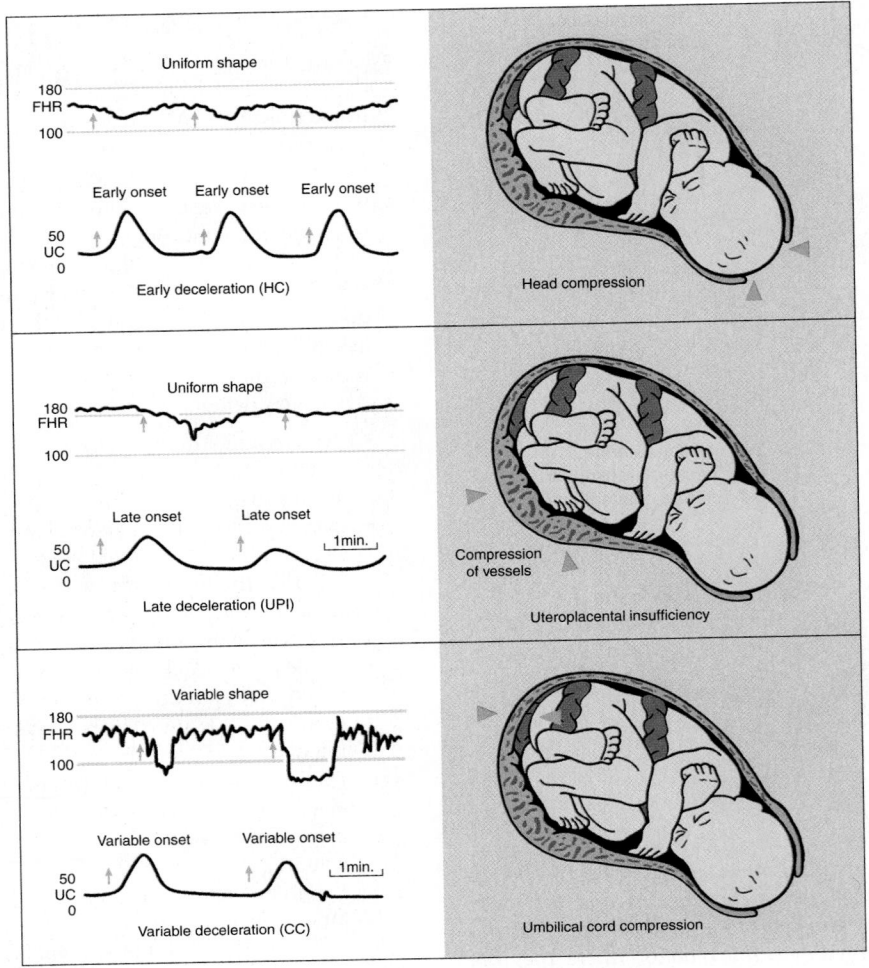

Figure 51-6 *Fetal Heart Rate Patterns from Continuous Electronic Fetal Monitoring*

may also be involved. The vomiting progresses to the point that the woman vomits everything swallowed. It does not subside at about 12 weeks' gestation as does "morning sickness."

Dehydration leads to fluid and electrolyte imbalance and alkalosis from the loss of hydrochloric acid. As the situation becomes worse, the client experiences tachycardia and may have hypovolemia, hypotension, an increase in hematocrit and blood urea nitrogen (BUN), and a decrease in urine output.

The starvation situation causes protein and vitamin deficiencies. Cardiac functioning may be disrupted by severe potassium loss. Untreated, the client may experience metabolic changes or death. Embryonic or fetal death may occur.

The treatment goals are to control vomiting, correct dehydration, restore electrolyte balance, and maintain adequate nutrition.

Medical–Surgical Management

Medical

The client is usually hospitalized and intravenous fluids containing glucose, vitamins, and electrolytes are started immediately. IV therapy is continued until all

vomiting has stopped for 48 hours. Psychotherapy may be recommended.

Pharmacological

A sedative may be given, but medications are kept to a minimum because of potential teratogenic (harmful) effects to the fetus.

Diet

The client is kept NPO until all vomiting has stopped for 48 hours. Small amounts of dry foods are then tried. Progression to a regular diet is done slowly.

Activity

Bed rest is usually maintained until the condition begins to improve. Visitors may be restricted for a few days to allow the client to rest.

Nursing Management

Provide opportunities for the client to express feelings and perceptions of the pregnancy and the fetus. Maintain a quiet environment. Administer IV fluids as ordered.

Assess skin turgor and mucous membranes. Maintain accurate I & O record. Ensure good oral hygiene.

NURSING PROCESS

Assessment

Subjective Data

Especially important is the client's emotional state and her feelings about the pregnancy, the fetus, and her mate. Ask what triggers her nausea and vomiting.

Objective Data

Check the amount and character of all emesis, intake and output, and fetal heart rate. Note signs of jaundice and vaginal bleeding.

Nursing diagnoses for a client with hyperemesis gravidarum may include the following:

Nursing Diagnoses	Planning/Goals	Nursing Interventions
Imbalanced Nutrition: Less Than Body Requirements, related to persistent vomiting	The client will cease vomiting.	Maintain relaxed, quiet environment. Monitor amount and character of all emesis, and maintain accurate I&O record. Ensure good oral hygiene after each vomiting episode. When vomiting stops, provide bland foods and oral fluids as ordered. Maintain cheerful, optimistic attitude.
Deficient Fluid Volume related to decreased fluid intake and excessive fluid loss.	The client will have fluid balance.	Administer IV fluids as ordered. Monitor laboratory reports for electrolyte levels. Assess skin turgor and mucous membranes. Provide small amounts of oral fluids when tolerated. Maintain accurate I&O record.
Fear, related to fetal well-being	The client will discuss fears with health caregivers.	Provide opportunities for client to express fears. Show acceptance of client's perceptions. Assist client to identify personal strengths. Listen to what the client says. Help client identify sources of support.

Evaluation Each goal must be evaluated to determine how it has been met by the client.

BLEEDING

Bleeding disorders include abortion, ectopic pregnancy, hydatidiform mole, placenta previa, abruptio placenta, and disseminated intravascular coagulation.

ABORTION

Abortion is the spontaneous (natural) or induced (purposeful) termination of a pregnancy before viability

of the fetus. A fetus is considered viable at 24 weeks' gestation. With medical intervention, a fetus between 20 and 24 weeks' gestation may survive. Some states have defined viability as 20 to 24 weeks' gestation and a weight of 500 g.

A spontaneous abortion is often called a **miscarriage.** Spontaneous abortions may be related to chromosomal abnormalities, faulty implantation, teratogenic substances, placental abnormalities, incompetent cervix, chronic maternal diseases, maternal infections, and endocrine imbalances. Clinically, spontaneous abortions are classified as:

Figure 51-7 *Types of Spontaneous Abortions:* **A,** *Threatened;* **B,** *Inevitable;* **C,** *Incomplete*

 • *Threatened*: Unexplained bleeding and cramping. The cervix is closed and membranes are intact (Figure 51-7A).

 • *Inevitable*: Increased bleeding and cramping. The cervix begins to dilate and the membranes may rupture (Figure 51-7B).

 • *Incomplete*: Some of the products of conception are expelled. Most often the placenta is not expelled. Bleeding is heavy and cramping severe (Figure 51-7C).

• *Complete*: All products of conception are expelled.

• *Missed*: Embryo or fetus dies but is retained. The cervix is closed. If the fetus is not expelled within 6 weeks, disseminated intravascular coagulation (DIC) may develop.

• *Habitual*: Any of the above occurring in three consecutive pregnancies. Most commonly, the cervix begins to dilate in the second trimester. This is called an **incompetent cervix.**

Medical–Surgical Management

Medical

For threatened abortion, the client is usually told to limit activities for 24 to 48 hours. If the bleeding is going to stop, it will usually do so in 48 hours. If the bleeding stops, the client is advised to avoid stress, fatigue, strenuous activity, and sexual intercourse. Having one or two rest periods during the day is also recommended until the pregnancy seems to be progressing normally.

PROFESSIONAL TIP

Spontaneous Abortion

The client who has a miscarriage may experience a wide spectrum of emotions, from shock, disbelief, and guilt to anger and despair. She may have difficulty managing these feelings as well as responding to the reactions of partner, family, and friends. The nurse can assist by answering the woman's questions, allowing her to express her emotions, and respecting her need to grieve.

Surgical

A client with an inevitable or incomplete abortion generally is hospitalized to remove the products of conception from the uterus. A dilation and curettage (D & C) or suction evacuation is performed. Depending on the amount of blood loss, the client may be given blood transfusions.

When the products of conception, in a missed abortion, are not expelled in 4 to 6 weeks, the client is hospitalized. For 12 weeks' gestation or less, a D & C is performed. If more than 12 weeks' gestation, induction of labor with oxytocin may be used.

When habitual abortions are caused by an incompetent cervix, it can be treated surgically by cerclage (Shirodkar procedure, Figure 51-8). Suture material is placed in the cervix in a purse-string fashion at the level of the internal os. This is done at about 16 weeks' gestation. The suture can be left in for future pregnancies and a cesarean birth planned, or the suture may be removed at term and a vaginal birth allowed. If the mother goes into labor or the membranes rupture, she must call her health care provider and go to the hospital immediately.

Nursing Management

Frequently assess the amount of bleeding, presence of clots, and any expelled tissue. Provide a calm environment and actively listen to the client. Provide information about the situation and prepare client for procedures and treatments.

NURSING PROCESS

Assessment

Subjective Data

The client may describe abdominal cramping and vaginal bleeding, and may have feelings of fear and guilt.

Figure 51-8 *Shirodkar Procedure: Purse-string sutures keep the cervix closed in an incompetent cervix.*

Objective Data

Note the amount of bleeding, presence of clots, and any tissue expelled. Vital signs may indicate excessive blood loss (hypovolemia).

Nursing diagnoses for a client having an abortion may include the following:

Nursing Diagnoses	Planning/Goals	Nursing Interventions
Situational Low Self-esteem, related to feelings of guilt for doing something to cause abortion	The client will maintain usual level of self-esteem.	Provide information about causes of a spontaneous abortion. Assist client to identify personal strengths. Actively listen to the client.
Aute Pain, related to contractions (cramping) of uterine muscle	The client will describe having less pain.	Administer analgesic as ordered. Monitor effect of analgesic.
Fear, related to potential loss of pregnancy	The client will discuss fear with family.	Provide opportunities for the client to express fears. Help client identify sources of support. Show acceptance of client's perceptions.

Evaluation Each goal must be evaluated to determine how it has been met by the client.

SAMPLE NURSING CARE PLAN

THE CLIENT HAVING AN ABORTION

Pat, age 25, G4, P3, T2, P1, A0, L3, is admitted to the hospital with some bleeding and cramping. She states, "I'm scared, I don't understand what's happening." Vital signs are BP 108/66, T 98.6, P 86, R 24. Her skin is cool. At her first prenatal visit 3 weeks ago, the fetus was 12 weeks' gestation. Crying, she says, "I don't know what I did to cause this to happen."

Two hours later, Pat's cramping is severe and the bleeding heavy, bright red. Vital signs are BP 88/60, P 100, and R 28. Her skin is cold and clammy.

Nursing Diagnosis 1 *Deficient Fluid Volume* related to heavy bleeding as evidenced by hypotension and decreased pulse pressure

Nursing Outcomes Classification (NOC)
Fluid Balance

Nursing Interventions Classification (NIC)
Vital Signs Monitoring

PLANNING/GOALS	NURSING INTERVENTIONS	RATIONALE
Pat will have vital signs return to baseline values.	Administer IV fluids and/or blood as ordered.	Replaces fluid volume lost by bleeding.
	Monitor Pat's vital signs every 15 minutes or less.	Clinical indicators of fluid volume.
	Save all vaginal pads and clots or tissue passed for physician to see.	Allows physician to estimate blood loss and identify any tissue passed.
	Administer analgesic as ordered.	Relieving pain will make Pat more comfortable.
	Prepare Pat for surgery as ordered.	Most likely, a D & C will be performed.

EVALUATION   After a D & C, Pat's vital signs returned to baseline values.

continues

SAMPLE NURSING CARE PLAN

Nursing Diagnosis 2 *Anxiety* related to changes in her pregnancy as evidenced by statement "I'm scared, I don't understand what's happening."

Nursing Outcomes Classification (NOC)
Coping

Nursing Interventions Classification (NIC)
Anxiety Reduction
Coping Enhancement

PLANNING/GOALS	NURSING INTERVENTIONS	RATIONALE
Pat will verbalize her feelings about bleeding and cramping while pregnant.	Speak slowly and calmly to Pat.	Conveys calmness and sense of security.
	Evaluate Pat's understanding of what is happening and possible treatment options.	Provides information for educational needs.
	Involve spouse/significant other in discussion.	Gives family information and a feeling of control.
	Be direct and focus on the specific topic.	Anxiety decreases ability to concentrate.
	Help Pat identify coping methods used in the past.	Important to know how Pat has coped in the past.

EVALUATION Pat shared feelings of fear and guilt about the bleeding and cramping.

Nursing Diagnosis 3 *Anticipatory Grieving* related to probable loss of pregnancy as evidenced by crying and statement "I don't know what I did to cause this to happen"

Nursing Outcomes Classification (NOC)
Grief Resolution

Nursing Interventions Classification (NIC)
Grief Work Facilitation

PLANNING/GOALS	NURSING INTERVENTIONS	RATIONALE
Pat will verbalize what losing a pregnancy means to her.	Allow Pat to express her feelings.	Releases energy and is calming.
	Assess Pat's coping skills.	Coping skills may need to be reinforced or adapted.
	Assist Pat to identify personal resources and strengths.	Promotes integrity of self.
	Provide privacy for Pat and her family.	Allows them a chance to discuss the situation and make plans.

EVALUATION Pat is having trouble talking about losing the pregnancy.

ECTOPIC PREGNANCY

An **ectopic pregnancy** occurs when a fertilized ovum implants outside the uterine cavity. The most common site is in the fallopian tube. This generally happens when the fertilized ovum is unable to move through the tube. Figure 51-9 illustrates other possible sites of implantation in an ectopic pregnancy.

In the United States, the rate of ectopic pregnancy in women ages 15-45 years is about 19.7 per 1,000 pregnancies (Tenore, 2000). Risk factors include pelvic inflammatory disease, in utero exposure to diethylstilbestrol, sexually transmitted diseases, pharmacologic treatment of infertility, and endometriosis (Minnick-Smith & Cook, 1997).

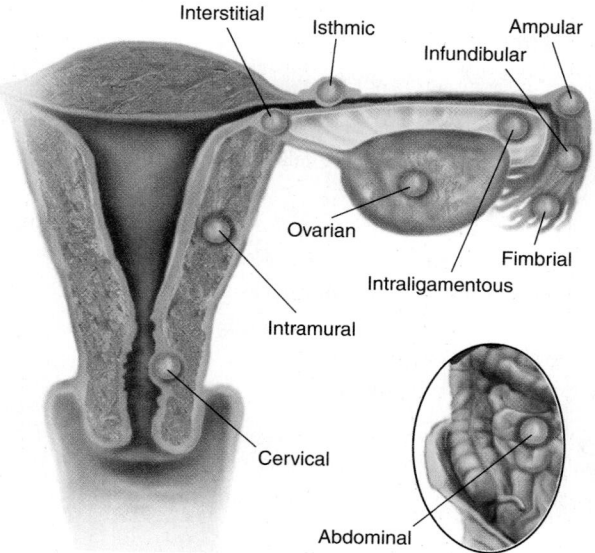

Figure 51-9 *Possible Sites of Implantation in Ectopic Pregnancy*

The pregnancy appears normal at first with the usual signs and symptoms, including the presence of hCG in the blood and urine. Symptoms of ectopic pregnancy begin gradually about 3 to 5 weeks after the first missed menstrual period. Pain is noted as the fallopian tube stretches with the growing embryo. The tube finally ruptures (a severe pain occurs) and bleeds into the peritoneal cavity. Some vaginal bleeding may be apparent. The client may rapidly show signs of hypovolemic shock. The signs of shock are out of proportion to the apparent blood loss. Ectopic pregnancy is a significant cause of maternal morbidity and mortality, and is nearly always fatal to the embryo.

Medical–Surgical Management

Medical

The menstrual history is reviewed and a pelvic examination performed to identify abnormal pelvic masses and tenderness. Severe pain occurs when the cervix is moved. A transvaginal ultrasound is also done. Serial testing of hCG shows a slower increase than in a normal pregnancy, in which the hCG level doubles every 48 to 72 hours. A serum progesterone level of 25 ng/mL strongly suggests a normal pregnancy, whereas a level of 5 ng/mL or less indicates a nonviable pregnancy. A level between 5 ng/mL and 25 ng/mL is uncertain, and a transvaginal ultrasound is needed.

Surgical

Rapid surgical treatment is generally necessary to remove the products of conception and to control bleeding. Laparotomy is seldom used now unless the client has orthostatic hypotension, tachycardia, or a falling hematocrit. Laparoscopic salpingostomy or salpingectomy are preferred. The procedure of choice is salpingostomy when future fertility is desired (Minnick-Smith & Cook, 1997). If the fallopian tube is badly damaged, a

salpingectomy is performed. The ovary is left in place if not damaged. Blood transfusions are often required.

Pharmacological

Methotrexate (Mexate, Folex) may be given to resolve an ectopic pregnancy.

Diet

If the client has surgery, she will be NPO before and after surgery.

Activity

The client is usually on bed rest until the situation is resolved.

Nursing Management

Administer analgesic as ordered. Provide information about an ectopic pregnancy. Actively listen to client. Encourage client to express feelings. Monitor vital signs. Prepare for surgery as ordered and begin preoperative teaching.

NURSING PROCESS

Assessment

Subjective Data

The client describes amenorrhea, nausea, breast tenderness, and a dull ache on one side that has increasingly become more severe. When the tube ruptures, the client will describe a single excruciating pain in the abdomen and may also have referred shoulder pain.

Objective Data

Some vaginal bleeding may be apparent. Laboratory reports may show a low hemoglobin and hematocrit, a rising leukocyte level, and a slowly rising hCG level. The RBC count is low and sedimentation rate elevated. The abdomen may be rigid and tender. Vital signs may indicate hypovolemic shock.

Nursing diagnoses for a client with an ectopic pregnancy may include the following:

Nursing Diagnoses	Planning/Goals	Nursing Interventions
Anticipatory Grieving related to the loss of the pregnancy	The client will understand that grieving may last several months.	Encourage client and family to talk about their feelings. Allow them privacy to grieve. Listen actively to concerns about this and future pregnancies. Provide information about causes of ectopic pregnancy. Refer to other professionals for help as needed.
Impaired Tissue Integrity, related to the rupture of a fallopian tube	The client will regain tissue integrity of the fallopian tube or it will be removed.	Prepare client for surgery as ordered. Begin preoperative teaching.
Acute Pain, related to tubal rupture and blood in the abdomen	The client will express less pain.	Administer analgesic as ordered and evaluate its effectiveness. Provide information about cause of pain.

Evaluation Each goal must be evaluated to determine how it has been met by the client.

HYDATIDIFORM MOLE ← Molar Pregnancy

Hydatidiform mole (trophoblastic disease) is an abnormality of the placenta. The chorionic villi become fluid-filled, grapelike clusters; the trophoblastic tissue proliferates; and there is no viable embryo. In effect, the fertilized ovum dies and the chorion develops into vesicles. There is a possibility of developing choriocarcinoma.

The complete mole has only paternal genetic material. There is no embryonic tissue, only the fluid-filled cystic villi. A large amount of hCG is produced because the chorionic villi are proliferating. The classic signs are bleeding (usually brownish but may be red), uterine enlargement greater than would be expected for the gestation, and no fetal heart tones (FHT) heard (Figure 51-10). If any of the grapelike clusters are passed, it is diagnostic.

The partial mole has only focal areas of the fluid-filled cystic villi; some chorionic villi are formed normally. There is a fetus with multiple chromosomal anomalies and little chance for survival. A partial mole may not be recognized until the products of conception are examined after a spontaneous abortion.

The client may experience hyperemesis gravidarum because of the higher serum hCG level. If symptoms of pregnancy-induced hypertension appear before 24 weeks' gestation, a molar pregnancy is very probable. The primary diagnostic tool is ultrasound.

Medical–Surgical Management
Medical

After surgery to remove the mole, the client must be followed for 1 to 2 years. The care includes chest x-rays to detect metastases, physical examinations with a pelvic examination, and regular (usually weekly) laboratory measurement of hCG level. The client is advised not to become pregnant during the follow-up time.

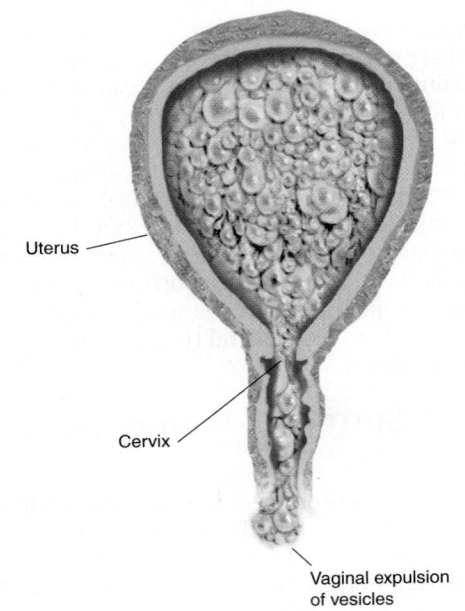

Uterus

Cervix

Vaginal expulsion of vesicles

Figure 51-10 *Hydatidiform Mole*

Surgical

The desire of the client for future fertility influences the surgical procedure to be used to empty the uterus. A D & C may be performed, but it is difficult to make certain that no fragment of the molar pregnancy is left in the uterus. A hysterotomy, cutting the uterus open (like cesarean birth), allows visual determination that the uterus is completely emptied. If the client is older and no future fertility is desired or there is excessive bleeding, a hysterectomy is performed.

CLIENT TEACHING

Methotrexate

- There is a risk of photosensitivity when taking methotrexate (Mexate, Folex) to reduce hCG levels following treatment for hydatidiform mole.
- Clients should avoid sun exposure while taking this medication.

Pharmacological

If the hCG level remains high or rises after the uterus is evacuated, methotrexate (Mexate, Folex) is given. Oxytocin is given to keep the uterus contracted to control bleeding. Typed and cross-matched blood must be available.

Activity

Bed rest is maintained until after surgery, then ambulation is progressively increased.

Nursing Management

Monitor vaginal bleeding. Assess uterine size and FHT (none heard). Prepare for ultrasound. Prepare for surgery as ordered.

NURSING PROCESS

Assessment

Subjective Data

The client may describe severe nausea and vomiting and may be having some brownish vaginal discharge.

Objective Data

There is vaginal bleeding, usually brownish but may be bright red. Uterine enlargement is greater than expected for gestational age. Ultrasound reveals a characteristic molar pattern. The client may have symptoms of pregnancy-induced hypertension (BP 140/90 or an increase of 30/15, proteinuria, and edema measured by sudden weight gain).

Nursing diagnoses for a client with hydatidiform mole may include the following:

Nursing Diagnoses	Planning/Goals	Nursing Interventions
Fear, related to the possible development of choriocarcinoma	The client will discuss fears with health care provider or other professional.	Provide opportunities for client to express fears. Help client identify sources of support. Refer to other professionals as needed.
Deficient Knowledge, related to lack of understanding for regular monitoring of hCG level and delaying pregnancy	The client will discuss reasons for regular monitoring of hCG level and why pregnancy should be delayed.	Present information as to how hCG level indicates whether choriocarcinoma is developing. Provide reasons for delaying another pregnancy. Allow client to express feelings about regular laboratory testing of blood.

Evaluation Each goal must be evaluated to determine how it has been met by the client.

PLACENTA PREVIA

Placenta previa occurs when implantation is in the lower uterine segment with the placenta lying over or very near the internal cervical os (Figure 51-11). The cause is unknown, but predisposing factors may be multiparity, uterine scarring from D & C or cesarean birth, or maternal advancing age and smoking.

The classic symptom is *painless bleeding* in the last half of pregnancy. There may be occasional bright red spotting or intermittent gushes of blood. Rarely is bleeding continuous. The uterus is relaxed and not tender.

Bleeding is unrelated to maternal activity. Placenta previa is classified in three ways:

- *Low-lying or Marginal:* Placenta is near the internal cervical os but does not cover any part of opening.
- *Partial:* Placenta covers part of internal cervical os opening.
- *Complete or Total:* Placenta completely covers internal cervical os opening.

Toward the last part of pregnancy, the cervix effaces (thins). This movement of the cervix pulls away from the placenta, and the exposed placental sinuses begin

Figure 51-11 *Placenta Previa:* **A,** *Low implantation (marginal);* **B,** *Partial placenta previa;* **C,** *Total placenta previa.*

to bleed. The earlier this happens, the more serious the situation.

Effects on the Fetus/Neonate

The gestational age of the fetus and the amount of bleeding determine the effects on the fetus/neonate. During profuse bleeding, the fetus may suffer from hypoxia. After delivery, the neonate should be checked to see if the bleeding resulted in anemia.

Medical–Surgical Management

Medical

The goal is to maintain the pregnancy until the fetus is mature enough to survive outside the uterus. Fetal maturity is assessed by checking the lecithin/sphingomyelin ratio for lung maturity. The mother is usually hospitalized. Hemoglobin and hematocrit (H & H) is usually determined every 12 hours. The laboratory will type and cross-match, and two units of blood will be kept on call in the event of severe blood loss.

Diagnosis is made with an ultrasound. Once the diagnosis is made, no vaginal examinations are performed because of the risk of causing more bleeding by disturbing the placenta. If an ultrasound is unavailable, vaginal bleeding profuse, and the pregnancy near term, the health care provider may examine the client vaginally. This is done in the delivery room with a setup for vaginal delivery and a setup for a cesarean delivery.

Surgical

If the maternal situation becomes worse or there is fetal distress, a cesarean birth is begun immediately.

Pharmacological

In an attempt to accelerate fetal lung maturity, a drug such as betamethasone (Celestone) may be given to the mother.

Activity

The client is on bed rest with bathroom privileges as long as no bleeding occurs. If bleeding begins, the client is on complete bed rest.

Nursing Management

Maintain the client on bed rest. Monitor vital signs and FHR. Prepare for ultrasound. Maintain a calm environment. Assess for uterine contractions.

NURSING PROCESS

Assessment

Subjective Data

The client describes painless bleeding.

Objective Data

Vaginal bleeding may range from spotting to profuse bleeding. The uterus remains soft and relaxes fully between contractions if labor begins. FHR generally remains stable unless bleeding is profuse and maternal shock occurs.

Nursing diagnoses for a client with placenta previa may include the following:

Nursing Diagnoses	Planning/Goals	Nursing Interventions
*Deficient **Fl**uid Volume,* related to blood loss	The client will maintain perfusion to placenta and vital organs.	Observe, report, and record blood loss (count and/or weigh pads). Monitor client's vital signs, FHR, I&O, and laboratory reports. Maintain comfortable environment to prevent diaphoresis. Inspect skin for pallor, cyanosis, clamminess, and coldness. Encourage client to maintain fluid intake
*Impaired **G**as Exchange, Fetal,* related to decreased maternal blood volume and hypotension	FHR will remain within normal limits.	Monitor FHR, baseline variability, and decelerations. Observe amniotic fluid for meconium. Instruct client in positions to promote placental perfusion.

Evaluation Each goal must be evaluated to determine how it has been met by the client.

Figure 51-12 *Abruptio Placenta:* **A,** *Central abruption, concealed hemorrhage;* **B,** *Marginal abruption, external hemorrhage;* **C,** *Complete abruption, external hemorrhage (could also be concealed)*

ABRUPTIO PLACENTA → C-SECTION

The premature separation from the wall of the uterus of a normally implanted placenta is called **abruptio placenta.** It occurs spontaneously after the 20th week of gestation in 1 of 75 to 90 pregnancies (Bougere, 1998). The cause is unknown. Contributing factors may include maternal hypertension, multiple pregnancy, abdominal trauma, smoking, use of alcohol, or use of cocaine. Generally, it occurs late in pregnancy or during labor. There are three types of abruptio placenta (Figure 51-12).

- *Central:* Center of the placenta separates with blood trapped between placenta and uterine wall; there is no apparent bleeding.
- *Marginal:* Edge of placenta separates and bright red bleeding is apparent vaginally.
- *Complete:* Entire placenta separates with profuse bleeding apparent vaginally.

A central abruption may progress to a complete abruption. In central and complete, blood invades the uterine muscle (bruising called *Couvelaire uterus*), causing a rigid, painful abdomen. After delivery, the uterus contracts poorly and the client may require a hysterectomy to control the bleeding. The damage to the uterine muscle and the retroplacental clotting can cause a large release of thromboplastin. This can trigger the develop-ment of disseminated intravascular coagulation (DIC). Maternal mortality is relatively low. Problems after the delivery depend on the severity of the bleeding. Table 51-3 compares placenta previa and the various types of abruptio placenta.

Effects on the Fetus/Neonate

Perinatal mortality is about one-third of the cases of abruptio placenta. The outcome depends on fetal maturity and severity of the abruption. Preterm labor, hypoxia, and anemia are the most serious complications. Irreversible brain damage or fetal death may occur if hypoxia is not reversed quickly.

Medical–Surgical Management
Medical

Intravenous fluids, generally lactated Ringer's solution, are given to prevent or reverse hypovolemia. Laboratory tests to evaluate client's status and the clotting mechanism are ordered: H & H, platelet count, fibrinogen level, fibrin split products, thrombin time, prothrombin time, partial thromboplastin time, and bleeding time. Also, a type and cross-match for three to four units of blood or packed cells is requested (Bougere, 1998). If the mother is Rh negative, she is checked for Rh sensitization. An indwelling urinary catheter is inserted.

If separation is small and the pregnancy near term, induction of labor and vaginal delivery may be possible. If labor is not progressing in 8 hours, a cesarean birth is performed. If separation is moderate or severe, a cesarean birth is performed as soon as possible.

Surgical

Cesarean delivery is performed in many cases to prevent fetal demise. A hysterectomy may be required to control hemorrhage.

Pharmacological

RhoGAM is given to the nonsensitized Rh-negative mother. Cryoprecipitate or plasma is given to treat hypofibrinogenemia. Analgesics are given as ordered.

Diet

No special diet or restrictions are required, although the client will be NPO if surgery is necessary.

TABLE 51-3	COMPARISON OF PLACENTA PREVIA AND ABRUPTIO PLACENTA			
CONDITION	**BLEEDING**	**ABDOMEN**	**PAIN**	**BP**
Placenta Previa	Bright red	No rigidity	None	Depends on amount of bleeding
Abruptio Placenta				
Central	None	Rigid	Acute	Decreased
Marginal	Dark red	No rigidity	Uterine tenderness	Decreased
Complete	Profuse	Rigid	Acute	Shock

Activity

The client will remain on bed rest until the situation is resolved.

Nursing Management

Monitor the client's bleeding, pain, vital signs, FHR, and fetal activity. Administer blood products or blood as ordered. Provide oxygen as ordered. If a cesarean delivery is to be performed, prepare the client for surgery. Maintain the client on bed rest. Accurately record I&O and insert indwelling urinary catheter as ordered. Have client lie on her side (left preferred) but not on her back.

NURSING PROCESS

Assessment

Subjective Data

The client may describe moderate to severe pain in the abdomen. Fetal movement may become hyperactive and then may cease.

Objective Data

Vaginal bleeding is assessed. External fetal monitor will show uteroplacental insufficiency, baseline changes, and reduced variability. The contraction pattern will change and the resting tone will increase. Vital signs show indications of shock.

Nursing diagnoses for a client with abruptio placenta may include the following:

Nursing Diagnoses	Planning/Goals	Nursing Interventions
Impaired Gas Exchange, Fetal related to altered uteroplacenta oxygen transfer due to placental separation	The fetus will not have hypoxia.	Watch external fetal monitor for decelerations, decreased baseline variability, and FHR. Provide nasal oxygen to mother. Have mother lie on left side.
Anticipatory Grieving, related to possible loss of pregnancy	The client will be able to verbalize feelings about possible loss of pregnancy.	Encourage client and family to talk about their feelings. Allow them some privacy to grieve. Contact minister, priest, or rabbi as requested by the client.
Acute Pain, related to retroplacental bleeding and possibly contractions	The client will verbalize an understanding of the cause of the pain.	Provide simple explanation for cause of pain. Encourage and assist client to relax.
Deficient Fluid Volume, related to blood loss	The client will regain fluid balance.	Monitor vital signs and assess for cold, clammy, cyanotic skin. Administer IV fluids as ordered and accurately record I&O. Evaluate client's state of consciousness.

Evaluation Each goal must be evaluated to determine how it has been met by the client.

DISSEMINATED INTRAVASCULAR COAGULATION

Disseminated intravascular coagulation (DIC) is an overstimulation of the normal clotting process. Rapid, massive fibrin formation causes small thrombi to form throughout the circulatory system, depleting the clotting factors and platelets. Generalized bleeding may then occur, leading to anemia or ischemia to vital organs because of the clots in the blood vessels.

DIC occurs as a complication of a primary problem. It is not only a complication of obstetrical situations, but also of many medical–surgical situations such as neoplasms, blood transfusion reaction, traumas, and infections. Men can also experience DIC. Obstetrical problems that may precipitate DIC include abruptio placenta, placenta previa, hydatidiform mole, PIH, retained products of conception, amniotic fluid embolism, and infections.

Effects on the Fetus/Neonate

The primary problem may require immediate delivery of the fetus, even if preterm. The fetus may experience hypoxia to varying degrees. Fetal death can occur.

Medical–Surgical Management

Medical

Symptom onset is sudden with the client complaining of dyspnea or chest pain and becoming very restless and cyanotic and spitting frothy, blood-tinged mucus.

The underlying cause must be identified and corrected. If the fetus is not yet born, delivery should be facilitated. Diagnostic tests that may be used are hemoglobin, hematocrit, fibrinogen level, platelet count, prothrombin time, and partial thromboplastin time.

Pharmacological

Intravenous administration of blood, fibrinogen, or cryoprecipitate is begun. Heparin given by continuous-infusion pump inhibits thrombin activity and thus prevents formation of microemboli. There is no effect on already existing clots.

Oxygen therapy is often begun.

Nursing Management

Closely monitor all clients with an obstetrical problem that may precipitate DIC for sudden onset of dyspnea or chest pain, restlessness, cyanosis, and spitting frothy blood-tinged mucus. Maintain a calm, positive manner. Administer IV fluids, blood, or other substance to help restore normal clotting. Give heparin as ordered. Provide oxygen as ordered. Monitor vital signs, lung sounds, and fetus (if not yet delivered) continuously with an electronic fetal monitor.

NURSING PROCESS

Assessment

Subjective Data

The client may describe dyspnea or chest pain.

Objective Data

The client may be extremely restless or cyanotic and be expectorating blood-tinged frothy mucus. Bleeding gums, epistaxis (nose bleed), petechiae under the blood pressure cuff around the client's arm, or bleeding from injection sites may also be present.

Nursing diagnoses for a pregnant client with DIC may include the following:

Nursing Diagnoses	Planning/Goals	Nursing Interventions
Anxiety, related to the sudden change in health status	The client will express understanding of what is happening to her and will feel less anxious.	Maintain a calm, positive manner. Explain to client what is happening, procedures, and treatment to be implemented. Remain with client. Allow client to express her anxiety. Answer client's questions.
Impaired **G**as Exchange, related to reduced oxygen-carrying capacity and ischemia of lung tissue	The client will maintain adequate gas exchange to prevent tissue death.	Administer IV fluids, blood, or other substance to help restore a normal clotting mechanism. Administer heparin and provide oxygen as ordered. Monitor lung sounds and respiratory rate. If fetus not yet delivered, monitor continuously with electronic fetal monitor.

Evaluation Each goal must be evaluated to determine how it has been met by the client.

Re-Read clubs

PREGNANCY-INDUCED HYPERTENSION

Pregnancy-induced hypertension (PIH), the most common hypertensive disorder in pregnancy, appears after 20 weeks' gestation. The classic symptoms are hypertension, edema, and proteinuria. It is seen most often in primigravidas, especially those younger than 20 or older than 35 years of age, who are in the lower socioeconomic group and have poor nutritional status. Diabetes, multiple pregnancy, or a family history of PIH also increase a client's risk.

Peripheral arteriole vasoconstriction and vasospasm lead to increased blood pressure and decreased perfusion of the uterus and placenta. Renal blood flow is lowered, renal glomerular filtration rate is lowered, and proteinuria results. Cerebral edema causes headaches and visual disturbances. Deep tendon reflexes become hyperactive. The liver enlarges, putting pressure on the liver capsule, which causes epigastric pain. The condition may progress to **eclampsia,** or convulsions.

Despite decades of research, the cause remains unknown. It was previously called *toxemia* because it was thought that a toxin was produced in a pregnant woman's body. This term is no longer used. The only cure is delivery of the baby. PIH may progress from mild to severe **preeclampsia** to eclampsia.

Effects on the Fetus/Neonate

Abruptio placenta and placental infarction may occur. Intrauterine growth retardation (IUGR) may occur as well as acute hypoxia and intrauterine death. A preterm infant may be born either because of spontaneous labor or obstetrical intervention.

Mild Preeclampsia

In mild preeclampsia, the blood pressure increases 30 mm Hg systolic or 15 mm Hg diastolic over the client's baseline blood pressure on two occasions at least 6 hours apart, or a BP of 140/90 is noted. For example, a client with a baseline BP of 92/64 would be considered hypertensive at 122/80. Thus it is very important to have a baseline BP early in pregnancy.

Edema may be noted in the face and hands. It is objectively defined as weight gain of more than 1 pound per week.

Urine may show 1+ or 2+ albumin on a dipstick or 300 mg/L in 24 hours. Proteinuria is usually the last of the three classic symptoms to appear.

Severe Preeclampsia

Blood pressure increases to 160/110 or higher on two occasions 6 hours apart in severe preeclampsia. Generalized edema is easily noted in the face, hands, sacral area, lower extremities, and abdomen. Weight gain may be 2 pounds in a few days to a week.

Urinary albumin is 3+ or 4+ on dipstick. Urine output may drop to less than 500 mL/24 hours. Hematocrit, uric acid, and serum creatinine levels are elevated. The client may exhibit other symptoms such as continuous headache, blurred vision, scotomata (spots before the eyes), nausea, vomiting, irritability, hyperreflexia, cerebral disturbances, pulmonary edema, dyspnea, cyanosis, and epigastric pain. Epigastric pain is often the last symptom identified before the client moves into eclampsia.

Eclampsia

The grand mal seizure experienced by the client has a tonic phase (pronounced muscular contractions) and a clonic phase (alternate contraction and relaxation of muscles). Then the client slips into a coma lasting from minutes to hours. With no treatment, the seizure/coma sequence may be repeated one or more times and death may follow.

Seizure activity may trigger uterine contractions, but the client in a coma is unaware of them and unable to let anyone know.

HELLP Syndrome

HELLP syndrome is a complication of preeclampsia/eclampsia with liver damage. It is characterized by **h**emolysis, **e**levated **l**iver enzymes, and **l**ow **p**latelet count.

- Hemolysis is caused when intra-arterial lesions develop as a result of vasospasm, causing platelets to aggregate and a fibrin network to be formed. The RBCs are forced through the fibrin network and lysed, resulting in a large drop in hematocrit.
- Elevated liver enzymes (AST and ALT) may be caused by microemboli in the vessels of the liver, causing ischemia.
- Low platelet count (must be less than 100,000/mm³) results when the platelets are entrapped at the intra-arterial lesions.

The result of this syndrome is ischemia and tissue damage. The client may also show signs of hypoglycemia. A blood sugar less than 40 mg/dL is often associated with maternal mortality. Up to 20% of women with PIH have HELLP syndrome (Ruddy, 2000).

Medical–Surgical Management

Medical

The goals of treatment are to lower blood pressure, prevent convulsions, and deliver a healthy baby.

A client with mild preeclampsia may be allowed to stay home but is advised to stay in bed, lying on either side. This increases renal and placental blood flow. The client generally feels well, so education is very important to improve compliance with the plan of care.

Laboratory tests may include hematocrit, platelet count, electrolytes, liver function (AST and ALT), estriol level, 24-hour urine for protein and creatinine, and serum creatinine.

Surgical

If the mother's condition continues to deteriorate or the environment within the uterus becomes harmful to fetal well-being, a cesarean birth may be necessary.

Pharmacological

Magnesium sulfate (MgSO₄) is a CNS depressant that decreases the possibility of convulsions. It also relaxes smooth muscles and may decrease blood pressure to some degree. MgSO₄ is usually given intravenously for greater accuracy of dosage, but may be given intramuscularly by Z-track. It is excreted by the kidneys and may reach a toxic level if the client has impaired renal function. Magnesium sulfate toxicity may lead to cardiac arrest. Common side effects are flushing, sweating, hy-

---

CLIENT TEACHING

Home Management of Mild Preeclampsia

- Bed rest is essential.
- Lie on either side but not on the back.
- Reduce anxiety.
- Take medications as prescribed.
- Eat a high-protein, moderate-sodium diet.
- Keep all prenatal appointments (may be two per week).
- Report immediately headache, visual disturbances, edema of face or hands, severe nausea and vomiting, and epigastric pain.

potension, hypothermia, muscle weakness, constipation, nausea, and vomiting. An indwelling catheter is generally inserted to accurately measure output.

Calcium gluconate, the antidote for MgSO$_4$ must be kept in a syringe at the bedside ready to be given if signs of magnesium toxicity are noted. MgSO$_4$ is usually given for 24 to 48 hours after delivery to ensure that convulsions do not occur.

An antihypertensive drug may be given. Hydralazine (Apresoline) is the drug of choice except for clients with cardiac dysfunctions, who are given labetalol hydrochloride (Normodyne, Trandate).

A sedative such as phenobarbital or diazepam (Valium) may be given to help the client rest quietly.

Oxytocin may be given to induce labor. It may be given along with magnesium sulfate.

Diet

A well-balanced, high-protein, moderate-sodium diet should be provided. Excessively salty foods should not be eaten, but sodium restriction is no longer recommended. If the client is nauseated or there are signs of impending convulsions, the diet is withheld.

Activity

Bed rest, lying preferably on the left side but not on the back, must be complete. *Takes pressure off vagus nerve.*

Nursing Management

Frequently monitor vital signs and FHT. Assess for edema (hands and face), proteinuria, headache, blurred vision, irritability, hyperreflexia (deep tendon reflexes), dyspnea, cyanosis, nausea, and epigastric pain. Involve client and family in decisions when possible. Assist client and family to identify sources of support. Encourage the client to express feelings about her situation. If magnesium sulfate is being given, assess for toxicity.

NURSING PROCESS

Assessment

Subjective Data

Ask the client about headache, visual disturbances, epigastric pain, swelling of hands and face, nausea, and dyspnea.

Objective Data

Check vital signs and weight and compare to previous figures, and check urine for protein. Edema may be found in the face, hands, sacral area, lower extremities, or abdomen. Check laboratory reports of electrolytes, platelet count, liver enzymes, and hematocrit. Monitor I&O.

Nursing diagnoses for a client with PIH may include the following:

Nursing Diagnoses	Planning/Goals	Nursing Interventions
Interrupted Family Processes, related to illness and bed rest or hospitalization of mother	The family will work together to maintain family functioning.	Involve client and family in decisions when possible. Encourage client and family to verbalize feelings about situation. Encourage family to visit client as client's condition allows. Assist client and family to plan how to deal with situation. Help client and family identify sources of support.
Deficient Knowledge, related to lack of information about PIH, its treatment, and implications for mother and baby	The client will verbalize an understanding of PIH, its treatment, and implications for herself and her baby.	Discuss PIH and implications with client. Explain the purpose and importance of each aspect of the plan of care. Encourage client to express feelings about her situation.

continues

Nursing Diagnoses	Planning/Goals	Nursing Interventions
Deficient **F**luid Volume, related to shift in fluids from intravascular to interstitial	The client will maintain intravascular fluid volume.	Assess BP and FHT every 1 to 4 hours. Weigh daily. Maintain client on bed rest, lying on side, especially the left side. Assess for edema. Accurately record I&O. Test urine for protein as ordered. Monitor laboratory test results.

Evaluation Each goal must be evaluated to determine how it has been met by the client.

CHRONIC MEDICAL PROBLEMS

Conditions in this group include diabetes mellitus, chronic hypertension, heart disease, and maternal phenylketonuria.

DIABETES MELLITUS

Diabetic clients who wish to become pregnant should have their diabetes well under control before conception.

Gestational diabetes mellitus (GDM) is an abnormal glucose metabolism that appears only during pregnancy. Many women with GDM will have diabetes later in life. Whether the mother has chronic diabetes or GDM, the effects during pregnancy are the same.

Pregnancy and Carbohydrate Metabolism

Insulin production is increased in early pregnancy because of the stimulation of the mother's pancreas by the increased levels of estrogen, progesterone, and other hormones. The tissue response to insulin is also increased along with increased storage of glycogen in the liver and muscles. An increased resistance to insulin develops in the last half of pregnancy because of hPL (an insulin antagonist), prolactin, and elevated levels of cortisol and placental enzymes called insulinases, which destroy insulin. This diabetogenic effect of pregnancy occurs after about 20 weeks' gestation. The result is a catabolic state after a meal is absorbed and also during the night. Fat, at this time, is more readily metabolized, and ketones may be found in the mother's urine. Glucose from the mother provides the growing fetus with energy, thus putting stress on the balance of glucose production and utilization. Diabetes already present is more difficult to control. In a case where the pancreas has little insulin reserve, gestational diabetes occurs.

Effects of Pregnancy on Diabetes

The insulin requirements change throughout pregnancy. The need for insulin may decrease during the first trimester. The risk of hypoglycemia or hyperinsulinemia are increased if nausea and vomiting are present. Placental maturation and the increasing production of hPL cause the insulin requirements to rise during the second trimester, and they may even be four times higher by the end of pregnancy. After the placenta is passed, removing the source of hPL, there is generally an immediate decrease in the amount of insulin required.

There is a physiological decrease in the renal threshold for glucose. The risk of ketoacidosis is greater during pregnancy, as is an acceleration of vascular disease.

Effects of Diabetes on Pregnancy

Pregnancy in a diabetic client has a higher risk of complications than for a nondiabetic client. If vascular changes already exist, the chance for PIH is greater.

Hydramnios, an excessive amount of amniotic fluid, may occur. This may lead to preterm labor or premature rupture of the membranes.

Hyperglycemia can result in ketoacidosis caused by increased fat metabolism. Often, ketoacidosis develops slowly, but can result in maternal and fetal death if untreated. Maternal complications are directly related to the degree of blood glucose control.

Effects on the Fetus/Neonate

Macrosomia, excessive fetal growth, results from maternal hyperglycemia. The hyperglycemia stimulates fetal insulin production to utilize the available glucose. After birth, there is no more maternal glucose, but the fetal pancreas continues to produce a high level of insulin. In 2 to 4 hours, the neonate is hypoglycemic. Fetal insulin production gradually decreases to an appropriate level.

Intrauterine growth retardation (IUGR) may result when the mother has vascular changes, which also occur in the placenta. This decreases perfusion of the placenta, and the fetus does not receive adequate amounts of nutrients.

A high fetal insulin level inhibits the production of surfactant in the lungs, making the possibility of respiratory distress syndrome very high. The decreased ability of maternal glycosylated hemoglobin (hemoglobin with glucose attached) to release oxygen causes the fetus to have polycythemia (excessive number of red blood cells). The polycythemia is a direct cause of hyperbilirubinemia because the immature liver is unable to metabolize the increased amount of bilirubin.

Congenital anomalies are several times higher in diabetic pregnancies and may be caused by hyperglycemia in early pregnancy. Many anomalies involve the heart, central nervous system, and skeletal system.

Medical–Surgical Management

Medical

The goals of care are to maintain **euglycemia** (normal blood glucose level) between 70 mg/dL and 120 mg/dL, and to have a healthy mother and baby. The client is usually followed by both her endocrinologist and obstetrician.

Clients are taught to monitor their blood glucose level and give themselves insulin according to a sliding scale. For clients with GDM, this may be very difficult because diabetes is new to them.

Fetal status is evaluated throughout the pregnancy. AFP screening is performed because diabetic pregnancies have an increased risk of fetal neural tube defects. Gestational age is established by ultrasound at about 18 weeks' gestation and repeated every 4 to 6 weeks to monitor fetal growth and assess for congenital abnormalities. The mother monitors fetal activity daily beginning about 28 weeks' gestation. An NST is often scheduled weekly beginning also at about 28 weeks. A CST may be performed at about 32 weeks and may be scheduled weekly until a positive result occurs, indicating that the fetus is having trouble handling the contractions.

Many clients with diabetes are hospitalized several times during the pregnancy. The timing of birth is based mainly on fetal well-being but should never be past 40 weeks' gestation. The L/S ratio and presence of PG in the amniotic fluid is usually checked about 38 weeks or earlier if an NST is nonreactive.

Surgical

If fetal well-being is deteriorating, a cesarean birth is often performed.

Pharmacological

Humalin is generally used because it is unlikely to cause an allergic reaction. Insulin is given, most commonly, by multiple injections. This may be scheduled twice a day or four to six times per day after a blood glucose check. Oral hypoglycemics should be discontinued, with the physician's knowledge, when the client plans to become pregnant, or immediately when she becomes pregnant.

Diet

Pregnant women should increase their caloric intake about 300 kcal/day (35 to 40 kcal/Kg/day of ideal weight is recommended). Total kilocalories for the day should be divided among three meals and three snacks. The bedtime snack, eaten as late as possible, should have complex carbohydrates and protein to prevent hypoglycemia during the night. There should be no more than 10 hours between the bedtime snack and breakfast. A dietician should assist the pregnant diabetic client with meal plans based on food preferences, lifestyle, and culture.

Activity

Activity should be maintained throughout pregnancy unless contraindicated by complications. Activity level is taken into account when the diet and insulin prescribed are determined.

Nursing Management

Listen actively to the client. Answer questions and provide support. Teach glucose monitoring and insulin self-injection as needed. Monitor fetal status through results of AFP screening, ultrasound, nonstress test, contraction stress test, and amniocentesis. Emphasize the importance of keeping all scheduled prenatal visits and testing appointments.

NURSING PROCESS

Assessment

Subjective Data

Ask questions regarding a family history of diabetes, congenital abnormalities, neonatal deaths, or unexplained stillbirths. At each prenatal visit, ask about diet, activity, and medication compliance. After 28 weeks, record maternal evaluation of fetal activity.

Objective Data

Check urine for sugar, and also measure vital signs and weight. Evaluate NST results and results of laboratory tests. Note signs of infection.

Nursing diagnoses for a client with diabetes during pregnancy may include the following:

Nursing Diagnoses	Planning/Goals	Nursing Interventions
Deficient **K**nowledge, related to disease process of diabetes, control of diabetes, and implications for pregnancy	The client will verbalize an understanding of the disease process of diabetes, control of diabetes, and implications for the pregnancy.	Present to or review with the client the pathophysiology of diabetes and clarify client misconceptions. Teach how to monitor blood glucose level, the desired range, and importance of good control.

continues

Nursing Diagnoses	Planning/Goals	Nursing Interventions
		Teach self-administration of insulin (if applicable) to client and significant other.
		Review effects of diabetes on client and fetus.
		Teach danger signs and whom to notify.
		Refer to diabetic support group in the community.
Risk for Injury, Fetus, related to decreased uteroplacental functioning	The client will verbalize an understanding of the various antepartal tests and what to expect during the procedures.	Teach client the possible effects of poor uteroplacental functioning.
		Explain purpose of periodic ultrasound, fetal activity record, weekly NST, amniocentesis for L/S ratio and PG level, and biophysical profile.
Noncompliance, related to need for close monitoring and extra prenatal visits	The client will perform blood glucose testing on schedule and attend all scheduled prenatal visits.	Review the importance of maintaining euglycemia.
		Assist client in making a chart on which to record results of blood glucose testing.
		Review importance of attending all scheduled prenatal visits.
		Work to schedule prenatal visits when most convenient for the client.

Evaluation Each goal must be evaluated to determine how it has been met by the client.

CHRONIC HYPERTENSION

A BP 140/90 or higher before pregnancy or before the 20th week of gestation that lasts longer than 6 weeks after delivery is termed chronic hypertension. A diastolic pressure of more than 80 mm Hg in the second trimester may indicate chronic hypertension.

A client with untreated or poorly controlled hypertension may show signs of hypertensive vascular disease such as arteriosclerosis and retinal hemorrhage. Renal, disease may be present. The placenta may have infarcts, and placenta abruptio may occur.

Effects on the Fetus/Neonate

A placenta with infarcts has reduced perfusion. This may cause IUGR and fetal hypoxia.

PIH Superimposed on Chronic Hypertension

Clients who have moderate to severe chronic hypertension are most at risk to develop PIH. In these women, PIH develops rapidly and moves to a crisis state faster than in women without chronic hypertension. More stillbirths, abruptio placenta, and severe renal failure are found in clients with chronic hypertension. Any of the classic signs indicate PIH. These clients are hospitalized for medical management and nursing care.

Medical–Surgical Management

Medical

The goals of care are to prevent development of preeclampsia and to ensure a healthy fetus. Prenatal visits are generally scheduled every 2 weeks. An ultrasound is performed early to establish, or verify, the EDB. Around 22 and 32 weeks' gestation, an ultrasound checks for IUGR. If renal disease is suspected, creatinine clearance is determined early and repeated every 2 months.

Pharmacological

Antihypertensive medication, such as methyldopa (Aldomet), is continued throughout the pregnancy.

Diet

A well-balanced diet providing 1.5 g/Kg/day of protein is recommended. Salt intake should remain as it was before pregnancy.

Activity

Daily rest periods, with the client preferably lying on her left side (never on the back), are important to maintain adequate perfusion to the placenta and relieve dependent edema.

Nursing Management

Provide information about hypertension and how it may affect a pregnancy. Answer client's questions. Encourage client to plan rest periods (lying on the side) throughout the day. Emphasize the importance of keeping all scheduled prenatal visits and testing appointments.

NURSING PROCESS

Assessment

Subjective Data

Most clients have no symptoms of hypertension until it becomes severe. Then headaches or visual disturbances may occur.

Objective Data

Blood pressure will be 140/90 or higher.

Nursing diagnoses for a pregnant client with chronic hypertension may include the following:

Nursing Diagnoses	Planning/Goals	Nursing Interventions
Risk for Injury, Fetus, related to placental infarcts and poor placental perfusion	The client will verbalize an understanding of possible placental changes leading to fetal injury and interventions to prevent this.	Teach client the possible placental changes related to hypertension. Assist client to plan for rest periods throughout the day. Administer antihypertensive medications as ordered.
Deficient Knowledge related to disease process and effects on pregnancy	The client will verbalize an understanding of the disease process and effects on pregnancy.	Provide the client with information about the disease process and how pregnancy may be affected. Allow opportunity for client to ask questions.

Evaluation Each goal must be evaluated to determine how it has been met by the client.

HEART DISEASE

The normal physiological increase in blood volume that peaks about 28 to 32 weeks' gestation, and the increased cardiac output and heart rate, may cause problems in the client with heart disease. The heart compensates at first by tachycardia, and ventricular dilation and hypertrophy. When these mechanisms fail, the heart is no longer able to compensate and congestive heart failure occurs.

The results of having had rheumatic fever often restrict cardiac output and cause pulmonary congestion. The effects of congenital heart disease on pregnancy depend on the specific defect. Hypertension may cause cardiac insufficiency.

Effects on the Fetus/Neonate

IUGR and hypoxia may occur.

Medical–Surgical Management

Medical

Many clients are cared for by both their cardiologist and obstetrician. Early diagnosis and ongoing management is assessed by the use of chest x-rays, auscultation of heart sounds, EKG, echocardiogram, and sometimes cardiac catheterization. Prenatal care appointments may be increased to two or three per week between 28 and 32 weeks' gestation, when blood volume is highest. Sometimes hospitalization is necessary.

Pharmacological

Antibiotics are often used as a prophylaxis for all pregnant women with heart disease. Heparin may be used if coagulation problems develop because heparin does not cross the placenta. Thiazide diuretics and furosemide (Lasix) may be used for congestive heart failure.

Diet

The diet should be high in iron and protein but low in sodium. Adequate kilocalories for normal weight gain should be provided.

Activity

Physical activity may be restricted depending on the client's symptoms. Eight to 10 hours of sleep and frequent rest periods throughout the day are important. The side-lying position is best to prevent compression of the inferior vena cava.

Nursing Management

Monitor vital signs, lung and heart sounds, and FHT. Emphasize the importance of keeping all scheduled prenatal visits and testing appointments. Encourage the client to eat a diet high in iron and protein, but low in sodium. Stress importance of side lying during daytime rest periods and during the night. Assist client to identify a support system to help with household chores.

NURSING PROCESS

Assessment

Subjective Data

Ask about activity level, amount of rest, increasing fatigue with activity, dyspnea, palpitations, cough, and anxiety. Inquire about the availability of household help and the support system, to ascertain the client's ability to rest and relax.

Objective Data

These data include weight gain (fluid retention), edema, vital signs, signs of infection, anemia, heart murmurs, or crackles in the lungs.

Nursing diagnoses for a pregnant client with heart disease may include the following:

Nursing Diagnoses	Planning/Goals	Nursing Interventions
Impaired Gas Exchange, related to pulmonary edema	The client will maintain adequate gas exchange.	Monitor and accurately record I&O. Assess vital signs frequently. Administer medications as ordered.
Activity Intolerance related to generalized decreased perfusion	The client will be able to tolerate some activity.	Assess activity tolerance frequently. Promote activity level established by the physician. Discuss activity limitations and the need for sleep and rest periods.
Fear related to effects of maternal cardiac condition on fetal well-being	The client will express her fears about fetal well-being.	Provide information on how fetal well-being may be affected by maternal cardiac condition. Listen to the client express her fears about fetal well-being.

Evaluation Each goal must be evaluated to determine how it has been met by the client.

MATERNAL PHENYLKETONURIA

Phenylketonuria (PKU) is an inborn error of metabolism in which there is a deficiency of the enzyme necessary to metabolize the amino acid phenylalanine. It is genetically inherited by a recessive gene. The accumulation of this amino acid and its metabolites leads to irreversible brain damage.

Since 1967, all newborns in the United States have had a screening blood test for PKU. The infants diagnosed with PKU were put on a phenylalanine-free diet. For years it was thought that the child treated with a phenylalanine-free diet outgrew the problem by about age 9. It is now known that the modified diet should be continued. When a woman with PKU keeps her phenylalanine level less than 2.0 mg/dL while pregnant, the outcome of pregnancy is better (Acosta & Wright, 1992).

Effects on the Fetus/Neonate

A poorly regulated maternal phenylalanine level causes an increase in the incidence of IUGR, mental retardation, microcephaly, and heart defects.

Medical–Surgical Management

Medical

The mother's blood phenylalanine level should be checked every 2 to 4 weeks during the first half of pregnancy. It may be checked every week in the last half of pregnancy, along with iron and zinc levels.

Diet

A very expensive modified protein supplement can be used before and during pregnancy. Fruits, vegetables, fats, and some low-protein cereals make up the rest of the diet.

Nursing Management

Encourage client to maintain a phenylalanine-free diet and to have her blood level checked throughout the pregnancy.

INFECTIONS

Any infection is a risk factor during pregnancy and should be diagnosed and treated promptly. Untreated infections may cause abortion, congenital anomalies, fetal infections, IUGR, preterm labor, mental retardation, or death.

TORCH GROUP

The TORCH group of infections include **t**oxoplasmosis, **r**ubella, **c**ytomegalovirus, and **h**erpesvirus type 2.

TOXOPLASMOSIS

Toxoplasmosis is caused by the protozoan *Toxoplasma gondii*. This disease goes almost unnoticed by adults because the symptoms are mild, vague, and flu-like. The organism may be ingested by eating undercooked, raw, or cured meat (Cook et al., 2000). Maternal toxoplasmosis before pregnancy seems to offer protection against fetal infection.

Effects on the Fetus/Neonate

There is an increased incidence of abortion, preterm birth, stillbirth, and neonatal death if the mother contracts toxoplasmosis when she is pregnant. Damage to the fetus is generally more severe if the disease is acquired before 20 weeks' gestation. The neonate may have microcephaly, hydrocephaly, and convulsions. Many infants die soon after birth. Those who survive may be blind, deaf, or severely retarded.

Medical–Surgical Management

Medical

The goals are to identify the pregnant client at risk and treat the disease promptly when diagnosed. The incubation period is 10 days.

Pharmacological

The client may be treated with sulfadiazine (Microsulfon) or pyrimethamine (Daraprim).

Diet

No raw or partially cooked meats should be eaten. Fruits and vegetables should be washed before they are eaten.

Activity

Gloves should be worn when gardening because contact with soil is a significant risk factor. Travel outside the United States, Canada, and Europe is also a significant risk factor (Cook et al., 2000).

Nursing Management

Encourage the client to eat only well-done meats, to wash all fruits and vegetables before eating them, and to wear gloves when gardening.

NURSING PROCESS

Assessment

Subjective Data

The client may have no symptoms or may have malaise and/or myalgia.

Objective Data

A rash may be evident as well as splenomegaly and enlarged cervical lymph nodes.

Nursing diagnoses for a pregnant client with toxoplasmosis may include the following:

Nursing Diagnoses	Planning/Goals	Nursing Interventions
Deficient Knowledge related to lack of knowledge about toxoplasmosis disease process	The client will verbalize an understanding of toxoplasmosis disease process.	Provide information about toxoplasmosis, incubation period, how acquired, and ways to prevent it. Allow time for client to ask questions and clarify misconceptions.
Anticipatory Grieving, related to effects of toxoplasmosis on fetus/neonate	The client will express feelings about possible effects on fetus/neonate.	Encourage client to discuss feelings about possible effects of toxoplasmosis on her fetus. Provide a private place for client and family to discuss the situation.

Evaluation Each goal must be evaluated to determine how it has been met by the client.

RUBELLA

Rubella, German measles, and three-day measles are all names for the same disease. After an incubation period of 14 to 21 days, a maculopapular rash appears and then vanishes in 3 days. Rubella is highly contagious and is spread by airborne droplets.

Effects on the Fetus/Neonate

The earlier in pregnancy the infection occurs, the more severe the fetal effects. Congenital rubella syndrome occurs in many of the infections that occur before 8 weeks' gestation. It is characterized by cataracts, deafness, and patent ductus arteriosus. The infant may also have IUGR, mental retardation, and hyperbilirubinemia. Sometimes a petechial rash may be seen. These infants are infectious and may shed the virus for months.

Medical–Surgical Management

Medical

Prevention is the best cure. The prenatal laboratory screening includes the hemagglutination inhibition (HAI). A titer of 1:16 or higher signifies immunity, while a titer of less than 1:8 signifies a susceptibility to rubella. The client who is susceptible should avoid exposure to rubella while pregnant.

A pregnant woman who becomes infected with rubella during the first trimester has a 90% chance of fetal infection with the accompanying anomalies (Schweon, 2001).

Pharmacological

All children should be immunized with the live attenuated vaccine by age 1. Susceptible pregnant women should be immunized very soon after delivery, and avoid becoming pregnant for 3 months following immunization to avoid the chance of infecting a fetus.

Nursing Management

Identify clients who are susceptible to rubella and provide information about avoiding exposure while pregnant. Encourage susceptible clients to receive the immunization very soon after delivery and then delay another pregnancy for 3 months. Encourage parents to have infants receive all immunizations as scheduled.

NURSING PROCESS

Assessment

Subjective Data

There may be no symptoms or the client may describe muscle aches and joint pain.

Objective Data

Temperature may be slightly elevated, and a maculopapular rash and lymphadenopathy may be present.

Nursing diagnoses for a pregnant client with rubella may include the following:

Nursing Diagnoses	Planning/Goals	Nursing Interventions
Ineffective Health Maintenance, related to lack of knowledge about her need for rubella immunization before becoming pregnant	The client will receive rubella vaccine soon after delivery.	Provide information about the implications of rubella when the HAI results are known. Provide information about rubella immunization. Answer client questions and clarify any misunderstandings.
Interrupted Family Processes, related to the probability of fetal anomalies caused by maternal rubella	The client and family will verbalize understanding of the probability of fetal anomalies and make a decision about continuing the pregnancy	Discuss with client and family the probability and types of fetal anomalies that generally occur with maternal rubella. Provide a private place for client and family to discuss the situation. Answer questions and clarify misconceptions.

Evaluation Each goal must be evaluated to determine how it has been met by the client.

CYTOMEGALOVIRUS

Cytomegalovirus (CMV) is a member of the herpesvirus group. More than half of all adults have antibodies for CMV, which is found in saliva, breast milk, cervical mucus, urine, and semen. It spreads by close contact. It is asymptomatic in adults and children but can affect the fetus in utero or during delivery.

Effects on the Fetus/Neonate

The fetus may have extensive damage leading to fetal death; however, the fetus may survive with hydro-

cephaly, microcephaly, mental retardation, cerebral palsy, or with no noticeable damage.

An infected newborn is usually small for gestational age (SGA). Mental retardation, auditory deficits, or learning disabilities may not be noticed right away.

Medical–Surgical Management

Medical

Diagnosis is made when CMV is found in the maternal urine and an elevated IgM level with CMV antibodies identified in the blood.

There is no treatment for the mother or neonate.

HERPES GENITALIS (HERPES SIMPLEX VIRUS TYPE 2)

Herpes simplex virus type 2 (HSV-2) causes painful, vesicular genital lesions. The lesions appear within a few hours to 20 days after exposure. The primary episode is the most severe. Women who have their first infection close to the time of delivery have a greater chance of neonatal infection. After the membranes rupture, the virus ascends from active lesions to the fetus, or the fetus comes in contact with the lesions during a vaginal delivery. HSV-2 is not found in breast milk, so the mother may breast-feed.

Effects on the Fetus/Neonate

When there is an active HSV-2 infection in the first trimester, about one-half will end in spontaneous abortion or stillbirth. Most infected infants have no symptoms at birth. Symptoms of poor feeding, jaundice, and seizures develop after a 2- to 12-day incubation period. Many of these infants will also have the vesicular lesions.

Medical–Surgical Management

Medical

Diagnosis is made by culturing active lesions. Treatment is mainly to relieve pain. When no lesions are visible at the time of delivery, a vaginal birth is acceptable. Pregnancy is one of many causes of recurrence. There is no known cure.

Surgical

When active lesions are visible at the time of delivery, a cesarean birth is best to prevent fetal contact with the lesions (virus).

Pharmacological

Cleansing with povidone-iodine (Betadine) may help prevent a secondary infection. Burow's solution may relieve discomfort.

Nursing Management

Inquire if client has ever had a herpes infection. Provide information regarding possible effect on the fetus/neonate, preventing spread of infection, and how to care for active lesions.

NURSING PROCESS

Assessment

Subjective Data

Ask whether the client or her partner have ever had a herpes infection. Client may describe pain and discomfort from the lesions if she has a herpes infection.

Objective Data

Lesions may be seen when infection is active. A cervical culture may indicate presence or absence of the virus.

Nursing diagnoses for the pregnant client with HSV-2 infection may include the following:

Nursing Diagnoses	Planning/Goals	Nursing Interventions
Acute *Pain* related to local, open vulvar lesions	The client will describe a decrease in pain after treatment is begun.	Administer medications as ordered. Suggest a sitz bath several times a day followed by air-drying of the vulva and wearing cotton underwear.
Ineffective *Sexuality Patterns*, related to unwillingness to engage in sexual intercourse	The client will maintain sexuality patterns.	Provide client with information about disease process, and the method of transmission. Refer client to community resources. Encourage client to engage in forms of sexual expression that do not involve genital contact.
Ineffective *Coping*, related to depression about risk to fetus if herpes lesions are present at birth	The client will verbalize an understanding about how decision is made regarding the type of delivery when herpes lesions are present.	Provide client with information about the factors relative to type of delivery performed. Encourage client to have appropriate cultures run as recommended by her health care provider. Encourage client to report any changes that may indicate a recurrence of lesions.

Evaluation Each goal must be evaluated to determine how it has been met by the client.

HIV/AIDS

Weight gain or even maintenance of weight during pregnancy is a challenge for an HIV-infected client. Counseling should be provided regarding optimum nutrition, exercise, rest, and sleep.

Pregnancy is considered to be a somewhat immunosuppressive state and may theoretically speed up the process of going from being HIV positive to an AIDS diagnosis.

Effects on the Fetus/Neonate

HIV may be transmitted to the fetus through the placenta, at the time of birth when exposed to maternal blood and vaginal secretions, or through breast milk. Infants often have a positive antibody titer for as long as 15 months after birth because of the transfer of maternal antibodies. Those infants who are not infected with HIV will seroconvert to a negative antibody titer.

Medical–Surgical Management

Medical

There is no cure for HIV or AIDS. Routine prenatal testing should be expanded to include a CD 4 lymphocyte count and serologic testing for changes indicating that AIDS is progressing. NST and ultrasound are performed at 32 weeks' gestation. NST is continued weekly to monitor fetal status, and ultrasound is performed every few weeks depending on what is seen.

Diet

Nutritional counseling and support regarding food handling, food preparation, and diet choices is often necessary.

Nursing Management

Follow Standard Precautions at all times. Discuss how HIV/AIDS can affect the pregnancy. Encourage an adequate food intake for fetal development. Emphasize the importance of attending all scheduled prenatal visits and testing appointments.

NURSING PROCESS

Assessment

Subjective Data

The client may be asymptomatic or may describe having fatigue, malaise, loss of appetite, or diarrhea.

Objective Data

Signs of anemia, cell-mediated immunodeficiency, progressive weight loss, lymphadenopathy, and neurologic dysfunction may be present. Purplish lesions may also be noted during assessment.

Nursing diagnoses for a pregnant client who has HIV/AIDS may include the following:

Nursing Diagnoses	Planning/Goals	Nursing Interventions
Risk for Infection, related to altered immune status	The client will not develop infections during pregnancy.	Use Standard Precautions at all times. Monitor client for signs of infection (fever, cough, sore throat). Teach client to report changes that may indicate infection.
Fear, related to outcome of pregnancy and disease	The client will verbalize fears about her pregnancy and HIV/AIDS.	Discuss HIV/AIDS disease process and how it can affect pregnancy. Provide opportunities for client to ask questions and clarify misconceptions. Assess client's support system and refer to community resources.
Imbalanced Nutrition: Less Than Body Requirements, related to lack of appetite	The client will maintain weight or gain weight.	Monitor client's weight. Obtain 24-hour diet recall from client. Provide information about nutritional needs. Assist client in planning a high-protein, high-calorie diet.

Evaluation Each goal must be evaluated to determine how it has been met by the client.

OTHER INFECTIONS

Maternal infections may result in spontaneous abortion, a preterm infant, or an infected infant. Table 51-4 provides a summary of other infections affecting pregnancy. These are covered in detail in the Reproductive Systems and Sexually Transmitted Diseases chapters.

HEMOLYTIC DISEASES

There are two types of hemolytic diseases: Rh incompatibility and ABO incompatibility. Rh incompatibility can be devastating to the fetus, but it can be prevented. ABO incompatibility is naturally occurring and much less severe, but it cannot be prevented.

RH INCOMPATIBILITY

Rh incompatibility can happen only when the mother is Rh negative and the fetus is Rh positive. That is, the mother does not have the Rh factor and the fetus does have the Rh factor. In this case, the father must be Rh positive for the fetus to be Rh positive. If the father is Rh negative, there is no problem because the fetus will also be Rh negative.

The placenta keeps the mother's blood and the fetus's blood separated. In cases of ectopic pregnancy, abortion, infection of the placenta, abruptio placenta, birth, or at the time of placental separation, small tears may occur in the placenta and fetal blood may enter maternal circulation. The mother is then sensitized by the fetal Rh-positive blood. She may also be sensitized by having a transfusion of Rh-positive blood, even the smallest amount.

Fetal (Rh-positive) blood in maternal (Rh-negative) circulation stimulates maternal production of Rh antibodies. The Rh antibodies, like many other antibodies, pass through the placenta and destroy fetal red blood cells (Figure 51-13). Because this usually occurs at the time of birth, the first infant is usually not affected.

Effects on the Fetus/Neonate

If a placental tear occurred and there was no treatment, the next Rh-positive fetus will have red blood cells destroyed by the maternal Rh antibodies. This causes anemia, which in turn causes fetal edema (hydrops fetalis).

The next step is congestive heart failure and severe jaundice, which can cause neurologic damage called **kernicterus.** This entire syndrome, the most severe of the two hemolytic diseases of the newborn, is called erythroblastosis fetalis.

TABLE 51-4	SELECTED INFECTIONS AND PREGNANCY		
INFECTION	**TREATMENT**	**MATERNAL EFFECTS**	**FETAL EFFECTS**
Sexually Transmitted			
Syphilis	penicillin G benzathin (Bicillin L-A) or doxycycline (Vibramycin). Sexual partner should also be treated.	Chancre, slight fever, malaise. Progresses through secondary and tertiary stages if untreated.	Spontaneous abortion, stillbirth, congenital syphilis, sniffling, peeling of soles and palms
Gonorrhea	ceftriaxone (Rocephin) plus erythromycin (Erythrocin Lactobionate). Partners must be treated.	Often no symptoms. May have purulent vaginal discharge, dysuria, or urinary frequency.	Ophthalmia neonatorum.
Chlamydia	erthromycin ethyl succinate (ABO-Erythro-ES)	Often no symptoms. May have purulent or thin vaginal discharge, burning on urination, preterm labor.	Conjunctivitis, chlamydial pneumonia, fetal death
Condylomata acuminata (venereal warts)	Cryosurgery, laser surgery, electrocautery, or trichloroacetic acid	Soft, grayish, raised lesions	Laryngeal papillomatosis if infection is present at birth
Hepatitis B (HBV)	Supportive. Vaccine available.	Often no symptoms.	Most become carriers.
Vaginal Infections			
Monilia	miconazole (Monistat), clotrimazole (Gyne-Lotrimin)	Thick, white, cheesy discharge Itching, dysuria	Thrush
Trichomoniasis	clotrimazole (Gyne-Lotrimin) in early pregnancy, metronidazole (Flagyl)	Foamy, green-gray discharge, prutitus	
Urinary Tract Infection			
Cystitis	Oral sulfonamides in early pregnancy, nitrofurantoin (Furadantin) in late pregnancy	Dysuria, urgency, low-grade fever. If not treated, may result in acute pyelonephritis.	Hyperbilirubinemia if sulfonamides taken in last few weeks of pregnancy

Figure 51-13 *Rh Sensitization and Prevention*

Medical–Surgical Management

Medical

One of the screening tests performed at the first prenatal visit determines the mother's Rh factor. When the mother is found to be Rh negative and the father is Rh positive or unknown, additional tests are run. An indirect Coombs' test detects Rh antibodies in maternal serum. The Rh antibody titer monitors what is happening when an Rh-negative woman is carrying an Rh-positive fetus. A rising titer may indicate the need for immediate intervention.

Ultrasound is performed at about 15 weeks to determine gestational age. It is repeated several times throughout the pregnancy to measure fetal growth and assess fetal heart size and for hydramnios.

Amniocentesis may also be performed several times to determine the bilirubin (product of red blood cell breakdown) level and lung maturity. A fetal intrauterine blood transfusion may be indicated to maintain the fetus in the uterus until the lungs are more mature. The fetus is given Rh-negative erythrocytes to replace those destroyed by the Rh-positive antibodies. The erythrocytes are put into the peritoneal cavity, where they are absorbed. Rh-positive antibodies will not harm the Rh-negative blood given to the fetus.

Pharmacological

Rh immune globulin (RhoGAM) is given to an Rh-negative mother who is not sensitized (has a negative indirect Coombs' and antibody titer) and whose Rh-positive infant has no antibodies on the infant's RBCs (negative direct Coombs'). RhoGAM must be administered within 72 hours of the infant's birth. It prevents the mother's body from making the Rh antibodies by providing temporary passive immunity.

It is recommended that RhoGAM be given at 28 weeks' gestation and after the delivery. RhoGAM is also given to an Rh-negative woman after an abortion (spon-

taneous or induced), an ectopic pregnancy, and amniocentesis. It is never given to an Rh-positive woman.

Nursing Management

Ensure that the client's Rh factor is known. If the client is Rh-negative and the father is Rh-positive or unknown, ensure that the client keeps all appointments to have her Rh antibody titer checked. At 28 weeks' gestation and after the delivery, administer RhoGAM as ordered.

ABO INCOMPATIBILITY

In ABO incompatibility, the way in which a tear in the placenta may occur and fetal and maternal blood mix is the same as for Rh incompatibility. In this situation, the problem occurs when maternal blood enters fetal circulation. Possible combinations for ABO incompatibility are given in Table 51-5. The most common type of ABO incompatibility occurs when the mother is type O and the fetus is either type A, B, or AB. The mother's plasma naturally contains anti-A and anti-B antibodies. These antibodies have a weaker hemolytic effect than Rh antibodies, and they only affect mature RBCs. The number of antibodies is limited to the amount of maternal blood that entered fetal circulation. There is not a continuous supply of antibodies. Because ABO incompatibility is naturally occurring, it may affect the fetus of the first pregnancy. The affected newborn will have a positive direct Coombs' and will become jaundiced in the first 3 days of life.

Nursing Management

Ensure that the client's blood type is known. Observe the newborn for jaundice within the first 3 days of life.

MULTIPLE PREGNANCY

Fundal height greater than expected for the weeks of gestation is often the first clue of a multiple pregnancy. An ultrasound will verify two or more fetuses. Two or more heartbeats that differ by 10 beats/minute may be heard. The alpha fetoprotein level may be elevated. The first trimester proceeds much the same as with a single fetus except that maternal blood volume has a greater increase. Some women have more severe nausea and vomiting as well as shortness of breath on exertion, dyspnea, and backache.

TABLE 51-5 POSSIBLE COMBINATIONS FOR ABO INCOMPATIBILITY

MOTHER	FETUS
A	B
B	A
O	A, B, AB

As the uterus grows, there is greater pressure on and displacement of the internal organs. Pressure on the ureters favors urinary stasis and possible infection. Digestive problems and constipation may be more disturbing, dependent edema more marked, and varicose veins more prominent. PIH is more frequent than with a single fetus.

Effects on the Fetus/Neonate

Each fetus may have a decreased intrauterine growth rate (low birthweight). There is a greater risk of fetal anomalies, abnormal presentations, and preterm birth. Perinatal mortality is much greater for twins than for a single fetus.

Medical–Surgical Management

Medical

The goals are to promote normal fetal development for all fetuses and to prevent delivery of preterm infants. Prenatal visits are more frequent, and serial ultrasounds assess the growth of each fetus. NST and FBPP testing usually begin about 30 weeks' gestation and are repeated every 3 to 7 days until delivery.

Surgical

The method of birth may not be determined until the mother is in labor. Depending on complications that may occur, a cesarean birth may be required.

🔲 Pharmacological

A prenatal vitamin/mineral preparation is doubly important with a multiple pregnancy. An extra calcium supplement and folic acid may be required.

Diet

A well-balanced diet of 4,000 kcal with 135 g of protein is recommended. A weight gain of 40 to 50 pounds is acceptable, with 15 to 20 pounds being gained by 20 weeks' gestation.

Activity

Frequent rest periods should be planned during the day. Resting in the side-lying position increases uteroplacental blood flow. The legs and feet should be elevated to reduce edema. Good posture should be maintained and good body mechanics used when lifting or moving objects.

Nursing Management

Actively listen to the client. Provide anticipatory guidance regarding the discomforts of pregnancy because they may be more intense with a multiple pregnancy. Encourage keeping scheduled prenatal visits and testing appointments. Emphasize the importance of taking the prescribed prenatal vitamin/mineral supplements and eating a well-balanced, high-protein diet. Assist the client to plan for rest periods in the side-lying position.

SUBSTANCE ABUSE

Drugs commonly abused include alcohol, cocaine, crack, marijuana, and heroin. The use of any of these substances is a threat to pregnancy. Substance abusers may not seek prenatal care, or they seek prenatal care very late in pregnancy. Most substance abusers do not voluntarily admit their addiction. These mothers may have an increased rate of PIH, abruptio placenta, poor nutrition, and sexually transmitted diseases. They often use available money for the drug habit instead of food.

Effects on the Fetus/Neonate

Alcohol may result in fetal alcohol syndrome, which manifests as both physical and mental abnormalities. Cocaine/crack increases the risk for IUGR, short body length, small head circumference, preterm birth, irritability, and low Apgar scores (an assessment of infant at 1 and 5 minutes after birth). Marijuana causes fine tremors and irritability. Heroin increases the risk for IUGR, hypoxia, preterm birth, irritability, and meconium aspiration. Irritability and poor consolability may interfere with maternal–infant bonding and attachment and increase the risk of infant abuse and neglect.

 –stool zwearth in.

Medical–Surgical Management

Medical

When a client is known or discovered to be a substance abuser, a multidisciplinary approach is best to manage the medical, legal, and socioeconomic considerations, and provide a safe labor and delivery. The client may require hospitalization for detoxification. "Cold turkey" withdrawal is not recommended during pregnancy because of possible fetal risks. Urine screening is performed regularly.

Nursing Management

Maintain a calm, nonjudgmental manner. Actively listen to the client. Provide information and care as needed.

NURSING PROCESS

Assessment

Subjective Data

Ask questions about the use of caffeine, tobacco, and over-the-counter drugs, and then about alcohol use and drug use. The client may have altered perceptions, so validation through other sources, if possible, is desirable.

CRITICAL THINKING

Substance Abuse

How would you handle the situation if you knew a client was a substance abuser but she would not tell anyone at the prenatal clinic?

Objective Data

Assess for irritability, psychomotor problems, poor nutrition, and possible infections.

Nursing diagnoses for a pregnant client who is a substance abuser may include the following:

Nursing Diagnoses	Planning/Goals	Nursing Interventions
*Imbalanced **N**utrition: Less than Body Requirements* related to inadequate intake of food	The client will gain appropriate weight during pregnancy.	Refer client to WIC (women, infant, and children) nutrition program. Monitor weight gain. Collect 24-hour diet recall from client. Explain foods client should include and why. Assist the client to plan meals.
*Deficient **K**nowledge* related to not understanding how substance abuse affects the fetus	The client will verbalize how substance abuse can affect the fetus.	Explain how substance abuse affects the fetus. Allow time for client questions and for clarification of misconceptions.
*Risk for **I**nfection,* related to use of dirty needles and syringes	The client will not have an infection from dirty needles and syringes.	Explain how client may pick up an infection from dirty needles and syringes. Refer client to community resources where clean syringes and needles may be available. Refer client to drug counseling program.

Evaluation Each goal must be evaluated to determine how it has been met by the client.

PRETERM LABOR

Preterm labor is labor that begins after viability but before 38 weeks' gestation. The causes of preterm labor may be maternal, fetal, or placental. Maternal factors that may cause preterm labor include PIH, diabetes, heart or renal disease, an incompetent cervix, premature rupture of membranes, and maternal infection. Fetal factors include fetal infection, multiple pregnancy, and hydramnios. Placental factors are placenta previa and abruptio placenta.

Effects on the Fetus/Neonate

Preterm labor may produce a neonate who is not able to cope well with extrauterine life.

Medical–Surgical Management

Medical

Preterm labor is confirmed by documented uterine contractions, ruptured membranes, and cervical dilation and effacement. No attempt is made to stop labor if any of the following conditions exist: the cervix dilated 4 cm or more, severe PIH, prolonged rupture of membranes, hemorrhage, abruptio placenta, fetal complications, or fetal death.

Pharmacological

The process of stopping labor with medications is called **tocolysis.** The drugs used in an attempt to stop preterm labor are called *tocolytics.*

Ritodrine hydrochloride (Yutopar) is a beta-adrenergic agonist that inhibits contractility of the uterus. Maternal pulse, BP, lung sounds, and fetal heart rate must be closely monitored.

Turbutaline sulfate (Brethine) is also a beta-adrenergic agonist that relaxes the uterine muscle. It is being used more frequently even though the FDA has not approved it for tocolysis.

Magnesium sulfate ($MgSO_4$) has fewer side effects than the beta-adrenergic agonists and is being used more in preterm labor. A loading dose is given and then continued at the lowest rate necessary to maintain a noncontracting uterus (Mandeville & Troiano, 1999). Tocolysis is usually maintained with a maternal serum level of 5 to 8 mg/dL.

Guinn et al. (2001) recommend that women who are at risk for preterm delivery be given a single injection of corticosteroids to enhance fetal lung maturity. Weekly injections gave no better results.

Nursing Management

Explain all treatments and procedures and keep the client informed of responses to them. Allow client time to ask questions. Monitor vital signs, FHT, and contractions. Administer medications as ordered.

NURSING PROCESS

Assessment

Subjective Data

Client may describe having contractions or that "my water broke." The client may also express concern about what is happening.

Objective Data

Contractions may be documented, cervix dilating and effacing, or membranes ruptured. The client may experience tension, restlessness, or vital sign changes.

Nursing diagnoses for a client in preterm labor may include the following:

Nursing Diagnoses	Planning/Goals	Nursing Interventions
Anxiety, related to perception of what is happening and not having time to prepare for labor	The client will express less anxiety about being in preterm labor.	Explain what is happening to client and all tests and procedures before beginning them. Spend time with client so she can express her anxieties and ask questions. Keep client informed about how the preterm labor is responding to treatment.
Deficient Knowledge, related to lack of information about preterm labor causes, determination, and treatment	The client will verbalize an understanding about preterm labor and treatments.	Explain what preterm labor is, possible/probable causes, and treatment. Allow client time to ask questions. Clarify any misunderstandings.
Fear, related to risk for fetus	The client will express her fears for fetal welfare.	Encourage client to express fears related to fetal well-being. Keep client informed about fetal status. Encourage family to spend time with client.

Evaluation Each goal must be evaluated to determine how it has been met by the client.

Summary

- High-risk factors can often be identified early in prenatal care.
- Continuing prenatal care allows for signs of complications to be identified as early as possible.
- Many procedures and tests are available to assess fetal well-being.
- When bleeding occurs in pregnancy, mothers often feel guilty that they may have done something to cause the bleeding.
- Mothers with chronic medical conditions are often cared for by both the medical physician and the obstetrician during pregnancy.
- Complications of pregnancy add to the emotional and financial stress for the client and family.

Review Questions

1. Judy is a 16-year-old primigravida at 38 weeks whose membranes ruptured spontaneously. Her chart indicates that she was seen by a physician for the first time 2 weeks ago. She is having contractions 10 to 12 minutes apart. The assessment finding indicating a high-risk pregnancy is:
   a. lack of prenatal care and age.
   b. she is not considered high risk.
   c. the membranes rupturing spontaneously.
   d. the contractions being 10 to 12 minutes apart.

CASE STUDY

Part A: Mary Jo, age 32, is G 3, P 2, T 1, P 1, A 0, L 2. The children are ages 1¹/₂ and 3. Bob, her husband, works 8 to 5. She is 32 weeks' gestation. Her BP has been 104/68 at her prenatal visits. Today her BP is 136/84. She has gained 6¹/₂ pounds in the 4 weeks since her last visit. There is edema in both feet.

Part B: Two weeks later, Mary Jo's BP is 140/90 and she has gained 4 more pounds. She states that she had to take her rings off because they were too tight. The physician admits her to the hospital with orders for bed rest in side-lying position, MgSO₄ IV drip, and a high-protein diet.

Part C: The electronic fetal monitor shows a sustained increase in the baseline fetal heart rate. Mary Jo's deep tendon reflexes are very reactive.

The following questions will guide your development of a nursing care plan for the case study:

Part A:

1. What other assessments should be made?
2. What advice would you anticipate the physician giving Mary Jo?
3. How can you assist Mary Jo to implement the physician's advice?

Part B:

4. What are the goals for Mary Jo's care?
5. What nursing assessments must now be obtained?
6. What diagnostic tests might be ordered?

Part C:

7. Identify three nursing diagnoses and goals for Mary Jo.
8. Identify nursing interventions for each nursing diagnosis.

---

2. The maturity of which organ is based on the ratio of lecithin to sphingomyelin?

   a. placenta
   b. fetal lungs
   c. acini glands
   d. fetal kidneys

3. In planning the care of a client with DIC, the nurse would include:

   a. giving coagulants.
   b. turning every 2 hours.
   c. watching for signs of bleeding.
   d. massaging the fundus frequently.

4. A pregnant client is receiving magnesium sulfate. The nurse observes that the client's respirations are 8 and her patellar reflexes have decreased. The nurse recognizes that these observations should be:

   a. considered to be the desired result.
   b. recorded and monitored to see if they continue.
   c. brought to the attention of the charge nurse immediately.
   d. considered as an indication that a higher dose of medication is needed.

5. A pregnant woman's blood is found to be Rh negative. Which of the following must be true for Rh incompatibility to be possible?

   a. father's blood is found to be Rh positive.
   b. father's blood is found to be Rh negative.
   c. mother does not develop a secondary anemia during pregnancy.
   d. mother has at least 2 blood transfusions during pregnancy.

References/Suggested Readings

Acosta, P., & Wright, L. (1992). Nurses' role in preventing birth defects in offspring of women with phenylketonuria. *JOGNN, 21*(4), 270.

Atassi, K., & Harris, M. (2001). Disseminated intravascular coagulation. *Nursing2001, 31*(3), 64.

Barton, J. B., & Sibai, B. M. (2001). HELLP syndrome. In B. M. Sibai (Ed.). *Hypertensive disorders in women.* Philadelphia: W. B. Saunders.

Bougere, M. (1998). Action stat: Abruptio placenta. *Nursing98, 28*(2), 47.

Carpenter, T. (2003). Is it morning sickness or something worse? *RN, 66*(10), 34–37.

Cook, A. J. C. et al. (2000). Undercooked meat the culprit in toxoplasmosis. *BMJ, 321*(7254), 142–147.

Dickason, E., Silverman, B., & Kaplan J. (1998). *Maternal-infant nursing care* (3rd ed.). St. Louis: MO: Mosby–Year Book.

Dochterman, J., & Bulechek, G. (2004). *Nursing Interventions: Classification (NIC)* (4th ed.). St. Louis, MO: Mosby.

Farrell, M. (2003). Improving the care of women with gestational diabetes. *MCN, 28*(5), 301–305.

Friedman, S. A., Lubarsky, S. L., and Lim, K. H. (2001). Mild gestational hypertension and preeclampsia. In B. M. Sibai (Ed.). *Hypertensive Disorders in Women*. Philadelphia: W. B. Saunders.

Guinn, D. A. et al. (2001). Corticosteroids for women at risk for preterm delivery. *JAMA, 286*(13), 1581–1587.

Harvey, C. (1997). A look at electronic fetal monitoring update; the new terms. *Lifelines, 1*(6), 49–51.

Irgens, J. U., Reisaeter, L. et al. (2001). Longterm mortality of mothers and fathers after preeclampsia: Population-based cohort study. *BMJ, 323*(7323), 1213.

Katz, V., Farmer, R., & Kuller, J. (2000). Preeclampsia into eclampsia: Towards a new paradigm. *American Journal of Obstetrics & Gynecology, 182*(6), 1389–1396.

Ladewig, P., Moberly, S., Olds, L., & London, M. (2001). *Contemporary maternal-newborn nursing care* (5th ed.). Menlo Park, CA: Addison-Wesley.

Littleton, L., & Engebretson, J. (2002). *Maternal, neonatal, and women's health nursing*. Clifton Park, NY: Thomson Delmar Learning.

Lu, J., & Nightengale, C. (2000). Magnesium sulfate in eclampsia and preeclampsia: Pharmokinetic principles. *Clinical Pharmacology, 38*(4), 305–314.

Mandeville, L. K., & Troiano, N. H. (1999). *High risk and critical care intrapartum nursing* (2nd ed.). Philadelphia: Lippincott Williams & Wilkins.

Minnick-Smith, K., & Cook, F. (1997). Current treatment options for ectopic pregnancy. *MCN, 22*(1), 21–25.

Montgomery, K. (2003). Health promotion for pregnant adolescents. *Lifelines, 7*(5), 432–444.

Moorhead, S., Johnson, M., & Maas, M. (2004). *Nursing Outcomes Classification (NOC)* (3rd ed.). St. Louis, MO: Mosby.

Morgan, E. (2002). Eclampsia. *Nursing2002, 32*(3), 104.

National Heart, Lung, and Blood Institute. (2000). *Working group report on high blood pressure in pregnancy*. Washington, DC: National Institutes of Health.

Neal, J. (2001). RhD isoimmunization and current management modalities. *JOGNN, 30*(6), 589–606.

Neuman, M., & Graf, C. (2003). Pregnancy after age 35: Are these women at high risk? *Lifelines, 7*(5), 422–430.

NICHD (1997). Electronic fetal heart monitoring: Research guidelines for interpretation. The National Institute of Child Health and Human Development Research Planning Workshop. *JOGNN, 26*(6), 635–640.

Nick, J. (2003). Deep tendon reflexes: The what, why, where, and how of tapping. *JOGNN, 32*(3), 297–306.

North American Nursing Diagnosis Association. (2003). *Nursing diagnoses: Definitions & classification 2003–2004*. Philadelphia: Author.

Reis, P., Sander, C., & Pearlman, M. (2000). Abruptio placentae after auto accidents: A case control study. *Journal of Reproductive Medicine, 45*(1), 6–10.

Ruddy, L. (2000). Preeclampsia. *AJN, 100*(8), 45–46.

Schweon, S. J. (2001). Protecting yourself during pregnancy. *Nursing2001, 31*(3), 72.

Simpson, K., & Creehan, P. (2001). *AWHONN perinatal nursing* (2nd ed.). Philadelphia: Lippincott Williams & Wilkins.

Spratto, G., & Woods, A. (2004). *2004 PDR for nursing*. Clifton Park, NY: Thomson Delmar Learning.

Tenore, J. (2000). Ectopic pregnancy. *American Family Physician, 61*(4), 1080–1088.

Urbanski, T., Higgins, P., Murray, M., & Joffe, G. (1996). Caring for a woman with a hydatidiform mole and coexisting pregnancy. *MCN, 21*(2), 85–89.

Resources

Association of Women's Health, Obstetric, and Neonatal Nurses (AWHONN), 2000 L Street NW, Suite 740, Washington, DC, 20036, 800-673-8499, www.awhonn.org

THE BIRTH PROCESS

MAKING THE CONNECTION

Refer to the following chapters to increase your understanding of the birth process:

Basic Nursing
- **Assessment**
- **Pain Management**

Adult Health Nursing
- **Anesthesia**

Maternal & Pediatric Nursing
- **Prenatal Care**
- **Complications of Pregnancy**

LEARNING OBJECTIVES

Upon completion of this chapter, you should be able to:
- Define key terms.
- Differentiate between true labor and false labor.
- Discuss signs of impending labor.
- Describe possible causes of labor.
- Identify the variables that affect the progress of labor.
- Describe the four stages of labor.
- Describe the mechanisms of labor.
- Discuss the maternal systemic responses to labor.
- Identify nursing actions necessary when admitting a woman to the labor unit.
- Discuss the specific assessments used when caring for a woman in labor: fetopelvic relationships, fetal assessment, contractions, Leopold's maneuvers, vaginal examination.
- Describe the most common complications of labor—dystocia and fetal distress
- Identify possible medical–surgical interventions for labor: cesarean birth, induction and augmentation of labor, amniotomy, episiotomy, forceps, vacuum extractor, and analgesia/anesthesia.
- Discuss possible nursing diagnoses and nursing interventions for a client during labor and delivery.
- Appropriately care for a client during labor and delivery.

KEY TERMS

acme	fontanelle
amniotomy	forceps
augmentation of labor	frequency
bloody show	fundus
Braxton Hicks	increment
contractions	induction of labor
cephalopelvic	intensity
disproportion	interval
cervical dilatation	lightening
cesarean birth	macrosomic
crowning	mechanism of labor
decrement	molding
duration	nuchal cord
dysfunctional labor	precipitate birth
dystocia	precipitate labor
effacement	presenting part
engagement	preterm birth
episiotomy	preterm labor
external version	prolapsed cord
false labor	pudendal block
Ferguson's reflex	restitution
fetal attitude	station
fetal lie	suture
fetal position	tocolytic agent
fetal presentation	uterine retraction

INTRODUCTION

The past decade has brought great changes in birthing practices. For hospital births, the concept of labor, delivery, recovery, postpartum (LDRP) rooms has given the expecting couple a more homelike environment, and the mother is not moved from the labor room to the delivery room, to the recovery room, to the postpartum room during the birthing process (Figure 52-1). Family and friends, even the baby's siblings, may be present in the LDRP room during the birth process.

Community birthing centers and other settings offer alternatives for the laboring couple. Many clients attend childbirth classes and have in mind a birthing plan or expectations of what they anticipate the birthing process will be like.

This chapter outlines the birth process, from the onset of labor through the birth of the infant.

ONSET OF LABOR

For 38 to 40 weeks, the pregnancy has been advancing and the fetus developing. Now, as the fetus reaches maturity, the birth process begins. Researchers are still trying to determine exactly what causes the onset of labor; however, there are two theories relative to why labor begins.

Theories Regarding Onset of Labor

The mechanical theory is based on the principle that as a hollow organ in the body becomes filled and distended, the organ tends to empty itself. Examples of this phenomenon are the bladder and sigmoid colon. This mechanism alone is not enough to fully explain the onset of labor because a woman can have a full-term $6^1/_2$-lb baby with one pregnancy and full-term twins each weighing $5^1/_2$ lb with the next pregnancy.

The hormonal theory of the onset of labor relates to the changes in maternal progesterone and estrogen levels, the maternal production of oxytocin and prostaglandin, and the increase in fetal production of cortisol. There seems to be a highly integrated relationship among these hormones.

As the pregnancy nears its end, the placental production of progesterone decreases, thus decreasing the relaxing effect of progesterone on the uterus. The estrogen level rises, causing an increased sensitivity of the myometrium to oxytocin. Oxytocin, now produced by the mother's posterior pituitary gland, stimulates the uterus to contract. As the pregnancy nears 40 weeks of gestation, the uterus becomes more sensitive to oxytocin. Fetal cortisol production increases as the pregnancy nears term. It is believed to decrease the placental production of progesterone and stimulate the precursors of prostaglandin.

Signs of Impending Labor

Several signs indicate that labor will soon begin. The signs are lightening, Braxton Hicks contractions, cervical softening, bloody show, rupture of membranes, gastrointestinal disturbance, and a sudden burst of energy.

Lightening

Lightening is the descent of the fetus into the pelvis. This may occur as early as 2 weeks before labor begins in the primigravida client but may not occur until a multigravida client is already in labor. The downward movement of the fetus and thus the uterus makes the upper part of the abdomen flatter. This relieves pressure on the diaphragm, allowing the mother to breathe easier, but she may experience:

- Leg cramps from pressure now on pelvic nerves
- Urinary frequency from pressure now on the bladder
- Increased venous stasis from pressure now on the veins, resulting in edema of the lower extremities

Braxton Hicks Contractions

Braxton Hicks contractions are irregular, intermittent contractions felt by the pregnant woman toward the end of pregnancy. The tightening sensation in the abdomen may become fairly regular and uncomfortable. The woman may go to the care provider's office or the hospital thinking she is in labor. If the cervix is not dilated and then the contractions stop, this is called **false labor.** Table 52-1 compares false labor and true labor.

Cervical Changes

At about 34 weeks of gestation, because of the changing ratio of estrogen to progesterone and the production or prostaglandin, the cervix begins to "mature" or "ripen." That is, the cervix becomes softer and more spongy. **Effacement,** thinning and shortening of the cervix, may begin, especially when the woman is a primigravida. These cervical changes increase during labor to allow delivery of the fetus.

Bloody Show

Bloody show consists of cervical secretion, blood-tinged mucus, and the mucous plug that blocked the

Figure 52-1 *The LDRP concept allows the laboring couple to remain in the same room throughout the birth experience.*

TABLE 52-1	COMPARISON OF FALSE LABOR AND TRUE LABOR

FALSE LABOR	TRUE LABOR
Contractions often irregular but may be regular for a short time (1 to 2 hours).	Contractions occur at regular intervals.
Interval between contractions stays the same.	Interval between contractions gradually shortens.
Contraction intensity and duration remain the same.	Contractions increase in intensity and duration.
Contractions frequently stop when the client ambulates or changes position.	Contractions continue and often become stronger when the client ambulates.
Contractions eventually cease with controlled breathing or other relaxation techniques.	Contractions are usually not stopped with controlled breathing, other relaxation techniques, or sedation.
Cervix may soften but does not efface or dilate.	Cervix softens, effaces, and dilates.

cervix during pregnancy. Labor often begins within 24 to 48 hours after the bloody show is noticed; however, a vaginal examination that includes cervical manipulation may result in a blood-tinged discharge. This may be confused with bloody show.

Rupture of Membranes — water breaking

Rupture of membranes (ROM) usually occurs after labor has begun; however, in about 12% of women, the amniotic membranes rupture before the onset of labor (Ladewig, Moberly, Olds, & London, 1998). When this occurs, the pregnant woman should notify her certified nurse midwife (CNM)/physician and proceed to the birthing facility. If **engagement** (when the widest diameter of the fetal presenting part [head] enters the inlet to the true pelvis) has not yet occurred, there exists the danger that the umbilical cord will wash out with the amniotic fluid (prolapsed cord).

Test

If labor does not begin spontaneously within 12 to 24 hours after the membranes rupture and the pregnancy is near term, labor is often induced to avoid infection.

It is sometimes difficult for the woman to determine whether the membranes have ruptured or whether urine has escaped from her bladder. A simple test with nitrazine paper is helpful. When moistened in the discharge, the nitrazine paper will turn blue (react) if the discharge is amniotic fluid; the paper will usually not react if the membranes are still intact.

 Litmus paper

Gastrointestinal Disturbance

Some women report having one or more of the following near the time of labor: indigestion, nausea, vomiting, and diarrhea. They may experience a 1- to 3-pound weight loss.

Sudden Burst of Energy

A few days before labor begins, some women will have a sudden burst of energy. The reason for this is unknown. The prospective mother should be careful not to tire herself. She will need the energy when labor begins.

MATERNAL SYSTEMIC RESPONSES TO LABOR

Knowing how the various systems of the mother's body respond to labor is important when making assessments and performing nursing interventions.

Cardiovascular System

Cardiac output increases because 400 mL of blood is squeezed from the uterus into maternal circulation with each contraction (Lowdermilk & Perry, 2003). The client's blood pressure increases during the first and second stages of labor because of the contractions. Blood pressure is highest during a contraction, so blood pressure should be taken *between* contractions. Anxiety and pain may also make the blood pressure increase. About 10% to 15% of women in labor will experience supine hypotensive syndrome, or decreased blood pressure when in a supine position (Burroughs & Leifer, 2001).

Respiratory System

Oxygen consumption during labor is equal to that of moderate to strenuous exercise. As long as the respiratory center is not depressed by medication, the increased respiratory rate continues with oxygen consumption almost double the normal amount. If the mother develops hypoxia or acidosis, the fetus may be compromised. Hyperventilation may decrease the level of carbon dioxide in the mother's blood.

CULTURAL CONSIDERATIONS

Regarding Childbirth

- In Malawi, Africa, women are advised not to stand in doorways or peep through windows because this will cause the fetus to be stuck in the pelvis (Gennaro et al., 1998).
- Muslim laws of modesty require that women's hair, arms to the wrist, and legs to the ankles be covered at all times. The women may not be alone with a man other than their husband or a blood relative (Hutchinson & Baqi-Aziz, 1994).
- Southeast Asian women must lie on their side with a pillow under the head during labor (Mattson, 1995).
- Some Native American tribes specify the appropriate dress, position, and who is in attendance for birth (Cesario, 2001).

Renal System

When engagement occurs, the bladder, now an abdominal organ, is pushed forward and upward. A distended bladder may impede fetal descent. Pressure from the presenting part, especially during a contraction, may cause edema of the tissues because of impaired blood and lymph drainage. Urinary flow is decreased, especially when the woman is supine, because the uterus compresses the ureters. Often there is a lessened urge to void, so the client must be encouraged to do so.

Gastrointestinal System

During labor, peristalsis and absorption decrease. Gastric emptying time is prolonged and gastric contents increase in acidity (Blackburn, 2003). The staff in many hospitals do not allow the client in labor to eat solid food because there is always a possibility of an obstetrical emergency requiring surgery. Eating solid food would increase the risk of aspirating vomitus. The absorption of liquid is unchanged during labor. The lips and mouth become dry as a result of mouth breathing.

Fluid and Electrolyte Balance

Because of the muscular activity of labor, the mother's body temperature increases and she perspires profusely. The normal increase in respiratory rate and the tendency of women in labor to hyperventilate both cause an increase in fluid loss. The hyperventilation also affects electrolyte balance. To prevent dehydration, the staff in many hospitals routinely have intravenous fluids running on all clients in labor.

Immune System

The white blood count (WBC) increases, sometimes up to 25,000/mm³, during labor and stays elevated during the early postpartum period. The natural increase makes it difficult to identify any infectious process the woman may have.

Integumentary System

The vagina and perineum have a great ability to stretch. The degree of stretching varies with each client; however, there may still be minute tears in the vagina and/or perineum after the birth of the baby.

Musculoskeletal System

The marked increase in muscle activity during labor is accompanied by increased body temperature, diaphoresis, fatigue, and some proteinuria (1+) (Lowdermilk & Perry, 2003). The relaxation of pelvic joints, caused by the influence of relaxin, may result in backache. Leg cramps also may be experienced.

Neurological System

The client may be euphoric at the beginning of labor. This often changes to seriousness and then to amnesia between contractions during the second stage of labor. Endogenous endorphins (a morphinelike chemical produced naturally by the body) increase the

CULTURAL CONSIDERATIONS

Pain in Childbearing Women

- Chinese believe they will dishonor themselves and their family by any wild or loud response to pain (Weber, 1996).
- Mayan women overcome with fatigue and pain may be scolded or physically restrained (Weber, 1996).
- South and Central American cultures believe that the more intense the pain, the stronger the love for the infant (Scott-Ramos, 1995).
- Muslim women either freely vocalize their pain and pray to Allah or stoically endure the pain. Some believe that the husband will be more concerned for them after delivery if the suffering was loud and obvious (Ahmed, 1994; Hutchinson & Baqi-Aziz, 1994).
- Korean women may stoically endure pain during labor because sanskin (goddess of three spirits) dislikes screaming (Howard & Berbiglia, 1997).
- In Malawi, Africa, women are considered a disgrace to the family and cultural group if they cry during labor (Gennaro et al., 1998).
- Guatemalan women may vocalize their pain by moaning rhythmically while rubbing their thighs and abdomen (Callister & Vega, 1998).

client's pain threshold and have a sedative effect. Pressure on the perineum, by the fetus descending through the birth canal, causes physiologic anesthesia in the perineal tissues.

Pain

The discomfort and pain of labor and birth are individual, subjective, very personal, and have a wide range of expression (Lowe, 1996). Visceral pain usually predominates the first stage of labor, with the stimuli originating in the uterus, cervix, adnexa, and pelvic ligaments. With fetal descent increasing during the late first stage and beginning second stage of labor, the traction and distention on the pelvic structures around the vagina are the primary stimuli for pain. The distention of the perineum is the stimulus for pain during the remainder of the second stage of labor and is transmitted primarily by the pudendal nerves. Figure 52-2 illustrates the intensity and distribution of discomfort during various stages of labor. Stages of labor are discussed later in this chapter.

The softness of pelvic tissues in parous women (women who have delivered at least one child) seems to cause less nociceptive stimuli than in nulliparous women (women who have never delivered a child) during the first stage of labor; however, during the second stage of labor, parous women have increased nociceptive stimuli because of the speed and the intensity of fetal descent (Lowe, 1996). As with pain from any other cause, individuals respond in ways that are acceptable in their

Severe discomfort
Moderate discomfort
Mild discomfort

Figure 52-2 *Intensity and Distribution of Discomfort during Various Stages of Labor:* **A,** *First stage;* **B,** *Early second stage;* **C,** *Late second stage and birth*

culture. Health care providers must be sensitive to the fact that expression of pain is rooted in cultural heritage.

VARIABLES AFFECTING LABOR

There are four major variables that affect labor. They are known as the four Ps: passage, passenger, powers, and psyche (Burroughs & Leifer, 2001; Murray, Gorrie, & McKinney, 2001).

Passage

The passage consists of the bony pelvis, uterus, cervix, vagina, and perineum.

Pelvis

The size and shape of the true pelvis must be adequate for the fetal head to pass through for a vaginal birth. The CNM/physician can use several methods to determine the adequacy of the true pelvis, such as:

- Palpation—Internally, the bony prominences can be felt; externally, the distance between the ischial tuberosities can be measured and then the distance between the ischial spines estimated.

- Ultrasound—An ultrasound is used to estimate pelvic adequacy as well as fetal growth, multiple pregnancy, placenta location, and fetal presentation.
- Pelvimetry—X-ray of the pelvis is seldom performed during pregnancy because of the radiation involved.

Uterus

The upper part of the uterus (fundus) becomes thicker with contractions and the lower section becomes thinner, forming a tube.

Cervix

The uterine contractions put pressure on the fetus, which in turn puts pressure on the cervix, causing the cervix to efface and dilate.

Vagina

The vagina sustains many changes throughout pregnancy. Various hormones cause an increase in vascularity, loosening of connective tissue, and hypertrophy of the smooth muscle cells. These changes allow the vagina to stretch enough for the fetus to pass through.

Perineum

The pressure of the fetus on the perineum causes stretching and thinning of the perineum.

Passenger

The size of the fetus as well as the fetal attitude, fetal lie, fetal presentation, and fetal position affects how easily the fetus can advance through the passage.

Size

The largest part of the fetal body is usually the head. Because the bones of the fetal skull are not fused, the bones can move, sometimes even overlap, as the fetus moves through the mother's bony pelvis. The shaping of the fetal head to adapt to the mother's pelvis during labor is called **molding.**

The major bones of the skull are two frontal bones, two temporal bones, two parietal bones, and the occiput. The bones are joined by thin, fibrous, membrane-covered spaces called **sutures.** Where the sutures meet, there are larger membranous areas called **fontanelles** (Figure 52-3). The largest is the diamond-shaped anterior fontanelle. The posterior fontanelle is triangular and smaller. The care providers can palpate the two fontanelles and the suture connecting them through the cervix and determine fetal position.

Fetal Attitude

Fetal attitude is the relationship of fetal body parts to one another. The ideal attitude of the fetus at term is flexion, with the head flexed onto the chest, the arms flexed over the chest, and the hips and knees flexed on the abdomen. If any part of the fetus is extended, especially the head or the legs, labor is usually more difficult. The attitude is then called extension.

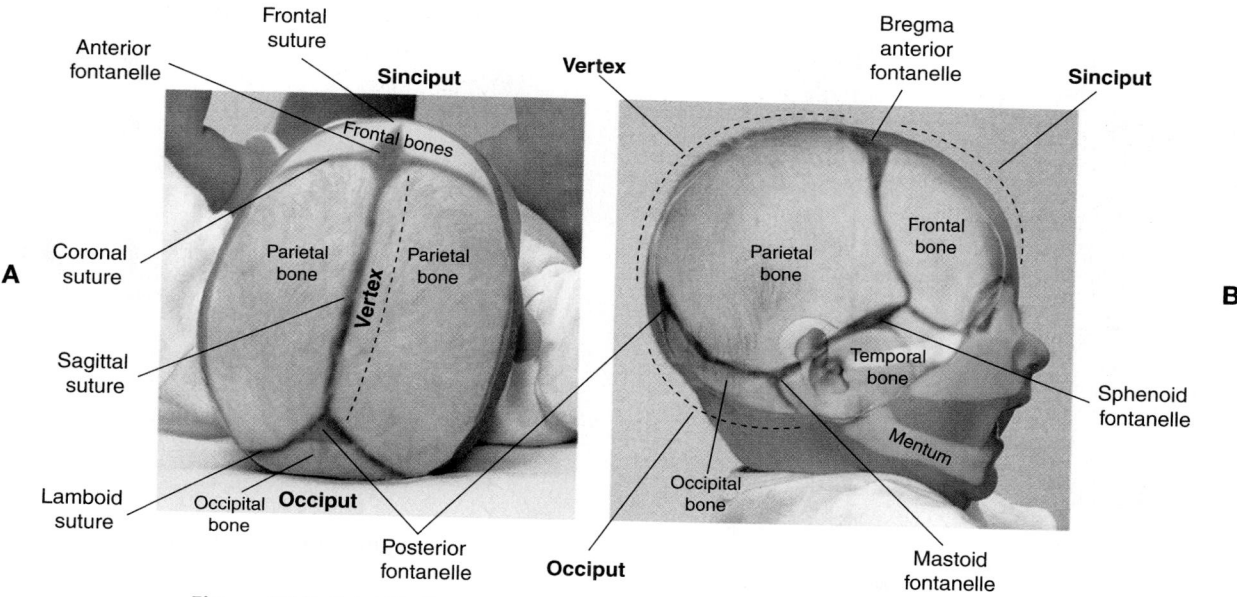

Figure 52-3 *Fetal Skull—Sutures and Fontanelles:* **A,** *Superior view;* **B,** *Lateral view*

Fetal Lie

The relationship of the cephalocaudal (head to foot) axis of the fetus to the cephalocaudal axis of the mother is called the **fetal lie.** When the fetal cephalocaudal axis is parallel to the mother's, it is called a longitudinal lie. At term, the fetus has a longitudinal lie in 99% of pregnancies (Dickason, Silverman, & Kaplan, 1998). When the fetal cephalocaudal axis is at a right angle to the mother's, it is called a transverse lie (Figure 52-4).

Fetal Presentation – what is coming out 1st.

Fetal presentation is determined by the fetal lie and the part of the fetus that enters the pelvis first. The part of the fetus in contact with the cervix is called the **presenting part.** The most common type of presentation is cephalic (head), in 95% of deliveries, with breech (buttocks) being 4%, and shoulder 1% of deliveries (Burroughs & Leifer, 2001) (Figure 52-5).

Cephalic Presentations
Cephalic presentations may be further differentiated by the part of the head entering the pelvis first. They may be:

- Vertex—with the occiput as the presenting part – most easiest common
- Brow—with the sinciput as the presenting part
- Face—with the face as the presenting part } more challenging

Breech Presentations
Breech presentations are differentiated by the attitude of the fetus's legs. The various breech presentations are as follows:

- *Complete breech:* Hips and knees are flexed on the abdomen in an attitude of flexion, with the buttocks as the presenting part.
- *Frank breech:* The hips are flexed, but the knees are extended with the buttocks as the presenting part.
- *Footling breech:* The hips and knees are extended with the foot as the presenting part (may be single footling or double footling).

Figure 52-4 *Fetal Attitude and Fetal Lie:* **A,** *Fetal attitude flexion, fetal lie longitudinal;* **B,** *Fetal attitude flexion, fetal lie transverse*

Figure 52-5 *Fetal Presentation:* **A,** *Complete breech;* **B,** *Frank breech;* **C,** *Footling breech;* **D,** *Shoulder;* **E,** *Vertex;* **F,** *Face*

RP-Right Posterior
LP-Left Posterior

RA-Right Anterior
LA-Left Anterior

Figure 52-6 *Pelvic Quadrants*

TABLE 52-2   IDENTIFIED LANDMARKS ON VARIOUS PRESENTING PARTS

PRESENTING PART	IDENTIFIED LANDMARK
Vertex	Occiput (O)
Face	Mentum (M)
Breech (all)	Sacrum (S)

Shoulder Presentation
A shoulder presentation occurs in a transverse lie. The presenting part is usually the shoulder but may be the arm, back, abdomen, or side.

Fetal Position

Fetal position refers to the relationship of the identified landmark on the presenting part of the four quadrants of the mother's pelvis (Figure 52-6). The identified landmarks on various presenting parts are shown in Table 52-2.

The brow presentation does not have an identified landmark. The brow usually changes either to a vertex or face presentation. Although the shoulder presenta-

tion cannot be delivered vaginally, there is still a landmark designated for it, which is SC (scapula).

There are six possible positions for each presenting part as follows:

- Right occiput anterior (ROA) mentum (RMA) sacrum (RSA)
- Right occiput transverse (ROT) mentum (RMT) sacrum (RST)
- Right occiput posterior (ROP) mentum (RMP) sacrum (RSP)
- Left occiput anterior (LOA) mentum (LMA) sacrum (LSA)
- Left occiput transverse (LOT) mentum (LMT) sacrum (LST)
- Left occiput posterior (LOP) mentum (LMP) sacrum (LSP)

Figure 52-7 illustrates the six positions of a vertex presentation. The same six positions apply to the face and breech presentations. The most common position is LOA, which is considered to be the most favorable for the welfare of both mother and baby.

Powers

The primary power during labor is the involuntary contractions of the uterus, which cause cervical effacement and dilatation during the first stage of labor. The secondary power is the voluntary use of the abdominal

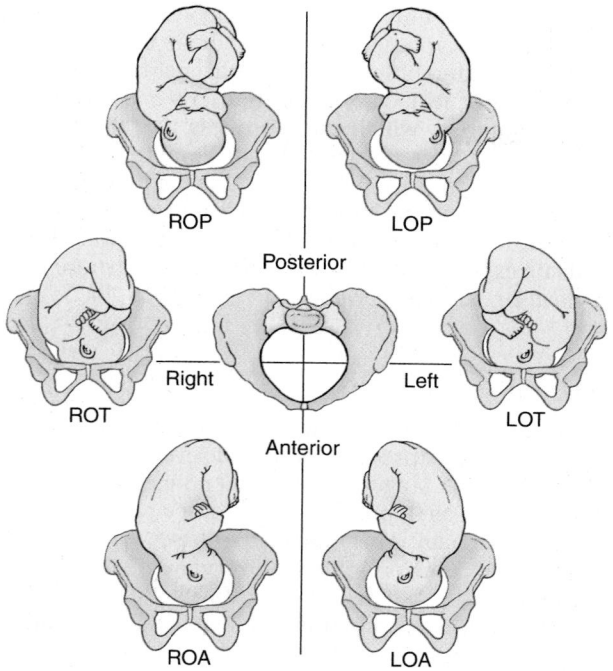

Figure 52-7 *Various Positions of a Vertex Presentation*

Figure 52-8 *Effacement and Dilatation:* **A,** *Primigravida;* **B,** *Multigravida*

PROFESSIONAL TIP

Fetal Positions
- The right or left and anterior, posterior, or transverse always refer to the mother's pelvis.
- The middle word or letter refers to the identified landmark on the fetus, either occiput, mentum, or sacrum.

---

muscles by the mother to push during the second stage of labor.

Uterine Contractions

The smooth muscle of the uterus has the ability to contract and relax rhythmically. The relaxation period between contractions allows the muscles and the mother to rest. Uterine relaxation also restores uteroplacental circulation, which is important to fetal oxygenation and effective circulation in the uterus. Contractions begin in the **fundus**, top of the uterus, and spread over the uterus in about 15 seconds (Burroughs & Leifer, 2001).

The muscle fibers of the uterus have the unique property of remaining permanently shortened to a small degree after each contraction. This is called **uterine retraction.** The shortening of the muscle fibers results in a gradual decrease in the uterine cavity size and a thickening of the muscle in the fundus. As the muscle fibers in the fundus retract, the lower uterine segment is pulled up. These two actions efface and dilate the cervix (Figure 52-8).

Each contraction has three phases:
1. **Increment:** increasing intensity of a contraction (the longest phase)
2. **Acme:** peak of a contraction
3. **Decrement:** decreasing intensity of a contraction

Contractions are described in terms of frequency, duration, and intensity. **Frequency** is the time from the beginning of one contraction to the beginning of the next contraction. It includes one contraction and one resting period between contractions **(interval). Duration** is the length of one contraction, from the beginning of the increment to the conclusion of the decrement. **Intensity** is the strength of the contraction at the acme. Figure 52-9A illustrates these aspects of a contraction while B shows the mother's abdomen before and during a contraction.

The duration of a contraction should not be longer than 90 seconds nor should the interval be less than 60 seconds. The uterus should completely relax between contractions. Contractions lasting longer than 90 seconds reduce uterine and placental circulation because of

Figure 52-9 A, *Aspects of a Contraction (frequency 2 minutes, duration 60 seconds, intensity moderate);* **B,** *Abdominal contour before and during a contraction*

the prolonged compression of the blood vessels. This in turn compromises the fetus.

Contractions are affected by the mother's position. When the mother lies on her back, the contractions are often more frequent but have less intensity. When she lies on her side, the contractions are usually less frequent but have greater intensity. Thus, a side-lying position improves progress in labor. Lying on the side also prevents supine hypotension syndrome in the mother and improves oxygenation of the uterus, placenta, and fetus because the heavy uterus is not compressing the inferior vena cava.

Mother's Pushing

Once the cervix has dilated completely, it is time for the fetus to navigate through the remaining mechanisms of labor. The accepted procedure has been for the mother to take a deep breath at the beginning of a contraction, hold her breath, and voluntarily push in a Valsalva-type bearing down throughout a contraction. This pushing technique is directed by the nurses and/or the CNM/physician.

The spontaneous onset of the urge to bear down is triggered when the presenting part reaches the pelvic floor where stretch receptors in the posterior vagina cause the release of oxytocin, which spontaneously increases the pushing sensation (Cosner & deJong, 1993). This spontaneous, involuntary urge to bear down is known as **Ferguson's reflex.**

Psyche

Psyche refers to the mother's attitude toward labor and her preparation for labor. The mother's attitude toward labor is shaped by her experiences and expectations.

Culture shapes values about and responses to childbirth. It provides the mother with ideas about how to behave during labor and how to interact with her baby.

Anxiety or fear causes the mother's body to secrete catecholamines, which can suppress uterine contractions and restrict placental blood flow. Relaxation increases the progress of labor. Childbirth preparation classes enhance the mother's ability to work with her body rather than working against it. When a woman has realistic expectations about childbirth, she is more likely to have a positive experience.

STAGES OF LABOR

For many years, labor was divided into three stages. In each of these three stages, specific events can be identified. A fourth stage has been acknowledged as being critical to the birth process: the recovery period after the birth of the baby. This chapter discusses four stages of labor. Table 52-3 presents an overview of the average duration of the first two stages. Stages 1 and 2 vary in average length for primigravida clients and multigravida clients. Stages 3 and 4 are approximately the same length for all clients and are not included in this table.

First Stage: Dilatation and Effacement

The first stage of labor begins with the onset of regular contractions and ends when **cervical dilatation,** the enlargement of the cervical opening (os), is complete (10 cm). This is usually the longest stage of labor and is divided into three phases: latent, active, and transition.

Latent Phase

The latent phase of the first stage of labor ends when the cervix is dilated 4 cm. Contractions occur every 10 to 20 minutes at first and become more frequent, every 5 to 7 minutes. The duration of the contractions begin at 15 to 20 seconds and progress to 30 to 40 seconds. The contraction intensity begins as mild and gradually becomes moderate.

The client is usually alert and often talkative. She is often relieved that labor has begun, yet anxious about what is ahead of her. This is a good time to review the client's preparations for labor and expectations of how labor and delivery will be handled (e.g., medications, persons present). Any needed teaching, especially breathing techniques, should be undertaken at this time. If the membranes have not ruptured, many women prefer to walk during this time.

Active Phase

The active phase of the first stage of labor begins when the cervix is dilated 4 cm and ends when the cervix is dilated 8 cm. Contractions occur every 3 to 5 minutes with a duration of 40 to 60 seconds. They are of moderate intensity, progressing to strong. Clients perceive varying degrees of discomfort. The client now focuses more on the breathing techniques during contractions and is less talkative.

TABLE 52-3	AVERAGE LENGTH OF LABOR STAGES 1 AND 2			
	FIRST STAGE			
CHARACTERISTIC	**Latent Phase**	**Active Phase**	**Transition Phase**	**SECOND STAGE**
Primigravida	8 to 10 hours	6 hours	2 hours	1 hour
Multigravida	5 hours	4 hours	1 hour	15 minutes
Cervical dilatation	0 to 4 cm	4 to 8 cm	8 to 10 cm	
Contractions				
Frequency	10 to 20 progressing to 5 to 7 minutes	3 to 5 minutes	2 to 3 minutes	2 to 3 minutes
Duration	15 to 20 progressing to 30 to 40 seconds	40 to 60 seconds	60 to 90 seconds	60 to 90 seconds
Intensity	Mild progressing to moderate	Moderate progressing to strong	Strong	Strong

Transition Phase

The transition phase of the first stage of labor begins when the cervix is dilated 8 cm and ends when the cervix is dilated 10 cm. Contractions occur every 2 to 3 minutes with a duration of 60 to 90 seconds. There is little rest for the client between contractions. The intensity of the contractions is strong. The client usually needs to be reminded to focus, relax, and breathe with each contraction. She is very aware of the increasing intensity of the contractions, may become very restless, and may fear being left alone. Requests for medication often accompany statements like "I can't take it anymore." Following are characteristics of the transition phase:

- Restlessness
- Hyperventilation
- Bewilderment and sometimes anger
- Difficulty following directions
- Focus on self
- Irritability
- Statements like "Don't touch me"
- Nausea, occasionally vomiting
- Very warm feeling
- Perspiration on upper lip
- Increasing rectal pressure

Safety: Use of Stirrups during Birth
Clients who are delivering in a modified lithotomy position may have their feet placed in stirrups to open the pelvis and facilitate access to the perineum.
- Stirrup height and lower leg length must be adjusted for each client.
- Both legs must be raised into the stirrups at the same time to prevent strain on the pelvic ligaments.

Second Stage: Birth of Baby

The second stage of labor begins when cervical dilatation is complete and ends with the birth of the baby. Contractions continue at a frequency of 2 to 3 minutes, duration of 60 to 90 seconds, and strong intensity. Now

that the cervix is completely dilated, the mother can actively assist in the descent of the fetus by contracting the abdominal muscles and bearing down with each contraction. This active participation in the process often gives her a sense of control.

As the fetal head descends, it puts pressure on the pelvic nerves and the mother has a greater desire to push. Pressure from the fetal head makes the perineum bulge, then flatten and move anteriorly. With each contraction, the labia begin to separate and the baby's head is seen, but the head recedes between contractions. When the largest diameter of the fetal head is past the vulva (head can be seen between contractions), **crowning** has occurred and the birth is imminent (Figure 52-10). At this time, an **episiotomy,** an incision in the perineum to facilitate passage of the baby, may be performed (Figure 52-11). A few more contractions will push the head out, and a few more will deliver the body.

As the fetus moves through the pelvis and birth canal, several changes in position must occur. This series of movements is collectively called the **mechanisms of labor** or cardinal movements.

Mechanisms of Labor

The mechanisms of labor are engagement, descent, flexion, internal rotation, extension, external rotation, and expulsion (Figure 52-12). The first three generally occur during the first stage of labor.

CLIENT TEACHING

Effective Pushing in Upright or Squatting Position
The mother can push more effectively if she:
- Flexes chin on her chest and bends over her uterus.
- With elbows *bent*, pulls on her flexed knees.
- Exhales and vocalizes when pushing.

Figure 52-10 *Crowning*

Figure 52-11 *Episiotomy: **A**, Midline, most common, directly toward anus; **B**, Right and left mediolateral, diagonal cut toward the side to prevent tearing into the rectum*

Engagement As explained earlier, engagement occurs when the presenting part of the fetus (usually head) fully enters the true pelvis. It generally happens before labor begins in primigravidas and after labor begins in multigravidas.

Descent Descent begins with engagement and continues with each contraction throughout the labor process.

Flexion The fetal head is bent forward as it meets resistance during descent, causing the chin to rest on the sternum. This allows the narrowest part of the head to enter the pelvic outlet.

Inernal Rotation Internal rotation takes place mainly during the second stage of labor. The head rotates so the occiput is next to the symphysis pubis.

Extension As the fetal head continues to descend, the occiput pivots under the symphysis pubis and the fetal head becomes unflexed (extended) and pushes upward out of the vagina. The head is actually born at this time.

Restitution and External Rotation Once the head has emerged, it rotates back to be in normal alignment with the shoulders. This is called **restitution.** Fetal position in the uterus can be identified by observing this turning of the head. The shoulders now rotate to be in an anteroposterior position under the symphysis pubis.

Expulsion The health care provider assisting with the birth applies gentle downward pressure on the baby's head to allow the anterior shoulder to emerge. Then the baby's head is gently raised so the posterior shoulder can be delivered. The rest of the baby's body then just slides out. This is called expulsion (Figure 52-13).

Third Stage: Delivery of Placenta

The third stage of labor begins with the birth of the baby and ends with the delivery of the placenta. This should occur in 30 minutes or less. After the baby is born, the uterus continues contracting, decreasing its capacity and thereby reducing the surface area of placental attachment. The reduced surface area causes the placenta to separate from the uterine wall. As it separates, bleeding occurs, causing the formation of a retroplacental (behind the placenta) hematoma. This

hematoma facilitates the separation process. The membranes are peeled from the uterine wall as the placenta slides into the vagina.

Signs that the placenta has separated should be observed about 5 to 10 minutes after the birth of the baby. These signs are:
• Globular shape of the uterus
• Gush of blood from the vagina
• More of the cord protrudes from the vagina (is visible)
When these signs of placental separation have appeared, the client is asked to push one last time to deliver the placenta. Figure 52-14 shows a placenta.

The birthing facility disposes of the placenta after the delivery. Occasionally, a client may request to have the placenta to uphold cultural expectations.

Fourth Stage: Recovery

The fourth stage of labor is the first 4 hours after the birth of the baby when the mother's body begins its physiological readjustments. Blood loss is usually between 250 mL and 500 mL. There is a moderate decrease in the

---

CRITICAL THINKING

Care Throughout Labor

How and why does the care of the client change as she moves through the phases and stages of labor?

Figure 52-12 *Mechanisms of Labor*

Figure 52-13 *Birth of an Infant*

Figure 52-14 A, *Fetal Side (note empty amniotic sac);* **B,** *Maternal Side*

CULTURAL CONSIDERATIONS

Placenta Disposal
- In Korea, the placenta is traditionally buried, burned, or submerged in the ocean at a time and place where there are no evil spirits (Howard & Berbiglia, 1997).
- In Malawi, Africa, the placenta is buried with the maternal side facing downward to prevent secondary sterility (Gennaro et al., 1998).
- To Native Americans, the placenta and umbilical cord (including the cord stump) are sacred and should not be discarded indiscriminately (Cesario, 2001).

PROFESSIONAL TIP

Prenatal Care and Childbirth Classes
- The client who has not had prenatal care or has not attended childbirth classes deserves the same care, support, and respect as the client who has had prenatal care and is prepared for childbirth.
- Nurses must be careful not to be judgmental toward clients who have not participated in prenatal care or childbirth classes.

CULTURAL CONSIDERATIONS

Client Beliefs
Most people believe that their own cultural beliefs are the best. The birth experience is given meaning by the client's cultural beliefs and practices. Incorporate cultural practices into care as much as possible as long as they are not detrimental to mother or fetus.

systolic and diastolic blood pressure and an increase in pulse rate. The uterus should remain contracted to control bleeding and be positioned in the midline of the abdomen about level with the umbilicus.

The new mother may be very hungry and thirsty. A shaking chill may be experienced in response to the ending of the physical work of labor. The bladder may be hypotonic due either to trauma during the second stage of labor and/or to decreased sensation from anesthesia. This may result in urinary retention.

ADMISSION OF CLIENT IN LABOR

Admission of a client in labor may be different for each person. Although there are standard nursing as-

sessments and interventions for a woman in labor, each client must be cared for individually based on her particular situation. The priorities of establishing a nurse–client relationship and assessing the condition of mother and fetus may be undertaken in a sequential order or may need to be performed simultaneously.

It is important to determine which stage of labor the mother may be in at the time of admission. A few specific questions might include the following:

- When did your labor begin?
- How frequent are the contractions and how long do they last?
- Have the membranes ruptured? (Has your water broken?)
- How many pregnancies is this for you? How long were your other labors (if this is not the first pregnancy)?

Depending on the answers to these questions, a determination is made about how to proceed with the admission. When a woman is admitted in early labor, time can be taken to establish the nurse–client relationship by:

- Making the woman and her partner or family feel welcome
- Determining their expectations about the birth (did they attend childbirth classes?)
- Identifying cultural values and preferences related to the birth process

Initial Assessment

After the nurse–client relationship has been established on admission, more specific assessments are made. Figure 52-15 shows a sample obstetric admitting record. A copy of the prenatal record is generally sent to the birthing facility and is added to the client's record when she is admitted. Information can be obtained from the prenatal record. Clients who have not received prenatal care will need a more extensive assessment.

A physical examination is performed, including the following:

- Vital signs
- Auscultation of heart and lungs
- Leopold's maneuvers (described in Prenatal Care chapter) to determine fetal lie and presentation
- Fetal heart rate (FHR) (described in Prenatal Care chapter), continuous electronic fetal monitoring may be used during the birthing process (described in Complications of Pregnancy chapter)
- Contractions for frequency, duration, and intensity
- Nitrazine test if mother is not sure whether the membranes have ruptured
- Vaginal examination (Figure 52-16) to determine cervical effacement and dilatation, fetal position, and station; usually done by the registered nurse (RN) or CNM/physician
- Inspection for signs of edema of face, hands, legs, and sacrum

The FHR may be heard in various places on the mother's abdomen depending on the position of the fetus (Figure 52-17).

Station is the relationship of the fetal presenting part to the ischial spines. It is measured in centimeters above (−) or below (+) the ischial spines (Figure 52-18).

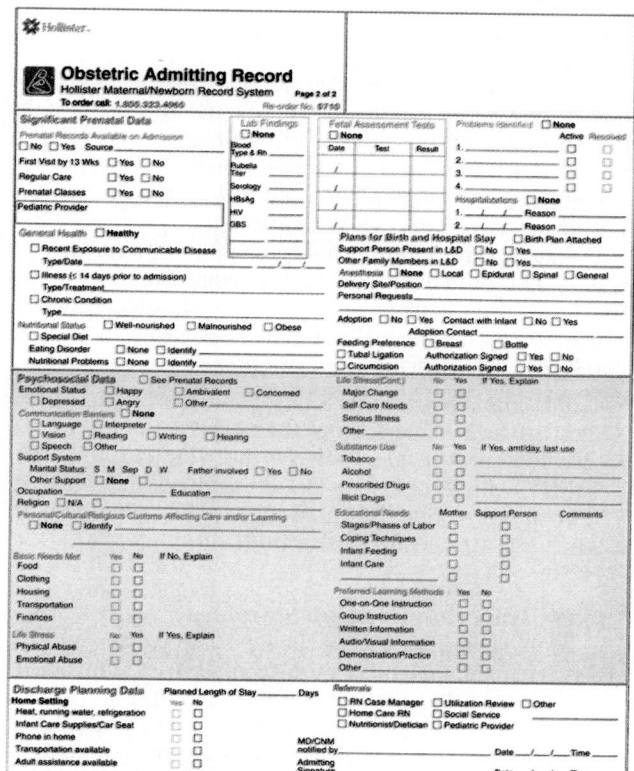

Figure 52-15 *Representative Obstetric Admitting Record (Permission to use this copyright material has been granted by the owner, Hollister Incorporated.)*

50% effaced, no dilatation

Effaced and partially dilated

Figure 52-16 *Vaginal Examination:* **A,** *50% effaced, no dilatation;* **B,** *100% effaced, partly dilated*

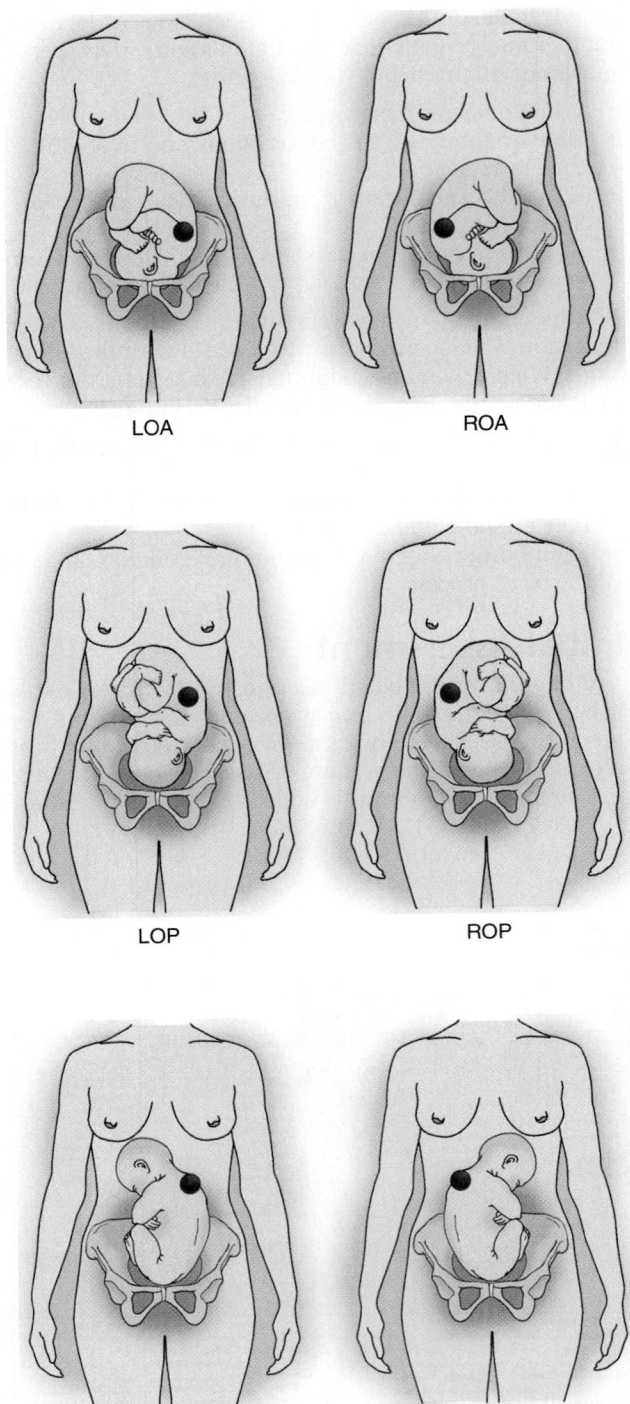

Figure 52-17 *Based on Leopold's maneuvers, FHR will best be heard in the marked areas for the various positions.*

Contractions are assessed by placing the fingers of one hand on the fundus of the uterus, and using light pressure to keep the fingers still. Contractions begin in the fundus and spread down the uterus. The person assessing the contractions can feel the tightening of the uterus before the mother is aware of it.

At least three contractions in a row should be assessed. The time each contraction begins and ends and the time lapse between contractions should be noted. The intensity can be estimated by how easily the uterus can be indented during a contraction.

- *Mild contraction:* Uterus is easily indented with the fingertips; feels like the tip of the nose.
- *Moderate contraction:* Uterus is more difficult to indent with the fingertips; feels similar to the chin.
- *Strong contraction:* Uterus unable to be indented with the fingertips; feels like the forehead.

Infection Control: Standard Precautions
- Disposable gloves should be worn any time hands might come in contact with amniotic fluid, blood, bloody show, urine, or feces.
- Wear a splash apron and eye covering (goggles or face mask) when the splashing of body fluids is possible.
- Wash hands before putting on gloves and immediately after removing them.

NURSING PROCESS

The nurse is an important member of the team that helps the mother successfully progress through the birth experience.

Figure 52-18 *Station: Relationship of the fetal presenting part to the ischial spines. The station illustrated is +2.*

Assessment

The nurse's role begins with a thorough assessment of the laboring woman and her progress.

Subjective Data

Subjective data to be gathered throughout labor and birth of the infant include the comfort of the mother, her ability to cope, and her desire to urinate or defecate.

Objective Data

Objective data include vital signs; FHR; frequency, duration, interval, and intensity of contractions; fetopelvic relationships, including fetal attitude, fetal lie, fetal presentation, and station; condition of membranes; maternal behavior, including tone of voice and facial expressions; and maternal verbalizations. Table 52-4 provides suggested time frames for selected assessments.

Nursing Diagnoses

Many different nursing diagnoses may be appropriate for a client during labor and the birthing process. Selected nursing diagnoses appropriate for the first three stages of labor are listed.

- **A**nxiety
- Impaired Verbal **C**ommunication
- Ineffective **C**oping
- Interrupted **F**amily Processes
- **F**atigue
- **F**ear
- Risk for Deficient **F**luid Volume
- **G**as Exchange Impaired (fetal)
- Risk for **I**nfection
- Risk for **I**njury
- Deficient **K**nowledge
- **P**ain
- Impaired **P**hysical Mobility
- **S**ocial Isolation
- Ineffective **T**issue Perfusion (maternal)
- Impaired **U**rinary Elimination

Planning/Outcome Identification

Based on the client's expectations of labor and the birthing process and the assessments performed by the facility staff, the planning and goals can be mutually set by the client and the nurse. Examples of possible goals may include that the client will:

- Demonstrate expected progress through labor.
- Express satisfaction with the assistance provided by her support person and facility staff.
- Maintain adequate hydration with oral and/or IV intake.
- Void at least every 2 hours to prevent bladder distention.
- Actively participate in the labor process.
- Not experience any injury during the labor and birthing process.

TABLE 52-4	SUGGESTED TIME FRAMES FOR SELECTED ASSESSMENTS			
ASSESSMENT	**LATENT PHASE**	**ACTIVE PHASE**	**TRANSITION PHASE**	**SECOND STAGE**
BP, P, R	q 1 h	q 1 h	q 30 min	q 5 min
Temperature	q 4 h	q 4 h	q 4 h	
(if ROM)	q 2 h	q 2 h	q 2 h	
FHR	q 1 h	q 30 min	q 15 min	q 5 min
Contractions	q 1 h	q 30 min	q 15 min	continuously

Nursing Interventions

Nursing interventions focus on continuing assessment of labor progress and fetal well-being, providing maternal physical care, assisting the client and her support person, and providing or assisting with pharmacologic comfort measures.

Continuing Assessment of Labor and Fetal Well-Being

Continuing assessment of labor progress and fetal well-being is performed as previously discussed. Any changes outside the normally expected changes must be reported immediately. Some facilities use continuous electronic fetal monitoring on all clients; however, the nurse should still personally assess and time contractions and listen to the FHR at regular intervals. Figure 52-19 presents a sample labor in progress record.

Providing Maternal Physical Care

Maternal physical care includes comfort measures, hygiene measures, ambulation and position, food and fluid intake, and elimination.

Comfort Measures Many comfort measures can be used with the client in labor. Some may work with one client and not the next, or may work for a while with one client and then she will not want that comfort measure used any more. Comfort measures to try include the following:

- Offering the client fluids and ice chips as ordered for per institutional policy
- Providing oral care
- Assisting the client with frequent position changes, encouraging side-lying or upright positions.
- Encouraging voluntary relaxation of specific muscle groups and the use of effleurage
- Suggesting the use of a cold washcloth on the forehead or nape of the neck
- Providing encouragement and praise
- Keeping the client informed of progress
- Checking the client's bladder and encouraging urination every 2 hours
- Giving a back rub or applying counterpressure to the sacrococcygeal area
- Assisting the client in walking and using a shower or Jacuzzi
- Offering the client analgesics as ordered

Hygiene Measures If showers or Jacuzzis are available and are not contraindicated for the client, their use should be offered to the client. The discomfort of labor is often reduced by these measures. Bed linens should be kept clean and dry. Linen savers should be changed frequently.

Ambulation and Position Ambulation may increase uterine activity, provide distraction from the discomforts of labor, and enhance maternal control of the situation. The client should be encouraged to walk only if the membranes are still intact, the presenting part is engaged after ROM, and if she has not had pain medication.

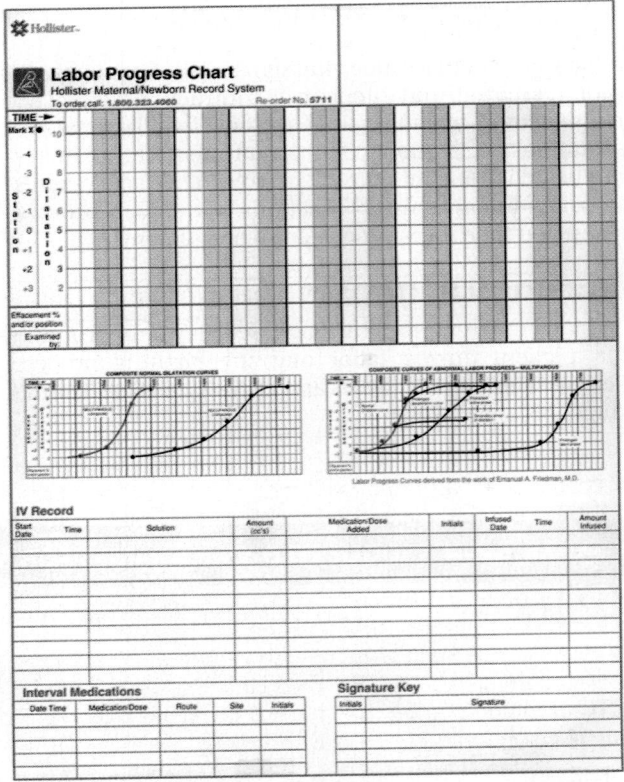

Figure 52-19 *Representative Labor Progress Record (Permission to use this copyright material has been granted by the owner, Hollister Incoporated.)*

The side-lying position promotes utero-placental blood flow (and thus fetal oxygenation) and renal blood flow. If the client wants to lie on her back, a pillow can be placed under one hip to keep the uterus from compressing the aorta and vena cava. Both the squatting position and the hands-and-knees position seem to facilitate an occiput posterior fetal position to rotate to an anterior position.

Food and Fluid Intake Clear liquids and ice chips are usually all that is offered to clients in labor. Because regional anesthesia has almost replaced general anesthesia in childbirth, the risk of aspiration is also almost eliminated, and the practice of giving clear liquids only is being challenged (Lowdermilk & Perry, 2003).

In some facilities, IV fluids are started on every client. It is very important to keep an accurate I&O when IV fluids are running because of the danger of hypervolemia.

Elimination The client should be encouraged to void every 2 hours. A distended bladder may impede descent of the presenting part, cause undue discomfort to the client, and lead to bladder atony after the birth.

If allowed, getting up to go to the bathroom may be the easiest for the client. Sitting on a bedpan at the edge of the bed with feet on a chair may be the next best option.

Catheterization may be required if the client cannot void and the bladder is distended. The vulva and perineum must be thoroughly cleaned to remove any amniotic fluid and bloody show before catheterization. If the catheter cannot be inserted, the presenting part is probably compressing the urethra; the procedure must be discontinued and the RN or CNM/physician notified.

Because of the decrease in intestinal motility, most women do not have a bowel movement during labor; however, the pushing and birth of the infant during the second stage of labor may cause some stool to be expelled from the rectum. This should be cleaned immediately and the client reassured that this is a normal and expected outcome.

Assisting Client and Support Person

The support person many times is the father, but it may be another woman or man. The person the mother has chosen to be the support person should be treated with the same respect as the mother, regardless of the relationship to the mother or the fetus.

The client who has participated in childbirth preparation classes with a support person already has some skills and a plan for coping with labor and birth. The nurse should determine what that plan is and assist, as needed, in carrying out that plan.

The client and support person who have not attended childbirth preparation classes should be taught the various techniques of coping with labor during the latent phase of labor. The nurse may actually provide more of the supportive care in this situation.

Breathing Techniques Three different breathing patterns are used. The first pattern is used until it is no longer effective, then the next pattern is used. Each breathing pattern begins and ends with a deep cleansing breath, with inhalation through the nose and exhalation through pursed lips, moving only the chest. The breathing techniques:

- Provide adequate oxygenation of mother and fetus.
- Provide a focus of attention.
- Decrease pain and anxiety.
- Increase mental and physical relaxation.

These breathing patterns are used only during a uterine contraction. Between contractions, breathing returns to the woman's regular breathing pattern.

Slow, Deep Chest Breathing For this pattern, the client takes a cleansing breath, then inhales through the nose and exhales through pursed lips, 6 to 9 breaths per minute. At the end of the contraction, she takes another cleansing breath. It takes concentration to breathe this slowly.

Shallow Breathing A cleansing breath is taken first. The client inhales and exhales through the mouth about 4 times every 5 seconds. This may be increased to 2 breaths per second, usually at the peak of a contraction.

Pant-Blow Breathing The pant-blow breathing is generally used when the contractions become very intense. This pattern is very similar to the shallow breathing except that every three or four breaths a forceful exhalation (blow) is made through pursed lips. A cleansing breath is taken at the beginning and end of the contraction. It takes great concentration to maintain this pattern during a contraction.

All clients should be kept informed of their progress in labor. Positive feedback to the client and support person regarding how they are coping with the labor process is also important.

If siblings are to be present for labor and the birth, another person should be there to watch over the children and provide them with explanations, diversions, and comfort as needed. Neither the support person nor the nurses should be responsible for the children. Their focus should be on the client.

Providing Pharamacological Comfort Measures

The nonpharmacological comfort measures may be all that is needed for some women in labor. For other women, the increasing discomfort interferes with their ability to relax, use the breathing techniques appropriately, and maintain a sense of control. Pharmacological comfort measures include systemic medications, regional blocks, and general anesthesia.

Systemic Medications Systemic medications should be administered only if:

- The client is willing to receive them and her vital signs are stable.

CRITICAL THINKING

Pushing in Labor

A client gravida 1 para 0 in labor is 7 cm dilated, station +1, and says that she wants to push. Her grandmother told her that she would have to push hard to have a baby, so the client wants to push and get it over with. How should the nurse respond?

- The fetus is at term, exhibits normal movement, has a FHR between 120 and 160 with no late or variable decelerations, and does not exhibit meconium staining of the amniotic fluid.
- Contractions are well established with the cervix dilated at least 4 to 5 cm in a nullipara or 3 to 4 cm in a multipara, the presenting part is engaged, and no complications are identified.

Effect on the fetus depends on the dosage given, timing and route of administration, and the pharmacokinetics of the drug. The intravenous (IV) route is generally preferred over the intramuscular (IM) route because the drug's effect is faster and more reliable. Table 52-5 lists drugs commonly used for pain management during labor.

Regional Blocks Several types of regional blocks may be used during labor and/or birth, including epidural block, intrathecal block, local infiltration, and pudendal block.

Epidural Block An epidural block may be used for pain control during labor and birth. It may be a continuous or intermittent infusion of a local anesthetic drug through a catheter placed in the epidural space. A very small dose of fentanyl (Sublimaze) or sufentanil (Sufenta) is often added to the local anesthetic drug for faster and longer-lasting relief of pain. Advantages are good pain control, yet the client can participate in the birth process and interact with her infant and support person. Disadvantages may include maternal hypotension, bladder distention, epidural catheter migration, nausea and vomiting, pruritis, and delayed respiratory depression.

Intrathecal Block Intrathecal injection of an opioid analgesic such as fentanyl (Sublimaze), sufentanil (Sufenta), or morphine (Duramorph) is a pain management option for labor that is gaining acceptance (Murray et al., 2001). A much smaller dose than is given systemically is injected into the subarachnoid space. Advantages are rapid onset yet no sedation, no hypotensive effect, and

TABLE 52-5 PAIN MANAGEMENT DRUGS COMMONLY USED DURING LABOR

DRUG	ROUTE	ONSET	PEAK EFFECT	LASTING
Narcotic Analgesics				
meperidine	IV	30 sec	5 to 10 min	2 to 4 hr
(Demerol)	IM	10 to 15 min	40 to 50 min	2 to 4 hr
fentanyl citrate	IV	1 to 2 min	3 to 5 min	$\frac{1}{2}$ to 1 hr
(Sulimaze)	IM	7 to 10 min	20 to 30 min	1 to 2 hr
Narcotic Agonist-Antagonists				
nalbuphine hydrochloride	IV	2 to 3 min	30 min	3 to 4 hr
(Nubain)	IM	15 min	60 min	3 to 6 hr
butorphanol tartrate	IV	2 to 3 min	$\frac{1}{2}$ to 1 hr	2 to 4 hr
(Stadol)	IM	10 to 30 min	$\frac{1}{2}$ to 1 hr	3 to 4 hr
pentazocine lactate	IV	2 to 3 min	15 to 30 min	2 to 3 hr
(Talwin)	IM	15 to 20 min	30 to 60 min	2 to 3 hr
Narcotic Antagonist				
naloxone	IV	1 to 2 min	unknown	depends on dose
(Narcan)	IM	2 to 5 min	unknown	longer than IV
Analgesic Potentiators				
promethazine hydrochloride	IV	3 to 5 min	unknown	12 hr
(Phenergan)	IM	20 min	unknown	12 hr
hydroxyzine hydrochloride Z-track	IM only	unknown	unknown	4 to 6 hr
(Atarax, Vistaril)				

no motor block, so the client may walk during labor. Disadvantages may include the short duration of action so that the client may require another injection and the inadequate relief of pain in late labor and during birth so that another pain relief measure is required.

Local Infiltration Local infiltration anesthesia of the perineum is achieved by injecting a local anesthetic into the perineum. This is used just before the time of birth in preparation for performing an episiotomy, suturing a laceration, or when a pudendal block cannot be performed. Local anesthetics such as procaine hydrochloride (Novocain), chloroprocaine hydrochloride (Nesacaine), and tetracaine hydrochloride (Pontocaine), which metabolize rapidly, and bupivacaine hydrochloride (Marcaine), lidocaine hydrochloride (Xylocaine), and mepivacaine hydrochloride (Carbocaine), which are more powerful and longer-acting, are often used. Advantages are that the procedure is technically uncomplicated and practically free of complications. A disadvantage is that a large amount of local anesthetic may be required.

Pudendal Block A **pudendal block** is the injection of a local anesthetic into the pudendal nerve to provide perineal, external genitalia, and lower vaginal anesthesia (Figure 52-20). The pudendal block may be performed during the transition phase of the first stage or the second stage of labor. The advantage is that there are no changes in maternal vital signs or the FHR. Disadvantages may include rectal puncture, sciatic nerve block, or a hematoma.

General Anesthesia Because general anesthesia involves loss of consciousness, it is rarely used in vaginal births. It may, however, be used for cesarean births, especially in emergency situations. The greatest danger is

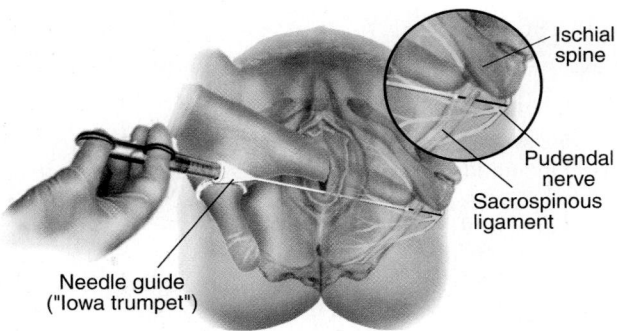

Figure 52-20 *Pudendal block provides anesthesia to the perineum, external genitalia, and lower vagina.*

fetal depression because most general anesthetics reach the fetus in about 2 minutes.

RISKS OF LABOR AND BIRTH

Most labors and births proceed as expected; however, there are complications that may be anticipated and some that happen unexpectedly. The most common risks—preterm labor and birth, premature rupture of membranes, dystocia, abnormal duration of labor, and prolapsed cord—are discussed.

Preterm Labor and Birth

Preterm labor is the onset of regular contractions of the uterus that cause cervical changes between 20 and 37 weeks of gestation. **Preterm birth** is a birth that takes place before the end of the 37th week of gestation. Only about half of the time can a precipitating cause be identified. The single most important factor predisposing to preterm labor and birth is having already had a preterm birth. Other factors often associated with preterm labor and birth include premature rupture of the membranes (PROM), multiple gestation, bacterial vaginosis, intraamniotic infection, bleeding, and uterine/cervical abnormalities.

Most women in preterm labor are admitted to the hospital for further evaluation. A urine specimen is examined for evidence of a urinary tract infection. Cervical or vaginal secretions are obtained during a sterile speculum examination to culture for *Chlamydia trachomatis*, group B streptococcus, or gonococcus infections.

If contractions are continuing and cervical changes are occurring, tocolytic agents may be prescribed. **Tocolytic agents** are medications that inhibit contractions. The most commonly used are ritodrine (Yutopar), terbutaline (Breathine), and magnesium sulfate. A corticosteroid may also be given to accelerate fetal lung maturation. There is greater fetal benefit if at least 24 hours elapse between the first dose and the birth.

If contractions subside and cervical dilatation and effacement remain the same, the client may be discharged with instructions to limit activities and medication to prevent labor.

Premature Rupture of Membranes

When the membranes rupture before labor begins, it is called premature rupture of membranes (PROM). This is the most common cause of preterm labor and occurs

in 2% to 18% of pregnancies (Varney, 1997). Contractions usually begin within 24 hours when the client is at term. In pregnancies of 28 to 34 weeks' gestation, labor may not start for a week or more.

In most cases of PROM, the cause is unknown. Besides preterm labor and birth, PROM can result in prolapse of the cord and intrauterine infection. A positive identification of amniotic fluid is made by observation of amniotic fluid escape from the cervix during a sterile speculum examination, a positive nitrazine test, or the presence of ferning when the fluid is viewed under a microscope (Gilbert & Harmon, 1998). The client may be hospitalized until after the birth of the infant, or if there are no signs of infections or fetal distress, she may be sent home. If hospitalized, continuing assessments include maternal vital signs; FHR; fetal movements; vaginal discharge for odor, color, and amount; and palpation of the uterus for tenderness.

Dystocia

Dystocia is a long, difficult, or abnormal labor caused by any of the four major variables (4 Ps) that affect labor. The following may be causes:

- Dysfunctional labor: ineffective contractions or maternal pushing efforts (powers)
- Pelvic structure variations (passage)
- Fetal variations: anomalies, abnormal presentation or position, very large size, or number of fetuses (passenger)
- Mother's responses: related to preparation for childbirth, past experiences, culture, and support persons (psyche)

Dysfunctional Labor

Dysfunctional labor is a labor with problems of the contractions or with maternal bearing-down efforts. The contractions may be hypertonic or hypotonic.

Hypertonic Uterine Contractions Hypertonic uterine contractions, usually occurring in the latent phase of labor, are very frequent and uncoordinated and have an increased resting tone. The mother has discomfort out of proportion to the intensity of the contractions, which do not dilate or efface the cervix. The excessive pain results from anoxia of the uterine muscle cells. A prolonged latent phase is generally the result.

The client may become fatigued and dehydrated and may express fear that she is losing control with the lack of progress. The fetus may experience distress because the hypertonic contractions and increased resting tone of the uterus interfere with uteroplacental blood flow. The increased and prolonged pressure on the fetal head may cause excessive molding, caput succedaneum, or cephalhematoma (discussed in Newborn chapter).

Bed rest and analgesics such as morphine sulfate or meperidine hydrochloride (Demerol) are given to relieve pain, promote relaxation, and induce sleep. When the client awakens, uterine contractions are often normal and labor proceeds.

Hypotonic Uterine Contractions Hypotonic uterine contractions, also called uterine inertia, usually occur in the active phase of labor. After normal progress through the latent phase of labor, the contractions become weak and inefficient in the active phase and may even cease. Common causes are cephalopelvic disproportion (CPD) (discussed later), malposition of the fetus, an overstretched uterus from multiple fetuses, a fetus of very large body size, hydramnios, or grand-multiparity (having delivered more than six infants).

The risks for the mother include intrauterine infection, especially if the membranes are ruptured and labor is prolonged; postpartum hemorrhage caused by inefficient uterine contractions after birth; exhaustion; and decreased coping ability. The fetus may experience distress because of the length of labor and sepsis from maternal pathogens ascending the birth canal.

An ultrasound is usually performed to rule out CPD. If all factors are normal, one or more measures for augmentation of (increasing) labor are instituted, including ambulation, enema, amniotomy, nipple stimulation, and oxytocin infusion (discussed later) (Varney, 1997).

Amniotomy An **amniotomy,** artificial rupture of membranes (AROM), is performed by the CNM/physician. Several linen savers and a folded bath towel are placed under the client to absorb the amniotic fluid. A disposable plastic hook is generally used (Figure 52-21). A vaginal examination is performed to determine dilatation, effacement, presenting part, and station, and FHR is assessed to determine that the fetus is doing well. If the presenting part is not engaged or if the presentation is not cephalic, the risk of a prolapsed cord is high and the amniotomy is generally not performed. Hall (2001) questions the frequency of performing amniotomy. The disadvantages seem to generally outweigh the advantages.

After an amniotomy, the FHR must be assessed for 1 full minute. A monitor pattern that is nonreassuring or has any significant changes must be promptly reported to the CNM/physician. If the cord is compressed, the FHR is usually less than 100 beats/minute, becoming even less during contractions. Amniotic fluid odor, color,

and quantity are documented. The fluid should be clear (sometimes flecks of vernix are present) with a mild odor. Greenish meconium-stained fluid may indicate placental insufficiency. Foul-smelling fluid or fluid with a strong odor with a cloudy appearance or yellow color often indicates chorioamnionitis. Maternal temperature should be taken every 2 hours after ROM and any elevation above 38°C (100.4°F) reported to the CNM/physician.

Maternal Bearing-Down Efforts Analgesia and/or anesthesia may block Ferguson's reflex and thus decrease the effectiveness of maternal bearing down. Lack of sleep, a long labor, inadequate hydration, and maternal position may also have an adverse effect on the mother's bearing-down efforts.

Pelvic Structure Variations

A woman with a small or abnormally shaped pelvis may experience a long and difficult labor. Only about 50% of women have the pelvic shape (gynecoid) most conducive to labor, fetal descent, and birth (Murray et al., 2001).

A distended bladder reduces the space available in the pelvis and is an obstruction to fetal descent. This greatly increases the client's discomfort. Other, less common obstructions are uterine fibroids or pelvic cysts.

Fetal Variations

Variations of the fetus that may cause dystocia include the following:

- Anomalies
- Abnormal presentation or position
- Size
- Number of fetuses

Anomalies Fetal anomalies such as hydrocephalus may prevent descent of the fetus. Anomalies are often discovered by an ultrasound during pregnancy. If a vaginal birth is not advisable or not possible, a cesarean birth is scheduled.

Abnormal Presentation or Position A cephalic presentation other than vertex makes a larger diameter of the fetal head move through the birth canal. Labor generally takes longer and is more difficult.

In a breech presentation, cervical effacement and dilatation are often slower because the buttocks are softer than the head and do not put firm pressure on the cervix to aid in dilatation. Following are risks to the fetus born in a breech presentation:

- Cord compression
- Aspiration of fluids in the vagina
- Head becoming stuck

External version (manipulation of the fetus through the mother's abdomen to a presentation facilitating birth) may be tried to change the presentation to cephalic.

It is not always possible to change the presentation of the fetus. Figure 52-22 illustrates the birth of a fetus in a complete breech presentation.

A position of occiput posterior or occiput transverse can contribute to dysfunctional labor. Labor is generally longer and causes more discomfort because the head has farther to rotate during internal rotation. Many women

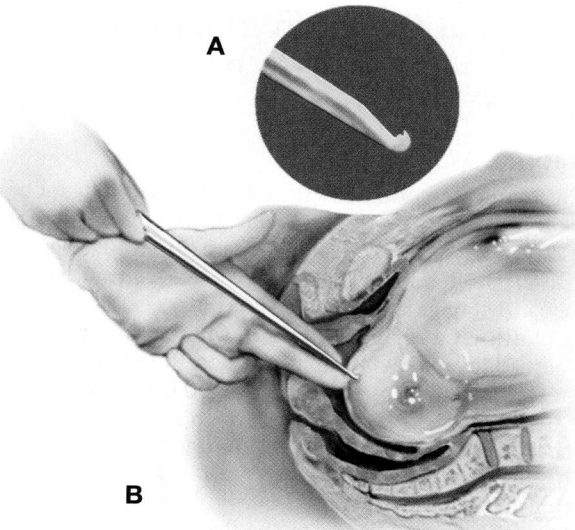

Figure 52-21 *A,* *Disposable plastic hook to rupture membranes: **B,*** *Technique for rupturing membranes*

Figure 52-22 *Birth of Fetus in Complete Breech Presentation:* **A,** *Descent and internal rotation;* **B,** *Extension of fetal back under symphysis (towel on legs used for traction);* **C,** *CNM/physician maintains head flexion by putting pressure on lower face with fingers of left hand (suprapubic pressure is applied by assistant to keep fetal head flexed);* **D,** *Assistant holds fetal legs with towel while CNM/physician assists the face and head over the perineum.*

Figure 52-23 *Fetus tends to rotate from occiput posterior to occiput anterior when mother is in a hands-and-knees position.*

describe severe back pain and have leg pain on the side where the head is positioned. A change in the mother's position may promote rotation of the fetal head. When the mother's abdomen is dependent to her spine, as in the hands-and-knees position, fetal rotation is encouraged (Figure 52-23).

Size An infant weighing more than 4,000 g (8.8 lb) is said to be **macrosomic**—having a very large body size. This may cause problems for a vaginal birth. As long as the mother's pelvis is of a size and shape to accommodate an infant this size, there is no problem. When the fetal head will not fit through the mother's pelvis, it is called **cephalopelvic disproportion** (CPD). The cause can be either fetal or maternal. The fetal head may be abnormally large and the mother's pelvis of normal size and shape, or the fetal head may be of average size and the mother's pelvis small or abnormally shaped. Whatever the cause, a cesarean birth is required.

Number of Fetuses When more than one fetus is present, the uterus is overdistended. One or more of the fetuses may be in a presentation less desirable than vertex. Twins often have a cesarean birth, and when there are three or more fetuses, birth is almost always cesarean (Murray et al., 2001).

Mother's Responses

The mother's perception of labor is more important than her actual experience in labor. Tales from family and friends, a bad experience with a previous labor, and cultural expectations can add to the stress of labor.

Excessive or prolonged stress experienced by the woman in labor may interfere with the progress of labor in several ways:

- Secretion of catecholamines (epinephrine and norepinephrine) by the adrenal glands in response to stress inhibits uterine contractions and decreases blood supply to the uterus and placenta while increasing blood supply to the skeletal muscles.
- Tense abdominal and pelvic muscles make contractions less effective.
- Contractions working against tense abdominal muscles increase pain, which adds stress to the situation and makes the mother more anxious.

The nurse can help allay the client's fears by offering encouragement, answering her questions honestly, and offering tips on how to make labor more successful. For instance, the nurse might suggest a change of position to a squatting bar to aid in fetal descent, or may offer a mirror so the mother can see the baby crown and be encouraged by her progress.

Abnormal Duration of Labor

Labor may be prolonged or abnormally short (precipitate).

Prolonged Labor

Many of the conditions previously discussed, such as hypotonic uterine contractions, CPD, abnormal fetal presentations or positions, or early use of analgesics may cause prolonged labor. Labor progress in either the first or second stage may be prolonged or arrested (stopped). The plotting of cervical dilatation on a labor graph, as found in Figure 52-19, helps in identifying these situations. Once the cause of the prolonged labor is identified, the CNM/physician can take steps to remedy the situation. A possible course of action might be induction of labor, a forceps- or vacuum-assisted birth, or cesarean birth (all discussed later).

When the active phase of the first stage of labor lasts more than 15 hours, the risk of fetal death increases sharply (Lowdermilk & Perry, 2003). With prolonged labor, maternal morbidity and mortality may result from infection, uterine rupture, serious dehydration, and postpartum hemorrhage.

Precipitate Labor/Precipitate Birth

A labor lasting less than 3 hours from the onset of contractions to the birth of the infant is considered a **precipitate labor.** Although a precipitate labor may end with a precipitate birth, they are not the same. Possible maternal complications during a precipitate labor include a loss of coping ability; an increased risk of uterine rupture; lacerations of the cervix, vagina, and perineum; and postpartum hemorrhage. Possible fetal complications include hypoxia, distress, and cerebral trauma.

A **precipitate birth** is a birth occurring suddenly and unexpectedly without a CNM/physician to assist. When a client says "the baby's coming" or words to that effect, the health care provider should always look to see whether she is correct. Most of the time a large part of the fetal head is visible, if not already crowning. In this situation the nurse should do the following:

- Stay with the mother.
- Call for assistance or send support person to get assistance. Other staff members can notify the CNM/physician.
- Remain calm and reassure mother.
- Open emergency birth pack.
- If time permits, scrub hands, put on sterile gloves, and place sterile drape under mother's buttocks.
- As the head crowns, instruct mother to pant.
- If membranes are still intact, tear the sac, allowing amniotic fluid to flow out.
- Apply gentle pressure to the fetal head with one hand to prevent it from popping out. *Do not hold the head back with force enough to prevent it from being born.*
- With the mother still panting, check at the back of the fetal head for the umbilical cord. If there is a **nuchal cord** (umbilical cord around the neck) and it is loose enough, slip the cord over the baby's head. If it is too tight, place two clamps on the cord, cut the

cord between the clamps, and unwind the cord from the neck.
- Suction the baby's mouth and throat first to prevent the infant from aspirating amniotic fluid and then the nose.
- With one hand on each side of the head, push gently downward until the anterior shoulder comes under the symphysis. Then gently raise the baby's head so the posterior shoulder is born.
- Ask the mother to push gently to assist in the birth of the rest of the infant's body.
- Hold the infant at the level of the uterus, being careful not to drop the slippery infant.
- Again, suction the mouth, throat, and nose of the infant.
- Dry the infant to prevent heat loss and place the infant on the mother's abdomen. Cover with a dry blanket.
- Document on the birth record the fetal position, nuchal cord, time of birth, Apgar scores (addressed later in this chapter) at 1 and 5 minutes after birth, gender, time and method of placental expulsion, and mother's condition.

Prolapsed Cord

When the umbilical cord lies below the presenting part of the fetus, it is termed a **prolapsed cord.** Prolapse of the cord may occur anytime and may be hidden (occult, not visible) or visible (Figure 52-24). It most commonly occurs with ROM, either spontaneous rupture of membranes (SROM) or AROM, as the cord washes down with the amniotic fluid. This happens in 1 of 400 births (Lowdermilk & Perry, 2003). Usta, Merier, and Sibai (1999) concluded that obstetrical intervention contributed to 47% of cord prolapse situations but found no increase in perinatal morbidity.

A cord below the presenting part is compressed between the fetus and the mother's pelvis, resulting in decreased blood flow to the fetus. The fetus will have bradycardia with variable decelerations during uterine contractions. Contributing factors include a long cord

Figure 52-24 *Prolapsed Cord:* **A,** *Hidden (occult, not visible);* **B,** *Prolapse with membranes still intact;* **C,** *Cord may be seen in vagina;* **D,** *Breech with prolapsed cord*

Figure 52-25 *Examiner's fingers relieve pressure on prolapsed cord in* **(A)** *vertex presentation and* **(B)** *breech presentation. Gravity relieves pressure on prolapsed cord with mother in* **(C)** *modified Sim's position and* **(D)** *knee-chest position.*

(greater than 100 cm or 40 in), unengaged presenting part, breech presentation, or transverse lie.

When a prolapsed cord is identified, pressure on the cord must be relieved immediately. The provider must call for assistance, don a sterile glove, insert two fingers into the vagina, and put pressure on the presenting part to relieve the compression of the cord. The client can then be assisted into a modified Sims' position with her hips up on pillows, the knee-chest position, or place the bed in Trendelenburg position. In these positions, gravity keeps the pressure of the presenting part off the cord (Figure 52-25). Occasionally, a vaginal birth may be possible, but generally a cesarean birth is preferred.

INDUCTION/AUGMENTATION OF LABOR

Induction of labor and augmentation of labor both relate to the stimulation of uterine contractions, but at different times in the labor process.

Induction of Labor

Induction of labor is the stimulation of uterine contractions *before* they begin spontaneously for the purpose of birthing an infant. Both chemical and mechanical methods can be used to induce labor. The most common methods used in the United States are intravenous oxytocin and amniotomy. Induction of labor may be considered in situations of preexisting maternal disease, PIH, PROM, postterm gestation, or fetal demise. Fetal maturity, especially lung maturity, must also be considered. Contraindications to induction are the same as those to spontaneous labor and vaginal birth (e.g., hydrocephaly, transverse lie).

If the cervix is "ripe" (soft), the probability of induction success is greater. If the cervix is not "ripe," prostaglandins are often used first to "ripen" the cervix. Dinoprostone (Prepidil) is often used, and the next day oxytocin infusion is begun. Frequently, oxytocin infusion and amniotomy are both used.

Oxytocin Infusion   Contruction of Uterus

A primary IV infusion of 1,000 mL of an electrolyte solution (e.g., lactated Ringer's) is started. A secondary infusion of 1,000 mL of the same solution is prepared with 10 units of oxytocin (Pitocin). The secondary infusion (with the oxytocin) is regulated by an infusion pump. The rate is very slow at the beginning with very small increases at regular intervals according to agency protocol or CNM/physician orders. The goal is to have contractions with a frequency 2 to 3 minutes, duration 40 to 60 seconds, and moderate intensity.

A fetal monitor is used to provide continuous data about FHR and contractions. Before each increase of the infusion rate, assessments of maternal blood pressure and pulse, FHR (bradycardia or decelerations), and contractions should be made and documented. An intake and output record is maintained throughout the induction process.

 Safety: Oxytocin Infusion
Discontinue the secondary infusion with the oxytocin if the following occur:
- Contractions are more frequent than every 2 minutes or the duration is more than 90 seconds.
- Uterus resting tone is more than 20 mm Hg.
- Fetal monitor shows:
  repeated late decelerations
  prolonged decelerations
  no variability

And then:
- Keep mother in side-lying position.
- Increase rate of primary IV fluid.
- Administer oxygen by face mask.
- Notify CNM/physician.

Augmentation of Labor

Augmentation of labor is the stimulation of uterine contractions *after* spontaneously beginning but the progress of labor is unsatisfactory. Intravenous oxytocin is used in the same manner as for induction of labor.

OBSTETRIC PROCEDURES

Sometimes a special obstetric procedure is needed to assist with the birth of an infant. These procedures are cesarean birth, forceps-assisted birth, and vacuum-assisted birth.

Cesarean Birth

Cesarean birth is the birth of an infant through an incision in the abdomen and uterus. Indications for cesarean birth include placenta previa, placenta abruptio, CPD, prolapsed cord, breech presentation, active genital herpes, dystocia, pregnancy-induced hypertension, hydrocephaly, multifetal pregnancy, and repeat cesarean birth.

Incisions

The skin incision and uterine incision are not necessarily the same. The skin incision may either be transverse (Pfannenstiel) or vertical. The uterine incision may be vertical in either the upper uterus (classic) or lower uterine segment or transverse in the lower uterine segment (Figure 52-26). Which incisions are used are determined by the client and physician depending on the time factor, reason for the cesarean birth, client's desire for future pregnancies, and physician preference.

Anesthesia

Regional block, epidural, or spinal anesthesia are the most popular because the mother is awake and aware of the birth of her infant. When time is of the essence or when an epidural or spinal cannot be used, general anesthetic is used.

Scheduled or Unscheduled Cesarean Birth

A cesarean birth may either be scheduled or unscheduled.

Scheduled Cesarean Birth A cesarean birth is scheduled if it is to be a repeat cesarean birth, if labor is contraindicated (e.g., complete placenta previa, hydrocephaly), or if labor cannot be induced and birth is necessary. These clients have some time to prepare for the cesarean birth.

Unscheduled Cesarean Birth Unscheduled cesarean births are usually the result of some difficulty in the labor process. Besides concern about the situation causing the need for a cesarean birth, the client and her support person often experience a sense of failure at not being able to have the baby "normally." The client is generally tired from the labor process and forgets or misunderstands any explanations given. After the infant's birth, it is important for the client to review with the nurse the events before the cesarean birth to ensure the client's understanding of what happened.

Preoperative procedures must be performed quickly. Generally, a Foley catheter is inserted to keep the bladder empty; an abdominal-mons surgical shave prep is completed; intravenous fluids are started (if not already running); blood and urine tests are ordered; and, if time is available, preoperative teaching may be instituted. The support person is encouraged to remain with the mother even in surgery to provide emotional support.

When the mother is awake during the cesarean birth, she is involved in seeing and holding her infant just as in a vaginal birth, unless infant resuscitation is required. A pediatrician is usually present to care for the infant. It is extremely important to keep the mother informed about what is happening.

Skin incision   **Uterine incision**

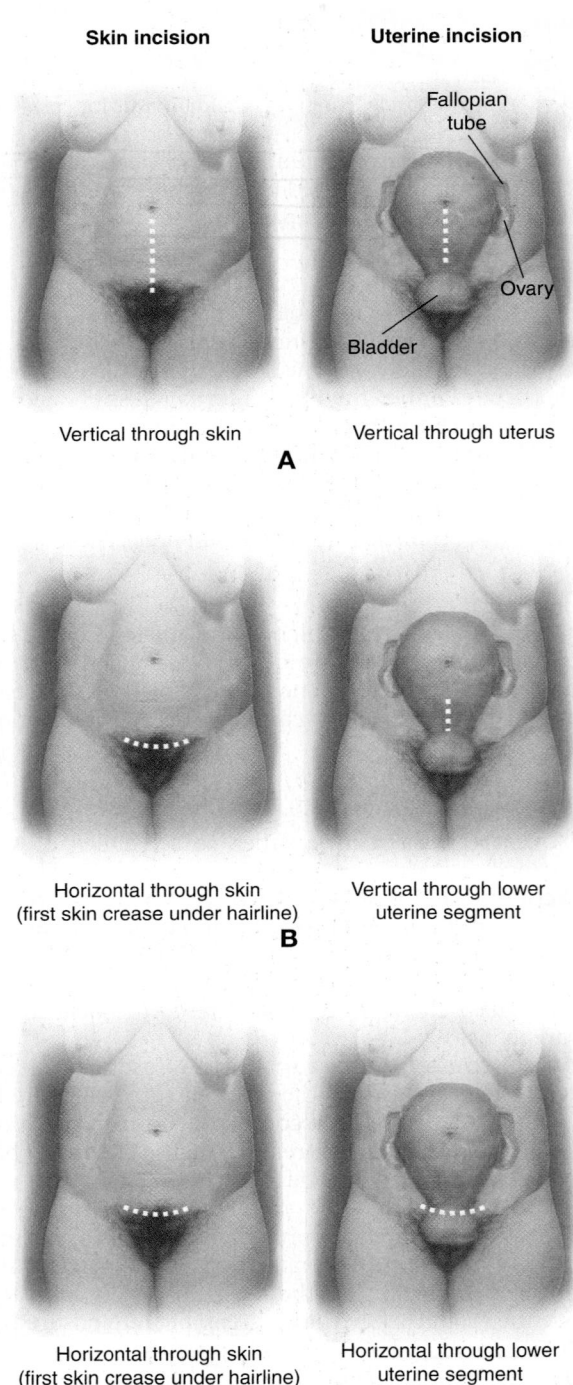

Vertical through skin   Vertical through uterus

A

Horizontal through skin   Vertical through lower
(first skin crease under hairline)   uterine segment

B

Horizontal through skin   Horizontal through lower
(first skin crease under hairline)   uterine segment

C

Figure 52-26 *Cesarean Birth: Skin and Uterine Incisions: A, Classic, vertical skin incision with high uterine incision; seldom used except in emergency situation; B, Horizontal skin incision with low vertical uterine incision; C, Horizontal skin incision with horizontal uterine incision*

Vaginal Birth after Cesarean

When the reason for the initial cesarean birth is a nonrecurring situation such as placenta previa, prolapsed cord, or breech presentation, the client may be able to have a vaginal birth with the next pregnancy. If a

Figure 52-27 *Types of Forceps*

low transverse uterine incision was made for the cesarean birth, a trial of labor is often recommended. If a classic uterine incision was made in the uterus, a trial of labor is contraindicated because the possibility of uterine rupture is very great. The possibility of a vaginal birth after cesarean (VBAC) is discussed throughout the pregnancy with the obstetrician.

Forceps-Assisted Birth

Forceps are metal instruments used on the fetal head to provide traction or to provide a method of rotating the fetal head to an occiput-anterior position. There are several types of forceps. Some forceps have fenestrated (open) blades and some solid blades, but they all have a locking mechanism that prevents the blades from compressing the fetal skull (Figure 52-27).

Forceps may be applied as:

· *Outlet forceps*—when head is crowning (Figure 52-28)
· *Low forceps*—when head is at +2 station or lower but not yet crowning
· *Midforceps*—when head is engaged but above +2 station

Indications

Any situation that threatens the mother or fetus that can be relieved by a vaginal birth is an indication for forceps use. Examples are an exhausted mother or one who has heart disease and a fetus in distress, in arrested rotation, or breech position (aftercoming head).

Application of Forceps

Before forceps are applied, the cervix must be completely dilated, membranes must be ruptured, and position and station of the fetal head must be known. The FHR must be checked, reported, and recorded *before* forceps are applied and again *after* forceps are applied to make sure the cord is not being compressed by the forceps. It may help the mother to understand about the forceps if it is explained that the forceps blades fit around the baby's head like two teaspoons fit around an egg (Lowdermilk & Perry, 2003). Traction is applied to the

Figure 52-28 *Outlet Forceps. Traction is applied downward and outward during contractions.*

Figure 52-29 *Vacuum-Assisted Birth*

forceps only during contractions. Rotation is performed between contractions.

After the birth of the infant, the mother must be assessed for vaginal and cervical lacerations, hematoma, and bruising. The newborn infant may have facial bruising or edema.

Vacuum-Assisted Birth

A cup connected to suction is placed over the occiput on the fetal head. After the suction (negative pressure) is attained, traction downward and outward is applied during contractions (Figure 52-29). Indications are the same as for forceps-assisted birth.

Maternal risks include vaginal and rectal lacerations. Fetal risks include cephalhematoma, brachial plexus palsy, retinal and intracranial hemorrhage, and hyperbilirubinemia (O'Brian & Cefalo, 1996).

IMMEDIATE INFANT/MOTHER CARE

During the first 20 to 30 minutes after the infant's birth, specific care is given to the infant and the mother.

 Infection Control: Standard Precautions
Disposable gloves should be worn when:
- Caring for the newborn until after the infant has received the initial bath
- Assessing the amount of lochia and the perineum
- Cleansing the perineum

Care of the Infant

Following are the immediate needs of the newborn infant:
- A—airway
- B—breathing
- C—circulation
- W—warmth

Infants born by cesarean delivery are at greater risk for respiratory distress because they do not receive the "vaginal squeeze" that aids in expelling amniotic fluid from the lungs.

Identification of the infant is the top priority after the immediate needs are met.

Airway

The CNM/physician suctions secretions from the mouth and nose of the infant at the time of birth. Shortly thereafter, the infant takes the first breath and may begin to cry. The mouth and nose of the infant are suctioned by the nurse as needed to maintain an open airway. The bulb syringe must be compressed before inserting into the mouth or nose of infant.

Breathing/Circulation

The infant's cardiopulmonary adaptation to extrauterine life is assessed by using the Apgar score (Table 52-6).

Each of the five items are assessed at 1 and 5 minutes after birth, providing a quick evaluation of how the heart and lungs are adapting. The five items to be assessed are arranged in priority from most important (heart rate) to least important (color). The infant is given a score, from 0 to 2, for each item. The five scores are then totaled.

When the Apgar score is 8 or higher, no special interventions are required. When the Apgar score is between 4 and 8, gentle rubbing of the infant's back for stimulation and administration of oxygen will usually result in an increase in the Apgar score at 5 minutes. It must be determined whether and when the mother received a narcotic for pain management during labor. Naloxone (Narcan) may be administered if the mother received a narcotic during laor.

When the Apgar score is between 0 and 4, the infant requires resuscitation. The infant must be kept on one side with the head flat or slightly elevated because a

TABLE 52-6	APGAR SCORE		
ITEM ASSESSED	SCORE		
	0	1	2
Heart rate	Absent	Slow (<100)	Over 100
Respiratory rate	Absent	Slow, weak cry	Good cry
Muscle tone	Flaccid	Some flexion of extremities	Well flexed
Reflex irritability	No response	Grimace	Cry, cough, or sneeze
Color	Blue, pale	Body pink, extremities blue	Completely pink (light skinned); absence of cyanosis (dark skinned)

A long band is applied to the mother's wrist. The other long band is usually applied to the father's wrist or other person serving as primary support. In multiple births, the mother and father have a band for each infant.

Most hospitals also footprint the newborn infant and either fingerprint or thumbprint the mother. The soles of the infant's feet must be dried and any vernix caseosa removed before footprinting.

Care of the Mother

If an oxytocic medication is to be given when the placenta is delivered, the blood pressure is taken both before and after the medication is administered. Maternal blood pressure is monitored every 5 to 15 minutes. The oxytocic medication may increase the BP. Excessive blood loss will cause the BP to fall.

The fundus of the uterus is palpated for firmness. It should be firm, about the size of a grapefruit, in the midline, below the umbilicus. The proper method of palpating the uterus is illustrated in Figure 52-31.

head-down position makes it more difficult to breathe as the intestines put pressure on the diaphragm.

Warmth

The infant must be dried to prevent heat loss by evaporation. A prewarmed radiant warmer is used while giving initial care. Skin-to-skin contact with a parent can also be used to provide warmth. A stockinette cap on the infant's *dry head* also helps prevent heat loss.

Identification

A set of four identification bands, two long and two short, imprinted with the same number are used. The mother's name, sex of infant, time of birth, and CNM/physician's name are written on each band. The two small bands are put on the infant (both ankles or a wrist and an ankle). The bands must fit the infant snugly but not too tightly (Figure 52-30).

Figure 52-31 *Palpation of Uterus after Delivery of Placenta*

Figure 52-30 *Matching identification bands are placed on infant, mother, and partner; infant is footprinted.*

After the CNM/physician has completed repairing the episiotomy (if one was made) and/or any lacerations, the perineum is washed with warm, sterile water and dried with a sterile towel. Maternity vaginal pads are then applied.

Safety: Removing Legs from Stirrups

If legs were in stirrups during the birth:
• Two persons are needed to remove them.
• Each person places one hand under the knee and one under the heel (the mother generally has little control over leg movement).

• At the same time, both legs are lowered to the bed.
• If the legs are numb, they may be bicycled to aid circulation return.

The mother may remain in the same bed (LDRP) or be moved to a recovery room bed. If the client is cold and begins to shiver, she should be covered with a warmed blanket, and a second blanket placed over it.

Mother, infant, and father or other support person are allowed time together to further the bonding and attachment process.

SAMPLE NURSING CARE PLAN

THE CLIENT IN LABOR

Anna Llanas, a 23-year-old gravida 1, para 0, is admitted in early labor. Her cervix is dilated 3 cm and is completely effaced. The fetus is at station 0. Contractions are every 5 minutes, duration 50 seconds, and of mild intensity. Her husband, Joe, is with her. They attend only the first two of the six childbirth preparation classes due to Joe's work schedule. Anna is tightly holding Joe's hand. Her voice is quivering as she says, "My water just broke. I'm scared. I don't know if I can do this. I've never done this before."

Nursing Diagnosis 1 *Anxiety* related to the situational crisis of labor and the birthing process at evidenced by gravida 1, para 0, attended only first 2 childbirth classes, voice quivering, statement that she is scared and doesn't know if she can do this

Nursing Outcomes Classification (NOC)
Anxiety Control
Coping

Nursing Interventions Classification (NIC)
Anxiety Reduction
Coping Enhancement

PLANNING/GOALS	NURSING INTERVENTIONS	RATIONALE
Anna will express less anxiety within an hour.	Maintain calm and confident manner.	Provides verbal and nonverbal message that labor is a normal process.
	Orient Anna and Joe to birthing room and explain admission procedure.	Allays feelings of anxiety regarding unfamiliar environment.
	Determine Anna's and Joe's knowledge and expectation of labor.	Establishes a baseline for intervention and enhances their sense of control.
	Discuss the expected progress of labor and what will happen during the process.	Lessens anxiety associated with the unknown.
	Involve Anna and Joe in decisions about care and share information on progress of labor.	Increases their sense of control.
	Involve Joe in the care of Anna.	Strengthens Anna's ability to cope.

EVALUATION Anna says she feels a little better and is now gently holding Joe's hand.

Nursing Diagnosis 2 *Risk for Infection* related to rupture of membranes as evidenced by statement "My water just broke."

Nursing Outcomes Classification (NOC)
Treatment Behavior: Illness or Injury

Nursing Interventions Classification (NIC)
Infection Protection
Labor Induction

continues

SAMPLE NURSING CARE PLAN

PLANNING/GOALS	NURSING INTERVENTIONS	RATIONALE
Anna will show no evidence of infection.	Assess amniotic fluid's color, odor, amount, and presence of meconium.	May indicate intrauterine infection or fetal distress.
	Monitor maternal vital signs and the FHR.	Evaluates for signs of infection and fetal distress.
	Maintain Standard Precautions by following good hand hygiene, wearing gloves when providing perineal care to Anna, and using aseptic technique when indicated.	Prevents spread of microorganisms.

EVALUATION   There are no signs of intrauterine infection or fetal distress.

Anna's vital signs are normal: T 98.6°F, P 84, R 20, and BP 114/70. FHR is 138. Anna reports back pain. Contractions are now every 3 to 4 minutes, duration 60 seconds, and of moderate intensity. The cervix is dilated 5 cm with station +1.

Nursing Diagnosis 3 *Acute Pain* related to increasing frequency, duration, and intensity as evidenced by contraction assessment

Nursing Outcomes Classification (NOC)
Pain Level
Pain: Disruptive Effects

Nursing Interventions Classification (NIC)
Pain Management
Anxiety Reduction

PLANNING/GOALS	NURSING INTERVENTIONS	RATIONALE
Anna will be able to cope with the discomfort.	Encourage Anna to change position frequently (every 30 minutes), using such positions as leaning forward when sitting or standing, side-lying, and hands and knees.	Shifts weight of fetus away from the back, relieving back pain; relieves strain and constant pressure; and helps fetus descend through pelvis.
	Instruct Anna and Joe to use focused breathing, effleurage, massage, sacral pressure, and conscious relaxation.	Increases relaxation and counteracts some of the discomfort.
	Offer the use of shower or Jacuzzi.	Increases ability to relax. Heat interferes with transmission of pain impulses.
	Palpate for distended bladder and encourage regular voiding (at least every 2 hours).	Prevents discomfort and the impediment of fetal descent.
	Share with Anna and Joe about the progress in labor.	Increases willingness to continue when Anna knows efforts are having desired results.
	Provide comfort measures such as oral care; ice chips; and cool, damp cloth to head or neck, and change damp gown and bed linens.	Relieves discomforts of dry mouth, diaphoresis, and leaking amniotic fluid.
	Inform Anna about the pharmacologic pain relief measures available to her.	Gives Anna a sense of control when she can choose when to use medication for pain.

EVALUATION   Anna is able to handle the discomfort with Joe's help with focused breathing and by applying counterpressure to her back.

continues

SAMPLE NURSING CARE PLAN

Nursing Diagnosis 4 *Risk for Impaired Urinary Elimination,* related to sensory impairment as evidenced by progress of labor, station +1

Nursing Outcomes Classification (NOC)
Neurological Status: Autonomic

Nursing Interventions Classification (NIC)
Urinary Catheterization

PLANNING/GOALS	NURSING INTERVENTIONS	RATIONALE
Anna's bladder will not exhibit signs of distention.	Palpate Anna's bladder at least every 2 hours.	Identifies a full bladder when Anna is unable to feel the urge to void.
	Encourage frequent voiding; catheterize if necessary.	Avoids bladder distention that may impede descent of fetus and result in trauma to bladder.

EVALUATION   Anna voids every 2 hours.

Anna's cervix is now 8 cm dilated, station is +2. Contractions are every 2 to 3 minutes, duration 70 seconds, and strong intensity. She is very uncomfortable, requests the pain medication, and says, "I can't take it anymore." Joe is concerned and asks, "Is she alright?" FHR and maternal vital signs remain close to the admission assessment. Anna is given meperidine (Demerol) 50 mg IV. She is now resting well between contractions. In 30 minutes Anna's cervix is completely dilated, station is +3. She pushes spontaneously several times during each contraction. When she pushes her back stiffens, her arms push on the bed, and she holds her breath. Anna prefers a semi-Fowler's position.

Nursing Diagnosis 5 *Deficient Knowledge (effective pushing technique)* related to lack of exposure to information since only attended first 2 prenatal classes, as evidenced by posture during pushing and breath holding

Nursing Outcomes Classification (NOC)
Knowledge: Labor and Delivery

Nursing Interventions Classification (NIC)
Teaching: Individual

PLANNING/GOALS	NURSING INTERVENTIONS	RATIONALE
Anna will push more effectively after instructions until birth of infant.	Teach Anna techniques to push more effectively.	Makes pushing more effective.
	During each contraction, Anna should do the following:	
	• Sit upright or squat	• Takes advantage of gravity; squatting slightly enlarges the pelvic outlet
	• Flex chin on chest and curl over uterus	• Directs force of push into pelvis
	• *With elbows bent,* pull on her flexed knees	• Provides more force to push
	• Exhale and vocalize when she pushes	• Prevents Valsalva maneuver, which causes a decrease in palcenta blood flow and thus oxygenation to the fetus
	Observe Anna's perineum for crowning.	Keeps everyone informed of progress.
	Allow Anna to rest between contractions (no unnecessary talking).	Allows Anna to gain strength for next contraction.

EVALUATION   In 30 minutes Anna and Joe have a 6 lb 10 oz (3,005 g) baby girl. The baby's Apgar scores are 8 at 1 minute and 9 at 5 minutes.

CASE STUDY

Peggy Kazmierski, a 30-year-old gravida 4, para 3, has been in labor 3 hours. Her cervix is 7 cm dilated, station is −1. The fetus is in a vertex presentation, LOA position. When the membranes rupture during a strong contraction, the umbilical cord prolapses from the vagina, and the head is making the perineum bulge. Peggy begins to cry and asks, "What is happening? I feel something hanging out of me."

The following questions will guide your development of a nursing care plan for the case study.

1. What are the first actions the nurse should take?
2. What assessments should be made?
3. Identify two nursing diagnoses and goals for Peggy.
4. Identify appropriate nursing interventions for the diagnoses.

Summary

- There are two theories relative to why labor begins: the mechanical theory and the hormonal theory.
- Signs of impending labor are lightening, Braxton Hicks contractions, cervical softening, bloody show, rupture of membranes, and a sudden burst of energy.
- The four major variables that affect labor are known as the four Ps: passage, passenger, powers, and psyche.
- Labor is divided into four stages, which include first stage (dilatation and effacement), second stage (birth of baby), third stage (delivery of placenta), and fourth stage (recovery).
- The mechanisms of labor describe how the fetus moves through the maternal pelvis and birth canal.
- There are many cultural aspects of labor and birth for the nurse to consider when caring for a client from another culture.
- Standard Precautions must be kept in mind when caring for a client during labor and birth because of the many opportunities for contact with body fluids and blood.
- Contractions are assessed for frequency, duration, interval, and intensity.
- Pain management is an important nursing intervention with both nonpharmacological and pharmacological measures.
- The most common risks of labor and birth are preterm labor and birth, premature rupture of membranes, dystocia, abnormal duration of labor, and prolapsed cord.
- Obstetric procedures that may be required to assist with the birth of an infant are cesarean birth, forceps-assisted birth, and vacuum-assisted birth.

Review Questions

1. Which of the following measures should the nurse take when supporting a prepared couple during labor?
   - a. verbally encouraging them
   - b. staying with them all the time
   - c. taking FHR after each contraction
   - d. leaving them alone to do "their own thing"

2. It is important for the nurse caring for a client in labor to make sure the bladder is kept empty because a full bladder may:
   - a. cause glucosuria.
   - b. cause proteinuria.
   - c. impede the progress of labor.
   - d. make the mother's back ache more.

3. Following rupture of membranes, the most appropriate action for the nurse is to:
   - a. listen to the FHR.
   - b. remove the wet linen.
   - c. time the contractions.
   - d. report the color and odor of the fluid.

4. A client is admitted for induction of labor with an oxytocic drug. She is 2 weeks past her EDB. Which of the following findings, if present, would it be essential to report to the CNM/physician before the oxytocic infusion is started?
   - a. low back ache
   - b. regular contractions of 60 seconds' duration
   - c. irregular contractions of 20 seconds' duration
   - d. a rise in blood pressure from 122/80 to 130/84

5. A client is having a precipitate birth. The most appropriate nursing action is to:
    a. stay with her and call for help.
    b. quickly move her to the delivery room.
    c. carefully monitor the FHR and contractions.
    d. assist her to change her position and breathe deeply.

References/Suggested Readings

Ahmed, S. (1994, December). *Culturally sensitive caregiving for Pakistani women.* Lecture presented at the Medical College of Virginia Hospitals, Richmond, VA.

Bergstrom, L., Seidel, J., Skellman-Hull, L., & Roberts, J. (1997). "I gotta push. Please let met push!": Social interactions during the change from first to second stage labor. *Birth, 24,* 173–180.

Blackburn, S. (2003). *Maternal, fetal, and neonatal physiology.* Philadelphia: W. B. Saunders.

Burroughs, A. (2001). *Maternity nursing* (8th ed.). Philadelphia: W. B. Saunders.

Callister, L., & Vega, R. (1998). Giving birth: Guatemalan women's voices. *JOGNN, 27*(3), 289–295.

Cesario, S. (2001). Care of the Native American woman: Strategies for practice, education, and research. *JOGNN, 30*(1), 13–19.

Chapman, L. (2000). Expectant fathers and labor epidurals. *MCN, 25*(3), 133–138.

Cosner, K., & deJong, E. (1993). Physiologic second stage labor. *MCN, 18*(1), 38–43.

D'Arcy, Y. (1999). Managing discomfort with a walking epidural. *Nursing99, 29*(6), 22.

DeSeve, M. (1997). Keeping the faith: Jewish traditions in pregnancy & childbirth. *Lifelines, 1*(4), 46–49.

Dickason, L., Silverman, B., & Kaplan, J. (1998). *Maternal–infant nursing care* (3rd ed.). St. Louis, MO: Mosby–Year Book.

Dochterman, J., & Bulechek, G. (2004). *Nursing Interventions Classification (NIC)* (4th ed.). St. Louis, MO: Mosby.

Dwyer, D., & Swayze, S. (2002). Problems after vacuum-assisted childbirth. *Nursing2002, 32*(1), 74.

Ferri, R., & Sofer, D. (2003). Do vaginal births need a good push? *AJN, 103*(4), 19.

Gennaro, S., Kamwendo, L., Mbweza, E., & Kershbaumer, R. (1998). Childbearing in Malawi, Africa. *JOGNN, 27*(2), 191–196.

Gilbert, E., & Harmon, J. (1998). *Manual of high risk pregnancy and delivery* (2nd ed.). St. Louis, MO: Mosby–Year Book.

Howard, J., & Berbiglia, V. (1997). Caring for childbearing Korean women. *JOGNN, 26*(6), 665–671.

Hutchinson, M., & Baqi-Aziz, M. (1994). Nursing care of the childbearing Muslim family. *JOGNN, 23*(9), 767–771.

Jordan, B. (1978). *Birth in four cultures.* St. Albans: Eden Press Women's Publications.

Ladewig, P., Moberly, S., Olds, S., & London, M. (2001). *Contemporary maternal–newborn nursing care* (5th ed.). Menlo Park, CA: Addison-Wesley.

Lambert, P. (2003). Laboring Lessons. *AWHONN Lifelines, 7*(2), 184.

Littleton, L., & Engebretson, J. (2002). *Maternal, neonatal, and women's health nursing.* Clifton Park, NY: Thomson Delmar Learning.

Lowdermilk, D., & Perry, S. (2003). *Maternity nursing* (6th ed.). St. Louis, MO: Mosby–Year Book.

Lowe, N. (1996). The pain and discomfort of labor and birth. *JOGNN, 25*(1), 82–92.

Martin, P., & Leaton, M. (2001). Amniotic fluid embolism. *AJN, 101*(3), 43–44.

Mattson, S. (1995). Culturally sensitive perinatal care for Southeast Asians. *JOGNN, 24*(4), 335–341.

McCartney, P. (1998a). The birth ball—Are you using it in your practice setting? *MCN, 23*(4), 218.

McCartney, P. (1998b). Caring for women with epidurals using the "laboring down" technique. *MCN, 23*(5), 274.

Moorhead, S., Johnson, M., & Maas, M. (2004). *Nursing Outcomes Classification (NOC)* (3rd ed.). St. Louis, MO: Mosby.

Murray, S., McKinney, E., & Gorrie, T. (2001). *Foundations of maternal–newborn nursing* (3rd ed.). Philadelphia, W. B. Saunders.

North American Nursing Diagnosis Association. (2003). *Nursing diagnoses: Definitions & classification 2003–2004.* Philadelphia: Author.

O'Brian, W. F., & Cefalo, R. C. (1996). Labor and delivery. In S. G. Gabbe, J. R. Niehyl, & J. L. Simpson (Eds.). *Obstetrics: Normal and problem pregnancies* (3rd ed.). New York: Churchill Livingstone.

Perez, P., & Herrick, L. (1998). Doulas: Exploring their roles with parents, hospitals & nurses. *Lifelines, 2*(2), 54.

Petersen, L., & Besuner, P. (1997). Pushing techniques during labor: Issues and controversies. *JOGNN, 26*(6), 719–726.

Schneiderman, J. (1998). Rituals of placenta disposal. *MCN, 23*(3), 142–143.

Scott-Ramos, I. (1995, January). *Culturally sensitive care giving for Latino women.* Lecture presented at the Medical College of Virginia Hospitals, Richmond, VA.

Sharts-Hopko, N. (1995). Birth in the Japanese context. *JOGNN, 24*(4), 343–351.

Simpson, K., & Creehan, P. (2001). *AWHONN perinatal nursing* (2nd ed.). Philadelphia: Lippincott Williams & Wilkins.

Tennyson, M. (2000). Labor at 20,000 feet. *AJN, 100*(9), 49–52.

Usta, M., Merier, B. M., & Sibai, B. M. (1999). Current obstetrical practice & umbilical cord prolapse. *AWHONN Lifelines, 5*(6), 10–13.

Varney, H. (1997). *Varney's midwifery* (3rd ed.). Sudberry, MA: Jones & Bartlett.

Weber, S. (1996). Cultural aspects of pain in childbearing women. *JOGNN, 25*(1), 67–72.

Resources

American College of Obstetricians and Gynecologists (ACOG), 409 12th Street S.W., P. O. Box 96920, Washington, DC, 20090-6920, 800-762-2264, www.acog.com

Association of Women's Health, Obstetric, and Neonatal Nurses (AWHONN), 2000 L Street N.W., Suite 740, Washington, DC, 20036, 800-673-8499, www.awhonn.org

Childbirth Graphics, P.O. Box 21207, Waco, TX, 76702, 800-229-3366, www.childbirthgraphics.com

C/SEC, Inc. (Cesarean/Support Education and Concern), 22 Forest Road, Framingham, MA, 01701, 508-877-8266

InterNational Association of Parents & Professionals for Safe Alternatives in Childbirth (NAPSAC), Box 646, Route #4, Marble Hill, MO, 63764-9725, 573-238-2010, www.napsac.org

Midwives Alliance of North America, 4805 Lawrence Ville Highway, Suite 116-279, Lilburn, GA, 30047, 888-923-6262, www.mana.org

National Association of Childbearing Centers, 3123 Gottschall Road, Perkiomenville, PA, 18074, 215-234-8068, www.BirthCenters.org

POSTPARTUM CARE

MAKING THE CONNECTION

Refer to the following chapters to increase your understanding of postpartum care:

Adult Health Nursing
- **Reproductive System**

Maternal & Pediatric Nursing
- **Prenatal Care**
- **Complications of Pregnancy**
- **The Birth Process**

LEARNING OBJECTIVES

Upon completion of this chapter, you should be able to:
- **Define key terms.**
- **Describe the various aspects of family adaptation.**
- **Discuss the mother's physiologic changes after the birth of her baby.**
- **Describe the expected and unexpected emotional/behavioral changes in the new mother.**
- **Demonstrate the postpartum assessments for every new mother and the additional assessments for a mother who has had a cesarean birth.**
- **Discuss the possible postpartum complications of hemorrhage and puerperal infection, including endometritis, mastitis, and thrombophlebitis.**
- **Explain the advantages and disadvantages of the various methods of family planning.**
- **Plan and provide the care of a woman who has had a baby.**

KEY TERMS

afterpains	mastitis
attachment	metritis
bonding	neonate
claiming process	oophoritis
colostrum	postpartum blues
disseminated	postpartum depression
intravascular	postpartum hemorrhage
coagulation	postpartum psychosis
dyspareunia	puerperal (postpartum)
engorgement	infection
engrossment	puerperium
entrainment	salpingitis
involution	subinvolution
let-down reflex	thrombophlebitis
lochia	

INTRODUCTION

Most problems occur

Postpartum period, or **puerperium,** is the term for the first 6 weeks after the birth of an infant. During this time, the mother and family will experience many changes, including changes in the structure and function of a family. The mother and, if she has one, her partner begin to establish a relationship with their newborn infant and adjust their lives to include the newborn. The mother and partner must also redefine their own relationship. If there are siblings, they must adjust to their new place in the family structure and the newborn's claim on the time and love of the parents.

Many factors influence family adaptation, including previous experience with a newborn and the convenience of a support system. Previously, postpartum care was focused on the mother and newborn, but now the father or partner, siblings, and sometimes grandparents are included. This chapter explores the events of the postpartum period, including the various ways a family adapts to the newborn; the physiologic and psychosocial changes the mother experiences; preparation for discharge; health promotion; postcesarean section care; and possible postpartum complications.

FAMILY ADAPTATION

Family roles and relationships must be reorganized with the birth of a baby. Bonding and attachment are the terms used to describe this process of becoming acquainted with the **neonate** (a newborn from birth to 28 days of life). The terms *bonding* and *attachment* are often used interchangeably, although they do have different meanings. *—4th stage of Delivery.*

3 HRS **Bonding** refers to a rapid process of attachment, parent to child only, taking place during the *sensitive period*, the first 30 to 60 minutes after the birth. The bonding is enhanced when parent and infant touch and interact with each other (Figure 53-1). Immediately after birth, the neonate generally is in a quiet, alert state and is ready for bonding and closeness.

Attachment, a long-term process that begins during pregnancy and intensifies during the postpartum period, establishes an enduring bond between parent and child and develops through reciprocal (parent-to-child and child-to-parent) behaviors. Becoming acquainted with the neonate is an important part of attachment. Touching, exploring, talking to, and using eye contact are all methods used to become acquainted.

The family identifies the infant's "likeness" to and the infant's "differences" from family members, and then the infant's unique qualities. This is often referred to as the **claiming process.**

Mother's Adaptation to Neonate

A mother's touch changes as she moves through a discovery phase with her infant. The mother usually begins by using her fingertips to explore her infant's face, fingers, and toes. This is called *finger-tipping.* The mother may then change to using her palm to stroke her infant's back, chest, arms, and legs. The mother uses her arms to enfold and bring her infant close to her body (Figure 53-2). She may smooth her infant's hair and rub her cheek on the infant's cheek or head. A parent's

CULTURAL CONSIDERATIONS

Touching an Infant

Nurses should be aware that in some cultures (Southeast Asian, Vietnamese, Cambodian, and Laotian), it is considered offensive to pat an infant on the head because the head is viewed as a sacred place where the soul resides (Mattson, 1995).

intense interest and preoccupation in the newborn is termed **engrossment.**

Most mothers speak in a high-pitched voice spontaneously to their infants, seeming to know intuitively that infants respond to higher-pitched voices. Soon after birth, infants can distinguish their mother's voice from others.

Father/Partner's Adaptation to Neonate

A father or partner may also exhibit engrossment and display an intense interest in how the baby looks and responds (Figure 53-3). The father also has a desire to touch and hold his baby.

Research has shown that, for fathers and partners, variables other than being an active participant in the birth process are important in developing attachment to the newborn. They include the father or partner's relationship with his own parents, relationship with the infant's mother, and previous experience with children.

Most fathers want to be involved, but many lack confidence in caring for an infant. Tiller (1995) suggests that information about child care be presented, or reviewed if the father attended prenatal classes, after the infant is born. At this time, the father is eager to learn because the information is now relevant.

Figure 53-1 *Bonding between Parents and Infant after the Birth*

Figure 53-2 *Mother Enfolding and Cuddling Her Infant*

Figure 53-3 *Father Displaying Engrossment*

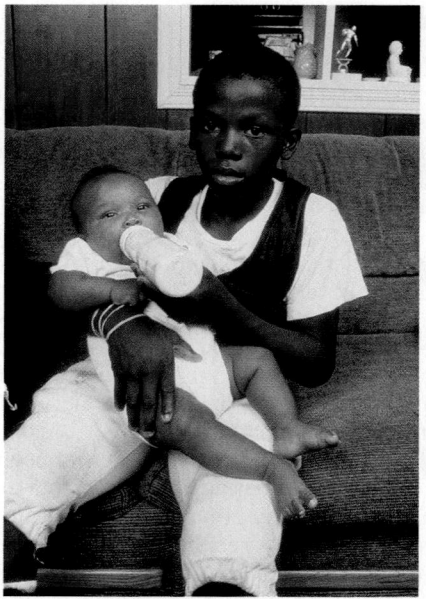

Figure 53-4 *An older sibling can hold or help feed the baby.*

LIFE CYCLE CONSIDERATIONS

Neonates' Reciprocal Behaviors

Neonates have the ability to:

- Make eye contact and move eyes to follow parent's face.
- Engage in intense, prolonged mutual gazing.
- Grasp parent's finger and hold on.
- Move in rhythm to the parent's voice. This is called **entrainment.**

Figure 53-5 *Grandparent Enjoying Grandchild*

Siblings' Adaptation to Neonate

The response of a sibling to the birth of a new sister or brother depends on age and developmental level of the older sibling. The adaptation is probably most difficult for toddlers, who often view the new baby as competition, someone who takes the parent's time and love. Negative behavioral changes may occur in the toddler, such as a return to thumb sucking or bed wetting; sleep problems; or hostility toward the mother, especially when she is caring for the new baby. Positive behavioral changes may be increased independence and taking an interest in the care of the newborn.

Parents' attitudes toward the newborn and their preparation of the siblings for the new arrival guide the older children's reactions. Parents can include each child in the care of the baby according to their capabilities. For example, toddlers may be able to bring a clean diaper to the parent; preschoolers may help prepare for the baby's bath; and older children may hold, carry, or feed the baby (Figure 53-4). Parents need to ensure that siblings are not left out. In addition to allowing the sibling to help with the new baby, parents should provide quality time with the older children.

Grandparents' Adaptation to Neonate

Grandparents go through a transition to grandparenthood just as parents go through a transition to parenthood. Practices and attitudes about childbirth and childrearing change from one generation to another, as do the roles of men and women. The extent to which grandparents understand and accept the current practices and attitudes affects their relationship with their children and how supportive they may be (Figure 53-5).

Factors Affecting Family Adaptation

Many factors affect family adaptation to the newborn:

- *Parental fatigue:* Not being able to sleep uninterrupted through the night may affect the caregivers' energy level.
- *Previous experience with a newborn:* First-time parents and parents with children will progress at different rates through the attachment process.
- *Parental expectations of the newborn:* The newborn's appearance, gender, and behaviors in relation to parental expectations may influence the attachment process.
- *Knowledge of and confidence in providing for newborn needs:* Parents have varying levels of experience in feeding, consoling, and providing care in general to newborns.
- *Temperament of the newborn:* Some infants are calm, easily consoled, and cuddly, whereas others are irritable, difficult to console, and do not like cuddling.
- *Temperament of parents:* Anxious, insecure, excitable parents have more difficulties than calm, secure, less anxious parents.
- *Age of parents:* Teenage, middle-age, and older parents will all react differently to the new family structure based on their life experiences.
- *Available support system:* Help with household tasks and help and encouragement with infant care can ease family adaptation to the newborn.
- *Unexpected events:* Cesarean birth may add stress and increase recovery time, therefore limiting time and energies available for newborn care.

Figure 53-6 *Uterine Involution. Uterine fundal descent is approximately 1 cm/day.*

MATERNAL PHYSIOLOGIC CHANGES

Many of the physiologic changes postpartum (following birth) are a reversal of the changes in the various body systems that occurred during pregnancy. The initiation of lactation and reestablishment of normal menstrual cycles also occur.

Reproductive System

Changes occur in the uterus, cervix, vagina, and perineum.

Uterus

Involution is the return of the uterus to its prepregnancy size and condition. There are three processes involved in involution:

- *Muscle fiber contraction:* With the uterus now empty, the uterus firmly contracts to control bleeding from the area of placental attachment; the muscle fibers gradually regain their former size and shape.
- *Catabolism:* The enlarged muscle cells of the uterus experience catabolic changes in protein cytoplasm

that reduce the size of each cell. Catabolic products are excreted as nitrogenous wastes in the urine.

- *Regeneration:* The endometrium is regenerated within 2 to 3 weeks, except for the placental site, which is healed and regenerated by approximately 6 weeks.

Uterine Fundal Descent Immediately following the birth, the uterus is about the size of a grapefruit, with the fundus about halfway between the umbilicus and symphysis pubis. The fundus then rises to the umbilicus and stays there about 12 hours. Then the fundus descends about 1 cm, 1 finger breadth, each day for about 10 days, when it is once again in the pelvis and unable to be palpated abdominally (Figure 53-6). A full bladder will push the uterus upward.

The contracting uterus may be a source of discomfort for some women after the infant's birth, especially for multiparas and those who are breastfeeding. Breastfeeding stimulates the release of oxytocin from the posterior pituitary, which stimulates strong uterine contractions as well as the "let-down" reflex. These contractions are known as **afterpains.**

Lochia Lochia is the uterine/vaginal discharge after childbirth. It is initially bright red, then changes to a

Lochia

Cultural norms may affect interpretation of postpartum events. For instance, women in Malawi, Africa, are considered "dirty" as long as they have a lochia discharge; sexual intercourse is therefore prohibited for 6 months following birth (Gennaro, Kamwendo, Mbweza, & Kershbaumer, 1998).

pink or pinkish brown, and then to a yellowish white. The odor of lochia is like a normal menstrual flow. A foul odor indicates infection.

For the first 3 days, the lochia is mostly blood with small pieces of decidua and mucus. This is called *lochia rubra.* About the fourth day, the amount decreases and the color changes to a pink or pinkish brown called *lochia serosa.* It is mostly a serous exudate with cervical mucus, erythrocytes, and leukocytes. After the 10th day, the erythrocyte level decreases and the discharge becomes yellowish white, *lochia alba.* Now the lochia consists of leukocytes, epithelial cells, decidua, mucus, serum, and bacteria. This discharge may last for 6 weeks or more (Visness, Kennedy, & Ramos, 1997).

Cervix

Within 18 hours after birth, the cervix has become firm, has shortened, and has regained its form (Lowdermilk & Perry, 2003). By the end of 2 weeks, the cervical os is closed, but after delivery the opening is more like a slit than a circle.

Vagina and Perineum

The vagina was greatly stretched during labor. It takes 6 weeks for the vagina to complete involution and regain the contour it had before pregnancy. It never does regain the size it had before pregnancy. The vaginal mucosa is atrophic in lactating women, at least until menstruation returns. The reduced level of estrogen causes a decrease in vaginal lubrication, which may cause **dyspareunia,** or coital discomfort.

The stretching and thinning of the perineum during labor may cause edema and bruising of the perineum after the birth. Many women have an episiotomy (surgical incision of the perineum) before the infant's birth. Lacerations of the perineum also may occur. Both lacerations and episiotomies are classified according to the tissues involved and will take time to heal:

- *First degree:* skin and mucous membrane
- *Second degree:* skin, mucous membrane, and muscle
- *Third degree:* skin, mucous membrane, muscle, and rectal sphincter

- *Fourth degree:* skin, mucous membrane, muscle, rectal sphincter, and rectal mucosa

Even when the episiotomy or laceration is small, it can cause a great deal of discomfort because the muscles of the perineum are used when sitting, stooping, bending, squatting, walking, and defecating.

Endocrine System

After the expulsion of the placenta, the levels of the placental hormones estrogen, progesterone, human placental lactogen (hPL), human chorionic gonadotropin (hCG), and relaxin rapidly decline. The decrease in hPL, estrogen, and cortisol causes a reversal of the diabetogenic effect of pregnancy. This rapid change necessitates frequent assessment of the diabetic mother's blood glucose level.

Lactation

The rapid decline of the estrogen and progesterone levels allows the prolactin to initiate milk production within 2 to 3 days after the infant's birth. Oxytocin, a posterior pituitary hormone, causes the milk to be expressed from the alveoli into the lactiferous ducts. This is called "let down." The **let-down reflex** is a neurohormonal reflex; that is, either neuro (the mind) or the hormone (oxytocin) may initiate "let down." A breastfeeding mother hearing a baby cry or thinking about feeding her infant often stimulates the let-down reflex, and milk will drip from the nipples (neuro). The release of oxytocin in response to the infant's sucking also stimulates the let-down reflex (hormonal). Many women describe a tingling/burning feeling in the breasts when the milk is "let down."

Menstrual Cycle

There is a great difference when ovulation and menstruation are reestablished based on whether the mother is breastfeeding or not breastfeeding. The level of follicle-stimulating hormone (FSH) is the same in both breastfeeding and nonbreastfeeding mothers. It is believed that the increased level of prolactin in breastfeeding mothers causes the ovaries to not respond to the FSH and ovulation does not occur (Bowes, 2001). The prolactin level remains high in breastfeeding women for approximately 6 weeks. The prolactin level is influenced by three factors: frequency and duration of feedings, supplemental feedings, and possibly the strength of the infant's sucking (Lowdermilk & Perry, 2003). In nonbreastfeeding mothers, the prolactin level returns to the prepregnant level within 2 weeks.

Ovulation in nonbreastfeeding mothers takes place as early as 27 days after the birth and usually has resumed by 2 months (Bowes, 2001). Most nonbreastfeeding mothers resume menstruating within 3 months after the birth.

The average time for ovulation to take place in breastfeeding mothers is approximately 190 days (Bowes, 2001). The return of ovulation and menstruation in breastfeeding mothers is determined, to a large measure, by the breastfeeding pattern. Approximately 25% of breastfeeding mothers ovulate before their menstrual

CULTURAL CONSIDERATIONS

Breastfeeding

- Some Hispanic, Southeast Asian, Vietnamese, Cambodian, and Laotian women may choose not to breastfeed until the milk comes in (Mattson, 1995).
- Many women will breastfeed until the child is 2 years old, based on cultural practices and expectations (Hutchinson & Baqi-Aziz, 1994).

CULTURAL CONSIDERATIONS

Foods in the Postpartum Period

A nurse must be sensitive to the fact that a new mother's food choices and preferences may have cultural or ethnic foundations. For instance:

- Women of Southeast Asia are taught that any food or drink must be hot in temperature and its effect on the body for at least 1 month. Foods are mainly rice and boiled chicken (Davis, 2001).
- Muslim women may request a vegetarian or kosher diet following childbirth (Hutchinson & Baqi-Aziz, 1994).

periods return (Zlatnik, 1999). This underscores the fact that breastfeeding is not a reliable form of birth control.

Breasts

During the last few weeks of pregnancy, the breasts begin to fill with a fluid called colostrum. **Colostrum** is a yellowish fluid rich in antibodies and high in protein. As milk production begins, 2 to 3 days after birth, the breasts feel firm, warm, and may be tender. This lasts about 48 hours. By day 3 or 4 after the birth, **engorgement** may occur; the breasts become quite distended (swollen), tender, and warm. This is caused mainly by vasocongestion, especially of the veins and lymphatics.

The changes in the breasts after the birth of a baby are partly determined by whether the mother is breastfeeding or not. For the nursing mother, frequent breastfeeding sessions will encourage milk production and sustain lactation.

If the mother does not intend to breastfeed, although milk is present it should not be expressed because this causes more milk to be produced. Engorgement spontaneously disappears and discomfort decreases in 24 to 48 hours if the breasts are not emptied of milk. If breastfeeding is never begun or is stopped, lactation ceases within a week.

Gastrointestinal System

Most new mothers are hungry and thirsty after giving birth because of the energy expended during labor. Following recovery from any analgesia or anesthesia the mother may have received, she may request extra food.

Mothers may encounter difficulty in having a bowel movement after giving birth. There are several reasons, including:

- Peristalsis has been decreased by the effects of the increased progesterone level during pregnancy; this may take several days to become normal again.
- Prelabor diarrhea
- Lack of food during labor
- Dehydration
- Perineal trauma, episiotomy repair, or hemorrhoids
- Mother's anticipation of discomfort

Cardiovascular System

The increase in blood volume during pregnancy allows a significant loss of blood without any ill effects to the mother. In a vaginal birth, blood loss averages 500 mL, whereas a cesarean birth averages a 1,000 mL blood loss.

Vital Signs

The new mother's temperature may rise to 100.4°F (38°C) during the first 24 hours because of dehydration during labor and the trauma of delivery. After 24 hours, the temperature should be normal, although it may rise again when milk production begins.

The pulse, which increased during pregnancy, remains elevated or may even rise for up to 24 to 48 hours, but should not exceed 100 beats per minute. Periods of bradycardia may also be experienced. The pulse returns to the prepregnant rate in approximately 8 weeks (Bowes, 2001).

The diaphragm descends when the uterus is emptied, making respirations much easier. In 6 to 8 weeks, respiratory function will return to the prepregnant rate. The blood pressure may have a small increase in both the systolic and diastolic aspects that lasts about 4 days (Bowes, 2001). The rapid decrease in intra-abdominal pressure after birth results in visceral blood vessel dilation, which may cause orthostatic hypotension.

Cardiac Output

Cardiac output, which increased during pregnancy, may increase even higher for up to 60 minutes following delivery. This increase occurs following both vaginal and cesarean births (Bowes, 2001). Cardiac output remains elevated for at least 48 hours, and then rapidly decreases in the first 2 weeks postpartum. The return of cardiac output to the prepregnancy level takes about 24 weeks (Simpson and Creehan, 2001).

Blood Volume

The changes in blood volume are rapid and dramatic. Three physiologic changes protect from excessive blood loss:

- Loss of the uteroplacental circulation (when the placenta is expelled) reduces the maternal vascular bed by 10% to 15%.
- Stimulus for vasodilation is removed with the loss of placental endocrine function.

• Movement of extravascular water, stored during pregnancy, into the blood vessels increases blood volume.

The excess plasma volume is eliminated from the body by both diuresis and diaphoresis. Diuresis (excessive urine excretion) results from a decrease in aldosterone, which was increased during pregnancy. It is not uncommon for a new mother to have a urinary output of 3,000 mL per day for 2 to 3 days (Murray, McKinney, & Gorrie, 2001). Diaphoresis (profuse perspiration), while not clinically significant relative to fluid elimination, may be uncomfortable for the mother, especially if she is not expecting it to occur. It often occurs at night for 2 to 3 nights following delivery.

Blood Values

The white blood cell count, which increased slightly during pregnancy (to 12,000/mm³), now increases to 20,000 or even 30,000/mm³ during the first 10 to 12 days after the infant's birth (Cunningham, Grant, Leveno, Gilstrap, and Cox, 2001). The neutrophil level increases the most for protection against invading organisms.

The large loss of plasma volume during the first 3 days after the birth results in a rise in both the hemoglobin and hematocrit levels by the seventh day, unless excessive blood loss has occurred.

Coagulation

The increased levels of clotting factors and fibrinogen during pregnancy remain elevated for a few days as protection against postpartum hemorrhage. Thus, there is an increased risk for thrombus (clot) formation. Mothers having varicose veins, a cesarean birth, or a history of thrombophlebitis are at greater risk for thrombus formation.

Varicosities

Varices of the legs, anus (hemorrhoids), and vulvar area empty rapidly immediately after the birth.

Urinary System

Physical changes take place in the structures of the urinary system; there are also chemical changes in the urine.

Physical Changes

The hypotonia of the bladder and dilation of the ureters during pregnancy take approximately 2 to 8 weeks to return to the prepregnant state (Cunningham et al., 2001). Also, the bladder, urethra, and tissue around the urinary meatus may have been traumatized and become edematous during labor and birth, which may result in difficulty in urination.

The mother may have a problem with overdistention and incomplete emptying of the bladder and residual retention of urine because the diuresis causes the bladder to fill quickly. Those mothers who received a regional anesthesia are especially at risk for bladder distention and difficulty voiding until the anesthesia wears off.

Postpartum hemorrhage and urinary tract infection are two complications related to urinary retention and bladder overdistention. Urinary stasis provides the bacteria with enough time to multiply and cause an infection. A full bladder displaces the uterus up and to the side, resulting in uterine atony (inability of the uterus to contract). This is the primary cause of excessive bleeding. Adequate emptying of the bladder helps the bladder regain its tone in 5 to 7 days after the birth (Lowdermilk & Perry, 2003).

Chemical Changes

The catabolic processes of uterine involution cause a mild proteinuria for 1 to 2 days in approximately 50% of new mothers (Simpson & Creehan, 2001). Ketonuria and elevated blood urea nitrogen (BUN) may also be present.

Musculoskeletal System

The musculoskeletal changes that occur during pregnancy are reversed during the postpartum period.

Joints, Ligaments, and Cartilage

As the level of the hormone relaxin decreases, the ligaments and cartilage, especially of the pelvis, begin to revert to their prepregnant positions. Hip or joint pain may be noticed as these changes take place. Joints, cartilage, and ligaments are stabilized by 6 to 8 weeks after the birth.

All joints return to their normal prepregnant state, except those in the feet. The new mother may discover a permanent increase in her shoe size (Lowdermilk & Perry, 2003).

Abdominal Muscles

Many new mothers, when they stand up, are dismayed when the abdominal muscles protrude, giving a still-pregnant appearance. It usually takes 6 weeks for the abdominal muscles to return almost to their prepregnant state (Lowdermilk & Perry, 2003). Previous muscle tone, proper exercise, and the amount of adipose tissue all influence the return of muscle tone.

Integumentary System

The level of melanocyte-stimulating hormone (MSH) declines rapidly after the birth, and the areas of hyperpigmentation begin to lighten in color. In some women, however, the linea nigra and the darkened nipple areola may remain dark. Most of the skin's elasticity returns, but some striae may still be visible as small or large silver streaks on the breasts, abdomen, buttocks, or thighs.

Spider angiomas (nevi) and palmar erythema usually fade with the decrease in the estrogen level. In some women, however, they do stay.

Any fine hair appearing during pregnancy usually disappears; however, any coarse or bristly hair appearing during pregnancy may remain.

Neurologic System

Any pregnancy-induced neurologic discomforts usually lessen after birth (Lowdermilk & Perry, 2003); however, fatigue, afterpains, muscle aches, episiotomy or abdominal incision pain, and breast engorgement all may create maternal discomfort. If the mother received an analgesic or anesthesia, she may experience a temporary loss of feeling in her legs and dizziness.

The mother who has a headache must be carefully assessed. If the mother had a regional anesthesia (epidural or spinal), the headache may be caused by a leakage of cerebrospinal fluid into the extradural space during needle placement; this is known as a spinal headache. This headache is generally more severe when the mother sits or stands and is relieved when she lies down. If the mother has blurred vision, photophobia, and abdominal pain with a headache, it may indicate that she is developing pregnancy-induced hypertension (PIH), or if she had PIH during pregnancy, that it is getting worse.

Weight Loss

Immediate weight loss is the sum of the infant's weight, placenta, amniotic fluid, and blood loss. Typically, this is approximately 13 lbs. During the next 6 weeks, an additional 8 to 9 lbs is lost as the result of diuresis, diaphoresis, and the involution of the reproductive organs. It takes most mothers approximately 6 months to return to their prepregnant weight, and some may take an entire year. The energy required for breastfeeding may assist in the weight loss process.

MATERNAL PSYCHOSOCIAL CHANGES

Both expected and unexpected emotional/behavioral changes may be encountered. The effects of early discharge must also be considered.

Expected Changes

Expected emotional/behavioral changes include those restorative/adaptive phases described by Reva Rubin, postpartum "blues," and those related to a cesarean birth.

Rubin's Restorative/Adaptive Phases

Rubin (1961) described three phases of maternal restoration/adaptation: *taking-in*, *taking-hold*, and *letting-go*.

Taking-In Phase This phase is focused mainly on the mother's need for food, fluid, and sleep. The mother's behavior is passive as she takes in the physical care and attention from others. She depends on others to meet her needs. Rubin (1961) described this as the phase of nurturing and protective care lasting 2 to 3 days. Studies by Ament (1990) and Wrasper (1996) confirmed the behavior described by Rubin but noted that the behavior was present only during the first 24 hours after birth.

Integration of the labor and birth experience into reality is the major task of the mother at this time. It is important for her to discuss the details of the labor and birth, especially with the nurse(s) who cared for her. She

---

COMMUNITY/HOME HEALTH CARE

Coping with Taking-Hold Phase

- Acknowledge parents' anxiety about caretaking abilities.
- Provide information about infant behaviors.
- Allow parents to provide infant care (nurse should not take over) even if performed awkwardly.
- Praise parents' caregiving efforts.
- Provide parents with a contact and phone number in the event they have questions.

---

is thus able to clarify details about her experience that she may not remember because of the effects of medication or the natural sleep and amnesia between contractions, especially in the second stage of labor. By describing to family and friends the birth experience, the mother realizes that the pregnancy is past and the infant is now a separate individual.

The father or partner may also experience a taking-in phase as he is congratulated on the birth of the infant. Family members often treat him in a special way.

Taking-Hold Phase In the taking-hold phase, the mother becomes more independent as she takes an interest in and responsibility for her own physical care. Her focus shifts to the care of her infant. She welcomes opportunities to learn about the behavior of infants and to practice caring for her infant. Martell (1996) and Wrasper (1996) believe that childbirth preparation classes, pain management practices, early newborn contact, rooming-in, and early discharge enhance taking-hold behaviors. Because most mothers are discharged during this phase, which lasts approximately 10 days, continued coping with the physical and emotional/behavioral changes at home is required.

The father or partner's interest in infant behaviors and care is similar to the mother's in the taking-hold phase. He may also be anxious but is usually willing to learn.

Letting-Go Phase If this is a first baby, the mother and father/partner must give up the role and carefree lifestyle of being only a couple. They are now a couple with a child.

The expected birth experience may not have been realized. For example, a planned vaginal birth with no anesthesia may have changed to a cesarean birth and/or use of regional anesthesia. The parents must let go of the planned experience and accept what really happened.

For some mothers and/or fathers, the newborn infant does not fit the expected baby they dreamed of and talked about during pregnancy. They may be disappointed in the gender, size, or other characteristics of the infant. Now they must let go of their expectations and accept the reality of their infant.

The mother and father let go of their role of "expecting" and move forward as a unit with a new member. They establish a lifestyle that includes the child and their role as parents. Time must be made for sharing adult activities and interests.

Postpartum Blues

Postpartum blues or "baby blues" is a mild, transient condition of emotional lability and crying for no apparent reason that affects up to 80% of women who have just given birth and lasts about 2 weeks (Albright, 1993). Other symptoms include fatigue, anxiety, restlessness, let-down feeling, headache, and sadness. The etiology is unknown. This is a self-limiting situation that begins about 3 days, peaks about 5 days, and disappears approximately 10 days after birth.

Cesarean Birth

When a cesarean birth is an emergency (unplanned), the taking-in phase may last longer because these mothers also need to accept and understand the events that made the cesarean birth necessary. It is important for the nurse to understand that these mothers are surgical clients requiring immediate physical care to restore or maintain physiologic health. When pain, bleeding, and incision care are under control, the nurse can help the mother understand the birth and incorporate the experience into her reality.

Some mothers may have feelings of frustration, anger, low self-esteem, or disappointment that they could not have their baby the "normal way" (vaginal birth). At the same time, they are relieved, happy, and filled with gratitude that the infant had a safe birth and is healthy. It may be a time of many, often opposing, emotions.

Unexpected Changes

Unexpected emotional/behavioral changes include postpartum depression, postpartum psychosis, and reaction to an infant with problems.

Postpartum Depression

Postpartum depression (PPD) is similar to postpartum blues but is more serious, intense, and persistent. Approximately 12% of new mothers experience a syndrome more severe than postpartum blues (Albright, 1993; Green & Adams, 1993; Lowdermilk & Perry, 2003). PPD may be mild, moderate, or severe, with symptoms becoming more numerous and intense as the severity increases.

The mother with mild PPD cares lovingly for her infant but is unable to feel the love. She may express feelings of irritability, guilt, shame, unworthiness, and a sense of loss of self. Symptoms persist past the first few weeks after the infant's birth.

Moderate PPD is characterized by spontaneous crying, insomnia or hypersomnia, fatigue, decreased concentration, and sometimes food cravings. *or not eating.*

With severe PPD, the irritability of the mother may explode into violent outbursts or uncontrollable crying often directed toward significant others. She often will not discuss her symptoms or negative feelings toward the infant, which may include disinterest, annoyance with care demands, or even thoughts of harming the infant.

Psychotherapy and pharmacological interventions are generally required. Sometimes, hospitalization is necessary.

Postpartum Psychosis

Postpartum psychosis is more severe than PPD and is characterized by delusions and thoughts of self-harm or infant harm. This condition is rare, occurring in 0.1% to 0.2% of births (Kaplan, Sadock, & Grebb, 1998). Symptoms usually begin within 2 to 3 weeks after the birth. The symptoms include fatigue, restlessness, insomnia, crying, labile emotions, inability to move, irrational statements, incoherence, confusion, and obsessive concerns about the infant's health. Approximately 50% have delusions and 25% have hallucinations (Lowdermilk & Perry, 2003).

Postpartum psychosis is a psychiatric emergency. Kaplan et al. (1998) report on a study in which 5% of clients with postpartum psychosis committed suicide and 4% committed infanticide. The mother is usually hospitalized and provided both pharmacological support and psychotherapy.

Infant with a Problem

It may be difficult for the mother and/or father to bond with and attach to an infant born preterm or with physical or functional anomalies (Figure 53-7). The parents may have feelings of guilt that they, somehow, caused the infant's problem. Either or both of the parents may not be able to accept an infant who does not look like a normal, healthy infant. When one parent's reaction to the infant

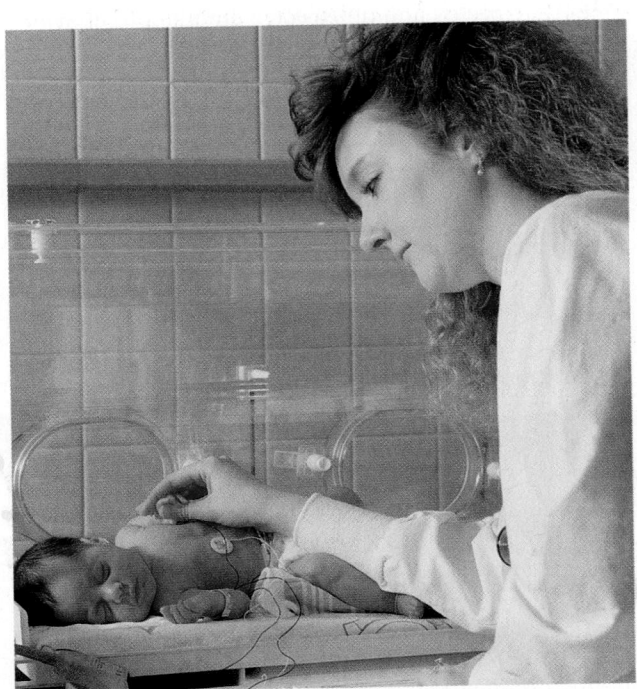

Figure 53-7 *Parents of an infant who requires special medical care should be encouraged to spend as much time with their child as possible.*

with a problem is opposite that of the other's, there may be a terrific strain on their relationship.

DISCHARGE

In an effort to reduce health care costs and meet consumer demand for a more family-centered experience with less medical intervention, the short hospital stay came into existence (Wilkerson, 1996). In the 1950s, most new mothers remained in the hospital 5 days for a vaginal birth and 7 days for a cesarean birth. The stays were gradually reduced to 3 days for a vaginal birth and 5 days for a cesarean birth. For several years in the early 1990s, third-party payers (health plans and insurance companies) mandated discharge within 24 hours for a vaginal birth and 72 hours or less for a cesarean birth.

Health care professionals became concerned about client (mother and infant) safety because many problems do not show up in the first 24 hours after birth. The time for assessing bonding/attachment and parenting behaviors was almost eliminated. Parents were barely acquainted with their infant and client teaching about newborn care, and identifying health problems such as dehydration, jaundice, and breastfeeding difficulties had to be rushed (Havens & Hannan, 1996).

The federal government passed the Newborns' and Mothers' Health Protection Act of 1996, which requires all health plans to allow a stay of 48 hours following vaginal birth and 96 hours following a cesarean birth (Health Care Financing Administration, 2002). Self-insured health plans must comply with this act. Group insurance plans and individual insurance may not have to comply if the client lives in a state having a law with certain protections for hospital stays after childbirth. More than 40 states and the District of Columbia have such laws (Health Care Financing Administration, 2002).

Follow-up home care is being utilized in many areas. This may be a telephone call or two to see how the mother and infant are doing, or it may include actual home visits.

NURSING PROCESS

Assessment

Assessments specific to the first few days postpartum include BUBBLE (breasts, uterus, bladder, bowel, lochia, and episiotomy), vital signs, lower extremities and Homans' sign, bonding/attachment, parenting, activity, comfort, and self-care. These assessments are usually performed, at least once a shift, until the mother is discharged. A sample initial postpartum profile sheet is shown in Figure 53-8.

Infection Control: Standard Precautions in Postpartum Care

Gloves should be worn when:
- Assessing the breasts if there is leakage of colostrum or milk
- Handling used breast pads
- Assessing lochia and the perineum

CLIENT TEACHING

Breast Assessment

- Explain the characteristics of the breast and what to expect depending on whether the mother is breastfeeding or not.
- Describe how to recognize problems such as mastitis and nipple fissures or cracks.

- Changing peripads or chux
- Handling anything on which there is lochia (bed linen, towels, washcloth, clothing, peripads, chux)

Subjective Data

Ask the mother whether the milk has come in or whether there is any breast discomfort; whether the bladder feels empty after urination; whether the mother is able to pass gas rectally or has the urge to have a bowel movement; whether any clots are passed vaginally and when the peripad was last changed; whether there is dizziness when getting up; whether contractions are felt during breastfeeding; or whether there is discomfort or pain, especially in the perineal area.

Objective Data

Breasts

Note the size and shape of the breasts and any abnormalities or reddened areas. The breasts should be gently palpated for softness, firmness, engorgement, warmth, or tenderness. Check the nipples for cracks, fissures, soreness, and inversion.

Uterus

Palpate the abdomen to find the top (fundus) of the uterus by pressing in and down with the side of one hand, and placing the other hand above the symphysis to support the uterus. The size, consistency, and placement (midline or off to one side) of the uterus is noted. It should be firm (not boggy) and in the midline. Each day it should descend approximately 1 cm (1 finger breadth). Fundal descent is documented in relation to the umbilicus (Figure 53-9).

CLIENT TEACHING

Assessing the Fundus

- Explain why it is important for the uterus to be firmly contracted.
- Demonstrate how to palpate the uterine fundus.
- Demonstrate the way to gently massage the fundus.

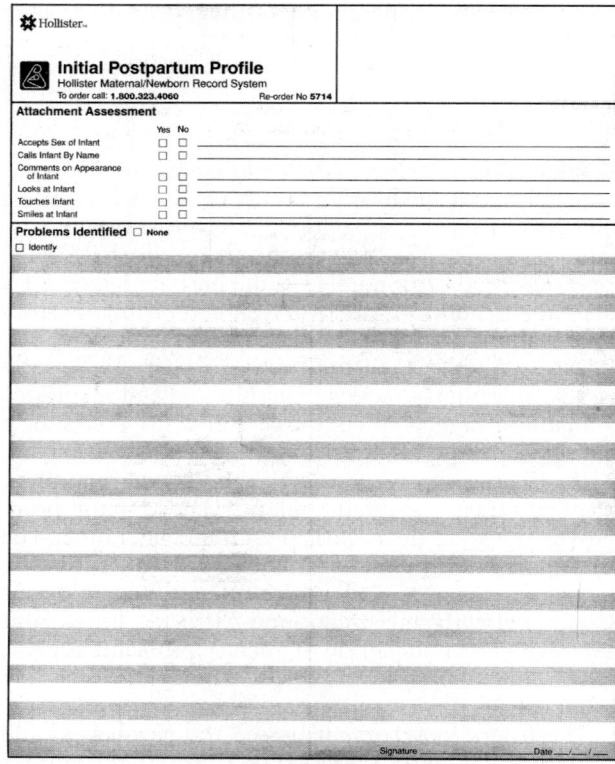

Figure 53-8 *Representative Initial Postpartum Profile (Permission to use this copyright material has been granted by the owner, Hollister Incorporated.)*

Figure 53-9 *The nurse supports the uterus with her left hand held beneath it while palpating the uterus to determine if it is firm or boggy and its position, midline or displaced.*

Bladder

When the abdomen is palpated for the uterine fundus, the bladder can also be palpated for distention. A full, distended bladder is very often the cause for the fundus to be higher than it should be and to be positioned off to one side (not in the midline) (Figure 53-10). An intake and output (I&O) record is kept during the first 24 hours, at least, to assist in identifying urine retention.

CLIENT TEACHING

Bladder and Bowel Elimination

Encourage the new mother to:

- Drink plenty of fluids.
- Ambulate frequently and use the bathroom, not a bedpan.
- Eat a well-balanced diet with increased fiber and fluids.
- Promptly answer nature's call to urinate or defecate.

Bowels

Inspect the abdomen for distention and auscultate for the presence of bowel sounds. The client's labor record should be reviewed to check whether she received an enema. The anus can be inspected when the episiotomy is checked.

Lochia

Ask the mother to lie on her back with knees flexed so the peripad can be lowered in the front. Lochia is assessed for color, amount, odor, and presence of clots. Then ask the mother to turn to her side to see whether any lochia has pooled under her buttocks.

CLIENT TEACHING

Lochia Assessment

- Describe the expected changes in the color and amount of lochia.
- Advise the mother that if the lochia changes from serosa back to rubra, she is either doing too much heavy work or the uterus is not firmly contracted. The mother should check fundal firmness and rest for a while.
- Instruct mother to notify her CNM/physician if clots are passed or if the lochia has an unusual or unpleasant odor.

Figure 53-10 *A full bladder displaces the uterus and prevents its contractions.*

Figure 53-11 *Assessment of lochia is based on the amount of blood saturation on a peripad.* **A,** Scant: *2-inch stain (10 mL).* **B,** Small: *4-inch stain (10-25 mL).* **C,** Moderate: *6-inch stain (25-50 mL).* **D,** Large: >6-inch stain (50-80 mL).

Amount It is difficult to estimate the amount of lochia on a perineal pad. Luegenbiehl, Brophy, Artigue, Phillips, and Flack (1990) identified a method to estimate the amount of lochia discharged in 1 hour (Figure 53-11).

The mother who has had a cesarean birth will have less lochia after the first 24 hours than a mother who had a vaginal birth. The lochia also usually changes from rubra to serosa sooner because the inside of the uterus is wiped with sponges during a cesarean birth, removing some of the endometrium.

Odor Lochia has a nonoffensive odor. If the lochia has a foul odor, an infection is present and the CNM/physician must be notified at once.

Presence of Clots A few small clots, which occur when blood pools in the vagina, are normal. Passing many or large clots is not normal and requires further investigation.

Episiotomy

Assess the episiotomy with the mother in Sims' position (Figure 53-12). This can be done when the mother is on her side for lochia assessment. With a gloved hand, very gently raise the upper buttock just enough to see the episiotomy. Changes in the episiotomy should be noted, such as the following:

- Redness—inflammation
- Ecchymosis—bruising
- Edema—swelling
- Discharge—from incision
- Approximation of suture line

ICE PACK SITZ BATH or WARM WATER

With the client in the same position, gently touch the external labia and note whether this causes pain. The labia should also be inspected for ecchymosis and edema. The anus can be inspected for hemorrhoids.

Figure 53-12 *The episiotomy is assessed with the mother lying on her side. The upper buttock is raised gently, just enough to see the episiotomy. The anal area can be assessed for hemorrhoids at the same time.*

Figure 53-13 *Homans' Sign Assessment. Discomfort experienced in the calf when the foot is sharply dorsiflexed is considered positive and may indicate thrombophlebitis.*

CLIENT TEACHING

Techniques to Decrease Episiotomy Discomfort

Instruct mother to:

- Tighten her buttocks and perineum before sitting to prevent pulling on the episiotomy and perineal area, and to release the tightening after being seated.
- Rest several times a day with feet elevated.
- Practice the Kegel exercise many times a day to increase circulation to the perineal area and to strengthen the perineal muscles.

Vital Signs

Assess vital signs every 15 minutes for the first 1 to 2 hours after birth. If no problems are identified, vital signs may then be checked every 8 hours.

Temperature   Temperature may increase to 100.4°F (38°C) during the first 24 hours. After the first 24 hours, a temperature over 100.4°F suggests an infection.

Pulse   After the first hour following the birth, the mother's pulse rate may decrease to 50 to 70 beats/minute for 6 to 8 days. An elevated pulse may indicate excessive blood loss, infection, anxiety, or pain.

Blood Pressure   Blood pressure should remain consistent with the baseline during pregnancy. An increase suggests PIH, whereas a decrease may indicate excessive bleeding.

Lower Extremities and Homans' Sign

Examine the mother's legs for signs of thrombophlebitis such as redness, heat, edema, and tenderness. Palpate the pedal pulses. Perform the assessment for Homans' sign.

To assess for Homans' sign, support the client's leg under the knee while sharply dorsiflexing the foot (Figure 53-13). Homans' sign is positive if the client experiences calf discomfort when the foot is dorsiflexed and negative if the client does not experience discomfort in the calf. When Homans' sign is positive, it must be reported at once to the CNM/physician because it may indicate thrombophlebitis.

Bonding/Attachment

Assess the interaction of the mother with her infant for the expected behaviors of bonding and beginning attachment. The manner in which the mother holds, examines, and speaks to the infant is important. For instance, the mother who cradles her infant, gazes at her infant's face, and speaks in a pleasant manner to the infant is exhibiting signs of bonding and attachment.

Parenting

Assess the skill with which the mother cares for her infant. For example, observe feeding, diapering, bathing, and consoling skills to determine whether additional teaching is required.

CULTURAL CONSIDERATIONS

Rest

Expectations of maternal activity during the postpartum period may be influenced by cultural norms. For example:

- Korean women rest an average of 21 days following birth (Howard & Berbiglia, 1997).
- Southeast Asian, Vietnamese, Cambodian, and Laotian women stay in bed without a pillow and keep warm for 2 days (Mattson, 1995).

Activity

Determine that the mother is ambulating, that is, getting up to go to the bathroom and frequently walking around. Many complications such as thromboses, emboli, and hypostatic pneumonia occur when the mother is in bed for extended periods.

Rest is just as important as activity. The mother expended a great deal of energy during labor and birth. Care should be planned so the mother has some uninterrupted periods of rest.

 Safety: First Ambulation
The first time a new mother gets out of bed, the nurse should be at her side and ready to assist in case the mother becomes lightheaded, weak, or dizzy.

Comfort

Comfort is essential to rest. Many new mothers never say anything about discomforts because they are so excited and pleased with their new infant. Be alert to any behavioral signs of discomfort. Most discomfort is related to perineal pain or afterpains.

Self-Care — *Teach about*

Assessment of self-care includes the mother's knowledge of how to care for herself and also whether she actually performs the care. Self-care includes showering, perineal care, checking the fundus, breast care, and rest. Support the client's recovery by encouraging her to bathe, toilet, and feed herself independently.

Nursing diagnoses for a postpartum mother may include the following:

Nursing Diagnoses	Planning/Goals	Nursing Interventions
Impaired **U**rinary *Elimination,* related to sensory motor impairment from bladder trauma during labor and birth	The mother will have appropriate urinary elimination (no bladder distention).	Monitor intake for adequate amount. Assess for bladder distention every 2 to 4 hours. Assist client to bathroom for elimination. Pour warm water over vulvar area or run water in the sink to stimulate urination. Catheterize, if necessary, as ordered.
Risk for **I**nfection related to episiotomy	The mother will have no signs of infection.	Assess episiotomy for redness and swelling. Teach mother pericare: wash hands, remove peripad from front to back, pour warm water over perineum, pat dry from front to back, apply clean peripad front first then toward the back, wash hands. Advise client to change peripad every 2 to 4 hours and every time she goes to the bathroom.
Acute **P**ain, related to episiotomy, engorged breasts, or involution of the uterus	The mother will state that discomfort has decreased.	*Episiotomy* Assess perineum for edema. Apply ice pack for 20 minutes; remove for at least 10 minutes before reapplying. Assist mother with Sitz bath as ordered, and watch for dizziness, floating feeling, or difficulty hearing (signs of possible fainting). Apply Dermoplast spray or Americain spray (topical anesthetics) to perineum after a sitz bath or pericare, as ordered. Emphasize the need to wash hands before and after any care of the episiotomy. Teach mother to squeeze buttocks together before sitting, release after sitting. Encourage mother to practice Kegel exercise 4 or 5 times a day. Administer analgesic as ordered. Avoid using rectal suppositories for clients with 3rd- or 4th-degree episiotomy *Engorged Breasts* (not breastfeeding) Encourage mother to wear a well-fitting supportive bra, removing it only for showers, to suppress lactation. Provide ice pack to axillary area and side of breast for 20 minutes 4 times a day to suppress lactation. Advise mother to avoid any stimulation to breast; stand with back to shower so warm water does not hit breasts. Administer analgesic as ordered.

Review

continues

Nursing Diagnoses	Planning/Goals	Nursing Interventions
		Engorged Breasts (breastfeeding)
		Encourage the mother to feed her infant approximately every 2 hours; empty (until soft) one breast; then feed from second breast or pump to soften.
		Administer antiinflammatory pain medication as ordered.
		Apply ice pack between feedings for 15 minutes on and 45 minutes off as ordered.
		Involution of Uterus (afterpains)
		Assess fundus for firmness and position.
		Determine when mother has pain.
		Explain, if mother is breastfeeding, that the oxytocin released in response to breastfeeding causes the uterus to contract. The discomfort lasts only a few minutes at the beginning of each breastfeeding session for the first 4 to 6 days.
		Administer analgesic as ordered.

Evaluation Each goal must be evaluated to determine how it has been met by the client.

HEALTH PROMOTION

The mother's record must be checked to determine the mother's need for Rh immune globulin (RhoGAM) and rubella immunization. When required, these two items protect the fetuses of future pregnancies.

Rh Immune Globulin

Rh immune globulin (RhoGAM) is given within 72 hours after birth to prevent sensitization of Rh-negative mothers who gave birth to Rh-positive infants. The RhoGAM promotes lysis of fetal Rh-positive red blood cells before the mother's body is able to form antibodies against them.

Rubella Immunization

It is recommended that all women who have not had rubella or who have a 1:8 rubella titer be given rubella vaccine in the immediate postpartum period. This will prevent fetal anomalies in future pregnancies if the mother is exposed to rubella. Breastfeeding is not a contraindication to receiving the immunization. Because the vaccine may be teratogenic, pregnancy must be avoided for 2 to 3 months.

PROFESSIONAL TIP

Rh Immune Globulin (RhoGAM) Administration

RhoGAM is administered intramuscularly to Rh-negative, antibody-negative (Coombs' negative) mothers who gave birth to an Rh-positive infant. It is never given to the infant.

CESAREAN BIRTH

All of the assessments just discussed are also performed on a mother who has had a cesarean birth. In addition, postoperative assessments are performed, including incision, respirations and breath sounds, abdomen and bowel sounds, fluid intake, urine output, and the degree of pain. *Respiratory status.*

Incision

Inspect the dressing for intactness and any bleeding or discharge. After the dressing is removed, assess the incision for signs of infection such as redness, heat, pain, or edema and the suture line for approximation.

Respirations and Breath Sounds *Respiratory*

If the mother received narcotics either epidurally or with patient-controlled analgesia (PCA), assess respirations frequently because narcotics depress the respiratory center. Assess respiratory rate and depth every 15 minutes for the first hour, every 30 minutes for the next 4 to 5 hours, and every hour for the remainder of the first 24 hours. Some institutions may use an apnea monitor. Auscultate breath sounds at each respiratory check to identify whether secretions are beginning to pool in the bronchioles. Assess the client's efforts of turning (changing position), coughing, deep breathing, and use of the incentive spirometer.

Abdomen and Bowel Sounds

In addition to the incision, assess the abdomen for softness or distention. Auscultate bowel sounds until peristalsis is noted in all four quadrants. Ask the mother whether she has been able to pass any flatus (gas) rectally.

SAMPLE NURSING CARE PLAN

THE POSTPARTUM CLIENT

Sophia and Jack Viernot have just participated in the birth of their first child, a daughter, weighing 6 lbs, 8 oz and measuring 21 inches long. A small episiotomy was made. Jack has "always wanted a son" and is "disappointed about having a daughter." He looks at the infant but does not touch her or speak to her.

Sophia is exhausted from the labor and birth, says she is too tired to hold the baby, and wants only to sleep. Her vital signs are within normal range, and the uterus tends to relax. Within $1^1/_2$ hours, she has saturated three peripads. A bulge is noted above the symphysis. Sophia is unable to urinate at this time.

Nursing Diagnosis 1 *Risk for Deficient Fluid Volume* related to early postpartum hemorrhage as evidenced by saturating three peripads in $1^1/_2$ hours

Nursing Outcomes Classification (NOC)
Fluid Balance

Nursing Interventions Classification (NIC)
Bleeding Reduction

PLANNING/GOALS	NURSING INTERVENTIONS	RATIONALE
Sophia's fluid volume will be maintained by reducing the amount of lochia discharge.	Palpate and monitor fundal height, location, and consistency.	Determines status of uterus (firm or boggy) and height and location relative to umbilicus.
	For boggy uterus, gently massage and assess muscle tone.	Promotes uterine contraction and increases uterine tone.
	Monitor lochia (amount and color), time peripad changed, and degree of peripad saturation.	Evaluates the amount of lochia.
	Assess for bladder fullness and encourage voiding.	A full bladder interferes with contracting of the uterus.
	Monitor intake and output.	Identifies potential need to urinate.
	Monitor vital signs, skin temperature, and color.	Detects signs of shock.
	Administer oxytocic agent as ordered.	Promotes uterine contraction.
	Explain involution process to Sophia and teach her to check and gently massage her uterus.	Involves Sophia in self-care.

EVALUATION   Sophia's fluid volume is maintained when voiding allows the uterus to contract and the amount of lochia to decrease.

Nursing Diagnosis 2 *Risk for Impaired Parenting* related to not gender desired as evidenced by Jack expressing a desire for a son, showing seeming disappointment with a daughter, not touching or speaking to the infant, and Sophia saying she is too tired to hold the baby

Nursing Outcomes Classification (NOC)
Parent–Infant Attachment

Nursing Interventions Classification (NIC)
Attachment Promotion
Environmental Management: Attachment Process

PLANNING/GOALS	NURSING INTERVENTIONS	RATIONALE
Sophia and Jack will demonstrate bonding and attachment behaviors with their daughter.	Assist Sophia in holding her daughter.	Emphasizes holding infant as important.
	Point out unique characteristics about the infant (e.g., dimple in right cheek, long fingers).	Helps Sophia and Jack get acquainted with their daughter.

continues

SAMPLE NURSING CARE PLAN

Ask Sophia and Jack who the infant looks like.	Assists Sophia and Jack in identifying family characteristics.
Model bonding and attachment behaviors for Sophia and Jack such as talking to infant, finger-tipping, and examining infant.	Shows Sophia and Jack how to interact with their daughter.
Describe infant's behavior and explain that the infant can see and hear her parents.	Enables Sophia and Jack to understand their infant and her abilities.

EVALUATION   Sophia follows nurse's example and strokes the infant's head and face with her fingertips and talks to her. Jack touches the infant's fingers but does not watch her intently or for longer than a few seconds.

Nursing Diagnosis 3 *Impaired Urinary Elimination* related to sensory motor impairment as evidenced by inability to urinate and bulge noted above the symphysis

Nursing Outcomes Classification (NOC)
Neurologic Status

Nursing Interventions Classification (NIC)
Urinary Retention Care
Urinary Catheterization

PLANNING/GOALS	NURSING INTERVENTIONS	RATIONALE
Sophia will have regular urinary elimination with no bladder distention.	Palpate bulge above symphysis while asking Sophia whether bladder feels full.	Confirms that bulge is a full bladder.
	Assist Sophia to the bathroom or onto bedpan if she is unable to ambulate.	Allows Sophia to empty her bladder.
	Run water in sink, place Sophia's hands in warm water, or pour water over her perineum.	Stimulates urination.
	Administer analgesic as ordered if Sophia has vulvar/perineal discomfort and is afraid to void.	Relieves discomfort; may help Sophia relax and void.
	Catheterize if necessary, as ordered.	Empties bladder, allowing uterus to contract and promoting comfort.

EVALUATION   Sophia empties her bladder when assisted to the bathroom.

Nursing Diagnosis 4 *Risk for Infection* related to inadequate primary defenses as evidenced by episiotomy and low pH of lochia

Nursing Outcomes Classification (NOC)
Tissue Integrity: Skin & Mucous Membranes

Nursing Interventions Classification (NIC)
Infection Protection

PLANNING/GOALS	NURSING INTERVENTIONS	RATIONALE
Sophia will have no evidence of infection.	Follow Standard Precautions, especially good hand hygiene before and after providing care, and wear gloves when contact with lochia or urine is possible.	Prevents spread of infection.
	Use strict aseptic technique when inserting a catheter or starting an intravenous infusion.	Reduces the risk of a nosocomial infection.

continues

SAMPLE NURSING CARE PLAN

Monitor vital signs.	If elevated, may indicate an infection.
Monitor for loss of appetite, malaise, and chills.	May indicate infection.
Assess episiotomy for redness, edema, drainage, and pain; and lochia for a foul odor.	Indicates infection.
Teach Sophia proper perineal care.	Keeps perineum clean and prevents contamination of episiotomy by anal organisms.

EVALUATION Sophia has no signs of infection.

Fluid Intake

Frequently assess the flow rate of intravenous fluids as well as the site. Record the amount of intravenous fluid and any oral fluid intake.

Urine Output

A Foley catheter is generally inserted into the bladder before the cesarean birth. Assess and record the amount of urine output as well as the clarity and color.

Pain

Most new mothers who have a vaginal birth are eager to interact with their newborn infant. This is no different following a cesarean birth; however, these mothers will need to be taught how to hold and carry the infant in a way that will not disturb or irritate their incisions. The mothers may not want pain medication because they want to stay awake with and enjoy their infants.

Breastfeeding mothers who have had a cesarean birth may also not admit to having pain because they are concerned that pain medication will be present in the breast milk. Pain medication is generally required for 24 to 48 hours following a cesarean birth. These mothers can be taught to support the baby with a pillow to avoid incisional pain while nursing.

COMPLICATIONS

The most common complications of childbirth are postpartum hemorrhage, infection, thromboembolic conditions, and disseminated intravascular coagulation.

POSTPARTUM HEMORRHAGE

Postpartum hemorrhage is defined as a blood loss of more than 500 mL after the third stage of labor or 1,000 mL after a cesarean birth. The hemorrhage is identified as either early, within the first 24 hours, or late, generally occurring 1 to 2 weeks after the birth, but may occur up to 6 weeks after the birth.

A postpartum hemorrhage can occur rapidly and may not be recognized until the client is in moderate to severe shock (Table 53-1).

EARLY POSTPARTUM HEMORRHAGE

Early postpartum hemorrhage has several possible causes: uterine atony, retained placental fragments, lacerations of the birth canal, and hematomas. Predisposing factors for postpartum hemorrhage include the following:

- Overdistention of the uterus (large infant, multiple gestation, or hydramnios)
- Grandmultiparity (more than 5)
- Precipitate labor or birth
- Prolonged labor
- Use of forceps or vacuum extractor
- Use of tocolytic drugs
- Use of oxytocin to augment or induce labor
- Cesarean birth
- Manual removal of the placenta
- Clotting disorders

Uterine Atony

Uterine atony is a lack of muscle tone in the uterus. The uterus feels soft and boggy. Hemorrhage from uterine atony is usually a steady flow. Blood pressure and pulse changes may not occur until the blood loss is severe because during pregnancy there is an increase in blood volume.

Retained Placental Fragments

Occasionally, small pieces of the placenta may not be expelled. These pieces prevent the uterus from contracting effectively, and bleeding continues.

TABLE 53-1   HEMORRHAGIC SHOCK

	BP	PULSE	RESP	SKIN	URINE OUTPUT	BLOOD LOSS	LEVEL OF CONSCIOUSNESS
Mild	Normal or increased	Increased be-coming weaker	Increased deep	Cool, pale	Normal 30 mL/hr	500–900 mL	Alert, oriented, anxious
Moderate	Systolic 60–90	Tachycardia be-coming irregular	Tachypnea becoming shallow	Cool, pale, moist	Decreased 10–22 mL/hr	1200–1500 mL	Oriented, increas-ing anxiety, restless
Severe	Systolic <60	120–160 irregular	30–50 shallow	Cool, clammy	Oliguric <10 mL/hr	1800–2100 mL	Lethargic
Very Severe	May not be detected	May be absent	>50	Cyanotic	Oliguria to anuria	>2400 mL	Slipping into unconsciousness

Lacerations of the Birth Canal

Factors predisposing a woman to lacerations of the birth canal include the following:

- Nulliparity
- Forceps-assisted or vacuum-assisted birth
- Precipitous birth
- Macrosomia
- Epidural anesthesia

Lacerations may occur in the perineum, vagina, cervix, or around the urethral meatus. Most lacerations are identified and repaired by the CNM/physician imme-diately following the birth. Occasionally, a laceration is overlooked and bright red bleeding persists when the uterus is firmly contracted.

Hematoma

A hematoma forms when there is bleeding into the tissues; there is no external laceration. Spontaneous or forceps-assisted births may result in hematoma forma-tion. The most common sites are the vulva, vagina, and retroperitoneal area (Figure 53-14). A hematoma is a bluish-purple mass that produces deep, severe, unrelent-ing pain and a feeling of great pressure. When the uterus is firmly contracted, the amount of lochia is within nor-mal limits, and the mother has a falling blood pressure or tachycardia and persistently describes severe pain, sus-pect a hematoma.

LATE POSTPARTUM HEMORRHAGE

A late postpartum hemorrhage usually occurs 1 to 2 weeks after the birth because of **subinvolution** (incom-plete return of the uterus to its prepregnant size and consistency) or retained placental fragments. Clots may form around the retained placental fragments immedi-ately postpartum, thus keeping lochia within normal limits. Several days later, when the clots slough, exces-sive bleeding occurs. There is usually no warning of a late postpartum hemorrhage.

Figure 53-14 *Hematoma of the Vulva*

Medical–Surgical Management

Medical

The CNM/physician carefully palpates the uterus to make sure it is contracting after the birth. A thorough ex-amination of the birth canal for lacerations or hematomas is also undertaken. A sonogram may be used to determine the presence of retained placental fragments.

Surgical

Cunningham et al. (2001) report that curettage, for-merly the usual treatment, is now believed to cause more bleeding because of trauma to the placental site. It now is performed when other methods have failed to control the bleeding.

Surgical evacuation of a large hematoma or one increasing in size may be necessary to attain hemostasis. The bleeding vessel is identified and ligated (tied).

Pharmacological

Oxytocin (Pitocin), methylergonovine maleate (Methergine), or prostaglandins may be given to contract the uterus. Methylergonovine maleate (Methergine) should not be given to a client with an elevated blood pressure. The strong contractions produced by these medications often loosen the retained placental fragments, which are then discharged with the lochia. Antibiotics are often used prophylactically to prevent infection. Blood transfusion or replacement of coagulation factors may be necessary depending on the amount of blood lost.

Activity

The mother is usually kept in bed until the bleeding is under control.

Nursing Management

Monitor vital signs; urine output; uterine height, firmness, and position; blood loss; and level of consciousness. Assess bladder for distension. Save all peripads, linen, and linen savers for estimate of blood loss.

For a hematoma, apply ice, assess pain using pain scale, and continue assessing the hematoma size.

CRITICAL THINKING

Contracted Uterus and Heavy Lochia

A client with a well-contracted uterus is having an extremely heavy lochia discharge. What assessments should be made? What nursing care should be provided?

NURSING PROCESS

Assessment

Subjective Data

The mother may either describe feeling like a lot of blood is coming from her vagina or a severe pain in the vulvar or perineal area.

Objective Data

Palpate the fundus for size, consistency, and position. Check how long the peripad has been in place, how much lochia is present, and whether the bladder is distended. Vital signs will probably be within the normal range.

Nursing diagnoses for a client with a postpartum hemorrhage may include the following:

Nursing Diagnoses	Planning/Goals	Nursing Interventions
*Deficient **F**luid Volume* related to blood loss from uterine atony, lacerations, retained placental fragments, or hematoma	The client will maintain adequate fluid volume.	Assess vital signs and the bladder for distention.
		Assess fundal height, firmness, and location as per agency protocol. If client has predisposing factors for postpartum hemorrhage, assess more frequently.
		Assess lochia amount and color and relate to firmness of fundus. Notify CNM/physician about excessive bleeding.
		Maintain mother on bed rest.
		Call for assistance; one nurse to monitor vital signs while a second nurse monitors fundus and lochia.
		Save all peripads, linen, and linen savers for more accurate estimate of blood loss.
		Document all assessments, interventions, and each time CNM/physician is notified.
		Administer medications as ordered.
*Acute **P**ain* related to tissue damage from hematoma formation	The client will describe having less pain.	Apply ice pack to hematoma.
		Continue assessment of hematoma size.
		Assess client's pain using 0 to 10 pain scale (0 = no pain, 10 = most pain).
		Notify CNM/physician of hematoma and pain assessment.
		Administer medications as ordered.
		Document all assessments, interventions, and each time CNM/physician is notified.

Evaluation Each goal must be evaluated to determine how it has been met by the client.

INFECTIONS

alkaline

Puerperal (postpartum) infection is an infection following childbirth occurring between the birth and 6 weeks postpartum. It is defined as a temperature of 38°C (100.4°F) or more on two separate occasions, after the first 24 hours, on any two of the first 10 postpartum days (Bowes, 1996).

Because all parts of the reproductive tract are connected to each other, it is easy for organisms to move from the vagina through the cervix, to the uterus, through the fallopian tubes, and out to the ovaries and peritoneal cavity. The increased blood supply to the reproductive tract during pregnancy provides more avenues for invading bacteria to be spread throughout the body with the possibility of causing a life-threatening septicemia.

Amniotic fluid and lochia are alkaline, so during labor and in the postpartum period, the normal acidity of the vagina is reduced, which encourages bacterial growth. Predisposing factors include the frequency of vaginal examinations during labor, the length of time membranes had been ruptured, and the length of labor. *PROM*

It is currently recommended that a prophylactic antibiotic be given to the mother having a cesarean birth *after* the cord is clamped. This prevents masking or partial treatment of any neonatal infections (Normand & Damato, 2001).

It is seldom necessary to keep the baby separated from the mother during maternal infection because they generally share the same organisms. Someone should be available to care for the infant because the mother is usually tired and does not have the energy to fully care for her infant.

Common postpartum infections are wound infection, metritis, mastitis, and urinary tract infection. Predisposing factors for puerperal infection are listed in Table 53-2.

WOUND INFECTION

The break in the skin from lacerations, episiotomies, and surgical incisions from cesarean birth provides an easy portal of entry for bacteria. Localized signs of infection (redness, warmth, edema, and tenderness) are assessed at the skin break, which, if untreated, will develop into generalized signs of infection, including an elevated temperature and malaise. Wound edges may separate and drainage may be evident.

METRITIS

Metritis, inflammation of the uterus, includes both endometritis (inflammation of the inside of the uterus, or endometrium) and parametritis (inflammation of the outside of the uterus, or parametrium, including the connective tissue of the broad ligaments). The usual causes are the organisms that normally inhabit the vagina and cervix. This infection easily spreads through the fallopian tubes **(salpingitis)** to the ovaries **(oophoritis).** The client may not appear ill except for chills and fever spikes (Ernest & Mead, 1998).

TABLE 53-2	PREDISPOSING FACTORS FOR POSTPARTUM INFECTION
PREDISPOSING FACTORS	**DESCRIPTION/ EXPLANATION**
Antepartum	
Medical conditions · Diabetes · Alcoholism · Drug abuse · Anemia · Poor nutrition/ malnutrition · Immunosuppression	Ability to defend against any infection is decreased
History of previous infections	Possibly more vulnerable to infections
Intrapartum	
Prolonged rupture of membranes	Provides direct access to interior of uterus
Chorioamnionitis	Organisms already in uterus
Prolonged labor	More time for bacteria to multiply
Excessive number of vaginal examinations	Increases opportunity for organisms from outside source or vagina to be introduced into the uterus
Internal fetal monitoring	Provides opportunity for introduction of organisms
Bladder catheterization	Possible introduction of organisms into bladder
Episiotomy, lacerations, and cesarean birth	Provide portals of entry for organisms
Postpartum	
Retained placental fragments	Good medium for bacterial growth
Hematoma	Makes tissues more susceptible
Hemorrhage	Infection-fighting components of blood are lost

MASTITIS

Mastitis is inflammation of the breast, generally during breastfeeding. The usual cause is *Staphylococcus aureus* but may also be *Candida albicans.* Symptoms appear between 2 and 4 weeks after birth. There is usually a crack or fissure in the nipple for the portal of entry. Nipple soreness may result in shorter breastfeeding times, allowing milk stasis, which is a good medium for bacterial growth.

URINARY TRACT INFECTION

Approximately 2% to 4% of new mothers will have a urinary tract infection (UTI) (Murray et al., 2001).

Trauma to the bladder and urethra during labor and birth, urinary stasis after the birth, and catheterization all contribute to the development of a UTI.

Medical–Surgical Management

Medical

The goal of treatment is to confine the infection and prevent it from spreading systemically.

A culture of drainage from a wound, the uterine cavity, or urine is performed to identify the causative agent of the infection. Breastfeeding should continue during an infection unless the antibiotic used is contraindicated during lactation. Even with mastitis, breastfeeding should continue; emptying the breast at regular intervals is beneficial. If an abscess forms and ruptures into the breast ducts, the breast should be pumped and the milk discarded. Breastfeeding should continue with the unaffected breast.

Surgical

Some sutures may be removed from the episiotomy, laceration repair, or abdominal incision to allow for drainage. If an abscess forms in mastitis, it may require an incision to allow drainage.

Pharmacological

As soon as a culture is taken, a broad-spectrum antibiotic is usually administered pending the results of the culture.

- *Wound infection:* Iodoform gauze may be placed in the open incision. An analgesic may be necessary.
- *Metritis:* Intravenous administration of antibiotics may be required initially. An antipyretic is given to reduce fever, and methylergonovine maleate (Methergine) is given to increase lochia drainage and promote involution.
- *Mastitis:* Early antibiotic therapy usually prevents abscess formation. An analgesic may be necessary.

Diet

A diet high in protein and vitamin C is needed for wound healing. Fluid intake should be increased to 3,000 mL/day for mothers with a urinary tract infection. Maintaining the increased fluid intake necessary for breastfeeding is essential even when the mother has mastitis.

Activity

Extra rest periods are necessary for all new mothers with an infection. This is especially important for mothers with metritis and mastitis, who should ambulate only enough for their own self-care initially. While in bed, the mother with metritis should be in Fowler's position to aid in lochial drainage from the uterus.

Health Promotion

Strict aseptic technique during labor and birth as well as frequent hand hygiene by those providing care to the mother are major factors in preventing postpartum infections.

Nursing Management

Monitor vital signs and assess pain level. Perform BUBBLE assessment at least every shift. Administer medications as ordered. Encourage client to stay in bed to rest and to increase fluid intake. Maintain client with metritis in Fowler's position. Assist client to feed and interact with her infant.

NURSING PROCESS

Assessment

Subjective Data

The mother may describe nausea, fatigue, malaise, pelvic pain or heaviness, leg tenderness, or breast tenderness.

Objective Data

The objective data may include fever; chills; foul-smelling lochia; redness, edema, drainage, or wound separation; dysuria, frequency, or urgency; cracked nipple; and redness and edema of the breast.

Nursing diagnoses for a client with a postpartum infection may include the following:

Nursing Diagnoses	Planning/Goals	Nursing Interventions
Deficient Knowledge related to lack of exposure to information about the etiology, management, or prevention of puerperal infections	The client will follow the management plan for her infection.	Teach client how changes after birth predispose to infection. Explain the specific management for client's infection. Answer client's questions.
Acute Pain related to wound infection, metritis, mastitis, or urinary tract infection	The client will describe less discomfort.	Administer analgesics and antibiotics as ordered. Continue assessing degree of pain using 0 to 10 pain scale (0 = no pain, 10 = worst pain).

continues

Nursing Diagnoses	Planning/Goals	Nursing Interventions
Interrupted Family Processes related to shift in health status of family member (mother)	The family will make adjustments for the mother's infection.	Assist family in understanding mother's limitations. Help family identify resources, people that can help out, until the mother is well.

Evaluation Each goal must be evaluated to determine how it has been met by the client.

THROMBOEMBOLIC CONDITIONS

Thrombophlebitis refers to the formation of a clot in an inflamed vein. Superficial thrombophlebitis is more common when the mother had preexisting varicose veins. Deep vein thrombosis (DVT) may or may not be related to vein inflammation and is seen more in women with a history of thromboses. Pulmonary embolism may be a complication of DVT. Septic pelvic thrombophlebitis is more commonly found in a mother with metritis as the inflammation spreads to the pelvic veins.

The incidence of thromboembolic conditions has decreased since early ambulation has become a standard practice after childbirth (Lowdermilk & Perry, 2003). Venous stasis and hypercoagulation, which are present during pregnancy, are the major causes. Other risk factors include maternal age older than 35, cesarean birth, prolonged time in stirrups during second stage of labor, obesity, smoking, and a history of varicosities or venous thromboses.

Medical–Surgical Management

Medical

Thrombophlebitis is usually managed with rest, elevation of the affected leg, and local application of heat. Elastic stockings are fitted for use when the mother is able to ambulate. Doppler ultrasound is an accurate diagnostic test for DVT. The mother who is receiving a broad-spectrum antibiotic for metritis and whose symptoms are not diminishing should be suspected of having septic pelvic thrombophlebitis.

⚙ Pharmacological

An analgesic is given to relieve discomfort. Antibiotics are often given if the mother has a fever. DVT and septic pelvic thrombophlebitis are usually treated with intravenous heparin for 5 to 7 days. During this time, warfarin sodium (Coumadin) is begun and is usually continued for several months.

Activity

Bed rest is required for all thromboembolic conditions. When the mother is allowed to ambulate, she must wear elastic stockings. In thrombophlebitis and DVT, the affected leg is elevated until symptoms decrease.

Health Promotion

Instruct the client to avoid prolonged standing or sitting. Legs are not to be crossed when sitting. Encourage walking to increase venous return. Pad stirrups and properly adjust for correct support and to prevent pressure on the legs.

Nursing Management

Maintain client on bed rest. Elevate the affected leg. Measure legs for elastic stockings for client to wear when able to ambulate. Administer medications as ordered. Teach client to avoid prolonged sitting or standing and to never cross her legs.

NURSING PROCESS

Assessment

Subjective Data

The mother may describe discomfort or pain in the leg affected with superficial thrombophlebitis or DVT and a fullness/heaviness or pain in the pelvis if septic pelvic thrombosis occurs.

Objective Data

Signs of superficial thrombophlebitis include redness, warmth, and swelling where the vein is inflamed. Deep vein thrombosis may manifest as edema and calf pain. A positive Homans' sign may be present, but may also be caused by a strained muscle or improper use of stirrups during the birth. The classic sign of septic pelvic thrombophlebitis is fever of unknown origin. When it is untreated, tachycardia, ileus, and an elevated white count develop.

A nursing diagnosis for clients with thromboembolic conditions may be:

Nursing Diagnosis	Planning/Goals	Nursing Interventions
Ineffective Tissue Perfusion Altered (peripheral), related to mechanical reduction of venous blood flow	The client will maintain adequate tissue perfusion.	Ensure affected leg is properly elevated. Apply heat to affected leg, as ordered. Measure client for antiembolic stockings and teach proper application when able to ambulate. Encourage fluid intake to prevent dehydration. Administer analgesics, antibiotics, heparin, and Coumadin as ordered. Assess for signs of pulmonary embolism (chest pain and dyspnea) and evidence of bleeding (i.e., petechiae, bruising, nosebleed, hematoma) related to heparin therapy. Emphasize importance of having prothrombin time checked while taking warfarin sodium (Coumadin). Keep protamine sulfate, the heparin antagonist, readily available.

Evaluation Each goal must be evaluated to determine how it has been met by the client.

DISSEMINATED INTRAVASCULAR COAGULATION

Disseminated intravascular coagulation (DIC) is an abnormal stimulation of the clotting mechanism, which consumes clotting factors, causing small clots throughout the vascular system and widespread bleeding internally, externally, or both. This results in platelet and clotting factor depletion. DIC may result from a missed abortion, abruptio placenta, amniotic fluid embolism, severe preeclampsia, hemorrhage, and a dead fetus. It is a complication of a preexisting problem.

Correction of the underlying cause is the main aspect of medical management. Blood replacement products including whole blood, packed red cells, or cryoprecipitate may be administered. Nursing care includes continued assessment for signs of bleeding and of complications from the blood products. Intake and output is recorded; urinary output must be maintained at more than 30 mL/hour.

CASE STUDY

Jeff and Meli Lahoti had their third child, a second son, yesterday. The baby weighed 8 lbs, 10 oz, the largest of their three children. The labor lasted 5 hours. An episiotomy was performed this time but had not been for the previous births.

Meli is having problems walking to the bathroom and says she feels faint and dizzy when she stands up. She talks constantly about the pain from the episiotomy. A bruised, edematous area is noted beside the episiotomy. Analgesics provide little relief. Plans were to breastfeed this infant as she had the first two. Today she does not want to feed the baby because she "hurts too much."

The following questions will guide your development of a nursing care plan for this case study.

1. What assessments should be made?
2. Identify three nursing diagnoses for Meli.
3. Identify planning/goals for Meli.
4. List nursing interventions to help Meli meet the goals.
5. How can the effectiveness of this plan be evaluated?

Summary

- The first 6 weeks after the birth of an infant is called the puerperium or postpartum period.
- Mothers, fathers, siblings, and grandparents all make special adaptations for the neonate.
- During the postpartum period, most of the physiologic changes of pregnancy are reversed and the mother's body returns to its prepregnant state.
- Immediate weight loss of the mother is 13 lbs with an additional 8- to 9-lb loss during the first 6 weeks postpartum.
- Rubin describes three phases of maternal restoration/adaptation—taking in, taking hold, and letting go.
- Unexpected emotional/behavioral changes include postpartum depression, postpartum psychosis, and reaction to an infant with problems.
- Specific assessments for the first few days postpartum include BUBBLE (breasts, uterus, bladder, bowel, lochia, and episiotomy), vital signs, Homans' sign, bonding/attachment, parenting, activity, comfort, and self-care.

Review Questions

1. The nurse observes passive and dependent behaviors displayed by a postpartum client. According to Reva Rubin, the client is in the:
   - a. taking-in phase.
   - b. letting-go phase.
   - c. taking-hold phase.
   - d. transitional phase.

2. A client has excessive vaginal bleeding after delivery. The assessment reveals a soft, boggy uterus located above the level of the umbilicus and displaced to the right side. The first action of the nurse should be to:
   - a. notify the CNM/physician.
   - b. massage the fundus and take vital signs.
   - c. initiate measures that encourage voiding.
   - d. put the client flat, take vital signs, and notify the CNM/physician.

3. A new mother tells the nurse that she is afraid of her baby and that she doubts she will be able to love the baby. The most appropriate action for the nurse would be to:
   - a. tell the client she will learn fast.
   - b. tell the client what a beautiful baby she has.
   - c. encourage the client to talk about her feelings.
   - d. have a psychiatrist visit the client immediately.

4. A client has excessive vaginal bleeding following the birth. The nurse should suspect a cervical or vaginal tear if client assessment reveals:
   - a. acute pelvic pain.
   - b. a hard, contracted uterus.
   - c. an elevation of blood pressure.
   - d. pieces of the placenta still attached to the uterine wall.

5. A client wants to know when she can begin breastfeeding and is anxious for her milk to start. The best response of the nurse would be:
   - a. "Ask your CNM/physician."
   - b. "Your baby will be brought to you at the next feeding time. Your milk will start right after that."
   - c. "We encourage you to breastfeed as soon as you wish. Your milk will probably 'come in' in about 3 days."
   - d. "The baby can breastfeed anytime after birth. After your colostrum is gone (3 to 4 days), your milk will come in (5 to 6 days)."

References/Suggested Readings

Albright, A. (1993). Postpartum depression: An overview. *Journal of Counseling Development 71*(3), 316.

Ament, L. (1990). Maternal tasks of the puerperium reidentified. *JOGNN, 19*(4), 330.

American Academy of Pediatrics (AP) & American College of Obstetricians and Gynecologists (ACOG). (1977). *Guide lines for perinatal care* (3rd ed.). Elk Grove Village, IL: American Academy of Pediatrics.

Beck, C., & Gable, R. (2001). Further validation of the Postpartum Depression Screening Scale. *Nursing Research, 50*(3), 155.

Beeber, L. (2002). The pinks and the blues. *AJN, 102*(11), 91–97.

Berger, D., & Loveland-Cook, C. A. (1998). Postpartum teaching priorities: The viewpoints of nurses and mothers. *JOGNN, 27*(2), 161–168.

Bowes, W. (2001). Postpartum care. In S. Gabbe, J. Niebyl, & J. Simpson (Eds.), *Obstetrics: Normal and problem pregnancies* (4th ed.). New York: Churchill Livingstone.

Brown, S. G., & Johnson, B. T. (1998). Enhancing early discharge with home follow-up. A pilot project. *JOGNN, 27*(1), 33–38.

Burroughs, A., & Leifer, G. (2001). *Maternity nursing* (8th ed.). Philadelphia: W. B. Saunders.

Callister, L., & Vega, R. (1998). Giving birth: Guatemalan women's voices. *JOGNN, 27*(3), 289–295.

Cesario, S. (2001). Care of the Native American woman: Strategies for practice, education, and research. *JOGNN, 30*(1), 13–19.

Cunningham, F. G., Grant, N. F., Leveno, K. J., Gilstrap, L. C., & Cox, S. (2001). *William's obstetrics* (21st ed.). Norwalk, CT: Appleton & Lange.

Davis, R. (2001). The postpartum experience for Southeast Asian women in the United States. *MCN, 26*(4), 208–213.

Dochterman, J., & Bulechek, G. (2004). *Nursing Interventions Classification (NIC)* (4th ed.). St. Louis, MO: Mosby.

Ernest, J. M., & Mead, P. B. (1998). Postpartum endometritis. *Contemporary OB/GYN, 43*(1), 33–38.

Ferguson, S., & Engelhard, C. (1996). Maternity length of stay and public policy: Issues and implications. *Journal of Pediatric Nursing, 11*(6), 392.

Ferketich, S. L., & Mercer, R. T. (1995). Paternal–infant attachment of experienced and inexperienced fathers during infancy. *Nursing Research, 44*(1), 31–37.

Gennaro, S., Kamwendo, L., Mbweza, E., & Kershbaumer, R. (1998). Childbearing in Malawi, Africa. *JOGNN, 27*(2), 191–196.

Green, S. E., & Adams, W. M. (1993). Chronic psychiatric illness and pregnancy: Nursing implications. *Journal of Perinatal, Neonatal Nursing, 7*(3), 7–18.

Ha, L. (1994, December). *Culturally sensitive caregiving for Vietnamese women.* Lecture presented at the Medical College of Virginia Hospitals, Richmond, VA.

Havens, D., & Hannan, C. (1996). Legislation to mandate maternal and newborn length of stay. *Journal of Pediatric Health Care, 10*(3), 141.

Health Care Financing Administration (2002). The Newborns' and Mothers' Health Protection Act of 1996. [Online]. Available: www.hcfa.gov/medicaid/hipaa/content/nmhpa.asp

Higgins, P. (2000). Postpartum complications. In S. Mattson & J. E. Smith (Eds.). *Core Curriculum for Maternal-Newborn Nursing* (2nd ed.). Philadelphia: W. B. Saunders.

Howard, J., & Berbiglia, V. (1997). Caring for childbearing Korean women. *JOGNN, 26*(6), 665–671.

Hutchinson, M., & Baqi-Aziz, M. (1994). Nursing care of the childbearing Muslim family. *JOGNN, 23*(9), 767–771.

Johnson & Johnson (1996). *Compendium of postpartum care* Skillman, NJ: Johnson & Johnson Consumer Products.

Kaplan, H., Sadock, B., & Grebb, J. (1998). *Kaplan and Sadock's synopsis of psychiatry* (8th ed.). Philadelphia: Lippincott Williams & Wilkins.

Kim-Godwin, Y. (2003). Postpartum beliefs & practices among non-western cultures. *MCN, 28*(2), 74–78.

Ladewig, P., Moberly, S., Olds, S., & London, M. (2001). *Contemporary maternal-newborn nursing care* (5th ed.). Menlo Park, CA: Addison-Wesley.

Littleton, L., & Engebretson, J. (2002). *Maternal, neonatal, and women's health nursing.* Clifton Park, NY: Thomson Delmar Learning.

Lowdermilk, D., & Perry, S., (2003). *Maternity nursing* (6th ed.). St. Louis, MO: Mosby–Year Book.

Luegenbiehl, D., Brophy, G., Artigue, G., Phillips, K., & Flack, R. (1990). Standardized assessment of blood loss. *MCN, 15*(4), 241–244.

Martell, L. (1996). Is Rubin's "taking-in" and "taking-hold" a useful paradigm? *Health Care Women International 17*(1), 1.

Mattson, S. (1995). Culturally sensitive perinatal care for Southeast Asians. *JOGNN, 24*(4), 335–341.

Moorhead, S., Johnson, M., & Maas, M. (2004). *Nursing Outcomes Classification (NOC)*(3rd ed.). St. Louis, MO: Mosby.

Murray, S., McKinney, E., & Gorrie, T. (2001). *Foundations of maternal–newborn nursing* (3rd ed.). Philadelphia: W. B. Saunders.

Neal, J. (2001). RhD isoimmunization and current management modalities. *JOGNN, 309*(6), 589–606.

Normand, M. C., & Damato, E. G. (2001). Postcesarean infection. *JOGNN, 30*(6), 642–647.

North American Nursing Diagnosis Association. (2003). *Nursing diagnoses: Definitions & classification 2003–2004.* Philadelphia: Author.

Placksin, S. (2000). *Mothering the new mother: Women's feelings and needs after childbirth. A support and resource guide.* New York: Newmark Press.

Rubin, R. (1961). Puerperal change. *Nursing Outlook, 9*(12), 743–755.

Ruchala, P., & Halstead, L. (1994). The postpartum experience of low-risk women: A time of adjustment and change. *MCN, 22*(3), 83.

Savoia, M. C. (1999). Bacterial, fungal, and parasitic disease during pregnancy. In G. N. Burrow, T. P. Duffy, & R. Kersey (Eds.). *Medical complications during pregnancy*(5th ed.). Philadelphia: W. B. Saunders.

Schneiderman, J. (1996). Postpartum nursing for Korean mothers. *MCN, 21*(3), 155–158.

Sharts-Hopko, N. (1995). Birth in the Japanese context. *JOGNN, 24*(4),343–351.

Simpson, K., & Creehan, P. (2001). *AWHONN perinatal nursing* (2nd ed.). Philadelphia, Lippincott Williams & Wilkins.

Smith-Hanrahan, C., & Deblois, D. (1995). Postpartum early discharge. *Clinical Nursing Research, 4*(1), 50.

Spratto, G. R., & Woods, A. L. (2004). *PDR nurse's drug handbook.* Clifton Park, NY: Thomson Delmar Learning.

Squires, A. (2003). Documenting surgical incision site care. *Nursing2003, 33*(1), 74.

Tiller, C. M. (1995). Father's parenting attitudes during a child's first year. *JOGNN, 24*(6), 508–514.

Troy, N. (2003). Is the significance of postpartum fatigue being overlooked in the lives of women? *MCN, 28*(4), 252–257.

Visness, C., Kennedy, K., & Ramos, R. (1997). The duration and character of postpartum bleeding among breast-feeding women. *Obstetrics and Gynecology, 89*(2), 159.

Wilkerson, N. (1996). Appraisal of early discharge programs. *Journal of Perinatal Education, 5*(2), 1.

Wrasper, C. (1996). Discharge and timing and Rubin's concept of puerperal change. *Journal of Perinatal Education, 5*(2), 13.

Zlatnik, F. (1999). The normal and abnormal puerperlium. In J. R. Scott, P. J. Di Saia, C. B. Hammond, & W. N. Spellacy (Eds.), *Danforths' obstetrics and gynecology* (8th ed.). Philadelphia: Lippincott Williams & Wilkins.

Resources

Association of Women's Health, Obstetric and Neonatal Nurses (AWHONN), 2000 L Street, N.W. Suite 740, Washington, DC, 20036, 800-673-8499. www.awhonn.org

Depression After Delivery (DAD), Inc., 91 East Summerset Street, Raritan, NJ, 08864, 800-944-4773, www.depressionafterdelivery.com

Health Science Consortium, 201 Silver Cedar Court, Chapel Hill, NC, 27514-1517, 919-942-8731

Hollister, Inc., 2000 Hollister Drive, Libertyville, IL, 60048, 800-323-4060, www.hollister.com

International Lactation Consultant Association (ILCA), 1500 Sunday Drive, Suite 102, Raleigh, NC 27607, 919-787-5181, www.ilca.org

Johnson & Johnson Consumer Products, Inc., 199 Grandview Road, Skillman, NJ, 08558-9418, 908-874-1000

Postpartum Support International, 927 North Kellogg Avenue, Santa Barbara, CA, 93111, 800-967-7636, www.chss.iup.edu/postpartum

MAKING THE CONNECTION

Refer to the following chapters to increase your understanding of newborn care:

Basic Nursing
- Life Cycle

Maternal & Pediatric Nursing
- Complications of Pregnancy
- The Birth Process
- Postpartum Care
- Basics of Pediatric Care
- Infants with Special Needs: Birth to 12 Months

Basic Procedures
- Hand Hygiene
- Use of Protective Equipment

- Taking a Temperature
- Taking a Pulse
- Counting Respirations
- Performing Cardiopulmonary Resuscitation (Infant)

Intermediate Procedures
- Administering an Intramuscular Injection
- Administering Oxygen
- Performing a Skin Puncture

LEARNING OBJECTIVES

Upon completion of this chapter, you should be able to:
- Define key terms.
- Describe the immediate needs of the newborn.
- Discuss what initiates breathing in the newborn.
- Describe the newborn's methods of heat production and heat retention.
- Identify the four ways heat is lost and nursing interventions to prevent heat loss.
- Describe the immediate care of the newborn.
- Discuss the Apgar score and how it is used.
- Describe the physical characteristics of the newborn.
- Identify the common variations in the newborn.
- Elicit the newborn's reflexes.
- Determine the gestational age of a newborn.
- Discuss the newborn's nutritional needs and how they can be met by breastfeeding and bottle feeding.
- Identify common problems the newborn may encounter and nursing interventions for each.
- Plan the care and then care for a newborn.

KEY TERMS

acrocyanosis
appropriate for
    gestational age
caput succedaneum
cephalhematoma
circumcision
cold stress
conduction
convection
cryptorchidism
Down syndrome
epispadias
Epstein's pearls
erythema toxicum
    neonatorum
evaporation
foremilk
hallux varus
hindmilk
hydrocele

hyperbilirubinemia
hypospadias
kernicterus
lanugo
large for gestational age
meconium
meningocele
milia
molding
mongolian spots
myelomeningocele
neonatal transition
neutral thermal
    environment
nevus flammeus
nevus vascularis
nonshivering
    thermogenesis
ophthalmia neonatorum
phimosis

continues

KEY TERMS—continued

pseudomenstruation
radiation
small for gestational
   age
spina bifida occulta
syndactyly
talipes equinovarus
   (clubfoot)

telangiectactic nevi
thermogenesis
thermoregulation
vernix caseosa
witch's milk

INTRODUCTION

At the time of birth, the newborn must quickly make changes in the respiratory system to allow gas exchange to take place in the lungs and also make changes in the circulatory system to support the change to respiratory gas exchange. These profound, vital changes are critical to maintaining extrauterine life. The first few hours after birth wherein the newborn makes these changes and stabilizes respiratory and circulatory functions is called the **neonatal transition** period. Other body systems also make changes in their functioning over a longer period, although they are not crucial to the immediate survival of the infant.

Nurses are instrumental in assisting the newborn and mother through the neonatal transition period.

IMMEDIATE NEEDS OF THE NEWBORN

The immediate needs of the newborn are airway, breathing, circulation, and warmth.

Airway

A clear airway is necessary for adequate gas exchange.

Breathing

In utero, the fetus relied on the placenta and the mother's respirations for gas exchange; however, fetal breathing movements, from approximately 11 weeks' gestation, help develop the chest wall muscles and the diaphragm (Ladewig, Moberly, Olds, & London, 2001). By approximately 35 weeks' gestation, the surfactant produced by the alveoli is sufficient in amount (L/S ratio 2 : 1) to allow the alveoli to remain partially expanded when the newborn begins to breathe at birth.

For the lungs to function, two changes must happen:

- Pulmonary ventilation must be established with lung expansion at the first breath.
- Pulmonary circulation must greatly increase.

The initiation of breathing is influenced by four factors— physical, chemical, thermal, and sensory—which work together.

Physical Factors

The physical (sometimes called mechanical) factors include the compression of the fetal chest as it moves through the birth canal, which squeezes fluid from the lungs and increases intrathoracic pressure; and the chest wall recoil, which occurs as the newborn's trunk emerges. The chest recoil creates negative intrathoracic pressure, which causes a small amount of air to replace the fluid that was squeezed out of the lungs and some of the lung fluid to move across the alveolar membranes into the interstitial tissue of the lungs. Each breath allows more air into the alveoli and more fluid into the interstitial tissue. Because the protein concentration is higher in the capillaries, the interstitial fluid is drawn into them. All of the alveolar fluid is absorbed within the first day after birth.

Chemical Factors (CO_2) – Increase to a level

When the cord is clamped, placental gas exchange ceases, causing an increase in $PaCO_2$ and a decrease in PaO_2 and pH (a transitory asphyxia). These changes stimulate the carotid and aortic chemoreceptors, which send impulses to the respiratory center in the medulla, which in turn stimulates respirations. A brief period of asphyxia stimulates respirations, whereas prolonged asphyxia is a central nervous system (CNS) respiratory depressant.

Thermal Factors

The change in temperature from the intrauterine environment to the extrauterine environment, a decrease of more than 20°F, is also a stimulus to breathing. The colder temperature stimulates the skin nerve endings and the newborn breathes as a response. Cold stress and respiratory depression result from excessive cooling of the newborn.

Sensory Factors

The comfortable, relatively quiet uterine environment is left behind for an environment full of sensory stimuli. The auditory and visual stimuli associated with birth, along with the tactile stimulation of being handled, assist in the initiation of respirations.

Circulation

Several circulatory changes are necessary for the successful change from fetal circulation to neonatal circulation. These changes involve the pulmonary blood vessels, ductus arteriosus, foramen ovale, and ductus venosus.

Pulmonary Blood Vessels

The dilation of these blood vessels begins with the first breath taken by the newborn. This results in lower pulmonary resistance, which allows the blood to freely circulate through the lungs to be oxygenated.

Ductus Arteriosus – reversal of Blood flow

Within minutes after birth, the ductus arteriosus has a reversal of blood flow caused by the increased pressure in the aorta and the increase of oxygen in the blood. This results in more blood flowing through the pulmonary arteries for oxygenation. Closure of the ductus arteriosus is complete within 24 hours and is permanent in 3 to 4 weeks.

Foramen Ovale

The foramen ovale closes within minutes after birth because of the higher pressure in the left atrium than in the right atrium. The increased blood flow in the lungs decreases pressure in the right atrium, and the return of blood from the lungs increases the pressure in the left atrium. Closure of the foramen ovale is permanent in approximately 3 months.

Ductus Venosus

When the cord is clamped, the blood ceases flowing through the umbilical vein to the ductus venosus and into the inferior vena cava. Blood now flows through the liver and is filtered as in adult circulation.

Warmth — Baby's cannot retain heat.

At birth the newborn must begin **thermoregulation,** maintenance of body temperature. Three factors are instrumental in thermoregulation: heat production, heat retention, and heat loss.

Heat Production

The newborn produces heat **(thermogenesis)** through general metabolism, muscular activity, and nonshivering thermogenesis (unique to the newborn). Newborns rarely shiver as adults do to increase heat production. Shivering seen in a newborn indicates that the metabolic rate has already doubled (Ladewig et al., 2001).

When the infant is in a cool environment and requires more heat, the metabolic rate increases, producing more heat. The newborn may cry and have muscular activity when cold, but there is no voluntary control of muscular activity.

If the infant's temperature is not adequately raised through increased metabolism, **nonshivering thermo-genesis,** the metabolism of brown fat, begins. Brown fat is a special fat found only in newborns. It appears at about 26 to 30 weeks of gestation and increases until 2 to 5 weeks of age (unless depleted by cold stress). The fat is highly vascularized, which gives it the brown color. The brown fat is located at the back of the neck, between the scapula, around the kidneys and adrenals, in the axilla, and around the heart and abdominal aorta (Figure 54-1). Once the brown fat has been metabolized, the infant no longer has this method of heat production available.

Heat Retention

Newborns retain heat by staying in a flexed position. This reduces the area of skin exposed to the environmental temperature, thus decreasing heat loss. They also use the mechanism of peripheral vasoconstriction to retain heat.

Heat Loss

The newborn has thin skin with blood vessels close to the surface and little subcutaneous fat to prevent heat loss. Heat moves from the warm internal areas to the cooler skin surface and then to the surrounding environment. Excessive heat loss is called **cold stress.** An increase in metabolism leads to a significant increase in the need for oxygen. When oxygen is used for metabolism (heat production), the infant may experience hypoxia. There may not be enough oxygen for the metabolic rate to increase, and the newborn will not be able to maintain body temperature. Prolonged cold stress causes respiratory difficulties and a decrease in surfactant production. Less surfactant hinders lung expansion, which in turn leads to more respiratory distress. Decreased blood oxygen may cause vasoconstriction of the pulmonary vessels with a return to fetal circulation patterns, which further increases respiratory distress.

The glucose necessary for increased metabolism is made available when glycogen stores are converted to glucose. If the glycogen is depleted, hypoglycemia results.

Brown fat metabolism results in the release of fatty acids. Continuous brown fat metabolism, when the newborn is in a cold stress situation for a considerable time, results in metabolic acidosis, which can be life-threatening. Excess fatty acids in the blood interfere with bilirubin transportation to the liver, which increases the risk of jaundice.

There are four methods by which the newborn loses heat: conduction, convection, evaporation, and radiation.

Figure 54-1 *Brown Fat Distribution in the Newborn*

PROFESSIONAL TIP

Effects of Cold Stress
- Oxygen need increased
- Respiratory distress
- Surfactant production decreased
- Hypoglycemia
- Metabolic acidosis
- Jaundice

Figure 54-2 *A radiant warmer keeps the air around the newborn warm, preventing heat loss by convection.*

Test

✗ **Conduction** **Conduction** is the loss of heat by direct contact with a cooler object. When a newborn is touched by cold hands or a cold stethoscope or is placed on a cold surface such as a scale, heat is lost. Heat loss can be prevented by warming objects touching the newborn. If a newborn is wrapped in a warmed blanket or placed against the mother's warm skin, heat will be lost by the blanket or mother's skin to the cooler newborn and the newborn is warmed.

✗ **Convection** **Convection** is the loss of heat by the movement of air. When air moves (air currents), heat is transferred to the air. Air currents from an open door or window, air conditioning, or from people moving around increase heat loss. A radiant warmer is often used for the newborn immediately after birth to prevent heat loss by convection (Figure 54-2). Heat loss in the newborn can be prevented by wrapping the infant in a blanket and placing a stocking cap on the head and by keeping the newborn out of any drafts.

✗ **Evaporation** **Evaporation** is the loss of heat when water is changed to a vapor. When a wet body dries, heat is lost, such as a newborn wet with amniotic fluid or during a bath. The insensible water loss from the skin and respiratory tract also results in heat loss. Heat loss can be prevented by immediately drying the newborn at birth and after receiving a bath, and by changing wet clothing and diapers promptly.

✗ **Radiation** **Radiation** is the loss of heat by transfer to cooler objects nearby, but not through direct contact. An infant placed near a cold window loses heat by radiation to the sides of the crib and the window. If the walls of an incubator are cold, the infant loses heat. Heat loss can be prevented by keeping cribs and incubators away from cold windows. *Best - skin to skin - to warm*

IMMEDIATE CARE OF THE NEWBORN

The immediate care of the newborn includes obtaining the Apgar score, resuscitation (if needed), providing a neutral thermal environment, proper identification of the infant, parent/infant bonding, and prophylactic care.

 Safety: Newborns and Standard Precautions
Penny-MacGillivray (1996) explains that blood and amniotic fluid, once believed to be sterile, are now considered contaminated with blood-borne pathogens. All newborns are now also considered contaminated until the first bath has removed all blood and amniotic fluid from the infant's body. The nurse performing the assessment and giving the first bath *must wear gloves*.

Apgar Score

The Apgar score, which assesses the infant's cardiopulmonary adaptations to extrauterine life, was discussed in the Birth Process chapter.

Resuscitation

Resuscitation is begun if no respirations are initiated by the infant. The LP/VN may be asked to use a bulb syringe to suction mucus from the infant's oropharynx, gently rub the infant's back for stimulation, or provide oxygen. More intense resuscitation would typically be performed by an RN or physician.

Neutral Thermal Environment

A **neutral thermal environment** is an environment in which the newborn can maintain internal body temperature with minimal oxygen consumption and metabolism. In this environment, the newborn's body does not have to focus on temperature maintenance but can focus on growth and development.

Identification

Proper identification of the newborn is vital. The identification bands must be checked and compared to the mother's band each time the baby is brought into the mother's room. The process of applying the identification bands is discussed in the Birth Process chapter.

Parent/Infant Bonding

Interaction between the parents and infant should be promoted as soon as the infant is stable. The nurse may need to assist the parents in holding their baby or to give them permission to examine the infant.

Prophylactic Care

Prophylactic care includes the administration of vitamin K and hepatitis B vaccine, instillation of an antibiotic ophthalmic ointment, and umbilical cord care.

Vitamin K

+ eye drops - for blood clotting

At birth, newborns lack vitamin K, which is necessary for the clotting process. Vitamin K is synthesized in the intestine and requires food and normal intestinal flora for the process. Because the intestines are sterile at birth, no vitamin K can be produced for several days. An intramuscular (IM) injection of vitamin K, phytonadione (aquaMEPHYTON), is generally given within the first hour after birth to prevent hemorrhagic disorders. A normal newborn is able to produce vitamin K by the eighth day (Lowdermilk & Perry, 2003).

Hepatitis B Vaccination *- upon Birth*

The Centers for Disease Control and Prevention (CDC), along with the Advisory Committee on Immunization Practices (ACIP), the American Academy of Pediatrics (AAP), and the American Academy of Family Physicians (AAFP), recommend that newborns be given the first dose of hepatitis B (Hep B) vaccine within 12 hours of birth. Infants whose mothers have hepatitis B should also receive hepatitis B immune globulin (HBIG) at the same time, but at a different site than the vaccine. The HBIG provides passive immunity until the newborn develops antibodies. In many agencies, the parents must give written permission for the infant to receive the hepatitis B vaccine.

Eye Prophylaxis

In the United States, it is mandatory that a prophylactic agent be instilled in the eyes of all neonates to prevent **ophthalmia neonatorum.** This is an inflammation of the newborn's eyes that results from passing through the birth canal when a gonorrheal or chlamydial infection is present. The medication used for prophylaxis varies with agency protocol but is generally erythromycin (Ilotycin Ophthalmic Ointment) or tetracycline (Achromycin Ophthalmic Ointment) (Lowdermilk & Perry, 2003). Silver nitrate 1% is now seldom used because it protects only against gonorrheal infection and not chlamydial infection. To promote parent/infant eye contact, bonding, and attachment, some agencies delay the eye prophylaxis for an hour or so.

Umbilical Cord Care *- Based on policy & procedure manual of facility.*

Umbilical cord care is the same as for any surgical wound (Krebs, 1998). The cord and the skin at its base are assessed for redness, edema, and purulent drainage each time the diaper is changed. The cord and skin are cleaned as per agency protocol (i.e., triple blue dye, alcohol, or erythromycin solution). The prevention of or early identification of any hemorrhage or infection is the goal of care. *- Keep dry - Keep diaper low*

Safety: Cord Hemorrhage
- When bleeding from the cord is noted, check the clamp and apply a second clamp on the body side of the first one.
- If the bleeding does not stop immediately, notify the health care provider.

PHYSICAL CHARACTERISTICS OF THE NEWBORN

The newborn infant is not just a miniature adult. Identification of the physical characteristics and common variations of the newborn found in the infant are documented. This provides a basis for nursing diagnoses and care. Agencies generally have a form to follow such as the one shown in Figure 54-3. This form incorporates data about the mother, the delivery, Apgar score, and gestational age along with the physical assessment of the infant.

Weight and Length

Most full-term newborns weigh between 2,500 g and 4,000 g or approximately 5 lb, 8 oz to 8 lb, 13 oz. Newborns lose 5% to 10% of their body weight in the first 3 to 4 days. This is a result of small fluid intake, volume of **meconium** (first bowel movements of newborn, black and tarry) (Figure 54-4), and urination. Birth weight is generally regained by 10 days of age.

Their head-to-heel length is 48 cm to 53 cm (approximately 19 in. to 21 in.), and crown-to-rump length is 31 cm to 35 cm (approximately 12 in. to 14 in.) or approximately equal to the head circumference.

chest 2-3 cm less than Head

Vital Signs

The axillary temperature should be between 36.5°C and 37.2°C (97.6°F and 98.9°F). A continuous skin probe is best for small newborns or those in a radiant warmer. Normal skin temperature is 36°C to 36.5°C (96.8°F to 97.6°F). Crying may slightly increase temperature.

The apical heart rate is 120 to 160 beats/minute. When the newborn is sleeping, the heart rate decreases, and when crying, the heart rate increases.

Respirations are 30 to 60 breaths/minute. As with the heart rate, sleep decreases respirations and crying increases respirations.

Blood pressure ranges between 60 and 80 mm Hg systolic and 40 and 45 mm Hg diastolic. By 10 days of age, it is 100/50 mm Hg. Activity and crying will increase the newborn's blood pressure.

General Appearance

Full-term newborns have a flexed posture. The head is flexed, the arms are flexed on the chest, and the legs are flexed on the abdomen.

Skin

At birth, the skin is red, puffy, and smooth. Some **vernix caseosa** (a white, creamy substance) may thinly cover the skin, with large amounts found in body creases. **Lanugo** (fine, downy hair) may still be seen on the forehead and shoulders, or it may all have disappeared. **Acrocyanosis,** blue coloring of the hands and feet, is generally present for several hours until the cardiopulmonary changes have stabilized and fully oxygenated blood has reached the hands and feet. Edema may be present around the eyes, face, dorsa of hands, legs, feet, and labia or scrotum.

Erythema Toxicum Neonatorum

Erythema toxicum neonatorum is a pink rash with firm, yellow-white papules or pustules found on the chest, abdomen, back, and buttocks of some newborns. This may appear 24 to 48 hours after birth and disappear in a few days without any treatment.

Telangiectactic Nevi

Telangiectactic nevi ("stork-bites") are birthmarks of dilated capillaries that blanch with pressure. They may appear on the eyelids, nose, occipital area, or nape of the neck and fade between 1 and 2 years of age.

Nevus Flammeus

Nevus flammeus (port-wine stain) is a large reddish-purple birthmark usually found on the face or neck that does not blanch with pressure. It is not raised above the skin. This does not spontaneously disappear but may be lightened with special laser treatments.

Nevus Vascularis

Nevus vascularis (strawberry mark) is a birthmark of enlarged superficial blood vessels. They are elevated, red, and of variable size and shape. They are most often found on the head, face, neck, and arms. By school age, they have generally disappeared.

Mongolian Spots

Mongolian spots are deep blue areas of coloration, usually in the sacral region, at birth. They are seen mainly in infants of African, Asian, American Indian, Hispanic, and Southern European descent.

Head

Three common variations in newborns involve the head: molding, caput succedaneum, and cephalhematoma.

Molding

Molding is the shaping of the fetal head to adapt to the mother's pelvis during labor. In 2 to 3 days the cranial bones typically return to their proper placement (Figure 54-7).

Caput Succedaneum

Caput succedaneum, edema of the newborn's scalp that is present at birth, may cross suture lines and is

Figure 54-7 *Molding:* **A,** *Movement of cranial bones during labor;* **B,** *Cranial bones return to their proper placement in 2 to 3 days;* **C,** *Infant exhibiting molding.*

caused by head compression against the cervix (Figure 54-8A). The edema disappears in 2 to 3 days. No treatment is needed.

Cephalhematoma

Cephalhematoma is a collection of blood between the periosteum and the skull of a newborn. It appears several hours to a day after birth, does not cross suture lines, and is caused by the rupturing of the periosteal bridging veins because of friction and pressure during labor and delivery (Figure 54-8B). It is usually the largest on the second or third day and spontaneously resorbs in 3 to 6 weeks. Table 54-1 compares caput succedaneum and cephalhematoma.

Eyes

The newborn's eyes may show signs of strabismus, which is caused by poor neuromuscular control. This usually disappears in 3 to 4 months. Subconjunctival hemorrhages are present in approximately 10% of newborns (Ladewig et al., 2001). Change in vascular tension or ocular pressure during birth causes these hemorrhages. They last for a few weeks and do not impair vision.

Ears

The ears may be of irregular shape and size. The pinna may be flat against the head.

Figure 54-8 A, *Caput Succedaneum;* **B**, *Cephalhematoma*

Mouth

Precocious teeth may be present at birth in the center of the lower gum. If loose, they should be removed to prevent aspiration. **Epstein's pearls,** small, whitish-yellow epithelial cysts, are found on the hard palate. They disappear within a few weeks.

Chest

Many newborns, both male and female, have engorged breasts as a result of maternal hormones. This occurs by the third day and may last 2 weeks. The nipples may secrete a whitish fluid, often called **"witch's milk."**

Genitalia

There are several variations in the female and male genitalia.

Female

Pseudomenstruation, a blood-tinged mucous discharge from the vagina, may be evident in the first week after birth. It is caused by the withdrawal of maternal hormones. A vaginal tag or hymenal tag may be present but will disappear in a few weeks.

Male

Hypospadias, placement of the urinary meatus on the underside of the penis, may be present. **Phimosis,** when the opening in the foreskin is so small that it cannot be pulled back over the glans, may interfere with urination. **Cryptorchidism,** failure of one or both testes to descend, may be evident. **Hydrocele,** fluid around the testes in the scrotum, usually disappears without any treatment. **Epispadias** is the placement of the urinary meatus on the top of the penis.

Extremities

There may be partial **syndactyly** (fusion of two or more fingers or toes) of the second and third toes. **Hallux varus,** placement of the great toe farther from other toes, may be present.

REFLEXES

Many of the newborn's movements are reflexive in nature. Some reflexes, such as sneezing, coughing, swallowing, blinking, yawning, and hiccupping, are present throughout life. Others disappear at various times throughout the first 2 years of life; these are discussed next. These neonatal reflexes must be lost before motor development can proceed (Estes, 2002). The presence of the reflexes indicates neurological integrity.

Rooting Reflex

The rooting reflex is elicited by stroking the skin at one corner of the infant's mouth. The infant will turn the head toward the side stroked (Figure 54-9). This reflex is present up until 3 or 4 months of age. Absence of the reflex during this time frame may indicate a frontal lobe lesion.

TABLE 54-1	COMPARISON OF CAPUT SUCCEDANEUM AND CEPHALHEMATOMA	
CHARACTERISTIC	**CAPUT SUCCEDANEUM**	**CEPHALHEMATOMA**
Fluid	Edema	Blood
Layer involved	Scalp	Between periosteum and skull
Relationship to suture lines	May cross suture lines	Does not cross suture lines
Appears	Present at birth	First or second day
Disappears	2 to 3 days	3 to 6 weeks

Sucking Reflex

Touching the newborn's lips elicits the sucking reflex (Figure 54-10). This reflex occurs until approximately 10 months of age. Preterm infants or an infant who is breastfed by a mother taking barbiturates will not exhibit the sucking reflex because of CNS depression.

Extrusion Reflex

When the tip of the tongue is touched or depressed, the infant will force the tongue outward. This reflex disappears at approximately 4 months of age. Feeding an infant food with a spoon before 4 months of age is difficult because of the extrusion reflex.

Palmar Grasp Reflex

When a finger is placed across the palm, the infant's fingers flex and grasp the examiner's finger (Figure 54-11). If the palmar grasp reflex is present after 4 months of age, frontal lobe lesions are suspected.

Plantar Grasp Reflex

When the infant's leg is held in one hand, and the plantar surface of the foot is touched below the toes with the other hand, the infant's toes will curl downward (Figure 54-12). This reflex lasts until 8 months of age. If the plantar grasp reflex is absent on one foot, an obstructive lesion is suspected. Absence of the reflex in both feet is seen with neurological alterations such as cerebral palsy.

Tonic Neck Reflex

The tonic neck reflex is sometimes referred to as the "fencing" reflex because of the position assumed by the infant. This reflex is elicited by placing the infant supine and rotating the head to one side. The arm and leg on the side to which the jaw is turned will extend and the opposite arm and leg will flex (Figure 54-13). Sometimes, this reflex may not be displayed until 6 to 8 weeks of age. If it is still seen after 6 months of age, cerebral damage is suspected.

Figure 54-9 *Rooting Reflex*

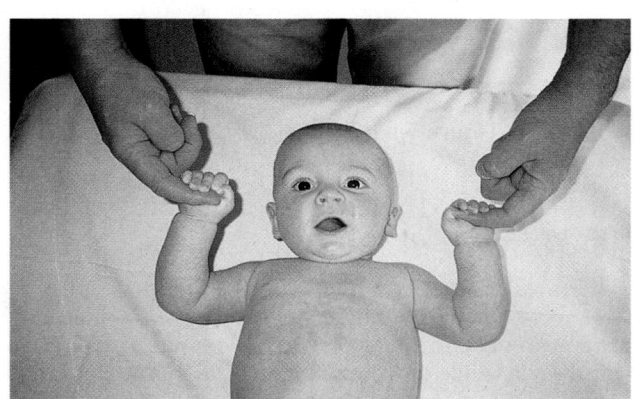

Figure 54-11 *Palmar Grasp Reflex*

Figure 54-10 *Sucking Reflex*

Figure 54-12 *Plantar Grasp Reflex*

Figure 54-13 *Tonic Neck Reflex*

Figure 54-15 *Gallant Reflex*

Figure 54-14 *Moro (Startle) Reflex*

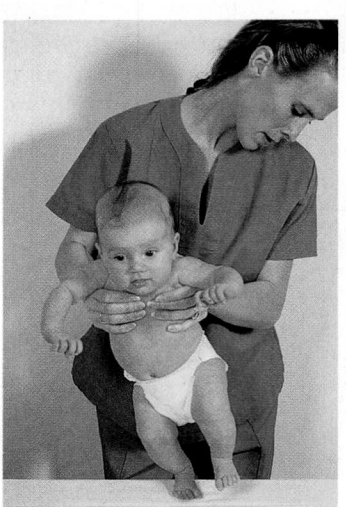

Figure 54-16 *Stepping Reflex*

Moro Reflex

The Moro reflex is sometimes called the startle reflex. It is elicited either by holding the newborn in a semisitting position and then allowing the head to fall backward to an angle of 30°, or having the infant lying on a flat surface and then hitting the surface to startle the infant. The response by the infant less than 4 months of age is to quickly extend and abduct the arms with the fingers fanning out. The thumb and forefinger form a "C" followed by adduction of the arms in an embracing motion. A slight tremor may be noted. The legs may also extend and then flex (Figure 54-14). The Moro reflex is present at birth and disappears between 4 and 6 months of age. Possible brain damage is indicated if the response persists after 6 months of age. An asymmetrical response may be caused by an injury to the clavicle, humerus, or brachial plexus.

Gallant Reflex

The Gallant reflex is elicited with the infant lying prone with the hands under the abdomen. The infant's skin is stroked along one side of the spine; the infant's shoulders and pelvis turn toward the stimulated side (Figure 54-15). A spinal cord lesion is suspected if there is no response from an infant younger than 2 months of age. This reflex is present from birth to age 2 months.

Stepping Reflex

To elicit the stepping reflex, the newborn is held under the arms with the feet placed on a firm surface. The in-

fant will lift alternate feet as if walking (Figure 54-16). This reflex disappears at about 3 months of age.

Babinski's Reflex

To elicit Babinski's reflex, the plantar surface of the infant's foot is stroked from the lateral heel area upward and across under the toes. The great toe should dorsiflex and the other toes fan out (Figure 54-17). The presence of Babinski's reflex after the infant has mastered walking (12 to 18 months of age) is abnormal.

Crossed Extension Reflex

The crossed extension reflex is elicited with the infant supine by holding one leg extended with the knee pressed down and stimulating the bottom of that foot. The other leg should flex, adduct, and then extend as if trying to push away the stimulus. This reflex should be present during the first 4 weeks of life.

Placing Reflex

To elicit the placing reflex, the infant is held under the arms from behind then brought to a standing position, touching the dorsum of one foot on the edge of

Figure 54-17 *Babinski's Reflex*

Babinski's Reflex

The expected response from an infant is opposite that of an older child or adult.

- The expected response from an infant (until walking is mastered) is dorsiflexion of the great toe and fanning of the other toes. This is a positive (normal) response.
- The expected response from a child who has mastered walking and for an adult is flexion of the great toe and other toes. This is a negative (normal) response.
- If an infant has a negative Babinski response or an older person has a positive Babinski response, a neurologic evaluation is required.

Figure 54-18 *Placing Reflex*

PROFESSIONAL TIP

Stepping Reflex and Placing Reflex

While fairly similar, the stepping and placing reflexes are two different reflexes and should not be tested at the same time.

First Period of Reactivity

During the first period of reactivity, the first 30 minutes after birth, the newborn is awake, alert, and active. It is a prime time for parent/infant interaction. The newborn may act hungry, with a strong sucking reflex evident. If the mother plans to breastfeed, this is the ideal time for her to begin. During this period, the newborn's heart rate and respirations are rapid, and bowel sounds are seldom heard.

Sleep Period

The newborn enters a sleep period that usually lasts from 2 to 4 hours. This is a time of deep sleep, from which it is difficult to awaken the newborn. The heart and respiratory rates return to baseline and bowel sounds become audible.

Second Period of Reactivity

The second period of reactivity lasts from 4 to 6 hours. The newborn is once again awake and alert. Physiologic responses vary. The heart and respiratory rates increase, yet there may be periods of apnea, which may cause the heart rate to decrease. During these fluctuations, the newborn may become mottled or slightly cyanotic.

The newborn may gag, spit up, or choke as gastric and respiratory mucus increases. Close observation is a must during this period of activity so that appropriate

the table. The tested leg will flex and lift onto the table (Figure 54-18). It is abnormal for there to be no response. An infant born in a breech presentation or one with paralysis or cerebral cortex difficulties may not respond to this stimulus.

BEHAVIORAL CHARACTERISTICS

During the first 6 to 10 hours after birth, the infant has a fairly predictable pattern of behavior called the periods of reactivity. Following that, the infant will exhibit various behavioral states, divided into sleeping and waking phases.

Periods of Reactivity

Two periods of reactivity occur during the first few hours of life, separated by a period of sleep.

interventions may be taken to maintain a clear airway for the infant.

The first meconium stool is often passed as the gastrointestinal tract becomes more active. The first voiding may now occur. The newborn may begin rooting, sucking, and swallowing, indicating a readiness for feeding.

Behavioral States

Brazelton (1995) identified that newborns have different states of being. He categorized them as sleep states and alert states.

Sleep States

Two sleep states have been identified for the newborn: quiet sleep and active sleep. At term, a newborn changes from one sleep state to the other approximately every 45 to 50 minutes during sleep. Of the total amount of sleep, 45% to 50% is active sleep, 35% to 45% is quiet sleep, and 10% is shifting between the two sleep states (Ladewig et al., 2001).

Quiet Sleep State In quiet sleep, the eyes are closed and there are no eye movements. Respirations are regular, quiet, and slower than in any other state. The heart rate is 100 to 120 beats/minute. There are startles or jerky movements at regular intervals. Stimuli in the environment are not likely to cause a change in the newborn's state.

Active Sleep State During active sleep, respirations are rapid and irregular and sucking movements may be observed. The infant stretches, moves extremities, makes faces, and may fuss briefly. Rapid eye movements (REM) occur. Environmental stimuli may startle the infant, who may then go back to sleep or awaken.

Alert States

There are four alert states: drowsy, quiet alert, active alert, and crying.

Drowsy State The transition between sleep and awake is called the drowsy state. The eyes open and then slowly close, as if unable to stay open. When open, the eyes appear glazed and unfocused. From this state, the infant may go back to sleep or awaken.

Quiet Alert State In the quiet alert state, the infant focuses on people or objects, responds with intense gazing, and seems very interested in the immediate environment. Body movements are minimal. When the infant is in the quiet alert state, it is a good time to enhance bonding. Parents should be made aware of this so they can take advantage of this opportunity.

Active Alert State The infant is often fussy and restless in the active alert state, with more rapid and irregular respirations. The awareness of discomfort from hunger or cold is more intense. Motor activity is quite frequent. The infant is less focused on visual stimuli than in the quiet alert state.

Crying State Crying is generally accompanied by jerky motor activity. Crying serves as a distraction from disturbing stimuli, allows a discharge of energy, and is a method of communication to elicit appropriate responses from parents or caregivers.

GESTATIONAL AGE

According to Alexander and Allen (1996), gestational age must be determined in the first 4 hours after birth so that age-related problems can be identified and appropriate care initiated.

The New Ballard Score is the most commonly used tool (Figure 54-19). It has two elements: external physical characteristics and neuromuscular maturity. If the findings of neuromuscular maturity are not in line with the findings of the external physical characteristics, a second assessment should be performed within 24 hours.

Assessment of External Physical Characteristics

The nurse should begin with resting posture, then skin, lanugo, plantar creases, breast, eye/ear, and then genitals.

Resting Posture

Although resting posture is a characteristic of neuromuscular maturity, it should be assessed first. The posture the newborn assumes when lying undisturbed is to be assessed. The very preterm infant has no flexion of the extremities, while the full-term infant is fully flexed.

Skin

The skin of a preterm infant is very transparent and thin. As gestation progresses, the veins disappear from view as subcutaneous fat is deposited. Vernix caseosa disappears near term but may remain in the creases. There may be some cracking and peeling of the skin, especially around the ankles and feet. As the skin loses moisture after birth, peeling is more apparent.

Lanugo

Lanugo is most abundant between 28 and 30 weeks' gestation. It disappears as the gestational age increases, first disappearing from the face, then the extremities and trunk. A small amount may remain on the shoulders, ears, and sides of the forehead at full term.

Plantar Creases

During the first 12 hours of life, the plantar creases are reliable signs of gestational age. Sole creases develop from the top (under toes) beginning about 32 weeks of gestation. The creases cover two-thirds of the sole by 37 weeks and cover the sole at 40 weeks' gestation.

CULTURAL CONSIDERATIONS

Lanugo

There may be more lanugo on infants with dark skin coloring than on fair-skinned infants with light-colored hair.

NEWBORN MATURITY RATING & CLASSIFICATION

ESTIMATION OF GESTATIONAL AGE BY MATURITY RATING

SYMBOLS: X - 1ST EXAM   O - 2ND EXAM

Gestation by Dates _____ wks

Birth Date _____ Hour_____ am/pm

APGAR _____ 1 min _____ 5 min

NEUROMUSCULAR MATURITY

	-1	0	1	2	3	4	5
Posture							
Square Window (wrist)	>90°	90°	60°	45°	30°	0°	
Arm Recoil		180°	140°-180°	110°-140°	90°-110°	<90°	
Popliteal Angle	180°	160°	140°	120°	100°	90°	<90°
Scarf Sign							
Heel to Ear							

MATURITY RATING

score	weeks
-10	20
-5	22
0	24
5	26
10	28
15	30
20	32
25	34
30	36
35	38
40	40
45	42
50	44

PHYSICAL MATURITY

Skin	sticky friable transparent	gelatinous red, translucent	smooth pink, visible veins	superficial peeling and/or rash few veins	cracking pale areas rare veins	parchment deep cracking no vessels	feathery cracked wrinkled
Lanugo	none	sparse	abundant	thinning	bald areas	mostly bald	
Plantar Surface	heel-toe 40 - 50mm:-1 <40 mm: -2	>50mm no crease	faint red marks	anterior transverse crease only	creases ant. 2/3	creases over entire sole	
Breast	imperceptible	barely perceptible	flat areola no bud	stippled areola 1-2mm bud	raised areola 3-4mm bud	full areola 5-10mm bud	
Eye/Ear	lids fused loosely: -1 tightly: -2	lids open pinna flat stays folded	sl. curved pinna; soft slow recoil	well curved pinna; soft but ready recoil	formed and firm instant recoil	thick cartilage ear stiff	
Genitals Male	scrotum flat, smooth	scrotum empty faint rugae	testes in upper canal rare rugae	testes descending few rugae	testes down good rugae	testes pendulous deep rugae	
Genitals Female	clitoris prominant labia flat	prominent clitoris small labia minora	prominent clitoris enlarging minors	majora & minora equally prominant	majora large minora small	majora cover clitoris and minors	

SCORING SECTION

	1st Exam=X	2nd Exam=O
Estimating Gest Age by Maturity Rating	Weeks	Weeks
Time of Exam	Date ___ Hour ___ am/pm	Date ___ Hour ___ am/pm
Age at Exam	Hours	Hours
Signature of Examiner	M.D.	M.D.

Figure 54-19 *New Ballard Score (Courtesy of Mead Johnson Nutritionals)*

PROFESSIONAL TIP

Ears

When caring for an infant of 32 weeks' gestation or less, be sure the infant's ears are flat to the head and not bent over. Lying on a bent ear can impair circulation to the ear.

Breast

The size of the breast bud tissue is measured by placing the forefinger and middle finger on each side of the breast tissue and measuring between the fingers. At term, the breast bud tissue should be 1 cm. This procedure should be performed gently to prevent tissue damage.

Eye/Ear

The eyelids are fused until 26 to 28 weeks of gestation. The upper pinna begins to curve over at about 33 to 34 weeks of gestation. The curving over continues until it is complete at 39 to 40 weeks of gestation.

The infant at less than 32 weeks of gestation has almost no ear cartilage. When folded, the ear remains

folded. By 36 weeks, there is enough cartilage for the ear to slowly return to its original state when folded. The ear of a full-term infant springs back quickly when folded.

Male Genitals

The male genitals are evaluated for descent of the testes, presence of rugae on the scrotum, and scrotal size. The testes are formed in the abdomen, move into the inguinal canal at 30 weeks of gestation, then into the upper scrotum by 37 weeks of gestation, and are fully descended by full term. Before 36 weeks, there are few rugae on the scrotum. By 38 weeks, rugae have formed on the anterior part of the scrotum and cover the scrotum by 40 weeks of gestation. The scrotum is large and pendulous by 40 weeks.

Female Genitals

Deposits of subcutaneous fat related to nutritional status as well as gestational age determine the appearance of the female genitals. The clitoris and labia minora seem large in comparison to the labia majora, which are small and widely separated at 30 to 32 weeks of gestation. By 36 to 38 weeks of gestation, the clitoris is mostly covered by the labia majora. By 40 weeks of gestation, the labia majora covers the labia minora and clitoris.

Neuromuscular Maturity

The five remaining neuromuscular characteristics to be evaluated are square window, arm recoil, popliteal angle, scarf sign, and heel to ear.

Square Window

The square window sign is elicited by bending the wrist so the palm is as flat against the arm as possible. If the angle between the palm and arm is 90 degrees and looks like a square window, the gestational age is 32 weeks or less and receives a score of 0. If the angle is greater than 90 degrees, the score is −1. The angle becomes smaller the more mature the infant is, until the palm can fold flat against the arm in a full-term newborn.

Arm Recoil

The infant's arms are held with the elbows fully flexed for 5 seconds. Then the arms are pulled straight down at the infant's sides and quickly released. The elbows of a full-term newborn, when released, rapidly recoil and have an angle less than 90 degrees. That infant is given a score of 4. Very preterm infants may not move their arms (no recoil) and receive a score of 0.

Popliteal Angle

The popliteal angle is measured when the thigh is flexed on the abdomen, the hips remain flat on the table, and the lower leg is straightened just until met by resistance. Then the angle behind the knee is scored. When the leg can be fully extended, a score of −1 is given, but if the popliteal angle is less than 90 degrees, a score of 5 is given.

Scarf Sign

The newborn's arm is drawn across the body toward the opposite shoulder until resistance is felt. The shoulder of the arm being tested should remain on the table. The relation of the elbow to the infant's midline is noted for scoring. If the elbow does not reach near the midline, it is a score of 4. When the elbow goes across and beyond the infant's body, a score of −1 is given.

Heel to Ear

With the hips remaining on the surface of the table, the newborn's foot is moved toward the ear on the same side. When resistance is felt, foot position relative to the ear and the degree of knee extension is noted. The preterm infant's leg will remain straight and the foot will be near the ear. The more mature the infant, the more resistance will be felt and more flexion will be noted.

Gestational Age Relationship to Intrauterine Growth

There is a normal range of birth weight for each week of gestation as well as for length, head circumference, and intrauterine weight–length ratio (Figure 54-20). Birth weight is classified as follows:

- **Large for gestational age** (LGA): Infant's weight falls above the 90th percentile for gestational age.
- **Appropriate for gestational age** (AGA): Infant's weight falls between the 90th and 10th percentile for gestational age.
- **Small for gestational age** (SGA): Infant's weight falls below the 10th percentile for gestational age.

The correlation of the infant's measurements for length and head circumference also documents the infant's level of maturity and appropriate classification of LGA, AGA, or SGA.

All of these determinations assist caregivers to expect possible physiologic complications, and together with the results of a physical assessment are the basis for preparing an appropriate care plan for the infant.

SLEEPING POSITION

Since 1992, most infants have been sleeping on their backs. That is when the American Academy of Pediatrics (AAP) recommended that babies be put to sleep on their back to prevent sudden infant death syndrome (SIDS). The incidence of SIDS has greatly decreased since this recommendation was made, but another easily prevented and treated condition, positional plagiocephaly, has increased. The recommendation for back sleeping still stands. Both conditions are discussed in the chapter on Infant with Special Needs: Birth to 12 Months.

FIRST BATH AND CORD CARE

The infant's first bath, and the type of bath for the next 10 days to 2 weeks, is a sponge bath. Newborns are not generally given a tub bath until after the cord has fallen off and healing is complete. Placing the infant under a radiant warmer during the bath helps prevent heat loss. Follow agency protocol for the order of the bath.

Nurses giving the first bath to newborns must wear gloves to comply with Standard Precautions regarding contact with blood or body fluids. A study by Varda and Behnke (2000) found that bathing could be done safely as soon as 1 hour after birth if the newborn's condition is stable and appropriate care is provided. Bathing newborns at 1 hour could decrease exposure of the family and health care providers to bloodborne pathogens (Varda and Behnke, 2000).

Wipe each eye with either a separate cotton ball or a separate place on a washcloth. The eyes are wiped from the inner to outer canthus. The entire face is washed. All of the creases of the ears are cleaned with a corner of a washcloth; a cotton-tipped applicator should *never* be used in the ears.

Using gauze squares and the approved soap, firmly wash the head to remove all blood and body fluids. Infants with a large amount of hair may require the use of a comb to remove all traces of substances in the hair. A second washing and rinsing of the head may be necessary. The head must be well dried when finished.

Soap or a cleansing agent is used on the rest of the body according to agency protocol. Creases must have special attention to be sure that all traces of blood and

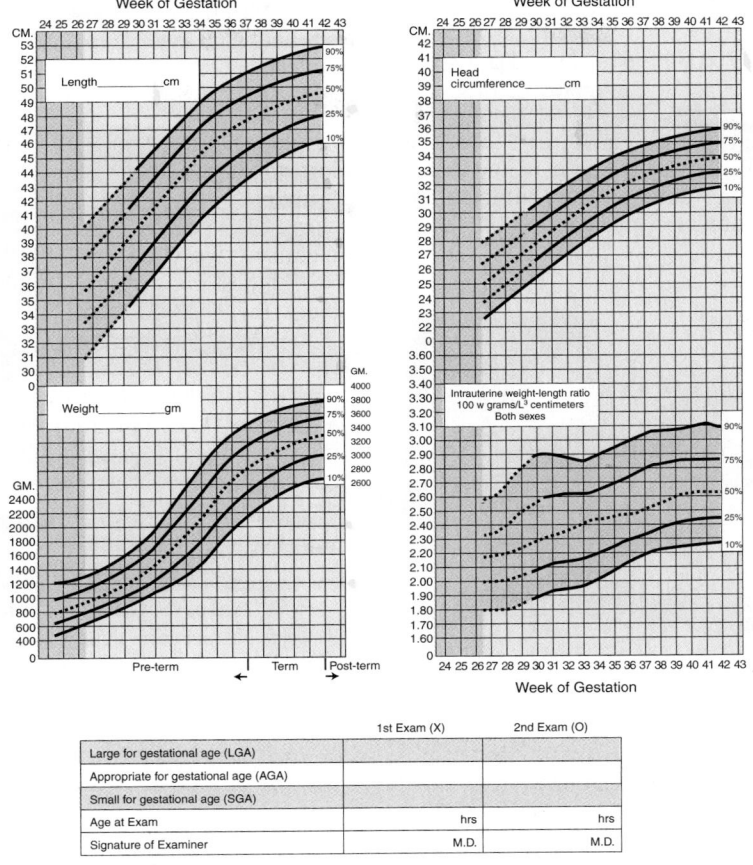

CLASSIFICATION OF NEWBORNS -
BASED ON MATURITY AND INTRAUTERINE GROWTH
Symbols: X - 1st Exam   O - 2nd Exam

	1st Exam (X)	2nd Exam (O)
Large for gestational age (LGA)		
Appropriate for gestational age (AGA)		
Small for gestational age (SGA)		
Age at Exam	hrs	hrs
Signature of Examiner	M.D.	M.D.

Figure 54-20 *Intrauterine Growth Grids (Courtesy of Mead Johnson Nutritionals)*

 CULTURAL CONSIDERATIONS

Umbilical Cord

In Malawi, Africa, infants are kept indoors and are not named until the umbilical cord falls off, typically within the first 2 weeks (Gennaro, Kamwendo, Mbweza, & Kershbaumer, 1998).

 CULTURAL CONSIDERATIONS

Infant Care

Nurses must be aware of different cultural practices in order to provide sensitive care. A few examples include:

- Korean tradition is to consider a newborn 1 year old at the time of birth.
- Korean parents will often tightly wrap a newborn in a blanket to prevent possible harm from the wind (Howard & Berbiglia, 1997).
- Japanese parents often choose to immerse the infant for a bath before the cord is healed (Sharts-Hopko, 1995).
- Muslim fathers traditionally call praise to Allah in the newborn's right ear before cleansing the infant.
- Most infants of Muslim parents are not named until they are 7 days old (Hutchinson & Baqi-Aziz, 1994).
- Babies of Southeast Asian parents are kept swaddled for the first few days (Mattson, 1995).

the majority of vernix caseosa are removed. The skin should be well rinsed to reduce the drying or potential irritating effect of the soap or cleansing agent (Lund et al., 1999). When completely washed and rinsed, the infant is dried and wrapped in a dry, warm blanket.

The infant may remain in the radiant warmer on dry linens or may be dressed, wrapped in a blanket with a hat on the head, and placed in a regular crib and covered with another blanket. Within 30 minutes to 1 hour, the infant's temperature should be checked.

Following the first bath, a bacteriostatic agent is applied to the cord stump and clamp according to agency protocol.

The cord should be cleaned, at least daily, with alcohol. The diaper should be folded under to allow the cord to dry and prevent urine from getting on the cord.

CIRCUMCISION —AFTER 8 days

Circumcision is the surgical removal of the prepuce (foreskin), which covers the glans penis. In 1999, the American Academy of Pediatrics made a policy statement on circumcision that "data are not sufficient to recommend routine neonatal circumcision. . . . If a deci-

sion for circumcision is made, procedural analgesia should be provided" (AAP, 1999). Circumcision is considered an elective procedure for which parents must give written consent. Only full-term, healthy newborns should be circumcised.

Procedure

The infant is placed on a circumcision board just before the procedure begins (Figure 54-21). Because infants prefer a flexed position, being placed on a circumcision board is frustrating to the newborn. Crying often begins at this point, before the procedure is started.

The best pain relief is provided by a penile nerve root block (Lenhart, Lenhart, Reid, & Chong, 1997; Pasero, 2001). A pacifier with 20% sucrose provides comfort and has been shown to be analgesic (Pasero, 2001). The physician then makes a slit in the prepuce and then uses either a Gomco (Yellen) clamp (Figure 54-22) or Plastibell (Figure 54-23) to control bleeding when the prepuce is cut off. After a circumcision with the Gomco clamp, A+D ointment or petroleum jelly is put on the penis to prevent the diaper from sticking to the site. At each diaper change, new ointment is applied for at least 24 to 48 hours.

Figure 54-21 *Circumcision Board. Infant is restrained just before the procedure begins.*

 Safety: Gomco (Yellen) Clamp
Inspect the clamp before use for inadequate closure or corrosion. Check the marks on component parts to make sure they match (Swayze, 1999).

Figure 54-22 *Gomco (Yellen) Clamp Used for Circumcision: A, After slit is made in prepuce, the cone is placed over the glans and the prepuce is pulled up around the cone; B, The cone is placed in the clamp, which is tightened to obliterate the blood vessels. This prevents bleeding. The prepuce is cut away and the clamp is removed in 3 to 5 minutes.*

Figure 54-23 *Plastibell Used for Circumcision. The plastibell is placed over the glans after a slit is made in the prepuce. A suture is tied around the ring. This prevents bleeding when the prepuce is cut away. The handle is removed, leaving the ring to fall off in 5 to 8 days, after healing.*

Nursing Management

The nurse ensures that the circumcision permit has been signed by a parent. Equipment and supplies are set up, and the infant is placed on the circumcision board with diaper removed. Most infants are not fed for 2 to 4 hours before the procedure to prevent regurgitation.

Safety: Circumcision Procedure
Keep a bulb syringe nearby in case the infant requires suctioning.

During the procedure, comfort the infant by talking to the infant, playing a tape of soft music or intrauterine sounds, or lightly stroking the infant. The infant should be kept warm during the circumcision procedure with a well-placed heat lamp. After the procedure, hold the infant to provide comfort. Care following a circumcision includes checking hourly for 12 hours to see if any bleeding is occurring and that the infant is voiding.

If the infant goes home within the first 12 hours after circumcision, bleeding must be minimal and the infant

must have voided. Ensure that the parents know how to care for the circumcision and that they have the physician's telephone number.

NUTRITION

Feeding the newborn is an important aspect of parenting. Nurses assisting in the choice of a feeding method must have knowledge of the newborn's nutritional needs. The American Academy of Pediatrics recommends breast milk for at least 12 months (AAP, 1997).

Nutritional Needs of Newborn

The full-term newborn needs a sufficient intake of calories to meet energy and growth requirements. There should be adequate carbohydrates and fats for energy so that proteins can be used for growth. A newborn requires 110 to 120 kcal/kg (50 to 55 kcal/lb) each day to meet these needs.

This equates to approximately 20 oz of breast milk or formula each day. Newborns lose weight the first few days of life partly because their intake of calories is less than their requirement. One reason is that the newborn's stomach capacity is only 20 mL (30 mL = 1 oz). This capacity increases rapidly, so that by 7 days of age the infant may consume 2 to 3 oz at each feeding. The infant regains birth weight by age 10 days.

Breast Milk and Infant Formula Composition

The compositions of breast milk and infant formula are different.

Breast Milk

Breast milk is biologically designed to meet the needs of human infants. Its composition changes to meet the changing nutritional and immunologic needs of the infant. Breast milk is easily digested.

The colostrum (first few days) is rich in immunoglobulins to protect the newborn's gastrointestinal tract from infection. Colostrum helps establish normal intestinal flora and has a laxative effect that assists in the passage of meconium.

In 2 weeks, mature milk is being produced. It contains sufficient nutrients to meet the infant's needs and has 20 kcal/oz. Breast stimulation and removal of milk from the breast stimulates the secretion of prolactin by the anterior pituitary of the mother. Prolactin increases milk production. As the demand becomes greater (infant feeding longer and more frequently), the milk supply increases.

The mother's diet makes little difference in the proportions of carbohydrates, protein, and most minerals in her breast milk, but fat content and the amount of vitamins are affected. The breastfeeding mother must eat a well-balanced diet to provide the most nutritious milk for her infant and to maintain her own health and energy level. An extra 500 calories per day is needed to support breastfeeding.

Infant Formula

Many infant formulas are modified to match the components in breast milk as nearly as possible. Most formulas are modified cow's milk. Protein is reduced, saturated fat is removed and replaced with vegetable fats, and vitamins and some minerals are added. Soy formulas are used for infants with allergies or who do not tolerate cow's milk–based formula. Nutramigen is a protein hydrolysate formula made from cow's milk but treated to be hypoallergenic.

Special formulas are made to meet special needs of some infants. Preterm infants need more calories but less quantity; these formulas provide 24 kcal/oz. Other formulas are modified to be low in the amino acid phenylalanine for infants with phenylketonuria (PKU), who cannot digest phenylalanine.

Feeding Method

Nutrition is provided for the newborn either through breastfeeding or bottle feeding. Whichever method the parents choose, nurses must support and assist the parents to make the experience meaningful. Some of the advantages and disadvantages of breastfeeding and bottle feeding are identified in Table 54-2.

Other factors besides the advantages and disadvantages of breastfeeding and bottle feeding enter into the decision of how to feed the newborn. These factors include support offered by the infant's father; support by other family members; the need to work outside the home by the mother; and age, educational level, and income level of the parents.

When the mother is breastfeeding (8 to 12 times a day at first), she is focused on the infant. Various tasks

TABLE 54-2 BREASTFEEDING/BOTTLE FEEDING, ADVANTAGES AND DISADVANTAGES

	BREASTFEEDING	BOTTLE FEEDING
Advantages	Nonallergenic Meets infant's specific nutritional needs Immunologic properties help prevent infections Easily digested Constipation unlikely (Figure 54-24) Overfeeding less likely Convenient, always available No formula or bottles to buy No formula and bottles to prepare Oxytocin release helps involution Mother more likely to eat well-balanced diet May help with mother's weight loss Enhances mother/infant attachment through skin-to-skin contact	Father or others may feed infant day or night Feed less frequently (3 to 4 hours) Amount of milk taken at each feeding known
Disadvantages	Feed more frequently (2 to 3 hours) More frequent diaper changes Amount of milk taken at each feeding unknown Medications taken by mother present in milk Discomfort of some mothers to nurse in public Expense of pumping and storing milk for periods when mother is unavailable (such as work hours)	Expense of formula, bottles Washing bottles Fixing and refrigerating formula Carrying bottles on outings May cause constipation

Figure 54-24 *Stool of a Breastfed Infant*

Figure 54-25 *Positions for Feeding Infant: **A,** Cradling, used for breast and bottle feeding; **B,** Football hold; **C,** Lying down; **D,** Across lap*

around the home may need to be left undone or the father will need to do them. Support from other family members may be based on how other family members have chosen to feed their infants.

Breastfeeding

Many factors influence breastfeeding, including positions for feeding, latching on, and length of feeding.

Positions for Feeding

— move than nipple needs to be in mouth. areola also

The infant should be held with the head slightly higher than the rest of the body. The cradle hold, with the infant's head in the bend of the mother's elbow and the arm supporting the infant's body, is probably the most common. It can be used whether breastfeeding or bottle feeding. Other positions that are particularly adaptable to breastfeeding are the football hold, side-lying position, and across-the-lap position (Figure 54-25). The mother's free hand should be in a "C" position, supporting the underside of her breast with the fingers.

Latching On

The mother should use the infant's rooting reflex to allow proper positioning of the nipple in the infant's mouth. Brushing the nipple against the infant's lower lip will cause the infant to open the mouth. When the mouth is wide open and the tongue is down, the mother

quickly brings the infant closer to the breast so the infant can latch on to the nipple and areola. When properly positioned, the tongue is on top of the lower gum and under the breast, with the lips flared outward. When the infant is properly latched on, the suction is strong. To remove the infant from the breast, the mother should insert a finger into the corner of the infant's mouth between the gums to break the suction and quickly remove the breast. The nipple should never be simply pulled out from the infant's mouth because this will cause the mother pain and may also result in tissue damage to the nipple.

Length of Feeding

Feeding length varies with each mother/infant unit; however, the feeding should be long enough to remove all of the **foremilk,** the watery first milk from the breast, which is high in lactose, like skim milk, and is effective in quenching thirst. This allows the infant to receive the **hindmilk,** which is higher in fat content, leads to weight gain, and is more satisfying.

CLIENT TEACHING

Timing of Feedings

Feedings should be given when the infant is hungry (demand feeding) rather than on a fixed schedule. The infant is ready to eat when wide awake, sucking on hands, rooting, and slightly fussy.

CRITICAL THINKING

Breastfeeding

Your client is trying to breastfeed her second child. With her first child, she gave up in three weeks because of cracked, sore nipples. What factors may affect her success or failure? What nursing interventions should be planned and implemented?

The average time for a feeding session is approximately 30 minutes. It is more important to know when the infant is finished feeding than to go by the clock. When an infant is satisfied, the sucking and swallowing will be much slower and the breast will be soft. The infant may fall asleep and release the nipple.

The first breast should be emptied (very soft) before moving the infant to the other breast. At the next feeding, the breast used last at the previous feeding should be used first. This ensures that each breast is emptied at least at every other feeding. As the infant grows and requires more milk, both breasts may be emptied at each feeding.

Bottle Feeding

Factors related to bottle feeding include bottles, formula preparation, and amount of feeding.

Bottles

Babies will generally feed well from any bottle and nipple, although many babies will eventually develop a preference and may refuse a new type of nipple. Whatever choice the parents make will be fine. Washing the bottles and nipples with a bottle and nipple brush in warm, soapy water is necessary for thorough cleaning. Rinsing thoroughly removes all traces of soap. Only if there is a question regarding the safety of the water supply (e.g., well water on a farm or ranch) is boiling of the bottles and nipples necessary.

Formula Preparation

Formulas are available in three forms: ready to feed, concentrated, and powdered. The latter two require addition of water. The choice of formula is generally left up to the parents. There is a great difference in price, so the choice may be made based on finances. Mixing of formula must be accurate to provide the 20 kcal/oz.

Amount of Feeding

Most newborns begin by drinking 7.5 mL to 15 mL ($1/4$ to $1/2$ oz) at a feeding but gradually increase to approximately 90 mL to 120 mL (3 to 4 oz) at each feeding in 2 weeks. The infant's appetite will generally increase during growth spurts at 2 weeks, 6 to 9 weeks, and 3 to 6 months, so the amount of formula should be increased by 30 mL (1 oz) in each bottle to meet this need.

Burping

All infants require burping, whether breastfed or bottle fed. Burping is needed to expel the air swallowed when the infant sucks. Some infants swallow more air than others and require more frequent burping.

To facilitate burping, the infant can be held upright on the feeder's shoulder, in a sitting position on the feeder's lap with the head and chest supported with one hand, or prone across the feeder's lap (Figure 54-26). The other hand is used to gently pat or rub the infant's back.

Burping should be done generally about halfway through the feeding for bottle feeding and when changing breasts for breastfeeding. Parents soon learn the infant's cues regarding the need to be burped.

Figure 54-26 *Burping Positions:* **A,** *Supported on the shoulder;* **B,** *Upright on the lap;* **C,** *Face down across the lap*

SAMPLE NURSING CARE PLAN

NEWBORN INFANT

Selena Sauve, born at 36 weeks' gestation, weighs 6 pounds 3 ounces and is 19 inches long. Her Apgar score was 8 at 1 minute and 9 at 5 minutes. Axillary temperature is 96.5°F (35.8°C), respirations 56, and apical pulse 148. The parents are very excited about Selena, their first child. Selena is very sleepy and is not breastfeeding well.

Nursing Diagnosis 1 *Ineffective **T**hermoregulation* related to immaturity as evidenced by birth at 36 weeks' gestation

Nursing Outcomes Classification (NOC)
Thermoregulation: Neonate

Nursing Interventions Classification (NIC)
Temperature Regulation

PLANNING/GOALS	NURSING INTERVENTIONS	RATIONALE
Selena's temperature will be between 97.5°F (36.4°C) and 98.9°F (37.2°C).	Keep Selena adequately clothed and covered.	Maintains her temperature.
	Maintain ambient room temperature between 77.2°F (25.1°C) and 78.1°F (25.6°C).	Is optimum environmental temperature.
	Keep Selena away from air conditioning vents, drafts, and fans.	Prevents heat loss by convection.
	Use warm water when bathing Selena, wrap her in a towel, and dry her quickly. Dry her head thoroughly and put a cap on her head.	Prevents heat loss by evaporation.
	Cover scales and examination area before Selena is laid down.	Prevents heat loss by conduction.
	Keep Selena's crib away from outside windows.	Prevents heat loss by radiation.
	Teach Selena's parents how to maintain a neutral thermal environment for Selena.	Prevents Selena from using her brown fat too fast.

EVALUATION   Selena's temperature is 97.8°F.

Nursing Diagnosis 2 *Risk for **I**nfection* related to risk factor of inadequate primary defenses as evidenced by cut umbilical cord and immature immune system

Nursing Outcomes Classification (NOC)
Tissue Integrity: Skin & Mucous Membranes

Nursing Interventions Classification (NIC)
Infection Control

PLANNING/GOALS	NURSING INTERVENTIONS	RATIONALE
Selena will have no signs of infection of the eyes, diaper area, or umbilical cord.	Use good hand hygiene technique (caregivers and parents) before and after caring for Selena.	Prevents spread of infection.
	Provide prescribed eye prophylaxis and keep eyes clean.	Prevents infection.
	Keep diaper area clean and dry.	Prevents skin irritation and infection.
	Place diaper below the umbilical cord.	Allows cord to dry and heal.
	Provide prescribed cord prophylaxis and clean umbilical cord daily with alcohol.	Prevents infection and removes exudate.

EVALUATION   Selena shows no signs of infection.

continues

SAMPLE NURSING CARE PLAN

Nursing Diagnosis 3 *Imbalanced Nutrition: Less than Body Requirements* related to limited nutritional intake as evidenced by being very sleepy and not breastfeeding very well

Nursing Outcomes Classification (NOC)
Nutritional Status: Food & Fluid Intake

Nursing Interventions Classification (NIC)
Lactation Counseling

PLANNING/GOALS	NURSING INTERVENTIONS	RATIONALE
Selena will lose only 5 to 10 ounces of weight during the first 3 days.	Assist mother in breastfeeding Selena.	Provides support for first time breastfeeding.
	Demonstrate use of rooting reflex to ensure proper latch on.	Uses natural response of infant for proper position of mouth and tongue.
	Explain that Selena will suck in spurts.	Assists mother in knowing that Selena has not finished breastfeeding when she rests.
	Explain that the breast has foremilk and hindmilk (needed for growth), so breasts must be emptied.	Ensures that mother will allow Selena to empty one breast before changing to the other breast.

EVALUATION   Selena lost 7 ounces during the first 3 days.

PROBLEMS OF THE NEWBORN

Problems of the newborn identified either at birth or before discharge include hyperbilirubinemia, respiratory distress, cleft lip/palate, hydrocephalus, spina bifida, Down syndrome, and talipes equinovarus. Newborn problems may also occur when the mother is diabetic, HIV positive, or a substance abuser. Phenylketonuria must be tested for as soon as possible so treatment can begin immediately.

HYPERBILIRUBINEMIA

Hyperbilirubinemia, an excess of bilirubin in the blood, may be related to physiologic jaundice or pathologic jaundice. Physiologic jaundice does not appear until after 24 hours of age and is more commonly seen after the infant has gone home. It is discussed in the Infants with Special Needs: Birth to 12 Months chapter.

Pathologic jaundice appears in the first 24 hours and may lead to **kernicterus** (deposits of bilirubin causing yellow staining in the brain, especially the basal ganglia, cerebellum, and hippocampus). The exact level of total bilirubin when kernicterus occurs is not known but may occur at 20 mg/dL in full-term infants and at a lower level in preterm neonates. The most common cause is Rh incompatibility.

Medical–Surgical Management

Medical

Phototherapy is the most common treatment for jaundice. The "bili" lights are special flourescent lamps (in the blue-light spectrum) placed over the infant. Only a diaper and an eye covering are on the infant to expose the most skin surface to the light. A fiber-optic phototherapy blanket and the BiliBed® with the Bilicombi™ blanket (Figure 54-27) have been designed to provide phototherapy without the eyes needing to be covered. Because the infant is covered, thermal regulation is no longer a problem, and interaction with the parents can take place. The infant may experience frequent, green, loose stools as the bilirubin is excreted.

Surgical

If the bilirubin level cannot be reduced quickly or maintained below 12 mg/dL with phototherapy treatment, exchange transfusion is necessary. Blood type O, Rh-negative blood is used. During this procedure, 5 mL to 10 mL of blood are removed from the infant and replaced with a like amount of donor blood. This is a very slow process. Complications of hypervolemia, hypovolemia, infection, cardiac arrhythmias, and air embolism may occur.

This procedure is seldom necessary today because of the widespread use of RhoGAM to prevent Rh incompatibility.

Figure 54-27 *BiliBed® with Bilicombi™ Blanket, 1999 Medela, Inc. (Photo courtesy of Medela, Inc.)*

Diet

Fluid intake is increased to assist in elimination of the bilirubin through the urine.

Nursing Management

Review record to identify factors predisposing the infant to jaundice. Assess infant for jaundice every 4 hours. Encourage adequate amount taken at each feeding. Provide extra water intake. Keep diaper area clean and protected.

NURSING PROCESS

Assessment

Subjective Data

None

Objective Data

Prenatal and perinatal records are reviewed to identify factors predisposing to jaundice. Jaundice in light-skinned infants is assessed by blanching the skin (pressing firmly with the thumb) over a bony prominence such as the forehead, nose, or sternum. When the thumb is removed, the area has a yellowish appearance before normal color returns if jaundice is present. In darker-skinned infants, the infant's oral mucosa, posterior aspect of the hard palate, or conjunctival sacs will have a yellow coloring when jaundice is present.

Nursing diagnoses for an infant with hyperbilirubinemia may include the following:

Nursing Diagnoses	Planning/Goals	Nursing Interventions
Risk for Deficient Fluid Volume related to increased insensible water loss and frequent loose stools secondary to phototherapy	The infant's intake will be at least 100 to 150 mL/kg/day.	Encourage adequate feedings of infant by mother. Provide extra water intake.
Risk for Impaired Skin Integrity related to frequent loose stools secondary to phototherapy	The infant's diaper area will maintain skin integrity.	Check diaper frequently and change as soon as soiled. Apply A+D ointment or petroleum jelly to diaper area after cleansing.

Evaluation Each goal must be evaluated to determine how it has been met by the client.

RESPIRATORY DISTRESS

Two types of respiratory distress may occur in a newborn: respiratory distress syndrome (RDS) and transient tachypnea of the newborn (TTN).

Respiratory distress syndrome is associated with preterm infants and surfactant deficiency. Verma (1995) describes respiratory distress syndrome as caused by alterations in surfactant quantity, composition, function, or production. These infants have hypoxia, respiratory acidosis, and metabolic acidosis.

Transient tachypnea of the newborn is found mainly in AGA and near-term infants (Ladewig et al., 2001). Either intrauterine or intrapartum asphyxia has been experienced by these infants. This results in the newborn's failure to clear the airway of lung fluid and mucus or aspiration of amniotic fluid. No respiratory difficulties are experienced at birth, but shortly after birth, the newborn may have flaring of the nares and expiratory grunting. By 6 hours of age, tachypnea is noted, with respirations as high as 100 to 140 breaths/minute.

Medical–Surgical Management

Medical

The goal is to determine which type of respiratory distress is affecting the newborn and begin treatment. For RDS, the goals of treatment are maintenance of adequate oxygenation and ventilation and correction of the respiratory and metabolic acidosis. Mild RDS is often treated only with increased, humidified oxygen concentration. Infants with moderate RDS may require continuous positive airway pressure (CPAP). Mechanical ventilation is required for severe RDS. The oxygen needs of infants with RDS increase over the first 48 hours.

Infants with TTN generally require ambient oxygen of 30% to 50% initially. This need for increased oxygen generally decreases over the first 48 hours. Treatment is usually required only for 4 days.

Nursing Management

Monitor respirations and pulse oximetry at least hourly. Use the Silverman-Anderson index to rate respiratory effort. Provide oxygen as ordered. Monitor oxygen concentration. Use strict aseptic technique when caring for the infant.

NURSING PROCESS

Assessment

Subjective Data

None

Objective Data

There will be cyanosis pallor or mottling of the skin, tachypnea, grunting respirations, retractions, and nasal flaring. To rate the infant's respiratory effort, the Silverman-Anderson index is often used (Figure 54-28). The heart rate is generally within normal limits.

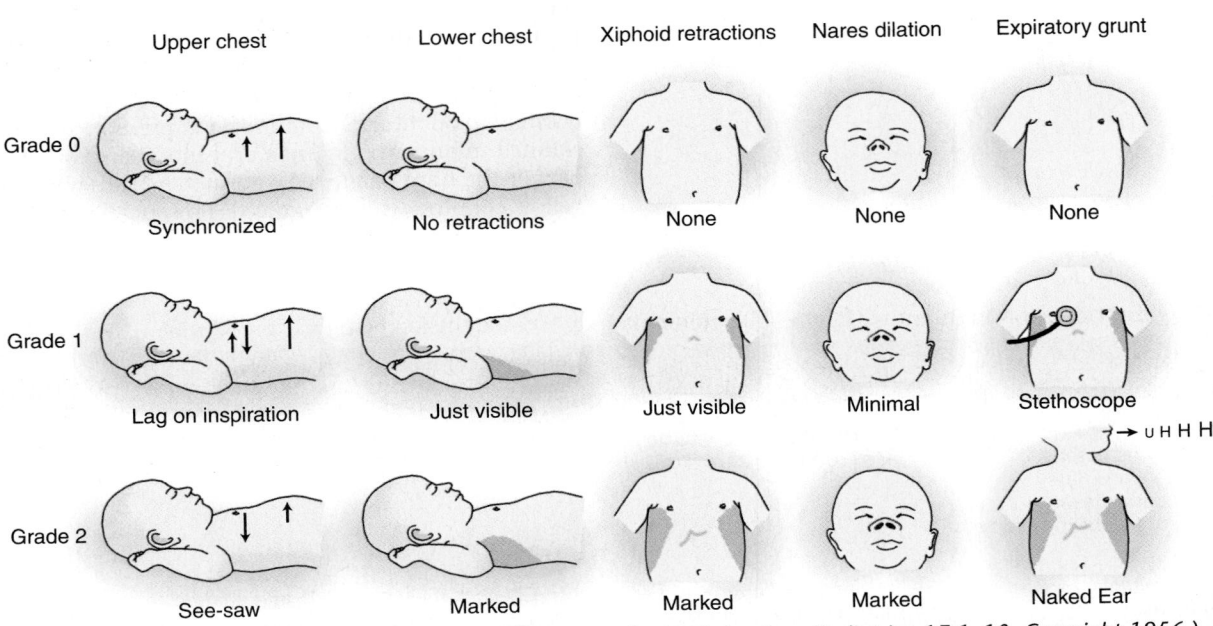

Figure 54-28 *Silverman-Anderson Index (Reproduced with permission from* Pediatrics *17:1–10. Copyright 1956.)*

Nursing diagnoses for an infant with respiratory distress may include the following:

Nursing Diagnoses	Planning/Goals	Nursing Interventions
Impaired Gas Exchange related to ventilation perfusion imbalance	The infant will have increased gas exchange as indicated by pulse oximetry.	Monitor pulse oximetry, respirations at least hourly. Provide oxygen as ordered. Monitor oxygen concentration.
Risk for Infection related to invasive procedures	The infant will have no signs of infection.	Maintain strict aseptic technique in the care of the infant.

Evaluation Each goal must be evaluated to determine how it has been met by the client.

CLEFT LIP/PALATE

The immediate concern with cleft lip/palate (Figure 54-29) is the problem of feeding the infant. The size of the cleft and whether the palate is also involved determine the difficulty of feeding. Special nipples and feeding devices are available. Hold the infant in an upright sitting position when feeding. Burp frequently because these infants swallow more air than usual. When sleeping, keep the infant in a side-lying position.

Parents of an infant with any congenital anomaly need support because they may need to grieve over the loss of a normal infant. The nurse must role model interacting with the infant. Complete coverage is found in the Infants with Special Needs: Birth to 12 Months chapter.

HYDROCEPHALUS

Hydrocephalus, excess cerebrospinal fluid in the cerebral ventricles, causes the infant's head to be enlarged. Head circumference is measured daily, fontanelles checked to see whether they are flat or bulging, and the infant's position changed frequently. The infant usually cannot move the head. Complete coverage is found in the Infant with Special Needs: Birth to 12 Months chapter.

SPINA BIFIDA

There are three types of spina bifida (neural tube defects): spina bifida occulta, meningocele, and myelomeningocele (Figure 54-30). **Spina bifida occulta** is a failure of the vertebral arch to close. There is a dimple on the back, which may have a tuft of hair in it. No care is required.

A **meningocele** is a saclike protrusion along the vertebral column filled with cerebrospinal fluid and meninges. Surgery is required to repair the defect, but there are no long-term effects.

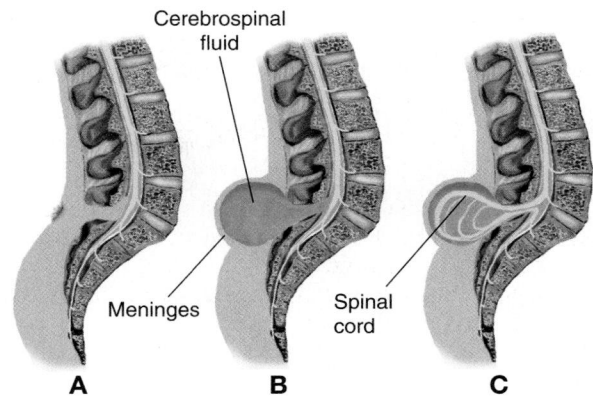

Figure 54-30 *Types of Spina Bifida:* **A,** *Spina bifida occulta;* **B,** *Meningocele;* **C,** *Myelomeningocele*

A **myelomeningocele** is a saclike protrusion along the vertebral column filled with spinal fluid, meninges, nerve roots, and spinal cord. Because of the nerve root and spinal cord involvement, there will be paralysis at some level after surgical repair.

The saclike protrusions must be kept covered with sterile saline dressings, and the infant handled carefully when changing position from side to side. The sac must be kept free from contamination by urine and stool. Head circumference is measured and fontanelles checked for bulging on each shift because hydrocephalus often develops. Complete coverage of myelomeningocele is found in the Infant with Special Needs: Birth to 12 Months chapter.

DOWN SYNDROME

Down syndrome is caused by a chromosomal abnormality, also called trisomy 21. Routine care is provided in the newborn period. Complete coverage is found in the Infant with Special Needs: Birth to 12 Months chapter.

TALIPES EQUINOVARUS

Talipes equinovarus, also called clubfoot, is a congenital deformity in which the foot and ankle are twisted inward and cannot be moved to a midline position (Figure 54-31). The foot or feet of some infants appear to turn inward, but if they can be moved to the midline, the cause is intrauterine position. Range-of-motion exercises will often correct this problem.

Infants with true clubfoot may have a cast on before going home. Complete coverage is found in the Infant with Special Needs: Birth to 12 Months chapter.

INFANT OF A DIABETIC MOTHER

The infant of a diabetic mother (IDM) requires close observation the first few hours to several days after birth. If the mother has vascular complications with the

Figure 54-29 *Types of Cleft Lip/Palate:* **A,** *Small notch in lip, palate normal;* **B,** *Cleft lip and cleft palate;* **C,** *Bilateral cleft lip and cleft palate;* **D,** *Lip normal, cleft palate*

Figure 54-31 **A,** *Talipes equinovarus (clubfoot);* **B,** *Foot moves to midline; positional, not clubfoot*

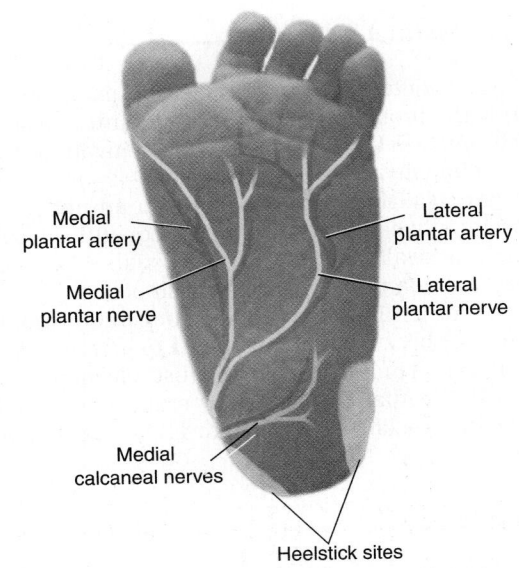

Figure 54-32 *Shaded areas are heelstick sites.*

diabetes, the infant is generally SGA. If the mother has gestational diabetes or diabetes without vascular changes, the infant is generally LGA, especially if the diabetes has not been well-controlled. The large size is the result of fat deposits and increased size of all organs except the brain. The IDM has less total body water, especially in the extracellular spaces. Following are complications seen most often in the IDM:

- *Hypoglycemia:* The loss of maternal glucose at birth and the high level of insulin produced by the infant decrease the infant's blood glucose within hours after birth. It takes a period of time for insulin production to be reduced in the newborn.
- *Respiratory distress:* Insulin is antagonistic to the cortisol-induced stimulation of lecithin (phospholipid necessary for lung maturation) synthesis. This results in less-mature lungs than would be expected for the gestational age. This does not seem to be a problem if the mother has vascular complications with her diabetes.
- *Hyperbilirubinemia:* Hepatic immaturity and a decreased extracellular fluid volume, which increases hematocrit, may be the cause of the hyperbilirubinemia seen 48 to 72 hours after birth (Ladewig et al., 2001). Any bruises from a difficult delivery may also be a cause.
- *Birth trauma:* The large size of many IDMs predisposes them to trauma during labor and delivery.
- *Congenital birth defects:* Birth defects may include patent ductus arteriosus, ventricular septal defect, transposition of the great vessels, small left colon syndrome, and sacral agenesis (Tyrala, 1996).

Medical–Surgical Management

Medical

Blood glucose monitoring is performed hourly during the first 4 to 6 hours of life and then every 4 hours for 24 hours, or per agency protocol. Blood is generally obtained by heelstick (Figure 54-32).

Pharmacological

An intravenous infusion of glucose may be necessary if early feeding does not keep the blood glucose at 45 mg/dL or above.

Diet

A feeding of 5% glucose water may be given soon after birth, followed in 1 hour by a breast or formula feeding, which is continued on a regular basis.

Nursing Management

Monitor blood glucose level as ordered. Ensure timely feedings. Administer glucose orally or IV as ordered. Prevent cold stress. Hold and comfort the infant after heelsticks.

NURSING PROCESS

Assessment

Subjective Data

None

Objective Data

Blood glucose screening of less than 45 mg/dL should be verified by laboratory analysis. The infant may show signs of jitteriness or tremors. Diaphoresis, although uncommon for a newborn, may occur with hypoglycemia. Poor muscle tone, low temperature, and rapid respirations may also be noted.

Nursing diagnoses for an infant with hypoglycemia may include the following:

Nursing Diagnoses	Planning/Goals	Nursing Interventions
*Imbalanced **N**utrition: Less Than Body Requirements* related to increased glucose use secondary to being IDM	The infant will maintain an adequate glucose level.	Ensure timely infant feedings. Monitor blood glucose level according to protocol. Prevent cold stress and identify other stressors (hypoxia, sepsis, RDS) that increase glucose use.
*Acute **P**ain* related to physical injury of heelsticks for glucose monitoring	The infant will decrease crying after each heelstick.	Properly perform heelstick to avoid nerves and arteries. Hold and comfort infant after heel stick procedure.

Evaluation Each goal must be evaluated to determine how it has been met by the client.

INFANT OF AN HIV-POSITIVE MOTHER

The transmission rate of HIV infection from mother to infant is 28% to 35% (Merenstein, Adams, & Weisman, 2002). This transmission may occur through the placenta at various gestational ages, through maternal blood and secretions during labor and birth, and through breast milk after the birth (Fanaroff & Martin, 2001).

Every infant born to an HIV-seropositive mother will have HIV antibodies that have crossed the placenta from the mother. By 8 to 15 months of age, uninfected infants have lost the maternal antibodies; but the infected infants have begun to develop their own antibodies and remain HIV seropositive (Fanaroff & Martin, 2001).

At birth, the HIV-infected infant typically has no symptoms. The appearance of an opportunistic disease between 3 and 6 months of age may alert caregivers to the presence of HIV infection. Lymphoid interstitial pneumonitis is considered a criterion for diagnosis (Fanaroff & Martin, 2001). As a basis for care, all infants of HIV-positive mothers must be presumed to be HIV positive.

Breastfeeding is not recommended.

INFANT OF A SUBSTANCE-ABUSING MOTHER

The infant of a substance-abusing mother (ISAM) is a substance abuser at birth. When the umbilical cord is cut at birth, the newborn experiences withdrawal. The severity of withdrawal symptoms depends on the substance(s) abused by the mother and the time and amount of the last dose. The symptoms may occur within the first 24 to 48 hours after birth or not until 4 or 5 days of age. Alcohol withdrawal symptoms often appear within 6 to 12 hours after birth or at least within the first 3 days. Infant alcohol dependence is physiologic. It may be very difficult for the substance-abusing mother to care for her infant initially and/or long term.

Complications commonly found in an ISAM include withdrawal, respiratory distress, jaundice, behavior

PROFESSIONAL TIP

Narcotic Antagonists

The use of naloxone (Narcan) is contraindicated for infants born to narcotic abusers. It may cause severe signs and symptoms of narcotic withdrawal, especially seizures.

problems, congenital anomalies, and growth retardation. Infants of alcohol-dependent mothers may also have fetal alcohol syndrome (FAS).

Medical–Surgical Management
Medical

Treatment is focused on management of the previously mentioned complications that may be present. Approximately 50% of these infants experience withdrawal symptoms severe enough to require treatment.

Pharmacological

Phenobarbital or tincture of opium may be used to control drug withdrawal symptoms. Phenobarbital or diazepam (Valium) may be used to control seizures in the alcohol-dependent infant.

Diet

Formula supplying 24 kcal/oz is recommended for the infant who experiences vomiting and diarrhea or who is excessively active.

Nursing Management

Monitor the infant's temperature, weight, skin turgor, and fontanells. Maintain strict intake and output. Provide small, frequent feedings. Provide a quiet environment and keep stimulation at a minimum. Administer medications as ordered. Role model interacting with the infant and encourage the mother to do so. Make referrals as necessary to social agencies and infant development programs.

NURSING PROCESS

Assessment

Subjective Data

None

Objective Data

The drug-dependent infant may experience hyperactivity, persistent high-pitched shrill cry, tremors, seizures, tachypnea, fever, disorganized sucking and swallowing, vomiting, diarrhea, stuffy nose, yawning, sneezing, and sweating. The alcohol-dependent infant may or may not have FAS, which includes mental retardation, hyperactivity, growth deficiency, distinctive facial abnormalities, and other congenital anomalies. This infant may also experience tremors, seizures, inconsolable crying, abdominal distention, great activity, and exaggerated rooting and sucking.

Nursing diagnoses for an infant experiencing withdrawal may include the following:

Nursing Diagnoses	Planning/Goals	Nursing Interventions
*Imbalanced **N**utrition: Less Than Body Requirements,* related to disorganized sucking and swallowing, vomiting, diarrhea, and hyperactivity	The infant will not lose excessive weight (more than 10% of birth weight).	Monitor infant's temperature so environment can be adjusted to maintain normal infant temperature. Provide small frequent feedings. Administer medications as ordered. Position infant on the side to avoid possible aspiration. Maintain strict intake and output. Weigh infant every 8 hours. Monitor for signs of dehydration (sunken fontanel, dry mucous membranes, poor skin turgor, weight loss).
*Risk for **I**njury* related to effects of substance withdrawal (seizures, hyperactivity)	The infant will not exhibit signs of seizures.	Administer medications as ordered. Decrease environmental activity. Plan care to necessitate minimum stimulation. Wrap infant snugly. Monitor activity level.
*Risk for Impaired **P**arenting* related to substance abuse and difficult temperament of the infant	The parent will show signs of bonding/attachment and an interest in infant care.	Explain effects of maternal substance abuse on infant and the process of withdrawal. Role model interacting with the infant. Encourage mother to interact with her infant. Explain and demonstrate infant care procedures, especially how to avoid excess stimulation of the infant. Make referrals to social agencies and infant development programs.

Evaluation Each goal must be evaluated to determine how it has been met by the client.

PHENYLKETONURIA

Most states require neonatal screening for the genetic disease phenylketonuria (PKU), an inborn error of metabolism in which the infant has a deficiency of the enzyme required to digest the amino acid phenylalanine.

The infant must ingest an ample amount of phenylalanine, found in both breast milk and regular infant formulas, for the PKU test to be reliable. The test is performed at least 24 hours after the initial breast or formula feeding.

PROFESSIONAL TIP

PKU

The time of the first breast or formula feeding is to be documented so at least 24 hours passes before the heelstick for the PKU test is performed.

CULTURAL CONSIDERATIONS

Phenylketonuria

The highest incidence of PKU is found in the white populations of Northern Europe and the United States; it is less common in populations of African, Chinese, and Japanese descent (AAP, 1996).

An infant with PKU must be put on a diet low in phenylalanine, preferably by 1 month of age. Infant formulas that are very low in phenylalanine are available. Without screening and diet modification, severe mental retardation results. Even with neonatal PKU screening, many affected children have some intellectual impairment (Lowdermilk & Perry, 2003).

CASE STUDY

Baby boy Hren, a full-term newborn, is 36 hours old. He has type B, Rh-positive blood and his mother has type O, Rh-positive blood. There is a small cephalhematoma on the right parietal bone. Routine assessment identified the appearance of jaundice when the skin was blanched on his forehead. His bilirubin level was 2 mg/dL on the cord blood and 4 mg/dL at 24 hours of age.

The following questions will guide your development of a nursing care plan for the case study.

1. What factors may be causing the jaundice?
2. What orders would you anticipate the physician would write?
3. What are the critical levels of bilirubin?
4. Phototherapy is begun using "bili" lights. What assessments and precautions must be taken when these lights are used?
5. Identify two possible nursing diagnoses and a goal for each for baby boy Hren.
6. Describe nursing interventions for meeting the goals.
7. How can the goals be evaluated?

Summary

- The immediate needs of the newborn are airway, breathing, circulation, and warmth.
- The initiation of breathing is related to physical, chemical, thermal, and sensory factors.
- Circulatory changes include the closing of the three fetal structures: the ductus arteriosus, foramen ovale, and the ductus venosus.
- Nonshivering thermogenesis, metabolism of brown fat, is the newborn's unique method of heat production.
- Infants lose heat through conduction, convection, evaporation, and radiation.

- The immediate care of the newborn includes obtaining the Apgar score, resuscitation (if required), providing a neutral thermal environment, identification, parent/infant bonding, and prophylactic care.
- Common variations of the newborn must be carefully documented, especially mongolian spots, to possibly prevent parents from being charged with child abuse.
- Neurologic integrity can be assessed through the many reflexes of the newborn. Most of these reflexes disappear during the first 2 years of life.
- Six states of being have been identified for the newborn: quiet sleep, active sleep, drowsy, quiet alert, active alert, and crying.

- Gestational age can be determined by assessing six physical characteristics and six neuromuscular maturity characteristics.
- Infants are considered contaminated with blood-borne pathogens until after the first bath.
- Problems of the newborn include hyperbilirubinemia, respiratory distress, cleft lip/palate, hydrocephalus, spina bifida, Down syndrome, talipes equinovarus, and phenylketonuria.
- Infants need special care when the mother is a diabetic, HIV positive, or a substance abuser.

Review Questions

1. The nurse is aware that survival of a newborn infant depends primarily on:

   a. the infant's regulation of body temperature.

   b. prompt expansion of the lungs and the establishment of gaseous exchange.

   c. the infant's energy provided from materials obtained from the environment.

   d. the rise in the infant's arterial oxygen tension and a rapid fall in carbon dioxide tension.

2. When assisting the establishment of respirations in a newborn, which of these actions should the nurse do first?

   a. tie the cord.

   b. provide continuous oxygen.

   c. use a resuscitation machine.

   d. remove mucus from the mouth, throat, and nose.

3. The nurse dries a newborn infant as soon after birth as possible, primarily to help:

   a. stimulate the infant's circulatory system.

   b. avoid excess heat loss from the infant's body.

   c. remove organisms from the infant's skin acquired during birth.

   d. remove the amniotic fluid so the infant is not so slippery.

4. A new mother asks the nurse about the bluish area on her infant's buttocks. The nurse's response is based on knowledge that this discoloration:

   a. is called mongolian spots.

   b. may need to be removed surgically.

   c. is a birthmark that the infant will have for life.

   d. should be checked about twice a year for precancerous cells.

5. The nurse is aware that the most generally accepted theory of the cause of physiologic jaundice is that it results from:

   a. dehydration fever.

   b. congenital obliteration of the bile ducts.

   c. rapid destruction of excess red blood cells.

   d. antibodies caused by the Rh negative factor in the maternal blood.

References/Suggested Readings

Alexander, G. R., & Allen, M. C. (1996). Conceptualization, measurement, and use of gestational age: I. clinical and public health practice. *Journal of Perinatology, 16*(1), 53.

Allard-Hendren, R. (2000). Alcohol use and adolescent pregnancy. *MCN, 25*(3), 159–162.

American Academy of Pediatrics (AAP). Committee on Pediatrics and Committee on Genetics (1996). Newborn screening fact sheets. *Pediatrics, 98*(3), 473.

American Academy of Pediatrics (AAP). Work Group on Breastfeeding (1997). Breastfeeding and the use of human milk. *Pediatrics, 100*(6), 1035.

American Academy of Pediatrics. (1999). Task force on circumcision. Circumcision policy statement. *Pediatrics, 103*(3), 686–693.

Armentrout, D., & Huseby, V. (2003). Polycythemia in the newborn. *MCN, 28*(4), 234–240.

Ballard, J. L., Khoury, J. C., Wedig, K., Wang, L., Eilers-Walsman, B. L., & Lipp, R. (1991). New Ballard Score, expanded to include extremely premature infants. *Journal of Pediatrics, 19*(3), 417–423.

Behrman, R. E., Kliegman, R.M., & Jenson, H. (Eds.). (2000). *Nelson's textbook of pediatrics* (16th ed.). Philadelphia: W. B. Saunders.

Blecher, M. (2001). *Cutting to the point on circumcision.* [Online]. Available: www.webmd.com/content/article/3609.220

Brazelton, T. B., & Nagent, J. K. (1995). *Neonatal behavioral assessment scale* (3rd ed.). London: Cambridge University Press.

Burroughs, A., & Leifer, G. (2001). *Maternity nursing* (8th ed.). Philadelphia: W.B. Saunders.

Callister, L., & Vega, R. (1998). Giving birth: Guatemalan women's voices. *JOGNN, 27*(3), 289–295.

Choudhry, U. (1997). Traditional practices of women from India: Pregnancy, childbirth, and newborn care. *JOGNN, 26*(5), 533–539.

Clinical Rounds. (2002). Why circumcision helps protect against infection. *Nursing2002, 32*(10), 33–34.

Dochterman, J., & Bulechek, G. (2004). *Nursing Interventions Classification (NIC)* (4th ed.). St. Louis, MO: Mosby.

Estes, M. E. Z. (2002). *Health assessment & physical examination* (2nd ed.). Clifton Park, NY: Thomson Delmar Learning.

Fanaroff, A., & Martin, R. (2001). *Neonatal-perinatal medicine: Diseases of the fetus and infant* (7th ed.). St. Louis, MO: Mosby–Year Book.

Gennaro, S., Kamwendo, L., Mbweza, E., & Kershbaumer, R. (1998). Childbearing in Malawi, Africa. *JOGNN, 27*(2), 191–196.

Hein, H. A., & Pettit, S. F. (2001). Back to sleep: Good advice for parents but not for hospitals? *Pediatrics, 107*(3), 537.

Howard, J., & Berbiglia, V. (1997). Caring for childbearing Korean women. *JOGNN, 26*(6), 665–671.

Hutchinson, M., & Baqi-Aziz, M. (1994). Nursing care of the childbearing Muslim family. *JOGNN, 23*(9), 767–771.

Kaufman, M., Clark, J., & Castro, C. (2001). Neonatal circumcision: Benefits, risks, and family teaching. *MCN, 26*(4), 197–201.

Krebs, T. (1998). Cord care: Is it necessary? *Mother Baby Journal, 3*, 5.

Ladewig, P., Moberly, S., Olds, S., & London, M. (2001). *Contemporary maternal–newborn nursing care* (5th ed.). Menlo Park: CA: Addison-Wesley.

Lenhart, J. G., Lenhart, N. M., Reid, A., & Chong, B. K. (1997). Local anesthesia for circumcision: Which techniques are more effective? *Journal of the American Board of Family Practice, 10*(1), 13–19.

Letko, M. (1996). Understanding the Apgar score. *JOGNN, 25*(4), 299.

Littleton, L., & Engebretson, J. (2002). *Maternal, neonatal, and women's health nursing.* Clifton Park, NY: Thomson Delmar Learning.

Lowdermilk, D., & Perry, S. (2003). *Maternity nursing* (6th ed.). St. Louis, MO: Mosby–Year Book.

Lund, C., Kuller, J., Lane, A., Lott, J., & Raines, D. (1999). Neonatal skin care: The scientific basis for practice. *JOGNN, 28*(3), 241–254.

Matsuura, T., Callister, L., & Schwartz, R. (2003). First-time mothers' views of breastfeeding support from nurses. *MCN, 28*(1), 10–15.

Mattson, S. (1995). Culturally sensitive perinatal care for Southeast Asians. *JOGNN, 24*(4), 335–341.

McCaffery, M. (2002). Circumcision: Is a local anesthetic appropriate? *Nursing2002, 32*(4), 24.

Merenstein, G., Adams, K., & Weisman, L. (2002). Infections in the neonate. In G. Merenstein & S. Gardner (Eds.), *Handbook of neonatal intensive care* (5th ed.). St. Louis, MO: Mosby–Year Book.

Moorhead, S., Johnson, M., & Maas, M. (2004). *Nursing Outcomes Classification (NOC)* (3rd ed.). St. Louis, MO: Mosby.

Murray, S., McKinney, E., & Gorrie, T. (2001). *Foundations of maternal–newborn nursing* (3rd ed.). Philadelphia: W. B. Saunders.

North American Nursing Diagnosis Association. (2003). *Nursing diagnoses: Definitions & classification 2003–2004.* Philadelphia: Author.

Pasero, C. (2001). Circumcision requires anesthesia and analgesia. *AJN, 101*(9), 22–23.

Penny-MacGillivray, T. (1996). A newborn's first bath: When *JOGNN, 25*(6), 481.

Queenan, J. (2001). *Positional plagiocephaly (flattened head).* [Online]. Available: http://kidshealth.org/parent/general/sleep/positional_plagiocephaly.html

Reifsnider, E., & Gill, S. (2000). Nutrition for the childbearing years. *JOGNN, 29*(1), 43–55.

Schneiderman, J. (1996). Postpartum nursing for Korean mothers. *MCN, 21*(3), 155–158.

Sharts-Hopko, N. (1995). Birth in the Japanese context. *JOGNN, 24*(4), 343–351.

Simpson, K., & Creehan, P. (2001). *AWHONN perinatal nursing* (2nd ed.). Philadelphia: Lippincott Williams & Wilkins.

Spratto, G. R., & Woods, A. L. (2004). *PDR nurse's drug handbook.* Clifton Park, NY: Thomson Delmar Learning.

Swayze, S. (1999). Clamping down on circumcision. *Nursing99, 29*(9), 73.

Thoyre, S. (2003). Technique for feeding preterm infants. *AJN, 103*(9), 69–73.

Tiedje, L., Schiffman, R., Omar, M., Wright, J., Buzzitta, C., McCann, A., & Metzger, S. (2002). An ecological approach to breastfeeding. *MCN, 27*(3), 154–161.

Tyrala, E. E. (1996). The infant of the diabetic mother. *Obstetric and Gynecologic Clinics of North America, 23*(1), 221.

Varda, K., & Behnke, R. (2000). The effect of timing of initial bath on newborn's temperature. *JOGNN, 29*(1), 27–32.

Verma, R. P. (1995). Respiratory distress syndrome of the newborn infant. *Obstetric Gynecologic Survey, 50*(7), 542.

Workman, E. (2001). Guiding parents through the death of their infant. *JOGNN, 30*(6), 569–573.

York, R., Bhuttarowas, P., & Brown, L. (1999). The development of nursing in Thailand. *MCN, 24*(3), 145–150.

Resources

Association of Women's Health, Obstetric and Neonatal Nurses AWHONN, 2000 L Street N.W., Suite 740, Washington, DC, 20036, 800-673-8499, www.awhonn.org

International Lactation Consultant Association (ILCA), 1500 Sunday Drive, Suite 102, Raleigh, NC 27607, 919-787-5181, www.ilca.org

La Leche League International, 1400 Meacham Road, Schaumburg, IL, 60173-4048, 847-519-7730, www.lalecheleague.org

Women, Infants, and Children (WIC), Supplemental Food Programs Division, Food and Nutrition Service—USDA, 3101 Park Center Drive, Alexandria, VA 22302, 800-545-2200, www.fns.usda.gov/wic

UNIT

18

Nursing Care of the Client: Childrearing

BASICS OF PEDIATRIC CARE

MAKING THE CONNECTION

Refer to the following chapters to increase your understanding of pediatric care:

Basic Nursing
- **Legal and Ethical Responsibilities**
- **Life Cycle**
- **Cultural Considerations**
- **Loss, Grief, and Death**
- **Wellness Concepts**

- **Medication Administration and IV Therapy**
- **Pain Management**

Adult Health Nursing
- **Anesthesia**
- **Surgery**

LEARNING OBJECTIVES

Upon completion of this chapter, you should be able to:
- Define key terms.
- Discuss the role of the nurse in preparing a child and family for hospitalization.
- Explain the role of the nurse in admission and discharge of the pediatric client.
- Prepare children at different developmental stages for procedures.
- Discuss various methods for assessing basic needs and planning daily care.
- Safely perform supportive pediatric procedures.
- Identify the child's concept of death at various developmental stages.
- Describe common responses (child, family, siblings, nurses) to a dying child.
- Discuss sources of support for the dying child.

KEY TERMS

assent	family-centered care
child life specialist	rooming-in
emancipated minor	

INTRODUCTION

Nursing care of children centers on promoting, maintaining, and restoring the health of the child and family. While families are very important to all clients in the health care area, parents are essential to the care and nurturing of the young child. For this reason, when providing care to children, inclusion of the family is essential. Family-centered care recognizes the family as the constant in a child's life. **Family-centered care** describes a philosophy of care recognizing the centrality of the family in the child's life and including the family's contribution and involvement in the plan of care and its delivery (Potts & Mandleco, 2002). An additional factor that impacts the health care of children is their rapidly evolving growth and development.

Children differ from adults in their physical, emotional, and cognitive responses. Physical, emotional, and cognitive immaturity will affect the child's response to comprehension of and reaction to illness or injury. For that reason, a child's developmental level must always be assessed and care plans based on that level. Nursing care of children covers the neonatal period (birth to 28 days), infancy (1 month to 1 year), toddlerhood (12 months to 3 years), preschool age (3 to 6 years), school age (6 to 10 years), preadolescence (10 to 12 years), and adolescence (13 to 20 years). For more detailed information on physical, emotional, cognitive, and moral development, refer to the life cycle chapter.

Trends in health care, such as shorter hospital stays, provision of care in the home, outpatient surgery, and managed care, have changed the settings in which children and their families receive care. These settings include the home, school-based and outpatient clinics, 24-hour observation and outpatient surgery areas, emergency rooms, rehabilitative care, hospitals, and intensive care units. Nurses must be able to rapidly assess, plan, implement, and evaluate care in these diverse settings.

Although any illness of a child is a major stressor for a family, it can also result in a positive experience. Nurses can maximize the client/family/nurse contact by fostering parent–child relationships, providing educational opportunities, promoting self-mastery, and providing socialization.

This chapter discusses preparing the child and family for hospitalization, pediatric procedures, and the dying child.

PREPARING THE CHILD AND FAMILY FOR HOSPITALIZATION

Foremost in the preparation of children for hospitalization on any unit is preparing the family. If the family has sound information about the child's illness, confidence in their medical recommendations, and the support of understanding nurses, then they are more likely to be able to assist in preparing the child for the hospital experience. Hospitalization may be planned or unexpected. When the hospitalization is planned, parents and child have time to prepare for the event. Many hospitals and agencies concerned with the care of the young child provide age-appropriate materials to assist parents and children to prepare for the experience of hospitalization. These materials include tours of the hospital with dress-up in surgical attire and playing with equipment, photographs and videotapes, health fairs to explain procedures, and books and films to explain in age-appropriate terms what to expect. Adolescents need different approaches in preparation for hospitalization; they not only learn from written materials, models, and films but also benefit from peers who have experienced the same procedures. Allowing them to ask questions of health care workers without their parents being present is also beneficial.

When hospitalization is unexpected, it is of utmost importance that children be given opportunities to explore their new surroundings and encouraged to view hospitalization as an adventure that they can handle. All children and their families need to be treated with respect. They need to know that the nurse will listen attentively, in an open-minded, nonjudgmental way.

Many hospitals have **child life specialists,** who are health care professionals with extensive knowledge of psychology and early childhood development, trained to prepare the child and family for hospitalization, surgery, and procedures. Their goals include maintaining normalcy, minimizing psychological trauma, and promoting optimal development of the child and family. A collaborative effort between the nurse, the child life specialist, and other health care providers helps ensure the best possible hospital experience for the child and family.

Many hospitals provide various educational programs such as an open house for well children and preadmission orientation. These programs are designed to orient the child and family to the environment and procedures and may incorporate such learning activities as audiovisuals, art, puppets, tours, and role-play.

The preparation of the child and family should be guided by consideration of the child's developmental level. Parents of infants and toddlers must be reassured of their important role as primary care providers, even during hospitalization (Figure 55-1). Parents must be encouraged to make the necessary arrangements that will allow them to room-in with the hospitalized child. **Rooming-in** is the practice of staying with a hospitalized client (child) 24 hours a day to provide care and comfort to that child. It may also be the method of choice when parents need to learn and practice specialized treatments that they will be performing at home for the child.

Admission

In the past, most care provided to ill children was in the hospital setting. The current trend is to utilize community-based areas such as clinics, free-standing surgical units, schools, and the home. Children admitted

Figure 55-1 *The nurse helps prepare the parents for an infant's hospitalization.*

to the hospital are more acutely ill, yet the time spent in the agency is shorter. Nursing's role in the care of children is changing and expanding. In planning care for children, prevention is a key component as well as teaching for the child and family. The nurse is frequently the first person who sees the child and family when they enter the health care system. The nurse's ability to assess the child and family for physical, psychosocial, cultural, spiritual, and growth and developmental factors sets the stage for the plan of care.

The plan of care begins with admission to the health care facility. The completion of admission information includes previous data regarding the child and family as well as information regarding peers and play patterns, eating patterns, sleeping patterns, school history, normal activity patterns, fears, habits, primary language spoken, language development and level of understanding, usual reaction to pain, special routines, and perception of parents regarding prior or present hospitalizations. In addition, an assessment of basic needs and daily care planning information will be obtained. Most agencies have policies and procedures for admission. Many institutions have a form for parents to complete regarding the child's routines, prior illnesses, current medications, and specific adaptations needed for the child and family. This form is usually signed by the parent and kept in the medical record. Although the agency may have a set policy for admission, the routine may need to be altered based on the needs of the child and family. For example, a fearful child in pain may need to have pain medication and support before being interviewed. Always focus on the needs of the client and family in order to support and assist in mobilizing coping mechanisms rather than data gathering.

The initial assessment determines the need for immediate care. After the family and child are made comfortable or stabilized, a more thorough physical assessment and health history may be obtained. The standard data collected are history of the client, allergies, nutritional intake, sleep, elimination, psychosocial information, spiritual and cultural factors, and the initial physical assessment. Data collected at the time of admission are

used to identify nursing diagnoses and to establish a plan of care; these are placed in the child's chart. Figure 55-2 shows an example of a pediatric admission form.

Many agencies have standardized care plans based on the most common problems identified by the assessment. These care plans are also placed on the chart and are the basis of care. In addition to standardized care plans, many agencies are developing clinical paths or care paths for specific disease states. These tools assist the nurse in giving care based on protocols that result in more rapid recovery, prevention of complications, reduction of length of stay, and cost-containing care for the client and family.

Protection/Safety

Situations may arise during hospitalization that may jeopardize the safety and well-being of the child. Be ever mindful of who has custody of the child, and screen visitors if there are threats to the child's safety. Issues of custody, disputes among family members, and kidnapping of children are no longer remote problems for hospital personnel. Security measures have been put in place in most pediatric units with visible identification of parents, approved visitors, and personnel. Many units utilize electronic surveillance for visitors and monitoring devices for hospitalized children.

Informed consent of the legal guardian is obtained at the time of admission for general treatment, including procedures such as IV insertions, specimen collection, and medication and oxygen administration. Separate informed consents of the legal guardian must be obtained for procedures such as lumbar punctures, chest tube insertion, and bone marrow aspirations. Federal guidelines state that children older than 7 years of age have the right to give **assent** (the child's voluntary agreement to participate in a research project or to accept treatment) for treatment and research procedures. In most states, clients older than 18 years of age can legally give informed consent. In addition, most states allow some exceptions for parental consent in cases involving emancipated minors. An **emancipated minor** is a child who has the legal competency of an adult because of circumstances involving marriage, divorce, parenting a child, living independently without parents, or enlistment in the armed services.

Choking and falls are also areas of concern with hospitalized children. To avoid choking, the environment

---

PROFESSIONAL TIP

ID Bands

It is very important for all clients to have a hospital identification (ID) band on at all times (Figure 55-3). It is equally important that all health care providers check the band for proper client identification before performing any procedure. Any child not having an ID band needs to have the band replaced before treatments.

ADMISSION FORM PART 1 OF 2
PARENT / PATIENT INFORMATION

Dear Parent,
We want to work with you to individually plan the care which your child will receive. You can help us by completing this form. The information will help us learn about your child's illness or condition and about his/her general health. If you have any questions or if you do not want to answer any or all of the questions, please return the form to the nurse. Your nurse will review your answers and together we will develop a plan for your child's care.
Thank you for your cooperation.
The DCH Nursing Staff

GENERAL INFORMATION

Primary language _____ Interpreter _____
Where will you be staying during your child's hospitalization? _____
Whom should we call in case of emergency: NAME: _____ RELATIONSHIP: _____
in case you are not available: _____ Phone, days _____ Phone, nights _____
What do you expect to happen during this hospitalization? _____
What childhood disease has your child had? ☐ measles, ☐ chicken pox, ☐ mumps, ☐ rubella;
Has your child been exposed to any of these within the past two weeks? ☐ Yes ☐ No
Do you have child's immunization card? ☐ Yes ☐ No

Are your child's immunizations current? ☐ Yes ☐ No   Check those which your child has had.
DPT ☐ 2 mo. ☐ 4 mo. ☐ 6 mo. ☐ 15 mo. ☐ 4-6 yrs.   OPV ☐ 2 mo. ☐ 4 mo. ☐ 15-18 mo. ☐ 4-6 yrs
HIB ☐ 2 mo. ☐ 4 mo. ☐ 6 mo. ☐ 12-15 mo.   MMR ☐ 15 mo. ☐ 11-12 yrs
Td ☐ 14-16 yrs.   Hepatitis ☐ Birth ☐ 1-2 mo. ☐ 6-18 mo.
TB Skin Test _____ Boosters _____

What is your child's grade in school? _____
(Patient only) Do you...smoke? ☐ No ☐ Yes _____ packs/day _____ use alcohol? ☐ No ☐ Yes _____
Previous hospitalization _____ Why? _____
Where? _____

Parent/Guardian: present ☐   Not available ☐   Telephone interview ☐

DISCHARGE PLANNING INFORMATION

Have you been receiving help from any agencies? ☐ Yes ☐ No
☐ Home Health ☐ Visiting Nurse ☐ WIC ☐ AFDC ☐ CIDCS ☐ Early Childhood Intervention
If you need help with your child at home, who can assist you? ☐ Yes ☐ No
Does your child require any special equipment or supplies in his/her daily home care? ☐ Yes ☐ No
(apnea monitor, oxygen, suction, etc....)
What information do you need regarding your child's illness and/or hospitalization? _____

IF YOU NEED HELP ARRANGING FOR POSTHOSPITAL SERVICES INFORM YOUR PHYSICIAN OR NURSE THAT YOU WOULD LIKE TO TALK TO A PROFESSIONAL STAFF MEMBER WHO HANDLES DISCHARGE PLANNING.

MEDICATION HISTORY

In this section, please list for each medication your child takes, the dose, how often taken, the time of the last dose, and you/your child's understanding of the reason the drug has been prescribed. If there are problems taking the drug, please describe those also. While your child is in the hospital, ALL medications will be provided. If you have brought medications with you, please do not leave them. Please take them home. Thank you.

Medication	Dose	Frequency	Last Taken	Purpose/Problems Taking

Allergies: Not known ☐   Medications ☐ _____   Foods _____   Other _____

DRISCOLL CHILDREN'S HOSPITAL
CHILDREN'S MEDICAL CENTER OF SOUTH TEXAS

ADMISSION ASSESSMENT

For the following questions, please check your answer – yes or no – and use the space provided to describe or provide more information.

NUTRITIONAL METABOLIC
YES ☐ NO ☐
Use a pacifier, bottle, cup, sippie/special nipple, feeding tube? _____
Type of diet? _____
Take formula? Type _____ Amount? _____ How often? _____
Has your child had any recent weight change? Loss _____ Gain _____
Any changes in appetite or thirst? _____
Any difficulties with eating, or swallowing food? _____
When did child last eat or drink? _____

ELIMINATION
Is child potty trained? Special words _____ Size _____
Diapers? Type _____
Has your child experienced any changes or difficulties with urination? _____
Does your child have a history of bed wetting? _____
Does your child often have diarrhea or constipation? _____
Are laxatives or other aids used for regularity? _____

ACTIVITY EXERCISE
Does your child have preferred play activities? _____
Does your child tire easily with play? _____
Does your child have appliances or need assistance for walking or mobility? (walker, wheelchair) _____
Briefly describe your child's usual daily routine: _____

COGNITIVE-PERCEPTUAL
YES ☐ NO ☐
Does your child have any difficulty hearing? Use a hearing aid? Type: _____
Does your child have any difficulty seeing? When were the eyes last checked? _____ Wear glasses? _____
Does your child sometimes have difficulty learning? _____
What is the easiest way for him/her to learn? (books, film watching, demonstrations) _____
What do you do special to comfort your child when having pain/discomfort? _____

COPING-STRESS
Are there any recent changes in family life that may affect this hospitalization? _____
How have your child/you and your family responded to these changes? _____
Are there other children in family? _____ Ages _____
Do you have family or friends in the Corpus Christi area? _____
Whom do you define as your family or support system? _____
Being in the hospital is stressful for many people. Is there anything we can do to make it easier for you or for your child? _____

ORIENTED TO
☐ Phone; ☐ Bed; ☐ Call light/Intercom; ☐ Parent bed/regulations (Recliners up by 8 a.m.) ☐ Patient Rights & Responsibilities
☐ Playroom; ☐ Mealtimes; ☐ Smoking policy; ☐ IV, VS routine, a.m. wts. ☐ Visitation Limits/hrs. ☐ Intake & Output Monitored
☐ Care of valuables; ☐ Side rails; ☐ TV; ☐ Isolation; ☐ ID Band ☐ Car seat for discharge ☐ Save diapers
☐ Bear Questionnaires ☐ No electrical appliances
Oriented by: _____

Parent Signature: _____ Date: _____ Time: _____

Figure 55-2 Pediatric Admission Form (Courtesy Driscoll Children's Hospital, Corpus Christi, TX)

ADMISSION FORM PART 2 OF 2

TO BE COMPLETED BY ADMITTING NURSE.   Attn. Physician/Time Notified _____ by _____
Arrival to RM _____ Date _____   Time _____   Resident _____ by _____
Brief History _____

GENERAL APPEARANCE: _____
_____

NEUROLOGICAL: Responds to: ☐ Verbal ☐ Pain ☐ Nonresponsive
Gait: ☐ N/A ☐ Walks ☐ Unable to stand ☐ Uncoordinated   LOC: ☐ Lethargic ☐ Semi-Comatose ☐ Comatose ☐ Alert
Movement: ☐ Coordinated ☐ Voluntary ☐ Involuntary; Speech _____   Head Circ _____
Anterior Fontanel _____
Seizures _____   Pupil   1 2 3 4 5 6 7 8
Developmental level: _____   Scale: • • • ● ● ● ⬤ ⬤
                                                         (mm)

CARDIO VASCULAR:
Apical pulse: rhythm _____ Peripheral pulses: RA _____ RL _____ LA _____ LL _____   HR _____
Clubbing: _____ Nailbed Color _____ Capillary Refill _____   BP _____
Comments: _____

RESPIRATORY:
Breath Sounds: ☐ Clear ☐ Crackles ☐ Wheezing ☐ Coarse ☐ Diminished _____   Temp. _____
Retractions: ☐ None ☐ Substernal ☐ Intercostal ☐ Subcostal _____   RR _____
Effort: ☐ Shallow ☐ Deep ☐ Labored ☐ Unlabored; Cough _____   Chest Circ _____
Chest Symmetry _____ Comments: _____   Sputum _____

GASTRO-INTESTINAL:
Abdomen: ☐ Soft ☐ Tender ☐ Nontender ☐ Rigid ☐ Distended; Last B.M. _____
Bowel Sounds: ☐ Active ☐ Hyperactive ☐ Hypoactive; Appetite _____   Wt _____
Tubes: ☐ OG ☐ NG ☐ GT ☐ JT _____   Ht _____
Comments: _____   Abd girth _____
GYNECOLOGICAL: ☐ No abnormalities reported ☐ Sexually active; LMP _____
Discharge _____ Lesions _____ Comments: _____

GENITOURINARY: Urine color _____ Amt. _____ Odor _____ Discharge _____
Incontinent _____ Last void _____
Comments: _____
MUSCULO-SKELETAL:
☐ Moves all extremities ☐ Limited ROM; Swelling _____
Contractures _____ Edema _____ Prosthetic devices _____
Comments: _____

INTEGUMENTARY: (on figure in box, note location of any items with the appropriate letter and check the box by the letter)
☐ Skin intact ☐ Warm ☐ Cool ☐ Cold ☐ Moist ☐ Dry; Color: ☐ Pale ☐ Pink ☐ Jaundiced ☐ Cyanotic ☐ Mottled
Turgor _____ Masses/Size _____ IV site, condition, fluids _____
Wounds/Dressings _____
Comments: _____

☐ B - Bruise
☐ D - Decubitus
☐ L - Laceration
☐ R - Rash
☐ S - Scar

Nursing Process/Plan of care initiated _____ Nurse initials
Allergies: Not Known _____ Medications _____
                Foods _____ Environmental _____
R.N. _____ Date/Time _____

Figure 55-2 *continued*

PROFESSIONAL TIP

Emancipated Minor

Emancipation laws vary from state to state, with some states *not* officially recognizing any form of emancipation.

Figure 55-3 *All hospitalized children will have an ID band placed on either the wrist or ankle.*

must be free of objects that could be placed in the mouth and possibly occlude the airway (e.g., broken balloons, syringe caps, toys, food). An adult should always be present when a young child is eating. Other safety concerns in the hospital setting include machinery (e.g., IV pumps and equipment, needles). Doors to treatment rooms, staircases, supply closets, and rooms containing extra equipment need to be equipped with locks preventing access by children.

Side rails on cribs must be up at all times. If a toddler is able to climb over the rails, a safety cover may need to be placed over the crib, or a regular bed may be used. Never turn your back to a child or reach for materials when the side rail is down if the child is not properly secured.

The Child Having Surgery

The child and family experience with surgery may be an elective procedure, planned in advance, or the result of an emergency with little time for planning. When possible, preadmission visits are an excellent way to prepare the child and family for surgery. Sessions should be scheduled within the week before admission. Table 55-1 contains suggestions for hospital preparation and surgery that are appropriate for planned procedures. As with any preparation, a multidisciplinary approach that includes parents, nursing staff, child life specialists, medical staff, and other involved professionals is best.

Preparation for surgery should include both psychosocial and physical preparation. The purpose of preoperative preparation is to reduce fear and anxiety associated with the surgical procedure and the surrounding environment. Play can facilitate preparation for hospitalization. Visits to units before the experience can familiarize the child and family with sights, sounds, smells, and equipment. Anatomically correct dolls and puppets, drawings, and models can be used to teach the child and family about the procedures. Through play, the child can experience the use of equipment to take vital signs and become familiar with other health care interventions.

Children need to be reassured that they will be transported to the operating room accompanied by parents and that their parents will be there when they wake up. Inform parents of the expected length of the surgery and inform them of the child's status throughout the procedure. It helps the child and parents if one nurse is designated to be the contact before, during, and after surgery.

Many hospitals and surgical units allow and encourage parents to be present during anesthesia induction. The presence of parents and familiar objects such as blankets and toys in the presurgical area decreases the child's and parents' anxiety. Decreased anxiety lessens the need for premedication for the child. Some common induction techniques for young children include concealing the breathing circuit in a play phone, behind a pacifier, or within a stuffed animal, and providing a choice of flavored gases (e.g., watermelon, grape, chocolate).

During the postoperative period, the child will be monitored for bleeding, pain level, and pulmonary and circulatory status. When the child awakens, it is important that the parents be present to calm and comfort the child. Comfort objects from home such as favorite toys may assist the child in feeling at ease. Use pain medication as necessary. Most health care facilities have instructions to follow for general and specific surgical procedures.

The child may be discharged home or admitted to an inpatient unit for further care. Because children recuperate more quickly in a familiar environment, they are discharged as soon as is safely possible following surgery. Discharge planning should be initiated at admission. The

---

TABLE 55-1   NURSING RESPONSIBILITIES TO THE CHILD HAVING SURGERY

PREPARATION FOR SURGERY	AGE CONSIDERATIONS
Psychological Explain surgery. Prepare for separation from family. Conduct preadmission visit.	*Infant:* Allow infant to remain on caregiver's lap as long as possible. *Toddler:* Use dolls, puppets, play hospital. *Preschooler:* Use books, videos, art. Assure toddlers and preschoolers that the surgery is not their fault and is not a punishment. *School-age Child:* Offer brief explanations with supporting visuals.
Physical Discontinue food and drink after specified time. Monitor fluid level (child has less fluid within body and can become dehydrated quickly). Perform specific preparation for procedure. Ensure that consent form is signed by guardian. Administer preoperative medication.	*Infant:* Explain to caregivers only. *Toddler:* Explain 3 days in advance. *Preschooler:* Prepare formally no more than 1 week in advance. *School-age Child:* Videos and tours.
Postoperative Care Make preparations for return of child. Obtain vital signs. Assess pain level. Inspect operative site. Check dressings for bleeding or other drainage. Check bowel and bladder function. Observe for signs of shock, dehydration, infection.	*Infant:* Maintain body warmth. Monitor intake and output. *Toddler and Preschooler:* Give favorite animal or try to provide comfort. *School-age Child:* Ask about comfort and preferred distraction activities. *All children:* Presence of parents on return to postop area and in child's room is important. Know the manifestations of pain and medicate as needed.

ability of the parents to provide adequate care at home determines the extent of education provided before discharge and the need for involvement of a home health agency after discharge.

Discharge/Discharge Planning

Use a multidisciplinary approach that includes the social service department, home care agencies, rehabilitation therapists, and the family to plan for equipment, procedures, and other home care needs. Discharge plans begin with admission of the child. Many agencies have a discharge planning nurse who coordinates the plans for home care. It is important for the nurse working with the client and family to take part in the planning and communicate frequently with the discharge nurse regarding information about the client and family.

Make the family aware that behavioral changes often occur after hospitalization. These changes are most evident in children 6 months to 6 years of age. The changes may include fear or anxiety about sleeping and separation, regression, withdrawal, aggression, and demanding behavior.

Assessment of the family's ability to manage the child's care and the ability of the home environment to support the care needed by the child is important. Early planning gives the health care providers and family time to investigate financial support by agencies such as Medicaid and private insurance. If the child is school-aged, the school district should be involved in order to plan for continued education. This may require special assessment by the school system and a plan of educational care developed to include home tutors, specialized services such as speech therapists and occupational therapists, and/or transportation to school with specialized medical care to be delivered at the school.

Parents may need to learn special or rehabilitative procedures for the child's care. Demonstrate, explain, and observe as the parents assume the care they will be responsible for at home. The education provided and the parents' ability to perform care are discussed with the public health nurse, home health nurse, or individual who will be managing the home care program. Assist parents in exploring options for relief from the child's care, such as respite care, relatives, church groups, or lists of caregivers with ability to give specialized care.

The family is the most important advocate and spokesperson for the child. When a child needs long-

CRITICAL THINKING

Preoperative Plan

Prepare a preoperative plan for a 3-year-old Hispanic male undergoing surgery for an inguinal hernia. What developmental, cultural, and physiological considerations for the child and his family should be included.

term care, the family will need the services of many agencies and numerous health care personnel. To coordinate health care and to prevent gaps and overlaps, one person needs to be identified as a case manager. The parent may decide to act as the child's case manager with support and education from discharge planners.

PEDIATRIC PROCEDURES

In preparing the child and family for procedures performed either at home or in an agency, it is important to take into consideration the child's growth and development, cognitive abilities, and physical and psychosocial factors. It is important that procedures be conducted effectively and efficiently with the least amount of discomfort to the client and family. The following procedures are common to the care of children. While they are similar to procedures performed on adults, they also may differ in several ways. Be knowledgeable about variations in preparation, equipment, positioning, and specific steps when performing procedures on children.

Physical Assessment

Physical assessments for the child are similar to those for the adult with a few differences. Measurements of physical size are significant in evaluating a child's health status. Deviation from the established norms may indicate a significant health problem.

Growth Measurements

Growth measurements for children are recorded at each well-child visit as well as visits for disease episodes. Take measurements correctly and accurately. Values for growth parameters are placed on percentile charts and evaluated with those of the general population. In general, percentiles from 5% to 95% are considered within normal ranges. All growth evaluations take into consideration a child's genetic predisposition. As well as genetic concerns, ethnic and socioeconomic background may influence growth norms. It is unknown whether the differences within the ethnic and socioeconomic backgrounds are from the cultural norms or the result of nutritional differences.

The growth charts most commonly used in the United States are those from the National Center for Health Statistics (NCHS) and are available for boys and girls of different ages. There are growth charts available for children 2 to 3 based on whether their height is measured in

COMMUNITY/HOME HEALTH CARE

Tips for Discharge

- Assess needs and resources.
- Plan for comprehensive care.
- Provide clear, concise written instructions.
- Link client with service provider.
- Coordinate services.
- Advocate for appropriate services.

General Instructions for All Pediatric Procedures

Preprocedure

Check physician's orders.

Review procedure in agency procedure manual.

Gather equipment and assistance if necessary.

Introduce yourself and assistants to child and parents.

Identify child by name band or approved identification method.

Give instructions and explanation to the child and parent and ask if there are any questions.

If parent is going to hold child, demonstrate exactly what you want done. Make sure the parent feels secure about assisting with the procedure. Make sure you know the agency policy regarding parents assisting with procedures by holding the child.

Wash your hands.

Don protective clothing if necessary.

During the Procedure

Maintain privacy.

Tell the child exactly what is expected of him or her, never threaten or tell a child you will have to "hold him/her down."

Have someone assist you if necessary and if it will facilitate the procedure being completed more quickly.

Maintain a conversation with parent and child, explaining what you are doing, in a calm soothing voice.

Keep the child and parent informed of the procedure's progress.

Tell the child when the procedure is nearly complete.

Support of Child and Family

Offer ways of coping with pain or discomfort (imagery, music). Give permission to cry.

Use developmentally appropriate words.

Give child as much choice over the procedure as possible.

Growth

Growth is a continuous and uneven process, and the most important point for monitoring the growth of children is comparison over time.

Figure 55-4 *Measuring Recumbent Length of an Infant*

3. Place a mark on the paper at the crown of the infant's head.
4. Extend the leg and place a mark on the paper at the base of the heel (toes pointing upward).
5. If a measuring board is used, place the infant's head against the board and extend the legs, placing the heels of the feet on the footboard.
6. Measure the distance between the two marks or on the measuring board.
7. Record the length.

Weight Infants are weighed on a platform scale. They may be placed in either a sitting or supine position, depending on their ability to sit unsupported. Before weighing the infant, make sure the scale is cleaned, a paper cover is placed on the scale, and the room is warm. The scale should always be balanced before weighing the infant. The method for weighing is as follows:

1. Place the nude child on the scale, making sure never to turn your back to the child on the scale. Hold your hand over the infant but do not touch the infant while obtaining the weight (Figure 55-5).
2. Measure to the nearest 10 grams or 2 ounces and record the weight.

Head Circumference During the first year or two of life, head circumference is measured as an important indication of brain growth. The method for obtaining head circumference is as follows:

1. Measure the head at its greatest circumference.
2. Wrap a measuring tape around the infant's head, placing it above the brows, the pinna of the ears, and around the occipital prominence. Make sure the tape is flat against the skin.
3. Record the circumference.

Chest Circumference The chest circumference is often measured during the first year of life as an indi-

a lying or standing position. Lying position is referred to as recumbent, and height while standing is referred to as stature. Most children younger than age 2 are measured in a recumbent position, and children older than 2 are measured in a standing position.

Children Younger Than Two Years of Age
Growth measurements for children younger than 2 differ in the procedure and types of measurements taken. Typical measurements taken for the child younger than 2 are length; weight; and head, chest, and abdominal circumferences.

Length Measurement of length is taken with the child in a supine position. The method for children younger than 2 is as follows:

1. Use a paper sheet to lay the infant in a recumbent (lying down) position. Extend the infant's body.
2. Ensure that the infant's head is in midline and legs are extended. Gently grasp knees and push toward table to fully extend legs (Figure 55-4).

Figure 55-5 *Measuring Weight of an Infant*

Figure 55-7 *Measuring Height of a Child*

cator of adequate growth. During the first year, head circumference is greater than chest circumference; after age 1, chest circumference exceeds head circumference. The method for obtaining chest circumference is as follows:

1. Measure the chest at its greatest circumference.
2. Wrap a measuring tape around the infant's chest, placing it under the axilla and over the nipple line (Figure 55-6).
3. Measure between inspiration and expiration.
4. Record the circumference.

 Safety: Paper Tape Measures
Use care when placing paper tape measures. Place under the infant and wrap around carefully. Do not slide the tape around an infant because this may result in paper cuts on the baby.

Abdominal Circumference The abdominal circumference is obtained on very young or preterm infants to detect abdominal distention. The method for measuring abdominal circumference is as follows:

1. Measure the abdomen at its point of greatest girth.
2. Place a paper tape around the infant's abdomen at the umbilicus.
3. Record the circumference.

Children Older Than Two Years of Age Typical measurements taken on children older than 2 years of age include height and weight.

Height After the age of 2 or 3, height is measured with the child standing upright. Remove the child's shoes before the measurement is taken, and have the child stand upright, with the back to the wall or scale. Ask the child to stand very straight with head in midline and shoulders, buttocks, and heels touching the wall or the attachment to a balance scale. The method for measuring height is as follows:

1. On the balance scale, lower the ruler device until it touches the top of the child's head (Figure 55-7). Take the measurement.
2. If measuring the child against a wall, place a flat edge such as a ruler on top of the child's head. Make a mark on the wall; measure from the floor to the mark.
3. Record the height.

Weight After a child can stand and balance well, weight is taken on a standing scale. Standing scales are digital or balance. Remove shoes for all children. Toddlers are weighed in their underclothes, older children are weighed in street clothes with heavy jackets removed. The method for weighing is as follows:

1. Keep the room warm and ensure privacy.
2. Balance the scale before asking the child to step on it.

Figure 55-6 *Measuring Chest Circumference of an Infant*

TABLE 55-2 NORMAL VITAL SIGNS BY AGE

AGE	TEMPERATURE	PULSE RATE	RESPIRATORY RATE	BLOOD PRESSURE
Newborn	98.8–99°F	100–170	30–50	Systolic: 65–95 Diastolic: 30–60
6 months–1 year	97.5–98.6°F	80–130	20–40	Systolic: 65–115 Diastolic: 42–80
3 years	97.5–98.6°F	80–120	20–30	Systolic: 72–122 Diastolic: 46–84
6 years	97.5–98.6°F	70–115	16–22	Systolic: 85–115 Diastolic: 48–64
10–14 years	97.5–98.6°F	60–110	14–20	Systolic: 93–137 Diastolic: 46–71
14–19 years	97.5–98.6°F	60–100	12–20	Systolic: 99–140 Diastolic: 51–80

3. Place child in center of scale and, with a balance scale, move the weights until the scale is balanced.
4. On digital scale, have child stand in center of scale and take reading.
5. Measure to the nearest 100 grams or $1/4$ pound and record the weight.

Vital Signs

Assessment of vital signs (temperature, pulse, respiratory rate, and blood pressure) is an important method for measuring and monitoring vital body functioning. In children, vital signs may change quickly and will provide the basis for decisions regarding care. Table 55-2 describes normal vital signs by age.

Body Temperature Temperature assessment is a simple, objective, inexpensive, and reliable indicator of illness and is part of the pediatric assessment. Currently, there are three types of thermometers utilized in pediatric agencies: electronic, digital, and tympanic membrane. The electronic and tympanic membrane thermometers are the most common types utilized in acute care agencies. Another type of thermometer known as a thermograph (plastic strips or dots) is used for screening only. Each agency will have guidelines to follow in taking temperatures.

Four routes are utilized for obtaining temperatures: axillary, oral, rectal, and tympanic. Axillary temperatures are usually taken on newborns, preterm infants, and infants and children younger than 3 years of age. The thermometer is placed in the axilla and the child's arm pressed close to the body for a minimum of 5 minutes if it is a mercury device or until the electronic thermometer registers.

An oral temperature may be taken in most children 6 years of age or older, including adolescents; the procedure is the same as for adults.

Because of the risk of rectal perforation, discomfort of the child and parent, concerns regarding sexual abuse, and difficulty comforting the child (Kai, 1993), rectal temperatures are taken only when no other route is available. The child is positioned supine, prone, or side-lying, and a well-lubricated thermometer is inserted no more than a maximum of 2.5 cm for 3 to 5 minutes. Rectal temperatures are contraindicated on preterm infants, immunosuppressed children, and children with rectal surgery or gastrointestional disorders (i.e., diarrhea and any bleeding disorder).

Tympanic temperature measurement is more quickly and easily obtained. The procedure appears to be less upsetting to children and is easy to learn by parents for home care. Tympanic temperatures and rectal temperatures appear to strongly correlate. Technique is very important in using the tympanic thermometer. Position of the thermometer enhances the accuracy of the reading. The ear canal must be straightened as when using an otoscope. With the ear tugged correctly and the probe tip pointing at the midpoint between the eyebrow and the sideburn on the opposite side of the face, more ac-

PROFESSIONAL TIP

Measuring Temperature

Regardless of the type of thermometer used, the child's temperature should be measured at the same site and with the same type of device to maintain consistency and allow for reliable comparison and tracking of temperatures over time.

curate temperature readings are obtained. Size of the probe also influences temperature. Using appropriately sized ear probes for children increases the accuracy of the reading.

The method for taking a temperature is as follows:

1. Prepare the child and family for the procedure and assure them that little discomfort will arise from the procedure.
2. Select the appropriate method for obtaining the temperature measurement based on the child's age and condition.
3. Provide an explanation of the procedure to the child and family.
4. Assist the child into a position of comfort. The child may remain on the parent's lap if preferred.
5. Wash hands.
6. Don gloves and use Standard Precautions.
7. Obtain the child's temperature using method chosen.
8. Offer praise to the child for cooperating.
9. Document and report core temperatures of less than 36°C (96.8°F) or greater than 38.5°C (101.4°F) or specified parameters for individual child.
10. Reassess the child's temperature every one-half to 1 hour, or per instructions.
11. Document method of temperature assessment, measurement obtained, and any resulting action.

 Safety: Thermometers
Regardless of the device utilized for temperature taking, *do not* lay it down in the child's bed for safety and for infection control reasons.

Heart Rate or Pulse For children younger than age 2 and those having irregular heart rhythms or congenital heart disease, apical pulse is the preferred site. Radial pulse is taken for children older than 3 years of age unless contraindicated. The method for taking a heart rate/pulse is as follows:

1. To count the pulse rate, place the stethoscope on the anterior chest at the fifth intercostal space in a midclavicular position (Figure 55-8).
2. Count the rate for 1 full minute.
3. Note whether the rhythm is regular or irregular.
4. Note whether the pulse is normal, bounding, or thready.
5. Compare the distal and proximal pulses for strength.

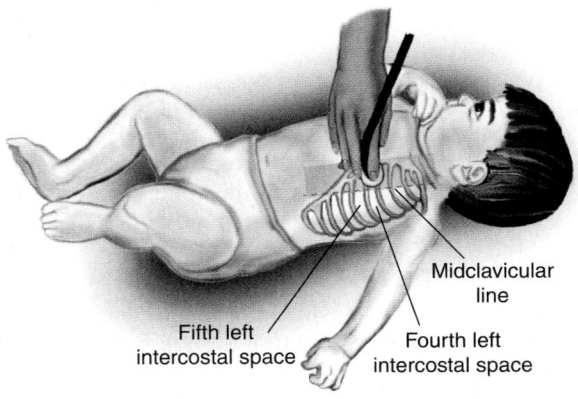

Midclavicular line

Fifth left intercostal space

Fourth left intercostal space

Figure 55-8 *Apical Pulse Position for Infant and Child*

6. Pulse rates may be checked at sites other than the apex of the heart, for example, the carotid, brachial, radial, femoral, and dorsal pedis sites.
7. Record rate, quality, and rhythm.

Respiratory Rate The rate, depth, and ease of respiration are observed in the child. Respiratory rate will vary by age of the child. Because respiratory rate is irregular, it needs to be counted for 1 full minute. It is best if the child is unaware that respirations are being counted. The method for obtaining a respiratory rate is as follows:

1. Children's respirations are diaphragmatic, so observe abdominal movement to count respirations.
2. Count respirations before obtaining temperature or pulse rates (expect abdominal respirations to be irregular).
3. Count for 1 full minute.
4. Record rate, quality, and rhythm.

Blood Pressure Blood pressure measurement for the child is basically the same as for an adult. The size of the cuff is determined by the size of the child's arm or leg. Generally, the bladder of the cuff is two-thirds of the width of the limb in which the BP is being measured. If the bladder is too small, the pressure will be falsely high; if it is too large, the pressure will be falsely low. Blood pressure may be taken on the upper or lower extremities. General instructions for BP measurement are as follows:

Electronic Monitoring:
1. Place the cuff around the desired extremity.
2. Activate the equipment according to the manufacturer's recommendations.
3. Stabilize limb during inflation and deflation because movement sometimes interferes with the device's ability to measure the blood pressure accurately.
4. For some devices, the first reading is a priming reading and the second reading is considered the true blood pressure reading. Refer to manual.
5. Record the reading.

Manual Cuff:
1. Position limb at level of heart.
2. Rapidly inflate cuff to about 20 mm Hg above point at which radial pulse disappears.
3. Release cuff pressure at a rate of about 2 to 3 mm Hg per second during auscultation of artery.
4. Record systolic value as onset of a clear tapping sound.
5. Record diastolic pressure as disappearance of all sounds. Record systolic, diastolic pressures, limb used, position, cuff size, and method.

Developmental Assessment

Developmental assessment for the growing child is an important measure. A tool that is frequently used for the child younger than 6 years of age is the Denver II (DDST). The test is composed of four sections: personal–social, fine motor-adaptive, language, and gross motor. Of the 125 items on the test, responses can be obtained by observing the child, asking the parent, and having the child perform a task.

Informing the parent that the DDST is not an I.Q. (intelligence quotient) test but a helpful measure of the child's growth and development begins the test. The parent and child are made comfortable in the testing environment. Age-appropriate communication and approaches are directed toward the child (e.g., very young children may prefer to sit on parent's lap). The child is then evaluated on a series of tasks, and rated on each with a "P" for pass, "F" for refuse, and "NO" for no opportunity. A caution is given when the child fails to perform an item that has been achieved by 75% to 90% of children of the same age. A delay indicates the child's inability to perform a task that would be expected to be mastered by children in the developmental stage just before the child's current developmental stage. A suspect test is one with one or more delays and/or two or more cautions.

Current illness, lack of sleep, anxiety, chronic disability, or sensory deficits can affect a child's performance. If these factors can explain a child's failure to successfully complete the DDST, then the test may be readministered in 1 month, providing resolution of the problem has occurred. If a developmental delay exists, early detection can lead to intervention and possible resolution.

Child Safety Devices

Restraints are used for many reasons with pediatric clients. Usually, restraints are used to protect and pre-

vent injury to the child. Restraints are regulated by the Omnibus Budget Reconciliation Act (OBRA), which states that restraints should be used only as a last resort for the protection of clients and others. The legislation further indicates that restraints may not be used for the convenience of the staff. Therefore, all possible alternatives should be considered before restraining the child. Some alternatives may be utilizing a person to sit with the child, using diversion with the child, and some behavior modification techniques. Physical restraints include safety vests, mittens, and ankle, elbow, and wrist restraints. The use of a restraint may require a physician's order stating why the restraint is needed and how long it will be left in place.

Before placing the restraint, check the extremity or area that will be restrained for any breaks in the skin, impaired circulation, and neurological deficits. Note any orthopedic problem. If these conditions exist, notify the physician before putting the restraint in place. General instructions for use of all restraints follow:

1. Explain to the child and family members why his/her body part will be restrained, where the restraint will be placed, what movement it will prevent, and how long it will be in place.
2. Puppets, dolls, or stories may be used to assist the child in understanding.
3. Always check the restraint 15 minutes after applying and at least every hour thereafter, or more often if the child is very active.
4. Check the restrained extremity for temperature, pulses, and capillary refill.
5. Remove the restraints every 2 hours to allow for range of motion and repositioning.
6. Restrain as little and as loosely as possible to maintain safety while allowing enough freedom so that the child can touch some part of the body.
7. Provide age-appropriate stimulation for the child while he/she is restrained.
8. Documentation will include:
   a. behavior that led to applying restraints
   b. attempts to calm client before restraining and client's response
   c. explanation to parent regarding restraint use
   d. circulatory and neuromuscular checks while restrained
   e. removal of the restraints, range of motion, and position changes every 2 hours

See Table 55-3 for a summary of the types of mechanical restraints used with children.

Specimen Collection

Specimens are collected from children the same as adults with a few modifications. Children require more specific explanations and directions in an age-appropriate format. Explain any sensation that may be felt. Regardless of the type of specimen collected, Standard Precautions must be used.

Urine

A urine sample is obtained to assess for infection and to determine levels of blood, protein, glucose, acetone,

TABLE 55-3 MECHANICAL RESTRAINTS USED WITH CHILDREN

TYPE OF RESTRAINT	DESCRIPTION	USES
Elbow restraint	Heavy fabric with compartments in which tongue blades are inserted; may also be heavy cardboard cylinders	Used to keep arms extended and away from target site; often used in head or neck surgery, and scalp vein infusion
Mummy restraint	Tightly wrapped blanket or sheet	Used for short procedures, usually on infant, to minimize movement
Jacket restraint	Jacket with ties that may be attached to bed	Used to keep child in bed after surgery
Crib top bubble restraint	Large plastic bubble attached to top of crib	Used for older infant and toddler to prevent falling and climbing out of bed

bilirubin, drugs, hormones, metals, and electrolytes excreted by the kidneys. Urine can also be assessed for concentration/specific gravity, pH, and other substances.

A collection bag is used to obtain a clean-catch urine sample from an infant and non-toilet-trained children. This collection method is not suitable for a culture because of the great possibility for contamination (Johnson, 1999). Older children, after being given clear instructions, are usually capable of collecting their own urine. Usually, 5-10 cc of urine is adequate.

The method of obtaining a urine sample for the infant is as follows:

1. Remove the diaper and clean the skin around the meatus; allow to dry thoroughly.
2. Attach the bag with the adhesive tabs, for girls, around the labia, and for boys, around the scrotum (Figure 55-9).
3. Make sure the seal is tight to prevent leakage.
4. Check the bag frequently for urine.
5. To remove the bag, pull away gently from the skin using moistened cotton balls to assist in releasing the adhesive.
6. Pour into container and cap tightly.
7. Send to lab immediately.
8. Document color, amount, clarity, and lab tests requested.

A clean-catch sample for a male older child is collected in the following manner:

1. Instruct the older child to clean the head of his penis (after retracting the foreskin, if not circumcised) three times, each time using a different towelette, moving from the urethral meatus outward.
2. Have the child urinate a small amount into the toilet, stop the flow, then urinate into the sterile container.
3. Proceed as above.

A clean-catch sample for a female older child is collected in the following manner:

1. Instruct the child to sit back on the toilet as far as possible with her legs apart. Have her spread her labia with her fingers and wipe each side with a

Figure 55-9 *Applying a Urine Collection Bag to a Child*

PROFESSIONAL TIP

Urine Specimen in Non-Toilet-Trained Child

- If collecting urine and blood specimens, place a urine bag on before drawing blood. Most stressful procedures will precipitate urination.
- Stroking the abdomen with an alcohol prep and fanning it dry will frequently cause urination (Ellis, 1989).
- Urine for most tests except culture and sensitivity may be obtained from the diaper. Using gloves, remove the diaper, tear out the wettest portion of the diaper, place in a syringe with plunger removed, insert plunger, and squeeze the urine out of the diaper.
- Before placing a paper diaper on an infant or incontinent child, cut a vertical slit in the front of the diaper. Place a urine bag, and then the diaper on the child, then gently pull the urine bag through the slit. This allows visualization of urination (James et al., 2002).

separate towelette using a front-to-back stroke. Tell the child to use a third wipe to clean the meatus, repeating the front-to-back motion.
2. Have the child urinate a small amount into the toilet, stop the flow, then urinate into the sterile container.
3. Proceed as above.

Stool

Stool specimens are used in pediatric clients to check for the presence of fat, blood, bacteria, parasites, or reducing substances. If the stool specimen is needed from an infant or incontinent child, scrape it from the diaper and place in the appropriate container. If the child is potty-trained, use a bedpan or container to collect the specimen. Record the time the specimen is obtained, color, consistency, any odor, and disposition.

Blood

Blood specimens are obtained from children by accessing veins of the hand or antecubital space, heelsticks, and femoral and jugular venipunctures. Collection of blood is very distressing to young children because of their lack of discrete body boundaries and the pain involved. The use of EMLA, a topical anesthetic cream, can reduce the discomfort of the needle penetrating the skin. EMLA contains lidocaine-prilocaine 5% and can be used to decrease pain associated with selected procedures: venipuncture, lumbar puncture, suture removal, immunizations, bone marrow aspiration, and removal of foreign bodies. EMLA is not approved for infants because of lack of testing and is not placed on skin that is broken. The cream is applied to the site liberally with an occlusive dressing and left in place 60 minutes before the procedure. The duration of the anesthesia is at least 2 and not more than 5 hours. Permission to use EMLA varies by institution; some may require a physician's order, and others allow the nurse to use it without an order. Children still may fear the needlestick; however, when the stick is not painful, they are more content. Venipunctures that are the same as those in adults are not covered in this section.

Jugular Venipuncture Jugular and femoral venipunctures are performed by a physician, with the nurse assisting and monitoring the child. The blood specimen is obtained from the large superficial external jugular vein. The nurse assists the physician by doing the following:

1. Place child in mummy restraint (possibly just hold child's arms).
2. Position child with head and shoulders extended over the edge of a table or small pillow with neck area hyperextended (Figure 55-10).
3. Take care that circulation and breathing during the procedure are not impaired.
4. Make sure that the nose and mouth are not covered by the restrainer's hand.
5. Document in the chart the amount of blood drawn, the site, condition of the site, and the type of dressing applied.

Femoral Venipuncture The nurse assists the physician by doing the following:

1. Place child in modified mummy restraint with legs exposed.
2. Position child's legs in a froglike position to provide extensive exposure of the groin area (Figure 55-11).
3. Restrain legs in frog position with hands while controlling the child's arm and body movements with downward and inward pressure of forearms.
4. Cover genitalia to avoid contamination if the child urinates.
5. Document in chart amount of blood drawn, site, condition of the site, and type of dressing applied.

Lumbar Puncture

Lumbar puncture (spinal tap) requires the infant or child to be held perfectly still. It is desirable to have an experienced staff member hold the child for the procedure. Lumbar puncture is performed as follows:

1. Place infant in sitting or side-lying position (neonates) with modified head extension to decrease respiratory distress during procedure.
2. Immobilize arms and legs with nurse's hands.

Figure 55-10 *Positioning for Jugular Venipuncture*

Figure 55-11 *Positioning for Femoral Venipuncture*

Figure 55-12 *Positioning for Lumbar Puncture*

3. Observe child for difficulty in breathing.
4. Place child on side with back close to or extended over the edge of examining table, head flexed, and knees drawn up toward the chest.
5. Reach over the top of the child and place one arm behind child's neck and the other behind the knees (Figure 55-12).
6. Stabilize this position by clasping own hands in front of the child's abdomen.
7. Observe carefully for compromise in circulatory or respiratory systems. The restrainer's body should not cover the nose and mouth of the child.
8. Document number of attempts to obtain spinal fluid, number of cc's to lab, lab tests requested, color and consistency of spinal fluid, and response of child to procedure.

Intake and Output

Most children in acute care agencies will be on intake and output, which is critical for children with the following conditions:

- Anyone receiving IV fluids or TPN
- Major surgery
- Prematurity
- Renal disease or dysfunction
- Congestive heart failure
- Heart disease or anomalies
- Endocrine disorders
- Gastrointestinal disorders
- Shock
- Burns
- Taking medications such as digoxin, lasix, or corticosteriods
- Neurological conditions

To measure output for infants, the nurse should:

1. Weigh the diaper before placing it on the infant and then again when wet. For each mg the diaper weighs, record 1 cc of urine. *Caution:* For those diapers that protect against wetness, the accuracy may be distorted because of the absorbent material embedded in the diaper.

2. A urine bag with adhesive may be placed on the child and the urine collected measured in this way. This is not usually done because of the irritation of the adhesive over time.

For toddlers and older children, measure urine and stool output in a bedpan or other container. All intake is measured and recorded on the intake and output sheet. If parents are present, instruct them to measure and record fluids taken in and those eliminated. Record all fluids from IVs and other sources. Measure drainage from stomas, colostomies, fistulas, and emesis and record.

Administration of Medications

Administration of medications to infants and children presents a number of adaptations. The medication dosage is determined by the physician; however, the nurse must observe the five rights of medication administration. Explain all procedures or treatments to the child and parents based on the child's developmental stage and the level of understanding of both parties. Explanations must be truthful, using nonthreatening words. All questions posed by the parents and child must be answered before giving the medication.

Approaches to Pediatric Clients

Children's reactions to medication administration are affected by developmental characteristics such as physical skills and cognitive understanding, environmental influences, past experiences, cultural influences, parental responses, current relationship with the nurse, and perception of the present situation.

Calculating Dosages for Children

Standardized doses of medication for children do not exist. The most common method of determining medication amounts is based on the child's weight. This method of determining the medication amount is more reliable because it allows for a more precise dose based on weight

---

LIFE CYCLE CONSIDERATIONS

Medication Administration in Children

Suggestions to facilitate successful medication administration in infants and children:

- Be honest with the child.
- Allow the child choices when possible.
- Provide distraction when appropriate.
- Praise the child for doing his/her best.
- Expect success; use a positive approach.
- Allow the child opportunity to express feelings.
- Involve the child in order to gain cooperation.
- Provide a developmentally appropriate explanation.
- Do not use basic foods such as milk to disguise medication.
- Spend some time with the child after administering the medication.

(see example in Professional Tip box). Medication doses also may be calculated by body surface area (BSA mg/m²). The formula to calculate dosage using surface area is:

$$\text{Approximate dose} = \frac{\text{BSA of child (m}^2)}{1.7} \times \text{Adult dose}$$

Oral Medications

The oral route of medication is the preferred method of administering medication to a child. Oral medications may come in liquids, pills, tablets, and caplets. Pediatric medications are frequently in a liquid suspension that tastes "good" and is colorful. Many medications have an unpleasant after-taste. Become aware of medications that are bitter or unpleasant and methods to decrease the unpleasant taste such as numbing the tongue before administration by giving a flavored ice popsicle or small ice cube. The method for administering oral medication to a child is as follows:

1. Select appropriate vehicle (e.g., calibrated cup, syringe, dropper, measuring spoon, nipple).
2. Prepare medication.
3. Measure into appropriate vehicle.
4. Avoid mixing medications with essential food items such as milk, formula, etc. (The child may later refuse the essential food item because of the association with medication.)
5. Administer the medication, employing safety precautions in identification and administration.

Specific instructions for administering oral medications to infants are as follows:

1. Hold infant in semi-reclining position.
2. Place syringe, measuring spoon, or dropper with medication in mouth well back on the tongue or to the side of the tongue.
3. Administer slowly and wait for the child to swallow to reduce likelihood of choking or aspiration.
4. Allow infant to suck medication placed in nipple.

Specific instructions for administering oral medications to the older infant or toddler are as follows:

1. Explain in developmentally appropriate terms what you are going to do.
2. Allow the child to sit on your lap or the parent's lap in a sitting or modified supine position.
3. Use mild or partial restraint.
4. Administer the medication slowly with a syringe or small medicine cup.

Figure 55-13 *Administering Oral Medication to a Child*

5. Never force actively resistive children because of the danger of aspiration; postpone 20 to 30 minutes and offer medication again.

Specific instructions for administering oral medications to a preschool child are as follows:

1. Use a straightforward approach.
2. For a reluctant child, use the following:
   • Simple persuasion (e.g., "When you take your medicine, we can go to the playroom.")
   • Reinforcement, such as stickers or other rewards for compliance

Intramuscular Injections

Intramuscular injections are used widely for pediatric clients. Medications given by the intramuscular route in-

Needle Threats

A child who has received multiple IM injections has a real fear of the "needle." The parents threaten the child that if he does not do what they say, the nurse will come and give him a "needle." How would you approach the parents? What interventions would assist the child to lessen his fear and regain control?

clude immunizations, antibiotics, and other drugs. Children have reported that injections are one of the most stressful and painful experiences of health care (Eland & Anderson, 1977; Gedaly-Duff & Burns, 1992). The task for nurses is to support the child while administering the medication quickly, safely, and with the least amount of pain and stress to the child. Pain perception is lessened with a distraction such as the child blowng bubbles or the skin being stroked around the injection site before and during the injection (Sparks, 2001).

Otic Medications

Otic medication is used frequently in children who have ear infections. Because of pain associated with cold coming in contact with the tympanic membrane, warm all otic medications to room temperature before administering. The child should receive an age-appropriate explanation regarding what will be felt and heard (e.g., "It may feel like a moth in your ear.") and what can be done to help. Assistance in restraining a young child may be needed.

Position the child on the side with the affected ear up, and clean any discharge with a clean gauze pad. Brace the administering hand above the ear on the head. To instill the solution in a child younger than 8 years of age, pull the pinna of the ear back and down; for an older child, the pinna is pulled back and up. After instillation, the tragus of the ear is massaged to ensure the drops reach the tympanic membrane. Cotton may be put loosely into the ear canal, if ordered.

Intravenous Medications

Children in acute care settings frequently receive intravenous (IV) medications. Children who have poor absorption as a result of dehydration, malabsorption syndromes, shock, and those in need of a high concentration of the drug quickly would receive IV fluids and medication. Children needing continuous pain relief benefit from IV medication administration. Advantages of IV medications are the immediate effect and the ability to control blood levels of the drugs used. Disadvantages are the same: side effects occur very quickly, and the drug may be very corrosive to the veins. Once the drug is administered into the bloodstream, further control is limited.

All drugs given by IV route require a specified minimum dilution and specific rate of flow. It is difficult to control the IV flow rate in children by gravity. Children

are at risk for fluid overload when IV rates are not controlled; therefore, all children receiving IV fluids or medications should receive those fluids through a volumetric infusion pump. IV medication may be delivered as a continuous infusion or intermittently. Syringe pumps are used in many agencies to deliver small amounts of medication.

Nursing care of the client receiving IV fluids and/or medication includes site assessment every hour for signs and symptoms of infiltration. Site assessment includes color of the site, tension of the skin, and skin temperature. When administering IV fluids and medications to the pediatric client, know the following:

- Type of fluid
- Compatibility of medication and IV solutions
- Recommended dilution of the drug
- Recommended time frame for administration
- Amount of flush needed
- Any precautions to observe before administration (e.g., for aminophylline [Aminophyllin], take apical pulse before administering)
- Side effects of the drug

THE DYING CHILD

Care of the dying child presents one of the greatest challenges to nurses. It involves sensitive, gentle physical care and comfort measures for the child as well as continuing emotional support for the family and caregivers.

Child

Children's understanding of death parallels their cognitive and psychosocial development. Preverbal infants and toddlers have no clear concept of death. Children between the ages of 3 and 5 may view death as a kind of sleep that is interchangeable with life. Because of their concrete thinking, school-age children begin developing the concept of death as final. Adolescents have a maturing understanding of death. In addition to their developmental level, children are greatly influenced by their life experiences and the attitudes of those around them.

Children can sense when they are seriously ill. They may realize they are dying because of the effects of disease and treatments on their body. The child usually experiences fear of death, of dying alone, and of pain. Nursing interventions include promoting socialization with family and peers, providing avenues for self-expression (i.e., drawings, fantasy play, storytelling), dealing directly with the child's questions, and allowing the death to occur in peace and with dignity.

Parents

When death is expected, the family begins a mourning process called anticipatory grieving. Manifestations of this process include denial, anger, and depression. It is important to acknowledge the parents' feelings, encourage expression, and guide them through the gradual process to reorganization. Spouses may need additional support when they are at different levels of grieving to prevent a sense of loneliness and isolation.

Explore options with the family concerning the child's care. The child and family have a right to request termination of treatment and to determine the care setting.

Parents who are caring for their dying child usually fear what the death will be like, not being present at the death, and pain the child will experience. The family needs to be encouraged to talk to the child about dying. Families need help to focus on the time that remains with the child. Openness and honesty allow the health care providers and the family to provide effective care, to avoid misunderstandings, to see that the child and the family resolve problems, and to share their love.

Siblings

Like their parents, siblings may experience anticipatory grief in the form of anger, denial, or fear. They may resent the attention given to the dying child. Siblings may fear that they caused their brother or sister to become ill or that the same thing will happen to them. They may need help in adapting to their parents' distraction, grief, and increased protectiveness.

Encourage parents to include siblings in the care of the dying child, in discussions about dying, and in the funeral. Like the dying child and the grieving parents, siblings need acknowledgment of their feelings and opportunities for expression.

Nurse

Caring for the dying is usually a team effort, but often the nurse is the coordinator of the care. Working effectively with dying children and their families requires confidence, empathy, and competence in addition to attention to managing personal stress. Nurses who are comfortable with their own mortality can help make the remainder of the child's life more meaningful and the family's mourning experience more healing.

Nurses experience reactions to caring for dying children including denial, anger, depression, guilt, and ambivalent feelings. Nurses may even cry in the presence of the child and the family. A grieving father wrote of a nurse caring for his son who had just died, "We were grateful for her kindness and her tears" (Brown, 1992). Learning to care for the dying involves talking with other professionals, sharing concerns, comforting each other in stressful times, maintaining good general health, using distancing techniques, and focusing on the positive aspects of the caregiver role.

Sources of Support

Hospice care may be an option for the dying child. Hospice services provide palliative care for the dying to live life to the fullest without pain, with choices of dignity, and with family support including follow-up care postdeath. Self-help groups such as Compassionate Friends, an international organization for bereaved parents and siblings, are available in many communities.

CASE STUDY

Tillie, a 5-year-old with an inoperable abdominal tumor, lives with her parents and a 7-year-old sister, Tammie. The decision has been made to discontinue chemotherapy. Tillie has been involved in decisions about her care throughout her illness. When asked about her condition, she states, "I'm very sick and I'm not getting better." Tillie spends much of her time curled in a fetal position with her favorite toy, a tattered rag doll named Dolly. Tillie refuses physical exams and pills and gets little sleep because of her pain.

The following questions will guide your development of a nursing care plan for the case study.

1. List subjective and objective data a nurse would want to know about Tillie and her family.
2. List three nursing diagnoses and goals for Tillie.
3. What would you expect a 5-year-old to understand about death?
4. What nursing interventions will be required for Tillie and her family?
5. List three successful outcomes for Tillie and her family.

Summary

- Even though hospitalization places great stress on children and their families, it can be a positive growth experience for the child.
- Teaching children and their families what to expect and explaining what is going to happen before, during, and after procedures helps reduce anxiety.
- Children's developmental stage and cognitive ability influence the preparation for treatments and procedures.
- Children must be protected from hazards that can cause harm to them.
- The child's stage of development, cognitive ability, and life experiences contribute to the child's understanding of death.

Review Questions

1. The major stressor of hospitalization for infants and young children is:
   a. pain.
   b. bodily injury.
   c. loss of control.
   d. separation anxiety.

2. Because of their stage of development, preschoolers may view hospitalization as:
   a. abuse.
   b. rejection.
   c. punishment.
   d. abandonment.

3. Before drawing blood on a 9-year-old, the nurse tells the child:
   a. a Band-Aid will not be necessary.
   b. the procedure will not be painful.
   c. not to worry about the tight tourniquet.
   d. the body will produce more blood to replace what is being taken.

4. An appropriate method for administering oral medication to a small child is to mix it with:
   a. milk.
   b. food from the child's plate.
   c. a large amount of water.
   d. sweet-tasting food or syrup.

References/Suggested Readings

Abbott, K., Fowler-Kerry, S. (1995). The use of a topical refrigerant anesthetic to reduce injection pain in children. *Journal Pain Symptom Management 10*(8), 584–590.

Ball, J., & Bindler, R. (2000). *Pediatric nursing* (2nd ed.). Norwalk, CT: Appleton & Lange.

Barnard, P., Morland, I., & Nagy, J. (1999). *Children, bereavement, and trauma; Nurturing resilience.* Philadelphia: Jessica Kingsley Publishers.

Bricher, G. (2000). Children in the hospital: Issues of power and vulnerability. *Pediatric Nursing, 20*(3), 277–282.

Brown, P. (1992). Saying goodbye. *Nursing Times, 89*(4), 26–29.

Deering, C., & Cody, D. (2002). Communicating with children and adolescents. *AJN, 102*(3), 34–40.

Eland, J. M., & Anderson, J. E. (1977). The experience of pain in children. In A. Jacox (Ed.), *Pain: A sourcebook for nurses and other health professionals.* Philadelphia: Lippincott Williams & Wilkins.

Eldridge, T. M. (2002). Preparation for painful procedures, hospitalization and surgery. In J. A. Fox (Ed.) *Primary health care of children.* St. Louis, MO: Mosby.

Ellis, R. (1989). Once more into the void. *Contemporary Pediatrics, 6*(8), 164.

Estes, M. E. Z. (2002). *Health assessment & physical examination* (2nd ed.). Clifton Park, NY: Thomson Delmar Learning.

Fennell, M. E. (1999). Parents in the OR: You bet! *RN, 62*(12), 38–39.

Frey, A. M. (2000). Pediatric IV insertion. *Nursing2000, 30*(12), 54–56.

Gedaly-Duff, V., & Burns, C. (1992). Reducing children's pain-distress associated with injection using cold: A pilot study. *Journal of the American Academy of Nurse Practitioners, 4*(3), 95–99.

Hamlin, J. J., & Coplein, G. E. (1998). Legal risks of pediatric nursing care and guidelines for documentation. *Journal of Nursing Law, 5*(3), 7–24.

Hockenberry, M., Wilson, D., Winkelstein, M., & Kline, N. (2003). *Wong's nursing care of infants and children* (7th ed.). St. Louis, MO: Mosby.

James, S., Ashwill, J. W., & Droske, S. C. (2002) *Nursing care of children: Principles and practice* (2nd ed.). Philadelphia: W. B. Saunders.

Johnson, C. (1999). New advances in childhood urinary tract infections. *Pediatrics in Review, 20*(10), 335–342.

Kai, J. (1993). Parents' perceptions of taking babies' rectal temperature. *British Medical Journal, 307*, 660–662.

Kliegman, R. M., Jenson, H. B., & Behrman, R. (2000). *Nelson textbook of pediatrics* (16th ed.). Philadelphia: W. B. Saunders.

LeDuc, K. (1999). Pediatric pharmacotherapeutics. In K. Guitierrez (Ed.), *Pharmacotherapeutics: Clinical decision-making in nursing.* Philadelphia: Saunders.

Marks, M. G. (1998). *Broadribb's introductory pediatric nursing* (5th ed.). Philadelphia: Lippincott Williams & Wilkins.

McEvoy, M. (2003). Culture & spirituality as an integrated concept in pediatric care. *MCN, 28*(1), 39–43.

Moldow, D., & Martinson, I. *Home care for seriously ill children: A manual for parents.* Children's Hospice International, 901 N. Washington Street, 7th Floor, Alexandria, VA 22314, (800) 24-CHILD.

Newton, M. S. (2000). Family-centered care: Current realities in parent-participation. *Pediatric Nursing, 26*(2), 164–168.

North American Nursing Diagnosis Association. (2003). *Nursing diagnoses: Definitions & classification 2003–2004.* Philadelphia: Author.

Potts, N., & Mandleco, B. (2002). *Pediatric nursing: Caring for children and their families.* Clifton Park, NY: Thomson Delmar Learning.

Schultz, T. (2000). Airing differences in pediatric nebulizer therapy. *Nursing2000, 30*(9), 55–57.

Shelton, T., & Stepanek, J. (1994). *Family-centered care for children needing specialized health and developmental services.* Association for the Care of Children's Health. Bethesda, MD.

Sparks, L. (2001). Taking the "Ouch" out of injections for children. *MCN, 26*(2), 72–78.

Spratto, G., & Woods, A. (2004). *2004 PDR nurses' drug handbook.* Clifton Park, NY: Thomson Delmar Learning.

Visintainer, M., & Wolfer, J. (1975). Psychological preparation for surgical pediatric patient: The effect on children's and parents' stress response and adjustment. *Pediatrics, 56*(2), 187–202.

Wong, D., Hockenberry-Eaton, M. (2001). *Wong's essentials of pediatric nursing* (6th ed.). St. Louis, MO: Mosby–Year Book.

Wu, T., & Daniel, L. (2001). Growth of immigrant Chinese infants in the first year of life. *MCN, 26*(4), 202–207.

Resources

Association for the Care of Children's Health, 19 Mantua Road, Mount Royal, NJ, 08061, 609-224-1742, www.acch.org

Children's Hospice International, 2202 Mt. Vernon Avenue, Suite 3-c, Alexandria, VA, 22301, 1-800-24-CHILD, 703-684-0330, www.chionline.org

Compassionate Friends, Inc., P. O. Box 3696, Oak Brook, IL, 60522-3696, 877-969-0010, www.compassionatefriends.org/index.html

National Association of Pediatric Home and Community Care, 40 University of Massachusetts Medical Center, Department of Pediatrics, Room S6-860, Worchester, MA 01655, 508-856-1908, www.gnofn.org

National Father's Network, The Kindering Center, 16120 N.E. 8th Street, Belleue, WA, 98008-3937, 425-747-4004, www.fathersnetwork.org

Sibling Support Project, Children's Hospital and Medical Center, CL-09, P.O. Box 5371, Seattle, WA, 98105-0371, 206-368-4911, www.chmc.org/departmt/sibsupp

INFANTS WITH SPECIAL NEEDS: BIRTH TO 12 MONTHS

MAKING THE CONNECTION

Refer to the following chapters to increase your understanding of infants with special needs:

Basic Nursing
- Life Cycle
- Cultural Considerations
- Loss, Grief, and Death
- Fluid, Electrolyte, and Acid–Base Balance
- Assessment
- Pain Management

Adult Health Nursing
- Anesthesia
- Surgery
- Respiratory System

- Cardiovascular System
- Hematologic and Lymphatic Systems
- Gastrointestinal System
- Urinary System
- Musculoskeletal System
- Neurological System
- Sensory System
- Integumentary System
- Immune System

Maternal & Pediatric Nursing
- Basics of Pediatric Care

LEARNING OBJECTIVES

Upon completion of this chapter, you should be able to:
- Define key terms.
- Differentiate the most common respiratory conditions affecting infants.
- Describe nursing care for infants with circulatory conditions.
- Discuss nursing considerations for infants with digestive conditions.
- Explain the evaluative techniques used for infants suspected of having musculoskeletal alterations.
- Differentiate among the skin disorders most commonly seen in infants.
- Explain the causes and effects of nervous system disorders seen in infants.
- Describe nursing care for infants with genitourinary conditions.
- Outline teaching strategies for parents of infants with visual and hearing impairments and cognitive disorders.
- Implement nursing interventions for infants who have been abused.
- Describe teaching guidelines for families of infants who have unsafe environments.

KEY TERMS

abduction	kernicterus
antipyretic	lecithin
atresia	meconium ileus
child abuse	meningitis
circumoral cyanosis	milia
colic	mongolian spots
dislocation	myelomeningocele
dysplasia	myringotomy
erythematous	projectile vomiting
hypotonia	pruritus
intussusception	stridor
jaundice	

INTRODUCTION

The immaturity of all body systems leaves infants vulnerable to numerous illnesses and disorders. Most health problems during infancy are caused by respiratory and gastrointestinal infections or congenital anomalies. Although infants can become ill rapidly, they usually recover quickly. This chapter describes common conditions and illnesses affecting all systems of the infant; typical medical and surgical management; and nursing care of infants.

RESPIRATORY SYSTEM

In the normal infant, breathing is quiet and shallow with variations in rate and rhythm. Respiratory movement is primarily abdominal. Respirations should be counted for 1 full minute while watching the rise and fall of the abdomen. The normal rate ranges from 30 to 50 breaths per minute. A persistent rate above 60 breaths per minute is an important sign of respiratory distress.

The child's respiratory tract is constantly changing and growing during the first 12 years of life. Differences between the respiratory tract of the adult and the infant contribute to the greater potential for obstruction, aspiration, infection, and airway resistance in the child (Table 56-1). In the infant, the most common respiratory disorders include otitis media, laryngotracheobronchitis, pneumonia, respiratory distress syndrome, cystic fibrosis, and sudden infant death syndrome.

OTITIS MEDIA

Otitis media, an inflammation of the middle ear, occurs bilaterally in 50% of diagnosed cases (Faden, Duffy & Boeve, 1998). The eustachian tubes, which allow for drainage from the middle ear to the nasopharynx, are shorter, wider, and more horizontal in infants than in adults (Figure 56-1). As a result, drainage is frequently impaired, resulting in retention of secretions and air in the middle ear. This positioning also facilitates the movement of bacteria up the eustachian tube from the pharynx into the middle ear. An upper respiratory infection often precedes the development of otitis media in infants. *Haemophilus influenzae* is a common causative agent of otitis media in infants.

Infants with otitis media may be irritable, pull at the infected ear, or have diarrhea, vomiting, fever, and hear-

TABLE 56-1	RESPIRATORY TRACT DIFFERENCES BETWEEN INFANTS AND ADULTS
DIFFERENCES IN CHILDREN	**SIGNIFICANCE**
Small nares, oral cavity, and nasopharynx; large tongue	Increases risk for obstruction
Obligatory nose breathers (<6 months) due to immature neurological function	Increases risk for obstruction
Rapid growth of lymph tissue	Increases risk for obstruction with infection
Larynx and glottis high in neck	Increases risk for aspiration
Large amount of soft tissues and loose, poorly anchored mucous membranes; long floppy epiglottis	Increases risk for obstruction with infection
Fewer functional airway muscles	Increases risk for aspiration
Immature cartilages that may collapse when neck is flexed	Increases risk for obstruction
Short neck resulting in structures being closer together	Increases risk for infection
Short, narrow airway	Increases risk for obstruction and aspiration; increases airway resistance/respiratory effort
Bifurcation of trachea at the third thoracic space	Increases risk for infection and aspiration
Immature intercostal muscles and cartilaginous ribs; primarily diaphragmatic breathers	Increases respiratory effort
Eustachian tube shorter, wider, and straighter	Increases risk for infection

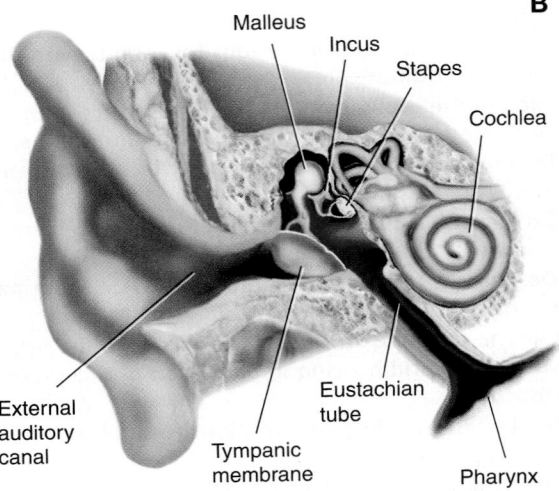

Figure 56-1 *Eustachian Tubes:* **A,** *Infant;* **B,** *Adult*

ing loss. Upon inspection, the ear drum will be red, bulging, and nonmobile. Prolonged otitis media may result in sensorineural and/or conductive hearing loss, which is further discussed in the hearing impairment section of this chapter.

Medical–Surgical Management

Medical

Medical treatment focuses on elimination of the infection and follow-up evaluation to determine the extent of hearing loss, if any.

Surgical

If infections recur, **myringotomy** (surgical incision of the eardrum) may be performed and tympanoplasty tubes inserted to drain the fluid from the middle ear.

Pharmacological

Treatment usually includes antibiotics, **antipyretics** (drug used to reduce an abnormally high temperature), and analgesics. Considerations when deciding which antibiotic to administer include compliance of parents in giving the medication, the child's willingness to take oral medications, and the pain involved with injections. Commonly used antibiotics include amoxicillin (Amoxil) and cefaclor (Ceclor). Newer antibiotics such as cefixime (Suprax) and loracarbef (Lorabid) are also used (Spratto & Woods, 2004).

Nursing Management

The primary nursing concerns are relieving fever and pain and teaching the parents about signs and symptoms, management, and prevention of otitis media. Acetaminophen (Tylenol) or ibuprophen (Motrin) may be used to reduce fever. In addition to analgesic administration, pain may be minimized by applying a heating pad on the low setting or an ice pack compress to the affected ear. Lying on the affected side will facilitate drainage, if the eardrum has ruptured or myringotomy has been performed. Providing liquids and soft foods may minimize pain caused by chewing.

Teach parents to have the infant examined at the first sign of a possible ear infection. Early possible signs of infection include hearing difficulties, pulling or rubbing of the ears, and irritability.

If antibiotics are prescribed, it is imperative that the child be given all of the medication. Failure to adhere to prescribed treatment may lead to the need for additional antibiotics; hearing loss; and potential speech and language problems.

Prevention of otitis media involves ensuring proper positioning during feeding. Infants who are bottle-fed should be held with the head slightly elevated to prevent formula from draining into the middle ear through the wide eustachian tube. Breastfed infants receive immunoglobulin A contained in the breast milk. Immunizations are also preventive (Potts & Mandleco, 2002).

Providing a smoke-free environment is another important element of prevention. Inform parents of the relationship between environmental tobacco smoke and

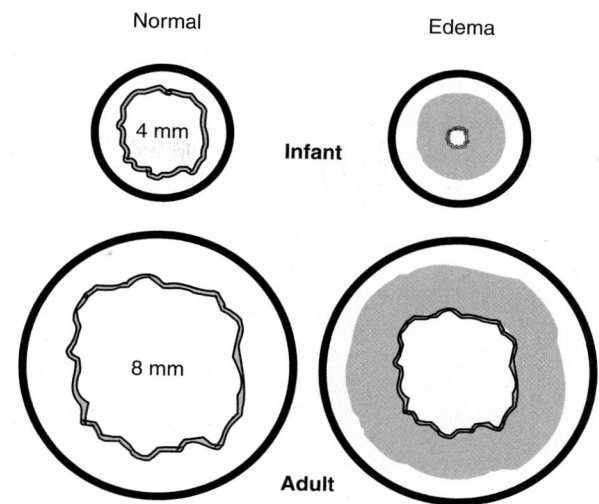

Figure 56-2 *Effect of Edema on Airway Resistance in the Infant versus the Adult: Whereas 1 mm of circumferential edema (on right) can cause a 75% decrease in the cross-sectional area of an infant's airway, it causes only a 44% decrease in the adult's.*

otitis media in young children. Passive smoking has been associated with an increase in blocked eustachian tubes, which can lead to nasopharyngeal congestion and upper respiratory infections (Faden et al., 1998).

LARYNGOTRACHEOBRONCHITIS

Laryngotracheobronchitis (LTB), the most common type of croup, is a viral illness that causes swelling (narrowing) of the upper airway (Figure 56-2).

Initial symptoms include inspiratory **stridor** (a high-pitched, harsh sound), a "barking" cough, and hoarseness. The child may have a persistent, low-grade fever and a history of profuse nasal drainage with increased respiratory effort for several days.

Medical–Surgical Management

Medical

Treatment is focused on maintaining a patent airway and improving respiratory effort by creating a highly humid, cool-mist environment.

PROFESSIONAL TIP

Throat Procedures

Procedures involving the throat (i.e., cultures and visual inspection) can cause laryngospasm and airway obstruction and should therefore be avoided when children present with symptoms such as inspiratory stridor, a barking cough, or hoarseness.

COMMUNITY/HOME HEALTH CARE

Managing LTB at Home

- Observe for early signs of respiratory distress, such as stridor at rest; lower rib retractions; difficulty swallowing; absence of cough; agitation; respiration >50; flaring nares
- Maintain high humidity with cool-air vaporizer, 10 to 15 minutes in the bathroom with steam from a hot shower, cool air through a window
- Hydrate with cool, noncarbonated, nonacidic beverages of choice; ice pops; jello; small pieces of ice
- Provide rest by holding, rocking, soothing, and staying calm

Pharmacological

[handwritten: when sleeping - moon face]

Use of medications such as bronchodilators, corticosteroids, and sedatives is controversial because of potential side effects. In severe cases caused by respiratory syncytial virus (RSV), ribavirin (Virazole), an aerosoled antiviral agent, may be used.

Nursing Management

[handwritten: - To manage, put mom or dad in w/ child.]

Children with mild croup (no stridor at rest, mild retractions, no cyanosis, and restlessness only when disturbed) are managed at home. Teach parents how to monitor for signs of respiratory distress and ways to maintain high humidity and hydration.

Care for the hospitalized infant includes a mist hood or tent with oxygen and, if the child is refusing oral fluids or respirations are greater than 60 breaths per minute, intravenous (IV) therapy. Infants may be held with the mist blowing in the face if being in the tent causes distress. Parents should remain with the child and provide routine care throughout hospitalization in an effort to keep the infant calm, quiet, and in the tent. The presence of favorite toys and items from home can also be comforting to the infant. It is important to keep linens and clothes dry and the child in a comfortable position (usually semireclined in an infant seat placed under the tent). If oxygen is administered, the concentration delivered is regulated to maintain arterial saturation above 95% (according to pulse oximetry).

[handwritten, left margin: (Hold diffuser of mouth, nebulize when sleeping) (Best Time)]

As with home care, monitoring for early signs of impending airway obstruction is paramount. Intubation equipment should be readily available at all times.

PNEUMONIA *[handwritten: - Frequent Turning.]*

An inflammation of the bronchioles and alveolar spaces of the lungs, pneumonia is most commonly caused by RSV in infants. Pneumonia is often preceded by an upper respiratory infection. Viral infections render the infant more susceptible to secondary bacterial invasion. Pneumococcal pneumonia is the most common form of bacterial pneumonia found in infants.

Onset is usually abrupt, with rapidly increasing fever, flaring nostrils, **circumoral cyanosis** (bluish discoloration surrounding the mouth), chest retractions, pulse rate of 140 to 180 beats per minute, respiratory rate of 60 to 80 breaths per minute, and nonproductive cough. Chest x-rays and secretion cultures are used to confirm the diagnosis.

Medical–Surgical Management

Medical

Treatment involves oxygen and cool-mist administration, chest physiotherapy, postural drainage, hydration, family support, antipyretics, antitussives, and antibiotics (if causative agent is bacterial).

Nursing Management

[handwritten: IV. site 1) scalp - side of Head 2) foot]

Monitor respiratory status, prevent further infection, and promote safety. Monitor hydration by accurate intake and output (I&O) measurement and assessment of skin turgor and anterior fontanel. Use a bulb syringe to suction the nose and nasopharynx as needed and before feeding. Saline nose drops may aid in clearing passages. Change the infant's position frequently to prevent both stasis of secretions in the lungs and secretion drainage into the eustachian tubes. Encourage parents to be active participants in their infant's routine daily care.

RESPIRATORY DISTRESS SYNDROME

[handwritten: possibly critical babies]

[handwritten: ← most frequent]

Preterm infants often have respiratory distress syndrome (RDS) because the lungs are deficient in surfactant, a soapy substance that reduces surface tension inside the air sacs. The lungs collapse after each breath, greatly reducing the infant's supply of oxygen. This, in turn, damages the lung cells, contributing to the formation of hyaline membrane. This membrane blocks gas exchange in the alveoli.

Clinical manifestations include tachypnea (70 to 120 breaths per minute in children), retractions, grunting, crackles, pallor, cyanosis, slow capillary refill, hypothermia, peripheral edema, flaccid muscle tone, gastrointestinal (GI) shutdown, jaundice, and acidosis. Chest radiographs confirm the diagnosis.

The first 96 hours are critical to the recovery of infants with RDS. Complications of RDS include complications of oxygen administration; intraventricular hemorrhage; bronchopulmonary dysplasia (BPD); and necrotizing enterocolitis.

Medical–Surgical Management

Medical

Treatment includes administration of surfactant through the endotracheal tube immediately at or soon after birth. In addition, continuous positive airway pressure (CPAP) helps keep the lungs partially expanded until they begin producing surfactant (approximately 5 days).

Health Promotion

Tx - maintain airway &/or surfactant towards baby.

Attempts may be made to prevent the occurrence of RDS. Surfactant may be administered to at-risk infants before the development of RDS. If preterm delivery is expected, **lecithin,** the major component of surfactant, may be measured to determine lung maturity. If insufficient lecithin is present, the mother may be given a glucocorticosteroid that crosses the placenta and causes the infant's lungs to produce surfactant within 72 hours.

Nursing Management

Closely monitor respirations, eliminate unnecessary physical stimulation and metabolic demands, and establish a positive relationship with the parents. Place the infant in a warmer under an oxygen hood or with mechanical ventilation.

CYSTIC FIBROSIS — *Baby salty = Bigger problem Respiratory problems*

Cystic fibrosis (CF), a major dysfunction of all exocrine glands, primarily affects the lungs, pancreas, liver, and reproductive organs. Characteristics of this disease include increased viscosity of mucous gland secretions, elevated sweat electrolytes, increased organic and enzymatic constituents of saliva, and abnormalities in autonomic nervous system function. This disease is transmitted as an autosomal-recessive trait, meaning that both parents must be carriers (Table 56-2). Therefore, it is common that infants with CF also have siblings with CF.

Most children show evidence of the disease by 1 year of age. The earliest manifestation of CF is **meconium ileus** (impacted feces in the newborn, causing bowel obstruction). **Intussusception** (telescoping of the bowel) may be another sign of the disorder. Rectal prolapse is a common problem resulting from difficulty passing the sticky, thick stools. These GI problems result from the lack of pancreatic enzymes. Most children have difficulty gaining and maintaining weight, despite a voracious appetite. Pulmonary complications, such as chronic moist, productive cough and frequent infections, are present in most children with CF. Many children develop barrel chests and clubbed fingers because of the chronic lack of oxygen. Fertility is low in females and males are usually sterile (Mickle & Cutting, 2000).

Parents frequently report that their infants taste like *salty* salt when they kiss them. This common manifestation is a result of the elevated sweat electrolytes. Diagnosis is confirmed with the sweat chloride test.

Although CF is a life-threatening illness, families must be encouraged to focus on positive outcomes. The life expectancy continues to rise, and the search for improved treatments continues.

Medical–Surgical Management

Medical

Treatment focuses on managing pulmonary complications, ensuring adequate nutrition, and assisting the child and family in adapting to a chronic disorder. Chest physiotherapy (CPT, postural drainage) is usually performed one to three times per day to maintain patent airways.

Pharmacological *test Sweat chloride Test*

Aerosol treatments and antibiotic therapy may be used as indicated. Commercially prepared pancreatic enzymes are given with meals and snacks to aid digestion and absorption of fats and proteins.

CPX (a chemical derivative of existing lead compounds) is a new protein repair therapy that may interact directly with the cystic fibrosis transmembrane regulator (CFTR) protein, the product of the CF gene. It appears to repair the faulty protein, thereby curing the basic CF defect. Clinical studies of this new drug began in August 1998. Researchers are evaluating the safety and pharmacodynamics of oral doses of CPX in as many as 50 adults with CF at multiple sites (Cystic Fibrosis Foundation, 1998).

Diet

Well-balanced, high-caloric diets should be maintained because children with CF often absorb only 50% of ingested foods.

Nursing Management

Monitor respiratory status, adventitious lung sounds, cough, stools, abdominal distension, and weight. Assess growth and development, hydration, and nutrition. Administer oxygen and medications as ordered. Encourage physical activity. Teach family skills needed to follow the prescribed therapeutic plan.

NURSING PROCESS

Assessment

Subjective Data

Assess the child and parents for indications of anxiety and fear. Interview the family about activities or events leading up to the crisis, effects of illness on day-to-day functioning, previous hospitalizations, and knowledge about the condition.

TABLE 56-2	AUTOSOMAL RECESSIVE INHERITANCE		
		MOTHER (CARRIER: HAS TRAIT)	
	GAMETES	A	a
Father (Carrier: Has Trait)	A	AA (no disease/trait)	Aa (has trait)
	a	Aa (has trait)	aa (has disease)

Objective Data

Physical assessment focuses on respiratory status, growth and development, hydration, and nutrition. Observe for adventitious lung sounds, cough, finger clubbing, barrel chest, frequency and nature of stools, abdominal distention, weight loss, fatigue, and pallor. Routinely plot height and weight on a growth chart, and assess developmental level using the Denver II test.

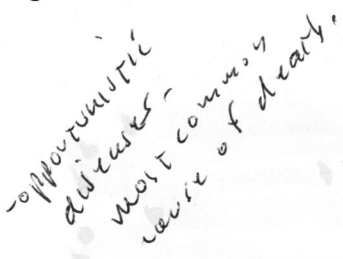

[handwritten margin note:] opportunistic diseases - most common cause of death.

Nursing diagnoses for the infant with CF may include the following:

Nursing Diagnoses	Planning/Goals	Nursing Interventions
Ineffective Airway Clearance, related to thick, tenacious secretions	The client will maintain a clear airway.	Initiate aerosol therapy, CPT, and breathing exercises as prescribed; schedule at least 1 hour before or after meals.
		Administer oxygen as prescribed and monitor closely for level of consciousness.
		Calculate and maintain required fluid intake.
		Observe for signs of infection.
		Assess respiratory status frequently.
		Administer antibiotics as prescribed.
Delayed Growth and Development related to inability to digest nutrients and possible loss of appetite	The client will exhibit signs of adequate growth and development.	Ensure high-caloric intake.
		Administer prescribed pancreatic enzymes with meals and snacks.
		Offer small, frequent feedings if appetite poor.
		Monitor weight and height (plot on growth chart).
		Assess developmental level (i.e., with the Denver II test).
		Encourage physical activity limited only by the child's endurance.
Fear (family) related to long term care and prognosis	The family will verbalize knowledge of disease and demonstrate proper techniques for care.	Teach the family the importance of carrying out prescribed therapeutic plan.
		Teach the family skills for carrying out prescribed therapeutic plan.
	The family will verbalize lessened fears and anxiety.	Provide numbers for CF Foundation and community resources.
	The family will utilize available support systems and community resources.	Encourage expression of feelings and concerns.
		Refer the family for genetic counseling.

Evaluation Each goal must be evaluated to determine how it has been met by the client.

SUDDEN INFANT DEATH SYNDROME

Sudden infant death syndrome (SIDS), commonly called "crib death," is the sudden, unexpected death of an apparently healthy infant in whom the postmortem fails to reveal an adequate cause. It is the leading cause of death in infants older than 1 month of age, with 90% of deaths occurring by 6 months of age (The American SIDS Institute, 1999). Although numerous theories have been proposed regarding the cause of SIDS (including airway obstruction, abnormal cardiorespiratory control, and hyperactive airway reflexes), no single cause has been identified.

Since 1992, when the American Academy of Pediatrics (AAP) recommended that infants be placed to sleep on their backs, the SIDS rate has decreased by more than 40% (AAP, 2000). Other modifiable risk factors to focus on are sleeping on a soft surface, maternal smoking, and overheating (AAP, 2000). Hersheberger (Dowshen, Hersheberger & Rutherford, 2001) states: "Parents need to know that SIDS is not caused by vomiting and choking or other minor illnesses. It is not caused by vaccines or other immunizations."

Typically, the infant is found huddled in the corner of a disheveled bed, with blankets over the head. Frothy, blood-tinged fluid fills the mouth and nose, and the infant may be lying face down in the secretions. The diaper is wet and full of stool. The hands may be clenched.

Nursing Management

Provide empathic support to the family. Ask parents only factual questions, with no suggestion of responsibility. It is vital to reassure them that death caused by SIDS is not predictable or completely preventable. Inform the family that an autopsy must be performed to confirm the diagnosis of SIDS. Encourage them to hold their child and say "good-bye." If the mother was breastfeeding, provide information about abrupt discontinuation of lactation. Refer to the SIDS Foundation.

Ideally, the family will receive a visit from a competent, qualified professional as soon after the death as possible. Areas needing to be discussed include expression of feelings, coping mechanisms, siblings' reactions, and birth of a subsequent child.

CARDIOVASCULAR SYSTEM

Indications that the heart is functioning normally include warm skin, pink mucous membranes, easily palpated pulses, symmetrical chest, normal growth and development, and high activity tolerance. Upon auscultation of a healthy heart at the point of maximum intensity (PMI), two sounds (S1 ["lub"] and S2 ["dub"]) are heard. Heart sounds should be clear and distinct, regular and even. The rate should be the same as the radial pulse. In many children, a *sinus arrhythmia*, wherein the heart rate increases on inspiration and decreases on expiration, is considered normal.

During fetal life, the lungs are inactive and require only a small amount of blood to nourish their tissues. Blood is circulated through the umbilical arteries to the placenta, where waste products and carbon dioxide are exchanged for oxygen and nutrients. The blood is then returned to the fetus through the umbilical vein.

At birth, the umbilical cord is cut, and the infant's own independent system is established. The ductus arteriosus, the foramen ovale, and the ductus venosus are no longer needed. They normally close and atrophy during the first several weeks after birth. Figure 56-3 illustrates the circulatory patterns of the healthy prenatal and postnatal heart.

Figure 56-3 *Circulation of the Heart:* **A,** *Prenatal;* **B,** *Postnatal*

Congenital cardiovascular defects range from mild to severe. They may be detected immediately at birth or may not be detected for several months.

CONGENITAL CARDIOVASCULAR DEFECTS

Congenital cardiovascular defects are among the leading causes of death during the first year of life (American Heart Association, 2001). Errors in formation of the heart or great vessels can occur prenatally, and persistence of fetal circulation can occur postnatally. Cardiovascular defects are best categorized according to blood flow patterns: (1) increased pulmonary blood flow, (2) decreased pulmonary blood flow, (3) obstructed blood flow out of the heart, or (4) mixed blood flow. Four of the most common cardiovascular defects in infants are listed in Table 56-3.

Rubella in the mother during the first trimester of pregnancy is a common cause of heart defects in infants. Other possible maternal causes include alcoholism, irradiation, ingestion of drugs, diabetes, malnutrition, and being more than 40 years old. Heredity is seldom a contributing factor.

TABLE 56-3   COMMON CARDIOVASCULAR DEFECTS IN INFANTS

	VENTRICULAR SEPTAL DEFECT (VSD)	ATRIAL SEPTAL DEFECT (ASD)	PATENT DUCTUS ARTERIOSUS (PDA)	TETRALOGY OF FALLOT (TOF)
Description	Opening between ventricles	Opening between atria; incompetent foramen ovale	Failure of fetal ductus arteriosus to close postnatally	Four defects: (VSD), pulmonic stenosis, overriding aorta, and right ventricular hypertrophy
Blood Flow Pattern	↑ Pulmonary flow, left-to-right shunting	↑ Pulmonary flow; left-to-right shunting	↑ Pulmonary flow, left-to-right shunting	↓ Pulmonary flow; right-to-left shunting
Manifestations	↑ Respiratory infections; normal growth and development; congestive heart failure (CHF), if defect large	Usually asymptomatic, possible dysrhythmias, CHF if defect large	Usually asymptomatic, CHF possible, machinery-like murmur	Hypoxia, murmur, delayed growth and development
Treatment	Surgical correction by 2 years of age; prognosis dependent on extent of defect	Surgical correction by 6 years of age; excellent prognosis	Possiblity indomethacin (Indocin) administration to premature babies; surgical correction by 2 years; excellent prognosis	Surgical correction by 1 year of age

Infants with severe cardiovascular defects may be born with obvious distress caused by hypoxia. Those with less serious defects may compensate and appear to be healthy at birth. Heart murmurs and delayed growth and development observed later may call attention to problems. Infants with severe defects will often manifest signs and symptoms of CHF, such as fatigability; orthopnea; failure to thrive; pale, mottled, or cyanotic skin; hoarse or weak cry; tachycardia; and signs of respiratory distress, such as rate over 60, costal retractions, orthopnea, wheezing, and coughing.

Medical–Surgical Management

Surgical

Surgical intervention to repair a defect may be postponed until the child develops CHF. Generally, the older the infant, the better the surgical outcome. Refer to Table 56-3 for treatments of common heart defects.

Pharmacological

Digoxin (Lanoxin) is the drug most often used to improve the heart's contractility and increase its output. Furosemide (Lasix) is the most commonly used diuretic. Because most diuretics cause potassium loss, serum potassium level is monitored, and potassium supplements may be ordered. Oxygen therapy and fluid management are also part of the treatment plan.

Diet

When infants experience significant dyspnea while feeding, special feeding techniques are needed, such as providing small, frequent feedings and softer nipples. Some infants need higher caloric formulas and diets to meet nutritional needs. Gavage feedings may be required if the infant becomes fatigued before taking an adequate amount of formula.

Nursing Management

Assess cardiac and respiratory function. Monitor behavioral patterns and growth and development. Administer oxygen and medications as ordered. Accurately record I&O. Weigh daily. Provide high-calorie feedings. If infant tires easily when eating, implement gavage feedings.

NURSING PROCESS

Assessment

Subjective Data

Take a history of the child's previous hospitalizations and assess the family's knowledge about the condition. Note the family's anxiety level, coping strategies, and economic status.

Objective Data

Assess the child's behavioral patterns, cardiac and respiratory function, fluid status, and growth and development. Obtain a detailed history of onset of symptoms and a typical day's activity schedule.

Nursing diagnoses for the infant with a heart defect may include the following:

Nursing Diagnoses	Planning/Goals	Nursing Interventions
Decreased Cardiac Output related to structural defect	The client will demonstrate sufficient cardiac output to meet metabolic demands.	Administer digoxin as prescribed. Monitor vital signs (including apical pulse for 1 minute), potassium level, urine output, cardiac rhythm, activity tolerance. Assess for signs of digoxin toxicity (vomiting, anorexia, dysrhythmias, bradycardia [pulse rate < 90 to 110]), peripheral perfusion. Provide periods of rest each hour.
Ineffective Breathing Pattern related to pulmonary congestion	The client will breathe effortlessly at rest.	Keep the client in semi-Fowler's position (i.e., use infant seat). Administer humidified oxygen as prescribed, assess respiratory rate and effort, color, and oxygen saturation. Employ comfort measures (i.e., holding, rocking, presence of parents). Respond quickly to crying.
Excess Fluid Volume related to fluid accumulation	The client will experience decreased edema.	Administer diuretics as prescribed. Measure I&O. Weigh daily (same time and scale). Assess skin for edema, breakdown. Turn every 2 hours and elevate edematous extremities. Monitor electrolytes.
Imbalanced Nutrition: Less than Body Requirements, related to fatigue and dyspnea	The client will demonstrate normal weight gain for age.	Give small, frequent, high-caloric feedings. Use soft nipple with large hole. Implement gavage feeding, if the infant tires before taking prescribed amount of formula. Make feeding time as stress free as possible. Hold the infant when bottle-feeding (preferably by primary caregiver).
Delayed Growth and Development related to low energy level	The client will meet developmental milestones for age.	Encourage age-appropriate activities, stimulation, and socialization. Allow the child to set own pace
Interrupted Family Processes related to child with life threatening illness/condition	The family will receive needed support.	Teach the family as needed about medication administration, signs and symptoms of CHF and when to report, feeding techniques, and appropriate activities for the child. Refer the family to appropriate community resources.

Evaluation Each goal must be evaluated to determine how it has been met by the client.

PROFESSIONAL TIP

Stress at Feeding Time

Ways to decrease stress at feeding time include the following:

- Decrease the noise level.
- Hold the infant while sitting in a rocker.
- Assess the infant's readiness to eat. (Infant is calm, demonstrates rooting, latches onto nipple eagerly, opens mouth voluntarily, looks at caregiver.)

HEMATOLOGIC AND LYMPHATIC SYSTEMS

The hematologic system regulates, directly or indirectly, the functions of all body tissues and organs. Some of the most common disorders occurring in infants include hyperbilirubinemia, iron-deficiency anemia, and sickle-cell anemia (SCA).

HYPERBILIRUBINEMIA

Hyperbilirubinemia, often referred to as jaundice, is a common occurrence in neonates. **Jaundice** is the yellow discoloration of the skin, sclera, mucous membranes, and body fluids resulting from excess bilirubin and deposition of bile pigments. Physiologically, hemoglobin is broken down by the liver into iron, protein, and bilirubin. The bilirubin binds to albumin and is transported to the liver, where it is conjugated. Conjugated bilirubin is then eliminated through the intestines. Neonates have an intestinal enzyme that can convert the conjugated bilirubin back to unconjugated bilirubin, which can be reabsorbed into the bloodstream. This process can contribute significantly to the amount of bilirubin that the immature liver must break down. As the bilirubin level rises, some of the excess bilirubin is deposited in body tissues, resulting in a temporary yellow discoloration of the skin and sclera. A high level of bilirubin can penetrate and damage brain cells, causing severe neural symptoms **(kernicterus)**. Hyperbilirubinemia develops during the first few days of life in 45% to 60% of term infants and in as many as 80% of preterm infants.

Medical–Surgical Management

Medical

The main objective of treatment is to reduce the amount of unconjugated bilirubin and aid in the conversion of bilirubin to a form that can be excreted by the body (urobilinogen). Full-term infants with jaundice may benefit from early and frequent breastfeeding (every 2 hours). Otherwise, treatment usually begins with a phototherapy light, called a bililight, or a fiber-optic blanket. This light causes a chemical reaction in the skin and converts unconjugated bilirubin to a form that can be excreted by the body (lumirubin). Therapy is usually continual, with short breaks for feeding and holding. Phototherapy may be done at home because it is less expensive than treatment in the hospital and the family will not have to be separated from their newborn.

Pharmacological

If the bilirubin level responds slowly to phototherapy, phenobarbital is sometimes given to enhance both the liver enzyme action and bilirubin excretion. Breastfeeding may have to be stopped for 24 to 48 hours if the level does not decrease with phototherapy. Ironically, breastfeeding and breast milk may cause hyperbilirubinemia as well as prevent it.

Nursing Management

Frequently assess for jaundice. Encourage frequent feedings. Maintain phototherapy as prescribed. Teach parents to do phototherapy at home.

NURSING PROCESS

Assessment

Subjective Data

Assess perinatal risk factors such as familial history of hyperbilirubinemia and induced delivery.

Objective Data

Assess for jaundice by applying light pressure to the skin over either the tip of the nose or the sternum in natural daylight. For dark-skinned infants, observe the sclera, conjunctiva, and oral mucosa for a yellow color. Bruising, petechiae, and pallor are also suggestive of hyperbilirubenemia.

Nursing diagnoses for the infant with hyperbilirubinemia may include the following:

Nursing Diagnoses	Planning/Goals	Nursing Interventions
Risk for Deficient Fluid Volume, related to insensible losses	The client will maintain fluid balance.	Assess skin for signs of dehydration. Calculate needed fluid intake to compensate for losses. Monitor I&O.
Risk for Impaired Skin Integrity related to use of phototherapy and diarrhea	The client's skin will remain intact.	Assess skin for breakdown. Monitor temperature every 2 to 4 hours. Keep skin clean and dry, do not apply any oils or lotions.
Interrupted Family Processes related to situational crisis	The family will receive needed support.	Encourage bonding by removing eye shields and allowing the parents to hold/feed the infant. Teach the importance of eye shields under light. Support the breastfeeding mother. Encourage pumping the breasts, if feeding must be stopped temporarily. Keep the parents informed.

Evaluation Each goal must be evaluated to determine how it has been met by the client.

IRON-DEFICIENCY ANEMIA

The incidence of iron-deficiency anemia is usually related to the infant's consuming large amounts of milk and foods that do not contain supplemental iron. These babies are often overweight because of excessive intake of cow's milk, which is a poor source of iron. In addition, cow's milk can cause loss of blood in the stool.

Because full-term infants have iron stores from fetal circulation that usually last for 5 to 6 months, iron-deficiency anemia usually surfaces between 9 and 24 months of age. Clinical manifestations may include extreme pallor (porcelain-like in fair-skinned infants), tachycardia, lethargy, irritability, and below-normal hemoglobin, hematocrit, and iron levels.

Medical–Surgical Management

Pharmacological

Iron therapy is usually prescribed and continued for 3 months after hemoglobin and hematocrit levels return to normal. An increase in hemoglobin level can be expected within 4 to 30 days. Ascorbic acid may also be prescribed in an attempt to facilitate iron absorption. Intramuscular (IM) or IV injections may be necessary if the level does not improve after 1 month of oral iron. Transfusions are indicated only for the most severe cases.

Diet

Long-term therapy is directed at increasing the dietary intake of iron and continuing the use of iron-fortified

---

PROFESSIONAL TIP

WIC

The federal supplemental food program called Women, Infants, and Children (WIC) is an excellent resource for nutritious food for low-income families with pregnant, postpartum, or lactating women and children up to 5 years of age. In addition to food, this program provides nutritional education and screening.

CLIENT TEACHING

Administration of Iron to Infants

When instructing caregivers in the administration of iron to infants, teach to:

- Administer with citrus fruit or juice in order to increase its absorption.
- Administer through a straw or medicine dropper placed at the back of the mouth, to decrease staining of the teeth.
- Brush or wipe the infant's teeth after administration.
- Expect dark, black stools.

---

formula until 12 months of age. At 4 to 6 months of age, iron-fortified cereal can be used (Grover, 2000).

Nursing Management

Prevent anemia by educating the family about administration of iron. It is important to explore any misconceptions parents may have, such as "milk is a perfect food" and "excessive weight gain equates to a healthy child and good mothering."

Encourage foods rich in iron, such as dried beans, iron-fortified cereals, apricots, prunes, egg yolks, and dark-green, leafy vegetables. Infants should remain on iron-fortified formulas until 12 months of age.

Instruct caregivers in the proper administration of oral iron. When administering IM preparations, no more than 1 mL should be given deep into the muscle using the Z-track method to prevent staining of tissues and to minimize irritation.

SICKLE-CELL ANEMIA

Sickle-cell anemia (SCA) is a genetic disorder characterized by the production of abnormal hemoglobin and resulting in red blood cells (RBCs) taking on a "sickle" shape (Figure 56-4). Because of the presence of fetal hemoglobin, clinical symptoms usually do not appear until 6 months of age. Episodes of sickling may be triggered by infection, dehydration, hypoxia, trauma, or general physical or emotional stress resulting in impaired circulation and increased RBC destruction.

The most common symptoms of SCA include abdominal pain (caused by sludging in the spleen and leading to its enlargement), fever, severe leg pain, and hot, swollen joints. In addition, growth retardation, chronic anemia, and increased susceptibility to infection may be experienced. This disease occurs primarily among African Americans and is transmitted as an autosomal-recessive trait wherein both parents are carriers (refer back to Table 56-2).

Medical–Surgical Management

Medical

Between episodes, the goal is to prevent crises with adequate hydration (1,500 to 3,000 mL/day). During crises, treatment may include bed rest, oxygen, analgesics (morphine), and fluids.

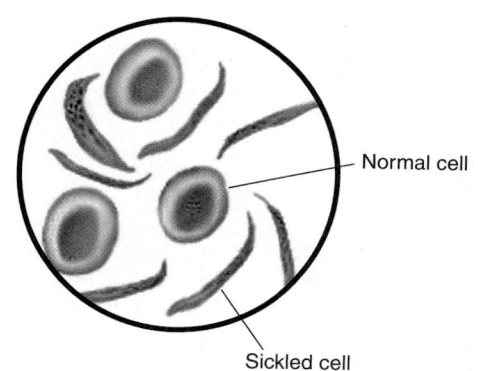

Normal cell

Sickled cell

Figure 56-4 *Sickling Cells*

CRITICAL THINKING

Immunizations

How should you respond to a parent who refused to have an infant immunized?

Pharmacological

Children with this disease must be immunized with influenza, pneumococcal, meningococcal, and hepatitis B vaccines because of increased susceptibility to infection and the likelihood of transfusion therapy. Prophylactic oral penicillin is often prescribed twice a day until age 5 or 6, and a daily supplement of folic acid is taken (Mayo Clinic, 2001).

Health Promotion

Avoid high altitudes, poorly pressurized airplanes, and exposure to extreme heat or cold. Maintaining hydration is of paramount importance. Neonatal screening, early intervention, prophylactic antibiotics, and parent education have allowed children with SCA to live into adulthood.

Nursing Management

Encourage continuous adequate hydration and immunizations. Prevent exposure to extreme heat or cold. Provide parent education. Monitor growth and development. When in crisis, administer analgesics, antibiotics, oxygen, and fluids as ordered. Apply heat to affected area.

NURSING PROCESS

Assessment

Subjective Data

Interview the family about activities or events leading up to the crisis, a history of child's health, and previous episodes. Evaluate the family's level of knowledge about the condition.

Objective Data

Assess all areas and systems that can be affected by circulatory obstruction, such as vital signs, vision, hearing, growth and development, and the respiratory, GI, renal, neurological, and musculoskeletal systems.

Nursing diagnoses for the infant with sickle-cell anemia may include the following:

Nursing Diagnoses	Planning/Goals	Nursing Interventions
Ineffective Tissue Perfusion related to vaso-occlusion and anemia	The client will maintain oxygen saturation levels at 95% or greater.	Administer oxygen as prescribed. Monitor oxygen saturation, capillary refill, and respiratory status. Maintain the client in a position of comfort (semi- to high-Fowler's). Administer packed RBCs as prescribed.
Acute Pain related to vaso-occlusion and tissue ischemia	The client will be pain free.	Apply heat to affected area; avoid cold compresses. Administer analgesics as prescribed (preferably morphine) and assess effectiveness by assessing behavior and vital signs. Reassure the family that opioids are appropriate, high doses may be needed, and addiction is rare. Position the client carefully and handle gently.
Risk for Infection related to splenic malfunction	The client will be infection free.	Provide one to one and one-half daily fluid requirement as determined by body weight. Provide daily food requirements as determined by body weight and length. Administer antibiotics as prescribed. Ensure that the infant avoids contact with known sources of infection. Ensure that immunizations are up-to-date.
Deficient Knowledge (family) related to cause and treatment of disease	The family will verbalize an understanding of the risk factors and ways to minimize them	Teach need for one to one and one-half times daily fluid requirement. Teach importance of hand hygiene and avoiding known sources of infection.

continues

Nursing Diagnoses	Planning/Goals	Nursing Interventions
		Reinforce importance of up-to-date immunizations for the infant.
		Teach to shield the infant from overexertion, emotional stress, and low-oxygen environments.
		Teach early intervention for any sign of infection (e.g., temperature of 101.5°F or greater) or dehydration (weight loss, dry skin and mucous membranes, sunken fontanel).
		Teach medication administration as ordered.
Interrupted **F**amily Processes related to child with chronic condition	The family will adjust to lifelong, potentially fatal hereditary disease.	Explain procedures and planned treatments.
		Allow the family to provide care in the hospital.
		Provide information about appropriate developmental activities.
		Encourage the family to talk about feelings and concerns.
		Stress positive outcomes (i.e., that most of the time, children are asymptomatic and can participate in appropriate activities without restrictions).
		Provide information regarding transmission of the condition; refer for genetic counseling.
		Provide numbers for American Sickle Cell Anemia Association and available support groups.

Evaluation Each goal must be evaluated to determine how it has been met by the client.

GASTROINTESTINAL SYSTEM

Infants have minimal saliva, no voluntary control of swallowing, a small stomach, rapid intestinal motility, a relaxed cardiac sphincter, deficiency of enzymes in the duodenum, and immature liver function. This accounts for the numerous GI problems that occur during the first 12 months of life, such as vomiting, diarrhea, **colic** (sudden, recurrent bouts of abdominal pain), and failure to thrive. In addition, because the immune system is also immature, the infant is highly susceptible to infection. Congenital defects resulting in **atresia** (absence or closure of a body orifice), malposition, nonclosure, or other abnormalities can occur in any area of the GI tract. Any GI problem, whether a lack of nutrients, an infection, or a congenital disorder, can quickly affect other parts of the body and ultimately affect general health and growth and development. The GI disorders discussed following include thrush, acute gastroenteritis, colic, failure to thrive, cleft lip/palate, esophageal atresia with tracheoesophageal fistula, pyloric stenosis, Hirschsprung's disease, gastroesophageal reflux, and intussusception.

THRUSH

Thrush (moniliasis, candidiasis) is an oral fungal infection that is transmitted from the vaginal canal of an infected mother to the newborn. Other contributing factors include poor hand hygiene by care providers, inadequate washing of bottles and nipples, and antibiotic therapy. Thrush is characterized by painless, white patches that look like curdled milk on the oral mucosa

Figure 56-5 *Thrush*

(Figure 56-5). The incidence is approximately 2% to 4%, with bottle-fed infants at greater risk than breastfed infants (Clayton, 2000).

Medical–Surgical Management

Pharmacological

Topical nystatin (Mycostatin) is the most commonly used treatment for thrush. It is applied to the oral mucosa four times per day with an applicator or a gloved finger and then swallowed. Rinse the mouth before medicating. In addition, if infants are breastfed, apply the medication to the breasts.

Nursing Management

Teach caregivers proper hand hygiene. Boiling bottles and nipples for 20 minutes will kill the spores.

ACUTE GASTROENTERITIS

Acute gastroenteritis (AGE) is an inflammation of the stomach and intestines that may be accompanied by diarrhea and vomiting. This common condition may be caused by malnutrition, lactose intolerance, chronic conditions, or infections by viruses, bacteria, and parasites.

The infant with AGE will have an increased number of green, liquid stools tinged with mucus or blood. In addition, symptoms of fluid and electrolyte imbalance, cramping, extreme irritability, and vomiting may be exhibited. Depending on age and nutritional status and on the severity and duration of the diarrhea, the infant may become severely dehydrated and gravely ill.

Medical–Surgical Management

Medical

Regaining and maintaining fluid balance is paramount. Use oral rehydrating fluids such as Pedialyte and Lytren for mild dehydration. For severe dehydration, IV solutions are needed to replace fluids and electrolytes. Antibiotics may be prescribed if bacterial infection is indicated from stool cultures.

Diet

Once rehydration is attained, the usual diet is continued. Research has indicated that early reintroduction of normal nutrients is desirable, and delayed introduction of food may be harmful in terms of nutritional status and duration of illness. Breastfed infants should continue on supplemental oral rehydrating solutions throughout the illness. If formula feedings are not tolerated, suggest lactose-free formulas. Complex carbohydrates, lean meats, fruits, and vegetables are well tolerated (AAP, 1996).

Nursing Management

Assess for dehydration. Monitor I&O and electrolyte levels. Administer fluids and electrolytes as ordered. Provide clear fluids and oral rehydrating solutions every 30 minutes. Follow proper hand hygiene and teach to parents. Keep diaper area clean and apply a barrier ointment.

NURSING PROCESS

Assessment

Subjective Data

Question caregivers regarding probable etiologic agents such as introduction of new food; exposure to infectious agents; travel to an area where the infectious agent is endemic; contact with foods that might be contaminated; crowded, dirty living conditions; and contact with pets that are known to be sources of enteric infections, such as pet turtles. Obtain allergy, drug, health, and diet histories.

Objective Data

Assessing for dehydration is paramount for infants with AGE (Table 56-4). Assess the diaper area for skin breakdown resulting from repeated contact with diarrheal stools.

Infection Control: Diaper Hygiene
- Change diapers as soon as they are soiled.
- Wear gloves when changing diapers.
- Fold the used diaper with soiled area to the inside and immediately place the diaper in a covered receptacle.
- Cleanse the skin and dispose of wipes along with the diaper.
- Remove gloves after disposal of wipes.
- Rediaper.
- Wash hands immediately after rediapering is complete.
- Store soiled clothing, cloth diapers, and washcloths in a covered receptacle.
- Cleanse surface of changing area.

TABLE 56-4	ASSESSING DEHYDRATION			
SIGNS AND SYMPTOMS	MILD		MODERATE	SEVERE
Weight loss	<5%		6–10%	>10%
Skin turgor	Taut		Tenting	Tenting
Skin color	Pale		Grey	Mottled
Mucous membranes	Slightly dry, pale		Very dry, grey	Parched
Urine output	Decreased		Absent	Absent
Blood pressure	Normal		Normal	Decreased
Pulse	Normal or increased		Increased	Increased/thready
Fontanelle	Flat		Depressed	Sunken

Nursing diagnoses for the infant with AGE may include the following:

Nursing Diagnoses	Planning/Goals	Nursing Interventions
Deficient Fluid Volume related to excessive GI losses	The client will be adequately hydrated (specify).	Monitor I&O and notify physician if output <1 mL/kg/h. Assess weight daily and compare with previous weights. Assess for degree of hydration. Monitor electrolyte levels. Administer fluids and electrolytes as prescribed. Encourage clear liquids and oral rehydrating solutions (Pedialyte, Lytren) in small doses every 30 minutes until rehydrated; after rehydration, alternate with water, breast milk, or half-strength formula, as needed.
Risk for Infection related to GI infection	The client and family will be infection free.	Teach proper hand hygiene and diaper hygiene to care providers. Wear gloves when handling diapers.
Risk for Impaired Skin Integrity related to frequent contact with diarrheal stools	The client's skin will remain intact.	Change diapers every 2 hours, as needed. Cleanse skin with mild soap (Dove) and water. Apply barrier (A&D Ointment). Teach the family proper techniques.

Evaluation Each goal must be evaluated to determine how it has been met by the client.

COLIC

Colic is a sudden, periodic attack of abdominal pain and cramping that is manifested by severe crying for several hours and by the drawing of the legs up to the abdomen. It usually occurs between birth and 3 months of age and at approximately the same time each day (late afternoon, early evening hours). During these episodes, the infant is generally inconsolable, which may interfere with parent–child attachment and family relations.

The child is usually eager to eat and is growing appropriately. There is no known cause of colic; however, speculation points to overfeeding, overly rapid feeding, improper burping, the swallowing of large amounts of air, and emotional stress between parent and child (Hockenberry et al., 2003).

Medical–Surgical Management
Medical

Sensitivity to formula, food allergies, peritoneal infection, and intestinal obstruction must be ruled out as specific causes of the distress. If sensitivity to formula is sus-

pected, another brand of formula may be substituted. In the case of breastfeeding mothers, avoid dairy products, onions, cabbage, and dry beans for several days in an attempt to relieve the infant's symptoms.

 Pharmacological

Sedatives, antispasmodics, antihistamines, and antiflatulents are sometimes recommended in an attempt to relieve symptoms.

CLIENT TEACHING

Suggestions for Alleviating Colic

- Provide rhythmic movement, such as rocking, swinging, and riding in the car.
- Alternate positions, such as placing the infant face down across the lap.
- Reduce environmental stimuli, especially during feedings.
- Provide a variety of tactile stimulation, such as rubbing the head or abdomen or placing prone on a warm heating pad.
- Provide small, frequent feedings.
- Burp during and after feedings.
- Respond immediately to crying.
- Provide background or "white" noise (vacuum cleaner, hair dryer) or play music.

Nursing Management

Assessing circumstances surrounding the colicky event, exploring techniques to relieve symptoms, and supporting parents during the colicky period are the primary nursing goals. Observe the feeding technique in order to assess the parent's sensitivity and response to the infant's cues of distress and evaluate the clarity of the infant's cues and the infant's responsiveness to the parent.

Reassure parents that colic usually resolves by 3 months of age and does not indicate poor or inadequate parenting. Encourage them to talk about their feelings toward the infant and any insecurities they may feel.

FAILURE TO THRIVE

Failure to thrive (FTT) is the label applied to infants who fail to gain weight and who show signs of delayed development. There are two categories of FTT: organic, which is caused by a physical defect or condition; and nonorganic, which is the result of psychosocial factors such as an impaired parent–child relationship. Manifestations of FTT include sustained growth failure (below the fifth percentile on the standardized growth chart), developmental delays in all areas, and poor feeding and sleeping patterns.

Medical–Surgical Management

Medical

If FTT is the result of a physical defect or condition, the condition is treated. Regardless of the cause, the primary goals are to provide adequate nutrition, promote growth and development, and assist parents in developing the skills needed to nurture their infant.

Health Promotion

In most cases of nonorganic FTT, a multidisciplinary health care team is needed to deal with the physical, psychosocial, mental, and emotional problems that may be occurring in the family. If the entire family is to become healthy, each member must be helped to change.

Nursing Management

Monitor weight gain and development. Provide adequate nutrition. Assist parents to develop nurturing skills.

NURSING PROCESS

Assessment

Subjective Data

Focus on the infant's routine, respiratory status, and diet history. Assess the family for depression, substance abuse, mental retardation, and psychosis as well as socioeconomic level, education, social isolation, stress factors, and support systems.

Objective Data

Focus on signs of malnutrition (skin, hair, nails, mucous membranes, energy level, developmental milestones) and on parent–infant interactions (parent's cues, infant's cues, and synchrony).

Nursing diagnoses for the infant with FTT may include the following:

Nursing Diagnoses	Planning/Goals	Nursing Interventions
Imbalanced **N**utrition: Less than Body Requirements, related to insufficient intake of calories and/or impaired parent/child interaction	The client will demonstrate growth curve above the 5th percentile.	Provide consistent nursing staff and develop a structured routine.
		Feed the infant on demand and increase intake as tolerated.
		Monitor I&O. Weigh daily.
		Encourage parental involvement in care, demonstrate and model appropriate care techniques, praise positive attempts at care, and provide for rooming-in.
		Use a variety of methods to teach child care to the parents.

continues

Nursing Diagnoses	Planning/Goals	Nursing Interventions
*Risk for Delayed **D**evelopment* related to inadequate stimulation	The client will attain age-appropriate developmental milestones.	Begin a program of play that stimulates interest and responsiveness. Teach the parents ways to play and interact with the infant and to cuddle the infant.

Evaluation Each goal must be evaluated to determine how it has been met by the client.

CLEFT LIP/PALATE

The most common facial malformations are cleft lip and cleft palate. They may occur separately or together. Failure of the palates and/or lip to fuse is evident at birth. The defect may occur unilaterally on either side or bilaterally and with varying degrees of severity. The cause is unclear, but some genetic component seems likely.

Clinical manifestations include nasal, lip, and palate distortions. The child born with a cleft palate and intact lip does not manifest the external disfigurement so potentially distressing to parents, but the physical problems are more serious. The infant with a cleft palate is at risk for aspiration, feeding difficulties, and respiratory infections (Figures 56-6 and 56-7).

Medical–Surgical Management

Medical

Care is directed toward closing the defects, maintaining adequate nutrition, preventing complications, and fostering normal growth and development of the child. Total care may involve many specialists, including pediatricians, nurses, plastic surgeons, orthodontists, prosthodontists, otolaryngologists, speech therapists, and psychiatrists. The extent of multidisciplinary care depends on the severity of the defect. Infants with cleft lip and palate are prone to recurrent otitis media, which will likely be treated with antibiotics.

Surgical

Closure of the lip precedes that of the palate, usually at 6 to 12 weeks of age. The palate is usually closed surgically at 12 to 18 months of age to facilitate speech development.

Health Promotion

Maternal use of multivitamin supplements containing folic acid around the time of conception has been reported to reduce the risk of cleft malformations by up to 50% (Shaw et al., 1995).

Nursing Management

Encourage parents to hold and interact with their infant and to participate in the care of the infant. Provide feedings as ordered using assistive devices. Keep infant in upright position for feeding. Burp frequently.

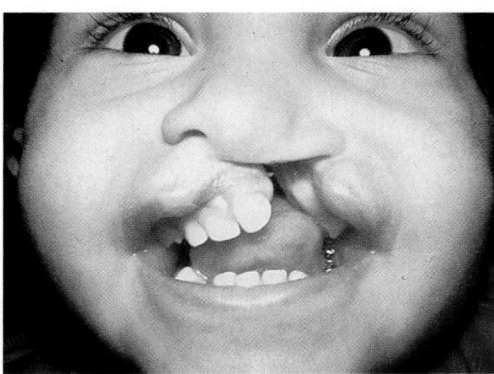

Figure 56-6 *Older Child with Unrepaired Cleft Lip (Courtesy of Dr. Joseph Konzelman, School of Dentistry, Medical College of Georgia)*

Figure 56-7 *Older Child with Unrepaired Cleft Palate (Courtesy of Dr. Joseph Konzelman, School of Dentistry, Medical College of Georgia)*

NURSING PROCESS

Assessment

Subjective Data

Assess immediately the emotional impact of the birth of an infant with a facial deformity. Assess the family's acceptance of the child periodically, at various appointments and hospital admissions.

Objective Data

Cleft lip and palate are observable at birth. A cleft palate is palpable with the finger. Document the degree of involvement. Evaluate the ability to suck, swallow, breathe, and handle secretions.

Nursing diagnoses for the infant with cleft lip or palate may include the following:

Nursing Diagnoses	Planning/Goals	Nursing Interventions
Compromised Family Coping related to birth of infant with visible and/or structural defect	The family will bond with the infant.	Encourage the parents to hold the infant.
		Point out positive attributes of the infant (e.g., hair, eyes, alertness); convey attitude of acceptance of the infant and family.
		Explain expected outcomes of surgical repair; show pictures of repaired children.
		Allow expression of feelings.
		Assess the parents' knowledge, degree of anxiety, level of discomfort, interpersonal relationships.
		Explore reactions of extended family.
		Encourage the parents to participate in care of the infant.
		Provide information.
		Refer to parental support groups and to other families in similar situations.
Imbalanced Nutrition: Less than Body Requirements related to infant's inability to form an adequate seal when sucking on the nipple	The infant will maintain a growth curve above the 5th percentile.	Provide 100 to 150 cal/kg/d and 100 to 130 mL/kg/d.
		Assess output daily.
		Weigh daily.
		Observe for respiratory impairment (i.e., for adventitious breath sounds, increased respiratory rate).
		Facilitate breastfeeding; refer for ongoing support (i.e., to La Leche League).
		Position the infant in an upright or semi-sitting position for feeding.
		Use effective assistive devices (i.e., longer, softer nipples; feeders).
		Feed small amounts slowly, allowing ample time for sucking and swallowing; burp after 15 to 30 mL.
		Initiate nasogastric feeding if infant is unable to ingest sufficient calories by mouth.
Impaired Tissue Integrity related to surgical correction of cleft	The client's tissue will heal with minimal scarring.	Position the infant on side or back.
		Use elbow restraints for 7 to 10 days as needed and teach proper application to parents.
		Medicate for pain around-the-clock for at least 24 hours postoperatively.
		Provide developmentally appropriate activities (e.g., music, mobiles, holding) to distract the infant's attention from the incision site.
		Do not use pacifiers, spoons, or straws for 7 to 10 days postoperatively.
		Progress to a soft diet appropriate to age and as ordered and tolerated within 48 hours.
Risk for Infection related to surgical procedure and accumulation of formula and secretions in oral cavity	The client's surgical site will be free of infection.	Assess vital signs and oral cavity every 2 hours.
		Cleanse suture line with normal saline or sterile water, as ordered.
		Give 5 to 15 mL water after each feeding to cleanse the mouth.
		Apply antibiotic cream as ordered.
		Ensure hand hygiene by all care providers.
		Include parents in care and prepare for home care.

Evaluation Each goal must be evaluated to determine how it has been met by the client.

ESOPHAGEAL ATRESIA WITH TRACHEOESOPHAGEAL FISTULA

Esophageal atresia and tracheoesophageal fistula are rare malformations that may occur alone or in combination and represent a failure of the esophagus to develop as a continuous passage (atresia) to the stomach and/or an unnatural connection between the esophagus and the trachea (fistula) (Figure 56-8). The cause is unknown.

Manifestations include excessive salivation, drooling, coughing, choking when feeding, and cyanosis. A history of polyhydramnios (excessive production of amniotic fluid) during the prenatal period is common.

Medical–Surgical Management

Medical

The primary goal is prevention and treatment of aspiration pneumonia. The infant will be designated NPO and administered IV fluids. Removal of secretions from the mouth and esophagus requires frequent or continuous suctioning through a nasogastric tube (NGT). Antibiotics are prescribed for any developing pneumonia.

Surgical

These defects represent a critical neonatal surgical emergency. Surgical correction may be accomplished in several stages depending on the size and condition of the infant and the extent of the defect. If closure of the gap requires staged repair, a gastrostomy tube will be placed for feeding. The prognosis is usually good with surgery.

Nursing Management

Nursing responsibility for detection of this malformation begins immediately after birth. Assess the newborn for color, amount of saliva, ability to swallow, respiratory distress, and abdominal distention. A maternal history of polyhydramnios necessitates assessment for the defect with insertion of an NGT. Do not initiate feedings until the infant has been assessed. When the defect is diagnosed, prepare the infant and the family for immediate surgery. Postoperative care is the same as that provided to any high-risk newborn.

PYLORIC STENOSIS

Pyloric stenosis is a common disorder that occurs when the circular muscle surrounding the pylorus hypertrophies and blocks gastric emptying (Figure 56-9). It is rarely diagnosed before the third week of life. Manifestations include **projectile vomiting** (ejection of stomach contents up to 3 feet), ravenous hunger, hyperactive bowel sounds, irritability, FTT, decreased number and volume of stools, an olive-shaped mass in the right upper quadrant, and visible peristaltic waves.

Medical–Surgical Management

Medical

Diagnosis is usually made before malnutrition, dehydration, and alkalosis are severe. It is unusual for the infant to require IV fluid therapy before surgery.

Figure 56-8 *Esophagus:* **A,** *Normal;* **B,** *Atresia/Fistula*

Figure 56-9 *Stomach:* **A,** *Normal opening;* **B,** *Pyloric stenosis*

Surgical

The defect usually is discovered early and repaired immediately. Most infants recover rapidly and completely with surgery.

Nursing Management

Recognize the signs and symptoms early. Pre- and postoperative care are the same as for any GI surgical client. Infants are allowed to resume feedings 4 to 6 hours postoperatively and may be discharged within 72 hours.

HIRSCHSPRUNG'S DISEASE/ MEGACOLON

Hirschsprung's disease is a congenital anomaly manifested as a partial or complete mechanical obstruction resulting from inadequate motility of part of the colon. There is an absence of parasympathetic ganglion cells and, thus, of peristalsis within the muscular wall of the distal colon and the rectum. As a result, the affected portion of the bowel narrows, and the portion directly above the affected area becomes greatly dilated and fills with feces and gas (Figure 56-10). Failure of the newborn to have a stool during the first 24 to 48 hours may indicate this defect. Older infants may have constipation or ribbonlike stools and an enlarged, distended abdomen.

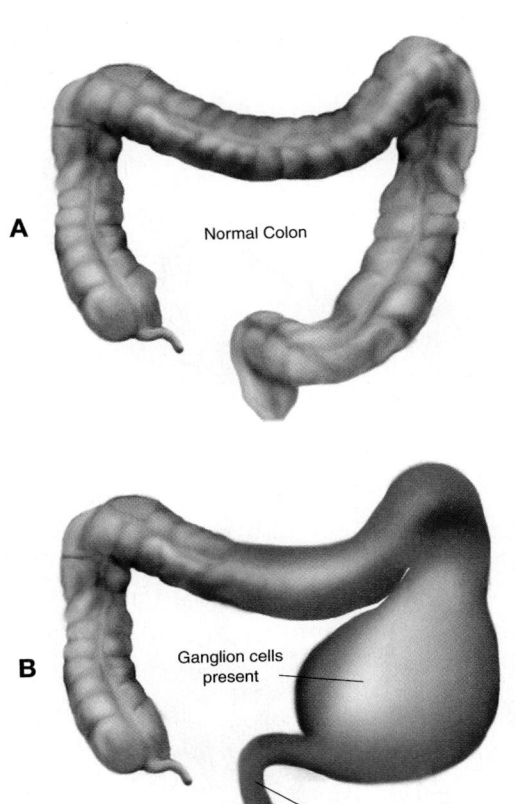

Figure 56-10 *Colon:* **A,** *Normal;* **B,** *Hirschsprung's disease/ Megacolon*

Medical–Surgical Management
Medical

For the child with a mild defect, management may involve dietary modification, stool softeners, and isotonic irrigations until the child is toilet trained. Most infants with Hirschsprung's require surgical intervention.

Surgical

Surgical intervention involves removal of the aganglionic bowel and creation of a temporary colostomy. Resection and colostomy closure are performed after the child reaches 10 kilograms.

Nursing Management

Assess the newborn for passage of stool during the first 24 to 48 hours and observe for signs of constipation and for malformed stools throughout infancy. Assess all infants with Hirschsprung's for weight gain, nutritional intake, and bowel habits. Teach parents both to ensure regular bowel habits with daily saline irrigations and a balanced diet and to observe for signs of fluid and electrolyte imbalances, such as dry mucous membranes and increased thirst.

Postoperative care may include reduction of anxiety and preparation for home care of the colostomy.

GASTROESOPHAGEAL REFLUX

Gastroesophageal reflux (GER) is the return of stomach contents into the esophagus caused by an immature sphincter. Manifestations such as hunger, irritability, FTT, vomiting, and frequent upper respiratory infections usually occur during the first 6 weeks of life.

Most infants have mild reflux and generally improve without surgical intervention by 1 year of age. Severe cases of GER that do not respond to therapy can result in esophageal strictures, respiratory distress, and FTT.

Medical–Surgical Management
Medical

Gastroesophageal reflux often resolves with dietary modifications, medication, and positioning. Small, frequent feedings and frequent burping are measures for minimizing reflux. Thickening formula with cereal (1 to 3 teaspoons of cereal for each ounce of formula) may be recommended if FTT persists.

Placing the infant prone and with the head elevated 30 degrees (Figure 56-11) is generally thought to be the most effective positioning for reducing the frequency of reflux (Orenstein, Izadnia & Khan, 1999). Positioning in an infant seat may cause increased intra-abdominal pressure and is not recommended.

Surgical

Severe cases of GER that do not respond to medical interventions may be treated with a surgical procedure called fundoplication, which involves loosely wrapping the gastric fundus around the lower esophagus.

Figure 56-11 *Thirty-degree Elevated Prone Position to Counter Gastroesophageal Reflux*

Pharmacological

Medications such as cimetidine (Tagamet), ranitidine (Zantac), or famotidine (Pepcid) may be effective in reducing gastric acid content.

Nursing Management

Recognize signs and symptoms of GER and educate parents regarding home care, including feeding, positioning, and medications. Pre- and postoperative care will be needed if the defect is surgically repaired.

INTUSSUSCEPTION

Intussusception is a disorder characterized by the telescoping of one portion of the bowel (usually the ileum) into a distal portion (usually the ascending colon). A previously healthy infant who develops intussusception will suddenly become pale, cry out sharply, and draw up the legs in a severe colicky spasm of pain. Such episodes last for several minutes and recur within 20 minutes. Vomiting and passage of "currant-jelly stools" (containing bloody mucus) also occur; however, these symptoms are present in fewer than 50% of infants with this condition (Kuppermann, O'Dea, Pincherry & Hoecker, 2000). Symptoms of shock, such as increased heart rate and changes in level of consciousness, appear quickly. If the intussusception is detected and reduced within 24 hours, morbidity is minimal; however, 5% to 10% of infants with intussusception die of complications such as perforation, peritonitis, and sepsis (Kliegman, Jensen & Behrman, 2000).

Medical–Surgical Management

Medical

Initial treatment involves hydrostatic reduction with barium or air enema at the time of diagnosis, with a success rate of 70% to 85% (Kleigman et al., 2000).

Surgical

If hydrostatic reduction fails or bowel damage is visualized during x-ray, surgical repair is done immediately. Surgery may consist of manual reduction of the telescoping, resection and anastomosis, or, possibly, colostomy, if the intestine is gangrenous.

Nursing Management

Recognize early the signs and symptoms of intussusception (i.e., abrupt onset of colicky pain and vomiting with currant-jelly stools). Help parents visualize telescoping by pressing the finger of an inflated rubber glove into the glove; pressing on the glove will then demonstrate hydrostatic reduction as the finger is pushed back to its normal position.

SAMPLE NURSING CARE PLAN

THE INFANT CLIENT WITH ABDOMINAL SURGERY

Eight-month-old Nathan was brought to the emergency room by his mother and father, who stated that he was perfectly fine until approximately 4 hours ago when he refused to eat lunch or take his bottle. He wanted to be held and became increasingly irritable. He began alternating between inconsolable crying and being quiet and limp. Physical examination revealed a palpable abdominal mass and passage of currant-jelly stool. Barium enema confirmed the diagnosis of intussusception, but attempts to reduce the blockage were unsuccessful. Nathan was admitted and prepared for surgery. Nathan weighs 8.8 kg and is maintaining a normal growth curve at the 50th percentile. He has attained all appropriate developmental milestones. This is Nathan's first illness and hospitalization. His mother begins to cry when she learns of the impending surgery and says, "What did I do wrong?" When the surgery is over, the doctor reports that Nathan has a temporary colostomy that will be closed in a few months. Nathan returns from surgery with an NGT and a urinary catheter in place and with dextrose 5% with normal saline being administered by IV at 40 cc per hour.

Nursing Diagnosis 1 *Risk for Injury* related to physical risk factors as evidenced by surgical procedure, loss of fluids, altered nutrition, and chemical risk factor of anesthesia

continues

SAMPLE NURSING CARE PLAN

Nursing Outcomes Classification (NOC)
Risk Control

Nursing Interventions Classification (NIC)
Surgical Precautions
Post-Anesthesia Care

PLANNING/GOALS	NURSING INTERVENTIONS	RATIONALE
Nathan will be free of injury, infection, and complications.	Assess vital signs, skin, hydration, and respiratory status every 4 hours.	Facilitates early detection of signs of complications.
	Administer antibiotics as prescribed.	Prevents infection.
Nathan will demonstrate required fluid I&O.	Provide mouth care at least every 4 hours.	Mucous membranes become dry when clients are NPO.
	Maintain NPO and monitor IV as prescribed, and record I&O.	An empty stomach prevents aspiration, and fluids maintain hydration.
	Assess bowel sounds every 2 hours.	Active bowel sounds indicate ability to tolerate food.
Nathan will maintain growth curve at 50th percentile.	When diet is ordered, offer small sips of water and advance as tolerated.	Small, frequent feedings decrease vomiting.

EVALUATION Surgical site is infection free and shows signs of healing. Mucous membranes are moist. Fluid requirements are maintained. Client loses less than 5% of admission weight.

Nursing Diagnosis 2 *Acute Pain* related to physical injury as evidenced by surgical procedure

Nursing Outcomes Classification (NOC)
Pain Level

Nursing Interventions Classification (NIC)
Post-Anesthesia Care
Pain Management

PLANNING/GOALS	NURSING INTERVENTIONS	RATIONALE
Nathan will be pain free.	Administer pain medications every 3 to 4 hours as prescribed and around-the-clock.	If child is able to sleep and rest, recovery is faster.
	Position for comfort; allow caregivers to hold and comfort.	
	Lubricate nostrils, if NGT present.	
	Perform procedures such as dressing changes and respiratory therapy after analgesia.	

EVALUATION Child sleeps quietly and shows no signs of restlessness.

Nursing Diagnosis 3 *Anxiety (parental)* related to hospitalization, colostomy, and home care as evidenced by parental reaction and questioning

Nursing Outcomes Classification (NOC)
Coping
Acceptance: Health Status

Nursing Interventions Classification (NIC)
Coping Enhancement
Anticipatory Guidance

continues

SAMPLE NURSING CARE PLAN

PLANNING/GOALS	NURSING INTERVENTIONS	RATIONALE
Nathan's parents will understand etiology, pathology, and treatment of illness.	Encourage expression of feelings.	Maintain positive family interaction during hospitalization.
	Explain procedures, keep informed of progress, and answer questions.	Facilitates development of rapport with the family.
Nathan's parents will provide comfort to their child.	Encourage parental presence and give positive reinforcement to client and family for cooperation and participation in care.	Active participation facilitates coping and decreases anxiety.
Nathan's parents will demonstrate proper techniques for home care procedures.	Teach parents to provide colostomy care, dressing changes, fluids, nutrition, and growth-fostering activities.	Provides parents with skills required to care for Nathan at home.
	Refer to appropriate community resources.	Decreases parents' anxiety and ensures proper care is provided.

EVALUATION Family care providers demonstrate skill and knowledge in caring for their child's needs. Parents verbalize decreased anxiety and return demonstrations of colostomy care and dressing changes.

MUSCULOSKELETAL SYSTEM

The musculoskeletal system provides protection to vital organs, supports weight, stores minerals, and supplies RBCs. Disorders may be congenital or acquired and require short- or long-term care. Most alterations of the arms and legs are mild variations of normal posturing, but some are severe anomalies. The two most common congenital skeletal defects are clubfoot and dislocated hip.

Figure 56-12 *Club Foot*

CONGENITAL TALIPES EQUINOVARUS (CLUB FOOT)

The equinovarus foot has a clublike appearance with the entire foot inverted, the heel drawn up, and the forefoot adducted (Figure 56-12). It can occur as a single anomaly or in connection with other defects such as **myelomeningocele** (a saclike protrusion situated along the vertebral column and filled with spinal fluid, meninges, nerve roots, and spinal cord). Club foot is apparent at birth and may be bilateral or unilateral. The degree of malformation and likelihood for complete correction varies. Even with correction, recurrence is common.

Medical–Surgical Management

Medical

Correction is usually started during the neonatal period with manipulation and casting of the foot. The long leg cast is changed every few days for the first few weeks and then every week or two for several months. Correction is confirmed by x-ray. Following casting, a splint with shoes attached is used for several months to maintain correction.

Surgical

Children who do not respond to nonsurgical treatment within 3 to 6 months need surgical correction. Following surgery, a cast is applied with the knee in a flexed position. After 6 to 12 weeks, casting is discontinued, and corrective shoes or bracing may be prescribed. Even with aggressive therapy, the foot is seldom entirely normal, and atrophy of the calf is common.

Nursing Management

Assess and explore the parents' feelings about their less-than-perfect newborn, the family's knowledge about the defect, treatment, and need for long-term care.

CLIENT TEACHING

Cast Care

Instruct parents in the following regarding cast care:

- Casts must be changed as prescribed to maintain growth and comfort.
- Wet casts should be handled with the palms (to prevent indentations).
- Hair dryers should not be used to facilitate drying of the cast.
- Plaster of paris casts should dry within 10 to 72 hours, depending on the size.
- Dry casts should be felt for "hot spots" and observed for visible stains due to drainage, which may indicate skin breakdown.
- Signs of swelling should be noted and reported immediately.
- Toes should be warm, pink, and moving.

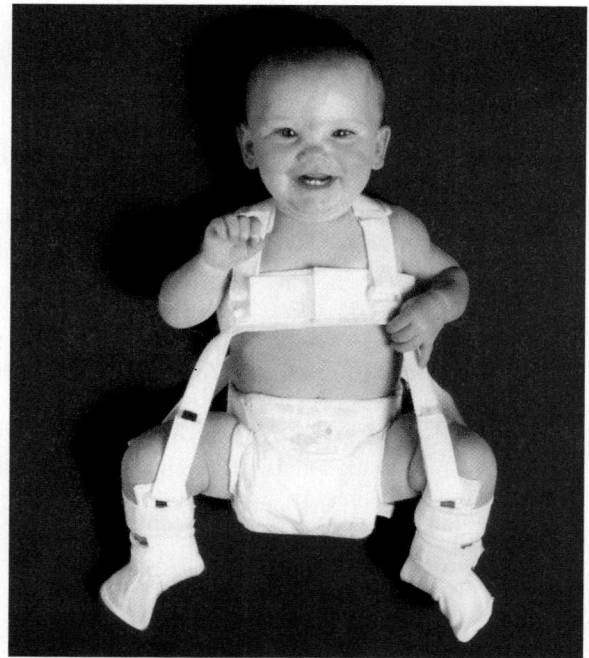

Figure 56-13 *A Pavlik harness is used to treat an infant with developmental dysplasia of the hip. (Courtesy Wheaton Brace Co., Carol Stream, IL)*

Nursing responsibilities include teaching the parents cast care, monitoring for complications, encouraging compliance with long-term follow-up, and facilitating normal development.

DEVELOPMENTAL DYSPLASIA OF THE HIP

Developmental **dysplasia** (abnormal development) of the hip (DDH) refers to a variety of conditions wherein the femoral head and the acetabulum are improperly aligned. These conditions include **dislocation** (displacement of the bone from its normal position in a joint), subluxation (partial dislocation), and acetabular dysplasia. These conditions can be congenital, but in some children, they develop after birth.

Manifestations include limited **abduction** (lateral movement away from body) of the affected hip, asymmetry of the gluteal and thigh fat folds, and telescoping or pistoning of the thigh. The walking infant may manifest minimal to pronounced variations in gait, with lurching toward the affected side. The longer the disorder goes untreated, the more pronounced the clinical manifestations become and the worse the prognosis.

Medical–Surgical Management

Early screening, detection, and treatment enable most affected children to attain normal hip function.

Medical

For young infants, the Pavlik harness is used to maintain flexion, abduction, and external rotation (Figure 56-13). This harness is highly effective when used as prescribed. A hip spica cast may be necessary when the

harness is ineffective. Older infants may require traction for weeks, either at home or in the hospital.

Surgical

The older infant may require closed reduction under anesthesia and/or open reduction followed by a hip spica cast.

Nursing Management

Teach parents how to use the Pavlik harness. If cast is necessary, teach parents cast care.

NURSING PROCESS

Assessment

Subjective Data

The nurse is alerted to the possibility of DDH when the infant has a history of being delivered by cesarean section or frank breech, is large for gestational age, or is a twin.

Objective Data

During the newborn assessment and routine nurturing activities, inspect the infant for limited abduction of the hip, a wide perineum, and unequal gluteal folds (Figure 56-14). The walking infant is assessed for a limp or an unusual gait.

Figure 56-14 *Assessing for DDH.* **A,** *Thighs and gluteal folds will show asymmetry.* **B,** *Flexion will show limited hip abduction.* **C,** *Knee height will show uneven level caused by shortened femur.*

Nursing diagnoses for the infant with DDH may include the following:

Nursing Diagnoses	Planning/Goals	Nursing Interventions
Anxiety (parental) related to having a less-than-perfect child and to the need to provide complex long-term care	The parents will verbalize feelings about their child and the condition. The parents will carry out prescribed therapy and provide daily care with confidence.	Explore the parents' feelings about their less-than-perfect newborn and their knowledge about the defect, treatment, and need for long-term care. Teach the parents about harness use (i.e., the hips should be flexed without being tight, the harness should be worn 23 hours per day). Explore options for the safe transport of the infant (i.e., use of a special car seat, adaptation of stroller).
Risk for Impaired Skin Integrity related to devices	The client's skin will remain intact.	Teach the parents to assess the infant's skin for irritation and to change the infant's position every 2 to 4 hours. Teach the parents ways of protecting the infant's skin from the brace (e.g., using a shirt that snaps at the crotch, long socks under the harness). Teach the parents to change diapers without removing the harness. Teach the parents to bathe the infant daily during the 1 hour that the harness is off.
Delayed Growth and Development related to immobility and difficulty in positioning	The client will attain milestones appropriate for age and limitations.	Teach the parents to provide activities that stimulate the infant's upper extremities and all five senses (e.g., blocks, musical toys, balls, bright mobiles) and to interact with the infant. Teach the parents methods of holding, nursing, feeding, and cuddling the infant when the harness is in use. Instruct the parents to include the infant in family activities and outings.

Evaluation Each goal must be evaluated to determine how it has been met by the client.

POSITIONAL PLAGIOCEPHALY

Positional plagiocephaly, also called flattened head syndrome, is a condition in which one side or the back of an infant's head is flattened. This can be caused when the infant is put to sleep in the same position repeatedly or by neck muscle problems. Queenan (2001) reports that the number of positional plagiocephaly cases increased six-fold from 1992 to 1994. These were the first two years following the American Academy of Pediatrics' (AAP) "Back to Sleep" promotion for infants to sleep on their backs to prevent sudden infant death syndrome (SIDS). SIDS has decreased, but positional plagiocephaly, which has an excellent corrective prognosis when treated early, has dramatically increased.

This head deformation is not self-correcting. Sometimes, after the infant's hair has grown, mild asymmetrical features may appear normal.

Medical–Surgical Management

Early identification and treatment allows time for re-shaping of the head before sutures and fontanels close.

Medical

When this positional deformity is detected, infants are generally placed in a light-weight plastic helmet or band, which redirects symmetrical growth of the infant's head (Figure 56-15).

Nursing Management

Prevention is the key through parental teaching. Parents should be taught to alternate the infant's head position during sleep (one sleep period with the right side of the head touching the mattress and the next sleep period the left). The infant is supine to sleep. Infants should not be left in an infant carrier, car seat, or swing for extended periods. Providing as much "tummy time" as possible when the infant is awake and supervised gives the back of the infant's head a rest and reduces the risk of developing positional plagiocephaly. This tummy position also strengthens neck muscles and arms and encourages learning and discovery of the world around.

INTEGUMENTARY SYSTEM

Normally, infants have soft, smooth, dry, cool, taut, elastic skin. Color is evenly distributed but may display variations such as freckles, **mongolian spots** (large patches of bluish skin on the buttocks of dark-skinned infants), small hemangiomas called "stork bites" (on eyelids or back of the neck), and **milia** (pearly white cysts on the face). Most of these blemishes disappear within months and require no treatment.

The infant's skin is immature and, thus, susceptible to disorders. The most frequently seen skin disorders include milia rubra, diaper dermatitis, seborrheic dermatitis, and atopic dermatitis.

MILIA RUBRA

Milia rubra, also known as prickly heat, is most noticeable on the folds of the skin, chest, and neck. This rash appears as pinhead-sized **erythematous** (reddishness of the skin) papules. It commonly occurs when infants are febrile or overdressed in summer heat. Infants may be irritable because of itching.

Nursing Management

Treatment is primarily preventive. Teach caregivers to avoid bundling infants in hot weather. Tepid baths may help alleviate itching.

DIAPER DERMATITIS

Diaper dermatitis, also called diaper rash, is characterized by erythema (redness), edema, vesicles, papules, and scaling on the perineum, genitals, buttocks, and skin folds. It is caused by repetitive exposure to an irritant such as urine, feces, soap, detergent, ointment, friction, or infection resulting from bacteria or yeast *(Candida albicans)* (Figure 56-16). The incidence is generally reported

Figure 56-15 *Child in DOC (Dynamic Orthotic Cranioplasty) Band for positional plagiocephaly. (Courtesy of Cranial Technologies, Inc.)*

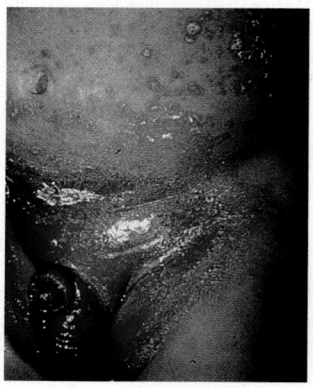

Figure 56-16 *Candidiasis (Courtesy of the Centers for Disease Control and Prevention [CDC])*

to be greater among bottle-fed than among breastfed infants (Wong et al., 1999).

Nursing Management

In order to prevent diaper rash, teach care providers to change diapers frequently and keep the infant's skin clean and dry. Use of disposable diapers and exposure of healthy skin to air, not heat, will help keep the skin dry. Ointments such as zinc oxide or petrolatum may be used to protect inflamed skin. Nystatin (Mycostatin) ointment or cream may be applied to treat *Candida*.

SEBORRHEIC DERMATITIS

Seborrheic dermatitis, also called cradle cap, is characterized by yellowish, scaly, or crusted patches on the scalp of infants up to 3 months of age (Figure 56-17). It typically results from excessive sebaceous gland activity.

Nursing Management

Teach caregivers that cradle cap is not caused by poor hygiene but, rather, by increased sebum production by the scalp. It will eventually disappear, although children with dry skin may continue to have flakes on the scalp. A mild shampoo or mineral oil may be left on the scalp for

Figure 56-17 *Seborrheic Dermatitis (Courtesy of the Centers for Disease Control and Prevention [CDC])*

a few minutes to help soften and loosen the crust. Then rinse and comb the hair with a fine-toothed comb to loosen and remove the crust. In most cases, no further treatment is needed. The crusting can usually be prevented by washing the infant's head with a washcloth and using a fine-toothed comb.

ATOPIC DERMATITIS

Atopic dermatitis, also called eczema, is a chronic, superficial inflammatory skin disorder characterized by intense **pruritus** (severe itching). It is considered to be at least in part an allergic reaction to irritants (wool, nylon, plastics, detergents, perspiration, cosmetics, and perfumed lotions and soaps) and allergens (dust, pollens, and foods). A strong family history of eczema, asthma, food allergies, or allergic rhinitis usually predisposes a child to eczema. The disorder is uncommon among breastfed infants before other foods are added to the diet.

Papules and vesicles usually begin forming on the cheeks and spread to the arms and legs and then to the trunk. Exudate and crust are often present.

Infantile eczema usually resolves by the age of 3 years; however, infants who have eczema tend to develop hay fever or asthma later in life.

Medical–Surgical Management
Medical

Treatment is aimed at relieving pruritus, hydrating skin, reducing inflammation, and preventing secondary infections. Baths and compresses may provide temporary relief.

Pharmacological

A variety of lotions, oral antihistamines, topical corticosteroids, and antibiotics may be prescribed.

Diet

A diet including a milk substitute such as soy formula, a vitamin supplement, and foods known to be hypoallergenic may be instituted to rule out offending foods. If the child's skin improves, foods are added back into the diet one at a time at intervals of approximately 1 week. The effects are then noted and any allergenic foods eliminated from the child's diet.

Health Promotion

Guidelines for preventing eczema include practicing breastfeeding; prohibiting cow's milk, eggs, fish, corn, citrus, peanuts, nuts, and chocolate for the first 12 months of life; and delaying introduction of solid foods until 6 months of age. Environmental control of dust, mold, animals, and cigarette smoke is also recommended.

Nursing Management

The major nursing goals are to soothe and relieve pruritus, maintain skin integrity, provide adequate nutrition and fluids, offer sensory stimulation, and teach the family about the condition. Parents may feel apprehensive or repulsed by their infant's appearance. They need to be encouraged to express their feelings but be assured that eczema, while potentially distressing, is a temporary condition.

NEUROLOGICAL SYSTEM

By the fourth week of gestation, the neural tube has closed, and the brain and the spinal cord have begun to form. By the second month of gestation, the brain is the most prominent part of the body. It grows rapidly and continues to grow through the fifth year of life. As myelinization of the peripheral nerves progresses, so do the child's coordination and fine motor abilities. The primitive reflexes (Moro, grasp, and rooting) disappear by 12 months of age. Alterations discussed following are spina bifida, hydrocephalus, febrile convulsions, **meningitis** (inflammation of the meninges), and cerebral palsy.

SPINA BIFIDA

Spina bifida is a neural tube defect wherein incomplete closure of the vertebrae and neural tube results in an opening through which meninges and spinal cord may protrude. Although the cause remains undetermined, genetic predisposition, maternal folic acid deficiency during pregnancy, and environmental factors such as pollution may be implicated. The severity of the defect can vary, with manifestations ranging from a dimple or small tuft of hair (which may be overlooked at birth) to a large, saclike protrusion anywhere along the

Figure 56-18 A, *Illustration of Myelomeningocele;* **B,** *Myelomeningocele*

lumbar or sacral area (Figure 56-18). The most severe form is myelomeningocele. The degree of neurological impairment depends on the location of the defect on the spinal cord and the size of the defect. The child may be asymptomatic or display neurological impairments varying from mild sensory loss to complete paralysis below the lesion. Associated defects may include hydrocephalus (present in 90% of clients) and genitourinary and orthopedic defects. Although these children often require lifelong therapy and care, many ultimately go on to live independently and become productive adults.

Medical–Surgical Management

Medical

Specialists such as neurologists, neurosurgeons, orthopedic specialists, pediatricians, urologists, and physical therapists may be needed to provide surgical repair and follow-up treatment.

Surgical

Surgery is required to close the defect but may not be performed immediately after birth. Waiting several days gives the family time to adjust to the initial shock and become involved in the decision-making process. Immediate closure reduces the risk of infection and allows for easier handling of the infant, which, in turn, facilitates earlier bonding.

Nursing Management

Preoperatively, monitor vital signs, neurological status, and behavior. Maintain infant in a prone position. Keep sac covered with moist, warm, sterile dressings and change every 2 hours. Administer medications as ordered.

Postoperatively, monitor vital signs, I&O, and provide prescribed wound care. Teach parents intermittent catheterization to keep infant's bladder empty until incision heals. Teach parents how to elicit sucking and to feed and cuddle infant, signs of increased intracranial pressure, and signs of constipation. Refer to Spina Bifida Association.

NURSING PROCESS

Assessment

Subjective Data

Assess the parents' feelings about their less-than-perfect newborn and their knowledge about the defect, the treatment, and the need for long-term care.

Objective Data

At birth, assess the intactness of the membranous sac. Assess neurological impairment by noting movement of the extremities; reflexes; anal reflex; urinary output; vital signs; fontanelles; and head circumference.

Nursing diagnoses for the infant with spina bifida may include the following:

Nursing Diagnoses	Planning/Goals	Nursing Interventions
Anxiety *(parental)*, related to having a less-than-perfect child and to the need to provide complex long-term care	The parents will verbalize their feelings about the child and condition.	Explore the parents' feelings about their less-than-perfect newborn and their knowledge about the defect, the treatment, and the need for long-term care.
		Teach the parents ways to elicit sucking and to feed and cuddle the infant.
	The parents will carry out prescribed therapy and provide daily care with confidence.	Teach the parents to assess for signs of constipation, such as abdominal distention, vomiting, and poor feeding.
		Teach the parents to recognize signs of increased intracranial pressure, such as irritability, restlessness, and vomiting.
		Explore options for mobility, such as splints, a walker, or a wheelchair.
		Refer the family to the Spina Bifida Association and to local resources and support groups.
*Risk for **I**nfection*, related to vulnerability of the sac, the surgical procedure, and the lack of bowel and bladder control	The client will be infection free.	***Preoperative:***
		Monitor the infant's vital signs, neurological status, and behavior.
		Administer prophylactic antibiotics, as ordered.
		Keep the sac covered with a moist, warm, sterile dressing and change every 2 hours.
		Maintain the infant in the prone position.
		Protect the sac from fecal contamination.
		Postoperative:
		Provide prescribed wound care.
		Instruct the parents in the use of intermittent, clean catheterization to keep bladder empty.
*Delayed **G**rowth and Development*, related to immobility	The client will attain milestones appropriate for age and limitations.	Teach the parents to provide activities that stimulate the infant's upper extremities and all five senses and to interact with the infant.
		Instruct the parents to include the infant in family activities and outings.
		Explore options for education and vocational training as the child grows older.

Evaluation Each goal must be evaluated to determine how it has been met by the client.

HYDROCEPHALUS

In hydrocephalus, the balance between the rate of cerebrospinal fluid (CSF) formation and absorption is disturbed. This disturbance may result from an obstruction in the circulation of CSF or from defective absorption. Hydrocephalus may be recognized at birth or weeks or months later. The condition may be congenital or occur as the result of a neoplasm, a head injury, or an infection.

Manifestations include an excessively large head at birth or rapid head growth along with widening cranial sutures. As pressure increases, the anterior fontanel becomes tense and bulges, and the eyes appear to be pushed downward, with the sclera visible above the iris ("sunset eyes"). Because of the increase in intracranial pressure, the infant may display irritability, restlessness, a high-pitched cry, vomiting, seizure, and change in level of consciousness.

Medical–Surgical Management

Surgical

Surgical intervention is the only effective means of relieving brain pressure and preventing further damage to the brain tissue. Surgery involves removing the obstruction or inserting a shunting device that bypasses the point of obstruction and drains the excess CSF into a body cavity, usually the peritoneum.

Nursing Management

Monitor vital signs, head circumference, and neurological signs. Prevent infections, provide loving care to the child and support to the family, and increase the family's knowledge about the condition. Set realistic growth and development goals. Many infants with hydrocephalus are able to ultimately live independently and become productive adults despite associated neurological disabilities.

FEBRILE CONVULSIONS

A convulsion or seizure involves involuntary muscle contraction and relaxation. Seizures may be a symptom of a wide variety of disorders. In infants and children, febrile seizures usually accompany such infections as otitis media, upper respiratory infections, and meningitis. Clinical manifestations include sudden occurrence, body stiffening, and loss of consciousness followed by quick, jerking movements of the arms, legs, and facial muscles. Breathing may be irregular, and swallowing ability may be absent.

Febrile seizures usually occur early in the course of a high fever. Usually, only one seizure occurs, and it will last less than 3 minutes. Febrile seizures carry little risk of neurological damage.

Medical–Surgical Management

Pharmacological

Most febrile seizures stop before the infant can be taken for medical attention. If the seizure continues, diazepam (Valium) is the drug of choice. Antipyretics such as acetaminophen (Tylenol) or ibuprophen (Motrin) may be used to reduce the infant's fever.

Nursing Management

Focus on teaching parents about febrile seizures and treating a fever. Parents are naturally extremely anxious when their child has experienced a seizure, especially the first time. Reassure the parents that febrile seizures are not life threatening, do not cause neurological damage, are common in children younger than 5 years of age who are experiencing infection, usually do not recur, and usually last less than 3 minutes.

MENINGITIS

The most common infection of the central nervous system (CNS) in infants is meningitis. The three main types of causative organisms are bacterial, tubercular, and viral. Meningitis may also occur as the result of complications of neurosurgery, trauma, systemic infection, or sinus or ear infection. Bacterial meningitis is the most common and serves as the focus of this discussion.

Clinical manifestations may occur suddenly or gradually and include neurological symptoms such as a high-pitched cry, fever, seizures, irritability, as well as vomiting, a bulging anterior fontanel, and poor feeding. Early diagnosis and treatment are essential for uncomplicated recovery.

Medical–Surgical Management

Medical

Meningitis is a medical emergency. A spinal tap (lumbar puncture) is performed promptly whenever symptoms are present and before administration of antibiotics. The causative organism usually can be ascertained from stained smears of the spinal fluid. Appropriate IV antibiotics are prescribed for bacterial meningitis. The infant is isolated from other clients for at least 24 hours.

Health Promotion

Current immunization schedules include the *Haemophilus influenzae* type b conjugate vaccine (HbCV). The incidence of *H. influenza* type B (Hib) has greatly decreased since the advent of this immunization.

CLIENT TEACHING

Tips for Treating a Fever

Teach parents to care for their febrile infant by:

- Administering acetaminophen or ibuprophen, but *never* aspirin
- Providing more clothing if the child is too cold and less clothing if the child is too warm, to prevent shivering
- Applying cool, moist compresses to the forehead 1 hour after administering an antipyretic
- Encouraging fluid intake (e.g., water, juice, ice, popsicles)

Nursing Management

After assisting with the spinal tap and starting the IV, complete the history and physical. It is important to note any food and fluid intake, nausea, vomiting, or loss of appetite, as well as recent immunizations, illnesses, surgery, and injuries and previous lumbar puncture.

Perform a complete neurological assessment and an evaluation of head circumference. Examine the fontanelles for bulging.

Maintain in isolation for at least 24 hours, administer antibiotics, monitor neurological status every 4 hours, maintain fluid balance, establish trust with the parents and infant, teach the parents about the disease and ways to care for their infant, and refer close contacts for possible prophylactic treatment.

CEREBRAL PALSY

Cerebral palsy (CP) is a nonprogressive motor disorder resulting from damage to the motor centers of the brain. This damage can occur during the prenatal, perinatal, or postnatal period.

Manifestations of CP vary in severity and may include delayed gross motor development (e.g., persistent head lag), alterations in muscle tone (e.g., body stiffness), abnormal motor performance (e.g., uncoordinated or involuntary movements), and reflex abnormalities (e.g., persistent tonic neck). In addition, the child may experience seizures, impaired vision and hearing, difficulty swallowing and speaking, and subnormal learning and reasoning. Less-severe cases of CP may not be diagnosed until 2 years of age.

Medical–Surgical Management

Medical

A multidisciplinary team including the family, pediatricians, neurologists, surgeons, nurses, nutritionists, therapists, social workers, and special education teachers is necessary to assist the child in developing maximum potential.

Surgical

Surgical intervention such as lengthening the Achilles' tendon and releasing the hamstrings may be necessary to improve ambulation.

Nursing Management

Encourage parents to stimulate and interact with their infant and participate in an infant-stimulation program. Refer to nutritionist, occupational therapist, and speech therapist as needed.

NURSING PROCESS

Assessment

Subjective Data

A history of conditions such as maternal diabetes, ABO or Rh incompatibilities, rubella in the first trimester, prematurity, prolonged labor, and postnatal infections or trauma may predispose an infant to brain damage and CP.

Objective Data

Further observe the infant who feeds poorly and is rigid, tense, or hypotonic. Assess for developmental delays with an instrument such as the Denver II test.

Nursing diagnoses for the infant with CP may include the following:

Nursing Diagnoses	Planning/Goals	Nursing Interventions
*Imbalanced **N**utrition: Less than Body Requirements,* related to difficulty chewing and swallowing and to increased muscle activity	The client will maintain a normal growth curve above the fifth percentile on the growth chart.	Encourage active swallowing by maintenance of a flexed sitting position, with the arms brought forward. Provide jaw stabilization from the front or side of the face. Provide a flexible feeding schedule with frequent, small feedings. Encourage use of adaptive utensils and foods to stimulate self-care (e.g., finger foods, foods that stick to utensils, spoon with padded handle). Refer to a nutritionist and an occupational therapist, as needed.
*Delayed **G**rowth and Development* related to neuromuscular impairment	The client will achieve maximum potential.	Teach the parents to stimulate the infant and to interact on the infant's functional level. Encourage early intervention and participation in infant-stimulation programs.
*Impaired Physical **M**obility* related to spasticity and muscle weakness	The client will attain mobility via assistive devices.	Refer to a physical therapist, as needed. Evaluate the need for special equipment. Ensure adequate rest. Perform prescribed range-of-motion and stretching exercises.

Nursing Diagnoses	Planning/Goals	Nursing Interventions
		Provide preoperative and postoperative care for the infant who requires corrective surgery.
		Select toys and activities that improve motor activity (e.g., place a desired toy such that the child must reach).
Impaired Verbal Communication, related to neuromuscular impairment and difficulty with articulation	The client will develop methods of communication	Refer to a speech therapist, as needed.
		Encourage the use of flash cards, articles, pictures, talking boards, a computer with a voice synthesizer.
		Encourage jaw-stabilization methods (as with feeding) to facilitate speech.

Evaluation Each goal must be evaluated to determine how it has been met by the client.

GENITOURINARY SYSTEM

During infancy, the kidneys are less able to concentrate urine, and output per kilogram of body weight is higher than that of an adult. Bladder capacity increases with age, from 20 to 50 mL at birth to 700 mL in adulthood, and the infant's urethra is shorter than the adult's. In addition, infants lack bladder control because of insufficient nerve development.

Most external defects of the genitourinary (GU) tract are not life threatening in the physical sense but may present social problems with lifelong implications for the child and family. More severe disorders such as exstrophy of the bladder and ambiguous genitalia lead to concerns about penis size, appearance of the genitalia, altered elimination, potential ability to procreate, and rejection by peers. These children and their families need emotional support in order to adjust to these permanent alterations. Hypospadias, hydrocele, cryptorchidism, vesicoureteral reflux, and Wilms' tumor are the most common types of urinary alterations.

HYPOSPADIAS

Hypospadias is a condition wherein the urethral opening is on the ventral (under) surface of the penis (Figure 56-19). It is often associated with undescended testes and inguinal hernia and is visible on inspection at birth.

Medical–Surgical Management

Surgical

Hypospadias is surgically corrected during the first year of life. The infant is not circumcised at birth because the foreskin may be used to correct the defect.

Nursing Management

Focus on preparing parents for the surgical procedure and for postoperative and home care. Assure parents that normal urination will be restored and that sexual function will not be impeded. Tell them that the penis

Figure 56-19 *Hypospadias (Courtesy of Dr. James Mandell, Chief Surgeon, Urology, Albany Medical College, Albany, NY)*

may never appear perfectly normal, even after the surgery. The infant may go home with a catheter in place until healing is complete. Have parents demonstrate catheter care before discharge.

HYDROCELE

Hydrocele is the result of the processus vaginalis failing to close, which allows fluid to enter the scrotum. The scrotum contains a palpable, round, nontender mass. This defect is often associated with inguinal hernia.

Medical–Surgical Management

Medical

Most hydroceles will close by 1 year of age without intervention.

COMMUNITY/HOME HEALTH CARE

Infant with External GU Defect Repair

Pain Management
- Medicate for pain as prescribed for 24 to 48 hours postoperatively.
- Protect the site by double diapering.

Infection Control
- Handwash before and after diapering.
- Carefully and thoroughly cleanse any area soiled with stool or urine.
- Watch for signs of infection, such as fever, irritability, drainage, and redness.
- Increase fluid intake.

Activity Restriction
- Do not allow the infant to play on riding toys.
- Do not allow the infant to straddle the caregiver's hip when being carried.

Surgical

If spontaneous closure does not occur by 1 year of age, surgical intervention may be done on an outpatient basis.

Nursing Management

Preoperative preparation and postoperative care are the focus of the nurse. Postoperatively, focus on pain management, infection control, and activity restriction. Alert parents to the potential for temporary swelling and discoloration of the scrotum.

CRYPTORCHIDISM

Cryptorchidism is a condition wherein one or both testes do not descend into the scrotal sac. One or both sides of the scrotum appear to be smaller than normal. When palpated, the scrotal sac is empty. This defect is often associated with inguinal hernia.

Medical–Surgical Management

Medical

The testes usually descend spontaneously by 1 year of age. If the testes have not descended after 1 year, hormone therapy may be prescribed.

Surgical

Surgical correction, if required, is performed by 3 years of age to prevent sterility.

Nursing Management

Preoperative preparation and postoperative care are the primary nursing concerns. Postoperative care focuses on pain management, infection control, and activity restriction.

VESICOURETERAL REFLUX

Vesicoureteral reflux refers to the backflow of urine from the bladder into the ureters and, possibly, the kidneys. Reflux can result from abnormal insertion of the ureters into the bladder or from a urinary tract infection (UTI). The primary manifestation of vesicoureteral reflux is recurrent UTIs. Specific clues of a UTI in the infant include poor feeding; vomiting; and failure to gain weight. A UTI is confirmed by detection of bacteria in the urine. Early diagnosis with radiological studies is important to prevent renal injury.

Medical–Surgical Management

Medical

The primary concern is preventing UTIs. Low-dose prophylactic antibiotic therapy is prescribed until the reflux is resolved. In addition, urine cultures, cystograms, and blood studies are necessary to monitor for UTI and kidney function. Less-severe refluxes will resolve spontaneously.

Surgical

Surgical reimplantation of the ureter(s) into the bladder may be necessary if UTIs persist.

Nursing Management

Nursing care includes treatment and prevention of UTIs (see the Urinary System chapter). Help parents understand that medical treatment may be needed for years and that compliance as well as follow-up is important. If surgery is required, provide pre- and postoperative care.

WILMS' TUMOR

Wilms' tumor (nephroblastoma) is found in the kidney region and is one of the most common early childhood cancers. The tumor arises from bits of embryonic tissue remaining after birth. The etiology is unknown, but Wilms' tumor is associated with other anomalies such as GU defects, microcephaly, and mental retardation. The most common manifestations are an abdominal mass located to one side of the midline, abdominal pain, malaise, anemia, and fever.

Medical–Surgical Management

Surgical

Surgical removal of the involved kidney and lymph node is the treatment of choice. Chemotherapy and radiation

PROFESSIONAL TIP

Wilms' Tumor
If a client has a Wilms' tumor, a sign stating, "Do not palpate the abdomen" should be posted at the head of the bed.

may be used pre- and postoperatively, depending on the stage and size of the tumor.

Nursing Management

If a mass is felt in a child's abdomen, stop palpation immediately because it is possible to dislodge cells and spread the tumor. Focus on pre- and postoperative care, chemotherapy administration, and family support.

COGNITIVE AND SENSORY SYSTEMS

Cognitive and sensory impairments result in a variety of lifelong challenges for infants and their families. Nursing care focuses on assessment of the degree of impairment and on appropriate interventions for individual and family adaptation. Some of the most common cognitive and sensory impairments occurring in infants include Down syndrome and visual and hearing impairments.

DOWN SYNDROME

Down syndrome is a chromosomal anomaly resulting in moderate to severe mental retardation. Evidence supports trisomy 21 (an extra chromosome); translocation of chromosomes 15, 21, and 22; and advanced parental age as possible causes of Down syndrome.

Manifestations include a variety of facial and body abnormalities and intellectual, language, and social alterations. Typically, the child with Down syndrome has upward- and outward-slanted (almond-shaped) eyes; a depressed nasal bridge; a protruding tongue; small, short, low-set ears; a short, broad neck; transverse palmar crease; broad, short hands with stubby fingers; a protruding abdomen; **hypotonia** (lax muscle tone); and a blunted affect (Figure 56-20). Numerous medical conditions may

Figure 56-20 *Young Girl with Down Syndrome. (From Down Right Beautiful 1996 calendar, Marijane Scott, Marijane's Designer Portraits.)*

CLIENT TEACHING

Feeding the Infant with Down Syndrome

- The tongue thrust represents a physiologic response rather than a refusal to eat.
- Use a long, straight-handled spoon to place food to the back and side of the mouth.
- Refeed food that is thrust out of the mouth.
- Increase fluids and fiber to prevent constipation.
- Monitor height and weight by plotting on a growth chart each month.

be associated with Down syndrome, including cardiac anomalies, GI defects, endocrine disorders, and leukemia.

Medical–Surgical Management

Medical

A multidisciplinary team of health care providers may be needed to assist the child with Down syndrome to reach personal maximum potential. During the first year, the focus is on monitoring for GI and cardiac disorders. Between the second and fourth years, medical emphasis is on sleep and behavioral difficulties, thyroid screening, and visual and dental assessment. Frequent infections are a common problem.

Surgical

Surgery may be required for correction of associated cardiac and GI anomalies.

Health Promotion

Prenatal diagnosis of Down syndrome is possible through genetic testing, alpha-fetoprotein (AFP) level, or amniotic fluid samples. As a result of increased prenatal diagnosis, approximately 40% of fetuses with Down syndrome in women older than 35 years of age are now electively terminated (James et al., 2002). Therefore, the number of children born with Down syndrome is decreasing.

Nursing Management

Assist parents to identify positive features and behaviors of infant. Emphasize that the infant needs play, discipline, and social interactions like every infant. Encourage the family to teach the child socially acceptable behaviors and to express their own fears and concerns.

NURSING PROCESS

Assessment

Subjective Data

At birth, it is especially important to elicit the family's health history, the results of amniocentesis (if done), and parental ages. As the infant grows, thoroughly evaluate interaction between the child and family, the family's coping abilities, and the degree to which the child is thriving.

Objective Data

During the initial physical examination at birth, assess for the unique features that indicate Down syndrome. As the child grows, assessment of developmental milestones will indicate delays in all areas (language, social, and motor).

Nursing diagnoses for the infant with Down syndrome may include the following:

Nursing Diagnoses	Planning/Goals	Nursing Interventions
Social Isolation, related to fear of and embarrassment about the child's behavior or appearance	The family will achieve optimal socialization.	Assist in identifying positive features and behaviors in the infant.
		Emphasize that the infant needs play, discipline, and social interaction, as does any infant.
		Encourage the family to teach the child socially acceptable behaviors (e.g., manners and appropriate touch).
		Encourage the family to express feelings and concerns.
		Refer the family to support groups.
Delayed Growth and Development related to poor sucking abilities and anomalies	The client will maintain a normal growth curve above the fifth percentile.	Explore options for ensuring optimal fluid and calorie intake (e.g., adaptive utensils).
		Encourage self-feeding, when age appropriate.
		Maintain routine.
		Refer to dietitian, as needed.

Evaluation Each goal must be evaluated to determine how it has been met by the client.

VISUAL IMPAIRMENT

The eye is not fully developed until approximately 10 to 12 years of age. Visual acuity normally increases from a range of 20/50 to 20/80 at birth to a range of 20/20 to 20/30 by age 5 years.

Visual impairments are classified as follows: sighted with eye problems, partially sighted (20/70 to 20/200), and legally blind (20/200 or less). Refractory errors are the most common type of childhood visual disorders.

Strabismus (crossed eye) is caused by lack of coordination of the extraocular muscles. When both eyes are unable to focus simultaneously, the brain suppresses the image from the deviating eye to prevent double vision (diplopia). Amblyopia (blindness from disuse) can develop if strabismus is not treated early. If untreated amblyopia occurs in a child younger than 4 years of age, permanent loss of vision in the deviated eye may result.

Manifestations of visual impairment may include failure to follow an object or to react to bright light, excessive rubbing of the eyes, squinting, tilting of the head, and crossed eyes (after 6 months of age). Visual impairments may be caused by perinatal and postnatal infections; conditions such as sickle-cell disease, juvenile rheumatoid arthritis, glaucoma, cataracts, and retinoblastoma; and injuries.

Medical–Surgical Management

Medical

Most visual disorders are treated with corrective lenses. Strabismus may require patching of the stronger eye to increase visual stimulation of the weaker eye. The earlier the treatment, the better the chances of normal development and function and adequate vision.

Surgical

Surgical intervention is required for glaucoma, cataracts, and, sometimes, strabismus.

Nursing Management

Early detection and referral are crucial in preventing childhood visual impairment. At birth, assess response to visual stimuli, ability to fixate and follow an object to midline, and ability to make eye contact. At 3 months of age, assess the infant for ability to follow moving objects. Crossed eyes after 6 months of age warrants further evaluation. Make referrals to available associations and support groups as needed (see the Resources listed at the end of this chapter).

Provide preoperative and postoperative care when surgical intervention is required. Educate the parents about the condition, the prescribed treatment, home care, and follow-up.

HEARING IMPAIRMENT

At birth, the ear is completely developed. Hearing impairments range from mild to profound and include deaf as well as hard of hearing. Hearing loss is divided into four categories. Conductive (middle-ear hearing loss) is the most common type of hearing impairment and results from interference of transmission of sound to the middle ear. It is usually caused by otitis media. Sensorineural hearing loss (nerve deafness) involves damage to the inner-ear structures and/or auditory nerves. Mixed hearing loss is a combination of conductive and sensorineural loss. It is usually caused by recurrent otitis media. Central hearing loss results from damage to the conduction system between the brainstem and the cerebral cortex.

Infants at risk for hearing loss include those with prenatal, perinatal, and postnatal conditions including a family history of hearing impairments; malformations; low birthweight; asphyxia; infection; CP; Down syndrome; or a history of being administered ototoxic drugs.

Manifestations of hearing impairment in the infant include failure to startle or awaken to a loud sound, to turn the head to sound by 4 months of age, and to babble by 3 months of age. As the child with a hearing impairment matures, language skills are affected, and the child may be perceived as having cognitive as well as behavioral problems.

Medical–Surgical Management

Medical

Treatment depends on the cause and type of loss. Antibiotics are prescribed for otitis media, which is the most common cause of conduction loss. Sensorineural loss is usually irreversible. Hearing aids or cochlear implants may be recommended.

Surgical

Insertion of tympanostomy tubes for chronic otitis media is controversial.

Nursing Management

Detection and prevention are the most important goals for the nurse. Assess all children for hearing acuity at birth, at well-child visits, and whenever there is a complaint specific to the ears. Developmental assessments reveal language delays in infants and children

CRITICAL THINKING

Altered Sensory Functioning
What can nurses do to decrease the incidence of alterations in sensory function among children?

with hearing impairments. When delays are noted, refer the child for further evaluation.

CHILD ABUSE

Child abuse is any intentional act of physical neglect or physical, emotional, or sexual abuse committed by a person responsible for the care of a child. Child abuse can be detected at any age, even in utero; however, adolescents experience the greatest incidence of abuse.

PHYSICAL NEGLECT

Physical neglect is failure to provide the adequate hygiene, health care, nutrition, love, nurturing, and supervision required for an infant's normal growth and development. Clinical manifestations of physical neglect in the infant may include inadequate weight gain, dental caries, poor hygiene, and lack of immunizations.

PHYSICAL ABUSE

Physical punishment that leaves marks, causes injury, or threatens the child's physical or emotional well-being is considered physical abuse. Typical clinical manifestations of physical abuse include bruises on the abdomen, buttocks, genitalia, thighs, and mouth; bruises with distinctive outlines indicative of such things as hangers, belt buckles, hands, teeth, and sticks; bone fractures at various stages of healing; spiral fractures; cerebral edema or hemorrhage; and burns (e.g., from immersion of feet in hot water or from cigarettes). The child may appear sad and forlorn or may actively seek to please.

Predisposing factors to physical abuse include characteristics of the parent, child, and environment. Parents who abuse their children may have been severely punished as children, have difficulty controlling aggressive impulses, be socially isolated, and have few supportive relationships. Children at greatest risk for abuse are those who are premature, illegitimate, unwanted, brain damaged, hyperactive, physically disabled, or "difficult" (James et al., 2002; Hockenberry et al., 2003). A stressful environment caused by divorce, poverty, unemployment, poor housing, frequent relocation, and drug addiction may contribute to physical abuse; however, abuse occurs at all educational, social, and economic levels.

A more unusual type of abuse is Munchausen syndrome, wherein one person either fabricates or induces illness in another to get attention. Usually, the mother has the syndrome and inflicts injury on her child.

EMOTIONAL ABUSE

Emotional abuse includes acts or omissions by the caregiver that could cause serious behavioral, cognitive, emotional, or mental disorders. Emotional abuse may involve shaming, ridiculing, embarrassing, or insulting the child and destruction of the child's personal property. Clinical manifestations in the emotionally abused child may include developmental delays, failure to thrive, disruptive behavior, extreme behavior (withdrawal, aggression), and unusual fearfulness, obsessions, and suicide attempts.

SEXUAL ABUSE

Sexual abuse is the exploitation of a child for the sexual gratification of an adult. Common forms of sexual abuse are oral–genital contact, fondling and caressing of the genitals, intercourse (vaginal or anal), rape, sodomy, and prostitution. Possible clinical manifestations in the infant include vaginal discharge; blood-stained diapers; genital redness, pain, itching, or bruising; lax rectal tone; difficulty sitting; and UTIs.

Medical–Surgical Management

Medical

Diagnosis of abuse is based on a careful history and thorough physical examination. Injuries are treated as needed. All health care providers are legally required to report any suspected child abuse to the local child protective agency.

Nursing Management

Monitor for inadequate weight gain; lack of immunizations; poor hygiene; bruises; bone fractures at different stages of healing; cerebral edema or hemorrhage; burns; developmental delays; failure to thrive; disruptive behavior; unusual fearfulness; vaginal discharge; blood-stained diaper; genital redness, pain, itching, or bruising; difficulty sitting; and UTIs. Assess child's history and physical examination, parent–infant interactions, child's response to surroundings and strangers, and developmental level.

Report all cases of suspected child abuse to the local child protective agency.

NURSING PROCESS

Assessment

Subjective Data

Obtain information about parental concerns; a general family history; and a specific child history. Begin with nonthreatening topics to demonstrate concern before asking about suspected abuse. Document verbatim details about the way the injuries occurred and use quotation marks.

Objective Data

Physical assessment and documentation must be thorough. Use figure diagrams to document skin injuries. Inconsistencies between what reportedly happened and the extent of injuries constitute a strong indicator of child abuse.

Nursing diagnoses for the abused child may include the following:

Nursing Diagnoses	Planning/Goals	Nursing Interventions
Risk for Injury related to family history of abuse/neglect	The client will be free from abuse/neglect.	Use a nonthreatening, nonjudgmental manner when interacting with the parents.
		Assess and document the child's history and physical examination results, family history, parent–child interactions, the child's response to surroundings and strangers, and the child's developmental level.
		Report all cases of suspected child abuse.
		Assist in removing the child from the unsafe environment.
		Refer the family to social services, as needed.
Impaired Parenting related to lack of knowledge	The family will respond to the child's needs appropriately.	Assess the family's strengths, weaknesses, coping mechanisms, and support systems.
		Assess the parents' expectations of the child; choice and use of comfort measures; responses to the child; and general knowledge about the child.
		Discuss the parenting that the parents received as children.
		Provide information regarding normal growth and development, nutrition, well-child care, and nurturing.

continues

Nursing Diagnoses	Planning/Goals	Nursing Interventions
		Role-model when interacting with the child.
		Encourage the parents to participate in the child's care.
		Reinforce positive behaviors on the part of the parents.
		Assist the family in identifying stressors and options for decreasing stress.
		Refer the parents to a support group such as Parents Anonymous.

Evaluation Each goal must be evaluated to determine how it has been met by the client.

ENVIRONMENTAL SAFETY

As infants develop and become mobile explorers, environmental safety becomes a major concern for all caregivers. An important role of the nurse is to educate caregivers regarding maintaining a safe environment and administering appropriate aid in the event of an accident. Common environmental safety hazards include poisoning, trauma, suffocation, and drowning.

POISONING

Poisonous substances can be found everywhere. Commonly ingested substances include cosmetics and other personal care products, medicines, cleaning products, plants, gasoline, toys, lead-based paint, and other miscellaneous foreign substances.

Medical–Surgical Management

Medical

The poison control center should be called initially and immediately to ascertain whether the child should be treated at home or taken to a treatment center. When the exact substance and amount are unknown, take the child to a treatment center, where complications can be anticipated and life support provided, if needed.

Vomiting is usually initiated immediately to the conscious child, unless the ingested substance is corrosive or highly irritating. Corrosives and irritants can cause further damage to mucous membranes of the esophagus and pharynx if vomited.

When emesis is contraindicated, gastric lavage is used to evacuate the stomach contents. In addition, activated charcoal may be administered to prevent further absorption of the poison.

Pharmacological

Activated charcoal may be administered orally or through an orogastric tube to absorb the poison and remove it from the body. Activated charcoal may be mixed with a cathartic such as magnesium sulfate (Epsom salts). An antiemetic is sometimes needed.

Magnesium sulfate may be prescribed to promote rapid elimination, thereby decreasing absorption of the

CLIENT TEACHING

Poison Prevention

Advise caregivers of the following poison prevention measures:

- Keep all medicines and household cleaners in original containers with childproof caps and out of reach of children.
- Do not treat medicine like candy *or* candy like medicine.
- Read labels carefully before using medicines and household cleaners.
- Attach the poison control center's phone number to the phone.
- Prevent children from chewing or ingesting plants.
- Be aware of those things at a child's eye level by crawling around the house on hands and knees.
- Mop floors and woodwork with a wet mop at least once a week (especially if the house was built before 1960).

poison. Mixing magnesium sulfate with a sweet liquid may enhance its palatability. Results should occur within 2 to 4 hours.

Nursing Management

Focus on poison prevention as well as on care of the poisoned child. Educate the public about ways to decrease the incidence of poisonings through printed materials such as checklists for poison proofing a home and illustrated first-aid guidelines. Consciousness-raising efforts should be included in each plan of care. Remind parents of the importance of keeping the phone number of the poison control center on the phone.

When confronted with a poisoning incident, focus on maintaining vital functions, preventing continued absorption of the poison, preventing complications related to the poisoning and treatment, reducing fear, and educating the caregiver about poison prevention. Once the child's condition is stabilized, exposure to the poison must be terminated. Substances should be removed from the mouth first manually and then by a sip of water; from the eye with a continuous flush of normal saline; and from the skin by removing contaminated clothing and washing the skin with soap and water.

Once exposure is terminated, identify the substance and consult the poison control center. Procedures to induce vomiting and prevent absorption are initiated as directed by the poison control center.

TRAUMA

Falls and motor vehicle injuries are the most common causes of trauma in infants. Medical–surgical management is dictated by the location and extent of the injury.

Nursing Management

Preventing trauma or injuries is of utmost importance. Parents must stay aware of their infant's abilities as the infant grows and develops and be prepared to provide a safe environment. Every time a nurse encounters a parent, provide developmentally appropriate safety information and reminders. Stress car seat safety.

SUFFOCATION/DROWNING

Suffocation occurs when air exchange is hindered by covering the mouth or nose, applying pressure to the throat and chest, or excluding air (e.g., via refrigerator entrapment).

Drowning can occur in only inches of water. Drowning is a great concern when an infant is in the tub.

Nursing Management

Educate parents and care providers. Safe cribs have no more than $2^3/_8$ inch space between the slats, and the crib mattress fits snugly against the slats. The crib is placed out of reach of windows and other furniture that may have cords or strings that could entrap or strangle a child. Other objects that may contribute to suffocation are electrical cords, toys with strings, plastic bags, pieces of balloons, crib mobiles, pieces of hard food, and restraining straps.

Drowning may occur in toilets, buckets of water, tubs, and pools. Remind caregivers that an infant or young child will not roll from the back to the stomach when the child's face is covered with water and that infants are top heavy and do not have the strength to pull themselves out of a bucket if they fall in head first.

CLIENT TEACHING

Tips for Maintaining a Safe Environment throughout Infancy

At 4 months, infants begin to roll and become very active:

- Keep crib side rails all the way up.
- Do not leave the infant unattended on raised areas such as beds, sofas, changing tables; instead, place on the floor or in a playpen.
- Use walkers away from the stairs.
- Never leave the infant unattended in the tub.
- Place car seat in the center of the back seat and facing backward until the infant is 20 pounds or 12 months old. *Always use a car seat.*

At 6 months, infants begin to crawl, reach, and put things in their mouths:

- Keep the floor swept and be alert for small objects that may be put in the mouth.
- Put gates at the tops and bottoms of stairways.
- Keep bathroom doors closed.
- Dress the infant in clothing that allows freedom of movement.
- Do not leave the infant unattended in highchair.
- Keep cords and plastic bags out of the infant's reach.

At 8 months, infants begin to pull up and walk around furniture:

- Ensure that furniture both inside and outside the house is sturdy enough for the infant to pull self to standing.
- Eliminate containers of water inside and outside the house.
- Avoid dressing the infant in socks without shoes.

At 10 to 12 months, infants may begin to walk:

- Keep exterior doors secure.
- Secure gates around swimming pools.
- Keep appliance doors closed at all times.
- Place the infant weighing more than 20 pounds in a front-facing car seat.

Summary

- The most common skin disorders of infancy are diaper rash, eczema, and cradle cap.
- The immaturity of the respiratory system creates hazards for the healthy infant and places the compromised infant at even greater risk of infection.
- Sudden infant death syndrome is the leading cause of death among infants.
- Signs of congenital heart disease in the infant include poor weight gain, poor feeding habits, fatigue, and respiratory infections.
- Iron-deficiency anemia can be prevented largely by teaching parents the importance of providing iron-fortified formula to infants until the age of 12 months.
- Possible signs of GI obstruction in the infant include abdominal pain, nausea and vomiting, abdominal distention, and decreased stool output.
- Treatment of colic may involve a change in feeding practices, correction of a stressful environment, and support of the parents.
- The most common defects of the GU tract include cryptorchidism, hydrocele, and hypospadias.
- The nursing goals when caring for infants with musculoskeletal impairments focus on preventing both skin breakdown and developmental delays.

CASE STUDY

Janie is a 10-month-old female who was brought to the clinic by her grandmother. The grandmother reports that Janie is irritable, refuses to eat, and does not want to be rocked or cuddled. Janie's temperature is 102°F. She had been treated for an upper respiratory infection 10 days ago. A spinal tap indicates that Janie has meningitis. An IV is started, and antibiotics are administered.

The following questions will guide your development of a nursing care plan for the case study.

1. List subjective and objective data a nurse should obtain about Janie.
2. List three nursing diagnoses and goals for Janie.
3. List three successful outcomes for Janie.
4. How can the spread of this infection be prevented?
5. What must be included in discharge planning if Janie's recovery is uneventful?

- Infants become feverish quickly and must be observed for febrile seizures and protected from injury.
- Routine immunization of infants against *H. Influenzae* type B infection has reduced the incidence of bacterial meningitis.
- Developmental assessment will reveal language and social delays in infants with hearing and visual impairments.
- Inconsistencies between what reportedly happened and the extent of injuries constitute a strong indicator of child abuse.

Review Questions

1. An appropriate nursing intervention when caring for an infant with an upper respiratory infection and elevated temperature is to:
   a. give tepid water baths to reduce fever.
   b. encourage food intake to maintain caloric needs.
   c. dress the infant in heavy clothing to prevent chilling.
   d. give frequent, small amounts of favorite fluids to prevent dehydration.

2. A 2-month-old breastfed infant with acute diarrhea is successfully rehydrated with oral solutions. The mother will now be instructed to:
   a. continue breastfeeding.
   b. stop breastfeeding until the breast milk can be cultured.
   c. stop breastfeeding until diarrhea is absent for 24 hours.
   d. express breast milk and dilute with sterile water before feeding.

3. During the first few days following surgical repair of an infant's cleft lip, the nurse will instruct the mother to:
   a. provide crib toys for distraction.
   b. remove restraints periodically to cuddle the infant.
   c. keep the infant heavily sedated to prevent suture strain.
   d. leave the infant in the crib at all times to prevent suture strain.

4. A new mother asks the nurse, "How can diaper rash be prevented?" The nurse's best response is:
   a. "Wash the area with soap and water after every diaper change."
   b. "Wash the area with mild soap and water and dry thoroughly after stools."
   c. "Wash the area with soap before applying a thin layer of oil after stools."
   d. "Wipe the buttocks with oil and apply powder to creases after every diaper change."

5. A clinical manifestation of increased intracranial pressure in infants is:
   a. irritability.
   b. diarrhea.
   c. photophobia.
   d. flat anterior fontanel.

References/Suggested Readings

American Academy of Pediatrics, Subcommittee on Acute Gatroenteritis, Provisional Committee on Quality Improvement. (1996). Practice parameter. The management of acute gastroenteritis in young children. *Pediatrics, 97*(3), 424–436.

American Academy of Pediatrics, Task Force on Infant Sleep Position and Sudden Infant Death Syndrome. (2000). Changing concepts of sudden infant death syndrome: Implications for infant sleeping environment and sleep position. *Pediatrics, 105*(3), 650–656. [Online]. Available: www.aap.org/policy/re9946.html

American Heart Association. (2002). *Congenital cardiovascular disease statistics.* [Online]. Available: http://216.185.112.5/presenter.jhtml?identifier=4576

American SIDS Institute. (1999). *SIDS information* [Online]. Available: www.sids.org/rsearch/test/sld003.htm

Anderson, R. N., Kochanek, K. D., & Murphy, S. L. (1997). Report of final mortality statistics, 1995. *Monthly Vital Statistics Report 4511* (Suppl. 2). Hyattsville, MD: National Center for Health Statistics.

Ball, J., & Bindler, R. (2000). *Pediatric nursing* (2nd ed.). Norwalk, CT: Appleton & Lange.

Barker, E., Sauline, M., & Caristo, A. (2002). Spina bifida. *RN, 65*(12), 33–38.

Castiglia, P. (1998). Trisomy 21 syndrome: Is there anything new? *Journal of Pediatric Health Care, 12*(1), 35–37.

Clayton, Y. M. (2000). Candidosis (candidiosis). In J. Harper, A. Orange, & N. Prose (Eds.), *Textbook of pediatric dermatology.* London: Blackwell Science, Ltd.

Clinical Rounds. (2002). SIDS linked to *E. coli. Nursing2002, 32*(7), 34–45.

Cystic Fibrosis Foundation. (1998). *CPX study in adult patients moves to phase II* [Online]. Available: www.cff.org/clinical03.htm

Dochterman, J., & Bulechek, G. (2004). *Nursing Interventions Classification (NIC)* (4th ed.). St. Louis, MO: Mosby.

Dowshen, S., Hersheberger, M., & Rutherford, K. (2001). *SIDS: Sudden and silent.* [Online]. Available: http://kidshealth.org/parent/general/sleep/sids.html

Duncan, B., Ey, J., Holberg, C. J., Wright, A. L., Martinez, F. D., and Taussig, L. M. (1993). Exclusive breast-feeding for at least 4 months protects against otitis media. *Pediatrics 91*(5), 867–872.

Eisenhauer, L. A., Nichols, L. W., Spencer, R. T., & Bergan, F. W. (1998). *Clinical pharmacology and nursing management* (5th ed.). Philadelphia: Lippincott.

Ellmers, K., & Criddle, L. (2002). Cystic fibrosis. *RN, 65*(9), 61–66.

Estes, M. E. Z. (2002). *Health Assessment & Physical Examination* (2nd ed). Clifton Park, NY: Thomson Delmar Learning.

Faden, H., Duffy, L., & Boeve, M. (1998). Otitis media: Back to basics. *Pediatric Infectious Disease Journal, 17*(12), 1105–1113.

Finesilver, C. (2002). Down syndrome. *RN, 65*(11), 43–48.

Gartner, L. M., & Greer, F. R. (2003). Prevention of rickets and vitamin D deficiency: New guidelines for vitamin D intake. *Pediatrics, 111*(4Pt1), 908.

Godshall, M. (2003). Caring for families of chronically ill kids. *RN, 66*(2), 30–34.

Gorman, K. (1999). Sickle cell disease. *AJN, 99*(3), 38–43.

Grover, G. (2000). Nutritional needs. In C. D. Berkowitz (Ed.), *Pediatrics: A primary care approach* (2nd ed.). New York: W. B. Saunders.

Hockenberry, M., Wilson, D., Winkelstein, M. L., & Kline, N. (2003). *Wong's nursing care of infants and children* (7th ed.). St. Louis, MO: Mosby.

James, S., Ashwill, J. W., & Droske, S. (2002). *Nursing care of children: Principles and practice* (2nd ed.). Philadelphia: W. B. Saunders.

Kaditis, A., & Wald, E. (1998). Viral croup: Current diagnosis and treatment. *Pediatric Infectious Disease Journal, 17*(9), 827–834.

Kitchens, G. G. (1995). Relationship of environmental tobacco smoke to otitis media in young children. *Laryngoscope. 105*(5, Part 2), 1–3.

Kliegman, R. M., Jensen, H., & Behrman, R. (2000). *Nelson's textbook of pediatrics* (16th ed.). Philadelphia: W. B. Saunders.

Kline, A. (2003). Pinpointing the cause of pediatric respiratory distress. *Nursing2003, 33*(9), 58–63.

Kuppermann, N., O'Dea, T., Pinchney, L., & Hoecher, C. (2000). Predictors of intussception in young children. *Archives of Pediatric and Adolescent Medicine, 154,* 250–255.

Marks, M. G. (1998). *Broadribb's introductory pediatric nursing* (5th ed.). Philadelphia: J. B. Lippincott Williams & Wilkins.

Mayo Clinic. (2001). *Sickle cell anemia* [Online]. Available: www.mayoclinic.com/invoke.cfm?id=DS00324

Medical College of Georgia. (2002). *Positional plagiocephaly.* [Online]. Available: www.mcg.edu/som/surgery/neuros/plagio.htm

Meekins, E. (2002). Would you recognize this pediatric disorder? *RN, 65*(4), 26–30.

Mera, K., & Hackley, B. (2003). Childhood vaccines: How safe are they? *AJN, 103*(2), 79–88.

Mickle, J., & Cutting, G. (2000). Genotype-phenotype relationships in cystic fibrosis. *Medical Clinics of North America, 84* 597–605.

Miles, M. (2003). Support for parents during a child's hospitalization. *AJN, 103*(2), 62–64.

Moorhead, S. C., Johnson, M., & Maas, M. (2004). *Nursing Outcomes Classification (NOC)* (3rd ed.). St. Louis, MO: Mosby.

North American Nursing Diagnosis Association. (2003). *Nursing diagnosis: Definitions & classification 2003–2004.* Philadelphia: Author.

Orenstein, S., Izadnia, F., & Khan, S. (1999). Gastroesophageal reflux disease in children. *Gastroenterology Clinics of North America, 28*(4), 947–969.

Potts, N., & Mandleco, B. (2002). *Pediatric nursing: Caring for children and their families.* Clifton Park, NY: Thomson Delmar Learning.

Queenan, J. (2001). *Positional plagiocephaly* (Flattened Head). [Online]. Available: http://kidshealth.org/parent/general/sleep/positional_plagiocephaly.html

Sassen, M. L., Brand, R., & Grote, J. J. (1997). Risk factors for otitis media with effusion in children 0 to 2 years of age. *American Journal of Otolaryngology 18*(5), 324–330.

Schuman, A. (1997). Disposable diapers? Definitely! *Contemporary Pediatrics 14*(11), 131–139.

Shaw, G., M., Lamamer, E. J., Wassernman, C. R., O'Malley, C. D., & Tolarova, M. M. (1995). Risks of orofacial clefts in children born to women using multivitamins containing folic acid periconceptionally. *The Lancet, 346*(8972), 393.

Simmerman, J. M., & Mauzy, C. (2001). Finally! Babies can get this vaccine. *RN, 64*(7), 28–32.

Spratto, G., & Woods, A. (2004). *2004 PDR nurses' drug handbook.* Clifton Park, NY: Thomson Delmar Learning.

Tinkle, M. (2002). Cystic fibrosis carrier screening: *AWHONN Lifelines, 6*(2), 134–139.

Tully, S., Bar-Haim, Y., & Bradley, R. (1995). Abnormal tympanography after supine bottle feeding. *Journal of Pediatrics, 1995*(126), S105–S111.

Van Riper, M. (2003). A change of plans. *AJN, 103*(6), 71–74.

Wahlgren, D., Hovell, M., Meltzer, S., Hofstetter, C., & Zakarian, J. (1997). Reduction of environmental tobacco smoke exposure in asthmatic children: A 2 year follow-up. *Chest, 111*(1), 81–88.

White, K. R., Munro, C. L., & Pickler, R. H. (1995). Therapeutic implications of recent advances in cystic fibrosis. *MCN, 20*(6), 58–64.

Wittmann-Price, R., & Pope, K. (2002). Universal newborn hearing screening. *AJN, 102*(11), 71–77.

Wong, D. L., Hockenberry-Eaton, M. (2001). *Wong's essentials of pediatric nursing* (9th ed.). St. Louis, MO: Mosby–Year Book.

Yetman, R., & Coody, D. (1997). Failure to thrive: A clinical guideline. *Journal of Pediatric Health Care, 11*(3), 134–137.

Zorb, S. (2002). Transplantation offers hope. *RN, 65*(9), 66–68.

Resources

American Cleft Palate–Craniofacial Association, 104 South Estes Drive, Suite 204, Chapel Hill, NC, 27514, 800-242-5338, www.cleftline.com

American Lung Association, 1740 Broadway, New York, NY, 10019 (800-586-4872), www.lungusa.org

American Sickle-Cell Anemia Association, 10300 Carnegie Avenue, Cleveland, OH, 44106, 216-229-8600, www.ascaa.org

American SIDS Institute, 2480 Windy Hill Road, Suite 380, Marietta, GA 30067, 770-612-1030, www.sids.org

American Society for Deaf Children, P. O. Box 3355, Gettysburg, PA 17325, 800-942-2732, www.deafchildren.org

American Speech-Language-Hearing Association, 10801 Rockville Pike, Rockville, MD 20852, 800-638-8255, www.asha.org

Automotive Safety for Children Program, 575 West Drive, Room 004, Indianapolis, IN, 46202-5109, 800-543-6227, www.preventinjury.org

Children's Nutrition Research Center, 1100 Bates Street, Houston, TX 77030, 713-798-4951, www.bcm.tmc.edu

Cystic Fibrosis Foundation, 6931 Arlington Road, Bethesda, MD, 20814, 800-344-4823, www.cff.org

Hydrocephalus Association, 870 Market Street, Suite 955, San Francisco, CA, 94102, 888-598-3789, www.hydroassoc.org

Kids Health, Nemours Foundation, 4600 Touchton Road East, Building 200, Suite 500, Jacksonville, FL 32246, 904-232-4100, www.kidshealth.org, www.nemours.org

La Leche League International, 1400 Meacham Road, Schaumburg, IL, 60173, 847-519-7730 (24-hour service), 800-LA-LECHE (for local number or catalog: 9 A.M.–3 P.M.)

National Association for Parents of Children with Visual Impairments, P. O. Box 317, Watertown, MA 02471, 800-562-6265, www.spedex.com

National Down Syndrome Society, 666 Brogg, New York, NY, 10012, 800-221-4602, www.ndss.org

Sickle Cell Disease Association of America, 200 Corporate Pointe, Suite 495, Culver City, CA 90230-8727, 800-421-8453, www.sicklecelldisease.org

Spina Bifida Association of America, 4590 MacArthur Boulevard, NW, Suite 250, Washington, DC, 20007-4226, 202-944-3285 or 800-621-3141, www.sbaa.org

United Cerebral Palsy National, 1600 L Street N.W., Suite 700, Washington, DC, 20036, 800-872-5827, www.ucpa.org, email: ucpnatl@ucpa.org

Women, Infants and Children (WIC), Supplemental Food Programs Division, Food and Nutrition Service—USDA, 3101 Park Center Drive, Alexandria, VA 22302, 800-545-2200, www.fns.usda.gov/wic

COMMON PROBLEMS: 1–18 YEARS

MAKING THE CONNECTION

Refer to the following chapters to increase your understanding of common pediatric problems:

Basic Nursing
- **Life Cycle**
- **Cultural Considerations**
- **Stress, Adaptation, and Anxiety**
- **Loss, Grief, and Death**
- **Wellness Concepts**
- **Basic Nutrition**
- **Safety/Hygiene**
- **Fluid, Electrolyte, and Acid–Base Balance**
- **Assessment**
- **Pain Management**

Adult Health Nursing
- **Anesthesia**
- **Surgery**

- **Oncology**
- **Respiratory System**
- **Cardiovascular System**
- **Hematologic and Lymphatic Systems**
- **Gastrointestinal System**
- **Urinary System**
- **Musculoskeletal System**
- **Neurological System**
- **Endocrine System**
- **Integumentary System**
- **Immune System**
- **Mental Illness**

Maternal & Pediatric Nursing
- **Basics of Pediatric Care**

LEARNING OBJECTIVES

Upon completion of this chapter, you should be able to:
- Define key terms.
- Discuss the common disorders of the integumentary system in children.
- Differentiate the pathophysiology, common diagnostic tests, treatment, and nursing care for skin conditions in children as compared to adults.
- Differentiate the etiology, medical–surgical management, and nursing care for respiratory conditions in children as compared to adults.
- Describe the causes, assessment, and management of rheumatic fever in children.
- Differentiate the pathophysiology, common diagnostic tests, treatment, and nursing care for digestive conditions in children as compared to adults.
- Differentiate the etiology, medical–surgical management, and nursing care for genitourinary conditions in children as compared to adults.

KEY TERMS

acanthosis nigricans
comedone
encopresis

epistaxis
Gowers' sign
rhinorrhea

- Discuss communicable and infectious diseases of childhood, including their causative agents, transmission, incubation periods, contagious periods, prevention, signs and symptoms, treatment, and nursing care.
- Differentiate the etiology, medical–surgical management, and nursing care for orthopedic conditions in children as compared to adults.
- Briefly describe behavioral problems in children, including symptoms, treatment, and nursing care.
- Plan care for a child with any of the common pediatric disorders.

INTRODUCTION

Pediatric nursing focuses on protecting children from illness and injury as well as assisting them to attain optimal levels of functioning, regardless of health status. The pediatric nurse must understand the phases of a child's growth and development (refer to the Life Cycle chapter) and be sensitive to the importance of family interactions. This chapter focuses on common childhood conditions and illnesses affecting all systems of the body; the typical medical and surgical management for these conditions; and nursing management of the child and family.

RESPIRATORY SYSTEM

Disorders of the respiratory system that occur most often in children include upper-respiratory infections, allergic rhinitis, tonsillitis, asthma, and foreign-body aspiration.

UPPER-RESPIRATORY INFECTIONS

Common upper-respiratory infections include nasopharyngitis (the common cold), pharyngitis, and influenza. Nasopharyngitis is usually credited with being the most common childhood respiratory illness. These disorders are generally responsive to supportive therapies, and symptoms typically improve within 3 days. Clinical manifestations, etiology, and management of these common upper-respiratory disorders are presented in Table 57-1.

Nursing Management

Maintaining fluid intake, providing comfort measures, and preventing spread of infection are the main goals of care for the child with an upper-respiratory infection. The child should not be forced to eat if appetite is decreased. An appropriate diet may include cool, bland fluids and soft foods such as gelatin, soup, mashed potatoes, puddings, hot cereals, and ice pops. Teach parents to observe for urinary output and for moist mucous membranes as signs of adequate hydration.

Comfort measures may include warm salt-water gargles ($1/_4$ tsp salt per 8 oz glass of water) and warm or cool compresses applied to the throat. Nasal decongestion may be relieved with normal saline drops before feedings and at bedtime. A cool-mist humidifier at the bedside may also relieve symptoms.

It is important that parents know how both to take a child's temperature and to safely administer nonsalicylate antipyretics, such as acetaminophen (Tylenol). Salicylates, such as aspirin, are not used because of the associated risk of Reye's syndrome.

Teach parents and children methods for preventing the spread of infection, such as conscientious hand hygiene, proper disposal of tissues, and covering of the nose and mouth when coughing and sneezing. Also avoid contact with infectious persons. Preventing the spread of infection is especially challenging in school and crowded living environments. Children in day care centers have a higher rate of infection than do children who spend their days in the home.

Untreated streptococcal infections may lead to complications such as rheumatic fever, meningitis, and glomerulonephritis. Emphasize to the parents of children with pharyngitis caused by streptococcal infection

TABLE 57-1	DISTINGUISHING CHARACTERISTICS OF COMMON URIs		
	NASOPHARYNGITIS	**PHARYNGITIS**	**INFLUENZA**
Manifestations	**Rhinorrhea** (watery nasal discharge), congestion, sneezing, fever, cough, sore throat, muscular aches, and possibly, enlarged lymph nodes	Sore throat, erythema and inflammation of the pharynx and tonsils, fever, enlarged, tender cervical lymph nodes *Viral:* gradual onset, hoarseness, cough, rhinitis, malaise *Bacterial:* abdominal pain, vomiting, headache	Chills, fever, flushed face, myalgia (pain in muscles), cough, rhinitis, headache, sore throat, photophobia, conjunctivitis
Etiology	Viral	Viral (80%) or bacterial (20%)	Influenza virus
Incidence	Typically 6 to 9 colds per year, most commonly in the fall and spring	Most common among 4 to 7-year-olds	Highest among school-age children
Management	Rest, fluids, nonsalicylate antipyretics, oral decongestants, sterile saline nose drops	Rest; fluids; nonsalicylate antipyretics or ibuprofen; warm salt-water gargles; cool, bland liquids; antibiotics for streptococcal infections	Rest, fluids, nonsalicylate antipyretics

CLIENT TEACHING

Administering Normal Saline Drops

1. Instill two drops.
2. Wait 5 minutes.
3. Instill two more drops.
4. Drops should not be used for more than 3 days.

PROFESSIONAL TIP

Throat Culture

The only reliable means of determining whether pharyngitis is viral or bacterial is with a throat culture. The nurse is most often the person who performs a throat smear for culture, which requires a physician's order. The applicator is swabbed across the tonsils, the posterior edge of the soft palate, and the uvula.

("strep throat") the importance of completing the course of prescribed antibiotics.

ALLERGIC RHINITIS

Allergic rhinitis ("hay fever") is an inflammatory disorder of the nasal mucosa. Most often, it is a seasonal, recurrent response to allergens such as animal dander, house dust, pollens, and molds. Manifestations include rhinorrhea, postnasal drip, sneezing, allergic conjunctivitis, sniffing, itchy nose and palate, dark circles under the eyes, and the "allergic salute" (transverse nasal crease that results from repeatedly pushing nose upward and backward to relieve itching).

Medical–Surgical Management

Pharmacological

Antihistamines, decongestants, and bronchodilators may be given to relieve symptoms of congestion and difficulty with breathing. Topical intranasal corticosteroids are quite effective in children who do not respond to antihistamines and decongestants. Systemic corticosteroids may be used in extreme cases. Immunotherapy or desensitization to allergens may be initiated if antihistamines and decongestants are not effective in relieving symptoms or are needed chronically. Desensitization is performed for those allergens that produce a positive reaction on skin testing. The allergist sets up a schedule for injections in gradually increasing doses until a maintenance dose is reached. Desensitization is considered to be a safe procedure with considerable benefit for some children. Severe reactions are uncommon. During immunotherapy, children must be observed for signs of anaphylaxis for 30 minutes after each injection.

Health Promotion

The treatment of choice is to eliminate the allergen from the child's environment. Recommendations for limiting the child's exposure to allergens include avoiding wool and down; using dust-proof covers on bedding; removing carpets, draperies, and blinds from the child's room, if not the whole house; keeping humidity lower than 50%; keeping pets outside; and using air filters.

Nursing Management

Focus on therapeutic management of the disease. After identification of the allergens, assist the family with allergy proofing the home and administering medications.

Drowsiness, dry mouth, and excitability are side effects of some antihistamines. Combining an antihistamine and decongestant may prevent drowsiness.

TONSILLITIS

Tonsillitis, a common illness among children, is an inflammation of the tonsils (two masses of lymphoid tissue located at the back of the mouth), resulting from pharyngitis. Tonsils filter and protect the respiratory and alimentary tracts from infection. They normally enlarge progressively between 2 and 10 years of age and reduce during preadolescence. If the tonsils become enlarged from infection, they can interfere with breathing and swallowing and cause partial deafness. Clinical manifestations of tonsillitis include sore throat; enlarged, bright-red tonsils; mouth breathing; halitosis; nasal speech; and snoring.

Medical–Surgical Management

Surgical

Tonsillectomy may be warranted in cases of abscesses, upper airway obstruction, and obstructive sleep apnea. Adenoidectomy (removal of lymphoid tissue in the nasal pharynx) is performed in cases of recurrent otitis media with eustachian tube obstruction or for persistent nasal or airway obstruction. If tonsillectomy can be postponed until 4 or 5 years of age, the apparent need often will have disappeared.

Pharmacological

Medical treatment includes analgesics for pain, antipyretics for fever, and antibiotics for streptococcal infections.

Nursing Management

Prepare child for surgery. Use dolls or puppets to assist the child in expressing fears and concerns and acting out the pending experience.

Postoperatively, monitor vital signs, I&O, and for signs of blood loss. Maintain child in prone or side-lying position. Encourage intake of cool or cold clear liquids when child is fully awake. Administer analgesic as ordered.

NURSING PROCESS

Assessment

Subjective Data

Be sensitive to the child's and family's level of anxiety and offer opportunities for expression of concerns. The use of puppets, dolls, and other materials may be an effective way to allow the child to act out the pending surgical experience and to express concerns and fears.

Objective Data

Presurgical assessments such as complete blood count (CBC), clotting time, and urinalysis are usually done on an outpatient basis.

Upon admission on the day of surgery, review vital signs and laboratory results for abnormalities, and assess the child for signs of infection (fever, elevated white blood count [WBC], and redness and exudate of the throat). Observe the child's mouth for loose teeth that could be aspirated during anesthesia.

Postoperatively, monitor vital signs and observe for hemorrhage, ability to swallow, and dehydration. The most obvious signs of bleeding from the surgical site are restlessness or anxiety, frequent swallowing, and rapid pulse. Each time vital signs are taken, use a flashlight to observe the pharynx for bleeding.

Nursing diagnoses for the child following a tonsillectomy may include the following:

Nursing Diagnoses	Planning/Goals	Nursing Interventions
Risk for **A**spiration related to unswallowed saliva and postoperative bleeding	The client's airway will remain patent.	Maintain the child in a prone or side-lying position. Monitor vital signs every 15 minutes for 1 hour and hourly for the next 4 hours. Ensure availability of suction equipment. Do not give oral fluids until the child is completely awake. Avoid hot liquids, irritating foods, and use of straws. Instruct the child to avoid coughing and clearing the throat; encourage the child to expectorate secretions into a tissue.
Deficient Risk for **F**luid Volume, related to blood loss and decreased oral intake	The client will maintain appropriate fluid intake and demonstrate minimal fluid loss.	Observe for signs of blood loss, such as frequent swallowing, elevated pulse and respirations, pallor, restlessness and anxiety; report to physician immediately. Maintain intravenous (IV) fluids until the child is taking oral fluids. Encourage intake of cold or cool liquids such as ice pops (no red), noncitric juices, gelatin (no red), and ice chips; introduce milk products only after clear liquids are tolerated. Record hourly intake and output (I&O).
Acute **P**ain related to surgical procedure	The client will have pain relief (<3 on a scale of 1 to 10).	Provide nonaspirin analgesic every 4 hours for at least the first 24 hours postoperative. Use age-appropriate pain assessment tools. Encourage the parents to stay at the child's bedside to provide reassurance and comfort.
Deficient **K**nowledge (family) related to discharge care	The caregivers will verbalize an understanding of discharge care.	Instruct the caregivers to: • Watch for signs of hemorrhage especially between the fifth and tenth postoperative days. • Watch for signs of infection (persistent earache, temperature over 102°F). • Call physician if bleeding or signs of infection occurs. • Encourage liquids and soft foods as tolerated for 10 days. • Avoid rough, scratchy foods for 3 weeks. • Maintain pain control with nonaspirin analgesics every 4 hours as needed during first week. • Restrict the child's activity for 10 days (i.e., no school or vigorous exercise).

continues

Nursing Diagnoses	Planning/Goals	Nursing Interventions
		• Expect the throat to be white in appearance and the mouth odor to be bad for the first week.
		• Bring child for follow-up visit in 1–2 weeks.

Evaluation Each goal must be evaluated to determine how it has been met by the client.

ASTHMA

Asthma, a reactive airway disease (RAD), is defined as narrowing or obstruction of the airway triggered by stimuli (such as cold air, smoke, viral infection, exercise, stress, drugs, or allergens) and inflammation that leads to mucosal edema and mucus hypersecretion. Asthma is the leading cause of school absenteeism and the most common admitting diagnosis in children's hospitals (Kliegman, Jenson, & Behrman, 2000). Clinical manifestations of asthmatic attacks or episodes include a dry, hacking cough; wheezing; and difficulty breathing. The child may need to sit up to breathe. Attacks may last for hours or days. Thick, tenacious mucus may be expectorated after a coughing episode. In children with repeated acute exacerbations, barrel chest and the use of accessory muscles of respiration are common findings. Chronic asthmatics are usually small according to the standard growth charts. In some cases, episodes no longer occur after puberty, and growth usually catches up in adolescence. There is evidence suggesting that RAD is hereditary (Kliegman et al., 2000). A definitive diagnosis of asthma can be made when the airway obstruction (indicated by pulmonary function tests) is reversed with bronchodilators.

Medical–Surgical Management
Medical

Medical treatment is aimed at preventing airway damage resulting from repeated and severe episodes of asthma. Care is focused on early recognition and treatment of episodes, identification and elimination of allergens, and education of the child and family. Allergy proofing the home along with skin testing followed by desensitization are methods used to control allergens (refer to the section on Allergic Rhinitis).

Educate families about the disease, including ways to prevent attacks; early signs of episodes; drug therapy; appropriate exercise; and chest physiotherapy (CPT), if needed. Early symptoms include increasing cough at night, in the early morning, or in conjunction with activity; respiratory retractions; and wheezing. Using a peak flowmeter is an objective way to measure airway obstruction: families must learn how both to use this device and to record the results.

Pharmacological

A combination of bronchodilators and anti-inflammatory agents is used to treat asthma. The most commonly prescribed bronchodilators are albuterol (Ventolin), metaproterenol sulfate (Alupent), and terbutaline (Brethine). These drugs cause relaxation of bronchial smooth muscle and inhibit the release of mediators from mast cells. Small doses by inhalation are the most effective mode of administration. Bronchodilators may be taken together by inhalation and be given parenterally for additional effect. Repetitive use may mask increasing airway inflammation and hyper-responsiveness. Correct use of the metered-dose inhaler (MDI) is important for maintaining control of asthma symptoms.

Theophylline is the oldest effective bronchodilator. It requires continuous oral or IV administration and is most therapeutic when the serum level measures 10–20 mcg/mL.

Anti-inflammatory drugs of choice include cromolyn sodium (Crolom) and corticosteroids such as prednisone (Deltasone). Cromolyn is an antiasthmatic, mast cell stabilizer that prevents asthma symptoms by blocking the release of mast cell mediators. Once symptoms start, however, cromolyn is ineffective. Adverse effects associated with cromolyn are airway irritation with mild cough and a bad taste. Corticosteroids effectively reduce mucosal edema and potentiate the effect of bronchodilators. Steroids may be given in inhaled form to reduce the oral dose required and to decrease systemic effects that accompany oral administration. Long-term use of oral steroids is reserved for chronic asthma that has not responded to other drugs. Adverse side effects of long-term oral therapy include Cushing's syndrome, growth suppression, osteoporosis, glaucoma, cataracts, peptic ulcer, hyperglycemia, and decreased resistance to infection (Eisenhauer, Nichols, Spencer & Bergan, 1998).

Activity

Children with asthma should not be automatically restricted from physical activity. With adequate treatment, a child with asthma can participate in most physical activities. Sports that do not require sustained exertion, such as gymnastics, baseball, and weight lifting, are well tolerated. Swimming is frequently recommended as an ideal sport because the air is humidified, and breathing increases end expiratory pressure.

SAMPLE NURSING CARE PLAN

THE CHILD WITH ASTHMA

Mikala, a 5-year-old girl, was admitted to the emergency room (ER) with severe coughing, fever, and difficulty breathing. Crackles and wheezing were evident in all fields upon auscultation. Vital signs were temperature 102°F; pulse, 160; and respirations, 40. Pulse oximetry was 90%. Her parents had given her Tylenol for what they thought was a "cold." When her condition worsened during the night, they brought her to the ER. Mikala has no history of asthma but has eczema. She has just started kindergarten. Her parents are extremely distraught and are asking many questions. Mikala cries every time anyone enters the room.

Nursing Diagnosis 1 *Ineffective Airway Clearance* related to secretions in the bronchi and exudate in the alveoli as evidenced by difficulty breathing, crackles, and wheezing

Nursing Outcomes Classification (NOC)
Respiratory Status: Airway Patency
Respiratory Status: Ventilation

Nursing Interventions Classification (NIC)
Medication Administration: Inhalation
Airway Management

PLANNING/GOALS	NURSING INTERVENTIONS	RATIONALE
Mikala will have effective airway clearance.	Monitor vital signs, auscultate breath sounds, assess respiratory effort and rate, assess skin color every 15 to 30 minutes, arterial blood gases (ABGs), pulse oximetry, and pulmonary function tests results.	Subtle changes may serve as an early warning of increased airway obstruction.
	Administer oxygen at the ordered flow rate (if chronic asthmatic, not to exceed 2 L/min).	Decreases hypoxia. Administration of oxygen to a child with chronic carbon dioxide retention may cause respiratory depression.
	Position the client upright or for comfort.	Enhances lung expansion.
	Ensure availability of suction equipment and tracheostomy tray.	Condition can deteriorate rapidly.
	Provide at least 1,600 cc fluids (IV/p.o.)/ 24 hours.	Liquefies secretions and replaces insensible fluid losses.
	Initiate nothing-by-mouth (NPO) status during periods of severe respiratory distress.	Oral fluid intake during periods of distress can cause aspiration.
	Administer ordered medications and assess for therapeutic effect.	Bronchodilators and steroids open airways and decrease edema.
	Assess breath sounds before and after CPT.	Theophylline level of >30 can cause serious complication.
	Encourage client to cough and deep breathe by blowing bubbles through a wand.	CPT, coughing, and deep breathing help loosen/eliminate secretions.

continues

SAMPLE NURSING CARE PLAN

EVALUATION   Mikala's airway is clear.

Nursing Diagnosis 2 *Anxiety* related to threat to or change in health status as evidenced by respiratory distress and hospitalization

Nursing Outcomes Classification (NOC)
Coping

Nursing Interventions Classification (NIC)
Allergy Management
Teaching: Individual

PLANNING/GOALS	NURSING INTERVENTIONS	RATIONALE
Mikala and her parents will be relaxed.	Maintain a calm, quiet environment and a reassuring manner.	Decreases oxygen demand and the work of breathing.
	Play with the child.	Builds rapport and trust.
	Keep the parents informed of procedures, treatments, and condition of their child.	Builds rapport and trust. Calming the parents can help calm child.

EVALUATION   Mikala cooperates with the staff. The parents participate in Mikala's care.

Nursing Diagnosis 3 *Deficient Knowledge* related to lack of exposure as evidenced by many questions

Nursing Outcomes Classification (NOC)
Knowledge Deficit: Disease Process
Knowledge Deficit: Treatment Regimen

Nursing Interventions Classification (NIC)
Teaching: Disease Process
Teaching: Prescribed Medication

PLANNING/GOALS	NURSING INTERVENTIONS	RATIONALE
Mikala's parents will verbalize accurate knowledge about asthma.	Teach the family about the disease, its triggers, and prescribed medications and treatment	Understanding increases compliance with treatment.
	Assess the family's knowledge about triggers, precipitating factors (such as colds), and allergen control.	Triggers may have been assessed. Knowledge of allergen control may decrease the likelihood of future episodes.
	Teach the importance of taking medications as prescribed.	Maintains therapeutic levels.
	Teach the importance of exercise and ways to choose appropriate activities based on the child's condition.	Promotes pulmonary and cardiovascular health, enhances self-esteem, and offers peer interaction.

EVALUATION   Mikala's parents verbalize accurate knowledge about the disease and its treatment. Mikala resumes normal activities.

FOREIGN-BODY ASPIRATION

Foreign-body aspiration is the inhalation of any object into the respiratory tract. Commonly aspirated items among children include nuts, grapes, popcorn, hard candy, dried beans, bones, coins, parts of toys, screws, and balloons. Aspiration may occur at any age but is most common between the ages of 6 months and 4 years. Clinical manifestations may include spasmodic coughing, respiratory distress, or gagging in the absence of fever or other symptoms of illness.

Medical–Surgical Management

Medical

Removal of foreign bodies from the respiratory tract is done by direct laryngoscopy or bronchoscopy. After the procedure, the child should remain hospitalized for observation of laryngeal edema and respiratory distress. Cool mist is provided and antibiotic therapy ordered if appropriate.

Health Promotion

It is important that parents and child care providers remain watchful as the child gains increased locomotor and manipulative skills and becomes more curious about the environment.

Nursing Management

After the object has been removed, the main focus of care is prevention. Assess the parents' knowledge of safety in relation to the child's developmental level. Encourage parents to keep cylindric, spheric, and pliable objects smaller than $1\frac{1}{4}$ inches out of children's reach. In addition, supervise children when eating, and cut food into small, irregular pieces.

CARDIOVASCULAR SYSTEM

A major threat to the child's cardiovascular system is rheumatic fever, which may lead to permanent heart damage and disability.

RHEUMATIC FEVER

Rheumatic fever is a chronic childhood disease affecting the heart, joints, lungs, and brain. It results from an autoimmune response to untreated group A *beta-hemolytic streptococcus* infections. Clinical manifestations are classified as minor and major. Minor clinical manifestations include fever, listlessness, anorexia, pallor, weight loss, and vague muscle, joint, or abdominal pain. Major clinical manifestations include polyarthritis, chorea (spasmodic twitchings), carditis, erythema marginatum (red skin lesions), and subcutaneous nodules. An elevated antistreptolysin-O (ASO) titer (indicative of recent streptococcal infection) is common among children with rheumatic fever.

Medical–Surgical Management

Medical

Diagnosis is made by evaluating presenting signs and symptoms and laboratory test results. A throat culture determines whether the infection is active. Erythrocyte sedimentation rate (ESR), C-reactive protein, and leukocyte count are elevated in the presence of inflammatory processes. Chest x-ray, electrocardiogram, and echocardiogram may demonstrate evidence of carditis.

The goals of medical management are to treat any existing strep infection, prevent recurrences and heart damage, and alleviate pain and fever. Bed rest is prescribed for the child with carditis until ESR and heart rate are within normal limits.

Pharmacological

Penicillin, salicylates, and corticosteroids are used to treat rheumatic fever. Long-term administration (as long as 5 years) of penicillin helps prevent the recurrence of rheumatic heart disease. Salicylates relieve pain, reduce inflammation of polyarthritis, and reduce fever. Corticosteroids are used in the presence of carditis. Residual heart disease (congestive heart failure) is treated as needed with digitalis and diuretics. Anticonvulsants may be prescribed to alleviate severe chorea.

Diet

A low-sodium diet may be prescribed in the presence of congestive heart failure.

Activity

Bed rest is essential to reduce the workload of the heart. The length of bed rest can range from weeks to months depending on the cardiac status.

Health Promotion

Continual health supervision for children is the key to prevention of rheumatic fever and resulting heart disease. It is important that children with upper respiratory infections be evaluated for group A *beta-hemolytic streptococcus* and treated with penicillin as prescribed.

Nursing Management

Maintain child on bed rest. Alternately apply heat and cold to affected joints. Provide distractions such as guided imagery, relaxation, board games, movies, books, or puzzles. Stress importance of evaluating children with upper-respiratory infections, and to take penicillin as prescribed even if symptoms disappear.

NURSING PROCESS

Assessment

Subjective Data

Initially, determine whether any family members have had a sore throat or unexplained fever within the past 2 months. Find out when symptoms began; what, if any, treatment was obtained; and if an antibiotic was prescribed, whether it was taken as directed.

Objective Data

Monitor the child for cardiac complications such as abnormal vital signs, shortness of breath, edema, and precordial pain. Assess joints for tenderness, small lumps, and rapid, purposeless movements. Use age-appropriate tools to assess pain.

Nursing diagnoses for the child with rheumatic fever may include the following:

Nursing Diagnoses	Planning/Goals	Nursing Interventions
*Acute **P**ain* related to inflamed joints	The client will be comfortable.	Alternate applying heat and cold to affected joints. Reposition the child every 2 hours, handle joints gently. Provide distraction such as guided imagery and relaxation.
***A**ctivity Intolerance* related to shortness of breath and pain	The client will tolerate restricted activities.	Limit activites to bed and chair, with bathroom privileges, and meals at the table. Include rest periods alternated with activities such as board games, computer use, movies, puzzles, books, art, and crafts.
*Risk for **I**njury* related to weakness and chorea	Child will be injury free.	If the child is experiencing chorea, the mattress may need to be placed on the floor and the child may require assistance going up and down stairs. Seizure precaution should be taken. Teach the importance of evaluating children with upper respiratory infections for streptococcus, and treating with penicillin.
*Deficient **K**nowledge* related to medication administration	The client and family understand the importance of antibiotic therapy in preventing recurrence of the disease and further heart damage.	Stress the importance of taking penicillin as prescribed even if symptoms disappear.

Evaluation Each goal must be evaluated to determine how it has been met by the client.

HEMATOLOGIC AND LYMPHATIC SYSTEMS

Leukemia, idiopathic thrombocytopenic purpura, and hemophilia are blood disorders that commonly occur during childhood.

LEUKEMIA

Leukemia, the most common childhood cancer, is the uncontrolled production of lymphocytes (immature white blood cells). The most common form of leukemia is acute lymphocytic leukemia (ALL). The prognosis has been improving dramatically thanks to vigorous therapy, but there is concern related to adverse effects of the ther-

apy. Clinical manifestations, the results of neutropenia and decreased red blood cells (RBCs) and platelets, include pallor, weakness, fever, excessive bruising, petechiae, purpura, bone or joint pain, and abdominal pain.

Medical–Surgical Management

Medical

In addition to the client's history, symptoms, and laboratory studies, bone marrow aspiration is done to confirm the diagnosis of leukemia. The goals of medical intervention are to eradicate the leukemic cells via chemotherapy and to provide supportive care during treatment.

Surgical

Bone marrow transplant may be recommended after the second remission.

Pharmacological

A combination of drugs is administered through a subclavian catheter and/or intrathecally to bring about remission. Treatment may last 2 to 3 years. After 30 days of initial treatment, remission can be verified via bone marrow aspiration and lumbar puncture. If remission occurs, the prognosis is good. For the child who suffers a relapse, different drugs are used in an attempt to reinduce a remission. Relapses decrease the probability of survival.

Nursing Management

Assess the emotional states of the child and the family members and identify needs so a plan can be made to assist them in working through and resolving their feelings and fears. Explore how the child and family are coping with the illness as well as the treatment.

IDIOPATHIC THROMBOCYTOPENIC PURPURA

Idiopathic thrombocytopenic purpura (ITP) is a blood disorder associated with a deficit of platelets in the circulatory system. An autoimmune disorder often preceded by a viral infection, ITP may be acute and self-limiting or be chronic and require therapy. The peak age of occurrence is 2 to 4 years. Manifestations include bruising and petechiae.

Medical–Surgical Management

Medical

Diagnostic evaluation involves gathering a history of viral illness, information about any medications, and a CBC, which will be normal except for a low platelet level. If the history and CBC suggest ITP, bone marrow aspiration may be done to rule out oncological disorders. Most cases are self-limiting, with the platelet count returning to normal within 6 months without therapy. Platelet transfusions may be necessary for the child with chronic ITP if active, uncontrolled bleeding occurs.

Surgical

When drugs no longer control the thrombocytopenia in a child with chronic ITP, a splenectomy may be indicated. Splenectomy is usually not performed before 5

years of age because of the immaturity of the child's immune system.

Pharmacological

Steroids and immune globulin are given to block the autoimmune destruction of platelets.

Nursing Management

Encourage the curtailing of physical activities and sports until condition is resolved. Observe for signs of bleeding. Advise to use soft-bristled toothbrush. Assist parents to establish a safe, age-appropriate home environment. Teach family the signs and symptoms of infection.

NURSING PROCESS

Assessment

Subjective Data

Parents may bring their child to the doctor because of a "red rash" or bruising. The child's activity level may be reported to be normal.

Objective Data

Observe for further bleeding (e.g., epistaxis, hematuria, blood in stools) and level of consciousness.

Nursing diagnoses for the child with ITP may include the following:

Nursing Diagnoses	Planning/Goals	Nursing Interventions
Risk for Injury related to low platelet count	The client will be free of injury.	Have the child curtail physical activities and sports until platelets return to normal.
		Encourage the use of a soft-bristled toothbrush to minimize gum bleeding.
		Observe for signs of bleeding.
		Flush the catheter with saline to confirm proper placement of an IV line.

continues

Nursing Diagnoses	Planning/Goals	Nursing Interventions
*Deficient **K**nowledge (family)* related to disorder and treatment	The family will verbalize an understanding of the disorder and treatment.	Teach the family that ITP should subside within 6 months. Teach the family side effects of steroids, such as edema, insomnia, mood changes, poor healing, peptic ulcers, and growth retardation. Establish a safe, age-appropriate home environment (e.g., pad table corners, crib rails, and knees and elbows to decrease injury). Instruct parents to use nonaspirin analgesics and antipyretics. Evaluate the child's platelet count weekly.
*Risk for **I**nfection* related to chronic use of steroids and/or splenectomy	The client will be free of infection.	Teach the family the signs and symptoms of infection. Administer pneumococcus vaccine and/or daily antibiotics, if the child has a splenectomy.

Evaluation Each goal must be evaluated to determine how it has been met by the client.

HEMOPHILIA

Neonatal bleeding from the umbilical cord or circumcision site may be an early manifestation of severe hemophilia. Mild hemophilia may not be detected until the toddler becomes mobile, and unusual bruising and bleeding occur from small injuries.

Nursing interventions center on prevention and teaching. Regular physical exercise strengthens muscles and joints and may decrease the number of bleeding episodes. Adolescents who have seroconverted to human immunodeficiency virus– (HIV-) positive status must be especially knowledgeable about safe sexual behavior (see the sexually transmitted diseases chapter).

GASTROINTESTINAL SYSTEM

Because many gastrointestinal (GI) problems mimic each other, a thorough history and assessment are extremely important (VanBoxel & Puhl, 2001).

Gastrointestinal disorders in children interfere with nutrition and fluid and electrolyte balance and have the potential for impairing growth. Common GI disorders of childhood include constipation and parasitic infections.

CONSTIPATION

Constipation is the infrequent or difficult passage of hard, dry stools. It is most common during the toddler

CRITICAL THINKING

Fluid Volume Deficit

What is the most important data to gather when assessing a child for fluid volume deficit?

CLIENT TEACHING

Guidelines for Preventing Constipation in Children

For toddlers and preschool children:

- Increase cereal, fruit, vegetable, and fluid intake.
- Encourage sitting on the toilet for 5 to 10 minutes after breakfast and after dinner.

For school-age children:

- Allow 1 hour to finish breakfast before leaving for school to allow sufficient time for bathroom use.
- Encourage children to take responsibility for including cereals, fruits, vegetables, and fluids in their diets.
- Encourage children to exercise daily.
- Decrease the anxiety of children by taking time each day to communicate about their days, activities, concerns, and fears.

and preschool years because of the child's (and parents') efforts at toilet training. School-age children may experience constipation as a result of busy schedules, hesitation to use unfamiliar bathrooms, and limited bathroom privileges. Other potential causes of constipation include lack of fresh fruit and vegetables and grains in the diet, dehydration, lack of exercise, emotional stress, certain drugs, pain from passage of hard stool, excessive milk intake, and a variety of GI tract and systemic disorders and spinal lesions.

Chronic constipation causes an enlarged rectum, which impairs sphincter control, resulting in **encopresis** (the passage of watery colonic contents around a hard fecal mass). Predisposing factors for encopresis include inadequate or inconsistent toilet training or psychological stress such as that related to starting school or the birth of a sibling. Clinical manifestations of constipation include abdominal pain and cramping without distention; palpable, movable fecal mass and a large amount of stool inside rectum; diarrhea; malaise; anorexia; and headache.

Medical–Surgical Management

Medical

Abdominal x-rays may reveal a rectum enlarged with stool and gas. The impaction is removed with enemas.

▨ Pharmacological

Stool softeners or laxatives may be prescribed in an effort to retrain the rectum after the impaction has been removed. Mineral oil may be prescribed to decrease the pain of defecation.

Diet

Increasing water and fiber intake and limiting milk intake will often decrease constipation and promote defecation.

Health Promotion

Counseling may be part of the treatment plan, if there is no evidence of physiologic disorders. Establishing and maintaining regular toileting habits, drinking fluids, eating a high-fiber diet, and participating in regular exercise will also help prevent constipation.

Nursing Management

Focus on teaching parents about normal bowel patterns in children and the importance of diet and exercise in maintaining those patterns. Assess the child's diet history and elicit a description of bowel patterns to provide clues to the cause of constipation. Dietary changes may be all that is required to resolve constipation.

Requiring the child to sit on the toilet for 10 minutes approximately 30 minutes after meals encourages regular bowel habits. Caution parents about the overuse of laxatives, stool softeners, and enemas. Use of mineral oil may cause soiling from leakage, which should not be mistaken for encopresis.

INTESTINAL PARASITIC INFECTIONS

Common parasitic infections include giardiasis (a protozoan) and helminths (i.e., pinworms, roundworms, hookworms). Children are more commonly infected than adults because they frequently put their hands in their mouths. Temperate climates, crowded conditions (i.e., day care centers, schools), untreated water, and poor hygiene practices may contribute to outbreaks of parasitic infections. Appearance, mode of transmission, and clinical manifestations vary, depending on the parasite (Table 57-2).

TABLE 57-2   COMMON INTESTINAL PARASITES

	APPEARANCE	MODE OF TRANSMISSION	CLINICAL MANIFESTATIONS
Giardiasis	Microscopic	Ingested cysts Person to person Untreated water Contaminated food Animals Soil Feces	Diarrhea Weight loss Abdominal cramping
Pinworm	White, threadlike worm	Person to person Ingested or inhaled eggs	Itching around the anus Irritability Distractibility
Roundworm	Pink worm, 9–12 inches in length	Eggs passed from hand to mouth (may migrate to liver and lungs)	Abdominal pain, distention, or obstruction Vomiting Jaundice Pneumonitis
Hookworm	Microscopic	Skin penetration by contact with contaminated soil (may migrate to lungs)	Dermatitis Anemia Pneumonitis Malnutrition

Medical–Surgical Management

Medical

Identification of a parasitic infection is done with fecal smear or a microscopic examination. Pinworms may be diagnosed by using cellophane tape to capture eggs from around the anus and then examining them under a microscope.

Pharmacological

Helminths are treated with oral anthelmintic medications such as pyrantel pamoate (Antiminth) or mebendazole (Vermox). Medication should be repeated 2 to 3 weeks later to eliminate any parasites that may hatch after the initial treatment. All family members should also be treated.

Metronidazole (Flagyl) or quinacrine hydrochloride (Atabrine HCl) are effective in treating giardiasis. Alert child care providers to the possibility of a yellow discoloration to the skin for the child on quinacrine hydrochloride (Atabrine HCl).

Diet

A well-balanced diet with additional protein and iron may be prescribed for the child with hookworms. These nutrients may be depleted from blood loss and malnutrition.

Health Promotion

Attention to meticulous sanitary practices is essential.

Nursing Management

Assist with collection of specimens, treatment of infections, and prevention of reinfection. Collect stool specimens from diapers, potty chairs, or a toilet covered with clear plastic wrap. Use a tongue blade to place the specimen into the designated and properly labeled container. Provide parents with detailed instructions for performing the tape test (see the accompanying Home Health Care box). Provide education regarding the course of treatment and home care.

ENDOCRINE SYSTEM

A common endocrine disorder in children is type 1, formerly called insulin-dependent, diabetes. The management of diabetes in children presents some unique challenges because of their physical immaturity and dependence on family for care. Stabilizing insulin needs during puberty requires vigilant monitoring of the glucose level and regulating diet, insulin, and exercise. The lifestyle of the entire family must change in order to effectively treat the child with diabetes. Family members should be familiar with and adhere to the prescribed regimen. Most school-age children are ready and able to learn to give their own injections and should be encouraged to do so.

For medical–surgical management and nursing management of the client with endocrine disorders, see the endocrine system chapter.

An increasing number of children, up to 45% of those with diabetes, have type 2 diabetes (American Diabetes Association, 2000). Most of these children are overweight or obese. Testing for type 2 diabetes in children is shown in Table 57-3. They are usually treated initially with nutrition therapy and an exercise program. Eventually, most will require drug therapy. Most pediatric diabetologists use oral agents for children with type 2 diabetes (American Diabetes Association, 2000).

MUSCULOSKELETAL SYSTEM

Maximizing bone mass in childhood reduces the impact of bone loss related to aging. It is also a critical time

TABLE 57-3	RECOMMENDATIONS FOR TESTING CHILDREN FOR TYPE 2 DIABETES

Overweight: BMI greater than 85th percentile for age and sex, weight for height greater than 85th percentile, or weight greater than 120% of ideal for height

plus

Any two of the following risk factors:
- Family history of type 2 diabetes in first- or second-degree relative
- Being Native American, African American, Hispanic, or Asian/Pacific Islander
- Show signs of insulin resistance or conditions associated with insulin resistance such as **acanthosis nigricans**, a velvety hyperpigmented patch on back of neck, in axilla, or antecubital area; hypertension; dyslipidemia, or polycystic ovarian syndrome (PCOS)

Age for Testing:
At age 10 years or at onset of puberty, whichever occurs first, and then every two years

Test: Fasting plasma glucose (FPG) preferred

Source: American Diabetes Association. (2000). Type 2 diabetes in children and adolescents. *Diabetes Care,* *22*(12), 381. [Online]. Available: www.diabetes.org

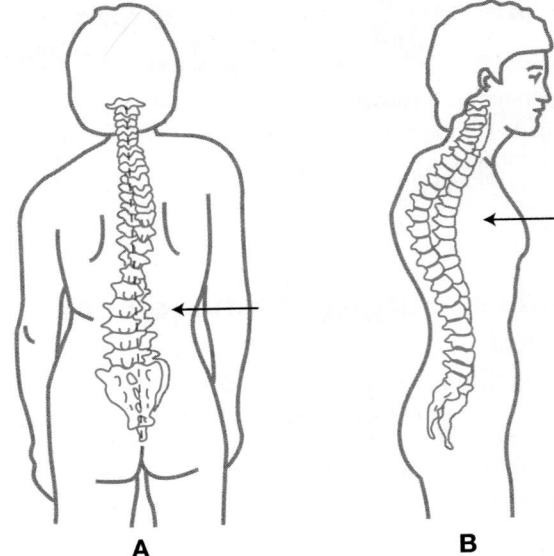

Figure 57-1 A, *Scoliosis;* **B,** *Kyphosis*

for developing lifestyle habits important to maintaining good bone health such as proper nutrition and physical activity (NIH, 2000).

Common musculoskeletal disorders in children include scoliosis, Legg-Calvé-Perthes disease, muscular dystrophy, juvenile arthritis, and fractures.

SCOLIOSIS

Scoliosis, the most common spinal deformity in children, involves lateral curvature greater than 20 degrees, spinal rotation, rib asymmetry, and thoracic hypokyphosis (Figure 57-1). It occurs most frequently in prepubescent girls and is usually not caused by any other injury or disease.

Clinical manifestations include visible curve of the spine, posterior rib hump when bending forward, asymmetrical rib cage, and uneven shoulder or pelvic heights. Parents may notice that the child's clothes do not fit properly (e.g., uneven hems).

Medical–Surgical Management

Medical

The goal of medical treatment is to stop the curvature of the spine. Early detection and treatment of scoliosis are essential to successful management. The treatment regimen depends on the degree and progression of the curvature and the reaction of the child and family. Children with mild curvatures may simply be monitored throughout the growth cycle. Electrical stimulation, bracing, and exercise may be prescribed for children with mild to moderate curvatures.

Surgical

Surgical intervention may be required for children with curvatures greater than 40 degrees. The goal of surgery is to correct the curvature of the spine with internal fixation and instrumentation.

Nursing Management

Involve child in the plan of care. Encourage child to perform exercises as prescribed. Provide suggestions to protect bony prominences when wearing a brace.

Postoperatively, assess extremities for color, capillary refill, warmth, sensation, and movement. Log roll the child every 2 hours. Monitor vital signs, for bowel distention, and urinary retention. Assess pain level and provide analgesics as ordered. Teach family about wound

---

LIFE CYCLE CONSIDERATIONS

Backpacks
A child should be able to stand up straight and maintain good posture when carrying a backpack. Therefore:

- Backpacks should be positioned above the child's buttocks.
- Both straps should be used instead of just one.
- The backpack should not be overloaded so the child has to lean forward when carrying it.

Source: Nemours. (2002). *School backpacks: How they affect your child's general health.* [Online]. Available: www.nemours.org/no/news/releases/2002/020206_backpack_study.html (accessed December 23, 2003) care. Discuss restrictions on activity. Emphasize importance of keeping follow-up appointments.

NURSING PROCESS

Assessment

Subjective Data

Initially, the child may complain of a sore back, improperly fitting clothing, or a slight limp. When being treated with a brace, assess the child for problems related to self-esteem and body image. Ask the child and parents to report on the degree of compliance with the prescribed regimen. If the child requires surgery, assess feelings and fears of the child and the family.

Objective Data

Screening for scoliosis is an important role of the nurse. Assess children 10 years of age and older. With clothes removed, observe the back for uneven shoulders and hips, prominent shoulder blade on one side, and curved spine. While bending at the waist and touching the toes, assess the child's back for a rib hump and curved spine (Figure 57-2).

When a brace is in place, continue monitoring the degree of curvature and assess the skin at pressure points

Figure 57-2 *Scoliosis screening reveals a rib hump and curved spine.*

for irritation. Progression of the curve may indicate either noncompliance with the prescribed treatment or the need for more aggressive therapy.

Postoperatively, the child is assessed for neurological status, pain, fluid balance, bleeding, and bowel and bladder function. Mobility and nutrition are quickly resumed if there are no complications.

Nursing diagnoses for the child with scoliosis may include the following:

Nursing Diagnoses	Planning/Goals	Nursing Interventions
*Deficient **K**nowledge (family and child)* related to lack of information about scoliosis, including treatment and surgery	The client and family will verbalize an understanding of and comply with the medical regimen.	Identify the client's and family's knowledge level and areas of concern. Inform the child and family that the brace must be worn for 16 to 23 hours/day for years. Inform the child and family that use of brace may eliminate need for surgery. If surgery is necessary, prepare the child and family for the need to log roll the child and the need for the child to cough and have them demonstrate preoperatively.
*Disturbed **B**ody Image* related to deformity, bracing, and surgical scar	The client will talk about feelings. The client will demonstrate self-confidence.	Involve the child in the plan of care. Provide the child with opportunities to ventilate feelings about being different. Encourage the child to talk about experiences with friends. Help the child select clothing that is stylish yet loose enough to fit over the brace. Help the child focus on positive body features (e.g., hair, complexion). Help the child select activities that will enhance abilities. Provide the child with privacy during hospitalization.
*Risk for Impaired **S**kin Integrity* related to wearing of a brace	The client's skin will remain intact.	Have the child wear a knit cotton shirt under the brace. Place a protective pad over bony prominences. Report reddened areas so that the brace can be adjusted.

continues

Nursing Diagnoses	Planning/Goals	Nursing Interventions
Impaired Physical **Mobility** related to restricted movement (brace/surgery)	The client will adjust to restricted movement.	Perform exercises as prescribed. Instruct the child in how to move with the brace (i.e., climb stairs, get in and out of a vehicle, chair, desk, and bed).
Risk for **Injury** related to neurovascular deficit secondary to instrumentation	The client will regain all body functions postoperatively.	Assess all extremities for color, capillary refill, warmth, sensation, and motion. Monitor signs of bowel distention and urinary retention. Maintain body alignment by logrolling every 2 hours and rolling from a side-lying position to a sitting position. Assist with early ambulation postoperatively.
Acute **Pain** related to operative procedure	The client will experience pain reduction to an acceptable level.	Assess pain level postoperatively, using pain scale. Provide prescribed analgesics around the clock for the first 24 to 48 hours. Explore alternate means of relieving pain (e.g., dim lights, music). Assess and document the child's response to relief measures.
Deficient **Knowledge** (family and child) related to home care	The client and family will successfully manage postoperative treatment at home.	Teach proper wound care. Discuss the importance of a well-balanced diet in maintaining healthy bones. Discuss activity restrictions (e.g., lifting no more than 10 pounds) and the length of time they will be in place. Have the child demonstrate moving without twisting or bending at the waist. Emphasize the importance of keeping follow-up appointments.

Evaluation Each goal must be evaluated to determine how it has been met by the client.

LEGG-CALVÉ-PERTHES DISEASE

Legg-Calvé-Perthes disease is necrosis of the head of the femur. The disease occurs most commonly in Caucasian boys between the ages of 4 and 8 years. The cause is unknown. Clinical manifestations include hip and knee soreness or stiffness, painful limp, and quadricep muscle atrophy.

Medical–Surgical Management

Medical

Diagnosis is made by x-ray. The goal of treatment is to maintain the shape of the femoral head and reduce the risk of permanent stiffness and degenerative arthritis. Methods used to accomplish this goal include traction, bracing, and surgery.

Initially, the child is hospitalized for non–weight-bearing range-of-motion exercises and bed rest. If there is no improvement within 10 days, alternate methods of treatment are usually begun.

Nonsurgical intervention may involve traction followed by the use of a non–weight-bearing abduction brace to position the femoral head in the acetabulum. Exercises maintain muscle integrity during the time that the child is required to wear the brace, for as long as 1 to 3 years.

Surgical

Surgical intervention is often the treatment of choice because it reduces treatment time and eliminates compliance problems. The child is usually able to resume normal activities in 3 to 4 months.

Nursing Management

Maintaining mobility and educating the child and family are the primary nursing goals. Encourage the family and child to adhere to treatment plans and keep follow-up visits. Demonstrate proper application of the abduction brace. Perform skin assessments daily. Encourage the child to maintain muscle integrity via prescribed exercises. Involvement in activities such as horseback riding and swimming may be permitted.

DUCHENNE MUSCULAR DYSTROPHY

Duchenne muscular dystrophy is an x-linked, recessive, hereditary, progressive, degenerative disease of the muscles. The disease occurs almost exclusively among males and is carried by females. Clinical manifestations include delayed motor development, difficulty standing or walking, progressive muscle weakness, increasing abnormalities in gait and posture, lordosis, pelvic waddling, frequent falling, **Gowers' sign** (walking the hands up legs to move from a sitting to a standing position), and a flat affect and smile. The disease continues into adolescence and young adulthood, when the client usually succumbs to respiratory failure. Children with Duchenne muscular dystrophy rarely live beyond 20 years of age. Complications include obesity, contractures, respiratory infections, and cardiac failure. Diagnosis is confirmed by serum enzyme assay, muscle biopsy, and electromyography.

Medical–Surgical Management

Medical

Initially, therapeutic management is aimed at maintaining ambulation and independence for as long as possible with bracing and physical therapy. Later, therapy is directed at maximizing sitting capabilities, respiratory function, and self-care. Genetic counseling is recommended for parents, female siblings, and maternal aunts and their female offspring.

Surgical

Contractures may be released surgically in order to keep the child as mobile as possible.

Nursing Management

Monitor children when there is a family history of muscular dystrophy. Encourage physical therapy exercise regimen and use of adaptive devices. Focus on the things the child can do.

NURSING PROCESS

Assessment

Subjective Data

When there is a family history of muscular dystrophy, monitor the child carefully. Assess both the family's ability to cope with a chronic, debilitating illness and the support systems available to the family.

Objective Data

Routinely monitor the child for mobility, self-care abilities, weight gain, and infections.

Nursing diagnoses for the child with Duchenne muscular dystrophy may include the following:

Nursing Diagnoses	Planning/Goals	Nursing Interventions
Impaired Physical Mobility related to progressive muscle wasting and contractures	The client will remain physically active.	Reinforce physical therapy exercise regimen. Encourage activity (e.g., school attendance, swimming). Encourage the use of adaptive equipment as needed (e.g., a back brace).
Self-Care Deficit (all) related to progressive weakness	The client will be able to perform activities of daily living (ADLs) as long as possible.	Instruct the family in ways to adapt the home as needed (e.g., grab bars, overhead sling, raised toilet, wheelchair access). Focus on those things the child can do to prevent frustration. Maintain the child's independence as long as possible (e.g., via an electric wheelchair and portable phone).
Compromised Coping, Family related to increased demands of care, financial burdens, and needs of other children	The family will cope effectively with the disease process.	Refer the family to resource and support groups. Assist the family in anticipating needs and coordinating services. Encourage involvement of extended family and friends. Encourage the family to express feelings.

Evaluation Each goal must be evaluated to determine how it has been met by the client.

JUVENILE ARTHRITIS

Juvenile arthritis (JA) is a systemic, multisystem disorder that affects the body's connective tissue; it is also known as an autoimmune inflammatory disease. There are many different forms of the disease, including juvenile rheumatoid arthritis.

Clinical manifestations include joint swelling accompanied by limited range of motion; pain; tenderness; and inflammation lasting longer than 6 weeks. Complications include blindness and disability. Prognosis is generally good with early detection and treatment.

Medical–Surgical Management

Medical

The goal of treatment is to maintain mobility and preserve joint function. The therapeutic regimen includes drugs, physical therapy, and/or surgery.

Surgical

Depending on the severity of the disease, surgery may be necessary to release contractures, correct leg-length discrepancies, and replace joints.

Pharmacological

Drug therapy includes aspirin, nonsteroidal anti-inflammatory drugs such as ibuprofen (Motrin) and naproxen (Naprosyn), slower-acting antirheumatic drugs such as gold sodium thiomalate (Myochrysine), and penicillamine (Cuprimine). Cytotoxic drugs may be used for severe disease that does not respond to other drugs. Corticosteroids may be used sparingly when the disease is life threatening.

Nursing Management

Refer to the Immune System chapter.

FRACTURES

Fractures in children tend to be less complicated and heal more quickly than do those in adults. The bones most commonly fractured in children include the clavicle, femur, tibia, humerus, wrist, and fingers. Fractures in the area of the epiphyseal plate (growth plate) can cause permanent damage and severely impair growth. Greenstick fractures are common among young children because of incomplete ossification. Evidence of old fractures in a young child suggests possible child abuse, whereas fractures in infants may indicate osteogenesis imperfecta (brittle bone disease).

Treatment usually involves realignment and immobilization using traction or closed manipulation and casting.

Refer to the Musculoskeletal System chapter for medical management and the nursing process.

IMMUNE SYSTEM

Infectious or communicable diseases are not life threatening to most children; however, children with immature or compromised immune systems are at greater risk of developing severe and even fatal complications as the result of communicable diseases.

COMMUNICABLE DISEASES

A communicable disease is an illness that is directly or indirectly transmitted from one person to another. Infants and young children are more susceptible to infectious diseases because their immune systems are not fully developed until 6 years of age, and their hygiene habits (e.g., covering the mouth when coughing) are lacking. Selected communicable diseases, along with causal agent, transmission mode, communicable period, incubation period, clinical manifestations, potential complications, treatment, and immunity conferment are listed in Table 57-4.

Nursing Management

Immunization is critical to the health of children. One of the goals of the U.S. government is to immunize 90% of children ages 15 to 35 months by the year 2010 (Healthy People 2010, 2000). Nurses and health care providers must be familiar with immunization schedules and the various frequent revisions to these schedules. The Advisory Committee on Immunization Practices (ACIP) of the U.S. Public Health Service Centers for Disease Control (CDC) and the American Academy of Pediatrics (AAP) Committee on Infectious Diseases are responsible for recommendations regarding vaccinations. Changes in recommendations are published in the *Morbidity and Mortality Weekly Report* for the ACIP and in *Pediatrics* for the AAP.

Recognize barriers to immunizations and be prepared to educate families about vaccine safety, administration, precautions, and contraindications. Barriers to immunization include long waiting lines, appointment-only systems, inaccessible clinic sites, and inability to speak English. Every opportunity must be taken to immunize children whenever they enter any health care facility.

Federal law requires health care providers to provide general information about immunizations before administration. This general information includes nature, prevalence, and risks of the disease; type of immunization product to be used; the expected benefits and the risk of side effects of the vaccine; and the need for accurate immunization records. If possible, provide this lengthy information before the immunization appointment so that families have time to read and understand the information and to ask questions. Otherwise, the health care provider must inform parents at the time of administration. Document informed consent of the parent(s).

Be knowledgeable about the safe administration of immunizations. This includes proper storage, reconstitution, sequence, injection site, and technique.

TABLE 57-4 SELECT COMMON COMMUNICABLE DISEASES

DISEASE (CAUSAL AGENT)	TRANSMISSION MODE AND COMMUNICABLE PERIOD	INCUBATION PERIOD	CLINICAL MANIFESTATIONS AND POTENTIAL COMPLICATIONS	TREATMENT AND IMMUNITY CONFERMENT
Chicken pox (varicella-zoster virus, Figure 57-3)	*Transmission mode:* direct contact, respiratory droplet, airborne particles *Communicable period:* 1 day before lesions appear until all lesions crust over	10–21 days	*Clinical manifestations:* Fever, malaise, irritability, and a rash that begins as macules and progresses to fluid-filled papules to crusted lesions. *Potential complications:* Reye's syndrome, skin infections, encephalitis	*Treatment:* antihistamines, baths, and lotions for itching *Immunity conferment:* Natural or with vaccine; may reactivate in adults as herpes zoster
Diphtheria (*Corynebacterium diphtheriae*)	*Transmission mode:* direct contact, contact with contaminated articles, or consumption of unpasteurized milk *Communicable period:* 2 to 4 weeks in presence of antibiotic treatment, months without treatment	2–5 days	*Clinical manifestations:* Fever, cough, pharyngitis, anorexia, membranous lesion on tonsils, pharynx, or larynx *Potential complications:* neuritis, carditis, congestive heart failure, respiratory failure	*Treatment:* Isolation, antitoxin, antibiotics, and analgesics *Immunity conferment:* diphtheria, tetanus, and acellular pertussis (DTaP) vaccine; passive immunity conferred by maternal antibodies
Erythema infectiosum, or Fifth disease (Parvovirus B19, Figure 57-4)	*Transmission mode:* Contact with respiratory secretions and blood *Communicable period:* unknown	4–20 days	*Clinical manifestations:* Fiery-red cheeks ("slapped face" appearance); erythematous, maculopapular, lacy rash on trunk then limbs *Potential complications:* none	*Treatment:* Supportive *Immunity conferment:* no vaccine
Hepatitis B, or serum hepatitis (hepatitis B virus [HBV])	*Transmission mode:* blood, secretions, prenatally, perinatally, sexual contact *Communicable period:* Throughout clinical course	50–180 days	*Transmission mode:* mild flulike symptoms, jaundice in adolescents *Potential complications:* Liver failure	*Treatment:* supportive care *Immunity conferment:* hepatitis B vaccine (Hep B)
Measles, or rubeola (measles virus, Figure 57-5)	*Transmission mode:* direct or indirect contact with respiratory droplets	10–21 days	*Clinical manifestations:* fever, runny nose, cough, enlarged lymph nodes, Koplik's spots (small, red spots with blue-white	*Treatment:* supportive care

continues

Figure 57-3 *Varicella (Courtesy of Robert A. Silverman, M.D., Clinical Associate Professor, Department of Pediatrics, Georgetown University)*

Figure 57-4 *"Slapped Face" in Erythema Infectiousum (Fifth Disease) (Courtesy of the Centers for Disease Control and Prevention [CDC])*

Figure 57-5 *Rubeola/Measles (Courtesy of the Centers for Disease Control and Prevention [CDC])*

TABLE 57-4 continued

DISEASE (CAUSAL AGENT)	TRANSMISSION MODE AND COMMUNICABLE PERIOD	INCUBATION PERIOD	CLINICAL MANIFESTATIONS AND POTENTIAL COMPLICATIONS	TREATMENT AND IMMUNITY CONFERMENT
	Communicable period: 4 days before to 5 days after appearance of rash		centers on oral mucosa, Figure 57-6), photophobia, maculopapular rash from hairline over entire body *Potential complications:* otitis media, pneumonia, encephalitis, airway obstruction	*Immunity conferment:* measles, mumps, rubella (MMR) vaccine *Active:* from infection with causative agent
Mononucleosis (Epstein-Barr virus)	*Transmission mode:* direct contact with saliva; blood transfusions; most common in adolescents and young adults *Communicable period:* Unknown	30–50 days	*Clinical manifestations:* fever, pharyngitis, fatigue, sore throat, enlarged lymph nodes *Potential complications:* splenic rupture, hepatitis, meningitis, encephalitis, Guillain-Barré syndrome	*Treatment:* supportive care, antipyretics, analgesics *Immunity conferment:* no vaccine
Mumps, or parotitis (paramyxovirus)	*Transmission mode:* direct or indirect contact with saliva *Communicable period:* 7 days before swelling until 2 to 3 days after swelling subsides	14–21 days	*Clinical manifestations:* fever; headache; malaise; anorexia; "earache" aggravated by chewing; enlarged parotid gland (Figure 57-7) *Potential complications:* orchitis, meningoencephalitis, hearing loss	*Treatment:* supportive care, antipyretics, analgesics *Immunity conferment:* MMR vaccine; natural; passive: mumps immune globulin
Pertussis, or whooping cough (*Bordetella pertussis*)	*Transmission mode:* direct contact or respiratory droplets *Communicable period:* 1 week after exposure until 4 to 6 weeks	5–21 days	*Clinical manifestations:* upper respiratory symptoms progressing to severe paroxysmal cough with inspiratory whoop *Potential complications:* pneumonia, otitis media, hemorrhage, convulsions	*Treatment:* antibiotics, supportive care with high humidity *Immunity conferment:* DTaP vaccine; active: from infection with causative agent

Figure 57-6 *Koplik's Spots in Rubeola (Courtesy of the Centers for Disease Control and Prevention [CDC])*

Figure 57-7 *Mumps (Courtesy of the Centers for Disease Control and Prevention [CDC])*

Figure 57-8 *Roseola (Courtesy of Robert A. Silverman, M.D., Clinical Associate Professor, Department of Pediatrics, Georgetown University)*

Figure 57-9 *Rubella (German measles/3-day measles) (Courtesy of the Centers for Disease Control and Prevention [CDC])*

TABLE 57-4 continued

DISEASE (CAUSAL AGENT)	TRANSMISSION MODE AND COMMUNICABLE PERIOD	INCUBATION PERIOD	CLINICAL MANIFESTATIONS AND POTENTIAL COMPLICATIONS	TREATMENT AND IMMUNITY CONFERMENT
Poliomyelitis, or infantile paralysis (poliovirus types I, II, III)	*Transmission mode:* fecal–oral, respiratory droplets *Communicable period:* unknown prior to symptoms, 1 week after symptoms for respiratory contact, up to 6 weeks for fecal contact	5–14 days	*Clinical manifestations:* fever, headache, adominal pain, stiff neck, pain and tenderness in lower extremities, paralysis *Potential complications:* permanent paralysis, respiratory arrest	*Treatment:* supportive, rehabilitative care *Immunity conferment:* poliovirus vaccine (inactivated) [IPV] or live oral [OPV]); active: immunity against a specific strain conferred by disease
Roseola, or exanthema subitum (herpesvirus type 6, Figure 57-8)	*Transmission mode:* unknown; Unknown appears between 6 months and 2 years of age *Communicable period:* unknown	Unknown	*Clinical manifestations:* rose-pink, nonpruitic maulopapules on trunk then face, neck, and limbs that fade on pressure *Potential complications:* febrile seizures	*Treatment:* antipyretics, supportive care *Immunity conferment:* no vaccine
Rubella, or German measles, 3-day measles (Rubella virus, Figure 57-9)	*Transmission mode:* airborne, direct contact with droplets, transplacental *Communicable period:* 10 days before symptoms and 15 days after rash appears	14–21 days	*Clinical manifestations:* fever, headache, malaise, runny nose, anorexia, maculopapular rash progressing from head to extremities *Potential complications:* risks for unborn fetus of infected mother; spontaneous abortion, stillbirth, ear, eye, and cardiac anomalies	*Treatment:* supportive care *Immunity conferment:* MMR vaccine
Scarlet fever, or scarlatina (group A *beta-hemolytic streptococci*, Figure 57-10)	*Transmission mode:* airborne respiratory droplets and contaminated articles *Communicable period:* from onset of symptoms until 24 hours after antibiotic therapy is initiated	1–7 days	*Clinical manifestations:* fever, headache, "strawberry tongue," abdominal pain, sore throat, skin on hands and feet peels in sheets after first week *Potential complications:* glomerulonephritis, rheumatic fever	*Treatment:* penicillin, antipyretics, analgesics *Immunity conferment:* no immunity
Tetanus, or lockjaw (*Clostridium tetani*)	*Transmission mode:* direct contact of skin wound with contaminated soil or implements *Communicable period:* not communicable	3–21 days	*Clinical manifestations:* stiffness of neck and jaw, difficulty breathing *Potential complications:* laryngospasm, death	*Treatment:* supportive care *Immunity conferment:* DTaP vaccine: passive: from tetanus antitoxin or immune globulin (TIG)

Figure 57-10 *Scarlet Fever (Courtesy of the Centers for Disease Control and Prevention [CDC])*

The nurse is responsible for documenting on the child's immunization record the type of vaccine, the date of administration, the manufacturer and lot number, the expiration date, and the administration site. Encourage parents to keep and provide immunization records at every health care visit.

INTEGUMENTARY SYSTEM

Because they are visible and often disfiguring, skin disorders can prove emotionally and psychologically stressful for the child and family. It is important to teach families and children strategies to maintain healthy skin. Skin disorders may be caused by infections (bacterial, fungal, viral), infestations (pediculosis, scabies), insects, substances (contact dermatitis), acne, and injuries such as burns.

BACTERIAL INFECTIONS

Bacterial infections of the skin are usually caused by staphylococci or streptococci. The two most common skin disorders of childhood resulting from bacterial infections are impetigo and cellulitis.

IMPETIGO

Impetigo, the most common skin infection of childhood, often begins in an area of broken skin, such as that caused by an insect bite or eczema. The face, mouth, hands, neck, and extremities are the most common sites.

Clinical manifestations include primary lesions (macules that change rapidly to form small, thin-walled vesicles with an erythematous halo), secondary lesions (ruptured vesicles covered by a honey-colored crust over an ulcerated base), pruritus, burning, and lymph node enlargement (Figure 57-11). Lesions usually resolve within 2 weeks. Because impetigo is commonly caused by streptococci, rheumatic fever or glomerulonephritis are possible complications.

Figure 57-11 *Impetigo (Courtesy of Robert A. Silverman, M.D., Clinical Associate Professor, Departments of Pediatrics, Georgetown University)*

COMMUNITY/HOME HEALTH CARE

Preventing Children from Scratching Lesions
To prevent children from scratching lesions:

- Cut the fingernails short.
- Give cool baths.
- Cover the lesions with clothing, when possible.
- At nighttime, cover the hands with socks or gloves.
- During the day, encourage activities that require use of the hands; and administer antihistamines or sedatives as needed to control itching.
- Keep the child cool.

Medical–Surgical Management
Pharmacological

A topical bactericidal ointment such as polymyxin B sulfate-neomycin (Neosporin) is applied for 5 to 7 days. Children with multiple lesions may require oral antibiotics such as erythromycin (AK-Mycin). In extreme and extended situations, parenteral antibiotics may be required.

Nursing Management

The primary nursing goals are to prevent the spread of infection and promote healing. The child with impetigo is treated at home and should not return to school for 2 days after antibiotics are initiated. Emphasize the importance of taking antibiotics as prescribed.

Encourage caregivers to employ preventive hygiene practices such as sleeping alone, bathing daily with antibacterial soap, using a separate towel, washing hands properly, and using separate eating utensils. Wash the lesions gently three times per day with a warm, soapy washcloth. Remove soaked crusts and apply topical bactericidal ointment. A small amount of bleeding after crust removal is common. Leave the lesions uncovered. Teach children to keep their fingers away from the lesions.

CELLULITIS

Cellulitis is a bacterial infection of the skin and subcutaneous tissue. The condition usually affects the face (buccal and periorbital regions) or lower extremities. Children with cellulitis have a history of trauma, impetigo, upper-respiratory infections, sinusitis, otitis media, or tooth abscess. Common causative organisms are staphylococci and streptococci. Clinical manifestations include rapid onset of red or lilac color; tender, hot, edematous skin; and enlarged lymph nodes. Possible complications of cellulitis include septic arthritis, osteomyelitis, meningitis, brain abscess, or blindness.

Medical–Surgical Management
Medical

Cellulitis of the extremities is usually treated at home with oral antibiotics and warm compresses. Cellulitis involving the joints or face is extremely serious, requiring hospitalization and IV antibiotics.

Surgical

Incision and drainage of the affected area may be necessary if the condition does not improve with treatment.

Nursing Management

Elevate the affected extremity and immobilize. Apply warm, moist soaks every 4 hours to increase circulation to the affected area, relieve pain, and promote healing. Inform parents that failure to administer the entire course of antibiotics as ordered may result in a more serious infection.

FUNGAL INFECTIONS

Fungal infections are named using the term *tinea* (ringworm) followed by the Latin word for the affected part of the body (Table 57-5).

Nursing Management

Adequate teaching is essential for successful treatment of tinea. Apply lotion and cream to the entire lesion and extending to approximately 1 inch beyond the lesion. Take oral medication for the full course of treatment, even if symptoms disappear. Proper hygiene is essential.

VIRAL INFECTIONS

Viral skin infections can produce lesions such as rashes, macules, papules, vesicles, urticaria (hives), and warts. Common communicable diseases of childhood that produce rashes and are preventable through immunizations include rubeola, rubella, and varicella (refer back to Table 57-3). Herpes simplex virus type 1 is a common, contagious skin infection for which there is no cure or prevention.

HERPES SIMPLEX VIRUS TYPE 1

Herpes simplex virus type 1 (HSV-1) is an often recurrent infection of the mouth ("cold sore," "fever blister"), throat, eyes, or fingers (Figure 57-12). After initial infection, the virus remains dormant within nerve cells and can be reactivated by fever, stress, trauma, sun exposure, menstruation, or immunosuppression. Children suffering from burns, eczema, diaper rash, or immunosuppression are particularly susceptible to HSV-1. Clinical manifestations include clusters of fluid-filled vesicles; ulcerations; swelling; inflammation; pruritus; and severe pain. Lesions usually dry and crust within 7 to 10 days.

Medical–Surgical Management
Medical

Given that there is no cure for HSV-1, treatment is directed toward relieving symptoms. Usually, children are

---

TABLE 57-5 COMMON FUNGAL INFECTIONS

INFECTION (SITES)	CLINICAL MANIFESTATIONS	AFFECTED POPULATION	TREATMENT AND PREVENTION
Tinea capitis (scalp)	Erythema, pruritus, scaly scalp with round patches of alopecia	2- to 10-year-old children	*Treatment:* oral griseofulvin (Fulvicin P/G, Grifulvin V) *Prevention:* avoid sharing combs, barber scissors, hats, and towels; avoid direct contact with infected scalp
Tinea corporis (trunk, face, extremities)	Ringlike, scaly plaques measuring $1/2$ to 1 inch and having pale centers and red margins	Young boys living in hot, humid climates	*Treatment:* antifungal cream applied three times per day until lesions have been gone for 1 week (usually 2 to 4 weeks). *Prevention:* treat infected pets
Tinea pedis (feet, toes; "athletes foot")	Fissures, red scaly lesions	Adolescents and adults	*Treatment:* daily washing and application of antifungal cream for up to 6 weeks. *Prevention:* avoid contaminated floors, sidewalks, and showers; nylon socks; plastic shoes; closed shoes
Tinea cruris (inner thighs, inguinal area; "jock itch")	Scaly lesions, erythema, pruritus, possible papules or vesicles	Most commonly, athletes and obese individuals	*Treatment:* oral griseofulvin (Fulvicin P/G, Grifulvin V), sitz baths to soothe *Prevention:* wear loose-fitting undergarments to promote dryness

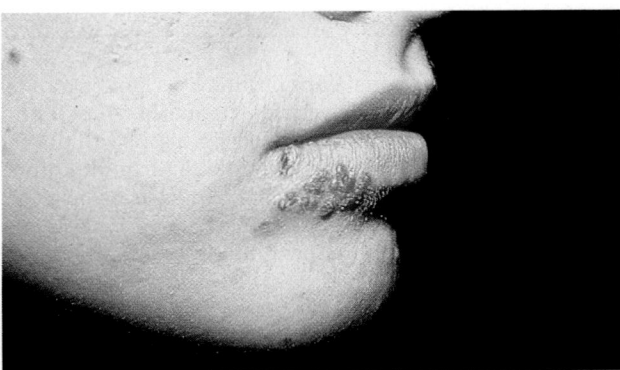

Figure 57-12 *Herpes Simplex Virus Type 1 (Courtesy of Robert A. Silverman, M.D., Clinical Associate Professor, Department of Pediatrics, Georgetown University)*

managed at home by ensuring adequate hydration, pain management, and secondary-infection prevention.

Pharmacological

Antibiotic ointment may be used to treat secondary infections. Acetaminophen (with or without codeine) and topical and mouth-rinse anesthetics may be prescribed for pain relief.

Nursing Management

Monitor for dehydration resulting from painful swallowing and for prevention of secondary infection. Offer frozen ice pops, Jell-O, noncitrus juices, milk, and flat sodas to help ensure adequate fluid intake despite painful swallowing. Encourage small, frequent feedings of bland, soft foods. Reassure parents that fluids are more important than solid food for the first few days.

Teach child to keep hands away from lesions to prevent spreading it to other areas.

Place the hospitalized child in contact isolation or under drainage and secretion precautions. The child is considered contagious until lesions have fallen off or mucous membrane ulcerations have healed.

INFESTATIONS

Infestations are one of the major health problems in schools. Common infestations are pediculosis and scabies.

PEDICULOSIS

Pediculosis (lice) is an infestation that most typically affects the head (capitis), body (corporis), or pubic area (pubis). Pediculosis of the head is the most common infestation seen in children. Lice attach their eggs (nits) to hair shafts close to the scalp. The nits then hatch in approximately 1 week. Clinical manifestations of head lice infestation include "dandruff" (nits) that is not easily removed, severe itching of the scalp, and "bugs" in the hair (usually behind the ears and at the back of the head) (Figure 57-13). Signs and symptoms of body lice infestation include intense pruritus and papular, rose-colored dermatitis in areas under tight-fitting clothing. Lice are easily passed from child to child in close-contact situations (e.g., the home, day care centers, and schools) via the sharing of headgear, hair-care products, pillows, blankets, and towels.

Medical–Surgical Management

Pharmacological

Several anti-lice products are available (Table 57-6).

COMMUNITY/HOME HEALTH CARE

Caring for the Child with HSV-1

- Wear gloves when suctioning or providing oral care and when handling soiled linens and clothing.
- Practice proper hand hygiene (remembering to wash hands after removing gloves).
- Wash all eating utensils and towels in hot, soapy water.
- Do not eat after the child.
- Prevent the child from putting the fingers in the mouth (using elbow restraints on infants, if needed).
- Use a protective cover such as a sheet when holding and cuddling the child.
- Provide oral fluids that do not irritate the mucous membrane, such as noncitrus juices, flat sodas, milk, and ice pops.
- Provide at least 100 mL (approximately $^1/_2$ cup) /kg/day for a child weighing less than 20 kg.
- Watch for signs of dehydration, such as dry skin and mucous membranes and decreased urine output (<3 to 4 times/day).
- Administer medications as prescribed.

PROFESSIONAL TIP

Checking for Lice

Because lice do not transmit from hair to hands, the use of gloves during head checks is neither necessary nor cost effective.

PROFESSIONAL TIP

Manual Removal of Lice

The National Pediculosis Association advocates early detection and manual removal of nits and lice to prevent the unnecessary use of chemical such as lindane.

Figure 57-13 *Nits (Courtesy of Hogil Pharmaceutical Corporation)*

TABLE 57-6   ANTI-LICE PRODUCTS

PRODUCT	TREATMENT	EFFECT
lindane (Kwell, Scabene)	Apply to hair, leave on for 4 to 5 minutes, and rinse out of hair with water; reapply in 1 week to kill hatched nits	Kills lice but does *not* effectively kill nits; may be reabsorbed through the skin and cause neurotoxicity
permethrin (Nix)	Apply to shampooed hair, leave on for 10 minutes, and rinse out of hair with water; do not re-shampoo for 24 hours	Safely kills lice and nits with one application
pyrethrins (TripleX, RID)	Apply to hair as directed; repeat treatment in 1 to 2 weeks, if live nits are present	Safely kills lice and nits; product of choice for those under 2 years of age and for pregnant adolescents

Nursing Management

Nursing care for children with pediculosis focuses on screening and education. Encourage parents and teachers to incorporate checking for lice into routine daily hygiene. Early detection facilitates immediate removal. There is no need to cut long hair or to shave the child's head, which only draws more attention to the fact that the child is infested.

Teach children that anyone can get lice and that taunting a child who has lice may hurt the child's feelings. Because lice are transmitted from person to person, children should be cautioned about using hair-care products, hats, pillows, blankets, and towels that do not belong to them.

SCABIES

Scabies results from the impregnated "itch mite" burrowing into the epidermis to lay her eggs. Clinical manifestations include intense pruritus and rash (papules, vesicles, and nodules) found most often on the wrists, finger webs, elbows, axillae, feet, ankles, head, neck, abdomen, waist, groin, and buttocks (Figure 57-14). Secondary infections often occur as a result of scratching the lesions.

Medical–Surgical Management
Pharmacological

Lindane (Kwell, Scabene) lotion (refer back to Table 57-6) is recommended for children and family members older than 2 years of age. Crotamiton (Eurax) lotion is used for children younger than 2 years of age because it is considered less toxic than lindane. An oral antihistamine such as diphenhydramine hydrochloride (Benadryl) or hydroxyzine (Atarax) may be prescribed to relieve pruritus.

Nursing Management

Nursing management for the child with scabies focuses on promoting healing, preventing secondary infections, and preventing further transmission of the condition. All persons having direct contact with the child, including care providers and those living in the child's

Figure 57-14 *Scabies (Courtesy of Robert A. Silverman, M.D., Clinical Associate Professor, Department of Pediatrics, Georgetown University)*

house, should be treated. Itching and rash may endure for 2 to 3 weeks.

BITES/STINGS

Animals (usually dogs), spiders, ticks, and insects (e.g., mosquitoes, fleas) account for the many bites and stings suffered by children. Bites and stings generally cause mild discomfort and are simple to treat; however, in some cases, life-threatening situations result.

ANIMAL BITES

Animal bites may result from domestic or wild animals but are most commonly caused by a familiar dog. Children younger than 4 years of age are bitten most frequently because of their height and the associated tendency to be near the dog's face. Dog bites usually occur on the face or extremities and can result in crushing and puncture wounds and lacerations.

Medical–Surgical Management

Medical

The primary medical concerns for the child who has suffered an animal bite are infections from rabies and tetanus and scarring, especially on the face. Generally, after the wound and surrounding area are thoroughly washed with mild soap and water, a clean dressing is applied.

Pharmacological

If the animal is unvaccinated for rabies, the child will be given a series of immunizations to prevent rabies. Antibiotics may be indicated if the wounds are deep. Tetanus toxoid may be administered, depending on the child's immunization history and the severity of the wound.

Nursing Management

Focus on prevention and wound care. It is important for children to learn "animal safety rules" in order to prevent bites.

CLIENT TEACHING

Animal Safety Rules

- Stay away from strange or wild animals such as raccoons, skunks, bats, and squirrels.
- Stay away from a dog's face.
- Pet animals by rubbing, stroking, scratching, and patting; never hit, bite, or pinch.
- Allow unfamiliar animals to smell you before attempting to touch them.
- Ask the permission of the owner before petting an animal.
- Never approach an animal while it is eating, sleeping, injured, or tending to its babies.

Teach parents and children to cleanse wounds properly and observe for signs of infection. Encourage parents to keep their child's immunizations up to date. If rabies immunizations are required, parents must understand the importance of returning for the injections on the appropriate days. Report animal bites to the community animal control agency.

SPIDER BITES

Bites from black widow and brown recluse spiders demand medical attention. Characteristically, these spiders are nonagressive, avoid light, and bite only in self-defense. Although both spiders inject toxic venom when they bite, the initial bite may go unnoticed. Within a few hours after the bite, however, manifestations such as swollen, painful erythema and systemic reactions surface. Black widow venom is neurotoxic and may cause dizziness, weakness, abdominal pain, paralysis, seizures, and, possibly, death from shock and renal failure. Brown recluse venom is necrotoxic, with the bite progressing to a necrotic ulcer within 1 to 2 weeks. Systemic reactions may include fever, nausea and vomiting, and joint pain. The recluse bite is not fatal, but the ulcer may take months to heal.

Medical–Surgical Management

Medical

The child with a black widow spider bite will be hospitalized for supportive care until neurological symptoms subside and renal function is confirmed. The child with a brown recluse bite will require wound care and pain management but will usually not require hospitalization.

Surgical

Skin grafting may be required for large ulcers resulting from the brown recluse spider bite.

Pharmacological

Antivenin (Lactrodectus mactans) is administered to the child with a black widow spider bite, if the child has no allergy to horse serum. In addition, analgesics, muscle relaxants, and tetanus prophylaxis may be required.

There is no antivenin for the brown recluse spider bite. Antibiotics, corticosteroids, analgesics, and tetanus prophylaxis may be prescribed for the time during which the wound is healing.

Nursing Management

Focus on wound care, proper administration of medications, and prevention. Teach parents and children to be cautious in areas where spiders are likely to live, such as woodpiles and closets.

TICK BITES

Ticks live in fields and woods. They feed on the blood of mammals (e.g., humans, dogs, livestock, and deer) by embedding their heads into the skin. Tick bites cause pruritic nodules at the site of attachment and, rarely, systemic reactions such as fever, rash, and paralysis.

Figure 57-15 *Contact Dermatitis (Courtesy of the Centers for Disease Control and Prevention [CDC])*

Lyme disease and Rocky Mountain spotted fever are caused by organisms that are transmitted by ticks.

Nursing Management

Preventing tick bites and removing embedded ticks are the primary focus. Remove ticks by applying vaseline or nail polish for 30 minutes to suffocate the tick. Then grasp the tick's body with tweezers and pull straight up in an attempt to remove the embedded head along with the body. Remove any remaining part of the head using a sterile needle. Then thoroughly cleanse hands.

INSECT BITES

Insects such as mosquitoes, flies, fleas, and gnats inject foreign proteins when they penetrate the skin to suck blood. Insect bites usually result in itching, erythema, and a small wheal. The severity of the reaction depends on the degree of the child's hypersensitivity.

Medical–Surgical Management

Medical

Medical management focuses on alleviating itching and preventing infection. Baths and cool compresses may relieve itching and prevent scratching, which can lead to bacterial infections.

Pharmacological

Antipruritics and antihistamines may be prescribed to control severe itching and facilitate sleep.

Nursing Management

Focus on preventing bites, alleviating itching, and preventing infection. Mattresses, carpets, furniture, and pets may require treatment with insecticides.

CONTACT DERMATITIS

Contact dermatitis is an inflammatory reaction of the skin to allergens, such as rubber, dyes, nickel, or poison ivy, or to irritants, such as soaps, wool, urine, or stool. Manifestations of allergic contact dermatitis include tiny, itching, weeping blisters over an area of skin (Figure 57-15). Manifestations of irritant contact dermatitis include localized, dry, inflamed, pruritic skin.

Medical–Surgical Management

Medical

Treatment involves discontinuing exposure to the offending agent, washing the skin thoroughly, and applying cool compresses.

Pharmacological

Steroid cream (1%) may be applied in a thin layer several times per day after the application of cool compresses. Oral steroids may be prescribed for severe cases.

Nursing Management

Nursing care is aimed at relieving itching, preventing infection, and identifying and removing offensive substances. In addition to cool compresses, oral antihistamines, antipruritic lotions, and tepid Aveeno baths may relieve itching. Avoid overheating. Teach children to recognize and avoid poison ivy, oak, and sumac.

ACNE

Acne, one of the most common health problems of adolescence, is a noninfectious, inflammatory disease of the skin involving the sebaceous glands and hair follicles (Figure 57-16). Pathophysiologic factors having the greatest influence on acne development are overproduction of sebum; formation of **comedones,** or whiteheads and blackheads (Figure 57-17); and proliferation of *Propionibacterium acnes* bacteria in the hair follicles (Hurwitz, 1995).

Manifestations include comedones, papules, pustules, and nodules on the face, neck, back, shoulders, and upper chest. Factors related to the development of acne include elevated hormone levels (especially androgens); predisposition; emotional stress; hot, humid environments; the premenstrual period, in females; and the growth of anaerobic bacteria. The visual lesions of acne, although usually temporary, may be extremely distressing to the adolescent, who is typically very concerned about appearance.

Figure 57-16 *Acne (From* Acne Vulgaris, *by G. Plewig and A. B. Klingmann (Eds.), 1975, Berlin/Heideberg, Germany: Springer-Verlag. Used with permission.)*

Figure 57-17 *Open Comedones (From* Acne Vulgaris, *by G. Plewig and A. B. Kligmann (Eds.), 1975, Berlin/Heideberg, Germany: Springer-Verlag. Used with permission.)*

Medical–Surgical Management

Pharmacological

Treatment is individualized, depending on the severity and types of lesions. The goal is to decrease sebum production and prevent infection with *P. acnes*. Topical agents benzoyl peroxide (Clearasil, Benoxyl) and tretinoin (Retin-A) are available as cleansers, lotions, creams, sticks, pads, gels, and bars and may be effective for mild cases. Other topical keratolytic agents containing sulfur, resorcinol, or salicylic acid may be prescribed for drying and peeling effects. Topical or oral antibiotics, such as erythromycin and tetracycline preparations, may be administered for infections.

CLIENT TEACHING

Isotretinoin (Accutane)

It is important that adolescent females on isotretinoin who are sexually active use contraceptives 1 month before treatment is started; during treatment; and 1 month after discontinuation of treatment. In addition, clients taking isotretinoin should not donate blood during this period.

Isotretinoin (Accutane) may be used for nodulocystic acne. Side effects of isotretinoin include dry lips and skin, eye irritation, temporary worsening of acne, **epistaxis** (nosebleed), bleeding and inflammation of the gums, itching, photosensitivity, and joint and muscle pain. In addition, isotretinoin may cause central nervous system, heart, thymus, and craniofacial abnormalities in the fetus.

If isotretinoin is to be prescribed, pregnancy tests are done 2 weeks before initiating, every month during, and 1 month after discontinuing the treatment. All women of childbearing potential are placed on contraception during treatment.

Nursing Management

A healthy lifestyle, including adequate rest, exercise, and diet, promotes healing of lesions. Be especially sensitive to the adolescent's feelings about the condition, no matter how mild the case may seem.

Educate the adolescent and family about acne and the prescribed treatment. Adolescents should take responsibility for implementing the prescribed care.

BURNS

Burns are the second leading cause of injury deaths among children between 1 and 14 years of age (James, Ashwill, & Droske, 2002). Carelessness of adults, the children's curiosity and increasing mobility, and caretakers' failure to adequately supervise children all contribute to the high incidence of burns among children. In addition, burns are a common form of child abuse (Herrin & Antoon, 2000). Thermal burns (e.g., from scalding liquids, house fires) are most common, followed by chemical (e.g., from touching or ingesting caustic agents) and electrical (e.g., from wires, curling irons, ovens), respectively.

The major manifestations of burns include severe wounds, pain, fluid and nutritional deficits, respiratory complications, and secondary infections. All systems of the burned child are at risk for complications.

Smoke inhalation can be fatal. Toxic fumes from burning plastics, polyurethanes, and many fabrics cause cyanide poisoning. Carbon monoxide and cyanide inhalation have the same signs and symptoms: nausea, vomiting, lethargy, confusion, tachycardia, metabolic acidosis, and possibly seizures and coma (Lewis, 1999).

Medical–Surgical Management

Medical

The severity of the burn injury is assessed on the basis of the percentage of surface burned and the depth of the wound. The Burn Wheel provides an accurate estimate of percentage of body surface area burn in children and by turning the wheel to align the correct values for weight and burns, it provides the amount of fluid resuscitation and continuation needed (Figure 57-18).

The involvement of specific body parts or certain specific burn distributions increase burn severity, regardless of body surface area affected. Burns to the face, hands, feet, perineal area, or anterior chest, and circumferential burns of the thorax or extremity are treated as major because of the potential for functional impairment. Regardless of the amount of tissue destroyed, if smoke inhalation is suspected, there is risk for airway obstruction.

Pharmacological

Tetanus antitoxin or toxoid should be ordered according to the child's immunization status. Intravenous morphine sulfate is the drug of choice for pain control. Analgesics must be administered 20 to 30 minutes before dressing changes and debridement to provide the most relief possible. Itching may persist for months and may be relieved with medication.

Figure 57-18 *The Burn Wheel (Invented by Stephen M. Milner)*

Health Promotion

Prevention of scarring and contractures is essential for optimal cosmetic and functional recovery. Pressure dressings and suits may need to be worn for more than 1 year to minimize scarring. Physical therapy, initiated at the time of admission and continued until the scars mature, prevents flexion contractures. These treatments add to the child's discomfort.

Nursing Management

Refer to the Integumentary System chapter for information on nursing management of the client who has been burned.

URINARY SYSTEM

Acute poststreptococcal glomerulonephritis, nephrotic syndrome, and enuresis are discussed following.

ACUTE POSTSTREPTOCOCCAL GLOMERULONEPHRITIS

Glomerulonephritis is an inflammation of the glomeruli of the kidneys. Acute poststreptococcal glomerulonephritis (APSGN) occurs as an immune reaction to streptococcal infection of the throat or skin.

Clinical manifestations of hematuria and periorbital edema usually appear 1 to 3 weeks after a streptococcal infection. Other possible manifestations include decreased urine output, hypertension, fever, and fatigue. The prognosis is excellent.

Medical–Surgical Management

Medical

The diagnosis of APSGN can be made based on history, presenting symptoms, and laboratory results. There is no treatment for APSGN. Medical management focuses on presenting signs and symptoms and the degree of renal dysfunction. Laboratory values usually return to normal within 6 to 12 weeks.

Pharmacological

Hypertension may be treated by limiting sodium and water intake or by administering diuretics or antihypertensives.

Nursing Management

Refer to the Urinary System chapter for information on nursing management of the client with APSGN.

NEPHROTIC SYNDROME

Nephrotic syndrome refers to kidney disorders characterized by proteinuria, hypoalbuminemia, and edema.

The most common childhood nephrotic disorder, minimal change nephrotic syndrome (MCNS), results from minimal alterations of the glomerulus. The cause of the alteration is unknown.

Clinical manifestations include pitting edema (periorbital and dependent), anorexia, fatigue, abdominal pain, increased weight, and normal blood pressure. Potential complications include respiratory compromise and peritonitis. Although the child may experience remissions and exacerbations for months, the prognosis in most cases is good.

Medical–Surgical Management

Medical

Diagnosis is made based on clinical presentation, age of the child, massive proteinuria (50 mg/kg/day), and hypoalbuminemia (below 27g/L).

Surgical

A kidney biopsy may be done if a lesion other than MCNS is suspected or the child does not respond as expected to pharmacological treatments.

Pharmacological

The use of corticosteroids such as prednisone (Cortan) induces remission in most cases. Corticosteroid therapy usually produces diuresis within 7 to 14 days. After diuresis occurs, prednisone is continued every other day for 3 days per week. Urine is tested daily for protein until protein has been absent from the urine for up to 7 days. The drug dosage is then gradually decreased and discontinued over a 4-week period. Repeat corticosteroid therapy is administered to children who have relapses after drug therapy is discontinued.

Alkylating agents such as cyclophosphamide (Cytoxan) may be used to reduce symptoms and prevent further relapses in children who do not respond adequately to repeated corticosteroid therapy. The risks and benefits of this therapy must be carefully considered.

When the child is in remission, administration of vaccines for pneumococci and flu should be considered because an exacerbation of nephrotic syndrome can occur following an infection.

Diet

A general "no-added-salt" diet is recommended. Offer appealing, small, frequent meals to the child, who typically has a poor appetite.

Nursing Management

Educate the child's family about the disease process. Monitor I&O hourly. Weigh the child daily. Measure abdominal girth and test urine albumin daily. Keep skin clean and dry. Inspect for skin breakdown and turn child every 2 hours. Screen visitors for signs of infection. Follow Standard Precautions carefully.

NURSING PROCESS

Assessment

Subjective Data

Question the family about symptom onset, appetite, urine output, irritability, and signs of fatigue.

Objective Data

Assess daily weight, abdominal girth, vital signs, and skin for pallor, irritation, breakdown, and edema.

Nursing diagnoses for the child with MCNS may include the following:

Nursing Diagnoses	Planning/Goals	Nursing Interventions
*Excess **F**luid Volume* related to compromised regulatory mechanism	The client will maintain fluid balance.	Monitor I&O hourly; report urinary output of <2 mL/kg/hr. Weigh daily. Measure abdominal girth daily at the level of the umbilicus. Test urine albumin daily with reagent strips.
*Risk for Impaired **S**kin Integrity* related to altered circulation	The client's skin will remain intact.	Inspect the child's skin for breakdown. Turn and reposition the child every 2 hours. Keep the child's skin clean and dry. Use a protective mattress (e.g., eggcrate).
*Risk for **I**nfection* related to immunosuppression	The client will remain infection free.	Screen visitors for signs of infection. Practice proper hand hygiene technique. Monitor the child for signs of infection, such as sore throat, cough, fever, abdominal pain. Monitor laboratory values daily.
*Deficient **K**nowledge (family)* related to treatment regimen	The family will follow through with the prescribed treatment.	Educate the family about the disease process. Instruct the family to test urine for albumin, assess for edema and infection, and administer drugs. Instruct the family to allow a return to ADLs once the child is free of edema.

Evaluation Each goal must be evaluated to determine how it has been met by the client.

ENURESIS

Enuresis is involuntary urination beyond the age when control of urination commonly is acquired. It is not unusual for nocturnal enuresis, or bedwetting, to occur until 8 years of age, because of small bladder capacity and delayed maturation of the neuromuscular system. Most children will outgrow bedwetting without therapeutic intervention.

When enuresis continues to occur beyond the eighth year or recurs in a child who has been dry both day and night for a prolonged period, there may be cause for concern. Possible causes of reoccurring enuresis include urinary tract infections, minor abnormalities of the urinary tract, pinworm infestation, constipation, diabetes, sickle-cell anemia, sexual abuse, stress, and sleep disorders.

Medical–Surgical Management

Medical

Urinalysis and urine culture are done to rule out infection. Other diagnostic studies are performed to rule out all possible causes. Common treatment approaches for enuresis without a physiologic cause include fluid restriction, bladder stretching exercises, behavioral conditioning (e.g., enuresis alarm), and reward systems.

Pharmacological

An anticholinergic such as oxybutynin chloride (Ditropan) may reduce uninhibited bladder contractions. Vasopressins such as desmopressin acetate (DDAVP) nasal spray may reduce nighttime urine output. Antidepressants such as imipramine hydrochloride (Tofranil) may be prescribed.

Other Therapies

If emotional factors are precipitating enuresis, psychosocial support may be an essential part of care. A multidisciplinary team approach is most effective.

PSYCHOSOCIAL DISORDERS

Psychosocial disorders are responses to stressors. Factors influencing an individual's response to stressors include temperament, developmental level, nature and duration of the stressors, past experiences, and coping and adaptive abilities of the family. Possible manifestations in children include depression, anxiety, encopresis, enuresis, passive–agressive behavior, and learning problems (James, et al., 2002). Some of the psychosocial disorders of childhood include obesity, anorexia nervosa and bulimia nervosa, autism, attention deficit hyperactivity disorder, and suicide.

OBESITY

Obesity is the excessive accumulation of fat resulting in an increase in body weight to 20% or more above ideal weight. Obesity can be a precursor of cardiovascular disease, hypertension, and diabetes. Factors contributing to obesity include an overconsumption of food; a sedentary lifestyle; a lack of parental knowledge regarding nutrition and food preparation; unstructured meals; genetic predisposition; and peer pressure.

The obese child may overeat to compensate for lack of parental love and to relieve stress. As a result of obesity,

the child may have low self-esteem, poor body image, difficulty in relationships, and recurring bouts of anxiety and depression.

Medical–Surgical Management

Medical

Obesity is difficult to treat. Positive outcomes are more likely when the child has a support system, understands the importance of weight reduction, and is actively involved in the plan of care.

Diet

Meals and snacks should consist of small servings of nutritional foods. Teach the family and child ways to select and prepare foods. Incorporate favorite foods into the menu whenever possible.

Activity

Incorporate physical exercise into the child's daily routine.

Nursing Management

Focus on meeting nutritional needs, managing related problems, and promoting self-esteem. Assess weight, exercise, and nutritional intake at predetermined intervals. Provide positive feedback for accomplishments, no matter how small. Discuss and revise goals as needed.

Support groups such as Weight Watchers and Overeaters Anonymous may be helpful. In addition, support groups may be available through schools, summer camps, or children's hospitals. A team approach utilizing a psychiatrist or psychologist, a nutritionist, and a nurse may be appropriate.

ANOREXIA NERVOSA AND BULIMIA NERVOSA

Anorexia nervosa and bulimia nervosa are two of the most common eating disorders among children. Anorexia nervosa is self-inflicted starvation; bulimia nervosa is binge-eating followed by purging. These disorders usually begin in middle to late adolescence and can last indefinitely, depending on response to treatment. The incidence is highest among caucasian girls in the higher socioecomonic classes (Hockenberry et al., 2003). Possible causes of these disorders include sensitivity to social pressure for thinness; distorted body image; and longstanding dysfunctional family patterns.

Clinical manifestations include body weight 15% below that expected for age and height, intense fear of gaining weight, dry skin, brittle nails, downy hair on the back and extremities, amenorrhea, constipation, hypothermia, bradycardia, low blood pressure, fluid and electrolyte imbalances, and anemia. Depression, crying spells, feelings of isolation and loneliness, and suicidal thoughts and feelings are common. Clues to frequent vomiting include dental caries and erosion and throat irritation. Callouses or abrasions may be noted on the back of the hands, from frequent contact with the teeth while inducing vomiting.

Medical–Surgical Management

Medical

The goal of medical treatment is to correct malnutrition and resulting complications. A weight gain of 0.1 to 0.2 kg/d is emphasized until the desired weight is attained. Enteral feedings or total parenteral nutrition (TPN) may be necessary to replace lost fluids, protein, and nutrients.

Pharmacological

Antidepressants such as imipramine hydrochloride (Tofranil) or desipramine hydrochloride (Norpramin) may be prescribed.

Other Therapies

Individual and family therapy are used to address dysfunctional family patterns and assist the adolescent in identifying and dealing with self-esteem and body image issues. Treatment is typically long-term.

Nursing Management

Refer to the Mental Illness chapter for possible nursing diagnoses for the client with anorexia or bulimia nervosa and to the Resources listing at the end of this chapter.

AUTISM

Autism is a complex disorder of brain function involving abnormal emotional, social, and linguistic development. The cause of autism is unknown; however, research suggests it may result from a disturbance in language comprehension, a biochemical problem involving neurotransmitters, or abnormalities in the central nervous system.

Possible clinical manifestations include lack of eye contact, aversion to touch, delayed language development, blank expression, lack of response to verbal stimulation, repetitive behaviors, bizarre body movements, and self-destructive behaviors. Manifestations may vary from mild to severe. The prognosis depends on early detection and the child's response to treatment.

Medical–Surgical Management

Medical

Diagnosis is based on the presence of specific criteria as listed in the *Diagnostic and Statistical Manual of Mental Disorders,* fourth edition (DSM-IV) (American Psychiatric Association, 1994). In addition, a complete physical and neurological examination is necessary to rule out other disorders such as lead poisoning, phenylketonuria, congenital rubella, and measles encephalitis.

Treatment is provided by a multidisciplanary team and focuses on promoting normal development, social interaction, and learning. Behavior-modification techniques are used to reward desirable behaviors and foster positive coping skills.

Nursing Management

Focus on early detection, decreasing environmental stimuli, providing supportive care, maintaining a safe environment, and giving parents anticipatory guidance. Monitor growth and development, especially language and social skills. When caring for a child with autism, ascertain the child's routines, rituals, and likes and dislikes. Because autistic children do not do well in unfamiliar environments, it is important that they be surrounded by familiar objects. The child

CLIENT TEACHING

Modifying Behavior in the Child Who Is Autistic

- Emphasize the child's positive skills.
- Provide immediate feedback for appropriate behavior.
- Continue social interactions even when the child is unresponsive.
- Provide tactile stimulation such as tickling, holding, cuddling, and shaking hands.
- Teach the child to embrace, kiss, and shake hands.
- Speak in short sentences.
- Use a firm but caring approach.
- Maintain daily routines.

may need assistance with self-care. Keep schedules and care providers as consistent as possible. Close supervision is usually required at all times.

Parents need a great deal of support to cope with the challenges of having an autistic child. Assist children to reach their maximum potential through enrollment in special education programs and participation in behavior modification. Some children may achieve independence by adulthood. Inform parents about local support groups and refer to the Autism Society of America for current information.

ATTENTION DEFICIT HYPERACTIVITY DISORDER

Attention-deficit hyperactivity disorder (ADHD) is a developmental disorder characterized by developmentally inappropriate degrees of inattention, overactivity, and impulsivity. The child is usually diagnosed between the ages of 3 and 6 years. Possible clinical manifestations include poor impulse control, distractibility, fidgeting with hands, squirming in seat, excessive talking, and difficulty following instructions.

Medical–Surgical Management
Medical

Diagnosis may be made based on diagnostic criteria in the *DSM-IV* (American Psychiatric Association, 1994) as well as a complete multidisciplinary evaluation. Treatment focuses on decreasing distractions, modifying behavior (e.g., setting limits, ensuring consistency, praising accomplishments), and/or initiating pharmacological therapy.

Pharmacological

The most commonly prescribed medications include methylphenidate (Ritalin), pemoline (Cylert), and dextroamphetamine (Dexedrine). These drugs stimulate the area of the child's brain that facilitates concentration.

CLIENT TEACHING

Caring for the Child with ADHD

- Praise positive behavior and set limits.
- Administer medication as prescribed and with meals.
- Give clear, simple instructions and provide frequent reminders to follow instructions.
- Reduce stimuli in the child's environment (e.g., turning off the TV when the child is trying to do homework).
- Allow for a shortened attention span by providing short teaching sessions and activities that allow for mobility.
- Consult with trained professional for behavior-modification therapy.

Potential side effects include loss of appetite resulting in delayed growth.

Nursing Management

Focus on improving the child's social interaction and educating the family and teachers.

SUICIDE

Suicide is the third leading cause of death among adolescents. Boys complete suicide four times more often than do girls, but girls attempt suicide five times more often than do boys. Males tend to use lethal methods such as guns, hanging, and jumping from high elevations, whereas girls more often overdose or cut the wrists. Adolescents who have attempted suicide once are at greatest risk for attempting again. Attempted suicide rarely occurs without warning (Centers for Disease Control and Prevention, 1997a).

Clinical manifestations in the suicidal adolescent may include depression, boredom, restlessness, concentration problems, irritability, lethargy, and intentional misbehavior. Children at high risk for committing suicide may be experiencing depression; pregnancy; failure in school; drug use; death of a friend or parent; problems with a relationship; sexual abuse; chronic illness; or a broken home.

Medical–Surgical Management
Medical

The child thought to be at high risk for suicide is usually admitted to a psychiatric unit for care. Treatment may include individual, group, and/or family therapy. Negotiating a "No-Suicide" contract is one method that may be used with a suicidal child. In this written and signed contract, the child agrees not to attempt suicide for a negotiated period (e.g., weeks, days, minutes). If at any time the child feels unable to keep the contract, the child agrees to contact help. Children with severe self-abusive behavior may need to be physically or chemically restrained.

Pharmacological

Drugs that may be used for chemical restraint include diphenhydramine hydrochloride (Benadryl), thioridazine hydrochloride (Mellaril), chlorpromazine (Thorazine), and lorazepam (Ativan). The suicidal child may also require antidepressant and/or antipsychotic medications.

Nursing Management

Assess risk factors, behaviors, attitude, how lethal is the proposed method of suicide, coping mechanisms, and support system. Be nonjudgmental and show empathy. Remove potentially harmful objects from the environment. Monitor the high-risk child at all times. Administer medications as prescribed. Encourage individual and group therapy for the entire family and keeping all follow-up appointments.

NURSING PROCESS

Assessment

Subjective Data

Assess the suicidal child for behaviors; attitudes; risk factors; lethality of the proposed method of suicide; coping mechanisms; and support systems.

Objective Data

Observe the child for signs of physical and sexual abuse, self-destructive behaviors, and sudden changes in behavior.

Nursing diagnoses for the child who is suicidal may include the following:

Nursing Diagnoses	Planning/Goals	Nursing Interventions
Risk for Self-directed Violence related to desire to ease emotional pain, solicit attention of others, or avoid responsibility	The client will be less likely to repeat the suicide attempt.	Use a nonjudgmental, empathic approach and a voice and demeanor that are clear, direct, and supportive to discuss feelings and the suicidal event. Remove potentially harmful objects from the environment (e.g., belts, scarves, shoestrings, matches, lighters). Monitor the high-risk child at all times, even during bathroom use and sleep. Administer prescribed medications. Suggest alternate activities for those times when impulsive behavior occurs. Restrain the child (as ordered) as an act of care, not punishment.
Interrupted Family Processes related to relational disturbance or abuse/neglect	The client will feel safe and receive support from others to meet needs.	Encourage individual and group therapy for the entire family to explore personal issues and the need for social support. Assist the parents to regain the ability to assist their child and manage the home environment. Foster parent–child interaction. Teach the family to monitor the child for sudden changes in behavior. Teach the family and child about medication administration. Encourage the family to keep follow-up appointments.

Evaluation Each goal must be evaluated to determine how it has been met by the client.

CASE STUDY

Jaime is a 14-year-old male. He was diagnosed with DMD at 5 years of age. His older brother also had DMD and died 2 years ago at the age of 16. Jaime lives with his parents and 10-year-old sister, Liza. Associated problems include confinement to a wheelchair; contractures of the hips, knees, and ankles; scoliosis requiring a brace; frequent respiratory infections; and obesity. Jaime attends the ninth grade, is a member of the chess club, and enjoys the youth group at his church.

The following questions will guide your development of a nursing care plan for the case study.

1. List the characteristic progression of DMD.
2. Cite three nursing diagnoses and goals for Jaime.
3. Identify interventions to help Jaime and his family address the nursing diagnoses identified in question 2.
4. How might genetic counseling benefit this family?
5. Identify resources available to help Jaime and his family cope with DMD.

Summary

- The most common skin disorders among toddlers and preschoolers are impetigo and dog bites.
- The most common skin disorders among school-age children are pediculosis and scabies.
- The most common skin disorder among adolescents is acne.
- Common respiratory tract infections of childhood include nasopharyngitis, pharyngitis, and influenza.
- Asthma is the leading cause of chronic illness among children.
- Treatment of asthma involves allergen control, drug therapy, controlled exercise, physical therapy, and desensitization.
- Prevention or treatment of group A streptococcal infection in turn prevents rheumatic fever.
- Nursing care of the child with leukemia focuses on preparing the child and family for diagnostic and therapeutic procedures, preventing complications of myelosuppression, managing problems of drug toxicity, and providing emotional support.
- Parents of a child with ITP must be able to detect signs of bleeding and know ways to prevent injuries.
- Constipation can be prevented by establishing and maintaining regular toileting habits, drinking fluids, eating a diet high in fiber, and participating in regular exercise.
- Children are more commonly infected with intestinal parasites than are adults because they put their fingers in their mouths more often.
- Obesity can be a precursor to cardiovascular disease, hypertension, and diabetes.
- Acute poststreptococcal glomerulonephritis occurs as an immune reaction to streptococcal infection of the throat or skin.
- Goals for the child with nephrotic syndrome include fluid balance, intact skin, freedom from infection, and compliance with urine testing and drug therapy.
- Goals for children with structural anomalies, such as scoliosis or Legg-Calvé-Perthes disease, and injuries may include preventing skin breakdown (due to casts and braces) and keeping follow-up appointments.
- Nursing care for the child with DMD focuses on maintaining physical activity, promoting respiratory function, managing weight, and encouraging age-appropriate social activities.
- Nursing care for the child with juvenile rheumatoid arthritis focuses on preventing injury, controlling pain, enhancing mobility, and encouraging age-appropriate activities.
- Nursing goals for the autistic child may include decreasing environmental stimuli, providing supportive care, maintaining a safe environment, and giving parents anticipatory guidance.
- Treatment for the child with ADHD focuses on decreasing distractions, modifying behavior, and initiating drug therapy.

- Suicide is the third leading cause of death among adolescents.
- Child abuse can be classified as physical abuse, physical neglect, emotional abuse, or sexual abuse.

Review Questions

1. Determining the causative agent and administering the proper treatment for skin and throat infections may prevent further complications such as:
   a. leukemia.
   b. mononucleosis.
   c. idiopathic thrombocytopenia purpura.
   d. acute post-streptococcal glomerulonephritis.

2. Children with leukemia are at high risk for infection because of:
   a. decreased lymphocytes.
   b. increased red blood cells.
   c. decreased platelets.
   d. decreased neutrophils.

3. Nursing diagnoses for the child with nephrotic syndrome may include:
   a. *Excess Fluid Volume* related to fluid retention.
   b. *Pain* related to operative procedure.
   c. *Impaired Physical Mobility*, related to use of a brace.
   d. *Disturbed Body Image* related to loss of hair.

4. A clinical manifestation of scoliosis is:
   a. lateral curvature of the spine.
   b. necrosis of the femoral head.
   c. quadricep muscle atrophy.
   d. Gower's sign.

5. Treatment for the child with ADHD includes:
   a. decreasing distractions.
   b. placing in special education class.
   c. prescribing sedatives.
   d. eating a special diet.

References/Suggested Readings

American Psychiatric Association. (1994). *Diagnostic and statistical manual of mental disorders* (4th ed.). Washington, DC: Author.

American Diabetes Association (ADA). (2000). Type 2 diabetes in children and adolescents. *Diabetes Care*, 22(12), 381. Also [Online]. Available: www.diabetes.org/ada/Consensus/pg381.htm

Ball, J., & Bindler, R. (2000). *Pediatric nursing* (2nd ed.). Norwalk, CT: Appleton & Lange.

Centers for Disease Control and Prevention. (1994). General recommendations on immunization: Recommendations of the Advisory Committee on Immunization Practices (ACIP), *MMWR, 43*(RR-1), 1–38.

Centers for Disease Control and Prevention. (1996). Update: vaccine side effects, adverse reactions, contraindications and precautions: Recommendations of the Advisory Committee on Immunization Practices (ACIP). *MMWR, 45*(RR-12), 1–35.

Centers for Disease Control and Prevention. (1997a). Rates of homicide, suicide, and firearm-related death among children—26 industrialized countries. *MMWR, 46*(5), 101–105.

Centers for Disease Control and Prevention. (1997b). Status report on the childhood immunization initiative; National, state, and urban area vaccination coverage levels among children aged 19–35 months—United States, 1996. *MMWR, 46*(29), 657–664.

Cooper, C. (2003). Would you recognize this syndrome? *RN, 65*(4), 49–52.

Dochterman, J., & Bulechek, G. (2004). *Nursing Interventions Classification (NIC)* (4th ed.). St. Louis, MO: Mosby.

Eisenhauer, L., Nichols, L., Spencer, R., & Bergan, F. (1998). *Clinical pharmacology & nursing management* (5th ed.). Philadelphia: Lippincott Williams & Wilkins.

Estes, M. E. Z. (2002). *Health assessment & physical examination* (2nd ed.). Clifton Park, NY: Thomson Delmar Learning.

Hayes, L. (2000). Poison emergency? *Nursing2000, 30*(9), 34–39.

Healthy People 2010. (2000). *Objectives* [Online]. Available: www.healthypeople.gov/document/html/objectives/14-22.htm

Herrin, J. T., & Antoon, A. Y. (2000). *Burn injuries*. In R. M. Kliegman, S. Jenson, & R. Behrman (Eds.), *Nelson textbook of pediatrics* (16th ed.). Philadelphia: W. B. Saunders.

Hockenberry, M., Wilson, D., Winkelstein, M., & Kline, N. (2003). *Whaley & Wong's nursing care of infants and children* (7th ed.). St. Louis, MO: Mosby.

Hurwitz, S. (1995). Acne treatment for the 90s. *Contemporary Pediatrics, 12*(8), 19–32.

James, S., Ashwill, J. W., & Droske, S. C. (2002). *Nursing care of children: Principles and practice* (2nd ed.). Philadelphia: W. B. Saunders.

Kamienski, M. (2003). Reye syndrome. *AJN, 103*(7), 54–57.

Kliegman, R. M., Jensen, H. S., & Behrman, R. (2000). *Nelson's textbook of pediatrics* (16th ed.). Philadelphia: W. B. Saunders.

Kline, A. (2003). Pediatric respiratory distress. *Nursing2003, 33*(9), 58–63.

Laskowski-Jones, L., & Salati, D. (2001). Responding to pediatric trauma. *Nursing2001, 31*(9), 36–41.

Lewis, A. M. (1999). Managing common pediatric emergencies. *Nursing99, 29*(1), 33–39.

Marks, M. G. (1998). *Broadribb's introductory pediatric nursing* (5th ed.). Philadelphia: J.B. Lippincott Williams & Wilkins.

Meleski, D. (2002). Families with chronically ill children. *AJN, 102*(5), 47–54.

Metules, T. (2002). Duchenne muscular dystrophy. *RN, 65*(10), 39–47.

Moorhead, S., Johnson, M., & Maas, M. (2004). *Nursing Outcomes Classification (NOC)* (3rd ed.). St. Louis, MO: Mosby.

Mulryan, K., & Cathers, P. (2000). Protecting the child. *Nursing2000, 30*(7), 39–43.

National Institutes of Health (NIH). (2000). Consensus Statement 111: Osteoporosis prevention, diagnosis, and therapy. [Online]. Available: http://consensus.nih.gov/con/111/111_statement.htm

Nemours. (2002). *School backpacks: How they affect your child's general health.* [Online]. Available: www.nemours.org/no/news/releases/2002/020206_backpack_study.html

North American Nursing Diagnosis Association. (2003). *Nursing diagnoses: Definitions & classification 2003–2004.* Philadelphia: Author.

Potts, N., & Mandleco, B. (2002). *Pediatric Nursing: Caring for children and their families.* Clifton Park, NY: Thomson Delmar Learning.

Ruiz, E. (2001). Type 2 disease in children. *RN, 64*(10), 44–48.

Schultz, T. (2000). Airing differences in pediatric nebulizer therapy. *Nursing2000, 30*(9), 55–57.

Siwula, C. (2003). Managing pediatric emergencies. *Nursing2003, 33*(2), 48–51.

Spratto, G., & Woods, A. (2004). *2004 PDR nurse's drug handbook.* Clifton Park, NY: Thomson Delmar Learning.

Thompson, S. (2003). When kids get CANCER. *RN, 66*(7), 29–33.

VanBoxel, A., & Puhl, P. (2001). Pediatric emergency: Assessing gut pain. *RN, 64*(4), 38–42.

Wong, D., Hockenberry-Eaton, M. (2001). *Wong's essentials of pediatric nursing* (6th ed.). St. Louis, MO: Mosby.

Resources

American Academy of Pediatrics (AAP), 141 Northwest Point Boulevard, Elk Grove Village, IL, 60007-1098, 800-433-9016; 847-228-5005, www.aap.org

American Diabetes Association (ADA), 1701 North Beauregard Street, Alexandria, VA 22311, 800-342-2383, www.diabetes.org

Autism Society of America (ASA), 7910 Woodmont Avenue, Suite 300, Bethesda, MD, 20814-3067, 301-657-0881, 800-3AUTISM, www.autism-society.org

Centers for Disease Control and Prevention, www.cdc.gov

Children with Diabetes, www.castleweb.com

Muscular Dystrophy Association of America, Inc., 3300 East Sunrise Drive, Tucson, AZ, 85718, 800-572-1717, www.mdausa.org

National Association of Anorexia Nervosa and Associated Disorders, Inc., P.O. Box 7, Highland Park, IL, 60035, 847-831-3438, www.anad.org

National Association of Pediatric Nurses Associates and Practitioners (NAPNAP), 20 Brace Road, Suite 200, Cherry Hill, NJ, 08034-2638, 856-852-9700, www.napnap. org

National Eating Disorders Association, 603 Stewart Street, Suite 803, Seattle, WA 98101, 206-382-3587, www.nationaleatingdisorders.org

National Hemophilia Foundation, 116 West 32nd Street, 11th Floor, New York, NY, 10001, 800-424-2634, www.hemophilia.org

The National Pediculosis Association, 50 Kearney Road, Needham, MA, 02494, 800-446-4NPA; 781-449-6487, www.headlice.org

National Scoliosis Foundation, Inc., 5 Cabot Place, Stoughton, MA, 02072, 800-673-6922, www.stepstn.com

Nemours Foundation, 1801 Rockland Road, Wilmington, DE 19803, 302-429-9400, www.nemours.org

Scoliosis Association, Inc., P.O. Box 811705, Boca Raton, FL, 33481-1705, 800-800-0669, www.scoliosis-assoc.org

Appendix A: NANDA Nursing Diagnoses 2003–2004

Activity Intolerance
Risk for Activity Intolerance
Impaired Adjustment
Ineffective Airway Clearance
Latex Allergy Response
Risk for Latex Allergy Response
Anxiety
Death Anxiety
Risk for Aspiration
Risk for Impaired Parent/Infant/Child Attachment
Autonomic Dysreflexia
Risk for Autonomic Dysreflexia
Disturbed Body Image
Risk for Imbalanced Body Temperature
Bowel Incontinence
Effective Breastfeeding
Ineffective Breastfeeding
Interrupted Breastfeeding
Ineffective Breathing Pattern
Decreased Cardiac Output
Caregiver Role Strain
Risk for Caregiver Role Strain
Impaired Verbal Communication
Readiness for Enhanced Communication
Decisional Conflict (Specify)
Parenteral Role Conflict
Acute Confusion
Chronic Confusion
Constipation
Perceived Constipation
Risk for Constipation
Ineffective Coping
Defensive Coping
Readiness for Enhanced Coping
Ineffective Community Coping
Readiness for Enhanced Community Coping
Compromised Family Coping
Disabled Family Coping
Readiness for Enhanced Family Coping
Risk for Sudden Infant Death Syndrome
Ineffective Denial
Impaired Dentition
Risk for Delayed Development
Diarrhea
Risk for Disuse Syndrome

Deficient Diversional Activities
Disturbed Energy Field
Impaired Environmental Interpretation Syndrome
Adult Failure to Thrive
Risk for Falls
Dysfunctional Family Processes: Alcoholism
Interrupted Family Processes
Readiness for Enhanced Family Processes
Fatigue
Fear
Readiness for Enhanced Fluid Balance
Deficient Fluid Volume
Excess Fluid Volume
Risk for Deficient Fluid Volume
Risk for Imbalanced Fluid Volume
Impaired Gas Exchange
Anticipatory Grieving
Dysfunctional Grieving
Delayed Growth and Development
Risk for Disproportionate Growth
Ineffective Health Maintenance
Health-Seeking Behaviors (Specify)
Impaired Home Maintenance
Hopelessness
Hyperthermia
Hypothermia
Disturbed Personal Identity
Functional Urinary Incontinence
Reflex Urinary Incontinence
Stress Urinary Incontinence
Total Urinary Incontinence
Urge Urinary Incontinence
Risk for Urge Urinary Incontinence
Disorganized Infant Behavior
Risk for Disorganized Infant Behavior
Readiness for Enhanced Organized Infant Behavior
Ineffective Infant Feeding Pattern
Risk for Infection
Risk for Injury
Risk for Perioperative-Positioning Injury
Decreased Intracranial Adaptive Capacity
Deficient Knowledge (specify)
Readiness for Enhanced Knowledge (specify)
Risk for Loneliness
Impaired Memory

Impaired Bed **M**obility
Impaired Physical **M**obility
Impaired Wheelchair **M**obility
Nausea
Unilateral **N**eglect
Noncompliance
Imbalanced **N**utrition: Less than Body Requirements
Imbalanced **N**utrition: More than Body Requirements
Readiness for Enhanced **N**utrition
Risk for Imbalanced **N**utrition: More than Body
    Requirements
Impaired **O**ral Mucous Membrane
Acute **P**ain
Chronic **P**ain
Readiness for Enhanced **P**arenting
Impaired **P**arenting
Risk for Impaired **P**arenting
Risk for **P**eripheral Neurovascular Dysfunction
Risk for **P**oisoning
Post-Trauma Syndrome
Risk for **P**ost-Trauma Syndrome
Powerlessness
Risk for **P**owerlessness
Ineffective **P**rotection
Rape-Trauma Syndrome
Rape-Trauma Syndrome: Compound Reaction
Rape-Trauma Syndrome: Silent Reaction
Relocation Stress Syndrome
Risk for **R**elocation Stress Syndrome
Ineffective **R**ole Performance
Bathing/Hygiene **S**elf-Care Deficit
Dressing/Grooming **S**elf-Care Deficit
Feeding **S**elf-Care Deficit
Toileting **S**elf-Care Deficit
Readiness for Enhanced **S**elf-Concept
Chronic Low **S**elf-Esteem
Situational Low **S**elf-Esteem
Risk for Situational Low **S**elf-Esteem
Self-Mutilation
Risk for **S**elf-Mutilation
Disturbed **S**ensory Perception (Specify: Visual,
    Auditory, Kinesthetic, Gustatory, Tactile, Olfactory)

Sexual Dysfunction
Ineffective **S**exuality Pattern
Impaired **S**kin Integrity
Risk for Impaired **S**kin Integrity
Sleep Deprivation
Disturbed **S**leep Pattern
Readiness for Enhanced **S**leep
Impaired **S**ocial Interaction
Social Isolation
Chronic **S**orrow
Spiritual Distress
Risk for **S**piritual Distress
Readiness for Enhanced **S**piritual Well-Being
Risk for **S**uffocation
Risk for **S**uicide
Delayed **S**urgical Recovery
Impaired **S**wallowing
Effective **T**herapeutic Regimen Management
Ineffective **T**herapeutic Regimen Management
Readiness for Enhanced **T**herapeutic Regimen
    Management
Ineffective Community **T**herapeutic Regimen
    Management
Ineffective Family **T**herapeutic Regimen Management
Ineffective **T**hermoregulation
Disturbed **T**hought Processes
Impaired **T**issue Integrity
Ineffective **T**issue Perfusion (Specify Type: Renal,
    Cerebral, Cardiopulmonary, Gastrointestinal,
    Peripheral)
Impaired **T**ransfer Ability
Risk for **T**rauma
Impaired **U**rinary Elimination
Readiness for Enhanced **U**rinary Elimination
Urinary Retention
Impaired Spontaneous **V**entilation
Dysfunctional **V**entilatory Weaning Response
Risk for Other-Directed **V**iolence
Risk for Self-Directed **V**iolence
Impaired **W**alking
Wandering

From *Nursing Diagnoses: Definitions & Classification, 2003–2004,* by North American Nursing Diagnosis Association, 2003.
Philadelphia: Author. Copyright 2003 by North American Nursing Diagnosis Association. Reprinted with permission.

Appendix B: Recommended Childhood and Adolescent Immunization Schedule

From Morbidity and Mortality Weekly Report (January 2004).

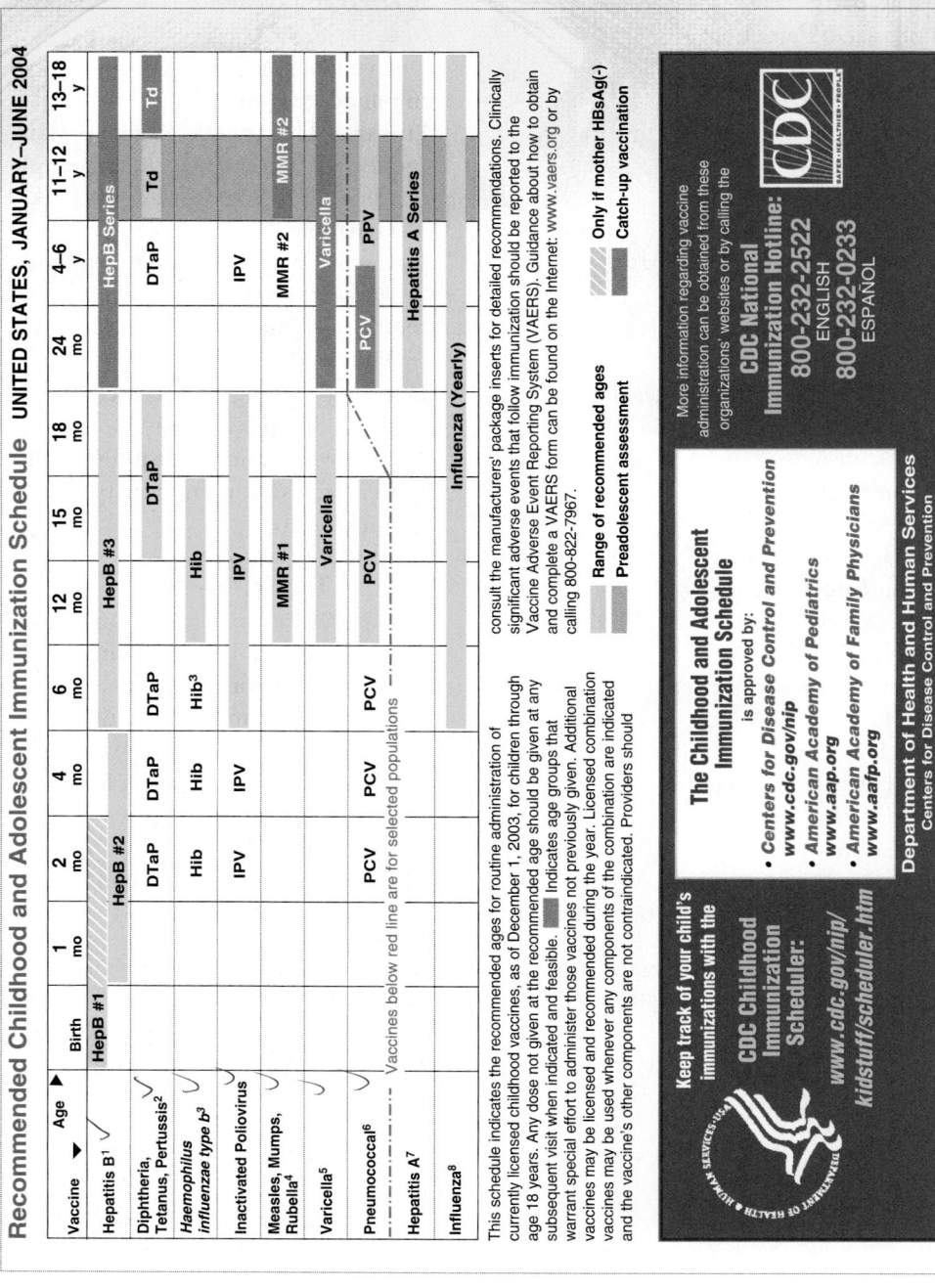

1. **Hepatitis B (HepB) vaccine.** All infants should receive the first dose of hepatitis B vaccine soon after birth and before hospital discharge; the first dose may also be given by age 2 months if the infant's mother is hepatitis B surface antigen (HBsAg) negative. Only monovalent HepB can be used for the birth dose. Monovalent or combination vaccine containing HepB may be used to complete the series. Four doses of vaccine may be administered when a birth dose is given. The second dose should be given at least 4 weeks after the first dose, except for combination vaccines which cannot be administered before age 6 weeks. The third dose should be given at least 16 weeks after the first dose and at least 8 weeks after the second dose. The last dose in the vaccination series (third or fourth dose) should not be administered before age 24 weeks.

Infants born to HBsAg-positive mothers should receive HepB and 0.5 mL of Hepatitis B Immune Globulin (HBIG) within 12 hours of birth at separate sites. The second dose is recommended at age 1 to 2 months. The last dose in the immunization series should not be administered before age 24 weeks. These infants should be tested for HBsAg and antibody to HBsAg (anti-HBs) at age 9 to 15 months.

Infants born to mothers whose HBsAg status is unknown should receive the first dose of the HepB series within 12 hours of birth. Maternal blood should be drawn as soon as possible to determine the mother's HBsAg status; if the HBsAg test is positive, the infant should receive HBIG as soon as possible (no later than age 1 week). The second dose is recommended at age 1 to 2 months. The last dose in the immunization series should not be administered before age 24 weeks.

2. **Diphtheria and tetanus toxoids and acellular pertussis (DTaP) vaccine.** The fourth dose of DTaP may be administered as early as age 12 months, provided 6 months have elapsed since the third dose and the child is unlikely to return at age 15 to 18 months. The final dose in the series should be given at age ≥4 years. **Tetanus and diphtheria toxoids (Td)** is recommended at age 11 to 12 years if at least 5 years have elapsed since the last dose of tetanus and diphtheria toxoid-containing vaccine. Subsequent routine Td boosters are recommended every 10 years.

3. ***Haemophilus influenzae* type b (Hib) conjugate vaccine.** Three Hib conjugate vaccines are licensed for infant use. If PRP-OMP (PedvaxHIB or ComVax [Merck]) is administered at ages 2 and 4 months, a dose at age 6 months is not required. DTaP/Hib combination products should not be used for primary immunization in infants at ages 2, 4 or 6 months but can be used as boosters following any Hib vaccine. The final dose in the series should be given at age ≥12 months.

4. **Measles, mumps, and rubella vaccine (MMR).** The second dose of MMR is recommended routinely at age 4 to 6 years but may be administered during any visit, provided at least 4 weeks have elapsed since the first dose and both doses are administered beginning at or after age 12 months. Those who have not previously received the second dose should complete the schedule by the 11- to 12-year-old visit.

5. **Varicella vaccine.** Varicella vaccine is recommended at any visit at or after age 12 months for susceptible children (i.e., those who lack a reliable history of chickenpox). Susceptible persons age ≥13 years should receive 2 doses, given at least 4 weeks apart.

6. **Pneumococcal vaccine.** The heptavalent **pneumococcal conjugate vaccine (PCV)** is recommended for all children age 2 to 23 months. It is also recommended for certain children age 24 to 59 months. The final dose in the series should be given at age ≥12 months. **Pneumococcal polysaccharide vaccine (PPV)** is recommended in addition to PCV for certain high-risk groups. See *MMWR* 2000;49(RR-9):1-38.

7. **Hepatitis A vaccine.** Hepatitis A vaccine is recommended for children and adolescents in selected states and regions and for certain high-risk groups; consult your local public health authority. Children and adolescents in these states, regions, and high-risk groups who have not been immunized against hepatitis A can begin the hepatitis A immunization series during any visit. The 2 doses in the series should be administered at least 6 months apart. See *MMWR* 1999;48(RR-12):1-37.

8. **Influenza vaccine.** Influenza vaccine is recommended annually for children age ≥6 months with certain risk factors (including but not limited to children with asthma, cardiac disease, sickle cell disease, human immunodeficiency virus infection, and diabetes; and household members of persons in high-risk groups [see *MMWR* 2003;52(RR-8):1-36]) and can be administered to all others wishing to obtain immunity. In addition, healthy children age 6 to 23 months are encouraged to receive influenza vaccine if feasible, because children in this age group are at substantially increased risk of influenza-related hospitalizations. For healthy persons age 5 to 49 years, the intranasally administered live-attenuated influenza vaccine (LAIV) is an acceptable alternative to the intramuscular trivalent inactivated influenza vaccine (TIV). See *MMWR* 2003;52(RR-13):1-8. Children receiving TIV should be administered a dosage appropriate for their age (0.25 mL if age 6 to 35 months or 0.5 mL if age ≥3 years). Children age ≤8 years who are receiving influenza vaccine for the first time should receive 2 doses (separated by at least 4 weeks for TIV and at least 6 weeks for LAIV).

Appendix C: Abbreviations, Acronyms, and Symbols

>	greater than
<	less than
ʒ	dram
℥	ounce
♏	minum
ā	before
AA	Alcoholics Anonymous
AAA	abdominal aortic aneurysm
AAFP	American Academy of Family Physicians
AaO₂	percentage saturation of hemoglobin with oxygen in arterial blood
AAOHN	American Association of Occupational Health Nurses
AAP	American Academy of Pediatrics
AAPB	Association of Applied Psychophysiology and Biofeedback
AARP	American Association of Retired Persons
AASM	American Academy of Sleep Medicine
AAT	animal-assisted therapy
AATH	American Association for Therapeutic Humor
ABC	airway, breathing, circulation
ABC	antigen-binding capacity
ABCD	asymmetry, border, color, diameter
ABD	abdominal
ABG	arterial blood gases
ABO	blood types
ABVD	A combination of chemotherapy drugs: doxorubicin (Adriamycin), bleomycin sulfate (Blenoxane), vinblastine (Velban), dacarbazine (DTIC-Dome)
a.c.	before meals
ACE	angiotensin-converting enzyme
ACIP	Advisory Committee on Immunization Practices
ACKD	acquired cystic kidney disease
ACR	American College of Rheumatology
ACS	American Cancer Society
ACTH	adrenocorticotropic hormone
AD	Alzheimer's disease
AD	right ear
ad lib	freely, as desired
ADA	American Diabetes Association
ADA	American Dietetic Association
ADA	Americans with Disabilities Act
ADAA	Anxiety Disorders Association of America
ADAMHA	Alcohol, Drug Abuse, and Mental Health Administration
ADC	AIDS dementia complex
ADD	attention deficit disorder
ADH	antidiuretic hormone
ADHD	attention deficit hyperactivity disorder
ADLs	activities of daily living
ADN	associate degree nurse (nursing)
AEB	as evidenced by
AFB	acid-fast bacillus
AFP	alpha-fetoprotein
AGA	appropriate for gestational age
AGE	acute gastroenteritis
AGF	angiogenesis factor
AHA	American Heart Association
AHA	American Hospital Association
AHCA	American Health Care Association
AHCPR	Agency for Health Care Policy and Research
AHNA	American Holistic Nurses' Association
AHRQ	Agency for Healthcare Research and Quality
AI	adequate intake
AID	artificial insemination by donor
AIDS	acquired immunodeficiency syndrome
AIH	artificial insemination by husband
AJN	*American Journal of Nursing*
AKA	above the knee amputation
ALFA	Assisted Living Federation of America
ALG	antilympocytic globulin
ALL	acute lymphocytic leukemia
ALS	amyotrophic lateral sclerosis
ALT	alanine aminotransferase
AMA	against medical advice
AMA	American Medical Association
AML	acute myelogenous leukemia
ANA	American Nurses Association
ANA	antinuclear antibody
ANS	autonomic nervous system
AoA	Administration on Aging
AORN	Association of Perioperating Registered Nurses
AP	anterior/posterior
AP	apical pulse
APA	American Psychiatric Association
APIC	Association for Practitioners in Infection Control and Epidemiology
APRN	advance practice registered nurse
APS	Adult Protective Services
APS	American Pain Society
APSGN	acute poststreptococcal glomerulonephritis
APTT	activated partial thromboplastin time
ARDS	adult respiratory distress syndrome
ARF	acute renal failure
AROM	active range of motion
AROM	artificial rupture of membranes
ARS	acute radiation syndrome
AS	left ear
ASA	acetylsalicylic acid
ASD	atrial septal defect
ASO	antireptolysin-O
ASPO	American Society for Psychoprophylaxis in Obstetrics
AST	aspartate aminotransferase
ATC	around the clock
ATG	antithymocytic globulin
ATN	acute tubular necrosis
ATP	adenosine triphosphatase
ATSDR	Agency for Toxic Substances and Disease Registry
AU	both ears
A-V	arteriovenous

AV	atrioventricular
AWHONN	Association of Women's Health, Obstetric, and Neonatal Nurses
AWS	alcohol withdrawal syndrome
B_1	thiamine
B_2	riboflavin
B_6	pyridoxine
B_{12}	cobolomine
BBA	Balanced Budget Act
BCG	bacilles *Calmette-Guérin*
BE	base excess
bid	twice a day
BKA	below the knee amputation
BMD	bone mineral density
BMI	body mass index
BMR	basal metabolic rate
BMT	bone marrow transplantation
B&O	belladonna and opium
BOW	bag of water
BP	blood pressure
BPD	biparietal diameter
BPD	bronchopulmonary dysplasia
BPH	benign prostatic hypertrophy
BPM	beats per minute
BRM	biologic response modifier
BSA	body surface area
BSE	breast self-examination
BSI	body substance isolation
BSN	bachelor of science in nursing
BUBBLE	breasts, uterus, bladder, bowel, lochia, and episiotomy
BUN	blood urea nitrogen
BVI	bladder volume indicator
c	cup
c̄	with
C	Celsius
Ca	calcium
Ca^+	calcium ion
C/A	complementary/alternative
CABG	coronary artery bypass graft
$CaCl_2$	calcium chloride
CAD	coronary artery disease
CAHD	coronary artery heart disease
CAI	computer-assisted instruction
C & S	culture and sensitivity
cap	capsule
CAPD	continuous ambulatory peritoneal dialysis
CARF	Commission on Accreditation of Rehabilitation Facilities
CAT	computed axial tomography
CAT	computerized adaptive testing
CATT	computerized axial transverse tomography
CBC	complete blood count
CBD	common bile duct
CBE	charting by exception
cc	cubic centimeter
CCNS	cell-cycle nonspecific
CCRC	continuing care retirement community
CCS	cell-cycle specific
CCU	coronary care unit
CDC	Centers for Disease Control and Prevention
CEA	carcinoembryonic antigen
CEPN-LTC™	Certification Examination for Practical and Vocational Nurses in Long-Term Care
CEU	continuing education unit

CF	cystic fibrosis
CFTR	cystic fibrosis transmembrane regulator
C-H	crown-heel
CHAP	Community health accreditation program
CHD	coronary heart disease
CHIP	Children's Health Insurance Program
CHO	carbohydrate (carbon, hydrogen, oxygen)
CHON	protein (carbon, hydrogen, oxygen, nitrogen)
CHOP	A combination of chemotherapy drugs: cyclophosphamide (Cytoxan), doxorubicin (Adriamycin), vincristine (Oncovin), and prednisone (Deltasone)
CIN	cervical intraepithelial neoplasia
CIS	carcinoma *in situ*
CK or CPK	creatine kinase or creatine phosphokinase
Cl	chlorine, chloride
Cl^-	chloride ion
CLL	chronic lymphocytic leukemia
CLTC	certified in long-term care
cm	centimeter
cmg	cystometrogram
CML	chronic myelogenous leukemia
CMS	circulation, movement, sensation
CMS	Centers for Medicare and Medicaid Services
CMV	cytomegalovirus
CN	cranial nerve
CNA	certified nursing assistant
CNM	certified nurse midwife
CNO	community nursing organization
CNS	central nervous system
CNS	clinical nurse specialist
Co	cobalt
CO_2	carbon dioxide
CO_2^-	carbon dioxide ion
COBRA	Comprehensive Omnibus Budget Reconciliation Act
COLD	chronic obstructive lung disease
COOH	carboxyl group
COPD	chronic obstructive pulmonary disease
COPP	A combination of chemotherapy drugs: cyclophosphamide (Cytoxan), vincristine (Oncovin), procarbazine (Matulanel), and prednisone (Deltasone)
CP	cerebral palsy
CPAP	continuous positive airway pressure
CPD	cephalopelvic disproportion
CPM	continuous passive motion
CPNP	Council of Practical Nursing Programs
CPR	cardiopulmonary resuscitation
CPR	computerized patient record
CPS	Child Protective Services
CPT	chest physiotherapy
C-R	crown-rump
Cr	chromium
CRE	chronic renal failure
CRNA	Certified Registered Nurse Anesthetist
CRP	C-reactive protein
CSF	cerebrospinal fluid
C&S	culture and sensitivity
CSM	circulation, sensation, motion
CST	contraction stress syndrome
CT	computed tomography
Cu	copper
CVA	cerebrovascular accident
CVC	central venous catheter
CVD	cardiovascular disease

CVP	A combination of chemotherapy drugs: cyclophosphamide (Cytoxan), vincristine (Oncovin), prednisone (Deltasone)
CVS	chorionic villi sampling
D_5W	dextrose 5% in water
DAI	diffuse axonal injury
D & C	dilatation and curettage
DAR	document, action, response
dc	discontinue
DDB	Disciplinary Data Bank
DDH	developmental dysplasia of the hip
DDS	doctor of dental surgery
DDST	Denver Developmental Screening Test
DEA	Drug Enforcement Agency
DES	diethylstilbestrol
DET	diethyltriptamine
DETOX	detoxification
DHHS	Department of Health and Human Services
DIC	disseminated intravascular coagulation
DICC	dynamic infusion cavernosometry and cavernosography
DJD	degenerative joint disease
DKA	diabetic ketoacidosis
dL	deciliter
DMARD	disease-modifying antirheumatic drug
DMD	doctor of dental medicine
DMD	Duchenne muscular dystrophy
DMT	dimethyltriptamine
DNA	deoxyribonucleic acid
DNR	do not resuscitate
DO	doctor of osteopathy
DOM	dimethyl-4-ethylamphetamine
DPAHC	durable power of attorney for health care
DPT	demerol, phenergan, thorazine
dr	dram, or ʒ
DRG	diagnosis-related group
DRI	dietary reference intake
DSM-IV	*Diagnostic and Statistical Manual of Mental Disorders,* 4th edition
DST	dexamethasone suppression test
DT	delirium tremens
DTaP	diphtheria, tetanus, acellular pertussis
DTP	diphtheria, tetanus, pertussis
DVT	deep vein thrombosis
EA	Emotions Anonymous
EABV	effective arterial blood volume
EAR	estimated average requirement
ECF	extended care facility
ECF	extracellular fluid
ECT	electroconvulsive therapy
ED	emergency department
EDB	estimated date of birth
EDD	estimated date of delivery
EEG	electroencephalograph
EENT	eyes, ears, nose, and throat
EFM	electronic fetal monitoring
EGD	esophagogastroduodenoscopy
EKG (ECG)	electrocardiogram
ELISA	enzyme-linked immunosorbent assay
elix	elixir
EMG	electromyogram
EMLA	eutectic (cream) mixture of local anesthetics
EMS	emergency medical services
EMT	emergency medical technician
EMT-P	emergency medical technician-paramedic
EPA	Environmental Protection Agency
EPO	exclusive provider organization
EPS	extrapyramidal symptom
ER	emergency room
ERCP	endoscopic retrograde cholangiopancreatogram
ERG	electroretinogram
ERT	estrogen replacement therapy
ESR	erythrocyte sedimentation rate
ESRD	end-stage renal disease
ESU	electrosurgical unit
ESWL	extracorporeal shock wave lithotripsy
ET	ear (tympanic) temperature
ETT	endotracheal tube
EVAD	explantable venous access device
F	fahrenheit
FAE	fetal alcohol effects
FAF	fibroblast activating factor
FAS	fetal alcohol syndrome
FAST	fetal acoustic stimulation test
FBD	fibrocystic breast disease
FBPP	fetal biophysical profile
FBS	fasting blood sugar
FCA	False Claims Act
FDA	Food and Drug Administration
Fe	iron
FHR	fetal heart rate
FHT	fetal heart tones
fl	fluid
Fl	fluorine
FOBT	fecal occult blood test
4 Ps	passage, passenger, powers, psyche
FSBG	finger stick blood glucose
FSH	follicle-stimulating hormone
ft	foot
FTA-ABS	fluorescent troponomal antibody-absorption test
FTT	failure to thrive
FVD	fluid volume deficit
g	gram
g/dL	grams per deciliter
GAD	generalized anxiety disorder
GAS	general adaptation syndrome
GCS	Glasgow Coma Scale
GDM	gestational diabetes mellitus
GED	general education development
GERD	gastroesophageal reflux disease
GFR	glomerular filtration rate
GGT	gammaglutamy transpeptidase
GH	growth hormone
GHB	glycosylated hemoglobin
GI	gastrointestinal
GIFT	gamete-intrafallopian transfer
GP/TPAL	gravida, para/term, preterm, abortions, living
GPA	Global Programme on AIDS
gr	grain
gtt	drop
GTT	glucose tolerance test
gtt/min	drops per minute
GU	genitourinary
Gy	gray
h	hour(s)
H^+	hydrogen ion
H_2CO_3	carbonic acid
H_2O	water
HAI	hemagglutination inhibition
H&H	hemoglobin and hematocrit
HAART	highly active antiretroviral therapy

HAV	hepatitis A virus
HB₅AG	hepatitis B surface antigen
HBIG	hepatitis B immune globulin
HBV	hepatitis B virus
HCFA	Health Care Financing Administration
hCG	human chorionic gonadotropin
HCl	hydrochloric acid, hydrochloride
HCO₃⁻	bicarbonate ion
Hct	hematocrit
HCV	hepatitis C virus
HD	Huntington's Disease
HDL	high density lipoprotein
HDV	hepatitis D virus
HELLP	**h**emolysis **e**levated **l**iver enzymes **l**ow **p**latelet count
Hep B	hepatitis B
HFA	Hospice Foundation of America
Hgb F	fetal hemoglobin
HF	heart failure
Hgb	hemoglobin
HHNS	hyperosmolar hyperglycemic nonketotic syndrome
HHV	human herpes virus
HiB	*haemophilus influenzae* type B
HICPAC	Hospital Infection Control Practices Advisory Committee
HIS	hospital information system
HIV	human immunodeficiency virus
HLA	human leukocyte antigen
HMO	health maintenance organization
hPL	human placental lactogen
HPV	human papillomavirus
hr	hour
HR	heart rate
HRSA	Health Resources and Services Administration
h.s.	hour of sleep
HSV-1	herpes simplex virus type 1
HSV-2	herpes simplex virus type 2
HTN	hypertension
I	iodine
IABP	intra-aortic balloon pump
IADL	instrumental activities of daily living
I&O	intake and output
IASP	International Association for the Study of Pain
IBD	inflammatory bowel disease
ICD	implantable cardioverter-defibrillator
ICEA	International Childbirth Education Association
ICF	intermediate care facility
ICF	intracellular fluid
ICN	International Council of Nurses
ICU	intensive care unit
ID	identification
ID	intradermal
IDM	infant of a diabetic mother
IFG	impaired fasting glucose
IgA	immunoglobulin A
IgD	immunoglobulin D
IgE	immunoglobulin E
IgG	immunoglobulin G
IgM	immunoglobulin M
IGT	impaired glucose tolerance
IHCT	interdisciplinary health care team
IHS	Indian Health Service
IM	intramuscular

in	inch
INR	International Normalized Ratio
I&O	intake and output
IOL	intraocular lens
IOM	Institute of Medicine
IOP	intraocular pressure
IPV	inactivated polio vaccine
IQ	intelligence quotient
ISAM	infant of a substance abusing mother
ITP	idiopathic thrombocytopenic purpura
ITT	insulin tolerance test
IUD	intrauterine device
IUGR	intrauterine growth retardation
IV	intravenous
IVAD	implantable vascular access device
IVF-ER	*in vitro* fertilization and embryo replacement
IVP	intravenous push, intravenous pyelogram
IVPB	intravenous piggyback
JA	juvenile arthritis
JCAHO	Joint Commission on Accreditation of Healthcare Organizations
JOGNN	*Journal of Obstetric, Gynecologic, and Neonatal Nursing*
K	potassium
K⁺	potassium ion
kcal	kilocalorie
KCl	potassium chloride
kg	kilogram
KS	ketosteroids
KUB	kidneys/ureters/bladder
KVO	keep vein open
L	liter
L/min	liters per minute
L/S	lecithin/sphingomyelin
LAAM	levo-alpha-acetyl-methadol
LAD	left anterior descending
LAS	local adaptation syndrome
lb	pound
LDH	lactic dehydrogenase
LDL	low density lipoprotein
LDRP	labor, delivery, recovery, postpartum
LE	lupus erythematosus
LES	lower esophageal sphincter
LFT	liver function test
LGA	large for gestational age
LH	lactate hydrogenase
LH	luteinizing hormone
LHRH	luteinizing hormone releasing hormone
LLQ	left lower quadrant
LMA	left mentum anterior
LMP	last menstrual period
LMP	left mentum posterior
LMT	left mentum transverse
LOA	left occiput anterior
LOC	level of consciousness
LOP	left occiput posterior
LOT	left occiput transverse
LP	lumbar puncture
LP/VN	licensed practical/vocational nurse
LPN	licensed practical nurse
L/S ratio	lecithin and ephingomyelin
LSA	left sacrum anterior
LSD	lysergic acid diethylamide
LSP	left sacrum posterior
LST	left sacrum transverse
LTB	laryngotracheobronchitis

LUQ	left upper quadrant
LVN	licensed vocational nurse
m²	square meter
MAC	*myobacterium avium* complex
MADD	Mothers Against Drunk Driving
MAO	monoamine oxidase
MAOI	monoamine oxidase inhibitor
MAP	mean arterial pressure
MAR	medication administration record
mcg (or μg)	microgram
MCNS	minimal charge nephrotic syndrome
MD	doctor of medicine
MDI	metered-dose inhaler
MDMA	methylene dioxyamphetamine
MDR	multidrug-resistant
MDR-TB	multidrug-resistant tuberculosis
MDS	minimum data set
MDT	maggot debridement therapy
mEq	milliequivalent
mEq/L	milliequivalents per liter
mg	milligram
mg/dL	milligrams per deciliter
MG	myasthenia gravis
Mg	magnesium
Mg⁺⁺	magnesium ion
MgCl	magnesium chloride
MgSO₄	magnesium sulfate
MI	myocardial infarction
m²	meter squared
min	minute
mL	milliliter
mm	millimeter
mm³	cubic millimeter
mm Hg	millimeters of mercury
mmol/L	millimoles per liter
MMR	measles, mumps, rubella
Mn	manganese
Mo	molybdenum
MOM	Milk of Magnesia
MOPP	A combination of chemotherapy drugs: mechlorethamine or nitrogen mustard (Mustargen), vincristine (Oncovin), procarbazine hydrochloride (Matulane), prednisone (Deltasone)
mOsm/kg	milliosmoles/kilogram
mOsm/L	milliosmoles per liter
MRI	magnetic resonance imaging
MRSA	methicillin-resistant *staphylococcus aureus*
MS	morphine sulfate
MS	multiple sclerosis
MSAFP	maternal serum alpha-fetoprotein
MSDS	material safety data sheet
MSG	monosodium glutamate
MSH	melanocyte-stimulating hormone
MUGA	multi-gated acquisition
MVC	motor vehicle collision
N₂	nitrogen
NA	Narcotics Anonymous
NA	not applicable
Na	sodium
Na⁺	sodium ion
Na₂SO₄	sodium sulfate
NAACOG	Nurses Association of the American College of Obstetricians and Gynecologists
NaCl	sodium chloride
NADSA	National Adult Day Services Associations
NaH₂PO₄	sodium dihydrogen phosphate

Na₂HPO₄	disodium phosphate
NAHC	National Association for Home Care
NaHCO₃	sodium bicarbonate
NaHPO₄	sodium monohydrogen phosphate
NANDA	North American Nursing Diagnosis Association
NaOH	sodium hydroxide
NAPNES	National Association for Practical Nurse Education and Services
NCAL	National Center for Assisted Living
NCCAM	National Center for Complementary and Alternative Medicine
NCHS	National Center for Health Statistics
NCLEX	National Council Licensure Examination
NCLEX-PN®	National Council Licensure Examination—Practical Nurse
NCLEX-RN®	National Council Licensure Examination—Registered Nurse
NCOA	National Council on Aging
NCSBN	National Council of State Boards of Nursing
NF	*National Formulary*
NFLPN	National Federation of Licensed Practical Nurses, Inc.
NG	nasogastric
NGT	nasogastric tube
NH₂	amino group
NHF	National Hemophilia Foundation
NHL	non-Hodgkin's lymphoma
NHO	National Hospice Organization
NIA	National Institute on Aging
NIAAA	National Institute on Alcohol Abuse and Alcoholism
NIAID	National Institute of Allergies and Infectious Diseases
NIAMS	National Institute of Arthritis and Musculoskeletal and Skin Diseases
NIC	Nursing Interventions Classification
NIDA	National Institute on Drug Abuse
NIDDK	National Institute of Diabetes and Digestive and Kidney Diseases
NIH	National Institute of Health
NINDS	National Institute of Neurological Disorders and Stroke
NIOSH	National Institute of Occupational Safety and Health
NIS	nursing information system
NKF	National Kidney Foundation
NLEA	Nutrition, Labeling, and Education Act
NLN	National League for Nursing
NLNAC	National League for Nursing Accrediting Commission
NMDS	nursing minimum data set
NMS	neuroleptic malignant syndrome
NNRTI	nonnucleoside reverse transcriptase inhibitor
NOC	Nursing Outcomes Classification
NOF	National Osteoporosis Foundation
NP	nurse practitioner
NPDB	National Practitioner Data Bank
NPO	*nil per os,* Latin for "nothing by mouth"
NPUAP	National Pressure Ulcer Advisory Panel
NREM	non-rapid eye movement
NRTI	nucleoside analog reverse transcriptase inhibitor
NS	normal saline
NSAID	nonsteroidal anti-inflammatory drug
NSF	National Sleep Foundation

NSR	normal sinus rhythm
NST	nonstress test
N/V	nausea/vomiting
O_2	oxygen
OA	osteoarthritis
OAM	Office of Alternative Medicine
O&P	ova and parasite
OBRA	Omnibus Budget Reconciliation Act
OCD	obsessive compulsive disorder
OD	right eye
OH⁻	hydroxyl
OHL	oral hairy leukoplakia
OPV	oral polio vaccine
OR	operating room
ORIF	open reduction/internal fixation
OS	left eye
OSHA	Occupational Safety and Health Administration
OT	occupational therapist
OTC	over-the-counter
OU	both eyes
oz	ounce
p̄	after
P	phosphorus
P	pulse
PA	physician's assistant
PAC	premature atrial contractions
$PaCO_2$	partial pressure of carbon dioxide
PACU	postanesthesia care unit
PaO_2	partial pressure of oxygen
Pap	Papanicolaou test
PAT	paroxysmal atrial tachycardia
PBI	protein bound iodine
p.c.	after meals
PCA	patient-controlled analgesia
PCO_2 ($PaCO_2$)	partial pressure of carbon dioxide
PCP	phencyclidine
PCP	*pneumocystis carinii* pneumonia
PCP	primary care provider
PCR	polymerase chain reaction
PCV	pneumococcal conjugate vaccine
PDA	patent ductus arteriosis
PDPH	postdural puncture headache
PEG	percutaneous endoscopic gastrostomy
PEM	protein energy manipulation
PERRLA	pupils equal, round, reactive to light and accommodation
PET	positron emission tomography
PFT	pulmonary function test
PG	phosphatidylglycerol
pH	potential hydrogen
PHS	Public Health Services
PI	peripheral intravenous
PICC	peripherally inserted central catheter
PID	pelvic inflammatory disease
PIE	problem, implementation, evaluation
PIH	pregnancy-induced hypertension
PKD	polycystic kidney disease
PKU	phenylketonuria
PLMS	periodic limb movement in sleep
PMI	point of maximum intensity
PMN	polymorphonuclear leukocyte
PMR	progressive muscle relaxation
PMS	premenstrual syndrome
PNI	psychoneuroimmunology
PNS	peripheral nervous system
po	*per os,* Latin for "by mouth"
PO_2 (PaO_2)	partial pressure of oxygen
PO_4^{--}	phosphate ion
POMR	problem-oriented medical record
POR	problem-oriented record
PPBS	post prandial blood sugar
PPD	postpartum depression
PPD	purified protein derivative
PPG	post prandial glucose
PPO	preferred provider organization
PPS	prospective payment system
PRL	prolactin level
PRN	*pro re nata,* Latin for "as required"
PRO	peer review organization
PROM	passive range of motion
PROM	premature rupture of membranes
PSA	prostate specific antigen
PSDA	Patient Self-Determination Act
PSP	phenolsulfonphtalein
PSVT	paroxysmal supraventricular tachycardia
pt	pint
PT	physical therapist
PT	prothrombin time
PTCA	percutaneous transluminal coronary angioplasty
PTH	parathyroid hormone
PTSD	post-traumatic stress disorder
PTT	partial thromboplastin time
PTU	propylthiouracil
PUVA	psoralen ultraviolet A-range
PV	polycythemia vera
PVC	premature ventricular contraction
PVD	peripheral vascular disease
q	*quaque,* Latin for "every"
qd	every day
qh	every hour
qid	four times a day
qod	every other day
qs	quantity sufficient
q2h	every 2 hours
qt	quart
R	respiration
RA	rheumatoid arthritis
RAD	reactive airway disease
RAIU	radioactive iodine uptake
RAST	radio allergosorbent test
RBC	red blood count, red blood cell
RD	registered dietician
RDA	recommended dietary allowance
RDD	radiation disperal device
RDS	respiratory distress syndrome
REM	rapid eye movement
Resp	respirations
RF	rheumatoid factor
RhoGAM	RH immune globulin
RICE	rest, ice, compression, elevation
RIND	reversible ischemic neurological deficit
RLQ	right lower quadrant
RLS	restless leg syndrome
RMA	right mentum anterior
RMP	right mentum posterior
RMT	right mentum transverse
RN	registered nurse
RNA	ribonucleic acid
RNFA	registered nurse first assistant
ROA	right occiput anterior
ROM	range of motion
ROM	rupture of membranes
ROP	right occiput posterior
ROS	review of systems

ROT	right occiput transverse
RPCH	rural primary care hospital
RPh	registered pharmacist
RPR	rapid plasma reagin
RR	recovery room
RSA	right sacrum anterior
RSP	right sacrum posterior
RST	right sacrum transverse
RSV	respiratory syncytial virus
R/T	related to
RT	respiratory therapist
RTI	respiratory tract infection
RUGS	resource utilization group system
RUQ	right upper quadrant
RWJF	Robert Wood Johnson Foundation
$\bar{s}$	without
S	sulfur
SA	sinoatrial
SADD	Students Against Drunk Driving
SaO$_2$	oxygen saturation
SBC	school-based clinic
SBP	systolic blood pressure
SC/SQ	subcutaneous
SCA	sickle-cell anemia
SCD	sequential compression device
SCI	spinal cord injury
Se	selenium
SGA	small for gestational age
SGOT	serum glutamic oxaloacetic transaminase
SGPT	serum glutamic pyruvic transaminase
SH	somatotropin hormone
SIADH	syndrome of inappropriate antidiuretic hormone
SIDS	sudden infant death syndrome
SL	sublingual
SLE	systemic lupus erythematosus
SMBG	self-monitor blood glucose
SNF	skilled nursing facility
SOAP	subjective data, objective data, assessment, plan
SOAPIE	subjective data, objective data, assessment, plan, implementation, evaluation
SOAPIER	subjective data, objective data, assessment, plan, implementation, evaluation, revision
SPF	sun protection factor
SROM	spontaneous rupture of membranes
$\bar{s}\bar{s}$	one half
SSA	Social Security Administration
SSKI	saturated solution potassium iodide
SSRI	selective serotonin reuptake inhibitor
STAT	*statim*, Latin for "immediately"
STD	sexually transmitted disease
supp	suppository
susp	suspension
SW	social worker
T	temperature
T$_3$	triiodothyronine
T$_4$	thyroxine
tab	tablet
TAC	tetracaine, adrenaline, cocaine
TB	tuberculosis
Tbsp	tablespoon
TD	tardive dyskinesia
Td	tetanus/diphtheria
TDD	telecommunication device for the deaf
TEE	transesophageal echocardiography
TEFRA	Tax Equity Fiscal Responsibility Act
TENS	transcutaneous electrical nerve stimulation

TF	tube feeding
THA	total hip arthroplasty
TIA	transient ischemic attack
TIBC	total iron binding capacity
t.i.d.	three times a day
TIG	tetanus immune globulin
TIPS	transjugular intrahepatic portosystemic shunt
TKA	total knee arthroplasty
TM	tympanic membrane
TMD	temporomandibular joint disease
TMJ	temporomandibular joint
TNM	tumor, node, metastasis
t.o.	telephone order
TOF	tetralogy of Fallot
TORCH	**to**xoplasmosis, **r**ubella, **c**ytomegalovirus, **h**erpesvirus
TPN	total parenteral nutrition
TPR	temperature, pulse, respirations
Tr or tinct	tincture
TRAM	transplantation of the rectus abdominis muscle
TRH	thyrotropin-releasing hormone
TSE	testicular self examination
TSH	thyroid-stimulating hormone
TSI	thyroid-stimulating immunoglobulin
tsp	teaspoon
TSS	toxic shock syndrome
TTN	transient tachypnea of the newborn
TULIP	transurethral ultrasound-guided laser-induced prostatectomy
TURP	transurethral resection of the prostate
U	unit
UA	routine urinalysis
UAP	unlicensed assistive personnel
UC	ulcerative colitis
UGI	upper gasrointestinal tract
UIS	Universal Intellectual Standards
UL	upper intake level
UMLS	Universal Medical Language System
UNOS	United Network for Organ Sharing
U-100	100 units insulin per cc
UPP	urethra pressure profile
UPSIT	University of Pennsylvania Smell Identification Test
URQ	upper right quadrant
USDHHS	United States Department of Health and Human Services
USP	*United States Pharmacopeia*
USPHS	United States Public Health Service
UTI	urinary tract infection
UV	ultraviolet
VA	Veterans Administration, Veterans Affairs
VAC	vacuum assisted closure
VAD	ventricular assist device, vascular access device
var	varicella
VAS	Visual Analog Scale
VBAC	vaginal birth after cesarean
VCD	vacuum constriction device
VDRL	venereal disease research laboratory
VF	ventricular fibrillation
VHF	viral hemorrhagic fevers
VLDL	very low-density lipoprotein
VMA	vanilymandelic acid
VRE	vancomycin-resistant enterococci
VS	vital signs
VSD	ventricular septal defect

VST	vibroacoustic stimulation test		**WPM**	words per minute
VT	ventricular tachycardia		**wt**	weight
WASP	white, Anglo-Saxon, Protestant		**YWCA**	Young Women's Christian Association
WBC	white blood cell, white blood count		**ZIFT**	zygote-intra-fallopian transfer
WHO	World Health Organization		**Zn**	Zinc
WIC	Women, Infants, and Children			
WNL	within normal limits			

Appendix D: English/Spanish Words and Phrases

Being able to say a few words or phrases in the client's language is one way to show that you care. It lets the client know that you as a nurse are interested in the individual. There are three rules to keep in mind regarding the pronunciation of Spanish words.

- If a word ends in a vowel, or in *n* or *s*, the accent is on the next to the last syllable.
- If the word ends in a consonant other than *n* or *s*, the accent is on the last syllable.
- If the word does not follow these rules, it has a written accent over the vowel of the accented syllable.

Courtesy phrases, names of body parts, and expressions of time and numbers are included in this section for quick reference. The English version will appear first, followed by the Spanish translation and Spanish pronunciation.

Courtesy Phrases

Please	Por favor	Por fah-**vor**
Thank-you	Grácias	**Grah**-the-as
Good morning	Buénos dias	Boo-**ay**-nos **dee**-as
Good afternoon	Buénas tardes	Boo-**ay**-nas **tar**-days
Good evening	Buénas noches	Boo-**ay**-nas **no**-chays
Yes/No	Si/no	See/no
Good	Bien	Be-en
Bad	Mal	Mahl
How many?	¿Cuántos?	¿Coo-**ahn**-tos?
Where?	¿Dónde?	¿**Don**-day?
When?	¿Cuándo?	¿Coo**ahn**-do?

Body Parts

abdomen	el abdomen	el ab-doh-men
ankle	el tobillo	el to-**beel**-lyo
anus	el ano	el **ah**-no
anvil (incus)	el yunque	el **yoon**-kay
appendix	el apéndice	el ah-**pen**-de-thay
aqueous humor	el humor acuoso	el oo-**mor** ah-coo-**o**-so
bladder	la vejiga	lah vay-**nee**-gah
brain	el cerebro	el thay-**ray**-bro
breast	el pecho	el **pay**-cho
buttock	la nalga	lah **nahl**-gah
calf	la pantorrilla	lah pan-tor-**reel**-lyah
cervix	la cerviz	lah ther-**veth**
cheek	la mejilla	lah may-**heel**-lyah
chin	la barbilla	lah bar-**beel**-lyah
choroid	la coroidea	lah co-ro-e-**day**-ah
ciliary body	el cuerpo ciliar	el coo-**err**-po the-le-**ar**
clitoris	el clítoris	el **clee**-to-ris
coccyx	el coxis	el **coc**-sees
conjunctiva	la conjuntiva	lah con-hoon-**tee**vah
cornea	la córnea	lah **cor**-nay-ah
penis	el pene	el **pay**-nay
prostate gland	la próstata	lah **pros**-ta-tah
pupil	la pupila	lah poo-**pee**-lah
rectum	el recto	el **rec**-to

retina	la retina	lah ray-**tee**-nah
sclera	la esclerótica	lah es-clay-**ro**-te-cah
scrotum	el escroto	el es-**cro**-to
seminal vesicle	la vesícula seminal	lah vay-**see**-coo-lah say-me-**nahl**
shoulder	el hombro	el **om**-bro
small intestine	el intestino delgado	el in-tes-**tee**-no del-**gah**-do.
spinal cord	la médula espinal	lah **may**-doo-lah es-pe-**nahl**
spleen	el bazo	el **bah**-tho
stirrup (stapes)	el estribo	el es-**tree**-bo
stomach	el estómago	el es-**toh**-mah-go
temple	la sien	lah se-**ayn**
testis	el testículo	el tes-**tee**-coo-lo
thigh	el muslo	el **moos**-lo
thorax	el tórax	el **to**-rax
tongue	la lengua	lah **len**-goo-ah
trachea	la tráquea	lah **trah**-kay-ah
upper extremities	las extremidades superiores	las ex-tray-me-**dahd**-es soo-pay-re-**or**-es
ureter	el uréter	el oo-**ray**-ter
uterus	el útero	el **oo**-tay-ro
vagina	el vagina	lah vah-**hee**-nah
vitreous humor	el humor vítreo	el oo-**mor vee**-tray-o
wrist	la muñeca	lah moo-**nyay**-cah

Expressions of Time, Calendar, and Numbers

after meals	después de comer	des-poo-**es** day co-**merr**
at bedtime	al acostarse	al ah-cos-**tar**-say
before meals	antes de comer	**ahn**-tes day co-**merr**
daily	el diario	el de-**ah**-re-o
date	la fecha	lah **fay**-chah
day	el dia	el **dee**-ah
every hour	a cada hora	ah **cah**-dah **o**-rah
hour (time)	la hora	lah **o**-rah
how often	cada cuánto tiempo	**cah**-dah coo-**ahn**-to te-**em**-po
noon	el mediodia	el may-de-o-**dee**-ah
now	ahora	ah-**o**-rah
once	una vez	**oo**-nah veth
today	hoy	**oh**-e
tomorrow	mañana	mah-**nyah**-nah
tonight	esta noche	**es**-tah **no**-chay
week	la semana	lah say-**mah**-nah
year	año	**a**-nyo
Sunday	el domingo	el do-**meen**-go
Monday	el lunes	el **loo**-nes
Tuesday	el martes	el **mar**-tes
Wednesday	el miércoles	el me-**err**-co-les
Thursday	el jueves	el hoo-**ay**ves
Friday	el viernes	el ve-**err**-nes
Saturday	el sábado	el **sah**-bah-do
zero	cero	**thay**-ro
one	uno	**oo**-no
two	dos	dose
three	tres	trays
four	cuatro	coo-**ah**-tro
five	cinco	**theen**-co
six	seis	**say**-ees
seven	siete	se-**ay**-tay
eight	ocho	**o**-cho
nine	nueve	noo-**ay**-vay
ten	diez	de-**eth**

Nursing Care Sentences and Questions

What is your name?
¿Como se llama usted?
¿**Co**-mo say **lyah**-mah oos-**ted?**

I am a student nurse.
Soy estudiente enfermera(o).
Soy es-too-de-**ahn**-tay en-fer-**may**-ra(o).

My name is . . .
Mi nombre es . . .
Mee **nom**-bray es . . .

Do you need a wheelchair?
¿Necesita usted una silla de rueda?
¿**Nay**-thay-**se**-ta oos-**ted oo**-nah **seel**-lyah day
    roo-**ay**-dah?

How do you feel?
¿Como se siente?
¿**Co**-mo say se-**ayn**-tah?

When is your family coming?
¿Cuándo viene su familia?
¿Coo-**ahn**-do vee-**en**-nah soo fah-**mee**-le-ah?

This is the call light.
Esta es la luz para llamar a la enfermera.
Es-tah es lah looth **pah**-ra lyah-**mar** a lah
    en-fer-**may**-ra.

If you need anything, press the button.
Si usted necesita algo, oprima el botón.
See oos-**ted** nay-thay-**se**-ta **ahl**-go o-pre-**ma** el
    bo-**tone.**

Do not turn without calling the nurse.
No se voltee sin llamar a la enfermera.
No say **vol**-tay seen lyah-**mar** a lah en-fer-**may**-ra.

The side rails on your bed are for your protection.
Los rieles del costado están para su protección.
Los re-**el**-es del cos-**tah**-do es-**tahn pah**-ra soo
    pro-tec-the-**on.**

Please do not try to lower or climb over the side rail.
Por favor no pretenda bajarlos (barjarlas) o treparse
    sobre ellos.
Por fah-**vor** no pray-**ten**-dah ba-**har**-los o
    tray-**par**-say **so**-bray **ayl**-lyos.

The head nurse is . . .
La jefa de enfermeras es . . .
La **hay**-fay day en-fer-**may**-ras es . . .

Do you need more blankets or another pillow?
¿Necesita usted más frazadas u orta almohada?
¿Nay-thay-**si**-ta oos-**ted** mahs frah-**thad**-dahs oo
    o-trah al-mo-**ah**-dah?

You may not smoke in the room.
No se puede fumar en el cuarto.
No say poo-**ay**-day foo-**mar** en el coo-**ar**-to.

Do you want me to turn on (turn off) the lights?
¿Quiere usted que encienda (apague) la luz?
¿Ke-**ay**-ray oos-**ted** day en-the-**en**-dah (a-**pah**-gay)
    lah looth?

Are you thirsty?
¿Tiene usted sed?
¿Tee-**en**-nah oos-**ted** sayd?

Are you allergic to any medication?
¿Es usted alérgico(a) a alguna medicina?
¿Es oos-**ted** ah-**lehr**-hee-co(a) ah ah-**goo**-nah nay-
    de-**thee**-nah?

You may take a bath.
Usted puede bañarse.
Oos-**ted** poo-**ay**-day bah-**nyar**-say.

Do not lock the door, please.
No cierre usted la puerta con llave, por favor.
No the-**err**-ray oos-**ted** lah poo-**err**-tah con **lyah**-vay
    por fah-**vor.**

Call if you feel faint or in need of help.
Llame si usted se siente débil o si necesita ayuda.
Lyah-mah see oos-**ted** say se-**ayn**-tah **day**-bil o see
    nay-thay-**se**-ta ah-**yoo**-dah.

Call when you have to go to the toilet.
Llame cuando tenga que ir al inodoro.
Lyah-mah coo-**ahn**-do **ten**-gah kay eer al in-o-**do**-
    ro.

I will give you an enema.
Le pondré una enema.
Lay pon-**dray oo**-nah ay-**nay**-mah.

Turn on your left (right) side.
Voltese a su lado izquierdo (derecho).
Vol-**tay**-say ah soo **lah**-do ith-ke-**er**-do(dah) (day-
    ray-cho[cha]).

Here is an appointment card.
Aqui tiene usted una tarjeta con la información
    escrito.
Ah-**kee** tee-**en**-nah oos-**ted oo**-nah tar-**hay**-tah con
    lah in-for-mah-the-**on** es-**cree**-to.

You are going to be discharged (released) today.
A usted le van a dar de alta hoy.
Ah oos-**ted** lay vahn ah dar day **ahl**-tah **oh**-e.

How did this illness begin?
¿Como empezó esta enfermedad?
¿**Co**-mo em-pa-**tho es**-tah en-fer-may-**dahd**?

Is the pain better after the medicine?
¿Siente usted alivio depués de tomar la medicina?
¿Se-**ayn**-tah oos-**ted** al-**lee**-ve-o des-poo-**es** day to-**mar** lah may-de-**thee**-nah?

Where is the pain?
¿Que la duele? (or) Dónde le duele?
¿**Kay** lah doo-**ay**-le? (or) **Don**-day lay doo-**ay**-le?

Do you have pains in your chest?
¿Tiene usted dolores in el pecho?
¿Tee-**en**-nah oos-**ted** do-**lor**-es en el **pay**-cho?

Are you in pain now?
¿Tiene usted dolores ahora?
¿Tee-**en**-nah oos-**ted** do-**lor**-es ah-**o**-rah?

Is it constant pain or does it come and go?
¿Es un dolor constante o va y vuelve?
¿Es oon do-**lor** cons-**tahn**-tay o vah ee voo-**el**-vah?

Is there anything that makes the pain better?
¿Hay algo que lo alivie?
¿**Ah**-ee **ahl**-go kay lo al-**le**-ve?

Is there anything that makes the pain worse?
¿Hay algo que lo aumente?
¿**Ah**-ee **ahl**-go kay lo ah-oo-**men**-tay?

Where do you feel the pain?
¿Dónde siente usted el dolor?
¿**Don**-day se-**ayn**-tah oos-**ted** el do-**lor**?

Point to where it hurts.
Apunte usted por favor, adonde le duele.
Ah-**poon**-tay oos-**ted** por fah-**vor** ah-**don**-day lay doo-**ay**-le.

Show me where it hurts.
Enséñeme usted donde le duele.
En-**say**-nah-may oos-**ted don**-day lay doo-**ay**-le.

Is the pain sharp or dull?
¿Es agudo o sordo el dolor?
¿Es ah-**goo**-do o **sor**-do el do-**lor**?

Do you know where you are?
¿Sabe usted donde esta?
¿Sah-**bay** oos-**ted don**-day es-**tah**?

You are in the hospital.
Usted está en el hospital.
Oos-**ted** es-**tah** en el os-pee-**tahl**.

You will be okay.
Usted va a estar bien.
Oos-**ted** vah a es-**tar** be-en.

Do you have any drug reactions?
¿Tiene usted alguna sensibilidad a productos químicos?
¿Te-**en**-nah oos-**ted** al-**goo**-nah sen-se-be-le-**dahd** a pro-**dooc**-tos **kee**-me-cos?

Have you seen another doctor or native healer for this problem?
¿Ha visto usted a otro médico o curandero tocante a este problema?
¿Ah **vees**-to oos-**ted** a o-tro **may**-de-co o coo-ran-**day**-ro to-**cahn**-tay a **es**-ah pro-**blay**-mah?

Have you vomited?
¿Ha vomitado usted?
¿Ah vo-me-**tah**-do oos-**ted**?

Do you have any difficulty in breathing?
¿Tiene usted alguna dificultad para respirar?
¿Te-**en**-nah oos-**ted** ah-**goo**-nah de-fe-cool-**tahd** **pah**-ra res-pe-**rar**?

Do you smoke?
¿Fuma usted?
¿Foo-**mar** oos-**ted**?

How many per day?
¿Cuántos al dia?
¿Coo-**ahn**-tos al **dee**-ah?

For how many years?
¿Por cuántos años?
¿por coo-**ahn**-tos **a**-nyos?

Do you awaken in the night because of shortness of breath?
¿Se despierta usted por la noche por falta de respiración?
¿Say des-pee-**err**-tah oos-**ted** por lah **no**-chay por **fahl**-tah day res-pe-rah-the-**on**?

Is any part of your body swollen?
¿Tiene usted alguna parte del cuerpo hinchada?
¿Te-**en**-nah oos-**ted** ah-**goo**-nah **par**-tay del coo-**err**-po in-**chah**-da?

How much water do you drink daily?
¿Cuántos vasos de agua bebe usted diariamente?
¿Coo-**ahn**-tos **vah**-sos day **ah**-goo-ah **bay**-be oos-**ted** de-ah-re-ah-**men**-tay?

Are you nauseated?
¿Tiene náusea?
¿Te-**en**-nah **nah**-oo-say-ah?

Are you going to vomit?
¿Va a vomitar?
¿Vah a vo-me-**tar**?

When was your last bowel movement?
¿Cuánto tiempo hace que evacúa usted?
¿Coo-**ahn**-to te-**em**-po **ah**-the kay ay-vah-**coo**-ah
   oos-**ted**?

Do you have diarrhea?
¿Tiene usted diarrea?
¿Te-**en**-nah oos-**ted** der-ar-**ray**-ah?

How much do you urinate?
¿Cuánto orina usted?
¿Coo-**ahn**-to o-**re**-nah oos-**ted**?

Did you urinate?
¿Orinó usted?
¿O-re-**no** oos-**ted**?

What color is your urine?
¿De qué color es la orina?
¿Day kay co-**lor** es lah o-**re**-nah?

Call when you have to go to the toilet.
Llame usted cuando tenga que ir al inodoro.
Lyah-mah oos-**ted** coo-**ahn**-do **ten**-gah kay eer al
   in-o-**do**-ro.

I need a urine specimen from you.
Necesito una muestra de orina de usted.
Nay-thay-**se**-to **oo**-nah moo-**ays**-trah day o-**re**-nah
   day oos-**ted**.

We will put a tube in your bladder so that you can
   urinate.
Le pondremos un tubo en la vejiga para que puede
   orinar.
Lay pon-**dray**-mos un **too**-be en lah vay-**hee**-gah
   pah-rah kay poo-**ay**-day o-re **nar**.

When was your last menstrual period?
¿Cuándo fue se última menstruación?
¿Coo-**ahn**-do foo-**ay** soo **ool**-te-mah
   mens-troo-ah-the-**on**?

Are you bleeding heavily?
¿Está sangrando mucho?
¿Es-**tah** san-**grahn**-do **moo**-cho?

Take off your clothes, please
Desvístase usted, por favor.
Des-**ves**-tah-say oos-**ted** por-fah-**vor**.

Just relax.
Relaje usted el cuerpo.
Ray-**lah**-he oos-**ted** el coo-**err**-po.

I am going to listen to your chest.
Voy a escucharle el pecho.
Voye a es-coo-**char**-lay el **pay**-cho.

Let me feel your pulse.
Déjeme tomarle el pulso.
Day-ha-me to-**bar**-lay el **pool**-so.

I am going to take your temperature.
Voy a tomarle la temperatura.
Voye a to-**mar**-lay lah tem-pay-rah-**too**-rah.

Lie down, please.
Acuéstese, por favor.
Ah-coo-**es**-tah-say por fah-**vor**.

Do you understand?
¿Me comprende usted?
¿May com-**pren**-day oos-**ted**?

That's right.
Así. Bien.
Ah-**see**. Be-en.

You are doing very well.
Usted va muy bien.
Oos-**ted** vah **moo**-e **be**-en.

Do not take any medicine from home.
No tome usted ninguna medicina traída de su casa.
No **to**-may oos-**ted** nin-**goon**-ay may-de-**thee**-nah
   trah-**ee**-dah day soo **cah**-sah.

I am going to give you an injection.
Voy a ponerle ana inyección.
Voye a po-**nerr**-lay **oo**-nah in-yec-the-**on**.

Take a sip of water.
Tome usted un traguito de agua.
To-may oos-**ted** un trah-**gee**-to day **ah**-goo-ah.

Very good. That was fine.
Muy bien. Excelente.
Moo-e **be**-en. Ex-thay-**len**-tay.

Don't be nervous.
No se ponga nervioso(a).
No say **pon**-gah ner-ve-o-so(ah).

Do you feel dizzy?
¿Se siente vertigo?
¿Say see-**ayn**-tah **verr**-to-go?

Please lie still.
Quédese inmóvil, por favor.
Kay-day-say in-**mo**-veel por fah-**vor.**

You must drink lots of liquids.
Usted debe tomar muchos líquidos.
Oos-**ted day**-bay to-**mar moo**-chos **lee**-ke-dos.

References

Kelz, R. K. (1982.) *Conversational Spanish for Medical Personnel.* Clifton Park, NY: Thomson Delmar Learning.

Velazquez de la Cadena, M., Gray, E., & Iribas, J. (1985). *New Revised Velazquez Spanish and English Dictionary.* Clinton, NJ: New Win Publishing, Inc.

Glossary

Abduction Lateral movement away from the body.

Ability Competence in an activity.

Abortion Termination of pregnancy before the age of fetal viability, usually 24 weeks.

Abruptio Placenta Premature separation, from the wall of the uterus, of normally implanted placenta

Absorption Passage of a drug from the site of administration into the bloodstream; Process whereby the end products of digestion pass through the epithelial membranes in the small and large intestines and into the blood or lymph system.

Abuse Incident involving some type of violation to the client; Misuse, excessive, or improper use of a substance, the absence of which does not cause withdrawal symptoms.

Acanthosis Nigricans A velvety hyperpigmented patch on the back of neck, in axilla, or anticubital area found in children with type 2 diabetes.

Acceleration Short increase in fetal heart rate caused by fetal movement.

Accommodation Process allowing for adjustment of thinking to take in new information and increase understanding.

Accountability Responsibility of actions and inactions performed by oneself or others.

Accreditation Process by which a voluntary, nongovernmental agency or organization appraises and grants accredited status to institutions and/or programs or services that meet predetermined structure, process, and outcome criteria.

Acculturation Process of learning beliefs, norms, and behavioral expectations of a group.

Acid Any substance that in a solution yields hydrogen ions bearing a positive charge.

Acidosis Condition characterized by an excessive number of hydrogen ions in a solution.

Acme Peak of a contraction.

Acquired Immunity Formation of antibodies (memory B cells) to protect against future invasions of an already experienced antigen.

Acquired Immunodeficiency Syndrome (AIDS) Progressively fatal disease that destroys the immune system and the body's ability to fight infection; caused by the human immunodeficiency virus (HIV).

Acrocyanosis Blue coloring of hands and feet.

Active Euthanasia Process of taking specific action to hasten a client's death.

Active Listening Process of hearing spoken words and noting nonverbal behaviors.

Actively Suicidal Descriptor of an individual intent upon hurting or killing self and who is in imminent danger of doing so.

Activities of Daily Living Basic care activities that include mobility, bathing, hygiene, grooming, dressing, eating, and toileting.

Actual Nursing Diagnosis Nursing diagnosis that indicates that a problem exists; composed of the diagnostic label, related factors, and signs and symptoms.

Acupressure Technique of releasing blocked energy within an individual when specific points (tsubas) along the meridians are pressed or massaged by the practitioner's fingers, thumbs, and heel of the hands.

Acupuncture Technique of application of needles and heat to various points on the body to alter the energy flow.

Acute Pain Has a sudden onset, relatively short duration, mild to severe intensity, with a steady decrease in intensity over several days or weeks.

Adaptation Ongoing process whereby individuals use various responses to adjust to stressors and change; change resulting from assimilation and accommodation.

Adaptive Energy Inner forces that an individual uses to adapt to stress (phrase coined by Selye).

Adaptive Measure Measure for coping with stress that requires a minimal amount of energy.

Addiction Overwhelming preoccupation with obtaining and using a drug for its psychic effects; used interchangeably with dependence.

Adhesion Internal scar tissue from previous surgeries or disease processes.

Adjuvant Medication Drug used to enhance the analgesic efficacy of opioids, treat concurrent symptoms that exacerbate pain, and provide independent analgesia for specific types of pain.

Administrative Law Law developed by those persons who are appointed to governmental administrative agencies and who are entrusted with enforcing the statutory laws passed by the legislature.

Adolescence Development from the ages of 13 years to 20 years that begins with the onset of puberty.

Adult Day Care Provision of a variety of services in a protective setting for adults who are unable to stay alone, but who do not need 24-hour care.

Advance Directive Written instruction for health care that is recognized under state law and is related to the provision of such care when the individual is incapacitated.

Adventitious Breath Sound Abnormal sound, including sibilant wheezes (formerly wheezes), sonorous wheezes (formerly rhonchi), fine and course crackles (formerly rales), pleural friction rubs, and stridor.

Affect Outward expression of mood or emotions.

Affective Domain Area of learning that involves attitudes, beliefs, and emotions.

Afferent Nerve Pathway Ascending spinal cord pathway that transmits sensory impulses to the brain.

Afferent Pain Pathway Ascending spinal cord.

Afterpains Discomfort caused by the contracting uterus after the infant's birth.

Age of Viability Gestational age at which a fetus could live outside the uterus, generally considered to be 24 weeks.

Agent Entity capable of causing disease.

Agglutination Clumping together of red blood cells.

Agglutinin Specific kind of antibody whose interaction with antigens is manifested as agglutination.

Agglutinogen Any antigenic substance that causes agglutination by the production of agglutinin.

Agnosia Inability to recognize, either by sight or sound, familiar objects such as a hairbrush.

Agnostic Individual who believes that the existence of God cannot be proved or disproved.

Agranulocytosis Acute condition causing a severe reduction in the number of granulocytes (basophils, eosinophils, and neutrophils).

Airborne Precautions Measures taken in addition to Standard Precautions and for clients known to have or suspected of having illnesses spread by airborne droplet nuclei.

Airborne Transmission Transfer of an agent to a susceptible host through droplet nuclei or dust particles suspended in the air.

Aldrete Score Scoring system for objectively assessing the physical status of clients recovering from anesthesia; serves as a basis for dismissal from the postanesthesia care unit (PACU) and ambulatory surgery; also known as the postanesthetic recovery score.

Algor Mortis Decrease in body temperature after death, resulting in lack of skin elasticity.

Alkalosis Condition characterized by an excessive loss of hydrogen ions from a solution.

Allergen Type of antigen commonly found in the environment.

Allergy Altered reaction of the tissues of some individuals to substances that in similar amounts are harmless to other people.

Allogeneic From a donor of the same species.

Alopecia Partial or complete baldness or loss of hair.

Alternative Therapy Therapy used instead of conventional or mainstream medical practices.

Ambulatory Surgery Surgical operation performed under general, regional, or local anesthesia involving less than 24 hours of hospitalization.

Amenorrhea Absence of menstruation.

Amnesia Inability to remember things.

Amniocentesis Withdrawal of amniotic fluid to obtain a sample for specimen examination.

Amnion Inner fetal membrane originating in the blastocyst.

Amniotomy Artificial rupture of the membranes.

Amphiarthrosis Articulation of slightly movable joints such as the vertebrae.

Amputation Removal of all or part of an extremity.

Anabolism Constructive process of metabolism whereby new molecules are synthesized and new tissues are formed, as in growth and repair.

Analgesia Pain relief without producing anesthesia.

Analgesic Substance that relieves pain.

Analysis Breaking down the whole into parts that can be examined.

Analyte Substance that is measured.

Anaphylaxis Type I systemic reaction to allergens.

Anasarca Generalized edema.

Anesthesia Absence of normal sensation.

Anesthesiologist Licensed physician educated and skilled in the delivery of anesthesia who also adds to the knowledge of anesthesia through research or other scholarly pursuits.

Anesthetist Qualified RN, dentist, or medical doctor who administers anesthetics.

Aneurysm Weakness in the wall of a blood vessel.

Anger Control Assistance Nursing intervention aimed at facilitating the expression of anger in an adaptive and nonviolent manner.

Angina Pectoris Chest pain caused by a narrowing of the coronary arteries.

Angiocatheter Intracatheter with a metal stylet.

Angioedema Allergic reaction consisting of edema of subcutaneous tissue, mucous membranes, or viscera.

Angiogenesis Formation of new blood vessels.

Angiography Visualization of the vascular structures through the use of fluoroscopy with a contrast medium.

Angioma Benign vascular tumor involving skin and subcutaneous tissue: most are congenital.

Anion Ion bearing a negative charge.

Annulus Valvular ring in the heart.

Anorexia Loss of appetite.

Anorexia Nervosa Psychiatric disorder of self-imposed starvation that results in a 15% or more loss of body weight.

Anosognosia Lack of awareness of own neurological deficits.

Anthropometric Measurements Measurements of the size, weight, and proportions of the body.

Antibiotic Resistance Resistance to a previously effective antimicrobial agent.

Antibody Immunoglobulin produced by the body in response to bacteria, viruses, or other antigenic substances. Destroys antigens.

Anticipatory Grief Occurrence of grief before an expected loss actually occurs.

Anticipatory Guidance Information, teaching, and guidance given to a client in anticipation of an expected event.

Antigen Any substance identified by the body as nonself.

Antineoplastic Agent that inhibits the growth and reproduction of malignant cells.

Antioxidant Substance that prevents or inhibits oxidation, a chemical process wherein a substance is joined to oxygen.

Antipyretic Drug used to reduce an abnormally high temperature.

Anxiety Subjective response that occurs when a person experiences a real or perceived threat to well-being; a diverse feeling of dread or apprehension.

Anxiolytic Antianxiety medication.

Aphasia Absence of speech; often the result of a brain lesion.

Apheresis Removal of unwanted blood components.

Appendicitis Inflammation of the vermiform appendix.

Appropriate for Gestational Age Infant's weight falls between the 90th and 10th percentile for gestational age.

Areflexia Absence of reflexes.

Aromatherapy Therapeutic use of concentrated essences or essential oils extracted from plants and flowers.

Arousal State of wakefullness and alertness.

Arterial Blood Gases Measurement of levels of oxygen, carbon dioxide, pH, partial pressure of oxygen (PO_2 or PaO_2), partial pressue of carbon dioxide (PCO_2 or $PaCO_2$), saturation of oxygen (SaO_2), and bicarbonate (HCO_3) in arterial blood.

Arteriography Radiographic study of the vascular system following the injection of a radiopaque dye through a catheter.

Arteriosclerosis Cardiovascular disease wherein plaque forms on the inside of artery walls, reducing the space for blood flow.

Arthroplasty Replacement of both articular surfaces within a joint capsule.

Ascites Abnormal accumulation of fluid in the peritoneal cavity.

Asepsis Absence of pathogenic microorganisms.

Aseptic Technique Collection of principles used to control and/or prevent the transfer of pathogenic microorganisms from sources within (endogenous) and outside (exogenous) the client.

Aspiration Procedure performed to withdraw fluid that has abnormally collected or to obtain a specimen; also inhalation of secretion or fluids into the pulmonary system.

Assault Threat to do something that may cause harm or be unpleasant to another person.

Assent Voluntary agreement to participate in a research project or to accept treatment.

Assessment First step in the nursing process; includes systematic collection, verification, organization, interpretation, and documentation of data.

Assessment Model Framework providing a systematic way to organize data.

Assign Transfer of a specific nursing task to unlicensed personnel capable of competently performing the task. The nurse remains accountable for the care.

Assimilation Process of taking in new experiences or information.

Assisted Living Combination of housing and services for persons who require assistance with activities of daily living.

Assisted Suicide Form of active euthanasia where another person provides a client with the means to end his own life.

Assumption Belief or attitude that one takes for granted in a situation that requires action or resolution.

Asthma Condition characterized by intermittent airway obstruction due to antigen–antibody reaction.

Astigmatism Asymmetric focus of light rays on the retina.

Ataxia Inability to coordinate voluntary muscle action.

Atelectasis Collapse of a lung or a portion of a lung.

Atheist Individual who does not believe in God or any other deity.

Atherosclerosis Cardiovascular disease of fatty deposits on the inner lining, the tunica intima, of vessel walls.

Atom Smallest unit of an element which still retains the properties of that element and which cannot be altered by any chemical change.

Atresia Absence or closure of a body orifice.

Attachment Long-term process that begins during pregnancy and intensifies during the postpartum period, which establishes an enduring bond between parent and child, and develops through reciprocal (parent to child and child to parent) behaviors.

Attitude Manner, feeling, or position toward a person or thing.

Attribute Characteristic that belongs to an individual.

Audible Wheeze Wheeze that can be heard without the aid of a stethoscope.

Auditory Hallucination Perception by an individual that someone is talking when no one in fact is there.

Auditory Learner Person who learns by processing information through hearing.

Augmentation of Labor Stimulation of uterine contractions after spontaneously beginning but having unsatisfactory progress of labor.

Aura Peculiar sensation preceding a seizure or migraine; may be a taste, smell, sight, sound, dizziness, or just a "funny feeling."

Auscultation Physical examination technique that involves listening to sounds in the body that are created by movement of air or fluid.

Autocratic Leadership style that is task oriented and based on the premise that the leader knows best.

Autoimmune Disorder Disease wherein the body identifies its own cells as foreign and activates mechanisms to destroy them.

Autologous From the same organism (person).

Automatism Mechanical, repetitive motor behavior performed unconsciously.

Autonomic Nervous System That part of the peripheral nervous system consisting of the sympathetic and parasympathetic nervous systems and controlling unconscious activities.

Autonomy Self-direction; Ethical principle based on the individual's right to choose and the individual's ability to act on that choice.

Autopsy Examination of a body after death by a pathologist to determine cause of death.

Autosomal Pertaining to a condition transmitted by a non-sex chromosome.

Awareness Capacity to perceive sensory impressions through thoughts and actions.

Azotemia Nitrogenous wastes present in the blood.

Bacteremia Condition of bacteria in the blood.

Bactericide Bacteria-killing chemicals; found in tears.

Balanced Budget Act Federal law enacted in 1997 that replaced cost-based reimbursement for care in skilled nursing facilities with a prospective payment system based on client assessment within a resource utilization group system.

Ballottement Rebounding of the floating fetus when pushed upward through the vagina or abdomen.

Bands Immature neutrophils.

Barium Chalky-white contrast medium.

Barrier Precautions Use of personal protective equipment, such as masks, gowns, and gloves, to create a barrier between the person and the microorganisms and thus prevent transmission of the microorganism.

Basal Metabolism Energy needed to maintain essential physiological functions when a person is at complete rest. It is the lowest level of energy expenditure.

Base Substance that when dissociated produces ions that will combine with hydrogen ions.

Baseline Level Lab value that serves as a reference point for future value levels.

Battery Unauthorized or unwanted touching of one person by another.

Behavioral Tolerance Compensatory adjustments of behavior made under the influence of a particular substance.

Beneficence Ethical principle based on the duty to promote good and prevent harm.

Benign Not progressive; favorable for recovery.

Bereavement Period of grief that follows the death of a loved one.

Bias Mental inclination or leaning.

Bioavailability Readiness to produce a drug effect.

Bioethics Application of general ethical principles to health care.

Biofeedback Measures physiological responses which assist individuals to improve their health by using signals from their own bodies.

Biologic Response Modifier Agent that destroys malignant cells by stimulating the body's immune system.

Biological Agent Living organism that invades a host, causing disease.

Biological Clock Internal mechanism in a living organism capable of measuring time.

Biopsy Excision of a small amount of tissue.

Blanching White color of the skin when pressure is applied.

Blastic Phase Intensified phase of leukemia that resembles an acute phase in which there is an increased production of white blood cells.

Blastocyst Cluster of cells that will develop into the embryo.

Bloody Show Expulsion of cervical secretions, blood-tinged mucus, and the mucus plug that blocked the cervix during pregnancy.

Body Image Individual's perception of physical self, including appearance, function, and ability.

Body Mass Index Measurement used to ascertain whether a person's weight is appropriate for height; calculated by dividing the weight in kilograms by the height in meters squared.

Body Mechanics Use of the body to safely and efficiently move or lift objects.

Bodymind Inseparable connection and operation of thoughts, feelings, and physiological functions.

Bonding Rapid process of attachment, parent to infant, that takes place during the sensitive period, the first 30 to 60 minutes after birth.

Borborygmi High-pitched, loud, rushing sounds produced by the movement of gas in the liquid contents of the intestine.

Bradycardia Heart rate less than 60 beats per minute in an adult.

Bradykinesia Slowness of voluntary movement and speech.

Bradypnea Respiratory rate of 10 or fewer breaths per minute.

Braxton-Hicks Contractions Irregular, intermittent contractions felt by the pregnant woman towards the end of pregnancy.

Breakthrough Pain Sudden, acute, temporary pain that is usually precipitated by a treatment, a procedure, or unusual activity of the client.

Brief Dynamic Therapy Short-term psychotherapy that focuses on resolving core conflicts deriving from personality and living situations.

Bronchial Sound Loud, high-pitched, hollow-sounding breath sound normally heard over the sternum. Longer on expiration than inspiration.

Bronchiectasis Lung disorder characterized by chronic dilation of the bronchi.

Bronchitis Inflammation of the bronchial tree accompanied by hypersecretion of mucus.

Bronchovesicular Sound Breath sound normally heard in the area of the scapula and near the sternum; medium in pitched blowing sound, with inspiratory and expiratory phases of equal length.

Bruxism Grinding of teeth during sleep.

Buffer Substance that attempts to maintain pH range, or hydrogen ion concentration, in the presence of added acids or bases.

Bulimia Nervosa Psychiatric disorder characterized by episodic binge-eating followed by purging.

Burnout State of physical and emotional exhaustion occurring when caregivers use up their adaptive energy.

Butterfly Needle Wing-tipped needle.

Cachectic Being in a state of malnutrition and wasting.

Cachexia State of malnutrition and protein wasting.

Calculus Concentration of mineral salts in the body leading to the formation of stone.

Calorie Amount of heat required to raise the temperature of 1 gram of water 1 degree Celsius.

Cancer Disease resulting from the uncontrolled growth of cells, which causes malignant cellular tumors.

Capitated Rate Preset fee based on membership rather than services provided; payment system used in managed care.

Caput Succedaneum Edema of the newborn's scalp which is present at birth, may cross suture lines, and is caused by head compression against the cervix.

Carcinogen Substance that initiates or promotes the development of cancer.

Carcinoma Cancer occurring in epithelial tissue.

Cardiac Cycle Cycle of an impulse going completely through the conduction system of the heart, and the ventricles contracting.

Cardiac Output Volume of blood pumped per minute by the left ventricle.

Cardiac Tamponade Collection of fluid in the pericardial sac hindering the functioning of the heart.

Carrier Person who harbors an infectious agent but has no symptoms of disease.

Caseation Process whereby the center of the primary tubercle formed in the lungs as a result of tuberculosis becomes soft and cheese-like due to decreased perfusion.

Catabolism Destructive process of metabolism whereby tissues or substances are broken into their component parts.

Cataplexy Sudden loss of muscle control.

Cataract Condition in which the lens of the eye loses its transparency and becomes opaque.

Categorical Imperative Concept that states that one should act only if the action is based on a principle that is universal.

Catharsis Process of talking out one's feelings; "getting things off the chest" through verbalization.

Cation Ion bearing a positive charge.

Cavitation Process whereby a cavity is created in the lung tissue through the liquefaction and rupture of a primary tubercle.

Ceiling Effect Medication dosage beyond which no further analgesia occurs.

Cellular Immunity Type of acquired immunity involving T-cell lymphocytes.

Centering Process of bringing oneself to an inward focus of serenity; done before beginning an energetic touch therapy treatment.

Central Line Venous catheter inserted into the superior vena cava through the subclavian or internal or external jugular vein.

Central Nervous System System of the brain and spinal cord.

Cephalalgia Headache; also known as cephalgia.

Cephalhematoma Collection of blood between the periosteum and the skull of a newborn; appears several hours to a day after birth, does not cross suture lines, and is caused by the rupturing of the periosteal bridging veins due to friction and pressure during labor and delivery.

Cephalopelvic Disproportion Condition in which the fetal head will not fit through the mother's pelvis.

Certification Voluntary process that establishes and evaluates standards of care; mandatory for any health care services receiving federal funds.

Cerumen Ear wax.

Cervical Dilatation Enlargement of the cervical opening (os) from 0 to 10 cm (complete dilatation).

Cesarean Birth Birth of an infant through an incision in the abdomen and uterus.

Chadwick's Sign Purplish-blue color of the cervix and vagina noted about the eighth week of pregnancy.

Chain of Custody Documentation of the transfer of evidence (of a crime) from one worker to the next in a secure fashion.

Chain of Infection Describes the development of an infectious process.

Chalazion Cyst of the meibomian glands.

Chancre Clean, painless, syphilitic primary ulcer appearing 2 to 6 weeks after infection at the site of body contact.

Change Dynamic process whereby an individual's response to a stressor leads to an alteration in behavior.

Change Agent Person who intentionally creates and implements change.

Charting by Exception Documentation method that requires the nurse to document only deviations from preestablished norms.

Chemical Agent Substance that interacts with a host, causing disease.

Chemical Name Precise description of the drug's chemical formula.

Chemical Restraint Medication used to control client behavior.

Chemoreceptor Receptor that monitors the levels of carbon dioxide, oxygen, and pH in the blood.

Chemotherapy Use of drugs to treat illness, especially cancer.

Cheyne-Stokes Respirations Breathing characterized by periods of apnea alternating with periods of dyspnea.

Child Abuse Any intentional act of physical, emotional, or sexual abuse or neglect committed by a person responsible for the care of a child.

Child Life Specialist Health care professional with extensive knowledge of psychology and early childhood development.

Chlamydia Sexually transmitted disease caused by the spherical bacterial organism *Chlamydia trachomatis*.

Chloasma Darkening of the skin of the forehead and around the eyes during pregnancy; also called the "mask of pregnancy."

Cholecystitis Inflammation of the gallbladder.

Cholelithiasis Presence of gallstones or calculi in the gallbladder.

Cholesterol Sterol produced by the body and used in the synthesis of steroid hormones.

Chorea Condition characterized by abnormal, involuntary, purposeless movements of all musculature of the body.

Chorion Outer fetal membrane formed from the trophoblast.

Chronic Acute Pain Discomfort that occurs almost daily over a long period, months or years, and may never stop; also known as progressive pain.

Chronic Nonmalignant Pain Discomfort that occurs almost daily, has been present for a least 6 months, and ranging from mild to severe in intensity; also known as chronic benign pain.

Chronic Pain Discomfort usually defined as long term (lasting 6 months or longer), persistent, nearly constant, or recurrent pain producing significant negative changes in a person's life.

Chronobiology Science of studying biorhythms.

Chvostek's Sign Abnormal spasm of the facial muscles in response to a light tapping of the facial nerve.

Chyme Acidic, semi-fluid paste found in the gastrointestinal tract.

Circadian Rhythm Biorhythm that cycles on a daily basis.

Circulating Nurse RN responsible and accountable for management of personnel, equipment, supplies, the environment, and communication throughout a surgical procedure.

Circumcision Surgical removal of the prepuce (foreskin) which covers the glans penis.

Circumoral Cyanosis Bluish discoloration surrounding the mouth.

Cirrhosis Chronic degenerative changes in the liver cells and thickening of surrounding tissue.

Civil Law Law that deals with relationships between individuals.

Claiming Process Process whereby a family identifies the infant's "likeness to" and the "differences from" family members, and the infant's unique qualities.

Clean Object Object on which there are microorganisms that are usually not pathogenic.

Cleansing Removal of soil or organic material from instruments and equipment used in providing client care.

Client Advocate Person who speaks up for or acts on behalf of the client.

Client Behavior Accident Mishap resulting from the client's behavior or actions.

Clinical Observing and caring for living clients.

Closed Reduction Repair of a fracture done without surgical intervention.

Coarse Crackle Moist, low-pitched crackling and gurgling lung sound of long duration.

Codependent Description for persons who live based on what others think of them.

Cognition Intellectual ability to think.

Cognitive Behavior Therapy Treatment approach aimed at helping a client identify stimuli that cause the client's anxiety, develop plans to respond to those stimuli in a non-anxious manner, and problem-solve when unanticipated anxiety-provoking situations arise.

Cognitive Domain Area of learning that involves intellectual understanding.

Cognitive Reframing Stress management technique whereby the individual changes a negative perception of a situation or event to a more positive, less threatening perception.

Coitus (Copulation) Sexual act that delivers sperm to the cervix by ejaculation of the erect penis.

Cold Stress Excessive heat loss.

Colic Condition of acute abdominal pain.

Colonization Multiplication of microorganisms on or within a host that does not result in cellular injury.

Colostomy Opening created anywhere along the large intestine.

Colostrum Antibody-rich yellow fluid secreted by the breasts during the last trimester of pregnancy and the first 2–3 days after birth; gradually changes to milk.

Combination Chemotherapy Administration of a combination of chemotherapy drugs over a set period of time.

Comedone Whitehead or blackhead.

Command Hallucination Perception by an individual of a voice or voices telling the individual to do something, usually to himself and/or someone else.

Communicable Agent Infectious agent transmitted to a client by direct or indirect contact, via vehicle, vector, or airborne route.

Communicable Disease Disease caused by a communicable agent.

Communication The sending and receiving of a message.

Comorbidity Simultaneous existence of more than one disease process within an individual.

Competency Specific skill or task needed for a particular position.

Complementary Therapy Therapy used in conjunction with conventional medical therapies.

Complete Protein Protein containing all nine essential amino acids.

Complicated Grief Grief associated with traumatic death such as death by accident, violence, or homicide; survivors often have more intense emotions than those associated with normal grief.

Compound Combination of atoms of two or more elements.

Comprehensive Assessment Type of assessment that provides baseline client data, including a complete health history and current needs assessment.

Compromised Host Person whose normal body defenses are impaired and is therefore susceptible to infection.

Computed Tomography Radiological scanning of the body with x-ray beams and radiation detectors to transmit data to a computer that transcribes the data into quantitative measurement and multidimensional images of the internal structures.

Concept Mental picture of abstract phenomena that serves to organize observations related to those phenomena.

Conditioning Teaching a person a behavior until it becomes an automatic response; method of conserving adaptive energy.

Conduction Loss of heat by direct contact with a cooler object.

Conductive Hearing Loss Condition characterized by the inability of sound waves to reach the inner ear.

Confabulation The making up of information to fill in memory gaps.

Confidential Private or secret.

Confidentiality Nondisclosure of the identity of or personal information about an individual.

Conflict Discord between two or more people that results from differences in ideas, values, or feelings.

Congruence Agreement between two things.

Conjunctivitis Inflammation of the conjunctiva.

Consciousness State of awareness of self, others, and surrounding environment.

Constipation Condition characterized by hard, infrequent stools that are difficult or painful to pass.

Constitutional Law Law that defines and limits the power of government.

Contact Precautions Measures taken in addition to Standard Precautions for clients known to have or suspected of having illnesses easily spread by direct client contact or by contact with fomites.

Contact Transmission Transfer of an agent from an infected person to a host by direct contact with that person, indirect contact with an infected person through a fomite, or close contact with contaminated secretions.

Contraception Measure taken to prevent pregnancy.

Contract Law Enforcement of agreements among private individuals.

Contracture Permanent shortening of a muscle.

Contrast Medium Radiopaque substance that facilitates roentgen (x-ray) imaging of the body's internal structures.

Convalescent Stage Time period in which acute symptoms of an infection begin to disappear until the client returns to the previous state of health.

Convection Loss of heat by the movement of air.

Copulation (Coitus) Sexual act that delivers sperm to the cervix by ejaculation of the erect penis.

Cotyledon Subdivision of the maternal side of the placenta.

Couvade Development of physical symptoms by the expectant father such as fatigue, depression, headache, backache, and nausea.

Crackle Abnormal breath sound that resembles a popping sound, heard on inhalation and exhalation; not cleared by coughing.

Crenation Condition wherein cells decrease in size, shrivel and wrinkle, and are no longer functional when in a hypertonic solution.

Crepitus Grating or crackling sensation or sound.

Cretinism Congenital lack of thyroid hormones causing defective physical development and mental retardation.

Criminal Law Law concerning acts of offense against the welfare or safety of the public.

Crisis Acute state of disorganization that occurs when usual coping mechanisms are no longer adequate. Stressor that forces an individual to respond and/or adapt in some way.

Crisis Intervention Specific technique used to help a person regain equilibrium.

Critical Pathway Comprehensive, standard plan of care for specific conditions.

Critical Period Time of the most rapid growth or development in a stage of the life cycle during which an individual is most vulnerable to stressors.

Critical Thinking The disciplined intellectual process of applying skillful reasoning, imposing intellectual standards and self-reflective thinking as a guide to a belief or action.

Cross-Tolerance Decreased sensitivity to other substances in the same category.

Crowning When the largest diameter of the fetal head is past the vulva.

Cryotherapy Use of cold applications to reduce swelling.

Cryptorchidism Failure of one or both testes to descend

Cultural Assimilation Process whereby members of a minority group are absorbed by the dominant culture taking on the characteristics of the dominant culture.

Cultural Diversity Differences among people resulting from ethnic, racial, and cultural variations.

Culture Integrated, dynamic structure of knowledge, attitudes, behaviors, beliefs, ideas, habits, customs, languages, values, symbols, rituals, and ceremonies that are unique to a particular group of people. Growing of microorganisms to identify a pathogen.

Curative To heal or restore health.

Curing Ridding one of disease.

Cutaneous Pain Discomfort caused by stimulating the cutaneous nerve endings in the skin.

Cyanosis Bluish discoloration of the skin and mucous membranes observed in lips, nail beds, and earlobes.

Cycling Alteration in mood between depression and mania.

Cystitis Inflammation of the urinary bladder.

Cystocele Downward displacement of the bladder into the anterior vaginal wall.

Cytology Study of cells.

Cytomegalovirus One of the herpes type viruses: inhabits saliva, urine, blood, semen, and vaginal secretions.

Data Clustering Process of putting data together in order to identify areas of the client's problems and strengths.

Dawn Phenomenon Early morning glucose elevation produced by the release of growth hormone.

Death Rattle Noisy respirations in the period preceding death caused by a collection of secretions in the larynx.

Debride To remove dead or damaged tissue or foreign material from a wound.

Decerebration Severing of the spinal cord.

Decidua The endometrium after implantation.

Decomposition Chemical reaction wherein the bonding between atoms in a molecule is broken and simpler products are formed.

Decrement Decreasing intensity of a contraction.

Defamation Using words to harm or injure the personal or professional reputation of another person.

Defense Mechanism Unconscious functions protecting the mind from anxiety.

Defining Characteristics Collected data; also known as signs and symptoms, subjective and objective data, or clinical manifestations.

Deglutition Swallowing of food.

Dehiscence Complication of wound healing wherein the wound edges separate.

Dehydration Condition wherein more water is lost from the body than is being replaced.

Delegation Process of transferring a select nursing task to a licensed individual who is compentent to perform that specific task.

Delirium Cognitive changes or acute confusion of rapid onset (less than 6 months).

Delusion False belief that misrepresents reality.

Dementia Organic brain pathology characterized by losses in intellectual functioning and a slow onset (longer than 6 months).

Democratic Leadership style in which all members have input in decision making.

Dental Caries Cavities.

Deontology Ethical theory that considers the intrinsic significance of an act as the criterion for determination of good.

Dependence Reliance on a substance to such a degree that abstinence causes functional impairment, physical withdrawal symptoms, and/or psychological craving for the substance. See also addiction.

Dependent Nursing Intervention Nursing action that requires an order from a physician or other health care professional.

Depersonalization Treating an individual as an object rather than as a person.

Depolarization Contraction of the heart.

Depression State wherein an individual experiences feelings of extreme sadness, hopelessness, and helplessness.

Detoxification Elimination of a substance from the body.

Development Behavioral changes in skills and functional abilities.

Developmental Tasks Certain goals that must be accomplished during each life cycle stage.

Dialysate Solution used in dialysis, designed to approximate the normal electrolyte structure of plasma and extracellular fluid.

Dialysis Mechanical means of removing nitrogenous waste from the blood by imitating the function of the nephrons; involves filtration and diffusion of wastes, drugs, and excess electrolytes and/or osmosis of water across a semipermeable membrane into a dialysate solution.

Diarthrosis Freely movable joint.

Didactic Systematic presentation of information.

Diet Therapy Treating disease or disorder with special diet.

Dietary Prescription/Order Order written by the physician for food, including liquids.

Differentiation Acquisition of characteristics or functions different from those of the original.

Diffusion Process whereby a substance moves from an area of higher concentration to an area of lower concentration.

Digestion Mechanical and chemical processes that convert nutrients into a physically absorbable state.

Diplopia Double vision.

Dirty Object Object on which there is a high number of microorganisms, some that are potentially pathogenic.

Disaster A situation or event of greater magnitude than an emergency that has unforeseen, serious or immediate threats to public health.

Discharge Planning Planning that involves anticipation of and planning for the client's needs after discharge.

Discipline Branch of learning, field of study, or occupation requiring specialized knowledge.

Disciplined Trained by instruction and exercise.

Disenfranchised Grief Grief not openly acknowledged, socially sanctioned, or publicly shared.

Disinfectant Chemical solution used to clean inanimate objects.

Disinfection Elimination of pathogens, with the exception of spores, from inanimate objects.

Dislocation Injury in which the articular surfaces of a joint are no longer in contact.

Disorientation State of mental confusion in which awareness of time, place, self, and/or situation is impaired.

Disseminated Intravascular Coagulation Abnormal stimulation of the clotting mechanism causing small clots throughout the vascular system and widespread bleeding internally, externally, or both.

Distraction Technique of focusing attention on stimuli other than pain.

Distress Subjective experience that occurs when stressors evoke an ineffective response.

Distribution Movement of drugs from the blood into various tissues and body fluids.

Diverticula Sac-like protrusion of the intestinal wall that results when the mucosa herniates through the bowel wall.

Diverticulitis Inflammation of one or more diverticula.

Diverticulosis Condition in which multiple diverticula are present in the colon.

Documentation Any printed or written record of activities.

Domestic Violence Aggression and violence involving family members.

Dominant Culture The group whose values prevail within a given society.

Down Syndrome Congenital chromosomal abnormality; also called trisomy 21.

Droplet Precautions Measures taken in addition to Standard Precautions for clients known to have or suspected of having serious illnesses spread by large particle droplets.

Drug Allergy Hypersensitivity to a drug.

Drug Incompatibility Undesired chemical or physical reaction between a drug and a solution, between a drug and the container or tubing, or between two drugs.

Drug Interaction Effect one drug can have on another drug.

Drug Tolerance Reaction that occurs when the body is accustomed to a specific drug that larger doses are needed to produce the desired therapeutic effects.

Ductus Arteriosus Fetal vessel connecting the pulmonay artery to the aorta.

Ductus Venosus Branch of the umbilical vein that enters the inferior vena cava.

Durable Power of Attorney for Health Care Legal document designating who may make health care decisions for a client when that client is no longer capable of decision making.

Duration Length of one contraction, from the beginning of the increment to the conclusion of the decrement.

Dysarthria Difficult and defective speech due to a dysfunction of the muscles used for speech.

Dysfunctional Grief Persistent pattern of intense grief that does not result in reconciliation of feelings.

Dysfunctional Labor Labor with problems of the contractions or of maternal bearing down.

Dysmenorrhea Painful menstruation.

Dyspareunia Painful intercourse.

Dysphagia Difficulty in swallowing.

Dysphasia Impairment of speech resulting from damage to the speech center in the brain.

Dysplasia Abnormal development.

Dyspnea Difficulty breathing as observed by labored or forced respirations through the use of accessory muscles in the chest and neck.

Dysrhythmia Irregularity in the rate, rhythm, or conduction of the electrical system of the heart.

Dystocia Long, difficult, or abnormal labor caused by any of the four major variables (4 Ps) that affect labor.

Dysuria Difficult or painful urination.

Early Deceleration Reduction in fetal heart rate that begins early in the contraction and virtually mirrors the uterine contraction.

Ecchymosis Large, irregular hemorrhagic area on the skin; also called a bruise.

Eclampsia Convulsion occurring in pregnancy induced hypertension.

Ectopic Pregnancy Pregnancy in which the fertilized ovum is implanted outside the uterine cavity.

Edema Detectable accumulation of increased interstitial fluid.

Effacement Thinning of the cervix.

Efferent Nerve Pain Pathway Descending spinal cord pathway that transmits sensory impulses from the brain.

Effluent Liquid output from an ileostomy.

Electrocardiogram Graphic recording of the heart's electrical activity.

Electroconvulsive Therapy Procedure whereby clients are treated with pulses of electrical energy sufficient to cause brief convulsions or seizures.

Electroencephalogram Graphic recording of the brain's electrical activity.

Electrolyte Compound that, when dissolved in water or another solvent, dissociates (separates) into ions (electrically charged particles).

Element Basic substance of matter.

Emancipated Minor Child who has the legal competency of an adult because of cicumstances involving marriage, divorce, parenting of a child, living independently without parents, or enlistment in the armed services.

Embolus Mass, such as a blood clot or an air bubble, that circulates in the bloodstream.

Embryonic Phase Development occuring during the first 2–8 weeks after fertilization of a human egg.

Emergency Medical or surgical condition requiring immediate or timely intervention to prevent permanent disability or death.

Emergency Medical Technician Health care professional trained to provide basic lifesaving measures prior to arrival at the hospital.

Emergency Nursing Care of clients who require emergency interventions.

Emotional Lability Loss of emotional control.

Empathy Capacity to understand another person's feelings or perception of a situation.

Emphysema Lung disease wherein air accumulates in the tissues of the lungs.

Empowerment Process of enabling others to do for themselves.

Empty Calories Calories that provide few nutrients.

Encephalitis Inflammation of the brain.

Encoding Laying down tracks in areas of the brain to enhance the ability to recall and utilize information.

Encopresis Passage of watery colonic contents around a hard fecal mass.

Endemic Occurring continuously in a particular population and having low mortality.

Endocrine Group of cells secreting substances directly into the blood or lymph circulation and affecting another part of the body.

Endometriosis Growth of endometrial tissue on structures outside of the uterus, within the pelvic cavity.

Endorphins Group of opiate-like substances produced naturally by the brain which raise the pain threshold, produce sedation and euphoria, and promote a sense of well-being.

Endoscopy Visualization of a body organ or cavity through a scope.

Energetic-Touch Therapy Technique of using the hands to direct or redirect the flow of the body's energy fields and enhance balance within those fields.

Engagement Condition of the widest diameter of the fetal presenting part (head) entering the inlet to the true pelvis.

Engorgement Distentions and swelling of the breasts in the first few days following delivery.

Engrossment Parents' intense interest in and peoccupation with the newborn.

Enriched Descriptor for food in which nutrients that were removed during processing are added back in.

Enteral Instillation Administration of drugs through a gastrointestinal tube.

Enteral Nutrition Feeding method meaning both the ingestion of food orally and the delivery of nutrients through a gastrointestinal tube, but generally meaning the latter.

Entrainment Infant's ability to move in rhythm to the parent's voice.

Enzyme Globular protein produced in the body that catalyzes chemical reactions within the cells.

Enzyme-Linked Immunosorbent Assay Basic screening test currently used to detect antibodies to HIV.

Epidemic Infecting many people at the same time and in the same geographic area.

Epidural Analgesia Analgesics administered via a catheter that terminates in the epidural space.

Episiotomy Incision in the perineum to facilitate passage of the baby.

Epispadius Placement of the urinary meatus on the top of the penis.

Epistaxis Hemorrhage of the nares or nostrils; also known as nosebleed.

Epstein's Pearls Small, whitish-yellow epithelial cysts found on the hard palate.

Equipment Accident Accident resulting from the malfunction or improper use of medical equipment.

Erythema Redness of the skin due to increased blood flow to the area.

Erythematous Characterized by redness of the skin.

Erythema Toxicum Neonatorum Pink rash with firm, yellow-white papules or pustules found on the chest, abdomen, back, and/or buttocks of a newborn.

Erythrocytapheresis Procedure that removes abnormal red blood cells and replaces them with healthy ones.

Erythropoiesis Production of red blood cells and their release by the red bone marrow.

Eschar Dry, dark, leathery scab composed of denatured protein.

Ethical Dilemma Where two or more ideals or values are in conflict.

Ethical Principle Widely accepted codes, generally based on the humane aspects of society, that direct or govern actions.

Ethical Reasoning Process of thinking through what one ought to do in an orderly, systematic manner based on principles.

Ethics Branch of philosophy concerned with determining right from wrong on the basis of knowledge.

Ethnicity Cultural group's perception of itself or a group identity.

Ethnocentrism Assumption of cultural superiority and inability to accept another cultures' ways.

Etiology Related cause of or contributor to a problem.

Euglycemia Normal blood glucose level.

Euphoric Characterized by elation out of context to the situation.

Eupnea Easy respirations with a rate that is age-appropriate.

Eustress Stress that results in positive outcomes.

Euthanasia Intentional action or lack of action that causes the merciful death of someone suffering from a terminal illness or incurable condition; derived from the Greek word *euthanatos,* which literally means "good or gentle death."

Evaluation Fifth step in the nursing process; determines whether client goals have been met, partially met, or not met.

Evaporation Loss of heat when water is changed to a vapor.

Evisceration Complication of wound healing characterized by a complete separation of wound edges accompanied by visceral protrusion.

Exacerbation Increase in the symptoms of a disease.

Exclusive Provider Organization Organization wherein care must be delivered by providers in the plan in order for clients to receive any reimbursement.

Excretion Elimination of drugs or waste products from the body.

Exophthalmos Marked protrusion of the eyeballs resulting from increased orbital fluid behind the eyeballs.

Expected Outcome Detailed, specific statement describing the methods to be used to achieve the goal. It includes direct nursing care, client teaching, and continuity of care.

Exposure Contact with an infected person or agent.

Expressed Contract Conditions and terms of a contract given in writing by the concerned parties.

External Respiration Exchange of gases between the atmosphere and the lungs.

External Version Manipulation of the fetus through te mother's abdomen to a presentation facilitating birth.

Extracellular Fluid Fluid outside of the cells; includes interstitial, intravascular, synovial, cerebrospinal, and serous fluids; aqueous and vitreous humor; and endolymph and perilymph.

Extravasation Escape of fluid into the surrounding tissue.

False Imprisonment Situation wherein a person is made to wrongfully believe that he cannot leave a place.

False Labor Contractions which do not cause the cervix to dilate.

Family-Centered Care A philosophy of caring recognizing the centrality of the family in the child's life and including the family's contribution and involvement in the plan of care and its delivery (Potts & Mandleco, 2000).

Fasciculation Involuntary twitching of muscle fibers.

Fat-Soluble Vitamin Vitamin requiring the presence of fats for its absorption from the gastrointestinal tract into the lymphatic system and for cellular metabolism: vitamins A, D, E, and K.

Fee for Service System in which the health care recipient directly pays the provider for services as they are provided.

Feedback Response from the receiver of a message so that the sender can verify the message.

Felony Crime of a serious nature that is usually punishable by imprisonment in a state penitentiary or by death.

Ferguson's Reflex Spontaneous, involutary urge to bear down during labor.

Fertilization Union of an ovum and a sperm.

Fetal Alcohol Syndrome Condition wherein fetal development is impaired by maternal consumption of alcohol.

Fetal Attitude Relationship of fetal body parts to one another, either flexion or extension.

Fetal Biophysical Profile Assessment of five variables: fetal breathing movement, fetal movements of body or limbs, fetal tone (flexion/extension of extremities), amniotic fluid volume, and reactive NST.

Fetal Lie Relationship of the cephalocaudal axis of the fetus to the cephalocaudal axis of the mother, either longitudinal or transverse.

Fetal Phase Intrauterine development from 8 weeks to birth.

Fetal Position Relationship of the identified landmark on the presenting part to the four quadrants of the mother's pelvis.

Fetal Presentation Determined by the fetal lie and the part of the fetus that enters the pelvis first.

Fibrinolysis Process of breaking fibrin apart.

Fidelity Ethical concept based on faithfulness and keeping promises.

Fight-or-Flight Response State wherein the body becomes physiologically ready to defend itself by either fighting or fleeing from the stressor.

Filtration Process of fluids and the substances dissolved in them being forced through the cell membrane by hydrostatic pressure.

Fine Crackle Dry, high-pitched crackling and popping ling sounds of short duration.

Flashback Rushing of blood back into intravenous tubing when a negative pressure is created on the tubing. Reliving of an original trauma as if the individual were currently experiencing it.

Flora Microorganisms which occur or have adapted to live in a specific environment, such as intestinal, skin, vaginal, or oral flora.

Flow Rate Volume of fluid to infuse over a set period of time.

Fluoroscopy Immediate, serial images of the body's structure or function.

Focus Charting Documentation method using a column format to chart data, actions, and responses (DAR).

Focused Assessment Type of assessment limited to a particular need, potential health care risks, or health care problem.

Fomite Object contaminated with an infectious agent.

Fontanelle Membranous area where sutures meet on the fetal skull.

Foramen Ovale Flap opening in the atrial septum that allows only right to left moevement of blood.

Foremilk Watery first milk from the breast, high in lactose, like skim milk, and effective in quenching thirst.

Forceps Metal instruments used on the fetal head to provide traction or to provide a method of rotating the fetal head to an occiput-anterior position.

Formal Contract Written contract that cannot be changed legally by an oral agreement.

Formal Teaching Teaching that takes place at a specific time, in a specific place, and on a specific topic.

Fortified Descriptor for food in which nutrients not naturally occurring in the food are added to it.

Fracture Break in the continuity of a bone.

Fraud Wrong that results from a deliberate deception intended to produce unlawful gain.

Free Radical Unstable molecule that alters genetic codes and triggers the development of cancer growth in cells.

Frequency Time for the beginning of one contraction to the beginning of the nect contraction.

Friction Force of two surfaces moving against one another.

Fulguration Procedure to destroy tissue with long, high-frequency electric sparks.

Functional Area Specialized area of the brain.

Fundus Top of the uterus.

Funic Souffle Sound of the blood pulsating through the umbilical cord; rate the same as the fetal heart beat.

Gastric Ulcer Erosion in the stomach.

Gastritis Inflammation of the stomach mucosa.

Gate Control Pain Theory Theory that proposes that the cognitive, sensory, emotional, and physiologic components of the body can act together to block an individual's perception of pain.

General Adaptation Syndrome Physiologic response that occurs when a person experiences a stressor.

General Anesthesia Method of producing unconsciousness; complete insensibility to pain; amnesia; motionlessness; and muscle relaxation.

Generic Name Name assigned by the U.S. Adopted Names Council to the manufacturer who first develops a drug.

Genogram A way to visualize family members, their birth and death dates, or ages and specific health problems.

Genuineness Sincerity.

Germicide Chemical that can be applied to both animate and inanimate objects for the purpose of eliminating pathogens.

Germinal Phase Development beginning with conception and lasts approximately 10 to 14 days.

Gerontological Nursing Specialty within nursing that addresses and advocates for the special care needs of older adults.

Gerontologist Specialist in gerontology in advanced practice nursing, geriatric psychiatry, medicine, and social services.

Gerontology Study of the effects of normal aging and age-related diseases on human beings.

Gingivitis Inflammation of the gums.

Glasgow Coma Scale Neurological screening test that measures a client's best verbal, motor, and eye response to stimuli.

Glucagon Hormone secreted by the alpha cells of the pancreas which stimulate release of glucose by the liver.

Gluconeogenesis Conversion of amino acids into glucose.

Glycogenesis Conversion of glucose into glycogen.

Glycogenolysis Conversion of glycogen into glucose.

Goal Aim, intent, or end.

Goiter Enlargement of the thyroid gland.

Gonorrhea Sexually transmitted disease caused by the gram-negative bacterial organism *Neisseria gonorrhea*.

Good Samaritan Law Law that provides protection to health care providers by assuring them of immunity from civil liability when care is provided at the scene of an emergency and the caregiver does not intentionally or recklessly cause the client injury.

Goodell's Sign Softening of the cervix noted about the eighth week of pregnancy.

Gower's Sign Walking hands up legs to get from sitting to standing position (as in Duchenne muscular dystrophy).

Granulation Tissue Delicate connective tissue consisting of fibroblasts, collagen, and capillaries.

Graphesthesia Ability to identify letters, numbers, or shapes drawn on the skin.

Gravida Pregnancy, regardless of duration, including present pregnancy.

Grief Series of intense psychological and physical responses occuring after a loss; these responses are necessary, normal, natural, and adaptive responses to the loss.

Growth Measurable changes in the physical size of the body and its parts.

Gynecomastia Abnormal enlargement of one or both breasts in males.

Half-life Time it takes the body to eliminate half of the blood concentration level of the original dose of medication.

Halitosis Bad breath.

Hallucination Sensory perception that occurs in the absence of external stimuli and that is not based on reality.

Hallux Varus Placement of the great toe farther from the other toes.

Hand Hygiene Rubbing together of all surfaces and crevices of the hands using a soap or chemical and water, followed by rinsing in a flowing stream of water.

Haustra Sac-like pouches of the colon.

Healing Process that activates the individual's recovery forces from within. To make whole.

Healing Touch Energy therapy using the hands to clear, energize, and balance the energy field.

Health According to the World Health Organization, the state of complete physical, mental, and social well-being, not merely the absence of disease or infirmity.

Health Care Delivery System Method for providing services to meet the health needs of individuals.

Health Care Surrogate Law Law enacted by some states that provides a legal means for decision making in the absence of advance directives.

Health Continuum Range of an individual's health, from highest health potential to death.

Health History Review of the client's functional health patterns prior to the current contact with a health care agency.

Health Maintenance Organization Prepaid health plan that provides primary health care services for a preset fee and focuses on cost-effective treatment methods.

Hearing Act or power of receiving sounds.

Heart Sound Sound heard by auscultating the heart.

Heberden's Nodes Enlargement and characteristic hypertrophic spurs in the terminal interphalangeal finger joints.

Hegar's Sign Softening of the uterine isthmus about the sixth week of pregnancy.

HELLP Syndrome Pregnancy-induced hypertension with liver damage characterized by **H**emolysis, **E**levated **L**iver enzymes, and **L**ow **P**latelet count.

Hemarthrosis Bleeding into the joints.

Hematemesis Vomiting of blood.

Hematocrit Percentage of red blood cells in a given volume of blood.

Hematopoiesis Process of blood cell production and development.

Hematuria Blood in the urine.

Hemiparesis Weakness of one side of the body.

Hemiplegia Paralysis of one side of the body.

Hemoconcentration Reduced volume of plasma water and the increased concentration of blood cells, plasma proteins, and protein-bound constituents.

Hemolysis Breakdown of red blood cells and the release of hemoglobin.

Hemopneumothorax Presence of blood and air within the pleural space.

Hemorrhagic Exudate Discharge that has a large component of red blood cells.

Hemorrhoid Swollen vascular tissue in the rectal area.

Hemostasis Cessation of bleeding.

Hemothorax Condition wherein blood accumulates in the pleural space of the lungs.

Hepatitis Chronic or acute inflammation of the liver.

Hesitancy Difficulty initiating the urinary stream.

Hindmilk Follows foremilk, is higher in fat content, leading to weight gain, and is more satisfying.

Hirsutism Excessive body hair in a masculine distribution.

Histamine Substance released during allergic reactions.

HIV-Wasting Syndrome Unexplained weight loss of more than 10% of body weight accompanied by weakness, chronic diarrhea, and fever in those infected with HIV.

Holistic Whole; includes physical, intellectual, sociocultural, psychological, and spiritual aspects as an integrated whole.

Homan's Sign Test to check for the presence of clots in the leg.

Homeostasis Balance or equilibrium among the physiologic, psychological, sociocultural, intellectual, and spiritual needs of the body; maintenance of internal environment.

Homonymous Hemianopia Loss of vision in half of the visual field on the same side of both eyes.

Hormone Substance that initiates or regulates activity of another organ, system, or gland in another part of the body.

Hospice Humane, compassionate care provided to clients who can no longer benefit from curative treatment, and have 6 months or less to live; allows individuals to die with dignity.

Host Organism that can be affected by an agent.

Human Immunodeficiency Virus (HIV) Retrovirus that causes AIDS.

Human Leukocyte Antigen Antigen present in human blood.

Humoral Immunity Type of immunity dominated by antibodies.

Hydatidiform Mole Abnormality of the placenta wherein the chorionic villi become fluid filled, grape-like clusters; the trophoblastic tissue proliferates; and there is no viable fetus.

Hydramnios (Polyhydramnios) Excess amount of amniotic fluid.

Hydrocele Fluid around the testes in the scrotum.

Hydrostatic Pressure Pressure that a fluid exerts against a membrane; also called filtration force.

Hygiene Study of health and ways of preserving health.

Hyperbilirubinemia Excess of bilirubin in the blood.

Hyperemesis Gravidarum Excessive vomiting during pregnancy.

Hypergylcemia Condition wherein the blood glucose level becomes too high as a result of the absence of insulin.

Hyperopia Farsightedness.

Hypersensitivity Excessive reaction to a stimulus.

Hypersomnia Alteration in sleep pattern characterized by excessive sleep, especially in the daytime.

Hyperthermia Condition in which the core body temperature rises above 106°F.

Hypertonic Solution Solution that has a higher molecular concentration than the cell; also called a hyperosmolar solution.

Hypertrophy Increase in muscle mass.

Hyperuricemia Increased uric acid blood level.

Hyperventilation Breathing characterized by deep, rapid respirations.

Hypervigilant Condition of constantly scanning the environment for potentially dangerous situations.

Hypervolemia Increased circulating fluid volume.

Hypnosis Altered state of consciousness or awareness resembling sleep and during which a person is more receptive to suggestion.

Hypoglycemia Condition wherein the blood glucose level is exceedingly low.

Hypomania Mild form of mania without significant impairment.

Hypospadias Placement of the urinary meatus on the underside of the penis.

Hypothermia Condition in which the core body temperature drops below 95°F.

Hypotonia Lax muscle tone.

Hypotonic Solution Solution that has a lower molecular concentration than the cell; also called hypo-osmolar solution.

Hypoventilation Breathing characterized by shallow respirations.

Hypovolemia Abnormally low circulatory blood volume.

Hypoxemia Decreased oxygen level in the blood.

Iatrogenic Caused by treatment or diagnostic procedures.

Idiopathic Occuring without a known cause.

Idiosyncratic Reaction Very unpredictable response that may be an overresponse, an underresponse, or an atypical response.

Ileal Conduit Implantation of the ureters into a piece of ileum, which is attached to the abdominal wall as a stoma so urine can be removed from the body.

Ileostomy Opening created in the small intestine at the ileum.

Illness Stage Time period when the client is manifesting specific signs and symptoms of an infectious agent.

Illusion Inaccurate perception or misinterpretation of sensory stimuli.

Imagery Relaxation technique of using the imagination to visualize a pleasant, soothing image.

Immune Response Body's reaction to substances identified as nonself.

Immunity Body's ability to protect itself from foreign agents or organisms.

Immunization Process of creating immunity or resistance to infection in an individual.

Immunotherapy Treatment to suppress or enhance immunological functioning.

Impaired Nurse Nurse who is habitually intemperate or is addicted to the use of alcohol or habit-forming drugs.

Implantable Cardioverter-defibrillator (ICD) Implantable device that senses a dysrythmia and automatically sends an electrical shock directly to the heart to defibrillate it.

Implantable Port Device made of a radiopague silicone catheter and a plastic or stainless steel injection port with a self-sealing silicone-rubber septum.

Implantation Embedding of a fertilized egg into the uterine lining.

Implementation Fourth step in the nursing process; performance of the nursing interventions identified during the planning phase.

Implied Contract Contract that recognizes a relationship between parties for services.

Impotence Inability of an adult male to have an erection firm enough, or to maintain it long enough, to complete sexual intercourse.

Incidence Frequency of disease occurrence.

Incident Report Risk-management tool used to describe and report any unusual event that occurs to a client, visitor, or staff member.

Incompetent Cervix Descriptor for when the cervix begins to dilate, usually during the second trimester.

Incomplete Protein Protein with one or more of the essential amino acids missing.

Increment Increasing intensity of a contraction.

Incubation Period Time between entry of an infectious agent in the host and the onset of symptoms.

Independent Nursing Intervention Nursing action initiated by the nurse and do not require direction or an order from another health care professional.

Induction of Labor Stimulation of uterine contractions before contractions begin spontaneously for the purpose of birthing an infant.

Infancy Development from the end of the first month to the end of the first year of life.

Infection Invasion and multiplication of pathogenic microorganims in body tissue that results in cellular injury.

Infectious Agent Microorganism that causes cellular injury.

Infertility Inability or diminished ability to produce offspring.

Infiltration Seepage of foreign substances into the interstitial tissue, causing swelling and discomfort at the IV site.

Inflammation Nonspecific cellular response to tissue injury.

Informal Teaching Teaching that takes place any time, any place, and whenever a learning need is identified.

Informed Consent Legal form signed by a competent client and witnessed by another person that grants permission to the client's physician to perform the procedure described by the physician and that demonstrates the client's understanding of the benefits, risks, and possible complications of the procedure, as well as alternate treatment options.

Ingestion The taking of food into the digestive tract, generally through the mouth.

Initial Planning Development of a preliminary plan of care by the nurse who performs the admission assessment and gathers the comprehensive admission assessment data.

Insensible Water Loss Water loss of which the person is not generally aware.

Insomnia Difficulty in falling asleep initially or in returning to sleep once awakened.

Inspection Physical examination technique that involves thorough visual observation.

Insulin Pancreatic hormone that aids in both the diffusion of glucose into the liver and muscle cells, and the synthesis of glycogen.

Intellectual Wellness Ability to function as an independent person capable of making sound decisions.

Intensity Strength of the contraction at the acme.

Interdependent Nursing Intervention Nursing action that is implemented in a collaborative manner with other health care professionals.

Internal Respiration Exchange of oxygen and carbon dioxide at the cellular level.

Interstitial Fluid Fluid in tissue spaces around each cell.

Interval Resting period between two contractions.

Intoxication Reversible effect on the central nervous system soon after the use of a substance.

Intracath Plastic tube for insertion into a vein.

Intracellular Fluid Fluid within the cells.

Intradermal Injection into the dermis.

Intramuscular Injection into the muscle.

Intraoperative Phase Time during the surgical experience that begins when the client is transferred to the operating room table and ends when the client is admitted to the postanesthesia care unit.

Intrathecal Analgesia Administration of analgesics into the subarachnoid space.

Intravascular Fluid Fluid consisting of the plasma in the blood vessels and the lymph in the lymphatic system.

Intravenous Injection into a vein.

Intravenous Therapy Administration of fluids, electrolytes, nutrients, or medications by the venous route.

Intravesical Within the urinary bladder.

Intussusception Telescoping of one part of the intestine into another.

Invasive Accessing the body tissues, organs, or cavities through some type of instrumentation procedure.

Involution Return of the reproductive organs, especially the uterus, to their pre-pregnancy size and condition.

Ion Atom bearing an electrical charge.

Ischemia Oxygen deprivation, usually due to poor perfusion.

Ischemic Pain Discomfort resulting when the blood supply to an area is restricted or cut off completely.

Isolation Separation from other persons, especially those with infectious diseases.

Isotonic Solution Solution that has the same molecular concentration as does the cell; also called an isosmolar solution.

Isotopes Atom of the same element that has a different atomic weight (i.e., different numbers of neutrons in the nucleus).

IV Push (bolus) The administration of a large dose of medication in a relatively short time, usually 1–30 minutes.

Jaundice Yellow discoloration of the skin, sclera, mucous membranes, and body fluids that occurs when the liver is unable to fully remove bilirubin from the blood.

Johnsonian Intervention Confrontational approach to a client with a substance problem that lessens the chance of denial and encourages treatment before the client "hits bottom."

Judgment Conclusion based on sound reasoning and supported by evidence.

Justice Ethical principle based on the concept of fairness extended to each individual.

Kaposi's Sarcoma Vascular malignancy that can occur any place in the body, including the internal organs.

Kardex A brief worksheet with basic client care information.

Keloid Abnormal growth of scar tissue that is elevated, rounded, and firm with irregular, clawlike margins.

Keratin Tough, fibrous protein produced by cells in the epidermis called keratinocytes.

Keratitis Inflammation of the cornea.

Kernicterus Severe neurologic damage resulting from a high level of bilirubin (jaundice).

Kernig's Sign Diagnostic test for inflammation in the nerve roots; the inability to extend the leg when the thigh is flexed against the abdomen.

Ketone Acidic byproduct of fat metabolism.

Ketonuria Presence of ketones in the urine.

Ketosis Condition wherein acids called ketones accumulate in the blood and urine, upsetting the acid–base balance.

Kilocalorie Equivalent to 1,000 calories.

Kinesthetic Learner Person who learns by processing information through touching, feeling, and doing.

Kwashiorkor Condition resulting when there is a sudden or recent lack of protein-containing foods.

Kyphosis Increased roundness of the thoracic spinal curve.

Laissez-faire Leadership style that is passive and non-direct.

Lanugo Fine hair covering the fetus's body.

Large for Gestational Age Infant's weight falls above the 90th percentile for gestational age.

Late Deceleration Reduction in fetal heart rate that begins after the uterus has begun contracting and increases to the baseline level after the uterine contraction has ceased.

Law That which is laid down or fixed.

Learning Act or process of acquiring knowledge and/or skill in a particular subject; process of assimilating knowledge resulting in behavior changes.

Learning Disability Heterogenous group of disorders manifested by significant difficulties in the acquisition and use of listening, speaking, reading, writing, reasoning, or mathematical abilities.

Learning Plateau Peak in the effectiveness of teaching and depth of learning.

Learning Style Individual preference for receiving, processing, and assimilating information about a particular subject.

Lecithin Major component of surfactant.

Leopold's Maneuvers Series of specific palpations of the pregnant uterus to determine fetal position and presentation.

Let-Down Reflex Neurohormonal reflex that causes milk to be expressed from the alveoli into the lactiferous ducts.

Lethargy Decreased energy level.

Leukemia Cancer occurring in blood-forming tissues.

Leukocytosis Increased number of white blood cells.

Leukopenia Decreased number of white blood cells.

Liability Obligation one has incurred or might incur through any act or failure to act.

Libel Written words that harm or injure the personal or professional reputation of another person.

Libido Sexual energy

Licensure Mandatory system of granting licenses according to specified standards.

Life Review Form of reminiscence wherein a client attempts to come to terms with conflict or to gain meaning from life and die peacefully.

Ligation Application of a band or tie around a structure.

Lightening Descent of the fetus into the pelvis, causing the uterus to tip forward, relieving pressure on the diaphragm.

Linea Nigra Dark line on the abdomen from umbilicus to symphysis during the pregnancy.

Lipid Organic compound that is insoluble in water but soluble in organic solvents such as ether and alcohol; also known as fats.

Lipodystrophy Atrophy or hypertrophy of subcutaneous fat.

Lipoma Benign tumor consisting of mature fat cells.

Lipoprotein Blood lipid bound to protein.

Liquefaction Necrosis Death and subsequent change of tissue to a liquid or semi-liquid state; often descriptive of a primary tubercle.

Listening Interpreting the sounds heard and attaching meaning to them.

Litholapaxy Procedure involving crushing of a bladder stone and immediate washing out of the fragments through a catheter.

Lithotripsy Method of crushing a calculus any place in the urinary system with ultrasonic waves.

Liver Mortis Bluish-purple discoloration of the skin that is a by-product of red blood cell destruction; it begins within 20 minutes of death.

Living Will Legal document that allows a person to state preferences about the use of life-sustaining measures should she be unable to make her wishes known.

Local Adaptation Syndrome Physiologic response to a stressor (e.g., trauma, illness) affecting a specific part of the body.

Localized Infection Infection limited to a defined area or single organ.

Lochia Uterine/vaginal discharge after childbirth; initially bright red, then changing to a pink or pinkish brown, then to a yellowish white.

Locomotor Pertaining to movement or the ability to move.

Logic Formal principles of a branch of knowledge (such as nursing).

Long-Term Care Facility Health care facility that provides services to individuals who are not acutely ill, have continuing health care needs, and cannot function independently at home.

Long-Term Goal Statement that profiles the desired resolution of the nursing diagnosis over a long period of time, usually weeks or months.

Lordosis Exaggeration of the curvature of the lumbar spine.

Loss Any situation, either potential, actual, or perceived, wherein a valued object or person is changed or is not accessible to the individual.

L/S Ratio Ratio of the surfactants lecithin and sphingomyelin; a 2:1 ratio indicates lung maturity in the fetus.

Lumbar Puncture Aspiration of cerebrospinal fluid from the subarachnoid space.

Lung Stretch Receptor Receptor that monitors the patterns of breathing and prevents overexpansion of the lungs.

Lymphokine Chemical substance released by sensitized lymphocytes (T cells) that assists in antigen destruction.

Lymphoma Tumor of the lymphatic system.

Macrosomia Excessive fetal growth characterized by a fetus weighing more than 4,000 g (8.8 lb.).

Magnetic Resonance Imaging Imaging technique that uses radiowaves and a strong magnetic field to make continuous cross-sectional images of the body.

Maladaptive Measure Measure used to avoid conflict or stress.

Malignant Becoming progessively worse and often resulting in death.

Malignant Hypertension Rapidly progressing form of hypertension with the diastolic pressure greater than 120 mm Hg.

Malpractice Negligent acts on the part of a professional; relates to the conduct of a person who is acting in a professional capacity.

Managed Care System of providing and monitoring care wherein access, cost, and quality are controlled before or during delivery of services.

Mania Extremely elevated mood with accompanying agitated behavior.

Marasmus Condition resulting from severe malnutrition; afflicts very young children who lack both energy and protein foods as well as vitamins and minerals.

Maslow's Hierarchy of Needs Theory of behavioral motivation based on needs; includes physiologic, safety and security, love and belonging, self-esteem, and self-actualization needs.

Mastication Chewing food into fine particles and mixing the food with enzymes in saliva.

Mastitis Inflammation of the breast, generally during breast feeding.

Material Principle of Justice Rationale for determining those times when there can be unequal allocation of scarce resources.

Matter Anything that occupies space and possesses mass.

Maturation Process of becoming fully grown and developed; involves physiologic and behavioral aspects.

Maturational Loss Loss that occurs as a person moves from one developmental stage to another.

Mechanism of Labor Series of movvements of the fetus as it passes through the pelvis and birth canal.

Meconium Fecal material stored in the fetal intestines.

Meconium Ileus Impacted feces in the newborn, causing intestinal obstruction.

Medicaid Government title program (XIX) that pays for health services for the aged, poor, disabled, and low-income families with dependent children.

Medical Asepsis Practices that reduce the number, growth, and spread of microorganisms.

Medical Diagnosis Clinical judgment by the physician that identifies or determines a specific disease, condition, or pathological state.

Medical Model Traditional approach to health care wherein the focus is on treatment and cure of disease not prevention.

Medicare Amendment (Title XVIII) to the Social Security Act that helps finace the health care of persons over 65 years old and for permanently disabled younger persons who receive Social Security disability benefits.

Medigap Insurance Insurance plan for persons with Medicare that pays for health care costs not covered by Medicare.

Meditation Quieting the mind by focusing attention on a sound, on an image, or on one's own breathing.

Melanin Pigment that gives skin its color.

Melena Stool containing partially broken down blood usually black, sticky, and tar-like.

Menarche Onset of the first menstrual period.

Ménière's Disease State of hearing loss characterized by tinnitus and vertigo.

Meningitis Inflammation of the meninges.

Meningocele Saclike protrusion along the vertebral column filled with cerebrospinal fluid and meninges.

Menopause Cessation of menstruation.

Menorrhagia Excessively heavy menstrual flow.

Mental Disorder Clinically significant behavior or psychological syndrome or pattern that occurs in an individual and is associated with present distress or disability or with a significantly increased risk of suffering, death, pain, disability, or an important loss of freedom (APA, 1994).

Mental Illness Condition wherein an individual has a distorted view of self, is unable to maintain satisfying personal relationships, and is unable to adapt to the environment.

Mentation Ability to concentrate, remember, or think abstractly.

Metabolic Rate Rate of energy utilization in the body.

Metabolism Sum total of all the biological and chemical processes in the body.

Metastasis Spread of cancer cells to distant areas of the body by way of the lymph system or bloodstream.

Metritis Inflammation of the uterus including the endometrium and parametrium.

Metrorrhagia Vaginal bleeding between menstrual periods.

Microthrombi Very small clots.

Micturition Process of expelling uring from the urinary bladder; also called urination or voiding.

Middle Adulthood Development from the ages of 40 years to 65 years.

Milia Pearly white cysts on the face.

Minority Group Group of people constituting less than a numerical majority of the population and are often labeled and treated differently from others in the society.

Miscarriage Spontaneous abortion.

Misdemeanor Offense that is less serious than a felony and may be punished by a fine or by sentence to a local prison for less than 1 year.

Misuse Use of a legal substance for which it was not intended, or exceeding the recommended dosage of a drug.

Mitosis Cell division.

Mixed Agonist-Antagonist Compound that blocks opioid effects on one receptor type while producing opioid effects on a second receptor type.

Mixture Substances combined in no specific way.

Mnemonic Method to aid in association and recall; a memorable sentence created from the first letters of a list of items to be used to recall the items later.

Mode of Transmission Process of the infectious agent moving from the reservoir or source through the portal of exit to the portal of entry of the susceptible "new" host.

Modulation Central nervous system pathway that selectively inhibits pain transmission by sending signals back down to the dorsal horn of the spinal cord.

Molding Shaping of the fetal head to adapt to the mother's pelvis during labor.

Molecule Atoms of the same element that unite with each other.

Mongolian Spots Large patches of bluish skin on the buttocks of dark-skinned infants.

Monounsaturated Fatty Acid Forms a glycerol ester with a double or triple bond; nuts, fowl, and olive oil.

Mood Subjective report of the way an individual is feeling.

Moral Maturity Ability to decide for oneself what is "right."

Morbidity Illness.

Mortality Death.

Mortuary Funeral home.

Morula Mass of cells resembling a mulberry.

Mourning Period during which grief is expressed and integration and resolution of the loss occur.

Mucous Fistula Stoma that secretes mucous.

Multigravida Condition of being pregnant two or more times.

Multipara Condition of having delivered twice or more after 24 weeks' gestation.

Myalgia Pain in muscles.

Myelomeningocele Saclike protrusion along the vertebral column that is filled with spinal fluid, meninges, nerve roots, and spinal cord.

Myocardial Infarction Necrosis (death) of the myocardium caused by an obstruction in a coronary artery; commonly known as heart attack.

Myocarditis Inflammation of the myocardium of the heart.

Myofascial Pain Syndrome Group of muscle disorders characterized by pain, muscle spasm, tenderness, stiffness, and limited motion.

Myopia Nearsightedness.

Myringotomy Surgical incision of the eardrum.

Myxedema Severe hypothyroidism in adults.

Narcolepsy Sleep alteration manifested as sudden uncontrollable urges to fall asleep during the daytime.

Narrative Charting Chronological account written in paragraphs describes the client's status, the interventions and treatments, and the client's response to treatments.

Necrosis Tissue death as the result of disease or injury.

Neglect Situation wherein a basic need of the client is not being provided.

Negligence General term referring to careless acts on the part of an individual who is not exercising reasonable or prudent judgement.

Neonatal Stage First 28 days of life following birth.

Neonatal Transition First few hours after birth wherein the newborn makes changes to and stabilizes respiratory and circulatory functions.

Neonate Newborn from birth to 28 days of life.

Neoplasm Any abnormal growth of new tissue.

Nephrotoxic Quality of a substance that causes kidney tissue damage.

Nesting Surge of energy late in pregnancy when the pregnant woman organizes and cleans the house.

Neuralgia Paroxysmal pain that extends along the course of one or more nerves.

Neurogenic Shock Hypotensive situation resulting from the loss of sympathetic control of vital functions from the brain.

Neuropeptide Amino acid produced in the brain and other sites in the body that acts as a chemical communicator.

Neurotransmitter Chemical substance produced by the body that facilitates or inhibits nerve-impulse transmission.

Neutral Thermal Environment Environment in which the newborn can maintain internal body temperature with minimal oxygen consumption and metabolism.

Nevi Pigmented areas in the skin; commonly known as bithmarks or moles.

Nevus Flammeus Large, reddish-purple birthmark usually found on the face or neck which does not blanch with pressure.

Nevus Vascularis Birthmark of enlarged superficial blood vessels, elevated and red in color.

Nociceptor Receptive neuron for painful sensations.

Nocturia Awakening at night to void.

Nocturnal Enuresis Incontinence that occurs during sleep.

Noninvasive Descriptor for procedure wherein the body is *not* entered with any type of instrument.

Nonmaleficence Ethical principle based on the obligation to cause no harm to others.

Nonshivering Thermogenesis Metabolism of brown fat; process unique to the newborn.

Nonverbal Communication Body language or a method of sending a message without words.

Nosocomial Infection Infection acquired in the hospital or other health care facility that was not present or incubating at the time of the client's admission.

Noxious Stimulus Underlying pathology that causes pain.

Nuchal Cord Condition of the umbilical cord being wrapped around the baby's neck.

Nuchal Rigidity Pain and rigidity in the neck.

Nulligravida Condition of never having been pregnant.

Nullipara Condition of never having delivered an infant after 24 weeks' gestation.

Nursing The art and science of assisting individuals in learning to care for themselves whenever possible; and of caring for them when they are unable to meet their own needs.

Nursing Audit Method of evaluating the quality of care provided to clients.

Nursing Care Plan Written guide of strategies to be implemented to help the client achieve optimal health.

Nursing Diagnosis Second step in the nursing process; a clinical judgement about individual, family, or community (aggregate) responses to actual or potential health problems/life processes.

Nursing Intervention Action performed by a nurse that helps the client achieve the results specified by the goals and expected outcomes.

Nursing Interventions Classification Standardized language for nursing interventions.

Nursing Minimum Data Set Elements that should be in clinical records and abstracted for studies on the effectiveness and costs of nursing care.

Nursing Outcomes Classification Standardized language for nursing outcomes.

Nursing Practice Act Statute that is enacted by the legislature of a state and that outlines the scope of nursing practice in that state.

Nursing Process Systematic method for providing care to clients, consisting of five steps: assessment, diagnosis, outcome identification and planning, implementation, and evaluation.

Nutrition All of the processes (ingestion, digestion, absorption, metabolism, and elimination) involved in consuming and utilizing food for energy, maintenance, and growth.

Nystagmus Constant, involuntary movement of the eye in various directions.

Obesity Weight that is 20% or more above the ideal body weight.

Objective Data Observable and measurable data that are obtained through standard assessment techniques performed during the physical examination and through laboratory and diagnostic tests.

Occult Blood Blood in the stool that can be detected only through a microscope or by chemical means.

Occult Blood Test (Guaiac) Test for microscopic blood done on stool.

Older Adulthood Development occurring from age 65 years until death.

Oligomenorrhea Decreased menstrual flow.

Oliguria Diminished production of urine.

Oncology Study of tumors.

Ongoing Assessment Type of assessment that includes systematic monitoring of specific problems.

Ongoing Planning Updates the client's plan of care.

Onset of Action Time for the body to respond to a drug after administration.

Oophoritis Inflammation of the ovary.

Open Reduction Surgical procedure that enables the surgeon to reduce (repair) a fracture under direct visualization.

Ophthalmia Neonatorum Inflammation of a newborn's eyes which results from passing through the birth canal when a gonorrheal or chlamydial infection is present.

Opinion Subjective belief.

Opioid Morphine-like compound that produces bodily effects such as pain relief, sedation, constipation, and respiratory depression.

Opisthotonos Complete arching of the body with only the head and feet on the bed.

Opportunistic Infection Infection in persons with a defective immune system that rarely causes harm in healthy individuals.

Oppression Condition wherein the rules, values, and ideals of one group are imposed on another group.

Orchiectomy Removal of a testis.

Orientation Person's awareness of self in relation to person, place, time, and, in some cases, situation.

Orthopedics (Orthopaedics) Branch of medicine that deals with the prevention or correction of the disorders and diseases of the musculoskeletal system.

Orthopnea Difficulty breathing while lying down.

Orthostatic Hypotension Significant decrease in blood pressure that results when a person moves from a lying or sitting (supine) position to a standing position.

Osmolality Measurement of the total concentration of dissolved particles (solutes) per kilogram of water.

Osmolarity Concentration of solutes per liter of cellular fluid.

Osmosis Movement of a solvent, usually water, through a semipermeable membrane, from a region of higher concentration to a region of lower concentration.

Osmotic Pressure Pressure exerted against the cell membrane by the water inside a cell.

Osteoporosis Increase in the porosity of bone.

Otitis Externa Bacterial infection of the external ear canal.

Otitis Media Inflammation of the middle ear.

Otosclerosis Conductive hearing loss secondary to a pathologic change of the bones in the middle ear.

Overflow Incontinence Leaking of urine when the bladder becomes very full and distended.

Oxidation Chemical process of combining with oxygen.

Oxidized Joined with oxygen.

Pain Unpleasant sensory and emotional experience associated with actual or potential tissue damage or described in terms of such.

Pain Threshold Level of intensity at which pain becomes appreciable or perceptible.

Pain Tolerance Level of intensity or duration of pain that a person is willing to endure.

Palliative Relief of symptoms, such as pain, without altering the course of disease.

Palliative Care Care that relieves symptoms, such as pain, but does not alter the course of disease.

Pallor Abnormal paleness of the skin, seen especially in the face, conjunctiva, nail beds, and oral mucous membranes.

Palpation Physical examination technique that uses the sense of touch to assess texture, temperature, moisture, organ location and size, vibrations and pulsations, swelling, masses, and tenderness.

Palpitation Fluttering or pounding sensation in the chest.

Pancreatitis Acute or chronic inflammation of the pancreas.

Papanicolaou Test Smear method of examining stained exfoliative cells.

Para Condition of having delivered after 24 weeks' gestation, whether infant is born alive or dead or number of infants born.

Paracentesis Aspiration of fluid from the abdominal cavity.

Paradoxical Reaction Opposite effect of that which would normally be expected.

Paramedic Specialized health care professional trained to provide advanced life support to the client requiring emergency interventions.

Paraplegia Paralysis of lower extremities.

Parasomnia Disorders that intrude on sleep in very active ways.

Parenteral Any route other than the oral-gastrointestinal tract.

Parenteral Nutrition Feeding method whereby nutrients bypass the small intestine and enter the blood directly.

Paresthesia Abnormal sensation such as burning, prickling, or tingling.

Paroxysmal Descriptor for a symptom that begins and ends abruptly.

Paroxysmal Nocturnal Dyspnea Condition of suddenly awakening, sweating, and having difficulty breathing.

Passive Euthanasia Process of working with the client's dying process.

Patency Being freely opened.

Pathogen Microorganism that causes disease.

Pathogenicity Ability of a microorganism to produce disease.

Patient-Controlled Analgesia Device that allows the client to control the delivery of intravenous or subcutaneous pain medication in a safe, effective manner through a programmable pump.

Peak Plasma Level Highest blood concentration of a single dose of a drug until the elimination rate equals the rate of absorption.

Peer Assistance Program Rehabilitation program that provides an impaired nurse with referrals, professional and peer counseling support groups, and assistance and monitoring back into nursing.

Peptic Ulcer Erosion formed in the esophagus, stomach, or duodenum resulting from acid/pepsin imbalance.

Perception Ability to experience, recognize, organize, and interpret sensory stimuli.

Percussion Physical examination technique that uses short, tapping strokes on the surface of the skin to create vibrations of underlying organs.

Percutaneous Balloon Valvuloplasty Insertion of a balloon in a stenosed valve to expand the narrowed valvular space.

Perfectionism Overwhelming expectation of being able to get everything done in a flawless manner.

Perfusion Blood flow through an organ or body part.

Pericardial Friction Rub Short, high-pitched squeak heard as two inflamed pericardial surfaces rub together.

Pericardiocentesis Removal of fluid from the pericardial sac.

Pericarditis Inflammation of the membrane sac surrounding the heart.

Perineal Care Cleansing of the external genitalia, perineum, and the surrounding area.

Perioperative Period of time encompassing the preoperative, intraoperative, and postoperative phases of surgery.

Peripheral Nervous System System of the cranial nerves, spinal nerves, and the autonomic nervous system.

Peripheral Resistance Pressure within a vessel that resists the flow of blood such as plaque buildup or vasoconstriction.

Peristalsis Rhythmic, coordinated, serial contraction of the smooth muscles of the gastrointestinal tract.

Peritonitis Inflammation of the peritoneum, the membranous covering of the abdomen.

Permeability Ability of a membrane to permit substances to pass through it.

Petechiae Pinpoint hemorrhagic spots on the skin.

Phantom Limb Pain Neuropathic pain that occurs after amputation with pain sensations referred to an area in the missing portion of the limb.

Pharmacokinetics Study of the absorption, distribution, metabolism, and excretion of drugs to determine the relationship between the dose of a drug and the drug's concentration in biological fluids.

Phimosis Condition wherein the opening in the foreskin is so small that it cannot be pulled back over the glans.

Phlebitis Inflammation in the wall of a vein without clot formation.

Phlebothrombosis Formation of a clot because of blood pooling in the vessel, trauma to the vessel's endothelial lining, or a coagulation problem with little or no inflammation in the vessel.

Phlebotomist Individual who performs venipuncture.

Phlebotomy Removal of blood from a vein.

Phospholipid Lipid composed of glycerol, fatty acids, and phosphorus; the structural component of cells.

Physical Agent Factor in the environment capable of causing disease in a host.

Physical Restraint Equipment that reduces the client's movement.

Physical Wellness Healthy body that functions at an optimal level.

Physically Aggressive Descriptor of an individual who threatens or actually harms someone.

Physiologic Anemia of Pregnancy Hemodilution caused by the increased maternal blood volume.

Phytochemical Physiologically active compound present in plants in very small amounts that gives plants flavor, odor, and color.

Pica Practice of eating substances not considered edible and which have no nutritive value, such as laundry starch, dirt, clay, and freezer frost.

PIE Charting Documentation method using the problem, intervention, evaluation (PIE) format.

Piggyback Addition of an intravenous solution to infuse concurrently with another infusion.

Placenta Membranous vascular organ connecting the fetus to the mother, which produces hormones to sustain a pregnancy, supplies the fetus with oxygena and food, and transports waste products of out the fetal system.

Placenta Previa Condition in which the placenta forms over or very near the internal cervical os.

Planning Third step of the nursing process; includes both the establishing of guidelines for the proposed course of nursing action to resolve the nursing diagnoses and developing the client's plan of care.

Plateau Level at which a drug's blood concentration is maintained.

Pleural Effusion Collection of fluid within the pleural cavity.

Pleural Friction Rub Abnormal breath sound that is creaky and grating in nature and is heard on inspiration and expiration.

Pleurisy Condition arising from inflammation of the pleura, or sac, that encases the lung.

Pneumonia Inflammation of the bronchioles and alveoli accompanied by consolidation, or solidification of exudate, in the lungs.

Pneumothorax Condition wherein air or gas accumulates in the pleural space of the lungs, causing the lungs to collapse.

Point-of-Care Charting Documentation system that allows health care providers to gain immediate access to client information at the bedside.

Poison Any substance that when taken into the body interferes with normal physiologic functioning; may be inhaled, injected, ingested, or absorbed by the body.

Polydipsia Excessive thirst.

Polymenorrhea Menstrual periods that are abnormally frequent, generally less than every 21 days.

Polyp Abnormal growth of tissue.

Polyphagia Increased hunger.

Polypharmacy Problem of clients taking numerous prescription and over-the-counter medications for the same or various disease processes, with unknown consequences from the resulting combinations of chemical compounds and cumulative side-effects.

Polyunsaturated Fatty Acid Forms a glycerol ester with many carbons unbonded to hydrogen atoms; fish, corn, sunflower seeds, soybeans, cotton seeds, and safflower oil.

Polyuria Increased urination.

Port-a-Cath Port that has been implanted under the skin with a catheter inserted into the superior vena cava or right atrium through the subclavian or internal jugular vein.

Portal of Entry Route by which an infectious agent enters the host.

Portal of Exit Route by which an infectious agent leaves the reservoir.

Post Void Residual Urine that remains in the bladder after urination.

Postictal After a seizure.

Post-mortem Care Care given immediately after death before the body is moved to the mortuary.

Postoperative Phase Time during the surgical experience that begins at the end of the surgical procedure and ends when the client is discharged, not just from the hospital or institution, but from medical care by the surgeon.

Postpartum Blues Mild transient condition of emotional lability and crying for no apparent reason, which affects up to 80% of women who have just given birth, and lasts about 2 weeks.

Postpartum Depression Condition similar to postpartum blues but which is more serious, intense, and persistent.

Postpartum Hemorrhage Bloos loss of more than 500 mL after the third stage of labor or 1,000 mL following a cesarean birth.

Postpartum Psychosis Condition more severe than postpartum depression and characterized by delusions and thoughts of self harm or infant harm.

Postprandial After eating.

Postterm Delivery after 42 weeks' gestation.

Preadolescence Development from the ages of approximately 10 years to 12 years.

Precipitate Birth Birth occurring suddenly and unexpectantly without a CNM/physician present to assist.

Precipitate Labor Labor lasting less than 3 hours from the onset of contractions to the birth of the infant.

Preeclampsia Phase of pregnancy-induced hypertension prior to convulsions.

Preferred Provider Organization Type of managed care model wherein member choice is limited to providers within the system for full reimbursement; other providers less reimbursement.

Prenatal Care Care of a woman during pregnancy, before labor.

Prenatal Stage Development beginning with conception and ending with birth.

Preoperative Phase Time during the surgical experience that begins when the client decides to have surgery and ends when the client is transferred to the operating table.

Presbycusis Sensorineural hearing loss associated with aging.

Presbyopia Inablility of the lens of the eye to change curvature to focus near objects.

Preschool Stage Development from the ages of 3 years to 6 years.

Prescriptive Authority Legal recognition of the ability to prescribe medications.

Presenting Part Part of the fetus in contact with the cervix.

Pressured Speech Rapid, intense style of speech.

Preterm Delivery after 24 weeks' gestation but before 38 weeks (full term).

Preterm Birth Birth that takes place before the end of the 37th week of gestation.

Preterm Labor Onset of regular contractions of the uterus that cause cervical changes between 20 and 37 weeks' gestation.

Prevention Obstructing, thwarting, or hindering a disease or illness.

Priapism Prolonged erection that does not occur in response to sexual stimulation.

Primary Care Care focused on promoting wellness and preventing illness or disability.

Primary Care Provider Health care provider whom a client sees first for health care, typically a family practitioner (physician/nurse), internist, or pediatrician.

Primary Health Care Client's point of entry into the health care system; includes assessment, diagnosis, treatment, coordination of care, education, prevention services, and surveillance.

Primary Hypertension High blood pressure, the cause of which is unknown; also known as essential hypertension.

Primary Prevention All practices designed to keep health problems from developing.

Primary Source Major provider of information about a client.

Primary Tubercle Nodule that contains tubercle bacilli and forms within lung tissue.

Privacy The right to be left alone, to choose care based on personal beliefs, to govern body integrity, and to choose when and how sensitive information is shared (Badzek & Gross, 1999).

Problem-Oriented Medical Record Documentation method employs a structured, logical format and focuses on the client's problem.

Procedure Step-by-step instruction describing the process for performing various nursing tasks.

Process Series of steps or acts that leads to the accomplishing some goal or purpose.

Procrastination Intentionally putting off or delaying something that should be done.

Prodromal Stage Time interval from the onset of nonspecific symptoms until specific symptoms of the infectious process begin to manifest.

Professional Boundaries Limits of the professional relationship that allow for a safe, therapeutic connection between the professional and the client.

Progressive Muscle Relaxation Stress management strategy in which muscles are alternately tensed and relaxed.

Projectile Vomiting Forceful ejection (up to 3 feet) of the contents of the stomach.

Prolapsed Cord Condition in which the umbilical cord lies below the presenting part of the fetus.

Prolapsed Uterus Downward displacement of the uterus into the vagina.

Prospective Payment Predetermined rate paid for each episode of hospitalization based on the client's age and principle diagnosis and the presence or absence of surgery or comorbidity.

Protocol Series of standing orders or procedures that should be followed under certain specific conditions.

Proxemics Study of the space between people and its effect on interpersonal behavior.

Pruritus Severe itching.

Pseudocyesis False pregnancy.

Pseudomenstruation Blood-tinged mucus discharge frohe vagina of a newborn caused by the withdrawal of maternal hormones.

Psychoanalysis Therapy focused on uncovering unconscious memories and processes.

Psychological Wellness Enjoyment of creativity, satisfaction of the basic need to love and be loved, understanding of emotions, and ability to maintain control over emotions.

Psychomotor Domain Area of learning that involves performance of motor skills.

Psychoneuroimmunology Study of the complex relationship among the physical, cognitive, and affective aspects of humans.

Psychoprophylaxis Mental and physical preparation for childbirth; synonymous with Lamaze.

Psychosis State wherein an individual has lost the ability to recognize reality.

Psychotherapy Treatment of mental and emotional disorders through psychological rather than physical methods.

Ptosis Drooping upper eyelid.

Puberty Emergence of secondary sex characteristics that signals the beginning of adolescence.

Public Law Law that deals with an individual's relationship to the state.

Pudendal Block Injection of a local anesthetic into the pudendal nerve to provide perineal, external genitalia, and lower vaginal anesthesia.

Puerperal (Postpartum) Infection Infection following childbirth occurring between the birth and 6 weeks postpartum.

Puerperium Term for the first 6 weeks after the birth of an infant.

Purpura Reddish-purple patches on the skin indicative of hemorrhage.

Purulent Exudate Discharge resulting from infection; also called pus.

Pulse Amplitude Measurement of the strength or force exerted by the ejected blood against the arterial wall with each heart contraction.

Pulse Deficit Condition in which the apical pulse rate is greater than the radial pulse rate.

Pulse Rate Indirect measurement of cardiac output obtained by counting the number of peripheral pulse waves over a pulse point.

Pulse Rhythm Regularity of the heart beat.

Pyelonephritis Bacteral infection of the renal pelvis, tubules, and interstitial tissue of one or both kidneys.

Pyorrhea Periodontal disease.

Pyuria Pus in the urine.

Quadriplegia Dysfunction or paralysis of both arms, both legs, and bowel and bladder.

Quickening Descriptor for when the mother first feels the fetus move, about 16 to 20 weeks' gestation.

Race A group of people with biological similarities.

Radiation Loss of heat by transfer to cooler near objects, but not through direct contact.

Radiography Study of x-rays or gamma ray-exposed film through the action of ionizing radiation.

Radiotherapy Treatment of cancer with high-energy radiation.

Rapport Mutual trust established between two people.

Readiness for Learning Evidence of willingness to learn.

Reasoning Use of the elements of thought to solve a problem or settle a question.

Reconstructive To rebuild or reestablish.

Rectocele Anterior displacement of the rectum into the posterior vaginal wall.

Recurrent Acute Pain Identified by repetitive painful episodes that recur over a prolonged period or throughout a client's lifetime.

Referred Pain Discomfort from the internal organs that is felt in another area of the body.

Reframing Technique of monitoring negative thoughts and replacing them with positive ones.

Regional Anesthesia Method of temporarily rendering a region of the body insensible to pain.

Rehabilitation Process designed to assist individuals to reach their optimal level of physical, mental, and psychosocial functioning.

Relapse Return to a previous behavior or condition.

Relaxation Technique Method used to decrease anxiety and muscle tension.

Religious Support System Group of ministers, priests, nuns, rabbis, shamans, mullahs, or lay persons who are able to meet clients' spiritual needs.

REM Movement Disorder Condition wherein the normal paralysis of REM sleep is absent or incomplete and the sleeper acts out the dream.

Remission Decrease or absence of symptoms of a disease.

Renal Colic Severe pain in the kidney that radiates to the groin.

Repolarization Recovery phase of the cardiac muscle.

Reservoir Place where the agent can survive.

Resident Flora Microorganisms that are always present, usually without altering the client's health.

Residual Urine Urine remaining in the bladder after the individual has urinated.

Respect Acceptance of an individual as is and in a nonjudgmental manner.

Respiration Process of exchanging oxygen and carbon dioxide.

Respite Care Care and service that provides a break to caregivers and is utilized for a few hours a week, for an occasional weekend, or for longer periods of time.

Responsiveness Person's ability to perceive environmental stimuli and body reactions and then to respond with thought and action.

Rest State of mental and physical relaxation and calmness.

Restitution Rotation of the fetal head back to be in normal alignment with the shoulders after delivery of the fetal head.

Restless Leg Syndrome Condition characterized by uncomfortable sensations of tingling or crawling in the muscles, and twitching, burning, prickling, or deep aching in the foot, calf, or upper leg when at rest.

Restraint Protective device used to limit the physical activity of a client or to immobilize a client or extremity.

Résumé Tool that summarizes employment qualifications.

Resuscitation Support measures implemented to restore consciousness and life.

Reticulocyte Immature red blood cell.

Retroperitoneal Behind the peritoneum outside the peritoneal cavity.

Retroplacental Behind the placenta.

Reverse Isolation Barrier protection designed to prevent infection in clients who are severely compromised and highly susceptible to infection; also known as protective isolation.

Reverse Tolerance Phenomenon whereby a smaller amount of substance will elicit the desired psychic effects.

Review of Systems Brief account of any recent signs or symptoms related to any body system.

Rhinorrhea Watery nasal discharge.

Rigor Mortis Natural stiffening of muscles after death. Begins about 4 hours after death.

Risk Nursing Diagnosis Nursing diagnosis indicating that a problem does not yet exist but that specific risk factors are present; composed of "Risk for" followed by the diagnostic label and a list of the risk factors.

Rooming-In Practice of staying with the client 24 hours a day to provide care and comfort.

Salpingitis Inflammation of the fallopian tube.

Salt Product formed when an acid and a base react with each other.

Sanguineous Bloody drainage from a wound or surgical drain.

Sarcoma Cancer occurring in connective tissue.

Satiety Feeling of adequate fullness from food.

School-Age Stage Development from the ages of 6 years to 10 years.

Sclerotherapy Treatment which involves injecting a chemical into the vein, causing the vein to become sclerosed (hardened) so blood no longer flows through it.

Sclerotic Hardened tissue.

Scoliosis Lateral curvature of the spine.

Scrub Nurse RN, LP/VN, or surgical technologist who provides services under the direction of the circulating nurse and who is qualified by training or experience to prepare and maintain the integrity, safety, and efficiency of the sterile field throughout an operation.

Sebaceous cyst Sebaceous gland filled with sebum.

Sebum Oily substance secreted by the sebaceous glands of the skin.

Secondary Care Care focused on diagnosis and treatment after the client exhibits symptoms of illness.

Secondary Hypertension High blood pressure occurring as a sequel to a pre-existing disease or injury.

Secondary Prevention Early detection, screening, diagnosis, and intervention, to reduce the consequences of a health problem.

Secondary Source Data source other than the client; can include family members, other health care providers, or medical records.

Sedation Reduction of stress, excitement, or irritability via some central nervous system depression.

Self-Awareness Consciously knowing how the self thinks, feels, believes, and behaves at any specific time.

Self-Care Deficit State wherein an individual is not able to perform one or more activities of daily living.

Self-Concept Individual's perception of self; includes self-esteem, body image, and ideal self.

Self-Efficacy Belief in one's ability to succeed in attempts to change behavior.

Semipermeable Membrane Membrane that allows passage of only certain substances.

Sensation Ability to receive and process stimuli received through the sensory organs.

Sensible Water Loss Water loss of which the person is aware.

Sensitivity Susceptibility of a pathogen to an antibiotic.

Sensorineural Hearing Loss Condition in which the inner ear or chochlear portion of cranial nerve VIII is abnormal or diseased.

Sensory Deficit Change in the perception of sensory stimuli; can affect any of the senses.

Sensory Deprivation State of reduced sensory input from the internal or external environment, manifested by alterations in sensory perception.

Sensory Overload State of excessive and sustained multisensory stimulation manifested by behavior change and perceptual distortion.

Sensory Perception Ability to receive sensory impressions and, through cortical association, relate the stimuli to past experiences and to form an impression of the nature of the stimulus.

Seroconversion Evidence of antibody formation in response to disease or vaccine.

Serosanguineous Exudate Discharge that is clear with some blood tinge; seen with surgical incisions.

Serous Exudate Discharge composed primarily of serum; is watery in appearance and has a low protein level.

Serum Lithium Level Laboratory test done to determine whether the client's lithium level is within a therapeutic range.

Shaman Folk healer-priest who uses natural and supernatural forces to help others.

Shamanism Practice of entering an altered state of consciousness with the intent to help others.

Shearing Force exerted against the skin by movement or repositioning.

Shift Report Report about each client between shifts.

Shock Condition of profound hemodynamic and metabolic disturbance characterized by inadequate tissue perfusion and inadequate circulation to the vital organs.

Short-Term Goal Statement that profiles the desired resolution of the nursing diagnosis over a short period of time, usually a few hours or days (less than a week).

Shroud Covering for the body after death.

Sibilant Wheeze Abnormal breath sound that is high pitched and musical in nature and is heard on inhalation and exhalation.

Sickle When red blood cells become crescent-shaped and elongated.

Single-Payer System Health care delivery model wherein the government is the only entity to reimburse health care costs.

Single Point of Entry Common feature of HMOs wherein the client is required to enter the health care system through a point designated by the plan.

Situational Loss Loss that takes place in response to external events generally beyond the individual's control.

Slander Words that are communicated verbally to a third party and that harm or injure the personal or professional reputation of another.

Sleep State of altered consciousness during which a person has minimal physical activity, changes in levels of consciousness; and a slowing of physiologic processes.

Sleep Apnea A period during sleep of not breathing; often associated with heavy snoring.

Sleep Cycle Sequence of sleep beginning with the four stages of NREM sleep, a return to stage 3 and then stage 2 (first phase), followed by the first REM sleep (second phase).

Sleep Deprivation Prolonged inadequate quality and quantity of sleep.

Small for Gestational Age Infant's weight falls below the 10th percentile for gestational age.

Snellen Chart Chart containing various-sized letters with standardized numbers at the end of each line of letters.

Snoring Noisy breathing during sleep.

SOAP Charting Documentation method using subjective data, objective data, assessment, and plan.

Sociocultural Wellness Ability to appreciate the needs of others and to care about one's environment and the inhabitants of it.

Somatic Nervous System Nerves that connect the central nervous system to the skin and skeletal muscles and control conscious activities.

Somatic Pain Nonlocalized discomfort originating in tendons, ligaments, and nerves.

Somnambulism Sleepwalking.

Somogyi Phenomenon In response to hypoglycemia, the release of glucose-elevating hormones (epinephrine, cortisol, glucose) which produces a hyperglycemic state.

Sonorous Wheeze Abnormal breath sound that is low pitched and snoring in nature and is louder on expiration.

Source-Oriented Charting Narrative recording by each member (source) of the health care team on a separate record.

Specific Order Order written in a client's medical record by a physician or nursing care plan written by a nurse especially for that individual client; not used for any other client.

Spermatogenesis Production of sperm.

Spina Bifida Occulta Failure of the vertebral arch to close.

Spinal Shock Cessation of motor, sensory, autonomic, and reflex impulses below the level of injury; characterized by flaccid paralysis of all skeletal muscles, loss of spinal reflexes, loss of sensation, and absence of autonomic function below the level of injury.

Spiritual Wellness Inner strength and peace.

Spiritual Care Recognition of and assistance toward meeting spiritual needs.

Spiritual Needs Individual's desire to find purpose and meaning in life, pain, and death.

Spirituality Relationships with one's self, with others, and with a higher power or divine source.

Spore Bacteria in a resistant stage that can withstand unfavorable environments.

Sprain Injury to ligaments surrounding a joint caused by a sudden twist, wrench, or fall.

Stable Alert with vital signs within the client's normal range.

Staff Development Delivery of instruction to assist nurses achieve the goals of the employer.

Standard Level or degree of quality.

Standard Precautions Preventive practices to be used in the care of all clients in hospitals regardless of their diagnosis or presumed infection status.

Standards of Practice Guidelines established to direct nursing care.

Standing Order Standardized intervention written, approved, and signed by a physician that is kept on file within health care agencies to be used in predictable situations or in circumstances requiring immediate attention.

Startle Response Overreaction to minor sounds or noises.

Stasis Dermatitis Inflammation of the skin due to decreased circulation.

Station Relationship of the fetal presenting part to the ischial spines.

Status Asthmaticus Persistent, intractable asthma attack.

Status Epilepticus Acute, prolonged episode of seizure activity that lasts at least 30 minutes and may or may not involve loss of consciousness.

Statutory Law Law enacted by legislative bodies.

Steatorrhea Fatty stool.

Stent Tiny metal tube with holes in it that prevents a vessel from collapsing and keeps the atherosclerotic plaque pressed against the vessel wall; any material used to hold tissue in place or provide support.

Stereognosis Ability to recognize an object by feel.

Stereotyping Belief that all people within the same ethnic, racial, or cultural group act the same way sharing the same beliefs and attitudes.

Sterile Without microorganisms.

Sterile Conscience Individual's personal sense of honesty and integrity with regard to adherence to the principles of aseptic technique, including prompt admission and correction of any errors and omissions.

Sterile Field Area surrounding the client and the surgical site that is free from all microorganisms; created by draping of the work area and the client with sterile drapes.

Sterilization Destroying all microorganisms including spores.

Stock Supply Medications dispensed and labeled in large quantities for storage in the medication room or nursing unit.

Stoma Surgical opening between a cavity and the surface of the body.

Stomatitis Inflammation of the oral mucosa.

Strabismus Inability of the eyes to focus in the same direction.

Strain Injury to a muscle or tendon due to overuse or overstretching.

Stress Nonspecific response to any demand made on the body (Selye, 1974).

Stress Incontinence Leakage of urine when a person does anything that strains the abdomen, such as coughing, laughing, jogging, dancing, sneezing, lifting, making a quick movement, or even walking.

Stress Test Measure of a client's cardiovascular response to exercise.

Stressor Any situation, event, or agent that produces stress.

Striae Gravidarum Reddish streaks frequently found on the abdomen, thighs, buttocks, and breasts; also called "stretch marks."

Stridor High-pitched, harsh sound heard on inspiration when the trachea or larynx is obstructed.

Stroke Volume Volume of blood pumped by the ventricle with each contraction.

Stye Pustular inflammation of an eyelash follicle or sebaceous gland on the eyelid margin.

Subacute Care Short-term, aggressive care for clients who are out of the acute stage of illness but who still require skilled nursing, monitoring, and ongoing treatment.

Subcutaneous Injection into the subcutaneous tissue.

Subinvolution Incomplete return of the uterus to its prepregnant size and consistency.

Subjective Data Data from the client's point of view, including feelings, perceptions, and concerns.

Subluxation Partial separation of an articlular surface.

Substance A drug, legal or illegal, that may cause physical or mental impairment.

Suicidal Ideations Thoughts of hurting or killing oneself.

Supine Hypotensive Syndrome Lowering of blood pressure in a pregnant woman when lying supine due to compression of the vena cava by the enlarged, heavy uterus.

Surfactant Phospholipids that are present in the lungs and lowers surface tension to prevent collapse of the airways.

Surgery Treatment of injury, disease, or deformity through invasive operative methods.

Surgical Asepsis Practices that eliminate all microorganisms and spores from an object or area.

Susceptible Host Person who has no resistance to an agent and thus is vulnerable to disease.

Suture Thin, fibrous, membrane-covered space between skull bones.

Synarthrosis Immovable joint.

Syndactyly Fusion of two or more fingers or toes.

Synergism Result of two or more agents working together to achieve a greater effect than either could produce alone.

Synthesiasis Hearing colors and seeing sounds.

Synthesis Chemical reaction when two or more atoms, called reactants, bond and form a more complex molecular product. Putting data together in a new way.

Syphilis Sexually transmitted disease caused by the spirochete *Treponema pallidum.*

Systemic Infection Infection that affects the entire body with involvement of multiple organs.

Tachycardia Heart rate in excess of 100 beats per minute in an adult.

Tachypnea Respiratory rate greater than 24 beats per minute.

Talipes Equinovarus A congenital deformity in which the foot and ankle are twisted inward and cannot be moved to a midline position; also known as clubfoot.

Teaching Active process wherein one individual shares information with another as a means to facilitate learning and thereby promote behavioral changes.

Teaching Strategy Technique to promote learning.

Teaching–Learning Process Planned interaction that promotes a behavioral change that is not a result of maturation or coincidence.

Telangiectasic Nevi Birthmarks of dilated capillaries that blanch with pressure; also called stork-bites.

Telangiestasia Permanent dilation of groups of superficial capillaries and venules; commonly known as "spider veins."

Telehealth Use of telecommunication equipment and communication networks to transfer health care information between participants at different locations.

Telemedicine An element of telehealth permitting physicians to provide care through a telecommunication system.

Telenursing An element of telehealth permitting nurses to provide care through a telecommunication system.

Teleology Ethical theory that states that the value of a situation is determined by its consequences.

Tenesmus Spasmodic contradiction of the anal or bladder sphincter, causing pain and a persistent urge to empty the bowel or bladder.

Teratogen Agent such as radiation, drugs, viruses, and other microorganisms capable of causing abnormal fetal development.

Teratogenic Causing abnormal development of the embryo.

Teratogenic Substance Substance that crosses the placenta and impairs normal growth and development.

Term Descriptor for a pregnancy between 38 and 42 weeks' gestation.

Tertiary Care Care focused on restoring the client to the state of health that existed before the development of an illness; if unattainable, then care directed to attaining the optimal level of health possible.

Tertiary Prevention Treatment of an illness or disease after symptoms have appeared so as to prevent further progression.

Tetany Sharp flexion of the wrist and ankle joints, involving muscle twitching or cramps.

Therapeutic Communication Communication that is purposeful and goal directed, creating a beneficial outcome for the client.

Therapeutic Massage Application of hand pressure and motion to improve the recipient's well-being.

Therapeutic Procedure Accident Accident that occurs during the delivery of medical or nursing interventions.

Therapeutic Touch Technique of assessing alterations in a person's energy fields and using the hands to direct energy to achieve a balanced state.

Thermogenesis Production of heat.

Thermoregulation Maintenance of body temperature.

Thoracentesis Aspiration of fluid from the pleural cavity.

Thrombectomy Surgical removal of a clot.

Thrombocytopenia Decrease in the number of platelets in the blood.

Thrombophlebitis Formation of a clot due to an inflammation in the wall of the vessel.

Thrombosis Formation of a clot due to an inflammation in the wall of the vessel.

Thrombus Formed clot that remains at the site where it formed.

Time Management System to help meet goals through problem solving.

Tinnitus Ringing sound in the ear.

Tocolysis process of stopping labor with medications.

Tocolytic Agent Medication that inhibits uterine contractions.

Toddler Stage Development begins at approximately 12 to 18 months of age, when a child begins to walk, and ends at approximately age 3 years.

Tolerance Decreased sensitivity to subsequent doses of the same substance; an increased dose of the substance is needed to produce the same desired effect.

Tophi Subcutaneous nodules of sodium urate crystals.

Tort Civil wrong committed by a person against another person or property.

Tort Law Enforcement of duties and rights among individuals and independent of contractual agreements.

Touch Means of perceiving or experiencing through tactile sensation.

Toxic Poisonous.

Toxic Effect Reaction that occurs when the body cannot metabolize a drug, and the drug accumulates in the blood.

Trade (Brand) Name Name assigned a drug by the pharmaceutical company. Always capitalized.

Transcutaneous Electrical Nerve Stimulation Process of applying a low-voltage electrical current to the skin through cutaneous electrodes.

Transducer Instrument that converts electrical energy to sound waves.

Transduction Noxious stimulus that triggers electrical activity in the endings of afferent nerve fibers (nociceptors).

Transesophageal Echocardiography Diagnostic ultrasonic imaging of the cardiac structures through the esophagus.

Transient Flora Microorganisms that attach to the skin for a brief period of time but do not continuously live on the skin.

Transmission Process whereby the pain impulse travels from the receiving nociceptors to the spinal cord.

Transmission-Based Precautions Practices designed for clients documented as, or suspected of, being infected with highly transmissible or epidemiologically important pathogens for which additional precautions beyond Standard Precautions are required to interrupt transmission in hospitals.

Trauma Wound or injury.

Traumatic Imagery Imagining the feelings of horror felt by the victim or reliving the horror of the incident.

Triage Classification of clients to determine priority of need and proper place of treatment.

Triglyceride Lipid compound consisting of three fatty acids and a glycerol molecule.

Trocar Sharply pointed surgical instrument contained in a cannula.

Trousseau's Sign Carpal spasm caused by inflating a blood pressure cuff above the client's systolic pressure and leaving it in place for 3 minutes.

Trust Ability to rely on an individual's character and ability.

Tumor Marker Substance found in the serum that indicates the possible presence of malignancy.

Turgor Normal resiliency of the skin.

Type and Cross-Match Laboratory test that identifies the client's blood type (e.g., A or B) and determines the compatibility of the blood between potential donor and recipient.

Ultrasound Use of high-frequency sound waves to visualize deep body structures; also called an echogram or sonogram.

Umbilical Cord Structure which connects the fetus to the placenta.

Uncomplicated Grief Grief reaction normally following a significant loss.

Unilateral Neglect Failure to recognize or care for one side of the body.

Unit Dose Form System of packaging and labeling each dose of medication by the pharmacy, usually for a 24-hour period.

Urethrocele Downward displacement of the urethra into the vagina.

Urethrostomy Formation of a permanent fistula opening into the urethra.

Urge Incontinence Inability to suppress the sudden urge or need to urinate.

Urinary Incontinence Involuntary loss of urine from the bladder.

Urinary Retention Inability to void when there is an urge to void.

Urobilinogen Colorless derivative of bilirubin formed by the normal bacterial action of intestinal flora on bilirubin.

Urolithiasis Calculus or stone formed in the urinary tract.

Urticaria Allergic reaction causing raised pruritic, red, nontender wheals on the skin; also called hives.

Uterine Retraction Unique ability of the muscle fibers of the uterus to remain shortened to a small degree after each contraction.

Uterine Souffle Sound of blood pulsating through the uterus and placenta.

Utility Ethical principle which states that an act must result in the greatest positive benefit for the greatest number of people involved.

Vaccination Inoculation with a vaccine to produce immunity against specific diseases.

Value System Individual's collection of inner beliefs that guides the way the person acts and helps determine the choices the person makes.

Values Influences on the development of beliefs and attitudes rather than behaviors.

Values Clarification Process of analyzing one's own values to better understand those things that are truly important.

Variable Deceleration Reduction in fetal heart rate that has no relationship to contractions of the uterus.

Variance Goals not met or interventions not performed according to the time frame.

Varicosities Visibly prominent, dilated, and twisted veins.

Vasectomy Surgical resecton of the vas deferens.

Vasoconstriction Decrease in the diameter of a vessel.

Vasodilate Increase in the diameter of a vessel.

Vector-Borne Transmission Transfer of an agent to a susceptible host by animate means such as mosquitoes, fleas, ticks, lice, and other animals.

Vehicle Transmission Transfer of an agent to a susceptible host by contaminated inanimate objects such as food, milk, drugs, and blood.

Vein Ligation Tying off an involved section of a vein with suture.

Vein Stripping Introducing a wire into a vein to strip the walls of the vein.

Venereal Disease Disease usually acquired as a result of sexual contact; the preferred term currently in use is sexually transmitted disease.

Venipuncture Puncturing of a vein with a needle to aspirate blood.

Ventilation Movement of gases into and out of the lungs.

Veracity Ethical principle based on truthfulness (neither lying nor deceiving others).

Verbal Communication Using words, either spoken or written, to send a message.

Verbally Aggressive Descriptor of an individual who says things in a loud and/or intimidating manner.

Vernix Caseosa White, creamy substance covering a fetus's body.

Vertigo Dizziness.

Vesicant Agent that may produce blisters and tissue necrosis.

Vesicular Sound Soft, breezy, low-pitched sound heard longer on inspiration than expiration resulting from air moving through the smaller airways over the lung periphery, with the exception of the scapular area.

Villi Finger-like projections that line the small intestine.

Viral Load Test Test that measures copies of HIV RNA.

Virchow's Triad Three factors (pooling of blood, vessel trauma, and a coagulation problem) that lead to the formation of a clot.

Virulence Frequency with which a pathogen causes disease.

Visceral Pain Discomfort felt in the internal organs.

Visual Hallucination Perception by an individual that something is present when nothing in fact is.

Visual Learner Person who learns by processing information through seeing.

Vitamin Organic compounds essential to life and health.

Vitiligo Depigmentation of the skin caused by destruction of melanocytes; appears as milk-white patches on the skin.

Void Process of urine elimination.

Volvulus Twisting of a bowel on itself.

Walking Rounds Reporting method used when members of the care team walk to each client's room and discuss care with each other and with the client.

Water Soluble Vitamin Vitamin that must be ingested daily in normal quantities because it is not stored in the body: vitamins C and B-complex.

Wellness State of optimal health wherein an individual maximizes human potential, moves toward integration of human functioning, has greater self-awareness and self-satisfaction, and takes responsibility for health.

Wellness Nursing Diagnosis Nursing diagnosis that denotes the client's statement of a desire to obtain a higher level of wellness in s ome area of function; composed of the diagnostic label which begins "Readiness for."

Western Blot Test Confirmatory test used to detect HIV infection.

Wharton's Jelly Thick substance surrounding and protecting the vessels of the umbilical cord.

Whistleblowing Calling public attention to unethical, illegal, or incompetent actions of others.

Windowing Cutting a hole in a plaster cast to relieve pressure on the skin or a bony area and to permit visualization of the underlying body part.

Witch's Milk A whitish fluid secreted by a newborn's nipples.

Withdrawal Symptoms produced when a substance on which an individual has dependence is no longer used by that individual.

Word Salad Nonsensical combination of words that is meaningless to others.

Wound Disruption in the integrity of body tissue.

Yin and Yang Opposing forces that, when in balance, yield health.

Young Adulthood Development from the ages of 21 years through approximately 40 years.

Zygote Fertilized ovum.

Index

Page numbers followed by "f" denote figures, "t" denote tables, and "b" denote boxes.

clinical features of, 1258f
nursing care plan for, 1261–1264
Scale
sling, 551–552
standing, 551
Scales (skin lesion), 1243f
Scalp
anatomy of, 446
injury to, 1069
Scar, 1243f
Scarf sign, 1560
Scarlet fever, 1661f, 1661t
Schedule
conflicts in, 10
rearranging of, 10–11
Scheduled medication orders, 410–411
Schiller test, 522t
Schilling test, 500t
Schizophrenia
antipsychotics for, 1327t–1328t, 1329b
description of, 1326–1327
hallucinations associated with, 1327
management of, 1327–1329
nursing process for, 1329–1330
teaching client about, 1327b
School-age child, 191–192
complementary and alternative therapies
for, 282t
death as viewed by, 237t
sleep patterns, 326–327
Schools, 96t
Sclerotherapy, 927
Scoliosis, 1037, 1037f, 1654–1656
Scope of practice, 25
Scrotum, 1177
Scrub nurse, 807
Scultetus binders, 630–632
Sebaceous cyst, 1258
Seborrheic dermatitis, 1625, 1625f
Sebum, 364, 1238
Seclusion, 1322
Secondary care, 83, 83t
Secondary prevention, 261
Second-degree burns, 1247, 1249f
Sedation
for anesthesia, 789–790
definition of, 789
Joint Commission on Accreditation of
Healthcare Organizations guidelines
for, 790
procedural, 478, 481
residual effects of, 790
uses of, 790
Sedative-hypnotics, 1351–1352
Seizures, 1077–1079
Selective serotonin reuptake inhibitors,
1318t, 1319b
Selenium, 299t, 384t
Self-actualization, 33–34
Self-attitude. see Attitude
Self-awareness, 34, 169
Self-care
client teaching and, 167
description of, 35–36
middle-age adults, 199b
physical wellness
alcohol use, 36
body mechanics, 35
definition of, 35
drug abuse effects, 36
exercise, 37
grooming, 35, 35f
nutrition, 36–37

posture, 35–36
relaxation, 37
rest, 37
sleep, 37
smoking cessation, 36
theory of, 130–131
Self-care deficits, 339–340, 340t
Self-concept, 34, 179
Self-discipline, 12
Self-disclosure, 116
Self-efficacy, 163
Self-esteem, 33
Self-examination
breast, 265–266, 1185, 1186f
testes, 1204, 1205f
Self-image, 4–5
Self-knowledge, 11–12
Self-nurturing, 38
Self-responsibility, 258
Self-talk, 124
Semen analysis, 522t
Semipermeable membrane, 388
Sensation
components of, 1108
definition of, 1107–1108
medications effect on, 1108b
Sensible loss of water, 289–290
Sensorineural hearing loss, 1114
Sensory alterations
diagnostic tests for, 1112t
disorientation, 1112
ear disorders. see Ear disorders
eye disorders. see Eye disorders
in older adults, 1405–1406
sensory deficit, 1113
sensory deprivation, 1113
sensory overload, 1113
Sensory block, 792
Sensory deficit, 1113
Sensory deprivation, 1113
Sensory overload, 1113
Sensory system. see also Ear(s); Eye(s)
age-related changes, 1113b
assessments of, 1067–1068, 1109–1112
chronic renal failure effects on, 1025t
congenital disorders of, 1632–1633
Sepsis, intravenous therapy-related, 427b
Septic shock, 1369, 1369t
Sequestrectomy, 1044
Seroconversion, 1295–1296
Seromycin. see Cycloserin
Seroquel. see Quetiapine fumarate
Serosanguineous exudate, 1246
Serotonin reuptake inhibitors (SSRIs), 1318t
Serous exudate, 1245
Sertraline hydrochloride, 1318t
Serum acid phosphatase, 496t
Serum alkaline phosphatase, 496t
Serum creatinine, 497t
Serum osmolality, 398
Serving meals, 1252–1253, 1252b
Servings, 301, 301t
Serzone. see Nefazodone hydrochloride
Seventh Day Adventists
description of, 212
dietary restrictions, 304
Severe acute respiratory syndrome, 867
Sexual abuse, 1635
Sexual assault, 1375
Sexual relationships, 264
Sexually transmitted diseases
acquired immunodeficiency syndrome,
1230
in adolescents, 195

antibiotic treatment for, 1223
characteristics of, 1224t–1225t
chlamydia, 1223, 1224t, 1226, 1479t
cytomegalovirus, 1224t, 1228–1229, 1298
definition of, 1223
diagnostic tests for, 1226t
gonorrhea, 1225t, 1226–1227, 1479t
Healthy People 2000 and 2010 goals for,
260t
hepatitis B, 1225t, 1230–1231, 1298
herpes simplex virus, 1224t, 1228
human papillomavirus, 1225t, 1229–1230
incidence of, 1223
nursing process for, 1231–1233
prevention of, 267, 1224
syphilis, 1225t, 1227–1228, 1479t
trichomoniasis, 1225t, 1230
Shaman, 272
Shamanism, 271–272
Sharps disposal container, 376f
Sharps injuries, 101b
Shaving, 351, 602–604
Shearing, 1269
Shiatsu, 277–278
Shift report, 123
Shingles. see Herpes zoster
Shirodkar procedure, 1458, 1458f
Shivering, 794–795
Shock
anaphylactic, 1369, 1369t
cardiogenic, 1369t, 1369–1370
definition of, 1368
description of, 1251
hemorrhagic, 1538t
hypovolemic, 1369, 1369t
management of, 1370
neurogenic, 1369t, 1369–1370
nursing process for, 1370
obstructive, 1369t, 1369–1370
septic, 1369, 1369t
signs and symptoms of, 1369–1370
Short bones, 1035
Short-term goals, 134, 134t
Shoulder exercises, 558
Shroud, 249
Shunts
peritoneal venous, 986
portosystemic, 967
transjugular intrahepatic portosystemic,
967, 987f
Sibilant wheezes, 448, 852
Siblings, 1435, 1522, 1596
Sickle-cell anemia
definition of, 940
description of, 267
epidemiology of, 940
in infants, 1609–1611
management of, 941, 1609–1610
nursing care plan for, 942–944
nursing process for, 941, 1610–1611
pathophysiology of, 940–941
Sickle-cell test, 497t
Side effects, 409
Side rails, 342, 342f, 1583
Side-lying position, 567–568
Sigmoid, 962f
Sigmoid colstomy, 974f
Sildenafil citrate, 1215, 1393
Silence, 117
Silverman-Anderson index, 1570f
Simmonds' disease, 1154
Simple carbohydrates, 290
Sims' position, 442f